DIAGNOSTIC PATHOLOGY
Genitourinary

SECOND EDITION

AMIN | TICKOO

MCKENNEY · PANER · SHEN · SMITH · AL-AHMADIE
VELAZQUEZ · CUBILLA · RO · REUTER

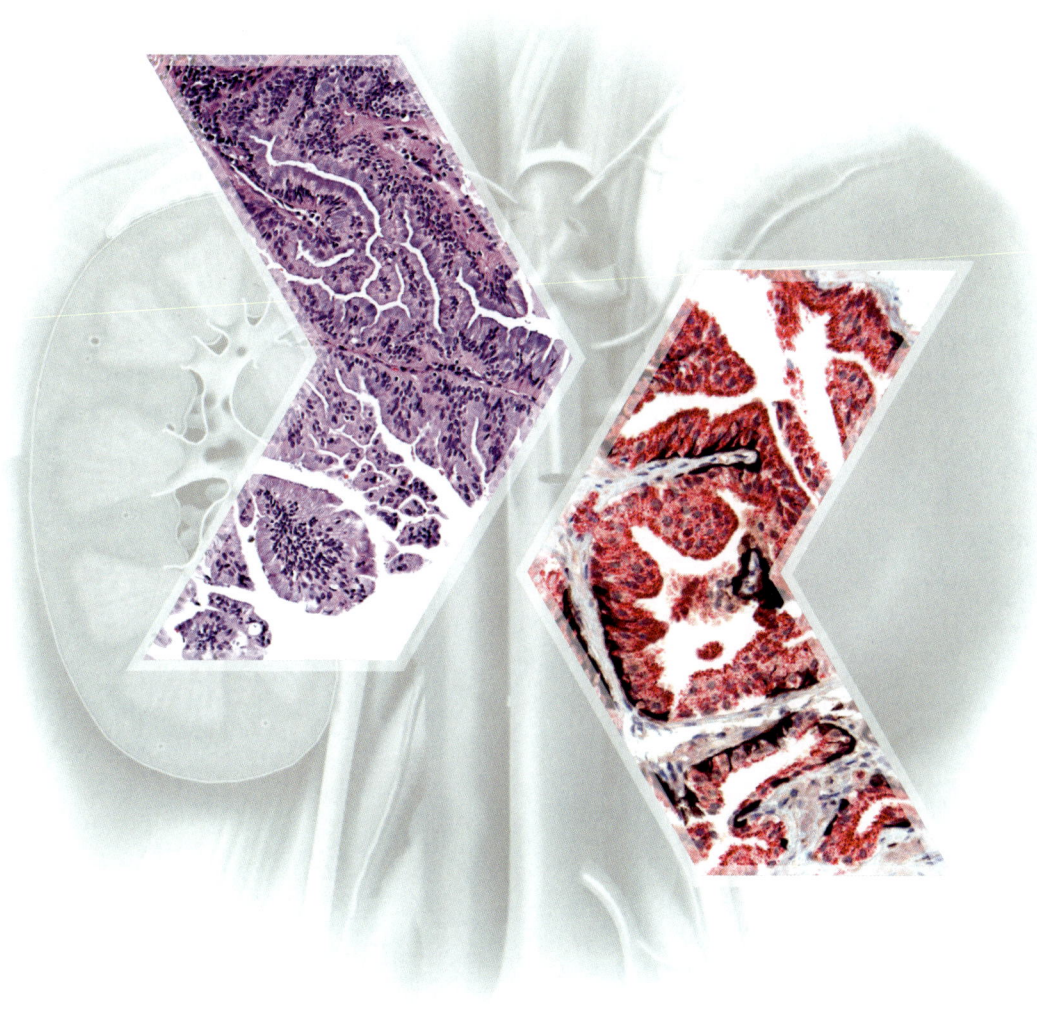

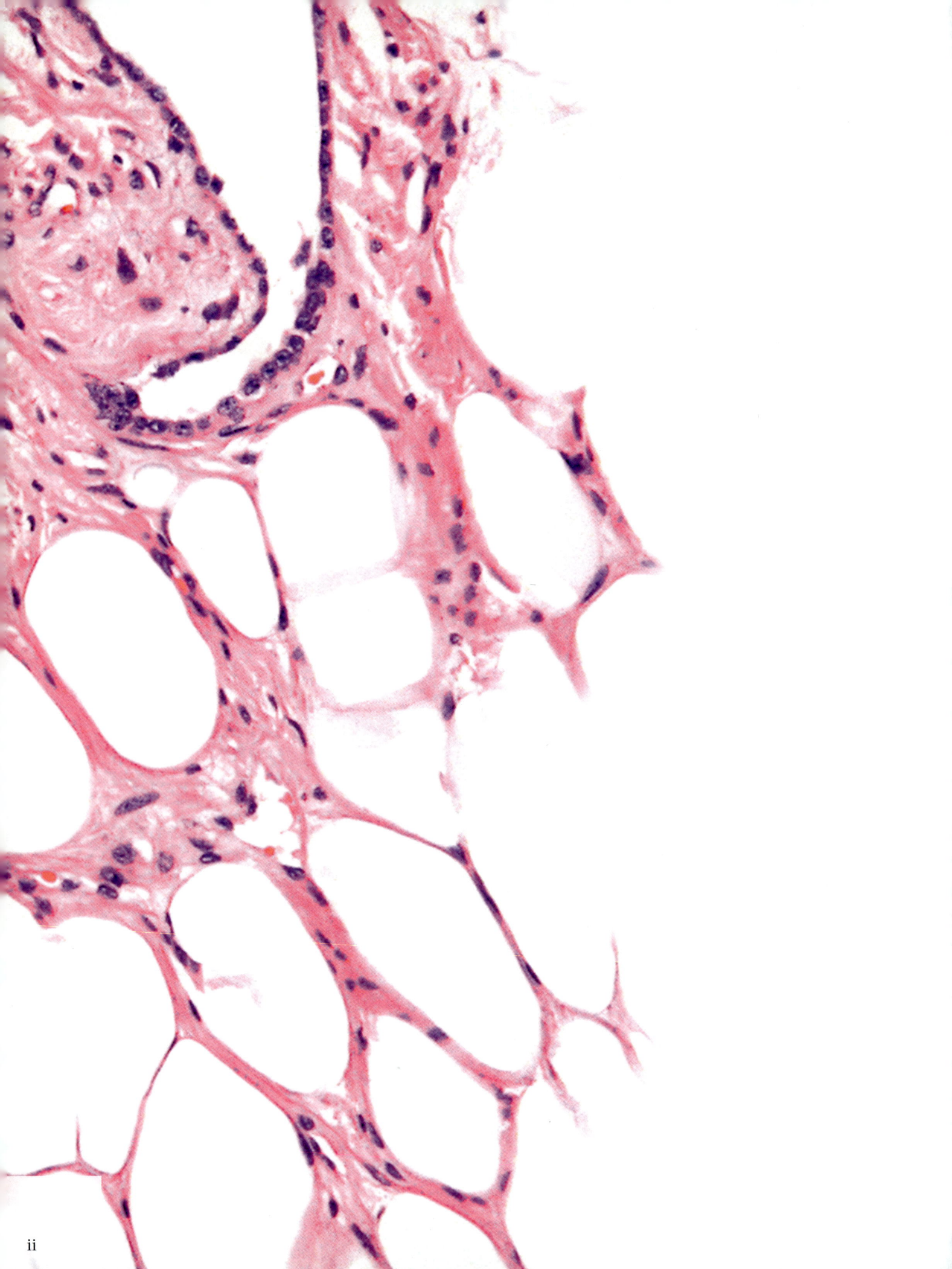
ii

DIAGNOSTIC PATHOLOGY
Genitourinary
SECOND EDITION

Mahul B. Amin, MD
Professor and Chairman Emeritus,
Pathology and Laboratory Medicine
Cedars-Sinai Medical Center
Professor of Pathology and Laboratory Medicine
UCLA David Geffen School of Medicine
Visiting Professor, Urology
USC Keck School of Medicine
Los Angeles, California
Visiting Professor, Pathology and Immunology
Baylor College of Medicine
Houston, Texas

Satish K. Tickoo, MD
Attending Pathologist
Department of Pathology
Memorial Sloan Kettering Cancer Center
New York, New York

ELSEVIER

1600 John F. Kennedy Blvd.
Ste 1800
Philadelphia, PA 19103-2899

DIAGNOSTIC PATHOLOGY: GENITOURINARY, SECOND EDITION   ISBN: 978-0-323-37714-0

Copyright © 2016 by Elsevier. All rights reserved.

No part of this publication may be reproduced or transmitted in any form or by any means, electronic or mechanical, including photocopying, recording, or any information storage and retrieval system, without permission in writing from the publisher. Details on how to seek permission, further information about the Publisher's permissions policies and our arrangements with organizations such as the Copyright Clearance Center and the Copyright Licensing Agency, can be found at our website: www.elsevier.com/permissions.

This book and the individual contributions contained in it are protected under copyright by the Publisher (other than as may be noted herein).

Notices

Knowledge and best practice in this field are constantly changing. As new research and experience broaden our understanding, changes in research methods, professional practices, or medical treatment may become necessary.

Practitioners and researchers must always rely on their own experience and knowledge in evaluating and using any information, methods, compounds, or experiments described herein. In using such information or methods they should be mindful of their own safety and the safety of others, including parties for whom they have a professional responsibility.

With respect to any drug or pharmaceutical products identified, readers are advised to check the most current information provided (i) on procedures featured or (ii) by the manufacturer of each product to be administered, to verify the recommended dose or formula, the method and duration of administration, and contraindications. It is the responsibility of practitioners, relying on their own experience and knowledge of their patients, to make diagnoses, to determine dosages and the best treatment for each individual patient, and to take all appropriate safety precautions.

To the fullest extent of the law, neither the Publisher nor the authors, contributors, or editors, assume any liability for any injury and/or damage to persons or property as a matter of products liability, negligence or otherwise, or from any use or operation of any methods, products, instructions, or ideas contained in the material herein.

Publisher Cataloging-in-Publication Data

Names: Amin, Mahul B. | Tickoo, Satish K.
Title: Diagnostic pathology. Genitourinary / [edited by] Mahul B. Amin and Satish K. Tickoo.
Other titles: Genitourinary.
Description: Second edition. | Salt Lake City, UT : Elsevier, Inc., [2016] | Includes bibliographical references and index.
Identifiers: ISBN 978-0-323-37714-0
Subjects: LCSH: Genitourinary organs--Diseases--Diagnosis--Handbooks, manuals, etc. | MESH: Male Urogenital Diseases--diagnosis--Atlases. | Male Urogenital Diseases--pathology--Atlases. | Kidney Neoplasms--diagnosis--Atlases. | Kidney Neoplasms--pathology--Atlases.
Classification: LCC RC874.D52 2016 | NLM WJ 17 | DDC 616.6'075--dc23

International Standard Book Number: 978-0-323-37714-0

Cover Designer: Tom M. Olson, BA

Printed in Canada by Friesens, Altona, Manitoba, Canada

Last digit is the print number: 9 8 7 6 5 4 3 2

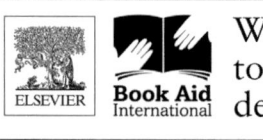

Dedications

To my wonderful family, Ushma, Anmol, and Aneri, for their everlasting warmth, love, and support; my late parents, who constantly motivated and inspired me to excel and serve; my residents and fellows, who support and challenge me to push the envelope of urologic pathology; my consultees, for sharing their difficult cases, which serve as a nidus for my educational and research efforts; my clinical and scientific colleagues, urologists, oncologists, and radiation oncologists, who constantly push me to try to be a better surgical pathologist; and my patients, who continually help engage me in a process of life-long learning and serve as a vivid and constant reminder that there is a lot more to be done for them.

Acknowledgments
I gratefully acknowledge the assistance of the visiting physician scholars to Cedars-Sinai (Dr. Ghee Yong Kwon, Korea; Dr. Nalan Nese, Turkey; and Dr. Anniah Chandrakanth, Canada) for going through my teaching files and helping to obtain innumerable pictures for this book, and the assistance of Dolores Ramirez, my Executive Administrative Assistant, for her efficient project management that kept this large initiative on track.
MBA

To my mother.
SKT

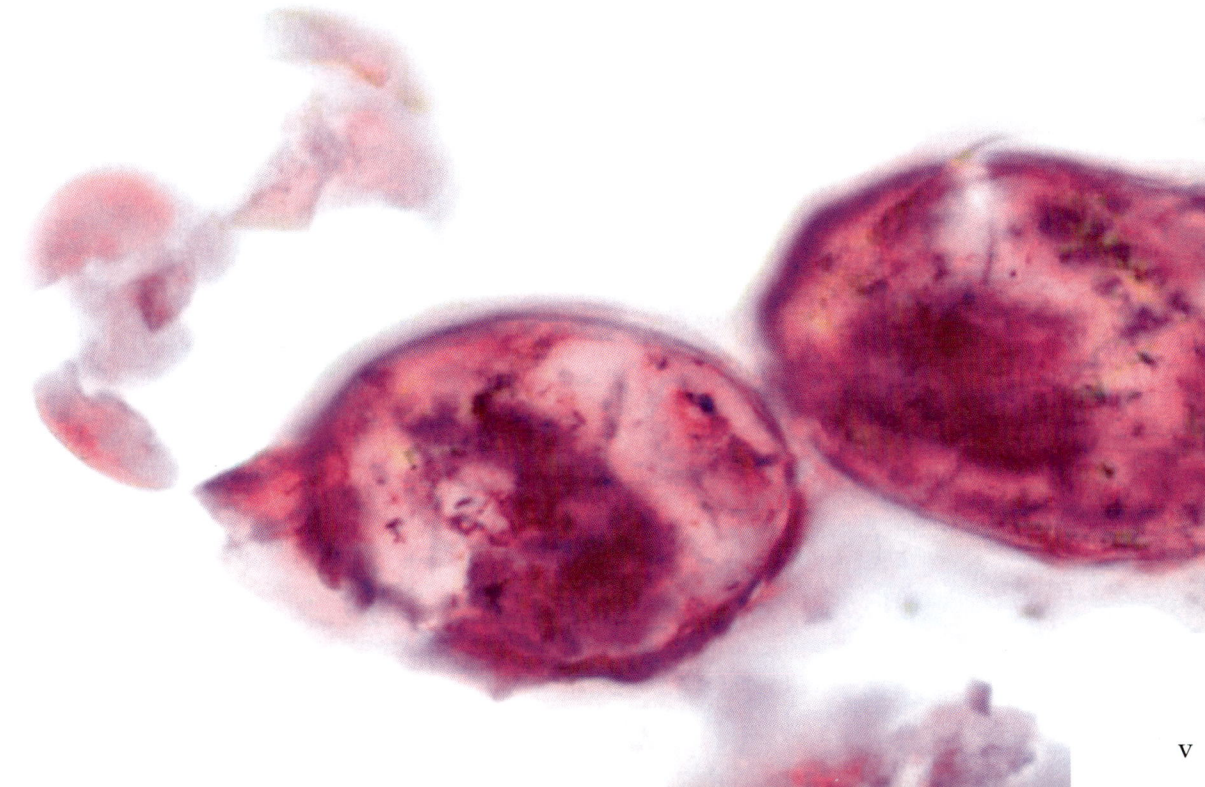

Contributing Authors

Jesse K. McKenney, MD
Section Head, Surgical Pathology
Cleveland Clinic
Cleveland, Ohio

Gladell P. Paner, MD
Associate Professor
Departments of Pathology and
Surgery Section of Urology
University of Chicago Medical Center
Chicago, Illinois

Steven S. Shen, MD, PhD
Associate Director, Surgical Pathology
Houston Methodist Hospital
Professor of Pathology and Laboratory Medicine
Weill Medical College of Cornell University
Houston, Texas

Steven Christopher Smith, MD, PhD
Assistant Director, Surgical Pathology
Department of Pathology
VCU Health System
Richmond, Virginia

Hikmat Al-Ahmadie, MD
Assistant Attending
Department of Pathology
Memorial Sloan Kettering Cancer Center
New York, New York

Elsa F. Velazquez, MD
Director of Dermatopathology
Miraca Life Sciences
Tufts University School of Medicine
Boston, Massachusetts

Antonio L. Cubilla, MD
Director
Instituto de Patología e Investigación
Emeritus Professor
School of Medicine, Universidad Nacional de Asunción
Asunción, Paraguay

Jae Y. Ro, MD, PhD
Director, Surgical Pathology
Department of Pathology and Genomic Medicine
Houston Methodist Hospital
Professor of Pathology and Laboratory Medicine
Weill Medical College of Cornell University
Houston, Texas

Victor E. Reuter, MD
Vice-Chairman
Department of Pathology
Memorial Sloan Kettering Cancer Center
New York, New York

Diego Fernando Sánchez Martínez, MD
Pathology Researcher
Instituto de Patología e Investigación
School of Medicine, Universidad Nacional de Asunción
Asunción, Paraguay

Maria José Fernández De Nestosa, PhD
Research Professor
Scientific and Applied Computing Laboratory
Facultad Politécnica, Universidad Nacional de Asunción
Asunción, Paraguay

Sofía Cañete Portillo, MD
Research Collaborator
Instituto de Patología e Investigación
Asunción, Paraguay
Pathology Resident
Department of Surgical Pathology
Instituto de Previsión Social
Asunción, Paraguay

Deepika Sirohi, MD
Clinical Fellow, Genitourinary Pathology
Department of Pathology and Laboratory Medicine
Cedars-Sinai Medical Center
Los Angeles, California

Chisato Ohe, MD
Visiting Postdoctoral Scientist
Department of Pathology and Laboratory Medicine
Cedars-Sinai Medical Center
Los Angeles, California

Mukul K. Divatia, MD
Staff Pathologist
Department of Pathology and Genomic Medicine
Houston Methodist Hospital
Houston, Texas

Judy Sarungbam, MD
Genitourinary Pathology Fellow
Department of Pathology
Memorial Sloan Kettering Cancer Center
New York, New York

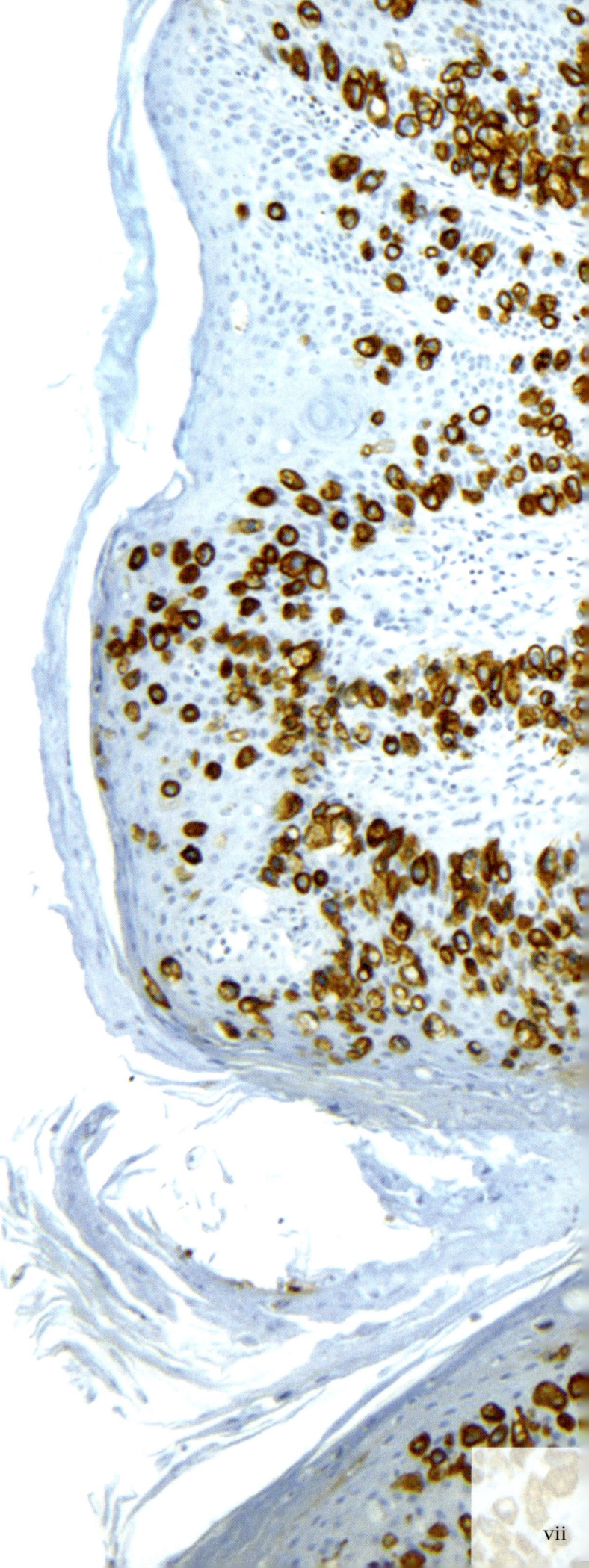

Preface

There could not be a more exciting time to publish the second edition of *Diagnostic Pathology: Genitourinary*. The subspecialty of genitourinary pathology (also called urologic pathology) continues to generate great clinical and academic interest, which results in a continued expansion in the knowledge base around entities encompassed within it. The World Health Organization (WHO) has just published the fourth edition of the WHO Classification of Tumours of the Urinary System and Male Genital Organs, and the nomenclature and classifications promulgated through this publication are largely consistent with this offering. Further, in recent years, the International Society of Urological Pathologists (ISUP) has been very active in publishing best practices and consensus and position statements. This book incorporates the approach promoted through these publications.

The second edition of *Diagnostic Pathology: Genitourinary* is therefore a considerably updated and revised edition, and through the authoring process, all authors have attempted five important goals. First, maintain the core goal established in the first edition of being a succinct, user-friendly, "one-stop" diagnostic compendium for the busy practicing pathologist as well as residents and fellows in training. The combination of pithy, factual, bulleted text along with rich and diverse illustrations is intended to help the pathologist arrive at the correct diagnosis, consider key differential diagnostic possibilities, and employ contemporary and judicious ancillary studies as appropriate, with reporting guidelines that enable generation of a complete and accurate surgical pathology report. Second, our very experienced author group, like other prominent academicians, travel and lecture frequently both within the United States and internationally. Our readers have been generous with compliments of the value of the book and importantly, during these educational forums, have provided feedback for improvement and refinement. We have incorporated their suggestions by including concurrent illustrations of a wide range of differential diagnoses, making our figure legends more didactic, educational, and practical, and emphasizing practical aspects about staging and assessment of prognostic factors. Third, we have updated the text in a manner reflecting the current understanding of the diseases in terms of diagnosis, prognosis, and approach to management. Fourth, we have added entirely new sections and chapters on recent entities or those previously not covered in the first edition. For example, new sections on the renal pelvis, ureter, urethra, urachus, and diverticular bladder disease, each with chapters within them, are added. Examples of new entities in the kidney include transcription elongation factor B (*TCEB1*)-mutated renal cell carcinoma and renal cell carcinomas occurring in the succinate dehydrogenase complex deficiency syndrome. In the bladder section, a new chapter on inverted neoplasms is included along with the aforementioned new sections. Other examples of new chapters include one on regressed (burnt-out) germ cell tumors of the testis and chapters on newer variants of penile cancer, including lymphoepithelioma-like and clear cell carcinoma. Finally, we have incorporated not only important advances in the literature, but also updated the book with recommendations from the ISUP and the WHO.

The overall organization of the book in terms of the five sections, Kidney Tumors and Tumor-Like Conditions, Urinary Bladder, Prostate Gland and Seminal Vesicles, Testis and Paratesticular Structures, and Penis and Scrotum, is maintained. The authors within the teams responsible for each section are very experienced, and, apart from drawing on their own clinical experiences, the entire authorship shared ideas, approaches, concepts, and classic teaching cases through face-to-face and phone discussions and e-mails to produce a synergistic offering. We, the editors, were additionally heavily involved over these attempts for consistency, easy readability, and practicality within each chapter at every level, from the text, tables, and illustrations to the didactic figure legends.

We hope that in this refined, updated, and expanded offering of the second edition, you continue to find value in the eBook version (available on the Expert Consult platform), which is intended to add another level of desktop user-friendliness and utility beyond what the hard copy of the book may bring. Finally, this second edition of content of *Diagnostic Pathology: Genitourinary* will also be part of the exciting new product, ExpertPath, which provides comprehensive decision support over all pathology sites searchable among other things by entity, pathological features, or immunohistochemical findings.

Mahul B. Amin, MD
Professor and Chairman Emeritus, Pathology and Laboratory Medicine
Cedars-Sinai Medical Center
Professor of Pathology and Laboratory Medicine
UCLA David Geffen School of Medicine
Visiting Professor, Urology
USC Keck School of Medicine
Los Angeles, California
Visiting Professor, Pathology and Immunology
Baylor College of Medicine
Houston, Texas

Satish K. Tickoo, MD
Attending Pathologist
Department of Pathology
Memorial Sloan Kettering Cancer Center
New York, New York

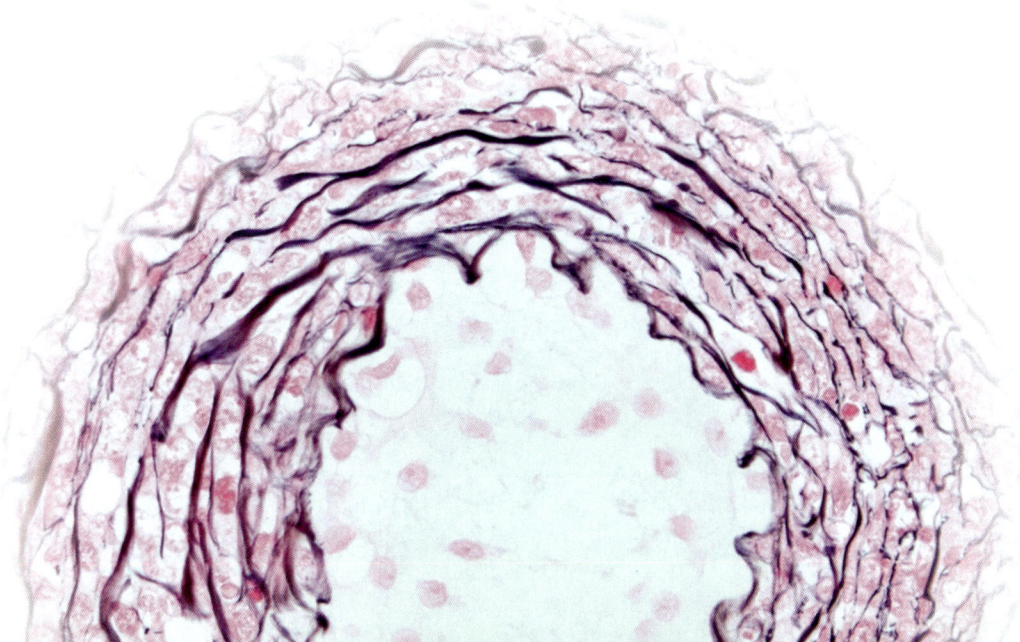

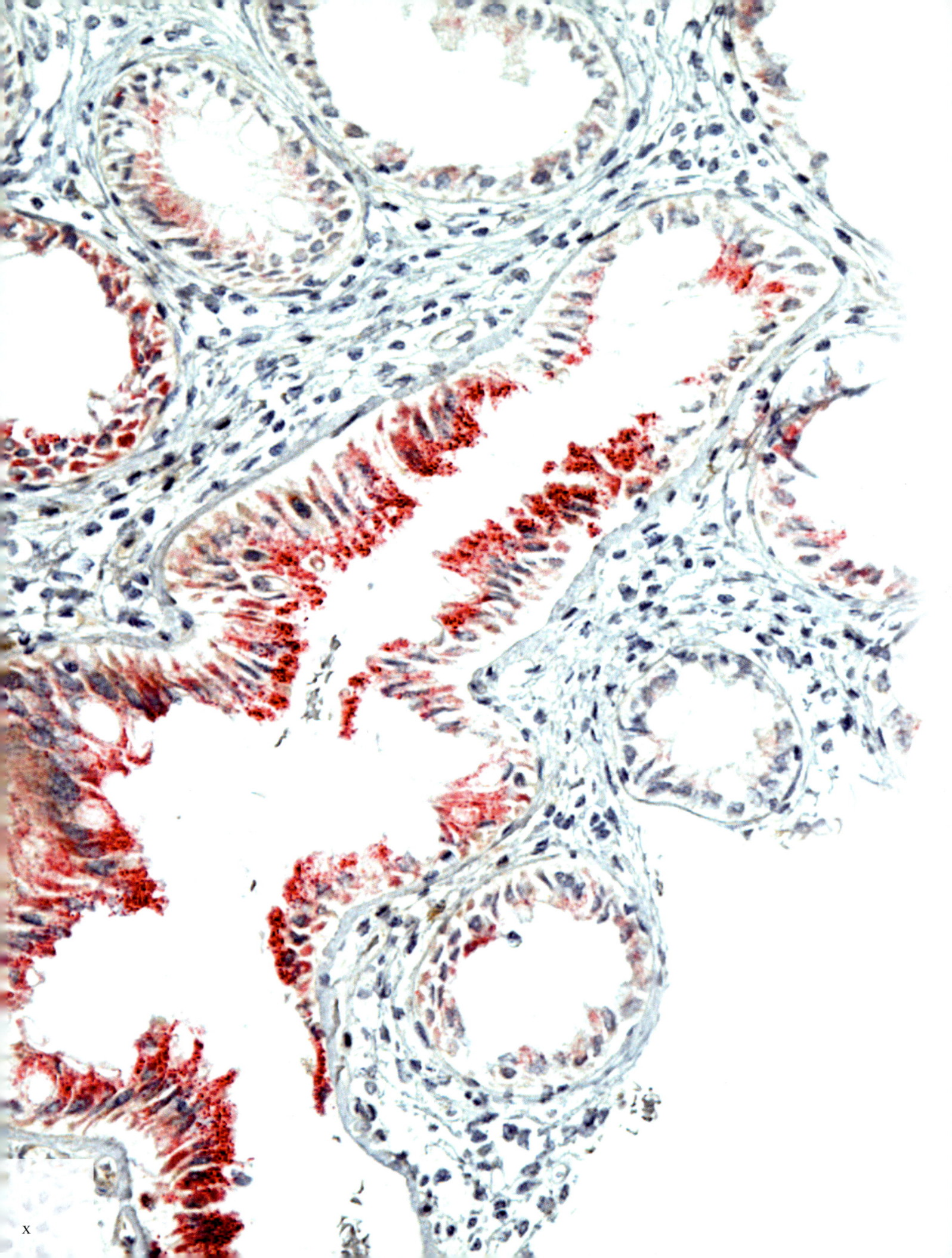

Acknowledgments

Text Editors

Arthur G. Gelsinger, MA
Nina I. Bennett, BA
Terry W. Ferrell, MS
Lisa A. Gervais, BS
Karen E. Concannon, MA, PhD
Emily C. Fassett, BA
Matt Hoecherl, BS
Tricia L. Cannon, BA

Image Editors

Jeffrey J. Marmorstone, BS
Lisa A. M. Steadman, BS

Illustrations

Laura C. Sesto, MA
Lane R. Bennion, MS
Richard Coombs, MS

Art Direction and Design

Tom M. Olson, BA
Laura C. Sesto, MA

Lead Editor

Sarah J. Connor, BA

Production Coordinators

Angela M. G. Terry, BA
Rebecca L. Hutchinson, BA

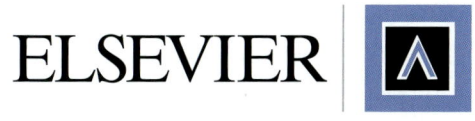

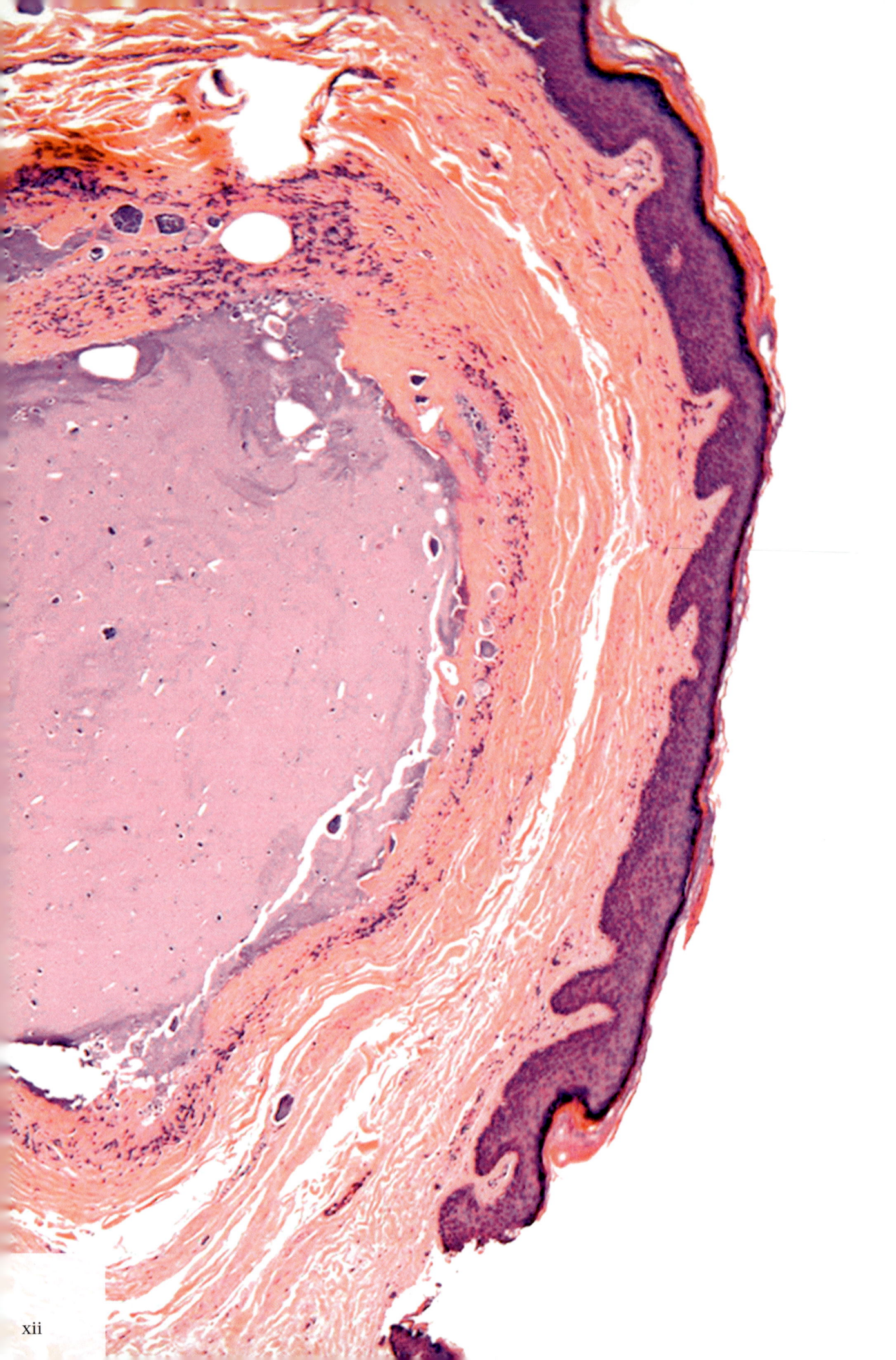

Sections

SECTION 1: Kidney Tumors and Tumor-Like Conditions

SECTION 2: Urinary Bladder

SECTION 3: Prostate Gland and Seminal Vesicle

SECTION 4: Testis and Paratesticular Structures

SECTION 5: Penis and Scrotum

TABLE OF CONTENTS

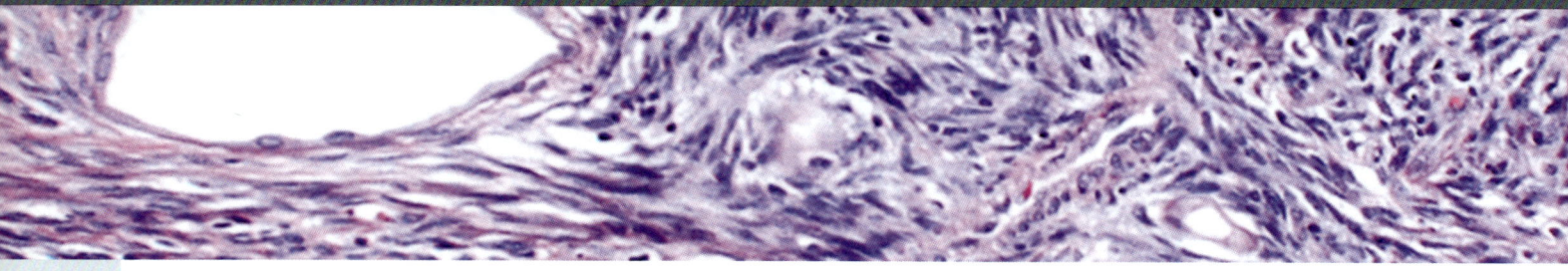

SECTION 1: KIDNEY TUMORS AND TUMOR-LIKE CONDITIONS

INTRODUCTION AND OVERVIEW

4 Classification of Kidney Tumors and Tumor-Like Lesions
Satish K. Tickoo, MD and Victor E. Reuter, MD

6 Introduction to Renal Cell Tumors
Satish K. Tickoo, MD and Victor E. Reuter, MD

FAMILIAL CANCER SYNDROMES

12 von Hippel-Lindau Syndrome
Satish K. Tickoo, MD and Victor E. Reuter, MD

16 Birt-Hogg-Dubé Syndrome
Satish K. Tickoo, MD and Victor E. Reuter, MD

20 Hereditary Leiomyomatosis Renal Cell Carcinoma Syndrome
Satish K. Tickoo, MD and Victor E. Reuter, MD

24 Tuberous Sclerosis Complex
Satish K. Tickoo, MD and Victor E. Reuter, MD

28 Succinate Dehydrogenase Complex Deficiency Syndrome
Satish K. Tickoo, MD and Victor E. Reuter, MD

32 Hereditary Papillary Renal Cancer and Miscellaneous Other Familial Cancer Syndromes
Satish K. Tickoo, MD and Victor E. Reuter, MD

NONNEOPLASTIC LESIONS

38 Renal Tuberculosis, Xanthogranulomatous Pyelonephritis, Renal Malakoplakia
Satish K. Tickoo, MD and Victor E. Reuter, MD

RENAL CELL TUMORS, BENIGN

44 Papillary Adenoma
Satish K. Tickoo, MD and Victor E. Reuter, MD

48 Renal Oncocytoma
Satish K. Tickoo, MD and Victor E. Reuter, MD

RENAL CELL CARCINOMA

54 Clear Cell Renal Cell Carcinoma
Satish K. Tickoo, MD and Victor E. Reuter, MD

64 Multilocular Cystic Clear Cell Renal Cell Neoplasm of Low Malignant Potential
Satish K. Tickoo, MD and Victor E. Reuter, MD

68 Transcription Elongation Factor B (*TCEB1*)-Mutated Renal Cell Carcinoma
Judy Sarungbam, MD, Satish K. Tickoo, MD, and Victor E. Reuter, MD

72 Clear Cell Papillary Renal Cell Carcinoma
Satish K. Tickoo, MD and Victor E. Reuter, MD

80 Papillary Renal Cell Carcinoma
Satish K. Tickoo, MD and Victor E. Reuter, MD

90 Chromophobe Renal Cell Carcinoma
Satish K. Tickoo, MD and Victor E. Reuter, MD

98 Collecting Duct Carcinoma
Satish K. Tickoo, MD and Victor E. Reuter, MD

104 Renal Medullary Carcinoma
Satish K. Tickoo, MD and Victor E. Reuter, MD

110 MiTF/TFE Family Translocation-Associated Carcinoma
Satish K. Tickoo, MD and Victor E. Reuter, MD

118 Mucinous Tubular and Spindle Cell Carcinoma
Satish K. Tickoo, MD and Victor E. Reuter, MD

124 Tubulocystic Carcinoma
Satish K. Tickoo, MD and Victor E. Reuter, MD

128 Thyroid-Like Follicular Carcinoma of Kidney
Satish K. Tickoo, MD and Victor E. Reuter, MD

132 Acquired Cystic Disease-Associated Renal Cell Carcinoma
Satish K. Tickoo, MD and Victor E. Reuter, MD

138 Subsequent Second Tumors
Satish K. Tickoo, MD, Chisato Ohe, MD, and Victor E. Reuter, MD

142 Renal Cell Carcinoma, Unclassified
Satish K. Tickoo, MD and Victor E. Reuter, MD

METANEPHRIC TUMORS

146 Metanephric Adenoma
Satish K. Tickoo, MD and Victor E. Reuter, MD

152 Metanephric Tumors Other Than Metanephric Adenoma
Satish K. Tickoo, MD and Victor E. Reuter, MD

NEPHROBLASTIC TUMORS

156 Nephrogenic Rests
Satish K. Tickoo, MD and Victor E. Reuter, MD

160 Nephroblastoma (Wilms Tumor)
Satish K. Tickoo, MD and Victor E. Reuter, MD

170 Cystic Partially Differentiated Nephroblastoma
Satish K. Tickoo, MD and Victor E. Reuter, MD

MESENCHYMAL TUMORS

172 Angiomyolipoma
Satish K. Tickoo, MD and Victor E. Reuter, MD

178 Epithelioid Angiomyolipoma
Satish K. Tickoo, MD and Victor E. Reuter, MD

TABLE OF CONTENTS

184 **Congenital Mesoblastic Nephroma**
Satish K. Tickoo, MD and Victor E. Reuter, MD

188 **Clear Cell Sarcoma of Kidney**
Satish K. Tickoo, MD and Victor E. Reuter, MD

192 **Malignant Rhabdoid Tumor**
Satish K. Tickoo, MD and Victor E. Reuter, MD

MIXED MESENCHYMAL AND EPITHELIAL TUMORS

196 **Mixed Epithelial and Stromal Tumor (MEST) Family Tumors and Pediatric Cystic Nephroma**
Satish K. Tickoo, MD and Victor E. Reuter, MD

204 **Synovial Sarcoma**
Satish K. Tickoo, MD and Victor E. Reuter, MD

NEUROENDOCRINE TUMORS

208 **Well-Differentiated Neuroendocrine Tumor (Carcinoid) and High-Grade Neuroendocrine Carcinoma**
Satish K. Tickoo, MD and Victor E. Reuter, MD

212 **Primitive Neuroectodermal Tumor**
Satish K. Tickoo, MD and Victor E. Reuter, MD

HEMATOPOIETIC TUMORS

216 **Hematopoietic Tumors**
Satish K. Tickoo, MD, Judy Sarungbam, MD, and Victor E. Reuter, MD

METASTATIC AND OTHER TUMORS

222 **Juxtaglomerular Cell Tumor (Reninoma)**
Satish K. Tickoo, MD and Victor E. Reuter, MD

226 **Renomedullary Interstitial Cell Tumor**
Satish K. Tickoo, MD and Victor E. Reuter, MD

230 **Other Rare Tumors**
Satish K. Tickoo, MD and Victor E. Reuter, MD

238 **Metastatic Tumors**
Satish K. Tickoo, MD, Deepika Sirohi, MD, and Victor E. Reuter, MD

IMMUNOHISTOCHEMICAL PROFILES FOR TUMORS INVOLVING KIDNEY

242 **Immunohistochemistry, Kidney**
Satish K. Tickoo, MD and Victor E. Reuter, MD

SECTION 2: URINARY BLADDER

INTRODUCTION AND OVERVIEW

250 **Classification of Bladder Tumors and Tumor-Like Lesions**
Jesse K. McKenney, MD

MICROSCOPIC ANATOMY

252 **Microscopic Anatomy of Urinary Bladder**
Hikmat Al-Ahmadie, MD

256 **Microscopic Anatomy of Urethra**
Gladell P. Paner, MD and Hikmat Al-Ahmadie, MD

260 **Microscopic Anatomy of Ureter**
Steven C. Smith, MD, PhD

262 **Microscopic Anatomy of Renal Pelvis**
Steven C. Smith, MD, PhD

NONNEOPLASTIC LESIONS OF URINARY TRACT

266 **Overview of Cystitis**
Jesse K. McKenney, MD

272 **Papillary-Polypoid Cystitis**
Jesse K. McKenney, MD

280 **Malakoplakia**
Jesse K. McKenney, MD

286 **Schistosomiasis**
Jesse K. McKenney, MD

288 **von Brunn Nests**
Jesse K. McKenney, MD

294 **Nephrogenic Adenoma (Metaplasia)**
Jesse K. McKenney, MD

302 **Fibroepithelial Polyp**
Jesse K. McKenney, MD

306 **Prostatic-Type Polyp (Ectopic Prostate)**
Jesse K. McKenney, MD

312 **Amyloidosis**
Jesse K. McKenney, MD

314 **Müllerian Lesions**
Jesse K. McKenney, MD

318 **Pseudocarcinomatous Hyperplasia**
Jesse K. McKenney, MD

326 **Hamartoma**
Jesse K. McKenney, MD

UROTHELIAL NEOPLASMS, GENERAL

328 **Overview of Urinary Bladder Neoplasms**
Hikmat Al-Ahmadie, MD

FLAT UROTHELIAL LESIONS

332 **Urothelial Carcinoma In Situ**
Jesse K. McKenney, MD

340 **Flat Urothelial Lesions Other Than Carcinoma In Situ**
Jesse K. McKenney, MD

UROTHELIAL NEOPLASMS, NONINVASIVE

344 **Urothelial Papilloma**
Jesse K. McKenney, MD

350 **Papillary Urothelial Neoplasm of Low Malignant Potential**
Jesse K. McKenney, MD

354 **Low-Grade Papillary Urothelial Carcinoma**
Hikmat Al-Ahmadie, MD

358 **High-Grade Papillary Urothelial Carcinoma**
Hikmat Al-Ahmadie, MD

364 **Inverted Urothelial Neoplasia**
Jesse K. McKenney, MD

UROTHELIAL NEOPLASMS, INVASIVE

374 **Invasive Urothelial Carcinoma**
Hikmat Al-Ahmadie, MD

382 **Overview of Invasive Carcinoma Subtypes**
Jesse K. McKenney, MD

TABLE OF CONTENTS

GLANDULAR LESIONS

- 404 Cystitis Cystica and Glandularis
  Hikmat Al-Ahmadie, MD
- 408 Villous Adenoma
  Hikmat Al-Ahmadie, MD
- 410 Invasive Adenocarcinoma
  Hikmat Al-Ahmadie, MD
- 416 Clear Cell Adenocarcinoma
  Hikmat Al-Ahmadie, MD

SQUAMOUS LESIONS

- 422 Squamous Proliferations Other Than Carcinoma
  Hikmat Al-Ahmadie, MD
- 426 Invasive Squamous Cell Carcinoma
  Hikmat Al-Ahmadie, MD

MESENCHYMAL LESIONS

- 432 Myofibroblastic Proliferations
  Jesse K. McKenney, MD
- 440 Smooth Muscle Tumors
  Jesse K. McKenney, MD
- 448 Skeletal Muscle Tumors
  Jesse K. McKenney, MD
- 454 Other Mesenchymal Tumors
  Jesse K. McKenney, MD

OTHER TUMORS OF URINARY BLADDER

- 462 Paraganglioma
  Jesse K. McKenney, MD
- 470 Metastatic and Secondary Carcinomas
  Jesse K. McKenney, MD

DIVERTICULA OF URINARY TRACT

- 478 Diverticula
  Hikmat Al-Ahmadie, MD
- 482 Diverticular-Associated Neoplasia
  Hikmat Al-Ahmadie, MD

URETHRA

- 486 Inflammatory Lesions of Urethra
  Steven C. Smith, MD, PhD
- 490 Carcinoma of Urethra
  Steven C. Smith, MD, PhD
- 494 Other Tumors and Tumor-Like Lesions of Urethra
  Steven C. Smith, MD, PhD

URETER

- 498 Urothelial Carcinoma of Ureter
  Hikmat Al-Ahmadie, MD
- 502 Other Tumors and Tumor-Like Lesions of Ureter
  Hikmat Al-Ahmadie, MD

RENAL PELVIS

- 506 Urothelial Carcinoma of Renal Pelvis
  Hikmat Al-Ahmadie, MD
- 514 Other Tumors and Tumor-Like Lesions of Renal Pelvis
  Hikmat Al-Ahmadie, MD

URACHUS

- 520 Urachal Remnants
  Steven C. Smith, MD, PhD
- 522 Tumors of Urachus
  Steven C. Smith, MD, PhD

IMMUNOHISTOCHEMICAL PROFILES FOR TUMORS INVOLVING URINARY BLADDER

- 528 Immunohistochemistry, Urinary Tract
  Steven C. Smith, MD, PhD

SECTION 3: PROSTATE GLAND AND SEMINAL VESICLE

INTRODUCTION AND OVERVIEW

- 536 Classification of Prostate Tumors and Tumor-Like Lesions
  Gladell P. Paner, MD
- 538 General Concepts, Prostate
  Gladell P. Paner, MD
- 544 Microanatomy and Zonal Variations
  Gladell P. Paner, MD

NONNEOPLASTIC LESIONS

- 554 Prostatitis
  Steven C. Smith, MD, PhD
- 558 Prostate Hyperplasia
  Gladell P. Paner, MD
- 566 Adenosis
  Hikmat Al-Ahmadie, MD
- 570 Atrophy and Its Variants
  Gladell P. Paner, MD
- 576 Hyperplasia of Mesonephric Remnants
  Steven C. Smith, MD, PhD
- 580 Verumontanum Mucosal Gland Hyperplasia
  Gladell P. Paner, MD and Deepika Sirohi, MD
- 582 Nephrogenic Adenoma (Metaplasia) of Prostatic Urethra
  Gladell P. Paner, MD

PUTATIVE PREMALIGNANT LESIONS AND LESIONS FALLING SHORT OF MALIGNANT DIAGNOSIS

- 590 Prostatic Intraepithelial Neoplasia
  Hikmat Al-Ahmadie, MD

PROSTATE NEOPLASMS

- 600 General Concepts, Prostate Carcinoma
  Steven C. Smith, MD, PhD
- 608 Acinar Adenocarcinoma
  Gladell P. Paner, MD
- 626 Acinar Adenocarcinoma Variants
  Gladell P. Paner, MD

TABLE OF CONTENTS

638 **Atypical Small Acinar Proliferations**
Steven C. Smith, MD, PhD

644 **Intraductal Carcinoma**
Hikmat Al-Ahmadie, MD

650 **Ductal Adenocarcinoma**
Gladell P. Paner, MD

658 **Urothelial Carcinoma Involving Prostate Gland**
Steven C. Smith, MD, PhD

664 **Prostate Carcinoma With Neuroendocrine Differentiation**
Steven C. Smith, MD, PhD

672 **Basal Cell Carcinoma**
Steven C. Smith, MD, PhD

678 **Sarcomatoid Carcinoma of Prostate**
Steven C. Smith, MD, PhD

684 **Carcinomas With Squamous Differentiation**
Gladell P. Paner, MD

690 **Stromal Tumors**
Gladell P. Paner, MD

698 **Mesenchymal Tumors of Prostate**
Gladell P. Paner, MD

706 **Melanocytic Lesions of Prostate**
Gladell P. Paner, MD

710 **Hematopoietic Neoplasms of Prostate**
Gladell P. Paner, MD

714 **Secondary Tumors of Prostate**
Gladell P. Paner, MD and Deepika Sirohi, MD

TUMORS OF SEMINAL VESICLE

718 **Cystadenoma and Epithelial Stromal Tumor**
Steven C. Smith, MD, PhD

722 **Seminal Vesicle Adenocarcinoma**
Gladell P. Paner, MD

IMMUNOHISTOCHEMICAL PROFILES FOR TUMORS AND TUMOR-LIKE LESIONS INVOLVING PROSTATE GLAND

724 **Immunohistochemistry, Prostate**
Steven C. Smith, MD, PhD

SECTION 4: TESTIS AND PARATESTICULAR STRUCTURES

INTRODUCTION AND OVERVIEW

732 **Classification of Testis and Paratestis Tumors and Tumor-Like Lesions**
Steven S. Shen, MD, PhD and Jae Y. Ro, MD, PhD

NONNEOPLASTIC LESIONS

734 **Cryptorchidism**
Steven S. Shen, MD, PhD and Jae Y. Ro, MD, PhD

738 **Sertoli Cell-Only Syndrome**
Steven S. Shen, MD, PhD and Jae Y. Ro, MD, PhD

742 **Nontuberculous Infections**
Steven S. Shen, MD, PhD and Jae Y. Ro, MD, PhD

744 **Nonspecific Granulomatous Orchitis**
Steven S. Shen, MD, PhD and Jae Y. Ro, MD, PhD

746 **Tuberculous Epididymo-Orchitis**
Steven S. Shen, MD, PhD and Jae Y. Ro, MD, PhD

GERM CELL TUMORS

748 **General Concepts, Germ Cell Tumors**
Steven S. Shen, MD, PhD and Jae Y. Ro, MD, PhD

GERM CELL TUMORS RELATED TO GERM CELL NEOPLASIA IN SITU

756 **Germ Cell Neoplasia In Situ**
Steven S. Shen, MD, PhD and Jae Y. Ro, MD, PhD

762 **Seminoma**
Steven S. Shen, MD, PhD and Jae Y. Ro, MD, PhD

770 **Embryonal Carcinoma**
Steven S. Shen, MD, PhD and Jae Y. Ro, MD, PhD

776 **Yolk Sac Tumor**
Steven S. Shen, MD, PhD and Jae Y. Ro, MD, PhD

784 **Choriocarcinoma and Variants**
Steven S. Shen, MD, PhD and Jae Y. Ro, MD, PhD

790 **Teratoma, Adult Type**
Steven S. Shen, MD, PhD and Jae Y. Ro, MD, PhD

794 **Mixed Germ Cell Tumors**
Steven S. Shen, MD, PhD and Jae Y. Ro, MD, PhD

798 **Somatic-Type Malignancy in Germ Cell Tumor**
Steven S. Shen, MD, PhD and Jae Y. Ro, MD, PhD

800 **Burnt-Out (Regressed) Germ Cell Tumor**
Steven S. Shen, MD, PhD and Jae Y. Ro, MD, PhD

GERM CELL TUMORS UNRELATED TO GERM CELL NEOPLASIA IN SITU

802 **Spermatocytic Tumor**
Steven S. Shen, MD, PhD and Jae Y. Ro, MD, PhD

806 **Teratoma, Prepubertal Type**
Steven S. Shen, MD, PhD and Jae Y. Ro, MD, PhD

810 **Yolk Sac Tumor, Prepubertal Type**
Steven S. Shen, MD, PhD and Jae Y. Ro, MD, PhD

814 **Carcinoid Tumor**
Steven S. Shen, MD, PhD and Jae Y. Ro, MD, PhD

SEX CORD-/GONADAL STROMAL TUMORS

818 **General Concepts, Sex Cord-/Gonadal Stromal Tumors**
Steven S. Shen, MD, PhD and Jae Y. Ro, MD, PhD

824 **Leydig Cell Tumors**
Steven S. Shen, MD, PhD and Jae Y. Ro, MD, PhD

828 **Sertoli Cell Tumors**
Steven S. Shen, MD, PhD and Jae Y. Ro, MD, PhD

834 **Large Cell Calcifying Sertoli Cell Tumor**
Steven S. Shen, MD, PhD and Jae Y. Ro, MD, PhD

838 **Granulosa Cell Tumor**
Steven S. Shen, MD, PhD and Jae Y. Ro, MD, PhD

842 **Juvenile Granulosa Cell Tumor**
Steven S. Shen, MD, PhD and Jae Y. Ro, MD, PhD

846 **Testicular Tumor of Adrenogenital Syndrome**
Steven S. Shen, MD, PhD and Jae Y. Ro, MD, PhD

850 **Sex Cord-Stromal Tumor, Mixed/Unclassified**
Steven S. Shen, MD, PhD and Jae Y. Ro, MD, PhD

TABLE OF CONTENTS

854 **Gonadoblastoma**
Steven S. Shen, MD, PhD and Jae Y. Ro, MD, PhD

HEMATOPOIETIC TUMORS

858 **Lymphoma/Leukemia/Plasmacytoma**
Steven S. Shen, MD, PhD and Jae Y. Ro, MD, PhD

TUMORS OF PARATESTICULAR STRUCTURES

864 **Adenomatoid Tumor**
Steven S. Shen, MD, PhD and Jae Y. Ro, MD, PhD

868 **Malignant Mesothelioma**
Steven S. Shen, MD, PhD and Jae Y. Ro, MD, PhD

872 **Adenocarcinoma of Rete Testis/Epididymis**
Steven S. Shen, MD, PhD and Jae Y. Ro, MD, PhD

874 **Papillary Serous Carcinoma, Müllerian Subtype**
Steven S. Shen, MD, PhD and Jae Y. Ro, MD, PhD

878 **Liposarcoma**
Steven S. Shen, MD, PhD and Jae Y. Ro, MD, PhD

882 **Melanotic Neuroectodermal Tumor**
Steven S. Shen, MD, PhD and Jae Y. Ro, MD, PhD

886 **Embryonal Rhabdomyosarcoma**
Steven S. Shen, MD, PhD and Jae Y. Ro, MD, PhD

890 **Other Sarcomas**
Steven S. Shen, MD, PhD and Jae Y. Ro, MD, PhD

METASTATIC TUMORS, TESTIS AND PARATESTICULAR STRUCTURES

894 **Metastatic Tumors, Testis and Paratesticular Structures**
Steven S. Shen, MD, PhD and Jae Y. Ro, MD, PhD

IMMUNOHISTOCHEMICAL PROFILES FOR TUMORS INVOLVING TESTIS AND PARATESTICULAR STRUCTURES

898 **Immunohistochemistry, Testis**
Steven S. Shen, MD, PhD, Mukul K. Divatia, MD, and Jae Y. Ro, MD, PhD

SECTION 5: PENIS AND SCROTUM

FREQUENT LESIONS OF UNCERTAIN RELATIONSHIP TO PENILE NEOPLASIA

908 **Condylomas**
María José Fernández De Nestosa, PhD

912 **Lichen Sclerosus et Atrophicus**
Elsa F. Velazquez, MD, Sofía Cañete Portillo, MD, and Antonio L. Cubilla, MD

914 **Squamous Hyperplasia**
Antonio L. Cubilla, MD, Diego Fernando Sánchez Martínez, MD, and Sofía Cañete Portillo, MD

918 **Lipogranuloma**
Elsa F. Velazquez, MD and Antonio L. Cubilla, MD

920 **Scrotal Calcinosis**
Elsa F. Velazquez, MD and Antonio L. Cubilla, MD

PENILE INTRAEPITHELIAL NEOPLASIA

922 **Penile Intraepithelial Neoplasia**
Elsa F. Velazquez, MD, Diego Fernando Sánchez Martínez, MD, and Antonio L. Cubilla, MD

PRIMARY EPITHELIAL TUMORS

928 **General Concepts, Squamous Cell Carcinoma**
Antonio L. Cubilla, MD, Diego Fernando Sánchez Martínez, MD, and Sofía Cañete Portillo, MD

938 **Squamous Cell Carcinoma, Usual Type**
Antonio L. Cubilla, MD, Diego Fernando Sánchez Martínez, MD, and Sofía Cañete Portillo, MD

VARIANTS OF SQUAMOUS CELL CARCINOMA

942 **Basaloid Squamous Cell Carcinoma**
Antonio L. Cubilla, MD, Diego Fernando Sánchez Martínez, MD, and Sofía Cañete Portillo, MD

946 **Basaloid Squamous Cell Carcinoma, Papillary Variant**
Diego Fernando Sánchez Martínez, MD and Antonio L. Cubilla, MD

948 **Warty (Condylomatous) Squamous Cell Carcinoma**
Elsa F. Velazquez, MD, Sofía Cañete Portillo, MD, and Antonio L. Cubilla, MD

952 **Warty-Basaloid Squamous Cell Carcinoma**
Diego Fernando Sánchez Martínez, MD and Antonio L. Cubilla, MD

954 **Verrucous Squamous Cell Carcinoma**
Elsa F. Velazquez, MD, Sofía Cañete Portillo, MD, and Antonio L. Cubilla, MD

958 **Papillary Squamous Cell Carcinoma, Not Otherwise Specified**
Antonio L. Cubilla, MD, Diego Fernando Sánchez Martínez, MD, and Sofía Cañete Portillo, MD

962 **Pseudoglandular Squamous Cell Carcinoma**
Diego Fernando Sánchez Martínez, MD and Antonio L. Cubilla, MD

964 **Pseudohyperplastic Squamous Cell Carcinoma**
Antonio L. Cubilla, MD, Diego Fernando Sánchez Martínez, MD, and Sofía Cañete Portillo, MD

966 **Cuniculatum Squamous Cell Carcinoma**
Antonio L. Cubilla, MD, Diego Fernando Sánchez Martínez, MD, and Sofía Cañete Portillo, MD

970 **Sarcomatoid Squamous Cell Carcinoma**
Elsa F. Velazquez, MD, Sofía Cañete Portillo, MD, and Antonio L. Cubilla, MD

974 **Mixed Squamous Cell Carcinoma**
Antonio L. Cubilla, MD, Diego Fernando Sánchez Martínez, MD, and Sofía Cañete Portillo, MD

978 **Lymphoepithelioma-Like Squamous Cell Carcinoma**
Diego Fernando Sánchez Martínez, MD and Antonio L. Cubilla, MD

980 **Clear Cell Carcinoma**
Diego Fernando Sánchez Martínez, MD and Antonio L. Cubilla, MD

TABLE OF CONTENTS

HPV- AND NON-HPV-RELATED TUMORS

982 **Overview of HPV- and Non-HPV-Related Tumors**
María José Fernández De Nestosa, PhD, Diego Fernando Sánchez Martínez, MD, and Antonio L. Cubilla, MD

OTHER NEOPLASTIC CONDITIONS

986 **Extramammary Paget Disease**
Elsa F. Velazquez, MD and Antonio L. Cubilla, MD

990 **Kaposi Sarcoma**
Elsa F. Velazquez, MD, Jesse K. McKenney, MD, and Antonio L. Cubilla, MD

992 **Myointimoma**
Jesse K. McKenney, MD, Mahul B. Amin, MD, and Elsa F. Velazquez, MD

METASTATIC TUMORS

994 **Metastatic Tumors, Penis**
Antonio L. Cubilla, MD, Diego Fernando Sánchez Martínez, MD, and Sofía Cañete Portillo, MD

IMMUNOHISTOCHEMICAL PROFILES FOR TUMORS INVOLVING PENIS

996 **Immunohistochemistry, Penis**
Antonio L. Cubilla, MD

DIAGNOSTIC PATHOLOGY
Genitourinary

SECOND EDITION

AMIN | TICKOO

MCKENNEY • PANER • SHEN • SMITH • AL-AHMADIE
VELAZQUEZ • CUBILLA • RO • REUTER

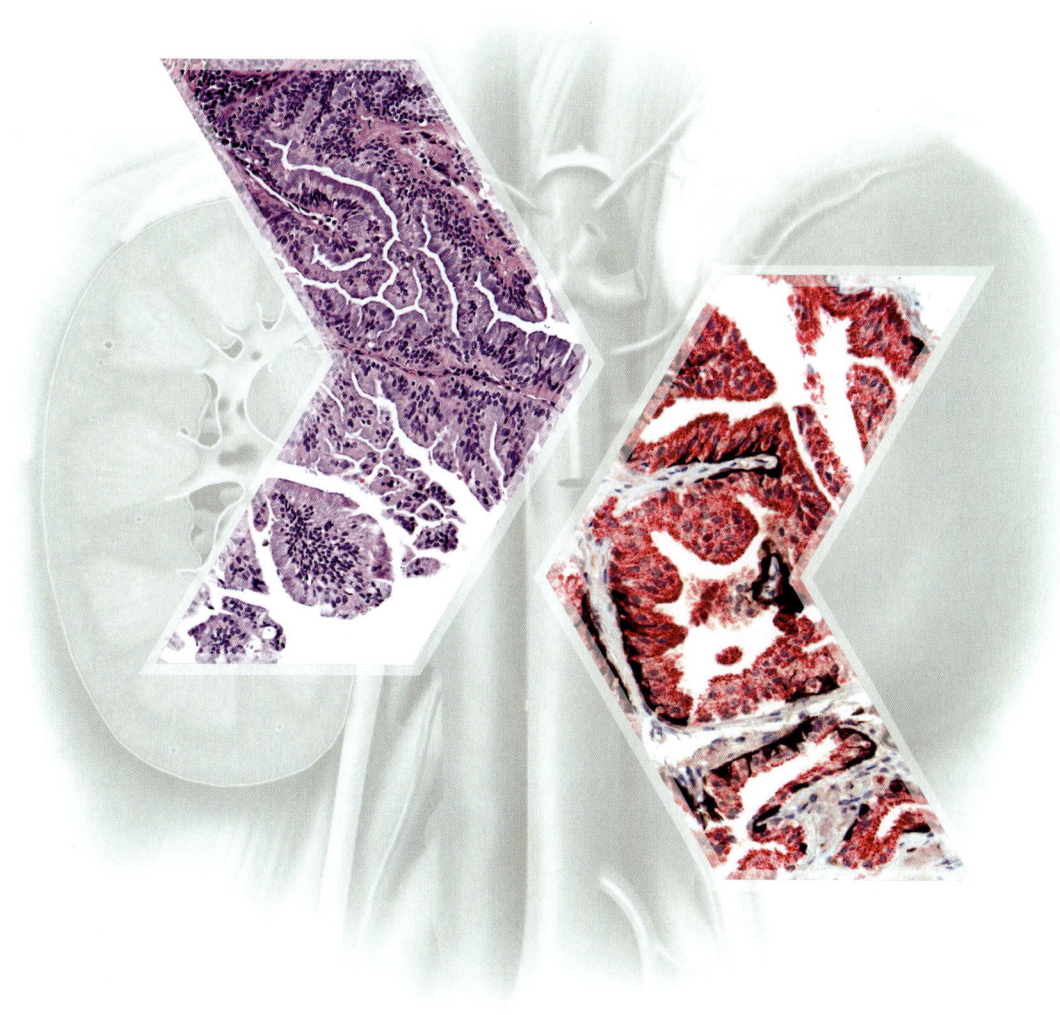

SECTION 1
Kidney Tumors and Tumor-Like Conditions

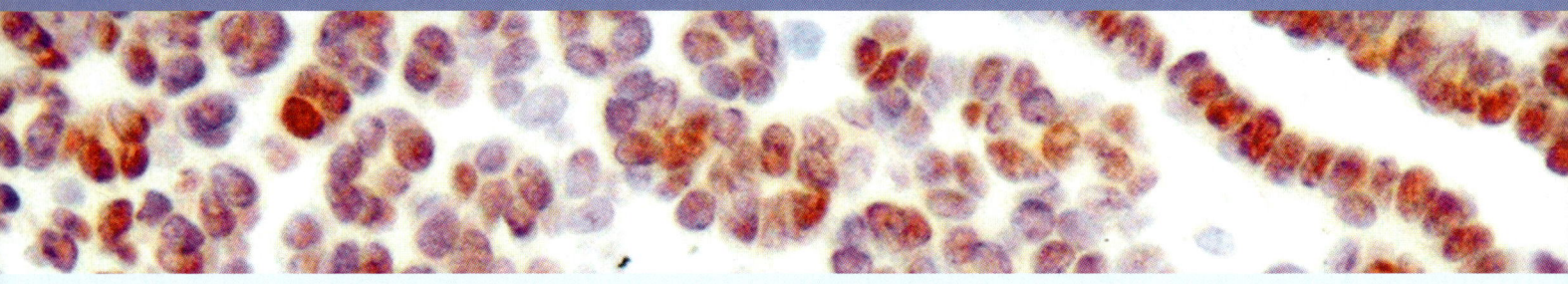

Introduction and Overview

Classification of Kidney Tumors and Tumor-Like Lesions	4
Introduction to Renal Cell Tumors	6

Familial Cancer Syndromes

von Hippel-Lindau Syndrome	12
Birt-Hogg-Dubé Syndrome	16
Hereditary Leiomyomatosis Renal Cell Carcinoma Syndrome	20
Tuberous Sclerosis Complex	24
Succinate Dehydrogenase Complex Deficiency Syndrome	28
Hereditary Papillary Renal Cancer and Miscellaneous Other Familial Cancer Syndromes	32

Nonneoplastic Lesions

Renal Tuberculosis, Xanthogranulomatous Pyelonephritis, Renal Malakoplakia	38

Renal Cell Tumors, Benign

Papillary Adenoma	44
Renal Oncocytoma	48

Renal Cell Carcinoma

Clear Cell Renal Cell Carcinoma	54
Multilocular Cystic Clear Cell Renal Cell Neoplasm of Low Malignant Potential	64
Transcription Elongation Factor B (*TCEB1*)-Mutated Renal Cell Carcinoma	68
Clear Cell Papillary Renal Cell Carcinoma	72
Papillary Renal Cell Carcinoma	80
Chromophobe Renal Cell Carcinoma	90
Collecting Duct Carcinoma	98
Renal Medullary Carcinoma	104
MiTF/TFE Family Translocation-Associated Carcinoma	110
Mucinous Tubular and Spindle Cell Carcinoma	118
Tubulocystic Carcinoma	124
Thyroid-Like Follicular Carcinoma of Kidney	128
Acquired Cystic Disease-Associated Renal Cell Carcinoma	132
Subsequent Second Tumors	138
Renal Cell Carcinoma, Unclassified	142

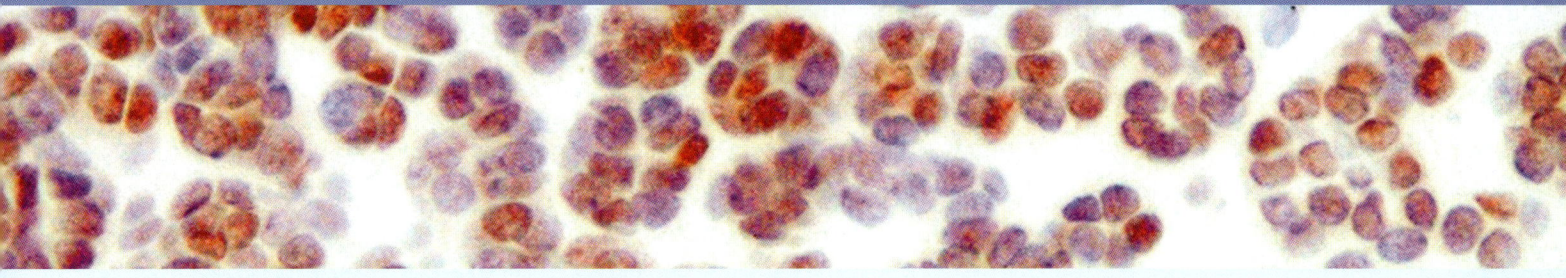

Metanephric Tumors

Metanephric Adenoma	**146**
Metanephric Tumors Other Than Metanephric Adenoma	**152**

Nephroblastic Tumors

Nephrogenic Rests	**156**
Nephroblastoma (Wilms Tumor)	**160**
Cystic Partially Differentiated Nephroblastoma	**170**

Mesenchymal Tumors

Angiomyolipoma	**172**
Epithelioid Angiomyolipoma	**178**
Congenital Mesoblastic Nephroma	**184**
Clear Cell Sarcoma of Kidney	**188**
Malignant Rhabdoid Tumor	**192**

Mixed Mesenchymal and Epithelial Tumors

Mixed Epithelial and Stromal Tumor (MEST) Family Tumors and Pediatric Cystic Nephroma	**196**
Synovial Sarcoma	**204**

Neuroendocrine Tumors

Well-Differentiated Neuroendocrine Tumor (Carcinoid) and High-Grade Neuroendocrine Carcinoma	**208**
Primitive Neuroectodermal Tumor	**212**

Hematopoietic Tumors

Hematopoietic Tumors	**216**

Metastatic and Other Tumors

Juxtaglomerular Cell Tumor (Reninoma)	**222**
Renomedullary Interstitial Cell Tumor	**226**
Other Rare Tumors	**230**
Metastatic Tumors	**238**

Immunohistochemical Profiles for Tumors Involving Kidney

Immunohistochemistry, Kidney	**242**

Classification of Kidney Tumors and Tumor-Like Lesions

NONNEOPLASTIC LESIONS

Tumor-Like Lesions
- Xanthogranulomatous pyelonephritis
- Renal malakoplakia
- Renal tuberculosis
- Inflammatory myofibroblastic lesion/tumor
- Perirenal and sinus cysts

NEOPLASMS

Kidney Tumors in Children
- Nephroblastic tumors
  - Nephroblastoma (Wilms tumor)
    - Favorable histology
    - Unfavorable histology (anaplasia)
  - Nephrogenic rests and nephroblastomatosis
  - Cystic, partially differentiated nephroblastoma
- Congenital mesoblastic nephroma
  - Classic
  - Cellular
  - Mixed
- Clear cell sarcoma
- Malignant rhabdoid tumor
- Renal cell tumors
  - MiTF/TFE family translocation-associated carcinoma
  - Renal medullary carcinoma
  - Papillary renal cell carcinoma
  - Clear cell renal cell carcinoma
  - Renal cell carcinoma, unclassified
- Metanephric tumors
  - Metanephric adenoma
  - Metanephric adenofibroma
  - Metanephric stromal tumor
- Pediatric cystic nephroma
- Rare tumors
  - Ossifying renal tumor of infancy

Kidney Tumors in Adults
- Benign epithelial tumors
  - Renal oncocytoma
  - Papillary adenoma
- Metanephric tumors
  - Metanephric adenoma
  - Metanephric adenofibroma
  - Metanephric stromal tumor
  - Metanephric adenosarcoma
- Renal cell carcinoma
  - Clear cell renal cell carcinoma
    - Multilocular cystic renal neoplasm of low malignant potential
  - Clear cell papillary renal cell carcinoma
  - Transcription elongation factor B (*TCEB1*)-mutated renal cell carcinoma
  - Papillary renal cell carcinoma
    - Type 1
    - Type 2
    - Oncocytic variant
    - Sarcomatoid
  - Chromophobe renal cell carcinoma
    - Classic
    - Eosinophilic variant
    - Sarcomatoid
  - Collecting duct carcinoma
  - Renal medullary carcinoma
  - Tubulocystic carcinoma
  - MiTF/TFE family translocation-associated carcinoma
    - Xp11.2 with *TFE3* gene fusion
    - t(6;11) with *TFEB* gene fusion
  - Mucinous tubular and spindle cell carcinoma
  - Thyroid-like follicular carcinoma of kidney
  - Renal cell carcinoma, unclassified
  - Tumors associated with end-stage kidney disease
    - Acquired cystic disease-associated renal cell carcinoma
    - Clear cell papillary renal cell carcinoma
    - Papillary renal cell carcinoma
    - Clear cell renal cell carcinoma
    - Chromophobe renal cell carcinoma
    - Collecting duct carcinoma
    - Renal oncocytoma
- 2nd tumors
  - Post neuroblastoma
  - Post transplant
  - Post chemotherapy

Mesenchymal Tumors: Benign
- Angiomyolipoma
- Medullary fibroma (renomedullary interstitial tumor)
- Leiomyoma
- Lipoma
- Hemangioma
- Lymphangioma
- Others

Mesenchymal Tumors: Malignant or Potentially Malignant
- Epithelioid angiomyolipoma (PEComa)
- Solitary fibrous tumor
- Leiomyosarcoma
- Synovial sarcoma
- Liposarcoma
- Fibrosarcoma
- Malignant fibrous histiocytoma
- Rhabdomyosarcoma
- Angiosarcoma
- Osteosarcoma
- Others

Rare Tumors With Epithelial &/or Parenchymal Differentiation
- Juxtaglomerular cell tumor (reninoma)
- Nephroblastoma and other "pediatric-type" renal tumors
- Renal epithelial and stromal tumor
  - Mixed epithelial and stromal tumor
  - Cystic nephroma

Neuroendocrine/Neural Tumors
- Well-differentiated neuroendocrine tumor (renal carcinoid tumor)
- Small cell neuroendocrine carcinoma
- Large cell neuroendocrine carcinoma

Classification of Kidney Tumors and Tumor-Like Lesions

- Ewing/primitive neuroectodermal tumor
- Paraganglioma
- Intrarenal schwannoma
- Pheochromocytoma
- Neuroblastoma

Hematopoietic Tumors
- Lymphoma
- Leukemia
- Plasmacytoma/multiple myeloma
- Posttransplantation lymphoproliferative lesions

Tumors Associated With Familial Syndromes
- von Hippel-Lindau syndrome
  - Clear cell renal cell carcinoma
  - Clear cell papillary renal cell carcinoma
- Hereditary papillary renal carcinoma syndrome
  - Papillary renal cell carcinoma, type 1
- Birt-Hogg-Dubé syndrome
  - Chromophobe renal cell carcinoma
  - Renal oncocytoma
  - Hybrid tumors
  - Others
- Hereditary leiomyomatosis and renal cell carcinoma syndrome (HLRCC)
  - HLRCC-associated renal cell carcinoma
- Tuberous sclerosis syndrome
  - Angiomyolipoma
  - Renal cell carcinoma
- Succinate dehydrogenase complex-deficiency syndrome
  - Succinate dehydrogenase B-deficient renal cell carcinoma
  - Others

Metastatic Tumors
- Prostate
- Lung
- Colon
- Female genital organs
- Salivary gland
- Others

Others
- Renal-adrenal fusion
- Intrarenal adrenal rests
- Intrarenal adrenal cortical neoplasms

Introduction to Renal Cell Tumors

TERMINOLOGY

Abbreviations
- Renal cell carcinoma (RCC)

EPIDEMIOLOGY

Incidence and Natural History
- RCC accounts for ~ 2% of all cancers, with 61,560 new cases expected in 2015 in USA
  o Worldwide: 338,000 cases in 2012
- In USA: 14,080 people expected to die from this disease in 2015
  o Worldwide: 143,000 deaths in 2012
- Incidence varies among countries
  o Highest rates in North America and Scandinavia
- Incidence of RCC increased substantially over last 2 decades, at least in part as result of improved diagnostic techniques
  o Most cases in larger medical centers now incidentally detected, mostly on radiologic investigations for unrelated conditions
- Up to 30% of patients with RCC present with metastatic disease
  o Recurrence develops in 40% of patients treated for localized tumor
- 5-year survival rates historically ~ 40%; median overall survival in patients with metastasis ~ 12 months
  o In more recent years, targeted therapies against various pathway molecules active in RCC show prolonged survival

Age Range
- RCCs show wide age spectrum
- Peak incidence, 6th and 7th decades of life
  o Occur 2x more frequently in men than in women

CLINICAL IMPLICATIONS

Anatomic Considerations
- Gerota fascia (renal fascia)
  o Layer of connective tissue encapsulating perirenal fat, kidney, and adrenal gland
    - Anterior to this fascia is anterior pararenal space, which contains pancreas, transverse colon, and parts of duodenum
    - Surgeons typically remove kidney along with its Gerota fascia
    - Microscopically, Gerota fascia does not have any distinctive features other than ill-defined, somewhat compressed connective tissue
      □ For practical purposes, tumors present at soft tissue (inked) margins of specimen equate Gerota fascia invasion (pT4)
- Protrusion vs. perinephric fat invasion
  o RCC frequently shows exophytic, often mushroom-like component protruding into perirenal fat
    - Usually capped by well-defined, smooth fibrous/fibromuscular capsule
    - Unless tumor shows irregular extensions, incomplete pseudocapsule, or single cells invading fat, not regarded as extracapsular extension (pT3a)
- Renal sinus
  o Constitutes extrarenal soft tissue lateral to imaginary vertical line joining medial-most aspects of upper and lower renal poles
  o Contains adipose tissue, lymphatics, veins, arteries, nerves, and pelvicalyceal system
  o Extends deep into kidney, even into renal cortex (intrarenal portion of sinus)
- Renal sinus vein and fat invasion
  o According to AJCC/TNM staging, sinus fat or extrarenal fat invasion, renal vein or large branches of renal vein in renal sinus invasion, all assigned same pT stage (pT3a)
  o Renal sinus fat or vein invasion occurs in overwhelming majority of tumors (clear cell RCCs) > 7 cm in diameter
  o Current AJCC/TNM staging designates tumors > 10 cm confined to kidney as pT2b; however, probability of tumors >10 cm limited to kidney very low
  o Sinus fat invasion may occur as direct tumor extension into fat or, more often, represents intravascular tumor penetrating through vessel wall

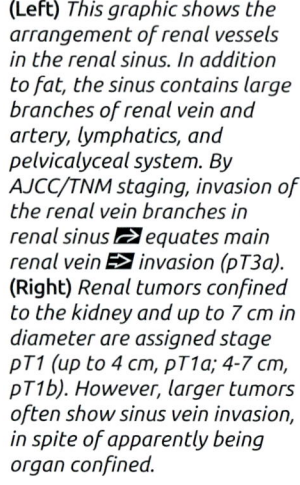

(Left) This graphic shows the arrangement of renal vessels in the renal sinus. In addition to fat, the sinus contains large branches of renal vein and artery, lymphatics, and pelvicalyceal system. By AJCC/TNM staging, invasion of the renal vein branches in renal sinus ➤ equates main renal vein ➡ invasion (pT3a). (Right) Renal tumors confined to the kidney and up to 7 cm in diameter are assigned stage pT1 (up to 4 cm, pT1a; 4-7 cm, pT1b). However, larger tumors often show sinus vein invasion, in spite of apparently being organ confined.

Graphic Image: Renal Sinus Anatomy

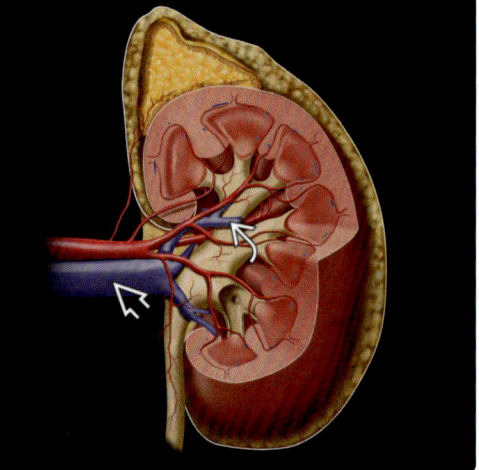

Graphic Image: pT1 Tumors

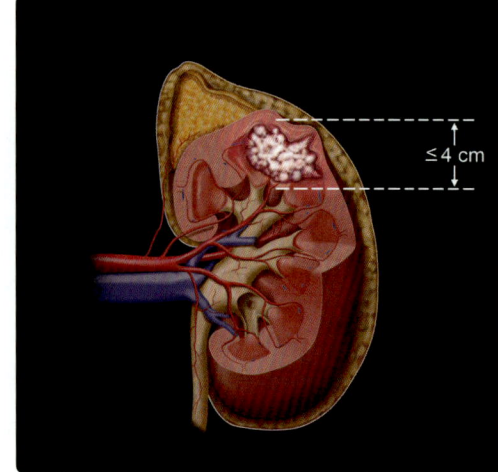

Introduction to Renal Cell Tumors

- Tissue sections including sinus areas may show tumor nodules with smooth outlines floating free in space
  - Such nodules invariably represent tumor in vessels or pelvicalyceal system
  - Deeper cuts into tissue blocks often reveal walls of veins or pelvicalyceal system that are not represented in the initial sections
  - When not apparent on deeper levels, further sampling of renal hilum is imperative
- Renal vein margin
  - Renal vein margin considered positive only if there is adherent tumor at actual margin, as confirmed microscopically

Intraoperative (Frozen-Section) Evaluation: Main Indications

- To determine whether tumor is renal cortical neoplasm or urothelial carcinoma of pelvicalyceal system
  - Distinction particularly important when partial nephrectomies being contemplated
    - For urothelial carcinoma, partial or total nephrectomy not adequate or acceptable option
      - Nephroureterectomy with bladder cuff is standard
    - For renal cortical neoplasms, no further intraoperative action may be needed
  - Specific intraoperative subtyping of cortical tumors not indicated, as surgical management not dependent on specific tumor type
- To evaluate surgical margins, particularly in partial nephrectomies

Staging Issues: Renal Cortical Tumors

- Renal cortical tumors confined to kidney is assigned stages pT1 or pT2 by AJCC/WHO
- Soft tissue or vascular spread beyond kidney (pT3) recognized as major prognostic factor
  - Before 6th edition of TNM/AJCC staging system (2002), no mention of renal sinus fat or renal vein branch invasion
  - Multiple recent studies report prognostic significance of renal sinus fat or large branches of renal vein invasion
    - Many publications have equated renal vein invasion with large sinus vein invasion
- Adrenal gland invasion: Involvement of ipsilateral adrenal gland by direct spread occurs in ~ 5% of cases
  - In current AJCC/TNM staging system, contiguous adrenal spread regarded as stage pT4
  - Discontinuous or contralateral involvement of adrenal gland considered metastasis (stage M1)

Specimen-Handling Issues: Radical and Total Nephrectomy Specimens for Renal Cortical Tumors

- Inking entire external surface often not required
  - However, inking required for cases with apparent extrarenal involvement on gross evaluation or on tumors with extrarenal bulging
- Specimen should be bisected in sagittal plane into anterior and posterior halves
  - Traditionally, specimens cut from lateral border toward hilum; however, opening renal vein and bisecting outward through vein is better option
    - This approach more often identifies gross sinus vein invasion

Specimen-Handling Issues: Partial Nephrectomy Specimens for Renal Cortical Tumors

- Inking of parenchymal resection margin a must
  - Inking external surface usually not required but should be performed in cases with apparent extrarenal involvement or bulging on gross evaluation

Sections to Be Submitted for Renal Cortical Tumors

- At least 1 block/cm of primary tumor
- Appropriate/variable number of blocks to identify extension into perirenal fat
- Multiple blocks from tumor-renal sinus interface
  - Such sampling important since renal sinus can extend deep into renal cortex, even when not recognized grossly
- Multiple blocks from identifiable or suspected venous or collecting system invasion
- At least 1 block from tumor-kidney interface
- 1 block from adrenal gland if away from tumor or multiple blocks if close to tumor
- All identified lymph nodes
- Blocks from all identifiable other renal abnormalities
- At least 1 block from macroscopically normal renal parenchyma, away from tumor

Grading Issues: Renal Cortical Tumors

- Multiple grading schemes have been proposed, and Fuhrman grading system has been most commonly used system
- However, primarily because of problems with reproducibility in Fuhrman system, WHO recommends WHO/International Society of Urological Pathology (ISUP) nucleolar grading system
- WHO /ISUP (nucleolar) grading system
  - Grade 1: Nucleoli absent or inconspicuous at 400 magnification
  - Grade 2: Nucleoli conspicuous and eosinophilic at 400 magnification and visible but not prominent at 100 magnification
  - Grade 3: Nucleoli conspicuous and eosinophilic at 100 magnification
  - Grade 4: Not based on nucleolar prominence but presence of
    - Extreme nuclear pleomorphism, multinucleated giant cells, &/or rhabdoid or sarcomatoid differentiation
- WHO/ISUP grading is only for clear cell and papillary renal cell carcinomas
  - Not found to be useful in chromophobe RCC
- Combination of nucleolar grade and presence of tumor necrosis recently reported as better grading scheme than nucleolar grade alone
- No role in grading of renal oncocytomas because of benign clinical behavior in all tumors

Management

- Renal cortical tumors
  - Partial, total, or radical nephrectomy is mainstay of treatment options

Introduction to Renal Cell Tumors

Primary Tumor (pT) Staging for Renal Cell Tumors (2010)

TNM	Definitions
pT1	Tumor ≤ 7 cm in greatest dimension, limited to kidney
pT1a	Tumor ≤ 4 cm in greatest dimension, limited to kidney
pT1b	Tumor > 4 cm but ≤ 7 cm in greatest dimension, limited to kidney
pT2	Tumor > 7 cm in greatest dimension, limited to kidney
pT2a	Tumor > 7 cm but ≤ 10 cm in greatest dimension, limited to kidney
pT2b	Tumor > 10 cm, limited to kidney
pT3	Tumor extends into major veins or perinephric tissues but not into ipsilateral adrenal gland and not beyond Gerota fascia
pT3a	Tumor grossly extends into renal vein or its segmental (muscle containing) branches, or tumor invades perirenal &/or renal sinus fat but not beyond Gerota fascia
pT3b	Tumor grossly extends into vena cava below diaphragm
pT3c	Tumor grossly extends into vena cava above diaphragm or invades wall of vena cava
pT4	Tumor invades beyond Gerota fascia (including contiguous extension into ipsilateral adrenal gland)

- Surgical resection of primary tumor is often performed to decrease tumor load even in patients with metastatic disease
  o In situ tumor ablations becoming more common now, particularly for smaller tumors
  o Active surveillance is management option in some cases, based on tumor subtype and other clinicopathological parameters (e.g., patient comorbidities)
  o Traditionally, immunotherapy using IL-2 and interferons was treatment of choice in metastatic settings
    - Chemotherapy not effective in most RCCs
    - 5-year survivals only ~ 20% with these therapeutic approaches
  o Targeted therapies against molecules of multiple pathways active in renal cancer have become treatment of choice in recent years
    - Besides their use in metastatic RCC, these therapies are currently also being evaluated in adjuvant setting in some high-risk tumors

Prognostic Factors
- Some established factors influencing clinical outcome in RCC include
  o Primary tumor stage, size, distant/nodal metastases, histologic subtype, nuclear grade (in clear cell RCC), sarcomatoid features, tumor necrosis, small vessel lymphovascular invasion
  o Performance status, presence or absence of systemic symptoms, thrombocytosis, anemia, elevated ESR, elevated C-reactive protein, etc.
- Molecular factors, including CA9, HIF-1-α, BAP1, SETD2, CXCR3, CXCR4, B7-H1, PTEN, Ki-67, survivin, vitamin D receptors, etc., reported to influence prognosis
  o Role of none of these is established yet

SELECTED REFERENCES

1. Raspollini MR et al: Unlike in clear cell renal cell carcinoma, KRAS is not mutated in multilocular cystic clear cell renal cell neoplasm of low potential. Virchows Arch. 467(6): 687-93, 2015
2. Siegel RL et al: Cancer statistics, 2015. CA Cancer J Clin. 65(1):5-29, 2015
3. Winters BR et al: Cystic renal cell carcinoma carries an excellent prognosis regardless of tumor size. Urol Oncol. 33(12):505.e9-505.e13, 2015
4. Tan PH et al: Renal tumors: diagnostic and prognostic biomarkers. Am J Surg Pathol. 37(10):1518-31, 2013
5. Trpkov K et al: Handling and staging of renal cell carcinoma: the International Society of Urological Pathology Consensus (ISUP) conference recommendations. Am J Surg Pathol. 37(10):1505-17, 2013
6. Luo JH et al: Analysis of long-term survival in patients with localized renal cell carcinoma: laparoscopic versus open radical nephrectomy. World J Urol. 28(3): 289-93, 2010
7. Srigley JR et al: Protocol for the examination of specimens from patients with invasive carcinoma of renal tubular origin. Arch Pathol Lab Med. 134(4):e25-30, 2010
8. Aubert S et al: MUC1, a new hypoxia inducible factor target gene, is an actor in clear renal cell carcinoma tumor progression. Cancer Res. 69(14):5707-15, 2009
9. Hagemann IS et al: A retrospective comparison of 2 methods of intraoperative margin evaluation during partial nephrectomy. J Urol. 181(2):500-5, 2009
10. Jain P et al: Renal cell carcinoma: Impact of mode of detection on its pathological characteristics. Indian J Urol. 25(4):479-82, 2009
11. Osunkoya AO et al: Diagnostic biomarkers for renal cell carcinoma: selection using novel bioinformatics systems for microarray data analysis. Hum Pathol. 40(12):1671-8, 2009
12. Sunela KL et al: Prognostic factors and long-term survival in renal cell cancer patients. Scand J Urol Nephrol. 43(6):454-60, 2009
13. Lane BR et al: Prognostic models and algorithms in renal cell carcinoma. Urol Clin North Am. 35(4):613-25; vii, 2008
14. Grignon D et al: Renal cell carcinoma and the renal sinus. Adv Anat Pathol. 14(2):63-8, 2007
15. Kirkali Z et al: What does the urologist expect from the pathologist (and what can the pathologists give) in reporting on adult kidney tumour specimens? Eur Urol. 51(5):1194-201, 2007
16. Berdjis N et al: Impact of resection margin status after nephron-sparing surgery for renal cell carcinoma. BJU Int. 97(6):1208-10, 2006
17. Bonsib SM: T2 clear cell renal cell carcinoma is a rare entity: a study of 120 clear cell renal cell carcinomas. J Urol. 174(4 Pt 1):1199-202; discussion 1202, 2005
18. Che M et al: Handling and reporting of tumor-containing kidney specimens. Clin Lab Med. 25(2):417-32, 2005
19. Fleming S et al: Best Practice No 180. Nephrectomy for renal tumour; dissection guide and dataset. J Clin Pathol. 58(1):7-14, 2005
20. Algaba F et al: Handling and pathology reporting of renal tumor specimens. Eur Urol. 45(4):437-43, 2004
21. Kubinski DJ et al: Utility of frozen section analysis of resection margins during partial nephrectomy. Urology. 64(1):31-4, 2004

Introduction to Renal Cell Tumors

Graphic Image: pT2

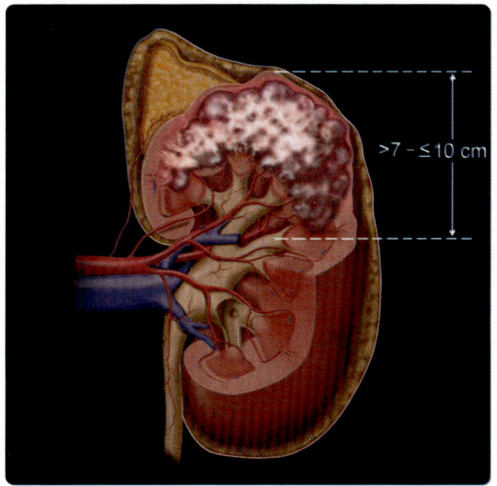

Graphic Image: pT3 and pT4

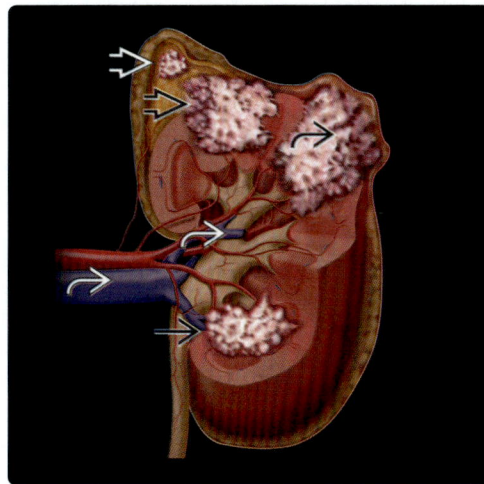

(Left) *Tumors > 7 cm in diameter, and confined to the kidney, are assigned pT2 stage by TNM/AJCC; pT2a, 7-10 cm, and 2b, > 10 cm. However for clear cell RCCs, it is extremely rare for > 7 cm tumors not to have sinus invasion.* **(Right)** *The size criterion does not apply to tumors with extrarenal extension. Tumors with renal sinus ➡ or perirenal ➡ fat or renal vascular ➡ invasion are all assigned stage pT3a. Tumors directly invading the adrenal ➡ are considered pT4, and those with discontinuous adrenal invasion ➡ as pM1.*

Sinus Vein Invasion

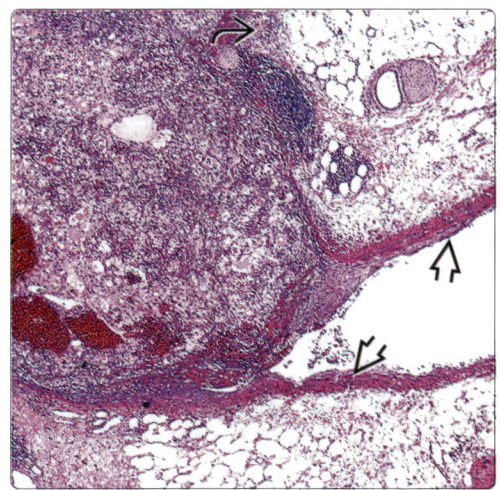

Sinus Vein Invasion

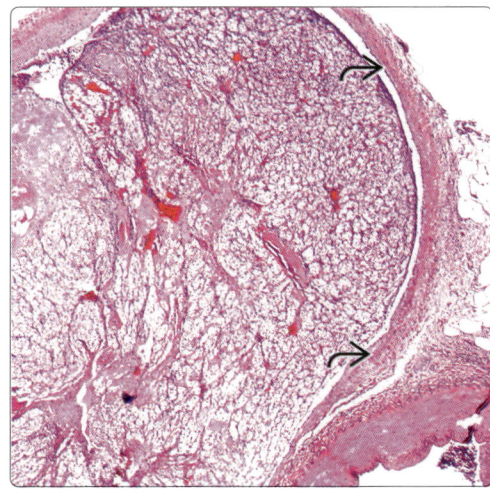

(Left) *Invasion of large renal vein branches ➡ in the renal sinus is equated with renal vein invasion (pT3a) by AJCC. Renal sinus fat invasion may occur as direct tumor extension, or by the invasion of tumor through the walls of the sinus veins ➡.* **(Right)** *Many, but not all, large branches of renal vein in the renal sinus possess prominent smooth muscle ➡ layer in their walls. Invasion of such veins has been shown to have clinical outcomes similar to the main renal vein invasion.*

Sinus Vein Invasion

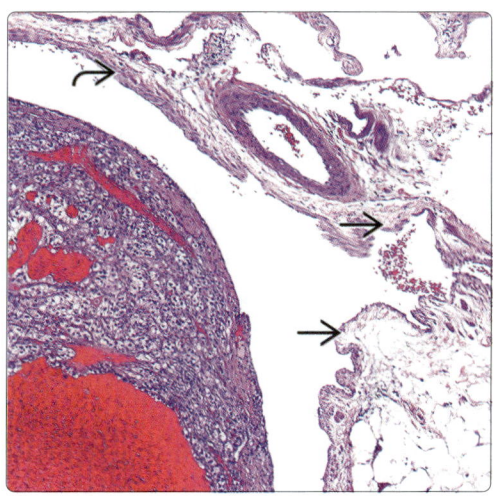

Sinus Vein Invasion

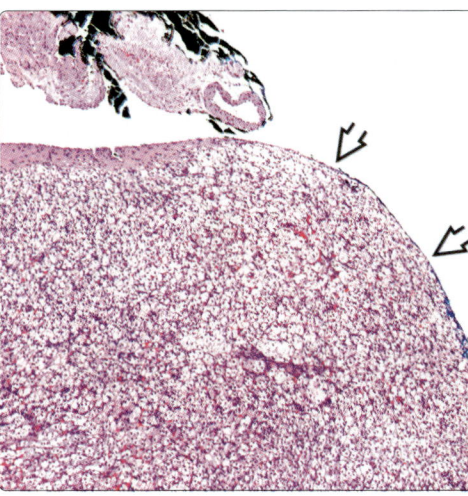

(Left) *The muscle layer ➡, in fact, is often discontinuous ➡, even in some of the largest of the veins in the renal sinus. Therefore, in the new AJCC staging system, the words "invasion of muscular branches" are being replaced by "invasion of large branches" of renal vein.* **(Right)** *In some cases, particularly in partial nephrectomy specimens, a tumor nodule with smooth outlines ➡ might appear "hanging free" in space. This almost invariably indicates tumor nodular in a vein or pelvicalyceal system.*

Introduction to Renal Cell Tumors

Sinus Vein Invasion

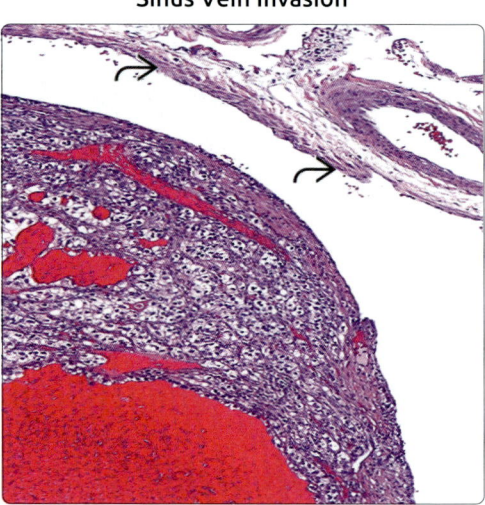

Tumor Capsule

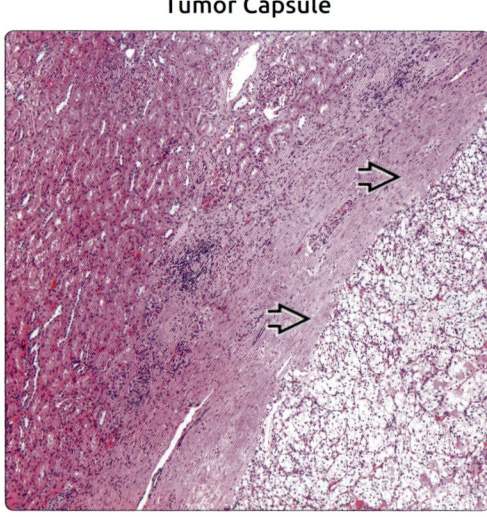

(Left) Deeper levels on sections with free-floating tumor nodules with smooth outlines often reveal the surrounding vessel walls ➡ that may not be present in the original sections. (Right) A number of renal cell tumors may have a fibrous capsule/pseudocapsule ➡. Among all renal cell carcinomas, papillary RCC is the most likely subtype to show a prominent fibrous pseudocapsule.

Tumor Capsule Penetration

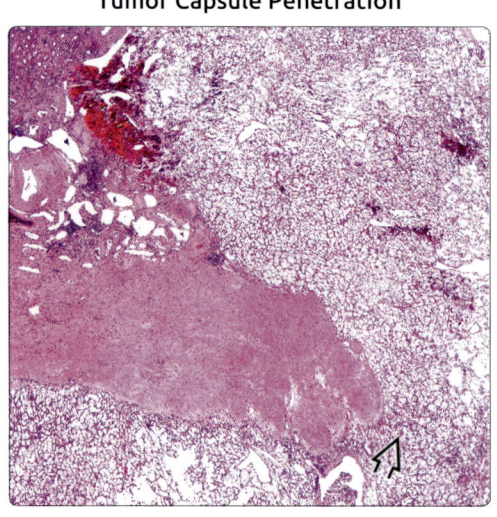

Renal Capsule Invasion

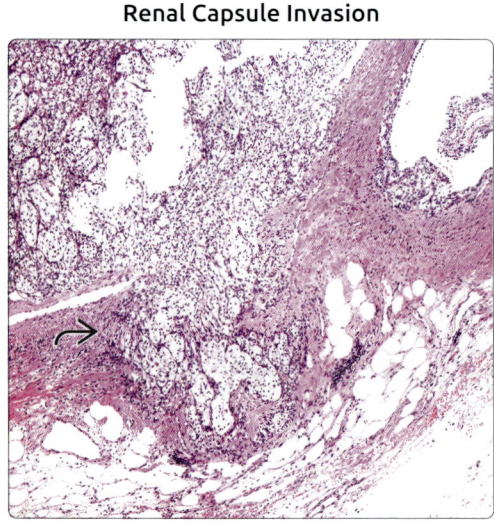

(Left) Penetration of the tumor through the tumor capsule ➡ is not a stage-defining occurrence in renal cell tumors. (Right) For a tumor to be regarded as stage pT3a because of capsular invasion, the tumor is required to penetrates the renal capsule ➡ and not the tumor capsule. pT3a stage is assigned to all tumors penetrating the renal capsule, invading the renal sinus fat, or invading renal vein or its large branches in the renal sinus.

Renal Sinus

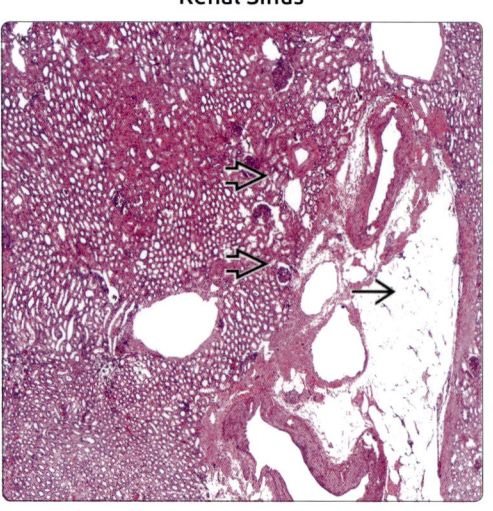

Renal Capsule

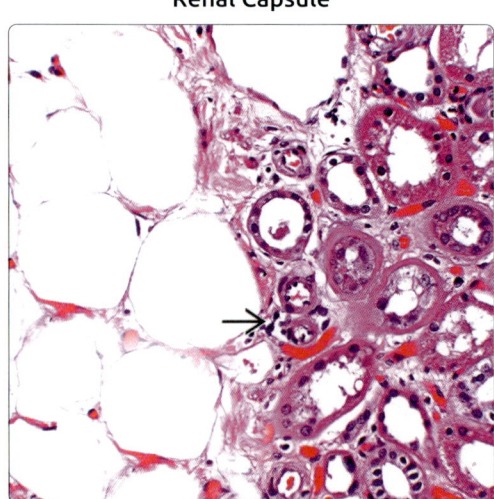

(Left) Renal sinus ➡ often extends deep into renal cortex ➡. Therefore, even tumors that grossly appear to be located within the cortex may also show sinus vein invasion. This is particularly true of tumors > 4-5 cm in maximum diameter. (Right) The renal capsule may be completely absent, and the tubules may be in direct contact ➡ with the sinus fat. This may result in an easy pathway for RCCs to invade the sinus fat, although such invasion more frequently occurs by penetration through vessel wall by intravenous tumors.

Introduction to Renal Cell Tumors

Sinus Vein and Sinus Fat Invasion

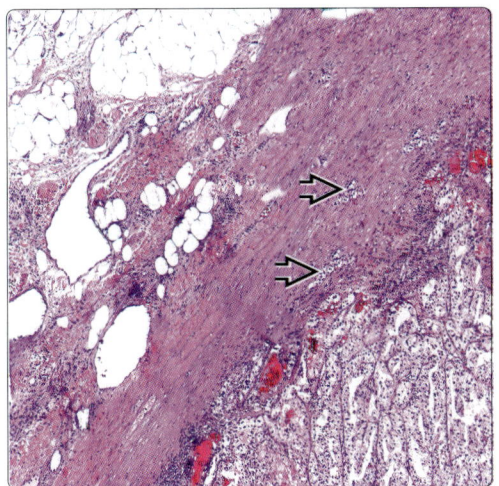

Fat Invasion: Is It Real?

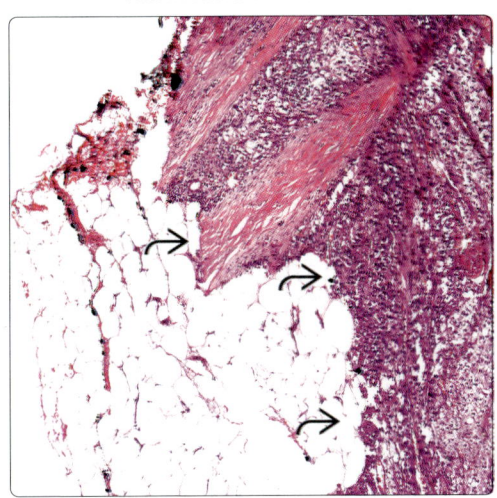

(Left) Nodules of tumor are often seen in the sinus fat in large tumors. While these are often regarded as sinus fat invasion, most in fact represent tumor completely filling large veins, destroying their walls ⇨, and extending into the surrounding soft tissue. (Right) This abrupt association of fat with tumor cells is not uncommon in nephrectomy specimens. Lack of tissue response, and the unnatural, abrupt relation of tumor capsule and tumor cells with the fat ⇨ indicates it to be an artifact and not a true pT3a tumor.

Renal Pelvis Invasion

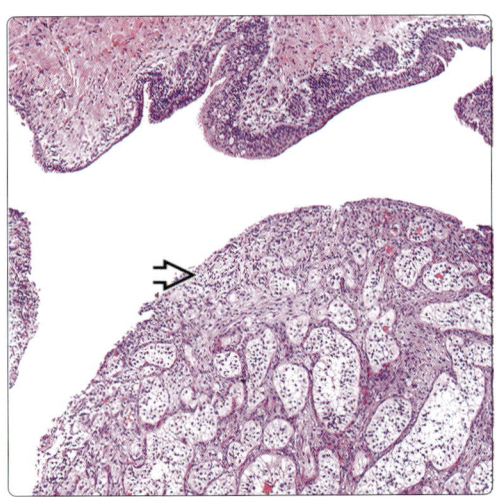

Tumor Arising in Cyst

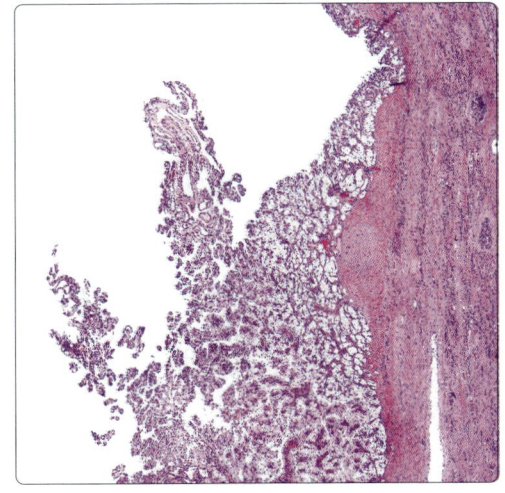

(Left) While invasion of the pelvicalyceal system by RCC may suggest an aggressive phenotype, renal pelvic or calyceal invasion ⇨ does not influence the pathological stage of the tumor according to AJCC. (Right) RCCs arising from a cyst wall raise the issue of assessment of true tumor size. Including the cyst in the size determination may overestimate the tumor size. It may be prudent to specify the size of solid area, as well as the size of the cyst, in such a case. TNM/AJCC does not specifically address this issue.

Prognostic Factors: Lymphovascular Invasion (LVI)

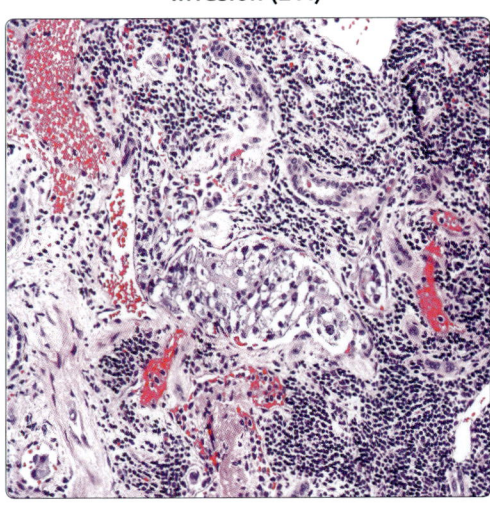

Prognostic Factors: Tumor Necrosis

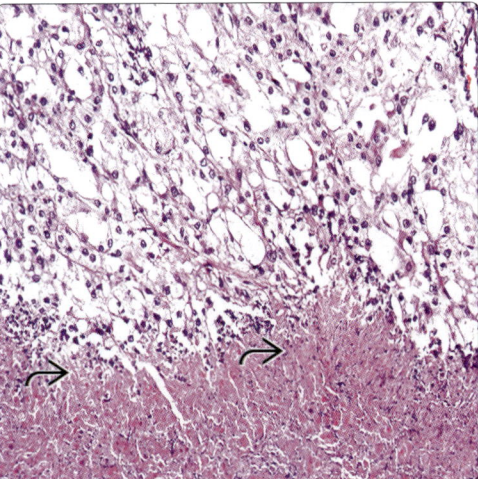

(Left) Small-vessel LVI appears to be an independent prognostic factor in clear cell, papillary and chromophobe RCC but likely not in other aggressive tumors, like HLRCC-associated, collecting duct and medullary carcinomas. (Right) Coagulative tumor necrosis ⇨ is considered to be an independent prognostic factor by some. Combination of nucleolar grade and the presence of tumor necrosis has recently been reported as a better grading scheme than nucleolar grade based on a large number of RCCs.

von Hippel-Lindau Syndrome

KEY FACTS

TERMINOLOGY
- Autosomal dominant syndrome, characterized by
  - Cerebellar, retinal and spinal hemangioblastomas, clear cell renal cell carcinomas (RCC) and multiple renal cysts, pheochromocytomas, pancreatic cysts and endocrine pancreatic tumors, endolymphatic sac tumors of ear, epididymal cystadenomas

ETIOLOGY/PATHOGENESIS
- Syndrome associated with alterations in tumor suppressor *VHL* gene, located at chromosome 3p25
  - *VHL* inactivated by various mutations, loss of heterozygosity (LOH), hypermethylations, or alterations in VHL modifier genes
    - Absence of functional gene product pVHL results in accumulation and overexpression of HIF-1α
    - Activated HIF-1 increases transcription of multiple genes by binding to hypoxia-responsive elements (HRE)
    - Many of these affected factors associated with angiogenesis, tumorigenesis, and tumor metastasis

CLINICAL ISSUES
- Depending on presence or absence of pheochromocytomas, VHL disease divided into types 1 and 2

MACROSCOPIC
- Renal lesions in VHL syndrome include multiple bilateral benign cysts, atypical cysts, cystic RCCs, and solid RCCs

MICROSCOPIC
- Almost all RCCs are clear cell RCC, morphologically similar to sporadic tumors
  - In addition to macroscopically identifiable tumors, numerous microscopic nodules of clear cells seen in VHL kidneys
- Occasional cysts and tumors morphologically similar to sporadic clear cell papillary RCC

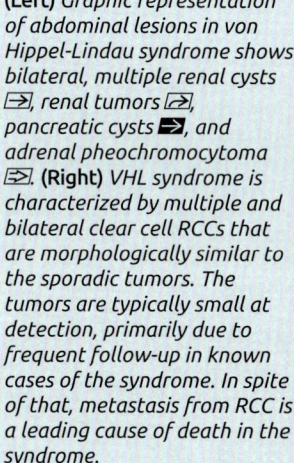

(Left) *Graphic representation of abdominal lesions in von Hippel-Lindau syndrome shows bilateral, multiple renal cysts ➡, renal tumors ➡, pancreatic cysts ➡, and adrenal pheochromocytoma ➡.* (Right) *VHL syndrome is characterized by multiple and bilateral clear cell RCCs that are morphologically similar to the sporadic tumors. The tumors are typically small at detection, primarily due to frequent follow-up in known cases of the syndrome. In spite of that, metastasis from RCC is a leading cause of death in the syndrome.*

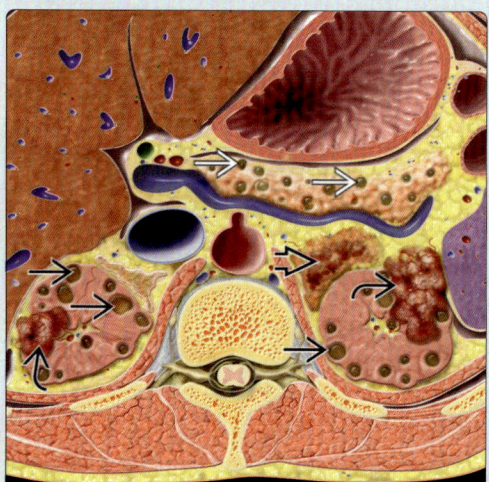

von Hippel-Lindau Syndrome: Abdominal Lesions

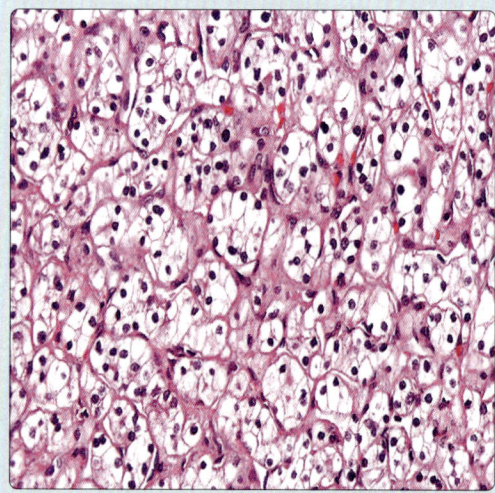

Clear Cell Renal Cell Carcinoma

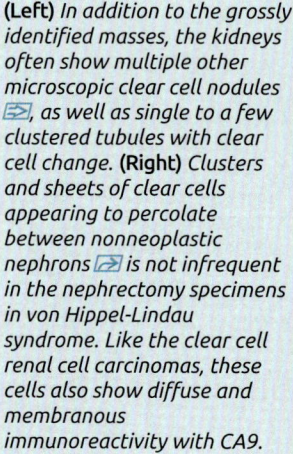

(Left) *In addition to the grossly identified masses, the kidneys often show multiple other microscopic clear cell nodules ➡, as well as single to a few clustered tubules with clear cell change.* (Right) *Clusters and sheets of clear cells appearing to percolate between nonneoplastic nephrons ➡ is not infrequent in the nephrectomy specimens in von Hippel-Lindau syndrome. Like the clear cell renal cell carcinomas, these cells also show diffuse and membranous immunoreactivity with CA9.*

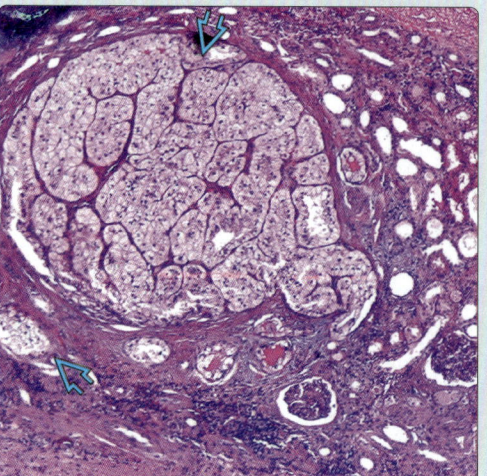

Microscopic Clear Cell Nodules

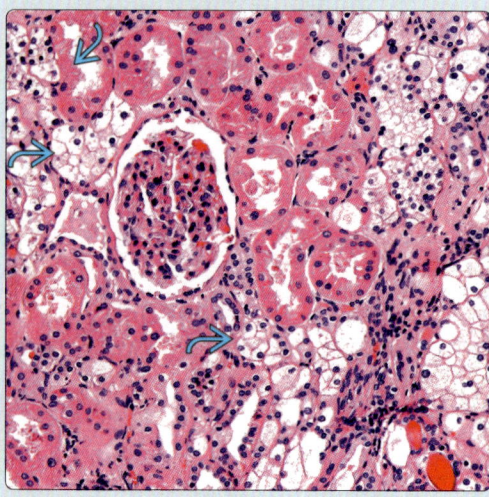

Percolating Clear Cells

von Hippel-Lindau Syndrome

TERMINOLOGY

Abbreviations
- von Hippel-Lindau syndrome (VHL)

Definitions
- Autosomal dominant syndrome, characterized by
  - Cerebellar and spinal hemangioblastomas
  - Retinal hemangioblastomas
  - Clear cell renal cell carcinomas (RCC) and multiple renal cysts
  - Pheochromocytomas
  - Pancreatic cysts and endocrine pancreatic tumors
  - Endolymphatic sac tumors of ear
  - Epididymal cystadenomas

ETIOLOGY/PATHOGENESIS

VHL Gene Alterations
- Syndrome associated with alterations in tumor suppressor *VHL* gene
- Gene located at chromosome 3p25
- Inactivated by various mutations, loss of heterozygosity (LOH), hypermethylations, or alterations in VHL modifier genes
- In VHL syndrome, germline mutation present in 1 allele of VHL gene
  - Clinical manifestations of disease result when mutations/silencing occur in other wild-type allele
  - *VHL* gene product pVHL essential for proteosomic degradation of hypoxia-inducible factor-1α (HIF-1α)
  - Absence of functional pVHL results in accumulation and overexpression of HIF-1α
  - Activated HIF-1 heterodimers localize to nucleus and regulate transcription of multiple genes by binding to hypoxia-responsive elements (HRE)
    – Targets activated include
      □ Vascular endothelial and platelet-derived growth factors (VEGF and PDGF) and receptors
      □ Glucose transporter protein-1 (GLUT1)
      □ Erythropoietin
      □ Carbonic anhydrase-IX (CA9)
      □ Transforming growth factor-alpha (TGF-α)
      □ C-X-C chemokine receptor type 4 (CXCR4)
      □ C-mesenchymal-epithelial transition factor (c-MET)
    – Many of these factors associated with angiogenesis, tumorigenesis, and tumor metastasis
- In addition to HIF degradation, VHL protein involved in multiple HIF-independent cellular processes
  - Directs proper deposition of fibronectin and collagen IV within extracellular matrix
  - Stabilizes microtubules and therefore helps in maintenance of primary cilia
  - Promotes stabilization and activation of p53 and promotes apoptosis by downregulation of Jun-B (in neurons)
  - VHL inactivation causes senescent-like phenotype dependent on retinoblastoma protein (Rb) and the SWI2/SNF2 chromatin remodeller p400

CLINICAL ISSUES

Presentation
- VHL, unlike most other familial renal cancer syndromes, shows high degree of genetic penetrance
- Estimated incidence: 1/36,000-1/45,500
- Depending on whether pheochromocytomas are present or not, VHL disease can be divided into 2 major types
  - Type 1: Not associated with pheochromocytomas
    – Involves loss of function mutations, including deletion, microinsertion, and nonsense mutations
  - Type 2 has high risk for pheochromocytomas and is divided into 3 subtypes
    – Type 2A: Associated with low risk for RCC
    – Type 2B: Associated with high risk for RCC
    – Type 2C: With pheochromocytomas only
    – Mutations that predispose to type 2 VHL are mainly of missense type that result in conformationally altered pVHL
    – These mutant pVHLs still may be able to retain some of their functions or may gain other novel functions
- VHL syndrome additionally comprises rare Chuvash polycythemia (familial erythrocythemia type 2)
  - Characterized by lack of solid tumors with high incidence in the Chuvash population in Volga river region

Treatment
- Options, risks, complications
  - Screening for renal tumors in VHL mutation-positive patients recommended after age 8, by annual ultrasound &/or MR of the abdomen
  - Current strategies advocate conservative management for all genetic, multifocal, bilateral tumors
    – Nephron-sparing surgery/tumor ablation strategy used with intent to remove all solid and partially cystic lesions from kidney
    – Procedure usually delayed until tumors grow beyond 3 cm in size
    – During follow-up, as new tumors develop, repeat procedures performed
    – Main intent of this approach to preserve renal function as much and as long as possible
  - Targeted therapies currently being investigated to potentially reduce tumor burden of even localized tumors in VHL

Prognosis
- In spite of relatively few patients developing metastasis, metastatic RCC is leading cause of death from VHL

MACROSCOPIC

General Features
- Renal lesions in VHL syndrome include
  - Multiple bilateral benign cysts, atypical cysts, cystic RCCs, and solid RCCs
- Kidneys are usually of normal size and weight, chiefly because most cysts and RCCs are small
- Mean age for development of renal carcinoma: 37 yr (range: 16-67 yr)
  - By age 70, chance of kidney cancer 70%

- However, renal lesions as earlier manifestation in only 7%
- Retinal and CNS hemangioblastomas usually manifest at earlier mean ages (25 and 30 yr)

Gross Features
- Cysts are usually few (3-30 in number; mean: 7.8 per kidney), usually small (almost all < 1.5 cm; mean size: 0.7 cm)
- Carcinomas multifocal and bilateral
  - Mostly solid, but some appear as solid nodules arising in cyst walls
  - Tumors often detected at small size due to frequent follow-up in known patients of syndrome

MICROSCOPIC
Histologic Features
- Renal cysts
  - Cysts may be unilocular or multilocular
  - Almost entirely lined by clear cells; focal or predominant granular cytoplasm rarely present
  - Cysts designated as
    - Benign cysts (1 layer of clear cells without atypia)
    - Atypical cysts (2 or 3 cells thick ± atypia)
      - Focal proliferations more than 3 cells thick regarded as cystic renal cell carcinoma
  - Increased vascularity often seen around cysts
- Renal cell carcinoma
  - Almost all RCCs are clear cell RCC, morphologically similar to sporadic tumors
  - In addition to macroscopically identifiable tumors, numerous microscopic nodules of clear cells seen in VHL kidneys
    - Some nodules well circumscribed
    - Others present as aggregates of clear cells, with irregular outlines
    - Clusters and sheets of clear cells appearing to percolate between nephrons are also common
  - Occasional cysts and tumors morphologically similar to sporadic clear cell papillary RCC
    - Reported to be similar to sporadic tumors by immunohistochemistry, and also lacking 3p losses
    - Others consider them different from sporadic clear cell papillary RCC, and similar to clear cell RCC
      - Differences likely a reflection of less rigorous morphological criteria applied for diagnosis of clear cell papillary RCC in these studies

DIFFERENTIAL DIAGNOSIS
Tuberous Sclerosis Complex
- Tuberous sclerosis complex (TSC) rarely with bilateral, multifocal RCC
  - Some RCCs have clear cell cytology and vasculature mimicking clear cell RCC
    - However, such clear cells often with voluminous cytoplasm and eosinophilic cytoplasmic strands
  - Frequently associated with angiomyolipomas and multiple cysts
    - Cyst lining often with abundant, eosinophilic granular cytoplasm, frequently with cytoplasmic vacuolization and hobnailing and large nuclei with prominent nucleoli
  - 3p or *VHL* gene-associated molecular alterations not found in TSC-associated RCC
    - *TSC1/TSC2* gene alterations present

Multifocal, Nonsyndromic Clear Cell Renal Cell Carcinoma
- Multifocality seen in ~ 5-10% of clear cell RCC
  - Many such tumors believed to represent intrarenal metastases
  - However, others shown to be of differing clonal origin, arising independently
- In general, number of multifocal tumors is quite small (2-5), not numerous as in VHL
- Not associated with other hallmarks of VHL, i.e., cysts, clusters of clear cells percolating between native nephrons, numerous clear cell nodules

Birt-Hogg-Dube (BHD) Syndrome
- ~ 9-12% of tumors in BHD syndrome are clear cell RCC
  - These clear cell tumors show *VHL* alterations
- Numerous oncocytic tumors and other features of renal oncocytosis in background

End-Stage Kidney Disease With Clear Cell Renal Cell Carcinoma
- Multifocal clear cell RCCs occasionally may be present in end-stage kidneys
- Often associated with other tumor types, both macroscopic and microscopic, often including
  - Clear cell papillary RCC, acquired cystic disease-associated RCC, papillary RCC, chromophobe RCC
- Background kidney invariably with end-stage renal disease, often with acquired cystic disease

SELECTED REFERENCES
1. Ben-Skowronek I et al: Von Hippel-Lindau Syndrome. Horm Res Paediatr. 84(3):145-52, 2015
2. Gossage L et al: VHL, the story of a tumour suppressor gene. Nat Rev Cancer. 15(1):55-64, 2015
3. Rao P et al: Clear cell papillary renal cell carcinoma in patients with von Hippel-Lindau syndrome--clinicopathological features and comparative genomic analysis of 3 cases. Hum Pathol. 45(9):1966-72, 2014
4. Richard S et al: Von Hippel-Lindau: how a rare disease illuminates cancer biology. Semin Cancer Biol. 23(1):26-37, 2013
5. Williamson SR et al: Clear cell papillary renal cell carcinoma-like tumors in patients with von Hippel-Lindau disease are unrelated to sporadic clear cell papillary renal cell carcinoma. Am J Surg Pathol. 37(8):1131-9, 2013
6. Maher ER et al: von Hippel-Lindau disease: a clinical and scientific review. Eur J Hum Genet. 19(6):617-23, 2011
7. Cheng L et al: Evidence for polyclonal origin of multifocal clear cell renal cell carcinoma. Clin Cancer Res. 14(24):8087-93, 2008
8. Gläsker S et al: Von Hippel-Lindau Syndrome. MDText.com, Inc. 2000

von Hippel-Lindau Syndrome

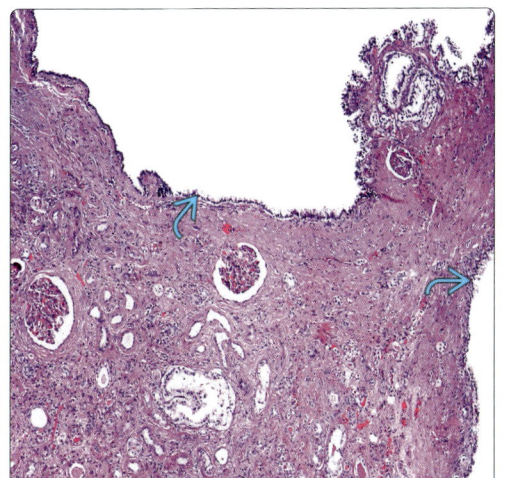

Cysts

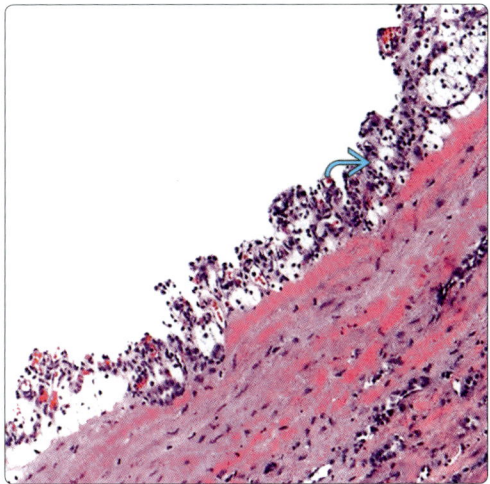

Atypical Cyst

(Left) A characteristic feature of the von Hippel-Lindau kidneys is the presence of multiple cysts that are usually lined by clear cells ⇨. In most cases, however, cysts are not numerous, and the average cyst count per kidney is approximately 8. (Right) Cysts lined by a single layer of cells without atypia are considered as benign cysts; those lined by 2-3 cells, ± cytological atypia, are designated as atypical cysts ⇨. Proliferations > 3 cells thick, even when focal, are regarded as cystic renal cell carcinoma.

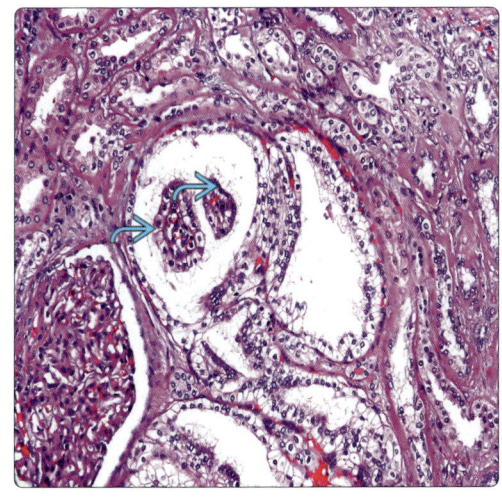

Atypical Cysts

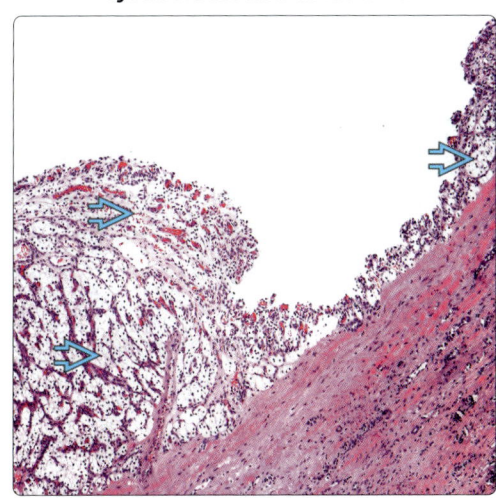

Cystic Renal Cell Carcinoma

(Left) This multilocular cyst with focal papillary proliferation ⇨ would be difficult to classify because of a single layer of epithelium. However, papillary proliferation with even minimal atypia is sufficient for it to be regarded as atypical cyst. (Right) Greater than 3 layers ⇨ lining a cyst are regarded as cystic carcinomas. Surgical management of von-Hippel Landau kidneys includes not only the enucleation of > 3 cm solid tumors, but also smaller identifiable solid and semisolid lesions like this.

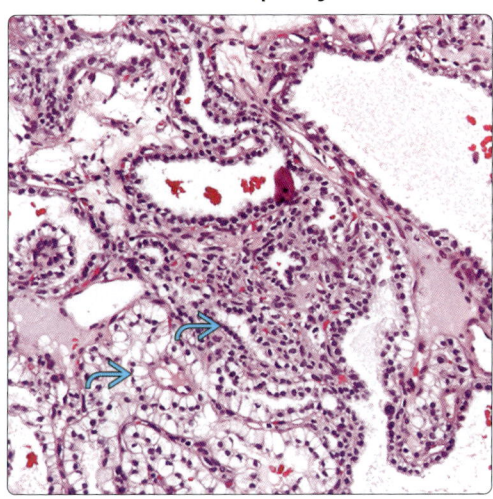

Clear Cell Papillary RCC

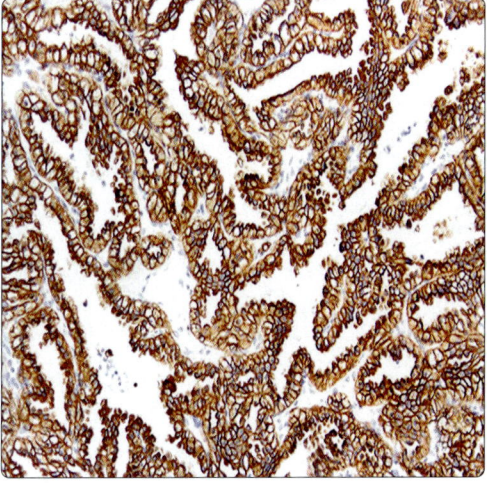

Clear Cell Papillary RCC

(Left) Some tumors and cysts in VHL show the features of clear cell papillary RCC, with typical linear arrangement of nuclei away from the basement membrane ⇨. Tumors with this predominant pattern are immunophenotypically similar to sporadic CCPRCC. However, such focal areas in otherwise typical CC-RCC show much more variable results, similar to that in sporadic CC-RCC with focal CCPRCC areas. (Right) Such CCPRCC show IHC features similar to sporadic tumors, including diffuse positivity for CK7 as seen here.

Birt-Hogg-Dubé Syndrome

KEY FACTS

TERMINOLOGY
- Autosomal dominant syndrome with incomplete penetrance, characterized by predisposition to development of cutaneous hamartomas, kidney neoplasms, lung cysts, and spontaneous pneumothorax

ETIOLOGY/PATHOGENESIS
- Birt-Hogg-Dubé (BHD) syndrome involves mutations in *BHD* gene that codes for folliculin protein
  - Folliculin binds to folliculin-interacting proteins 1 and 2 (FNIP1, FNIP2); combination acts as negative regulator of mTOR
    - Absence of this combination activates mTOR pathway that plays important role in tumorigenesis

CLINICAL ISSUES
- Skin lesions occur more frequently, and earlier, in BHD syndrome
  - Kidney tumors occur in ~ 20-25% of patients with syndrome; mean age: 54 years
- Multiple, bilateral renal tumors in BHD syndrome and renal oncocytosis often associated with chronic renal insufficiency at presentation and on follow-up

MICROSCOPIC
- Renal tumors in BHD syndrome usually have oncocytic cytoplasm
  - Most tumors show features of chromophobe renal cell carcinoma (RCC), hybrid chromophobe and oncocytoma, or renal oncocytoma
    - Clear cell, papillary, or unclassified RCC may also be present
    - Many oncocytic tumors characteristically show scattered clusters of cells with clear cytoplasm in background of oncocytoma-like histology

REPORTING
- Multiple oncocytic neoplasms &/or features of oncocytosis in nonneoplastic parenchyma should always raise possibility of BHD syndrome

Multiple Tumors in Birt-Hogg-Dubé
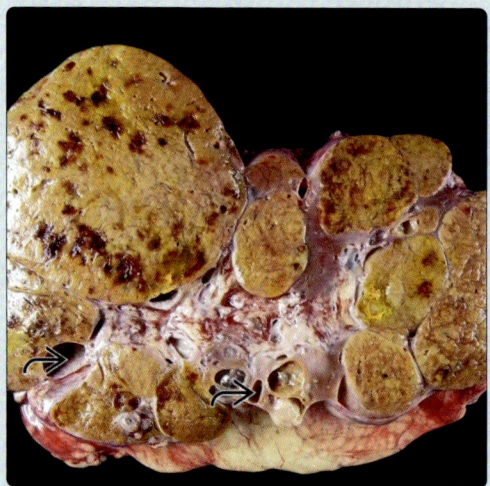

Multiple Tumor Types in Birt-Hogg-Dubé
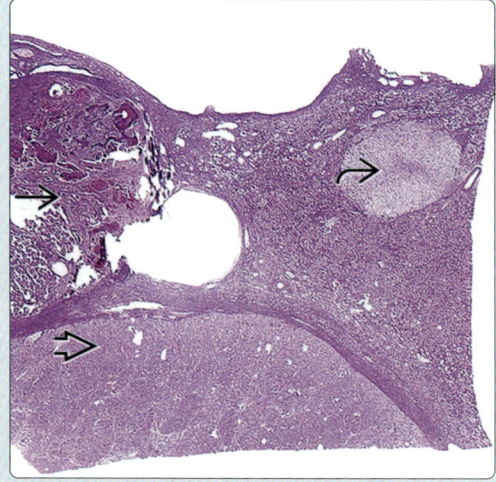

(Left) Cut surface of a nephrectomy specimen from a case of BHD syndrome shows the renal parenchyma studded with multiple solid tumors with yellow-brown appearance, indicative of oncocytic cell phenotype. Multiple cysts ⇨ are also evident. (Right) This whole-mount image from a BHD kidney shows different tumor types. The largest ⇨ is an oncocytic tumor, the medium ⇨ with papillary features, and the smallest ⇨ with clear cell features. Combination of different tumor subtypes is not uncommon in BHD.

Oncocytoma in Birt-Hogg-Dubé
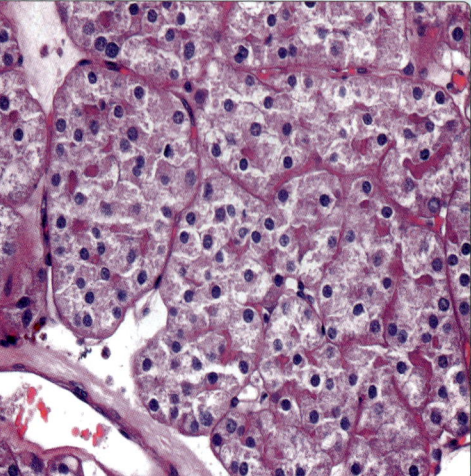

Chromophobe Renal Cell Carcinoma in Birt-Hogg-Dubé
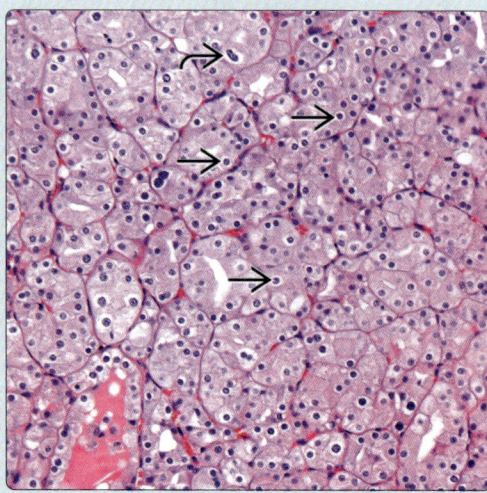

(Left) Most tumors in BHD syndrome show oncocytic features. This tumor has the morphology of a renal oncocytoma. (Right) Eosinophilic variant of chromophobe renal cell carcinoma (RCC) is among the more common RCC subtypes seen in BHD syndrome. Presence of perinuclear halos ⇨, even with relatively uniform nuclear contours, is diagnostic of chromophobe RCC. Evaluation at high magnification almost invariably shows some nuclear irregularities ⇨.

Birt-Hogg-Dubé Syndrome

TERMINOLOGY

Abbreviations
- Birt-Hogg-Dubé (BHD) syndrome

Definitions
- Autosomal dominant syndrome with incomplete penetrance, characterized by
  o Renal tumors
  o Cutaneous lesions (fibrofolliculomas, trichodiscomas, angiofibroma, perifollicular fibroma, and acrochordons)
  o Pulmonary cysts, spontaneous pneumothorax, bronchiectasis, and bronchospasm
  o Other associations
    – Colonic neoplasms, medullary thyroid carcinoma, lipomas

ETIOLOGY/PATHOGENESIS

BHD Gene
- BHD syndrome involves mutations in *BHD* gene
  o *BHD* gene maps to chromosome 17p12-q11.2
  o Gene codes for folliculin protein
  o Germline mutation in 1 allele is inherited, followed by somatic-type mutation in the other allele that may result in tumorigenesis
    – Supports role of *BHD* as tumor suppressor gene
    – Folliculin binds to folliculin-interacting proteins 1 and 2 (FNIP1, FNIP2)
      □ Interaction with folliculin leads to binding of FNIP1 to 5'-AMP activated protein kinase, negative regulator of mTOR
    – Kidney tumorigenesis in human BHD syndrome likely triggered by loss of interactions among folliculin, FNIP1, and FNIP2
      □ Leads to activation mTOR signaling pathways and tumorigenesis

Loss of Heterozygosity at *BHD* Locus and Promoter Methylation
- Rarely also been reported in sporadic renal cell carcinoma (RCC) of various histologic subtypes

CLINICAL ISSUES

Presentation
- **Diagnostic criteria for BHD syndrome (European BHD Consortium)**
  o Major criteria
    – At least 5 adult-onset fibrofolliculomas or trichodiscomas, and at least 1 of them confirmed histologically
    – Pathogenic *BHD* germline mutation
  o Minor criteria
    – Bilateral basally located multiple lung cysts with no other apparent cause, ± spontaneous primary pneumothorax
    – Early onset (< 50 years) or multifocal bilateral renal cancer, or renal tumors composed of mixed chromophobe and oncocytic morphology
    – 1st-degree relative with BHD syndrome
  o Presence of any 1 major criterion or 2 minor criteria required for diagnosis of BHD syndrome
- Pulmonary findings are most common feature of BHD syndrome
  o > 80% of BHD syndrome patients have lung cysts on CT imaging
    – ~ 40% of individuals with BHD have history of spontaneous pneumothorax
- Skin tumors usually appear before renal manifestations
- Renal tumors usually diagnosed in 6th decade of life (range: 31-73 years)
  o Skin lesions often appear in 3rd decade
- Renal tumors occur in 15-27% of patients with syndrome

Natural History
- Presence of bilateral numerous enlarging tumor nodules may compromise renal function
  o Chronic renal failure observed in large proportion of patients with renal oncocytosis and BHD syndrome

Treatment
- Members of families with history of syndrome with no renal lesions at initial screening
  o Radiological follow-up every 36 months
- Once renal tumors identified, interval imaging studies until largest tumor reaches 3 cm in maximal diameter
  o At this point, nephron-sparing surgery

Prognosis
- In patients with known syndromic conditions, tumors usually small at presentation
  o Therefore, minimal metastatic potential
    – However, synchronous or metachronous metastases described (in up to 12% cases)
      □ Particularly in patients with RCC (often large tumors with nononcocytic histologies) diagnosed without prior knowledge of the syndrome
- Development of chronic renal dysfunction also common feature
  o ~ 1/2 of patients with renal oncocytosis/BHD syndrome-associated multifocal renal tumors have chronic kidney disease at diagnosis
    – Additional ~ 1/4 of cases develop new onset chronic kidney disease on follow-up

MACROSCOPIC

General Features
- ~ 50% of patients with bilateral and multifocal tumors at presentation
- Most tumors with homogeneous, brown cut surface, indicative of oncocytic histology
  o Some tumors with gross characteristics suggestive of clear cell or papillary phenotype
- Occasional smooth-walled cysts frequently seen
  o Rare kidneys with multiple cysts

MICROSCOPIC

Histologic Features
- Renal tumors in BHD syndrome usually have oncocytic cytoplasm

- Most common tumor type displays hybrid features of renal oncocytoma and chromophobe RCC
  - Characteristically, many oncocytic tumors show scattered clusters of cells with clear cytoplasm
- Pure chromophobe RCC and renal oncocytomas other common tumor types
- Oncocytic tumors may occasionally have variable, but often focal, papillary architecture
- Other types of renal cell carcinoma also seen, including clear cell (9-12% tumors), papillary, or unclassified RCC
  - Clear cell RCC in BHD syndrome associated with von Hippel-Lindau (VHL) alterations, similar to that in sporadic setting
- Presence of wide spectrum of renal tumor morphologies suggests that *BHD* may play role in tumorigenesis across spectrum of RCC, regardless of histologic subtype
• Renal oncocytosis is evident in surrounding renal parenchyma in many, but not all, cases
  - Morphologic spectrum of renal oncocytosis includes
    - Numerous microscopic oncocytic nodules: May have features of chromophobe RCC, oncocytoma, or hybrid tumors
    - Cysts lined by oncocytic cells
    - Oncocytic changes in nonneoplastic renal tubules
    - Clusters and sheets of oncocytic cells percolating between nonneoplastic nephrons

ANCILLARY TESTS

Immunohistochemistry

• No specific immunohistochemical pattern known in oncocytic tumors of BHD syndrome; often show overlapping features between oncocytoma and chromophobe RCC
  - CD117, diffusely (+)
  - Like chromophobe RCC, most (+) for CD82
  - CK7, often focal cells or patchy clusters of cells (+)
  - S100A1 and Ksp-cadherin, often diffusely (+)

DIFFERENTIAL DIAGNOSIS

Renal Oncocytoma

• Renal oncocytoma has uniform, round nuclei, except for in pleomorphic, degenerate-appearing foci
  - Oncocytic tumors in BHD often, but not always, contain clusters of cells with clear cytoplasm
• Sporadic renal oncocytomas may be multifocal, as are rare familial oncocytomas, but should not have other features of oncocytosis in background kidney
  - At same time, BHD syndrome may show pure oncocytoma-like tumors
    - Essential to evaluate renal parenchyma for other features of oncocytosis/BHD, particularly in multifocal oncocytomas

Chromophobe Renal Cell Carcinoma

• Pure chromophobe RCC may be only tumor type present in some cases of BHD
• Most tumors show features of eosinophilic variant of chromophobe RCC
  - However, focal clusters of cells with clear cytoplasm may be present

• Tumors are often multifocal in BHD
  - Essential to evaluate renal parenchyma for other features of oncocytosis/BHD, particularly in multifocal chromophobe RCC

Oncocytic Renal Cell Carcinoma, Unclassified

• Oncocytic tumors with nuclear pleomorphism not acceptable for renal oncocytoma, or lacking perinuclear halos of chromophobe RCC may be seen in BHD
• Are often associated with other types of oncocytic tumors in BHD syndrome
• Essential to evaluate renal parenchyma for other features of oncocytosis/BHD, particularly in multifocal oncocytic RCC, unclassified

DIAGNOSTIC CHECKLIST

Pathologic Interpretation Pearls

• Presence of multiple oncocytic neoplasms should always initiate search for other microscopic features of oncocytosis in nontumorous renal parenchyma
• Multiple oncocytic neoplasms &/or features of oncocytosis in nonneoplastic parenchyma should always raise possibility of BHD syndromes and requires clinical assessment for features of BHD; findings may prompt genetic counseling
  - Renal oncocytosis not always associated with BHD syndrome; may be sporadic
  - Kidneys in BHD syndrome do not always show features of renal oncocytosis

SELECTED REFERENCES

1. Hasumi H et al: Folliculin-interacting proteins Fnip1 and Fnip2 play critical roles in kidney tumor suppression in cooperation with Flcn. Proc Natl Acad Sci U S A. 112(13):E1624-31, 2015
2. Iribe Y et al: Immunohistochemical characterization of renal tumors in patients with Birt-Hogg-Dubé syndrome. Pathol Int. 65(3):126-32, 2015
3. Benusiglio PR et al: Renal cell tumour characteristics in patients with the Birt-Hogg-Dubé cancer susceptibility syndrome: a retrospective, multicentre study. Orphanet J Rare Dis. 9:163, 2014
4. Luijten MN et al: Birt-Hogg-Dubé syndrome is a novel ciliopathy. Hum Mol Genet. 22(21):4383-97, 2013
5. Przybycin CG et al: Hereditary syndromes with associated renal neoplasia: a practical guide to histologic recognition in renal tumor resection specimens. Adv Anat Pathol. 20(4):245-63, 2013
6. Srigley JR et al: The International Society of Urological Pathology (ISUP) Vancouver Classification of Renal Neoplasia. Am J Surg Pathol. 37(10):1469-89, 2013
7. Stamatakis L et al: Diagnosis and management of BHD-associated kidney cancer. Fam Cancer. 12(3):397-402, 2013
8. Adamy A et al: Renal oncocytosis: management and clinical outcomes. J Urol. 185(3):795-801, 2011
9. Menko FH et al: Birt-Hogg-Dubé syndrome: diagnosis and management. Lancet Oncol. 10(12):1199-206, 2009
10. Toro JR et al: BHD mutations, clinical and molecular genetic investigations of Birt-Hogg-Dubé syndrome: a new series of 50 families and a review of published reports. J Med Genet. 45(6):321-31, 2008
11. Adley BP et al: Birt-Hogg-Dubé syndrome: clinicopathologic findings and genetic alterations. Arch Pathol Lab Med. 130(12):1865-70, 2006
12. Pavlovich CP et al: Renal tumors in the Birt-Hogg-Dubé syndrome. Am J Surg Pathol. 26(12):1542-52, 2002
13. Tickoo SK et al: Renal oncocytosis: a morphologic study of fourteen cases. Am J Surg Pathol. 23(9):1094-101, 1999

Birt-Hogg-Dubé Syndrome

Hybrid Oncocytic Tumor

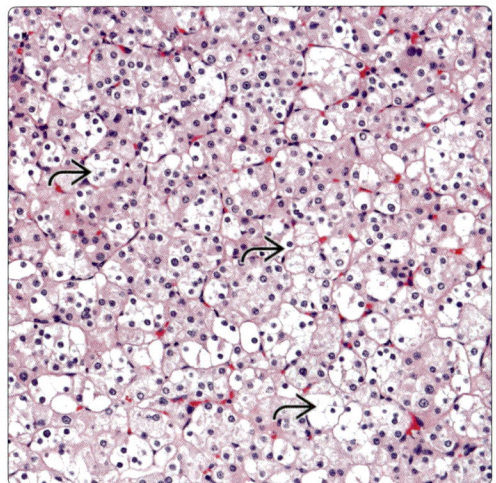

Clear Cells in Oncocytic Birt-Hogg-Dubé Tumors

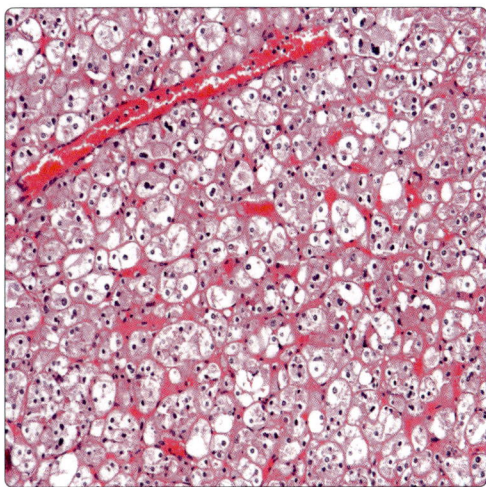

(Left) Tumors with hybrid oncocytoma-chromophobe histology often constitute the majority of tumors in BHD syndrome. Presence of single or clusters of cells with clear cytoplasm ➔ in a background of renal oncocytoma-like histology is quite characteristic. (Right) The presence of clear cell nests in an oncocytic tumor should raise the possibility of BHD syndrome and merits thorough evaluation of surrounding renal parenchyma for renal oncocytosis/features compatible with BHD syndrome.

Rare Papillary Architecture

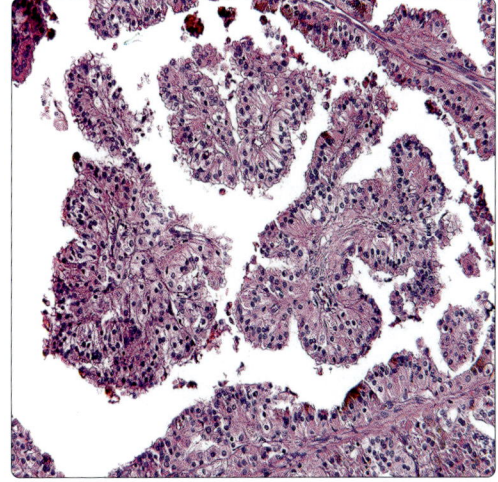

Clear Cell Renal Cell Carcinoma in Birt-Hogg-Dubé Syndrome

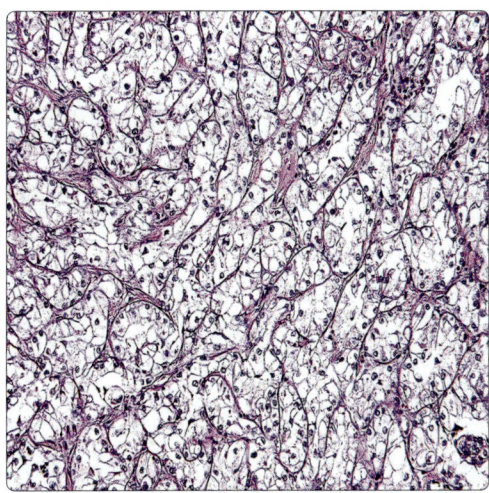

(Left) While the oncocytic tumors in BHD syndrome usually show the morphology of chromophobe RCC, renal oncocytoma, or hybrid oncocytoma-chromophobe tumor, papillary architecture is not uncommon. (Right) Clear cell, papillary, and unclassified RCC may also be seen in cases of BHD syndrome. Clear cell RCC constitute ~ 10% of the tumors in BHD syndrome, and these tumors usually show von Hippel-Lindau-related alterations. Such findings suggest that BHD may play role in tumorigenesis across the spectrum of RCC types.

Cysts

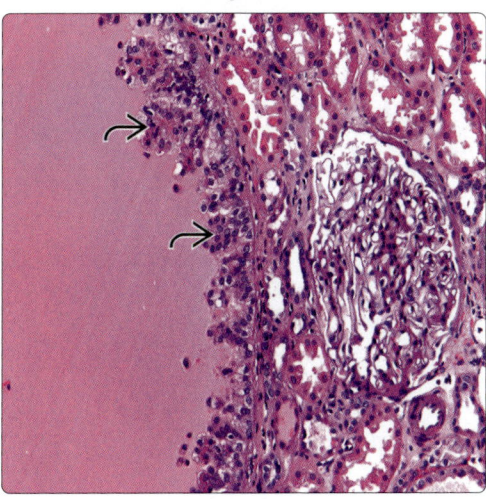

Multiple Oncocytic Lesions

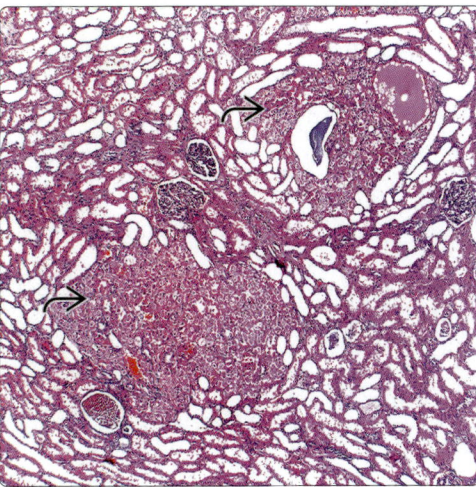

(Left) Many kidneys in BHD syndrome show multiple cysts lined by cells with eosinophilic cytoplasm. Rarely, the lining may appear proliferative, with multilayering or papillary infoldings ➔. (Right) The presence of multifocal oncocytic tumors, or tumors with hybrid histology, should always raise the suspicion of a syndromic association. Careful evaluation of the surrounding renal parenchyma for other features of oncocytosis (like oncocytic nodules ➔ or oncocytic cells infiltrating between native nephrons) is essential.

Hereditary Leiomyomatosis Renal Cell Carcinoma Syndrome

KEY FACTS

TERMINOLOGY
- Autosomal dominant disorder with presence of leiomyomatous tumors and renal cell carcinoma (RCC)
  - Renal carcinomas are highly aggressive, characterized by presence of large nucleoli surrounded by halo (CMV inclusion-like); this feature may be focal

ETIOLOGY/PATHOGENESIS
- Genetic basis of tumor is germline inactivating mutations in fumarate hydratase (*FH*) gene, located at 1q42.3-q43, encoding for fumarate hydratase
  - Absence of FH leads to accumulation of fumarate which, by competitive inhibition of prolyl hydroxylase, prevents degradation of HIF-1, resulting in its overexpression and tumorigenesis

CLINICAL ISSUES
- Patients often present with wide-spread metastatic disease even when renal tumor is quite small

MICROSCOPIC
- Predominant or prominent papillary architecture, often mimicking type 2 papillary RCC
  - Other common architectural patterns include, solid alveolar, tubular/glandular, tubulocystic, sheet-like, and sarcomatoid
- Presence of large nuclei with very prominent nucleoli surrounded by clear perinucleolar halo (CMV inclusion-like), most characteristic microscopic feature

ANCILLARY TESTS
- IHC
  - Fumarate hydratase (complete loss of expression)
  - 2SC (cytoplasmic and nuclear expression)
- Confirmation of diagnosis by germline genetic testing

TOP DIFFERENTIAL DIAGNOSES
- Type 2 papillary RCC, collecting duct carcinoma, tubulocystic carcinoma

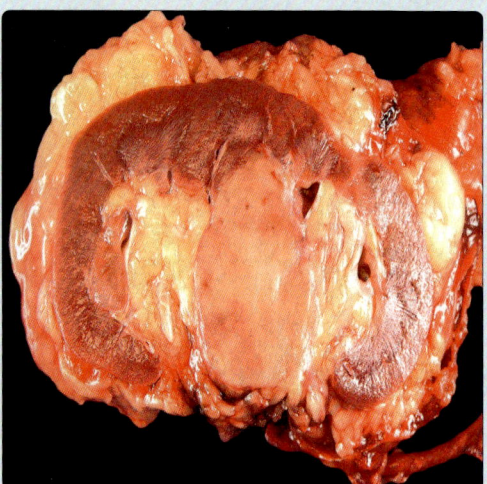

Gross: HLRCC-Associated RCC

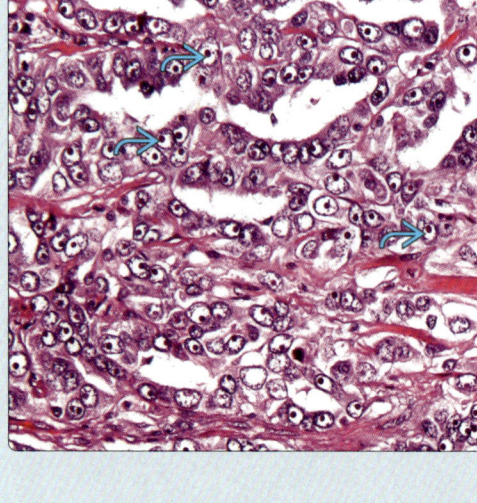

Characteristic Prominent Nucleoli

(Left) Hereditary leiomyomatosis renal cell carcinoma (HLRCC)-associated RCC can have variable gross features. Most appear solid and homogeneous, but some show cystic areas or areas of necrosis and hemorrhage. Often the tumors are small in size but show extensive metastases at presentation. (Right) Diagnostically, the most characteristic feature of HLRCC-associated RCC is the presence of large nucleoli and perinucleolar halos (CMV inclusion-like) 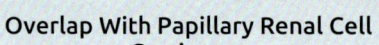. The feature is generally, but not always, present throughout the tumor.

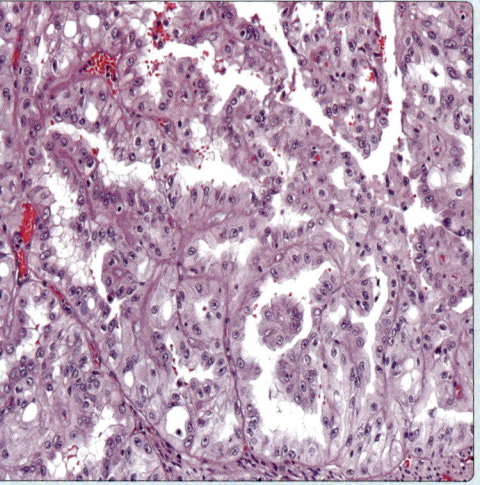

Overlap With Papillary Renal Cell Carcinoma

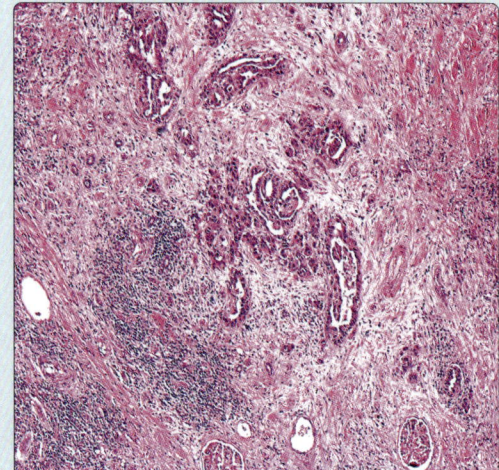

Overlap With Collecting Duct Carcinoma

(Left) HLRCC-associated RCCs show quite variable architectural patterns. The presence of frequent papillary architecture resulted in their designation as type 2 papillary RCC in the past. (Right) Infiltrative tubular and papillary patterns with desmoplastic stromal response has led to some tumors being regarded as collecting duct carcinoma. However, HLRCC-associated carcinoma is a distinct entity, with specific clinical, immunohistochemical, and molecular features.

Hereditary Leiomyomatosis Renal Cell Carcinoma Syndrome

TERMINOLOGY

Abbreviations
- Hereditary leiomyomatosis and renal cell cancer syndrome-associated renal cell carcinoma (HLRCC-associated RCC)

Definitions
- Autosomal dominant syndrome, characterized by leiomyomas of skin and uterus, occasional leiomyosarcoma of uterus, and RCCs
  - Renal tumors aggressive even when small, with high-grade nuclei containing characteristic, and diagnostically important, large nucleoli with perinucleolar halos (CMV inclusion-like)

ETIOLOGY/PATHOGENESIS

Genetic Basis of Tumor Is Germline Inactivating Mutations in Fumarate Hydratase Gene
- Fumarate hydratase (*FH*) gene located at 1q42.3-q43
  - *FH* gene encodes for enzyme fumarate hydratase
- Fumarate hydratase required to convert fumarate to malate in Krebs (tricarboxylic acid) cycle
  - Germline mutations in *FH* gene on 1 allele accompanied by mutations or deletions of other wild-type *FH* allele in tumors
  - Most common germline mutations are missense mutations
    - Truncation and whole-gene deletion other less common type of germline mutations
  - Loss of FH function results in increased levels of fumarate in cells
- Increased fumarate acts as competitive inhibitor of prolyl hydroxylase domain-containing proteins or PHDs (EGLN, HPH)
  - Inhibition of these proteins prevents hydroxylation, and therefore pVHL-mediated proteosomic degradation, of HIF-1
    - This results in HIF-1 overexpression and consequent transcription of multiple downstream products and carcinogenesis

CLINICAL ISSUES

Presentation
- Average age at diagnosis of renal tumor: 36-46 years (range: 17-75 years)
- Aggressive type of RCC, very often associated with widespread metastases at presentation even when small in size
  - Previously regarded as type 2 papillary RCC or collecting duct carcinoma
    - But, now regarded as specific entity distinct from type 2 papillary RCC and collecting duct carcinoma
- Renal tumors often solitary and unilateral, unlike most syndromic tumors
  - Only rare multifocal tumors described
- Penetrance for RCC lower than cutaneous and uterine manifestations
  - Only 20-35% of patients with *FH* mutations develop RCC
- Most patients with history of cutaneous leiomyomas
- In women, most have uterine leiomyomas and, rarely leiomyosarcoma, at young age
  - Many have had hysterectomy prior to diagnosis of HLRCC-associated RCC

Treatment
- Currently, no specific therapy against metastatic tumors is available
  - Drugs affecting Krebs cycle molecules are being investigated at this stage

Prognosis
- Metastases often present at time of diagnosis
  - Common metastatic sites include: Regional lymph nodes, lungs, liver

MACROSCOPIC

General Features
- Mostly solid, homogenous cut surface, but cystic areas and hemorrhage not uncommon
  - Sieve- or Swiss cheese-like cut surface present in occasional tumors
  - Few appear to arise from cyst wall as mural and infiltrative nodules

MICROSCOPIC

Histologic Features
- Renal tumors with variable, but often prominent, papillary architecture
  - Not to be considered type 2 papillary RCC, but separate distinct entity
  - Cores of papillae often hyalinized
- Other common architectural patterns include: Solid alveolar, tubular/glandular, tubulocystic, and sheet-like
  - Tubulocystic carcinoma-like areas often associated with other more glandular, solid, or papillary areas
    - Some consider as dedifferentiation in tubulocystic carcinoma
      - More likely, these represent de novo HLRCC-associated RCC with prominent tubulocystic areas
- Desmoplasia and multinodularity are also common
  - These features mimic those seen in collecting duct carcinoma
- Occasionally, may arise from cyst lined by cells morphologically similar to that in more solid areas
- Tumor cells are large and usually with abundant eosinophilic cytoplasm
  - Rarely, focal clear cell change also observed
- Most diagnostic and consistent feature
  - Large nuclei with very prominent orangeophilic or eosinophilic nucleoli, surrounded by clear perinucleolar halo
    - Appearance somewhat resembles CMV inclusions
    - This feature may be very focal in some cases
  - Possibility of HLRCC tumor should always be considered if these features present in kidney tumor
- Sarcomatoid and rhabdoid features may be present
- Cutaneous leiomyomas often have prominent nucleoli
- Uterine leiomyomas often cellular and atypical

Hereditary Leiomyomatosis Renal Cell Carcinoma Syndrome

- Nuclear and nucleolar features similar to that in renal tumors
- Background kidney may show cysts lined by single or multiple layers of atypical cells

ANCILLARY TESTS

Immunohistochemistry

- Fumarate hydratase expression completely lacking in almost all tumors
- Overexpression of S-(2-succino)-cysteine (2SC) most sensitive IHC test
  - Presence of both cytoplasmic and nuclear positivity characteristic and requirement
    - Focal cytoplasmic positivity, without nuclear staining, may occur in other high-grade tumors
  - 2SC overexpression related to
    - High levels of fumarate accumulated in HLRCC tumor cells causing aberrant succination of proteins with formation of stable chemical modification, S-(2-succino)-cysteine (2SC)
- Immunostain for CK7 often negative, or only very focally positive
- pax-8 frequently positive
- Stain for mucin may be positive in rare tumors

Genetic Testing

- Germline genetic testing required for final diagnosis of hereditary syndromic association

DIFFERENTIAL DIAGNOSIS

Type 2 Papillary Renal Cell Carcinoma

- All papillary RCCs are usually well circumscribed, often with prominent capsule
  - Markedly infiltrative edges should always raise possibility of alternate diagnoses, including HLRCC-associated RCC
- Presence of perinucleolar halos not feature
- Accompanying metastases at presentation relatively rare in true type 2 papillary RCC
- Papillary RCC shows retained FH reactivity; does not show diffuse cytoplasmic and nuclear positivity for 2SC

Collecting Duct Carcinoma

- Diffuse perinucleolar halos not feature
- Tumors show retained FH reactivity
  - Tumors do not show diffuse cytoplasmic and nuclear positivity for 2SC

Tubulocystic Renal Cell Carcinoma

- By definition, tubulocystic carcinomas well circumscribed tumors
- No solid or papillary areas present
  - Do not show show infiltrative borders
- Tumors show retained FH reactivity
  - Do not show diffuse cytoplasmic and nuclear positivity for 2SC

DIAGNOSTIC CHECKLIST

Pathologic Interpretation Pearls

- Tumors with papillary architecture, but extensive infiltrative borders, most likely are not type 2 papillary RCC
  - Differential diagnostic possibilities in this scenario include, among others
    - Collecting duct carcinoma
    - MiTF/TFE family translocation-associated RCC
    - HLRCC-associated RCC
  - Papillary cores in HLRCC-associated RCC are variably hyalized
    - In tumors with papillary architecture, prominent nucleoli and hyalinized cores should always raise suspicion of HLRCC-associated tumor
      - If not readily apparent, careful search for typical nucleolar features should be made
      - Characteristic nucleolar features not always uniformly present in tumor
- IHC staining for fumarate hydratase, 2SC, and TFE3 and TFEB should always be performed in such instances to establish diagnosis
  - Genetic testing is required for confirmation or definitive diagnosis
  - In absence of clinical history or genetic tests, but with FH loss, term FH deficient RCC may be used

SELECTED REFERENCES

1. Chen YB et al: Hereditary leiomyomatosis and renal cell carcinoma syndrome-associated renal cancer: recognition of the syndrome by pathologic features and the utility of detecting aberrant succination by immunohistochemistry. Am J Surg Pathol. 38(5):627-37, 2014
2. Llamas-Velasco M et al: Fumarate hydratase immunohistochemical staining may help to identify patients with multiple cutaneous and uterine leiomyomatosis (MCUL) and hereditary leiomyomatosis and renal cell cancer (HLRCC) syndrome. J Cutan Pathol. 41(11):859-65, 2014
3. Menko FH et al: Hereditary leiomyomatosis and renal cell cancer (HLRCC): renal cancer risk, surveillance and treatment. Fam Cancer. 13(4):637-44, 2014
4. Schmidt LS et al: Hereditary leiomyomatosis and renal cell carcinoma. Int J Nephrol Renovasc Dis. 7:253-60, 2014
5. Udager AM et al: Hereditary leiomyomatosis and renal cell carcinoma (HLRCC): a rapid autopsy report of metastatic renal cell carcinoma. Am J Surg Pathol. 38(4):567-77, 2014
6. Al-Hussain TO et al: Tubulocystic carcinoma of the kidney with poorly differentiated foci: a series of 3 cases with fluorescence in situ hybridization analysis. Hum Pathol. 44(7):1406-11, 2013
7. Linehan WM et al: Molecular pathways: Fumarate hydratase-deficient kidney cancer--targeting the Warburg effect in cancer. Clin Cancer Res. 19(13):3345-52, 2013
8. Sanz-Ortega J, Vocke C, Stratton P, Linehan WM, Merino MJ. Morphologic and molecular characteristics of uterine leiomyomas in hereditary leiomyomatosis and renal cancer (HLRCC) syndrome. Am J Surg Pathol. 37(1):74-80, 2013
9. Tolvanen J et al: Strong family history of uterine leiomyomatosis warrants fumarate hydratase mutation screening. Hum Reprod. 27(6):1865-9, 2012
10. Bardella C et al: Aberrant succination of proteins in fumarate hydratase-deficient mice and HLRCC patients is a robust biomarker of mutation status. J Pathol. 225(1):4-11, 2011
11. Garg K et al: Morphologic features of uterine leiomyomas associated with hereditary leiomyomatosis and renal cell carcinoma syndrome: a case report. Am J Surg Pathol. 35(8):1235-7, 2011
12. Merino MJ et al: The morphologic spectrum of kidney tumors in hereditary leiomyomatosis and renal cell carcinoma (HLRCC) syndrome. Am J Surg Pathol. 31(10):1578-85, 2007
13. Wei MH et al: Novel mutations in FH and expansion of the spectrum of phenotypes expressed in families with hereditary leiomyomatosis and renal cell cancer. J Med Genet. 43(1):18-27, 2006

Hereditary Leiomyomatosis Renal Cell Carcinoma Syndrome

Hyalinized Core
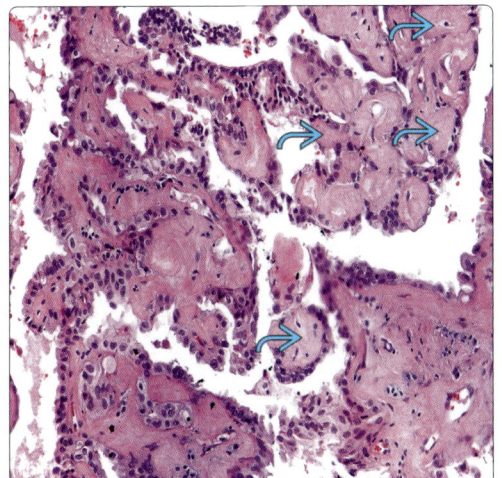

Tubulocystic Areas
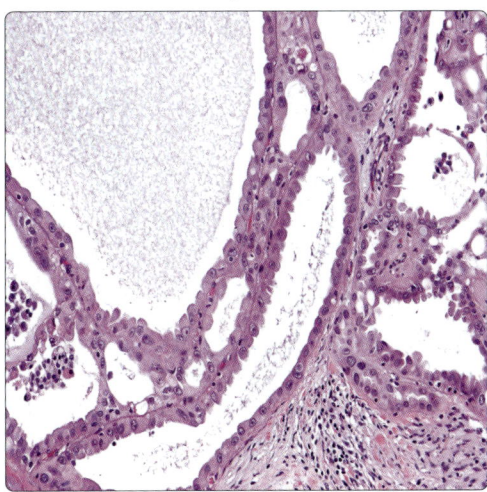

(Left) Papillae in HLRCC-associated RCC often show hyalinization ➡ in the cores. This feature in a carcinoma with papillary architecture and prominent nucleoli must alert one to the possibility of HLRCC. Careful search for typical nucleolar features that may not be diffuse in all tumors should be made. (Right) Many tumors show tubulocystic areas. Although, regarded as tubulocystic RCC with dedifferentiation by some, these more likely represent HLRCC-associated tumors with prominent tubulocystic architecture.

Sarcomatoid Features
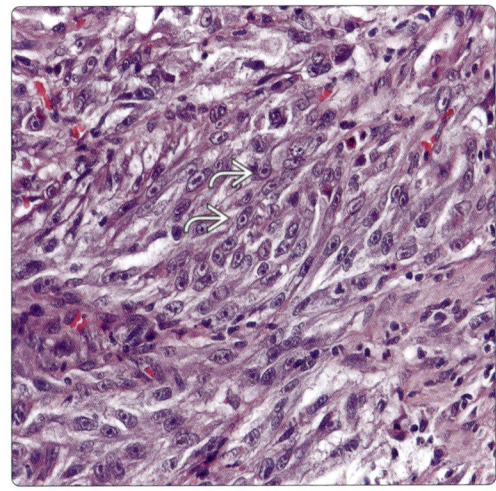

Lymphovascular Invasion
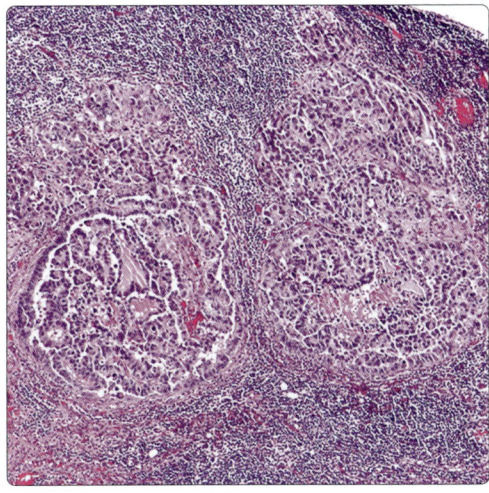

(Left) This example of HLRCC-associated RCC shows sarcomatoid features. The characteristic nuclear and nucleolar features ➡ are retained in the spindle cell component. However, these typical features may not be present throughout in all the tumors. (Right) The image shows metastasis in a regional lymph node from a 2.5-cm HLRCC-associated RCC. Widespread metastasis at presentation, even when the tumor may be quite small, is frequent in this entity.

Fumarate Hydratase IHC: Diffuse Loss
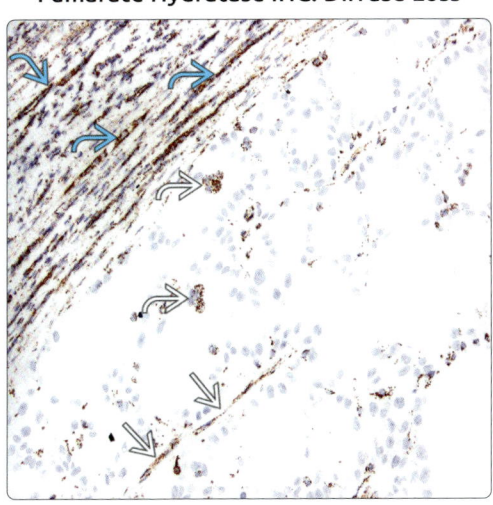

2SC IHC: Diffuse Positivity
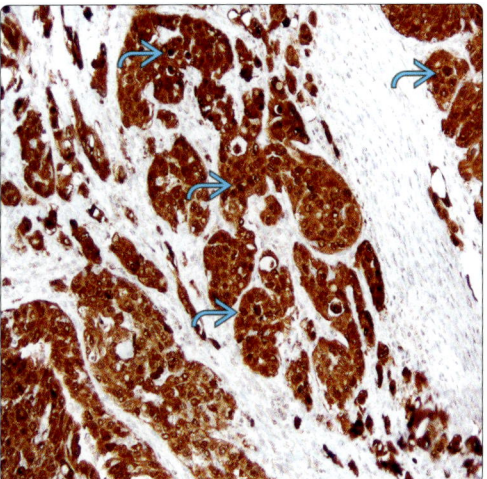

(Left) IHC for fumarate hydratase shows complete loss of immunoreactivity in the tumor. Notice retained immunoreactivity in the vessels ➡ and macrophages ➡ within the tumor, and the benign tubules ➡ and other nonneoplastic elements outside the tumor. (Right) IHC staining for 2SC shows diffuse cytoplasmic and nuclear ➡ positivity in HLRCC-associated RCC. Although, 2SC appears to be a more sensitive antibody, its commercial nonavailability at this time makes fumarate hydratase a more practical initial test for the tumor.

Tuberous Sclerosis Complex

KEY FACTS

TERMINOLOGY

- Autosomal dominant syndrome, usually affecting central nervous system, resulting in combination of neurological symptoms
- Also characterized by tumors or tumor-like lesions in multiple sites, including
  - Cortical tubers, subependymomas, and giant cell astrocytomas of brain, retinal hamartomas, cardiac rhabdomyomas, angiomyolipomas/PEComas of kidney and other organs, and renal cell carcinomas

ETIOLOGY/PATHOGENESIS

- Associated with inactivating mutations in tumor suppressor genes, tuberous sclerosis complex 1 and 2 (*TSC1* and *TSC2*)
- Few cases also associated with large deletions in polycystic kidney disease 1 (*PKD1*) gene that lies adjacent to and co-involves *TSC2* locus on chromosome 16

CLINICAL ISSUES

- Most common renal manifestation is angiomyolipoma (AML) (80%); RCC rare occurrence in TSC (2-3%)

MICROSCOPIC

- TSC-associated RCC shows variety of histologies; including
  - Tumors with voluminous, variably granular eosinophilic and clear/vacuolated cytoplasm and large nuclei with prominent nucleoli, tumors with uniform eosinophilic cells, mimicking chromophobe RCC, and tumors with TCEB1-mutated or RAT-like RCC features
    - Combination of patterns present in many tumors
- Background renal parenchyma often with multiple cysts and multiple angiomyolipomas

TOP DIFFERENTIAL DIAGNOSES

- Clear cell RCC; TCEB1-mutated RCC; renal angiomyoadenomatous tumor (RAT)-like RCC

Multiple Angiomyolipomas

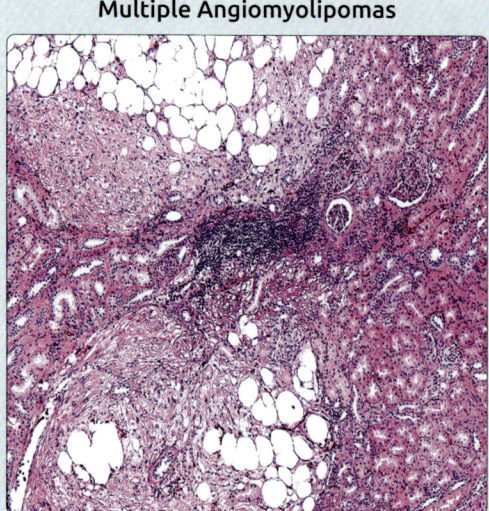

Angiomyolipoma in Lymph Nodes

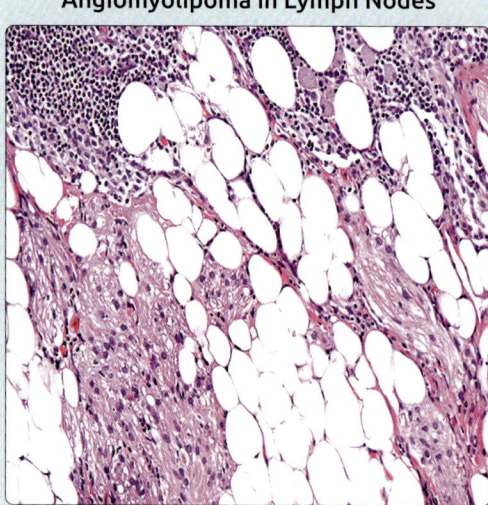

(Left) Tuberous sclerosis syndrome (TSC) is associated with multiple renal angiomyolipomas in the overwhelming majority of patients. Often, the lesions and the subsequent diagnosis of the syndrome are recognized only after evaluation of nephrectomy specimens removed for other reasons. **(Right)** AMLs in the kidney, along with their presence in resected lymph nodes, may be indicative of the syndrome. When observed, suggesting the possibility of TSC in pathology reports is highly recommended.

Epithelioid Angiomyolipoma

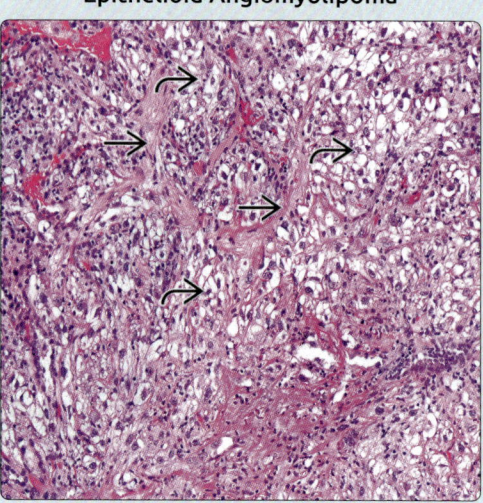

RCC in TSC

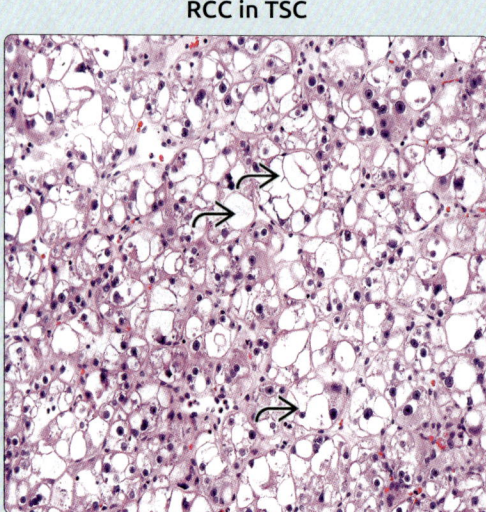

(Left) Before accepting an epithelioid tumor as an RCC, the possibility of epithelioid AML needs to be excluded. Some epithelioid AMLs have prominent clear cell cytology ⟹, and the vasculature ⟹ may also mimic that in clear cell RCC. **(Right)** RCCs in TSC often show nested or solid architecture with intricately branching vasculature. Frequently, tumors show cells with voluminous ⟹, variably granular eosinophilic &/or clear cytoplasm, cytoplasmic vacuolization, large nuclei, and prominent nucleoli.

Tuberous Sclerosis Complex

TERMINOLOGY

Abbreviations
- Tuberous sclerosis complex (TSC)

Synonyms
- Bourneville disease

Definitions
- Autosomal dominant syndrome, usually affecting central nervous system, resulting in combination of symptoms including
  - Seizures, developmental delay, behavioral problems
- Also characterized by tumors or tumor-like lesions in multiple sites, including
  - Cortical tubers, subependymomas, and giant cell astrocytomas of brain
  - Retinal hamartomas
  - Cardiac rhabdomyomas
  - Angiomyolipomas (AML) of kidney and other organs
  - PEComas of other viscera and soft tissues
  - Clear cell "sugar" tumors of lung, pancreas, and uterus
  - Lymphangioleiomyomatosis of lung
  - Renal cell carcinomas (RCC)

ETIOLOGY/PATHOGENESIS

Tuberous Sclerosis Complex (*TSC1* and *TSC2*) Genes
- TSC associated with inactivating mutations in these tumor-suppressor genes
- *TSC1* localized to chromosome 9q34; *TSC2* to 16p13.3
  - Prevalence of mutations in *TSC1* and *TSC2* roughly equal in TSC syndrome;
    - In sporadic angiomyolipomas, *TSC2* mutations more frequent
- Proteins encoded by *TSC1* (hamartin) and *TSC2* genes (tuberin) function as complex to negatively regulate mTOR signaling
  - Negative regulation done through activation of Ras homologue expressed in brain (Rheb)
    - Rheb-specific GTPase is located downstream of tuberin
    - Altered *TSC* gene functions generate excessive RhebGTP
  - Abnormal/absent hamartin/tuberin complex leads to increased activated mTOR and possible tumorigenesis
    - Activated mTOR pathway markers overexpressed in AML and related tumors
- About 2/3 of cases of TSC sporadic, as result of new mutations
  - Siblings of such patients with risk of TSC in 1-2%
    - Likely due to gonadal/germline mosaicism in parent, with genetic change confined solely to germline (gamete-producing cells)
- Chromosome 3p and *VHL* gene-associated alterations not present in TSC-associated RCC, irrespective of morphological features

Polycystic Kidney Disease 1 (*PKD1*) Gene Deletions
- *PKD1* gene lies adjacent to *TSC2* locus on chromosome 16
  - Large *PKD1* deletions often involve adjacent *TSC2* gene
  - Syndrome termed TSC2/PKD1 contiguous gene syndrome (CGS)
    - CGS present in 2-3 % of patients with TSC
    - CGS often associated with early onset polycystic kidney disease and renal impairment

CLINICAL ISSUES

Epidemiology
- TSC affects 25,000-40,000 individuals in United States and ~ 1-2 million worldwide
  - Estimated prevalence of 1 in 6,000 newborns
- Occurs in all races and ethnic groups and in both genders

Presentation
- Most common renal manifestation is AML (80%)
  - AMLs often show typical triphasic histology
    - However, as in sporadic tumors, any variant histology may be present
    - Epithelioid AMLs reportedly more likely to occur in TSC than in sporadic settings
      - However, many recent studies do not support this hypothesis
    - Multiple, bilateral tumors and multiple organ involvement hallmarks of tuberous sclerosis
- RCC rare occurrence in TSC (2-3%)
  - Diagnosed more frequently at younger age than sporadic RCC (range: 7-65 yr; mean: 42 yr); often multifocal and bilateral
  - More commonly reported in females; (F:M = 2-3:1)

Treatment
- Drugs
  - mTORC1 inhibitors used in some patients with metastatic disease with variably positive results

Prognosis
- Most tumors small at diagnosis, although rare tumors as large as 22 cm also described
- Rare metastases, particularly to regional lymph nodes, reported
  - Deaths due to RCC extremely uncommon

MICROSCOPIC

Histologic Features
- TSC-associated RCC shows variety of histologies
  - Feature common to most includes intricate, branching fibrovascular septations similar to clear cell RCC
  - However, many other distinctive features, including
    - Nested, solid, often multi(micro)cystic, with large cells showing voluminous, variably granular eosinophilic &/or clear to vacuolated cytoplasm, large nuclei and prominent nucleoli
      - Some cells with cytoplasm condensed around nuclei with peripheral clarity; tumor giant cells not infrequent
      - Cells with clear-appearing cytoplasm often with delicate cobweb-like eosinophilic strands
    - Nests and sheets of round to cuboidal uniform cells with eosinophilic cytoplasm, mimicking chromophobe RCC, or tumors with mixed chromophobe and oncocytoma-like features in some cases

- Nests, acini, and often branching tubules with abundant clear cytoplasm and prominent intratumoral fibromuscular septations, imparting nodular growth pattern at low magnification
  - Such tumors mimic *TCEB1*-mutated tumors and so-called renal angiomyoadenomatous tumor (RAT)
- Although nested growth pattern most frequent, variable papillary architecture often present
- Combination of above patterns present in many tumors
- Psammomatous calcifications present in occasional tumors
- Background renal parenchyma often with multiple cysts (40%)
  - Cysts usually lined by single layer of eosinophilic cells, frequently with cytoplasmic vacuolization and hobnailing
    - Most lining cells with large nuclei and prominent nucleoli
- AMLs, ranging in size from microscopic to grossly recognizable, often present in surrounding renal parenchyma
  - Multiple AMLs may be present in regional lymph nodes
  - Presence of multiple AMLs in kidney or regional lymph nodes strong indicator of TSC in kidneys resected for RCC

ANCILLARY TESTS

Immunohistochemistry

- Immunoprofile not consistent
  - Varies according to tumor morphology
    - Tumors with TCEB1/RAT, or eosinophilic chromophobe-like features, often CK7(+)
    - Tumors with TCEB1/RAT-like features usually CA9(+)
    - CD10, variably (+) in all morphologic patterns
    - pax-8(+) in all morphologic patterns
    - CD117, usually (-), but may be (+) in occasional tumor with chromophobe/oncocytic eosinophilic features
    - AMACR (-) in tumors with TCEB1/RAT-like features, but variably (+) in other morphologies
  - mTOR pathway markers, p-4EBP1 and p-S6, strongly expressed in all tested tumors

Genetic Testing

- Germline *TSC1/TSC2* gene mutations, with LOH of other allele, common underlying mechanism in TSC-associated RCC
  - Mutations present in all tumors irrespective of tumor morphology

DIFFERENTIAL DIAGNOSIS

Clear Cell RCC

- Usually unifocal and unilateral, occurring at older age
- Cells with voluminous clear cytoplasm and eosinophilic cytoplasmic strands very unusual
- AMACR and CK7 usually (-)
- Association with AML and multiple cysts in surrounding parenchyma very rare
- 3p or *VHL* alterations in overwhelming majority; such changes not found in TSC-associated RCC

TCEB1-Mutated RCC

- Usually unifocal and unilateral tumors
- Not associated with AML and cysts in surrounding parenchyma
- No TSC gene-related molecular alterations
- Tumor-specific LOH of chromosome 8 and *TCEB1* gene mutations always present

Renal Angiomyoadenomatous Tumor (RAT)-Like RCC

- RAT as specific entity is not recognized
  - Many such tumors regarded to be with morphological spectrum of clear cell papillary RCC
    - Such tumors have the immunoprofile of clear cell papillary RCC, including
      - CK7(+) in almost 100% cells, CA9(+) (cup-shaped), and CD10/AMACR(-)
- Some others may in fact be TSC-associated or *TCEB1*-mutated RCC
  - Such possibilities need to be considered and excluded

DIAGNOSTIC CHECKLIST

Pathologic Interpretation Pearls

- Multifocal tumors with morphological variability and features not common for clear cell RCC should raise possibility of syndromic associations
- Multiple cysts &/or multiple AMLs in surrounding renal parenchyma, or in regional lymph nodes should alert pathologists to possibility of TSC

SELECTED REFERENCES

1. Tyburczy ME et al: A shower of second hit events as the cause of multifocal renal cell carcinoma in tuberous sclerosis complex. Hum Mol Genet. 24(7):1836-42, 2015
2. Guo J et al: Tuberous sclerosis-associated renal cell carcinoma: a clinicopathologic study of 57 separate carcinomas in 18 patients. Am J Surg Pathol. 38(11):1457-67, 2014
3. Yang P et al: Renal cell carcinoma in tuberous sclerosis complex. Am J Surg Pathol. 38(7):895-909, 2014
4. He W et al: Epithelioid angiomyolipoma of the kidney: pathological features and clinical outcome in a series of consecutively resected tumors. Mod Pathol. 26(10):1355-64, 2013
5. Przybycin CG et al: Hereditary syndromes with associated renal neoplasia: a practical guide to histologic recognition in renal tumor resection specimens. Adv Anat Pathol. 20(4):245-63, 2013
6. Linehan WM: Genetic basis of kidney cancer: role of genomics for the development of disease-based therapeutics. Genome Res. 22(11):2089-100, 2012
7. Borkowska J et al: Tuberous sclerosis complex: tumors and tumorigenesis. Int J Dermatol. 50(1):13-20, 2011
8. Duffy K et al: Mutational analysis of the von hippel lindau gene in clear cell renal carcinomas from tuberous sclerosis complex patients. Mod Pathol. 15(3):205-10, 2002
9. Bjornsson J et al: Tuberous sclerosis-associated renal cell carcinoma. Clinical, pathological, and genetic features. Am J Pathol. 149(4):1201-8, 1996

Tuberous Sclerosis Complex

RCC in TSC
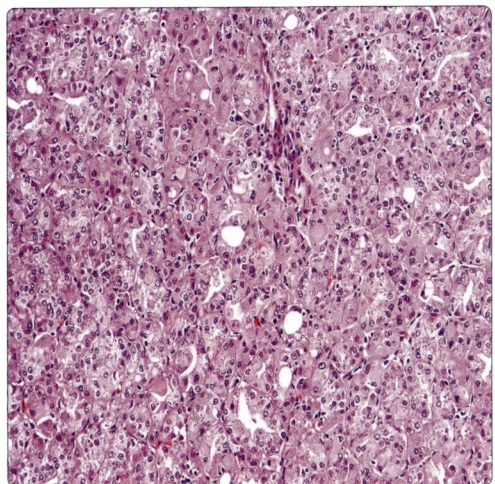

RCC in TSC
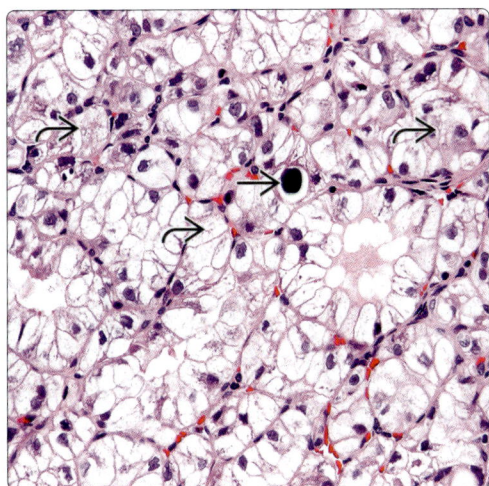

(Left) Many RCCs are composed of cells with pure eosinophilic cytoplasm, mimicking chromophobe RCC or renal oncocytoma, but most tumors do not fit the classic description of chromophobe RCC or oncocytoma. (Right) Clear cell cytology is also not unusual, but these clear cells often show fine eosinophilic cytoplasmic strands ⇨. Although mimicking clear cell RCC, marked morphological variability and the presence of psammomatous calcifications ⇨ is unusual for clear cell RCC.

Papillary Architecture
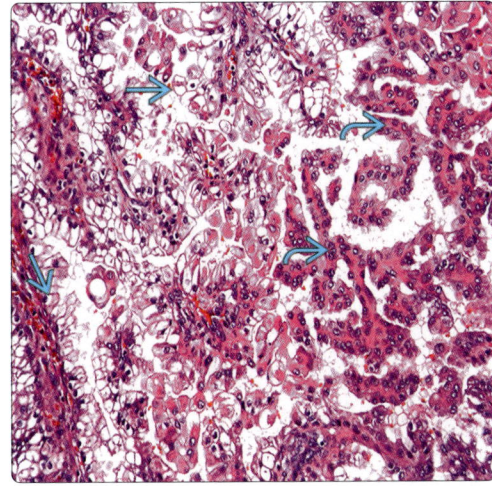

RCC in TSC
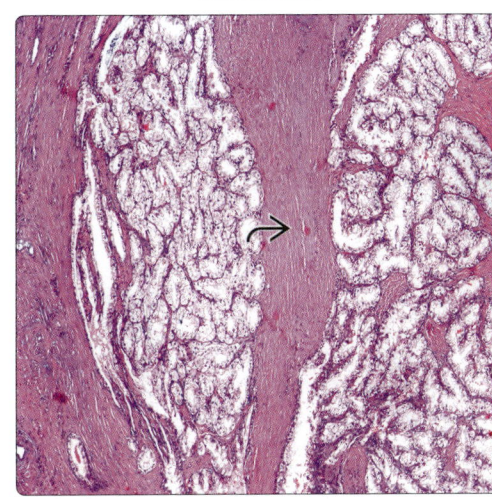

(Left) While nested pattern is frequent, variable papillary architecture ⇨ is not uncommon. A characteristic feature is the presence of cells with voluminous clear cytoplasm ⇨, often with fine fibrillary eosinophilic cytoplasmic strands. (Right) Some tumors show prominent fibromuscular septations ⇨, raising the differential diagnostic possibility of the recently described TCEB1-mutated or RAT-like tumors. Multifocality, variability in architecture, and presence of cysts or AML should merit molecular investigations.

Multifocal RCC and Multiple Cysts
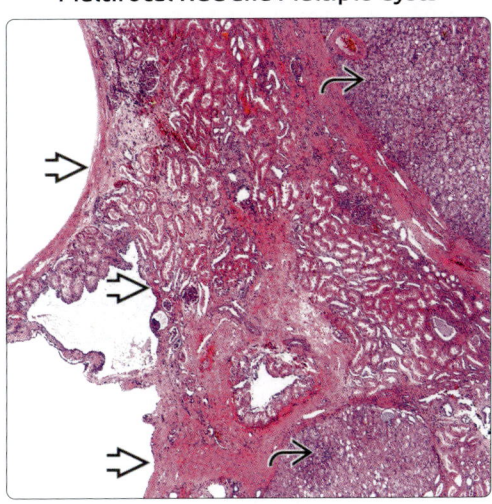

Renal Cysts in TSC
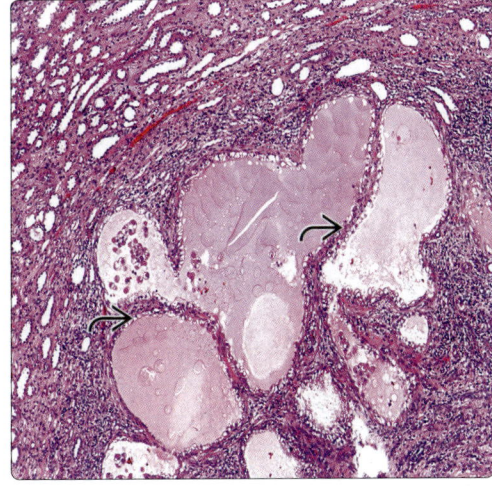

(Left) RCCs in TSC are often multifocal ⇨. The tumors may show variable morphologies. Variable morphologies, and the presence of multiple cysts ⇨ in the renal parenchyma, particularly if associated with AMLs in the kidney or lymph nodes, are highly suggestive of TSC syndrome. (Right) The renal cysts in TSC syndrome are often lined by large cells with eosinophilic cytoplasm or cells with clear cytoplasm with eosinophilic cytoplasmic strands ⇨. Nuclei are often large, and contain prominent nucleoli.

Succinate Dehydrogenase Complex Deficiency Syndrome

KEY FACTS

TERMINOLOGY
- Autosomal dominant syndrome with incomplete penetrance due to mutations in SDH gene or SDH gene assembly factor (SDHAF)
- Characterized by multiple tumor types, including
  - Head and neck and other extraadrenal paragangliomas, adrenal pheochromocytomas, gastrointestinal stromal tumors (GISTs), thyroid tumors, testicular seminoma, and neuroblastomas

ETIOLOGY/PATHOGENESIS
- Germline mutation in any of 4 genes encoding succinate dehydrogenase (SDH) enzyme (SDHA, SDHB, SDHC, and SDHD), or SDH gene assembly factor (SDHAF2)

CLINICAL ISSUES
- Extrarenal manifestations such as pheochromocytomas, paragangliomas, carotid body tumors, and gastrointestinal stromal tumors more common than RCC
- Risk of developing RCC ~ 14% by age 70

MACROSCOPIC
- SDH-deficient RCC: Mostly well circumscribed, often with pushing border; mean tumor size: 4.6 cm (range: 0.7-20 cm)

MICROSCOPIC
- Architecture predominantly nested or solid sheet-like; other patterns, micro-/macrocystic, tubular, papillary, sarcomatoid, and rhabdoid
- Most characteristic feature: Cytoplasmic inclusions containing pale eosinophilic or flocculent to completely clear material and neuroendocrine-like nuclei

ANCILLARY TESTS
- Loss of SDHB protein by immunohistochemistry a sensitive and specific marker; absent SDHB staining in tumors with mutations of SDHB, SDHA, SDHC, SDHD, or SDHAF2

TOP DIFFERENTIAL DIAGNOSES
- Renal oncocytoma; eosinophilic variant chromphobe RCC; RCC, unclassified, oncocytic type; HLRCC-associated RCC

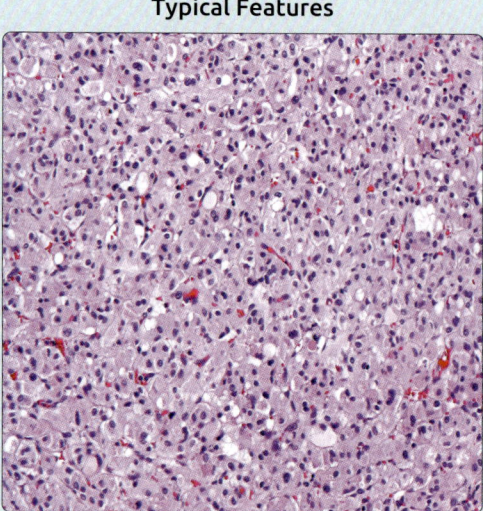

Typical Features

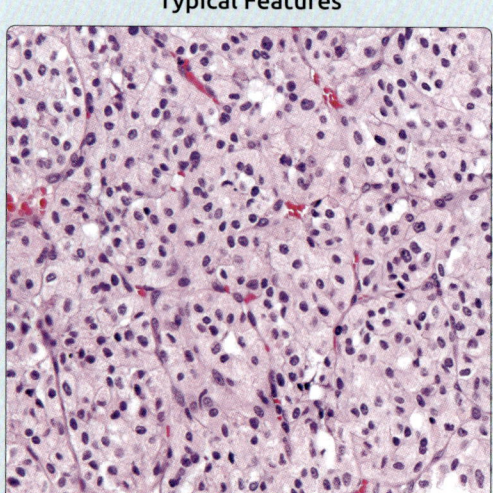

Typical Features

(Left) SDHB-deficient RCC often shows sheet-like or nested growth pattern, frequently mimicking renal oncocytoma. However, even at low magnification, the nuclear atypia is often beyond that acceptable for oncocytoma. *(Right)* Nuclear variability not typical of renal oncocytoma often leads to diagnostic consideration of oncocytic low-grade unclassified RCC. Such morphological features in younger patients merit considerations of SDHB-deficient tumors and additional investigations.

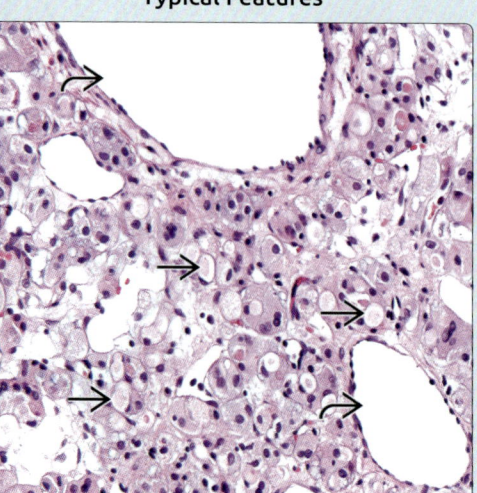

Typical Features

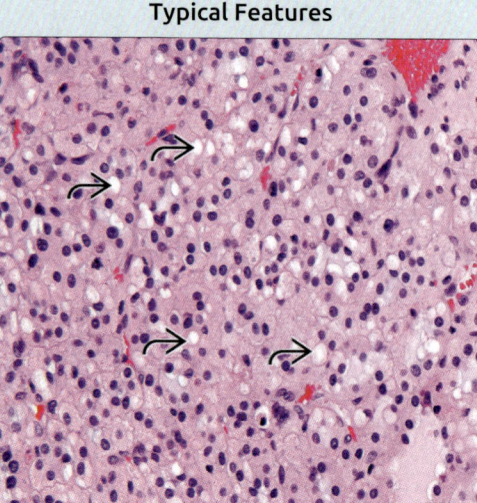

Typical Features

(Left) Architectural patterns in SDHB-deficient tumors may be quite variable, and cystic components ➔ are not uncommon. Presence of cytoplasmic inclusions that range from eosinophilic ➔ to completely clear is highly characteristic. *(Right)* In some tumors, the cytoplasmic inclusions may appear predominantly clear ➔. The inclusions are believed to represent giant mitochondria. Presence of such cytoplasmic inclusions in all oncocytic neoplasms strongly merits investigations for SDH-deficient RCCs.

Succinate Dehydrogenase Complex Deficiency Syndrome

TERMINOLOGY

Synonyms
- Hereditary paraganglioma/pheochromocytoma syndrome

Definitions
- Autosomal dominant syndrome with incomplete penetrance due to mutations in SDH gene or SDH gene assembly factor (SDHAF)
- Characterized by multiple tumor types, including
  o Head and neck and other extraadrenal paragangliomas
  o Adrenal pheochromocytomas
  o Renal cell carcinomas
  o Gastrointestinal stromal tumors (GISTs)
  o Others, including thyroid tumors, testicular seminoma, and neuroblastomas

ETIOLOGY/PATHOGENESIS

Germline Loss-of-Function Mutation in Any of 4 Genes Encoding Succinate Dehydrogenase Enzyme
- SDHA, SDHB, SDHC, and SDHD, or SDH gene assembly factor (SDHAF2)
- Genes located on chromosomes 5p15, 1p36, 1q21 and 11q23, and 11q12, respectively
- SDH enzyme comprises mitochondrial complex II; involved in Krebs cycle and in electron transport chain
  o Complex II couples oxidation of succinate to fumarate in Krebs cycle with electron transfer to terminal acceptor ubiquinone in electron transfer chain (ETC)
- Tumorigenesis involves mutation in one allele and LOH of other wild type allele, leading to complete loss of function of enzyme
- Due to SDH dysfunction, succinate cannot be converted to fumarase
  o Accumulated succinate leaves mitochondria into cytosol and causes competitive inhibition of enzyme HIFα prolyl hydroxylase
    – Leads to prevention of hydroxylation of HIF
      □ Hydroxylation of HIF an essential requirement for its proteosomic degradation by pVHL complex
    – Therefore, HIF gets overexpressed and induces multiple downstream molecules and possible tumorigenesis
- Mutations in complex II enzymes also shown to contribute to some accumulated reactive oxygen species, oxidative stress, genomic instability, and tumorigenesis
- Patients with SDH-deficient RCC most often (75%) associated with mutation in SDHB
  o Rarely, mutations also reported in SDHA, SDHC, and SDHD

CLINICAL ISSUES

Epidemiology
- Overall estimated incidence of RCC: 0.05-0.1% of all resected renal cell tumors

Presentation
- Extrarenal manifestations such as pheochromocytomas, paragangliomas, carotid body tumors, and GISTs more common than RCC
  o Pheochromocytomas and paragangliomas may occur quite early in life, even by 3 years of age
- Based on mutations and the affected organs, paraganglioma (PGL) syndrome divided into 5 types (PGL1-5)
  o Specific genes involved
    – PGL1: SDHD
    – PGL2: SDHAF2
    – PGL3: SDHC
    – PGL4: SDHB
    – PGL5: SDHA
  o In general, renal tumors associated in order of frequency
    – PGL4 > PGL1 > PGL3 > PGL5
  o Adrenal pheochromocytomas occur mostly in
    – PGL4 > PGL1 > PGL5
  o Head and neck paragangliomas occur mostly in
    – PGL2 > PGL1 > PGL4 > PGL5
  o Thoraco-abdominal paragangliomas in
    – PGL4 > PGL1 > PGL4 and PGL5
- Risk of developing RCC in SDH syndrome approximately 14% by age 70
- Mean age at presentation for RCC: 37 years (range: 14-76)
  o Bilateral RCCs in approximately 25% of patients with renal tumors

Prognosis
- Previously believed to be mostly with indolent clinical behavior
  o However, up to 1/3 of tumors with metastases and aggressive clinical behavior
    – Tumors with metastases often show high nuclear grade and coagulative necrosis
      □ Metastases occasionally develop long after primary tumor diagnosis
    – Tumors without high nuclear grade or coagulative necrosis only rarely reported to metastasize

MACROSCOPIC

General Features
- SDH-deficient RCC
  o Mean tumor size: 4.3-5.1 cm (range: 0.7-20 cm)
  o Mostly well circumscribed, often with pushing border sometimes associated with pseudocapsule
    – Rarely, tumors with infiltrative edges
      □ Such tumors often exhibit high-grade histology
  o Cut surface often solid, variegated, tan-brown or red-brown, sometimes hemorrhagic
  o Occasional tumors with grossly identified cystic change
    – Cystic change appreciated more often on histologic evaluation

MICROSCOPIC

Histologic Features
- Architecture predominantly nested or solid sheet-like
  o Other architectural patterns uncommonly present include
    – Micro- or macrocystic
    – Tubular and glandular
    – Papillary
    – Rhabdoid

Succinate Dehydrogenase Complex Deficiency Syndrome

- Sarcomatoid
- Most tumors with smooth outlines without encapsulation; partial encapsulation in occasional tumors
  - Rare tumors with irregular, infiltrative edges, and multinodularity
- Tumors predominantly composed of cells with eosinophilic, variably granular cytoplasm
- Nuclei typically uniform and round, with smooth nuclear contours, finely clumped chromatin, and small or absent nucleoli (neuroendocrine-like)
  - Rare tumors with high-grade nuclei, with prominent nucleoli
    - Such cases often with rhabdoid features
    - Frank sarcomatoid differentiation also present in occasional tumor
- Most characteristic feature
  - Presence of cytoplasmic inclusions containing pale eosinophilic or flocculent to completely clear material
  - These inclusions correspond to giant mitochondria by ultrastructural examination
    - Inclusions often readily detected, although in cases with higher nuclear grade, may be only focally present
  - Rare SDH-deficient tumors may not show inclusions even after careful examination
    - Such cases often only identified after immunohistochemical evaluation based on clinical history or atypical features in an oncocytic neoplasm
- Tumor necrosis very uncommon; but often present in cases with high nuclear grade
  - In one large series, all metastatic cases with tumor necrosis in primary tumors
- Many, but not all, tumors with prominent intratumoral mast cells
  - Mast cells more commonly visualized on CD117 stain, and may not be clearly identified on H&E evaluation

ANCILLARY TESTS

Immunohistochemistry
- Loss of SDHB protein by immunohistochemistry a sensitive and specific marker
  - Lack of SDHB staining highly suggestive of germline mutation in *SDHB* gene
  - SDHB staining also absent in tumors with mutations of *SDHA*, *SDHC*, *SDHD*, or *SDHAF2*
- Tumors with *SDHA* mutation also with loss of staining for SDHA
  - SDHA positivity retained in tumors associated with *SDHB*, *SDHC*, *SDHD*, and *SDHAF2* mutations
- CD117(-), but highlights intratumoral mast cells
  - CK7(-), CA9(-), S100A1(-)
  - Other keratins and EMA also often (-), or only focally (+)
- pax-8, Ksp-cadherin (+) in all cases

DIFFERENTIAL DIAGNOSIS

Renal Oncocytoma
- Uniform nuclei, with nuclear pleomorphism only in degenerate-appearing foci
- Lack the intracytoplasmic inclusions
- CD117(+); retained SDHB immunoreactivity

Eosinophilic Variant Chromophobe RCC
- At least some irregular nuclei with perinuclear halos
- Lack the intracytoplasmic inclusions
- CK7 often at least focally (+); CD117(+); Ksp-cadherin (+); retained SDHB immunoreactivity

Renal Cell Carcinoma, Unclassified, Oncocytic Type
- Lack the intracytoplasmic inclusions
- Often CD117(+); retained SDHB immunoreactivity

HLRCC-Associated Renal Cell Carcinoma
- Rare SDHB-deficient RCC with very prominent nucleoli, raising possibility of HLRCC-associated carcinoma
- SDHB-deficient tumors with intracytoplasmic inclusions
  - Retained fumarate hydratase and absence of 2SC positivity
  - Lack SDHB immunoreactivity, unlike HLRCC tumors

DIAGNOSTIC CHECKLIST

Pathologic Interpretation Pearls
- In renal oncocytoma-like tumors, presence of nuclear and architectural variability mandates careful search for intracytoplasmic inclusions
  - Even when inclusions not present or not prominent, immunohistochemical staining for SDHB in such cases needs to be performed
- Prior history of pheochromocytoma, paraganglioma or GIST in patient with oncocytic renal neoplasm should always raise possibility of *SDH* mutations

SELECTED REFERENCES

1. Benn DE et al: 15 years of paraganglioma: clinical manifestations of paraganglioma syndromes types 1-5. Endocr Relat Cancer. 22(4):T91-T103, 2015
2. Williamson SR et al: Succinate dehydrogenase-deficient renal cell carcinoma: detailed characterization of 11 tumors defining a unique subtype of renal cell carcinoma. Mod Pathol. 28(1):80-94, 2015
3. Gill AJ et al: Succinate dehydrogenase (SDH)-deficient renal carcinoma: a morphologically distinct entity: a clinicopathologic series of 36 tumors from 27 patients. Am J Surg Pathol. 38(12):1588-602, 2014
4. Papathomas TG et al: Non-pheochromocytoma (PCC)/paraganglioma (PGL) tumors in patients with succinate dehydrogenase-related PCC-PGL syndromes: a clinicopathological and molecular analysis. Eur J Endocrinol. 170(1):1-12, 2014
5. Gill AJ: Succinate dehydrogenase (SDH) and mitochondrial driven neoplasia. Pathology. 44(4):285-92, 2012
6. Ricketts CJ et al: Succinate dehydrogenase kidney cancer: an aggressive example of the Warburg effect in cancer. J Urol. 188(6):2063-71, 2012
7. Bardella C et al: SDH mutations in cancer. Biochim Biophys Acta. 1807(11):1432-43, 2011
8. Gill AJ et al: Renal tumors associated with germline SDHB mutation show distinctive morphology. Am J Surg Pathol. 35(10):1578-85, 2011
9. Ricketts CJ et al: Tumor risks and genotype-phenotype-proteotype analysis in 358 patients with germline mutations in SDHB and SDHD. Hum Mutat. 31(1):41-51, 2010
10. Ricketts C et al: Germline SDHB mutations and familial renal cell carcinoma. J Natl Cancer Inst. 100(17):1260-2, 2008

Succinate Dehydrogenase Complex Deficiency Syndrome

Uncommon Features

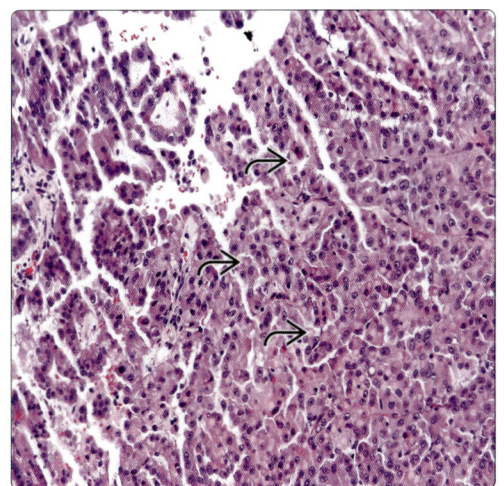

Uncommon Features

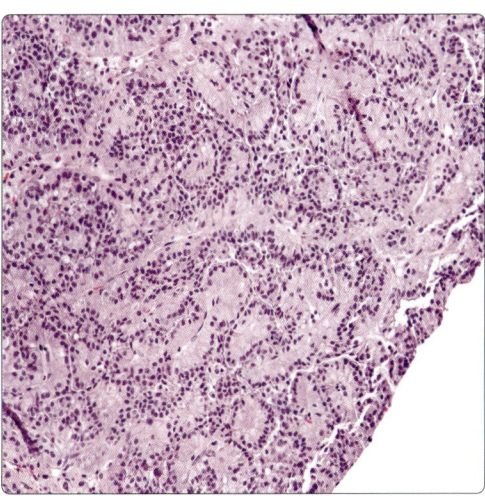

(Left) In addition to to the usual nested or solid patterns, some SDHB-deficient RCCs may have variable, and occasionally extensive, papillary architecture. The characteristic cytoplasmic inclusions ➡ are often still identifiable in such variant morphologies. (Right) Very occasionally, SDHB-deficient tumors show true glandular differentiation; this architectural pattern is generally very focal. Presence of the more typical features in the rest of the the tumor will often lead to the proper diagnostic considerations.

Uncommon Features

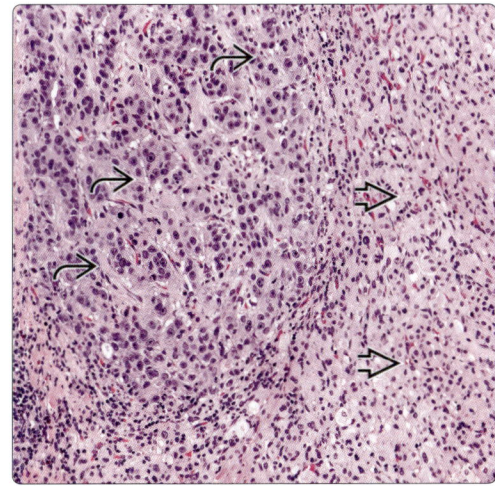

Uncommon Features

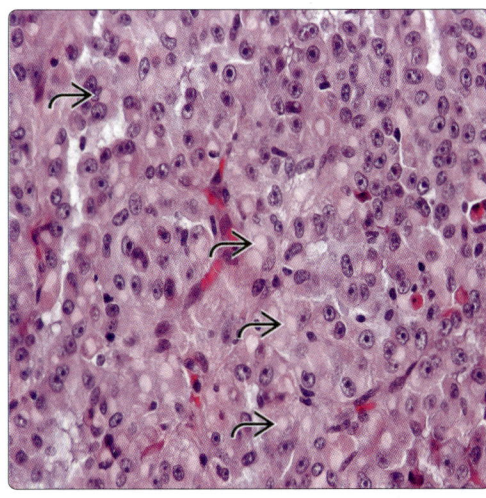

(Left) Most SDHB-deficient RCCs show low-grade nucleolar (WHO/ISUP grade 1 or 2) features ➡. However, tumors with high-grade features ➡ are not uncommon and may be seen closely apposed to low-grade areas in some tumors (seen here). (Right) Tumors with prominent nucleoli, particularly in young patients, may sometimes raise possibility of HLRCC-associated RCC. Lower grade typical areas & characteristic inclusions even in high-grade areas ➡ should point toward the correct diagnosis.

Mast Cells

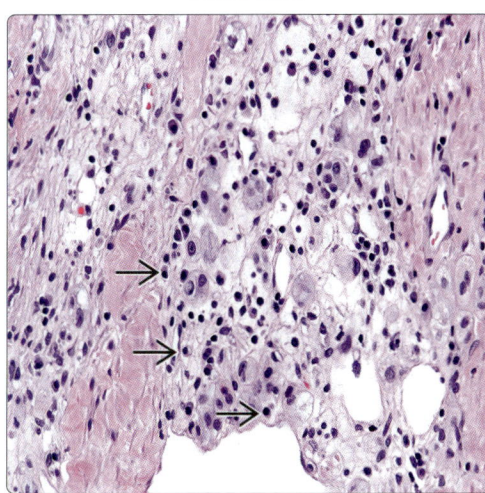

Loss of SDHB Staining

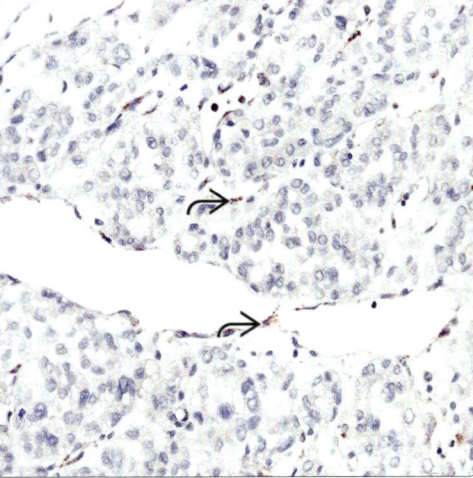

(Left) Intratumoral mast cells ➡ are a frequent feature in SDHB-deficient RCC. However, mast cells may be present in many other renal tumors with eosinophilic cytoplasm. Thus, while useful in the differential diagnosis, mast cells in an eosinophilic tumor should not be considered diagnostic for SDHB-deficient tumors. (Right) SDHB-deficient tumors lack the immunohistochemical positivity for SDHB in the tumor cells. Intratumoral vasculature ➡ and inflammatory cells are positive and act as internal positive controls.

Hereditary Papillary Renal Cancer and Miscellaneous Other Familial Cancer Syndromes

KEY FACTS

TERMINOLOGY
- Hereditary papillary renal cancer syndrome (HPRC); hyperparathyroidism-jaw tumor syndrome (HPT-JT); other familial renal cell carcinoma syndromes (OFRC)
- HPRC: Autosomal dominant syndrome characterized by multiple, bilateral papillary renal cell carcinomas (RCCs)
- HPT-JT: Autosomal-dominant syndrome, characterized by primary hyperparathyroidism, ossifying fibroma of maxilla and/or mandible, renal and uterine tumors
- OFRC: Include autosomal-dominant Cowden or PTEN hamartoma tumor syndrome; BRCA-associated protein 1 (BAP1) hereditary cancer predisposition syndrome; constitutional balanced chromosome 3 translocation RCC

ETIOLOGY/PATHOGENESIS
- Mutations present: *c-MET* protooncogene in HPRC; *CDC73* tumor suppressor gene in HPT-JT; *PTEN* gene in Cowden or PTEN hamartoma tumor syndrome; *BAP1* gene in BAP1 cancer predisposition syndrome
- In constitutional balanced chromosome 3 translocation RCC, loss of rearranged chromosome during mitosis leads to greater errors during chromosomal segregation

MICROSCOPIC
- HPRC: Renal tumors associated are all type 1 papillary RCC
- HPT-JT: Mixed epithelial and stromal tumor, adult Wilms tumor and papillary RCC
- Cowden or PTEN hamartoma tumor syndrome: Papillary RCC (types 1 and 2), chromophobe and clear cell RCC
- Constitutional balanced chromosome 3 translocation and BAP1 hereditary cancer predisposition syndromes: Both with clear cell RCC

TOP DIFFERENTIAL DIAGNOSES
- Multifocal sporadic papillary RCC
- Sporadic mixed epithelial and stromal tumor
- Multifocal, bilateral clear cell RCC

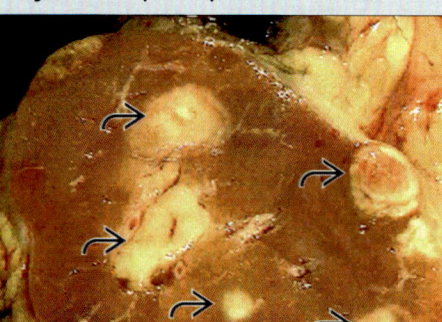

Hereditary Papillary Renal Cancer Syndrome (HPRC): Gross Features

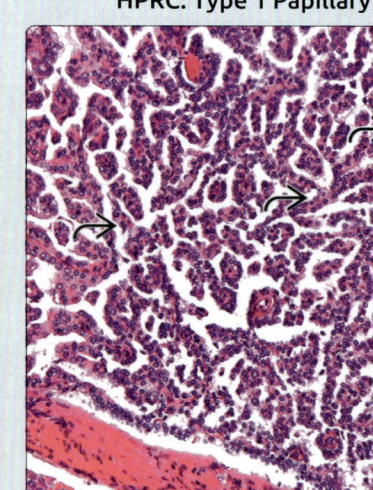

HPRC: Type 1 Papillary RCC

(Left) Hereditary papillary renal cancer syndrome (HPRC) is characterized by the presence of numerous bilateral type 1 papillary renal cell carcinomas (RCCs) ⇨, as seen in this gross picture from one such patient. The tumors are often well circumscribed and of low stage. *(Right)* All tumors in HPRC show the morphological features similar to sporadic type 1 papillary RCC. Thus, all architectural patterns that are observed in sporadic setting may be seen. This slide depicts thin, elongated, branching papillary architecture ⇨.

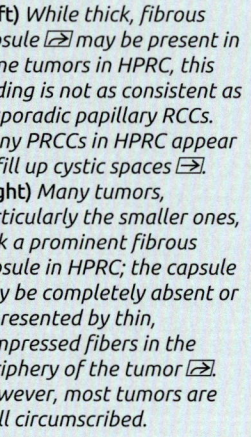

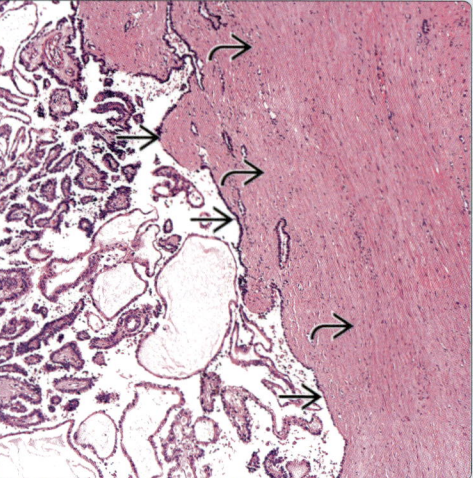

HPRC: Encapsulation

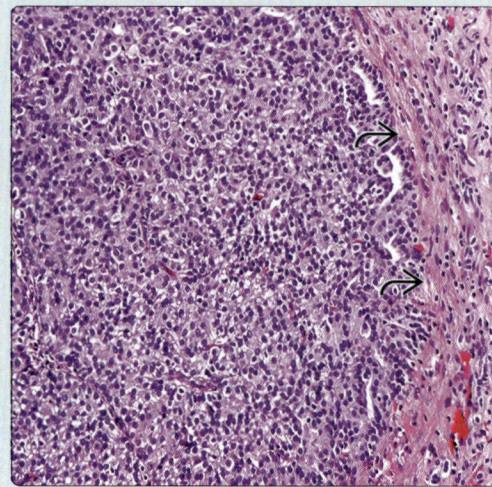

HPRC: Tumor Circumscription

(Left) While thick, fibrous capsule ⇨ may be present in some tumors in HPRC, this finding is not as consistent as in sporadic papillary RCCs. Many PRCCs in HPRC appear to fill up cystic spaces ⇨. *(Right)* Many tumors, particularly the smaller ones, lack a prominent fibrous capsule in HPRC; the capsule may be completely absent or represented by thin, compressed fibers in the periphery of the tumor ⇨. However, most tumors are well circumscribed.

Hereditary Papillary Renal Cancer and Miscellaneous Other Familial Cancer Syndromes

TERMINOLOGY

Abbreviations
- Hereditary papillary renal cancer syndrome (HPRC); hyperparathyroidism-jaw tumor syndrome (HPT-JT); other familial renal cell carcinoma syndromes (OFRC)

Definitions
- HPRC: Autosomal dominant syndrome, with incomplete but very high penetrance, characterized by
  o Multiple, bilateral papillary renal cell carcinomas (RCCs)
    – Hundreds to thousands of tumors known to occur in each kidney
- HPT-JT: Rare autosomal dominant syndrome, characterized by
  o Primary hyperparathyroidism (PHPT), ossifying fibroma of maxilla and/or mandible, renal and uterine tumors
    – Associated with increased risk of parathyroid cancer
- OFRC: Include autosomal dominant Cowden or PTEN hamartoma tumor syndrome; BRCA-associated protein 1 (BAP1) hereditary cancer predisposition syndrome; constitutional balanced chromosome 3 translocation RCC

ETIOLOGY/PATHOGENESIS

HPRC: Mutations in *c-MET* Gene
- Syndrome associated with activating mutations of *c-MET* protooncogene
  o Gene is located at chromosome 7q31
  o Hepatocyte growth factor (a.k.a. scatter factor) acts as ligand for MET transmember tyrosine kinase protein
  o Normally, binding to hepatocyte growth factor activates MET tyrosine kinase protein
    – Tyrosine phosphorylation induces proliferation and differentiation of epithelial and endothelial cells, cell branching, and invasion
  o *c-MET* mutations result in ligand-independent constitutive activation of MET tyrosine kinase
  o Activated tyrosine kinase then binds to and activates several signal transducers and adaptors, such as
    – Phosphatidylinositol 3 kinase (PI3K)
    – pp60src
    – Growth factor receptor-bound protein 2 (Grb2)
    – GRB2-associated binding protein 1 (Gab1)
  o This constitutive activation of *c-MET* results in tumorigenesis

HPT-JT: Mutations in *CDC73* Gene
- Cell division cycle 73(*CDC73*), tumor suppressor gene
  o Located at 1q25- q32 and encodes parafibromin
  o Parafibromin constituent of transcriptional regulator, RNA polymerase II-associated factor I complex
    – Suppresses mitogenic activities of cyclin D1 and c-myc pathways

Other Familial RCC Syndromes
- Germline mutations in *PTEN* gene (located on chromosome 10q22-23) occurring in > 70% of patients with Cowden syndrome
- Mutations in *BAP1* gene (located on 3p21.1); *BAP1* encodes nuclear ubiquitin carboxyterminal hydrolase, enhances BRCA1-mediated cell growth suppression by chromatin modification
- In constitutional balanced chromosome 3 translocation RCC, loss of rearranged chromosome during mitosis leads to greater errors during chromosomal segregation

CLINICAL ISSUES

Epidemiology
- Families with *c-MET* mutations and HPRC quite rare
  o Not only von Hippel-Lindau (VHL), but even other inherited renal cancer syndromes, such as hereditary leiomyomatosis and RCC and BHD much more common
- PHPT with prevalence of 40 per 100,000 individuals; association with HPT-JT even rarer (< 1-2 per 100,000)
- Other familial RCC syndromes even more rare

Presentation
- HPRC
  o Tumors often manifest at relatively late age (50-70 years)
    – Recently, early onset form of disease has also been described
  o High likelihood of person developing papillary RCC by age 80, supporting its high penetrance
    – ~ 50% of members of affected families develop disease
  o Tumors are multifocal and bilateral
  o No extrarenal manifestations of HPRC known at present
- HPT-JT
  o Characterized by hyperparathyroidism secondary to parathyroid adenoma or carcinoma
    – Other associations of syndrome include fibroosseous lesions of jaw bones and renal tumors
- Cowden or PTEN hamartoma tumor syndrome
  o Frequently with multiple hamartomas, macrocephaly, increased risk for breast, endometrial, thyroid, and genitourinary (prostate and kidney) cancers, and dermatologic conditions such as acral keratosis and facial trichilemmomas
- BAP1 hereditary cancer predisposition syndrome
  o Associated with uveal and cutaneous melanomas, mesothelioma, melanocytic *BAP1*-mutated atypical intradermal tumors and clear cell RCC
- Constitutional balanced chromosome 3 translocation
  o Bilateral and multifocal clear cell RCC, detected in individuals older than in VHL disease
  o No known extrarenal manifestations

Treatment
- Partial nephrectomy/nephrectomies and tumor enucleation or ablation when tumors reach size of 3 cm, standard management similar to cases of VHL syndrome

Prognosis
- Most tumors small and identified incidentally
- Only rare metastases reported in HPRC, particularly to regional lymph nodes
- Others, too few cases for definitive prognostication

Hereditary Papillary Renal Cancer and Miscellaneous Other Familial Cancer Syndromes

MACROSCOPIC

General Features

- HPRC: Grossly, multifocal and bilateral tumors, usually well circumscribed
  - Number of tumors in each kidney may run in dozens to hundreds or more
- HPT-JT: Mostly reported as unilateral tumors
- Constitutional balanced chromosome 3 translocation and BAP1 hereditary cancer predisposition syndromes, often bilateral and multifocal

MICROSCOPIC

Histologic Features

- HPRC
  - Renal tumors associated with syndromic c-MET mutations are all type 1 papillary RCC
  - Tumors show papillary or tubulopapillary architecture, similar to type 1 sporadic carcinomas
    - Foamy macrophages and calcifications commonly present
  - Occasional tumor with areas mimicking type 2 histology described
    - Tumors with type 1 and type 2 areas behave like type 1 tumors
  - Surrounding renal parenchyma with numerous papillary adenomas
    - All tumors < 1.5 cm in size considered papillary RCC in past now regarded as papillary adenoma
- HPT-JT
  - Mixed epithelial and stromal tumor, most commonly reported renal neoplasm; adult Wilms tumor and papillary RCC other reported tumors
  - Background kidney with multiple cysts, resembling polycystic kidney disease
- Cowden or PTEN hamartoma tumor syndrome
  - Papillary RCC (types 1 and 2) most common subtype; chromophobe and clear cell RCC other reported subtypes
- Constitutional balanced chromosome 3 translocation and BAP1 hereditary cancer predisposition syndromes: Both with clear cell RCC

DIFFERENTIAL DIAGNOSIS

Multifocal Sporadic Papillary Renal Cell Carcinoma

- Needs distinction from HPRC
  - Multifocal nonsyndromic papillary RCC rarely show > 10-12 tumors
    - Tumors in HPRC often present with numerous, even hundreds or more of tumors
  - In general, family history of multiple papillary renal tumors lacking
  - Morphological or immunohistochemical features of individual tumors not helpful in distinction
  - Enumerable papillary adenomas unlikely in sporadic tumors
  - Diagnosis of HPRC may be positively excluded only by negative genetic testing results
  - Syndrome associated with activating mutations of c-MET proto-oncogene, whereas such mutations present in only 10-13% of sporadic tumors

Sporadic Mixed Epithelial and Stromal Tumor

- HPT-JT with mixed epithelial and stromal tumor (MEST) may raise differential diagnosis of sporadic MEST
- Syndrome characterized by hyperparathyroidism in > 85% of cases
  - Also often associated with fibroosseous lesions of mandible and maxilla

Multifocal, Bilateral Clear Cell Renal Cell Carcinoma

- Multifocal and bilateral clear cell RCCs may be seen in VHL, constitutional balanced chromosome 3 translocation and BAP1 hereditary cancer predisposition syndromes
  - VHL and BAP1 hereditary cancer predisposition syndromes often with other characteristic syndromic associations
    - Nuclear staining for BAP1 IHC completely lost in tumor in BAP1 syndrome
      - However, BAP1 may be lost in clear cell RCC in some sporadic and VHL cases as well
  - Constitutional balanced chromosome 3 translocation RCC shows no extrarenal manifestations
  - Differentiation may require molecular evaluation in some cases

SELECTED REFERENCES

1. Popova T et al: Germline BAP1 mutations predispose to renal cell carcinomas. Am J Hum Genet. Clin Genet. 92(6):974-80, 2013
2. Ho TH et al: Genetic kidney cancer syndromes. J Natl Compr Canc Netw. 12(9):1347-55, 2014
3. Przybycin CG et al: Hereditary syndromes with associated renal neoplasia: a practical guide to histologic recognition in renal tumor resection specimens. Adv Anat Pathol. 20(4):245-63, 2013
4. Mester JL et al: Papillary renal cell carcinoma is associated with PTEN hamartoma tumor syndrome. Urology. 79(5):1187, 2012
5. Wadt KA et al: Novel germline c-MET mutation in a family with hereditary papillary renal carcinoma. Fam Cancer. 11(3):535-7, 2012
6. Dharmawardana PG et al: Hereditary papillary renal carcinoma type I. Curr Mol Med. 4(8):855-68, 2004
7. Tan MH et al: Renal neoplasia in the hyperparathyroidism-jaw tumor syndrome. Curr Mol Med. 4(8):895-7, 2004
8. Chen JD et al: Hyperparathyroidism-jaw tumour syndrome. J Intern Med. 253(6):634-42, 2003
9. Lindor NM et al: Papillary renal cell carcinoma: analysis of germline mutations in the MET proto-oncogene in a clinic-based population. Genet Test. 5(2):101-6, 2001
10. Lubensky IA et al: Hereditary and sporadic papillary renal carcinomas with c-met mutations share a distinct morphological phenotype. Am J Pathol. 155(2):517-26, 1999
11. Schmidt L et al: Germline and somatic mutations in the tyrosine kinase domain of the MET proto-oncogene in papillary renal carcinomas. Nat Genet. 16(1):68-73, 1997
12. Teh BT et al: Autosomal dominant primary hyperparathyroidism and jaw tumor syndrome associated with renal hamartomas and cystic kidney disease: linkage to 1q21-q32 and loss of the wild type allele in renal hamartomas. J Clin Endocrinol Metab. 81(12):4204-11, 1996
13. Zbar B et al: Hereditary papillary renal cell carcinoma. J Urol. 151(3):561-6, 1994

Hereditary Papillary Renal Cancer and Miscellaneous Other Familial Cancer Syndromes

HPRC: Foamy Macrophages
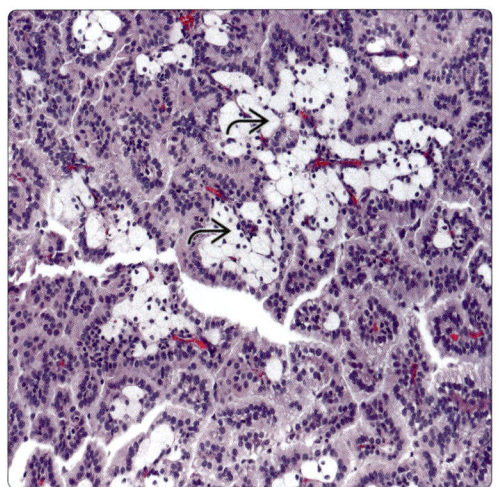

HPRC: Solid, Tubular Architecture
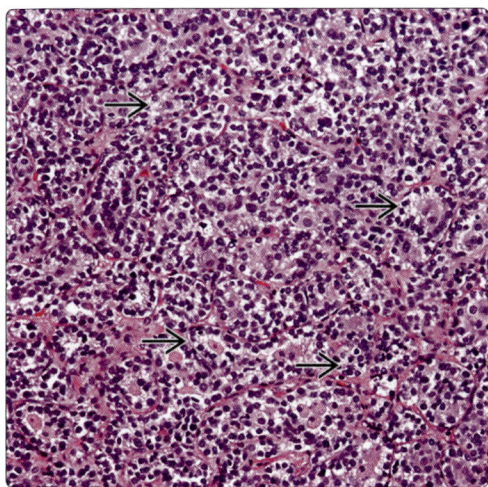

(Left) Foamy macrophages predominantly occupying the papillary cores are quite common in the papillary RCCs in HPRC. Similar to sporadic tumors, occasionally these macrophages are also present in the tumor stroma ➔, outside the papillary cores. (Right) Many papillary RCCs in HPRC show solid-appearing architecture. Careful evaluation reveals this appearance to be mostly created by closely packed tubules ➔.

HPRC: Solid-Glomeruloid Architecture
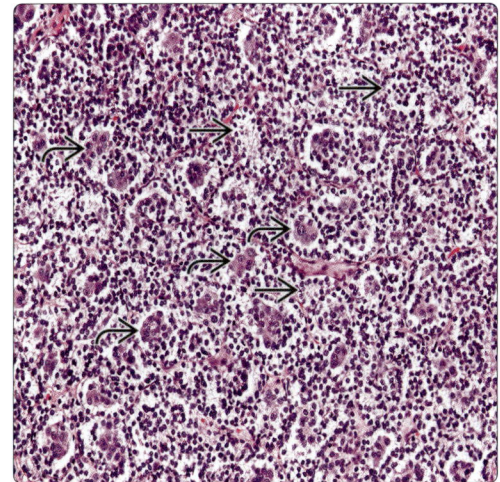

HPRC: Cytoplasmic Clarity
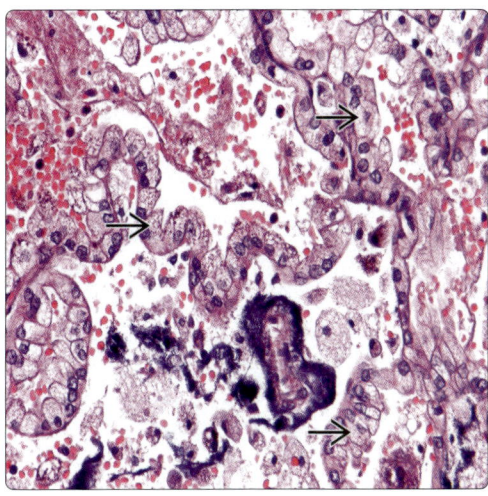

(Left) This papillary RCC from a case of HPRC shows solid-glomeruloid architectures. While the tubules in the background show low nuclear grade and amphophilic to clear cytoplasm ➔, the glomeruloid tufts show larger cells with eosinophilic cytoplasm and large prominent nucleoli ➔. (Right) As in sporadic type 1 PRCC, the tumors in HPRC also show focal cytoplasmic clarity; however, these clear-appearing cells are not optically transparent but, in fact, contain finely granular and reticulate cytoplasm ➔.

HPRC: Papillary Adenoma
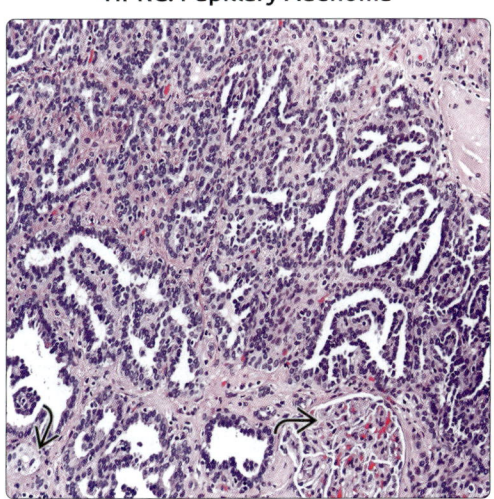

HPRC: Intracystic Papillary Adenoma
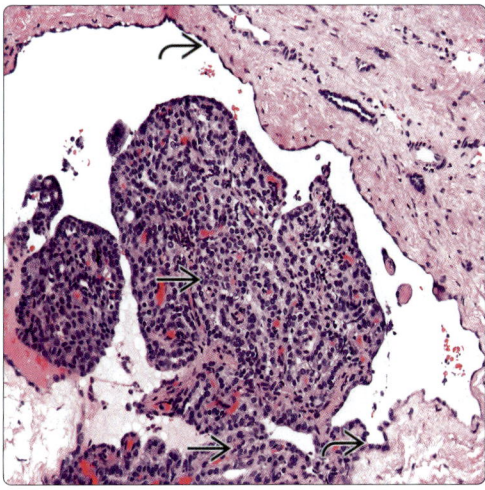

(Left) One of the most characteristic features of HPRC kidneys is the presence of numerous (often enumerable) papillary adenomas. In some cases, papillary adenomas leave only small proportion of background nonneoplastic parenchyma dispersed among adenomas ➔. (Right) Some of the papillary adenomas ➔ in HPRC arise from, and are continuous with, the lining of cystic spaces ➔. When the cyst lining is flat, this can raise the suspicion of tumor emboli in vascular spaces and may require exclusion by IHC.

Hereditary Papillary Renal Cancer and Miscellaneous Other Familial Cancer Syndromes

HPRC: Cystic Papillary Adenoma

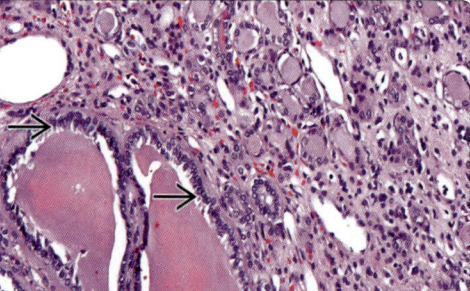

HPRC: Surgical Approach

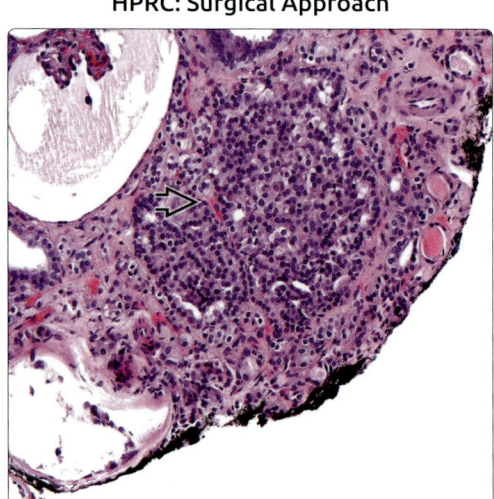

(Left) Many adenomas may be composed of only 2 or 3 tubules and at times appear as clusters of cystically dilated tubules lined by cytologically atypical epithelium ⇛. (Right) Surgical approach to the tumors in HPRC is similar to that for tumors in VHL syndrome. To preserve renal function, surgery is usually delayed until tumors grow beyond 3 cm in size. Repeat procedures are performed as new tumors develop and grow. This image shows a papillary adenoma ⇛ in a wedge of renal parenchyma, removed for 2 larger tumors.

HPRC: CK7

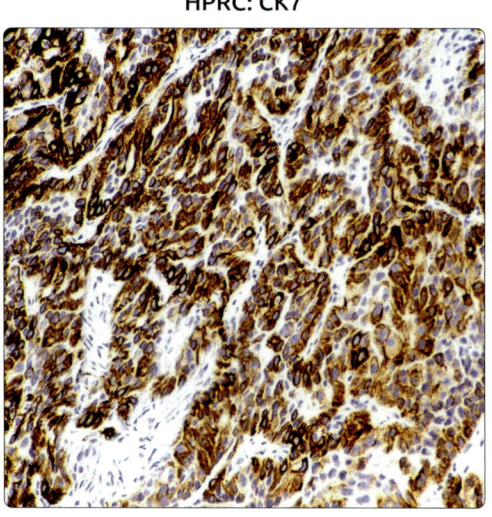

HPRC: CK7

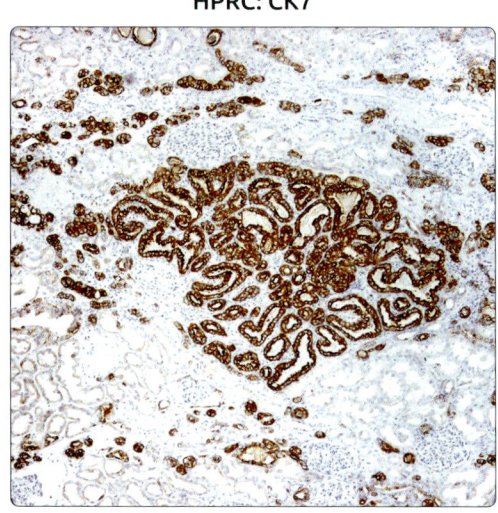

(Left) Immunohistochemistry does not differentiate between the papillary tumors of HPRC syndrome and papillary RCC of sporadic setting. As seen here, diffuse CK7 positivity in this papillary RCC does not point toward either one of these conditions. (Right) Similarly, papillary adenomas in either the familial or sporadic setting cannot be discriminated by CK7 IHC, as it is diffusely positive in overwhelming majority of lesions in both the settings.

HPRC: AMACR

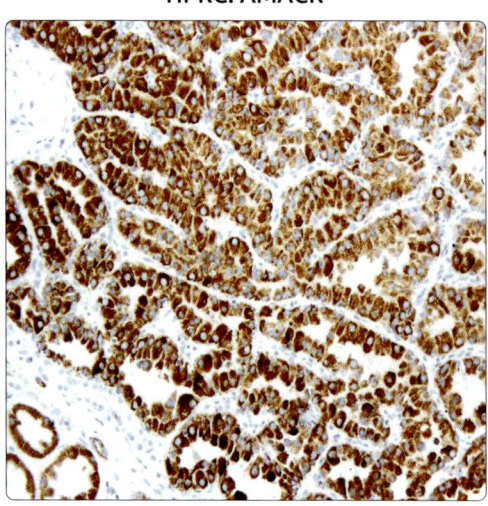

HPRC: CD10

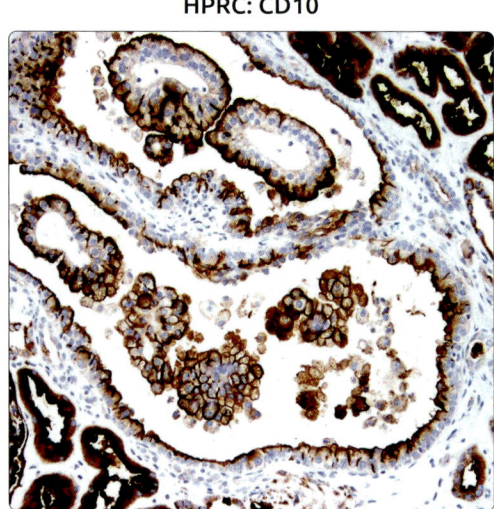

(Left) As in sporadic tumors, AMACR shows diffuse cytoplasmic, granular positivity in the vast majority of papillary RCCs, as well as papillary adenomas in HPRC. (Right) This image shows a papillary adenoma with positivity for CD10. The staining is membrane-predominant, with mostly a luminal or inverted cup-like pattern; only focal box-like staining pattern is seen. Such staining pattern is seen in tumors in both the sporadic and syndromic settings.

Hereditary Papillary Renal Cancer and Miscellaneous Other Familial Cancer Syndromes

HPT-JT: Mixed Epithelial and Stromal Tumor (MEST)

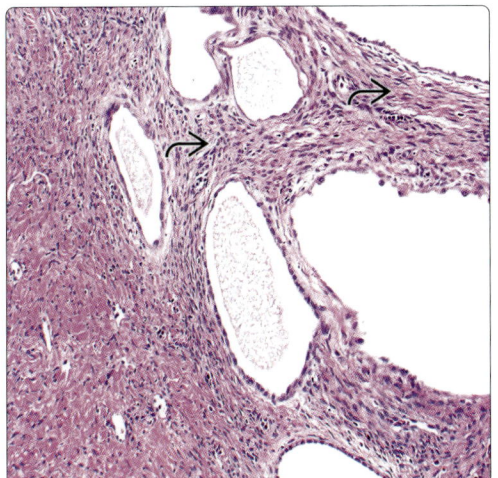

Cowden or PTEN Hamartoma Tumor Syndrome: Papillary RCC, Type 1

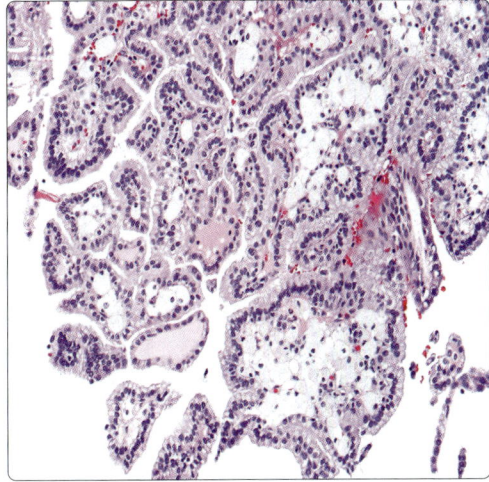

(Left) MEST is the most commonly described renal tumor in HPT-JT. Other renal tumors reported in the syndrome include adult Wilms tumor and papillary RCC. MEST of the syndrome has the same morphologic features, including the ovarian-type stroma ⊟, as in the sporadic tumors. (Right) Papillary RCC is the most common subtype of RCC reported in Cowden or PTEN Hamartoma Tumor Syndrome. This image shows a type 1 papillary RCC, which is morphologically similar to that seen in sporadic settings.

Cowden or PTEN Hamartoma Tumor Syndrome: Papillary RCC, Type 2

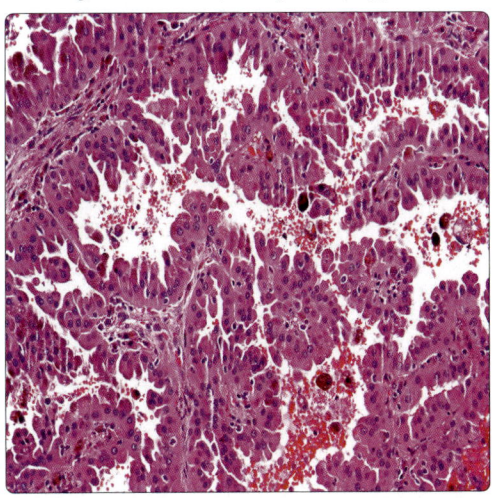

Cowden or PTEN Hamartoma Tumor Syndrome: Chromophobe RCC

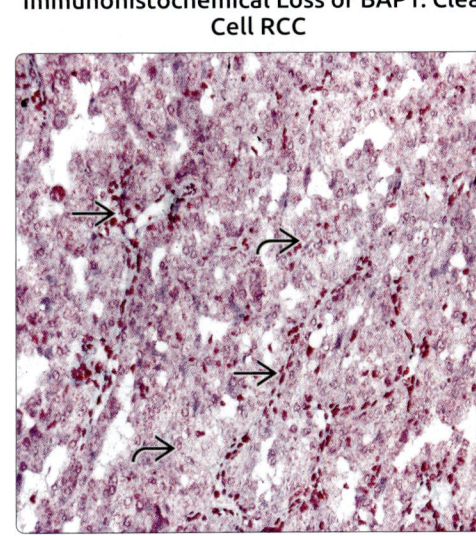

(Left) Both the type 1 and type 2 papillary renal cell carcinomas are described in Cowden or PTEN hamartoma tumor syndrome. Overall, Cowden syndrome is rare, with estimated incidence of 1 in 200,000 individuals; 70% of these patients have germline mutations in the PTEN gene. 1/3 of patients with PTEN mutations develop RCC. Thus, in absolute terms this syndrome-associated RCCs are very uncommon. (Right) Chromophobe, as well as, clear cell renal cell carcinomas are also described in the syndrome.

BAP1 Hereditary Cancer Predisposition Syndrome: Clear Cell RCC

Immunohistochemical Loss of BAP1: Clear Cell RCC

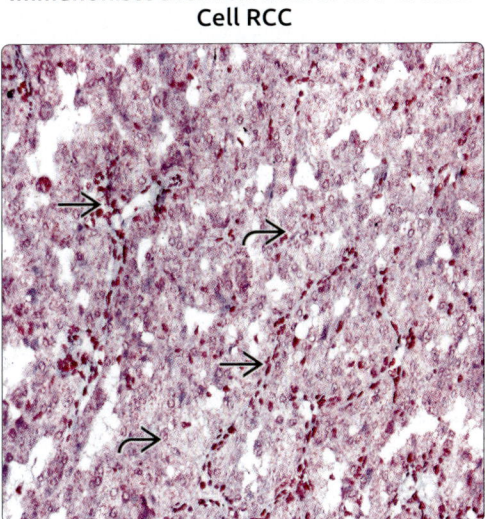

(Left) Uveal and cutaneous melanomas, mesothelioma, and atypical melanocytic intradermal tumors are more common than clear cell RCC in BAP1 hereditary cancer predisposition syndrome. All the RCCs described to-date in the syndrome have been clear cell RCC. (Right) Nuclear staining for BAP1 is completely lost ⊟ in the tumor cells in BAP1 syndrome. However, BAP1 may also be lost in clear cell RCC in some sporadic and VHL cases. Notice the retained positivity in the endothelial and inflammatory cells ⊟.

Renal Tuberculosis, Xanthogranulomatous Pyelonephritis, Renal Malakoplakia

KEY FACTS

TERMINOLOGY
- Renal tuberculosis (RTB), xanthogranulomatous pyelonephritis (XGP), renal malakoplakia (RMP)

ETIOLOGY/PATHOGENESIS
- RTB caused by members of *Mycobacterium tuberculosis* complex, mostly *Mycobacterium tuberculosis*, but rarely *M. bovine*, and occasionally by Bacille Calmette-Guérin (BCG) as complication of intravesical treatment of bladder cancer
- XGP and RMP: Most often, associated with gram-negative bacteria
- RMP: Due to defective macrophage lysosomal digestion of phagocytized bacteria

CLINICAL ISSUES
- Genitourinary TB 3rd most common form of extrapulmonary TB after pleural and lymph node TB worldwide, including North America
- XGP present in approximately 20% of nephrectomy specimens performed for chronic pyelonephritic renal disease; RMP very uncommon; mostly as case reports
- Both XGP and RMP affect more females than males

MACROSCOPIC
- RTB part of disseminated infection or localized renal disease; XGP and RMP, diffuse, segmental, or focal

MICROSCOPIC
- RTB: Disseminated disease with miliary foci of epithelioid granulomata, ± caseation, particularly in renal cortex
- In localized tuberculosis, confluent epithelioid granulomata with caseous necrosis preferentially in renal medulla
- XGP: Aggregates of foamy histiocytes forming small clusters below urothelium to large, destructive, nodular lesions
- RMP: Dominant feature is aggregates of histiocytes with eosinophilic cytoplasm (von Hansemann histiocytes) and Michaelis-Gutmann bodies

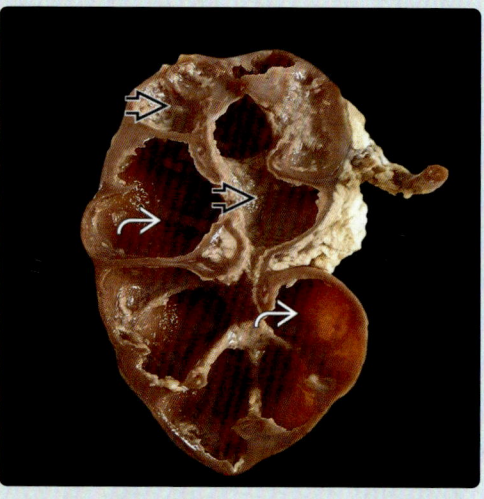

Tuberculous Pyonephrosis: Gross Features

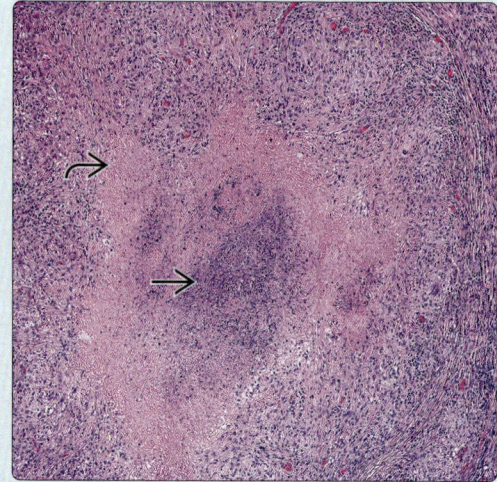

Renal Tuberculosis: Necrotizing Granulomas

(Left) Gross image from a TB kidney shows a markedly dilated pelvicalyceal system ⇨ with adherent necrotic debris covering the urothelial lining ⇨. These features are indicative of pyonephrosis. (Courtesy N. Singh, MD.) (Right) The histological hallmark of RTB is the necrotizing granulomas ⇨. TB granulomas often show nuclear debris within necrosis ⇨. Atypical mycobacterial infections and miliary TB generally lack necrosis.

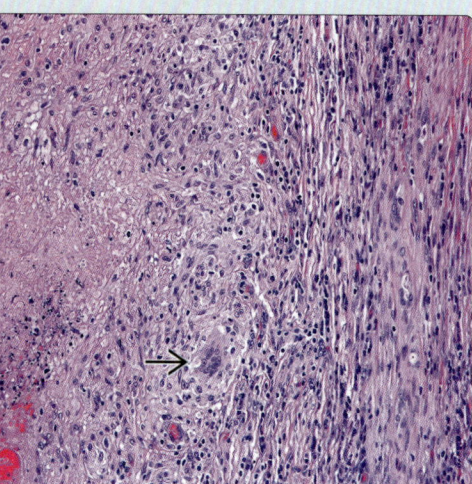

Renal Tuberculosis: Necrotizing Granulomas

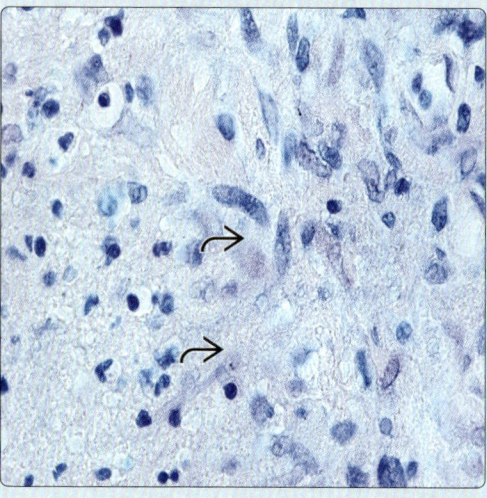

AFB Stain Positivity

(Left) The epithelioid granulomas in tuberculosis characteristically show the presence of Langhans giant cells ⇨. (Right) AFB stain positivity in granulomatous inflammation, in the form of positive microorganisms showing beaded configuration ⇨, is highly specific but with very low sensitivity for mycobacteria. Thousands of bacilli per g by weight of tissue are needed for AFB stain to be positive in tissue sections. PCR testing is much more sensitive. (Courtesy J. Sarungbam, MD.)

Renal Tuberculosis, Xanthogranulomatous Pyelonephritis, Renal Malakoplakia

TERMINOLOGY

Abbreviations
- Renal tuberculosis (RTB), xanthogranulomatous pyelonephritis (XGP), renal malakoplakia (RMP)

Definitions
- RTB: *Mycobacterium tuberculosis* complex disease; often with necrotic, fibrotic, cavitary granulomatous lesions associated with ureteric/calyceal distortion
- XGP: Subacute and chronic pelvicalyceal and renal parenchymal inflammatory mass-like lesion predominantly composed of histiocytes
- RMP: Mass-like lesion showing histiocytes with abundant eosinophilic cytoplasm and Michaelis-Gutmann bodies

ETIOLOGY/PATHOGENESIS

Infectious Agents
- RTB caused by members of *Mycobacterium tuberculosis* complex, mostly *Mycobacterium tuberculosis*, but rarely *M. bovine*, and occasionally by Bacille Calmette-Guérin (BCG) as complication of intravesical treatment of bladder cancer
  - Very rare cases by *M. avium-intracellulare* in AIDS and other immunosuppressed individuals
  - Unlike other bacterial urinary infections, TB is descending infection resulting from hematogenous spread of bacilli in corticomedullary junction: Areas of high blood perfusion and blood oxygen saturation
    - Granulomas latent for many years, with mycobacteria reactivated after immune suppression, spilling into nephrons, getting trapped in narrow loops of Henle and causing caseating papillary lesions
      - Bacilli shed into urine, spreading TB to downstream urothelium and adjacent genital organs
- XGP and RMP: Most often, associated with gram-negative bacteria
  - *Escherichia coli* found in most cases, with other gram-negative bacilli as less common pathogens
  - XGP: Consistently associated with obstruction, calculi, and recurrent urinary tract infections
  - RMP: Believed to be due to defective macrophage lysosomal digestion of phagocytosed bacteria (particularly coliforms)
    - Decreased levels of intracellular cyclic guanosine monophosphate (cGMP) might be cause of defective phagocytosis in RMP
      - Inadequate elimination leads to accumulation of partially digested bacteria or bacterial glycolipids
      - Deposition of calcium and iron occurs on residual bacterial glycolipid in monocytes or macrophages, forming Michaelis-Gutmann bodies
- Patients with XGP usually with underlying systemic disease, e.g., SLE, diabetes mellitus, myotonic dystrophy, or chronic active hepatitis

CLINICAL ISSUES

Epidemiology
- General features
  - Genitourinary TB 3rd most common form of extrapulmonary TB after pleural and lymph node TB worldwide, including North America
  - Kidney most common genitourinary organ to be afflicted, but very rare with rate of 3 cases/100,000 in USA; immunocompromised patients, particularly with HIV, at higher risk
  - XGP present in approximately 20% of nephrectomy specimens performed for chronic pyelonephritic renal disease; RMP very uncommon; mostly as case reports
  - Typically, patients in their 40s or 50s, with all entities described between ages 4 weeks to 84 years
  - No sex predilection for RTB, but F > M in XGP and RMP

Presentation
- RTB: Systemic symptoms in disseminated type
  - Systemic symptoms less common in patients with localized RTB, may present with hematuria, flank pain, or nonspecific urinary symptoms
- XGP and RMP: Most patients symptomatic with fever, flank or abdominal pain, anorexia, weight loss, lower urinary tract symptoms, and gross hematuria

Treatment
- Reactivated genitourinary TB treated with 6-month course of antituberculous therapy; rarely, surgery for nonfunctional kidneys with extensive disease, particularly with hypertension and ureteropelvic junction obstruction
- XGP and RMP: Most patients receive antibiotics before nephrectomy
  - Improving immunodeficient states and use of bethanechol chloride (Urecholine) medical treatment options for RMP
    - Urecholine (cholinergic agonist) improves bactericidal activity of monocytes against *E. coli*

Prognosis
- Response to treatment in RTB based on eradication of mycobacteria on subsequent cultures
- For XGP and RMP, if unilateral or localized, usually cured by surgery, but primary causes for both need to be addressed

MACROSCOPIC

General Features
- RTB can be part of disseminated infection or localized renal disease
  - Renal specimens in disseminated disease with miliary or multifocal tuberculosis usually autopsy finding
  - Nephrectomy for localized disease usually performed for mass lesion under clinical impression of tumor, or nonfunctional kidney ± hydro-/pyonephrosis
    - Often with extensive involvement by necrotic (caseous) masses with extensive fibrosis, extending to perirenal areas, or with pyonephrosis associated with ureteropelvic or ureteric stenosis
- In XGP and RMP, changes diffuse, segmental, or focal
  - Irregular, ill-defined yellow masses, at least partly necrotic, usually centered on renal medulla
  - Pelvicalyceal system usually outlined by thick bands of often friable, partially necrotic yellow tissue, with associated hydronephrosis or pyonephrosis
- Renal calculi, often staghorn type, very frequent in XGP and RTB

Renal Tuberculosis, Xanthogranulomatous Pyelonephritis, Renal Malakoplakia

MICROSCOPIC

Histologic Features

- Renal tuberculosis
  - Disseminated disease with miliary foci of epithelioid granulomata, ± caseation, particularly in renal cortex
    - With severe immunosuppression, mycobacteria-like *M. avium-intracellulare* may be causation; lesions more diffuse and poorly formed with histiocytes packed with organisms, without caseous necrosis
      - In some patients, interstitial nephritis, usually but not always with granulomata
  - In localized tuberculosis, confluent epithelioid granulomata with caseous necrosis preferentially in renal medulla
    - Papillary necrosis and tuberculous pyelonephritis and pyonephrosis; ureteric involvement often with irregular strictures and segmental dilation
  - Keratinizing squamous metaplasia as late complication, with potential risk for squamous cell carcinoma
- Xanthomatous pyelonephritis
  - Foamy histiocytes with abundant clear cytoplasm, or rarely with focal eosinophilic cytoplasm, present as small clusters under urothelium, to large destructive nodular lesions with secondary renal parenchymal involvement
    - Admixed polymorphous inflammation with lymphocytes, plasma cells, and neutrophils and variable number of multinucleated giant cells, and microabscesses
  - Extension of process to ureter &/or perirenal fat is commonly present
- Malakoplakia
  - Dominant feature as aggregates of histiocytes often with PAS(+) eosinophilic cytoplasm (von Hansemann histiocytes)
  - Some histiocytes contain concentrically lamellar or targetoid, basophilic, often calcified inclusions (Michaelis-Gutmann bodies), the most characteristic feature of RMP
    - Prussian blue (iron), PAS, and von Kossa stains may be needed to visualize Michaelis-Gutmann bodies, when rare
  - Admixed polymorphous inflammation with presence of lymphocytes, plasma cells, and neutrophils, and variable number of multinucleated giant cells
  - Microscopically, malakoplakia evolves through 3 phases
  - Early (prediagnostic) phase; with plasma cells and von Hansemann histiocytes in edematous stroma, and absent Michaelis-Gutmann bodies
  - Classic phase; with histiocytes containing easily identifiable Michaelis-Gutmann bodies and few lymphocytes and plasma cells
  - Fibrosing phase; with fibroblasts and collagen interspersed between foci of histiocytes, with occasional Michaelis-Gutmann bodies
- Both XGP and RMP often multifocal, associated with variable degrees of fibrosis, with irregular outlines and without pseudocapsule

Ultrastructure

- Bacilliform microorganisms, either intact or in different stages of disintegration within phagolysosomes in macrophages in RMP

DIFFERENTIAL DIAGNOSIS

Other Granulomatous Inflammations

- Many conditions other than RTB, including foreign bodies, fungal infections, cat-scratch disease, sarcoidosis, etc. can show granulomatous inflammation
  - Necrotizing granulomas with AFB positivity highly supportive of tuberculosis

Clear Cell Renal Cell Carcinoma

- Cells arranged in nests, alveoli, tubules, and cysts, with intricate, branching, vascular septations
- Presence of brisk inflammatory infiltrate intimately admixed with sheets of clear cells should raise possibility of XGP over RCC
- Nuclei round or oval, with dark and granular chromatin in carcinoma; nuclear membranes often with angulations, and nuclear chromatin usually pale in XGP and RMP
- Immunohistochemistry rarely required but invariably decisive in differentiation
  - Cytokeratins and EMA/MUC1 positive in carcinoma, vs. histiocytic markers positive in XGP and RMP

DIAGNOSTIC CHECKLIST

Pathologic Interpretation Pearls

- XGP and RMP are pseudotumorous lesions that closely mimic malignancy clinically, radiographically, and pathologically
- Main differential diagnostic consideration for XGP is clear cell RCC with associated extensive inflammation
- Carcinoma with clear cell cytology is usually of lower grade
  - Typical intricately branching vasculature is particularly prominent in such lower grade tumors

SELECTED REFERENCES

1. Sourial MW et al: Genitourinary tuberculosis in North America: A rare clinical entity. Can Urol Assoc J. 9(7-8):E484-9, 2015
2. Daher Ede F et al: Renal tuberculosis in the modern era. Am J Trop Med Hyg. 88(1):54-64, 2013
3. Li L et al: Xanthogranulomatous pyelonephritis. Arch Pathol Lab Med. 135(5):671-4, 2011
4. Korkes F et al: Xanthogranulomatous pyelonephritis: clinical experience with 41 cases. Urology. 71(2):178-80, 2008
5. Yiğiter M et al: Renal parenchymal malacoplakia: a different stage of xanthogranulomatous pyelonephritis? J Pediatr Surg. 42(7):E35-8, 2007
6. Eastwood JB et al: Tuberculosis and the kidney. J Am Soc Nephrol. 12(6):1307-14, 2001
7. Evans NL et al: Renal malacoplakia: an important consideration in the differential diagnosis of renal masses in the presence of Escherichia coli infection. Br J Radiol. 71(850):1083-5, 1998
8. August C et al: Renal parenchymal malacoplakia: ultrastructural findings in different stages of morphogenesis. Ultrastruct Pathol. 18(5):483-91, 1994
9. Mittal BV et al: Xanthogranulomatous pyelonephritis–(a clinicopathological study of 15 cases). J Postgrad Med. 35(4):209-14, 1989

Renal Tuberculosis, Xanthogranulomatous Pyelonephritis, Renal Malakoplakia

Xanthogranulomatous Pyelonephritis: Gross Features

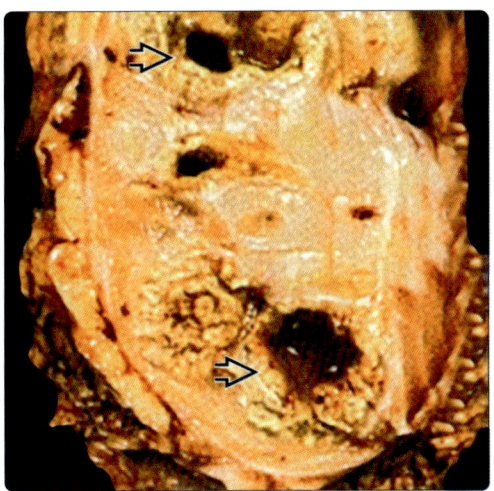

Xanthogranulomatous Pyelonephritis: Gross Features

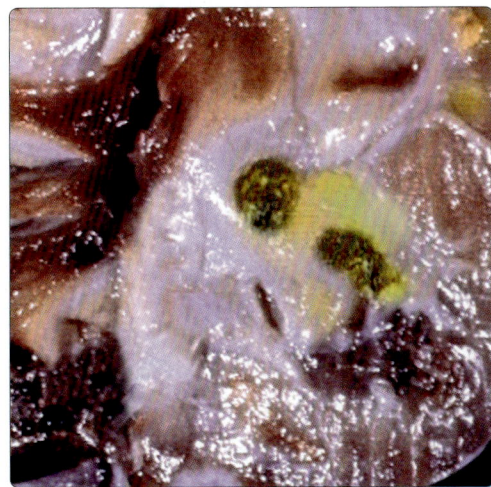

(Left) Gross photograph depicts the characteristic appearance of xanthogranulomatous pyelonephritis. The dilated calyces are surrounded by an irregular band of yellow, necrotic material ⇨. The yellow coloration is reflective of lipid-containing (foamy) histiocytes in the lesion. *(Right)* While XGP is usually diffuse, some cases may show only segmental or focal involvement. Such nondiffuse appearance is usually due to the involvement of only individual calyces.

Xanthogranulomatous Pyelonephritis: Microscopic Features

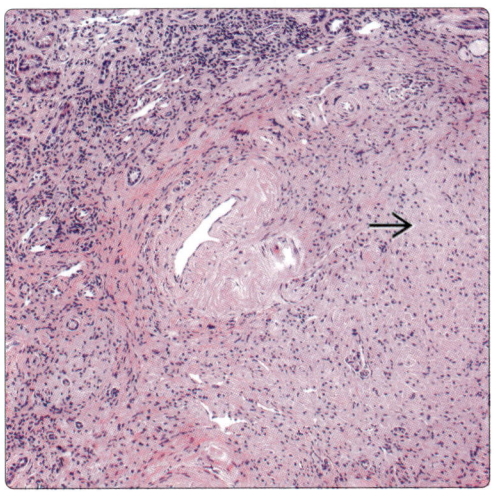

Xanthogranulomatous Pyelonephritis: Microscopic Features

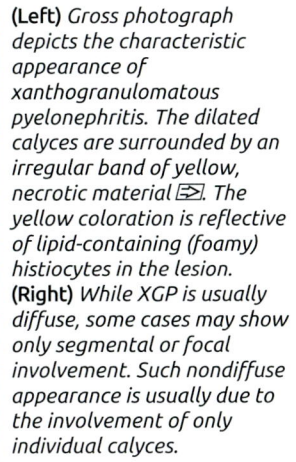

(Left) H&E section shows a nonencapsulated mass-like lesion. Although it appears circumscribed in this image, multifocal appearance ⇨ of the lesions should alert to the possibility of XGP. *(Right)* Sheets of histiocytes devoid of circumscription, with finger-like projections ⇨ and entrapped medium-sized arteries ⇨, go against the diagnosis of RCC. Close evaluation of cytology reveals absence of distinct epithelial features, pale nuclear chromatin, and angulations of nuclear membranes in XGP.

Xanthogranulomatous Pyelonephritis: Calcifications

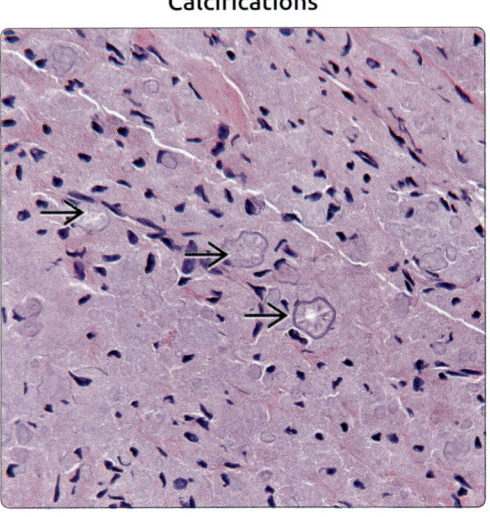

Xanthogranulomatous Pyelonephritis: Microscopic Features

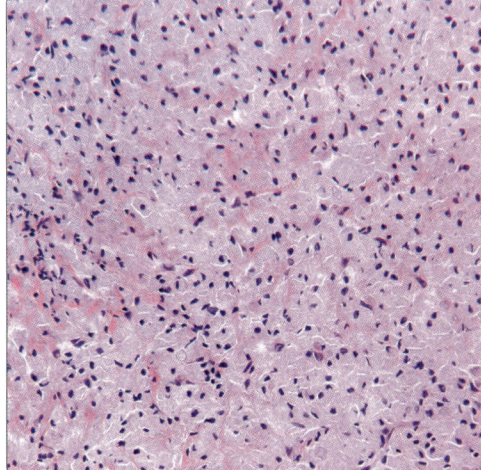

(Left) XGP shows a collection of histiocytes with focal calcification ⇨. Calcifications suggest a longstanding process and are not specific for either XGP or RMP. *(Right)* Large collection of cells with clear or foamy cytoplasm and forming a mass lesion may raise doubts sometimes. Use of cytokeratin immunostaining will exclude the possibility of neoplastic epithelium. However, caution is required in interpreting entrapped tubules in such areas.

Renal Tuberculosis, Xanthogranulomatous Pyelonephritis, Renal Malakoplakia

Xanthogranulomatous Pyelonephritis: Nuclear Features

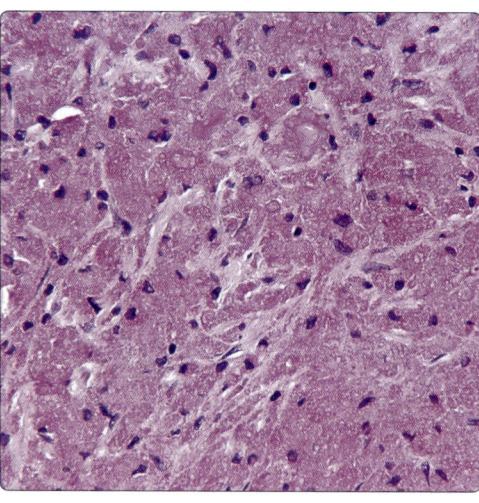

Xanthogranulomatous Pyelonephritis: Differential Diagnosis

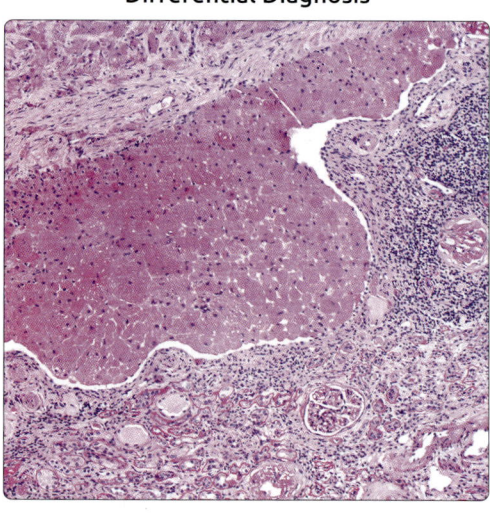

(Left) Periodic acid-Schiff stain shows diffuse positivity in the lesional cells. The histiocytic nuclei usually show uniform pale chromatin, unlike that in carcinoma, which has hyperchromatic and often irregular nuclei. (Right) Periodic acid-Schiff shows a collection of histiocytes in a cortical cyst. The presence of sheets of histiocytes in renal parenchyma is not always diagnostic of XGP or malakoplakia. By definition, the diagnosis requires involvement of the pelvicalyceal system.

Renal Malakoplakia: Pelvicalyceal Involvement

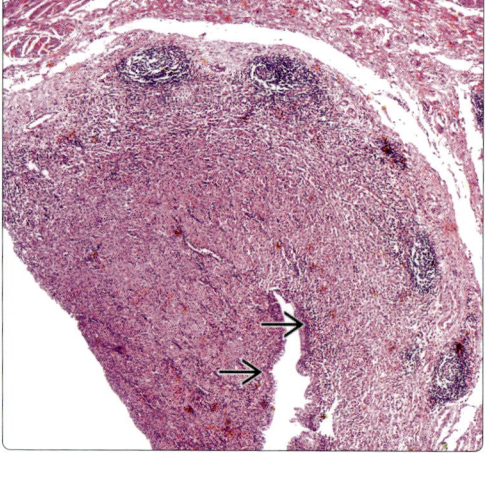

Renal Malakoplakia: Pelvicalyceal Involvement

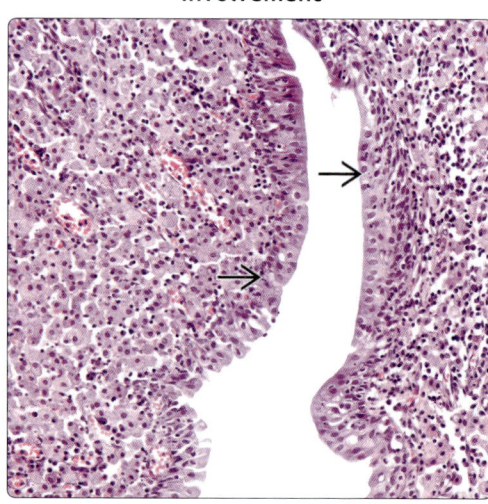

(Left) Low-power view of renal malakoplakia shows that the lesion has its epicenter in the pelvicalyceal system ➡. (Right) As seen at higher magnification, the histiocytic proliferation surrounds and invades the urothelial lining ➡ in renal malakoplakia. Both XGP and RMP involve the pelvicalyceal system, the lining of which is usually markedly roughened and irregular on gross evaluation. On microscopic examination, most of the lining appears ulcerated or with reactive changes.

Renal Malakoplakia: Polymorphous Infiltrate

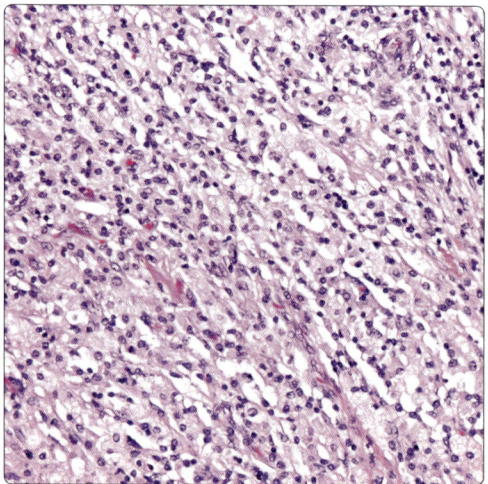

Renal Malakoplakia: Michaelis-Gutmann Bodies

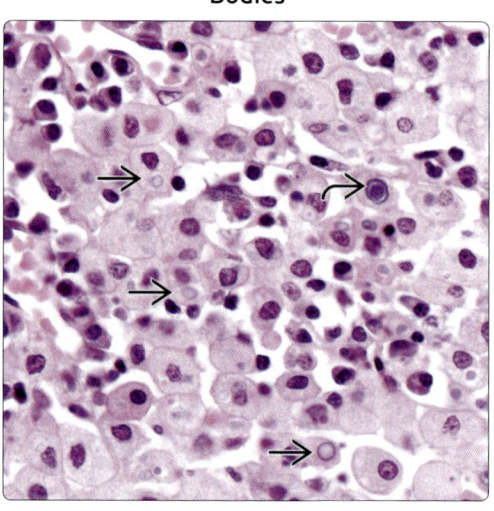

(Left) Most XGP cases show mixed inflammatory infiltrate, including lymphocytes, plasma cells, and neutrophils. Polymorphous inflammatory infiltrate is common in both xanthogranulomatous pyelonephritis and malakoplakia. (Right) RMP shows multiple Michaelis-Gutmann bodies in the histiocytes ➡. Characteristically, these appear as concentrically lamellar or targetoid, basophilic structures ➡.

Renal Tuberculosis, Xanthogranulomatous Pyelonephritis, Renal Malakoplakia

Renal Malakoplakia: Michaelis-Gutmann Bodies

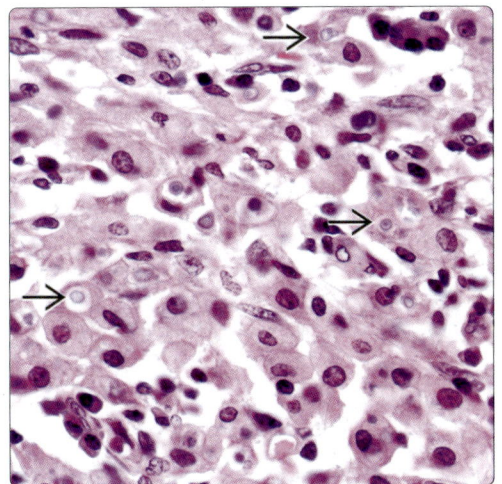

Renal Malakoplakia: von Hansemann Histiocytes

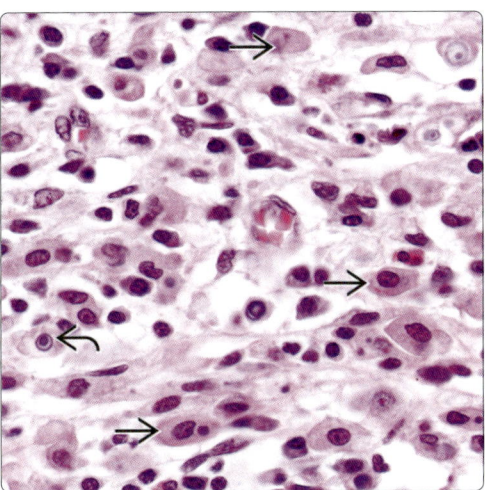

(Left) H&E shows the typical features of renal malakoplakia. Sheets of histiocytes are seen, many containing the characteristic Michaelis-Gutmann bodies ➡. (Right) Renal malakoplakia shows the typical morphology of von Hansemann histiocytes. Unlike the foamy, clear macrophages in XGP, the histiocytes in malakoplakia have predominantly eosinophilic cytoplasm ➡. A Michaelis-Gutmann body is present in 1 of the histiocytes ➡.

Renal Malakoplakia: Classic Phase

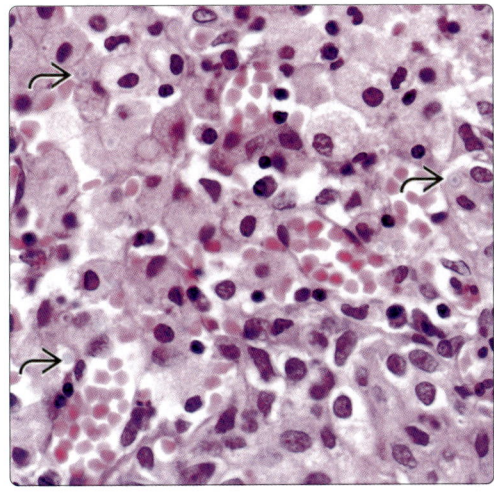

Renal Malakoplakia: Nuclear Details

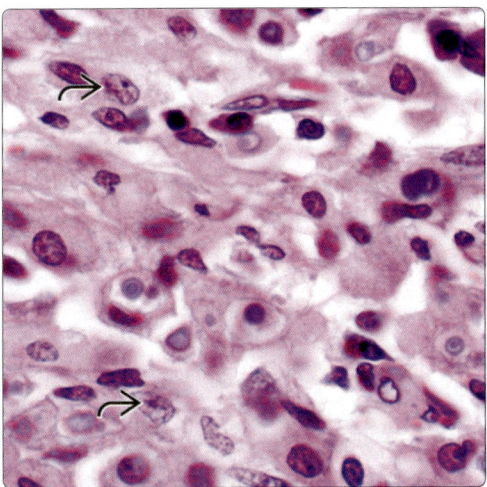

(Left) This image demonstrates the classic phase of malakoplakia. Sheets of histiocytes are admixed with relatively few plasma cells and lymphocytes in this phase. Michaelis-Gutmann bodies are abundant ➡. In the early (prediagnostic) phase, Michaelis-Gutmann bodies may be absent or very difficult to find. (Right) High-magnification view of renal malakoplakia shows the typical nuclear features of the histiocytes, including pale chromatin and nuclear membrane irregularities ➡.

Renal Malakoplakia: PAS Stain

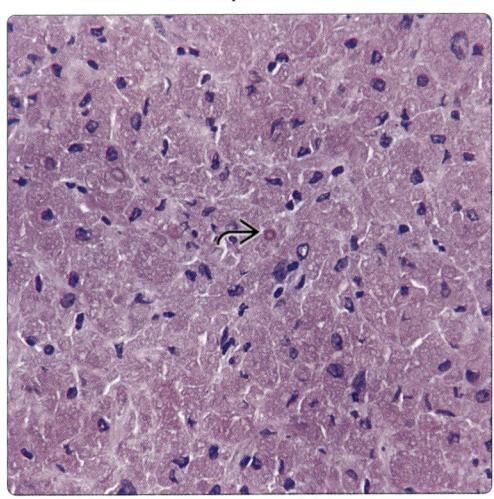

Renal Malakoplakia: CD68

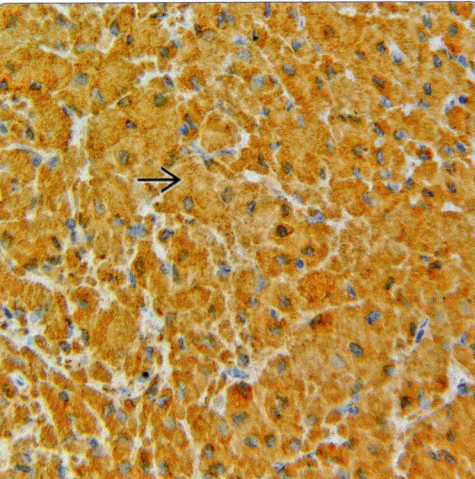

(Left) Periodic acid-Schiff (seen here), von Kossa, or iron stains highlight the Michaelis-Gutmann bodies ➡ and may be needed in cases with paucity of such bodies. Note the diffuse granular cytoplasmic stain in the histiocytes, which may be seen in both xanthogranulomatous pyelonephritis and RMP. (Right) While the histiocytic nature of the clear cells in XGP is quite apparent on H&E in most cases, sometimes immunohistochemistry may be needed. CD68 ➡ and CD163 histiocytic markers diffusely stain these cells.

Papillary Adenoma

KEY FACTS

TERMINOLOGY
- Benign epithelial proliferations with papillary, tubular, or tubulopapillary configuration; ≤ 15 mm by current definition
  - Size criterion change allows more rational use of donor kidneys
    - Prevents kidneys being rejected as transplant donors due to presence of benign, small, well-differentiated papillary lesions

ETIOLOGY/PATHOGENESIS
- Trisomy 7 and 17 and loss of Y chromosome very frequently observed

CLINICAL ISSUES
- Incidence of 7-40% in autopsy studies
  - Higher incidence in patients with chronic renal disease, particularly acquired cystic disease of kidney
- Reported incidence of 7% in nephrectomy specimens resected for other tumors
  - More common in kidneys harboring papillary renal cell carcinoma (RCC)

MACROSCOPIC
- Well-circumscribed, grayish-white to yellow nodules
- By definition, all tumors ≤ 15 mm in diameter

MICROSCOPIC
- Resembles papillary RCC (usually type 1)
- Have papillary, tubular, or tubulopapillary architecture; usually with low-grade nuclei; lack capsule by definition

ANCILLARY TESTS
- Most are CK7 and AMACR positive
  - CD10 often shows luminal staining pattern

TOP DIFFERENTIAL DIAGNOSES
- Papillary RCC

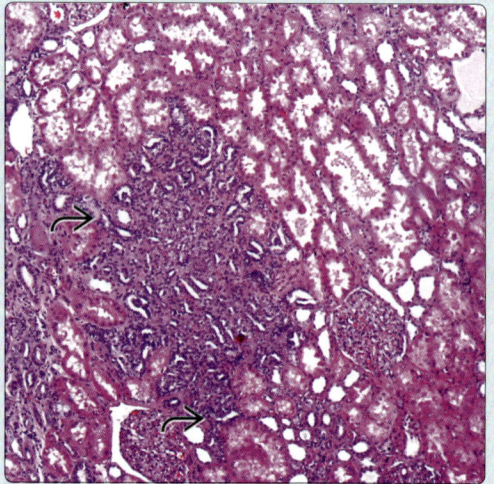

Low-Magnification Appearance

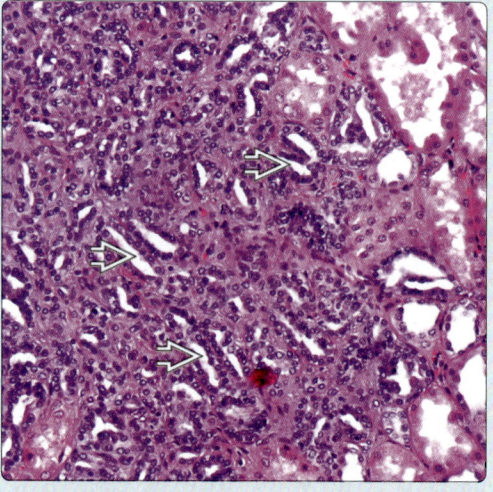

Tubular Architecture

(Left) Most papillary adenomas are well circumscribed and, by definition, nonencapsulated; however, irregular extensions ⇒ into surrounding parenchyma are not uncommon. Notice the prominent tubular architecture in this example. (Right) In spite of the nomenclature of papillary adenoma, many of these small tumorous lesions show variable, but sometimes predominant or exclusive, tubular architecture ⇒.

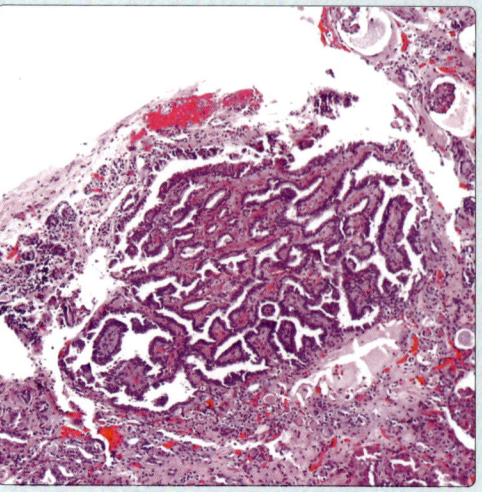

Absence of Capsule

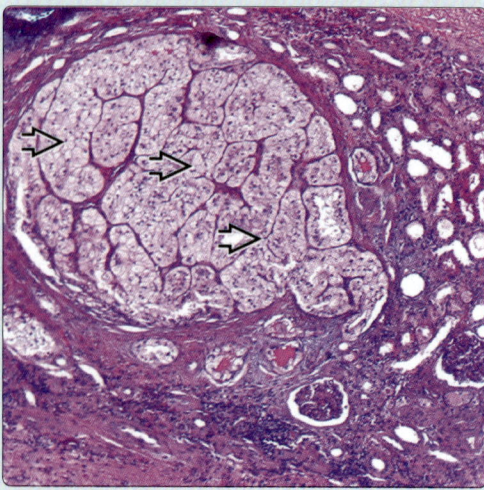

Small Clear Cell Renal Cell Carcinoma

(Left) Papillary adenomas show papillary &/or tubular architectural features similar to that seen in larger papillary renal cell carcinomas (RCCs). By current definition, these are 15 mm or less in maximum diameter and are unencapsulated. (Right) Microscopic lesions with features of clear cell ⇒ or other subtypes of RCC are not designated as adenomas, even when < 15 mm in size, although, there is little evidence that such small tumors ever metastasize.

Papillary Adenoma

TERMINOLOGY

Synonyms
- Renal cortical adenoma

Definitions
- ≤ 15 mm benign unencapsulated epithelial proliferations with papillary, tubular, or tubulopapillary configuration
  - Clinically important recent change in size criterion from 5 mm to 15 mm

ETIOLOGY/PATHOGENESIS

Genetic Features
- Trisomy 7 and 17 and loss of Y chromosome very frequent; gains of chromosomes 12, 16, and 20 also seen
- Frequent association with papillary renal cell carcinoma (RCC) raises question of adenomas representing intrarenal metastases from papillary RCC
  - Loss of heterozygosity assays on multiple tumors in kidney show discordant allelic loss patterns
    - Therefore, likelihood of adenomas representing intrarenal metastases from papillary RCC is very low

CLINICAL ISSUES

Epidemiology
- Incidence
  - 7-40% in autopsy studies; frequency increases with age (10% < 40 years vs. 40% > 70 years)
  - Higher incidence in patients with chronic renal disease
  - Reported incidence of 7% in nephrectomy specimens resected for other tumors

Presentation
- Incidental finding in kidneys removed for larger tumors or other causes and at autopsy
- More common in kidneys harboring papillary RCC (> 25%), compared to other types of renal tumors
- When papillary adenomas are bilateral and multifocal (numerous), they are called renal adenomatosis

Treatment
- Surgical approaches
  - Determined by other presenting lesions (tumor or nontumorous condition)

Prognosis
- Benign, considered to be putative precursor of papillary RCC
  - However, marked differences in incidences of papillary adenomas vs. papillary RCC raises doubts about this presumption

MACROSCOPIC

General Features
- Larger lesions may be apparent grossly, as well-circumscribed, usually subcapsular, grayish-white to yellow nodules

Size
- By current definition, all tumors are ≤ 15 mm in diameter
- Change in size criterion from 5 mm to 15 mm based on
  - Reported absence of metastasis in tumors < 15 mm; prevents denial of transplant donor kidneys due to presence of small, well-differentiated papillary lesions

MICROSCOPIC

Histologic Features
- Resembles papillary RCC, usually type 1
- Tumors do not show capsule and are in direct contact with surrounding renal parenchyma
- Cytoplasm often amphophilic/basophilic and scant
  - Rare tumors with more abundant eosinophilic cytoplasm
  - Occasional tumors with cytoplasmic clarity: Not optically transparent, but with fine cytoplasmic granularity, similar to that seen in some papillary RCCs
- Papillary, tubular, or tubulopapillary architecture
- Usually with low-grade nuclei; by current definition grade 1 or 2 nuclei
  - Rare tumors with nuclei showing prominent nucleoli; such tumors may not be regarded papillary adenomas by some
- Foam cells and calcification may be present (rare)
- Very small examples may consist of only very few neoplastic tubules clustered together
- Lesions with clear cell carcinoma-like features, even if < 15 mm, not considered adenomas

ANCILLARY TESTS

Immunohistochemistry
- Similar to papillary RCC: CK7 and AMACR positive; CD10 often with luminal or inverted cup-like staining pattern

DIFFERENTIAL DIAGNOSIS

Papillary Renal Cell Carcinoma
- Size &/or presence of capsule definitive distinguishing criterion

DIAGNOSTIC CHECKLIST

Pathologic Interpretation Pearls
- By new definition (WHO), upper limit of size acceptable in papillary adenomas is 15 mm
  - No capsule or high-grade nuclei are allowed

SELECTED REFERENCES

1. Lohse CM et al: Outcome prediction for patients with renal cell carcinoma. Semin Diagn Pathol. 32(2):172-83, 2015
2. Eccher A et al: Donor kidneys with miliary papillary renal cell neoplasia: the role of the pathologist in determining suitability for transplantation. Ann Transplant. 19:362-6, 2014
3. Srigley JR et al: The International Society of Urological Pathology (ISUP) Vancouver Classification of Renal Neoplasia. Am J Surg Pathol. 37(10):1469-89, 2013
4. Umbreit EC et al: Metastatic potential of a renal mass according to original tumour size at presentation. BJU Int. 109(2):190-4; discussion 194, 2012
5. Wang KL et al: Renal papillary adenoma–a putative precursor of papillary renal cell carcinoma. Hum Pathol. 38(2):239-46, 2007
6. Jones TD et al: Molecular genetic evidence for the independent origin of multifocal papillary tumors in patients with papillary renal cell carcinomas. Clin Cancer Res. 11(20):7226-33, 2005
7. Brunelli M et al: Gains of chromosomes 7, 17, 12, 16, and 20 and loss of Y occur early in the evolution of papillary renal cell neoplasia: a fluorescent in situ hybridization study. Mod Pathol. 16(10):1053-9, 2003

Papillary Adenoma

Solid Architecture

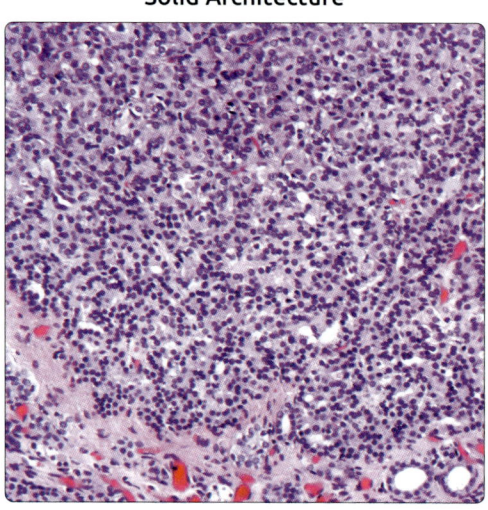

Clear Cell Change

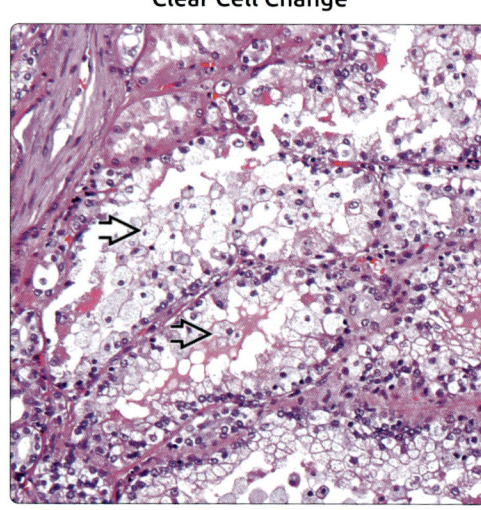

(Left) Like papillary renal cell carcinoma, some papillary adenomas may appear to have solid architecture. In most such cases, evaluation at higher magnification reveals this appearance primarily to be because of tightly packed tubules. (Right) H&E shows a papillary adenoma with cytoplasmic clarity and abundant foamy macrophages ➡. Psammomatous calcifications may be observed. In contrast to papillary renal cell carcinoma, a fibrous capsule is absent in papillary adenomas.

Clear Cell Change

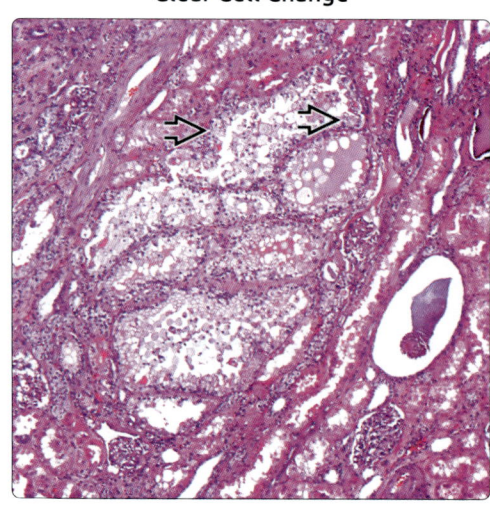

Size Criterion

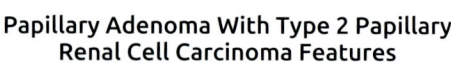

(Left) Papillary adenomas showing cytoplasmic clarity ➡, similar to that occasionally seen in some papillary renal cell carcinomas, do not have optically transparent cytoplasm, but show fine and irregular cytoplasmic granularity. (Right) The current definitional criterion of up to 15 mm size for papillary adenoma by WHO is arbitrary, as almost all small tumors, even up to 20 mm in size, have shown a benign outcome. This photomicrograph depicts a papillary neoplasm that was 10 mm in size.

Small Papillary Adenoma

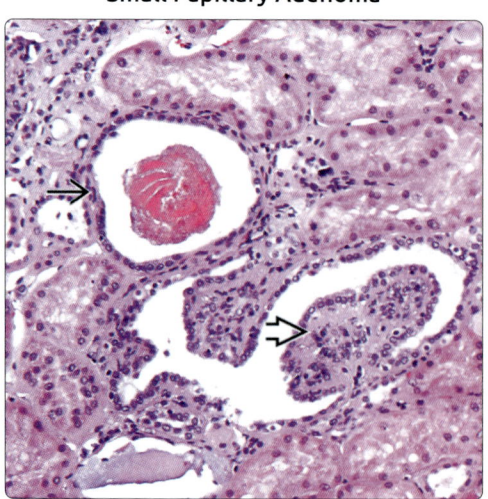

Papillary Adenoma With Type 2 Papillary Renal Cell Carcinoma Features

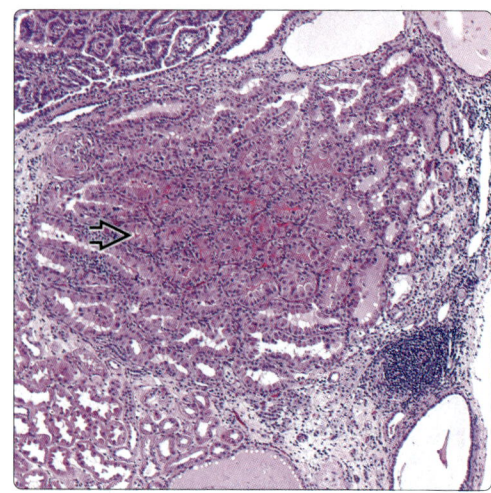

(Left) This minute papillary adenoma consists of a collection of only 3 neoplastic tubules. Notice the combined papillary ➡ and tubular ➡ architecture of the lesion, a frequent finding in most papillary adenomas. (Right) While most papillary adenomas are similar to minute type 1 papillary carcinomas, rare examples, as depicted here, have prominent eosinophilic cytoplasm ➡, larger nuclei, and may have more prominent nucleoli. The lesion lacks a capsule.

Papillary Adenoma

Immunohistochemistry: CK7

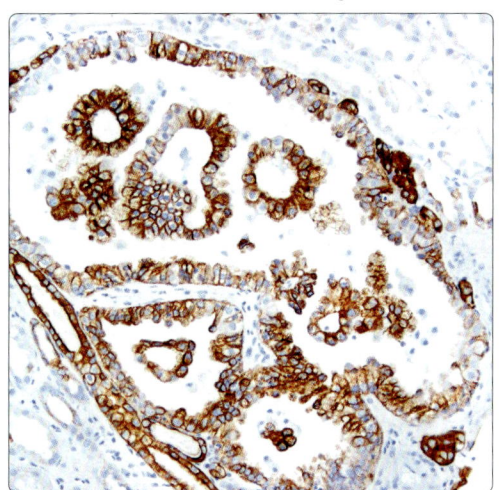

Immunohistochemistry: AMACR

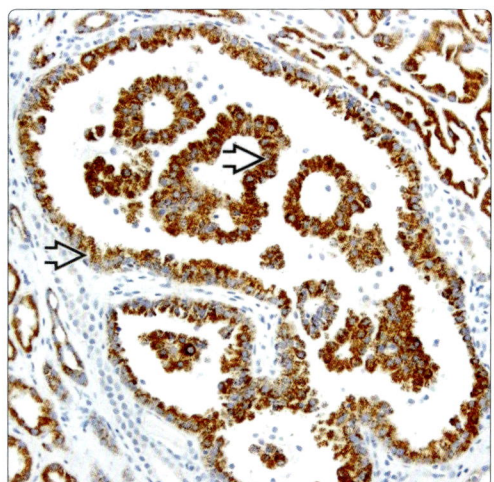

(Left) Minute papillary adenoma with diffuse positivity for CK7 is shown. As is usual in papillary RCC, particularly type 1, almost all papillary adenomas show such diffuse immunoreactivity for CK7. *(Right)* Most papillary adenomas also stain diffusely and strongly for AMACR. Similar to papillary RCC, the positivity is in the form of diffuse, cytoplasmic, granular staining ⇨.

Immunohistochemistry: CD10

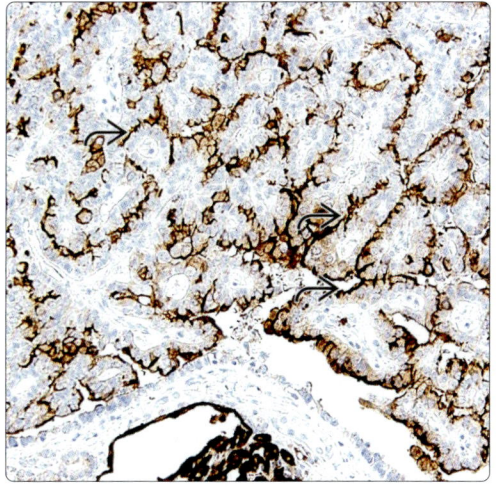

Immunohistochemistry: CD10

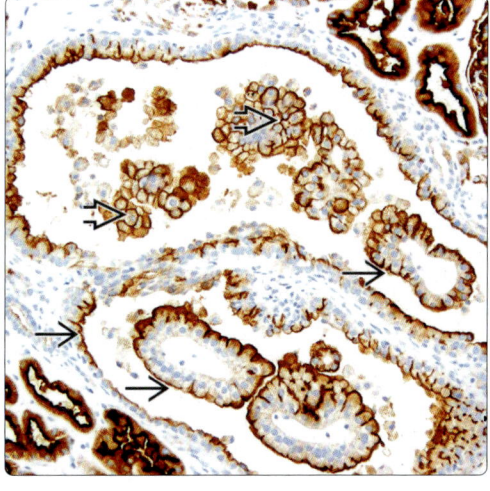

(Left) CD10 usually shows extensive and diffuse staining pattern in papillary adenomas and RCCs; however, the staining is typically luminal in location ⇨. *(Right)* Papillary adenoma shows positive immunoreactivity for CD10. The positivity is membrane predominant. While it focally stains the membranes on all sides of the cell (box-like pattern) ⇨, in most of the lesion only a luminal or inverted cup-like pattern ⇨ is present, similar to what is present in most papillary RCCs.

Oncocytic Papillary Adenoma

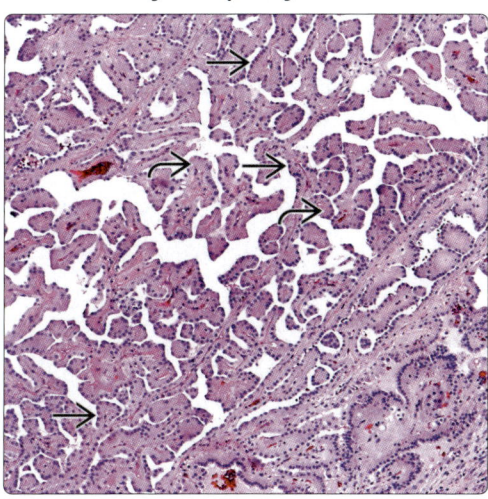

Papillary Adenoma vs. Papillary Renal Cell Carcinoma

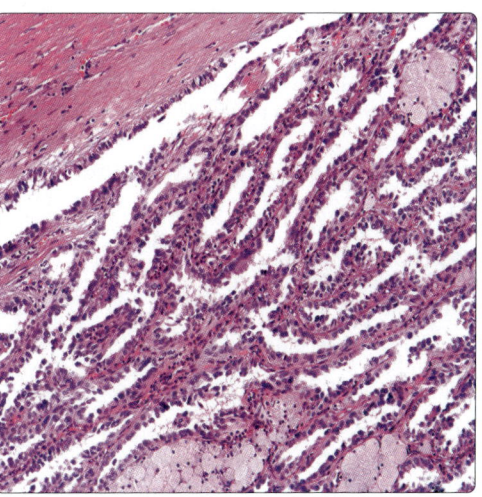

(Left) Some unencapsulated papillary tumors < 1.5 cm may have oncocytic cytoplasm ⇨ with linear arrangement of nuclei away from the basement membrane ⇨. Such papillary adenomas resemble the larger oncocytic papillary RCCs. *(Right)* By the currently accepted criteria, presence of a fibrous capsule/pseudocapsule in a papillary neoplasm excludes it from the category of papillary adenoma. Such tumors < 1.5 cm are best regarded as papillary RCC.

Renal Oncocytoma

KEY FACTS

ETIOLOGY/PATHOGENESIS
- Loss of chromosomes Y and 1; Ch 11q13 alterations; Ch 14 deletions; mtDNA mutations
- Many tumors with normal karyotype

CLINICAL ISSUES
- Benign

MACROSCOPIC
- Well circumscribed, nonencapsulated
- Mahogany brown to yellow-tan color
- Central stellate scar: 33%

MICROSCOPIC
- Architecture: Typically solid nests, but micro- and macrocysts or tubules also common
- Abundant granular eosinophilic cytoplasm; uniform, round nuclei with vesicular chromatin and frequently prominent central nucleoli

- CD117, E-cadherin, Ksp-cadherin, S100-A (+); CK7 usually (-), occasionally focal (+); claudin-7 (-) or focal (+)
- Occasional isolated cells or groups of cells with marked degenerative-appearing hyperchromasia and pleomorphism; rarely diffuse symplastic atypia

ANCILLARY TESTS
- EM: Cytoplasm packed with mitochondria
- Round nucleus; cytoplasm packed with mitochondria mostly showing lamellar cristae

TOP DIFFERENTIAL DIAGNOSES
- Chromophobe RCC (eosinophilic variant)
- Clear cell RCC (eosinophilic variant)
- Epithelioid (oncocytoma-like) angiomyolipoma
- RCC, unclassified (oncocytic, low-grade type)
- Succinate dehydrogenase-deficient RCC
- Tubulocystic RCC
- Tuberous sclerosis-associated RCC

Gross Features

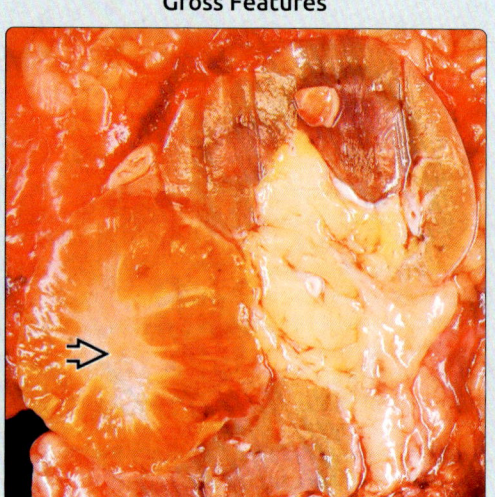

Histological Features

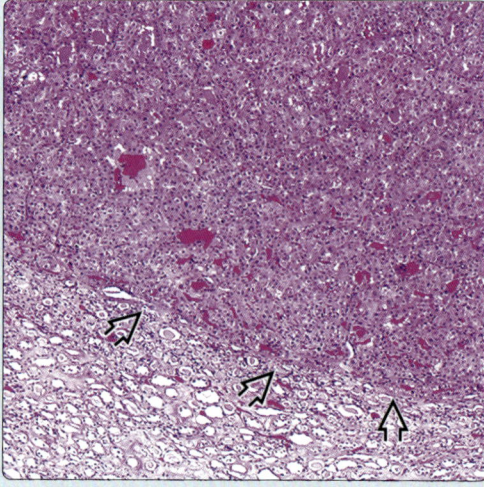

(Left) Renal oncocytoma (RO) is typically well circumscribed with tan-brown cut surface. A central scar ⇨ is present in about 30% of the tumors. Such scars may also be seen in other low-grade, slow-growing tumors. (Right) Although ROs, both grossly and on microscopic evaluation, are well circumscribed, they usually lack a pseudocapsule. In this H&E image, notice the advancing edge of the tumor ⇨ that directly abuts the surrounding renal parenchyma.

Histological Features

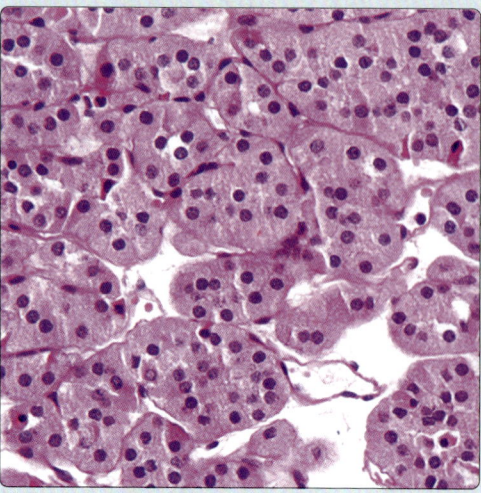

Histological Features

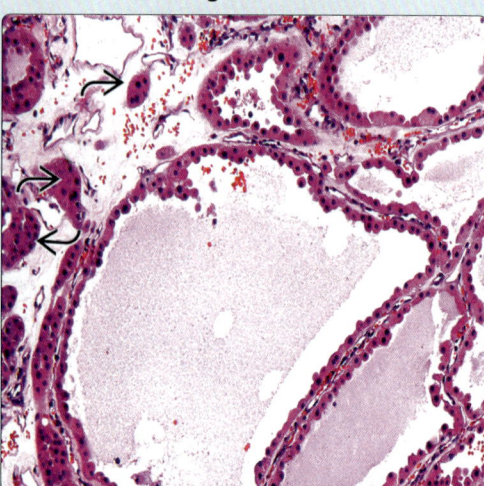

(Left) The typical histologic features of RO include solid nests of cells with oncocytic cytoplasm and uniform, round nuclei, in a background of variable, but often loose, stroma. (Right) Some ROs may show variable tubulocystic architecture. When extensive, this may even raise the possibility of tubulocystic carcinoma. However, the presence of round and uniform nuclei with evenly distributed chromatin, as well as solid nests ⇨, supports RO over tubulocystic carcinoma.

Renal Oncocytoma

TERMINOLOGY

Definitions
- Benign, oncocytic renal neoplasms with prominent or exclusive nested architecture and uniform round nuclei

ETIOLOGY/PATHOGENESIS

Molecular Abnormalities
- Loss of chromosome 1 (whole or partial) and chromosome Y
- Chromosome 11q13 alterations, including translocations
  - 11q13 alterations involve mostly translocation t(5;11)(q35;q13)]
  - Also, 11q13 translocations often involve *CCDN1* gene, with overexpression of gene product cyclin-D1
- Chromosome 14 deletions
- Mitochondrial DNA (mtDNA) mutations, particularly with losses of genes for respiratory chain complex I
- Many tumors with normal karyotype and no known FISH abnormalities
- Rare familial cases described; later, many of these found to have Birt-Hogg-Dubé (BHD) syndrome

CLINICAL ISSUES

Epidemiology
- Incidence
  - 6-9% of renal tumors
- Age
  - Mean: 62 yr (range: 32-89 yr)
- Sex
  - M:F = 2:1

Presentation
- Usually asymptomatic, detected on radiologic investigations for unrelated symptoms

Prognosis
- Benign

MACROSCOPIC

General Features
- Well circumscribed, nonencapsulated
  - Usually solitary mass; sometimes multifocal (17%) and bilateral (4%)
- Mahogany brown to yellow-tan color
- Central stellate or peripheral scars in up to 1/3 of cases
  - Scars more common in larger tumors
- Uncommon features
  - Variably cystic cut surface
  - Gross extension into perinephric fat
  - Invasion into large veins of renal sinus

Size
- Mean: 4.4 cm (range: 0.6-26 cm)

MICROSCOPIC

Histologic Features
- Well circumscribed: Usually no pseudocapsule with tumor directly abutting surrounding renal parenchyma
  - Rare tumors with partial or complete pseudocapsule
- Architecture
  - Typically solid nests, but micro- and macrocysts or tubules also common
  - Closely packed nests sometimes superficially imparting solid appearance
  - Occasional tumors with "archipelagic" or trabecular foci
  - Rarely, single oncocytic cells, usually in loose clusters, also present
  - Presence of papillae very rare
    - Mostly within dilated tubules or cysts
    - More than focal papillations not compatible with diagnosis of oncocytoma
- Cells with deeply eosinophilic, granular cytoplasm
  - Nuclei uniform and round
    - Chromatin uniform and vesicular
    - Prominent central nucleoli often present
  - Cytoplasmic clearing rare, usually restricted to areas of scarring
  - Sometimes cells at periphery of nests, oncoblasts, have scant cytoplasm
    - Rare tumors almost entirely composed of such oncoblast-like smaller cells
      - Such tumors may be associated with pseudorosette-like structures with cells arranged around basement membrane-like material
- Occasional isolated or groups of cells with marked degenerative-appearing hyperchromasia and pleomorphism
  - These pleomorphic cells nonproliferative on Ki-67 staining
    - Supports degenerative nature of such pleomorphic foci
- Stroma hypocellular, often hyalinized
- Mitotic activity, very low
  - Atypical mitoses not seen
- Hemorrhage occasionally present, but necrosis not seen
  - Hemorrhage often seen within lumina of tubules and cysts
  - Some tumors composed exclusively of hemorrhage-filled cysts and tubules
    - Term telangiectatic oncocytoma used for such tumors by some
- Some tumors with perinephric fat (20%) or vascular (5%) invasion
  - Occasional tumors with atypical features of invasion into large renal sinus veins
  - Perinephric fat invasion shows no stromal response
  - Fat or vascular invasion has no influence on benign nature of renal oncocytomas

Renal Oncocytosis
- Rarely, kidneys with numerous oncocytomas or small oncocytic nodules
- Often associated with
  - Clusters of oncocytic cells percolating within interstitium between normal nephrons
  - Cysts lined by oncocytic cells
  - Oncocytic change in nonneoplastic tubules

Renal Oncocytoma

- Chromophobe renal cell carcinomas (RCCs) &/or tumors with hybrid oncocytic/chromophobe morphology also found
- Most cases now believed to be manifestation of Birt-Hogg Dubé syndrome

Hybrid Oncocytic Tumors

- While regarded by some as distinct entity, term best used in syndromic settings only
  - Such tumors common in setting of Birt-Hogg-Dubé, succinate dehydrogenase or tuberous sclerosis (TSC) syndromes, and non-BHD renal oncocytosis
  - Most sporadic cases represent either chromophobe RCC or are best regarded as unclassified RCC, low-grade oncocytic type

ANCILLARY TESTS

Immunohistochemistry

- CD117, E-cadherin, Ksp-cadherin, S100-A, CK-PAN, and low molecular weight cytokeratins (+)
- CK7(-), or scattered focally (+) cells
- Vimentin (-); however, focal strong positivity in areas around scar or in oncoblasts

Electron Microscopy

- Round nucleus
- Cytoplasm packed with mitochondria
  - Mitochondria with mostly lamellar cristae

DIFFERENTIAL DIAGNOSIS

Chromophobe RCC (Eosinophilic Variant)

- Nuclear irregularities, with perinuclear halos
- Variety of growth patterns, including solid with incomplete fibrovascular septations, and broad alveoli
- CK7 often, but not always, positive
- S100-A1 often, but not always, negative
- Microvesicles and mitochondria with tubulovesicular cristae on EM

Clear Cell RCC (Eosinophilic Variant)

- Fine arborizing vascularity
- Nuclear atypia, chromatin irregularities
- CA9 and CD10, diffuse membranous positivity
- CD117 negative

Epithelioid (Oncocytoma-Like) Angiomyolipoma

- Nuclear pleomorphism is common
- Smooth muscle and adipose component may be present
- Melanocytic markers HMB-45 and Melan-A(MART-1), and Cathepsin-K positive
  - Epithelial markers, negative

RCC, Unclassified (Oncocytic, Low-Grade Type)

- Nuclear pleomorphism
- At least focal solid architecture in most cases
- Easily identifiable mitotic figures may be present
- CD117 does not help in this differentiation
  - Often positive in such tumors

SDHB-Deficient RCC

- Nuclear pleomorphism, enlarged tubules
- Characteristic cytoplasmic eosinophilic to clear inclusions
- Loss of SDHB on immunohistochemical staining
- CD117, usually negative
- Epithelial markers, negative or only focally positive

TSC-Associated RCC

- Rare RCCs in TSC with oncocytoma or chromophobe RCC-like, or hybrid oncocytic features
- Often associated with RCCs of other type, and angiomyolipomas
- Multiple cysts usually lined by cells with abundant eosinophilic cytoplasm and large, pleomorphic nuclei

DIAGNOSTIC CHECKLIST

Pathologic Interpretation Pearls

- Renal oncocytoma and eosinophilic variant of chromophobe RCC biologically different tumor types (benign vs. malignant)
- However, both show molecular similarities and mutations in mtDNA genes
  - This raises some questions about their exact relationship
- Nonetheless, based on their biological outcomes, pathological distinction between 2 remains essential

SELECTED REFERENCES

1. Davis CF et al: The somatic genomic landscape of chromophobe renal cell carcinoma. Cancer Cell. 26(3):319-30, 2014
2. Hes O et al: Renal hybrid oncocytic/chromophobe tumors - a review. Histol Histopathol. 28(10):1257-64, 2013
3. Srigley JR et al: The International Society of Urological Pathology (ISUP) Vancouver Classification of Renal Neoplasia. Am J Surg Pathol. 37(10):1469-89, 2013
4. Xiao GQ et al: Telangiectatic oncocytoma: a previously undescribed variant of renal oncocytoma. Am J Clin Pathol. 140(1):103-8, 2013
5. Petersson F et al: Renal small cell oncocytoma with pseudorosettes A histomorphologic, immunohistochemical, and molecular genetic study of 10 cases. Hum Pathol. 42(11):1751-60, 2011
6. Sukov WR et al: CCND1 rearrangements and cyclin D1 overexpression in renal oncocytomas: frequency, clinicopathologic features, and utility in differentiation from chromophobe renal cell carcinoma. Hum Pathol. 40(9):1296-303, 2009
7. Tickoo SK et al: Pathologic features of renal cortical tumors. Urol Clin North Am. 35(4):551-61; v, 2008
8. Hornsby CD et al: Claudin-7 immunohistochemistry in renal tumors: a candidate marker for chromophobe renal cell carcinoma identified by gene expression profiling. Arch Pathol Lab Med. 131(10):1541-6, 2007
9. Rohan S et al: Gene expression profiling separates chromophobe renal cell carcinoma from oncocytoma and identifies vesicular transport and cell junction proteins as differentially expressed genes. Clin Cancer Res. 12(23):6937-45, 2006
10. Skinnider BF et al: An immunohistochemical approach to the differential diagnosis of renal tumors. Semin Diagn Pathol. 22(1):51-68, 2005
11. Amin MB et al: Prognostic impact of histologic subtyping of adult renal epithelial neoplasms: an experience of 405 cases. Am J Surg Pathol. 26(3):281-91, 2002
12. Tickoo SK et al: Ultrastructural observations on mitochondria and microvesicles in renal oncocytoma, chromophobe renal cell carcinoma, and eosinophilic variant of conventional (clear cell) renal cell carcinoma. Am J Surg Pathol. 24(9):1247-56, 2000
13. Füzesi L et al: Cytogenetic analysis of 11 renal oncocytomas: further evidence of structural rearrangements of 11q13 as a characteristic chromosomal anomaly. Cancer Genet Cytogenet. 107(1):1-6, 1998
14. Tickoo SK et al: Discriminant nuclear features of renal oncocytoma and chromophobe renal cell carcinoma. Analysis of their potential utility in the differential diagnosis. Am J Clin Pathol. 110(6):782-7, 1998
15. Amin MB et al: Renal oncocytoma: a reappraisal of morphologic features with clinicopathologic findings in 80 cases. Am J Surg Pathol. 21(1):1-12, 1997

Renal Oncocytoma

Pseudocapsule
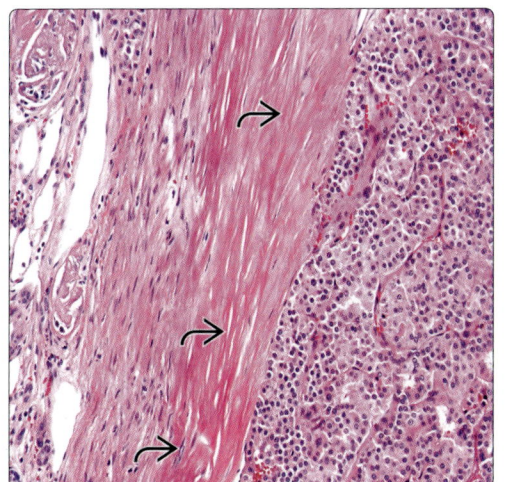

Typical Nested Architecture
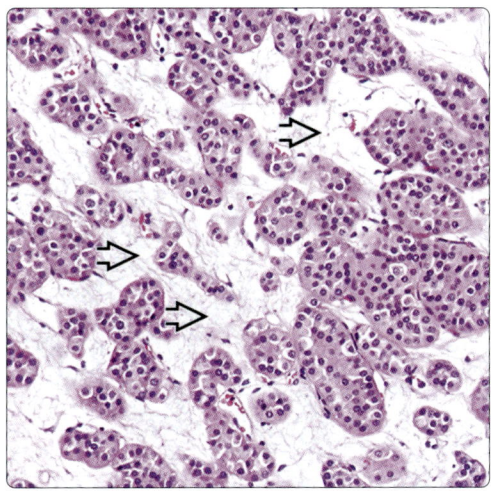

(Left) ROs, in spite of being well circumscribed, usually show no pseudocapsule. However, rare cases may not follow that paradigm and may show prominent encapsulation ⇨. (Right) Typically the nests of cells, arranged in discrete islands or interconnected archipeligenous pattern, are separated by loose stroma ⇨ in most cases of RO.

Hyalinized Areas
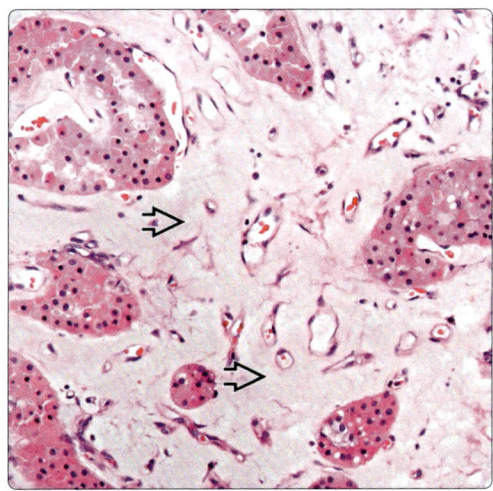

Telangiectatic Pattern
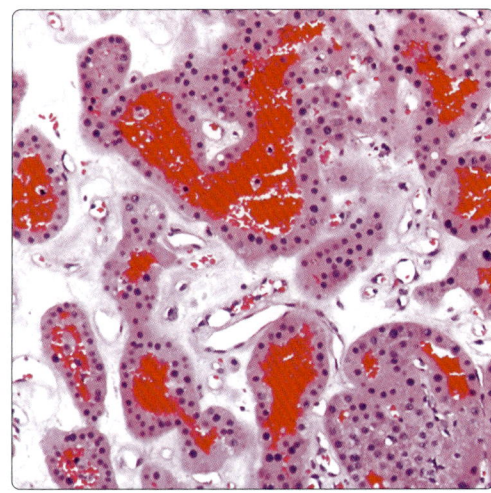

(Left) In some ROs, variable proportions of the stroma may be fibrotic and hyalinized ⇨. Fibrotic stroma is particularly evident in and around the grossly identifiable scars in the tumor but may be evident only on microscopic evaluation in some cases. (Right) Tubules and microcysts in oncocytomas frequently show the presence of fresh blood in the lumina. Tumors with such a predominant pattern have been designated as telangiectatic ROs by some authors. However, this represents only a morphologic variation in RO.

Prominent Nucleoli
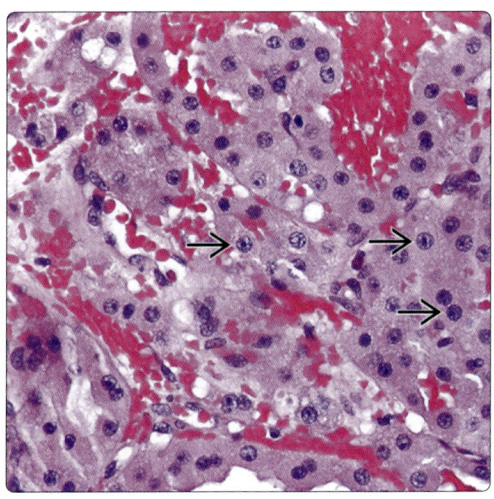

Oncoblasts
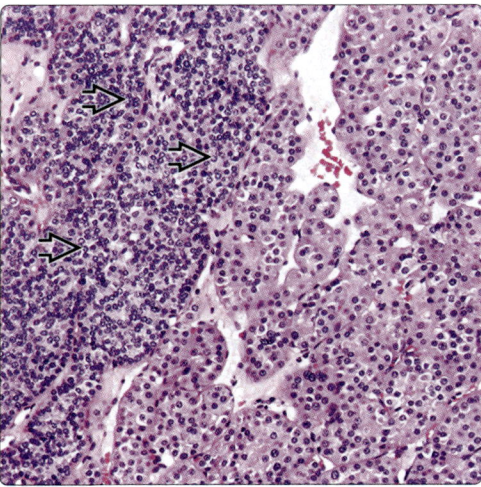

(Left) Uniformity of the shape and size of the nuclei is a prerequisite for rendering the diagnosis of RO in an oncocytic renal tumor. A significant proportion ROs possess prominent nucleoli ⇨. (Right) Many ROs show collections of darker-appearing cells, the so-called oncoblasts ⇨. These cells possess scant cytoplasm, but nuclear details are somewhat similar to those in the larger oncocytic cells. Rare tumors show predominance of such small cell morphology.

Renal Oncocytoma

(Left) Some oncocytomas show closely compressed nests, giving the impression of solid architecture. However, careful evaluation reveals the thin fibrovascular septations ⇨ separating the solid nests, supporting the nested growth pattern typical of RO. (Right) Some ROs reveal single oncocytic cells in the stroma, often clustered in small foci ⇨ in a background of typical histology.

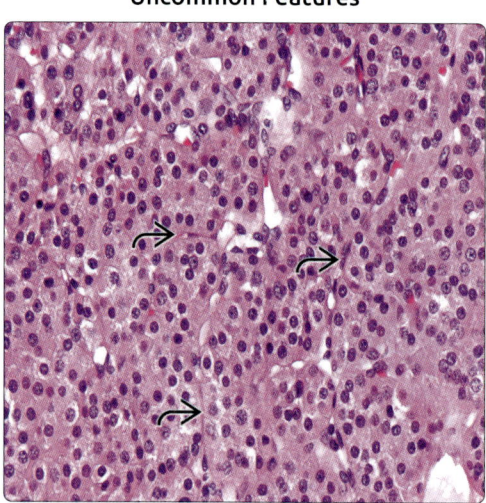
Uncommon Features

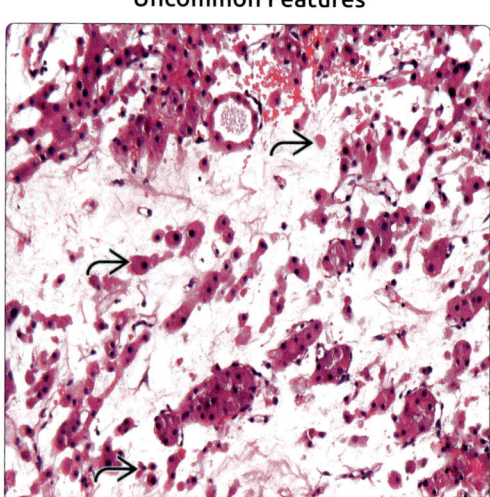
Uncommon Features

(Left) Rarely, oncocytomas show a trabecular and archeplagic architectural pattern with irregularly branching and communicating columns of cells. Such architecture is usually focal but may be quite prominent in some tumors. (Right) Focal papillations ⇨, particularly within the dilated tubules and cysts, are occasionally present in RO. However, prominent papillary architecture is not a feature of the tumor.

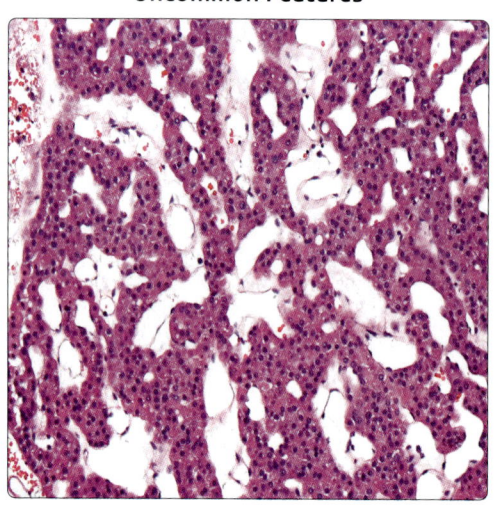
Uncommon Features

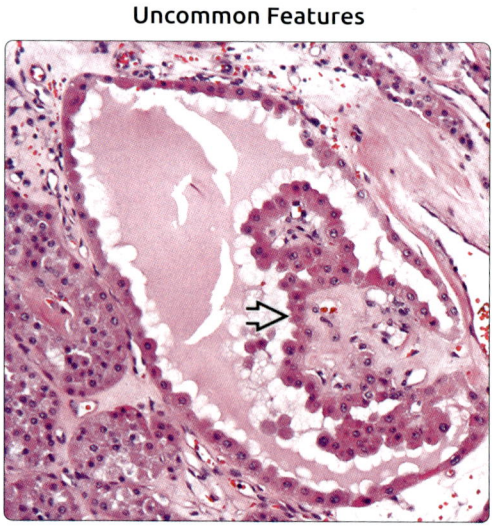
Uncommon Features

(Left) Up to 20% of ROs show extension into perinephric fat. Usually, no desmoplastic response is present in these areas. Presence of neoplastic cells in fat in a tumor with features otherwise typical of RO does not merit histologic grading or pathologic staging. (Right) Vascular invasion, including that of large muscle-bearing vessels ⇨ in the renal sinus, may be present in up to 5% of cases. Neither the vascular invasion nor extrarenal extension influences the benign nature of otherwise typical oncocytoma.

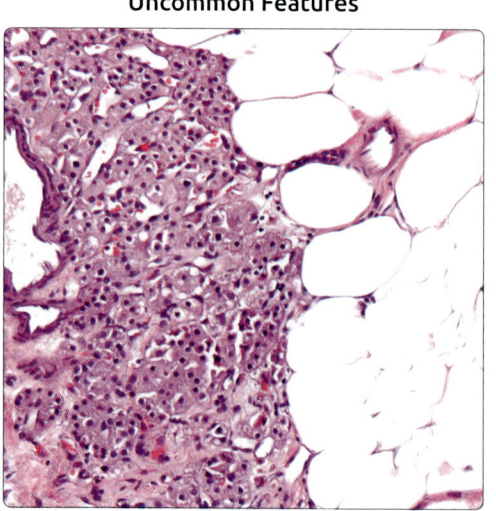
Uncommon Features

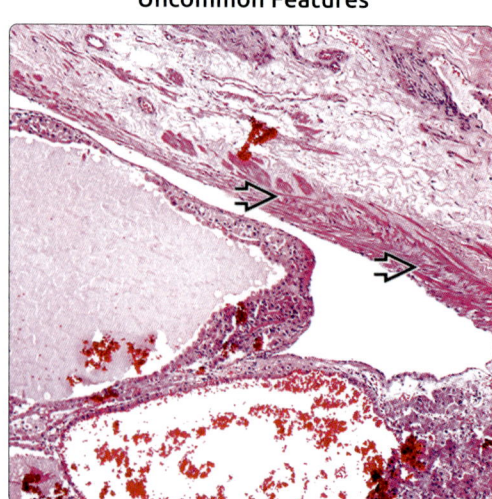
Uncommon Features

Renal Oncocytoma

Degenerate Atypia
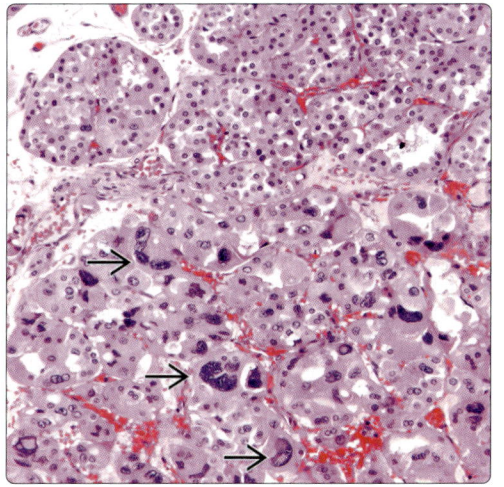

Ki-67 Immunohistochemistry
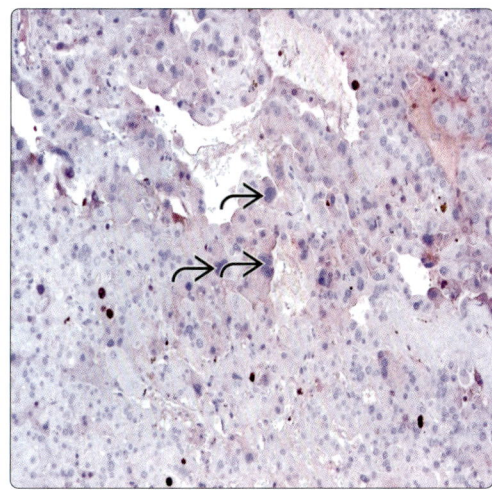

(Left) Foci with marked nuclear hyperchromasia and pleomorphism ⇨ are quite common in RO. Such nuclear atypia is believed to be a degenerative phenomenon. (Right) Immunohistochemical staining for Ki-67 is always completely negative in these pleomorphic, hyperchromatic cells ⇨ in RO. This confirmation of nonproliferation of the pleomorphic nuclei supports the degenerative nature of this phenomenon.

Clear Cell Change: Areas of Scarring
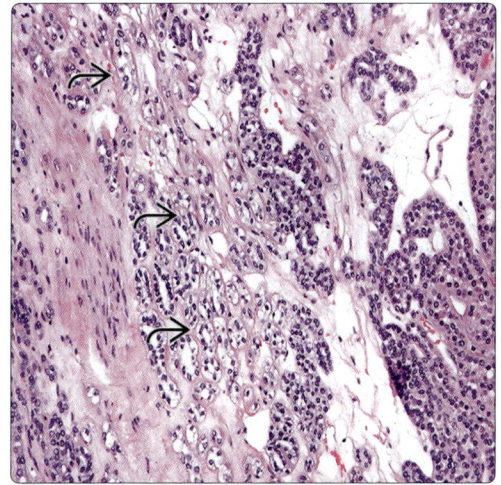

CK7 Immunohistochemistry
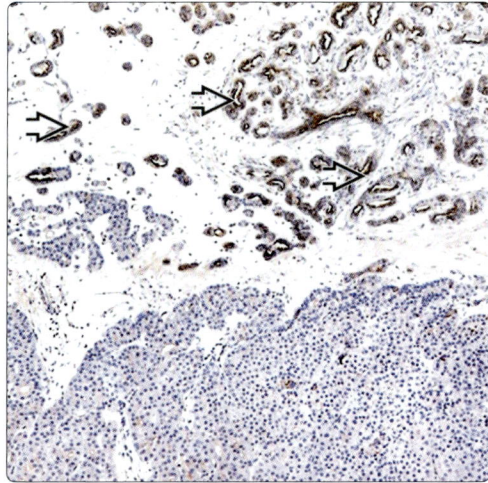

(Left) Clear cell cytology is generally not compatible with the diagnosis of RO. However, prominent clear cell change may be noted in and adjacent to the area of scars ⇨. (Right) Such clear cell areas around scars are often diffusely positive for CK7 ⇨. This diffuse positivity on limited material, such as needle core biopsies, may lead to misdiagnosis, unless the nature of the sampled areas is appreciated.

Hybrid Oncocytic Tumor or Chromophobe RCC
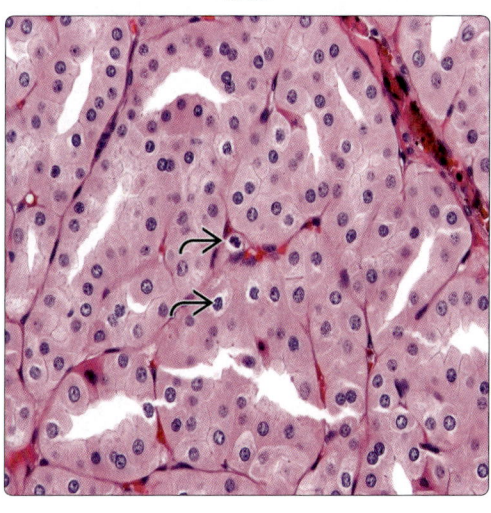

Cytologic Atypia: Unclassified RCC, Low Grade
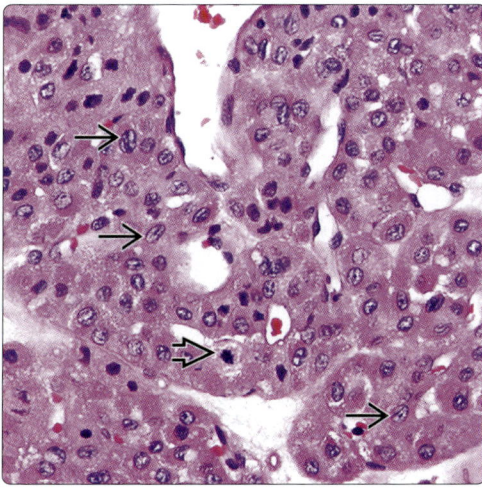

(Left) Some tumors may show predominance of RO-like nuclear features, with focal nuclear irregularities and perinuclear halos ⇨. These considered as hybrid oncocytic tumors by some are called chromophobe renal cell carcinoma (RCC) by others. (Right) Other than degenerate foci, only minimal nuclear atypia is allowable in RO. Diffuse nuclear irregularities ⇨ and frequent mitoses ⇨ are not permissible. The term unclassified RCC low grade, oncocytic may be used in cases with diffuse atypia but with other features of RO.

Clear Cell Renal Cell Carcinoma

KEY FACTS

ETIOLOGY/PATHOGENESIS
- Mutations in *VHL* gene (3p25-26) or chromosome 3p losses in all VHL syndrome cases and > 90% of sporadic tumors
- Mutations also frequent in chromatin remodeling complex genes *PBRM1, SETD2* and *BAP1,* genes in PI3K-AKT-mTOR pathway, and *FHIT* gene
- Copy number gains of chromosome 5q in up to 70% of clear cell renal cell carcinomas (CC-RCCs)

CLINICAL ISSUES
- Currently, most cases are asymptomatic; diagnosed as result of radiologic investigations for unrelated symptoms
- Nephrectomy most common mode of management in clinically localized disease, with partial nephrectomy becoming standard of care
- Targeted therapies against HIF and mTOR pathway markers, and more recently, novel immunotherapies, with some promising clinical responses
- Most aggressive subtype among common subtypes of renal cell carcinoma, with 5- and 10-year survival of 75% and 62%, respectively

MACROSCOPIC
- Cut surface typically golden-yellow (due to presence of intracytoplasmic lipid); areas of necrosis, fibrosis, cystic change, hemorrhage are quite common

MICROSCOPIC
- Cells arranged in nests, micro or macrocysts, or solid sheets, surrounded by intricate, branching fibrovascular septations
- Areas with granular/eosinophilic cytoplasm usually higher grade

TOP DIFFERENTIAL DIAGNOSES
- MiTF/TFE family translocation RCC, clear cell papillary RCC, epithelioid angiomyolipoma, chromophobe RCC, TSC-associated RCC, TCEB1-mutated RCC, adrenal cortical tumors, papillary RCC

Gross Features

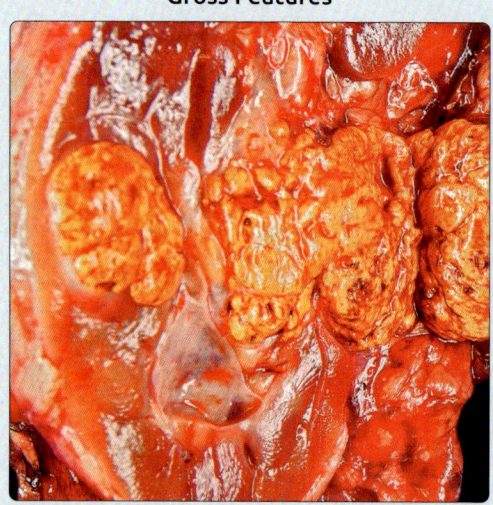
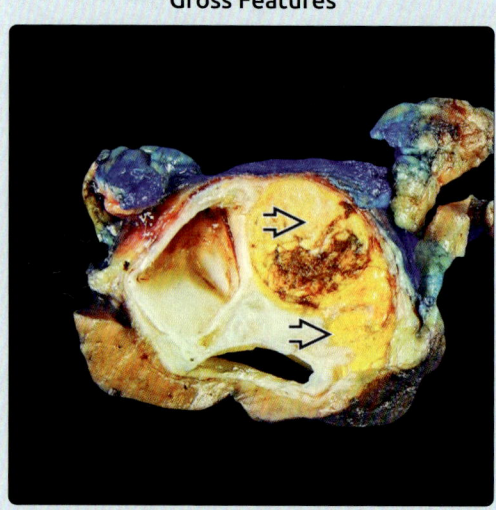

(Left) A clear cell renal cell carcinoma (CC-RCC) typically shows a golden-yellow cut surface. This gross appearance is a reflection of abundant intracytoplasmic lipid in these tumors. Tumors with golden-yellow cut surface are microscopically rich in clear cell cytology. (Right) Gross photograph of another CC-RCC shows a markedly cystic cut surface. Some tumors may be predominantly cystic with only focal solid areas. The solid areas in the tumor reveal the characteristic golden-yellow appearance ⊇.

Microscopic Features / Immunohistochemical Feature

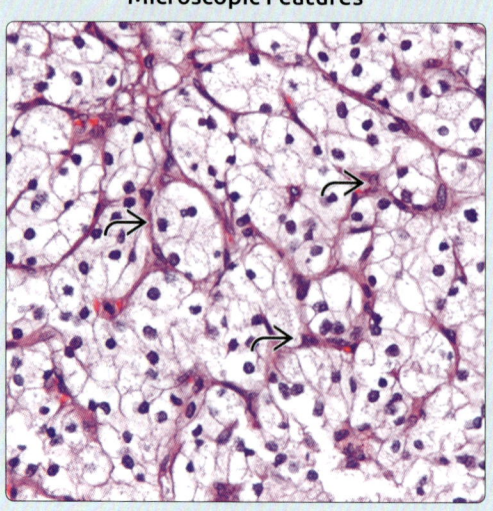
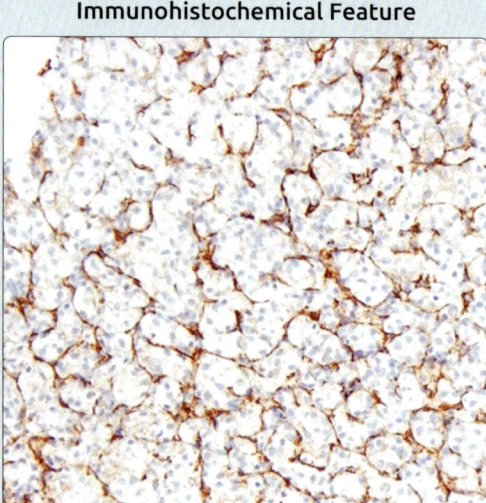

(Left) The delicate, prominent interconnecting vascular framework, as seen here ⇗, is identified in most CC-RCCs and is diagnostically the most important feature of the tumor. This characteristic vascular pattern is lost only in the very high-grade and sarcomatoid areas. (Right) Intricately branching fibrovascular septations that surround the tumor cell nests are highlighted here by a CD31 immunohistochemical stain.

Clear Cell Renal Cell Carcinoma

TERMINOLOGY

Abbreviations
- Clear cell renal cell carcinoma (CC-RCC)

Synonyms
- Conventional (clear cell) renal cell carcinoma

ETIOLOGY/PATHOGENESIS

Mutations in *VHL* Gene (3p25-26) or Chromosome 3p Losses
- Present in virtually all cases of von Hippel-Lindau (VHL) syndrome
- Somatic mutations/losses/promoter hypermethylation in > 80% of sporadic CC-RCC
  - Overall, chromosome 3p copy number loss in more than 90% of tumors

Hypoxia-Inducible Factor (HIF) and von Hippel-Lindau Pathways
- Normal VHL gene product, pVHL, required to target and degrade hydroxylated HIF-1 in normoxemic states
- In states of hypoxia (as in ischemic/perinecrotic areas in any tumor), or when pVHL is absent or abnormal (as in all VHL cases and most sporadic CC-RCC), HIF1-α escapes degradation
- Overexpressed HIF1-α activates number of downstream molecules, including
  - VEGF
  - GLUT1
  - CA9
  - EDGF and PDGF
  - Many of these factors believed to have role in tumor initiation and progression in CC-RCC

Other Common Mutations
- Mutations also frequent in chromatin remodeling complex genes *PBRM1* (polybromo 1), *SETD2* (SET domain containing 2), and *BAP1* (BRCA1-associated protein-1) (~ 41%, 11%, and 10% tumors, respectively)
  - All 3 genes located at 3p21
  - Exact role of these mutations in pathogenesis or biology of CC-RCC not completely clear at this time
  - *PBRM1* and *BAP1* mutations almost always mutually exclusive
  - *SETD2* mutations often occur alone or together with *PBRM1*, but not with *BAP1* mutations
  - *BAP1* mutation typically associated with high-grade tumors and with poor outcome
- Other common mutations involve genes in PI3K-AKT-mTOR pathway (> 25%)
- Copy number gains of chromosome 5q in up to 70% of CC-RCCs
  - Relevant target gene on chromosome 5q identified as *SQSTM1* (sequestosome 1)
    - Gene product, p62, serves as adaptor molecule that facilitates degradation of multiple proteins by autophagy
- Potential tumor suppressor gene *FHIT* (fragile histidine triad protein), located at 3p14.2, epigenetically silenced in ~ 50% of CC-RCC
- Also, inactivating mutations of the *NF2* tumor suppressor gene in small subset of CC-RCCs, all of which with no mutations for *VHL*

CLINICAL ISSUES

Presentation
- Currently, most cases asymptomatic; diagnosed as result of radiologic investigations for unrelated symptoms
- Classical triad of hematuria, mass lesion, and pain present in < 30% of cases

Treatment
- Surgical approaches
  - Nephrectomy still most common mode of management in clinically localized disease
  - Partial nephrectomy becoming standard of care in many cases (> 70% of cases in some institutions)
  - Total or radical nephrectomies associated with long-term higher incidence of deteriorating renal function compared to partial nephrectomies
  - Partial nephrectomy replacing more radical procedures in overwhelming majority, including centrally occurring tumors and tumors > 4 cm
- Drugs
  - Response to chemotherapy &/or radiation for advanced disease is unsatisfactory
  - Immunotherapies, including interleukins and cytokines, were major therapeutic options in metastatic disease until recently, with only limited positive responses
  - Targeted therapies against VEGF/HIF and mammalian target of rapamycin (mTOR) pathway markers have recently become standard of care
    - In spite of prolongation of survivals with these therapies, resistance develops or tumors regrow when the drugs stopped
  - Targeted therapies now being investigated as adjuvant therapies for high-risk, locally advanced, nonmetastatic tumors
- Novel immunotherapies
  - Given the fact that rare CC-RCC show spontaneous regression (immune effect) and IL-2/interferon resulted in durable responses in rare cases, immunotherapy being revisited now
  - Therapies under investigation include
    - Personalized product derived from patient-derived tumor RNA and dendritic cells (DCs) as subcutaneous injections
    - DC-Ad-GM-CA9, product of patient dendritic cells, adenovirus vector, granulocyte monocyte colony stimulating factor (GM-CSF), and carbonic anhydrase IX (CA9), as vaccine
    - Antibodies against programmed cell death receptor (PD-1) and PD-1 ligands (PD-L1 and PD-L2)

Prognosis
- Most aggressive subtype among common subtypes of renal cell carcinoma
- Overall 5- and 10-year survival of 75% and 62%, respectively
- Most important indicators of prognosis include pathologic stage, nuclear grade, sarcomatoid features, and Memorial Sloan Kettering Cancer Center clinical status

Clear Cell Renal Cell Carcinoma

MACROSCOPIC

Size
- 1-24 cm

Gross Features
- May be well circumscribed but usually unencapsulated
- Cut surface typically golden-yellow (due to presence of intracytoplasmic lipid); areas of necrosis, fibrosis, cystic change, hemorrhage are quite common
- Tumors may be variegated in appearance with variable degrees of aforementioned features
- Cystic change may vary from focal to extensive multicystic
- In high-grade/sarcomatoid areas, solid gray, tannish-white to fleshy-appearing cut surface
- Most tumors limited to renal parenchyma
    - Larger tumors, particularly those > 7 cm, very often involve renal sinus veins and sinus fat
        - Careful sampling of sinus essential to demonstrate sinus fat or large segmental branches of renal vein invasion
        - Stromal response/pseudoencapsulation may make determination of fat invasion difficult in some cases, requiring careful interpretation

MICROSCOPIC

Histologic Features
- Cells arranged in nests, solid alveoli, tubules, micro or macro cysts, or solid sheets, surrounded by intricate, branching fibrovascular septations
- Typical vascularity retained in most cases except in high-grade solid or sarcomatoid areas
- Focal papillary architecture acceptable; most often related to tumor cell dropout and pseudopapillary architecture; rare cases with focal true papillations
    - Prominent papillation should raise possibility of alternative diagnoses, including translocation-associated, clear cell papillary, or unclassified RCC
- Lower grade areas usually with clear cell (optically transparent) cytology; related to abundant intracytoplasmic glycogen and fat
- Areas with granular/eosinophilic cytoplasm usually higher grade
- Grading
    - Fuhrman nuclear grading is most commonly used grading scheme of tumor
        - Associated with clinical outcome
        - Nuclear grade assigned according to highest grade in tumor, even if focal
        - Tumors with sarcomatoid areas assigned grade 4
        - However, marked interobserver variability, and most tumors regarded Grade 2 or 3 making discrimination difficult
    - Recently, International Society of Urological Pathology (ISUP)/WHO grading recommended as easier and better scheme for CC-RCC and papillary renal cell carcinoma (PRCC)
        - Better correlation with clinical outcomes
        - Grades 1-3 based on greatest nucleolar prominence in the tumor, even when focal
            - Grade 1: Inapparent nucleoli at 400x magnification
            - Grade 2: Nucleoli easily identifiable at 400x, often eosinophilic
            - Grade 3: Eosinophilic nucleoli easily identifiable at 100x
        - Grade 4 based on rhabdoid or sarcomatoid features, or markedly pleomorphic nuclei with lobulations or multinucleation
    - Grading based on nucleolar scheme in association with presence or absence of tumor coagulative necrosis considered even better by some
- Some tumors may have prominent cell borders superficially resembling chromophobe RCC
- Focal CC-RRCC-like nuclear alignment present in some tumors
    - Represents morphological variation in CC-RCC and not mixed CC-RCC and CC-PRCC
- Sarcomatoid features in ~ 5% tumors
    - Indicator of more aggressive clinical behavior

Predominant Pattern/Injury Type
- Alveolar

Predominant Cell/Compartment Type
- Epithelial

ANCILLARY TESTS

Immunohistochemistry
- CK-PAN(AE1/AE3), EMA/MUC1, and vimentin are positive
- CD10, RCC, pax-2, pax-8, and CA9 are positive
    - CA9 often positive even in high-grade and sarcomatoid areas
    - CA9 shows diffuse membranous staining highlighting all the cell membranes (box-like pattern)
- CK7, AMACR, CD117, and Ksp-cadherin are mostly negative
    - CK7 may be focally positive in tumors with cystic features or high-grade areas in some
- Loss of BAP1 and PBRM1 staining in tumor cells highly correlates with mutations in these genes

DIFFERENTIAL DIAGNOSIS

Papillary Renal Cell Carcinoma
- Prominent papillary architecture
- Foamy histiocytes within fibrovascular stalks and stroma and hemosiderin deposition
- IHC: Usually CK7 and AMACR diffusely positive; CA9 negative to focal perinecrotic/papillary tip positive

Translocation-Associated Renal Cell Carcinoma
- Usually combination of prominent papillary architecture and clear cell cytology
- High nuclear grade
- IHC: Cytokeratins and EMA/MUC1 negative to focally positive; strong and diffuse nuclear immunoreactivity for TFE3 or TFEB

Clear Cell Papillary Carcinoma
- Prominent papillary or branching tubular architecture with exclusive clear cell cytology
- Usually low nuclear grade
- Nuclei arranged in linear manner away from basement membrane in most of the tumor

Clear Cell Renal Cell Carcinoma

- IHC: CK7 and CA9 diffusely positive, CA9 mostly with absent luminal staining (cup-shaped pattern) ; HMWCK(+); AMACR(-); CD10 usually negative

Epithelioid Angiomyolipoma
- Usually high nuclear grade even in areas with clear cell cytology; multilobulated/multinucleated polymorphous cells often present
- Vasculature usually not as intricate or branching as in CC-RCC
- May be associated, at least focally, with typical angiomyolipoma areas, or focal fat &/or dysmorphic vessels
- IHC: Cytokeratin/EMA/MUC1(-); HMB-45/Melan-A(MART-1)/MITF/Cathepsin K(+)

Chromophobe Carcinoma
- Characteristic nuclear and cytoplasmic features
- Plant cell appearance and koilocytoid atypia
- Fibrovascular septations most often incomplete
- 2 cell populations (eosinophilic and clear cell) in predictable arrangement
- IHC: CK7 and CD117 usually (+); Ksp-cadherin (+); CA9(-)

Adrenal Cortical Tumors
- Correlation with imaging findings crucial
- Clear cells with bubbly cytoplasm
- IHC: EMA/MUC1 and cytokeratins (-); inhibin, Melan-A(MART-1) (+)

Other Tumors With Clear Cell Features
- Tuberous sclerosis-associated RCC
  o Often multifocal
    - Variable histologies among different tumors and often within same tumor
  o Usually associated with cysts and angiomyolipomas in surrounding parenchyma
  o Germline *TSC1/TSC2* gene mutations
    - Associated with loss of heterozygosity (LOH) of other allele
- TCEB1-mutated RCC
  o Prominent fibromuscular stroma imparting vaguely nodular configuration to tumor
  o Cells with abundant clear cytoplasm
  o Often CK7(+)
  o *TCEB1* mutations and 8q21 LOH of other allele
    - No *VHL* mutations

DIAGNOSTIC CHECKLIST
Clinically Relevant Pathologic Features
- Currently, tumors invading renal sinus or perinephric fat assigned the same pT stage
- Similarly, tumors invading segmental branches of renal vein assigned same pT stage as renal vein invasion
- Probability of sinus vein/fat invasion in CC-RCCs > 5 cm is > 60%
  o In tumors > 7 cm in size, this likelihood increases to > 90%
    - Therefore, careful reevaluation of all such tumors for sinus vessel and fat invasion is mandatory if they appear organ-confined on initial assessment

Pathologic Interpretation Pearls
- Intricate, branching vasculature most important diagnostic pathological feature
  o Clear cell cytology not present in all cases
    - Therefore, not essential for diagnosis
- Some tumors may contain high-grade areas that are unrecognizable as CC-RCC
  o Presence of even focal classical, low-grade CC-RCC areas in such tumors confirms their true nature

SELECTED REFERENCES
1. Abel EJ et al: Risk factors for recurrence after surgery in non-metastatic RCC with thrombus; a Contemporary multicenter analysis. BJU Int. ePub, 2015
2. Thomas JS et al: Metastatic clear cell renal cell carcinoma: A review of current therapies and novel immunotherapies. Crit Rev Oncol Hematol. 96(3):527-3, 2015
3. Cancer Genome Atlas Research Network: Comprehensive molecular characterization of clear cell renal cell carcinoma. Nature. 499(7456):43-9, 2013
4. Hakimi AA et al: Clinical and pathologic impact of select chromatin-modulating tumor suppressors in clear cell renal cell carcinoma. Eur Urol. 63(5):848-54, 2013
5. Hakimi AA et al: Adverse outcomes in clear cell renal cell carcinoma with mutations of 3p21 epigenetic regulators BAP1 and SETD2: a report by MSKCC and the KIRC TCGA research network. Clin Cancer Res. 19(12):3259-67, 2013
6. Sato Y et al: Integrated molecular analysis of clear-cell renal cell carcinoma. Nat Genet. 45(8):860-7, 2013
7. Feifer A et al: Prognostic impact of muscular venous branch invasion in localized renal cell carcinoma cases. J Urol. 185(1):37-42, 2011
8. Bertini R et al: Renal sinus fat invasion in pT3a clear cell renal cell carcinoma affects outcomes of patients without nodal involvement or distant metastases. J Urol. 181(5):2027-32, 2009
9. Nese N et al: Renal cell carcinoma: assessment of key pathologic prognostic parameters and patient characteristics in 47,909 cases using the National Cancer Data Base. Ann Diagn Pathol. 13(1):1-8, 2009
10. Rini BI et al: Renal cell carcinoma. Lancet. 373(9669):1119-32, 2009
11. Simmons MN et al: Laparoscopic radical versus partial nephrectomy for tumors >4 cm: intermediate-term oncologic and functional outcomes. Urology. 73(5):1077-82; discussion 1082, 2009
12. Thompson RH et al: Contemporary use of partial nephrectomy at a tertiary care center in the United States. J Urol. 181(3):993-7, 2009
13. Al-Ahmadie HA et al: Carbonic anhydrase IX expression in clear cell renal cell carcinoma: an immunohistochemical study comparing 2 antibodies. Am J Surg Pathol. 32(3):377-82, 2008
14. Pfaffenroth EC et al: Genetic basis for kidney cancer: opportunity for disease-specific approaches to therapy. Expert Opin Biol Ther. 8(6):779-90, 2008
15. Thompson RH et al: Patients with pT1 renal cell carcinoma who die from disease after nephrectomy may have unrecognized renal sinus fat invasion. Am J Surg Pathol. 31(7):1089-93, 2007
16. Tickoo SK et al: Immunohistochemical expression of hypoxia inducible factor-1alpha and its downstream molecules in sarcomatoid renal cell carcinoma. J Urol. 177(4):1258-63, 2007
17. Bonsib SM: Renal lymphatics, and lymphatic involvement in sinus vein invasive (pT3b) clear cell renal cell carcinoma: a study of 40 cases. Mod Pathol. 19(5):746-53, 2006
18. Reuter VE: The pathology of renal epithelial neoplasms. Semin Oncol. 33(5):534-43, 2006
19. Bonsib SM: T2 clear cell renal cell carcinoma is a rare entity: a study of 120 clear cell renal cell carcinomas. J Urol. 174(4 Pt 1):1199-202; discussion 1202, 2005
20. Skinnider BF et al: An immunohistochemical approach to the differential diagnosis of renal tumors. Semin Diagn Pathol. 22(1):51-68, 2005
21. Bonsib SM: The renal sinus is the principal invasive pathway: a prospective study of 100 renal cell carcinomas. Am J Surg Pathol. 28(12):1594-600, 2004
22. Cheville JC et al: Comparisons of outcome and prognostic features among histologic subtypes of renal cell carcinoma. Am J Surg Pathol. 27(5):612-24, 2003
23. Amin MB et al: Prognostic impact of histologic subtyping of adult renal epithelial neoplasms: an experience of 405 cases. Am J Surg Pathol. 26(3):281-91, 2002

Clear Cell Renal Cell Carcinoma

Gross Features

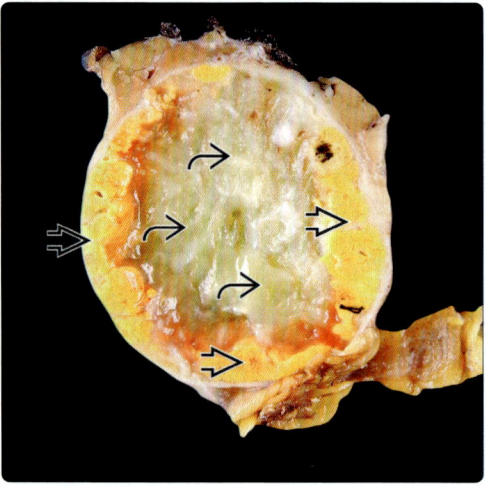

(Left) This gross photograph shows a large central scar ⮕ in a CC-RCC surrounded by a rim of viable tumor ⮕. A central scar can be seen in a number of slow-growing renal tumors, including CC-RCC, renal oncocytoma, and chromophobe RCC.

Gross Features

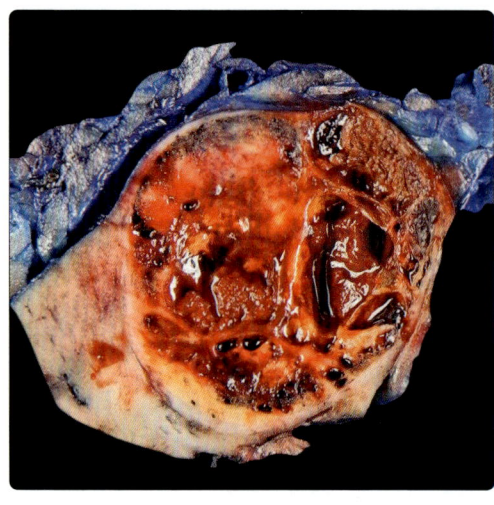

(Right) This gross photograph shows a cystic, necrotic, and hemorrhagic cut surface of a CC-RCC. Gross necrosis, hemorrhage, and cystic changes are frequently observed in these tumors.

Morphological Features

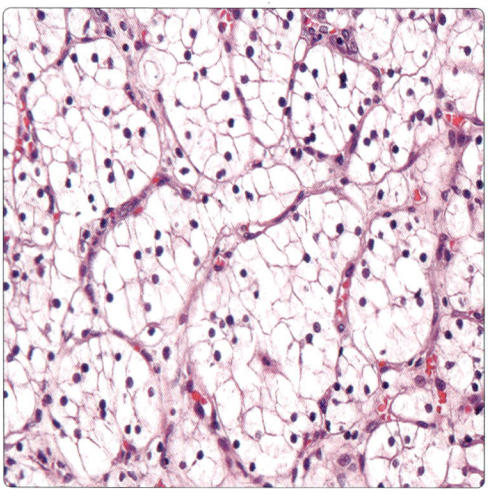

(Left) Hematoxylin and eosin shows a prototypic example of CC-RCC with nests of clear cells surrounded by intricately branching vascular septa. Since nucleoli are inconspicuous at this high magnification (x400), this is a Grade 1 tumor using the International Society of Urological Pathology (ISUP)/WHO grading scheme.

Microscopic Features

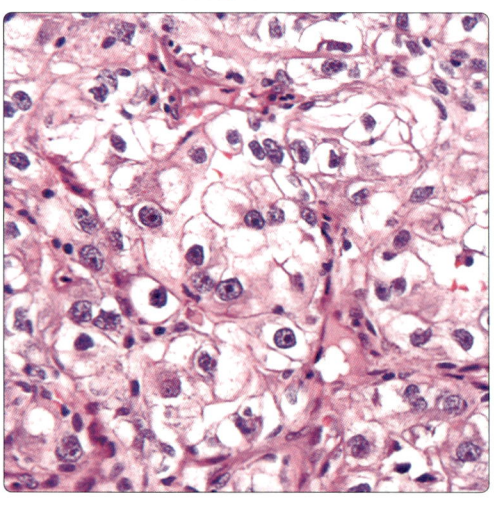

(Right) Hematoxylin and eosin stained section shows a CC-RCC with grade 3 nuclei by ISUP/WHO grading. Such nucleoli should be easily visible at 100x magnification.

Microscopic Features

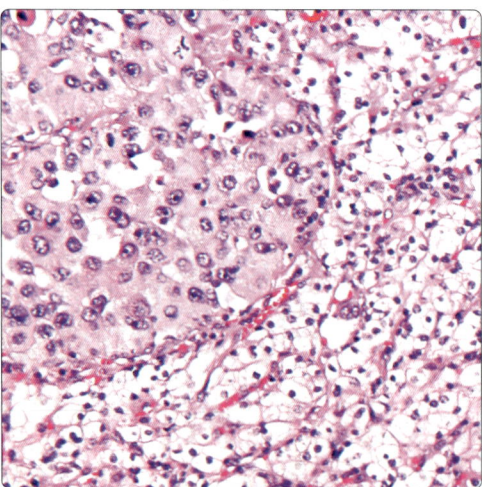

(Left) Many tumors show a combination of cells with clear and eosinophilic cytoplasm, either intimately admixed or as separate, discrete foci. Note the higher nuclear grade (3) in the cells with eosinophilic cytoplasm, a finding that is quite common in CC-RCC.

Microscopic Features

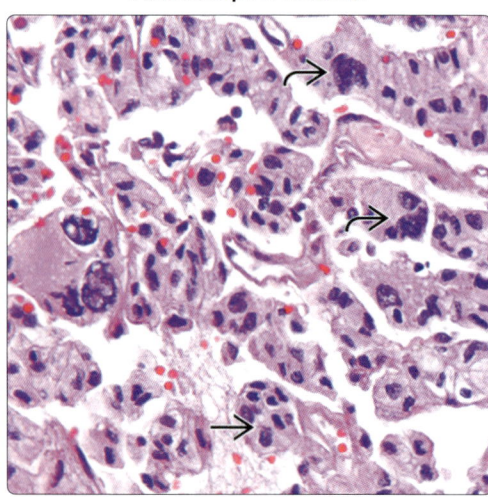

(Right) A nuclear grade 4 CC-RCC shows multilobulated and hyperchromatic nuclei ⮕. Some cells contain multiple nuclei ⮕. Grade heterogeneity is common, and the tumor is graded by the highest grade, even if focal.

Clear Cell Renal Cell Carcinoma

Gross Features

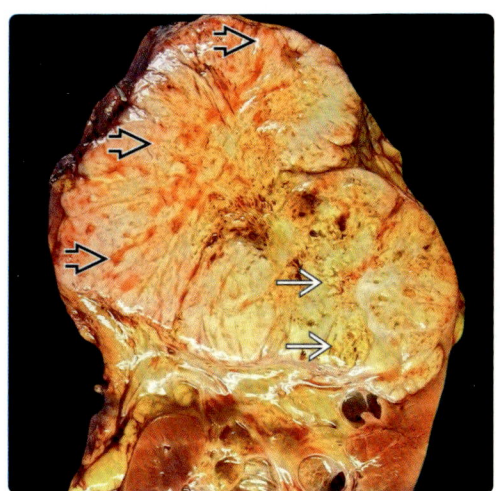

Microscopic Features

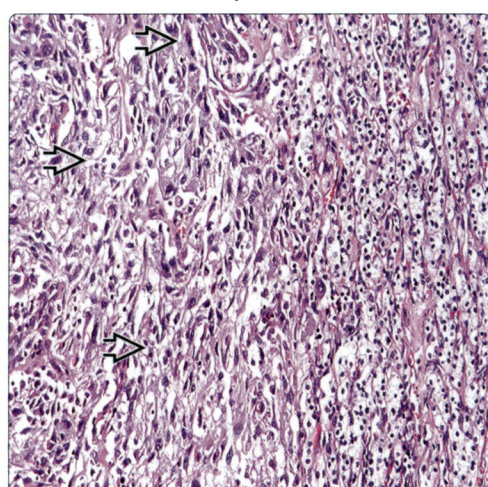

(Left) Gross photograph shows a CC-RCC with large sarcomatoid areas. Compared to the golden-yellow cut surface in the lower grade ➡ epithelial areas, the sarcomatoid ➡ areas show a pale tan to fleshy appearance. Sampling of areas with a grossly fleshy and gray-tan appearance is a key to identifying sarcomatoid and higher grade areas in a tumor. (Right) Sarcomatoid features ➡ in CC-RCC portend an aggressive clinical behavior. All tumors with sarcomatoid areas are considered high grade (grade 4).

Immunohistochemical Features

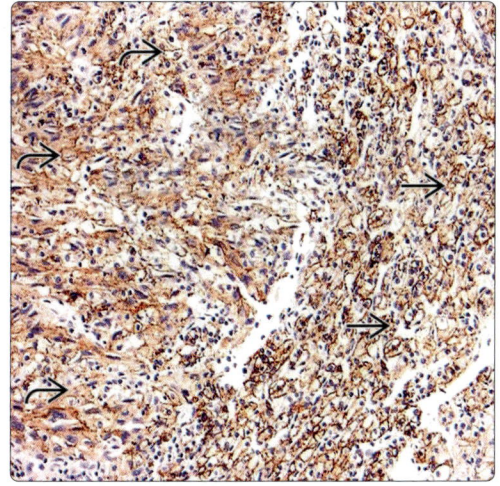

Microscopic Features

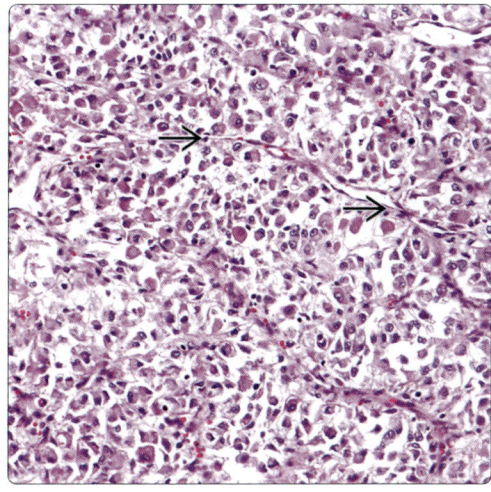

(Left) Some tumors may have extensive sarcomatoid features, with very focal identifiable clear cell epithelial areas. Diagnosis of CC-RCC with sarcomatoid features is appropriate in that situation. Immunostain for CA9, which is mostly positive even in sarcomatoid areas ➡ of CC-RCC ➡, is very useful in difficult cases. (Right) This photomicrograph shows a high-grade CC-RCC with rhabdoid cytology. The typical CC-RCC vascular pattern is retained ➡. Rhabdoid morphology is assigned grade 4 in the ISUP/WHO scheme.

Microscopic Features

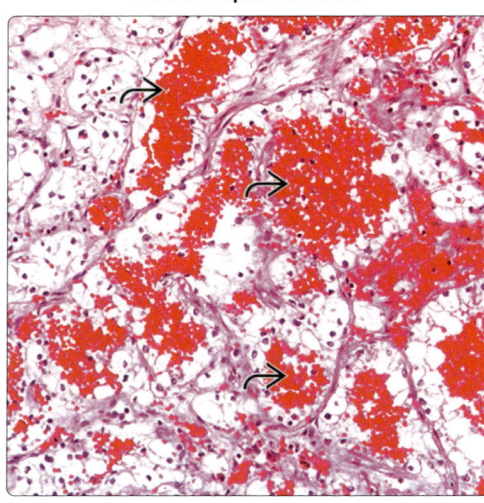

Microscopic Features

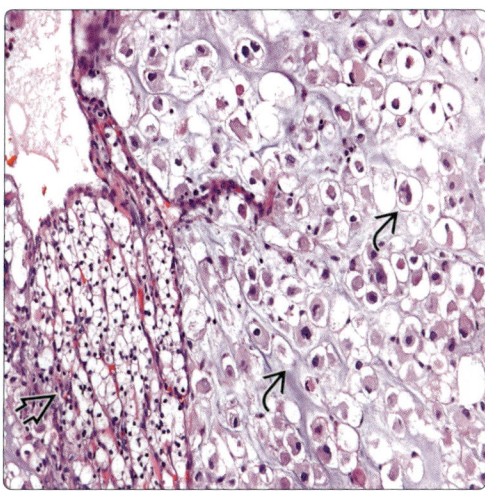

(Left) CC-RCC frequently shows fresh hemorrhage into the glandular lumina ➡. This feature is also often retained in the metastatic sites. (Right) This CC-RCC ➡ shows a markedly myxoid/chondroid background ➡. Such features are uncommon, but when typical CC-RCC foci are present in a tumor with high-grade areas with variable morphologic features, it is still a CC-RCC. Such tumors should not be regarded as collision tumors, or RCC, unclassified.

Clear Cell Renal Cell Carcinoma

Microscopic Features

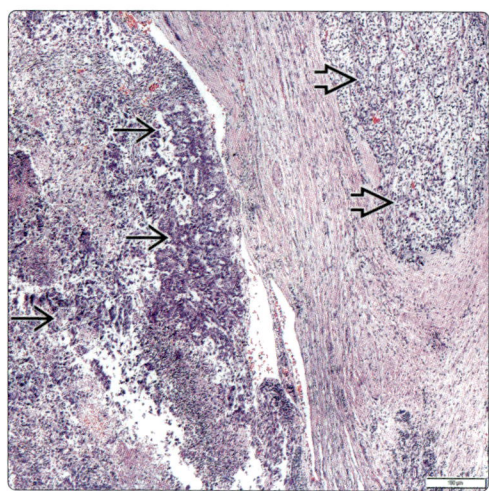

Immunohistochemical Features

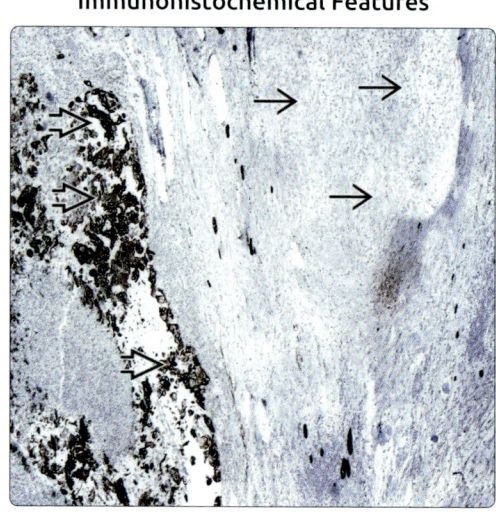

(Left) Presence of predominant or exclusive solid and pseudopapillary areas ⇾ would make rendering the diagnosis of CC-RCC in this tumor very difficult. However, the typical low-grade foci ⇾ clearly indicates this to be a CC-RCC. (Right) High-grade, poorly differentiated areas in CC-RCC may also show aberrant antigenicity, as demonstrated by the CK7 positivity ⇾ in high-grade areas of this tumor. Notice the lack of staining in the typical low-grade areas ⇾.

Microscopic Features

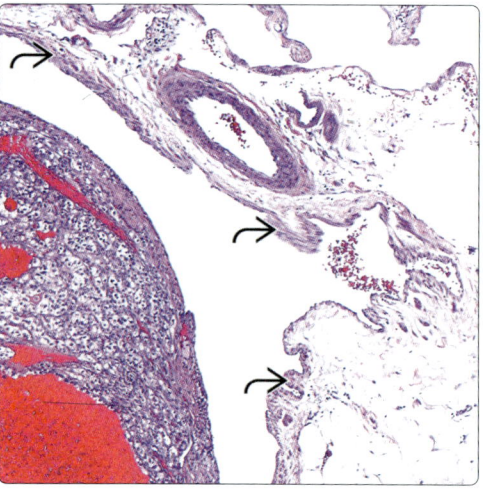

Microscopic Features

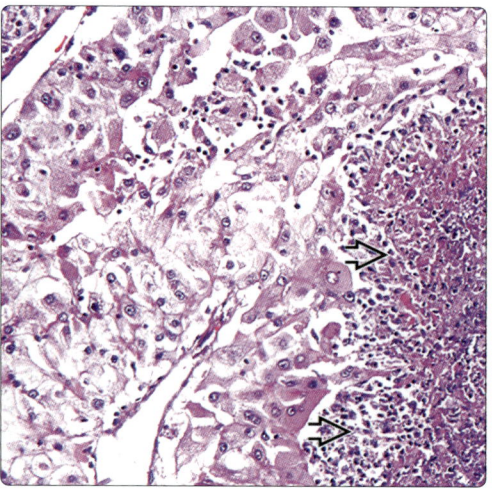

(Left) This image shows the tumor invading a muscle-containing branch of the renal vein ⇾ in the renal sinus. Such a finding is equivalent to renal vein invasion for pT staging purposes. Careful sampling of renal sinus, even when the tumor grossly appears away from it, is essential to identify this feature. (Right) This image shows microscopic tumor necrosis ⇾ in a CC-RCC. Microscopic tumor necrosis is usually associated with high-grade tumors and has been considered by some to be an independent prognostic indicator in CC-RCC.

Microscopic Features

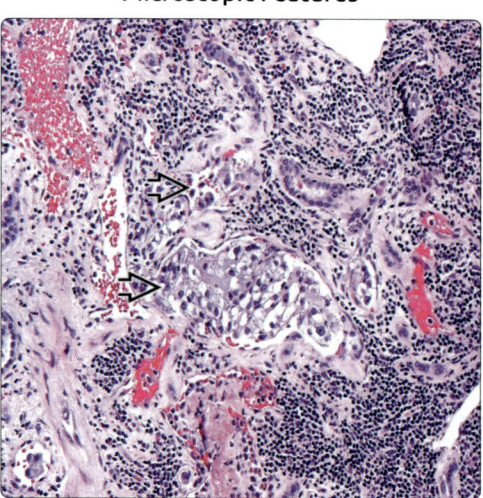

Immunohistochemical Features

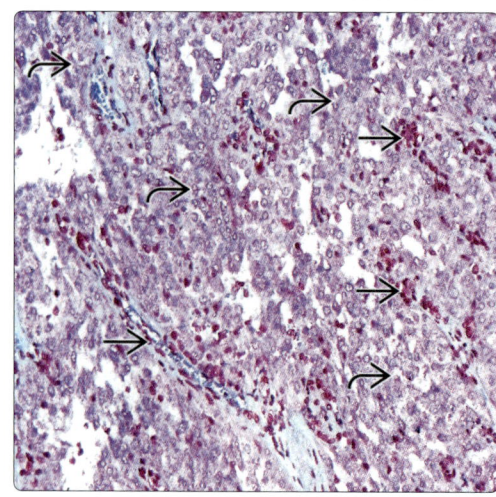

(Left) Small vessel lymphovascular invasion ⇾ is uncommon in CC-RCC. Such vascular invasion has been associated with aggressive clinical behavior and reported to be an independent prognostic indicator in some studies. (Right) BAP1 mutations and loss of BAP1 immunohistochemical nuclear staining ⇾ is associated with high-grade tumors in CC-RCC and often predicts aggressive clinical behavior. Notice the retained positivity in the endothelial and inflammatory cells ⇾.

Clear Cell Renal Cell Carcinoma

HIF-1-α
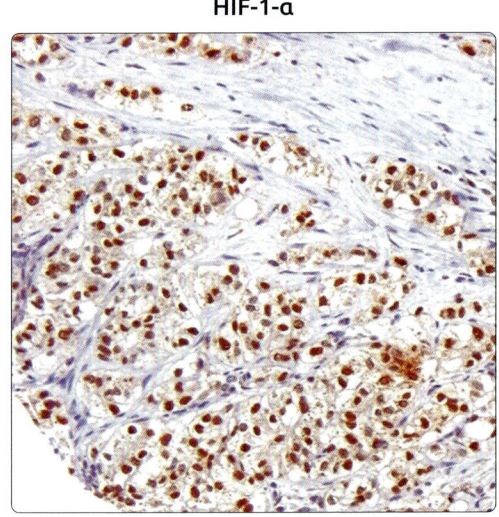

CA9
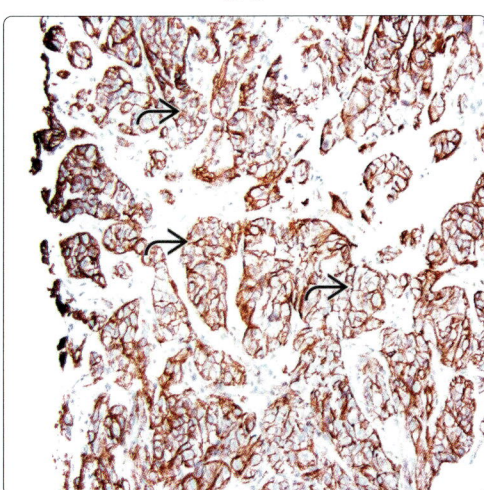

(Left) Immunohistochemical staining shows diffuse nuclear immunoreactivity for HIF-1-α in CC-RCC. Diffuse overexpression of HIF is a consequence of the absence/mutation of VHL gene in most of CC-RCCs. (Right) Diffuse, membrane-predominant (box-like) ➡ immunostaining for CA9 is present in > 90% of CC-RCC. This staining pattern contrasts from the cup-shaped staining in clear cell papillary RCC. Diffuse overexpression of CA9, a downstream molecule for HIF, indicates defective/absent VHL.

CD10
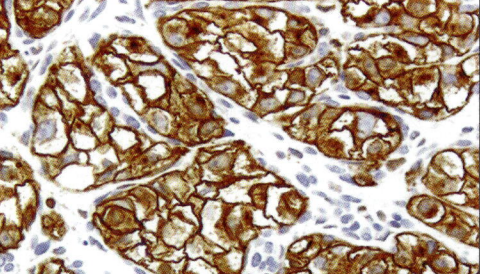

CD10
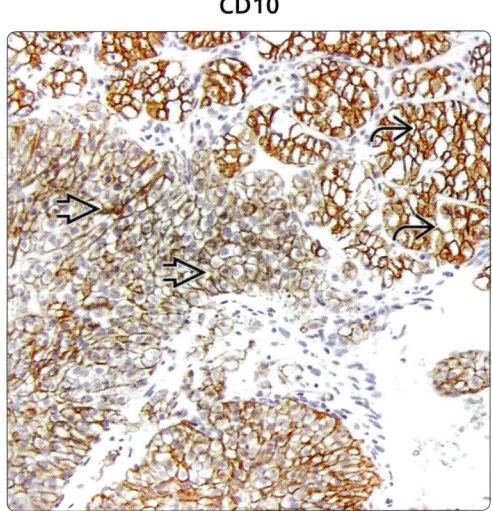

(Left) Immunohistochemical staining for CD10 typically shows diffuse membranous positivity. Any other pattern of staining (e.g., in metastasis of unknown primary) should not be considered characteristic of CC-RCC. (Right) However, CD10 positivity generally tends to be lost or become focal and weaker in higher grade ➡ compared to lower grade areas ➡. A combination of markers CA9, CD10, pax-8, and vimentin is helpful, particularly in a metastatic setting.

EMA
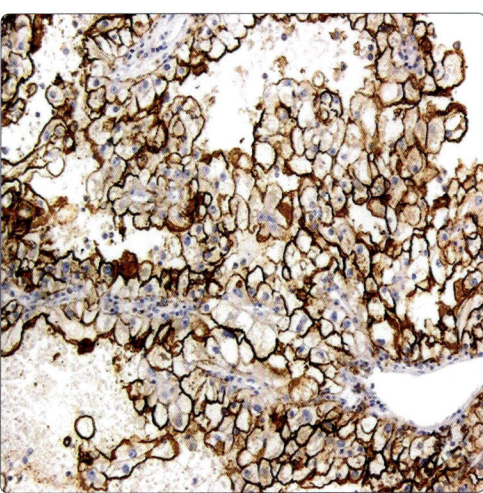

Vimentin
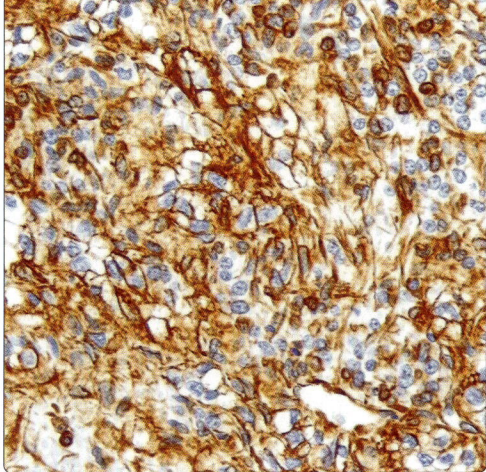

(Left) EMA is a more sensitive epithelial marker than cytokeratin in CC-RCC. Although usually not required for other diagnostic considerations in most cases, EMA negativity in an RCC favors translocation-associated RCC over CC-RCC in the appropriate morphological context. (Right) Staining for vimentin is usually positive in CC-RCC. However, the diffuse positivity, as depicted here, is seen in < 2/3 of tumors. Vimentin is more often positive in high-grade tumors and sarcomatoid areas in a tumor.

Clear Cell Renal Cell Carcinoma

Metastatic Considerations

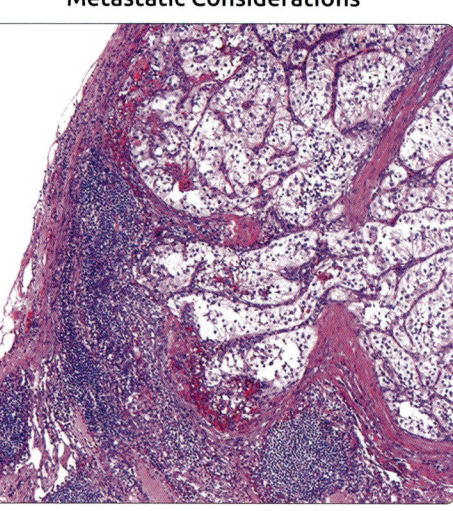
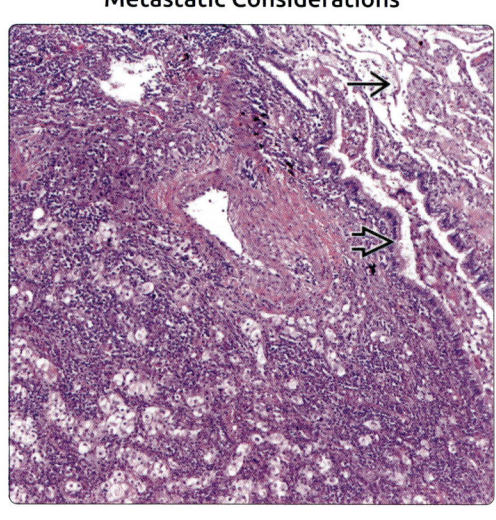

(Left) The image shows a CC-RCC metastatic to a regional lymph node. Clinical history or imaging findings of renal mass are helpful if metastasis is the primary presentation. A combination of CA9, CD10, pax-2 and pax-8, and vimentin is a useful immunohistochemical panel. (Right) CC-RCC frequently metastasizes to the lungs. Notice the background alveolar parenchyma ⇨ and bronchial tissue ⇨ in the image.

Metastatic Considerations

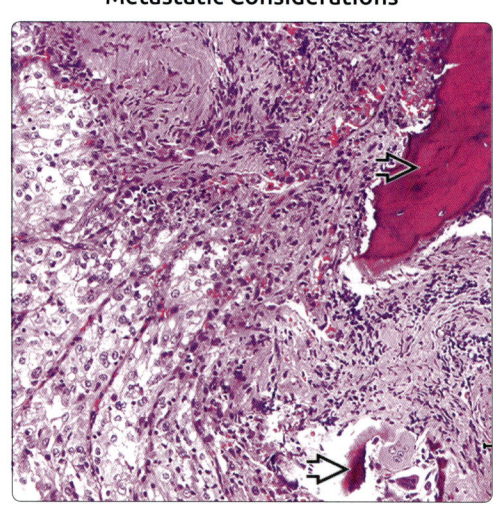
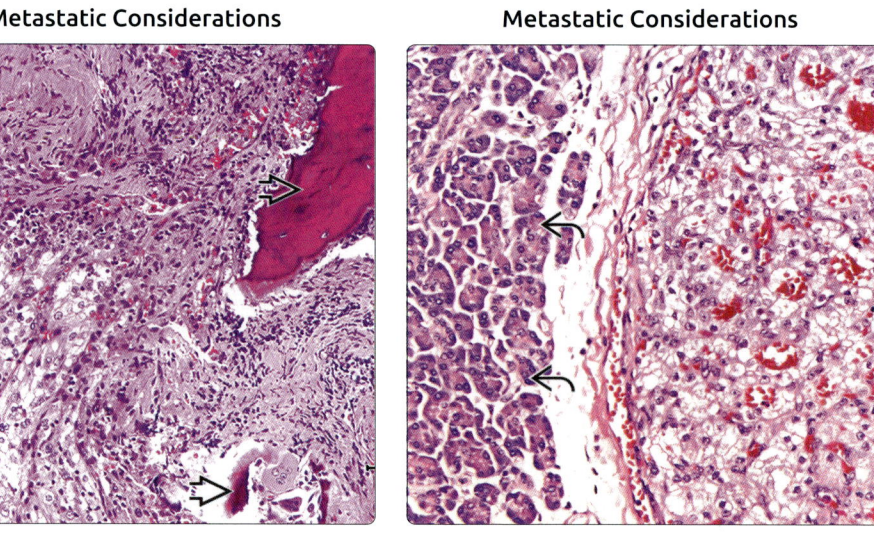

(Left) Besides the lymph nodes, lungs and bone are the most common sites of metastases from CC-RCC. Distorted bony trabeculae ⇨ are identified in this image. CC-RCC does not infrequently show metastasis to unusual sites, sometimes long after the primary diagnosis. (Right) Hematoxylin and eosin section shows CC-RCC metastatic to the pancreas. Note the native pancreatic parenchyma (acini) ⇨.

Metastatic Considerations

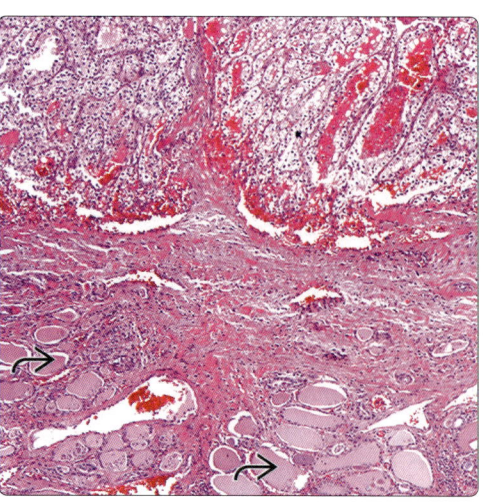
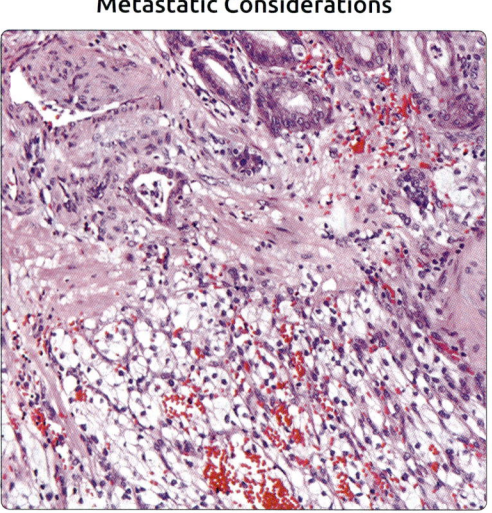

(Left) This image shows CC-RCC metastatic to the thyroid gland. The residual thyroid tissue is seen in the lower 1/2 of the figure ⇨. CC-RCC is only 1 of the differential diagnostic possibilities in a metastasis of unknown primary, as many other neoplasms can have clear cytoplasm. (Right) This image shows a gastric metastasis from CC-RCC. CC-RCC shows a remarkable predilection of metastasizing to unusual sites. RCC should always be in the differential diagnosis of an unusual clear cell tumor at any site.

Clear Cell Renal Cell Carcinoma

Differential Diagnostic Considerations

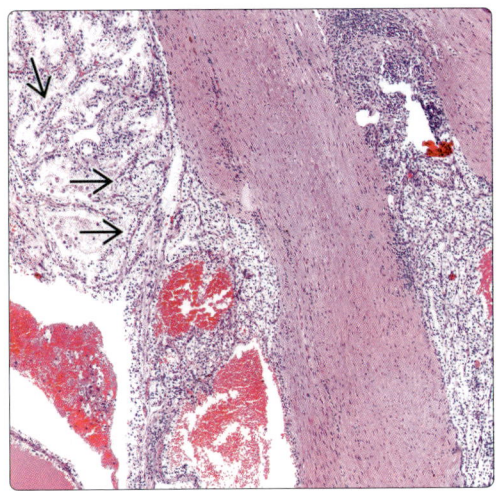

Differential Diagnostic Considerations

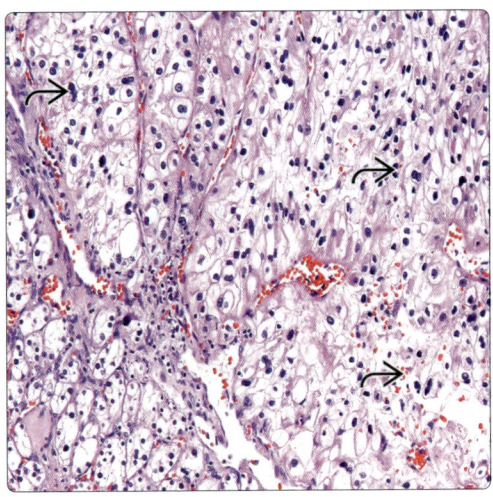

(Left) CC-RCC may show focal areas with linear arrangement of the nuclei ➡, raising the differential diagnostic consideration of CC-PRCC. However, CK7 is either negative or only focally positive in such tumors, unlike that in CC-PRCC. (Right) Some CC-RCCs contain areas superficially resembling chromophobe RCC ➡. However, typical clear cell areas are almost invariably present. Immunostaining for CA9, CD117, and CK7 is also useful in the differentiation.

Differential Diagnostic Considerations

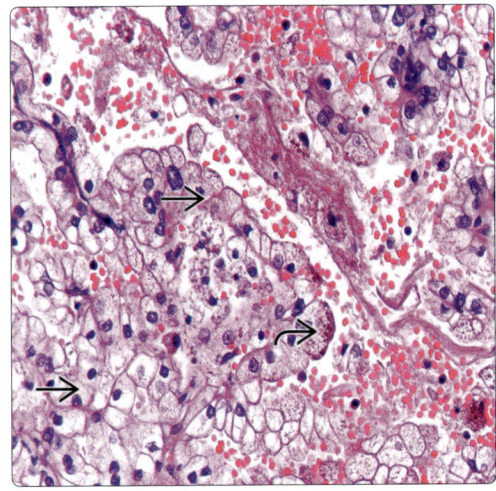

Differential Diagnostic Considerations

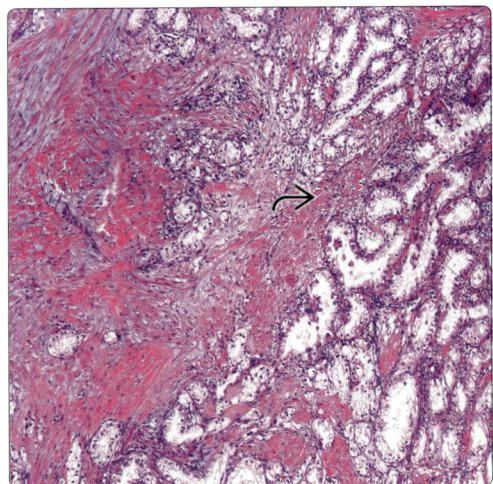

(Left) PRCC may show areas with clear cell cytology ➡. The clear cells in PRCC often show fine cytoplasmic, including hemosiderin ➡, granules, and fibrillations. Similarly, CC-RCC may also contain focal papillary or pseudopapillary foci, often associated with cell breakdown. (Right) Rarely, proven VHL-mutant CC-RCC contains prominent fibromuscular septations ➡. More often, such features should raise the differential diagnostic possibility of TCEB1-mutated or TSC-associated RCC.

Differential Diagnostic Considerations

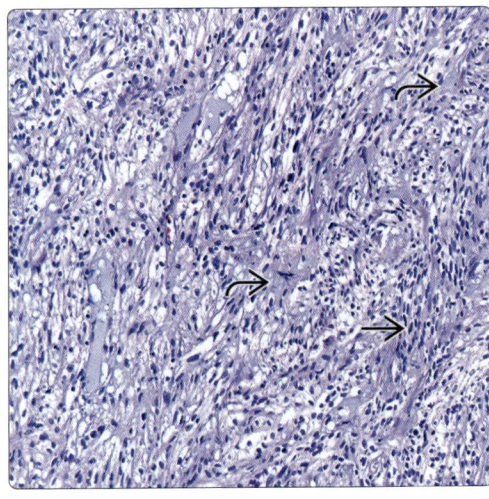

Differential Diagnostic Considerations

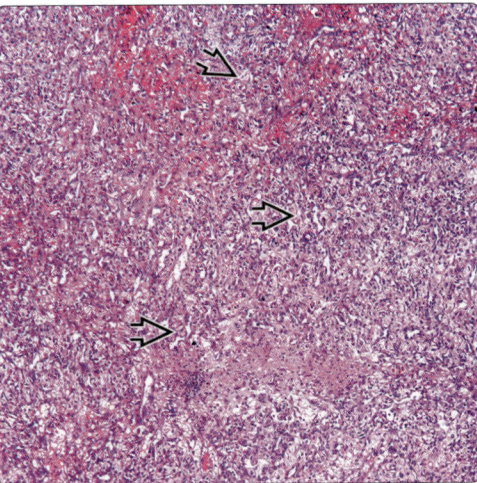

(Left) Rare CC-RCC shows areas with myxoid stroma ➡ and spindle cell areas ➡, mimicking mucinous tubular and spindle cell RCC. Typical CC-RCC histology is often present in other areas. CA9 immunostaining will be useful in more difficult cases. (Right) Some CC-RCC contain foci resembling cerebellar hemangioblastoma, with prominent vascularity ➡ and few clear cells that look like stromal cells. Such areas are often adjacent to foci of sclerosis, and almost always show pax-8 positivity.

Multilocular Cystic Clear Cell Renal Cell Neoplasm of Low Malignant Potential

KEY FACTS

TERMINOLOGY
- Multilocular cystic renal cell neoplasm of low malignant potential (MC-LMP)
- Renal cortical neoplasm composed of numerous clear cell-lined cysts with small clusters of clear cells in tumor septa

ETIOLOGY/PATHOGENESIS
- Presence of *VHL* alterations similar to that in clear cell renal cell carcinoma (RCC)

CLINICAL ISSUES
- On mean follow-up of > 6.5 years, no recurrences or metastases described
- > 80% cases with stage pT1 disease at presentation

MACROSCOPIC
- Well circumscribed, almost always with fibrous pseudocapsule
- Multicystic cut surface with marked variation in size of cysts
- No solid or expansile masses are present in tumor

MICROSCOPIC
- Cyst lining usually consisting of 1 or several layers of neoplastic cells
  - Nonetheless, in many areas epithelial lining may be absent
  - Focal papillations of the cyst lining occasionally present
  - Nuclei randomly distributed in the clear cells
    - Linear arrangement of nuclei not compatible with this diagnosis (suggests clear cell papillary RCC)
- Clusters of tumor cells with clear cytoplasm always present within fibrous septa or in adjacent pseudocapsule
- No expansile or solid masses of tumor evident

TOP DIFFERENTIAL DIAGNOSES
- Cystic nephroma, benign multiloculated renal cortical cysts, cystic clear cell papillary renal cell carcinoma, cystic clear cell renal cell carcinoma with regression, cystic partially differentiated nephroblastoma

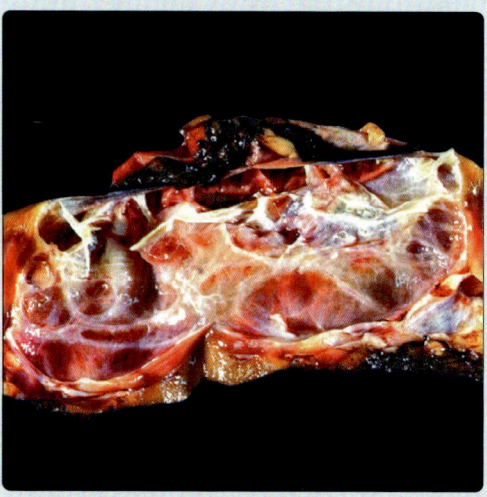

Gross Features

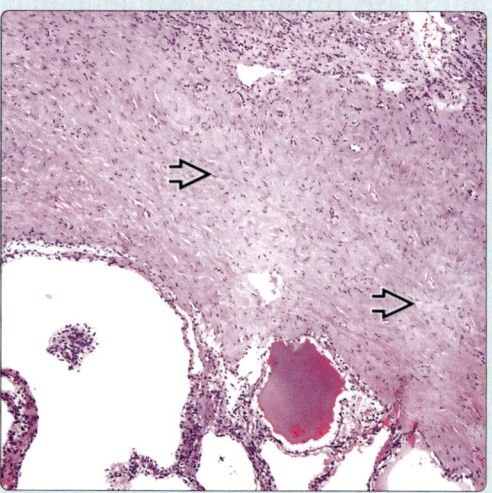

Microscopic Features

(Left) Multilocular cystic clear cell renal cell neoplasms of low malignant potential (MC-LMP) typically show a well-circumscribed tumor almost entirely composed of cysts with thin walls, a prominent fibrous capsule, and no solid expansile areas. (Right) Variably prominent fibrous pseudocapsule ⇒ separating the tumor from the surrounding renal parenchyma, as seen here, is present in all MC-LMP.

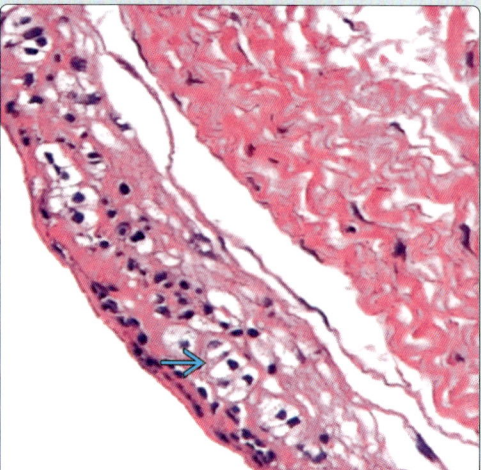

Microscopic Features

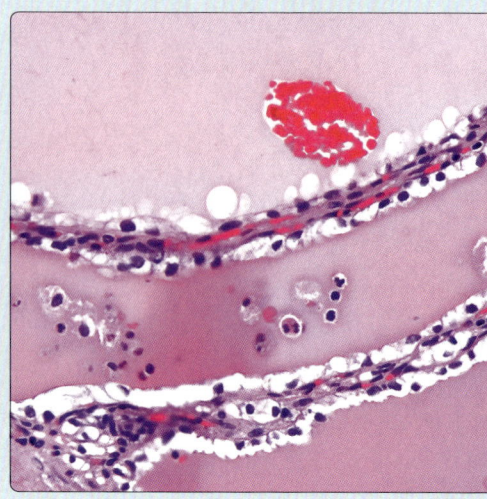

Microscopic Features

(Left) The cysts in MC-LMP are composed of cysts lined by clear cells with small clusters in tumor septa ⇒. (Right) Other tumors may be almost entirely composed of large cysts. Grossly, such tumors will show spongy to predominantly macrocystic features, often filled with serous or hemorrhagic fluid, and occasionally clotted blood.

Multilocular Cystic Clear Cell Renal Cell Neoplasm of Low Malignant Potential

TERMINOLOGY

Abbreviations
- Multilocular cystic renal cell neoplasm of low malignant potential (MC-LMP)

Synonyms
- Multilocular cystic renal cell carcinoma (RCC) (no longer recommended)

Definitions
- Renal cortical neoplasm composed of numerous clear cell-lined cysts with small clusters of clear cells in tumor septa
  - Solid, grossly recognizable areas of clear cells or hyalinization in tumor inconsistent with diagnosis

ETIOLOGY/PATHOGENESIS

Genetic Features
- Presence of VHL alterations similar to that in clear cell RCC; hence, regarded variant of clear cell RCC

CLINICAL ISSUES

Epidemiology
- Incidence
  - Constitute ~ 4% of all clear cell tumors; ~ 200 cases reported in literature
- Age
  - Range: 30-80 years
- Sex
  - M:F = 1.2-2.1:1

Presentation
- 51-90% of cases discovered incidentally on radiologic evaluation for nontumor-related conditions
- Unifocal and unilateral, with only rare exceptions

Prognosis
- On mean follow-up > 6.5 years, no recurrences or metastases described
- > 80% cases with stage pT1 disease at presentation
  - Very rare cases pT3, and even these with benign outcome
  - Because of such outcomes, redesignated by ISUP and WHO as neoplasm of low malignant potential rather than RCC

MACROSCOPIC

General Features
- Well circumscribed, almost always with fibrous pseudocapsule
- Multicystic cut surface containing variably sized cysts with smooth lining
  - May contain serous or bloody fluid, or blood clots
- Septations usually quite thin, with no solid or expansile masses
  - Calcifications in septa occasionally observed

Size
- Range: 1-14 cm (mean: 4.9 cm)

MICROSCOPIC

Histologic Features
- Multilocular cysts with thin fibrous septa and cysts lined by 1 or several layers of neoplastic cells
  - In many areas, epithelial lining may be absent, or be lined by foamy macrophages; focal papillations may be present
  - Tumor cells with clear cytoplasm and Fuhrman/WHO ISUP (nucleolar) grade 1 or 2 nuclei
- Presence of clusters of tumor cells within fibrous septa or in adjacent pseudocapsule with no expansile or solid masses, a definitional requirement

ANCILLARY TESTS

Immunohistochemistry
- CK7(+); CA9(+) in box-like pattern; CD10(-) to focally luminal (+); HMWCK often (+)

DIFFERENTIAL DIAGNOSIS

Cystic Clear Cell Renal Cell Carcinoma With Regression
- Predominantly cystic with fibrosis, hyalinization and occasional calcification
  - Such features suggest tumor regression, and not inherent multilocular cystic nature of tumor

Cystic Clear Cell Papillary Renal Cell Carcinoma
- Linear arrangement of nuclei away from basement membrane
- CA9 characteristically with cup-shaped positivity; CK7, HMWCK and CD10, similar staining patterns in both

Cystic Nephroma
- Multiloculated cysts, often lined by flat to cuboidal or hobnailed cells; rarely with clear cell cytology; no clear cell nests in septa
- ER and PR (+); ovarian-type stroma commonly present

Cystic Partially Differentiated Nephroblastoma
- Primarily lesion of childhood; clusters of blastemal or primitive epithelial elements present in septa

Benign Multiloculated Renal Cortical Cysts
- Multiloculated cysts, usually lined by flat to cuboidal, nonclear cells; no clear cell nests in septa

SELECTED REFERENCES

1. Brimo F et al: Cystic clear cell papillary renal cell carcinoma: is it related to multilocular clear cell cystic neoplasm of low malignant potential? Histopathology. ePub, 2015
2. Srigley JR et al: The International Society of Urological Pathology (ISUP) Vancouver Classification of Renal Neoplasia. Am J Surg Pathol. 37(10):1469-89, 2013
3. Williamson SR et al: Cystic partially regressed clear cell renal cell carcinoma: a potential mimic of multilocular cystic renal cell carcinoma. Histopathology. 63(6):767-79, 2013
4. Gong K et al: Multilocular cystic renal cell carcinoma: an experience of clinical management for 31 cases. J Cancer Res Clin Oncol. 134(4):433-7, 2008
5. Suzigan S et al: Multilocular cystic renal cell carcinoma : a report of 45 cases of a kidney tumor of low malignant potential. Am J Clin Pathol. 125(2):217-22, 2006
6. Murad T et al: Multilocular cystic renal cell carcinoma. Am J Clin Pathol. 95(5):633-7, 1991

Multilocular Cystic Clear Cell Renal Cell Neoplasm of Low Malignant Potential

Microscopic Features

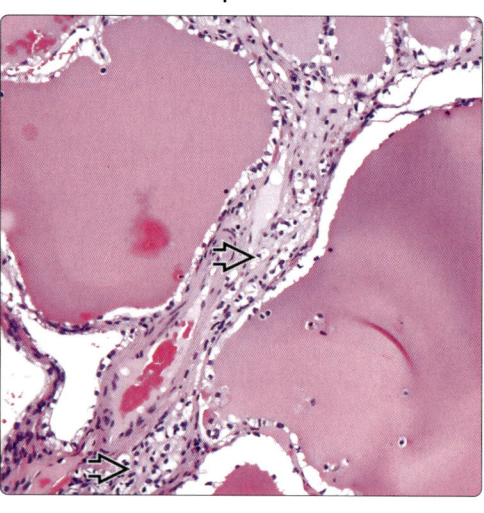

(Left) By definition, MC-LMP always show the presence of clusters of clear cells ⇨ within the fibrous septations. Notice that these clear cells do not alter the smooth profiles of the septa. (Right) Most tumors on microscopic evaluation are composed of variably sized cysts, lined by clear cells with low nuclear grade, and lacking solid or expansile masses. Nuclei are randomly distributed in the clear cells.

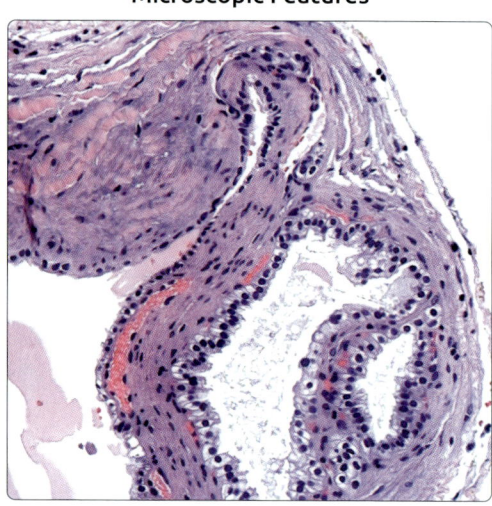

Immunohistochemical Features

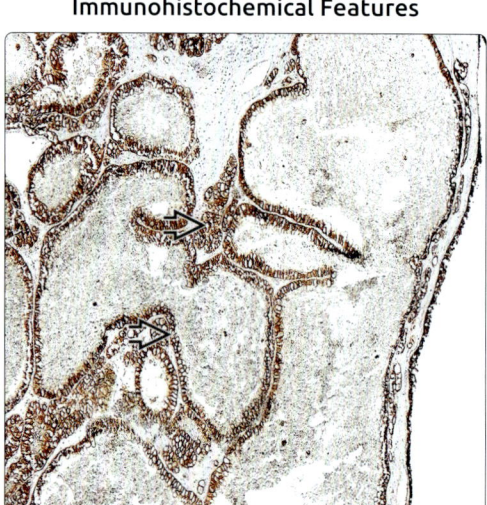

(Left) MC-LMPs show diffuse membranous positivity ⇨ with box-like staining pattern for CA9, similar to that seen in clear cell renal cell carcinoma (RCC). (Right) Most MC-LMPs show positivity for CK7, highlighting the differential diagnostic consideration of clear cell papillary RCC. However, the positivity is often (though not always) patchy, similar to that in clear cell RCCs with cystic features.

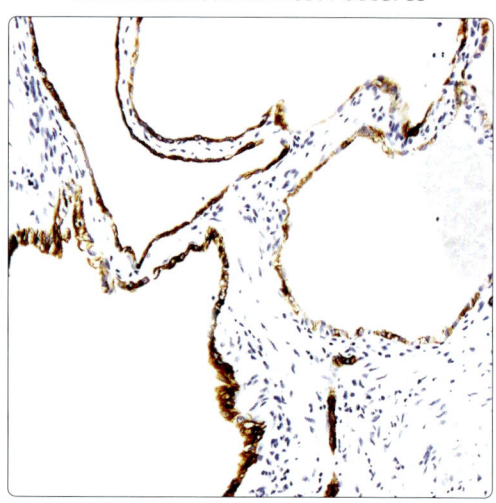

Immunohistochemical Features

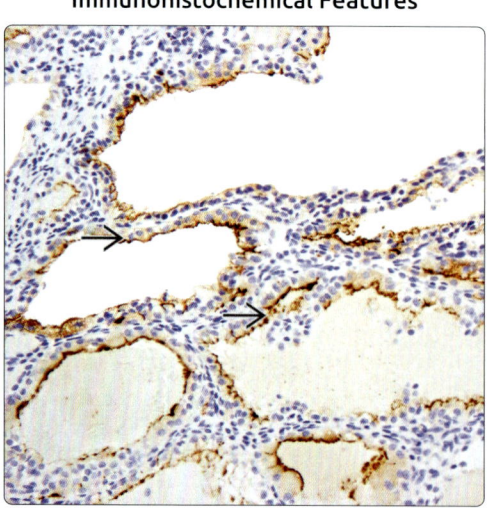

(Left) CD10 immunoreactivity is frequent in MC-LMP. In most cases it is patchy and luminal ⇨, unlike the diffuse membranous reactivity seen in most clear cell RCCs. (Right) Similar to clear cell papillary RCC, staining with HMCK(34βE12) is often positive ⇨ in MC-LMP, thus the relationship of these with clear cell papillary RCC remains indeterminate.

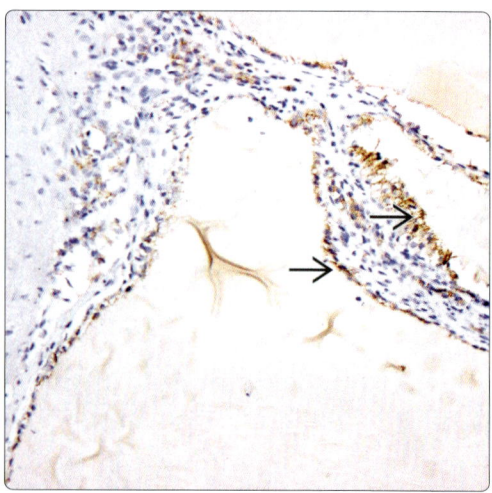

Multilocular Cystic Clear Cell Renal Cell Neoplasm of Low Malignant Potential

Differential Diagnosis: Clear Cell RCC

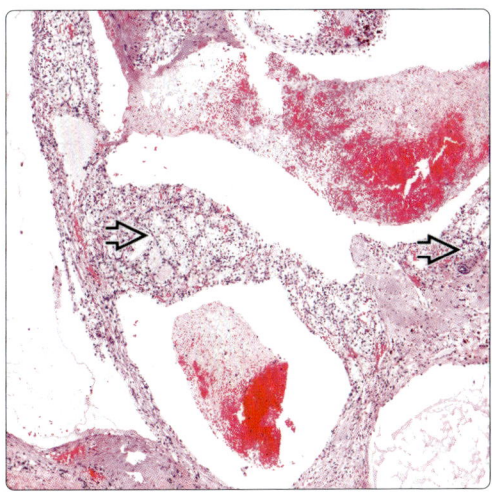

Differential Diagnosis: Clear Cell RCC

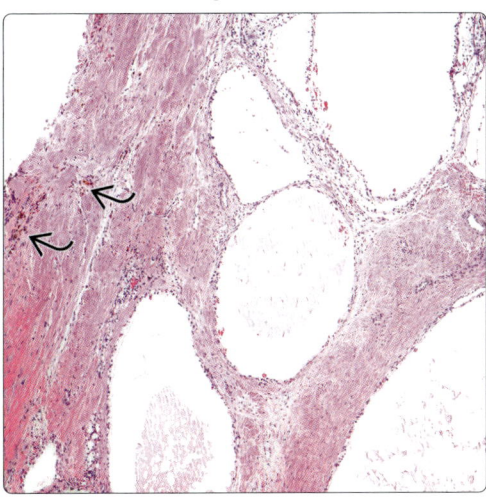

(Left) *Predominantly cystic clear cell tumors with the septations expanded by clear cells ⇒ are not regarded as MC-LMP. These are considered as clear cell RCC with extensive cystic features.* **(Right)** *Tumors composed of predominantly clear cell-lined cysts, but with areas of sclerosis, hemosiderin-laden macrophages ⇒ and dystrophic calcification are best classified as clear cell RCC with regressive changes, and not MC-LMP.*

Differential Diagnosis: Clear Cell Papillary RCC

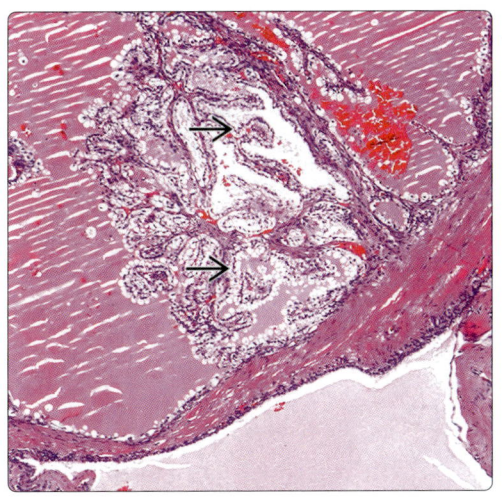

Differential Diagnosis: CPDN

(Left) *Clear cell papillary RCC (CC-PRCC) with cystic features is another close differential diagnostic consideration. The papillary proliferations in CC-PRCC typically show a linear arrangement of nuclei away from basement membrane ⇒. Other than the cup-shaped pattern of positivity for CA9, IHC may not be helpful in this distinction.* **(Right)** *Cystic partially differentiated nephroblastoma (CPDN) can also be mistaken for multilocular cystic clear cell neoplasm, particularly when the blastemal elements in the septate ⇒ are not prominent.*

Differential Diagnosis: Cystic Nephroma

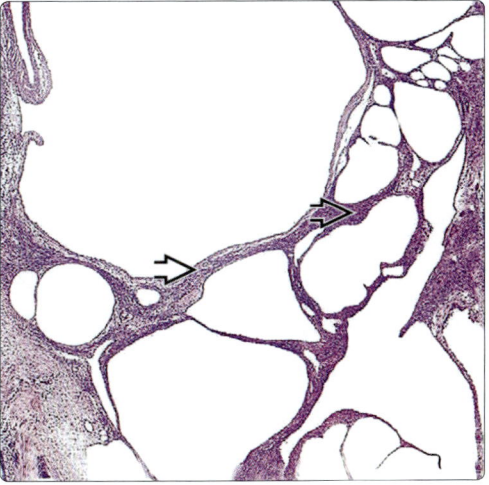

Differential Diagnosis: Segmental Obstructive Dilatation

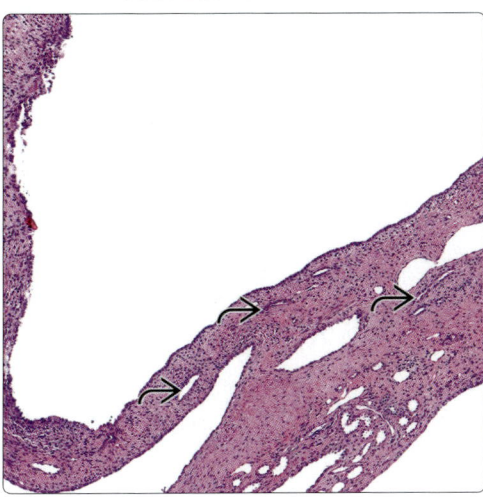

(Left) *Cystic nephroma is also a close differential diagnostic consideration. These tumors often have cellular spindle cell histology ⇒ in the septa. Immunostains for ER and PR are positive.* **(Right)** *Rarely, the collecting system in the kidneys may show segmental dilatation and mimic multilocular cystic neoplasm. This is often related to localized obstruction. The lining of the cystic spaces is often multilayered, urothelial type. Collecting ducts are frequently seen in the septations ⇒.*

Transcription Elongation Factor B (*TCEB1*)-Mutated Renal Cell Carcinoma

KEY FACTS

TERMINOLOGY
- Morphologically, clear cell RCC-like tumor with thick, fibromuscular bands, voluminous cytoplasm, and mutations in *TCEB1* gene

ETIOLOGY/PATHOGENESIS
- Mutations in *TCEB1* gene; gene encodes protein elongin C, subunit of transcription factor B (SIII) complex
  - von Hippel-Lindau tumor suppressor protein binds to elongins B and C, along with other molecules, helping formation of VHL complex
  - Lack of complex prevents degradation and stabilization of HIF
- All tumors with loss of heterozygosity of chromosome 8 at the location of *TCEB1* (8q21.11) in other allele

CLINICAL ISSUES
- Mostly small, pT1a, tumors

MICROSCOPIC
- Well circumscribed with at least partial encapsulation
- Thick fibromuscular bands traversing (and at least partially surrounding) tumor, imparting multinodular appearance to tumor on low-power evaluation
- Variable architectural patterns, often in combination, including small acinar, solid alveolar, tubular (often branching with infoldings, mimicking papillary architecture), focal papillary
- Some tumors with focally linear arrangement of nuclei similar to clear cell papillary RCC

ANCILLARY TESTS
- Diffuse (+) CA9 (membranous, box-like), & HIF-1; CK7 often (+) but not 100% cell positivity as in clear cell papillary RCC

TOP DIFFERENTIAL DIAGNOSES
- Clear cell RCC, clear cell papillary RCC, TSC-associated RCC, other renal tumors with fibromuscular stroma and CK7 positivity

Gross Features
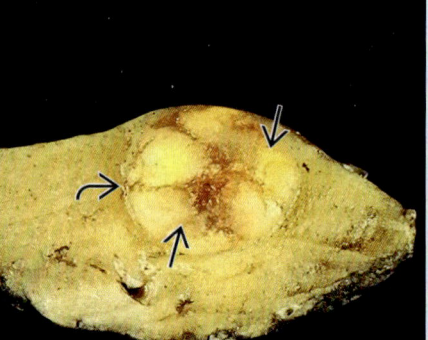

Encapsulation
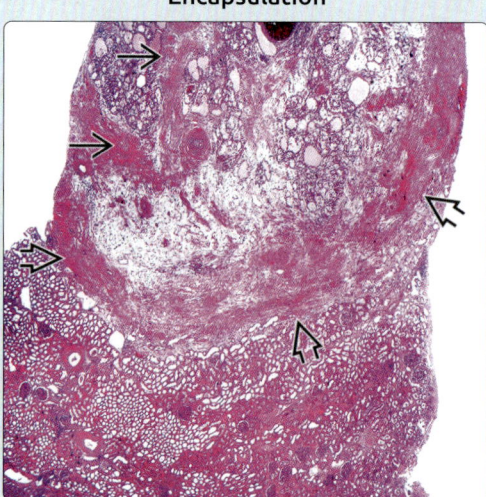

(Left) Grossly, transcription elongation factor B (TCEB1)-mutated RCC is usually a small, well-circumscribed, and often encapsulated ➡ tumor. Cut surface is pale-tan with fibrous bands traversing the tumor, occasionally imparting a grossly nodular appearance ➡. (Right) Low-magnification image of TCEB1-mutated RCC highlights the circumscription and encapsulation ➡ that is present in all tumors described to date. Notice the prominent fibromuscular stroma ➡ that is a characteristic feature of the tumor.

Multinodular Appearance
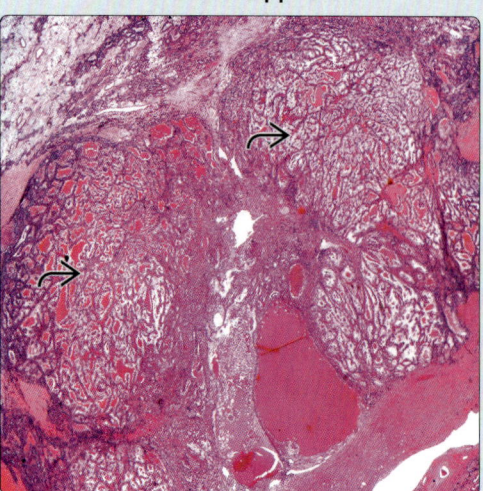

Prominent Fibromuscular Stroma
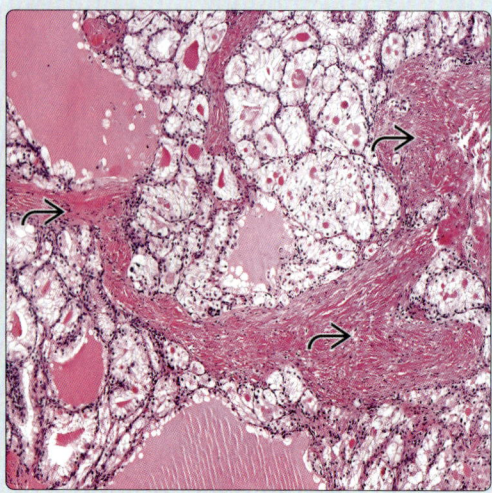

(Left) All described TCEB1-mutated tumors have shown prominent fibromuscular stroma transecting the tumor parenchyma. Such stroma often imparts a vaguely nodular ➡ appearance to the tumor, when viewed by scanner or low magnification under the microscope. (Right) This high-magnification view of the tumor shows variably thick fibromuscular bands ➡ in the tumor parenchyma. The fibromuscular stroma is always present in the tumor, but may be less than prominent in some.

Transcription Elongation Factor B (TCEB1)-Mutated Renal Cell Carcinoma

TERMINOLOGY

Abbreviations
- Transcription elongation factor B (TCEB1)-mutated renal cell carcinoma (RCC)

Definitions
- Morphologically, clear cell RCC-like tumor with thick, fibromuscular bands, voluminous cytoplasm, and mutations in TCEB1 gene

ETIOLOGY/PATHOGENESIS

All Tumors With Mutations in TCEB1 Gene
- This gene encodes protein elongin C, subunit of transcription factor B (SIII) complex
- Located at chromosome 8q21.11
- von Hippel-Lindau tumor suppressor protein binds to elongins B and C, along with other molecules, helping formation of VHL complex
- Complete VHL complex is prerequisite for binding to hydroxylated HIF and its subsequent proteosomic degradation
- Lack of complex prevents degradation and, therefore, stabilization of HIF with activation of downstream products, similar to that in clear cell RCC (CC-RCC)
  - However, mechanism of HIF stabilization different in TCEB1-mutated carcinoma compared to clear cell RCC
- All tumors with loss of heterozygosity (LOH) of chromosome 8 at location of TCEB1 (8q21.11) in other allele
- All tumors lack clear cell RCC signature 3p loss, VHL or other related gene mutations

CLINICAL ISSUES

Presentation
- To date, all tumors identified incidentally on radiological evaluation for unrelated symptoms
- Mostly small, pT1a tumors with only rare tumor with perinephric fat invasion (pT3a)

Treatment
- Size and location dependent, most are amenable to partial nephrectomy

Prognosis
- No metastases reported to date

MACROSCOPIC

General Features
- Grossly, small, well-circumscribed, and often encapsulated tumors, with pale-tan cut surface showing fibrous bands traversing it, occasionally with nodular appearance

MICROSCOPIC

Histologic Features
- Well circumscribed with at least partial encapsulation, with variable amount of cystic change in all
- Thick, fibromuscular bands traversing and surrounding (at least partially) tumor, imparting multinodular appearance to tumor on low-power evaluation
- Variable architectural patterns, in combination, including
  - Small acinar with intricately branching vascular septations (similar to clear cell RCC), solid alveolar, tubular (often branching with infoldings, mimicking papillary architecture), focal true long papillations
- Cytologically, most cells appear to have clear cytoplasm at low-magnification evaluation
  - At higher magnification, however, many of these clear cells show finely granular or reticulate cytoplasm
- All tumors have voluminous cytoplasm, at least focally, with prominent cell membranes
- Nuclei are mostly low grade (equal to nucleolar grade 2)
- Some tumors with focal linear arrangement of nuclei similar to clear cell papillary RCC (CC-PRCC)
- No tumor necrosis, lymphovascular invasion, or histiocytes

ANCILLARY TESTS

Immunohistochemistry
- Diffusely (+) for CA9 (membranous, box-like); CK7 (+), but may be focal to diffuse, but not in 100% of cells
- CD10 variable, (-) to diffusely (+); HMW-CK usually (-), rarely (+)

Genetic Testing
- All tumors with LOH of chromosome 8 at location of TCEB1 (8q21.11)
- All tumors with mutations in TCEB1 gene

DIFFERENTIAL DIAGNOSIS

Clear Cell RCC
- Combination of prominent fibromuscular stroma, nodular appearance within tumor, voluminous cells, and CK7 positivity should raise possibility of TCEB1-mutated RCC
- Molecular testing for 3p loss, or VHL and related gene mutations characteristic

Clear Cell Papillary RCC
- CC-PRCC has diffuse linear nuclear arrangement
- CK7 stains almost 100% of cells; CA9 cup-shaped (+), and HMW-CK is almost always diffusely (+)

Tuberous Sclerosis Complex (TSC)-Associated RCC
- Some TSC-associated RCC may resemble TCEB1-mutated carcinoma
  - TSC-associated RCC often multifocal and bilateral, usually associated with family history
  - Surrounding renal parenchyma and lymph nodes often with angiomyolipomas

Other Renal Tumors With Fibromuscular Stroma and CK7 Positivity
- Since not investigated for TCEB1 mutations, difficult to determine their true nature

SELECTED REFERENCES

1. Argani P: MiT family translocation renal cell carcinoma. Semin Diagn Pathol. 32(2):103-13, 2015
2. Hakimi AA et al: TCEB1-mutated renal cell carcinoma: a distinct genomic and morphological subtype. Mod Pathol. 28(6):845-53, 2015
3. Williamson SR et al: Renal cell carcinoma with angioleiomyoma-like stroma: clinicopathological, immunohistochemical, and molecular features supporting classification as a distinct entity. Mod Pathol. 28(2):279-94, 2015

Transcription Elongation Factor B (*TCEB1*)-Mutated Renal Cell Carcinoma

Branching Tubules

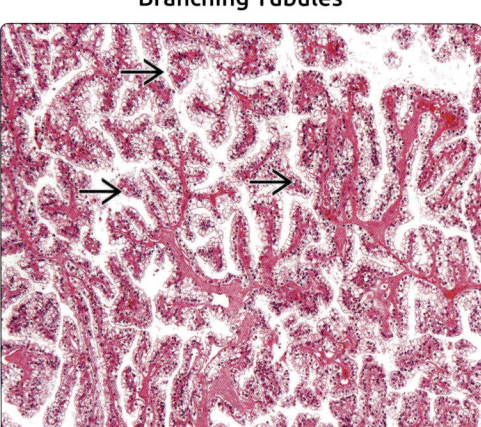

Branching Tubules

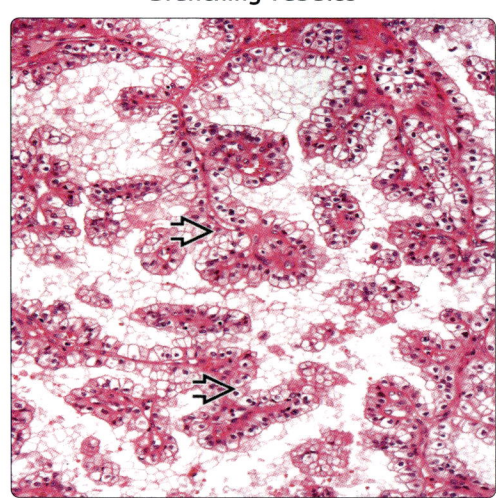

(Left) In addition to small acinar and alveolar patterns, cystic branching tubules with infoldings that mimic papillary architecture ⇒ are characteristic. Tubular or branching tubular architecture is the most common pattern in TCEB1-mutated carcinoma. **(Right)** In this higher magnification view, exaggerated branching of tubules has given rise to papillations ⇒ that may at times be difficult to differentiate from a true papillary architecture.

Papillary Architecture

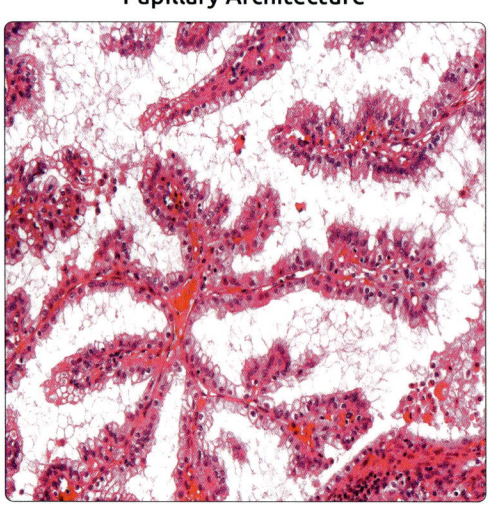

Voluminous Cytoplasm

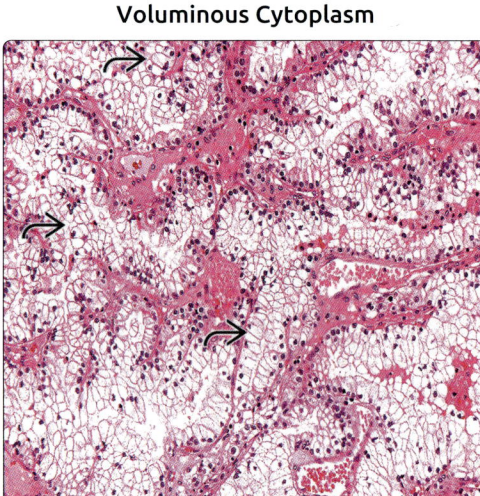

(Left) Papillary architecture is focally present in a number of TCEB1-mutated renal cell carcinomas. However, unlike the papillae of a true papillary renal cell carcinoma, no macrophages are noted in the papillary cores, and the tumor also lacks any necrosis. **(Right)** Another characteristic feature of TCEB1-mutated carcinomas is the presence of cells with voluminous cytoplasm with prominent cell membranes ⇒, at least focally, in all tumors.

Voluminous Cytoplasm With Fine Granularity

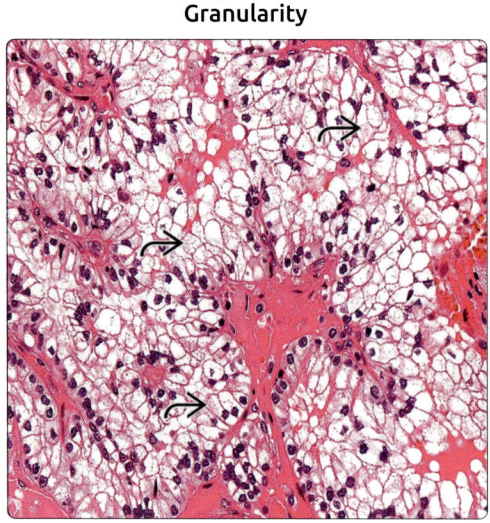

Linear Arrangement of Nuclei

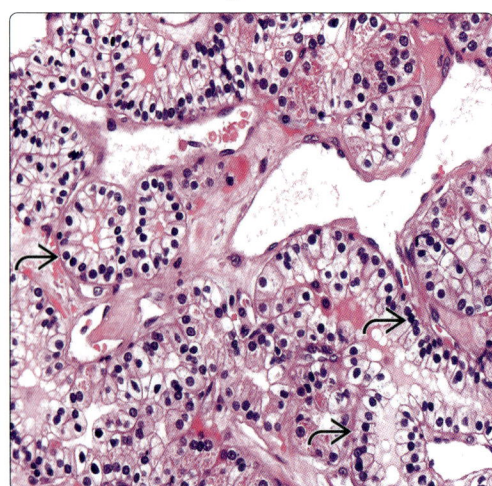

(Left) Cytologically, most cells in TCEB1-mutated RCCs appear to have a clear cytoplasm at low-power evaluation. However, at higher magnification many such clear cells show finely granular cytoplasm ⇒. Focally, a greater degree of cytoplasmic eosinophilia may also be present. **(Right)** Some tumors show linear arrangement of the nuclei ⇒ similar to that seen in CC-PRCC; however, this is always focal. Branching tubular architecture and linear nuclear arrangement may raise the suspicion of a CC-PRCC.

Transcription Elongation Factor B (*TCEB1*)-Mutated Renal Cell Carcinoma

Cystic and Nested Architecture

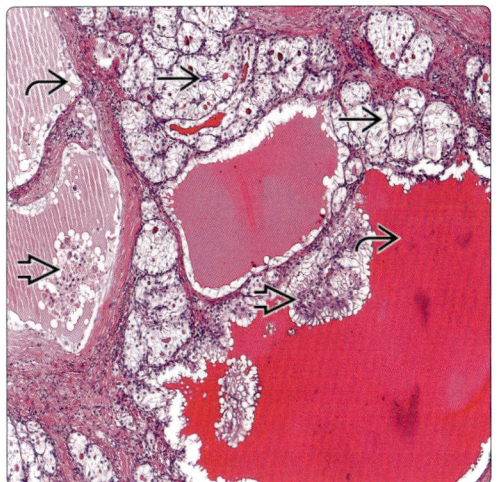

Box-Shaped Pattern: CA9

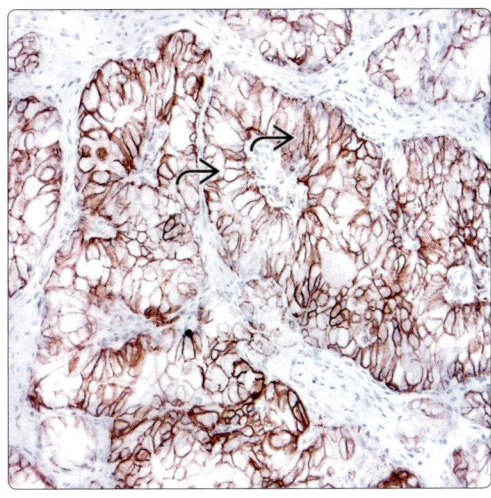

(Left) At least focal cystic architecture is present in most of TCEB1-mutated renal cell carcinomas. This image shows a combination of cystic ➡ and nested ➡ architectures. Cyst lining also shows papillary proliferation ➡, not uncommon in the tumor. **(Right)** CA9 staining pattern in TCEB1-mutated renal cell carcinoma is the same as in clear cell renal cell carcinoma (diffuse membranous, box-shaped ➡). This is in distinction from the cup-shaped pattern seen in clear cell papillary renal cell carcinoma.

CK7 Positivity

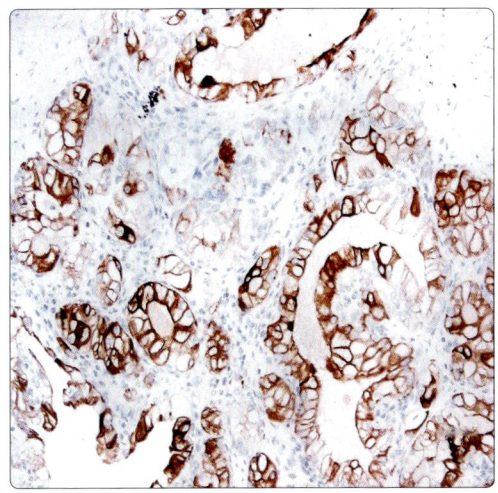

Differential Diagnosis: Clear Cell Papillary RCC

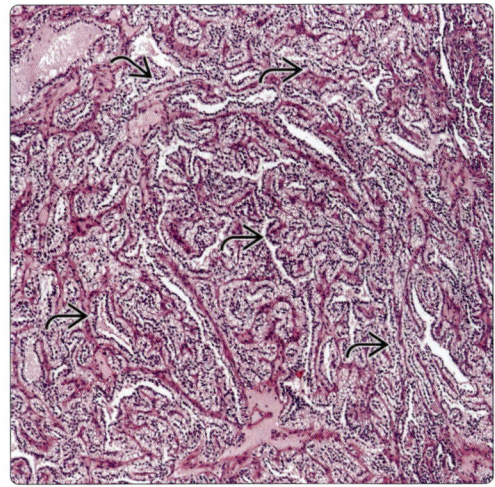

(Left) All TCEB1-mutated carcinomas show positive staining for CK7. The immunoreactivity ranges from focal, patchy to more diffuse. However, the staining is not reported to be positive in 100% of tumor cells in any case, as of today. **(Right)** This image of a clear cell papillary RCC shows the prominent branching tubular architecture, similar to that in TCEB1-mutated tumors. However, the linear arrangement of the nuclei is present throughout ➡, unlike such focal presence in the latter tumor.

Differential Diagnosis: CA9

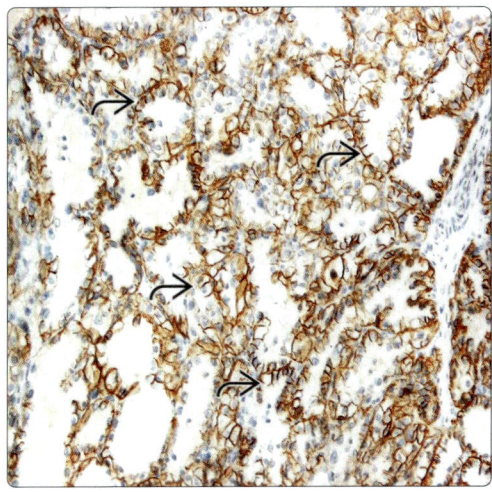

Differential Diagnosis: CK7

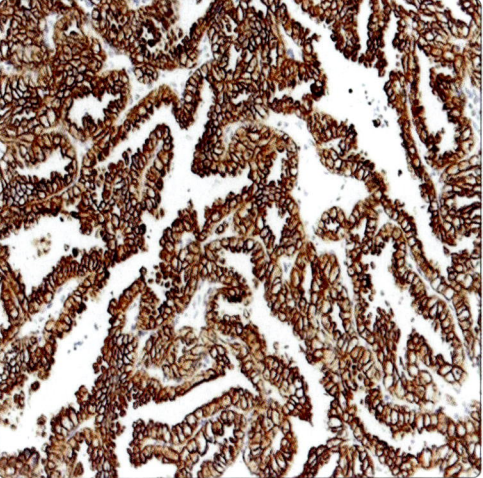

(Left) Unlike the box-shaped staining pattern with CA9 in TCEB1-mutated carcinomas, clear cell papillary RCC shows the characteristic cup-shaped staining pattern, with lack of positivity along the luminal aspects of the cells ➡. **(Right)** CK7 stains 100% of the tumor cells in almost all clear cell papillary RCCs. Thus, the immunohistochemical staining patterns for CA9 and CK7 can easily help in differentiation of most TCEB1-mutated tumors from clear cell papillary renal cell carcinoma.

Clear Cell Papillary Renal Cell Carcinoma

KEY FACTS

TERMINOLOGY
- Carcinoma with clear cell cytology, low nuclear grade, papillary and tubular/branching tubular/acinar architecture, and nuclei in linear arrangement away from basal aspect of cells includes tumor previously called RAT
  - Characteristic immunoprofile: Diffuse CK7(+), CA-IX(+) (with cup-shaped positivity), 34BE12(+), CD10(-)

ETIOLOGY/PATHOGENESIS
- No 3p25.3 losses
- No *VHL* gene mutations or trisomies of chromosome 7 or losses of Y
- Sorbitol pathway likely mechanism of HIF activation

CLINICAL ISSUES
- Most tumors small, pT1 stage
- Likely biologically indolent; no metastases reported to date

MICROSCOPIC
- Often cystic
- Usually prominent papillary architecture
  - Tubular, branching tubular and collapsed acinar solid-appearing architecture is also common
- Almost all cells with clear cytoplasm
- Nuclei, almost always low grade
- Diagnostically essential, diffuse nuclear arrangement in linear alignment, away from basal aspect of cells, usually in center of cytoplasm or more apical
- CK7(+), CA9(+) (cup-like pattern), HMCK (34βE12)(+), CD10 (-) or focally (+), AMACR(-)

TOP DIFFERENTIAL DIAGNOSES
- Clear cell renal cell carcinoma (RCC) with clear cell papillary-like areas
- Papillary RCC
- Translocation-associated renal carcinoma
- Other CK7(+) clear cell tumors with prominent fibromuscular stroma

Gross: Cystic
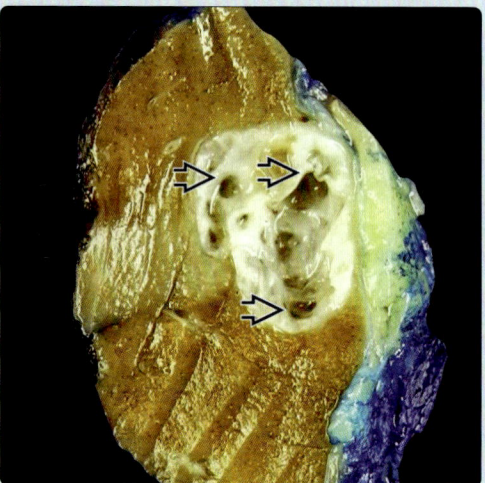

Gross: Solid
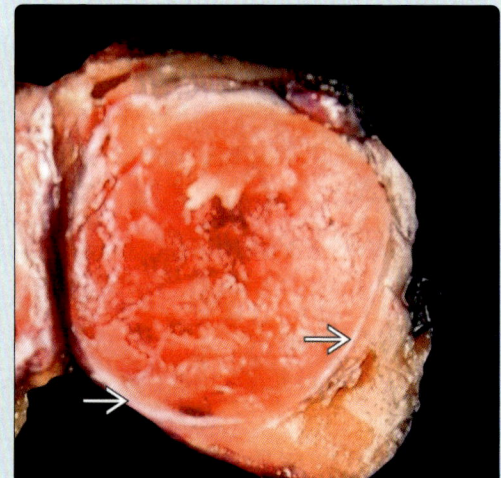

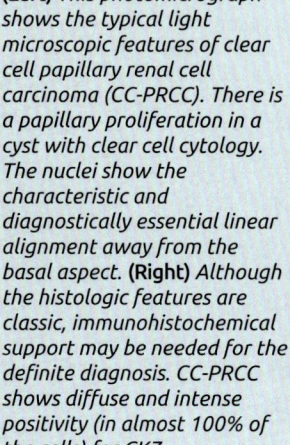

(Left) Clear cell papillary RCCs of the kidney are prominently or predominantly cystic ➡. The tumors are often small in size and well circumscribed with a well-defined capsule. Multifocal tumors may occasionally be seen, more often in the setting of end-stage kidneys. (Right) Some tumors appear more solid. Notice the prominent capsule ➡. This is a typical finding in clear cell papillary RCC. CC-PRCC shares this gross feature with papillary renal cell carcinoma. On the other hand, it lacks necrosis, a common finding in papillary RCC.

Microscopic Features
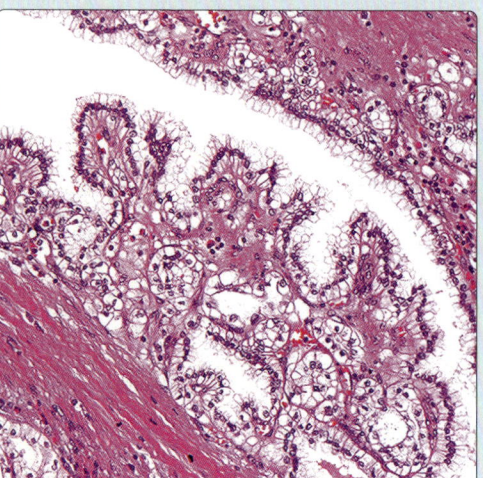

Immunohistochemical Features
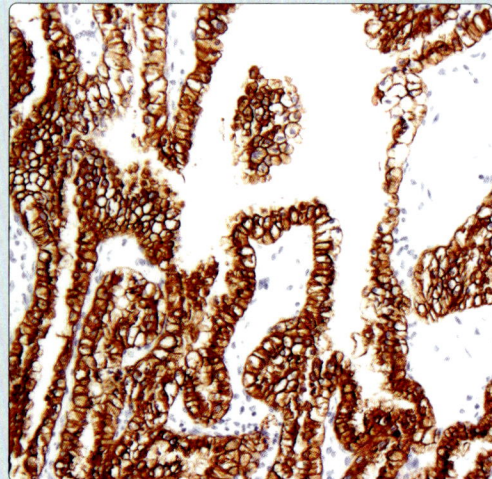

(Left) This photomicrograph shows the typical light microscopic features of clear cell papillary renal cell carcinoma (CC-PRCC). There is a papillary proliferation in a cyst with clear cell cytology. The nuclei show the characteristic and diagnostically essential linear alignment away from the basal aspect. (Right) Although the histologic features are classic, immunohistochemical support may be needed for the definite diagnosis. CC-PRCC shows diffuse and intense positivity (in almost 100% of the cells) for CK7.

Clear Cell Papillary Renal Cell Carcinoma

TERMINOLOGY

Abbreviations
- Clear cell papillary renal cell carcinoma (CC-PRCC)

Definitions
- Carcinoma with clear cell cytology, mostly low nuclear grade, branching tubular/acinar/papillary architecture, linear alignment of nuclei away from basal aspect of cells
  o Diagnostically important characteristic immunoprofile
  o Includes tumors previously called renal angiomyoadenomatous tumor (RAT), which contain prominent smooth muscle stroma

ETIOLOGY/PATHOGENESIS

End-Stage Kidneys
- Often associated with end-stage renal disease
  o But more commonly seen in nonend-stage setting ± impaired renal function

Molecular Features
- No 3p25.3 losses, *VHL* gene mutations, or trisomies of chromosome 7 or losses of Y
- Activation of HIF pathway by non-VHL-dependent mechanisms
  o Elevated intracellular sorbitol, causing hypertonic/hyperosmotic stress, likely mechanism of HIF pathway activation
- MicroRNA (miR)200 family overexpressed in CC-PRCC
  o Low levels present in clear cell renal cell carcinoma (RCC) and papillary RCC

CLINICAL ISSUES

Presentation
- Initially reported in setting of end-stage renal disease ± acquired cystic disease
  o However, now more often recognized in nonend-stage setting
- Estimated to account for up to 4.3% of all renal cell tumors
  o Considered 4th most common type of RCC in 1 recent study
- In addition to clear cell RCC, CC-PRCC-like tumors also seen in patients with VHL syndrome
  o Whether these represent true sporadic-like CC-PRCC or another distinct entity remains to be settled
- Mostly unifocal, occasionally multifocal at presentation
- Most tumors small, pT1 stage; rarely invade perinephric fat, pT3a
- No lymph node or other metastases reported to date

Treatment
- Surgical approaches
  o Due to smaller size and nonaggressive radiologic appearance, usually treated by partial nephrectomy or tumor ablation

Prognosis
- Biologically indolent tumor
  o No metastases reported to date

IMAGING

CT Scan Reveals Low Density With Cystic Change or Cystic Formation
- MR shows isointensity on T1WI and hypointensity on T2WI

MACROSCOPIC

General Features
- Usually well circumscribed
- Variably, but often prominently, cystic
- Some tumors entirely solid

Size
- Usually small
  o Mean size: 2.6 cm; largest described tumor: 6 cm

MICROSCOPIC

Histologic Features
- Well circumscribed, often encapsulated
  o Some tumors with prominent myoid metaplasia of capsule with intratumoral fibromuscular stroma
- Often cystic
  o However, some tumors predominantly solid with very few cystic areas
- Common architectural patterns include tubular with frequent branching, papillary, tubulocystic, and compact nested
  o Tubular branching often imparts pseudopapillary appearance
- Many tumors with true and occasionally prominent papillary architecture with fibrovascular cores
  o Some with tightly packed papillae giving rise to solid appearance
- Tightly packed, very small, collapsed acini give tumor solid, sheet-like appearance
- Some other tumors with clear cell cytology, CK7 positivity, and prominent fibromuscular stroma mimic CC-PRCC
  o Many such tumors with CC-PRCC features (nuclear arrangement) in only focal/patchy areas now regarded as not representing CC-PRCC
- Necrosis is not feature of the tumor
  o However, degenerative changes with foamy macrophages, cholesterol clefts, and foreign body giant cell reaction may be rarely present
- Almost all cells have clear cytoplasm
  o Except in solid collapsed acinar areas
    – Scant cytoplasm in these areas makes cells appear somewhat amphophilic
- Nuclei almost always low grade (equivalent or lower than Fuhrman/nucleolar grade 2)
- Most characteristic feature is arrangement of nuclei
  o Nuclei in linear arrangement, away from basal aspect of cells, usually in center of cytoplasm or more apical
  o Such arrangement present in most of the tumor, even in areas with acinar growth pattern
  o In solid, collapsed acinar areas, such pattern may not be easily discernible
- Proteinaceous, colloid-like secretions frequently observed within lumina of tubules, acini, and cystic spaces

Clear Cell Papillary Renal Cell Carcinoma

ANCILLARY TESTS

Immunohistochemistry

- CK7
  - Diffusely and strongly positive (almost always 100% of cells)
- CA9
  - Diffusely positive; with almost invariable absence of staining along luminal aspect of cells (cup-like pattern)
- HMCK (34βE12)
  - Often diffusely positive
- AMACR: Negative
- CD10: Negative or very focally positive
- B-RAF: Often positive
- Parafibromin and hKIM-1: More often positive, compared to clear cell or papillary RCC
- c-MET: Positive in > 90%

DIFFERENTIAL DIAGNOSIS

Clear Cell Renal Cell Carcinoma With Clear Cell Papillary-Like Areas

- Papillary areas uncommon
- Only focal or patchy linear nuclear arrangement
  - Random nuclear arrangement in rest of tumor
    - Tumors with only focal or patchy linear nuclear arrangement are often clear cell or other types of RCC
    - Such tumors not to be regarded as CC-RCC or hybrid CC-RCC and clear cell RCC
- Usually diffuse CD10 immunoreactivity; CK7 patchy or negative; CA-IX, box-like; 34βE12, usually negative
  - Rare CC-PRCC reported in literature to show 3p losses or VHL mutations
    - These tumors very likely do not represent true CC-PRCC

Papillary Renal Cell Carcinoma

- Optically transparent clear cytoplasm not seen
  - Clear cells when present, show finely reticulated, granular cytoplasm
    - Such clear cells often contain finely granular hemosiderin pigment
- Foamy macrophages, areas of necrosis very common
- IHC: CK7(+), AMACR(+), and CA9(-) or only focally positive

Other CK7(+) Renal Tumors With Prominent Fibromuscular Stroma

- Other tumors with variable tubular architecture, prominent fibromuscular septations, and diffuse CK7 positivity are now recognized as being distinct
  - Some with CC-PRCC-like areas considered to be within morphologic spectrum of CC-PRCC, e.g., RAT
  - Others with such features, but with at the most only focal true CC-PRCC-like areas, include
    - Newly described *TCEB1*-mutated RCC
    - Some cases of *TSC1*-associated RCC
    - Rare, MiTF/TFE family translocation-associated RCC
      - Unlike CC-PRCC, these tumors show
      - At most, only very focal linear arrangement of nuclei
- Patchy CK7 positivity; and not virtually diffuse tumor cell positivity as in CC-RCC
- CA9, if positive, with box-like staining pattern
- CD10 positivity
- Negative staining for 34βE12
- Specific clinical, IHC, or genetic features characteristic of condition

MiTF/TFE-Family Translocation-Associated Renal Cell Carcinoma

- Predominant clear cell histology is rare
- Often associated with cells containing eosinophilic cytoplasm
  - Clear cells with ballooned out cytoplasm frequently seen
- Combination of nested and papillary architecture
- Psammoma bodies often present
- Usually high nuclear grade
- Cytokeratins and EMA/MUC1 usually negative or very focally positive
- TFE (TFE3 or TFEB) immunostains positive depending on cytogenetic profile

SELECTED REFERENCES

1. Aron M et al: Clear cell-papillary renal cell carcinoma of the kidney not associated with end-stage renal disease: clinicopathologic correlation with expanded immunophenotypic and molecular characterization of a large cohort with emphasis on relationship with renal angiomyoadenomatous tumor. Am J Surg Pathol. 39(7):873-88, 2015
2. Deml KF et al: Clear cell papillary renal cell carcinoma and renal angiomyoadenomatous tumor: two variants of a morphologic, immunohistochemical, and genetic distinct entity of renal cell carcinoma. Am J Surg Pathol. 39(7):889-901, 2015
3. Hakimi AA et al: TCEB1-mutated renal cell carcinoma: a distinct genomic and morphological subtype. Mod Pathol. 28(6):845-53, 2015
4. Parihar A et al: Xp11 translocation renal cell carcinoma morphologically mimicking clear cell-papillary renal cell carcinoma in an adult patient: report of a case expanding the morphologic spectrum of xp11 translocation renal cell carcinomas. Int J Surg Pathol. 23(3):234-7, 2015
5. Guo J et al: Tuberous sclerosis-associated renal cell carcinoma: a clinicopathologic study of 57 separate carcinomas in 18 patients. Am J Surg Pathol. 38(11):1457-67, 2014
6. Kuroda N et al: Clear cell papillary renal cell carcinoma: a review. Int J Clin Exp Pathol. 7(11):7312-8, 2014
7. Aydin H et al: Clear cell tubulopapillary renal cell carcinoma: a study of 36 distinctive low-grade epithelial tumors of the kidney. Am J Surg Pathol. 34(11):1608-21, 2010
8. Michal M et al: Difference between RAT and clear cell papillary renal cell carcinoma/clear renal cell carcinoma. Virchows Arch. 454(6):719, 2009
9. Verine J: Renal angiomyoadenomatous tumor: morphologic, immunohistochemical, and molecular genetic study of a distinct entity. Virchows Arch. 454(4):479-80, 2009
10. Gobbo S et al: Clear cell papillary renal cell carcinoma: a distinct histopathologic and molecular genetic entity. Am J Surg Pathol. 32(8):1239-45, 2008
11. Tickoo SK et al: Pathologic features of renal cortical tumors. Urol Clin North Am. 35(4):551-61; v, 2008
12. Tickoo SK et al: Spectrum of epithelial neoplasms in end-stage renal disease: an experience from 66 tumor-bearing kidneys with emphasis on histologic patterns distinct from those in sporadic adult renal neoplasia. Am J Surg Pathol. 30(2):141-53, 2006

Clear Cell Papillary Renal Cell Carcinoma

Gross
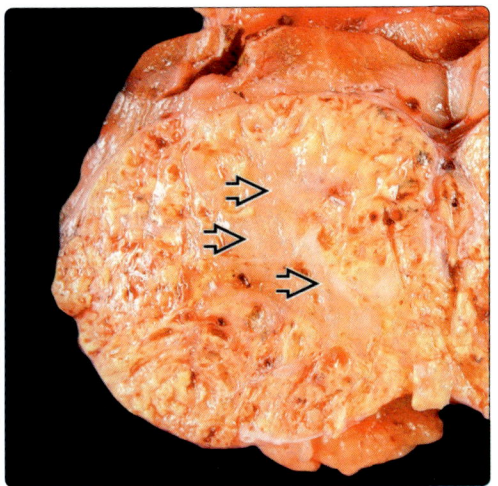

Capsule
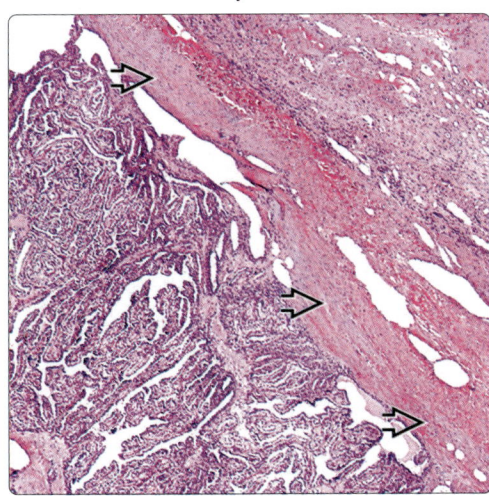

(Left) Some CC-PRCCs show a combination of solid and cystic appearance with a spongy cut surface or even more solid cut surface without any gross cysts. Irregular scars ⇨ may occasionally be seen in the center of the lesion. (Right) Hematoxylin and eosin-stained section shows a thick fibrous capsule in a CC-PRCC ⇨. The tumor is composed of elongated tubules with frequent branching and tightly packed papillae. The architecture overlaps considerably with papillary RCC.

Intracystic Growth
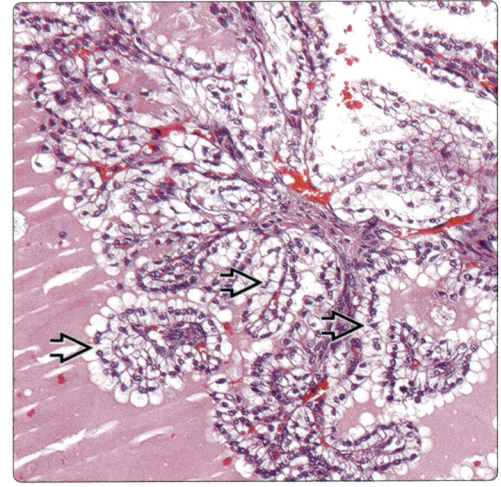

Compact Architecture
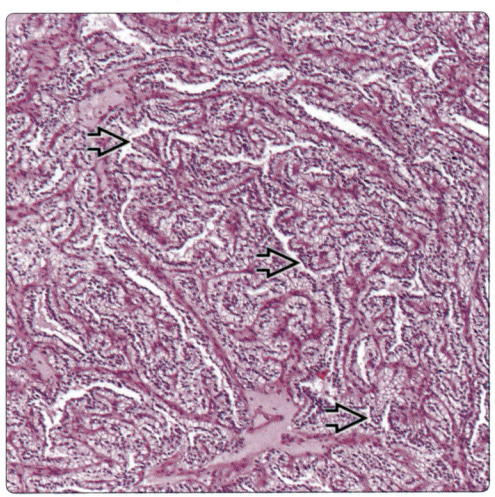

(Left) Many CC-PRCCs contain a prominent cystic component. In many such areas, as seen here, the walls of the cysts show papillary proliferations lined by cells with clear cytoplasm. The nuclei are aligned in a single layer away from the basal aspect of the cells ⇨. (Right) Section from a noncystic component of the tumor shows more solid areas with tightly packed branching tubules. Branching of tubules, a characteristic feature of the tumor, often imparts pseudopapillary architecture in CC-PRC ⇨.

Tubular and Cystic Architecture
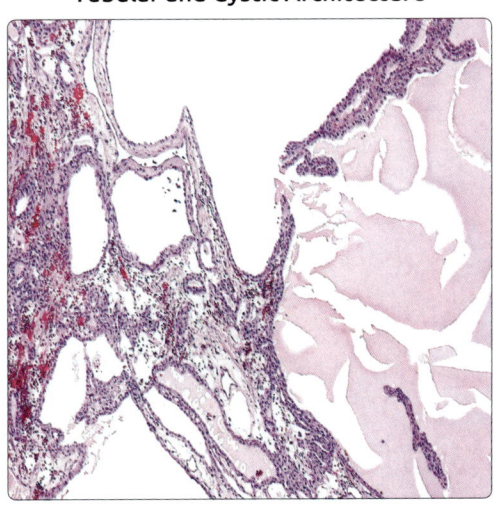

Architectural Patterns
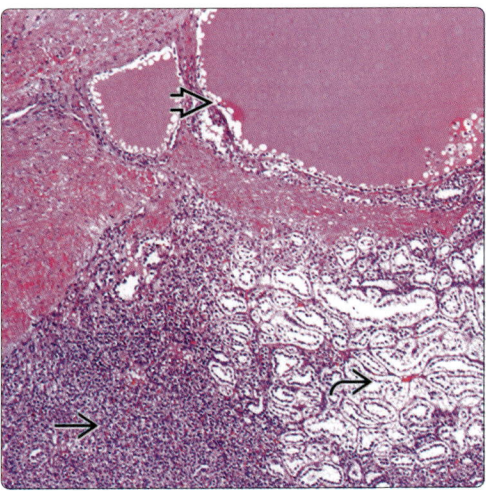

(Left) Some tumors show prominent tubular and cystic architecture. The tubules often contain eosinophilic secretions or hemorrhagic material. In these areas, the tumor may resemble a clear cell RCC. Distinction between these 2 is primarily based on the linear arrangement of the nuclei in most of the tumor in CC-PRCC. (Right) A combination of architectural patterns is often seen in CC-PRCC. In this paraffin section, the tumor shows mixed cystic ⇨, tubular ⇨, and solid collapsed acinar ⇨ architectural patterns.

Clear Cell Papillary Renal Cell Carcinoma

Architectural Patterns
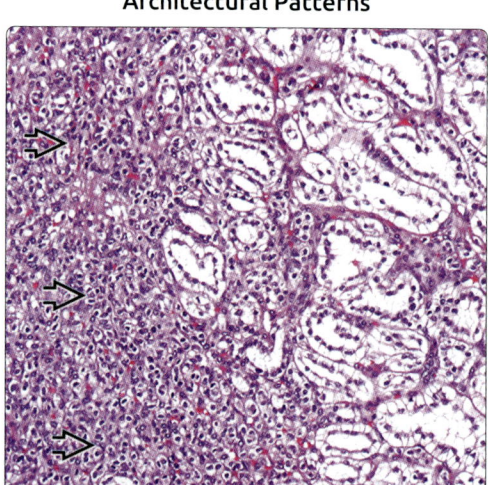

Branching Tubules
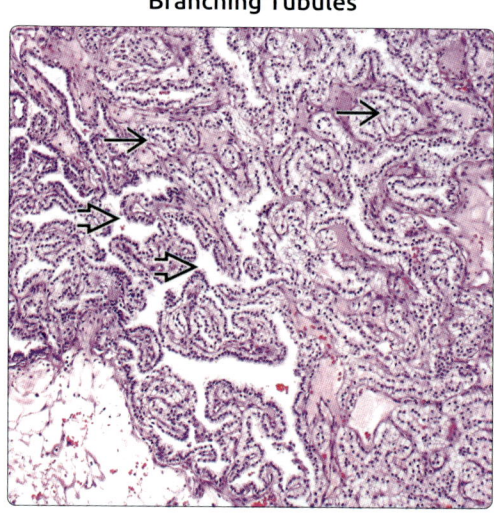

(Left) While the term angiomyoadenomatous tumor has been proposed for similar lesions with myoid metaplasia, features in the tumor that are otherwise typical for CC-PRCC, including solid acinar pattern ⇒, do not support a separate designation. IHC and molecular findings also support this diagnosis. (Right) A CC-PRCC shows prominently branching tubular ⇒, and some nonbranching tubular, ⇒ architectural patterns. Prominent branching of the tubules, a frequent finding, often gives the impression of a papillary architecture.

Fibromuscular Septations
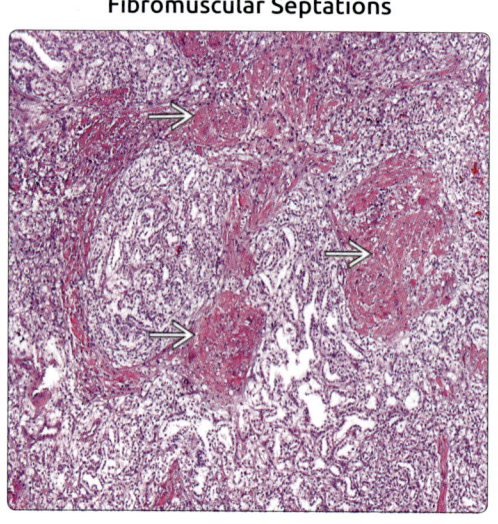

Collapsed Acini
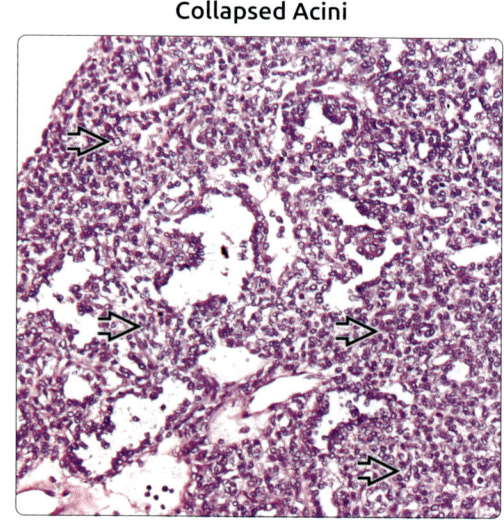

(Left) The presence of a fibromuscular capsule is a distinctive feature of clear CC-PRC. Occasionally, this smooth muscle proliferation extends deep into the tumor ⇒. This finding is not specific and may be seen in other RCCs, including clear cell RCC. (Right) Some CC-PRCs may show areas of collapsed, tightly packed acinar growth patterns ⇒. Such areas in a needle biopsy may be mistaken for clear cell RCC. Immunohistochemistry is often of value in such settings.

Linear Nuclear Alignment
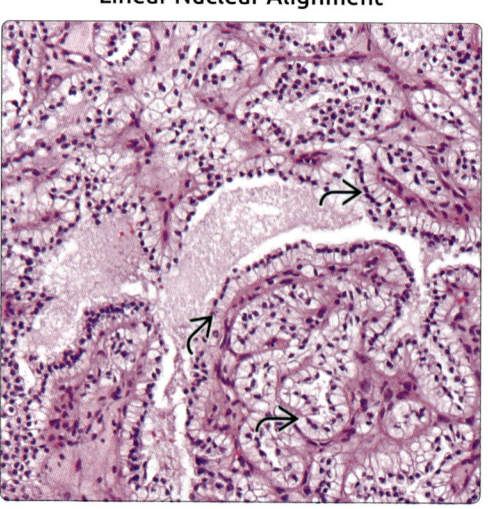

Linear Nuclear Alignment
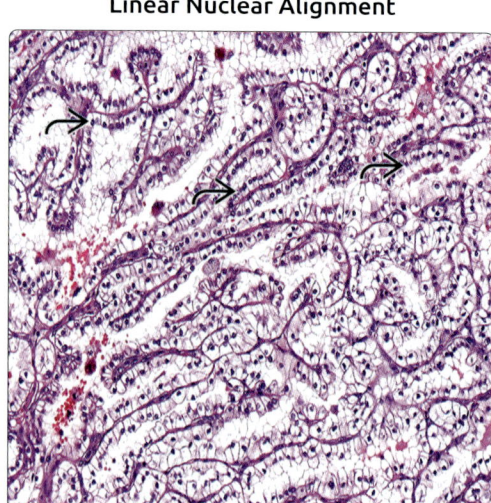

(Left) Whether cystic, solid, tubular, or papillary, the most characteristic and diagnostically important feature of CC-PRCC is the diffuse linear alignment of the nuclei away from the basal aspects of the cells ⇒. Often these nuclei approach the luminal surface but sometimes may be arranged in the middle of the cells. (Right) Such a diffuse, linear arrangement of the nuclei ⇒ is a consistent feature in all CC-PRCCs. Focal or patchy presence of this finding does not qualify a tumor as a CC-PRCC.

Clear Cell Papillary Renal Cell Carcinoma

Linear Nuclear Alignment
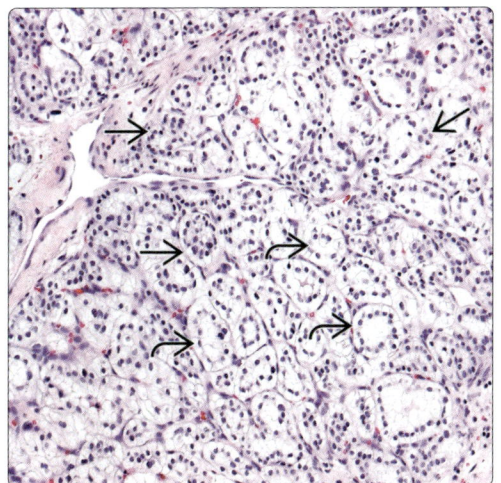

Linear Nuclear Alignment
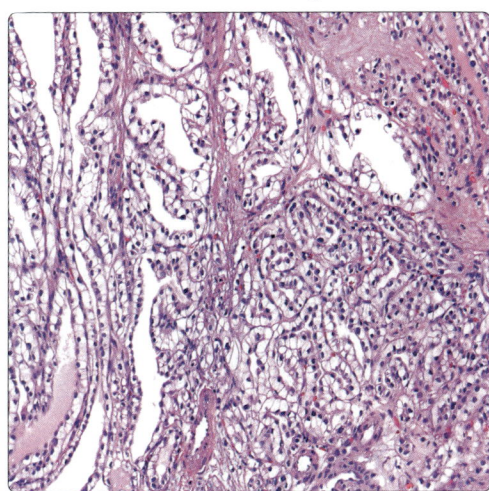

(Left) While diffuse, linear arrangement of nuclei ➡ is a diagnostic prerequisite for CC-PRCC; sometimes this arrangement may not be obvious in acinar areas of the tumor. However, such areas still show a tendency toward such an arrangement in all cases ➡. *(Right)* The characteristic nuclear alignment is present in all architectural patterns, as seen here. However, in the areas with collapsed acini, such arrangement may not always be obvious due to the paucity of cytoplasm and close packing of cells.

Diffuse CK7
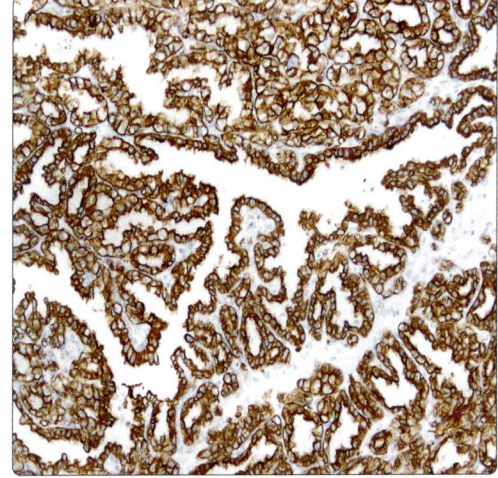

Diffuse CK7
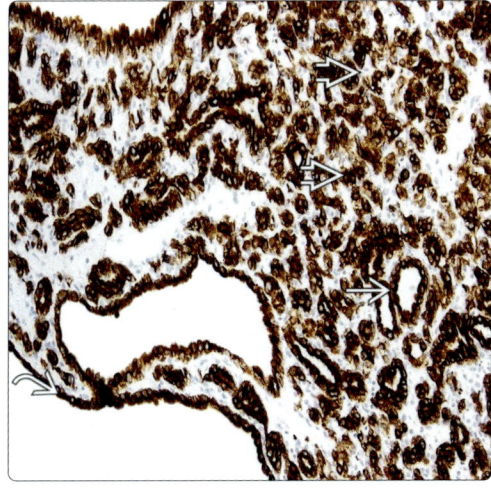

(Left) CC-PRCC shows CK7 positivity in almost 100% of the tumor cells. Focal or patchy CK7 positivity may also be seen in mimickers of CC-PRCC; such patchy positivity should raise the possibility of other differential diagnoses. *(Right)* CK7 shows diffuse and strong immunoreactivity in all architectural patterns, as illustrated here in the cystic ➡, tubular ➡, and the collapsed tightly packed acinar areas ➡. This is quite unlike what is observed in CC-PRCC and other mimics of CC-RCC.

CA9: Cup-Shaped
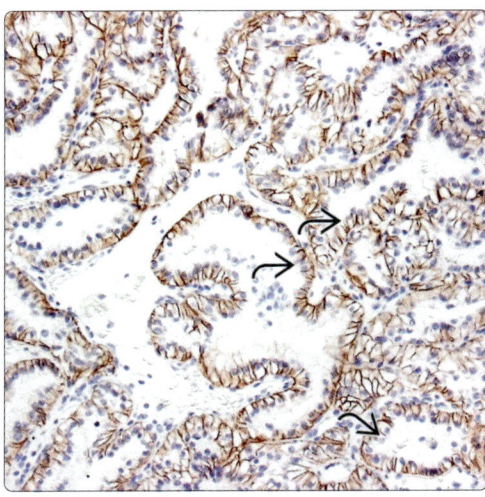

CA9: Cup-Shaped
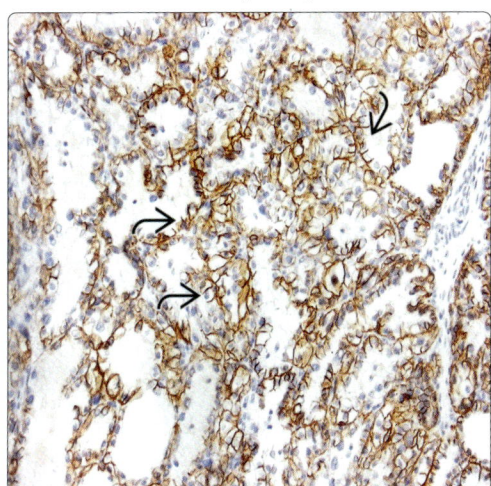

(Left) CA9 marks the tumor in a diffuse membranous staining pattern. This immunoreactivity overlaps with that of CC-RCC; however, the reactivity is mostly and characteristically absent in the luminal aspects of CC-RCC (cup-shaped pattern) ➡. *(Right)* Cup-shaped pattern of immunoreactivity with CA9 ➡ is present in all architectural patterns in CCP-RCC, whether papillary, tubular, cystic, or solid. However, this staining pattern may sometimes be difficult to be discerned in collapsed acinar areas.

Clear Cell Papillary Renal Cell Carcinoma

CA9: Cup-Shaped

CA9: Box-Shaped in Clear Cell Renal Cell Carcinoma

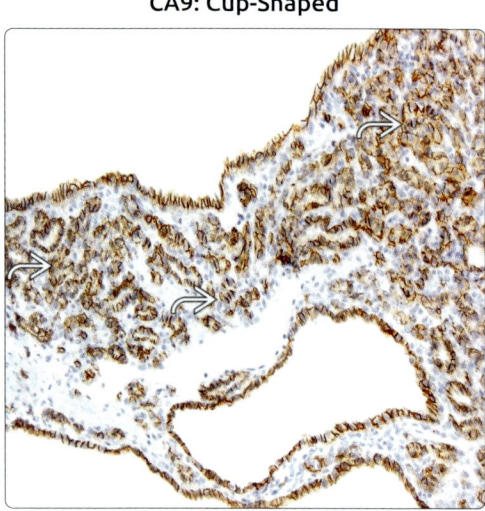

(Left) Although often difficult to interpret in the collapsed acinar areas of the tumor, the cup-shaped immunoreactivity for CA9 may occasionally be quite obvious, as illustrated here ➡. Such cup-shaped CA9 positivity is almost never the predominant pattern in other RCCs with clear cell cytology. (Right) In comparison, CA9 stains all aspects of the cell membrane in CC-RCC, and other mimickers of CC-PRCC, as illustrated here in a microacinar architectural area in a CC-RCC.

HMCK

CD10

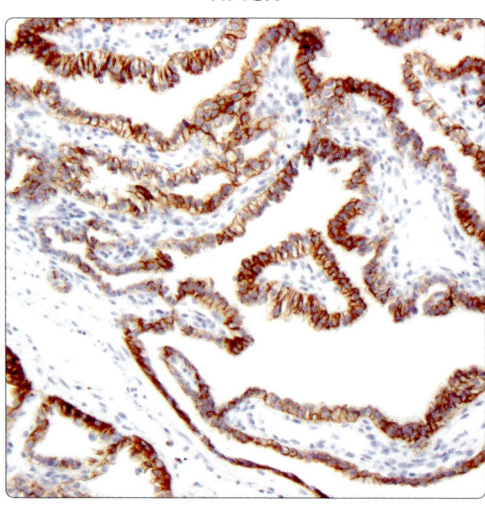
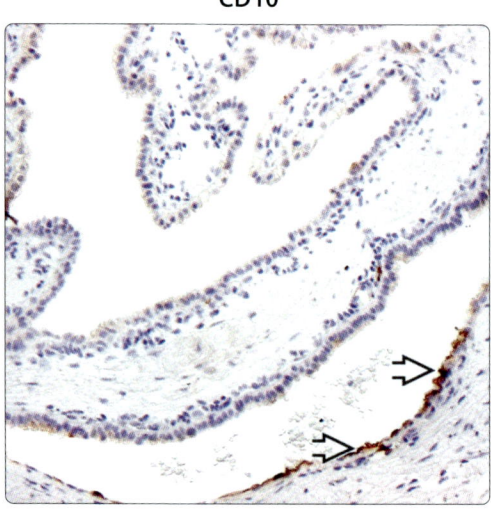

(Left) CC-PRCC often shows diffuse immunoreactivity for HMCK(34βE12). In general, expression of this marker is limited in the more common subtypes of RCC, particularly in those with clear cell cytology. However, clear cell RCCs with cystic features and multilocular clear cell neoplasms of low malignant potential may also be positive. (Right) In contrast to CC-RCC, CD10 is usually negative or only focally positive ➡ in CC-PRCC. Cytogenetically, these tumors are also distinct from CC-RCC and papillary RCC.

AMACR

Clear Cell Renal Cell Carcinoma With CC-PRCC-Like Areas

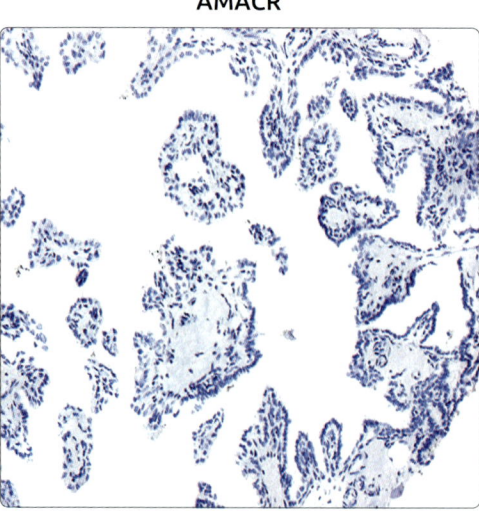
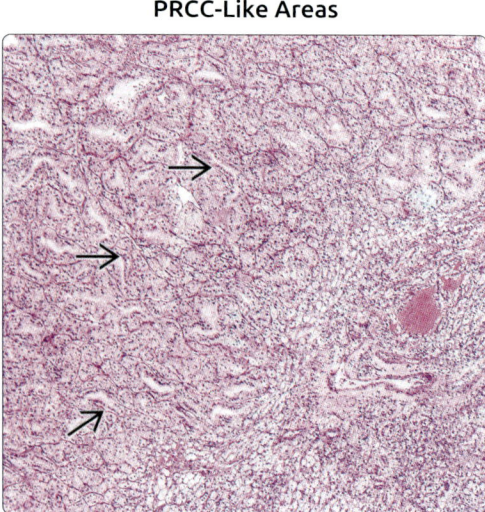

(Left) Immunoreactivity for AMACR is consistently negative in CC-PRCC, particularly in resection specimens. However, focal positivity may occasionally be seen, particularly in biopsy specimens. (Right) CC-PRCC-like linear arrangement of the nuclei ➡ may be seen in focal areas, or even larger patches, in CC-RCC and some other tumors. Unless diffuse, such nuclear patterns should not be considered diagnostic of CC-PRCC. In difficult cases, IHC is very often helpful.

Clear Cell Papillary Renal Cell Carcinoma

CA9 in Pseudo-Clear Cell Papillary Areas

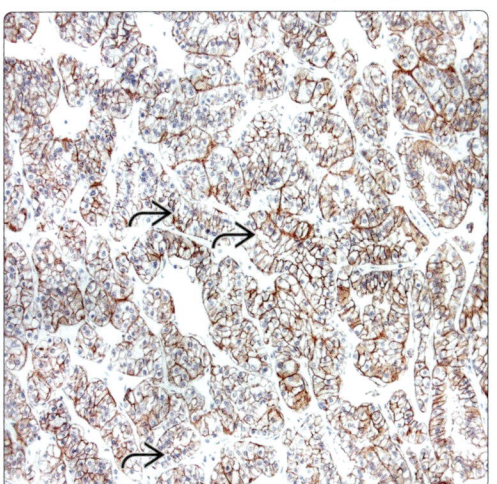

CD10 in Pseudo-Clear Cell Papillary Areas

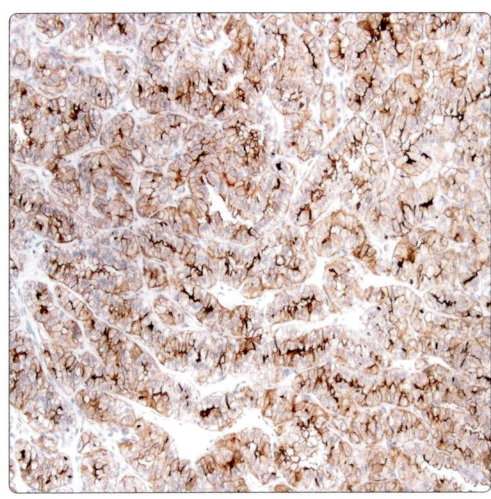

(Left) *CA9 shows diffuse membranous immunoreactivity in a box-shaped pattern in this case of CC-RCC with clear cell papillary-like foci ➦, unlike the cup-like pattern that is seen in true CC-PRCC.* **(Right)** *Unlike what is expected in CC-PRCC, CD10 is diffusely positive in this CC-RCC with CC-PRCC-like areas. CK7 positivity is also variable and usually patchy (not in 100% of the cells) in such cases.*

HMWCK in Pseudo-Clear Cell Papillary-Like Areas

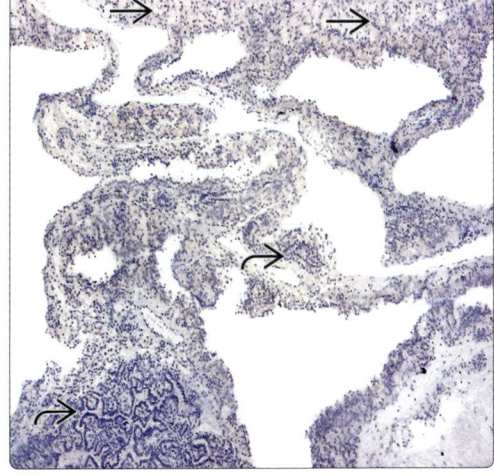

Biopsy Diagnosis of Clear Cell Papillary Renal Cell Carcinoma

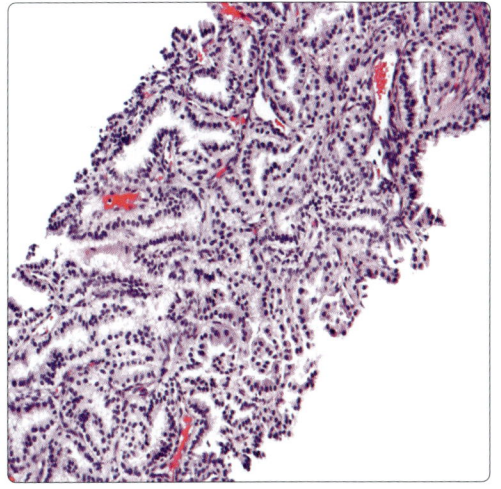

(Left) *Tumors usually lack immunoreactivity for 34βE12, in both the typical clear CC-RCC ➦ as well as CC-PRCC-like ➦ areas, unlike what is seen in true CC-PRCC.* **(Right)** *In spite of the fact that clear cell papillary-like areas may be seen in other tumor types, the diagnosis of CC-PRCC can be made on needle core biopsies with the classical morphological features throughout the biopsy material. We are of the opinion that IHC support is essential in biopsy cases.*

Biopsy Diagnosis of Clear Cell Papillary Renal Cell Carcinoma

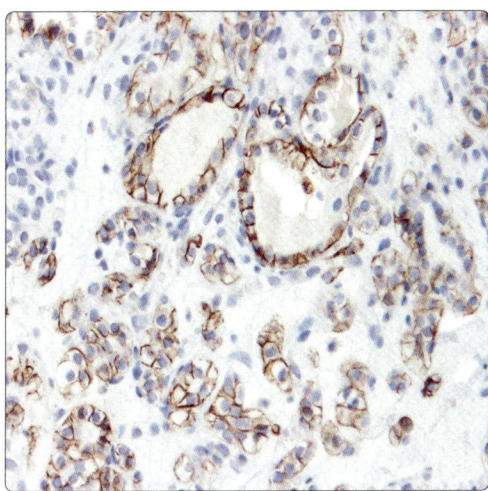

Biopsy Diagnosis of Clear Cell Papillary Renal Cell Carcinoma

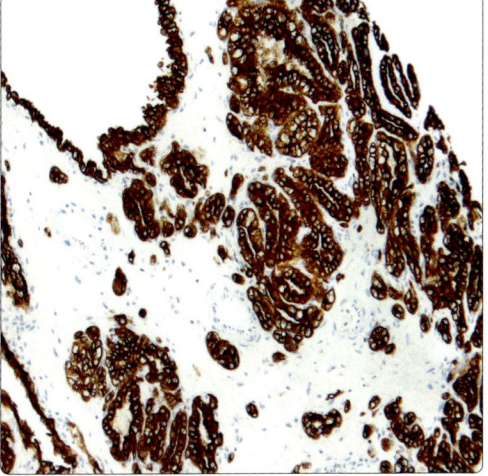

(Left) *The characteristic cup-shaped pattern of immunoreactivity for CA9 is seen in a biopsy of clear CC-PRCC. It is imperative that this pattern of staining be present in the biopsy before a diagnosis of CC-PRCC can be made on a biopsy.* **(Right)** *This figure illustrates diffuse CK7 positivity in a biopsy from clear cell papillary RCC. Almost 100% of the tumor cells are typically immunoreactive. Positivity for 34βE12, and absent to very focal staining for CD10, also support the diagnosis on core biopsy material.*

Papillary Renal Cell Carcinoma

KEY FACTS

TERMINOLOGY
- Papillary renal cell carcinoma (PRCC)
- 2nd most common subtype of renal cell carcinoma (RCC), usually showing predominant or exclusive papillary architecture, frequently with well-formed tumor capsule

ETIOLOGY/PATHOGENESIS
- Majority of sporadic PRCCs are characterized by trisomy of chromosomes 7 and 17, as well as loss of chromosome Y

CLINICAL ISSUES
- Although majority of patients with unilateral tumors, PRCC is more often bilateral and multifocal compared to other common renal cell tumors

MACROSCOPIC
- Often surrounded by fibrous pseudocapsule on gross evaluation
- Most exhibit variegated cut surface

MICROSCOPIC
- Majority of PRCCs exhibit broad morphologic spectrum, including papillary, tubular, and solid patterns
- Areas containing papillary architecture seen in most cases
- Cores of papillae are mostly loose and fibrovascular, often containing variable amount of foamy macrophages
- WHO divides papillary RCC into type 1 and type 2

TOP DIFFERENTIAL DIAGNOSES
- Clear cell RCC exhibiting papillary or pseudopapillary growth, collecting duct carcinoma (CDC), MiTF/TFE family translocation-associated renal carcinomas (TFE carcinoma)
- Hereditary leiomyomatosis RCC (HLRCC)-associated RCC, clear cell papillary RCC (CC-PRCC), metanephric adenoma, tuberous sclerosis-associated RCC
- *TCEB1*-mutated RCC, mucinous tubular spindle cell carcinoma (MTSCC), urothelial carcinoma of pelvicalyceal system, chromophobe RCC with papillary architecture, juxtaglomerular cell tumor with papillary architecture

Gross Features

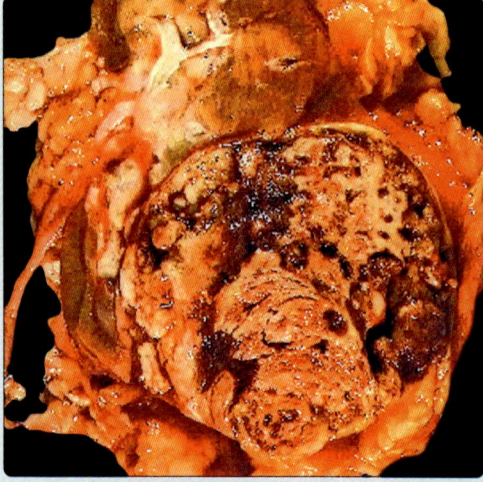

Microscopic Features

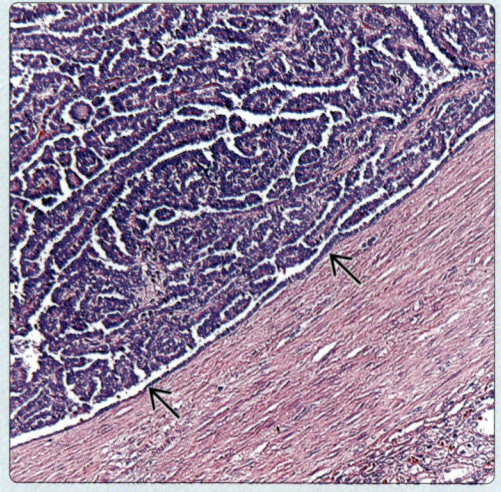

(Left) Gross photograph of a papillary renal cell carcinoma (PRCC) shows an encapsulated mass with a necrotic and hemorrhagic cut surface. Among the common renal cell tumors, PRCC is the most likely to have a capsule. (Right) As is usually evident on gross appearance, most PRCCs show a prominent capsule on microscopy. The capsule is often lined by epithelial cells resembling those in the tumor ⇒. This at times gives the impression of the tumor filling a large cyst.

Microscopic Features

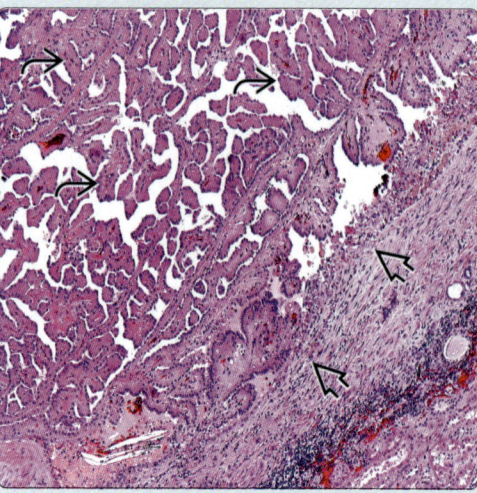

Microscopic Features

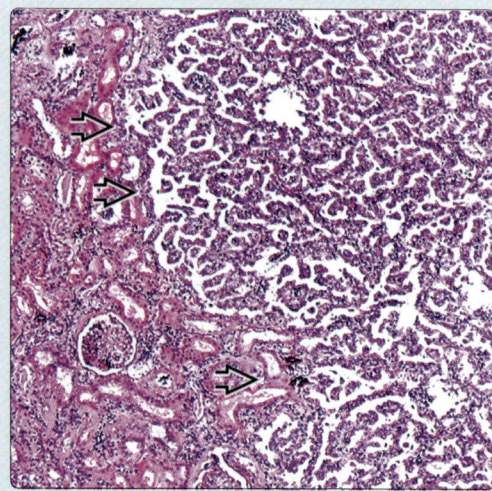

(Left) A prominent capsule, by definition, is a common feature in PRCC. Such encapsulation is present in most tumors, irrespective of morphological variation. This image depicts an oncocytic papillary variant ⇒ with a prominent fibrous capsule ⇒. (Right) Rarely, papillary RCCs may also show no encapsulation, with the tumor directly abutting surrounding renal parenchyma ⇒. This is usually, but not always, associated with smaller tumors.

Papillary Renal Cell Carcinoma

TERMINOLOGY

Abbreviations
- Papillary renal cell carcinoma (PRCC)

Definitions
- 2nd most common subtype of renal cell carcinoma (RCC), usually showing predominant or exclusive papillary architecture, frequently with well-formed tumor capsule
  - Tumors with papillary architecture but showing features of other recognized subtypes of RCC (e.g., MiT family translocation RCC, hereditary leiomyomatosis and RCC-associated RCC, collecting duct carcinoma, tuberous sclerosis-associated RCC, clear cell papillary RCC, etc.) are not PRCC

ETIOLOGY/PATHOGENESIS

Molecular Characteristics
- Majority of PRCCs characterized by trisomy of chromosomes 7 and 17, as well as loss of chromosome Y
- Trisomies of chromosomes 8, 12, 16, and 20, and loss of 1p, 4q, 6q, 7, 9p, 13q, Xp, and Xq also observed in some cases
  - Some investigators suggest that tumors with trisomy 7/17 alone are likely to have indolent behavior
    - Whereas those with additional genetic abnormalities behave aggressively
- More gains of 7p and 17p by comparative genomic hybridization reported by some in type 1, compared to type 2 tumors
- Activating mutations of *MET* oncogene, located at 7q31, present in all cases of hereditary papillary renal carcinoma syndrome
  - Similar mutations observed in ~ 13% sporadic papillary RCCs
- Mutations in *BAP1, SETD2, ARID2, and KEAP1* genes also present in some PRCCs
  - Thus, mutations in *BAP1 and SETD2* genes similar to that in clear cell RCC; but no *VHL* mutations present in PRCC

CLINICAL ISSUES

Epidemiology
- Incidence
  - Comprise 11-15% of renal cell neoplasms
- Age
  - Ranges from 3rd-8th decades of life with peak incidence in 6th-7th decades
  - Similar to other renal cell tumors
- Sex
  - Reported M:F = 1.8:1-4:1

Presentation
- > 50% of cases present as incidental masses, detected on radiologic investigation for unrelated conditions
- Reported size ranges from 1-18 cm (median: 6.4 cm)
  - However, downward size migration seen in modern times due to incidental discovery on imaging
- Although majority of tumors unilateral, PRCC is more often bilateral and multifocal compared to other common renal cell tumors

Treatment
- Surgical approaches
  - Partial nephrectomy preferred option
    - Total or radical nephrectomy rarely performed now at some institutions even for tumors > 4 cm in size
- Drugs
  - Resistance to systemic therapy characterizes patients with metastatic papillary RCC
  - Targeted therapies against VEGF tyrosine kinases and mTOR inhibitors in metastatic PRCC with clinical responses in occasional case
    - Inhibiting MET signaling pathway and combined inhibitors with MET and VEGFR-2 activity (foretinib) also under active investigation
  - Targeted immunotherapy using PD-1/PD-L1 [Programmed Death-1 and its ligand (PD-L1) and CTLA-4 (cytotoxic-lymphocyte associated antigen-4)] inhibitors also being used in multiple trials

Prognosis
- Overall, 5- and 10-year survivals better than clear cell RCC and possibly worse than chromophobe RCC
  - However, some studies show no significant prognostic differences between PRCC and chromophobe RCC

MACROSCOPIC

General Features
- Well-circumscribed mass
- Often surrounded by fibrous pseudocapsule on gross evaluation
  - Of all common renal cell tumor types, PRCC most likely to be surrounded by fibrous pseudocapsule
- Most exhibit variegated cut surface
  - Color related to microscopic findings
    - Tumors with abundant foamy macrophages, tan to yellow
    - Tumors with intratumoral hemorrhage, dark tan to brown
- Grossly visible areas of necrosis, hemorrhage, and cystic change very common, present in 32-70% of tumors
  - Some tumors almost entirely necrotic
- Multifocality present in > 45% of cases
  - In some, this is reported to be only microscopic finding; many such microscopic tumors may be considered papillary adenomas now

MICROSCOPIC

Histologic Features
- Majority of PRCCs exhibit broad morphologic spectrum, including papillary, tubular, and solid patterns
  - Papillary patterns include
    - Classic papillary with discrete papillary fronds lined by neoplastic cells with central fibrovascular core
    - Papillary-trabecular with delicate, elongated papillations arranged in parallel fashion
    - Papillary-solid with closely packed papillae, sometimes masking their true growth pattern
  - Areas containing papillary architecture seen in most cases

Papillary Renal Cell Carcinoma

- However, > 50% show variable proportion of solid, tubular, &/or glomeruloid growth patterns
  - Glomeruloid growth pattern composed of tubular structures with intraluminal tufting of tumor cells
    - Cells lining tubules cuboidal with scant to moderate amphophilic cytoplasm
    - Cells tufting into lumen with abundant eosinophilic cytoplasm and usually higher grade nuclei
  - Rarely, sarcomatoid growth or rhabdoid features may be seen; both associated with aggressive behavior
- Cores of papillae are mostly composed of loose, fibrovascular tissue, often containing variable number of foamy macrophages
  - However, variations in morphology not uncommon, and may include
    - Cores with no macrophages
    - Branching papillae
    - Some papillae with no distinct cores, as in tumors with micropapillary features
    - Marked hyalinization of cores
    - Variable degree of edema, sometimes leading to fluid-filled, grape-like polypoid structures
- WHO divides papillary RCC into 2 types
  - Type 1 with papillae covered by smaller cells with scant, amphophilic cytoplasm and single cell layer
  - Type 2 with larger tumor cells, often with higher nuclear grade, eosinophilic cytoplasm, and nuclear pseudostratification
    - Type 1 tumors more often (+) for CK7 than type 2 PRCC
    - Reportedly worse prognosis in type 2 compared to type 1 tumors
    - Trisomies 7 and 17 more often reported in type 1 than type 2 PRCC
    - *MET* gene mutations only present in type 1 PRCC
- Psammoma bodies, hemosiderin-laden macrophages, hemosiderin deposition within tumor cells often present in PRCC
- Some PRCC with mixture of type 1 and type 2 morphologic features
  - Tumors with any type 1 component, irrespective of amount of type 2 areas, clinically behave similar to pure type 1 PRCC
- Molecular evaluation suggests classification of PRCC not exactly the same as proposed by WHO
  - Type 1: Similar to type 1 of WHO
  - Type 2A: Tumors with eosinophilic cytoplasm but low-grade nuclei
  - Type 2B: Tumors with mixture of type 1 and type 2A features
  - Type 2C: Tumors with high-grade nuclei; these often with topoisomerase II-α overexpression
- Nuclear grading
  - Many believe Fuhrman grading system to be well suited for PRCC; others disagree and do not use Fuhrman grading scheme in PRCC
  - WHO considers International Society of Urological Pathology (ISUP)/WHO nucleolar grading scheme to be better option for grading papillary RCC
- Tumors with oncocytic cytoplasm, low-grade, nonoverlapping nuclei with linear arrangement towards cell apices considered as oncocytic PRCC
  - Immunohistochemically CK7(+)
  - Show trisomies 7 and 17
  - Show biologic behavior similar to type 1 PRCC
    - Features suggest that eosinophilic PRCC with low-grade nuclei are molecularly and biologically similar to type 1 tumors

ANCILLARY TESTS

Immunohistochemistry

- Diffuse positivity for CK7 very frequent; more common in type 1 than type 2 tumors
- AMACR diffusely (+), with cytoplasmic granular staining
- CD10 often (+), usually with luminal membranous staining
- CA9 mostly (-) or focally (+); positivity usually limited to papillary tips or perinecrotic areas
- RCC, pax-8, and pax-2(+)

DIFFERENTIAL DIAGNOSIS

Clear Cell Renal Cell Carcinoma Exhibiting Papillary or Pseudopapillary Growth

- Focal papillary architecture may be seen in clear cell RCC
  - Usually result of cell drop-off in areas away from feeding vessels, often creating pseudopapillitis
    - Adequate sampling and presence of typical cytoarchitectural features of clear cell RCC in other areas should clarify issue
  - Prominent psammoma bodies and hemosiderin deposition within tumor cells are not present in clear cell RCC
  - Any fibrovascular cores would be unusual in clear cell RCC and, if present, would be focal
  - Clear cells in clear cell RCC usually have optically transparent, completely clear cytoplasm
    - In papillary RCC, clear-appearing cells usually with variable granularity and often fine hemosiderin
  - CA9 with diffuse membranous reactivity in majority of clear cell RCCs; CK7 and AMACR usually (-) or very focal

Collecting Duct Carcinoma

- Has variable amount of papillary growth pattern
- Invariably widely infiltrative and associated with pronounced desmoplastic stroma
- Virtually always high grade
- Shows prominent multinodular growth pattern and glandular and sheet-like architecture; focal intracytoplasmic and luminal mucin common feature
- Often reactive for CEA, PNA, soybean agglutinin, ULEX-1, *Ulex europaeus*, and HMCK (34βE12)
  - CK7 may be expressed in both tumors
- Cytogenetic studies may be needed to solve difficult diagnostic problems

MiTF/TFE Family Translocation-Associated Renal Carcinomas

- More common in young patients
- Admixture of solid, nested, and papillary growth

Papillary Renal Cell Carcinoma

- Usually with high nuclear grade and often with cells showing voluminous cytoplasm
  - Cytoplasm varies from clear to eosinophilic
- (-) or only focally (+) for cytokeratins and EMA/MUC1
  - Characteristically exhibit nuclear immunoreactivity for TFE3 or TFEB, depending on translocation

Hereditary Leiomyomatosis Renal Cell Carcinoma-Associated Renal Carcinoma

- Tumors show variable, but often prominent, papillary architecture
  - Considered to be type 2 PRCCs in past
- Other architectural patterns, including glandular, alveolar, and solid are often present
- Most characteristic morphologic feature: Very prominent nucleoli with perinucleolar halos
- History of leiomyomas, both uterine and others, is common
- Fumarate hydratase lost in the tumor; 2SC with diffuse, cytoplasmic and nuclear positivity; CK7 usually (-)
- Molecular evidence of fumarate hydratase (FH) gene alterations

Clear Cell Papillary Renal Cell Carcinoma

- Variable amount of papillary and tubular architecture and cystic change
- Clear cell cytology, almost exclusive
- Most characteristic feature: Nuclei in linear alignment away from basal aspect of cells
- Almost 100% cells diffusely (+) with CK7; CA9 diffusely (+) (cup-shaped pattern); HMCK(34βE12) often (+)
  - (-) for AMACR and CD10 (most often)

Metanephric Adenoma

- vs. solid-architecture PRCC
  - Metanephric adenoma mostly without pseudocapsule
  - Most important feature in PRCC
    - PRCC has more abundant cytoplasm, along with prominent nucleoli
    - These nuclear features are not acceptable in metanephric adenoma
- CK7 and AMACR immunostaining usually (-) or only focally (+)
- CD57 and WT1 usually (+)

Mucinous Tubular Spindle Cell Carcinoma

- vs. PRCC with low-grade spindle cell areas
  - 1 of the more difficult differential diagnoses
  - Luminal surfaces in mucinous tubular spindle cell carcinoma (MTSCC) are regular and smooth
    - Glands and papillae in such PRCCs often with very irregular luminal outlines
- Myxoid or mucinous stroma in MTSCC
  - Not present in PRCC
- Trisomies of chromosomes 7 and 17 and loss of Y chromosomes in PRCC
  - Not present in MTSCC

Other Tumors With Papillary Architecture

- Tuberous sclerosis-associated RCC
  - Some with papillary architecture, lined by variably clear and eosinophilic cells often with voluminous cytoplasm
  - Presence of multifocal tumors and angiomyolipomas and cysts in the surrounding renal parenchyma
- TCEB1-mutated RCC
  - Well-circumscribed tumors with prominent fibromuscular septations imparting vaguely nodular configuration, branching tubular and acinar pattern, abundant clear cytoplasm
    - Diffuse, membranous (+) for CA9 (box-like), and often prominent CK7 (+)
- Papillary urothelial carcinoma of pelvicalyceal system
  - Papillae lined by transitional epithelium; usually CK7, CK20, HMCK (34βE12), GATA3, and p63(+)
- Chromophobe RCC with papillary architecture
  - Papillations focal; raisinoid nuclei with perinuclear halos; accompanying other architectural patterns almost always present
- Juxtaglomerular cell tumor with papillary architecture
  - Tumor cells with uniform round nuclei; papillary lining, entrapped native tubules, CK(+), rest of cells CK(-)

DIAGNOSTIC CHECKLIST

Pathologic Interpretation Pearls

- Many renal cell tumors besides papillary RCC show variable, often prominent, papillary architecture
- Prominent multinodular growth pattern and more than focal desmoplasia are not usual features in papillary RCC, including type 2 PRCC
- Alternative diagnosis in nonclassic cases should always be considered, and diagnosis should be based on overall cytoarchitectural features

SELECTED REFERENCES

1. Alomari AK et al: Clinicopathological and immunohistochemical characteristics of papillary renal cell carcinoma with emphasis on subtyping. Hum Pathol. 46(10):1418-26, 2015
2. Bigot P et al: The subclassification of papillary renal cell carcinoma does not affect oncological outcomes after nephron sparing surgery. World J Urol. ePub, 2015
3. Cornejo KM et al: Papillary renal cell carcinoma: correlation of tumor grade and histologic characteristics with clinical outcome. Hum Pathol. 46(10):1411-7, 2015
4. Courthod G et al: Papillary renal cell carcinoma: a review of the current therapeutic landscape. Crit Rev Oncol Hematol. 96(1):100-12, 2015
5. Kovac M et al: Recurrent chromosomal gains and heterogeneous driver mutations characterise papillary renal cancer evolution. Nat Commun. 6:6336, 2015
6. Reuter VE et al: Best practices recommendations in the application of immunohistochemistry in the kidney tumors: report from the International Society of Urologic Pathology consensus conference. Am J Surg Pathol. 38(8):e35-49, 2014
7. Warrick JI et al: Papillary renal cell carcinoma revisited: a comprehensive histomorphologic study with outcome correlations. Hum Pathol. 45(6):1139-46, 2014
8. Srigley JR et al: The International Society of Urological Pathology (ISUP) Vancouver Classification of Renal Neoplasia. Am J Surg Pathol. 37(10):1469-89, 2013
9. Tickoo SK et al: Differential diagnosis of renal tumors with papillary architecture. Adv Anat Pathol. 18(2):120-32, 2011
10. Klatte T et al: Cytogenetic and molecular tumor profiling for type 1 and type 2 papillary renal cell carcinoma. Clin Cancer Res. 15(4):1162-9, 2009
11. Kunju LP et al: Papillary renal cell carcinoma with oncocytic cells and nonoverlapping low grade nuclei: expanding the morphologic spectrum with emphasis on clinicopathologic, immunohistochemical and molecular features. Hum Pathol. 39(1):96-101, 2008
12. Hes O et al: Oncocytic papillary renal cell carcinoma: a clinicopathologic, immunohistochemical, ultrastructural, and interphase cytogenetic study of 12 cases. Ann Diagn Pathol. 10(3):133-9, 2006
13. Yang XJ et al: A molecular classification of papillary renal cell carcinoma. Cancer Res. 65(13):5628-37, 2005

Papillary Renal Cell Carcinoma

Gross Features

Gross Features

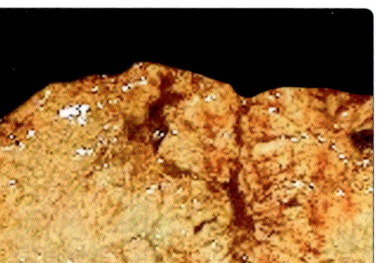

(Left) This PRCC shows a prominent yellow cut surface. Yellow color is often indicative of prominent lipid-laden (foamy) macrophages in the tumor. (Right) This PRCC shows a homogeneous tan cut surface. The appearance of the cut surface is reflective of the microscopic features, indicating a relative lack of necrosis and paucity of lipid-laden macrophages in this case. Solid, homogeneous-appearing PRCC are frequently type 1 tumors.

Type I Histology

Foam Cells

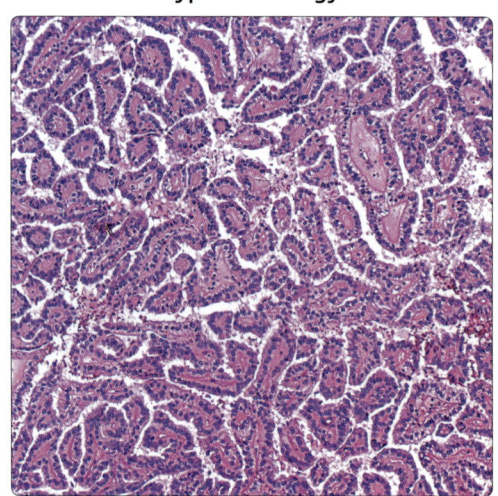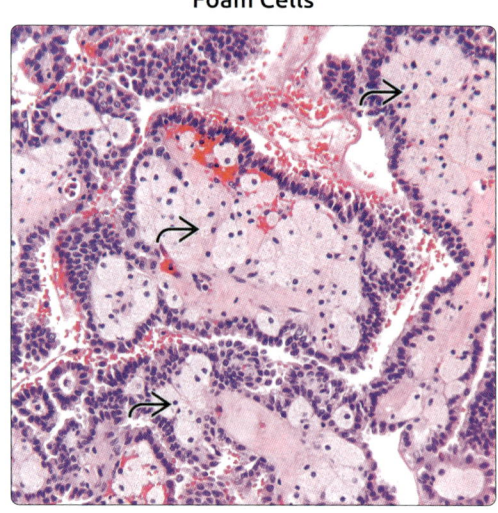

(Left) This hematoxylin and eosin stained section of PRCC shows discrete papillary fronds lined by neoplastic cells, with central fibrovascular cores. (Right) This photomicrograph shows 1 of the typical features of a PRCC, prominent papillary architecture and abundant foamy macrophages ⮕ in the papillary cores. The lining cells are amphophilic and cuboidal in this case.

Papillae With Foam Cells

Papillae With Edematous Fluid

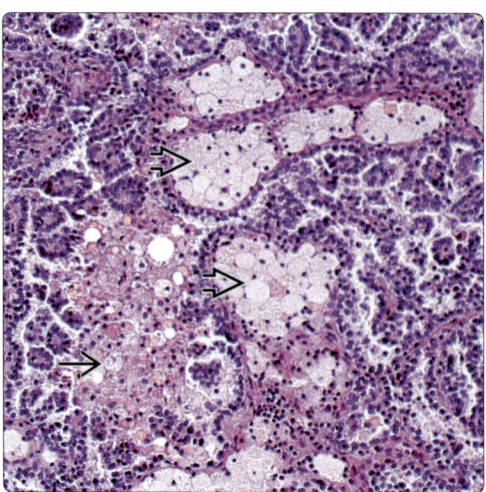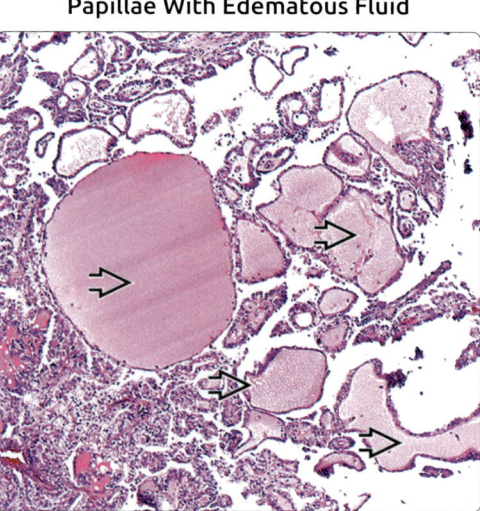

(Left) While the cores of the papillae in PRCC commonly show variable amounts of foamy macrophages ⮕, occasionally, these foam cells may also be observed in the spaces between papillae ⮕. (Right) This hematoxylin and eosin of PRCC shows papillary cores with marked edema ⮕. Variable degrees of edematous fluid collection within the cores is sometimes present and occasionally may lead to presence of grape-like, polypoid structures.

Papillary Renal Cell Carcinoma

Microscopic Features

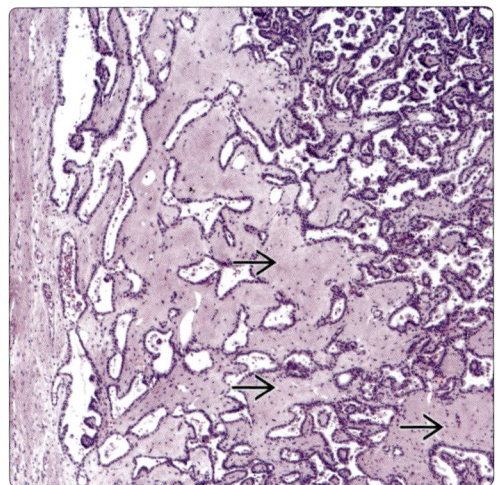

Microscopic Features

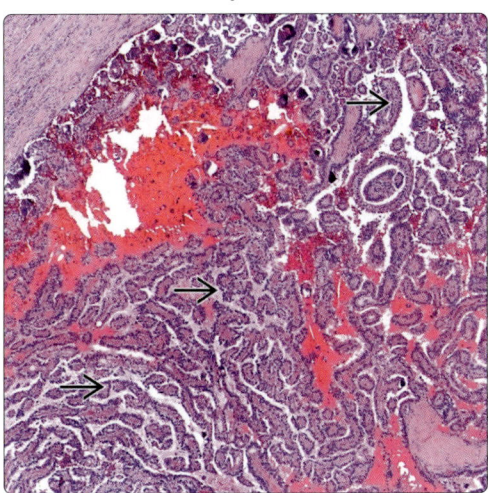

(**Left**) Hematoxylin and eosin stained section shows expanded but hyalinized papillary cores ➡ in a PRCC. This pattern of sclerotic appearance in the cores is relatively uncommon and is usually only seen in type 1 PRCC. (**Right**) The papillae may be lined by smaller cells with scant, amphophilic cytoplasm ➡ and a single layer. PRCC with these features are regarded as type 1 by WHO.

Microscopic Features

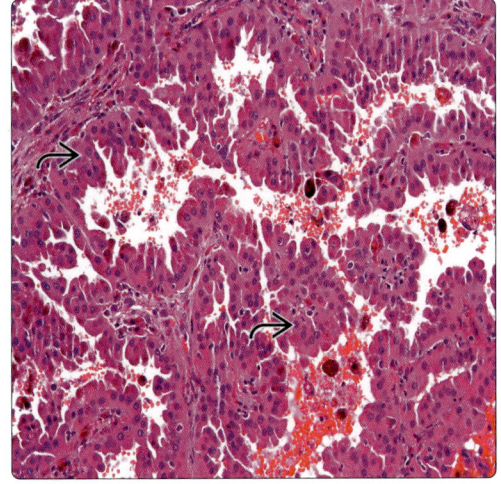

Microscopic Features

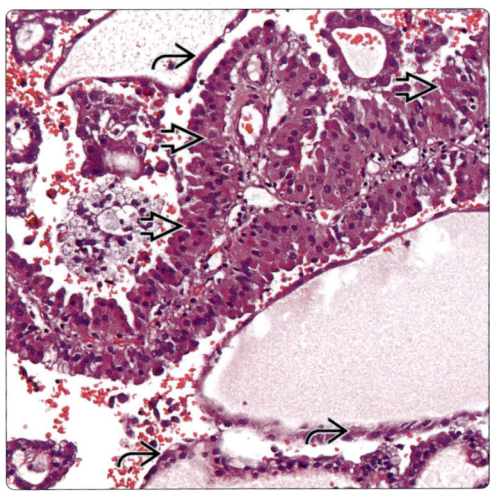

(**Left**) Some PRCCs show abundant eosinophilic cytoplasm, large nuclei with prominent nucleoli, and pseudostratification of the nuclei. Eosinophilic cytoplasm with nuclear pseudostratification ➡ are considered to be a prerequisite for the diagnosis of type 2 PRCC. (**Right**) Some PRCCs show an admixture of type 1 ➡ and type 2 ➡ areas. Such tumors with mixed features are biologically known to behave like pure type 1 PRCC.

Microscopic Features

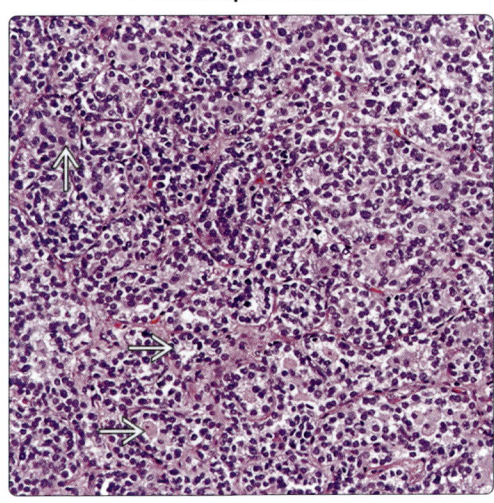

Microscopic Features

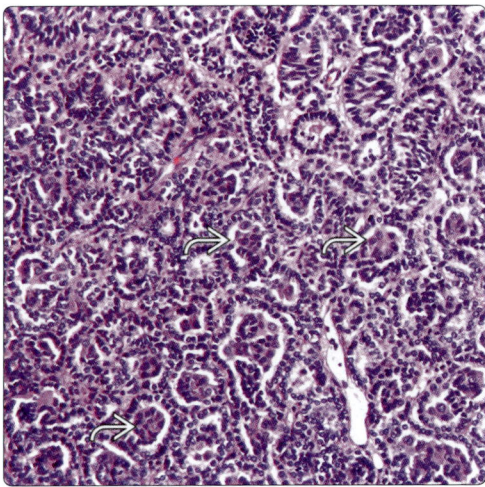

(**Left**) Some PRCCs show tightly packed papillae, resulting in a solid appearance. Note the multiple tubular structures ➡ in this tumor. Many of these tubules represent cross-sectional profiles of papillae. When the papillae are arranged in long parallel arrays, a papillary-trabecular appearance may be appreciated. (**Right**) Glomeruloid architecture ➡ may be present in some PRCCs. This finding may be focal and is often linked with solid and tubular architecture. Some tumors show entirely glomeruloid features.

Papillary Renal Cell Carcinoma

(Left) PRCC may also show variable or often prominent clear cell areas. These clear-appearing cells are not optically transparent, as in clear cell RCC, show finely granular and reticulate cytoplasm, and often contain finely granular hemosiderin ⇨. (Right) This image shows a type 1 PRCC with solid and tubular architecture and somewhat clear cytoplasm in a needle core biopsy. Correct interpretation is quite possible on limited material but may need immunohistochemical support.

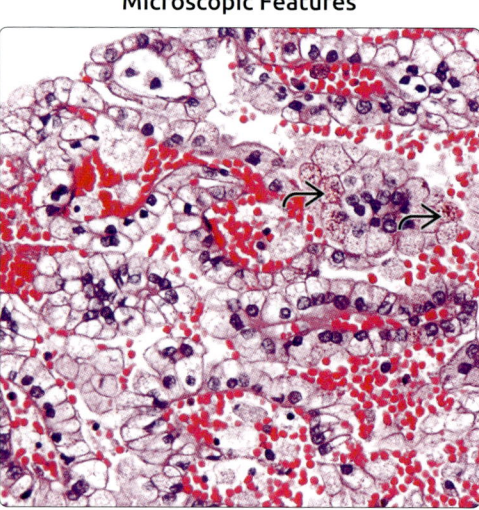

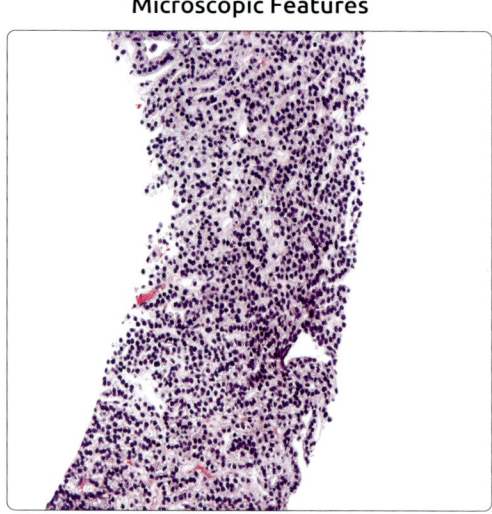

(Left) One of the other common findings in PRCC is the presence of hemosiderin in the macrophages as well as tumor cells ⇨. While this finding may be seen in tumors with type 1 histology, it is more common in tumors with abundant eosinophilic cytoplasm. (Right) Type 2 PRCC usually shows a paucity of foamy macrophages. CK7 positivity is less frequent in such tumors compared to type 1 cases, and the tumors are also often absent for MET gene mutations.

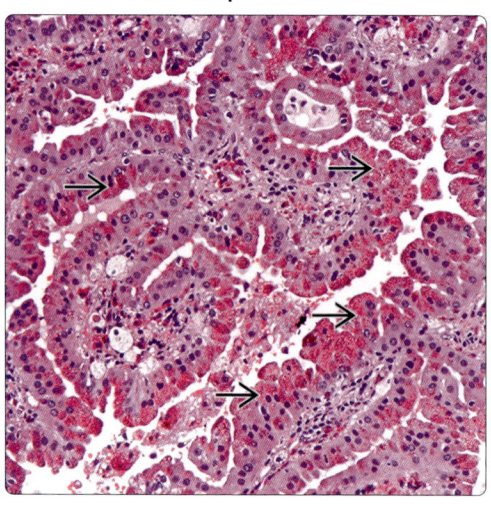

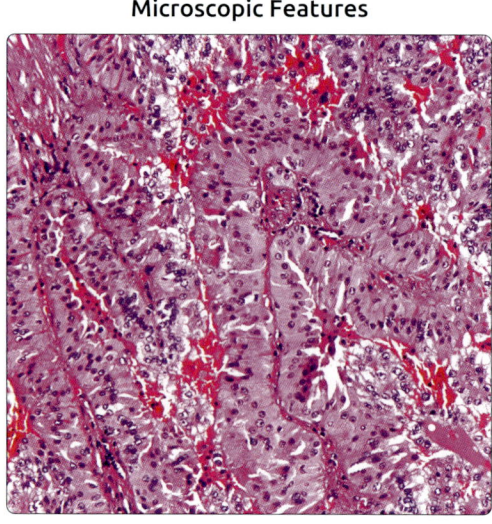

(Left) Rarely, PRCC may show low-grade spindle cell foci ⇨ mimicking mucinous tubular spindle cell carcinoma. Usually, the glands in such tumors have irregular, shaggy lumina ⇨ and lack stromal mucin. Such tumors show trisomies 7/17, as in type 1 PRCC. (Right) Oncocytic PRCC with abundant pink cytoplasm may be mistaken for type 2 tumors. However, such tumors show low-grade nuclei with linear arrangement, lack of nuclear pseudostratification, and immunohistochemical and biological features similar to type 1 RCC.

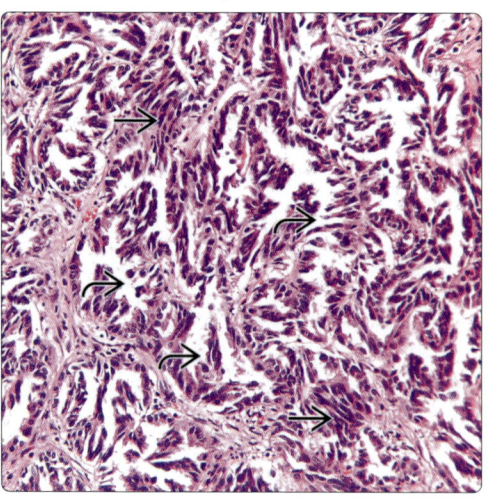

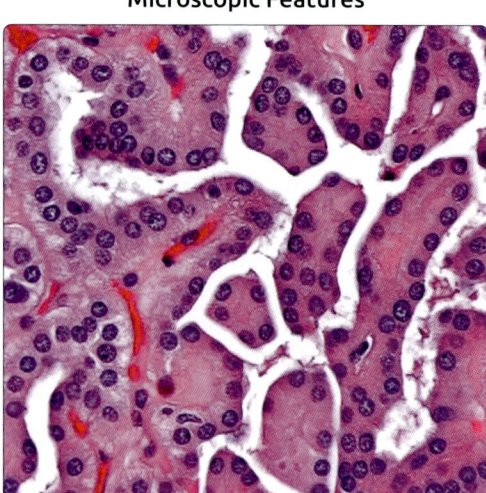

Papillary Renal Cell Carcinoma

CK7

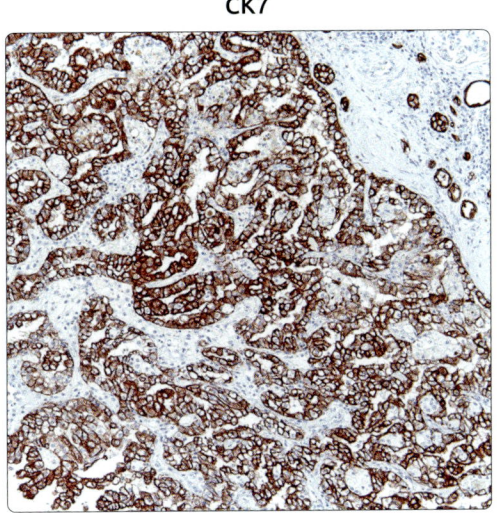

AMACR

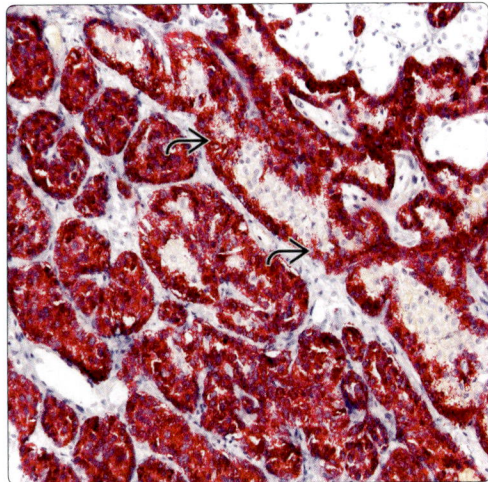

(Left) CK7 shows diffuse, cytoplasmic, and membranous positivity in PRCC. Such diffuse staining is more often seen in tumors with type 1, rather than type 2, features. Other positive markers include RCC, pax-8, pax-2, and CD10. **(Right)** PRCCs are usually diffusely positive for AMACR. The staining is characteristically cytoplasmic and granular ➔.

CD10

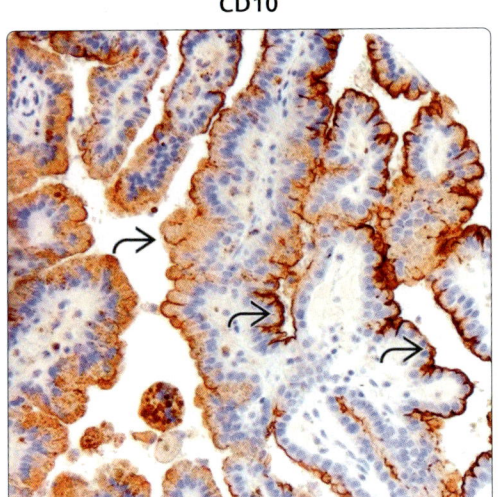

CA9

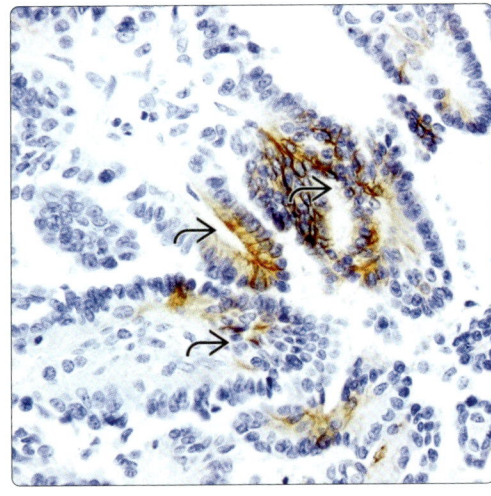

(Left) Similar to clear cell RCC, PRCC also shows diffuse, membrane-predominant immunoreactivity for CD10. However, the pattern of positivity is usually different. CD10 often highlights the luminal aspects of the cells in PRCC ➔, whereas it usually stains all the cell membranes in clear cell RCC in a box-like pattern. **(Right)** Unlike clear cell RCC, PRCC is usually negative for CA9 by immunohistochemistry. Less often, it may show focal positivity in the papillary tips ➔.

CA9

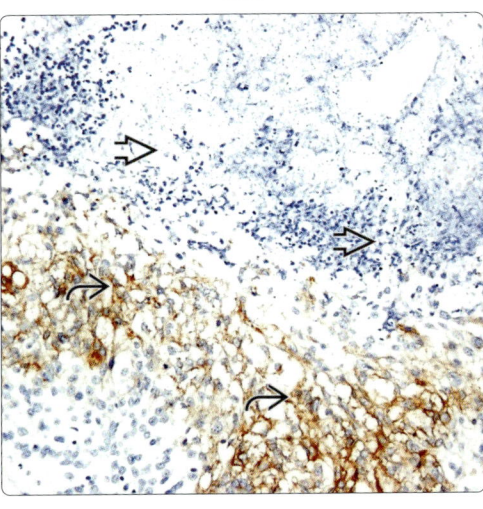

Iron Stain

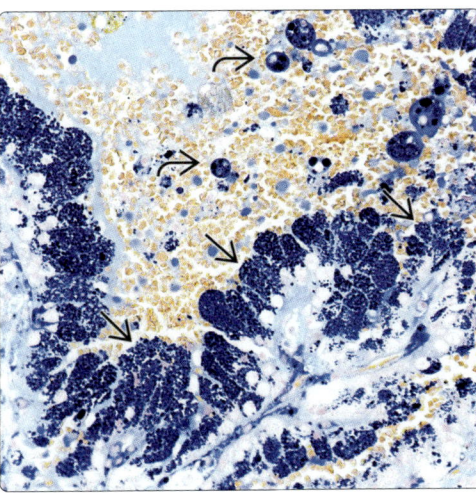

(Left) In addition to staining the papillary tips, CA9 often shows patchy reactivity ➔ around foci of necrosis ➔. This pattern of staining reflects hypoxic areas and is related to overexpressed HIF in such areas. **(Right)** Perl iron stain confirms the presence of hemosiderin in the tumor cells ➔ as well as in the macrophages ➔ between the papillae. Such positivity is present not only in the easily identifiable hemosiderin-containing cells but frequently also in areas with clear cell cytology.

Papillary Renal Cell Carcinoma

(Left) Some PRCCs may show areas with micropapillary features. Such papillations are often small and do not show fibrovascular cores ⮕. Micropapillary architecture does not have any special biological implications in the tumor and are present only in type 1 tumors. (Right) Rare PRCC may also show rhabdoid features ⮕. As expected, tumors with rhabdoid features in general are aggressive in behavior, even when showing type 1 histology ⮕ in the majority of the tumor.

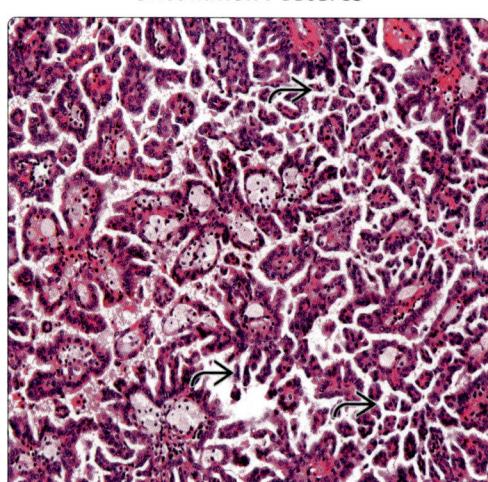
Uncommon Features

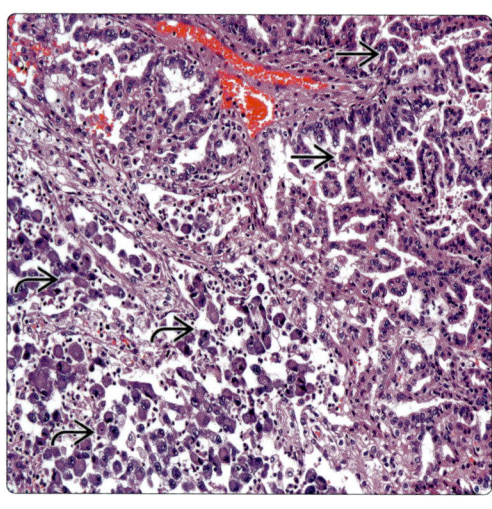
Uncommon Features

(Left) About 5% of PRCC show sarcomatoid features ⮕. Sarcomatoid areas always show high-grade cytology. Presence of sarcomatoid areas in PRCC, as in other tumor types, predicts an aggressive behavior. (Right) On the other hand, low-grade spindle cell foci may be present in some tumors. Distinction from high-grade sarcomatoid features is not difficult as they lack nuclear pleomorphism, necrosis, and mitotic activity. However, distinction from mucinous tubular and spindle cell carcinomas may be more difficult.

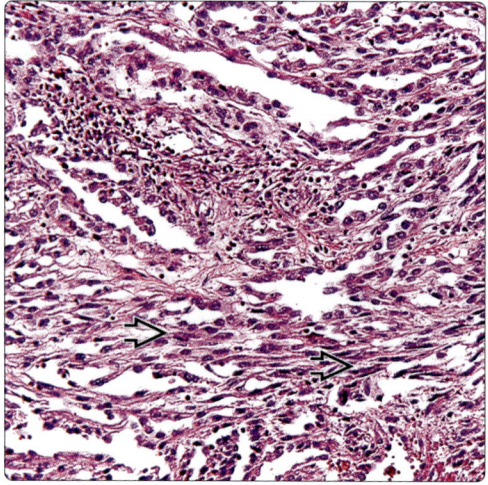
Uncommon Features

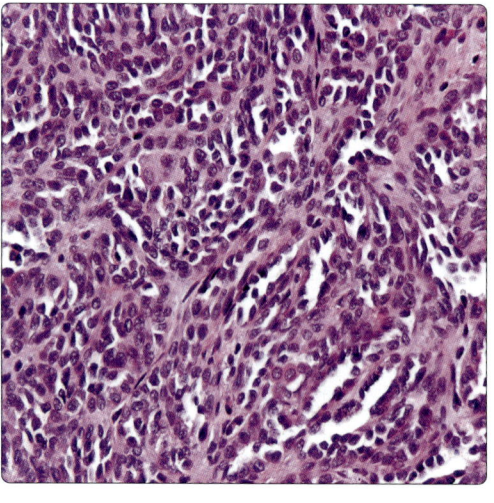
Uncommon Features

(Left) Like other subtypes of RCC, PRCC may show perinephric or sinus fat invasion ⮕. However, this feature is less common than in clear cell RCC. (Right) Lymphovascular invasion ⮕ in PRCC, while uncommon, shows very significant association with clinical outcome. In 1 large study of more than 200 cases of PRCC with type 1 features, all case with lymphovascular invasion were dead of disease.

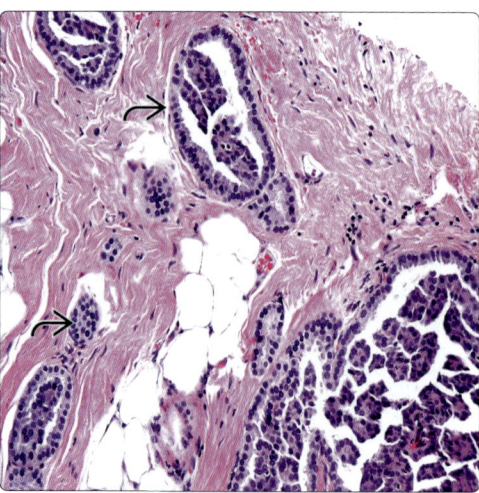
Uncommon Features

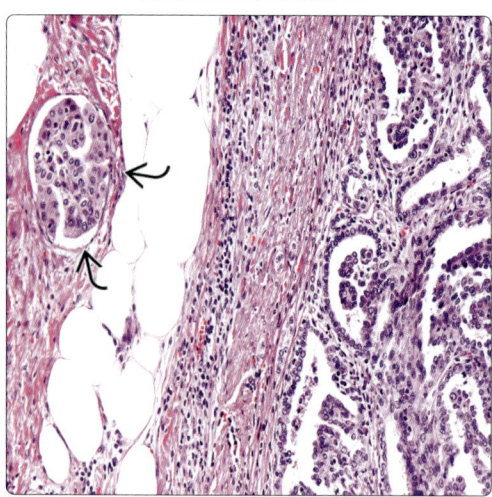
Uncommon Features

Papillary Renal Cell Carcinoma

Collecting Duct Carcinoma

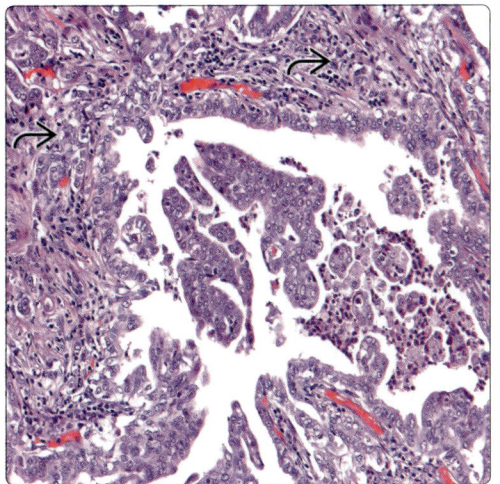

Hereditary Leiomyomatosis RCC-Associated RCC

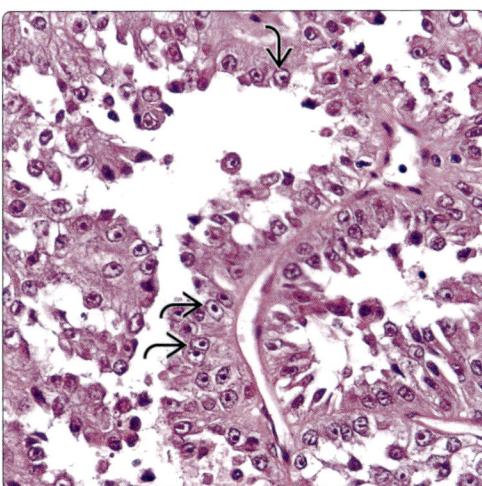

(Left) *All tumors with predominant or exclusive papillary architecture are not PRCC. Careful evaluation of all histomorphological features is imperative. This case represents a collecting duct carcinoma with stromal desmoplasia ⇨ and multinodular growth pattern.* (Right) *Hereditary leiomyomatosis RCC-associated RCC also often shows features of type 2 PRCC. The characteristic feature is the presence of prominent nucleoli with perinucleolar halos ⇨.*

Clear Cell Papillary RCC

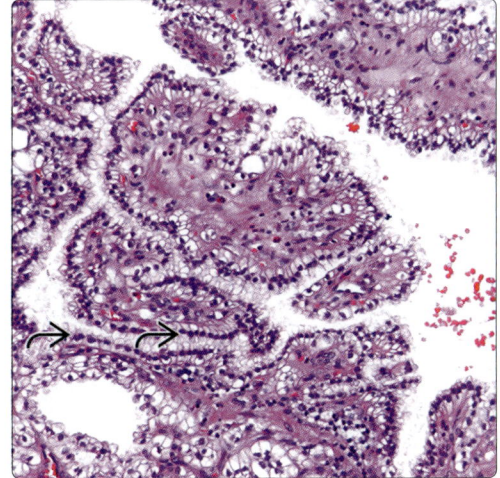

MiTF Family Tumor

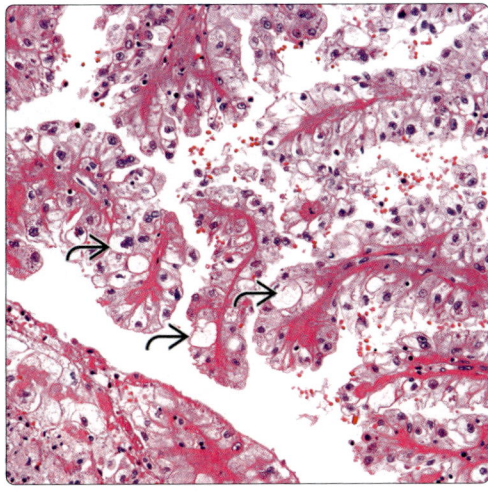

(Left) *Clear cell PRCC can show prominent papillary architecture. It has almost exclusive clear cell cytology and nuclei aligned in a linear fashion away from the basal aspect ⇨. They are AMACR(-) and CA9 diffusely (+) (cup-shaped).* (Right) *MiTF/TFE translocation RCCs often show prominent papillary architecture. However, they usually have clear cells, show high nuclear grade, and some cells with voluminous cytoplasm ⇨. Epithelial markers are usually negative, and TFE stains and FISH are positive.*

Tuberous Sclerosis Family Tumor

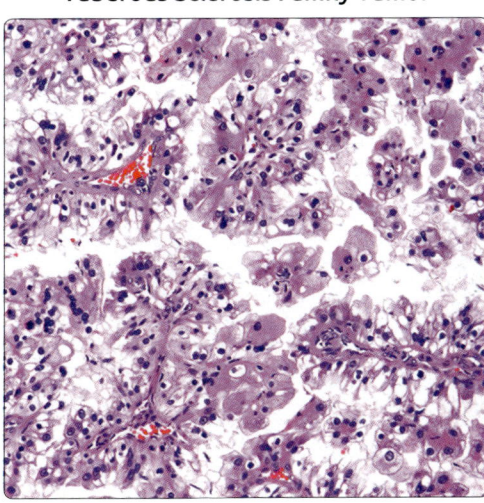

Chromophobe RCC

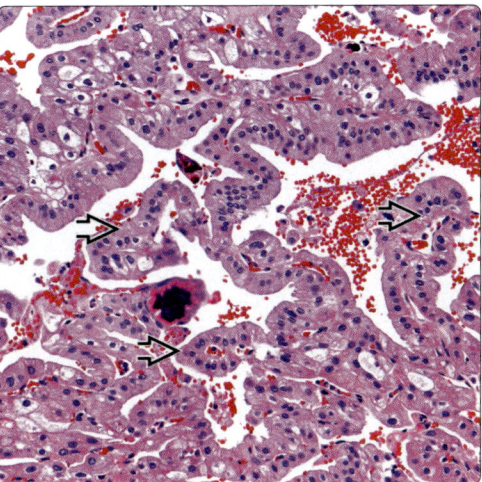

(Left) *Tumors associated with tuberous sclerosis syndrome may also show extensive papillary architecture. They are often multifocal, with different tumors often showing variable histologies, and are frequently associated with the presence of angiomyolipomas and cysts in the surrounding renal parenchyma.* (Right) *Variable papillary architecture may also be seen in many other tumors. This image shows focal papillations ⇨ in an otherwise typical chromophobe RCC.*

Chromophobe Renal Cell Carcinoma

KEY FACTS

TERMINOLOGY
- Chromophobe renal cell carcinoma (Ch-RCC)
- Characterized by large pale and smaller eosinophilic tumor cells in variable proportions, with wrinkled nuclei and perinuclear halos

ETIOLOGY/PATHOGENESIS
- Ch-RCC typically shows combined chromosomal losses usually affecting chromosomes 1, 2, 6, 10, 13, and 17
- Mutations in mitochondrial DNA (mtDNA) seen in 20% of tumors, predominantly in eosinophilic variants

CLINICAL ISSUES
- Prognosis of Ch-CRC much better than clear cell RCC, and somewhat better than papillary RCC in some studies
- Sarcomatoid features in tumor, most frequent association with aggressive clinical behavior

MICROSCOPIC
- Pattern of growth is predominantly solid, separated by thin, incomplete fibrovascular septa
- In classic-type tumors, predominant cell type with pale, somewhat clear-appearing cytoplasm
- In eosinophilic variants, predominance of tumor cells with densely eosinophilic, granular cytoplasm
- Most tumors show admixture of pale and eosinophilic cells
- Most characteristic histological feature: Hyperchromatic nuclei showing irregular, wrinkled outlines (raisinoid nuclei) with perinuclear halos
- Presence of cytoplasmic microvesicles unique and consistent ultrastructural feature of Ch-RCC

TOP DIFFERENTIAL DIAGNOSES
- Renal oncocytoma
- Renal cell carcinoma, unclassified, low grade
- Clear cell renal cell carcinoma, eosinophilic variant
- SDHB-deficient renal cell carcinoma

Gross Features

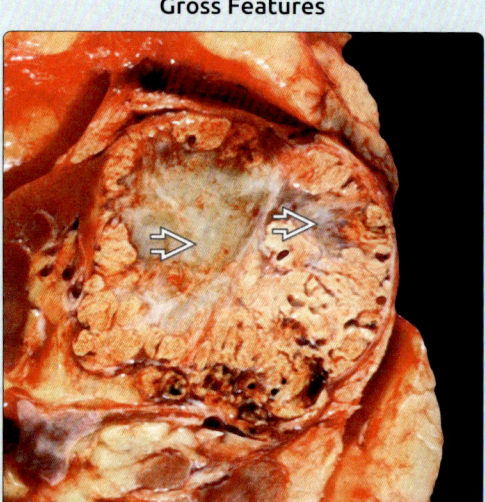

Microscopic Features

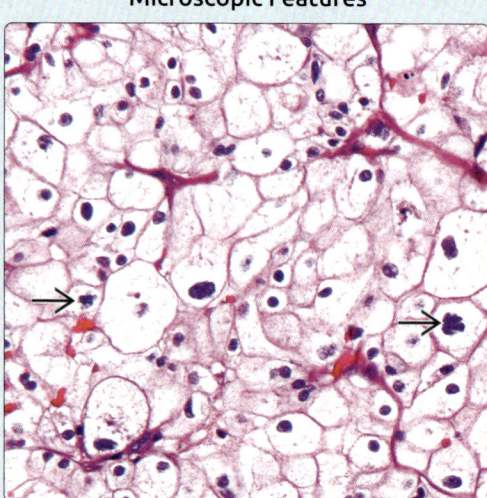

(Left) Gross features of chromophobe renal cell carcinoma vary according to the cell type. This example of a tumor with classical histology shows a yellow-tan cut surface. A macroscopic central scar ⇨ is observed in ~ 15% of Ch-RCCs. Such a scar is indicative of a slowly growing tumor; scars are also seen in some renal oncocytomas and low-grade clear cell RCCs. (Right) The nuclei in Ch-RCC are typically hyperchromatic, with markedly irregular nuclear membranes ➡, as seen in this classical histology of the tumor.

Gross Features

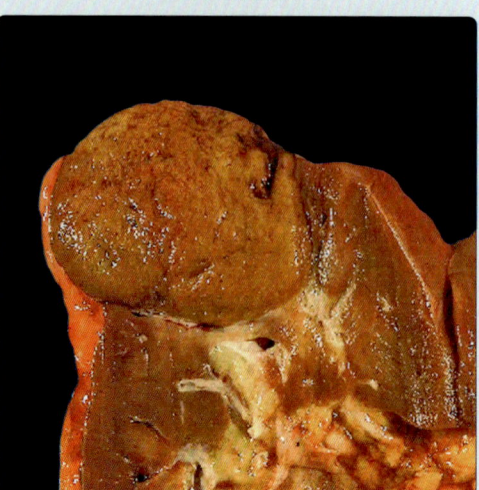

Microscopic Features

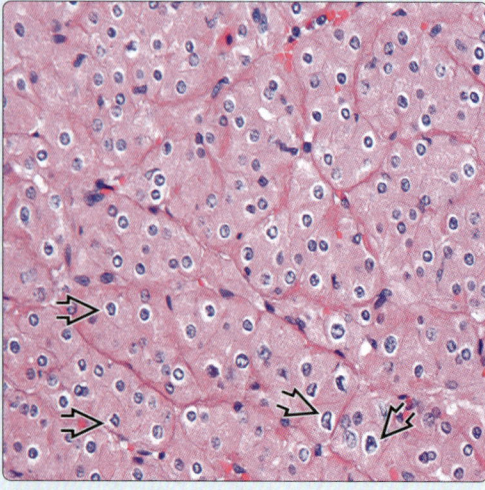

(Left) The brown cut surface of this chromophobe renal cell carcinoma suggests prominence of cells with eosinophilic cytoplasm in this tumor. Such a gross appearance also raises the possibility of a renal oncocytoma. (Right) In this section taken from tumor on the left, all the cells show granular, eosinophilic cytoplasm. Perinuclear halos ⇨ around irregular, raisinoid nuclei seen in this eosinophilic variant are the most diagnostic feature of chromophobe renal cell carcinoma.

Chromophobe Renal Cell Carcinoma

TERMINOLOGY

Abbreviations
- Chromophobe renal cell carcinoma (Ch-RCC)

Definitions
- 3rd most common subtype of RCC
  - Characterized by large pale and smaller eosinophilic tumor cells in variable proportions, with wrinkled nuclei and perinuclear halos

ETIOLOGY/PATHOGENESIS

Genetic Features
- Ch-RCC shows loss of 1 copy of chromosomes 1, 2, 6, 10, 13, and 17 in > 85% of tumors
  - Other less frequent losses of chromosomes 3, 5, 8, 9, 11, 18, 21, and Y also seen
    - All classic cases show the characteristic copy losses
      - Such losses less frequent or absent in eosinophilic variants
- TP53 and PTEN mutations other significant single somatic mutations (in 32% and 9% cases, respectively), as observed in The Cancer Genome Atlas (TCGA) cohort
- Mutations of different genes in mammalian target of rapamycin (mTOR) pathway also frequent (together, in > 20%)
- Recurrent rearrangements in promoter region of telomerase reverse transcriptase (TERT) also noted in TCGA cohort
- Mutations in mitochondrial DNA (mtDNA) seen in 20% of the tumors, mostly involving electron transport chain (ETC) complex I
  - Such mutations observed predominantly in eosinophilic variants
- Upregulation of number of genes encoding proteins integrated to membranes also reported
  - Many of these upregulated gene products related to vesicle-mediated transport
- Expression levels of microRNAs, mir-191, 19a, 210, and 425 significantly associated with recurrence-free and overall survival
  - mir-210 most independent prognostic factor in terms of recurrence-free survival
- Morphologically chromophobe or chromophobe RCC-like tumors also observed in BHD, renal oncocytosis or SDHB deficient RCC
  - Such tumors with distinct other genetic alterations characteristic of the specific entity

Cell of Origin
- Ch-RCC thought to arise from intercalated cells of renal cortex, similar to renal oncocytoma

CLINICAL ISSUES

Epidemiology
- Incidence
  - Comprise 5-11% of renal epithelial tumors
- Age
  - Mean: 59 years; range: 21-92 years
- Sex
  - M:F = 1.2:1

Presentation
- Usually present as unilateral renal mass
- Large proportion of patients asymptomatic, with incidentally detected tumors following investigations for unrelated symptoms

Treatment
- Surgical approaches
  - Partial nephrectomy surgical treatment of choice, whenever feasible
- Drugs
  - No specific chemotherapeutic agent consistently effective in metastatic cases
  - Targeted therapies against vascular growth factor tyrosine kinase receptors and mTOR pathway molecules with some rare responses

Prognosis
- Prognosis of Ch-RCC better than clear cell RCC and somewhat better than papillary RCC in some studies
- Overall, 96% and 94% disease-free survival rates at 5 and 10 years after nephrectomy
- Sarcomatoid features, microscopic tumor necrosis, and small vessel invasion associated with aggressive clinical behavior
  - Pathological tumor stage another factor correlating with adverse clinical outcome in some studies
  - Significance of nuclear (including modified Fuhrman nuclear grades)/nucleolar grade have not shown consistent results
- Overall, patients with metastatic Ch-RCC tend to do better than patients with metastasis from other common subtypes of RCC

IMAGING

Radiographic Findings
- Usually large, well-circumscribed, unicentric renal mass; often with features of hypovascularity; may show central scar

MACROSCOPIC

General Features
- Characteristically, well circumscribed but not encapsulated
- Cut surface homogeneous beige or pale-tan; occasionally dark brown or mahogany
  - Gross appearance reflection of microscopic cell types; more brown with increasing proportion of eosinophilic cells
- Central scar present in ~ 15% of tumors
- Gross hemorrhage and necrosis present in 25-30%; cystic change less common
- Multifocality in < 10%
- Gross involvement of renal vein seen in small number of cases

Size
- Mean: ~ 8 cm (range: 1-30 cm)
  - Largest among common subtypes of RCC
    - Mean size progressively decreasing because of earlier incidental detection on radiologic investigations for unrelated causes

Chromophobe Renal Cell Carcinoma

MICROSCOPIC

Key Descriptors

- Predominant pattern/injury type
  - Neoplastic
- Predominant cell/compartment type
  - Epithelial
- Key microscopic features
  - Pattern of growth predominantly solid, separated by thin incomplete fibrovascular septa
  - Some tumors with variable nested, broad alveolar, solid, cystic, tubular, trabecular, or even papillary/pseudopapillary patterns
    - Nested/alveolar and tubular pattern usually associated with eosinophilic variants
  - Small percentage (~ 5%) exhibit sarcomatoid pattern of growth
  - Microscopic foci of necrosis present in 15-25% of cases
  - In classic-type tumors, predominant cell type is that with pale, somewhat clear-appearing cytoplasm
    - Unlike clear cell RCC, cytoplasm not optically transparent but finely reticulated and granular
    - Frothy or soap bubble appearance in well-fixed specimens primarily due to ultrastructurally identified microvesicles
    - Larger cells with more voluminous clear to foamy (hydropic) cytoplasm often present among other clear cells
  - In eosinophilic variants (40% of tumors), predominance of tumor cells with densely eosinophilic, granular cytoplasm
  - Most show admixture of pale and eosinophilic cells
    - Both cell types often randomly juxtaposed to one another; more frequently clear cells arranged along septations and eosinophilic cells away from septations
  - Most characteristic feature is hyperchromatic nuclei with irregular, wrinkled nuclear membranes (raisinoid nuclei)
    - Proportion of such nuclei variable from case to case
    - Wrinkled nuclei more prevalent in classic types than in eosinophilic variants
  - Another characteristic feature is presence of perinuclear cytoplasmic clarity (perinuclear halos)
    - While usually prominent, perinuclear halos may be only focal in some eosinophilic variants, requiring careful search
  - Binucleated cells present in virtually all cases
  - Cell membranes usually appear prominent due to peripheral displacement of other organelles by abundant microvesicles (plant cell appearance)
  - Foci with bizarre, hyperchromatic, degenerate atypia similar to those in renal oncocytoma not infrequent
  - Mitotic activity uncommon in Ch-RCC but may be prominent in sarcomatoid and rarely in some epithelial tumors
  - Fuhrman nuclear grading not appropriate for Ch-RCC
    - Recently proposed modified nuclear grading and nucleolar grading schemes show correlation with outcome in some studies
      - But not confirmed on multivariate analyses

ANCILLARY TESTS

Histochemistry

- Colloidal iron stain; not always diagnostically useful
  - Variable granular or reticular and diffuse cytoplasmic staining with Hale colloidal iron in majority of cases
  - Difficult stain to perform well and highly laboratory-dependent
    - Focal, weak, or luminal-type staining, as seen in some oncocytomas, observed in some eosinophilic variants

Immunohistochemistry

- General comments
  - CK7 shows diffuse expression in > 75% Ch-RCC typically with membranous accentuation
    - In eosinophilic variants, positivity is often less diffuse
      - Occasionally, may be present only in few clusters of cells
  - CD117 and Ksp-cadherin diffusely positive in overwhelming majority
  - Most cases also show positivity with MOC-31, claudin-7, and EpCAM/BER-EP4/CD326
  - CA9 is negative or only focally positive in perinecrotic areas
  - RCC and CD10 are usually negative but may show focal positivity in some cases
  - S100A1, CD82, AMY1A considered useful in some publications but not confirmed on large number of cases

Electron Microscopy

- Cytoplasmic microvesicles unique and consistent ultrastructural feature of Ch-RCC
  - These vesicles lack affinity for H&E stain, resulting in cells with clear or flocculent cytoplasmic appearance on light microscopy
  - Origin is uncertain but likely related to defective mitochondriogenesis
  - Microvesicles often concentrated in perinuclear location, corresponding to perinuclear halos on light microscopy
- Abundant mitochondria present in cells with eosinophilic cytoplasm
  - Mitochondria often show tubulocystic cristae

DIFFERENTIAL DIAGNOSIS

Renal Oncocytoma

- Eosinophilic variant of Ch-RCC closely mimics renal oncocytoma, particularly in cases with solid and nested growth patterns
  - Separation of these entities is essential, as renal oncocytoma is benign tumor
- Distinction primarily histomorphological
- Nuclei in renal oncocytoma are round and uniform
  - Lack nuclear membrane irregularities that are always present, at least focally, in Ch-RCC
- Perinuclear halos are absent in renal oncocytomas
- Immunohistochemistry may help
  - CK7 negative or shows rare single cell positivity in oncocytoma
  - Other markers claimed to help in this distinction (EpCAM/BER-EP4/CD326, claudin-7, MOC-31, MAI1, and S1001A)

Chromophobe Renal Cell Carcinoma

- Not proven helpful in difficult cases yet
  - Presence of microvesicles in Ch-RCC on ultrastructural evaluation most distinctive feature
  - Cytogenetic investigations excluding combined multiple chromosomal losses, typical of Ch-RCC, may be helpful
    - However, some eosinophilic chromophobe RCCs may not show multiple chromosomal losses
      - These cases raise questions about biological relationship between eosinophilic Ch-RCC and oncocytoma

Clear Cell Renal Cell Carcinoma

- Both classic and eosinophilic variants may have overlapping features with clear cell RCC
  - Distinction less problematic than its separation from renal oncocytoma
- Separation is essential because of relatively indolent clinical behavior of Ch-RCC
- Cytoplasm in clear cells of clear cell RCC usually optically transparent (lipid and glycogen)
  - In Ch-RCC, cytoplasm is not entirely optically clear in clear cells but is finely reticulated or irregularly granulated; acid mucopolysaccharide in microvesicles
- Clear cell RCC shows intricate, branching vasculature
- Clear cell RCC may show foci with perinuclear clearing (or prominent cell membrane), but this is not prominent feature
- Immunohistochemical stains show diffuse membranous reactivity for CA9, RCC, and CD10; but negativity for CK7 in most cases
- Ultrastructurally, clear cell RCC lacks prominent microvesicles and tubulovesicular cristae in mitochondria
- 3p losses and *VHL* gene alterations in clear cell RCC will prove conclusive in very rare cases where genetic evaluation may be needed

Renal Cell Carcinoma, Unclassified (Low-Grade Oncocytic Type)

- Usually shows solid nests/alveoli with oncocytoma-like architecture, similar to some Ch-RCCs
- Tumors demonstrate nuclear pleomorphism and mitotic index beyond that acceptable for oncocytoma
- Do not show nuclear wrinkling and perinuclear halos as seen in Ch-RCC, eosinophilic variant
- Immunophenotypic differentiation, not conclusive
- Term hybrid oncocytic tumor used by some authors to express overlap with, but also to separate it from, oncocytoma, which has benign outcome

Epithelioid Angiomyolipoma (Oncocytoma-Like)

- Nuclear pleomorphism is usually significant
- Perinuclear halos are not observed
- Presence of fat cells &/or dysmorphic vessels if present, helpful
- Tumors negative for cytokeratin and CK7
  - Positive for melanocytic markers HMB-45 and melan-A (MART-1), and cathepsin-K

DIAGNOSTIC CHECKLIST

Pathologic Interpretation Pearls

- Renal cell tumors with clear cell cytoplasm may raise differential diagnostic possibilities of Ch-RCC and clear cell RCC
- Predominant acinar growth pattern with clear cytoplasm more indicative of clear cell RCC
  - Ch-RCC with clear cells is more likely to show sheet-like architecture
- Intricate arborizing vascular pattern and optically clear cytoplasm is feature of clear cell RCC
  - Ch-RCC with clear cells almost always shows incomplete septa not completely surrounding cell nests or alveoli
  - Cytoplasm is not optically transparent in Ch-RCC; it shows fine reticulations or irregularly clustered granules
- Tumors with pink cytoplasm and nested/solid alveolar growth often raise possibility of oncocytoma, Ch-RCC (eosinophilic), SDHB-deficient, or unclassified RCC/hybrid tumors
- Uniform nuclei throughout tumor, with exception of markedly pleomorphic symplastic foci, are indicative of oncocytoma
- Nuclear irregularities may be present in Ch-RCC or RCC, unclassified
  - Important to look for foci with perinuclear halos to make diagnosis of Ch-RCC
    - If such foci are absent and there is no intratumoral fat/dysmorphic vessels, it is prudent to consider tumor as unclassified RCC (low-grade oncocytic type)

SELECTED REFERENCES

1. Davis CF et al: The somatic genomic landscape of chromophobe renal cell carcinoma. Cancer Cell. 26(3):319-30, 2014
2. Jain S et al: Amylase α-1A (AMY1A): a novel immunohistochemical marker to differentiate chromophobe renal cell carcinoma from benign oncocytoma. Am J Surg Pathol. 37(12):1824-30, 2013
3. Cheville JC et al: Chromophobe renal cell carcinoma: the impact of tumor grade on outcome. Am J Surg Pathol. 36(6):851-6, 2012
4. Volpe A et al: Chromophobe renal cell carcinoma (RCC): oncological outcomes and prognostic factors in a large multicentre series. BJU Int. 110(1):76-83, 2012
5. Przybycin CG et al: Chromophobe renal cell carcinoma: a clinicopathologic study of 203 tumors in 200 patients with primary resection at a single institution. Am J Surg Pathol. 35(7):962-70, 2011
6. Paner GP et al: A novel tumor grading scheme for chromophobe renal cell carcinoma: prognostic utility and comparison with Fuhrman nuclear grade. Am J Surg Pathol. 34(9):1233-40, 2010
7. Amin MB et al: Chromophobe renal cell carcinoma: histomorphologic characteristics and evaluation of conventional pathologic prognostic parameters in 145 cases. Am J Surg Pathol. 32(12):1822-34, 2008
8. Choueiri TK et al: Efficacy of sunitinib and sorafenib in metastatic papillary and chromophobe renal cell carcinoma. J Clin Oncol. 26(1):127-31, 2008
9. Delahunt B et al: Fuhrman grading is not appropriate for chromophobe renal cell carcinoma. Am J Surg Pathol. 31(6):957-60, 2007
10. Brunelli M et al: Eosinophilic and classic chromophobe renal cell carcinomas have similar frequent losses of multiple chromosomes from among chromosomes 1, 2, 6, 10, and 17, and this pattern of genetic abnormality is not present in renal oncocytoma. Mod Pathol. 18(2):161-9, 2005
11. Motzer RJ et al: Treatment outcome and survival associated with metastatic renal cell carcinoma of non-clear-cell histology. J Clin Oncol. 20(9):2376-81, 2002
12. Tickoo SK et al: Ultrastructural observations on mitochondria and microvesicles in renal oncocytoma, chromophobe renal cell carcinoma, and eosinophilic variant of conventional (clear cell) renal cell carcinoma. Am J Surg Pathol. 24(9):1247-56, 2000
13. Tickoo SK et al: Colloidal iron staining in renal epithelial neoplasms, including chromophobe renal cell carcinoma: emphasis on technique and patterns of staining. Am J Surg Pathol. 22(4):419-24, 1998

Chromophobe Renal Cell Carcinoma

(Left) Clear cells in Ch-RCC are not optically clear and show reticular/irregularly granular cytoplasm. Many clear cells appear ballooned out and hydropic ⇨. Also note a mitotic figure ⇨. The apparent thick, plant-like ⇨ cell wall appearance results from abundant microvesicles pushing other organelles to the periphery. (Right) Most Ch-RCC typically show a mixture of larger, pale ⇨, and smaller, eosinophilic ⇨ cells. The clear cells tend to concentrate along the septa ⇨, and the eosinophilic cells are toward the center.

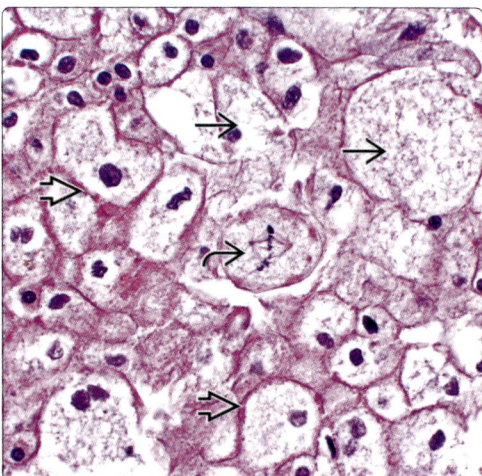
Microscopic Features

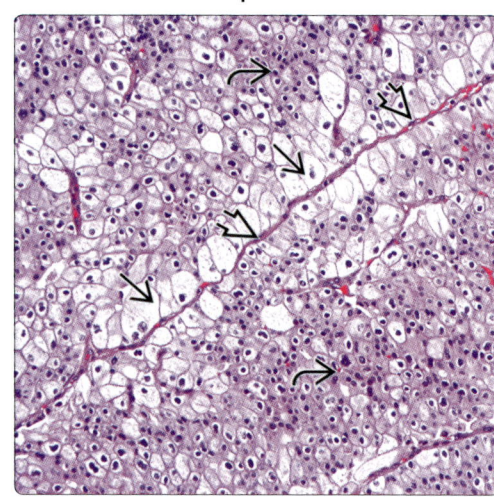
Microscopic Features

(Left) Occasionally, Ch-RCC shows well-defined foci with either pure eosinophilic ⇨ or clear cells ⇨ adjacent to each other. In spite of cytologic differences, both the classic and eosinophilic variants share many cytogenetic features and, to a great extent, immunophenotypic profiles. (Right) Most typically, Ch-RCC shows solid sheets of clear and eosinophilic cells, separated by thin and incomplete ⇨ vascular septations that do not completely encircle cell nests.

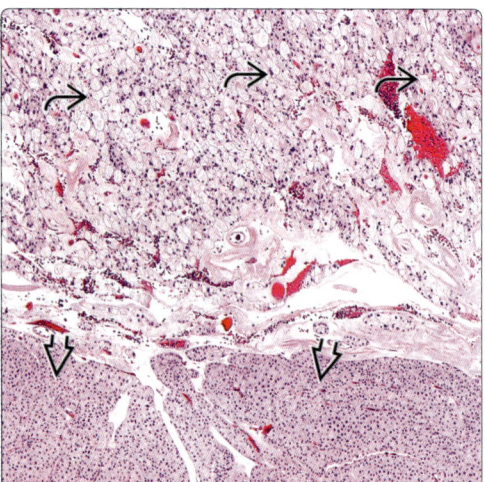
Microscopic Features

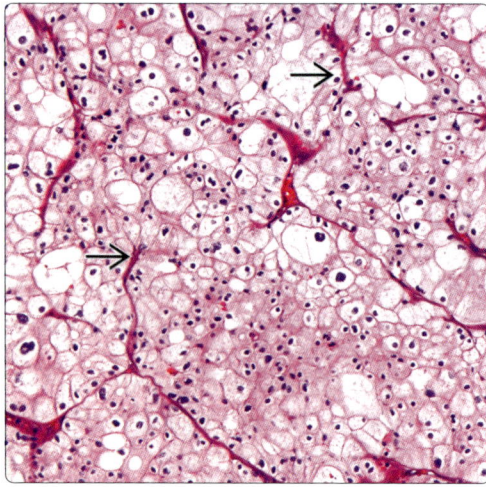
Microscopic Features

(Left) Architectural pattern in some tumors is often entirely acinar. Such architecture is particularly more common in tumors composed almost exclusively of cells with eosinophilic cytoplasm (eosinophilic variants). The eosinophilic variants constitute ~ 30-40% of all Ch-RCCs. (Right) Occasionally, Ch-RCCs may show focal to predominant tubular architecture. Tumors with predominant tubular architecture are often the eosinophilic variants.

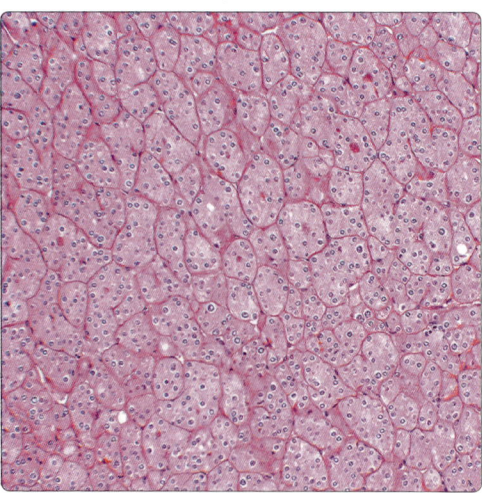
Microscopic Features

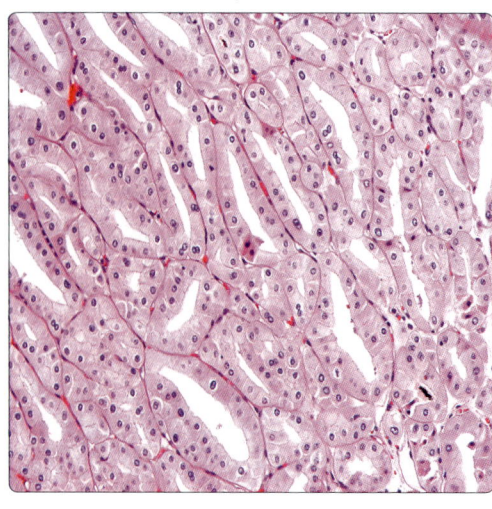
Microscopic Features

Chromophobe Renal Cell Carcinoma

Uncommon Microscopic Features

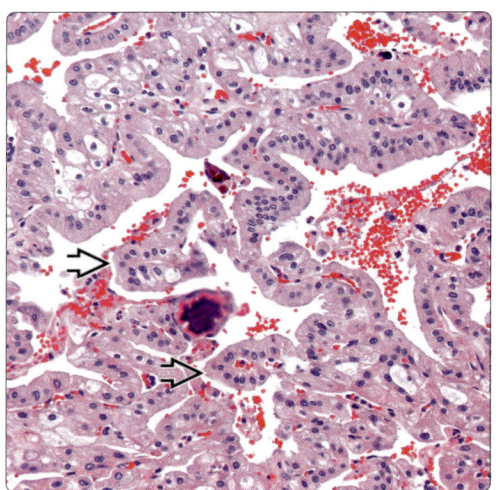

Uncommon Microscopic Features

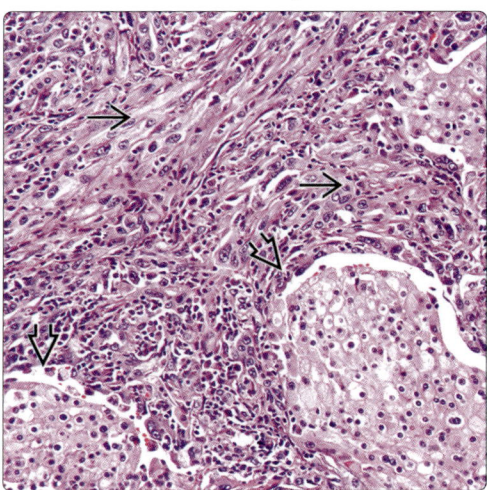

(Left) Focal papillations ⇨ may be present in some Ch-RCCs and are often seen in areas that show tubulocystic architecture. (Right) Approximately 5% of Ch-RCCs show sarcomatoid features ⇨. Typically, sarcomatoid areas appear juxtaposed to the epithelial components of the tumor ⇨, without gradual transition that is often present in other tumor types. Sarcomatoid features are often associated with aggressive clinical behavior.

Uncommon Microscopic Features

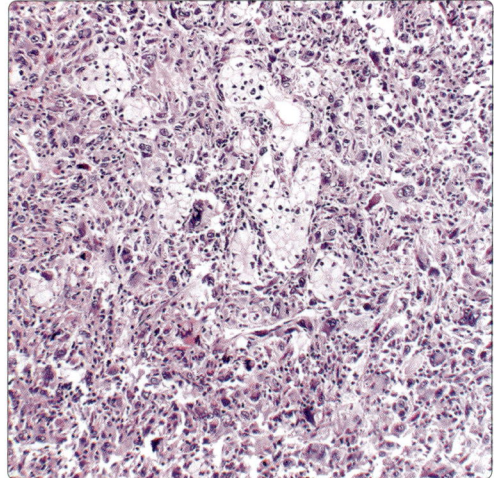

Uncommon Microscopic Features

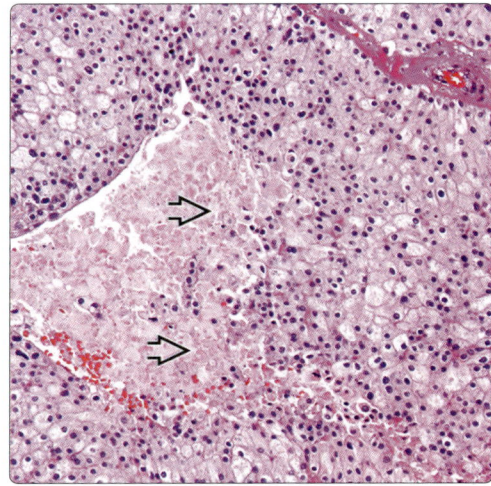

(Left) Rhabdoid and sarcomatoid features may sometimes coexist in a tumor. Both features indicate the aggressive phenotype of a Ch-RCC. (Right) Approximately 15% or more of Ch-RCCs show microscopic foci of tumor necrosis ⇨. Even in tumors without sarcomatoid features, microscopic tumor necrosis in Ch-RCC has been shown to be associated with aggressive clinical behavior in multiple studies.

Uncommon Microscopic Features

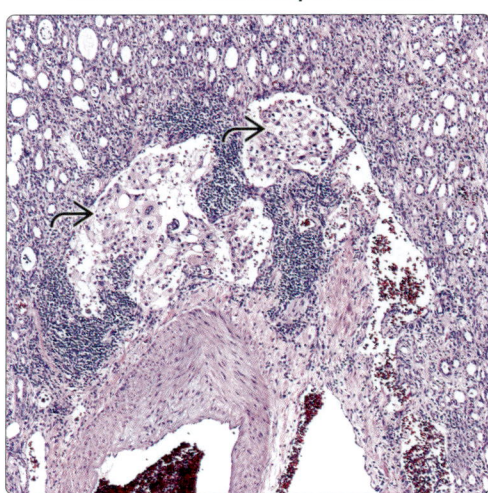

Uncommon Microscopic Features

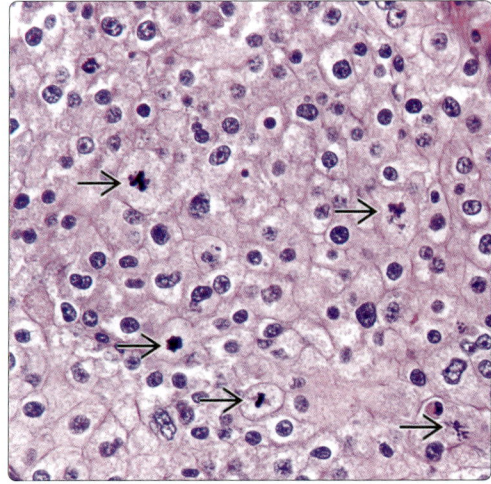

(Left) Lymphovascular invasion ⇨ in Ch-RCC is another feature that shows significant association with adverse clinical outcome. (Right) Other than in tumors with sarcomatoid features, mitotic figures are unusual in Ch-RCC; however, rare cases with pure epithelial histology may also show brisk mitotic activity ⇨. While intuitively brisk mitotic rates would be expected as a marker of aggressive behavior, none of the recent large studies have been able to confirm this.

Chromophobe Renal Cell Carcinoma

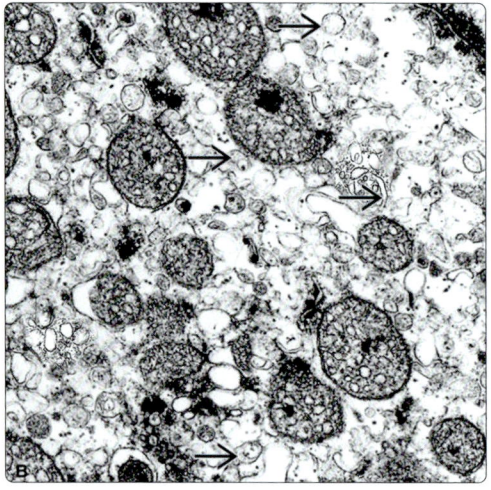

Ultrastructural Features

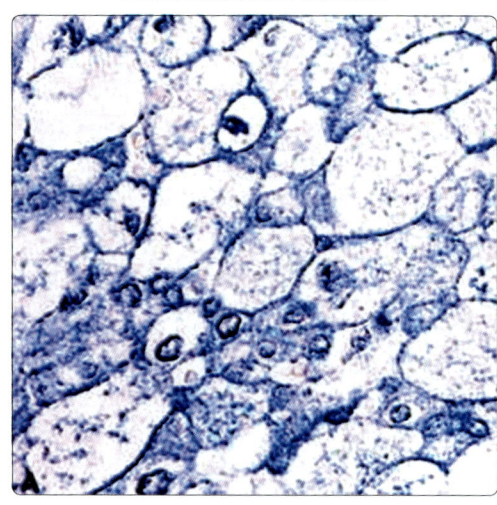

Histochemical Features

(Left) Numerous cytoplasmic microvesicles are the ultrastructural hallmark of Ch-RCC ➡. Their predominant perinuclear location results in the light microscopic perinuclear halos. Microvesicles also displace other organelles to the cell periphery, leading to the apparently prominent cell membranes. (Right) Hale colloidal iron often shows diffuse, reticular cytoplasmic staining in Ch-RCC. Occasional oncocytomas may also show luminal positivity. Some eosinophilic Ch-RCC may also label like renal oncocytoma.

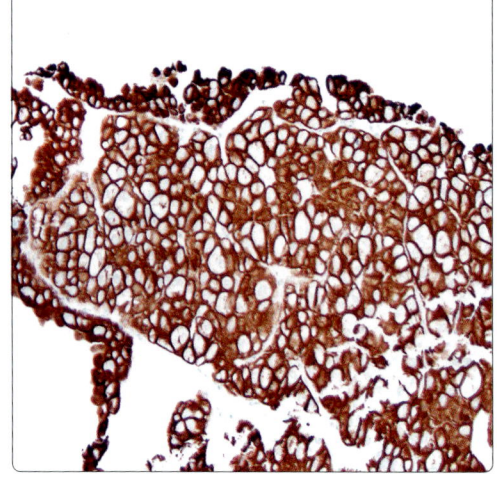

Immunohistochemistry

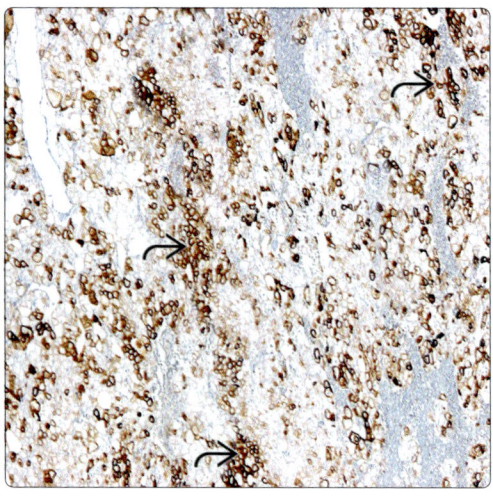

Immunohistochemistry

(Left) CK7 often shows diffuse membrane-predominant positivity in Ch-RCC, a pattern different from that in renal oncocytoma. CK7 is either negative or usually only stains rare single cells in renal oncocytoma. (Right) However, CK7 positivity may be patchy ➡ or focal, particularly in eosinophilic variants of Ch-RCC. In rare eosinophilic variants, only rare cells or clusters of cells may be positive, making distinction from oncocytoma difficult based on IHC alone.

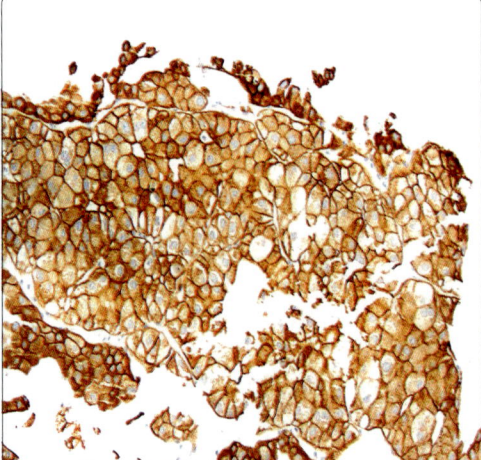

Immunohistochemistry

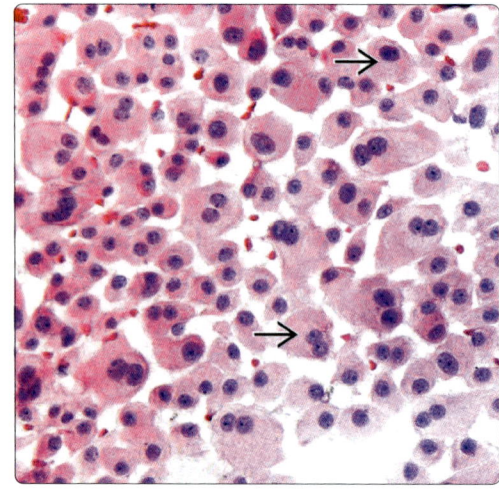

Cytology

(Left) CD117 stains both Ch-RCC and renal oncocytoma in a diffuse fashion, usually with membrane accentuation in Ch-RCC. The diffuse positivity may help in distinguishing these tumors from eosinophilic variants of clear cell RCC. Vimentin is negative in most CH-RCCs. (Right) Cytologic preparations often do not show the perinuclear halos, but significant nuclear atypia and minimal paleness of perinuclear cytoplasm ➡ is quite characteristic.

Chromophobe Renal Cell Carcinoma

Uncommon Microscopic Features

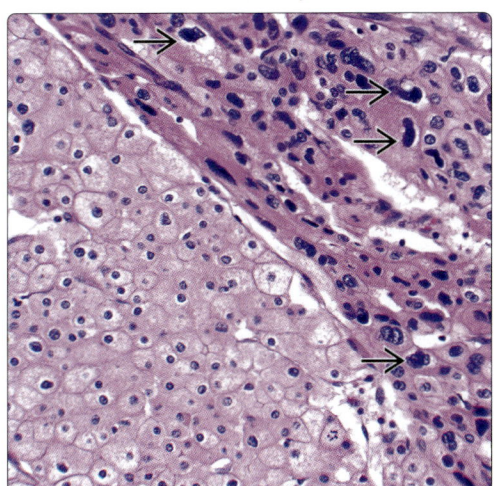

Uncommon Microscopic Features

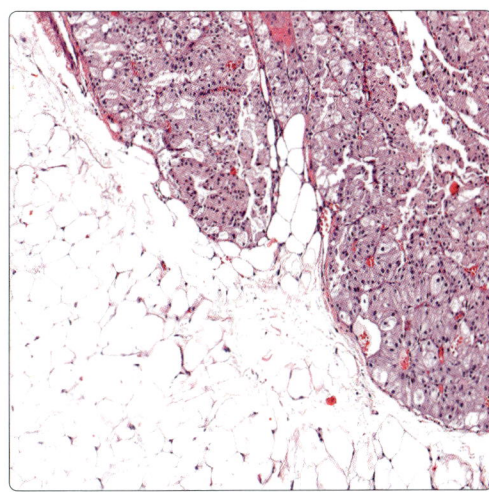

(Left) This image shows an area with markedly pleomorphic, hyperchromatic, and polyploid nuclei ➡. Such degenerate-appearing foci may occasionally be seen in Ch-RCC, but are more commonly seen in renal oncocytoma. **(Right)** Like renal oncocytoma, Ch-RCC may show perinephric fat invasion without any reactive desmoplasia. This is more often seen in the eosinophilic variants of Ch-RCC. Fat invasion without desmoplastic response may also be seen in oncocytic RCC, unclassified.

Metastasis

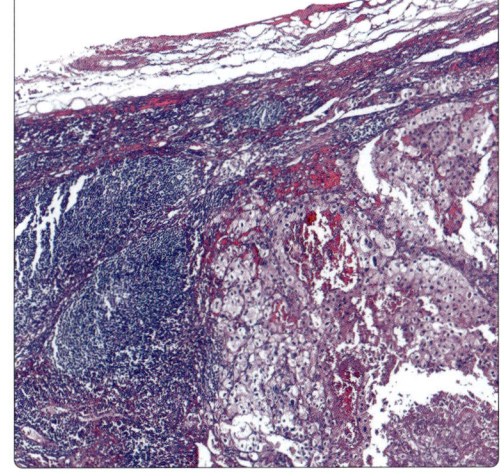

Metastasis

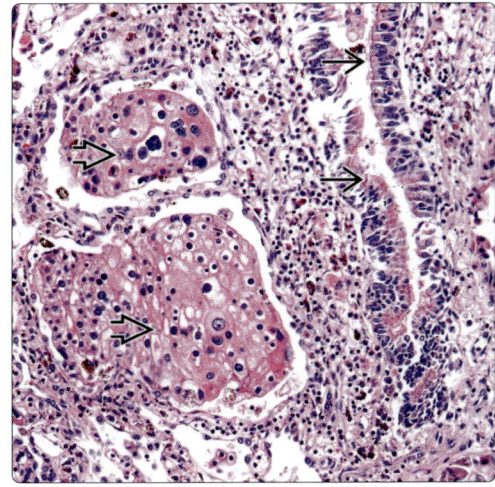

(Left) Stage for stage, Ch-RCC has better prognosis than clear cell RCC (and possibly papillary RCC). Metastases most often involve the regional lymph nodes, as shown here. **(Right)** This image shows a Ch-RCC metastatic to the lung ➡. Notice the adjacent benign bronchial epithelium ➡ and alveolar parenchyma. The overall survival with metastatic Ch-RCC seems to be better than that with other metastatic nonclear cell renal cell carcinomas, supporting its inherently more indolent nature.

Biopsy Diagnosis

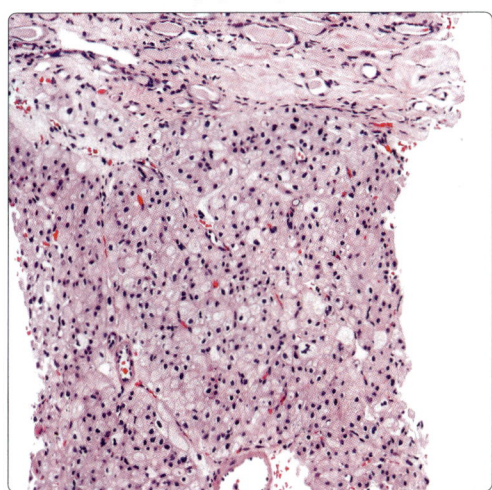

Biopsy Diagnosis

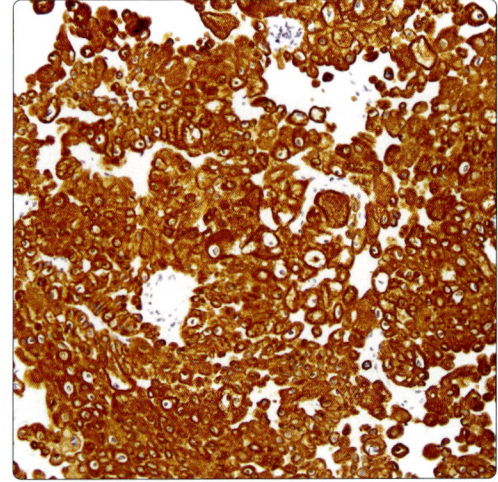

(Left) Classical and most cases of eosinophilic variants can easily be diagnosed on needle core biopsies if the characteristic morphological features are present. **(Right)** The distinction from renal oncocytoma on needle core biopsies may be difficult in some cases. In the differential diagnostic considerations between oncocytoma and eosinophilic variant of Ch-RCC, diffuse immunoreactivity for CK7, as seen here, supports Ch-RCC.

Collecting Duct Carcinoma

KEY FACTS

TERMINOLOGY
- Collecting duct carcinoma (CDC)
- Rare, high-grade renal cell carcinoma (RCC) likely arising from cells of collecting ducts of renal medulla
- Diagnostic features still evolving, with characteristic, but not entirely specific, morphologic and immunophenotypic features

CLINICAL ISSUES
- Wide age range of 13-83 years (mean: 50 years)
- Predominantly centered in medulla of kidney
- ~ 1/2 of patients die of disease within 2 years
  - Median survival: 44 weeks

MICROSCOPIC
- Primarily high-grade adenocarcinoma
  - Variable architectural patterns, usually in various combinations, including tubular, papillary, solid, cribriform
- Typically with multinodular growth pattern, desmoplastic stroma, and intratumoral inflammatory infiltrate
- Lymphovascular invasion present in majority of cases
- Metastases to regional nodes frequent (> 50% cases at presentation)

ANCILLARY TESTS
- Often positive for lectins, ULEX-1, PNA, and soybean agglutinin

TOP DIFFERENTIAL DIAGNOSES
- Papillary renal cell carcinoma
- Urothelial carcinoma with glandular features
- Renal medullary carcinoma
- Hereditary leiomyomatosis renal cell cancer syndrome-associated RCC
- Metastatic carcinoma
- Renal cell carcinoma, unclassified

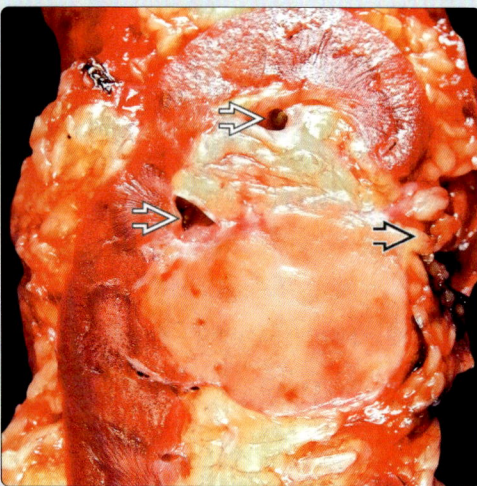

Gross Features

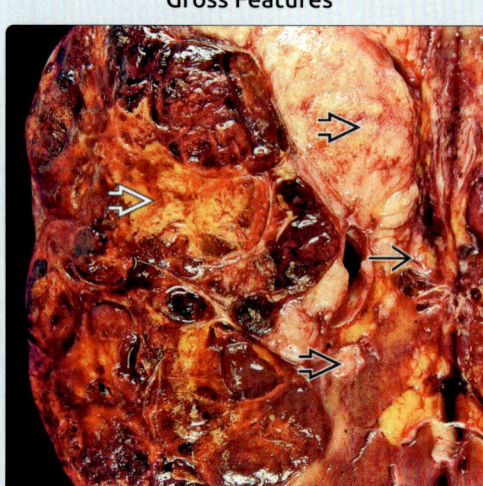

Gross Features

(Left) This example of collecting duct carcinoma (CDC) centered in the renal medullary region of a kidney shows a somewhat homogeneous cut surface. Extension into sinus fat ➡ and pelvicalyceal system ➡ are common. (Right) Gross and microscopic variability is frequent in CDC. This multinodular tumor shows a combination of solid, tan ➡, and hemorrhagic necrotic ➡ areas. Note the invasion of the renal sinus fat ➡, a frequent finding. Urothelial carcinoma is always in differential grossly.

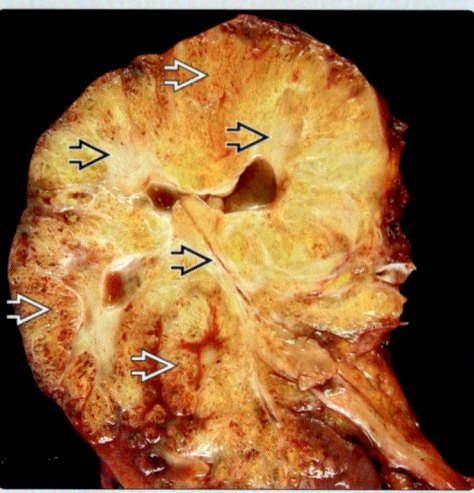

Gross Features

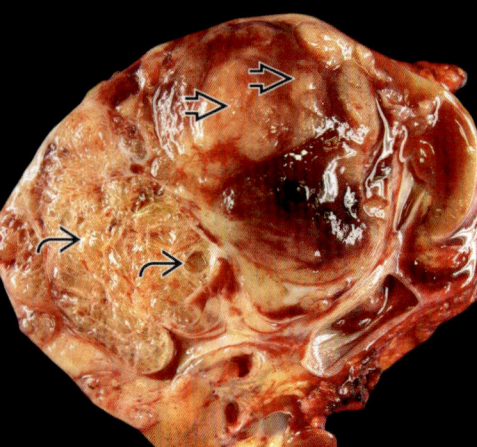

Gross Features

(Left) This CDC shows fleshy solid areas of sarcomatoid differentiation ➡. The epithelial component in this tumor reveals a fine, sieve-like microcystic growth pattern ➡. In large tumors, it may be difficult to ascertain whether the tumor is centered in the renal medulla. (Right) This tumor shows 2 distinct gross features, one with a fleshy tan cut surface ➡ with hemorrhage and the other with soap bubble-type, multicystic appearance ➡. The latter on microscopy corresponds to tubulocystic histology.

Collecting Duct Carcinoma

TERMINOLOGY

Abbreviations
- Collecting duct carcinoma (CDC)

Synonyms
- Carcinoma of collecting ducts of Bellini

Definitions
- Rare, high-grade renal cell carcinoma (RCC), likely arising from cells of collecting ducts of renal medulla
  - Diagnostic features still evolving, with characteristic, but not entirely specific, morphologic and immunophenotypic features

ETIOLOGY/PATHOGENESIS

Genetic Features
- Monosomies of chromosomes 1, 6, 14, 15, and 22 consistently observed in few tumors tested
- Loss of heterozygosity (LOH) of multiple chromosomal arms, including 1q, 6p, 8p, 13q, and 21q present in most cases
  - Minimal area of deletion located at 1q32.1-32.2 also identified
  - 8p LOH postulated to be associated with particularly aggressive behavior
- Amplification of HER2 present in some cases
- Trisomies of 7 and 17 (typical of papillary RCC), or chromosome 3 losses (typical of clear cell RCC) are absent
- Recently, alterations involving NF2 (29% cases), SETD2 (24%), SMARCB1 (18%), and CDKN2A (12%) genes described, based on small number of evaluated cases
- Also, role of polyoma family BK virus under investigation

CLINICAL ISSUES

Epidemiology
- Incidence
  - Constitute < 1% of malignant renal cell tumors
    - M:F = 2.3:1
  - Recently, largest multiinstitutional series in literature included 39 cases
  - Nationwide survey study from Japan was able to include 81 cases in report
- Age
  - Wide range: 13-83 years (mean: 50 years)

Site
- Predominantly centered in medulla of kidney
  - In larger tumors, site of origin difficult to determine

Presentation
- Most patients present with hematuria
- Palpable flank mass, pain, and weight loss other presentations
- Symptoms related to metastases also frequent
  - Unlike what is usual in more common RCC subtypes, ~ 2/3 cases symptomatic at presentation

Treatment
- Currently, surgical excision and urothelial carcinoma-like chemotherapeutic options commonly followed
  - Responses to any therapy very limited and of short duration
  - Recently, targeted therapies against tyrosine kinase receptors of VEGF-related molecules have been used
    - Results with combination of VEGF-A inhibitor, bevacizumab, with gemcitabine and cisplatin shown be promising

Prognosis
- Unfavorable outcomes very common
  - ~ 1/2 of patients die of disease within 2 years, with median survival of 44 weeks
- Frequently metastatic at presentation, commonly with multiple organ involvement, including
  - Lymph nodes, various viscera (lungs being most common), and bone

MACROSCOPIC

General Features
- Predominantly located in medulla, but larger tumors often involve cortex secondarily
- Classically, gray-pale with invasive borders
- Typically has multinodular growth pattern
- Areas of necrosis, hemorrhage, and cystic change are frequently present
- Grossly, majority of tumors invade renal sinus and perinephric fat
- Well-circumscribed tumors with purely cystic appearance previously considered low-grade CDC
  - These now regarded as separate entity (tubulocystic carcinoma)
  - Some CDCs with otherwise typical high-grade features also show variable amount of tubulocystic areas

Size
- 1-15 cm (median: 6 cm)

MICROSCOPIC

Histologic Features
- Primarily high-grade adenocarcinoma, widely infiltrative and often multinodular
- Variable architectural patterns, usually in various combinations
  - Including tubular, solid tubular/acinar, papillary, solid sheet-like, and cribriform
  - Like other RCCs, CDCs may also show sarcomatoid features
    - Biologic significance of such features not as dramatic as in other RCCs, as usual CDC by itself is very aggressive tumor
  - Rarely, with prominent rhabdoid or signet ring cell features
- Multinodular growth pattern with marked desmoplastic stroma and intratumoral inflammatory infiltrate, including microabscesses
  - Inflammatory infiltrate often lymphoid, and only infrequently neutrophilic
- Surrounding renal collecting ducts often show dysplastic cytologic features
- High-grade cytology (grade 3 or 4), often with marked nuclear pleomorphism and brisk mitotic activity

Collecting Duct Carcinoma

- Sometimes cytoplasmic mucin may be seen, highlighted by Alcian blue or mucicarmine stain
- Lymphatic/vascular invasion
  - Present in majority of cases
- Lymph nodes
  - Metastases to regional nodes frequent (> 50% cases at presentation) in CDC

ANCILLARY TESTS

Immunohistochemistry

- General comments
  - Generally positive for
    - HMCK(34βE12), EMA, CK7, CEA, pax-8, S100A1, INI1
  - Very often stain positive with lectins, ULEX-1, PNA, and soybean agglutinin
  - Usually negative for
    - CD10, AMACR, E-cadherin, CA9, OCT3/4

DIFFERENTIAL DIAGNOSIS

Papillary Renal Cell Carcinoma

- Usually well circumscribed; stromal desmoplasia rare
- Papillary cores often contain foamy macrophages
- Usually CK7 and AMACR positive; HMCK(34βE12) and lectin stains often negative

Urothelial Carcinoma With Glandular Features

- Often with intrapelvic papillary or flat in situ carcinoma component
- Presence of squamous morphology and sheets or other typical patterns of urothelial carcinoma
- GATA3, uroplakin-2 positive

Renal Medullary Carcinoma

- Cribriform architecture, intratumoral neutrophils more common
- Typically with sickle cell trait, and presence of sickled red cells in specimen
- Baf47 (INI1) loss, OCT3/4 positive

Hereditary Leiomyomatosis Renal Cell Cancer Syndrome-Associated Renal Cell Carcinoma

- Presence of prominent nucleoli and perinucleolar halos characteristic
- Loss of fumarate hydratase, and diffuse nuclear and cytoplasmic staining for 2SC

Renal Cell Carcinoma, Unclassified

- Morphologic features of CDC may be shared by many other high-grade tumors, and CDC may show marked variability in morphology
  - In such situations, dependence on immunoprofile, even though not highly specific, is prudent
  - In absence of typical immunophenotype, such tumors should be considered RCC, unclassified

Metastatic Carcinoma

- History of primary tumor
- Most often bilateral
- *Ulex europaeus* and PNA staining depends on type of primary (e.g., enteric tumors may be positive); other tumor specific characteristics also helpful
- CDX2, TTF1, GATA3 and other markers may be helpful

DIAGNOSTIC CHECKLIST

Pathologic Interpretation Pearls

- Stromal desmoplasia, multinodular growth pattern, intratumoral inflammation, and renal tubular dysplasia common to both CDC and urothelial carcinoma
- Immunophenotyping may also not be helpful in their separation
  - Finding of in situ urothelial component is only reliable differentiating feature
  - Adequate sampling of urothelium, including that of urothelium away from tumor mass, is therefore absolute requirement
- Collecting duct carcinomas with prominent papillary architecture often misdiagnosed as papillary RCC, type 2
  - In papillary tumors with mixture of other architectural patterns, desmoplasia, and multinodularity, possibility of CDC must always be considered
- HLRCC (new subtype of RCC) must also be ruled out

SELECTED REFERENCES

1. Pal SK et al: Characterization of clinical cases of collecting duct carcinoma of the kidney assessed by comprehensive genomic profiling. Eur Urol. S0302-2838(15)00522-9, 2015
2. Amin MB et al: Collecting duct carcinoma versus renal medullary carcinoma: an appeal for nosologic and biological clarity. Am J Surg Pathol. 38(7):871-4, 2014
3. Pécuchet N et al: Triple combination of bevacizumab, gemcitabine and platinum salt in metastatic collecting duct carcinoma. Ann Oncol. 24(12):2963-7, 2013
4. Gupta R et al: Carcinoma of the collecting ducts of Bellini and renal medullary carcinoma: clinicopathologic analysis of 52 cases of rare aggressive subtypes of renal cell carcinoma with a focus on their interrelationship. Am J Surg Pathol. 36(9):1265-78, 2012
5. Elwood H et al: Immunohistochemical analysis of SMARCB1/INI-1 expression in collecting duct carcinoma. Urology. 78(2):474.e1-5, 2011
6. Albadine R et al: PAX8 (+)/p63 (-) immunostaining pattern in renal collecting duct carcinoma (CDC): a useful immunoprofile in the differential diagnosis of CDC versus urothelial carcinoma of upper urinary tract. Am J Surg Pathol. 34(7):965-9, 2010
7. Choueiri TK et al: Sunitinib in renal-cell carcinoma: expanded indications. Lancet Oncol. 10(8):740, 2009
8. Osunkoya AO et al: Comparison of gene expression profiles in tubulocystic carcinoma and collecting duct carcinoma of the kidney. Am J Surg Pathol. 33(7):1103-6, 2009
9. Wright JL et al: Effect of collecting duct histology on renal cell cancer outcome. J Urol. 182(6):2595-9, 2009
10. Kobayashi N et al: Collecting duct carcinoma of the kidney: an immunohistochemical evaluation of the use of antibodies for differential diagnosis. Hum Pathol. 39(9):1350-9, 2008
11. Oudard S et al: Prospective multicenter phase II study of gemcitabine plus platinum salt for metastatic collecting duct carcinoma: results of a GETUG (Groupe d'Etudes des Tumeurs Uro-Génitales) study. J Urol. 177(5):1698-702, 2007
12. Tokuda N et al: Collecting duct (Bellini duct) renal cell carcinoma: a nationwide survey in Japan. J Urol. 176(1):40-3; discussion 43, 2006
13. Polascik TJ et al: Molecular genetics and histopathologic features of adult distal nephron tumors. Urology. 60(6):941-6, 2002
14. Steiner G et al: High-density mapping of chromosomal arm 1q in renal collecting duct carcinoma: region of minimal deletion at 1q32.1-32.2. Cancer Res. 56(21):5044-6, 1996
15. Fleming S et al: Collecting duct carcinoma of the kidney. Histopathology. 10(11):1131-41, 1986

Collecting Duct Carcinoma

Microscopic Features

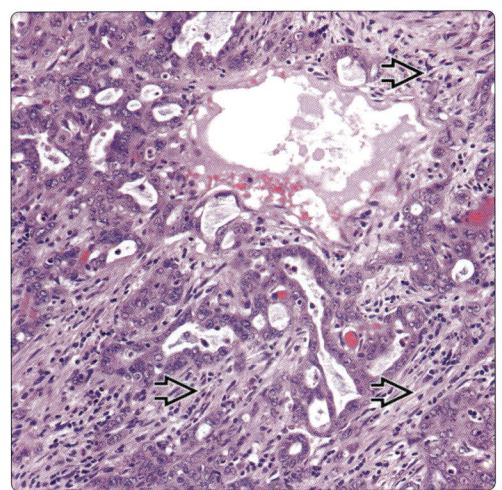

Microscopic Features

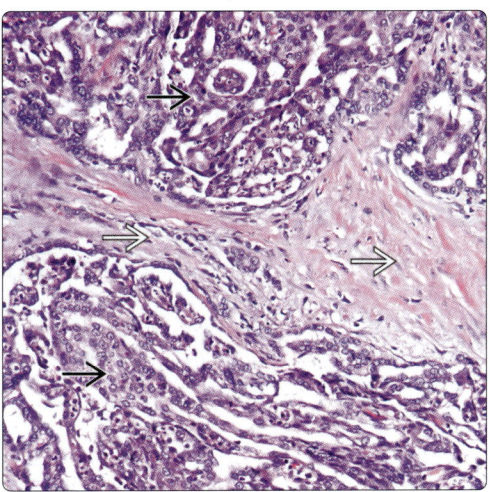

(Left) Microscopically, CDC is a high-grade adenocarcinoma that may show variable architectural patterns. Multinodularity and abundant stromal desmoplasia ⇨ are common. (Right) Some CDCs show variable, and occasionally extensive, papillary architecture. However, high-grade cytology ⇨, marked stromal desmoplasia ⇨, and multinodular growth pattern are maintained, and these features should differentiate such tumors from type 2 papillary renal cell carcinoma (RCC).

Microscopic Features

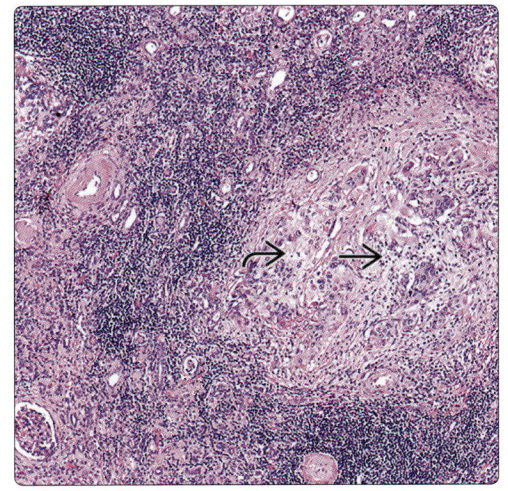

Microscopic Features

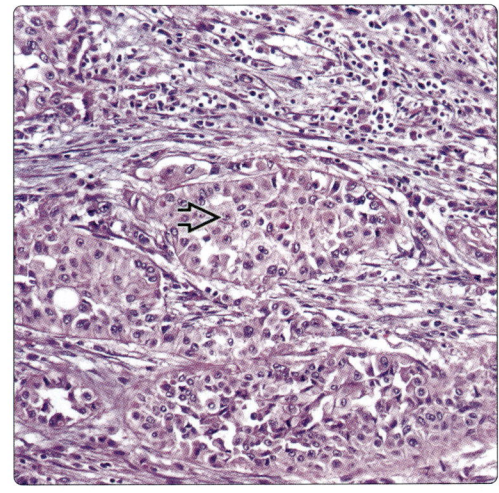

(Left) Tubular, glandular, or tubulopapillary architecture are most common in CDC. Notice the prominent desmoplastic stroma ⇨ and lymphocytic response ⇨, both characteristic features of the the tumor. (Right) Although glandular features are common in CDC, solid areas ⇨ or nests, as depicted in this photomicrograph, are not uncommon. Such architecture makes distinction from invasive urothelial carcinoma difficult in some cases.

Microscopic Features

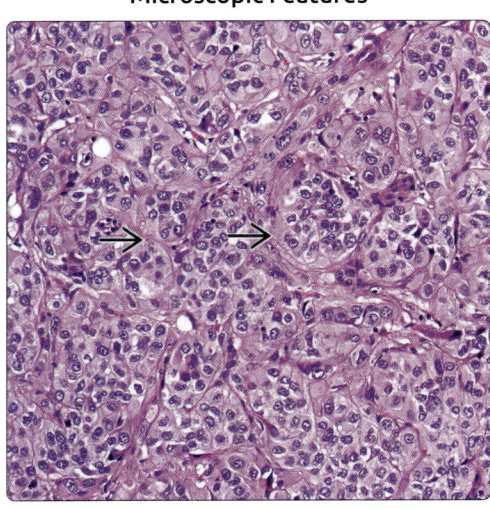

Microscopic Features

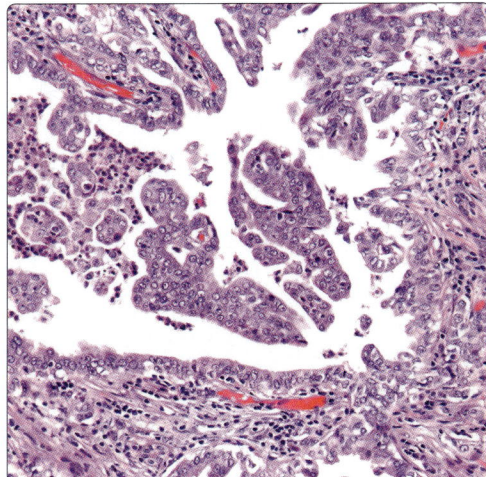

(Left) Some cases of CDC may have a prominent solid tubular architecture, with tubules surrounded by basement membrane-like material ⇨. Extensive sampling of urothelium is a must to exclude urothelial carcinoma. (Right) Almost exclusive papillary architecture may be present in some tumors. However, papillary architecture alone is no reason for regarding a renal tumor as papillary RCC. Attention to all gross and microscopic findings is essential to mislabel such CDCs as type 2 papillary RCC.

Collecting Duct Carcinoma

Microscopic Features

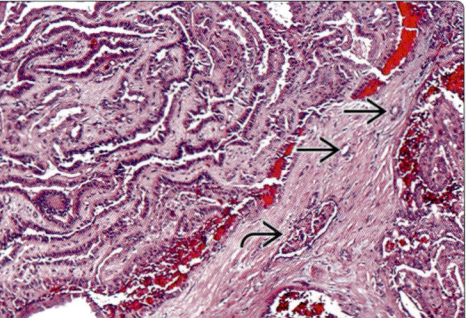

Microscopic Features

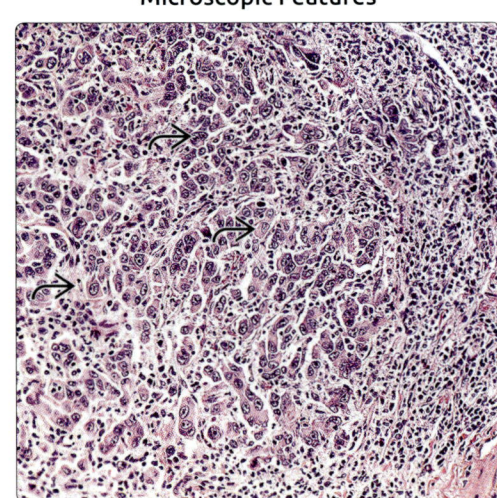

(Left) *Multinodular growth pattern is a frequent finding in CDC. The intervening fibrotic renal parenchyma in this image contains sclerotic glomeruli ⇨, as well as atrophic renal tubules ⇨.*
(Right) *Rarely, CDC may show prominent rhabdoid ⇨ or even signet ring cell features. Almost all tumors are nuclear or International Society of Urological Pathology (ISUP)/WHO grade 3 or 4.*

Histological Features

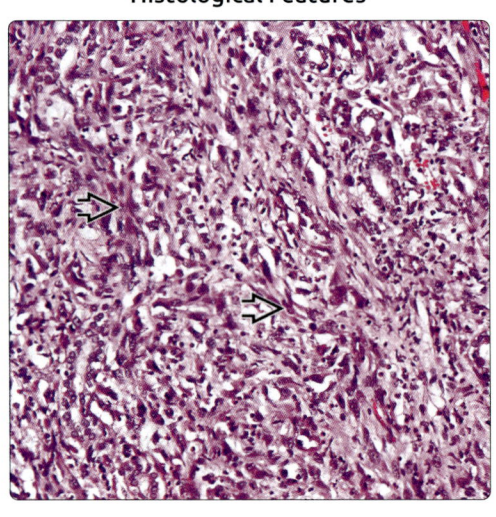

Microscopic Features

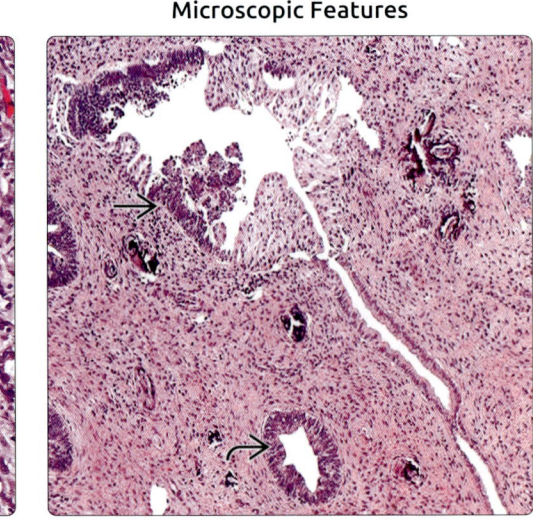

(Left) *Like other renal cancers, CDC may show sarcomatoid differentiation ⇨. This finding does not necessarily portend a more aggressive clinical behavior, as even the nonsarcomatoid tumor is inherently clinically aggressive.* (Right) *Surrounding renal collecting ducts often show dysplastic cytologic features ⇨ in CDC. This image also shows intratubular growth pattern ⇨ of the tumor. Although characteristic, this is not specific to CDC and may be seen even in some cases of papillary RCC.*

Microscopic Features

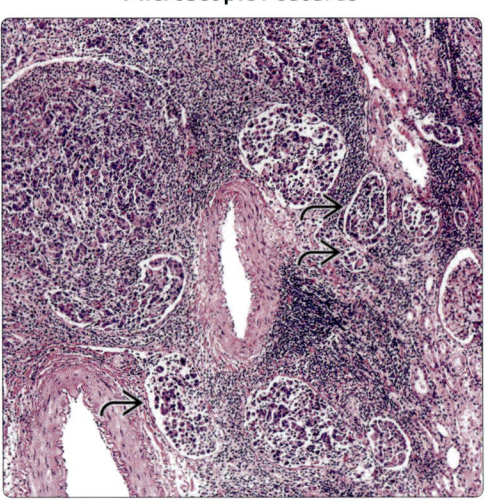

Microscopic Features

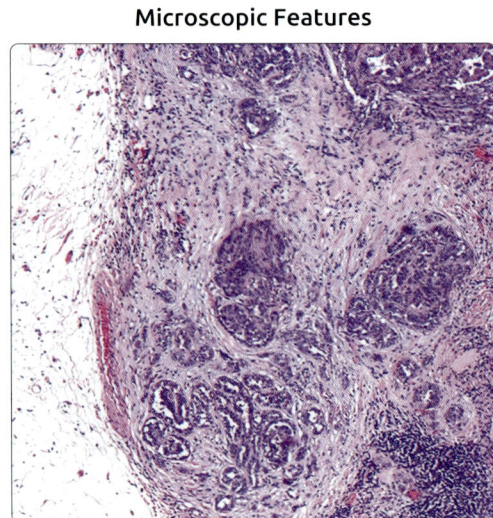

(Left) *CDC is among the most aggressive subtypes of RCC. Lymphovascular invasion ⇨ is present in almost all cases.*
(Right) *This image shows perinephric fat invasion in a CDC. Most tumors show perinephric or sinus fat invasion, or invasion into the venous system. An overwhelming majority of CDCs present with pT3 or pT4 disease.*

Collecting Duct Carcinoma

Histological Features
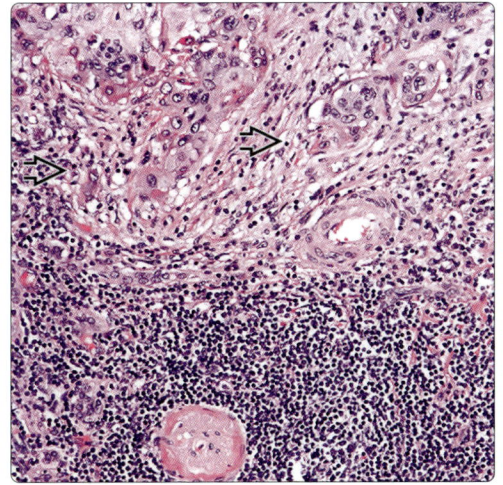

Immunohistochemical Features
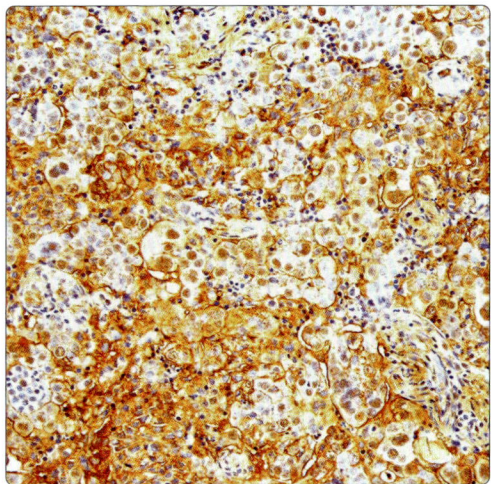

(Left) Lymph node metastasis ➲ is present in >50% of the cases of CDC at the time of presentation. Other common sites of metastasis at presentation include lungs and skeletal system. (Right) ULEX-1 often stains positive in CDC. However, some tumors completely lack staining. ULEX-1 may also stain other renal tumors related to the distal nephron and urothelial carcinoma. It has limited role diagnostically. pax-8 is consistently positive.

Immunohistochemical Features
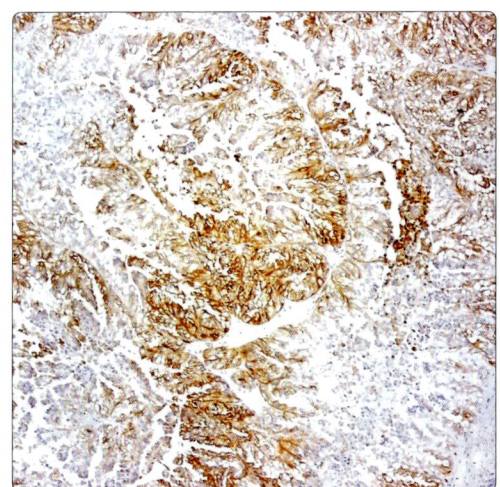

Differential Diagnosis
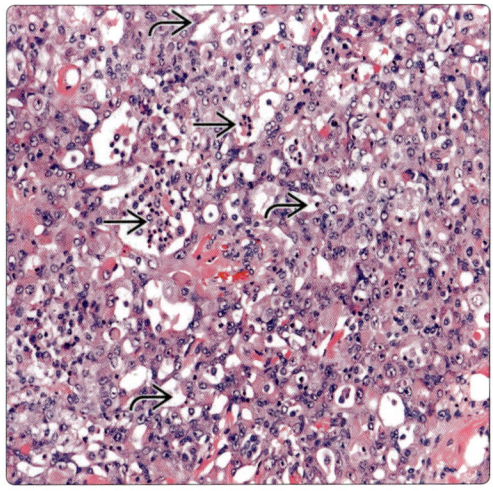

(Left) While HMCK(34βE12) immunostaining is often positive in CDC, the positivity may be quite focal or entirely absent in some cases. In general, immunohistochemical staining patterns are often not reliable in the distinction of CDC from urothelial carcinoma invading the renal parenchyma. (Right) CDC and renal medullary carcinoma show significant morphological overlap. However, cribriform architecture ➲, and intratumoral neutrophils ➲, instead of lymphocytes, are more common in the latter.

Differential Diagnosis
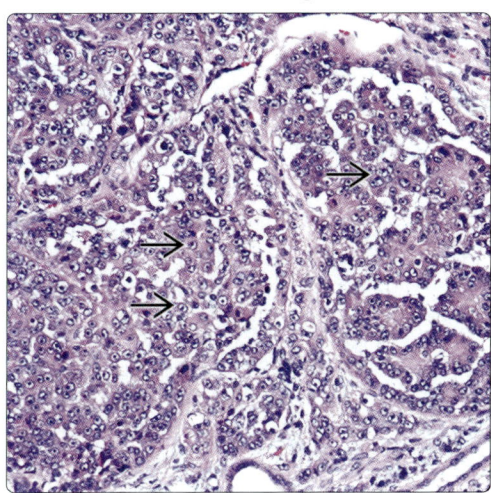

Differential Diagnosis
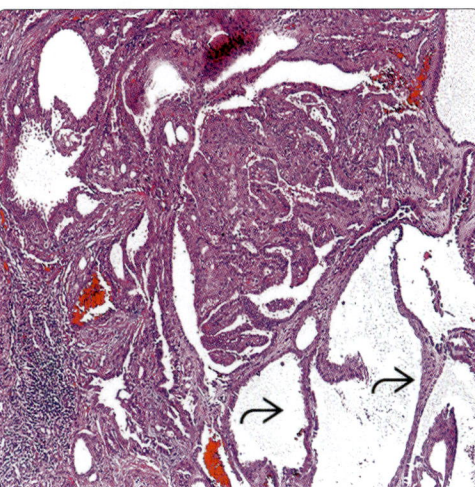

(Left) Renal tumors hereditary leiomyomatosis and renal cell cancer syndrome also show many similarities with CDC. However, these characteristically show very prominent nucleoli with perinucleolar halos ➲. (Right) CDCs may also show tubulocystic RCC-like areas ➲. Many such tumors are now known to be in-fact hereditary leiomyomatosis RCC-associated tumors. Immunohistochemical staining for fumarate hydratase & 2SC is important in their distinction from CDC. Metastasis should also be ruled out clinically.

Renal Medullary Carcinoma

KEY FACTS

TERMINOLOGY
- Distinctive clinicopathologic entity in patients with sickle cell hemoglobinopathies (HbS)
- Consistent immunohistochemical loss of hSNF5/INI1/Baf47

ETIOLOGY/PATHOGENESIS
- Presence of HbS in virtually all cases, suggesting some cause-effect relationship between hemoglobinopathy and this tumor
- Loss of immunohistochemical nuclear expression of hSNF5/INI1/Baf47 protein consistent finding, similar to pediatric rhabdoid tumor of kidney, but through different mechanisms

CLINICAL ISSUES
- Usually male and African American
- Medullary region of kidney
- Patients with sickle cell trait (Hb-AS), Hb-SC, and rarely Hb-SS
- Very aggressive tumor with metastases at presentation in almost all and mean survival of 4 months

MACROSCOPIC
- Gray-white, possessing infiltrative borders and extending into perihilar fat

MICROSCOPIC
- Reticular, cribriform, solid, tubular, or adenoid cystic-like growth patterns
- Marked desmoplastic stroma and intratumoral inflammatory infiltrate, usually neutrophilic
- Sickled RBCs frequently observed, both within tumor and surrounding parenchymal vessels

TOP DIFFERENTIAL DIAGNOSES
- Collecting duct carcinoma; urothelial carcinoma with prominent glandular features; *VCL-ALK* fusion carcinoma; unclassified renal cell carcinoma, with medullary phenotype

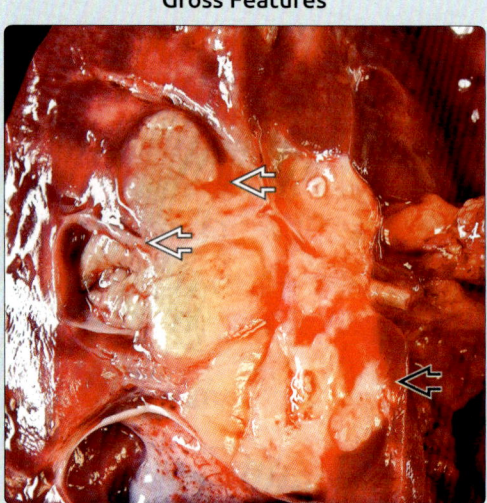

Gross Features

(Left) The photograph demonstrates the gross appearance of a renal medullary carcinoma (RMC). The tumors, particularly the smaller ones, are renal medulla based, with infiltrative borders ⇨. Here, it also invades the renal pelvis ⇨.

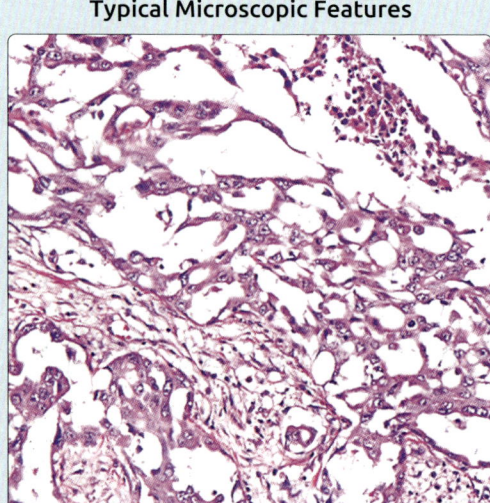

Typical Microscopic Features

(Right) RMC often shows a mixture of architectural patterns, reticular and cribriform patterns being the most common. The tumor invariably shows high nuclear grade.

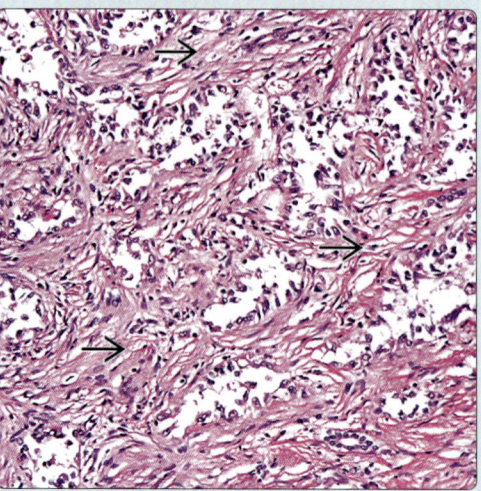

Stromal Desmoplasia

(Left) This RMC shows a prominent tubular architecture. Some tumors may be predominantly tubular. Irrespective of the architectural patterns, stromal desmoplasia ⇨ is a consistent finding.

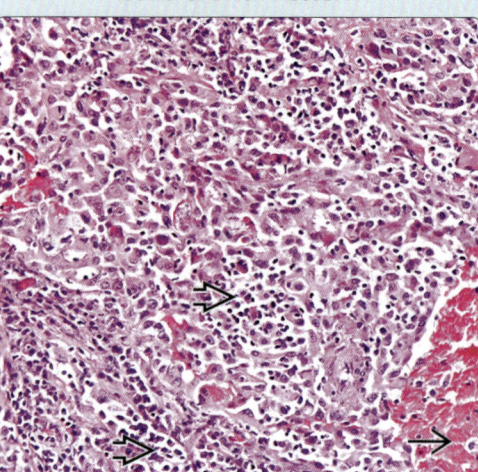

Solid Growth Pattern

(Right) Solid growth pattern in RMC is also common and is usually associated with other growth patterns within the same tumor. Notice the intratumoral inflammatory infiltrate ⇨ and agglutinated red blood cells ⇨, both consistent features in RMC.

Renal Medullary Carcinoma

TERMINOLOGY

Abbreviations
- Renal medullary carcinoma (RMC)

Synonyms
- Medullary renal cell carcinoma

Definitions
- Distinctive clinicopathologic entity occurring almost exclusively in patients with sickle cell (SC) trait
  - Rare cases in patients with hemoglobin SC disease and very occasionally in sickle cell disease (SS)
- Consistent immunohistochemical loss of hSNF5/INI1/Baf47

ETIOLOGY/PATHOGENESIS

Sickle Cell Hemoglobinopathies
- Presence of HbS in virtually all cases, suggesting some cause-effect relationship between hemoglobinopathy and this tumor
  - Exact mechanism unknown
    - Role of tissue hypoxia and hypoxia-inducible factor (HIF) in tumorigenesis or tumor viability/tumor progression is suggested

SMARCB1
- Loss of immunohistochemical nuclear expression of hSNF5/INI1/Baf47 protein, similar to pediatric rhabdoid tumor of kidney, consistent finding
  - CGH analysis demonstrates complete loss of 1 allele of *SMARCB1*, with no mutations in other allele
    - In contrast, both germline-mutated and sporadic renal and extrarenal rhabdoid tumors show bi-allelic alterations in gene
    - Alterations in *SMARCA4* gene, a gene closely related to *SMARCB1*, also seen in some rhabdoid or related tumors
      - Alterations in this gene not reported in renal medullary carcinoma

ABL1-BCR Amplifications
- Amplification of both *ABL1* and *BCR* genes described in few cases
- *ABL1-BCR* translocation described in 1 case but not in 3 others tested

Relationship to Collecting Duct Carcinoma
- Some consider RMC to be particularly aggressive form of collecting duct carcinoma
- Various clinicopathological differences, including age, survival, hSNF5/INI1/Baf47 loss, ethnicity etc., makes that possibility less likely
- May represent different entities with morphological overlap
  - Such morphological overlaps not unusual in renal carcinomas; examples include
    - Clear cell features in clear cell renal cell carcinoma (RCC), clear cell-papillary RCC, translocation-associated RCC
    - Type 2 papillary RCC, collecting duct carcinoma (CDC), hereditary leiomyomatosis RCC-associated RCC

CLINICAL ISSUES

Epidemiology
- Incidence
  - Uncommon tumor
    - ~ 225 cases described to date
- Age
  - Range: 5-39 yr
    - Only occasionally in older patients
- Sex
  - Predominantly male, especially in patients < 25 yr
    - M:F, 10:1 in some series
- Ethnicity
  - Mostly African American
    - Occasional cases in people of Mediterranean ancestry; rarely others

Presentation
- Often with hematuria or flank pain
  - Many presenting with symptoms related to metastases
  - One of rare renal tumors with symptomatic presentations

Laboratory Tests
- Most with sickle cell trait (Hb-AS) or Hb-SC on hemoglobin electrophoresis
- Rarely with homozygous sickle cell anemia (Hb-SS)
  - Hemoglobinopathy occasionally only recognized after pathological diagnosis of renal tumor

Treatment
- No consistently effective therapy to date
  - Most undergo surgical resection
  - Rare cases with some response to gemcitabine-cisplatin-based chemotherapy
    - However, overall prognosis and outcomes remain dismal

Prognosis
- Biologic behavior very aggressive
  - Mean survival ~17 weeks
  - Most cases with metastases at presentation

MACROSCOPIC

General Features
- Medullary based, gray-white cut surface, infiltrative borders often with extension into sinus fat
- Satellite nodules in adjacent parenchyma frequently observed
  - Often representing tumor emboli in large vessels

MICROSCOPIC

Histologic Features
- Most common architectural features: Reticular or cribriform glands
  - Other patterns include
    - Glandular
    - Solid nests and tubular, often angulated
    - Undifferentiated sheet-like
    - Yolk sac tumor-like

Renal Medullary Carcinoma

- Adenoid cystic-like
- Stroma almost always fibrotic or desmoplastic
- Intratumoral inflammatory infiltrate, mostly neutrophils, very frequent
  - Rarely predominantly lymphocytic/lympho-plasmacytic
- Tumor margins always infiltrative
- Cytoplasmic mucin commonly observed (> 70% cases)
- Cytology usually high grade, often with marked nuclear atypia
  - Occasional cases with rhabdoid or sarcomatoid features
- Sickled RBCs frequently observed, both within tumor and surrounding renal parenchymal vessels
  - In most cases, round outlines even in rare RBCs difficult to find
  - Many cases with agglutinated RBCs in vessels, with no clearly discernible outlines of individual red cells
- Often with high pT and pN stage
  - Satellite tumor nodules in kidney due to frequent vascular spread

Predominant Pattern/Injury Type
- Neoplastic

Predominant Cell/Compartment Type
- Epithelial

ANCILLARY TESTS

Immunohistochemistry
- Loss of hSNF5/INI1/Baf47 nuclear expression, consistent and diagnostically important finding
- Most cases with OCT3/OCT4 expression
- CK7 often positive
  - Usually HMCK (34βE12) negative
- CK20 frequently positive
- pax-8/pax-2 often negative

DIFFERENTIAL DIAGNOSIS

Collecting Duct Carcinoma
- Medullary carcinoma believed by some to be particularly virulent variant of CDC
  - Medullary carcinoma very often with cribriform architecture; uncommon in CDC
- No hemoglobinopathy
- Usually HMCK (34βE12) positive

Urothelial Carcinoma
- Intrapelvicalyceal papillary component or in situ urothelial carcinoma

VCL-ALK Renal Cell Carcinoma
- Tumors with HbS hemoglobinopathy, but no loss of hSNF5/INI1/Baf47
- Strong ALK expression by immunohistochemistry
  - *Vinculin-ALK* fusion on molecular analysis
- Described tumors with medullary epicenter, dyscohesive polygonal or spindle-shaped cells with prominent cytoplasmic vacuoles
  - Published tumors only in children with nonaggressive clinical behavior
- However, rarely observed in older individuals with more aggressive clinical features

Unclassified RCC, With Medullary Phenotype
- Proposed terminology for
  - Tumors with morphological features of RMC
  - Immunohistochemical loss of hSNF5/INI1/Baf47
  - Absence of sickling of RBCs on histological sections
    - Absence of HbS hemoglobinopathy
  - Await further molecular assessment for proper characterization and classification

DIAGNOSTIC CHECKLIST

Clinically Relevant Pathologic Features
- RMC regarded as tumor with HbS hemoglobinopathy and loss of hSNF5/INI1/Baf47
- Some tumors with medullary carcinoma-like histology with loss of hSNF5/INI1/Baf47, but no evidence of HbS hemoglobinopathy
  - Such tumors better regarded as RCC, unclassified with medullary carcinoma phenotype
    - Additional molecular studies required to ascertain true nature and relation with RMC
- For tumors with hSNF5/INI1/Baf47 loss, in proper morphological perspective, RMC to be excluded before accepting as CDC or other tumor types

SELECTED REFERENCES

1. Alvarez O et al: Renal medullary carcinoma and sickle cell trait: A systematic review. Pediatr Blood Cancer. 62(10):1694-9, 2015
2. Iacovelli R et al: Clinical outcome and prognostic factors in renal medullary carcinoma: A pooled analysis from 18 years of medical literature. Can Urol Assoc J. 9(3-4):E172-7, 2015
3. Amin MB et al: Collecting duct carcinoma versus renal medullary carcinoma: an appeal for nosologic and biological clarity. Am J Surg Pathol. 38(7):871-4, 2014
4. Smith NE et al: VCL-ALK renal cell carcinoma in children with sickle-cell trait: the eighth sickle-cell nephropathy? Am J Surg Pathol. 38(6):858-63, 2014
5. Liu Q et al: Renal medullary carcinoma: molecular, immunohistochemistry, and morphologic correlation. Am J Surg Pathol. 37(3):368-74, 2013
6. Srigley JR et al: The International Society of Urological Pathology (ISUP) Vancouver Classification of Renal Neoplasia. Am J Surg Pathol. 37(10):1469-89, 2013
7. Calderaro J et al: SMARCB1/INI1 inactivation in renal medullary carcinoma. Histopathology. 61(3):428-35, 2012
8. Gupta R et al: Carcinoma of the collecting ducts of Bellini and renal medullary carcinoma: clinicopathologic analysis of 52 cases of rare aggressive subtypes of renal cell carcinoma with a focus on their interrelationship. Am J Surg Pathol. 36(9):1265-78, 2012
9. Rao P et al: Expression of OCT3/4 in renal medullary carcinoma represents a potential diagnostic pitfall. Am J Surg Pathol. 36(4):583-8, 2012
10. Bell MD: Response to paclitaxel, gemcitabine, and cisplatin in renal medullary carcinoma. Pediatr Blood Cancer. 47(2):228, 2006
11. Ronnen EA et al: Medullary renal cell carcinoma and response to therapy with bortezomib. J Clin Oncol. 24(9):e14, 2006
12. Strouse JJ et al: Significant responses to platinum-based chemotherapy in renal medullary carcinoma. Pediatr Blood Cancer. 44(4):407-11, 2005
13. Davis CJ Jr et al: Renal medullary carcinoma. The seventh sickle cell nephropathy. Am J Surg Pathol. 19(1):1-11, 1995

Renal Medullary Carcinoma

Inflammatory Infiltrate

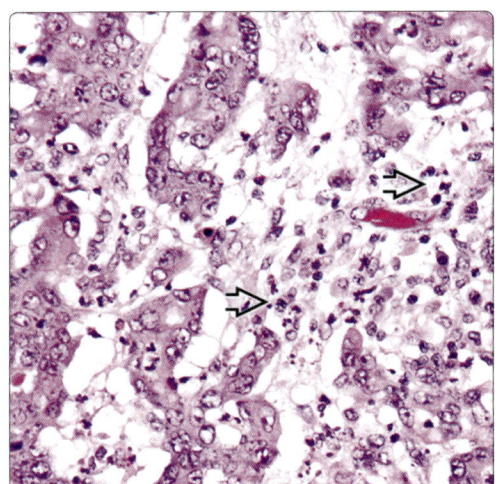

Micropapillary Architecture

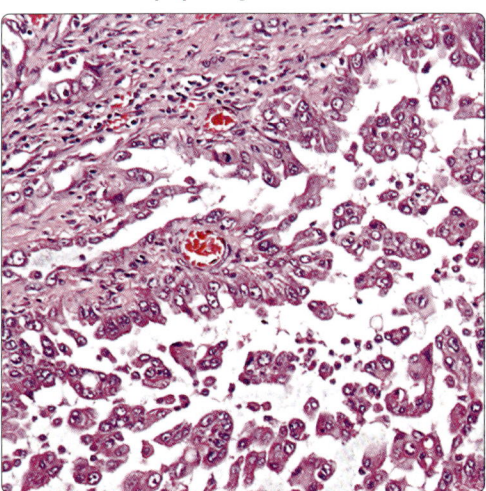

(Left) The photomicrograph shows an RMC with prominent inflammatory infiltrate within the tumor ⇒. Intratumoral inflammatory infiltrate is typical and is often neutrophilic but sometimes may be predominantly lympho-plasmacytic. (Right) This intermediate magnification view of an RMC shows a micropapillary architecture in the tumor. Papillary and micropapillary features are often present focally, usually in combination with other architectural patterns.

Yolk Sac Tumor-Like Features

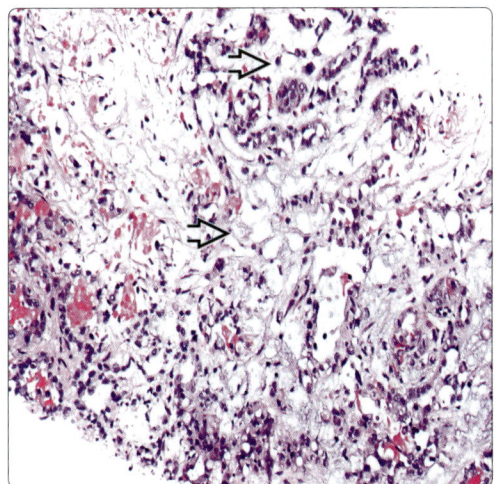

Adenoid Cystic Carcinoma-Like Features

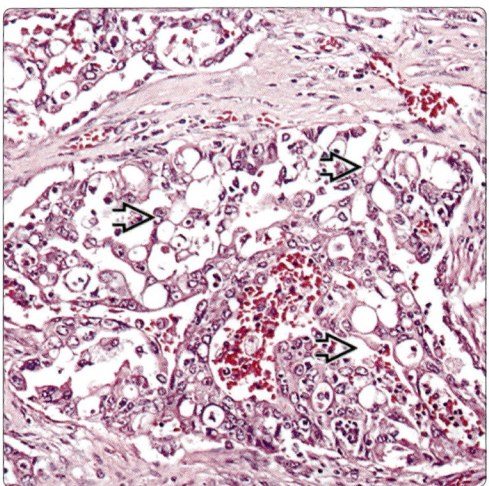

(Left) This photomicrograph from a renal needle core biopsy shows an RMC with loose and myxoid stroma ⇒ and microcystic-like appearance. This appearance in some cases is reminiscent of yolk sac tumor. (Right) This H&E image shows cribriform architecture ⇒ in an RMC. Cribriform architecture with small lumina may sometimes give an impression of adenoid cystic carcinoma-like areas.

Stromal Desmoplasia

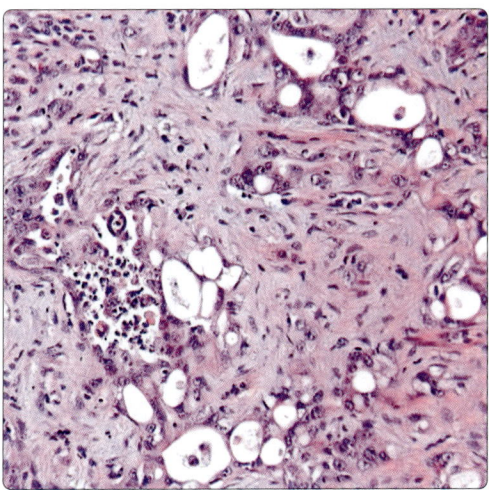

Sickled Red Blood Cells

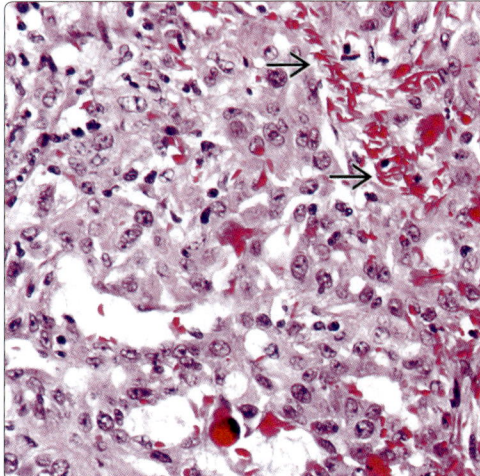

(Left) Stromal desmoplasia with stromal hyalinization is the norm in RMC. Other tumors in the kidney that consistently demonstrate this feature include CDC, invasive urothelial carcinoma, metastatic carcinoma to the kidney, and unclassified high-grade renal cell carcinoma, NOS. (Right) One of the characteristic features of RMC is the presence of sickled red blood cells ⇒. Such cells are seen both within the tumor and in the nonneoplastic parenchyma. Many times, the RBCs appear agglutinated within small capillaries.

Renal Medullary Carcinoma

(Left) Crenated or sickled red blood cells both within the tumor and in the benign parenchymal vasculature ⇨ are an almost consistent finding in RMC. (Right) Sometimes the solid areas in RMC may show rhabdoid features ⇨, raising the possibility of a rhabdoid tumor of the kidney. The negative nuclear reactivity for SNF5 in both may further compound the confusion. However, other areas of the tumor will usually show more classic morphology. Diffuse staining for CK7 may also help.

Sickled Red Blood Cells
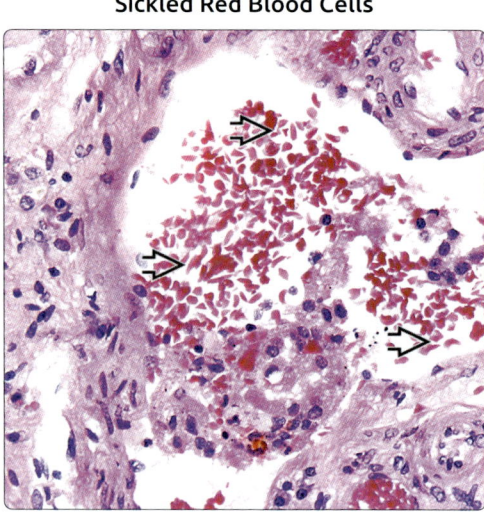

Rhabdoid Features
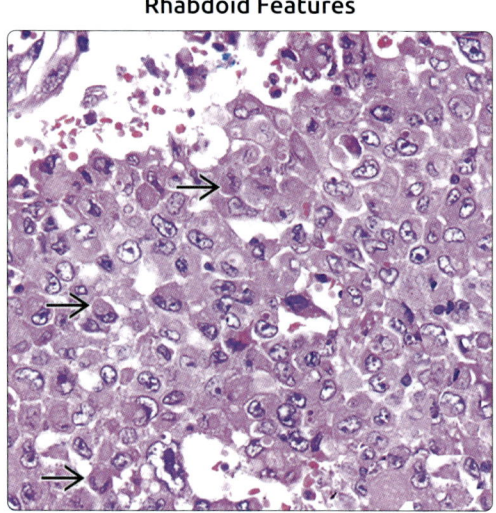

(Left) Microscopic foci of tumor necrosis ⇨ are frequent in RMC. The cytologic features of this aggressive tumor are always high grade. (Right) Similarly, vascular invasion, including that of large muscular ⇨ vessels, is also very common in RMC. This feature, along with the high nuclear grade and extensively infiltrative margins, are in keeping with high metastatic potential for this tumor.

Necrosis
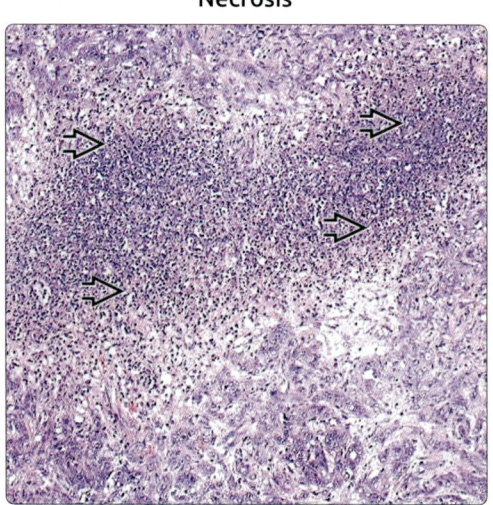

Vascular Invasion
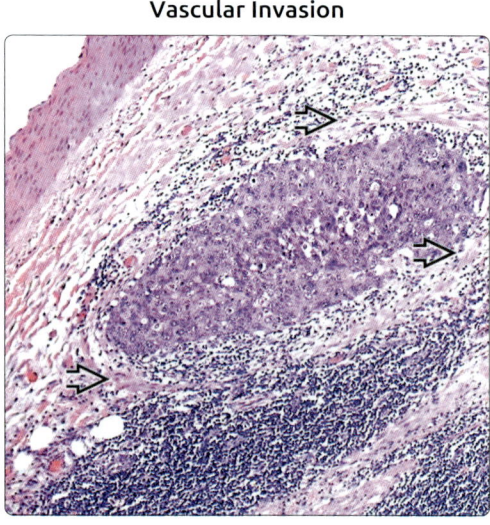

(Left) RMC characteristically shows high pT stage and invades perinephric fat ⇨ in > 80% of the tumors. (Right) RMC shows focal intracellular ⇨ and intraluminal mucin highlighted by mucicarmine stain in > 70% of the tumors. Glandular features and positivity for CK7 and CK20 may raise the suspicion of urothelial carcinoma. Lack of in situ disease, age, clinical history, or sickling of RBCs in tissue sections should lead to the correct interpretation.

Perinephric Fat Invasion
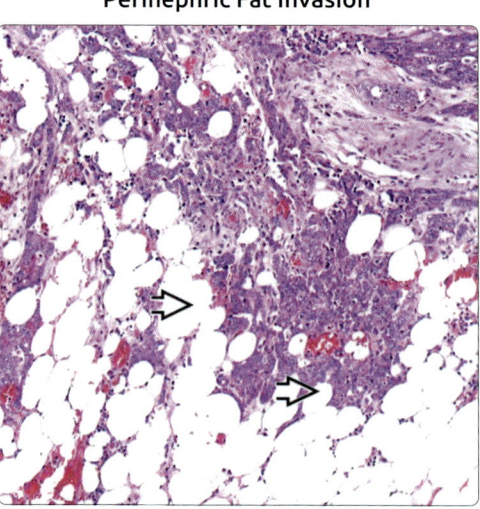

Intracellular Mucin
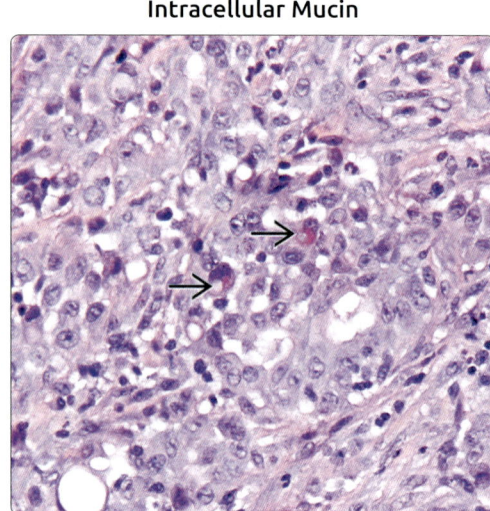

Renal Medullary Carcinoma

Metastatic Features

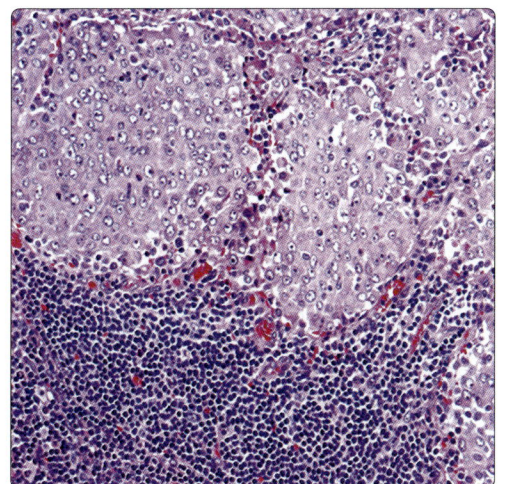

Metastatic Features

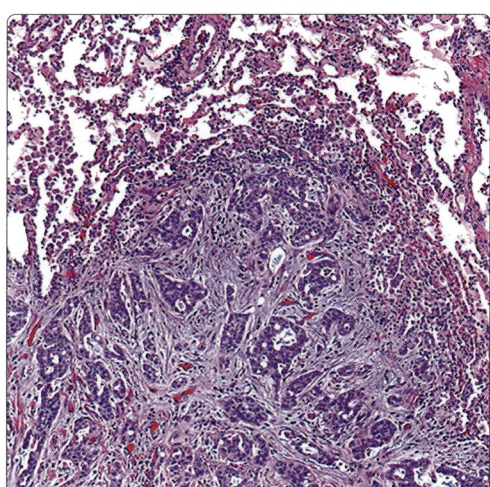

(Left) This image shows RMC metastatic to a regional lymph node. Most cases of RMC show metastatic disease at presentation, and, in many, it is the metastasis that brings the presence of a renal tumor into focus. (Right) This H&E image shows RMC metastatic to the lung. The presence of crenated/sickled red cells in a metastatic focus, and in the surrounding tissues, may bring to notice the presence of the hemoglobinopathy for the 1st time in some cases.

Immunohistochemical Features

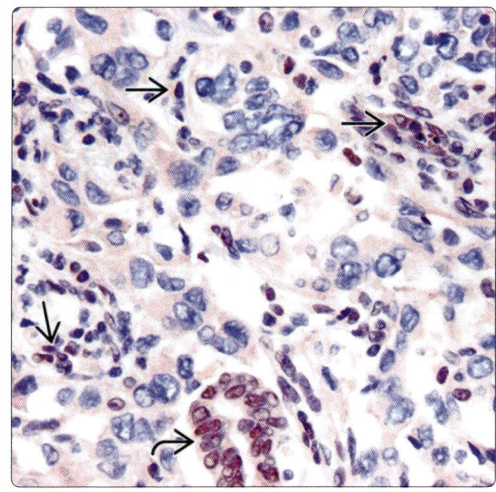

Immunohistochemical Features

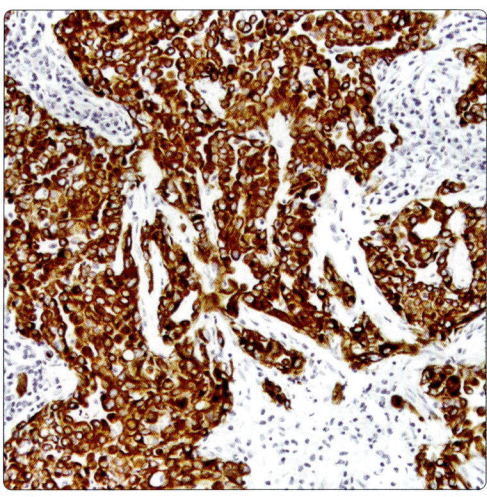

(Left) RMCs consistently lack immunohistochemical nuclear reactivity for SNF5 (INI1), similar to that seen in renal rhabdoid tumor. Notice the retained reactivity in the stromal cells and lymphocytes ➡, as well as a benign renal tubule ➡. (Right) Immunohistochemical staining with CK7 usually shows a diffuse and strong immunoreactivity in RMCs. pax-8 is frequently negative, OCT3/OCT4 in ~ 30-50% of cases.

Immunohistochemical Features

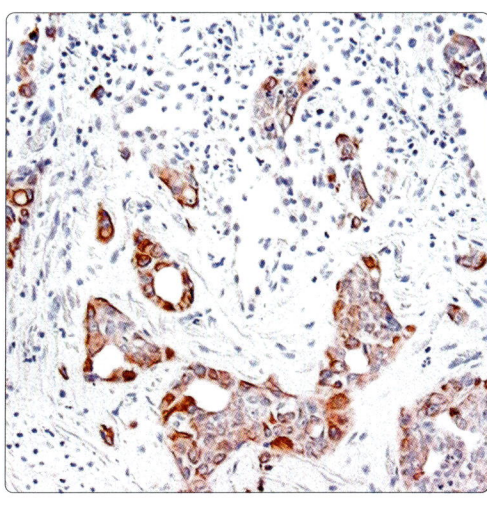

Immunohistochemical Features

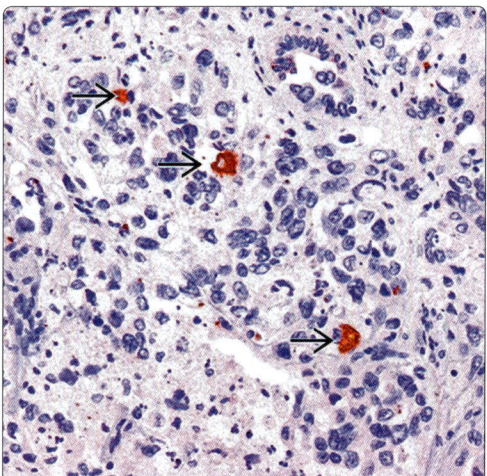

(Left) Immunostaining for CK20 is also often focally to more diffusely positive in RMC. Thus, immunostaining profiles for CK7 and CK20 can usually not distinguish RMC from urothelial carcinoma. (Right) On the other hand, staining for HMCK (34βE12) is either negative or very focal ➡ in RMC. Lack of reactivity for HMCK (34βE12) has been considered by some as a feature suggesting that RMC is unrelated to collecting duct carcinoma.

MiTF/TFE Family Translocation-Associated Carcinoma

KEY FACTS

TERMINOLOGY
- Renal carcinomas characterized by translocations involving MiTF/TFE family genes (*TFE3* or *TFEB*) and with fusions to different, mostly well-characterized genes at a number of different chromosomal locations, including
  - For TFE3: 17q25 (*ASPSCR1* or *ASPL*), 1q21 (*PRCC*), 1p34 (*PSF*), Xq12 (*nonO*), 17q23 (*CLTC*), 17q25 (*RCC17*), 3q23 (unknown), and for TFEB: 11q12 (*MALAT1* or *a*)

CLINICAL ISSUES
- Uncommon, but constitute large proportion of RCCs in pediatric age groups
- Among children, TFE3 renal carcinomas, particularly ASPSCR1 or ASPL-TFE3 carcinomas, usually present at advanced stage
  - In spite of such locally advanced presentation, clinical behavior usually less aggressive
- In adults, clinical course more aggressive, with multiple reported deaths due to disease

MICROSCOPIC
- Carcinoma with high nuclear grade, prominent papillary &/or solid alveolar growth patterns, and composed of clear cells with psammomatous calcifications, most distinctive histopathologic appearance in Xp11 tumors
  - However, presence of cells with granular eosinophilic cytoplasm not uncommon

ANCILLARY TESTS
- Negative or only focally positive for epithelial markers and vimentin
- TFE3 and TFEB highly sensitive and specific immunohistochemical markers for TFE3 and TFEB renal carcinomas
  - Suffer from technical and fixation issues
- TFE3 and TFEB break-apart FISH assays proven to be very useful for diagnosis
  - Technical and fixation issues associated with IHC assays less common

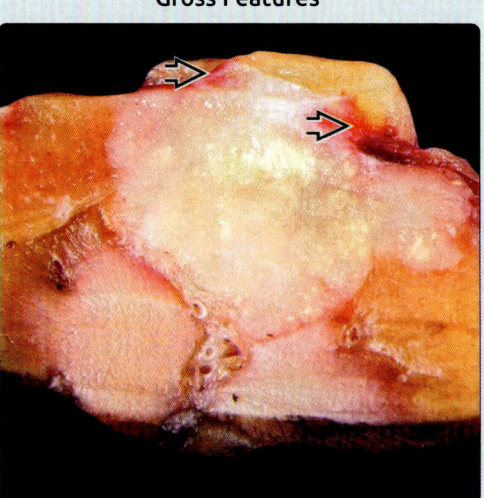

Gross Features

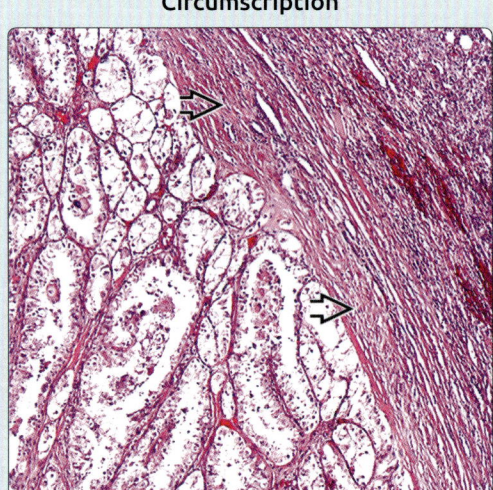

Circumscription

(Left) *Typical gross appearance of a TFE3 renal carcinoma that shows a well-circumscribed tumor with tan-yellow cut surface. Many tumors, however, show invasion into perinephric fat* ➡. (Right) *Well-circumscription of a TFE3 renal carcinoma is shown. While most MiTF renal carcinomas are well circumscribed, without a distinct tumor capsule, some show a pseudocapsule* ➡ *that may show microcalcifications.*

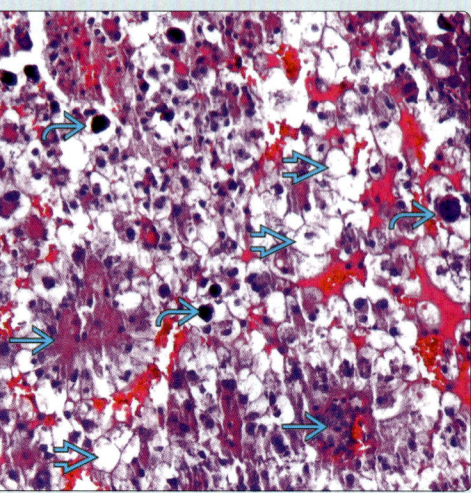

TFE3 Carcinoma: Papillary Architecture

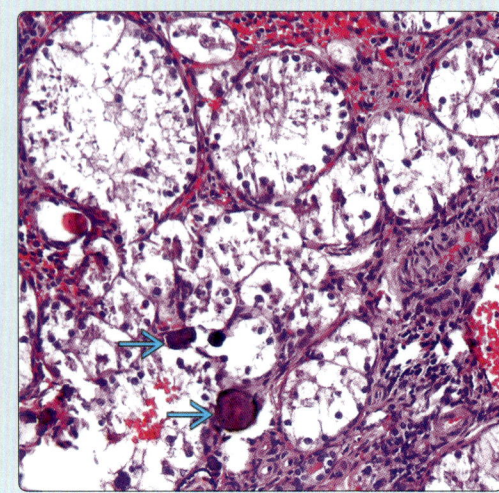

TFE3 Carcinoma: Typical Histology

(Left) *Papillary architecture in TFE3 renal carcinoma is quite common. Clear cell cytology with papillary architecture* ➡, *psammomatous calcifications* ➡, *and cells with voluminous cytoplasm* ➡ *strongly point toward the diagnosis of a TFE3 carcinoma.* (Right) *Hematoxylin & eosin stain shows characteristic light microscopic features of a TFE3 renal carcinoma. The presence of numerous psammomatous calcifications* ➡ *in a tumor resembling high-grade clear cell renal cell carcinoma (RCC) should always be investigated for a TFE carcinoma.*

MiTF/TFE Family Translocation-Associated Carcinoma

TERMINOLOGY

Abbreviations
- Microphthalmia-associated transcription factor (*MiTF*), transcription factor binding to IGHM enhancer 3 (*TFE3*), transcription factor EB (*TFEB*) translocation-associated carcinoma

Synonyms
- Translocation-associated carcinoma, Xp11.2 and t(6;11) renal carcinomas, *TFE3* (Xp11.2) and *TFEB* [t(6;11)] carcinomas

Definitions
- Renal carcinomas characterized and defined by translocations involving MiTF/TFE family genes (*TFE3* or *TFEB*), with fusions to different genes at number of different chromosomal locations, including
  o For TFE3: 17q25 (*ASPSCR1* or *ASPL*), 1q21 (*PRCC*), 1p34 (*PSF*), Xq12 (*NONO*), 17q23 (*CLTC*), 17q25 (*RCC17*), 3q23 (unknown); and for TFEB: 11q12 (*MALAT1* or *α*)

ETIOLOGY/PATHOGENESIS

Molecular Abnormalities
- *TFE3*, *TFEB*, *TFEC*, and *MiTF* are members of MiTF-TFE family of basic helix-loop-helix zipper (bHLH-Zip) factors that bind DNA as homo- and heterodimers
- Members of this family believed to be involved in developmental and cellular processes in various cell types
  o *MiTF* in maturation of melanocytes of neural crest origin, retinal pigment epithelium, and bone marrow-derived mast cells and osteoclasts; *TFEB* in placental vascularization; *TFE3* in transforming growth factor β (TGF-b)-activated signal transduction and B-cell activation, as well as cooperation with *MiTF* and *TFEC* in osteoclast development
- *TFE3* gene localized to chromosome Xp11.2
- Reported chromosomal translocations and corresponding gene fusion identified in *TFE3* carcinomas
  o Alveolar soft part sarcoma chromosome region, candidate 1 gene (*ASPSCR1* or *ASPL*)-TFE3; t(X;17)(p11.2;q25)
    – ASPL (a.k.a. *ASPSCR1* or *PRCC2*) is novel gene of unknown function
    – Translocation similar to that in alveolar soft part sarcoma (ASPS); but, translocation balanced in TFE3 renal carcinoma, and unbalanced (loss of some genetic material) in ASPS
  o Papillary renal cell carcinoma (RCC) (translocation-associated) gene *(PRCC)-TFE3*; t(X;1)(p11.2;q21)
    – *PRCC* is novel gene encoding major subunit of clathrin, multimeric cytoplasmic organelle protein
  o PTB-associated splicing factor gene *(PSF)-TFE3*; t(X;1)(p11.2;p34)
  o Non-POU domain-containing, octamer-Binding (*NONO*)-*TFE3*; Inv(X)(p11;q12)
    – *PSF* and *NONO* are splicing factor genes
  o Clathrin heavy chain 1 gene *(CLTC)-TFE3*; t(X;17)(p11.2;q23)
    – *CLTC* encodes major subunit of clathrin
  o *RCC17-TFE3*; t(X;17)(p11.2;q25.3)
  o Unknown gene: *TFE3*; t(X;3)(p11;q23)
  o Different *TFE3* gene fusions consistently lead to overexpression of fusion protein relative to native TFE3, such that protein becomes detectable by immunohistochemical assay
- *TFEB* gene localized to chromosome 6p21
  o *TFEB* gene fused to metastasis-associated lung adenocarcinoma transcript 1 (*MALAT1*) (also called α), gene transcribed into long noncoding RNA of unknown function located at 11q13
    – Translocation fuses *MALAT1* with 1st intron of *TFEB*
  o *MALAT1-TFEB* fusion gene results in dysregulated expression of full-length TFEB protein detectable by IHC

Postchemotherapy
- ~ 15% of cases in children associated with prior exposure to chemotherapy
  o Exposure usually during 1st and 2nd decades of life for other childhood malignancies or SLE
  o Interval between chemotherapy and development of (RCC), between < 2-13 yr
  o All reported patients received either DNA topoisomerase II inhibitor &/or alkylating agent
  o Exact mechanism for postchemotherapy development of these tumors not known

CLINICAL ISSUES

Epidemiology
- Incidence
  o RCCs account for < 5% of pediatric renal neoplasms
    – Although uncommon, Xp11 renal carcinomas constitute approximately 40% of RCC in children
  o Fewer cases described in adults; oldest 78 yr
    – Reported to comprise 1.6 to 4% of all RCCs in adults
    – Because of marked differences in number of RCCs in adults and children, absolute total number of cases in adults much > in children
  o t(6;11) RCCs less common than Xp11 carcinoma; ~ 50 cases reported in literature; age range: 3-68 yr (median: 31 yr)
- Sex
  o No sex predilection

Presentation
- Pediatric and young adult patients usually symptomatic at presentation; only a few cases discovered incidentally
- Most common symptom, hematuria, followed by abdominal mass, abdominal pain, and weight loss
- Rare atypical presentations in adults include heavily calcified renal mass, outflow obstruction with consequent pyelonephritis, and misdiagnosis as renal cyst or nephrolithiasis

Treatment
- Optimal treatment approach remains to be determined
- Reported cases managed similar to conventional RCC
- mTOR inhibitors tried in metastatic cases with no significant efficacy

Prognosis
- TFE3 renal carcinomas among children, particularly *ASPSCR1-TFE3* carcinomas, usually present at advanced stage

MiTF/TFE Family Translocation-Associated Carcinoma

- In spite of locally advanced presentation, including lymph node metastasis, clinical behavior usually less aggressive
- Among adults, clinical course more aggressive with multiple reported deaths due to disease
- Only advanced stage (distant metastasis) and older age at diagnosis independent predictors of death
- Sites of metastasis include lymph nodes, lung, liver, spine, and adrenal gland
- Of the ~ 50 *TFEB* published cases, 4 have developed metastases, leading to death in 3
- Both, Xp11, 6;11 translocation RCCs with potential to metastasize late (8-30 yr after diagnosis)

MACROSCOPIC

General Features

- Mostly well circumscribed but nonencapsulated
  - Some tumors with irregular infiltrative outlines, with perirenal and renal sinus extensions
  - Rarely, pseudocapsule is present, which may show calcifications
- Cut surface tan-yellow, often showing hemorrhage and necrosis; similar to clear cell RCC

Size

- 2.7-21 cm, mean: 6.8 cm

MICROSCOPIC

Histologic Features

- While morphologic features often correlate with translocation type, significant morphologic overlap between different translocation groups
- Carcinoma with high nuclear grade, prominent papillary &/or solid alveolar growth patterns, and composed of clear cells is most distinctive histopathologic appearance in Xp11 tumors
- However, presence of cells with granular eosinophilic cytoplasm is not uncommon
- Histology of Xp11 translocation carcinomas with specific chromosomal translocations often have characteristic features
  - ASPSCR1-TFE3 carcinoma usually shows
    - Large cells with voluminous cytoplasm, discrete cell borders, vesicular chromatin, and prominent nucleoli
    - Tumor cells often dyscohesive, leading to alveolar and pseudopapillary architecture
    - True papillary formations also not uncommon and rarely predominant architectural pattern
    - Psammoma bodies almost universal and sometimes extensive; usually form upon characteristic hyaline nodules
  - PRCC-TFE3 carcinoma typically shows
    - Less abundant cytoplasm
    - More nested and compact architecture with some nests having central lumina forming acinar pattern; psammoma bodies and hyaline nodules uncommon
    - Papillary architecture common; present either merging with or sharply defined from acinar areas
    - Usually, but not always, lower nuclear grade than *ASPL-TFE3* tumors
- Uncommon histologic features
  - Solid or nested growth with clear-to-eosinophilic cytoplasm mimicking clear cell RCC, or multilocular cystic renal neoplasms of low malignant potential-like features
  - Tubular growth pattern mimicking collecting duct carcinoma
  - Biphasic population of larger clear cells and smaller cells clustered around nodular hyaline material similar to t(6;11) translocation renal cell carcinoma
  - Pleomorphic giant cells, or hobnailed pattern
  - Sarcomatoid features, or fascicles of bland-appearing spindle cells with focal myxoid stroma mimicking MTSCC
  - Clear cell-papillary RCC-like area
  - Oncocytic areas mimicking oncocytoma, or oncocytic spindled areas resembling epithelioid angiomyolipoma
  - Trabecular patterns mimicking carcinoid tumor
- Morphologic features of other Xp11 translocation carcinomas (PSF–TFE3, nonO–TFE3, CLTC–TFE3) not well defined because of few reported cases
- MALAT1 or α-TFEB carcinomas with t(6;11)(p21;q12) usually with
  - Nests, sheets, and tubules of cells separated by thin vascular septa
  - Papillary architecture uncommon but may be focally to extensively present in some tumors
  - Most tumor cells with abundant clear cytoplasm, well-defined cell borders, and usually round nuclei with prominent nucleoli
  - Some tumors with variable proportion of granular eosinophilic cytoplasm
  - Usually minor subpopulation of smaller cells with high nuclear/cytoplasmic ratio and dense nuclear chromatin
    - Typically clustered around nodules of hyaline basement membrane material
    - Hyaline material may be entirely absent in some of such smaller cell areas
  - Similar, biphasic morphology rarely also seen in TFE3 carcinoma

ANCILLARY TESTS

Immunohistochemistry

- Unlike common RCCs, often negative or only focally positive for cytokeratins and epithelial membrane antigen (EMA/MUC1)
- Vimentin usually negative but may be weakly and focally positive
- CD10, RCC antigen, AMACR, and E-cadherin usually positive in TFE3 carcinomas; but, CD10 and RCC antigen usually absent or only focally positive in TFEB tumors
- Cathepsin-K highly specific for diagnosis of translocation RCC among all RCCs; however, sensitivity < that for TFE IHC or FISH
- Melanocytic markers melan-A (MART-1) and HMB-45 frequently positive in TFEB carcinoma, and rarely expressed in TFE3 tumors
- TFE3 highly sensitive and specific marker for Xp11 translocation-associated carcinomas
  - Diffuse, strong nuclear labeling reported with 97.5% sensitivity and 99.6% specificity; similar staining also in ASPS
  - Other renal cell tumors and large number of tested nonrenal tumors negative

MiTF/TFE Family Translocation-Associated Carcinoma

- TFEB highly sensitive and specific marker for 6;11 carcinomas
  - Lymphocytes sometimes may show weak nuclear reactivity
- Major drawbacks of immunohistochemical assays: Technically challenging, and suboptimal fixation resulting in weak and patchy nonspecific staining

Electron Microscopy
- In TFE3 carcinomas, evidence of epithelial differentiation present varying from cell junctions, well-formed glandular lumina containing microvilli, and basement membranes
  - Rare instance of well-formed rhomboid crystals characteristic of alveolar soft part sarcoma reported
- TFEB renal carcinomas show occasional cell junctions; true desmosomes not prominent
  - Distinctive extracellular pools of duplicated basement membrane material surrounded by smaller tumor cells

FISH Assays
- TFE3 and TFEB break-apart FISH assays proven to be very useful for diagnosis
  - Suffer less from technical and fixation issues associated with IHC assays

DIFFERENTIAL DIAGNOSIS
Clear Cell Renal Cell Carcinoma
- High-grade clear cell carcinoma with large solid alveoli vs. ASPSCR1-TFE3 carcinoma
  - Transition to more typical lower grade, smaller acinar growth pattern often present
  - Cells with voluminous cytoplasm uncommon; psammomatous calcifications rarely, if ever, seen
  - Immunostains for CK-PAN (AE1/AE3), CAM5.2, and EMA/MUC1 positive, and Cathepsin-K and TFE3 negative
- Clear cell carcinoma vs. TFEB renal carcinoma
  - Clear cell carcinoma lacks biphasic pattern of large epithelioid cells and clusters of smaller cells
  - Immunostains for CK-PAN (AE1/AE3), CAM5.2, EMA/MUC1, CD10, and vimentin usually positive; Cathepsin-K and TFEB negative

Papillary Renal Cell Carcinoma
- Foamy macrophages frequent in papillary cores
- CK-PAN (AE1/AE3), CAM5.2, CK7, and AMACR positive; TFE3 and TFEB negative

Clear Cell Papillary Renal Cell Carcinoma
- Nuclei low grade and arranged in linear pattern away from basement membrane
- Tumors often cystic
- CK7, CA9, and HMCK (34βE12) positive; AMACR and CD10 mostly negative

Epithelioid Angiomyolipoma (E-AML)/PEComa
- In some E-AML nests, alveoli, and sheets of cells separated by thin vascular septa may raise possibility of TFE carcinoma
  - HMB-45, Cathepsin-K, and cytokeratins may not help in distinction
  - TFE3 or TFEB stain will be useful
    - However, rare PEComas in extrarenal sites have shown aberrant strong TFE3 expression by IHC; no such cases reported in kidneys
  - Also, E-AML may contain focal fat &/or rare dysmorphic vessels; sm-actin may also be useful in most cases

DIAGNOSTIC CHECKLIST
Pathologic Interpretation Pearls
- Renal tumors with clear cell cytology with voluminous cytoplasm should always raise differential diagnostic consideration of translocation-associated carcinoma
  - The possibility is particularly high in younger patients
  - Immunohistochemical staining for epithelial markers (cytokeratins and EMA/MUC1) in such cases must be performed
    - Negative or only focal positivity of these stains further strengthens possibility of translocation-associated carcinoma
- Tumors resembling high-grade clear cell renal cell carcinoma, but showing prominent psammomatous calcifications, also require exclusion of translocation-associated renal carcinoma
  - Psammomatous calcifications, particularly when numerous, very unusual finding in clear cell renal cell carcinoma

SELECTED REFERENCES
1. Argani P: MiT family translocation renal cell carcinoma. Semin Diagn Pathol. 32(2):103-13, 2015
2. Magers MJ et al: MiT family translocation-associated renal cell carcinoma: a contemporary update with emphasis on morphologic, immunophenotypic, and molecular mimics. Arch Pathol Lab Med. 139(10):1224-33, 2015
3. Srigley JR et al: The International Society of Urological Pathology (ISUP) Vancouver Classification of Renal Neoplasia. Am J Surg Pathol. 37(10):1469-89, 2013
4. Martignoni G et al: Cathepsin K expression in the spectrum of perivascular epithelioid cell (PEC) lesions of the kidney. Mod Pathol. 25(1):100-11, 2012
5. Geller JI et al: Translocation renal cell carcinoma: lack of negative impact due to lymph node spread. Cancer. 112(7):1607-16, 2008
6. Argani P et al: Xp11 translocation renal cell carcinoma in adults: expanded clinical, pathologic, and genetic spectrum. Am J Surg Pathol. 31(8):1149-60, 2007
7. Argani P et al: Translocation carcinomas of the kidney after chemotherapy in childhood. J Clin Oncol. 24(10):1529-34, 2006
8. Argani P et al: Renal carcinomas with the t(6;11)(p21;q12): clinicopathologic features and demonstration of the specific alpha-TFEB gene fusion by immunohistochemistry, RT-PCR, and DNA PCR. Am J Surg Pathol. 29(2):230-40, 2005
9. Argani P et al: Primary renal neoplasms with the ASPL-TFE3 gene fusion of alveolar soft part sarcoma: a distinctive tumor entity previously included among renal cell carcinomas of children and adolescents. Am J Pathol. 159(1):179-92, 2001
10. de Jong B et al: Cytogenetics of a renal adenocarcinoma in a 2-year-old child. Cancer Genet Cytogenet. 21(2):165-9, 1986

MiTF/TFE Family Translocation-Associated Carcinoma

TFE3 Carcinoma: Solid Alveolar Architecture

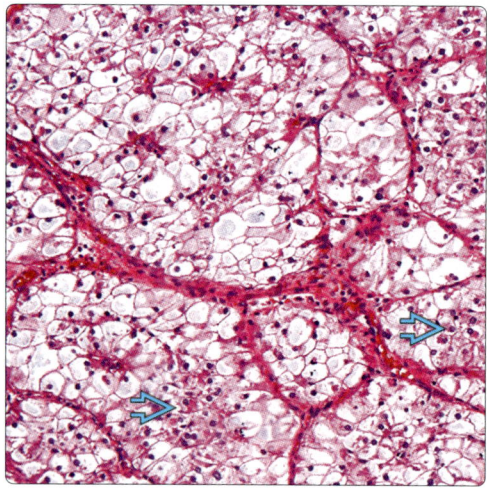

TFE3 Carcinoma: Typical Features

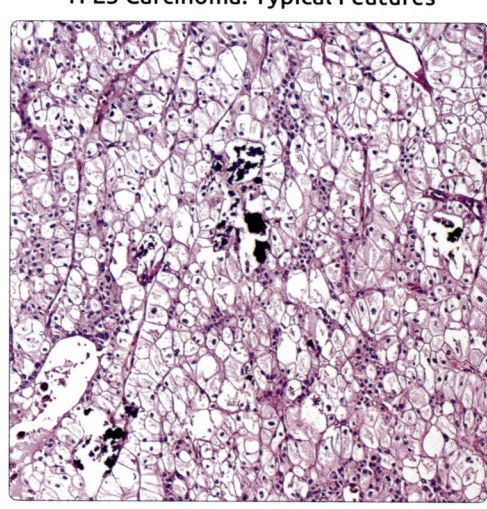

(Left) Solid alveolar growth pattern is not uncommon in TFE3 renal carcinoma. The solid alveoli often show central cell dyscohesion ⇨ and morphologically mimic alveolar soft part sarcoma. Such a growth pattern is commonly associated with *ASPSCR1-TFE3* gene fusion. (Right) Photomicrograph of a TFE3 renal carcinoma shows nests of clear cells separated by delicate vasculature. Voluminous cytoplasm and psammomatous calcifications are quite typical.

TFE3 Carcinoma: Alveolar Architecture

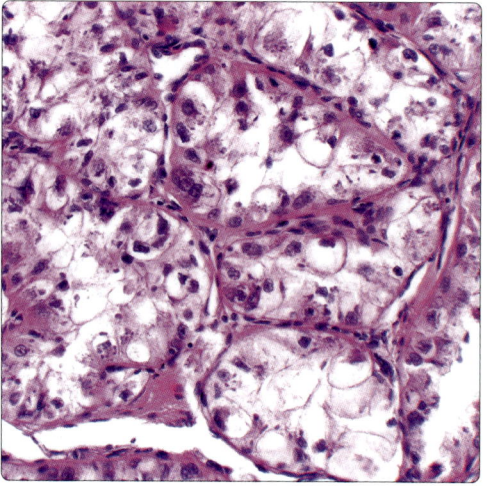

Papillary Architecture

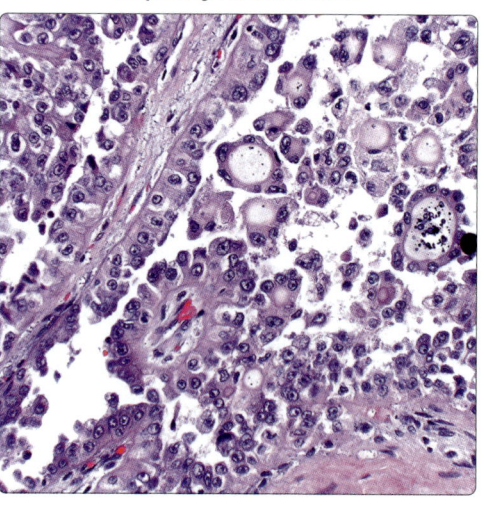

(Left) Solid alveolar architectural pattern in a TFE3 translocation-associated carcinoma, as seen here, is quite common, and the thin branching septations may raise the possibility of a high-grade clear cell renal cell carcinoma. Presence of clear cell RCC-like features in younger patients always merits investigations for a TFE carcinoma. (Right) Prominent papillary architecture may be observed in some TFE3 tumors. Such architectural pattern is less common in TFEB translocation-associated carcinomas.

TFE3 Carcinoma: Papillary Architecture

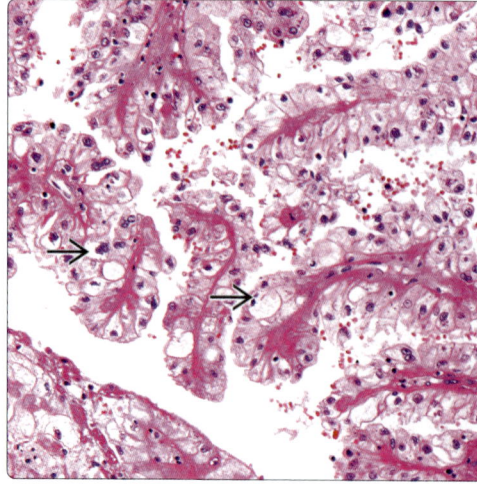

TFE3 Carcinoma: Papillary Architecture and Clear Cells

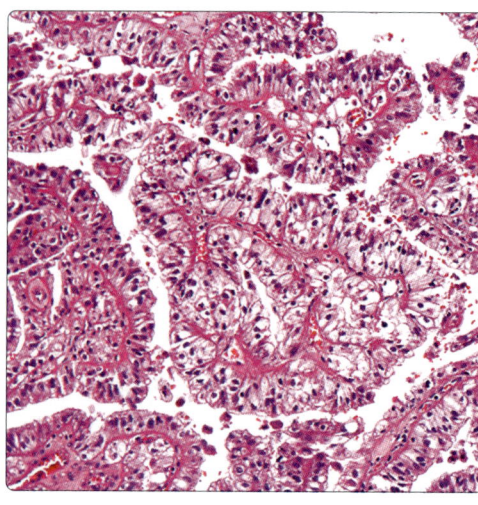

(Left) Most TFE3 tumors may show pseudopapillary architecture with dyscohesive solid acini, but true papillary architecture is not uncommon. The voluminous cytoplasm in some of the cells ⇨ is a pointer toward translocation-associated carcinoma. (Right) Presence of papillary architecture with prominent clear cell and high-grade cytology should always raise the differential diagnostic possibility of a translocation-associated renal carcinoma, particularly when seen in younger patients.

MiTF/TFE Family Translocation-Associated Carcinoma

TFE3 Carcinoma: Voluminous Cytoplasm

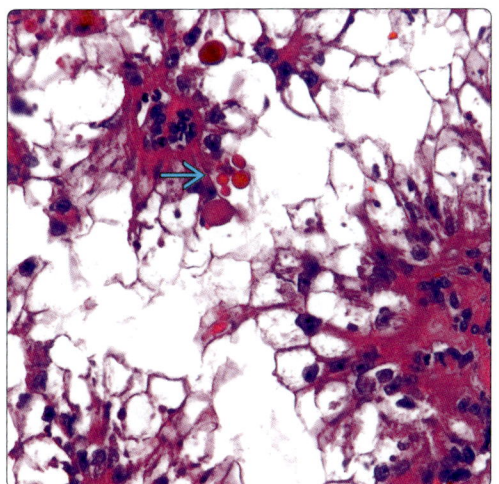

TFE3 Carcinoma: Eosinophilic Cytoplasm

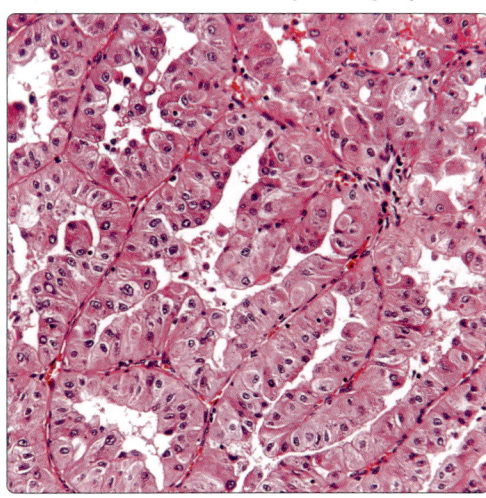

(Left) A high magnification view of TFE3 carcinoma with papillary architecture shows voluminous clear cytoplasm and high-grade nuclei. Intra- and inter-cellular hyaline globules ➡ are also occasionally seen, and these may act as nidus for psammomatous calcifications. (Right) While clear cell cytology is common in TFE3 carcinomas, some tumors may show prominent to predominant, and, rarely, almost exclusive cytoplasmic eosinophilia. Rarely, renal oncocytoma-like appearance may also be present.

Tumor Necrosis

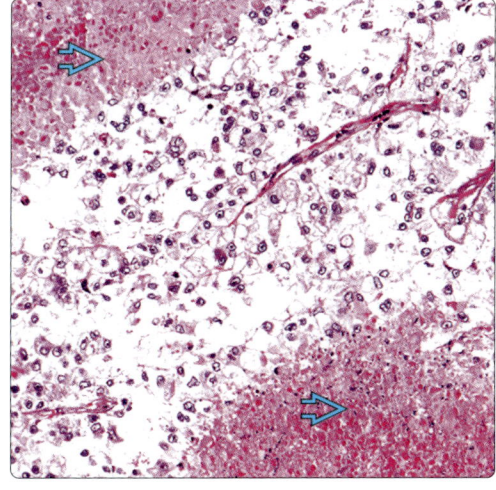

High pT Stage

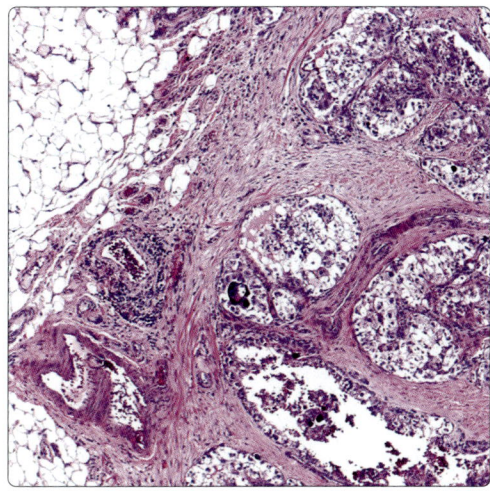

(Left) Coagulative tumor necrosis ➡ and hemorrhage are commonly observed in TFE renal carcinoma. These findings are often noted even in gross specimens. This photomicrograph is a reflection of such commonly observed gross findings. (Right) This photomicrograph shows perinephric fat invasion in a TFE3 carcinoma. TFE3 renal carcinomas often present at high tumor stage. However, compared to the adults, high pT stage does not necessarily predict aggressive outcome in children.

Cytological Atypia

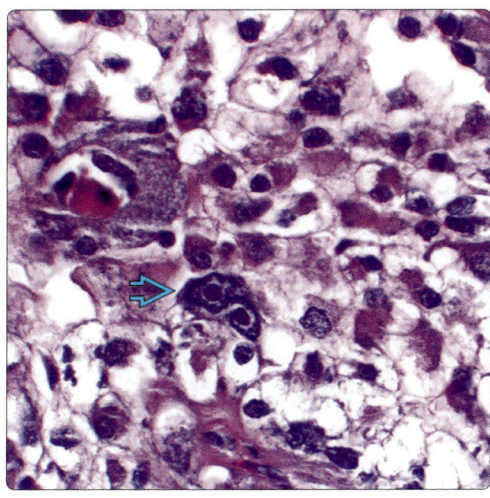

TFEB Carcinoma: Nested Architecture and Clear Cells

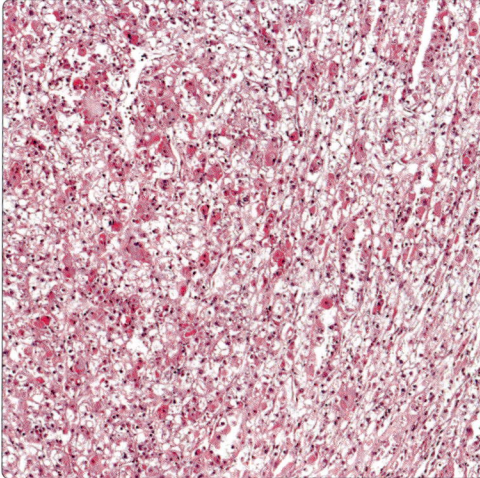

(Left) Some translocation-associated carcinomas may occasionally show marked focal cytologic atypia ➡ and presence of pleomorphic giant cells. While such features are not associated with adverse clinical outcome, distant metastases and older age are independent predictors of death. (Right) A low magnification view of a TFEB t(6;11) renal carcinoma shows nests, sheets, and tubules of cells, predominantly with clear cytoplasm, separated by thin vascular septa.

MiTF/TFE Family Translocation-Associated Carcinoma

TFEB Carcinoma: Most Typical Features

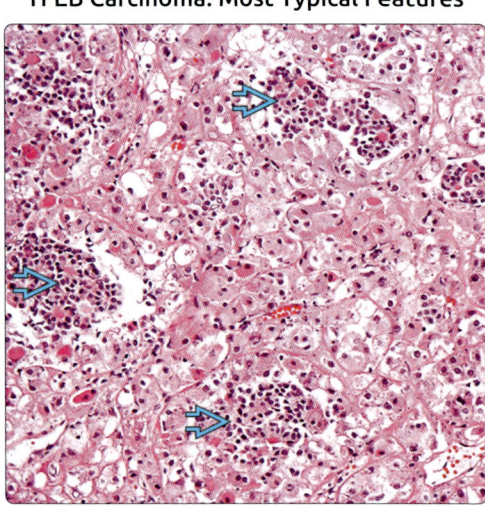

TFEB Carcinoma: Biphasic Histology

(Left) The most characteristic feature of TFEB carcinoma is a biphasic morphology. Dispersed among the larger cells are clusters and islands of smaller cells ⇨ with high nuclear/cytoplasmic ratio and somewhat denser-appearing nuclear chromatin. (Right) This smaller cell population in a TFEB carcinoma is present within a tubular structure ⇨ lined by larger epithelioid cells similar to rest of the tumor. The smaller cells are arranged around small nodules of hyaline material ⇨ ultrastructurally shown to be basement membrane material.

TFEB Carcinoma: Biphasic Histology

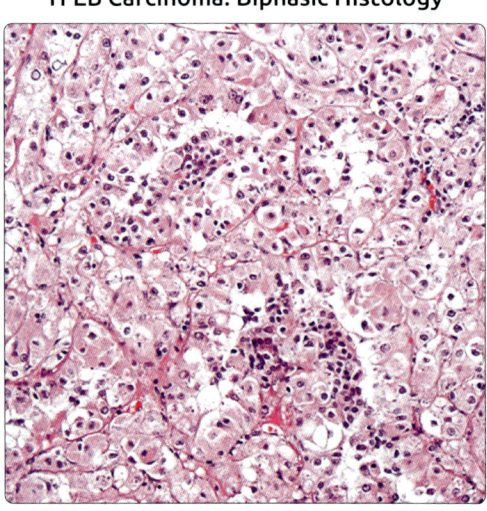

TFEB Carcinoma: Psammomatous Calcifications

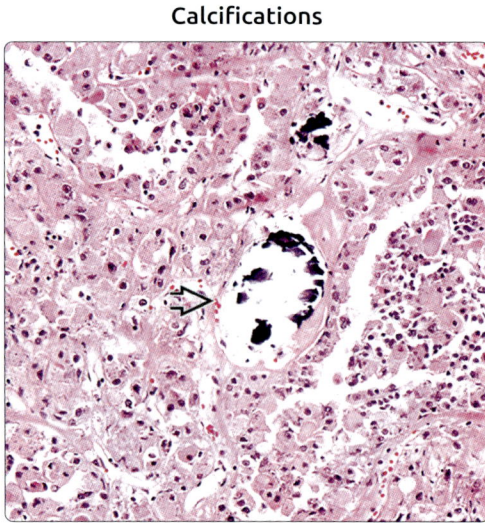

(Left) While the nodules of basement membrane material within the smaller cell clusters are typically abundant in a given tumor, in some cases such hyaline nodules may be quite rare and difficult to find. (Right) Focal calcification is seen in a t(6;11) renal carcinoma ⇨. Compared to the TFE3 tumors, psammomatous calcifications in TFEB carcinoma are quite rare and may be completely absent.

TFEB Carcinoma: Eosinophilic Cytoplasm

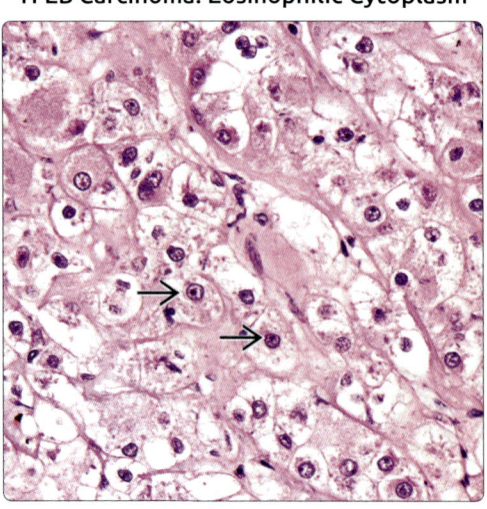

TFEB Carcinoma: Papillary Architecture

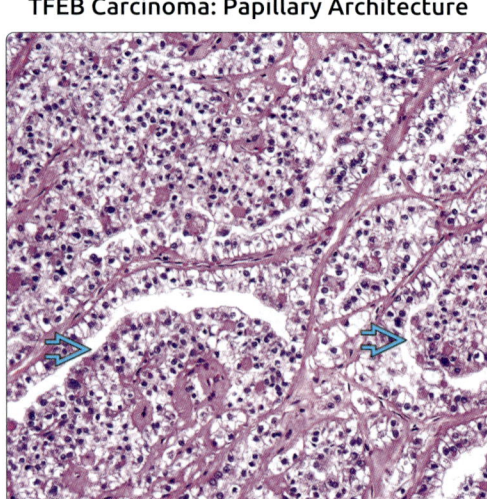

(Left) While most tumors show an admixture of clear and eosinophilic cells, some TFEB tumors are predominantly or almost exclusively composed of cells with eosinophilic cytoplasm. Most tumors do not show significant nuclear pleomorphism, but the presence of prominent nucleoli ⇨ is not uncommon. (Right) This TFEB renal carcinoma has focal papillations ⇨ in a background of a predominantly nested growth pattern.

MiTF/TFE Family Translocation-Associated Carcinoma

Epithelial Markers

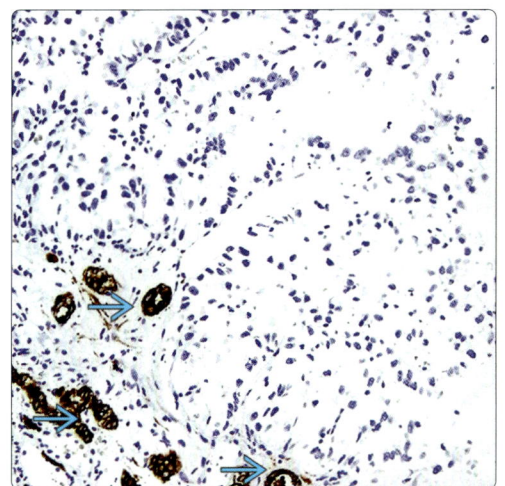

TFE3 Immunohistochemistry

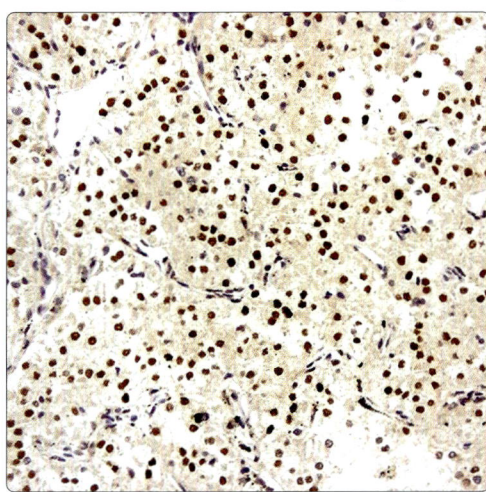

(Left) Translocation-associated renal carcinomas are negative or only focally and weakly positive for cytokeratins and EMA/MUC1. Tumors with clear cells, voluminous cytoplasm, ± papillary architecture, and lacking staining for epithelial markers point toward TFE3 renal carcinoma. Note the positive internal control ➡. (Right) Diffuse and strong nuclear positivity for TFE3 IHC is characteristic of all types of Xp11 renal carcinomas, irrespective of the fusion gene partner.

TFEB Immunohistochemistry

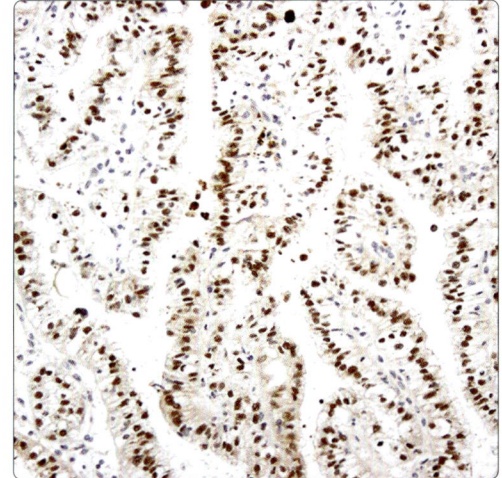

HMB-45

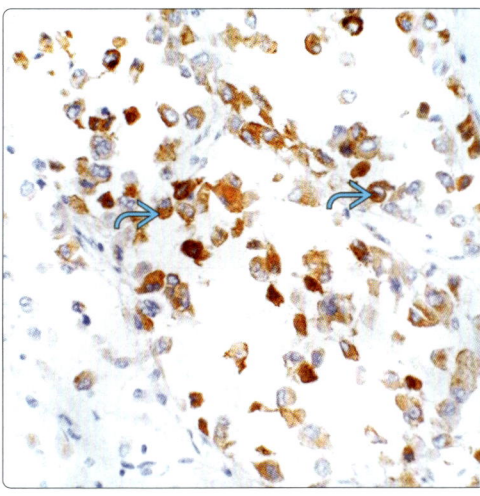

(Left) TFEB immunostaining shows diffuse nuclear positivity in a TFEB renal carcinoma. As with TFE3 immunostain in Xp11.2 carcinomas, TFEB immunostain is highly specific for t(6;11) tumors. TFEB immunostain may also show focal nuclear staining in some lymphocytes. (Right) While melanocytic markers HMB-45 ➡ and Melan-A (MART-1) are frequently positive in TFEB renal carcinomas, rare cases of TFE3 tumors may also show focal positivity.

TFE3 FISH: Break-Apart Probe

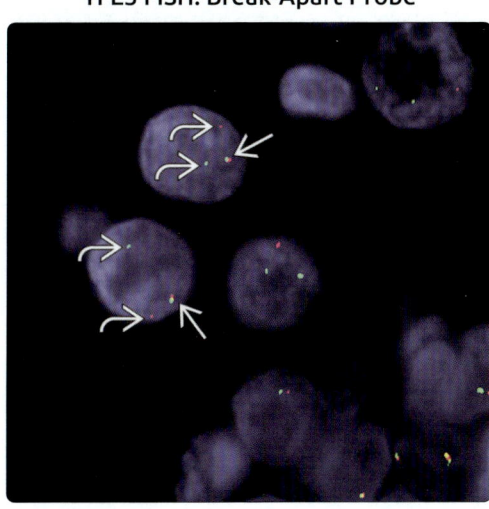

Biopsy Diagnosis

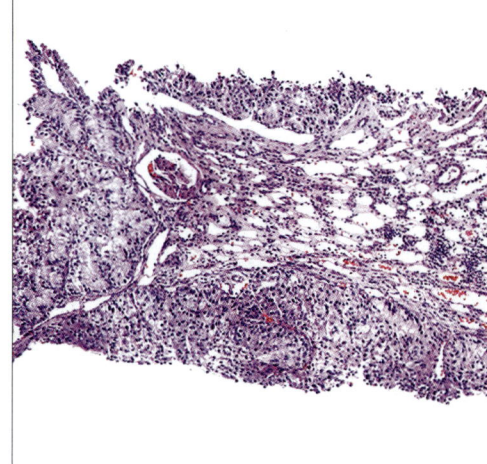

(Left) Break-apart FISH assays suffer less from the technical and fixation issues and sometimes non-specific weak staining associated with the IHC assays. Here, TFEB assay shows separated red and green ➡ signals (positive result), along with 1 fused red-green ➡ signal present in each cell in this female patient. (Right) Attention to the morphological features, should alert one to the possibility of a translocation carcinoma even on needle core biopsies. IHC or FISH will be confirmatory.

Mucinous Tubular and Spindle Cell Carcinoma

KEY FACTS

TERMINOLOGY
- Low-grade biphasic carcinoma usually associated with favorable prognosis

ETIOLOGY/PATHOGENESIS
- Loss of Chr 1, 4, 6, 8, 9, 13, 14, 15, and 22
- Gains of 11q, 16q, 17, and 20q
- No trisomies 7 and 17

CLINICAL ISSUES
- Majority discovered incidentally
- Show predominantly indolent behavior
  - Very occasional cases with epithelial anaplasia, sarcomatoid differentiation, or metastases reported

MACROSCOPIC
- Well-circumscribed mass
- Gray-white to tan or yellow cut surface
- Tumor usually well circumscribed, occasionally encapsulated, and often centered in medulla

MICROSCOPIC
- Tightly packed elongated, often branching, tubules
- Basophilic extracellular mucin separating tubules
- Variable low-grade spindled cell appearance

ANCILLARY TESTS
- IHC results: Significant overlap with papillary renal cell carcinoma (RCC)
  - AMACR and CK7 often (+); CD10 often (-) or focal (+)

TOP DIFFERENTIAL DIAGNOSES
- Papillary RCC
  - Usual type with sarcomatoid differentiation
  - With low-grade spindle cell foci
  - With overlapping mucinous tubular and spindle cell carcinoma (MTSCC)-like features
- Other RCCs with myxoid stroma

Gross Features

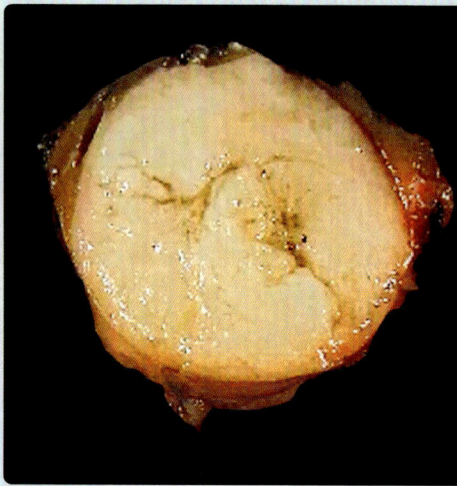

Microscopic Features

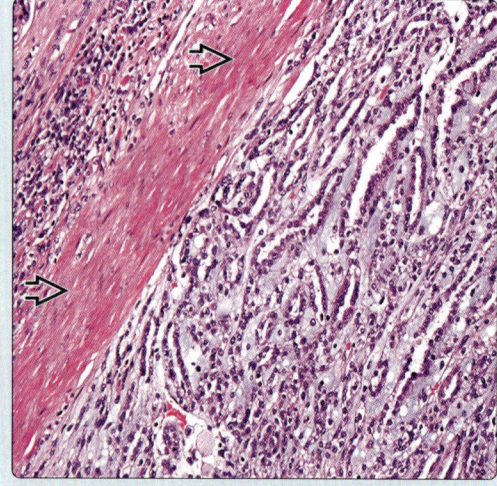

(Left) Gross photo of mucinous tubular and spindle cell carcinoma (MTSCC) shows a well-circumscribed mass with typical homogeneous tan-white, glistening cut surface. Some tumors may possess a distinct capsule. (Right) Most, but not all, MTSCCs are well circumscribed, &/or partly encapsulated ➡, similar to most papillary renal cell carcinomas (RCCs). Myxoid stroma in a predominantly long tubular pattern is seen. Unlike most papillary RCCs, prominent papillary architecture is very unusual in MTSCC.

Microscopic Features

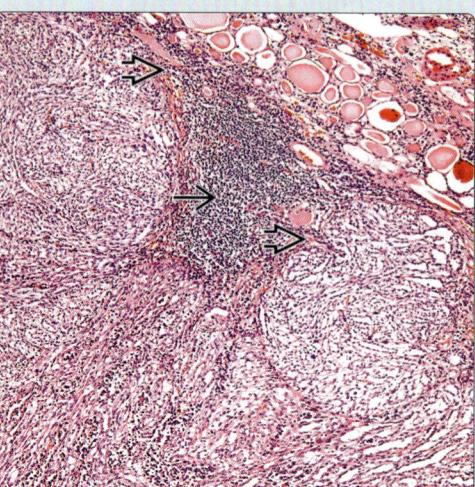

Microscopic Features

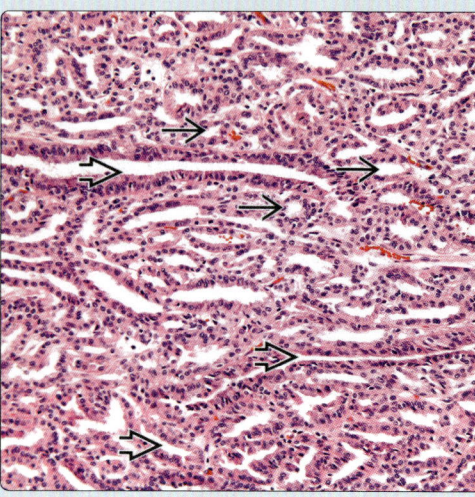

(Left) Some MTSCCs may be nonencapsulated and show irregular tumor borders. The tumor front in some of such tumors appears multi-nodular ➡ and may be associated with lymphoid aggregates ➡. (Right) Most of the tubules show narrow slit-like lumina ➡. Other tubules may be small and have more rounded contours ➡. The cells lining the tubules are low columnar or cuboidal, with uniform, low-grade, round nuclei. Significant nuclear pleomorphism occurs in only very rare cases.

Mucinous Tubular and Spindle Cell Carcinoma

TERMINOLOGY

Abbreviations
- Mucinous tubular and spindle cell carcinoma (MTSCC)

Definitions
- Low-grade biphasic neoplasm with epithelial and spindle cell components usually associated with favorable prognosis

ETIOLOGY/PATHOGENESIS

Molecular Abnormalities
- Loss of Chr 1, 4, 6, 8, 9, 13, 14, 15, and 22
- Gains of 11q, 16q, 17, and 20q
- No trisomies 7 and 17
  - Most common mimickers of MTSCC, i.e., papillary renal cell carcinoma (RCC) with MTSCC-like areas, show molecular signature similar to papillary RCC and not MTSCC
- Tumors with sarcomatoid change with multiple other losses and gains, including reported gains of Chr 2, 5, 7, 9, 10, 12, 17, 19, 20, and X

CLINICAL ISSUES

Epidemiology
- Incidence
  - Relatively rare, accounting for less than 1% of all renal neoplasms
- Age
  - Range: 13-81 yr
    - Mean: 58 yr
- Sex
  - Female preponderance
    - M:F = 1:3

Presentation
- Majority are asymptomatic and discovered incidentally on radiological evaluation for other conditions

Prognosis
- Show predominantly indolent behavior
  - Rare reported cases with local lymph node metastasis
  - Very occasional cases with epithelial anaplasia or sarcomatoid differentiation and metastases have been reported
    - Even rarer MTSCC with typical features with metastases described

MACROSCOPIC

General Features
- Tumor usually well circumscribed, occasionally encapsulated, and often centered in medulla, which may be difficult to demonstrate in large tumors and tumor enucleations
  - Gray-white to tan or yellow, often glistening, cut surface
  - Hemorrhage or necrosis unusual, except in sarcomatoid areas

Size
- 2-18 cm (mean: 4.2 cm)

MICROSCOPIC

Histologic Features
- Architectural details
  - Tubules with slit-like lumina
    - Often show branching
    - Some tubules small and more rounded
    - Sometimes tubules with whorling
    - Luminal surfaces of tubules, generally smooth
  - Low-grade spindle cell areas with nuclei similar to epithelial areas
    - Spindle cells appear to originate from and be continuous with tubular lining
    - Occasionally spindle cells may form solid sheets
  - Presence of variable amounts of basophilic extracellular mucin
    - Extracellular mucin positive for alcian blue histochemistry
  - Focal papillations quite frequent
- Cytologic details
  - Cells with cuboidal to low-columnar cytology lining tubules
  - Usually scant cytoplasm with relatively uniform nuclei usually bearing inconspicuous nucleoli
- Uncommon morphologic features include
  - Predominant spindle cell or epithelial components
  - Very scant mucin
  - Focal clear cell or eosinophilic cytology
  - Presence of foamy macrophages
  - Multifocal papillary areas
    - However, many such tumors with classical papillary RCC-like areas turn out to be papillary RCC on molecular analysis
  - High-grade epithelial areas
  - High-grade sarcomatoid differentiation
    - Such high-grade sarcomatoid areas often with associated necrosis, prominent mitotic activity and pleomorphism
- Tumors often contain background inflammatory infiltrate, including plasma cells

Predominant Pattern/Injury Type
- Neoplastic

Predominant Cell/Compartment Type
- Epithelial, biphasic or mixed

ANCILLARY TESTS

Immunohistochemistry
- Significant overlap with papillary RCC
  - CK7, positive
  - AMACR, positive
  - HMWK (34be12), often negative or focal positive
  - CD10, often negative or very focal positive

DIFFERENTIAL DIAGNOSIS

Papillary Renal Cell Carcinoma
- Usual type, including that with sarcomatoid differentiation
  - Predominant papillary architecture
  - Necrosis and hemorrhage common

Mucinous Tubular and Spindle Cell Carcinoma

- Frequently prominent foamy macrophages and psammoma bodies
- Absent stromal mucin
- Presence of trisomy Chr 7 and Chr 17; loss of Chr Y
- With low-grade spindle cell foci
  - Absent stromal mucin
  - Presence of trisomy Chr 7 and Chr 17; loss of Chr Y
  - Male sex
  - More commonly CD10 positive
  - Luminal surface of tubules usually irregular, shaggy
- With overlapping MTSCC-like features
  - Typical papillary RCC-like features often present in at least some parts of the tumor
  - MTSCC-like areas variable, but often not diffuse
  - Presence of trisomy Chr 7 and Chr 17; loss of Chr Y
  - In general, in tumors with mixed features, presence of classic papillary areas favors diagnosis of papillary RCC rather than MTSCC

Other Renal Cell Carcinomas With Myxoid Stroma

- Mere presence of mucinous or myxoid stroma not specific for MTSCC
- Diffuse, or more often focal, myxoid stroma present in a variety of RCCs
  - Such tumors, among others, include
    - Clear cell RCC
    - Collecting duct carcinoma
    - Papillary RCC
    - RCC, unclassified
    - Renal medullary carcinoma
    - SDHB-deficient RCC
  - All morphological and immunophenotypic features need to be taken into consideration before diagnosing or excluding MTSCC

DIAGNOSTIC CHECKLIST

Pathologic Interpretation Pearls

- Key reason to be aware of MTSCC is to avoid mistaking it for sarcomatoid papillary carcinoma
- Immunohistochemical stains usually do not differentiate MTSCC from papillary RCC
  - However, CD10 is often negative in MTSCC and positive in papillary RCC
- Close attention to morphologic features is essential and useful in most instances
- In rare difficult cases, molecular evaluation may be employed for this distinction
- More recent and detailed molecular evidence further supports the distinctness of MTSCC from papillary RCC
  - Some earlier publications raised doubts regarding their relationship or separation from PRCC
  - More recent studies show no molecular overlap in typical cases
  - Tumors with overlapping features in most instances turn out to be papillary RCC by molecular analysis
    - Tumors with overlapping features often show following morphological findings
      - Distinct papillary RCC-like areas with other separate areas mimicking MTSCC; or
      - Papillary RCC-like areas intimately admixed with typical MTSCC areas including presence of elongated tubules and extracellular mucin
- Mere presence of myxoid stroma not specific for MTSCC
  - Myxoid stroma occasionally seen in variety of other RCCs, including
    - Clear cell RCC
    - Collecting duct carcinoma
    - Papillary RCC
    - RCC, unclassified
    - Renal medullary carcinoma
    - Rare cases of SDHB-deficient RCC, etc.
- Sarcomatoid change may very rarely occur in MTSCC
- Rare cases with rhabdoid features also reported

SELECTED REFERENCES

1. Ren Q et al: Mucinous tubular and spindle cell carcinoma (MTSCC): A genome-wide copy number analysis of MTSCC and Its histologic mimickers. Mod Pathol. 28: 2 (Suppl.):254A, 2015
2. Peckova K et al: Mucinous spindle and tubular renal cell carcinoma: analysis of chromosomal aberration pattern of low-grade, high-grade, and overlapping morphologic variant with papillary renal cell carcinoma. Ann Diagn Pathol. 19(4):226-31, 2015
3. Srigley JR et al: The International Society of Urological Pathology (ISUP) Vancouver Classification of Renal Neoplasia. Am J Surg Pathol. 37(10):1469-89, 2013
4. Ursani NA et al: Mucinous tubular and spindle cell carcinoma of kidney without sarcomatoid change showing metastases to liver and retroperitoneal lymph node. Hum Pathol. 42(3):444-8, 2011
5. Larkin J et al: Metastatic mucinous tubular and spindle cell carcinoma of the kidney responding to sunitinib. J Clin Oncol. 28(28):e539-40, 2010
6. Dhillon J et al: Mucinous tubular and spindle cell carcinoma of the kidney with sarcomatoid change. Am J Surg Pathol. 33(1):44-9, 2009
7. Argani P et al: Papillary renal cell carcinoma with low-grade spindle cell foci: a mimic of mucinous tubular and spindle cell carcinoma. Am J Surg Pathol. 32(9):1353-9, 2008
8. Kuroda N et al: Mucinous tubular and spindle cell carcinoma with Fuhrman nuclear grade 3: a histological, immunohistochemical, ultrastructural and FISH study. Histol Histopathol. 23(12):1517-23, 2008
9. Cossu-Rocca P et al: Renal mucinous tubular and spindle carcinoma lacks the gains of chromosomes 7 and 17 and losses of chromosome Y that are prevalent in papillary renal cell carcinoma. Mod Pathol. 19(4):488-93, 2006
10. Fine SW et al: Expanding the histologic spectrum of mucinous tubular and spindle cell carcinoma of the kidney. Am J Surg Pathol. 30(12):1554-60, 2006
11. Kuroda N et al: Frequent expression of neuroendocrine markers in mucinous tubular and spindle cell carcinoma of the kidney. Histol Histopathol. 21(1):7-10, 2006
12. Paner GP et al: Immunohistochemical analysis of mucinous tubular and spindle cell carcinoma and papillary renal cell carcinoma of the kidney: significant immunophenotypic overlap warrants diagnostic caution. Am J Surg Pathol. 30(1):13-9, 2006
13. Ferlicot S et al: Mucinous tubular and spindle cell carcinoma: a report of 15 cases and a review of the literature. Virchows Arch. 447(6):978-83, 2005
14. Kuroda N et al: Review of mucinous tubular and spindle-cell carcinoma of the kidney with a focus on clinical and pathobiological aspects. Histol Histopathol. 20(1):221-4, 2005
15. Eble JN: Mucinous tubular and spindle cell carcinoma and post-neuroblastoma carcinoma: newly recognised entities in the renal cell carcinoma family. Pathology. 35(6):499-504, 2003

Mucinous Tubular and Spindle Cell Carcinoma

Microscopic Features

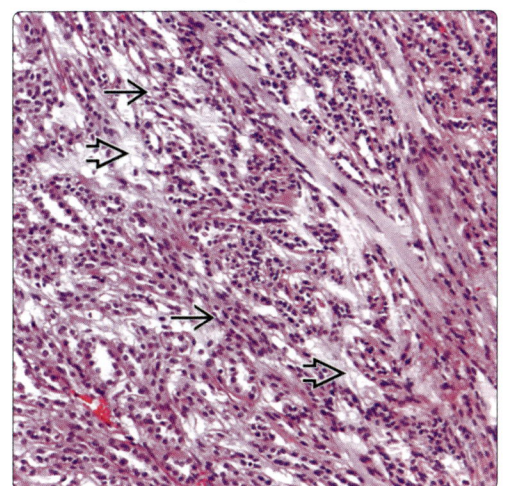
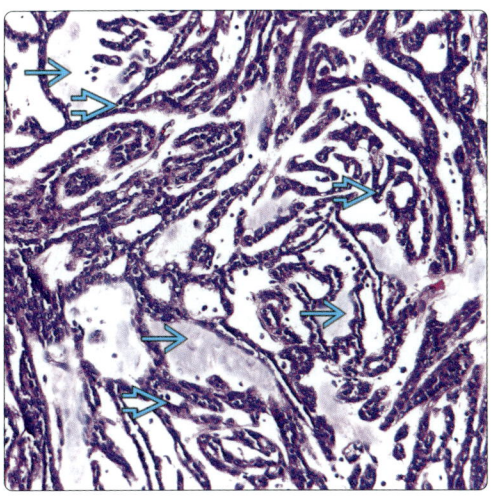

(Left) Typical microscopic appearance of MTSCC shows variably shaped tubules, low-grade spindle cell areas ⇨, and stromal mucin ⇨. Any of these 3 features may be focal or rare in some tumors. (Right) Extensive tubular branching is shown here. While the tubules show some branching in most cases, in some mucinous tubular and spindle cell carcinomas this branching is exquisite and may be associated with marked interconnecting tubular architecture ⇨. In such areas, the myxoid background may be quite prominent ⇨.

Microscopic Features

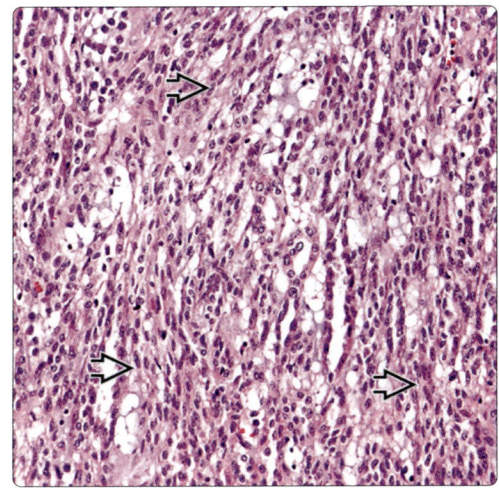
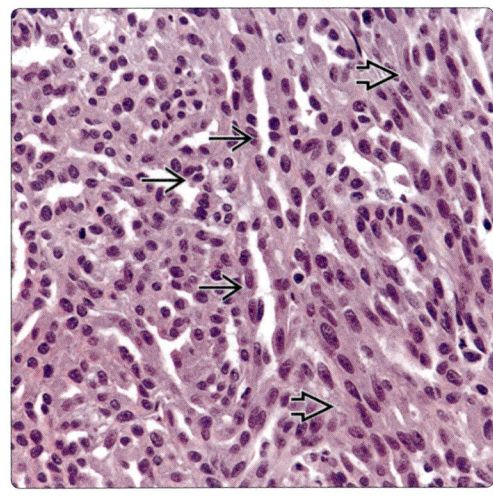

(Left) The banal-appearing spindle cells ⇨ appear to be intimately admixed with the tubular component. The juxtaposition or the imperceptible blending of these 2 features is typical in mucinous tubular and spindle cell carcinoma. (Right) The spindle cells often appear to emerge from the epithelial component and show low-grade nuclear features ⇨, morphologically almost identical to the nuclei in the epithelial component ⇨. Mitotic activity is rare in most cases.

Microscopic Features

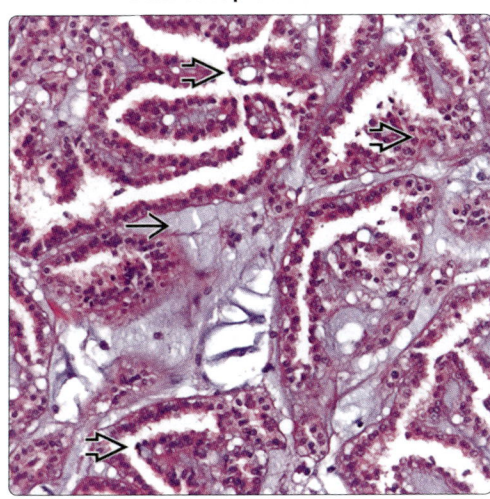
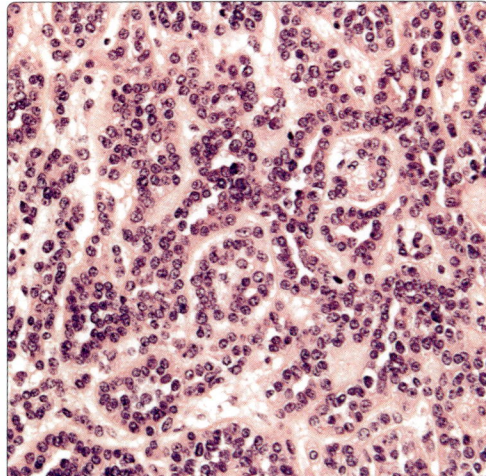

(Left) While the epithelial component in MTSCC predominantly consists of elongated, sometimes branching, or more rounded tubules, focal ill-defined papillations are not uncommon ⇨. The typical mucinous stroma ⇨ is seen. (Right) In some areas, the tubules may be short and round, bearing superficial resemblance to those seen in metanephric adenoma or solid PRCC. At the same time, prominent papillary architecture is extremely uncommon and should raise the differential of PRCC.

Mucinous Tubular and Spindle Cell Carcinoma

(Left) Typically, the cells lining the tubules in mucinous tubular and spindle cell carcinoma are cuboidal, with a small amount of amphophilic cytoplasm ⇨. Rarely, foci with more abundant and clear cytoplasm may also be observed ⇨, and such cells are often closely associated with the other more typical cell types. **(Right)** In some cases, the stromal mucin shows prominent vacuolization that may lead to a mistaken belief of the presence of clear and signet ring cells.

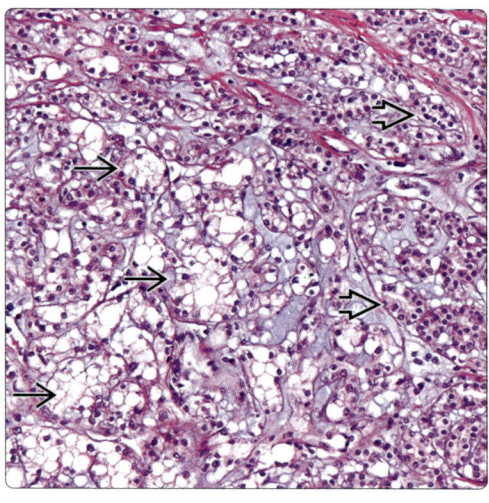
Microscopic Features

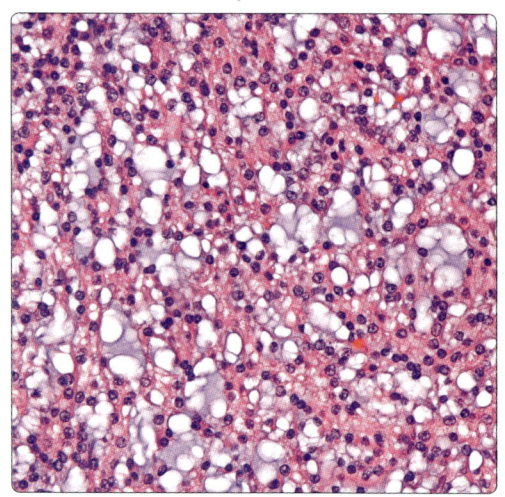
Microscopic Features

(Left) Some mucinous tubular and spindle cell carcinomas show marked paucity of epithelial component. Such spindle cell predominant tumors may be mistaken for a sarcoma, but the cytologic features are low grade, necrosis is absent, and some epithelial component is invariably seen on careful search. **(Right)** In very occasional cases, tubules with clear cell cytoplasm may be clustered together ⇨, forming small, usually ill-defined nodular areas. Appreciation of all the 3 diagnostic features in rest of the tumor is important.

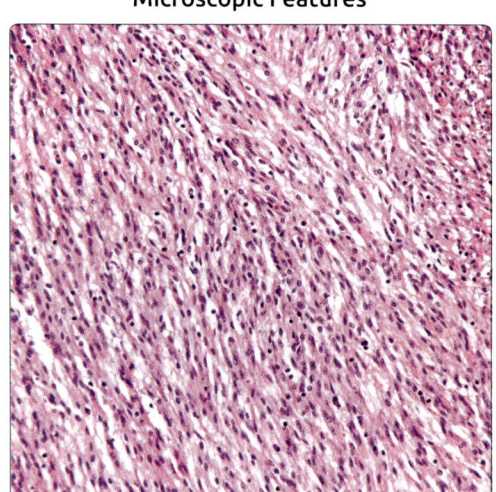
Microscopic Features

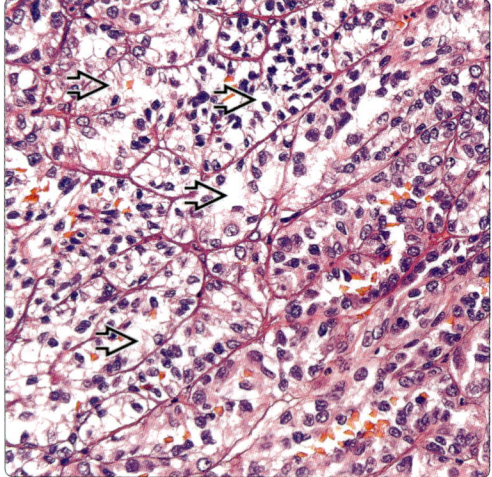
Microscopic Features

(Left) Mucinous stroma, while characteristic, is not specific for MTSCC. Focal areas resembling MTSCC may be present in other tumors, as in this example of a clear cell RCC. Typical histology in the rest of the tumor should point towards the true diagnosis. **(Right)** Appropriate immunohistochemistry may be required in some cases to confirm the alternate diagnosis. CA9 in the case of clear cell RCC, with focal MTSCC-like areas, shown in this H&E image, confirms the appropriate diagnosis.

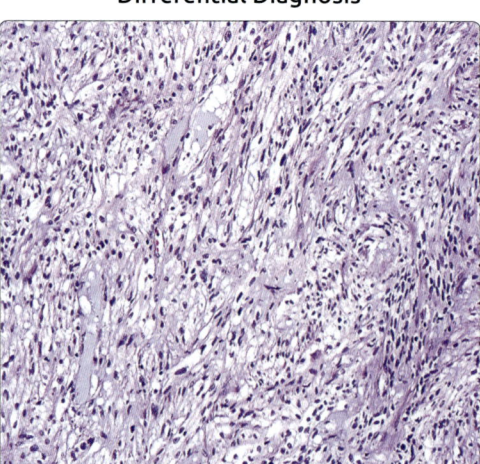
Differential Diagnosis

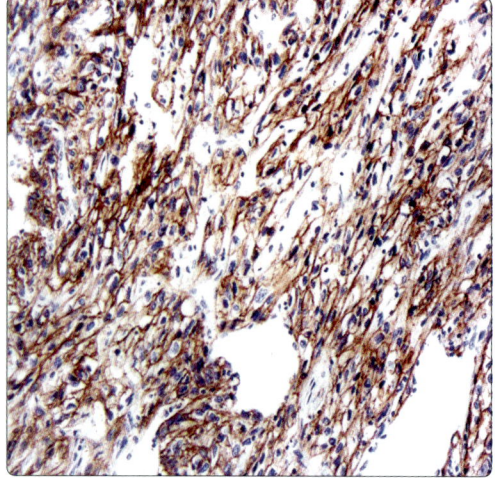
Differential Diagnosis and Immunohistochemistry

Mucinous Tubular and Spindle Cell Carcinoma

Uncommon Features

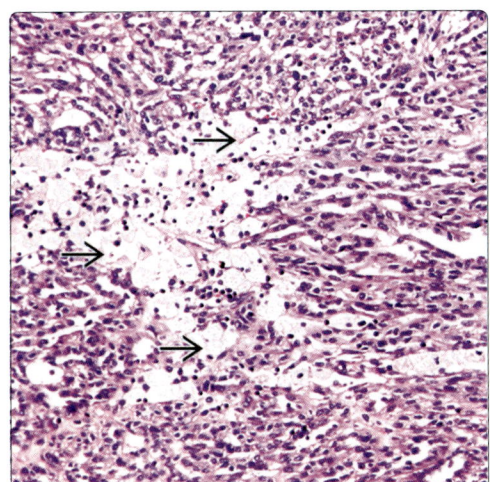

Uncommon Features

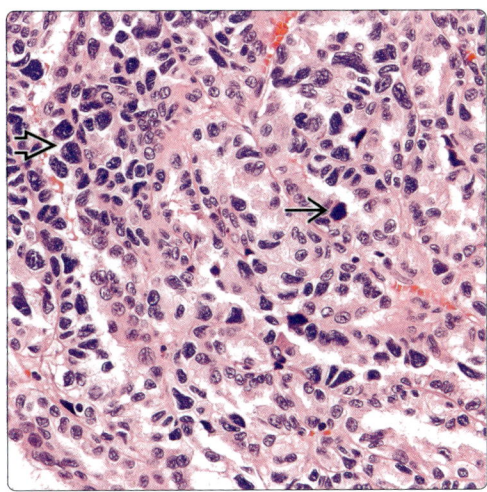

(Left) Occasionally the tumors may show focal to rarely more diffuse foamy macrophages ⇒, raising the differential diagnostic possibility of papillary RCC. However, unlike papillary RCC, the foam cells are usually randomly distributed, and are not related to papillary cores in MTSCC. (Right) This image of a MTSCC shows significant nuclear pleomorphism ⇒ and brisk mitotic activity ⇒ in the epithelial component of the tumor. Appreciation of other typical features of these tumors is necessary in such rare cases.

Uncommon Features

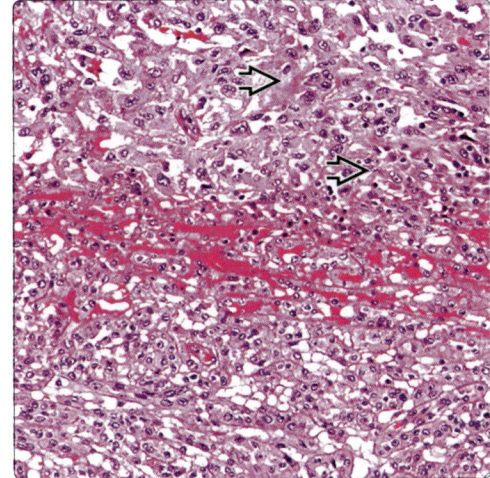

Uncommon Features

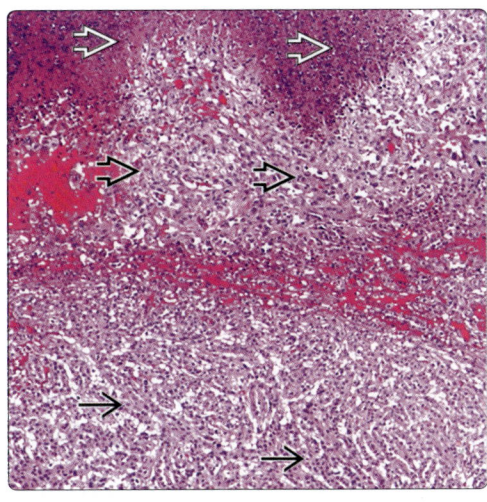

(Left) Unlike the low-grade spindle cell elements that are common in MTSCC, true sarcomatoid areas ⇒ are high grade, mitotically active, and may show areas of necrosis. True sarcomatoid features are extremely uncommon in mucinous tubular and spindle cell tumors. (Right) This MTSCC ⇒ shows sarcomatoid features ⇒ with a large area of necrosis ⇒. Compared to the usual low-grade MTSCC, tumors with sarcomatoid features usually show infiltrative borders and gross necrosis.

Immunohistochemical Features

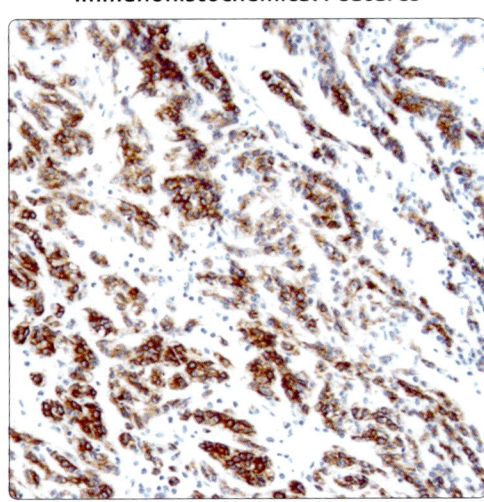

Immunohistochemical Features

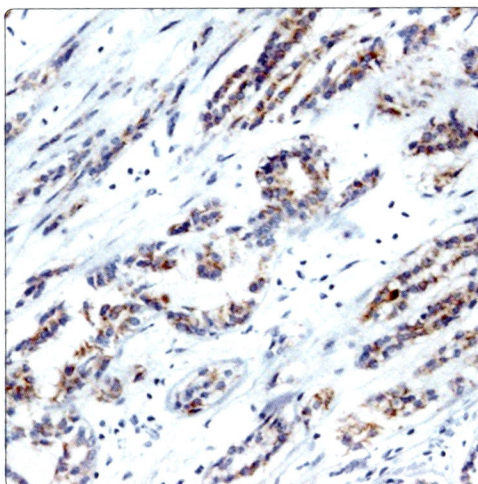

(Left) Similar to papillary RCC, CK7 is diffusely positive in mucinous tubular and spindle cell carcinoma, staining both the epithelial and spindle cell components. (Right) Immunostaining with AMACR is usually diffusely positive in both the epithelial and spindle cell components. Thus, CK7 and AMACR do not help in the differentiation between mucinous tubular and spindle cell carcinoma and papillary RCC. Careful attention to the presence of a low-grade spindle cell morphology and myxoid features may be more helpful in this distinction.

Tubulocystic Carcinoma

KEY FACTS

TERMINOLOGY
- Tubulocystic carcinoma (TC) of kidney
  - Well-circumscribed carcinoma with pure tubular and cystic architectural growth
  - Cysts and tubules lined by single layer of atypical cells with abundant eosinophilic cytoplasm and variable hobnailed appearance

CLINICAL ISSUES
- Tumors with potentially low malignant behavior; < 100 cases reported in literature
- Strong male preponderance (M:F = 7:1 or greater)

MACROSCOPIC
- Well-circumscribed tumors with spongy bubble wrap appearance; no solid areas

MICROSCOPIC
- Composed of small to intermediate-sized tubules admixed with cystically dilated tubules, dispersed evenly in frequently fibrotic stroma
- Tubule and cyst lining composed of single layer of flat, hobnail, or cuboidal to columnar cells; no solid areas

ANCILLARY TESTS
- Majority are positive for CK7, CK19, parvalbumin, CD10, AMACR, Ksp-cadherin, and FH

TOP DIFFERENTIAL DIAGNOSES
- Hereditary leiomyomatosis and renal cell carcinoma-associated carcinoma with TC-like areas
- Collecting duct carcinoma with TC-like areas
- Other adult renal epithelial tumors with predominant tubules and cysts

Gross Features

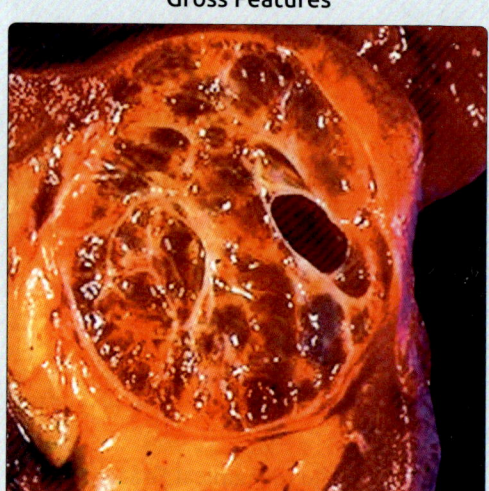

Typical Features

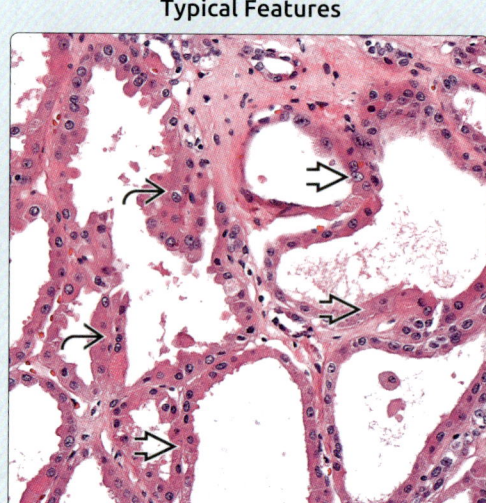

(Left) Gross photograph demonstrates a well-circumscribed tumor with a spongy cut surface and variable-sized cysts, the typical gross appearance of a tubulocystic carcinoma. **(Right)** Tubulocystic carcinoma consists of tubules and variably sized cysts lined by cells with abundant eosinophilic cytoplasm ⇨. Lining cells often have large nuclei with open chromatin and prominent nucleoli. Sometimes incomplete septations may appear hanging free in the cyst lumina ⇨.

Circumscription

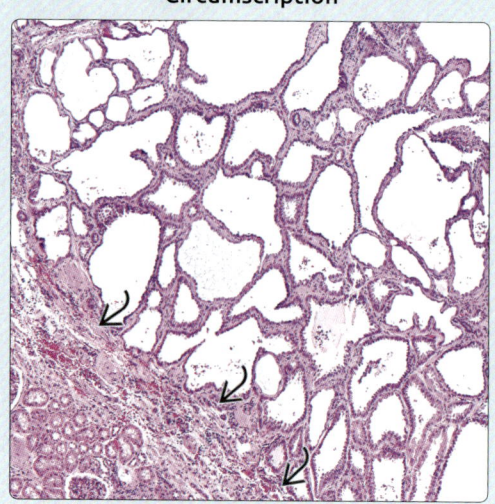

Hyalinized Stroma

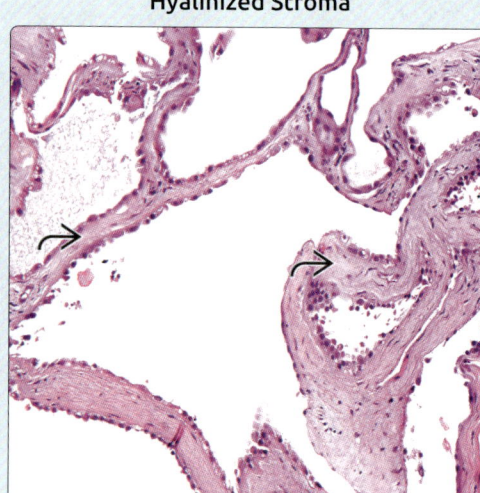

(Left) By definition, tubulocystic carcinomas are well circumscribed. Partial to incomplete encapsulation may be present, but more often the tumor is in direct contact ⇨ with surrounding renal parenchyma without any encapsulation. **(Right)** Characteristically, the intervening stroma between the tubule and cysts in tubulocystic carcinoma is fibrotic and paucicellular ⇨. In rare instances, the stroma might be relatively more cellular.

Tubulocystic Carcinoma

TERMINOLOGY

Abbreviations
- Tubulocystic carcinoma (TC) of kidney

Definitions
- Well-circumscribed renal cell carcinoma (RCC) with pure tubular and cystic architectural growth
  - Cysts and tubules lined by single layer of atypical cells with abundant eosinophilic cytoplasm and variable hobnail appearance

ETIOLOGY/PATHOGENESIS

Historic Perspective
- Previously regarded as low-grade collecting duct carcinoma (CDC)
- Now considered as distinct entity
  - Areas with TC-like morphology occasionally observed in otherwise typical hereditary leiomyomatosis and renal cell carcinoma (HLRCC)-associated carcinoma &/or CDC

Molecular Abnormalities
- Unique molecular signature distinct from clear cell and chromophobe RCC; overexpression of genes related to amino acid metabolism and cell cycle
- Loss of chromosomes 9, 15, and 18, and copy neutral LOH in the region of 6p22.1 also described
- Based on single case, using clustering analysis, molecular signature reported to be closely related to papillary RCC
  - However, association or relationship with papillary RCC not confirmed by any subsequent studies
- Recent molecular studies suggest HLRCC tumors with tubulocystic areas or so-called "TC with dedifferentiation" unrelated to true TC

CLINICAL ISSUES

Epidemiology
- Uncommon; < 100 cases reported in literature; age range: 34-94 years (mean: 60); male preponderance (M:F = 7:1)

Presentation
- Majority asymptomatic and incidentally discovered

Treatment
- Often amenable to surgical treatment due to low tumor stage at presentation
- Rare reported cases of metastatic disease

Prognosis
- Tumor with relatively less aggressive clinical behavior; overwhelming majority pT1 tumors
  - < 10% reported with stage pT3 disease
- Disease progression, including local recurrence and metastasis to lymph nodes, bone, and liver in ~ 10% of cases

MACROSCOPIC

General Features
- Well-circumscribed, usually unifocal, spongy bubble wrap appearance with multiple variable-sized cysts containing clear serous fluid

Size
- Range: 0.2-17 cm (mean: 4.2 cm)

MICROSCOPIC

Histologic Features
- Well-circumscribed with small to intermediate-sized, cystically dilated tubules
- Tubule and cyst lining composed of single layer of flat, hobnail, or cuboidal to columnar cells
  - Cellular stratification and papillations very focal and uncommon
- Cells with abundant eosinophilic cytoplasm and large nuclei, often with regular nuclear membranes and prominent nucleoli
- Mitotic activity and tumor necrosis rare to absent
- Stroma intervening between tubules and cysts usually fibrotic and often paucicellular

ANCILLARY TESTS

Immunohistochemistry
- Majority positive for CK7, AMACR (racemase), CD10, and Ksp-cadherin
  - Occasional tumors immunoreactive with HMCK(34βE12), usually only focal
- Unlike HLRCC carcinomas with TC areas, fumarate hydratase (FH) retained and 2SC negative in the few tested tumors

DIFFERENTIAL DIAGNOSIS

HLRCC-Associated Carcinoma With TC-Like Areas
- High-grade tumors with solid, papillary and glandular areas, and characteristic large nucleoli with perinucleolar halos
  - Mutations in *FH* gene; immunohistochemistry with loss of FH, and diffuse cytoplasmic and nuclear positivity for 2SC

Collecting Duct Carcinoma With TC-Like Areas
- Multinodular growth pattern with extensive desmoplasia; solid, papillary, and glandular areas common; frequent intratumoral inflammation

Other Adult Renal Epithelial Tumors With Predominant Tubules and Cysts
- Focal or prominent area with tubules and cysts; lining cells and background typical of primary histologic subtype

SELECTED REFERENCES

1. Chen YB et al: Hereditary leiomyomatosis and renal cell carcinoma syndrome-associated renal cancer: recognition of the syndrome by pathologic features and the utility of detecting aberrant succination by immunohistochemistry. Am J Surg Pathol. 38(5):627-37, 2014
2. Al-Hussain TO et al: Tubulocystic carcinoma of the kidney with poorly differentiated foci: a series of 3 cases with fluorescence in situ hybridization analysis. Hum Pathol. 44(7):1406-11, 2013
3. Sangle NA et al: Novel molecular aberrations and pathologic findings in a tubulocystic variant of renal cell carcinoma. Indian J Pathol Microbiol. 56(4):428-33, 2013
4. Srigley JR et al: The International Society of Urological Pathology (ISUP) Vancouver Classification of Renal Neoplasia. Am J Surg Pathol. 37(10):1469-89, 2013
5. Amin MB et al: Tubulocystic carcinoma of the kidney: clinicopathologic analysis of 31 cases of a distinctive rare subtype of renal cell carcinoma. Am J Surg Pathol. 33(3):384-92, 2009

Tubulocystic Carcinoma

Cytological Features

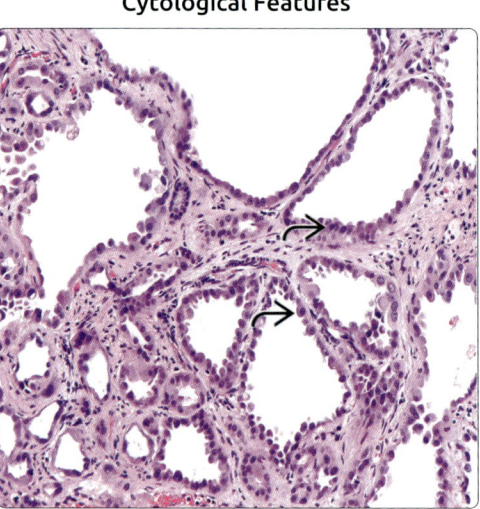

Cytological Features

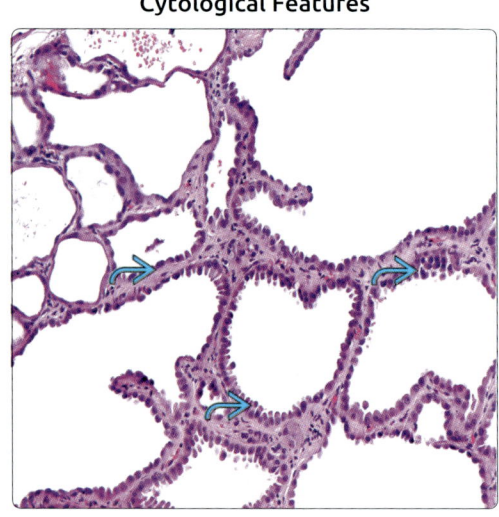

(Left) The lining cells in tubulocystic carcinoma typically have abundant eosinophilic cytoplasm, with relatively uniform large nuclei and prominent nucleoli ⮕. However, nuclear membrane irregularities are uncommon, and when present are at the most focal. (Right) Most tubulocystic carcinomas also show variable hobnailing of the lining epithelium ⮕. This feature may not be prominent or may even be absent in rare cases.

Cytological Features

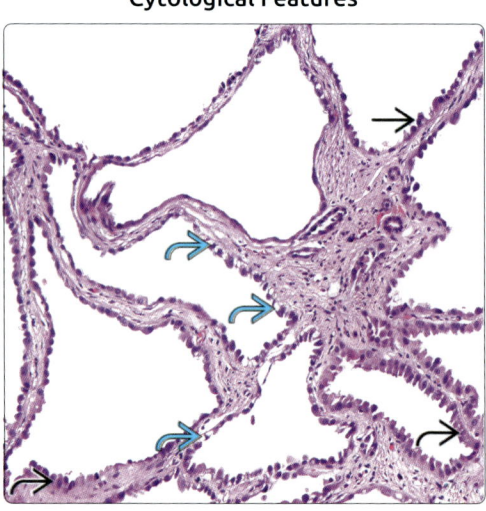

Stromal Features

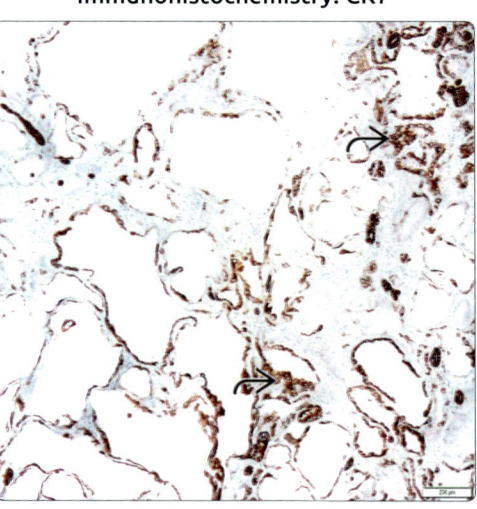

(Left) While the presence of lining cells with abundant eosinophilic cytoplasm ⮕ is a consistent feature in all tubulocystic carcinomas, cells with hobnailing ⮕ are also frequent. Rare tumors may also focally contain cells with cytoplasmic vacuoles ⮕. (Right) Characteristically, the intervening stroma between the tubule and cysts in tubulocystic carcinomas is fibrotic and paucicellular. In rare instances, the stroma might be slightly more cellular ⮕, as seen in this case.

Immunohistochemistry: CK7

Immunohistochemistry: Fumarate Hydratase

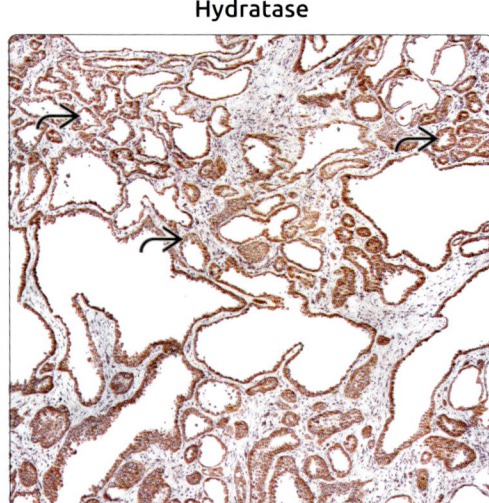

(Left) Tubulocystic carcinomas often show CK7 positivity, which frequently is patchy ⮕. Immunoreactivity for CK7 may, however, be completely negative in some cases. (Right) HLRCC-associated RCC with tubulocystic carcinoma (TC)-like areas is the closest differential diagnosis for TC. Unlike what is seen in HLRCC tumors, true TC shows retained diffuse cytoplasmic immunoreactivity for fumarate hydratase ⮕. Because FH is a mitochondrial antigen, the positivity is always finely granular.

Tubulocystic Carcinoma

Differential Diagnosis: Renal Oncocytoma
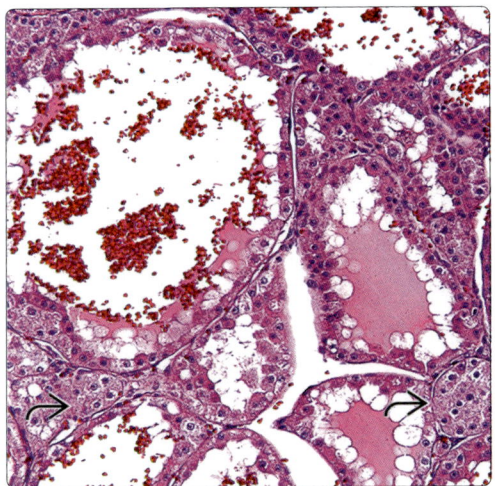

Differential Diagnosis: Chromophobe RCC
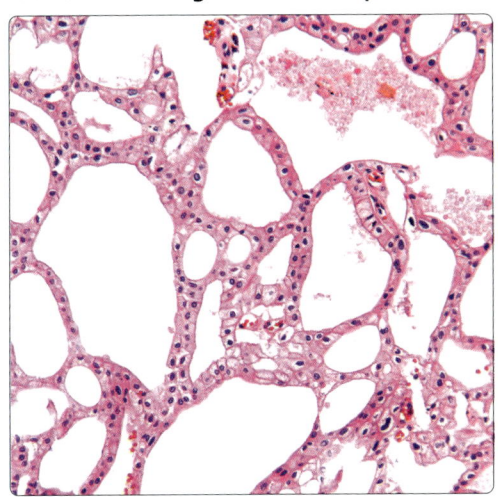

(Left) A close differential diagnosis of tubulocystic carcinoma is renal oncocytoma with prominent tubular and cystic areas, as seen here. Oncocytoma has uniform round nuclei, a variable number of solid tumor nests ⇨, and frequently loose stroma. It lacks the prominent CK7 positivity. (Right) Although this chromophobe RCC has cystic areas architecturally resembling a tubulocystic carcinoma, its cytologic features (binucleation, koilocytoid atypia, and 2 cell types) would suggest the correct diagnosis.

Differential Diagnosis: HLRCC-Associated RCC
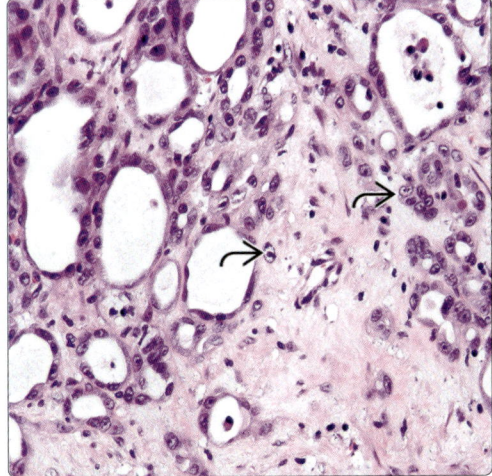

Differential Diagnosis: HLRCC-Associated RCC
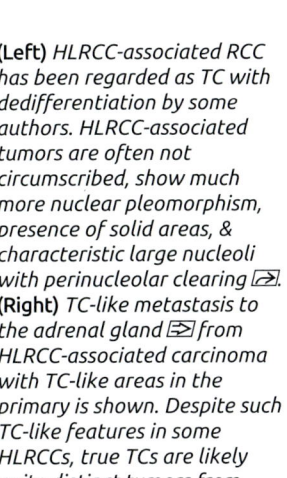

(Left) HLRCC-associated RCC has been regarded as TC with dedifferentiation by some authors. HLRCC-associated tumors are often not circumscribed, show much more nuclear pleomorphism, presence of solid areas, & characteristic large nucleoli with perinucleolar clearing ⇨. (Right) TC-like metastasis to the adrenal gland ⇨ from HLRCC-associated carcinoma with TC-like areas in the primary is shown. Despite such TC-like features in some HLRCCs, true TCs are likely quite distinct tumors from HLRCC-associated carcinoma.

Differential Diagnosis: HLRCC-Associated RCC
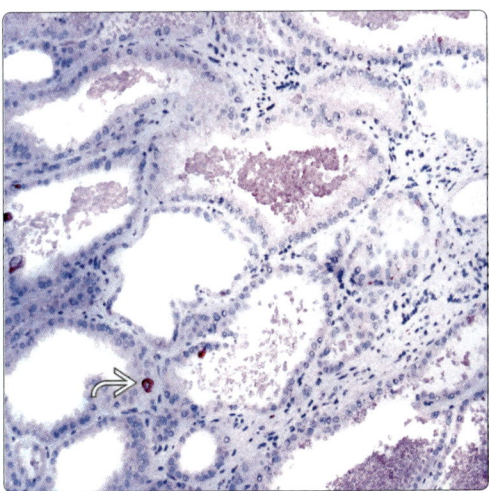

Differential Diagnosis: HLRCC-Associated RCC
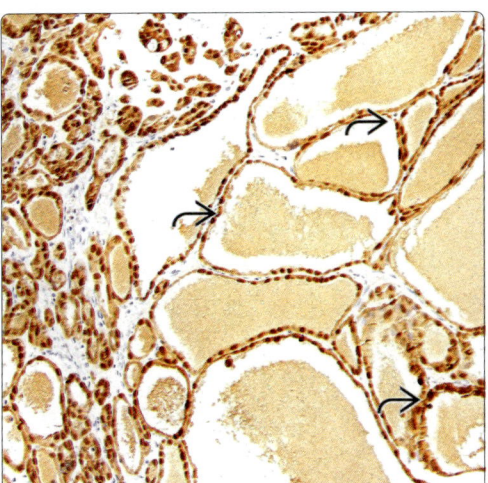

(Left) Unlike what is seen in true HLRCC-associated RCCs, 2SC immunohistochemistry reveals absent, or at the most only focal ⇨, cytoplasmic staining in true TC. (Right) The immunohistochemical staining for 2SC in fumarate hydratase-mutated HLRCC tumors consistently reveals a diffuse cytoplasmic and nuclear positivity, as seen in this tumor with prominent TC-like areas ⇨. Such nuclear and cytoplasmic positivity is highly characteristic of HLRCC tumors, although focal cytoplasmic staining may be rarely present in other RCCs.

Thyroid-Like Follicular Carcinoma of Kidney

KEY FACTS

TERMINOLOGY
- Thyroid-like follicular carcinoma of kidney (TLFC-K)
- Recently described primary renal cell carcinoma closely mimicking well-differentiated thyroid follicular neoplasms

ETIOLOGY/PATHOGENESIS
- Multiple losses involving chromosomes 1p, 3, 9p, 9q, 12, 17, and X; gains involving 7q, 8q, 12, 16, 17p, 17q, 19q, 20, 21q, and Xp described in case reports

CLINICAL ISSUES
- Extremely uncommon; < 20 cases described
- Based on few cases described, possibly renal cell carcinoma of low malignant potential
- Only 1 case known to have regional lymph node metastasis at presentation

MACROSCOPIC
- Well circumscribed
- Homogeneous, tan brown-to-dark brown cut surface
- Size: 1.9-11.8 cm (mean: 2.8 cm)

MICROSCOPIC
- Well circumscribed with distinct fibrous capsule
- Prominent follicular architecture composed of microfollicles and macrofollicles
- Clear cell change or spindle cells not observed
- Follicles lined by cells with moderate amount of amphophilic-to-eosinophilic cytoplasm
- Tumors lack histologic features seen in papillary carcinoma of thyroid, including prominent papillations, nuclear clearing, inclusions or grooves
- Mostly negative for CK7
- While most cases positive for pax-8, all cases negative for thyroglobulin and TTF-1

TOP DIFFERENTIAL DIAGNOSES
- Metastatic thyroid carcinoma

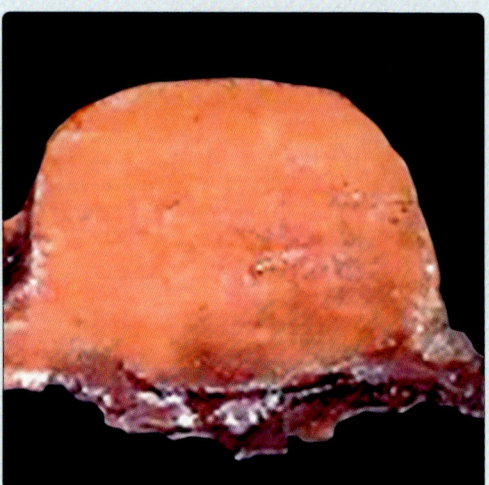

Gross Features

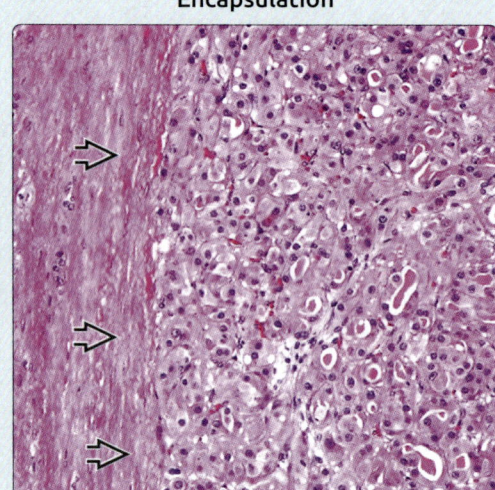

Encapsulation

(Left) Thyroid-like follicular carcinoma (TLFC) is typically a well-circumscribed tumor with homogeneous, tan-brown cut surface. The tan-brown color resembles thyroid parenchyma. Gross hemorrhage or necrosis are extremely uncommon. (Right) Reported thyroid-like follicular carcinoma have all been well circumscribed, with a well-defined fibrous capsule ➡. However, the thickness of the capsule is quite variable.

Typical Histologic Features

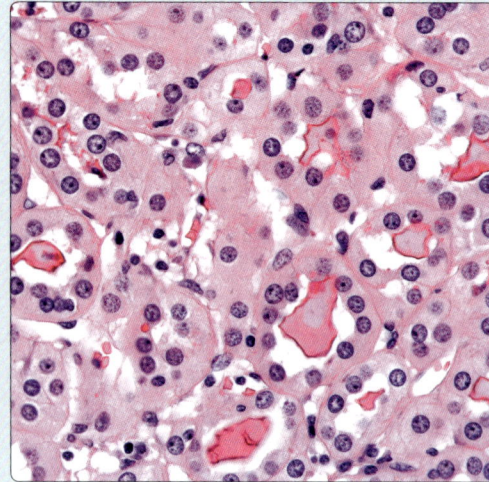

Typical Nuclear Features

(Left) The characteristic histologic features of thyroid-like follicular carcinoma of the kidney (TLFC-K) include a prominent micro- or macrofollicular architecture with colloid-like material ➡ in the follicles. (Right) Unlike the typical nuclear features in papillary thyroid carcinoma, the nuclei in thyroid-like follicular carcinomas usually lack grooves, inclusions, and clearing of chromatin. Nucleoli are usually not prominent, and at the most approach ISUP/WHO nucleolar grade 2.

Thyroid-Like Follicular Carcinoma of Kidney

TERMINOLOGY

Abbreviations
- Thyroid-like follicular carcinoma of kidney (TLFC-K)

Definitions
- Recently described primary renal cell carcinoma closely mimicking well-differentiated thyroid follicular neoplasms

ETIOLOGY/PATHOGENESIS

Genetic Features
- Gene expression profiling comparing with clear cell and chromophobe RCC overexpressed 135 (including multiple cell cycle regulatory genes) and underexpressed 46 genes
- Multiple losses involving chromosomes 1p, 3, 9p, 9q, 12, 17, and X; gains involving 7q, 8q, 12, 16, 17p, 17q, 19q, 20, 21q, and Xp described in case reports

CLINICAL ISSUES

Presentation
- Extremely uncommon; < 20 cases described
- Age range: 29-83 yr
- Most incidentally discovered during radiologic work-up for other medical conditions

Prognosis
- Based on few cases described, mostly renal cell carcinoma of low malignant potential
  - Only rare cases with metastasis at presentation, with no known deaths due to disease

MACROSCOPIC

General Features
- Well circumscribed, unifocal tumor
  - Size range: 1.9-11.8 cm (mean: 2.8)
- Homogeneous, tan brown to dark brown cut surface; necrosis or hemorrhage very rare

MICROSCOPIC

Histologic Features
- Well circumscribed
  - Distinct fibrous capsule of variable thickness present in all cases
- All described tumors organ confined
  - Only 2 tumors reported to be > 7 cm in size; all others pT1 (< 4 cm)
- Prominent follicular architecture composed of microfollicles and macrofollicles
  - Follicles filled with inspissated colloid-like material, occasionally focally calcified
- Patchy intratumoral lymphoid aggregates
  - Occasional tumors with lymphoid follicles, &/or widely distributed mast cells
- Clear cell change or spindle cells not observed
  - Focal papillary architecture described in 1 case
- Necrosis or lymphovascular invasion usually absent
- Follicles lined by cells with moderate amount of amphophilic-to-eosinophilic cytoplasm
  - Nuclei mostly round to oval, with mild nuclear membrane irregularities and uniform chromatin
  - Nucleoli inconspicuous, at most similar to nucleolar grade 2
  - Rare mitotic figures may be present
  - Tumors lack histologic features typical in papillary carcinoma of thyroid, including
    - Prominent papillations, nuclear clearing or pseudoinclusions and grooves

ANCILLARY TESTS

Immunohistochemistry
- Typically negative for CK7; but rare cases positive for CK7
- Usually, but not always, negative for pax-2, RCC, CD10, WT1, Ksp-cadherin, AMACR, vimentin, CD56, and CD57
- All cases negative for thyroglobulin and TTF-1

DIFFERENTIAL DIAGNOSIS

Metastatic Thyroid Carcinoma
- Rare event, although more reported cases than primary thyroid-like follicular carcinoma of kidney described
- About 1/2 of metastatic cases from thyroid carcinoma with architectural &/or nuclear features of papillary thyroid carcinoma
  - Others follicular, morphologically similar to thyroid-like follicular carcinoma of kidney
- Most metastatic thyroid carcinoma cases present with disseminated metastatic disease, in addition to renal involvement
- All reported cases of metastatic thyroid carcinoma with immunoreactivity for thyroid markers, including thyroglobulin &/or TTF-1
- All cases with confirmed thyroid neoplasms

DIAGNOSTIC CHECKLIST

Pathologic Interpretation Pearls
- Before accepting diagnosis of primary thyroid-like follicular carcinoma of kidney, possibility of metastatic thyroid carcinoma must be excluded
- In addition to clinical history, immunostaining for thyroglobulin and TTF-1 prerequisites for rendering this diagnosis
- pax-8 positivity not helpful in distinction from primary renal tumors

SELECTED REFERENCES

1. Dawane R et al: Thyroid-like follicular carcinoma of the kidney: one case report and review of the literature. Am J Clin Pathol. 144(5):796-804, 2015
2. Dhillon J et al: Thyroid-like follicular carcinoma of the kidney with metastases to the lungs and retroperitoneal lymph nodes. Hum Pathol. 42(1):146-50, 2011
3. Amin MB et al: Primary thyroid-like follicular carcinoma of the kidney: report of 6 cases of a histologically distinctive adult renal epithelial neoplasm. Am J Surg Pathol. 33(3):393-400, 2009
4. Sterlacci W et al: Primary thyroid-like renal tumor or renal metastasis from the thyroid? Virchows Arch. 455(1):97-8, 2009
5. Gupta R et al: Metastatic papillary carcinoma of thyroid masquerading as a renal tumour. J Clin Pathol. 61(1):143, 2008
6. Angell SK et al: Primary thyroidlike carcinoma of the kidney. Urology. 48(4):632-5, 1996

Thyroid-Like Follicular Carcinoma of Kidney

Typical Histological Features

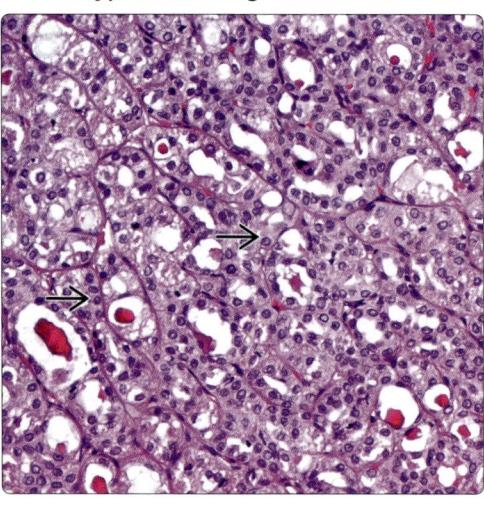

(Left) The cells lining the follicles ➡ in TLFC-K show a moderate amount of amphophilic-to-eosinophilic cytoplasm. The nuclei are round and occasionally oval with mild nuclear membrane irregularities. Mitotic activity is rare, and necrosis and vascular invasion are very uncommon. **(Right)** While follicular architecture is the most characteristic and defining feature of the tumor, rarely more solid and irregular nests ➡ may be focally present. Focal intratumoral desmoplasia ➡ may be present in rare tumors.

Intratumoral Desmoplasia

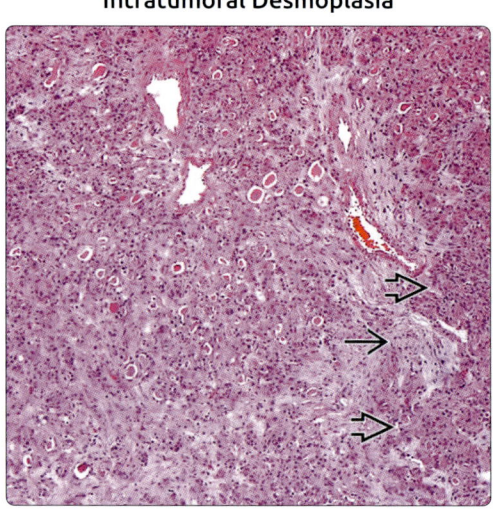

Lymphoid Infiltrates

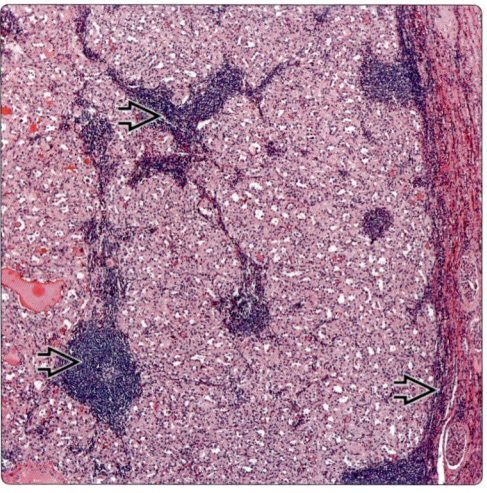

(Left) Marked lymphocytic infiltration ➡ may occasionally be observed in TLFC-K. The infiltrate is often present as prominent intratumoral collections but may sometimes be seen predominantly surrounding the tumor. **(Right)** Occasionally, the lymphoid infiltration in TLFC-K may show prominent lymphoid follicle formation ➡. Also, note the complex follicular architecture ➡ in this tumor.

Lymphoid Infiltrates

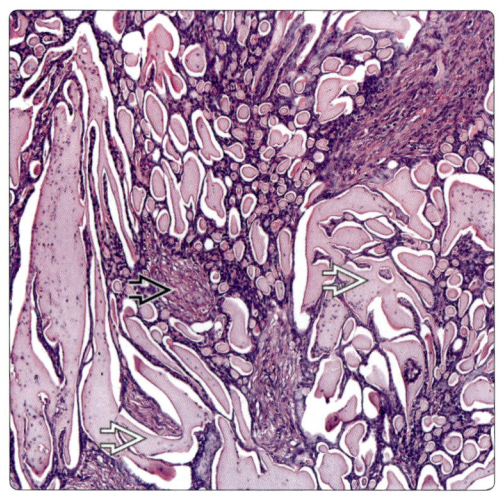

Macrofollicular Features

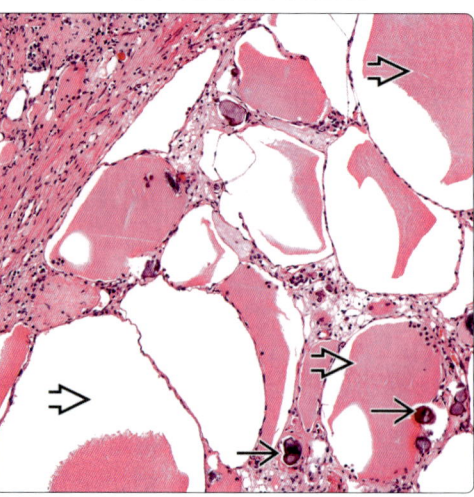

(Left) Some TLFC-K have a prominent macrofollicular pattern ➡. The colloid-like material in such follicles usually appears less dense and is often retracted from the lining cells. Occasionally, this colloid-like material may show calcifications ➡. **(Right)** While most thyroid-like follicular renal cancers are characterized by the presence of lymphoplasmacytic infiltrates, some tumors show widely distributed mast cells ➡.

Mast Cells

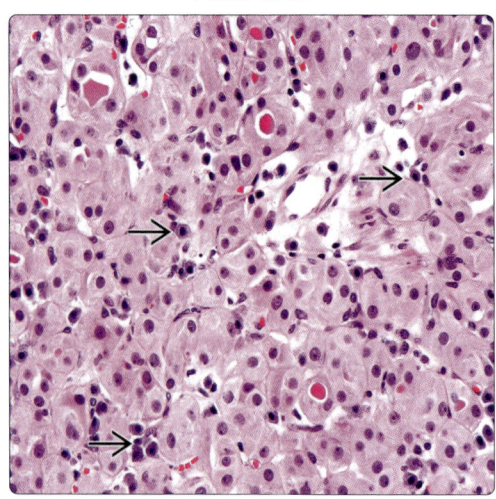

Thyroid-Like Follicular Carcinoma of Kidney

Follicular Carcinoma Thyroid

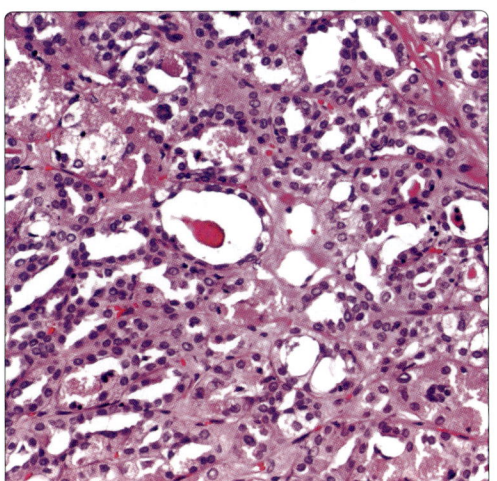

Papillary Thyroid Carcinoma

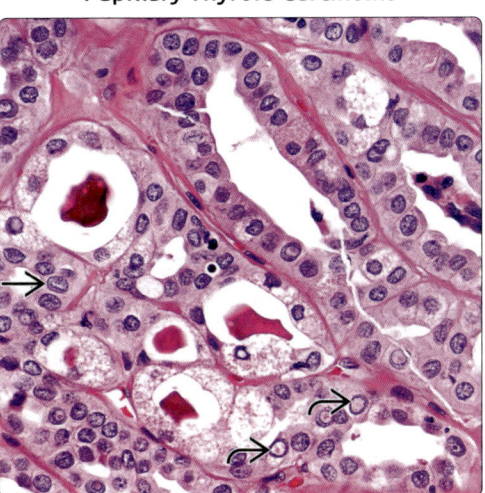

(Left) Microscopic features of a TLFC-K are reminiscent of a follicular carcinoma of the thyroid. Based on the relative incidences, the probability of a tumor with such histologic features representing a metastasis from thyroid is at least equal to, if not greater than, a renal primary. (Right) Follicular variant of papillary thyroid carcinoma metastatic to the kidney morphologically closely mimics the primary renal tumors. However, the characteristic nuclear features of grooves ⇨ and pseudoinclusions ⇨ are distinctive.

CK7

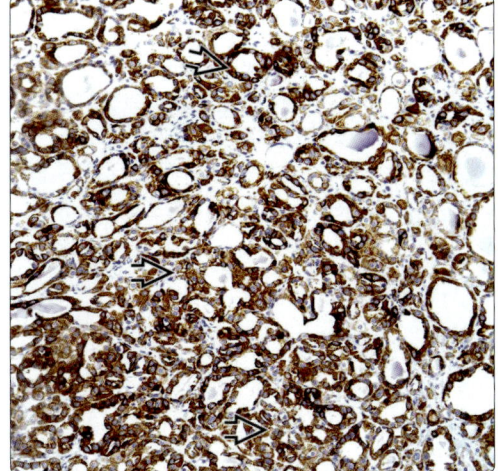

AMACR

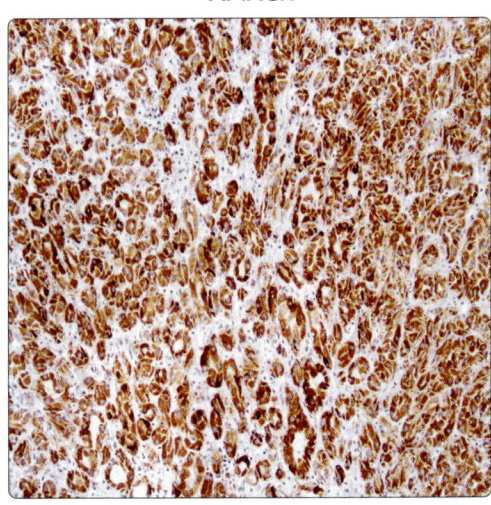

(Left) TLFC-K is usually negative for CK7. However, rare cases show variable, and sometimes diffuse, CK7 positivity ⇨. Thus, C7 immunoreactivity cannot be used for distinction from its mimics. (Right) Most TLFC-K are negative for AMACR. However, some tumors may show diffuse immunoreactivity for AMACR/p504s. Therefore, the commonly used immunomarkers like CK7 and AMACR may not be very helpful in distinction from metastatic PTC.

pax-8

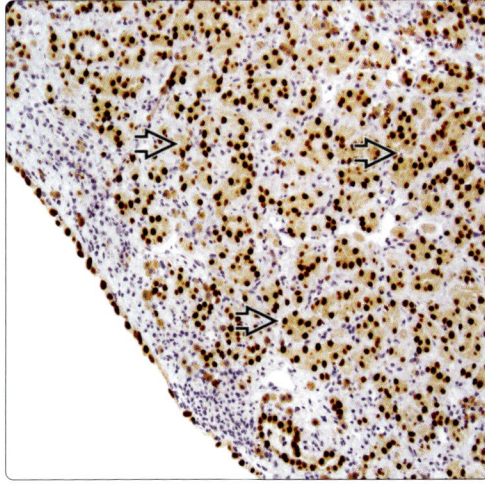

TTF-1 and Thyroglobulin

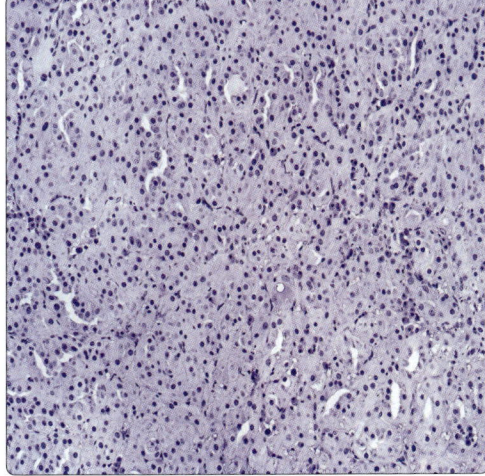

(Left) pax-8 shows diffuse nuclear immunoreactivity both in most primary renal tumors, including TLfC-K ⇨, and thyroid tumors. Thus, diffuse immunoreactivity will not help in the distinction of primary tumors and metastasis to the kidney. (Right) TTF-1 and thyroglobulin immunohistochemical stains most useful in the distinction of TLfC-K and metastatic thyroid carcinomas, being usually positive in thyroid cancers and negative in the morphologically similar primary renal tumors.

Acquired Cystic Disease-Associated Renal Cell Carcinoma

KEY FACTS

TERMINOLOGY
- Most common subtype of renal cell carcinoma occurring in end-stage kidneys, specifically with acquired cystic disease
  - Now recognized as distinct entity by WHO and ISUP

ETIOLOGY/PATHOGENESIS
- ACD-associated RCC mostly but not always seen in patients on dialysis
- Overall, incidence of renal cancer markedly increased (3-7%) in patients with end-stage kidneys
- Most common subtype of RCC in end-stage kidneys
- Other subtypes commonly occurring in both cystic and noncystic end-stage kidneys include clear cell papillary, papillary, clear cell, and chromophobe renal cell carcinoma

MICROSCOPIC
- Combination of acinar, solid alveolar, solid sheet-like, micro- or macrocystic, and papillary architecture in various combinations
- Intra- and intercytoplasmic microscopic lumina ("holes"), imparting cribriform/sieve-like appearance
- Presence of intratumoral oxalate crystals in majority of tumors
  - Some tumors may lack intratumoral oxalate crystals
- Cells usually large with abundant eosinophilic cytoplasm and prominent nucleoli
  - Areas with clear cell cytology not uncommon

DIAGNOSTIC CHECKLIST
- Presence of multiple small lumina/sieve-like, cribriform architecture, and intratumoral oxalate crystals diagnostic
- Variable proportions of papillary architecture and clear cell or eosinophilic cell cytology
- Background kidney with diagnostically essential end-stage features with multiple cysts
- AMACR positive, CA9 negative, and CK7 very focal to negative by IHC

Gross Features
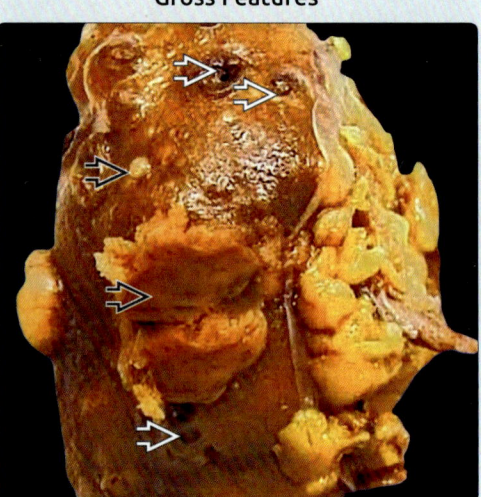

Gross Features
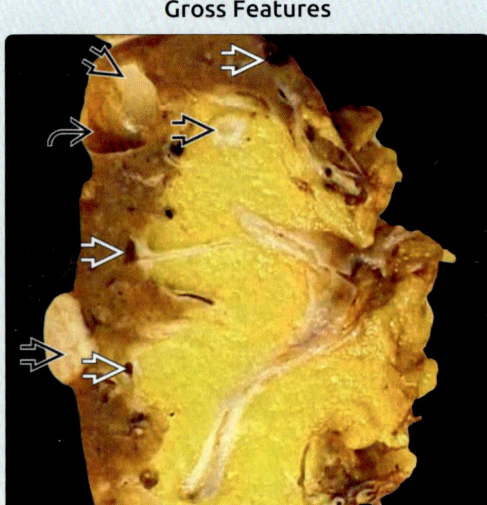

(Left) Gross photograph shows multiple cysts ⇨ and solid tumors ⇨ in an end-stage kidney. Unless almost totally occupied by large tumors, such kidneys are often small in size. (Right) Multiple cysts ⇨ and solid ⇨ or partly cystic ⇨ tumors are identified in the cut surface of this specimen. The marked cortical thinning and blunting of the papillae are hallmarks of an end-stage kidney. Gross examination is very important to identify gross solid and complex cystic lesions.

Sieve-Like Appearance
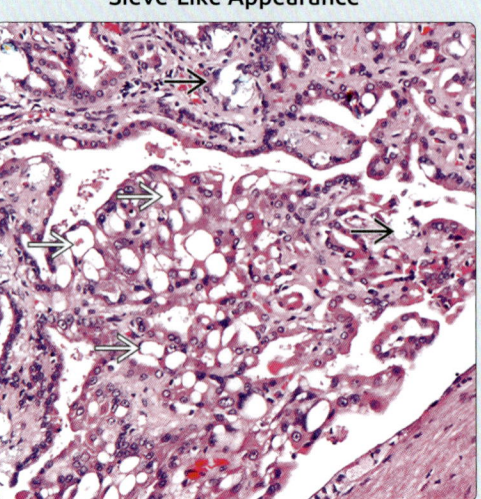

Intracystic Growth
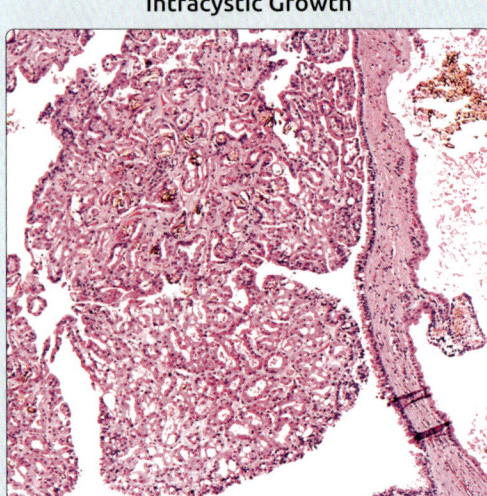

(Left) Typical microscopic appearance of acquired cystic disease-associated RCC (ACD-associated RCC) shows papillary and tubular architecture, small lumina ("holes") ⇨, large cells with eosinophilic cytoplasm, and intratumoral oxalate crystals ⇨. (Right) ACD-associated RCCs are often seen arising from the wall of a cyst, and many such tumors may have prominent papillary architecture. Because of architectural similarity, such tumors in the past may have been considered papillary renal cell carcinoma by some.

Acquired Cystic Disease-Associated Renal Cell Carcinoma

TERMINOLOGY

Abbreviations
- Acquired cystic disease-associated renal cell carcinoma (ACD-associated RCC)

Definitions
- Most common subtype of RCC occurring in end-stage kidneys, specifically those with acquired cystic disease
  - Now recognized as distinct new entity by WHO and International Society of Urologic Pathology (ISUP)
- Tumor composed of cells with eosinophilic cytoplasm, cribriform/sieve-like appearance, and oxalate crystals in setting of end-stage kidney disease

ETIOLOGY/PATHOGENESIS

Role of Dialysis and End-Stage Renal Disease
- Acquired cystic kidney disease (ACKD) usually but not always seen in patients on dialysis
  - Incidence of cystic disease progressively higher with longer durations of dialysis
    - 10-20% for dialysis up to 3 years
    - 40-60% at 5 years
    - > 90% at 10 years or more
- Type of dialysis, hemodialysis or peritoneal, is not important
- Causes of increased tumorigenesis in end-stage and ACKD are possibly multifactorial, and include
  - Depressed cellular and humoral immunity in renal failure
  - Impaired antioxidant defense and increased synthesis of reactive oxygen species
  - Release of free radicals with resultant DNA damage, mutations, and cancer
  - Use of immunosuppressive medications
  - Oxalate crystal-induced tubular proliferative activity

CLINICAL ISSUES

Epidemiology
- Incidence
  - Incidence of renal tumors up to 100x greater in patients with end-stage kidney disease, particularly ACDK, compared with that in general population
    - Overall incidence of renal cancer 3-7% in end-stage kidneys
  - Previously, papillary RCC believed to be most common RCC subtype in end-stage kidneys
  - In reality, ACD-associated RCC is most common subtype of RCC in end-stage kidneys
    - ACD-associated RCC accounts for dominant mass in 36% of end-stage kidneys overall and 46% of end-stage kidneys with acquired cystic disease
    - ACD-associated RCC also most common tumor type among other, often multiple, small tumor nodules dispersed within end-stage kidneys
    - Proportion of ACD-associated RCC, compared to other RCC subtypes, reported to increase with increasing duration of dialysis
      - However, this has not been confirmed in largest reported series to date
  - Other subtypes commonly occurring in both cystic and noncystic end-stage kidneys include
    - Clear cell papillary RCC
    - Papillary RCC
    - Clear cell RCC
    - Chromophobe RCC
    - Rare cases of hemangioma, collecting duct carcinoma, renal oncocytoma, renal capsuloma also described

Presentation
- ACD-associated RCC seen exclusively in end-stage kidneys with acquired cystic disease
- Most cases diagnosed incidentally on radiologic follow-up in patients with chronic renal disease

Prognosis
- Most tumors with nonaggressive biologic behavior
  - Likely because diagnosed at small size with low pT stage
    - Usual small size because of constant care due to underlying renal medical condition and resultant earlier radiologic detection
- Very few cases with aggressive features, including pT3 stage or rhabdoid/sarcomatoid differentiation
- Rare deaths due to tumor reported; only in those with sarcomatoid features and metastatic disease

MACROSCOPIC

Background Kidney
- Usually with numerous cysts
- Frequently small, shrunken, and granular

Tumors
- Often multifocal (> 50%) and bilateral (> 20%)
- Carcinomas usually well circumscribed, many appearing to arise within cysts
- Larger tumors with thick fibrous capsule, often with foci of calcification

MICROSCOPIC

Histologic Features
- Acinar, solid alveolar, solid sheet-like, micro- or macrocystic, and papillary architecture in various combinations and proportions
- Intra- and intercytoplasmic microscopic lumina ("holes"), imparting cribriform/microcystic/sieve-like appearance
- Presence of intratumoral oxalate crystals in majority of tumors
  - Only tumor type in end-stage kidneys consistently displaying intratumoral oxalate crystals
- Most tumor cells are large with abundant eosinophilic cytoplasm and prominent nucleoli
  - Foci with clear cytoplasm are also seen
- Rare cases of ACD-associated RCCs with sarcomatoid or rhabdoid features
  - Aggressive behavior observed in some cases with sarcomatoid features, including
    - Widespread metastases
    - Death due to disease

Cytologic Features
- Clusters of cells with papillary configuration
- Cells polygonal to columnar with abundant eosinophilic granular cytoplasm and round, centrally located nuclei

Acquired Cystic Disease-Associated Renal Cell Carcinoma

- o Finely granular nuclear chromatin
- o Prominent central nucleoli
- Differentiation from type 2 eosinophilic papillary renal cell carcinoma difficult on cytologic basis

Lymph Nodes
- Rare cases with metastasis reported

Predominant Pattern/Injury Type
- Neoplastic

Predominant Cell/Compartment Type
- Epithelial

Pathology of Background Kidney
- Features of end-stage kidney
- Numerous cysts in renal parenchyma, some multiloculated
  - o In some, cyst lining resembling cells of ACD-associated RCC
    - Large cells with granular, eosinophilic cytoplasm and prominent nucleoli
    - Focal proliferation, sometimes with papillary architecture may be present
      - □ CA9(-), CK7(-), CD10(+/-), AMACR(+)
  - o In some, cyst lining resembling cells of clear cell papillary RCC
    - Clear cells with uniform nuclei often with linear alignment away from basement membrane
      - □ CA9(+), CK7(+), CD10(-), AMACR(-)
  - o Other cysts with foamy-appearing cell lining, occasionally with papillary infoldings
- Sometimes groups of cysts clustered together

ANCILLARY TESTS

Immunohistochemistry
- Diffusely positive for AMACR
- Negative/very focally positive for CK7
- Negative for CA9
- Also positive for CD10, RCC, and GST-α

Genetic Testing
- ACD-associated RCC lacks trisomies 7 and 17, or 3p losses
  - o Array CGH or FISH studies show gains of chromosomes 3, 7, 16, 17, and Y
    - Genotype quite different from that of papillary and clear cell RCC
      - □ Frequent gains of chromosomes 3, 16, and Y distinguish it from papillary RCC
      - □ Frequent gain, and not loss, of chromosome 3 distinguishes it from clear cell RCC
  - o Rare cases with loss of chromosome 7, 17, or Y

DIFFERENTIAL DIAGNOSIS

Papillary Renal Cell Carcinoma
- Lacks "holes" and sieve-like areas
- Intratumoral oxalate crystals extremely uncommon
- Usually show abundant foamy macrophages in cores of papillae
- Typically CK7 and AMACR positive by immunohistochemistry
- Often with trisomies/polysomies 7 and 17

Clear Cell Renal Cell Carcinoma
- Lacks "holes," sieve-like areas, and intratumoral oxalate crystals
- Arborizing, branching vascular septations are distinctive
- Mostly negative for CK7 and negative/only focally positive for AMACR
  - o Diffuse membranous positivity for CA9 and CD10 characteristic for clear cell renal cell carcinoma

DIAGNOSTIC CHECKLIST

Pathologic Interpretation Pearls
- Papillary architecture in ACD-associated RCC may suggest diagnosis of papillary renal cell carcinoma
- Similarly, clear cell cytology may raise possibility of clear cell renal cell carcinoma
- In background of acquired cystic disease, attention to morphologic features in entire tumor essential for correct diagnosis
- Presence of multiple small lumina/sieve-like, cribriform architecture and intratumoral oxalate crystals diagnostic
- Diffuse AMACR positivity with CK7 negativity characteristic

SELECTED REFERENCES

1. Hosseini M et al: Pathologic spectrum of cysts in end-stage kidneys: possible precursors to renal neoplasia. Hum Pathol. 45(7):1406-13, 2014
2. Kryvenko ON et al: Haemangiomas in kidneys with end-stage renal disease: a novel clinicopathological association. Histopathology. 65(3):309-18, 2014
3. Ahn S et al: Acquired cystic disease-associated renal cell carcinoma: further characterization of the morphologic and immunopathologic features. Med Mol Morphol. 46(4):225-32, 2013
4. Srigley JR et al: The International Society of Urological Pathology (ISUP) Vancouver Classification of Renal Neoplasia. Am J Surg Pathol. 37(10):1469-89, 2013
5. Sassa N et al: Renal cell carcinomas in haemodialysis patients: does haemodialysis duration influence pathological cell types and prognosis? Nephrol Dial Transplant. 26(5):1677-82, 2011
6. Pan CC et al: Immunohistochemical and molecular genetic profiling of acquired cystic disease-associated renal cell carcinoma. Histopathology. 55(2):145-53, 2009
7. Kuroda N et al: Sarcomatoid acquired cystic disease-associated renal cell carcinoma. Histol Histopathol. 23(11):1327-31, 2008
8. Schwarz A et al: Renal cell carcinoma in transplant recipients with acquired cystic kidney disease. Clin J Am Soc Nephrol. 2(4):750-6, 2007
9. Cossu-Rocca P et al: Acquired cystic disease-associated renal tumors: an immunohistochemical and fluorescence in situ hybridization study. Mod Pathol. 19(6):780-7, 2006
10. Tickoo SK et al: Spectrum of epithelial neoplasms in end-stage renal disease: an experience from 66 tumor-bearing kidneys with emphasis on histologic patterns distinct from those in sporadic adult renal neoplasia. Am J Surg Pathol. 30(2):141-53, 2006
11. Sule N et al: Calcium oxalate deposition in renal cell carcinoma associated with acquired cystic kidney disease: a comprehensive study. Am J Surg Pathol. 29(4):443-51, 2005
12. Cheuk W et al: Atypical epithelial proliferations in acquired renal cystic disease harbor cytogenetic aberrations. Hum Pathol. 33(7):761-5, 2002
13. Denton MD et al: Prevalence of renal cell carcinoma in patients with ESRD pre-transplantation: a pathologic analysis. Kidney Int. 61(6):2201-9, 2002
14. Koul HK et al: COM crystals activate the p38 mitogen-activated protein kinase signal transduction pathway in renal epithelial cells. J Biol Chem. 277(39):36845-52, 2002
15. Gronwald J et al: Chromosomal abnormalities in renal cell neoplasms associated with acquired renal cystic disease. A series studied by comparative genomic hybridization and fluorescence in situ hybridization. J Pathol. 187(3):308-12, 1999

Acquired Cystic Disease-Associated Renal Cell Carcinoma

Papillary Architecture

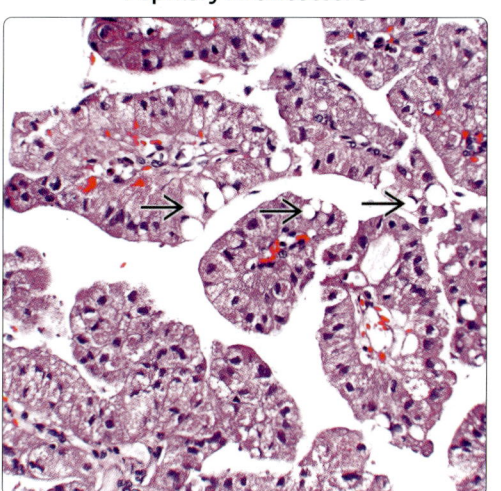

Tubular Architecture

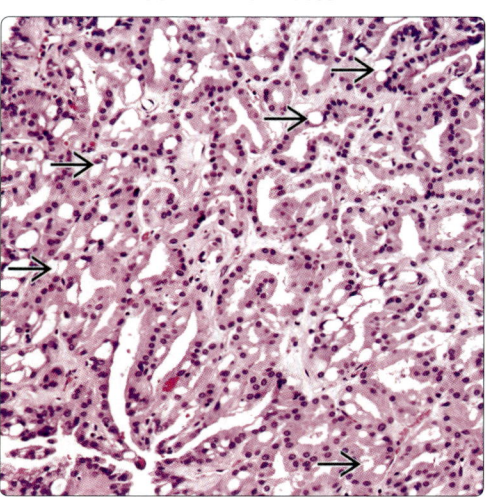

(Left) This photomicrograph shows prominent papillary architecture in an ACD-associated RCC. Differential diagnostic considerations in tumors with prominent papillary architecture include papillary RCC; however, papillary RCC does not typically show the intracytoplasmic lumina ⇨ as seen here. (Right) This hematoxylin & eosin section highlights predominant tubular features in an ACD-associated RCC. The small intra- and intercellular lumina ⇨ are easily identified.

Oxalate Crystals

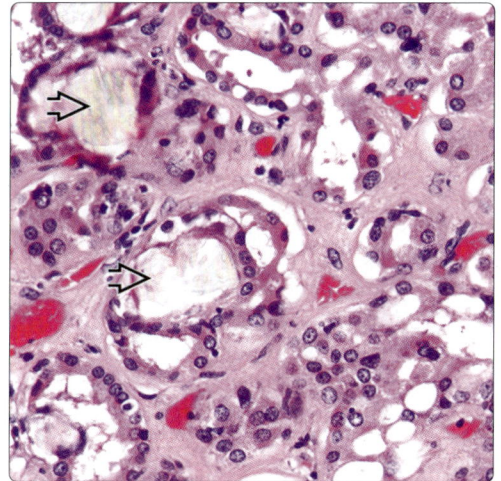

Oxalate Crystals

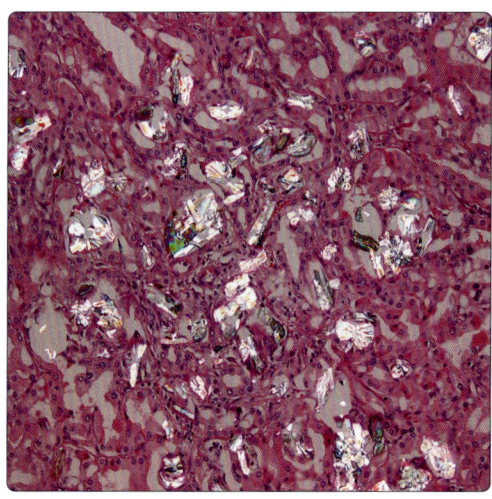

(Left) ACD-associated RCC almost invariably shows cells containing abundant eosinophilic cytoplasm. The oxalate crystals are also easily identifiable ⇨ even without using polarized light. (Right) Partial polarization highlights the intratumoral oxalate crystals in this photomicrograph. Although oxalate crystals are often present in nonneoplastic parenchyma, ACD-associated RCC is the only carcinoma arising in acquired cystic disease that consistently contains oxalate crystals.

Cytological Features

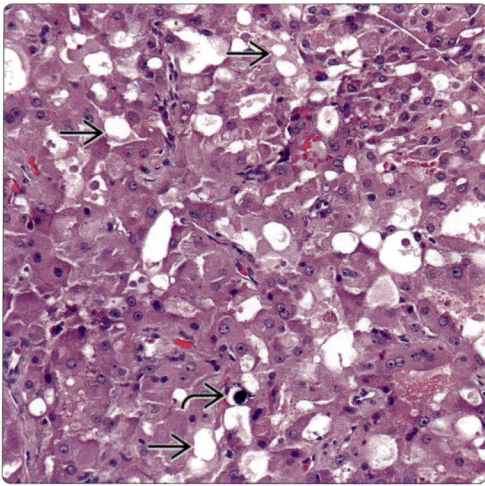

Cytological Features

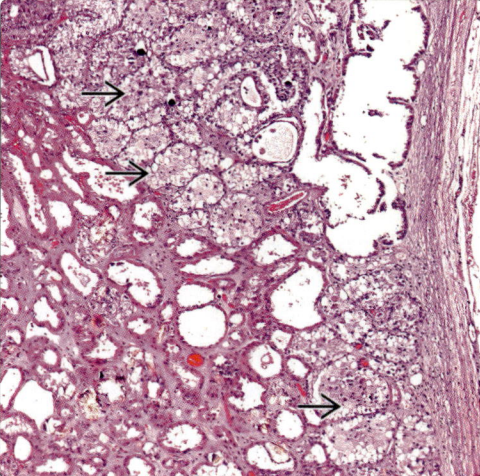

(Left) Typical cytologic features of ACD-associated RCC include cells with abundant eosinophilic cytoplasm and large nuclei with prominent nucleoli. Notice the prominent inter- and intracellular lumina ⇨, a characteristic feature of the tumor. Presence of calcifications ⇨ is also common. (Right) Areas with clear cell cytology in ACD-associated RCC ⇨ may raise the possibility of clear cell RCC, and this may be one of the reasons for the reported high incidence of clear cell RCC in end-stage kidneys.

Acquired Cystic Disease-Associated Renal Cell Carcinoma

Clear Cell Change and Calcification
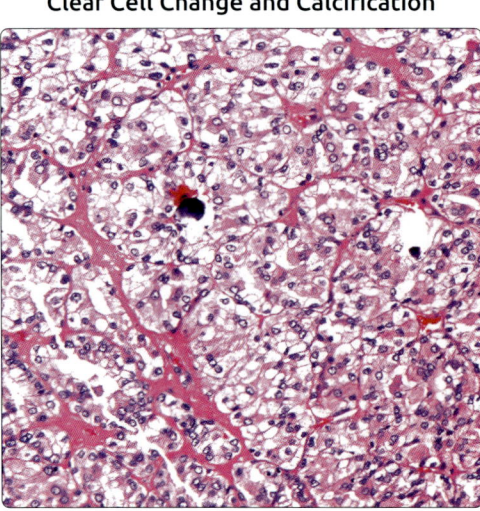

Intra- and Intercellular Lumina
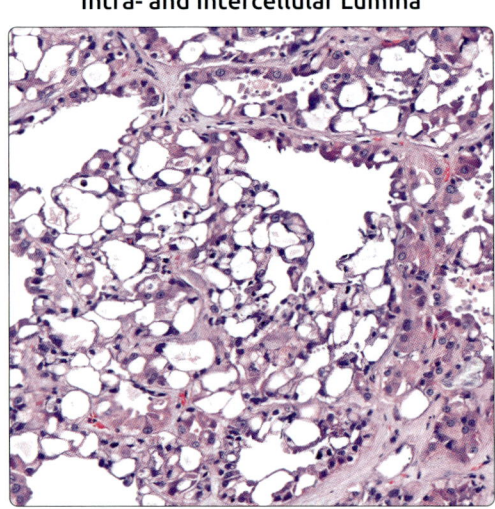

(Left) This higher magnification view highlights clear cell cytology in an ACD-associated RCC. Predominance of such areas in a tumor may lead to the misdiagnosis of clear cell RCC. Careful evaluation of the rest of the tumor is required. **(Right)** A higher magnification view shows the characteristic lumina imparting a cribriform/sieve-like appearance to the tumor. Such lumina are present, at least focally, in all architectural and cytological patterns of ACD-associated RCC.

AMACR Staining
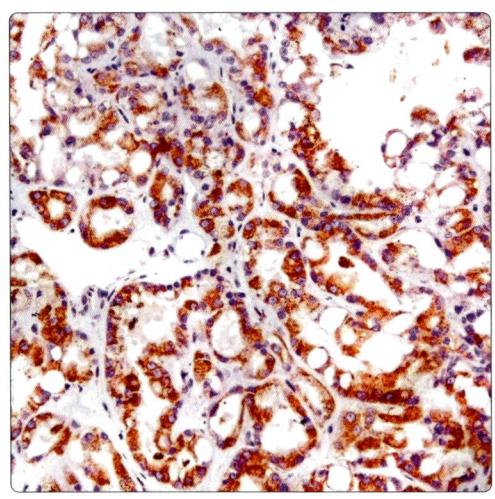

CK7 Staining
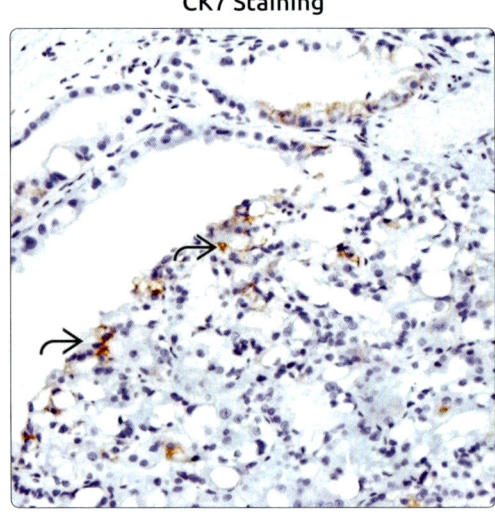

(Left) Diffuse AMACR positivity, similar to that seen in papillary RCC, is typical. Variable levels of positivity for AMACR are observed even in areas that show clear cell cytology in ACD-associated RCC. **(Right)** In spite of prominent papillary architecture in some cases, immunoreactivity for CK7 is absent or very focal ⇨ in almost all ACD-associated RCC. This staining pattern is unlike what is typical in papillary RCC, and is quite important in differentiating these tumors from papillary RCC.

Prominent Tubular and Cystic Architecture
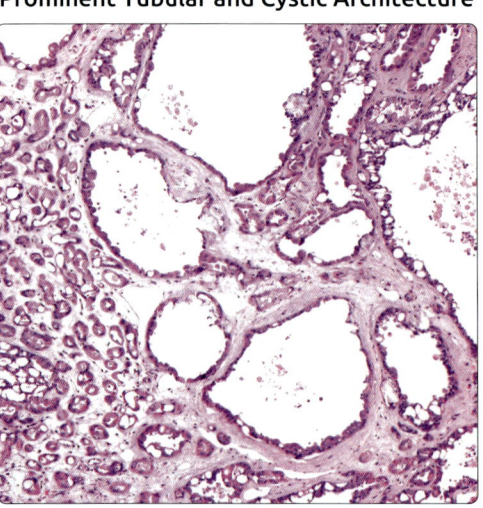

Hemorrhage and Hemosiderin
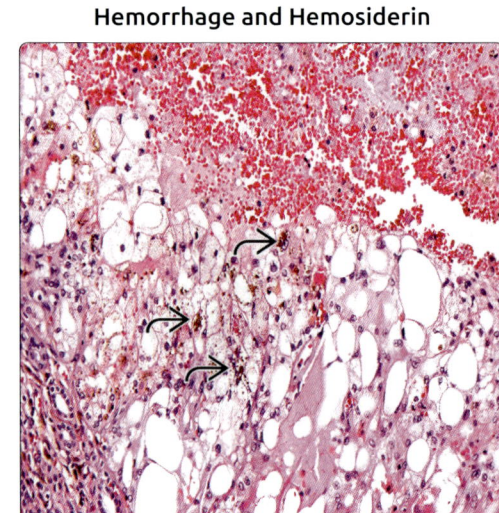

(Left) Cystic and tubular architecture is quite common in ACD-associated RCC. Most tumors show a combination of architectural patterns, but predominance of any one architectural pattern is not uncommon. This may lead to mistaken alternate diagnosis. **(Right)** Intratumoral hemorrhage is very frequent in ACD-associated RCC. Consequently, the presence of hemosiderin-laden macrophages and intracellular hemosiderin ⇨ granules within the tumor cells is not uncommon in the tumor.

Acquired Cystic Disease-Associated Renal Cell Carcinoma

Metastatic ACD-Associated RCC

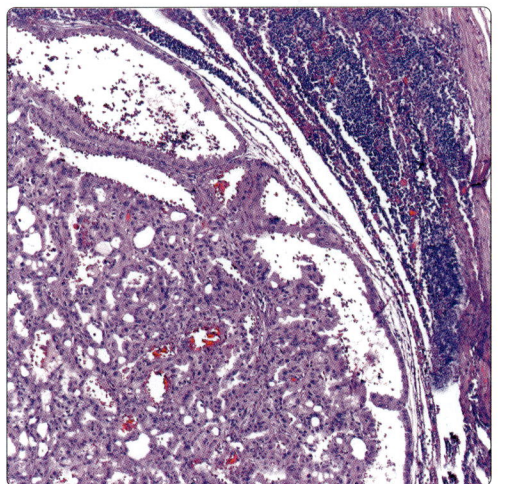

Metastatic ACD-Associated RCC

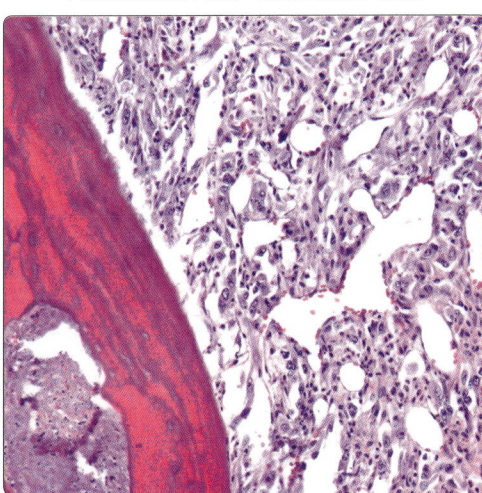

(Left) This hematoxylin & eosin section shows a metastasis to a lymph node. Metastasis rarely occurs in ACD-associated RCC, and in most cases, the metastasis is reported in regional lymph nodes. Metastatic tumors are often sarcomatoid but may also have typical epithelial histology. (Right) This microphotograph shows acquired cystic disease-associated RCC metastatic to bone. In addition to lymph nodes and bones, metastases have been reported in unusual sites, including myocardium.

Sarcomatoid Change

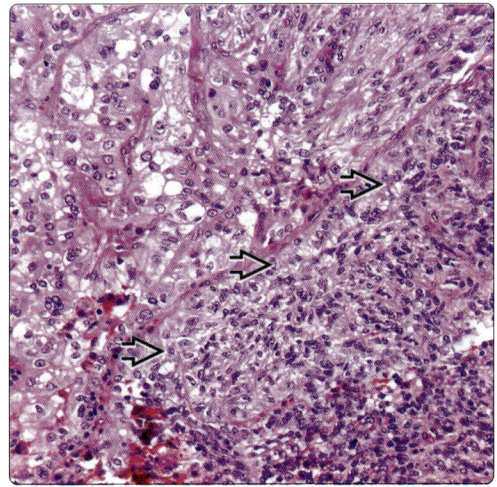

Adjacent Renal Parenchyma

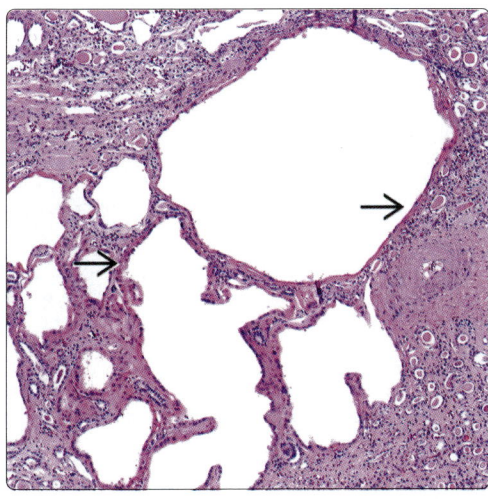

(Left) ACD-associated RCC occasionally may show sarcomatoid ⇒ features, but sarcomatoid differentiation is very rare in this tumor. Tumors with such features show aggressive biological behavior and have resulted in death with widespread metastases. (Right) This photomicrograph shows clustered cysts in the surrounding renal parenchyma. Such cysts are often lined by large cells with abundant eosinophilic cytoplasm ⇒, morphologically similar to the cells of ACD-associated RCC.

Clustered Atypical Cysts

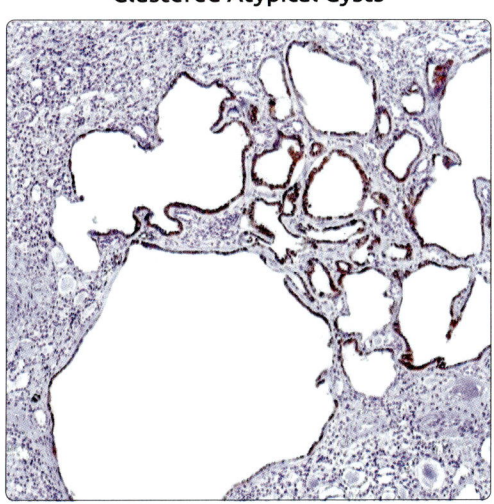

Clustered Atypical Cysts

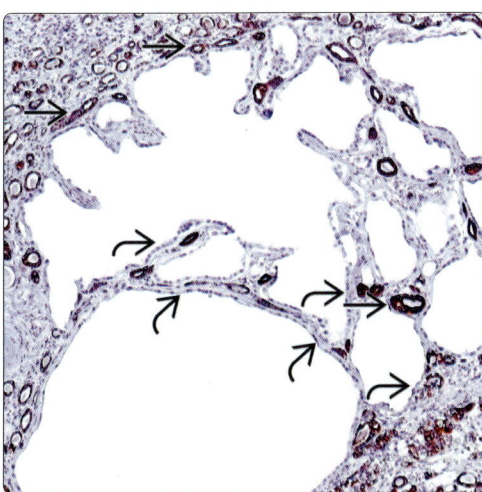

(Left) The eosinophilic cells lining the cysts in the surrounding renal parenchyma often show an immunohistochemical profile that is similar to that of ACD-associated RCC. This AMACR preparation shows diffuse positivity in the clustered cysts. Such cysts are likely the precursor lesion for the tumor. (Right) Similarly, such clustered cysts in the surrounding renal parenchyma often do not stain for CK7 ⇒. Notice the strong and diffuse positivity in the surrounding renal tubules ⇒.

Subsequent Second Tumors

KEY FACTS

TERMINOLOGY
- Renal cell tumors that develop following earlier renal or nonrenal tumor or autoimmune conditions
- Most of these tumors develop after prior chemotherapy or renal-directed radiotherapy

ETIOLOGY/PATHOGENESIS
- Best recognized prior tumors are neuroblastoma and Wilms tumor
- Lupus is most common associated autoimmune disease
- 2nd tumors in most cases have developed after platinum-based chemotherapy; suggests possible role for chemotherapy-induced chromosomal instability

MICROSCOPIC
- Initially described to be characteristic for specific tumor-associated 2nd tumors
  - However, similar morphologic features are seen in 2nd tumors developing after variety of 1st tumors

- Most postneuroblastoma carcinomas with eosinophilic and focally reticular cytoplasm reminiscent of oncocytic neoplasms, with solid and papillary architecture
  - More recently, tumors with more variable cytoarchitectural features including clear cell or papillary also described
  - Rare cases confirmed to be MiTF/TFE family translocation-associated carcinomas in postneuroblastoma setting
- Rarely, postneuroblastoma carcinoma-like tumors and PNET also reported after therapy for other tumors

DIAGNOSTIC CHECKLIST
- 2nd tumors of similar morphologic type may develop after variety of initial tumor types or autoimmune diseases
- Tumors often with oncocytic, clear cell, or papillary morphology
  - Most with high nuclear grade

Gross Features
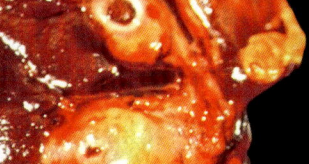

Solid and Papillary Architecture
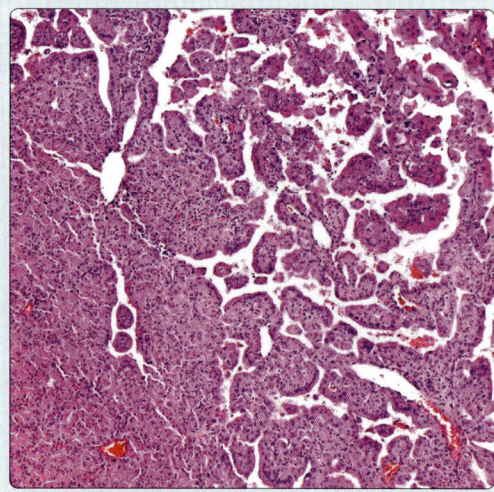

(Left) This postchemotherapy renal cell carcinoma has oncocytoid features similar to neuroblastoma-associated renal carcinoma. In addition to neuroblastoma, such tumors may develop after therapy for other tumors as well. (Right) This low-power image shows a postneuroblastoma renal tumor that has a solid and papillary architecture, and is composed of pleomorphic oncocytic cells. It is now known that a variety of RCC types can develop after childhood neuroblastoma.

Papillary Architecture
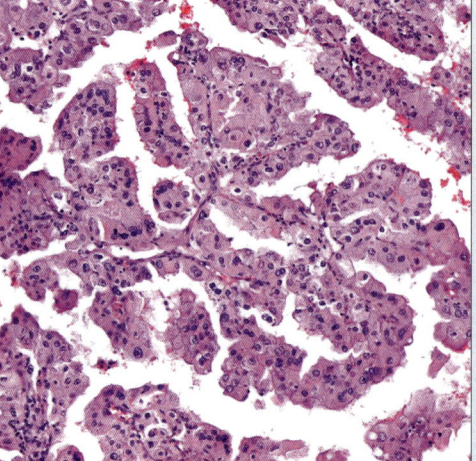

Solid Sheets of Oncocytic Cells
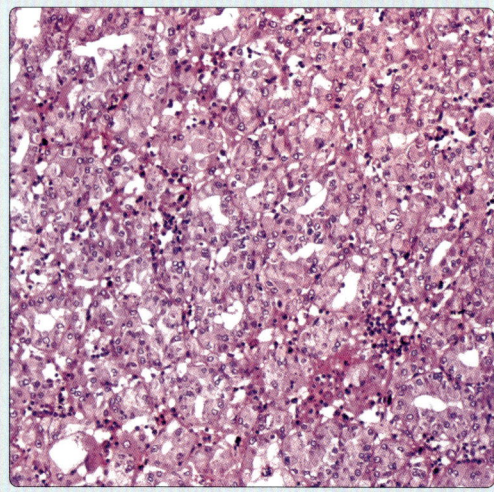

(Left) This intermediate magnification of a postneuroblastoma therapy renal cell carcinoma depicts a prominent papillary architecture with oncocytic cells and moderate nuclear pleomorphism. Such histology is not limited to tumors following neuroblastoma, but has also been reported following leiomyo- and rhabdomyosarcoma. (Right) Typical features of a post-neuroblastoma RCC include solid sheet-like architecture, with cells showing abundant oncocytic cytoplasm and nuclei with prominent nucleoli.

Subsequent Second Tumors

TERMINOLOGY

Definitions
- Renal cell tumors that develop following earlier renal or nonrenal tumor or other treated autoimmune conditions
  - Usually develop after prior chemotherapy or renal-directed chemotherapy
  - Can occur spontaneously

ETIOLOGY/PATHOGENESIS

Prior Tumors
- Neuroblastoma is best recognized prior tumor
  - 2nd tumors in most cases have developed after platinum-based chemotherapy; suggests possible role for chemotherapy-induced chromosomal instability
  - Rare tumors present synchronously without prior chemotherapy; suggests possible genetic predisposition in some cases
- Rare 2nd tumors reported in cases with prior Wilms tumor
  - Many of these, in addition to receiving chemotherapy, also received radiation
- Other entities recognized to be associated with chemotherapy include
  - TFE-translocation-associated renal carcinoma
  - Prior conditions: Leukemias, Wilms tumor, leiomyosarcoma, rhabdomyosarcoma, neuroendocrine tumors

Autoimmune Conditions
- Renal tumors described in autoimmune diseases: Lupus most common, followed by Wegener granulomatosis
- Other conditions: Polyarteritis nodosa, polymyositis/dermatomyositis and Crohn disease
- Alteration in cellular immunity &/or treatment with cyclophosphamide considered as underlying cause
- Persistent microscopic hematuria may be only presenting sign

Genetic Features
- Few postneuroblastoma tumors tested have often been aneuploid, with multiple allelic imbalances in different chromosomes, including 14q31 and 20q13 abnormalities
- Translocation-associated renal carcinomas show molecular alterations similar to cases with no prior history of therapy
- *TP53* and *SDHB* mutations reported in some cases

CLINICAL ISSUES

Epidemiology
- Incidence
  - Following childhood cancer, incidence of 2nd cancer in survivors is higher than in general population
    - Incidence is about 1% without any therapy, 3% with chemo- or radiotherapy alone, > 8% and with both together
    - Last incidence is roughly 20x greater than in general population
  - 2nd tumors involving kidney are quite rare
    - ~ 20 cases postneuroblastoma and < 10 cases post-Wilms tumor reported in literature
    - However, ~ 15% of cases with TFE carcinoma have history of prior cytotoxic chemotherapy
- Age
  - Patients with neuroblastoma-associated and postchemotherapy TFE carcinomas
    - Younger; range: 2-36 yr
      - Mean interval between prior tumor and RCC: 7 yr (range: Few months to 13 years)
  - Patients with renal tumors post-Wilms tumor
    - Older; range: 34-50 yr
      - Reported intervals after prior therapy: Often > 30 yr

Prognosis
- RCC associated with neuroblastoma: > 25% of cases reported to develop metastases
- Postchemotherapy TFE renal carcinoma
  - In children, often present at advanced stage with unusually aggressive behavior in some cases

MACROSCOPIC

General Features
- Can be unifocal, multifocal, or bilateral

MICROSCOPIC

Histologic Features
- Initially, 2nd tumors described to be with characteristic features after specific primary tumor
  - Many postneuroblastoma carcinomas with eosinophilic and focally reticular cytoplasm: Oncocytic neoplasms with solid and papillary architecture
    - High nuclear grade with extensive renal infiltration
- Subsequently, greater overlap in morphology of 2nd tumors, as well as associated primary tumors described
  - Many with papillary or clear cell RCC-like features
    - Some cases confirmed to be MiTF/TFE family translocation-associated carcinomas (both TFEB and TFE3) in postneuroblastoma setting
  - More recently, tumors with more variable cytoarchitectural features, including renal PNET, also been described
- Tumors developing after therapy for Wilms tumor reported predominantly as clear cell, and rarely papillary RCC and oncocytomas
  - However, these have not been systematically investigated for TFE translocations
    - One case reported to be TFE carcinoma
- Rarely, postneuroblastoma carcinoma-like tumors and PNET also reported after therapy for other tumors

SELECTED REFERENCES

1. de Menezes JL et al: Renal primitive neuroectodermal tumor as a second malignancy after chemotherapy and radiation for Non-Hodgkin's Lymphoma - treatment-related or just poor old bad luck?: A case report. J Cancer Res Ther. 11(3):649, 2015
2. Shnorhavorian M et al: Genitourinary long-term outcomes for childhood cancer survivors. Curr Urol Rep. 10(2):134-7, 2009
3. Dhall D et al: Pediatric renal cell carcinoma with oncocytoid features occurring in a child after chemotherapy for cardiac leiomyosarcoma. Urology. 70(1):178, 2007
4. Argani P et al: Translocation carcinomas of the kidney after chemotherapy in childhood. J Clin Oncol. 24(10):1529-34, 2006

Subsequent Second Tumors

(Left) Neuroblastoma is the most well known, but relatively uncommon, tumor associated with the development of 2nd renal tumors. A variety of other tumors are now known to bear association with such 2nd tumors. (Right) Neuroblastoma-associated renal carcinoma is typically composed of large oncocytic cells, with large, mildly pleomorphic nuclei with prominent nucleoli ⇨. Rare dispersed cells may have somewhat clear, bubbly cytoplasm ⇨.

Neuroblastoma

Postneuroblastoma Oncocytic RCC

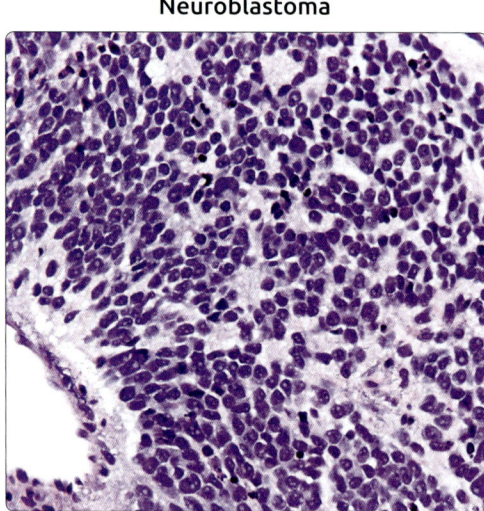

(Left) Morphologic features similar to neuroblastoma-associated RCC may also be seen in 2nd tumors developing after other neoplasms. This tumor arose in kidney of child previously treated for leiomyosarcoma. Notice focal papillations ⇨, finding frequent in post-neuroblastoma carcinomas. (Right) Tumors with various histologic features are now known to arise after neuroblastoma, including those with predominantly papillary architecture. Some such tumors are known as TFE translocation RCC.

Postleiomyosarcoma Oncocytic RCC

Postneuroblastoma RCC: Papillary Architecture

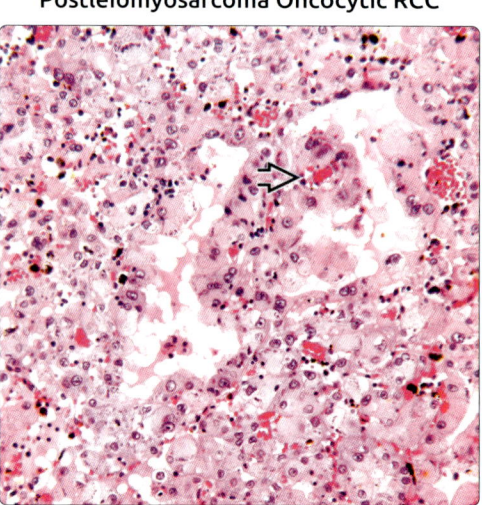
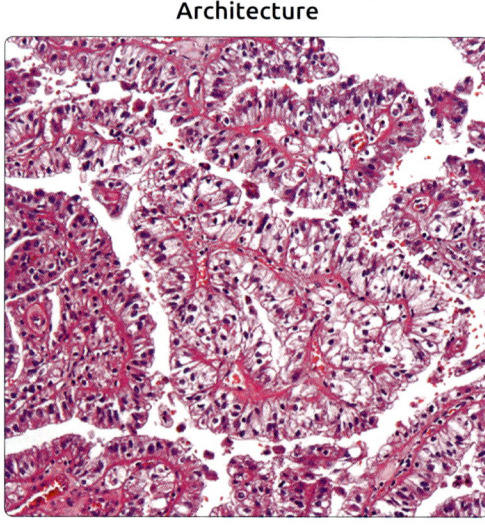

(Left) Although most of the 2nd tumors arising after neuroblastoma have not been studied for TFE translocations, such translocations have been confirmed in some. Such postneuroblastoma carcinomas have had the typical morphologic features of TFE renal carcinomas; solid alveolar architecture is seen here in one such tumor. (Right) Neuroblastoma-associated TFE carcinomas may show morphologic features of TFE3 or TFEB (as seen here) carcinomas, and immunostaining is confirmatory.

Postneuroblastoma RCC: Alveolar Architecture

Postneuroblastoma TFE-B Carcinoma

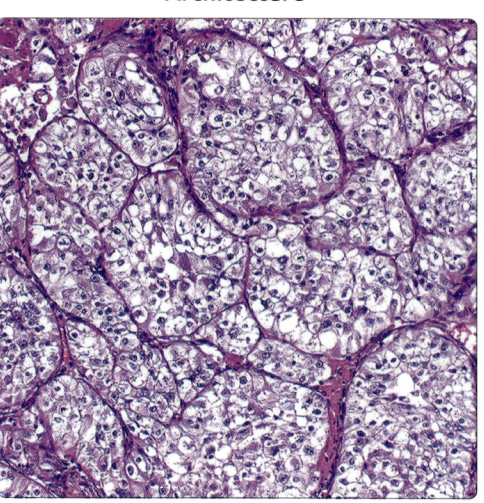
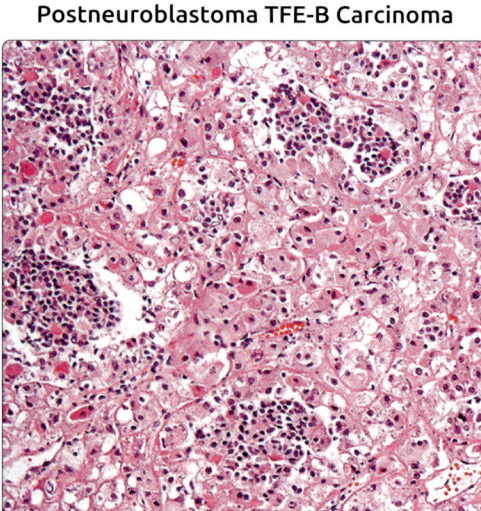

Subsequent Second Tumors

Clear Cell Morphology
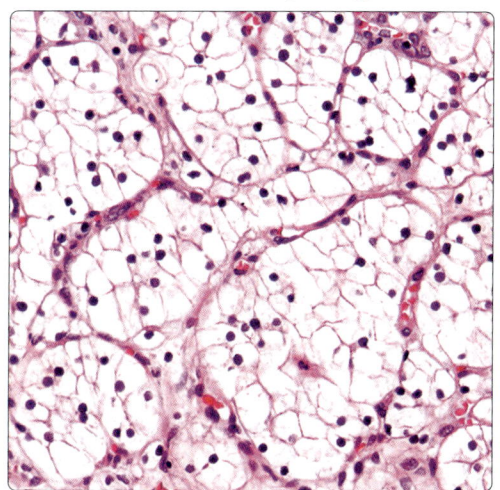

Primitive Neuroectodermal Tumor
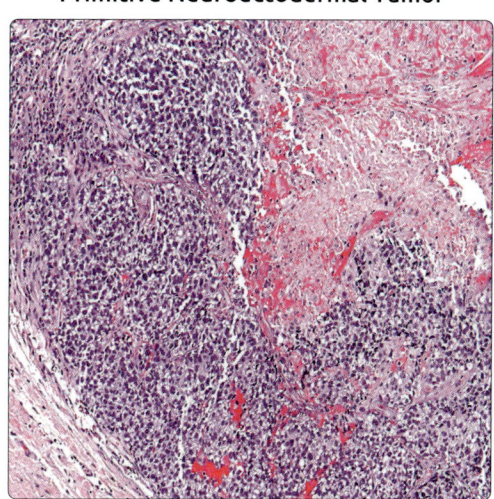

(Left) Number of postneuroblastoma 2nd tumors are regarded as clear cell RCC. However, many tumors with such features in children are MITF/TFE family-associated RCC. Also, most postneuroblastoma 2nd tumors arise in children, making it prudent to investigate all post-neuroblastoma tumors with clear cell/papillary features for TFE translocations. (Right) Rare PNET as 2nd tumors following therapy for leukemia, Hodgkin, or NHL are also described. (Courtesy J. Sarungbam, MD.)

Wilms Tumor
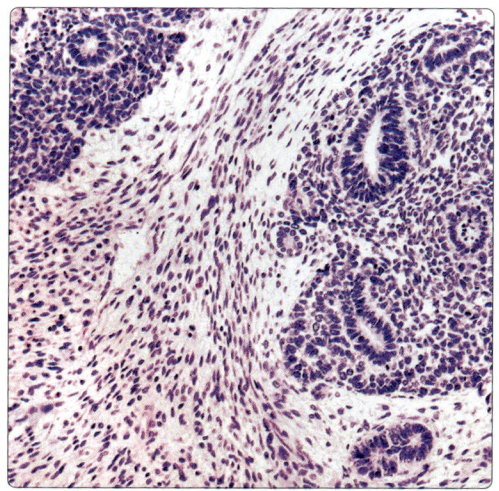

Papillary Architecture in Post-Wilms Tumor
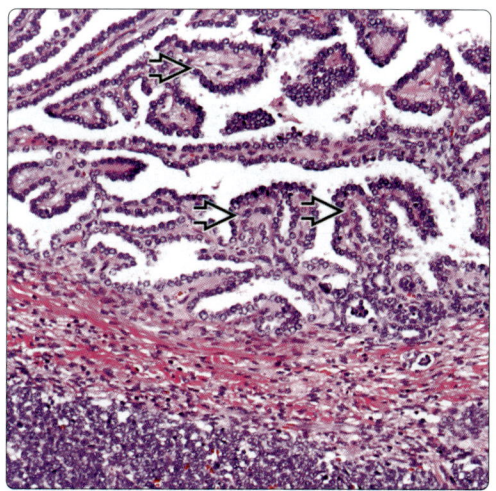

(Left) Some 2nd tumors are known to arise following Wilms tumor (shown here). (Right) Wilms tumors after chemotherapy often show large areas with differentiating epithelium, particularly with papillary architecture ➡. These areas, taken out of context, may closely resemble papillary RCC. Such synchronous epithelial differentiation likely does not play a big role in 2nd tumors arising after Wilms tumor, as most 2nd tumors arise many years, often > 30, after a Wilms tumor.

Post-Wilms RCC: Papillary Renal Cell Carcinoma
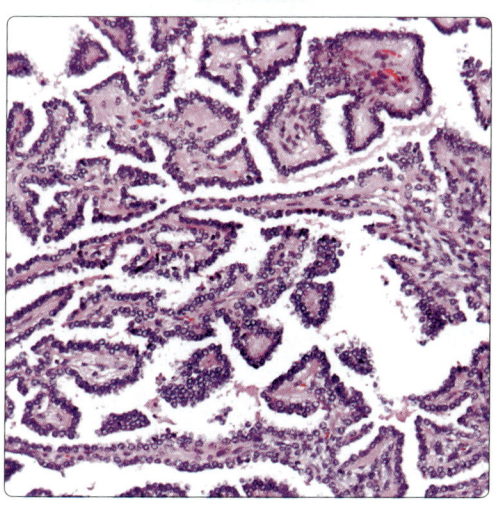

Post-Wilms RCC: Papillary Architecture
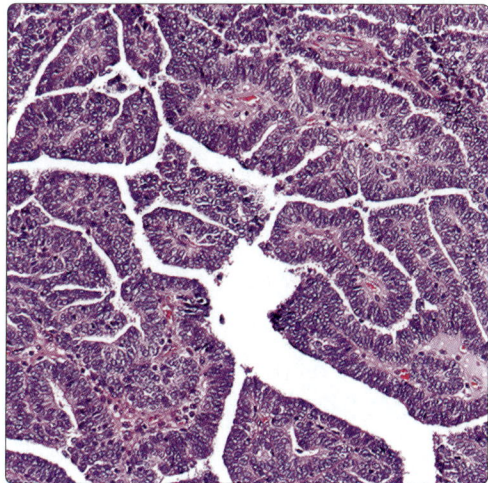

(Left) Occasionally, papillary renal cell carcinoma has also been reported as the 2nd tumor following a Wilms tumor. One case of post-Wilms MITF family-associated renal cell carcinoma has been reported and the frequency is likely to be higher if more tumors are tested, as 15% of translocation-associated carcinomas arise following chemotherapy. (Right) Other post-Wilms papillary tumors may demonstrate a high nuclear grade. Some of these 2nd tumors may have the features suggestive of adult-onset Wilms.

Renal Cell Carcinoma, Unclassified

KEY FACTS

TERMINOLOGY

- Renal cell carcinoma, unclassified (RCC-U)
- Unclassified renal cell carcinoma (RCC) not distinct subtype but diagnostic category for tumors that do not readily fit into any recognized subtypes of RCC, including
  - Tumors with combination of features of > 1 recognized subtype, unrecognized epithelial cell subtypes, low- or high-grade unclassified oncocytic neoplasms, or renal cell tumors with pure sarcomatoid histology
- Histologically, could be low or high grade

CLINICAL ISSUES

- RCC, unclassified category prevents inclusion of unusual tumors into common subtypes
- Placing of tumors in unclassified category, and gaining more experience with them, enables extraction of groups of tumors with similar features
  - These may then be reclassified as distinct entities
- Prognosis depends on tumor type, pathologic stage, and metastatic status

MICROSCOPIC

- High-grade tumors may have sheet-like, rhabdoid, large solid-alveolar, papillary, unusual tubulopapillary, glandular, or sarcomatoid architecture
  - Often with high-grade nuclei
- Some other tumors with cytoarchitectural features closely resembling renal oncocytoma

TOP DIFFERENTIAL DIAGNOSES

- Collecting duct carcinoma/hereditary leiomyomatosis RCC-associated RCC/renal medullary carcinoma
- Renal oncocytoma/chromophobe renal cell carcinoma, eosinophilic variant/succinate dehydrogenase-deficient RCC
- Tuberous sclerosis-associated RCC
- Metastatic carcinoma

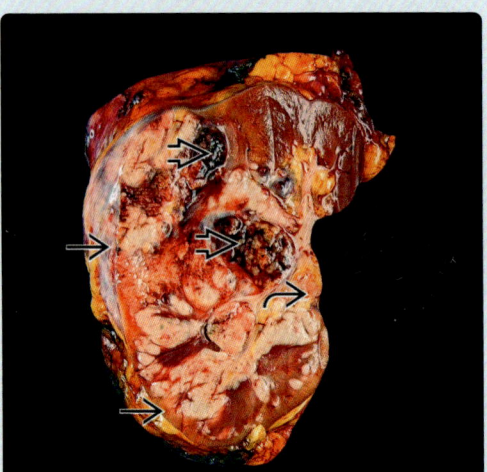

Gross Features

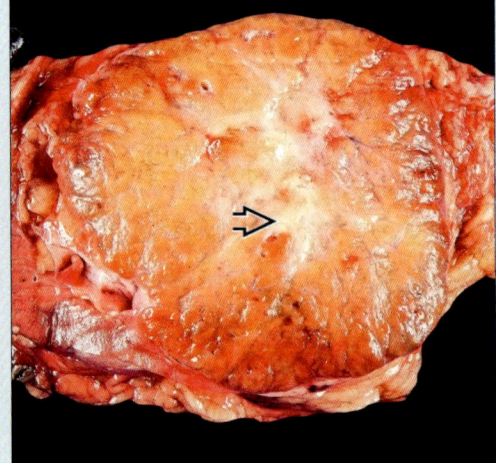

Gross Features

(Left) Some renal cell carcinomas (RCCs), unclassified, show grossly apparent aggressive features, including large size, infiltrative borders ➔, sinus fat invasion ➔, areas of hemorrhage, and necrosis ➔. Such tumors often show high nuclear grade. (Right) Other RCCs, unclassified, may have gross features that do not suggest aggressive behavior. They are well circumscribed and lack gross vascular/fat invasion or necrosis. Central scar ➔ in some suggests slow growth. Such tumors often mimic renal oncocytoma.

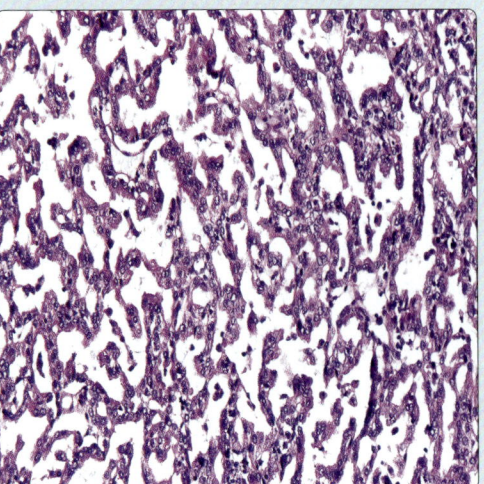

Trabecular/Microcystic Architecture

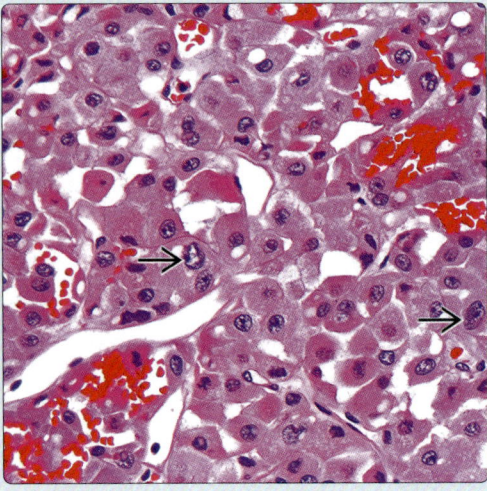

Oncocytoma-Like Features

(Left) Aggressive unclassified RCCs often show trabecular, sheet-like, or microcystic growth pattern. Most show high nuclear grade and high tumor stage. (Right) Some other unclassified RCCs show superficial resemblance to renal oncocytoma. Many such oncocytic renal cell carcinomas, unclassified, show sheet-like architectural pattern, at least focally, with nuclear pleomorphism ➔ beyond that acceptable in renal oncocytoma. Only anecdotal cases of metastasis from such tumors exist.

Renal Cell Carcinoma, Unclassified

TERMINOLOGY

Abbreviations
- Renal cell carcinoma (RCC), unclassified (RCC-U)

Definitions
- Not distinct subtype but includes
  - Tumors with combination of features of > 1 recognized subtype, unrecognized epithelial cell subtypes, low- or high-grade unclassified oncocytic neoplasms, or renal cell tumors with pure sarcomatoid histology

ETIOLOGY/PATHOGENESIS

Category of Unknown Pathogenesis
- Since these include variety of tumor types, no definite defined pathogenetic mechanisms or molecular features

CLINICAL ISSUES

Main Advantages for Creating Category
- Prevents forcible inclusion of unusual tumors into common subtypes; averts dilution of well-known clinicopathological features of recognized subtypes
- Placing of tumors in unclassified category, and gaining more experience with them, enables
  - Extraction of groups of tumors with similar features, reclassifying as distinct entities with more experience and data collection
- Examples of success of such approach include, among others, clear cell papillary, acquired cystic disease-associated, hereditary leiomyomatosis renal cell carcinoma (HLRCC)-associated, succinate dehydrogenase (SDHB)-deficient, translocation-associated RCCs, etc.

Presentation
- High-grade, morphologically aggressive-appearing tumors often present with high pT stage, regional lymph node (> 30%), and distant metastasis (> 50%)
- Low-grade tumors, particularly those with oncocytic features, often detected incidentally

Treatment
- High-grade, aggressive-type tumors often treated with surgery and variety of chemotherapeutic/immunotherapeutic agents
- Low-grade, indolent tumors usually managed by surgical resection alone

Prognosis
- Depends on tumor type, pathologic stage, and metastatic status; > 50% of patients with aggressive type dead of disease within 2 years
  - In lower grade indolent tumors, only anecdotal incidence of metastasis observed

MACROSCOPIC

General Features
- Tumors with aggressive morphologic features usually large and often multinodular
  - Areas of hemorrhage and necrosis, extension into veins &/or perinephric and sinus fat often present
- Tumors with nonaggressive morphologic features, variable size, often organ confined; frequently with tan-brown or brown cut surface, suggesting eosinophilic cell histology

MICROSCOPIC

Histologic Features
- High-grade tumors with sheet-like, rhabdoid, large solid-alveolar, papillary, unusual tubulopapillary, glandular, or sarcomatoid architecture, high-grade nuclear features, and often with necrosis, brisk mitotic activity, small vessel invasion, and perirenal and renal vein invasion
- Some tumors with cytoarchitectural features closely resembling renal oncocytoma
  - However, often with more solid architecture, nuclear pleomorphism, more than occasional mitoses, and rarely focal necrosis; no chromophobe-like perinuclear clearing

DIFFERENTIAL DIAGNOSIS

Collecting Duct Carcinoma/HLRCC-Associated RCC/Renal Medullary Carcinoma
- Rigid, consistent, and well-established morphologic features not well established in collecting duct carcinoma, hence distinction may be difficult
- HLRCC-associated RCC with prominent nucleoli surrounded by perinucleolar halos; lack of fumarate hydratase and positive for 2SC staining
- Renal medullary carcinoma with red cell sickling, history of sickle cell trait, and loss of staining for INI1

Renal Oncocytoma/Chromophobe Renal Cell Carcinoma, Eosinophilic Variant/SDHB-Deficient RCC
- Renal oncocytoma has uniform, round nuclei and often nested growth pattern, and chromophobe RCC shows perinuclear halos; usually diffusely positive for CD117 and focal positivity for CK7
- SDHB-deficient RCC with cytoplasmic inclusions, and loss of staining for SDHB

Tuberous Sclerosis-Associated RCC
- Often bilateral and multifocal with associated angiomyolipomas and positive family history

Metastatic Carcinoma
- Clinical history, multifocal, interstitial growth

SELECTED REFERENCES

1. Amin MB et al: Collecting duct carcinoma versus renal medullary carcinoma: an appeal for nosologic and biological clarity. Am J Surg Pathol. 38(7):871-4, 2014
2. Srigley JR et al: The International Society of Urological Pathology (ISUP) Vancouver Classification of Renal Neoplasia. Am J Surg Pathol. 37(10):1469-89, 2013
3. Talento R et al: Evaluation of morphologically unclassified renal cell carcinoma with electron microscopy and novel renal markers: implications for tumor reclassification. Ultrastruct Pathol. 37(1):70-6, 2013
4. Lopez-Beltran A et al: Unclassified renal cell carcinoma: a report of 56 cases. BJU Int. 110(6):786-93, 2012
5. Kim HJ et al: Virtual-karyotyping with SNP microarrays in morphologically challenging renal cell neoplasms: a practical and useful diagnostic modality. Am J Surg Pathol. 33(9):1276-86, 2009
6. Karakiewicz PI et al: Unclassified renal cell carcinoma: an analysis of 85 cases. BJU Int. 100(4):802-8, 2007
7. Zisman A et al: Unclassified renal cell carcinoma: clinical features and prognostic impact of a new histological subtype. J Urol. 168(3):950-5, 2002

Renal Cell Carcinoma, Unclassified

Rhabdoid Features

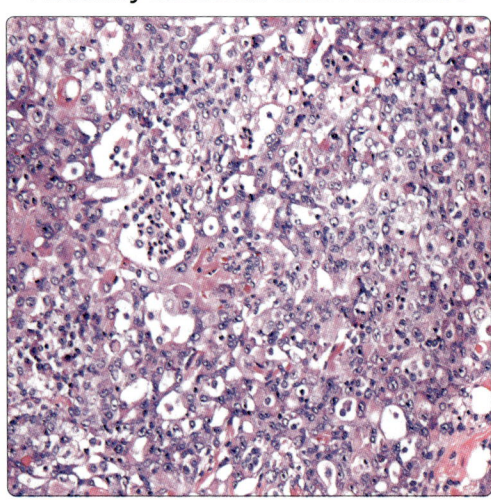

Medullary Carcinoma-Like Architecture

(Left) Occasional tumors may have pure rhabdoid features ➡. In such tumors, common subtypes, including clear cell RCC, need to be excluded by thorough sampling, as well as immunohistochemical staining for CA9. (Right) Tumors with cribriform and microcystic growth pattern raise the possibility of renal medullary carcinoma. However, in the absence of a history of sickle trait or disease, or the absence of RBC sickling in the tumor, the alternate nomenclature of RCC, unclassified, with renal medullary phenotype is suggested.

Combined Morphological Features

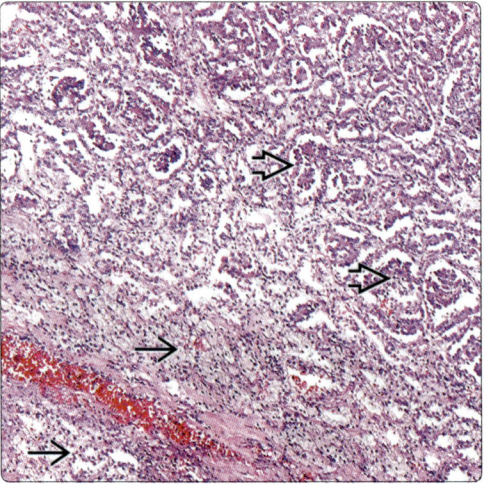

Combined Morphological Features

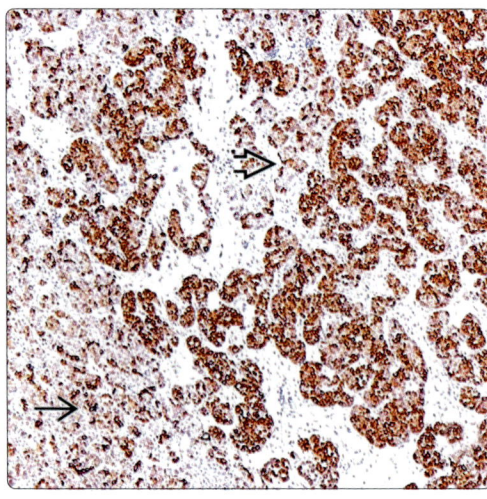

(Left) Renal tumors with a combination of > 1 type of the usual subtypes are also considered RCC, unclassified. Note papillary ➡ and clear cell-like ➡ features. (Right) Immunostain for CK7 in this RCC, unclassified, shows strong and diffuse immunoreactivity in both papillary ➡ and clear cell-like ➡ areas, and CA9 was negative. This staining pattern would not support a clear cell RCC. Histologic evidence of morphologic transitions and unusual immunopatterns help in excluding the possibility of collision tumors.

Oncocytic Features

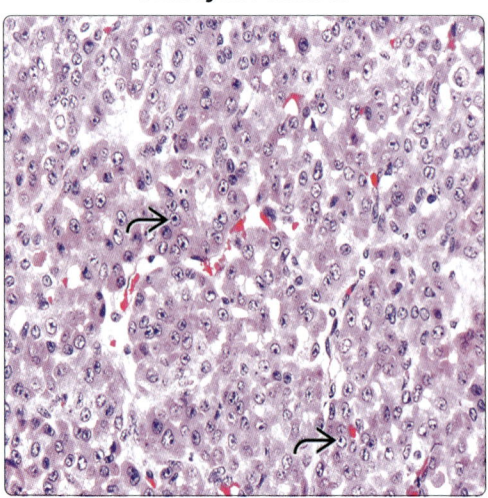

SDHB-Deficient RCC

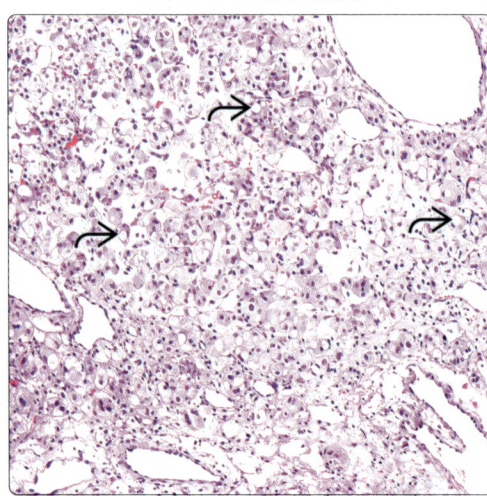

(Left) Some RCC, unclassified may show high-grade nuclear details with oncocytic cytoplasm. This example shows prominent nucleoli and perinucleolar clarity ➡. In such cases, the possibility of SDHB-deficient and HLRCC-associated RCC needs to be excluded. (Right) Although morphologically resembling the tumor on the left, this tumor shows cytoplasmic inclusions ➡, raising the possibility of SDHB RCC. In the presence of retained SDHB immunoreactivity, even such tumors are regarded as RCC, unclassified.

Renal Cell Carcinoma, Unclassified

Large Ballooned-Out Pleomorphic Cells
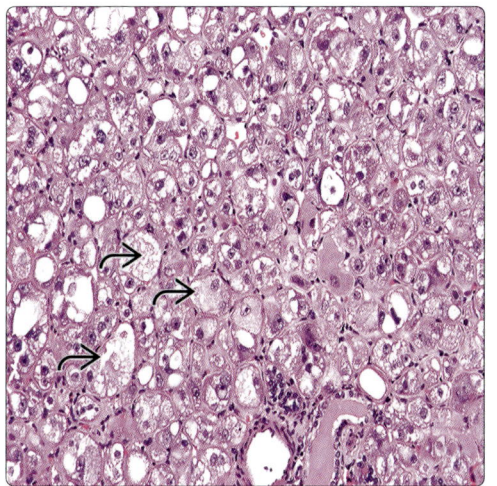

Sarcomatoid Features
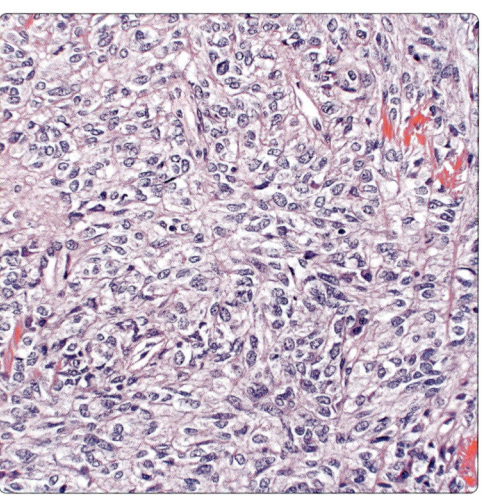

(Left) Tumors with dispersed large cells with ballooned-out cytoplasm ➔ should raise the possibility of epithelioid angiomyolipoma and tuberous sclerosis-associated RCC. Lack of IHC or other morphological or historical supports will put many such tumors in the RCC, unclassified category. (Right) RCC, unclassified shows a predominantly sarcomatoid histology. Tumors with the absence or presence of unrecognizable epithelial components are included in the unclassified category after specific sarcomas are ruled out.

Branching Papillary Architecture
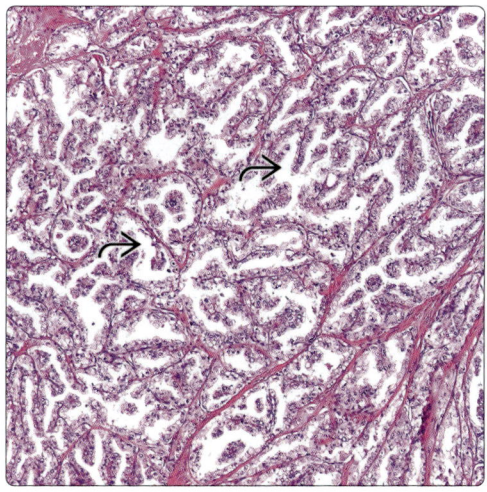

Papillary Architecture With Large Clear and Eosinophilic Cells
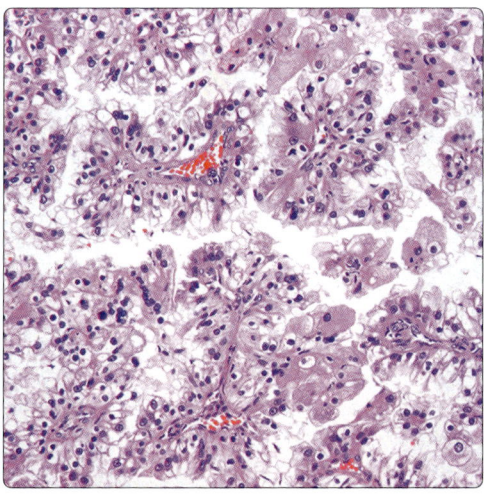

(Left) Branching papillations ➔ with clear cell cytology raise the diagnostic possibility of clear cell papillary and translocation-associated RCC. Careful attention to histology and immunophenotype is needed to exclude such possibilities. (Right) This RCC, unclassified shows a combination of prominent papillary architecture and clear and eosinophilic cell cytology. Such features will often raise the possibility of translocation-associated and TSC-associated RCC, particularly if keratins are only focally positive.

Extreme Multifocality
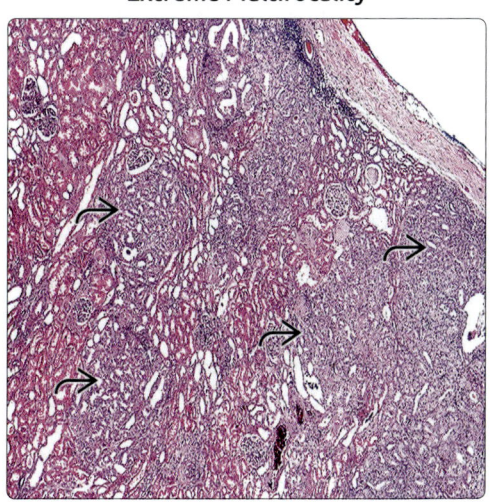

Metastasis
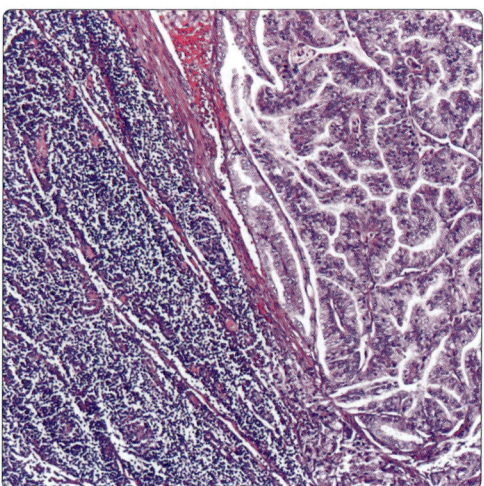

(Left) Rarely, the kidney may be occupied by numerous tumor nodules not fitting any specific entities like renal oncocytosis, BHD, or VHL syndromes ➔. While a syndromic condition is quite likely, lack of association of the morphology with any known syndromes will result in the interpretation of unclassified RCC with carcinomatosis. (Right) In spite of the morphology suggestive of translocation-associated RCC, lack of IHC and FISH support in this case metastatic to a lymph node results in the diagnosis of RCC, unclassified.

Metanephric Adenoma

KEY FACTS

TERMINOLOGY
- Benign neoplasm composed of small primitive cells resembling early metanephric tubular differentiation
  - Part of spectrum of neoplasms that includes metanephric adenofibroma and metanephric stromal tumor

ETIOLOGY/PATHOGENESIS
- Microsatellite allelotyping has shown potential tumor suppressor gene on chromosome 2p13 in 56% of informative cases
- Recently, *BRAF V600E* mutations found in ~ 90% of metanephric adenoma (MA)
  - By immunohistochemistry, BRAF V600E positivity with overall 88% sensitivity and 100% specificity for mutation

CLINICAL ISSUES
- Age range: 11 months to 83 years (reported mean: 41 years)
- Female preponderance (M:F = 1:2)
- ~ 12% with symptoms related to polycythemia
- Benign course with no reported metastasis

MICROSCOPIC
- Cellular tumor composed of crowded small acini of primitive blue cells in paucicellular intervening stroma
- Papillary component, including glomeruloid appearance, fairly common
- Tumor cells have minimal cytoplasm with uniform, round to ovoid nuclei, slightly larger than size of lymphocyte

ANCILLARY TESTS
- Often positive for WT1 (diffuse nuclear), AMACR (cytoplasmic, granular), CD57, and BRAF V600E (diffuse cytoplasmic)

TOP DIFFERENTIAL DIAGNOSES
- Papillary renal cell carcinoma
- Epithelial predominant Wilms tumor

Gross Features

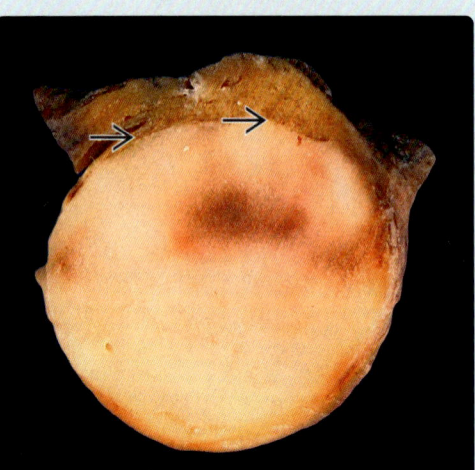

Gross Features

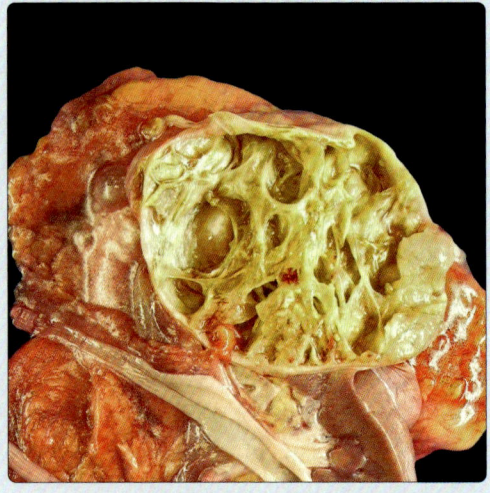

(Left) This gross image shows the typical gross features of a metanephric adenoma (MA): A well-circumscribed tumor ⇒, without a capsule, and with a cut surface that is homogeneous and tan-yellow. (Right) This gross image shows a relatively uncommon gross appearance of MA. While cystic areas are often seen, extensive cyst formation, as seen here, is very rare. Microscopically, besides cystic degeneration, tumors with this change frequently show extensive sclerosis and prominent calcifications.

Tumor Circumscription

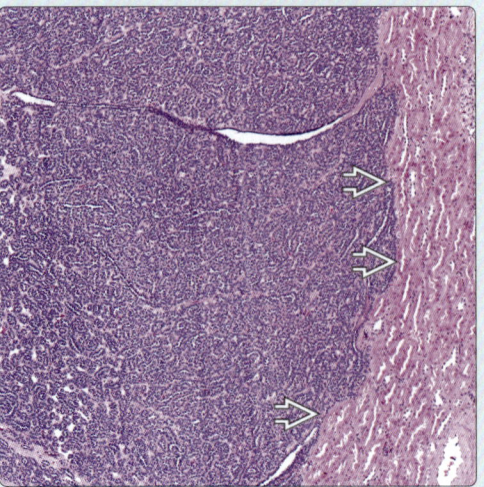

Rare Pseudocapsule

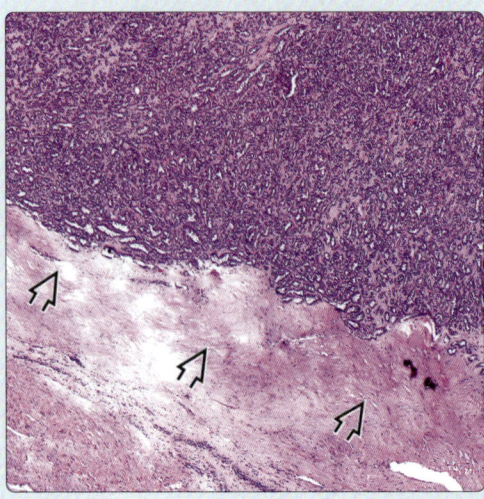

(Left) MAs are typically well circumscribed and most often (not always) without a capsule, with the tumor in direct contact with renal parenchyma ⇒. In such cases, there are usually no features of compression in the surrounding renal parenchyma. (Right) Rarely, MA may be surrounded by a variably well-formed fibrous capsule ⇒. In some of such cases, distinction from a papillary renal cell carcinoma (RCC) might be difficult, and the diagnosis depends on careful morphologic evaluation.

Metanephric Adenoma

TERMINOLOGY

Abbreviations
- Metanephric adenoma (MA)

Synonyms
- Embryonal adenoma

Definitions
- Benign neoplasm composed of small primitive cells resembling early metanephric tubular differentiation
  - Part of spectrum of neoplasms that includes metanephric adenofibroma and metanephric stromal tumor

ETIOLOGY/PATHOGENESIS

Molecular Abnormalities
- Recently, *BRAF V600E* mutations found in ~ 90% of MA
  - By immunohistochemistry, BRAF V600E positivity with overall 88% sensitivity and 100% specificity for mutation
    - Diffuse cytoplasmic staining in vast majority of MAs
      - Other tumors only very rarely positive and staining often very focal
- Microsatellite allelotyping shows potential tumor suppressor gene on chromosome 2p13 in 56% of informative cases
- No allelic changes in Wilms tumor 1 (*WT1*) gene region at chromosome 11p13 or in papillary renal cell tumor (*PRCC*) gene region at chromosome 17q21.32
- No trisomies for 7 and 17 or Y chromosomes
  - Prior reported trisomies 7 and 17 possibly related to solid PRCC misdiagnosed as MA

CLINICAL ISSUES

Epidemiology
- Age
  - 11 months to 83 years (mean: 41 years)
    - More often reported in adults, compared to that in pediatric age range
- Sex
  - Female predominance
    - M:F = 1:2

Presentation
- Considered by some as hyperdifferentiated, benign end of the Wilms tumor spectrum
  - Occasionally seen in association with differentiating epithelial-predominant Wilms tumors
  - However, recently found *BRAF* mutations in MA and not in Wilms tumor make such assumptions suspect
    - Potentially likely that it represents morphological similarity in distinct tumor types
    - Examples of similar morphological similarities exist in other different renal cell tumors, including
      - Papillary type 2 features in papillary renal cell carcinoma (RCC) and collecting duct carcinoma (CDC), HLRCC-associated RCC, etc.
      - Tuberous sclerosis complex (TSC)-associated RCC and clear cell RCC
      - Tubulocystic RCC and HLRCC-associated RCC with tubulocystic areas
- \> 50% of cases detected incidentally
  - Most symptomatic cases show abdominal or flank pain, hematuria, and palpable mass
  - ~ 12% with symptoms related to polycythemia

Prognosis
- Benign course with no reported metastasis in tumors with typical morphology
  - Single case reported with lymph node metastasis in a child
    - Case probably represents Wilms tumor
      - Case with reported high atypical mitotic activity

IMAGING

General Features
- Calcifications seen in up to 43% of cases

MACROSCOPIC

General Features
- Typically unilateral, solitary, well circumscribed, and well delineated
- Majority are unencapsulated
  - But, discontinuous or continuous capsule present in some
- Cut surface solid tan-pink, gray to yellow
  - Gross cystic change in ~ 12% of tumors
- Hemorrhage and necrosis infrequent findings
  - More common in tumors with cystic features
- Gross calcifications in up to 20%
  - Rare cases with grossly entirely calcified tumor

Size
- Range few mm to 20 cm; mean: 5.5 cm

MICROSCOPIC

Histologic Features
- Most tumors with no pseudocapsule
  - Show well-circumscribed margins in direct contact with surrounding renal parenchyma
  - Usually no significant compression-related alterations in adjacent parenchyma
    - Rare tumors with presence of partial or complete pseudoencapsulation
    - Such tumors need differentiation from type 1 papillary RCC
- Cellular tumor composed of crowded small acini of primitive blue cells in paucicellular intervening stroma
  - Presence of elongated tubules, often with branching, not infrequent
- Focal papillary component, including glomeruloid structures, fairly common
  - Rare tumors with prominent papillary architecture
    - Such tumors most difficult to differentiate from type 1 papillary RCC
    - Presence of foamy macrophages usually not feature
      - However, such macrophages present in rare cases
      - When present, foamy macrophages extremely focal occurrence
- Cells with minimal cytoplasm and relatively uniform, round to ovoid nuclei

Metanephric Adenoma

- Nuclear folds and grooves fairly common
- Nucleoli inconspicuous; mitoses rare to absent
  - Chromatin distribution uniform
- Rare cysts and blastemal-like, sheet-like patterns
- Many tumors with regressive features, including
  - Hyalinization
  - Calcifications, when present, often psammomatous, both in capsule and within tumor parenchyma
  - Necrosis and hemorrhage
  - Dystrophic ossification

ANCILLARY TESTS

Immunohistochemistry

- Often positive for
  - WT1
    - Diffuse, nuclear
  - AMACR
    - Cytoplasmic, granular
  - pax-8, pax-2
    - Diffuse, nuclear
  - CD57
    - Positivity for CD57 important differential diagnostic consideration
- Usually negative for CK7 except in branching large tubules and papillary areas
- Most tumors with diffuse cytoplasmic positivity for BRAF V600E antigen
  - Such positivity correlates with mutations in *BRAF V600E* gene in overwhelming majority of cases
  - BRAF positivity very rare in other related renal cell tumors
    - Therefore, diffuse cytoplasmic positivity for BRAF is important consideration in favor of MA
- Molecular (FISH) evaluation for chromosomes 7, 17, and Y recommended for tumors with unexpected immunophenotype
  - Many of these in fact represent type 1 papillary RCC with tubular architecture and low nuclear grade

Electron Microscopy

- Clusters of cells occasionally forming microlumen and surrounded by smooth, basal lamina matrix
- Junctional complexes at apical end of luminal lining cells with florid microvilli

DIFFERENTIAL DIAGNOSIS

Papillary Renal Cell Carcinoma

- PRCC type 1, solid variant and tubular predominant, closest differential diagnosis
  - PRCC often with fibrous pseudocapsule
  - Nuclei higher grade, often with more pleomorphism and prominent nucleoli
  - Amount of cytoplasm usually exceeds minimal cytoplasm of MA
  - Diffusely positive for AMACR, CK7, and EMA/MUC1
    - WT1 and CD57(-)
  - BRAF immunoreactivity extremely rare
  - Trisomy 7 and 17 and loss of Y chromosome very frequent

Epithelial Predominant Wilms Tumor

- Pseudocapsule usually present
- Nuclei primitive-appearing and hyperchromatic
  - Mitotic activity usually brisk
  - Nuclear overlap quite frequent
- Other components of Wilms tumor (stromal and blastemal) may be present
- Usually negative or only focally positive for CD57
- BRAF immunoreactivity not present

DIAGNOSTIC CHECKLIST

Pathologic Interpretation Pearls

- Rare but distinctive benign renal tumor that may appear alarming at low-power microscopy due to primitive round blue cells or tubular appearance
- Attention to bland nuclear features without significant hyperchromasia, nuclear overlap, or prominent mitotic activity is key
- Scant cytoplasm also norm
- Immunohistochemical reactivity for BRAF V600E antigen often diagnostically confirmatory

SELECTED REFERENCES

1. Chami R et al: BRAF mutations in pediatric metanephric tumors. Hum Pathol. 46(8):1153-61, 2015
2. Kinney SN et al: Metanephric adenoma: the utility of immunohistochemical and cytogenetic analyses in differential diagnosis, including solid variant papillary renal cell carcinoma and epithelial-predominant nephroblastoma. Mod Pathol. 28(9):1236-48, 2015
3. Ritterhouse LL et al: BRAF V600E mutation-specific antibody: a review. Semin Diagn Pathol. 32(5):400-8, 2015
4. Udager AM et al: Molecular and immunohistochemical characterization reveals novel BRAF mutations in metanephric adenoma. Am J Surg Pathol. 39(4):549-57, 2015
5. Yakirevich E et al: Cadherin 17 is a sensitive and specific marker for metanephric adenoma. Am J Surg Pathol. 39(4):479-86, 2015
6. Zhu B et al: Immunoexpression of napsin a in renal neoplasms. Diagn Pathol. 10:4, 2015
7. Choueiri TK et al: BRAF mutations in metanephric adenoma of the kidney. Eur Urol. 62(5):917-22, 2012
8. Burger M et al: Metanephric adenoma of the kidney: a clinicopathological and molecular study of two cases. J Clin Pathol. 60(7):832-3, 2007
9. Argani P: Metanephric neoplasms: the hyperdifferentiated, benign end of the Wilms tumor spectrum? Clin Lab Med. 25(2):379-92, 2005
10. Muir TE et al: Metanephric adenoma, nephrogenic rests, and Wilms' tumor: a histologic and immunophenotypic comparison. Am J Surg Pathol. 25(10):1290-6, 2001
11. Pesti T et al: Mapping a tumor suppressor gene to chromosome 2p13 in metanephric adenoma by microsatellite allelotyping. Hum Pathol. 32(1):101-4, 2001
12. Davis CJ Jr et al: Metanephric adenoma. Clinicopathological study of fifty patients. Am J Surg Pathol. 19(10):1101-14, 1995
13. Jones EC et al: Metanephric adenoma of the kidney. A clinicopathological, immunohistochemical, flow cytometric, cytogenetic, and electron microscopic study of seven cases. Am J Surg Pathol. 19(6):615-26, 1995

Metanephric Adenoma

Tightly Packed Small Tubules

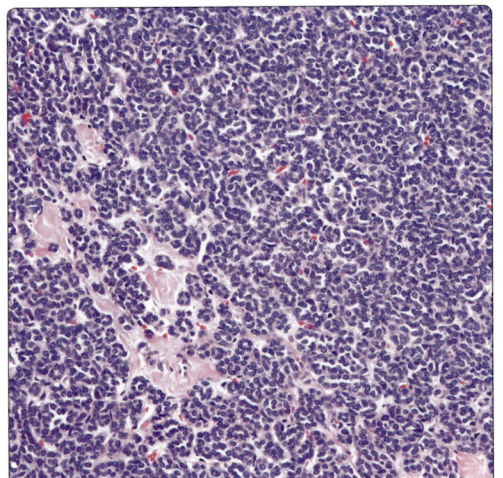

Cytological Features

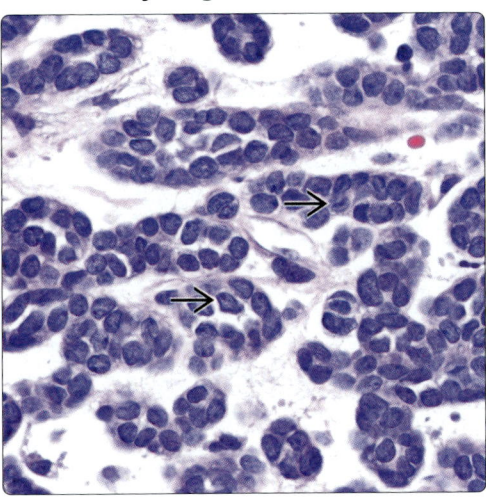

(Left) A low-magnification evaluation of MA characteristically reveals tightly packed small tubules separated by a modest amount of stroma. The scant stroma is usually paucicellular. (Right) Careful evaluation and higher magnification assessment reveals the nuclei to be uniform, round to ovoid, often overlapping, and sometimes with central folds ➡. Unlike blastema, nucleoli are inconspicuous, and mitotic figures are rare.

Glomerulations and Branching Tubules

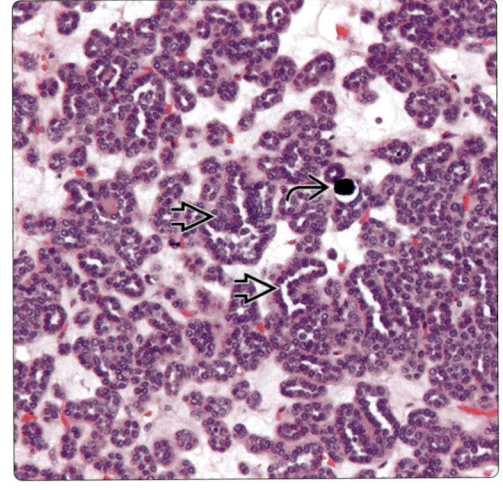

Degenerative Features

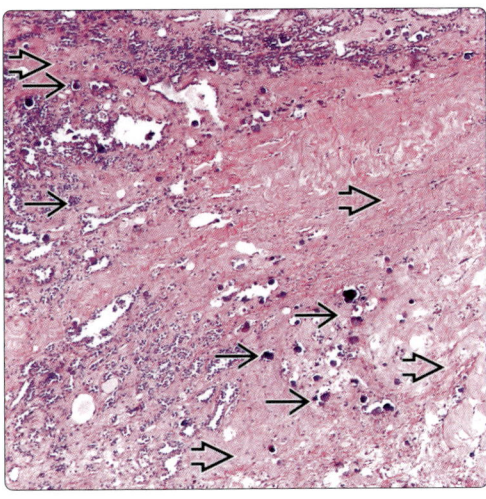

(Left) At low magnification, in addition to the small tubules, glomeruloid formations ➡ and elongated tubules with branching are also commonly observed in MA. Psammomatous calcifications ➡ are quite common and may be diffuse and extensive. (Right) Rarely, MAs show extensive degenerative changes. Such tumors are often grossly cystic and on microscopy show a background of extensive sclerosis ➡, often with prominent calcifications ➡.

Prominent Branching Tubules

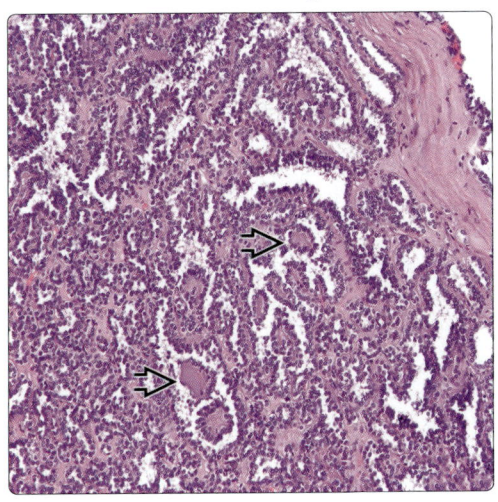

Rare Prominent Papillary Architecture

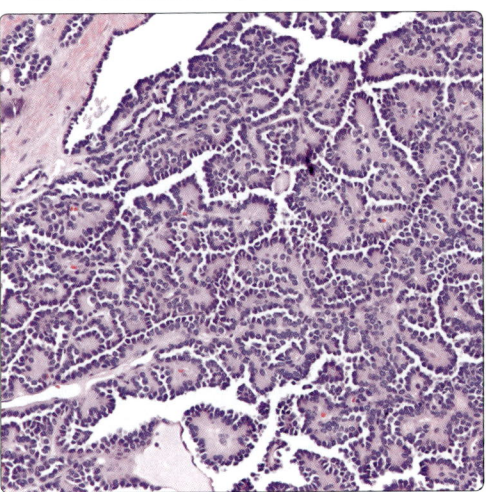

(Left) Some MAs show prominent branching tubules and focally papillary ➡ structures lined by cells with monotonous small nuclei and minimal cytoplasm. (Right) Occasional MAs have prominent papillary architecture. Small primitive tubules, focal papillations, and glomerulations may raise the possibility of a Wilms tumor. The low-grade nuclear features and minimal mitotic activity are helpful in distinction from Wilms tumor. MAs lack significant cytoplasm, which helps in the distinction from papillary RCC.

Metanephric Adenoma

(Left) Some MAs may show more mature-appearing tubules with hobnailing ⇒. This pattern is often focal, and the more common small primitive-appearing tubules are invariably present. **(Right)** In addition to the presence of a pseudocapsule, papillary architecture, and occasional CK7 and AMACR positivity, another reason for confusing rare MA with type 1 papillary RCC is the focal presence of foamy macrophages in the tumor ⇒. This is a very rare occurrence in MA.

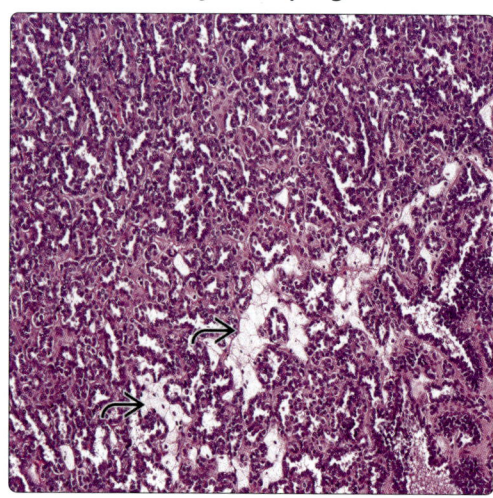

(Left) Immunohistochemical staining for CK7 is either negative or may show very focal ⇒ to patchy positivity in some MAs. Note the diffuse positive staining in the surrounding renal tubules ⇒. **(Right)** WT1 usually shows diffuse nuclear staining in MA. Thus, by itself, WT1 immunostaining cannot distinguish MA from an epithelial Wilms tumor.

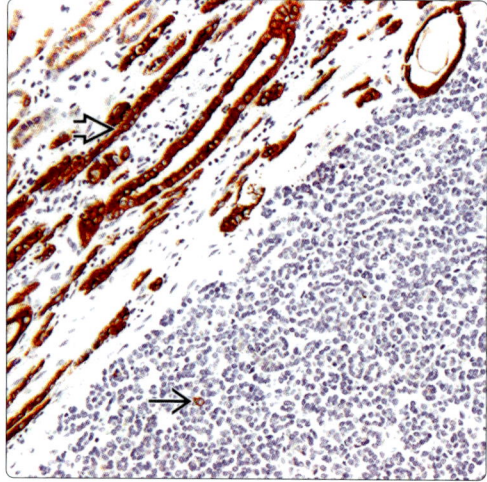
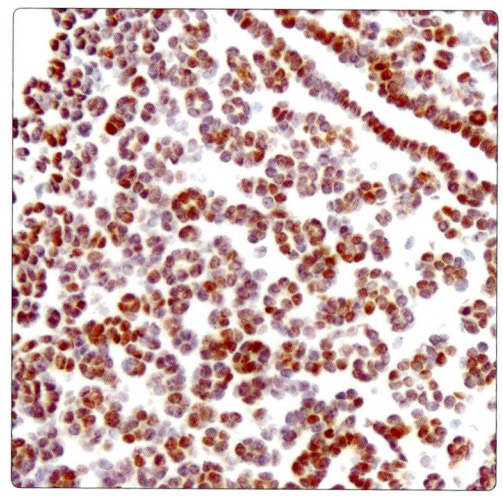

(Left) MAs are usually negative for AMACR; however, up to 10% may show focal positivity. Strong CK7 and AMACR positivity in the same tumor argues against the diagnosis of MA, and in appropriate morphologic context, favors a papillary RCC. **(Right)** CD57 is usually diffusely positive in MA; papillary RCC and epithelial Wilms tumor at the most are only focally positive. Therefore, a panel that includes AMACR, CK7, WT1, and CD57 is useful in differentiating MA from these close morphologic mimics.

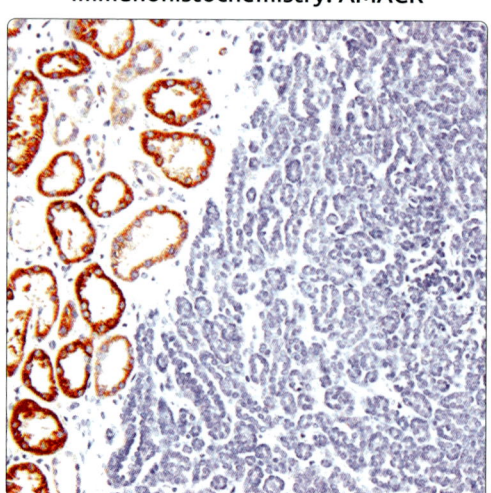
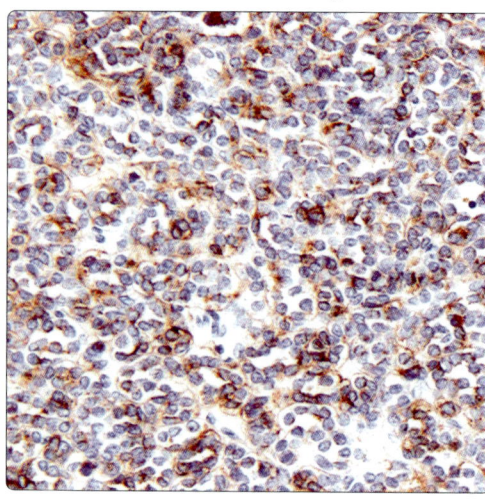

Metanephric Adenoma

Immunohistochemistry: BRAF

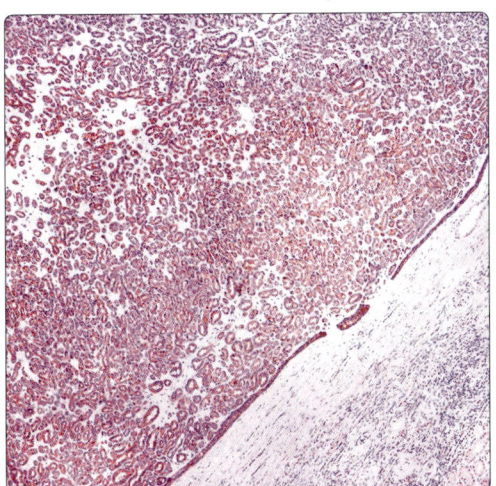

Immunohistochemistry: BRAF

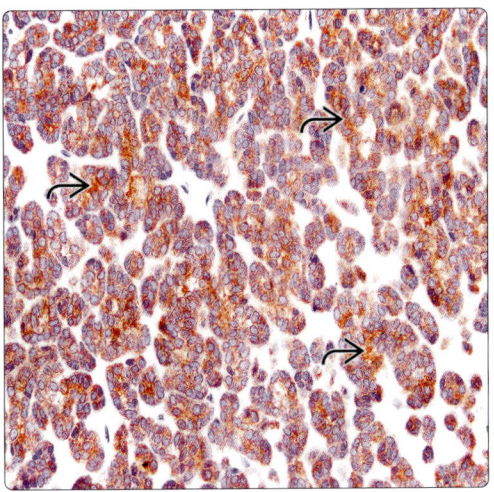

(Left) Greater than 90% of metanephric adenomas show BRAF V600E mutations. The mutation closely correlates with diffuse positivity for the mutated BRAF V600E antigen on immunohistochemistry in MA. Staining for this antibody is very rare in other close mimics of MA, and at the most may be focal in an occasional papillary RCC. (Right) This high-power image shows the typical diffuse cytoplasmic expression pattern of BRAF V600E in an MA ⇨.

Needle Biopsy Diagnosis

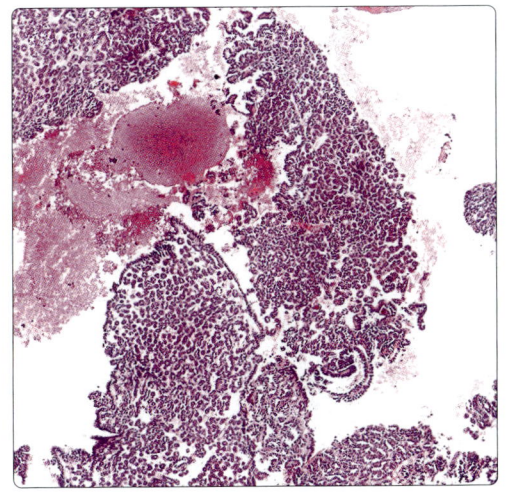

Needle Biopsy Diagnosis

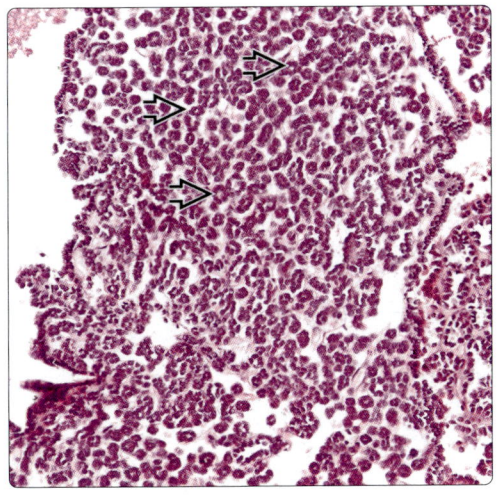

(Left) This needle core biopsy of the kidney shows a MA. Caution is warranted in making an outright diagnosis on a biopsy if the classic features are absent. (Right) A higher magnification details the typical small tubules ⇨, lined by monomorphic cells, with no nucleoli or significant mitotic activity. These morphologic features, even on limited material, are sufficiently diagnostic of an MA and may be supported by appropriate immunohistochemistry.

Needle Biopsy Diagnosis

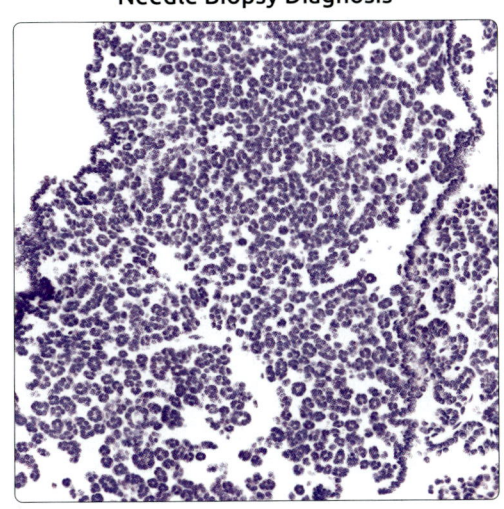

Needle Biopsy Diagnosis

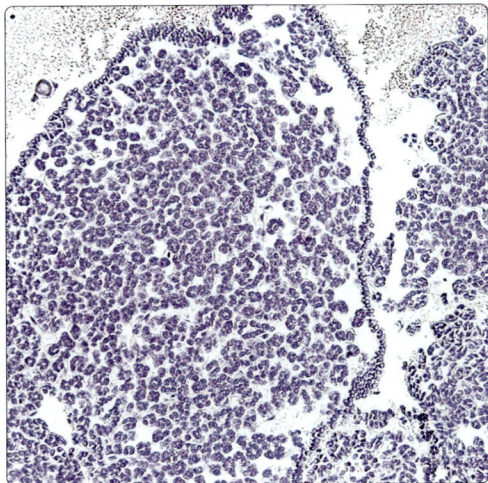

(Left) Immunostain for CK7 is also negative in this tumor. While morphology is sufficiently diagnostic in most cases, in rare instances, and if the pathologist has less experience with these tumors, a panel of stains may help distinguish MA from its mimics, which include solid, tubular papillary RCC and epithelial-predominant Wilms tumor. (Right) Immunohistochemical stain for AMACR on this needle core biopsy specimen is completely negative. These stains argue against papillary RCC.

Metanephric Tumors Other Than Metanephric Adenoma

KEY FACTS

TERMINOLOGY
- Metanephric stromal tumor (MST), metanephric adenofibroma (MAF)
- MST: Benign, purely stromal pediatric tumor
- MAF: Biphasic tumor composed of metanephric adenoma-like epithelial and MST-like stromal components

ETIOLOGY/PATHOGENESIS
- Similar to metanephric adenoma, *BRAF V600E* mutations described in both stromal and epithelial components in few MAF tested: Status not known in MST

CLINICAL ISSUES
- Mean age
  - MST: 2 years (range: 4 days to 15 years)
  - MAF: 72 months (range: 5 months to 36 years)
- Often asymptomatic and incidental findings; hypertension due to juxtaglomerular apparatus hyperplasia (JGAH) in some MST cases; polycythemia in some MAF; hematuria in both due to of renal pelvis involvement
- Both lesions with benign outcome

MICROSCOPIC
- Stroma similar in both tumors
- MSTs often show JGAH within entrapped glomeruli; this feature not seen in MAF
- Epithelium in MAF usually mitotically inactive metanephric adenoma-like, with other rarer variant features
- Stromal components immunoreactive for CD34, usually patchy

ANCILLARY TESTS
- MAF may be positive for BRAF V600E by IHC

TOP DIFFERENTIAL DIAGNOSES
- Congenital mesoblastic nephroma, classical variant

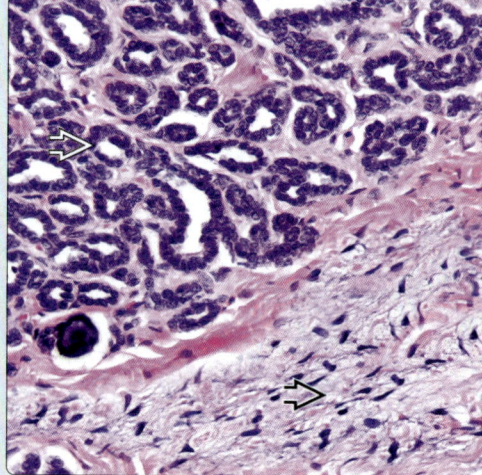

Metanephric Adenofibroma: Epithelium and Stroma

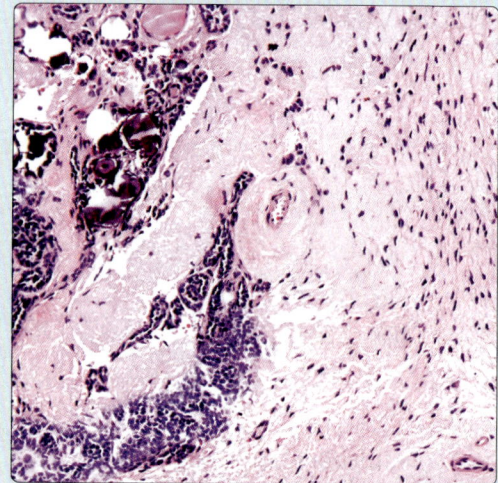

Metanephric Adenofibroma: Epithelium and Stroma

(Left) *Metanephric adenofibroma shows a mixture of stromal elements similar to a metanephric stromal tumor ⇨ and primitive-appearing epithelial components ⇨ similar to that in metanephric adenoma.* (Right) *The epithelial component in metanephric adenofibroma may closely resemble packed tubules in metanephric adenoma. However, some tumors may show brisk mitotic activity, or even epithelial-predominant Wilms tumor-like areas. Calcification may be a prominent feature.*

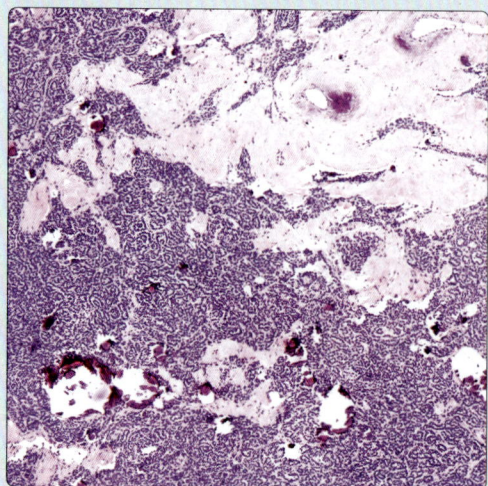

Metanephric Adenofibroma: Epithelium

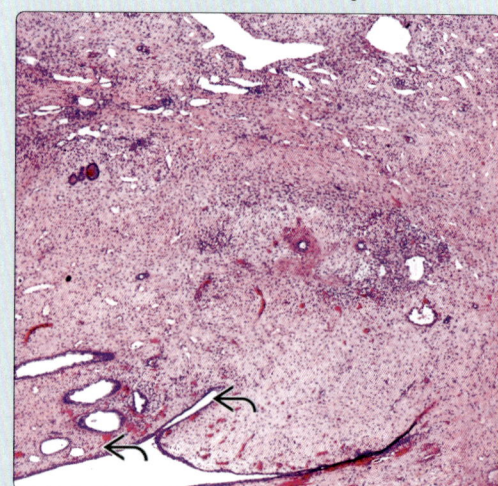

Medulla Centricity

(Left) *Metanephric adenofibroma may almost completely resemble a metanephric adenoma based on the predominance of the epithelial component. However, the presence of at least a small stromal component is a prerequisite for the diagnosis. Conversely, some MAF may be predominantly stromal, with very minute epithelial foci.* (Right) *Most metanephric adenofibromas and metanephric stromal tumors are medulla centric and may invade the pelvicalyceal system ⇨.*

Metanephric Tumors Other Than Metanephric Adenoma

TERMINOLOGY

Abbreviations
- Metanephric stromal tumor (MST), metanephric adenofibroma (MAF)

Definitions
- MST: Benign, purely stromal pediatric tumor
- MAF: Biphasic tumor composed of metanephric adenoma-like epithelial and MST-like stromal components

ETIOLOGY/PATHOGENESIS

BRAF V600E Mutation
- Similar to metanephric adenoma, BRAF V600E mutations described in both stromal and epithelial components in few MAF tested: Status not known in MST

Relationship With Wilms Tumor
- Some believe metanephric tumors represent hyperdifferentiated Wilms tumors or intralobar nephrogenic rests (ILNR) due to
  o Presence of epithelial-predominant Wilms tumor-like areas in some MAF and occurrence of ILNR in renal parenchyma in rare cases
    – Presence of BRAF mutations in metanephric tumors, but not in Wilms tumor, does not favor this theory

CLINICAL ISSUES

Epidemiology
- Incidence
  o Both tumors very rare
    – < 70 MAFs reported in literature
    – MST < 1/10 as common as congenital mesoblastic nephroma, which is by itself rare entity
- Age
  o MAF: Mean: 72 months (range: 5 months to 36 years)
  o MST: Mean: 2 years (range: 4 days to 15 years); only very rare cases reported in adults
- Sex
  o MAF: M:F = 2:1
  o MST: Equal representation in both

Other Features
- Both usually based in renal medulla
- Often asymptomatic and incidental findings; hypertension due to juxtaglomerular apparatus hyperplasia (JGAH) in some MST cases; polycythemia in some MAF; hematuria in both due to of renal pelvis involvement
- Surgical resection treatment of choice in both
- Both tumors with benign outcome

MACROSCOPIC

General Features
- Usually solitary, but rarely multifocal (particularly MST)
- Predominantly solid with variable cystic components; indistinct tumor borders, with usually yellow-tan to fibrous-appearing cut surface; hemorrhage and necrosis very rare, usually when associated with Wilms tumor

Size
- Mean for both: 3.8 cm (range: 1.8-11 cm)

MICROSCOPIC

Histologic Features
- Stroma similar in both tumors
  o Spindled to stellate cells with thin, hyperchromatic nuclei and slender, indistinct cytoplasmic extensions, often surrounding and entrapping renal tubules/blood vessels to form concentric onion skin rings or collarettes around these structures
  o More cellular, less myxoid spindle cell areas at periphery of collarettes yielding vaguely nodular architecture
  o Epithelioid transformation of medial smooth muscle of intratumoral arterioles (angiodysplasia of vessels); heterologous differentiation (glia or cartilage)
  o MSTs often show JGAH within entrapped glomeruli; this feature not seen in MAF
- Epithelium in MAF most often metanephric adenoma-like; mitotically inactive, and rarely with brisk mitoses (> 5/20 HPF); or as composite metanephric adenoma with epithelial predominant Wilms tumor, or tubulopapillary carcinoma-like areas

ANCILLARY TESTS

Immunohistochemistry
- Stromal components immunoreactive for CD34, often patchy; desmin, keratins, and S100 negative, but glial foci label for GFAP and S100
- Epithelial components usually positive for keratins; AMACR usually negative
- MAF may be positive for BRAF V600E by IHC

DIFFERENTIAL DIAGNOSIS

Congenital Mesoblastic Nephroma, Classical Variant
- Differentiation has to be made from MST
- Congenital mesoblastic nephroma (CMN) shows markedly infiltrative borders with entrapment of large clusters of native nephrons; MST only superficially infiltrative with entrapped single tubules or glomeruli
- MST shows angiodysplasia, concentric peritubular growth pattern, and JGAH
- CD34 positive in MST but not in CMN

DIAGNOSTIC CHECKLIST

Pathologic Interpretation Pearls
- Stroma similar in MST and MAF
  o Exception: No JGAH seen in MAF
- MST needs extensive sampling to exclude focal epithelial components of MAF

SELECTED REFERENCES

1. Chami R et al: BRAF mutations in pediatric metanephric tumors. Hum Pathol. 46(8):1153-61, 2015
2. Mangray S et al: Application of BRAF V600E mutation analysis for the diagnosis of metanephric adenofibroma. Am J Surg Pathol. 39(9):1301-4, 2015
3. Arroyo MR et al: The spectrum of metanephric adenofibroma and related lesions: clinicopathologic study of 25 cases from the National Wilms Tumor Study Group Pathology Center. Am J Surg Pathol. 25(4):433-44, 2001

Metanephric Tumors Other Than Metanephric Adenoma

Metanephric Stromal Tumor

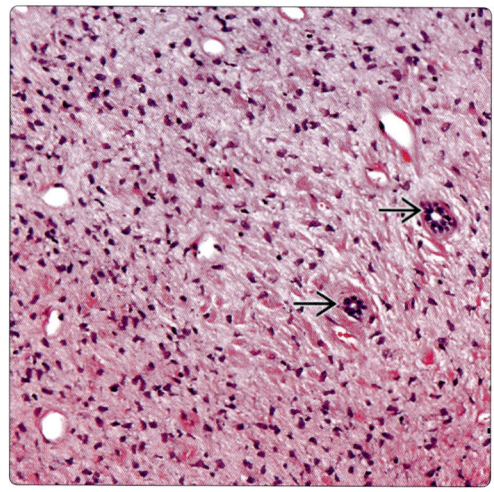

Metanephric Tumors: Stroma

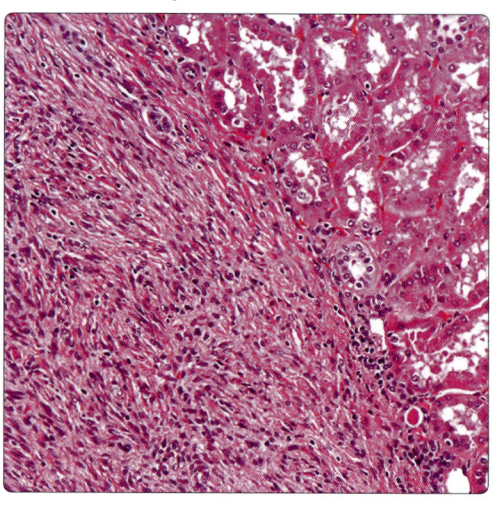

(Left) Metanephric stromal tumor is a benign, pediatric stromal neoplasm, usually with entrapped renal tubules ⇨ and glomeruli. Most cases were previously misdiagnosed as congenital mesoblastic nephroma. (Right) Although the stroma in both metanephric stromal tumor and metanephric adenofibroma shows marked similarities, MAF lacks the juxtaglomerular cell hyperplasia commonly seen in MST. The epithelial component in MAF remains the most distinctive feature between the 2.

Metanephric Tumors: Stroma

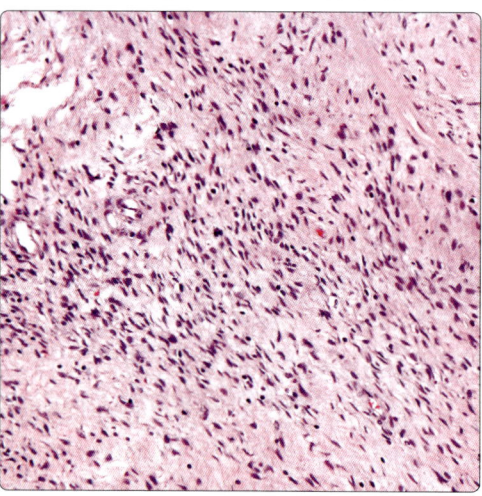

Metanephric Tumor: Angiodysplasia

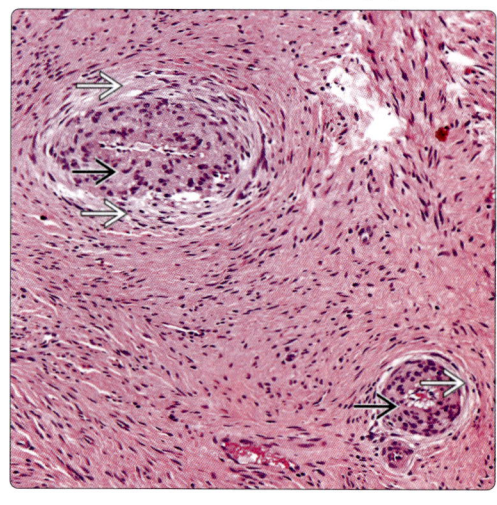

(Left) Based on this photomicrograph alone, which depicts the stroma in a metanephric tumor, it is not possible to discriminate between a metanephric stromal tumor and adenofibroma because of the similarities between the 2. (Right) The stroma in both metanephric stromal tumors and metanephric adenofibromas shows tumor vessels with epithelioid transformation of medial smooth muscle (so-called angiodysplasia) ⇨. This image also shows the typical myxoid stroma around the vessels ⇨.

Metanephric Stromal Tumor: Angiodysplasia

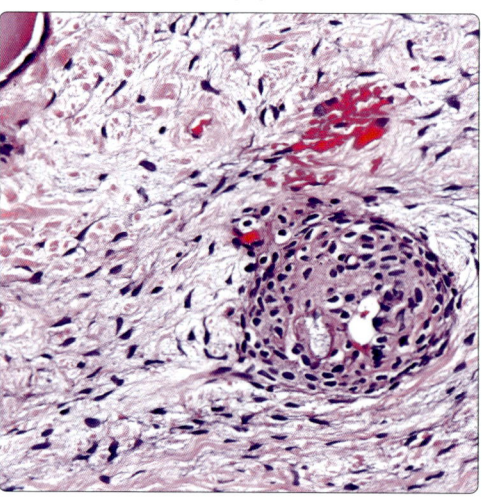

Metanephric Tumor: Cellular Stroma

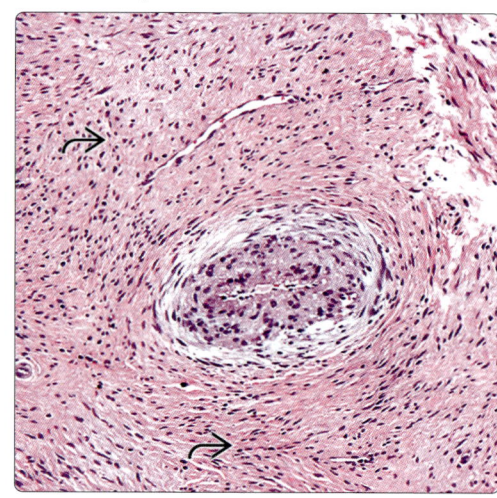

(Left) Myxoid stroma around this vessel with angiodysplastic features shows the typical concentric arrangement of the stromal cells. This often leads to what has been called an onion skin appearance. (Right) More cellular ⇨, less myxoid spindle cell areas at the periphery of collarettes of loose stroma often lead to vaguely nodular architecture. Such nodularity is a characteristic of MST. Note the epithelioid transformation of medial smooth muscle of an arteriole (angiodysplasia of vessels) seen here.

Metanephric Tumors Other Than Metanephric Adenoma

Metanephric Stromal Tumor: Vaguely Nodular Appearance

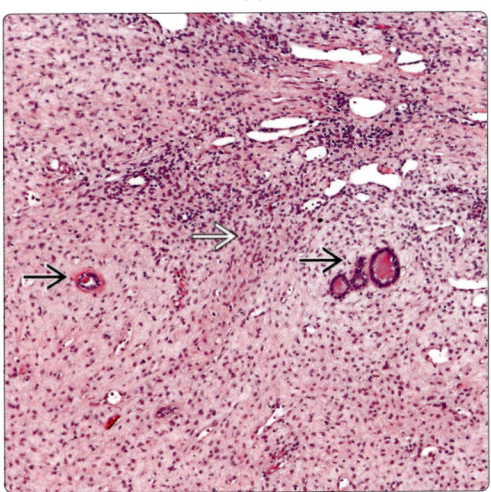

Metanephric Stromal Tumor: Angiodysplasia and Onion Skin Stroma

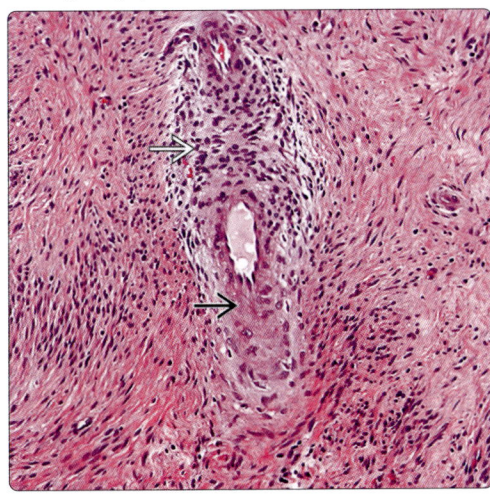

(Left) Most MSTs show vaguely nodular cellular patterns, primarily a result of loose myxoid stroma surrounding the entrapped tubules ➡ and blood vessels, separated by more dense stromal cellularity ➡. (Right) Morphologically, the stromal cells in MST are not much different from the cells in the classic variant of congenital mesoblastic nephroma, with which most metanephric stromal tumors were confused in the past. Note the angiodysplasia ➡ and perivascular onion skin stromal pattern ➡.

Metanephric Stromal Tumor: Reverse Cellular Stromal Pattern

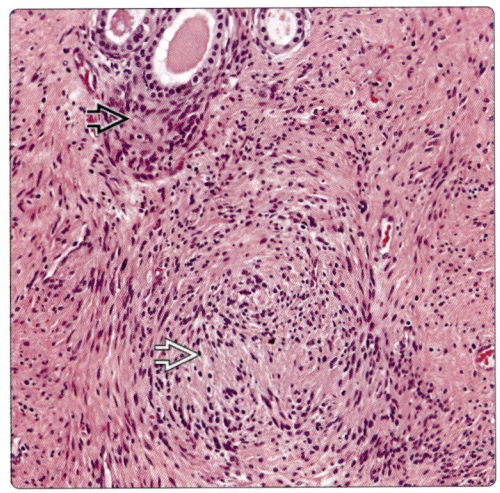

Metanephric Stromal Tumor: Embryonal Hyperplasia

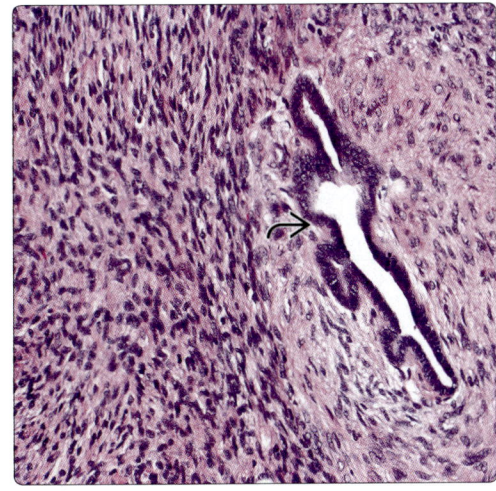

(Left) Some metanephric stromal tumors, as well as adenofibromas, show a reverse cellular pattern, with the tubules ➡ and vessels ➡ surrounded by more cellular stroma, compared to less dense stroma in between. (Right) The entrapped tubules in some metanephric stromal tumors may show a somewhat primitive appearance ➡. This is regarded as embryonal hyperplasia of the tubules. Sometimes such tubules are seen in close association with glial tissue forming glial-epithelial complexes.

Metanephric Stromal Tumor: Relative Circumscription

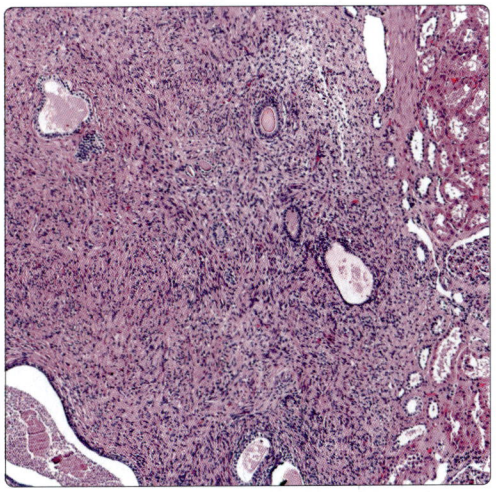

Congenital Mesoblastic Nephroma

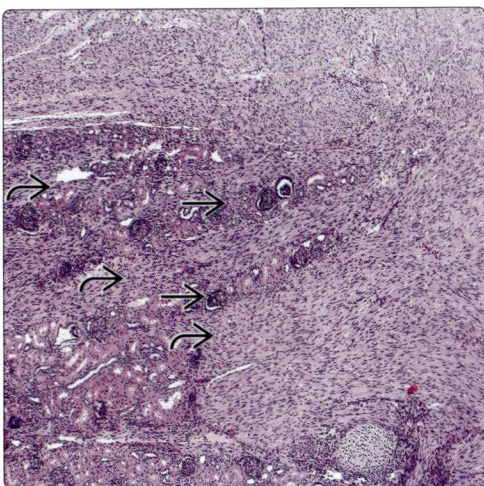

(Left) Most metanephric stromal tumors show superficially invasive borders entrapping individual native tubules and glomeruli. This is in contrast with what is seen in a mesoblastic nephroma with which this tumor has often been confused in the past. (Right) Unlike what is usually observed in metanephric stromal tumors, the advancing edges of the classic type of congenital mesoblastic nephroma invariably show extensive finger-like extensions ➡, entrapping large collections of native renal nephrons ➡.

Nephrogenic Rests

KEY FACTS

TERMINOLOGY
- Abnormally persistent nephrogenic cells, capable of developing into nephroblastomas

ETIOLOGY/PATHOGENESIS
- Mutations in *WT1* present in ILNR
- Insulin growth factor 2 loss of paternal imprinting (LOI) (in putative *WT2* gene region) present in PLNR of all types

CLINICAL ISSUES
- Encountered in up to 40% of patients with Wilms tumor and > 95% in patients with bilateral tumors
- Both PLNR and ILNR are observed in patients in Western countries, but PLNR are rarely, if ever, seen in Asian countries

MICROSCOPIC
- PLNR usually multifocal, located at periphery of renal lobes and sharply demarcated from surrounding renal parenchyma
- ILNR usually unifocal, localized within renal lobes, and poorly circumscribed with interdigitations into surrounding nephrons
- Dormant NR, small rests without evidence of proliferation
- Sclerosing and obsolete rests consist predominantly of tubules in fibrotic background
- Hyperplastic NR, showing signs of proliferation with abundant blastemal elements and increased size
- Neoplastic NR, arising within dormant, sclerosing, or hyperplastic rests
- Presence of pseudocapsule important in distinguishing hyperplastic or neoplastic (adenomatous) rest from nephroblastoma
- Designation of **nephroblastomatosis** is used for multifocal and diffuse, perilobar, interlobar, combined, or panlobar (replacing entire lobe) NRs

TOP DIFFERENTIAL DIAGNOSES
- Papillary adenoma

Perilobar Nephrogenic Rest
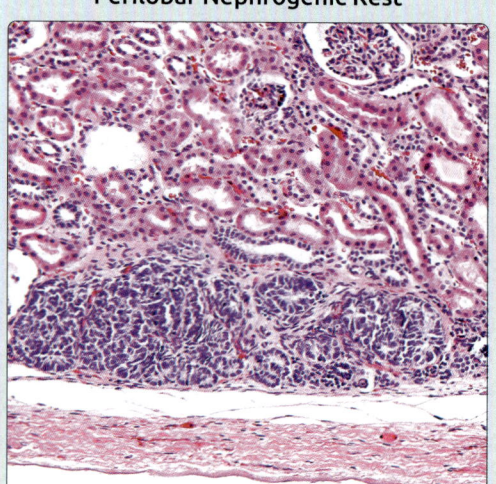

Intralobar Nephrogenic Rest (ILNR)
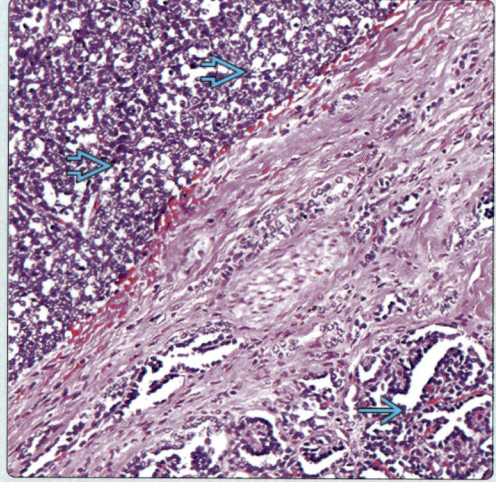

(Left) *Perilobar nephrogenic rests (PLNRs) are located at periphery of the renal lobes, well delineated from adjacent nephrons, and composed of blastema and tubules without any significant stromal components.* (Right) *This interlobar nephrogenic rest is present adjacent to a Wilms tumor ➡. Intralobar nephrogenic rests ➡ are located within the renal lobes, have irregular outlines, and often show prominent stromal components. Rests occurring in the renal sinus and pelvicalyceal system are also considered ILNR.*

Perilobar Nephrogenic Rest
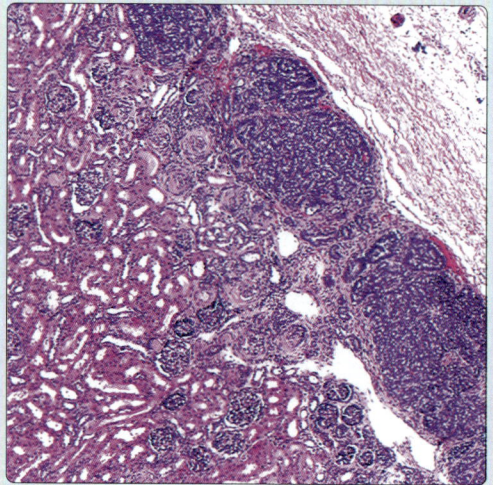

Interlobar Nephrogenic Rest
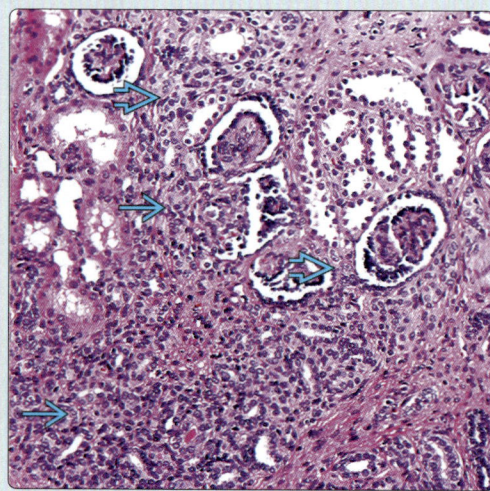

(Left) *Multiple PLNRs show features in between dormant and hyperplastic rests. Dormant NR are rests without proliferation, and hyperplastic NR are those with increased size and proliferative activity. However, these features represent a continuum rather than absolute static entities, as demonstrated in this image.* (Right) *An ILNR shows the typical irregular outlines and interdigitatons with surrounding glomeruli and tubules ➡. Prominent stromal component ➡, a characteristic of ILNR, is present.*

Nephrogenic Rests

TERMINOLOGY

Abbreviations
- Nephrogenic rest (NR), perilobar nephrogenic rest (PLNR), intralobar nephrogenic rest (ILNR)

Definitions
- Abnormally persistent nephrogenic cells associated with and capable of developing into nephroblastomas

ETIOLOGY/PATHOGENESIS

Molecular Alterations
- Like those in Wilms tumor (WT), alterations in *WT1* (11p13), *WT2* (11p15), and *WT3* (16q) genes present in accompanying NRs
  - Mutations in *WT1* present in ILNR
  - Insulin growth factor 2 loss of paternal imprinting (LOI) (in putative *WT2* gene region) present in PLNR of all types (sclerosing, hyperplastic, etc.)

CLINICAL ISSUES

Epidemiology
- Incidence
  - Encountered in up to 40% of WT cases, and > 95% in patients with bilateral tumors
  - Observed in 1% of infant autopsies
- Age
  - Median: WT and ILNR = 18.5 months; WT and PLNR = 35.5 months
- Sex
  - WT and NR show equal sex distribution or slight female preponderance in West, but significant male preponderance in Asia
- Ethnicity
  - PLNR somewhat more common than ILNR in West, but PLNR extremely uncommon in Asia

Treatment
- Hyperplastic rests difficult to distinguish from WT on biopsy; these and later forms treated similar to stage 1 WT [National Wilms Tumor Study Group (NWTS)]
  - Treating hyperplastic rests prevents compression and damage to native kidney, and diminishes targets for neoplastic transformation

Prognosis
- NRs in WT-bearing kidneys associated with higher incidence of synchronous or metachronous WT in other kidney
  - Higher incidence of concurrent bilateral Wilms tumor in patients with NRs, particularly PLNR
  - Risk of metachronous WT 15x higher in children < 1 yr of age with WT and NR (particularly PLNR)
  - Identifying NR on nephrectomy for WT leads to increased frequency of ultrasonographic follow-up for child

MICROSCOPIC

Histologic Features
- Based primarily on location, classified as perilobar or intralobar types
- Perilobar nephrogenic rests
  - Usually multifocal, located at periphery of lobes, sharply demarcated from surrounding parenchyma; predominantly consist of blastema and tubules, with scant stroma
- Intralobar nephrogenic rests
  - Usually unifocal, localized within renal lobes, and poorly circumscribed with interdigitations into surrounding nephrons; rich in stromal component
    - Rests occurring in renal sinus and pelvicalyceal system are also considered ILNR
- PLNR and ILNR subclassified as
  - **Dormant** (small rests without proliferation), **sclerosing** [mainly with differentiated blastema (usually tubular) with associated fibrosis], **obsolete** (predominantly with fibrosis, rare tubules)
  - **Hyperplastic**, showing signs of proliferation with abundant blastemal elements and increased size, usually grossly visible, showing significant proliferative activity
    - Represents generalized hyperplasia in the rest, with all cells in NR participating in proliferation; therefore, shape of rests maintained
  - **Neoplastic**, arising within dormant, sclerosing, or hyperplastic rests; usually grossly visible spherical nodule
    - Believed to represent proliferation from single cell; therefore, spherical shape with pushing borders compressing surrounding structures
    - No pseudocapsule present; absence of pseudocapsule important in distinguishing hyperplastic/neoplastic rest from nephroblastoma
  - Designation of **nephroblastomatosis** used for multifocal and diffuse, perilobar, interlobar, combined, or panlobar (replacing entire lobe) NRs
    - All or any stage of rests (dormant, hyperplastic, neoplastic) can be present
    - No quantitative criteria to determine definition of nephroblastomatosis, but usually present as thick cortical rind of nephrogenic tissue encasing kidney

DIFFERENTIAL DIAGNOSIS

Papillary Adenoma
- Frequently encountered in adults; shows mature epithelial component; lacks blastema

DIAGNOSTIC CHECKLIST

Pathologic Interpretation Pearls
- Intraoperative renal biopsies are often of limited utility in distinguishing between WT and mitotically active NR in small samples
  - Requires abundant tissue at periphery of lesion for distinction

SELECTED REFERENCES
1. Al-Hussain T et al: Wilms tumor: an update. Adv Anat Pathol. 21(3):166-73, 2014
2. Fukuzawa R et al: Molecular pathology and epidemiology of nephrogenic rests and Wilms tumors. J Pediatr Hematol Oncol. 29(9):589-94, 2007
3. Hennigar RA et al: Clinicopathologic features of nephrogenic rests and nephroblastomatosis. Adv Anat Pathol. 8(5):276-89, 2001
4. Beckwith JB et al: Nephrogenic rests, nephroblastomatosis, and the pathogenesis of Wilms' tumor. Pediatr Pathol. 10(1-2):1-36, 1990

Nephrogenic Rests

Interlobar Nephrogenic Rest

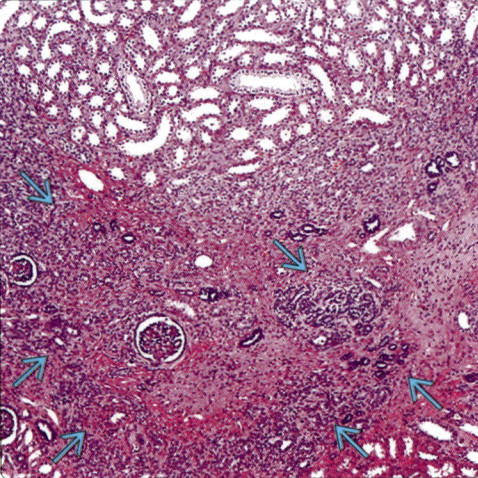

Wilms Tumor vs. NR

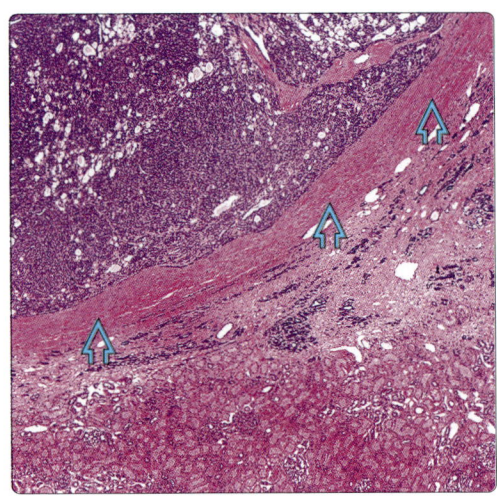

(Left) Low-magnification view shows a large intralobar nephrogenic rest ⇨. Unlike PLNR, ILNRs are usually single. Isolated ILNRs are much less common than PLNRs in pediatric autopsies. However, these are the predominant type of NR found in Asia. (Right) Unlike all types of nephrogenic rests, Wilms tumor (WT) usually shows the presence of a pseudocapsule ⇨. Encapsulation is an important distinguishing feature that separates Wilms tumor from all forms of NRs.

Dormant and Sclerosing NR

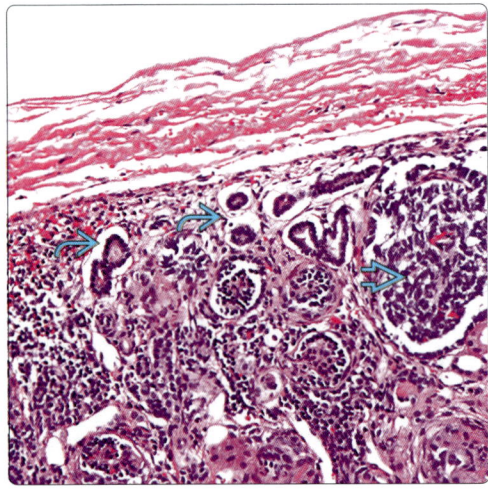

Hyperplastic Perilobar NR

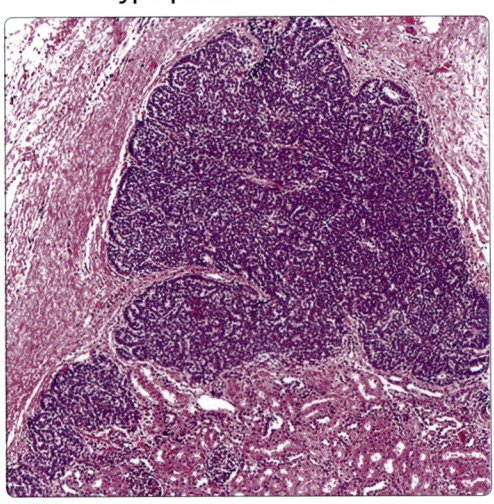

(Left) A dormant ⇨ and sclerosing ⇨ perilobar NR are shown side-by-side. Sclerosing NRs show variable proportion of fibrosis and usually consist of tubules separated by a fibrous background. (Right) A hyperplastic perilobar NR, by definition, represents an enlarged, proliferating rest. Proliferation involves all cells in the rest; therefore, the shape of the rest is preserved. (Courtesy P. Argani, MD.)

Hyperplastic Perilobar NR

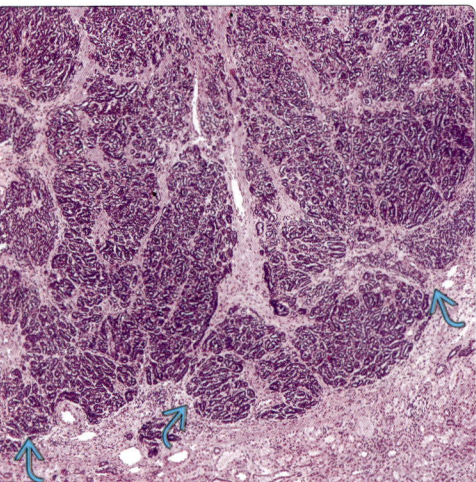

Neoplastic/Adenomatous Nephrogenic Rest

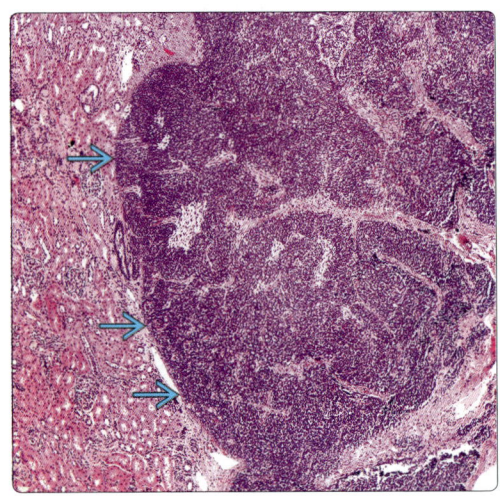

(Left) This image shows a large hyperplastic NR. Because its outlines are irregular, and the overall outline is not smooth and rounded ⇨. This rest does not qualify as a neoplastic or adenomatous NR. (Right) A smooth rounded-off front ⇨ in this NR is helpful in designating this rest as a neoplastic or adenomatous NR. A close differential diagnosis is an early WT, but lack of a fibrous capsule favors the diagnosis of an NR.

Nephrogenic Rests

Neoplastic Perilobar NR
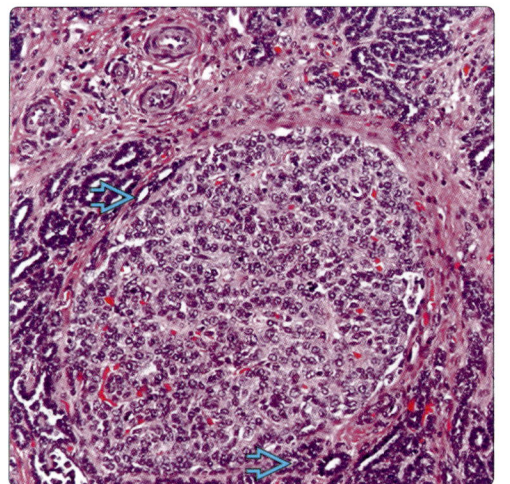

Neoplastic Perilobar NR
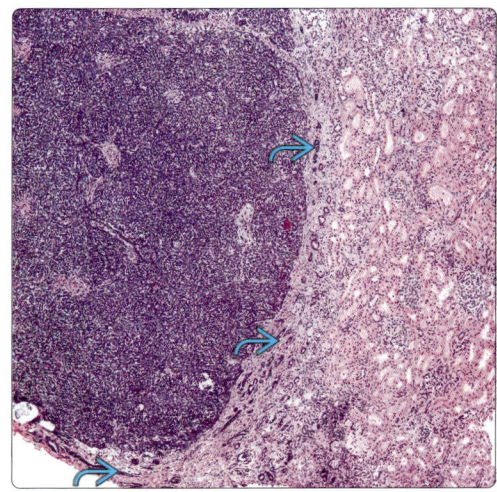

(Left) This image shows a neoplastic NR, occurring in a postchemotherapeutic setting. Neoplastic rests are believed to arise from the proliferation of a single cell; therefore, these are spherical and compress the surrounding NR remnants ⇨. (Right) This small nodule of predominantly blastemal cells can represent either a neoplastic NR or early WT. Lack of a fibrous capsule favors the former. Notice the residual sclerosing PLNR ⇨ along the periphery of the nodule.

Neoplastic/Adenomatous Perilobar NR
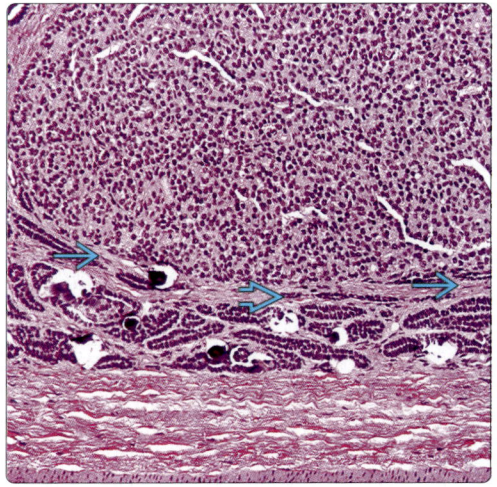

Nephroblastomatosis
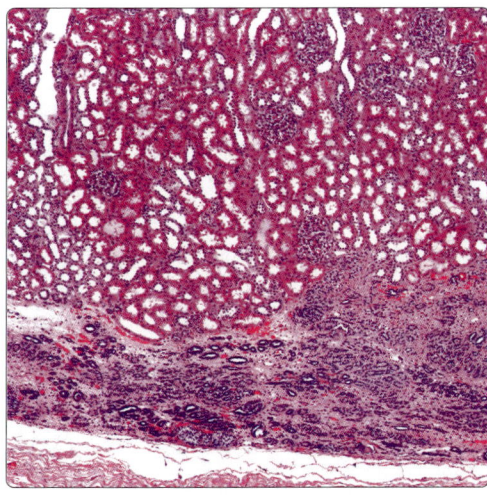

(Left) This image shows a postchemotherapy nephrogenic nodule with compression of residual NR components ⇨ and early pseudocapsule formation ⇨. Such nodules may be considered adenomatous/neoplastic by some and early WT by others. (Right) Low-magnification view shows nephroblastomatosis, which is characterized by the presence of a thick cortical rind of nephrogenic tissue encasing the kidney.

Nephroblastomatosis
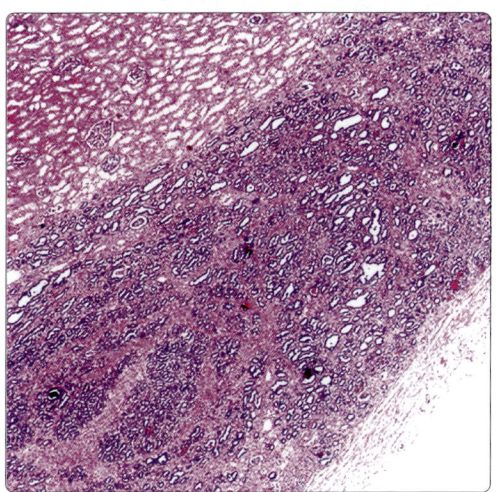

Posttherapy Nephroblastomatosis
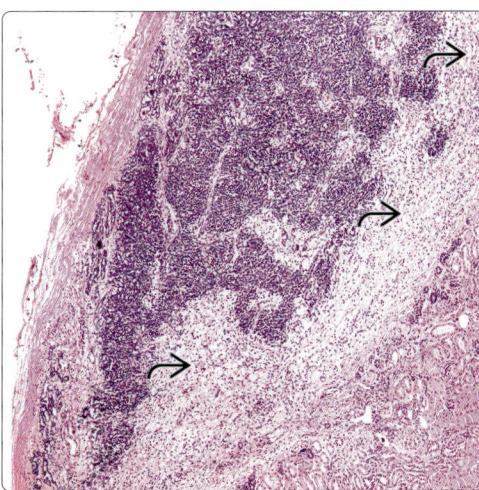

(Left) There are no quantitative criteria to determine how many rests would constitute nephroblastomatosis. However, diffuse radiologic thickening of the renal cortex is typical of nephroblastomatosis. (Right) This hyperplastic rest shows chemotherapy-related changes ⇨. Treating hyperplastic rests by chemotherapy similar to stage 1 WT prevents compression and damage to native kidney and diminishes the number of cells that may undergo neoplastic transformation.

Nephroblastoma (Wilms Tumor)

KEY FACTS

TERMINOLOGY
- Malignant embryonal neoplasm derived from nephrogenic blastema cells often, but not always, showing multiphasic patterns of differentiation

ETIOLOGY/PATHOGENESIS
- ~ 10% associated with syndromic conditions

CLINICAL ISSUES
- 98% of cases in children < 10 years of age
- Peak incidence: 2-3 years
- In general, Children's Oncology Group advocates primary resection followed by further therapy; International Society of Pediatric Oncology advocates preoperative therapy followed by surgical resection and further therapy
- Overall survival currently > 90%
- Most significant unfavorable factors include high stage at presentation and diffuse anaplasia (unfavorable histology)

MICROSCOPIC
- Most characteristic: Triphasic pattern consisting of undifferentiated blastemal, epithelial, and stromal components
- Features of anaplasia include markedly increased (3x) tumor cell nuclei with hyperchromasia and multipolar mitotic figures
- Only diffuse anaplasia clinically/therapeutically important; therefore, differentiation from focal anaplasia essential
- Anaplasia correlates with resistance to chemotherapy, and with *p53* mutations in tumor

TOP DIFFERENTIAL DIAGNOSES
- Other small blue cell tumors
- Immature teratoma
- Metanephric adenoma
- Papillary renal cell carcinoma (type 1, solid glomeruloid variant)

Gross Features

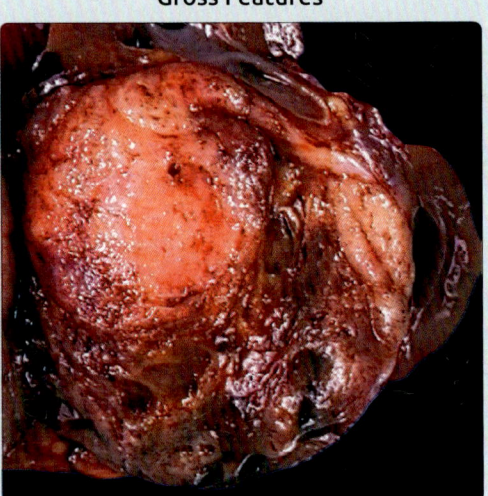

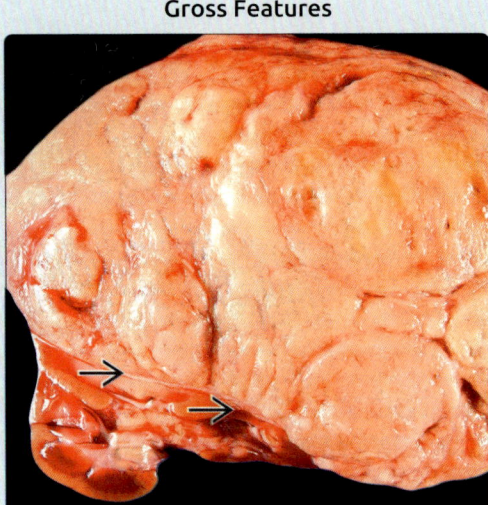

(Left) Gross appearance of a Wilms tumor shows a sharply circumscribed, soft, tan mass with an encephaloid cut surface bulging from the native renal parenchyma. Sharp circumscription is an important radiological feature for the presumptive diagnosis, and considered sufficient for initiating preoperative Wilms chemotherapy when indicated. (Right) Most Wilms tumors are well delineated, often with a prominent capsule ➡. The only notable exception to sharp circumscription is diffuse blastemal Wilms tumor.

Triphasic Histology

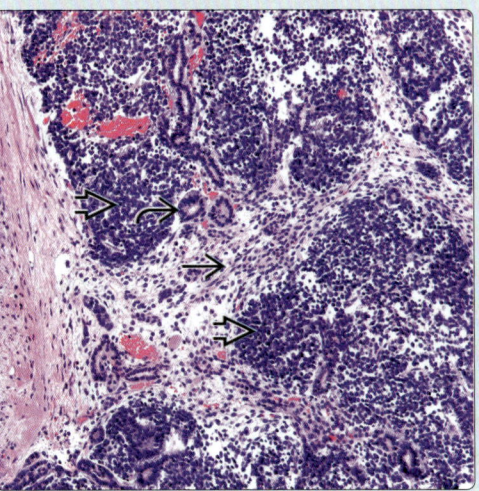

Encapsulation

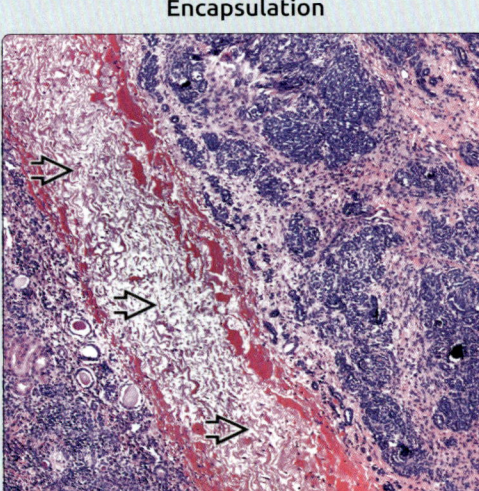

(Left) Triphasic patterns (blastemal ➡, epithelial ➡, and stromal ➡) are characteristic of Wilms tumors but are not essential; some tumors may only be biphasic or monophasic. Within the epithelial and stromal components, considerable heterogeneity in histology may be present. (Right) The usual well-circumscribed nature of a Wilms tumor with a prominent capsule ➡ is seen in this image. Tumors with diffuse blastemal pattern, however, often show infiltrative borders.

Nephroblastoma (Wilms Tumor)

TERMINOLOGY

Abbreviations
- Wilms tumor (WT)

Synonyms
- Nephroblastoma

Definitions
- Malignant embryonal neoplasm derived from nephrogenic blastema cells often, but not always, showing multiphasic patterns of differentiation

ETIOLOGY/PATHOGENESIS

Developmental Anomaly
- ~ 10% associated with syndromic conditions, including
  o WAGR syndrome (**W**ilms tumor, **A**niridia, **G**enitourinary malformations, mental **R**etardation), Denys-Drash syndrome (WT, mesangial sclerosis, pseudohermaphroditism), Beckwith-Wiedemann syndrome (WT, hemihypertrophy, macroglossia, omphalocele, visceromegaly), familial nephroblastoma, or others such as Trisomy 18, Perlman syndrome, Bloom syndrome, Frasier syndrome, Klippel-Trenaunay syndrome

WT1 Gene Deletions or Point Mutations
- *WT1* gene is localized to chromosome 11p13; *WT1* gene alterations consistently present in WAGR and Denys-Drash syndromes
- Among sporadic nephroblastomas, deletions in focus present in 1/3 and mutations in 10% of cases only
  o *WT1*-mutant tumors also show *β-catenin* (*CTNNB1*) mutations, activating Wnt signaling pathway
- Tumors with *WT1* mutations usually with stromal-prominent histology and rhabdomyogenesis, and associated with intralobar nephrogenic rests (ILNR)
- Such tumors common in both East Asians and whites

WT2 Gene Alterations
- 11p15 is location for putative *WT2* gene; 11p15 alterations common in Beckwith-Wiedemann syndrome
  o Insulin growth factor 2 (*IGF2*) gene and closely related H19 locus located within *WT2* region
  o Normally, only paternal allele-specific *IGF2* expressed (imprinting), because of differential methylation status of *H19* in paternal and maternal alleles
- Loss of imprinting (LOI) of *IGF2* and hypermethylation of *H19*-related genes identified in 33-50% of WTs
- Tumors with LOI usually stroma poor; often associated with perilobar nephrogenic rests (PLNR)
- Such tumors are rare in East Asians

Tumor-Specific LOH for Chromosomes 1p and 16q, and 1q Gains
- Loss of heterozygosity (LOH) for chromosomes 1p and 16q present in proportion of WT with favorable histology
  o These LOHs with significantly increased risk of aggressive behavior in such WT; 1q gains associated with higher tumor recurrences; favorable histology WT with LOH receive more aggressive treatment

CLINICAL ISSUES

Epidemiology
- Incidence
  o 1/8,000 children, constituting ~ 85% of pediatric renal malignancies
- Age
  o Peak incidence: 2-3 years; 98% of cases in children < 10; very uncommonly reported in adults

Presentation
- Most common: Abdominal mass, often detected by parents while bathing or clothing child; other common presentation: Pain, hematuria, hypertension, and acute abdominal crisis

Treatment
- In general, Children's Oncology Group (COG), which now includes National Wilms Tumor Study (NWTS), advocates primary resection; further therapy determined by stage and favorable or unfavorable histology of resected tumor
  o Vincristine, dactinomycin, doxorubicin, cyclophosphamide and etoposide, and radiation used in different combinations in favorable histology tumors depending on stage and presence of LOH
  o Patients with stage II to IV WT with diffuse anaplasia treated more aggressively
    – Stage I tumors with diffuse anaplasia treated like nonanaplastic tumors
  o Adjuvant chemotherapy now avoided for young patients (< 2 years) with small (< 550 g nephrectomy weight) stage I favorable histology tumors
    – Pathologic evaluation of lymph nodes essential requirement for this approach
- International Society of Pediatric Oncology (SIOP) advocates preoperative therapy followed by surgical resection; further therapy determined by response to prior therapy
  o Before resection, cases without metastasis receive vincristine and dactinomycin, and those with metastases receive vincristine, dactinomycin, and doxorubicin
  o Additional therapy given based on residual tumor in nephrectomy specimen

Prognosis
- Survival similar with both the NWTS and SIOP protocols (overall survival > 90%)
- Most significant unfavorable factors include
  o High stage at presentation and diffuse anaplasia (unfavorable histology)
- Majority of pretherapy WTs with blastemal predominance very sensitive to therapy
  o But, blastemal-type posttherapy tumors considered resistant to chemotherapy; managed similar to anaplastic tumors (SIOP)

MACROSCOPIC

General Features
- Most tumors unicentric; 7% multicentric, 5% bilateral
- Usually sharply demarcated from surrounding renal parenchyma, very often encapsulated

Nephroblastoma (Wilms Tumor)

- Cut surface often uniformly pale gray or tan with soft consistency, or with whorled, firm tumors with prominent stromal component

Specimen Handling and Sections to Be Submitted

- All pediatric renal tumor specimens must be weighed
  - Weight determines decisions about therapy in some cases, e.g., no chemotherapy in younger patients with stage I tumor and total kidney weight < 550 g
- Before opening specimen, perihilar and perirenal lymph nodes should be identified and sampled
  - Lack of pathologic evaluation of lymph nodes excludes some (otherwise qualifying) patients from "no chemotherapy required" approach
- In addition to inking entire surface of specimen, areas with suspected ruptures may be inked in different colors
- After opening specimen and sampling cut surface for tumor banking and other special studies, specimen should be fixed overnight
- Sampling from renal sinus and margins of resection essential for adequate staging
- Most sections taken from tumor must include tumor-renal parenchyma interface in order to evaluate tumor borders
- Documenting exact site from which each block is obtained is necessary
  - This is often critical for evaluating focal vs. diffuse anaplasia and for addressing staging issues in some cases

MICROSCOPIC

Histologic Features

- Most characteristic: Triphasic pattern consisting of undifferentiated blastemal, epithelial and stromal components; some tumors only biphasic or monophasic
- **Blastemal cells**: Small, closely packed, mitotically active cells with scant cytoplasm, overlapping nuclei, evenly distributed coarse chromatin, and usually small nucleoli
  - Tumors with diffuse blastemal pattern, often have infiltrative margins, unlike most other types of WTs
- **Epithelial components**: Ranging from primitive rosette-like tubules to well-formed maturing and mature tubules, ill-formed glomerular structures, variable papillary architecture
  - Mucinous or squamous differentiation occasionally present
    - Tumors with extensive heterologous differentiation designated teratoid Wilms tumor by some
- **Stromal component**: Nondescript spindle cells, smooth muscle, skeletal muscle, or fibroblastic differentiation
  - Occasionally, fat, cartilage, bone, ganglion cells, or neuroglia also seen
- Typical therapy-induced changes include coagulative tumor necrosis, fibrosis, foamy, &/or hemosiderin-laden macrophages (regressive changes)
- Posttherapy tumors often regressive type or completely necrotic
  - Complete necrosis not seen in pretherapy specimens
    - Tumors with necrosis and < 1/3 viable area considered completely necrotic
- Tumors with at least 1/3 viable area typed according to predominant (> 2/3 of viable areas) component
  - Those with > 1/3 viable area and < 2/3 of dominant histology in viable area considered mixed type
- If regressive changes occupy > 2/3 of tumor, considered regressive-type tumor
- Postchemotherapy nephroblastomas subclassified into 3 prognostic groups
  - Further therapy depends on risk assessment (SIOP), is divided into
    - Tumors with low, intermediate, or high risk
    - Posttherapy blastemal-type tumor [blastemal component constituting < 2/3 of viable tumor (SIOP)] considered high-risk tumor
- Tumors with anaplasia only type with unfavorable histology by NWTS/COG
  - ~ 5% WTs show anaplasia
    - Features of anaplasia include markedly enlarged tumor cell nuclei with hyperchromasia and multipolar mitotic figures
  - Anaplasia rare before 2 years of age and involves 13% of tumors beyond age 5
  - Anaplasia correlates with resistance to chemotherapy and with *p53* mutations in tumor
  - Only diffuse anaplasia clinically/therapeutically important; therefore, differentiation from focal anaplasia essential
  - Anaplasia considered focal when only present
    - In single/multiple sharply localized regions; when intrarenal, surrounded by nonanaplastic tumor; with no severe nuclear unrest (pleomorphism and hyperchromasia) in rest of tumor, and not present in intravascular tumor

Lymphatic/Vascular Invasion

- Invasion of renal sinus veins or lymphatics considered stage II in both COG and SIOP staging systems

ANCILLARY TESTS

Immunohistochemistry

- Immunoreactive for WT1 protein
  - Immunoreactivity usually limited to blastemal and epithelial elements; stroma negative
- Blastemal cells may label for desmin, but not other muscle markers like actin, myogenin, MYOD1
- Vimentin and cytokeratin negative or focal positive in blastema: Cytokeratin usually positive in epithelial components
  - CK7 may also be positive in more differentiated epithelial cells
- pax-8, pax-2 usually positive

DIFFERENTIAL DIAGNOSIS

Other Small Blue Cell Tumors

- Require differentiation from blastemal WT
  - Presence of nuclear molding, early tubular differentiation with organized nuclear alignment around early lumina typical of blastema
    - Presence of true tubular lumina always favors WT
  - Immunostains may be required in small biopsies to exclude other possibilities, including neuroblastoma, rhabdomyosarcoma, and primitive neuroectodermal tumor

Nephroblastoma (Wilms Tumor)

Staging of Pediatric Renal Tumors (Children's Oncology Group)

Stage	Main Pathologic Feature	Details of Pathologic Findings
I	Tumor limited to kidney and completely resected	Renal capsule intact; no prior biopsy
		No invasion of lymphatics or veins of renal sinus; margins negative
		No metastases
II	Tumor extends beyond kidney but completely resected	Tumor penetrates renal capsule, or lymphatics or veins in renal sinus
		Tumor invades renal vein, but all margins, including renal vein margin, are negative
		No metastases
III	Residual tumor or nonhematogeneous metastases confined to abdomen	Involves abdominal lymph nodes
		Tumor spillage of any degree occurring before or during surgery; biopsy of tumor (including fine-needle aspiration); peritoneal implants
		Gross residual tumor in abdomen
		Resection margin involved by tumor
IV	Hematogenous metastases or spread beyond abdomen	
V	Bilateral renal tumors	Tumor on each side to be staged separately and reported as substage on that side [e.g., stage V; substage III (right), substage I (left)]

Revised SIOP Working Classification of Nephroblastoma After Neoadjuvant Therapy

Stage	Risk Level	Residual Tumor Type
I	Low-risk tumors	Cystic partially differentiated nephroblastoma
		Completely necrotic nephroblastoma
II	Intermediate-risk tumors	Nephroblastoma, epithelial type, stromal type, mixed type, or regressive type
		Nephroblastoma, focal anaplasia
III	High-risk tumors	Nephroblastoma, blastemal type
		Nephroblastoma, diffuse anaplasia

Immature Teratoma

- Requires differentiation from WT with extensive heterologous differentiation (so-called teratoid WT)
  - Teratoma shows organized (organ-like) differentiation (e.g., ciliated epithelium with smooth muscle and cartilage, etc.)

Metanephric Adenoma

- Requires differentiation from epithelial-predominant WT
  - Uniform, nonoverlapping nuclei with delicate chromatin and inconspicuous nucleoli and lack of mitotic figures in MA; CD57 and B-raf positive

Papillary Renal Cell Carcinoma (Type 1, Solid Glomeruloid Variant)

- Requires differentiation from epithelial-predominant WT with papillary areas
  - Papillary renal cell carcinoma (RCC) often with foamy macrophages; often with higher-grade cytology, including more prominent nucleoli; AMACR and CK7 diffuse and strongly positive

DIAGNOSTIC CHECKLIST

Pathologic Interpretation Pearls

- Reporting of presence or absence of anaplasia is essential component of surgical pathology report on WT
  - Diffuse anaplasia, when present, usually apparent in most tumor sections; presence at any margin, or in extrarenal sites, considered diffuse anaplasia; presence in random biopsy (although rarely performed) also considered diffuse anaplasia

SELECTED REFERENCES

1. Dome JS et al: Advances in Wilms tumor treatment and biology: progress through international collaboration. J Clin Oncol. 33(27):2999-3007, 2015
2. Al-Hussain T et al: Wilms tumor: an update. Adv Anat Pathol. 21(3):166-73, 2014
3. Davidoff AM: Wilms tumor. Adv Pediatr. 59(1):247-67, 2012
4. Vujanic GM et al: The pathology of Wilms' tumour (nephroblastoma): the International Society of Pediatric Oncology approach. J Clin Pathol. J Clin Pathol. 63(2):102-9, 2010
5. Huang CC et al: Predicting relapse in favorable histology Wilms tumor using gene expression analysis: a report from the Renal Tumor Committee of the Children's Oncology Group. Clin Cancer Res. 15(5):1770-8, 2009
6. Cerrato F et al: Different mechanisms cause imprinting defects at the IGF2/H19 locus in Beckwith-Wiedemann syndrome and Wilms' tumour. Hum Mol Genet. 17(10):1427-35, 2008
7. Beckwith JB: Nephrogenic rests and the pathogenesis of Wilms tumor: developmental and clinical considerations. Am J Med Genet. 79(4):268-73, 1998

Nephroblastoma (Wilms Tumor)

Triphasic Histology

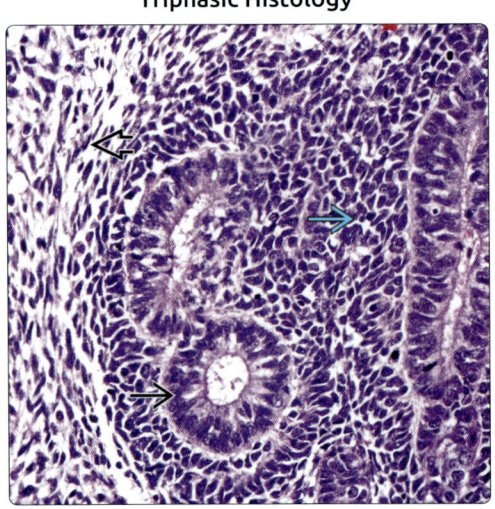

Blastemal Component

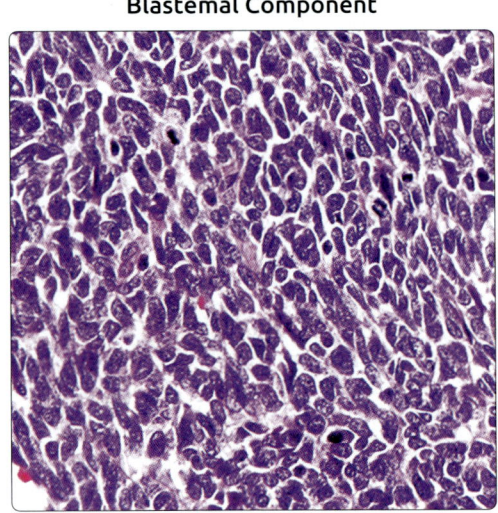

(Left) The typical triphasic morphology of a Wilms tumor is shown with blastemal ⇨, epithelial ⇨, and stromal ⇨ components. **(Right)** Blastema consists of small, closely packed, mitotically active cells with scant cytoplasm, overlapping nuclei, evenly distributed coarse chromatin, and usually small nucleoli. In pure blastemal Wilms, differentiation from other small round blue cell tumors may be difficult, and requires immunohistochemical support. However, tubular formation in this setting is highly supportive of a Wilms tumor.

Blastemal Wilms

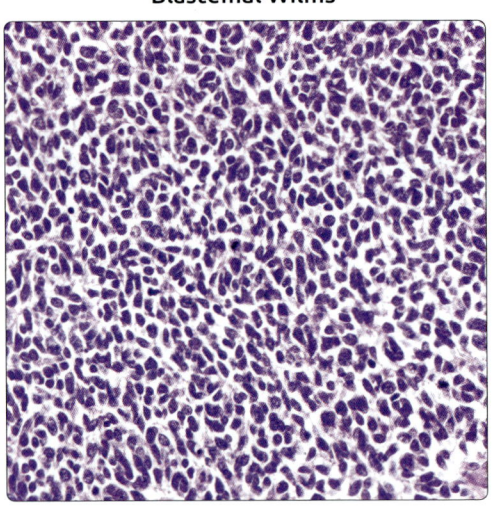

Blastemal Wilms

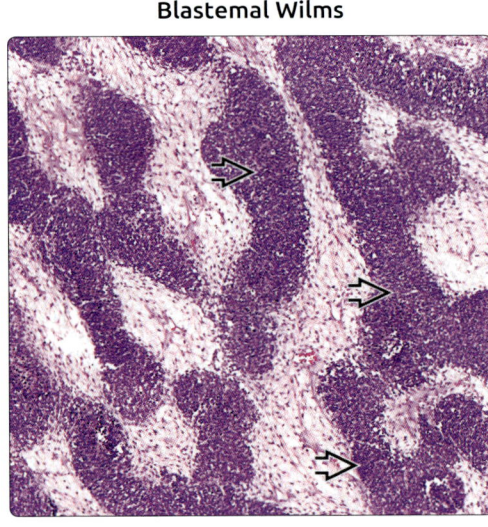

(Left) A purely blastema Wilms tumor is shown. Some tumors may be composed of sheets of blastemal elements alone. This is known as a Wilms tumor with a diffuse blastemal pattern & is considered an aggressive pattern in the tumor. At the same time, most tumors with blastemal pattern are responsive to current therapeutic approaches. **(Right)** In addition to the diffuse pattern, blastemal patterns may show more organized, serpentine ⇨, or nodular growth patterns often associated with myxoid stroma.

Nodular Blastemal Wilms

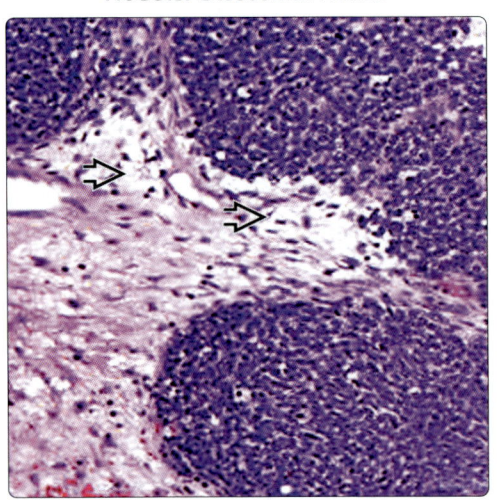

Epithelial Component

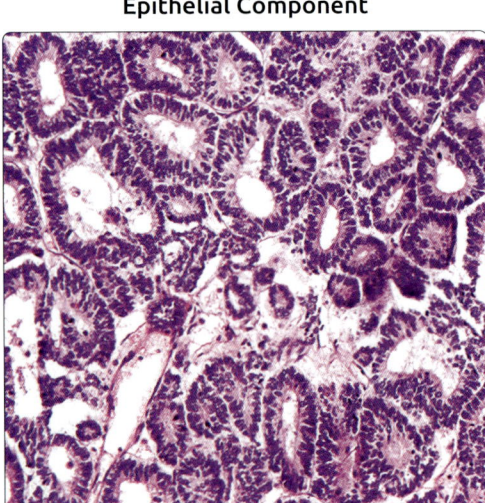

(Left) In tumors with nodular growth pattern, the blastema consists of variable-sized nodules in a usually loose, myxoid mesenchymal background ⇨. Tumors with such blastemal patterns usually lack invasive front that is seen in diffuse blastemal pattern tumors. **(Right)** Epithelial areas in Wilms tumors may show tubular differentiation of variable degrees, ranging from poorly developed tubular structures embedded in blastema to more differentiated tubules, usually lined by primitive & mitotically active cells.

Nephroblastoma (Wilms Tumor)

Triphasic Wilms With Differentiated Tubules

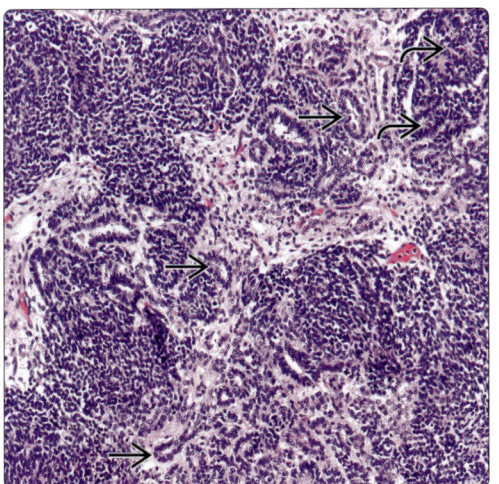

Epithelial Wilms

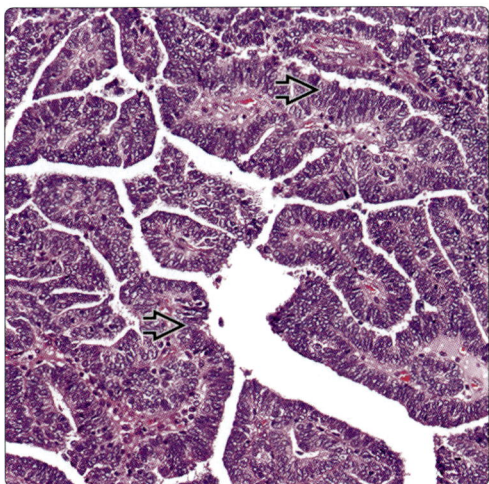

(Left) This image of a triphasic Wilms tumor shows tubular differentiation of variable degrees, ranging from poorly developed tubular structures embedded in blastema ⇒ to more differentiated tubules, lined by more organized and mature lining cells ⇒. *(Right)* Papillary formations are also common in epithelial areas. Very often, the lining cells appear primitive ⇒ but differentiation to more mature cells may also be seen, particularly in patients who have received prior chemotherapy.

Epithelial Patterns

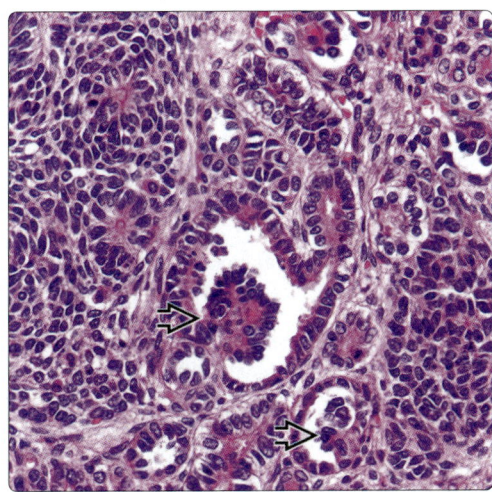

Epithelial Pattern

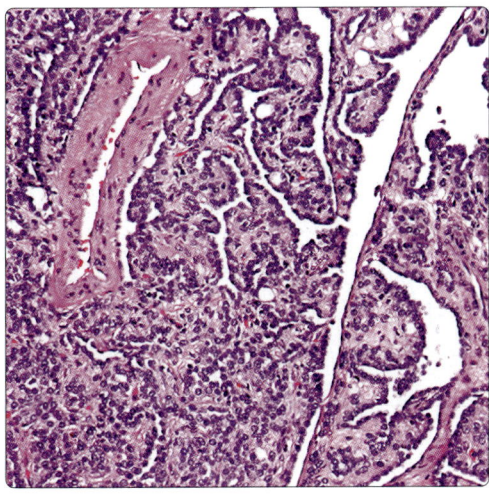

(Left) Glomerular differentiation in a Wilms tumor may range from primitive or attempted glomerular formations ⇒ to almost mature glomeruli closely resembling those of normal kidneys. *(Right)* Prominent papillary formations that appear well differentiated may be present in untreated cases of Wilms tumor. However, these features are more common in posttherapy Wilms and may raise the possibility of a papillary renal cell carcinoma.

Stromal Components: Skeletal Muscle

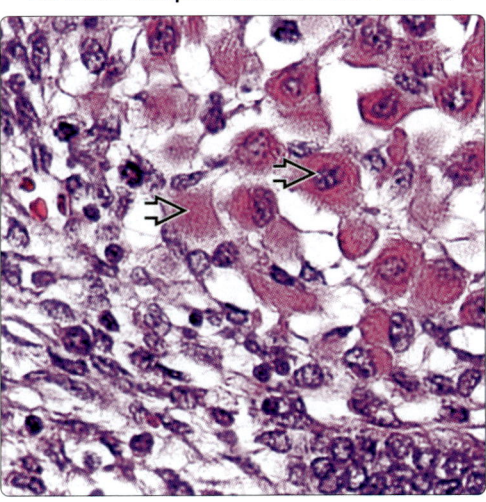

Stromal Components: Skeletal Muscle

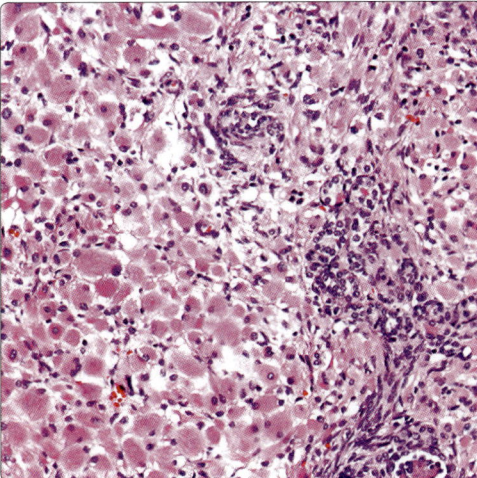

(Left) Among the stromal components, rhabdomyoblastic differentiation ⇒ is quite common & is the most frequent heterologous mesenchymal differentiation type in Wilms tumor. *(Right)* Extensive rhabdomyomatous differentiation is more common in posttherapy Wilms tumor. Postchemotherapy Wilms are mostly regressive or completely necrotic. About 10% are the blastemal type. Such blastemal Wilms are considered chemoresistant and regarded as high risk by the SIOP.

Nephroblastoma (Wilms Tumor)

Stromal Components: Spindle Cells NOS

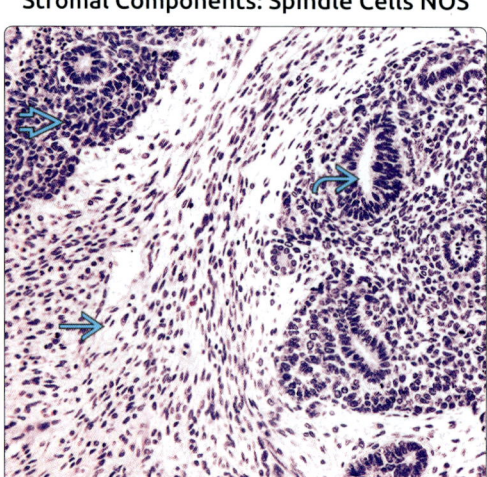

Stromal Components: Adipose Tissue

(Left) Triphasic patterns (blastemal ⇨, epithelial ⇨, and stromal ⇨) are characteristic of Wilms tumor but not essential. The stromal component in most cases is the nonspecific spindle cell type, and many tumors may be predominantly the stromal type. (Right) Undifferentiated, myxoid, fibroblastic, myofibroblastic, adipocytic ⇨, smooth muscle, cartilage, bone, and neuroglial type cells are the other stromal components that may be present in Wilms tumor.

Stromal Components: Skeletal Muscle & Fat

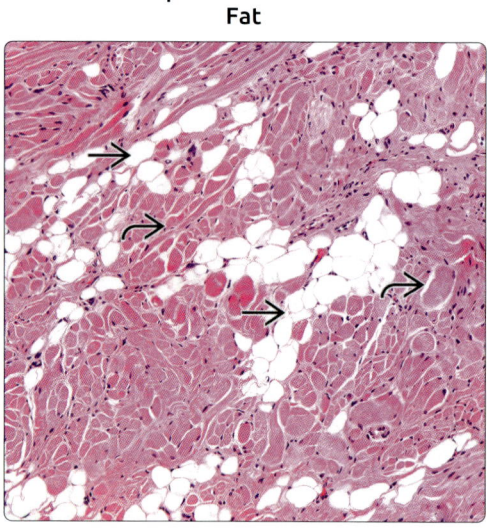

WT1 Immunohistochemistry

(Left) This Wilms tumor shows a combination of skeletal muscle ⇨ and adipose tissue ⇨ as the stromal components. Presence of even focal skeletal muscle differentiation in a small blue round cell tumor strongly favors the diagnosis of Wilms tumor. (Right) WT1 staining usually shows diffuse nuclear positivity in the blastemal and epithelial areas of the tumor, with the stroma being negative. Note the positive reaction in the glomerular mesangium and Bowman capsule lining ⇨ that acts as an internal control for WT1.

Anaplasia

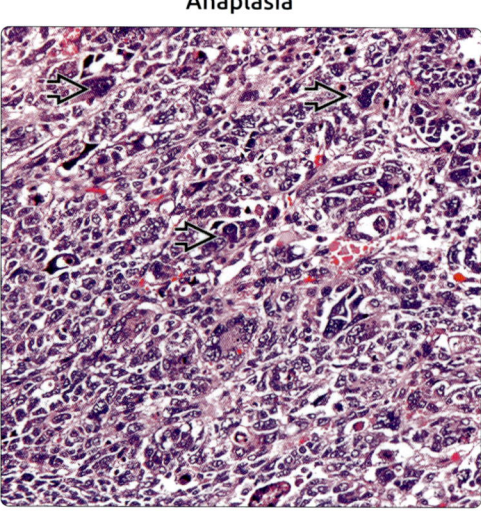

Anaplasia

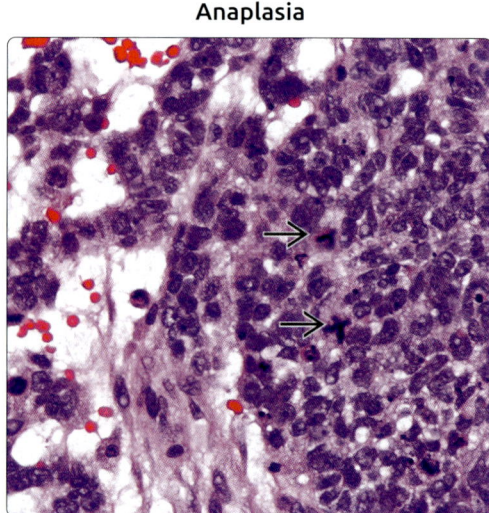

(Left) Tumors showing anaplasia are considered to be the only tumor type with unfavorable histology. Features of anaplasia include markedly enlarged ⇨ tumor cell nuclei (3x in size compared to the rest of the tumor cells), hyperchromasia, & multipolar mitotic figures. (Right) Multipolar mitotic figures ⇨ are considered a diagnostic feature of anaplasia in Wilms tumor. Only diffuse, not focal, anaplasia is used in making therapeutic decisions. Also, diffuse anaplasia in stage I tumors does not influence therapy.

Nephroblastoma (Wilms Tumor)

Anaplasia

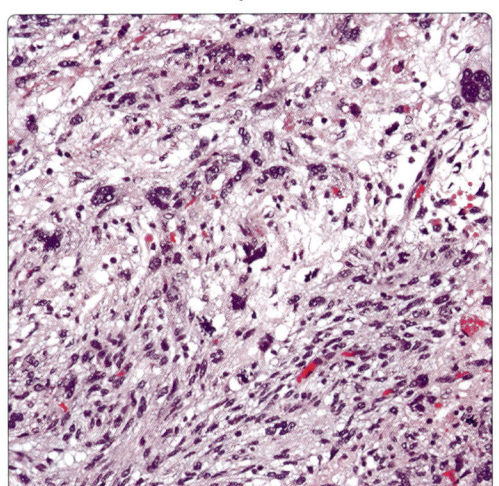

Anaplasia: p53

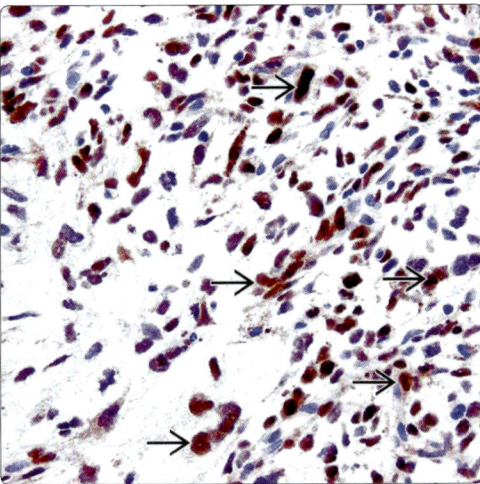

(Left) Anaplasia may be present in any or all 3 of the components of Wilms tumor. This image shows anaplastic features in the mesenchymal element of a tumor. Focal vs. diffuse anaplasia does not necessarily convey the relative amount, but the distribution & location, of anaplasia. (Right) Most anaplastic tumors show p53 gene mutations, corresponding to immunohistochemical overexpression ➡ in a majority of such tumors. p53 mutations have been associated with resistance to chemotherapy.

Posttherapy: Gross

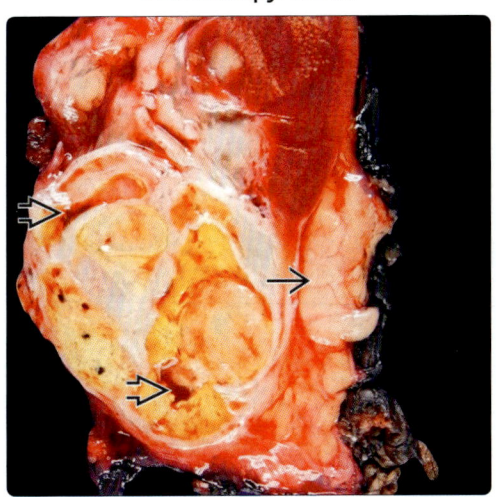

Posttherapy: Gross

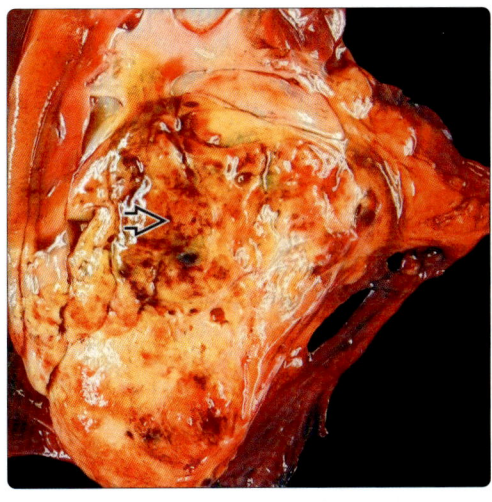

(Left) While NWTS/COG recommends pretherapy resection of most tumors, SIOP protocols (Europe) advocate chemotherapy before resection. Most posttherapy tumors show areas of necrosis and cystic change ➡. Note the separate nonaffected tumor nodule in perinephric fat ➡. (Right) Another gross photograph of a posttherapy Wilms tumor shows extensive necrosis ➡. While focal necrosis is common, extensive or total necrosis is very uncommon in specimens without prior treatment.

Posttherapy: Necrosis

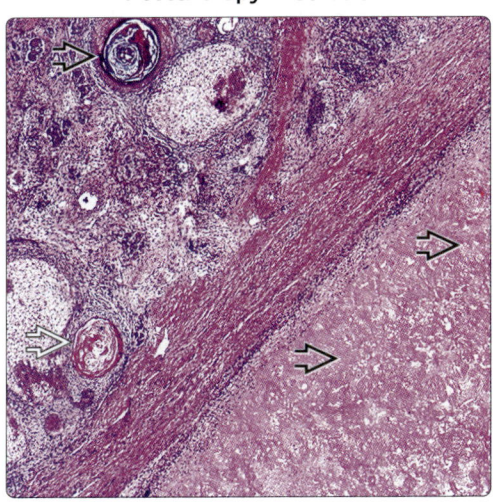

Posttherapy: Necrosis

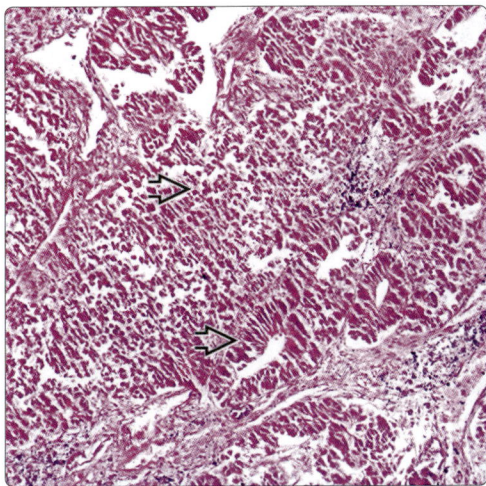

(Left) Posttherapy Wilms tumors often show necrosis ➡ and squamous differentiation ➡. (Right) Coagulative-type necrosis is common in posttherapy Wilms tumor. While dying tumor cells with vaguely recognizable nuclear details ➡ may help in diagnosis of a Wilms tumor, these areas of incompletely necrotic outlines are included among the necrotic component of posttherapy specimens & are considered as a part of "completely necrotic" Wilms tumors in tumors with > 2/3 of necrotic areas (SIOP).

Nephroblastoma (Wilms Tumor)

Posttherapy: Regressive Tumor

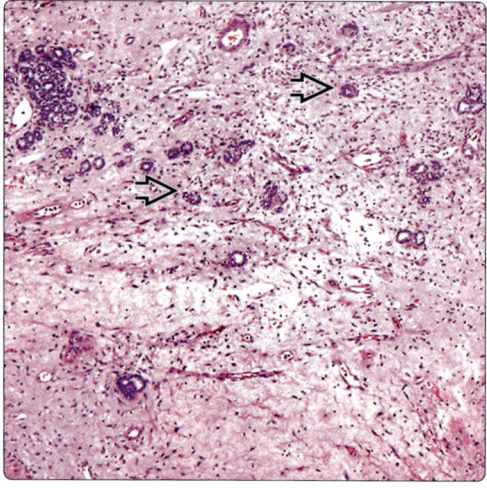

Posttherapy: Regressive Tumor

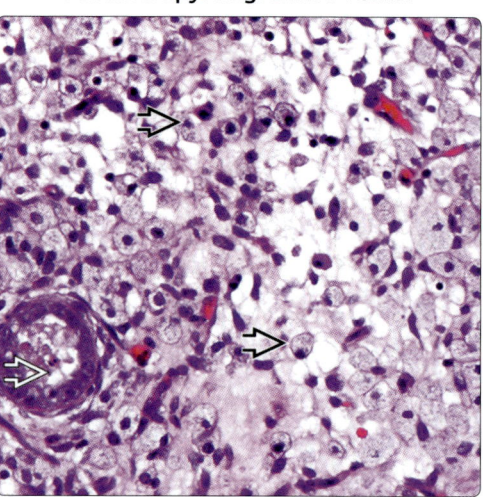

(Left) *A majority of posttherapy Wilms tumors show extensive fibrosis. Relatively mature-appearing tubules in such a background are regarded as epithelial rests ⇒ and are not included as viable epithelial component for the classification of posttherapy tumors.* (Right) *Posttherapy tumors often show large areas with foamy ⇒ or hemosiderin-laden macrophages. Rare, differentiated tubules may be present in such areas, and these are regarded as regressive changes ⇒.*

Posttherapy: Regressive & Blastemal Tumor

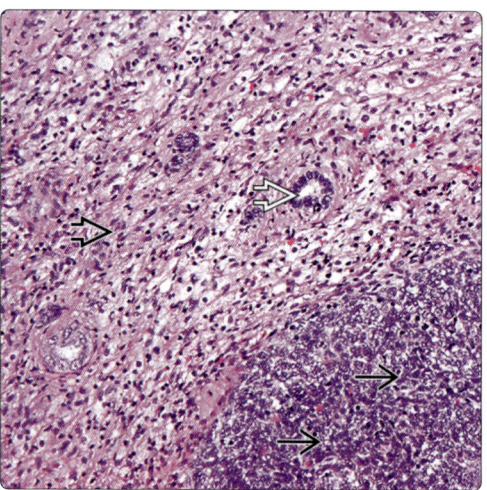

Posttherapy: Teratoid Tumor

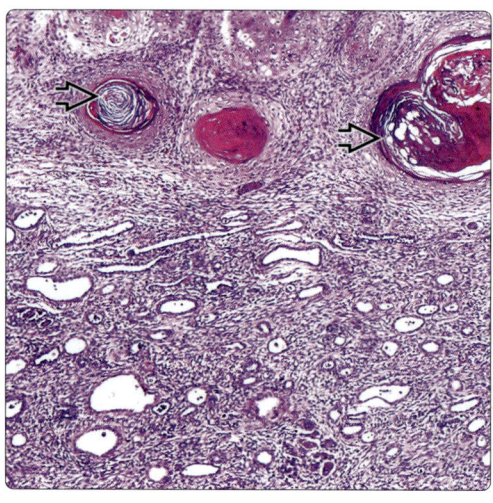

(Left) *Posttherapy Wilms tumor shows histiocytic response ⇒, few "cell rests" ⇒, and residual blastemal elements ⇒. SIOP requires determination of total viable component & proportion of blastemal elements in the viable areas for risk stratification and further therapy.* (Right) *While squamous differentiation may be seen in pretreatment cases, this is a more common feature in postchemotherapy residual tumors ⇒. Tumors with such extensive features have been regarded as "teratoid Wilms tumor" by some authors.*

Posttherapy: Cystic Partially Differentiated Nephroblastoma (CPDN)-Like Features

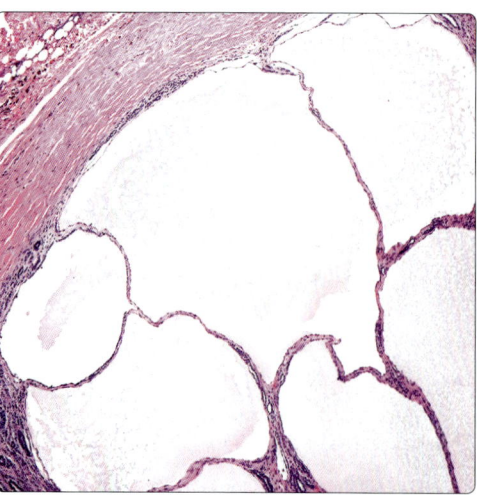

Complications of Biopsy

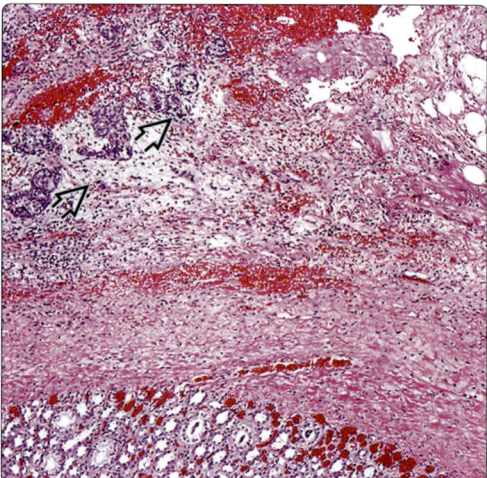

(Left) *Many postchemotherapy Wilms tumors show predominant or exclusive cystic, CPDN or cystic nephroma-like architecture. Such posttherapy tumors are regarded as low risk in SIOP classification. Similar features may be focally present in Wilms tumors without any chemotherapy.* (Right) *Prior biopsies (including FNA) result in upstaging the tumors to stage III (COG) with the presumption that biopsies lead to tumor spillage ⇒, as seen in this case. Initial biopsies of these tumors are not performed as a routine.*

Nephroblastoma (Wilms Tumor)

Vascular Invasion

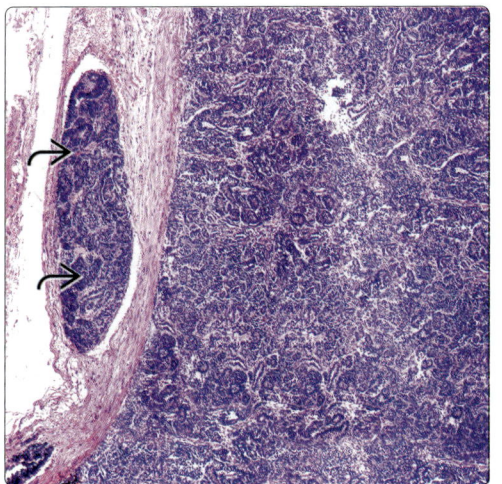

Peritoneal Implants

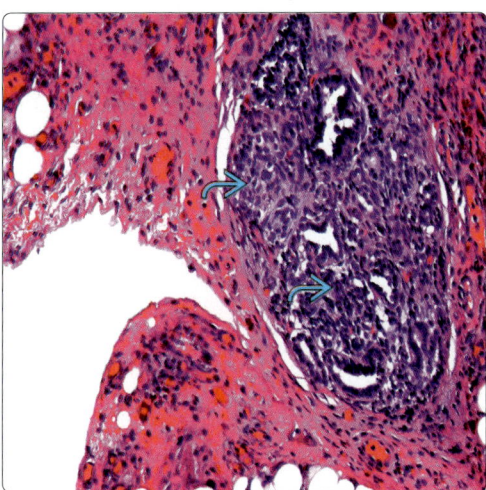

(Left) While perinephric or intrarenal vascular invasion is not stage-determining, any lymphovascular invasion in the renal sinus upstages a tumor to stage II, by both the COG and SIOP criteria. (Right) Peritoneal implantation of Wilms tumor is regarded as stage III disease in both the COG and SIOP staging systems. Such a tumor stage will result in radiotherapy, in addition to aggressive chemotherapy in Wilms tumor.

Metastasis: Lymph Nodes

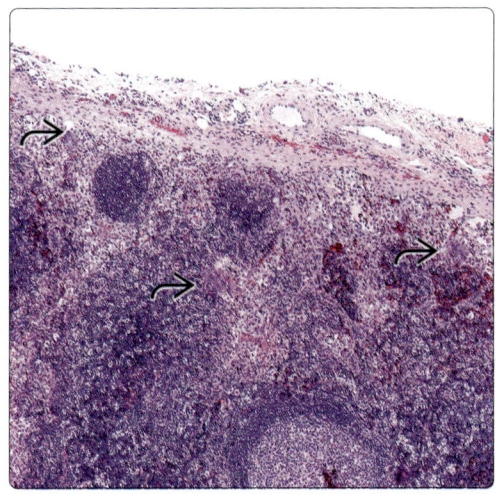

Metastasis: Lymph Nodes IHC

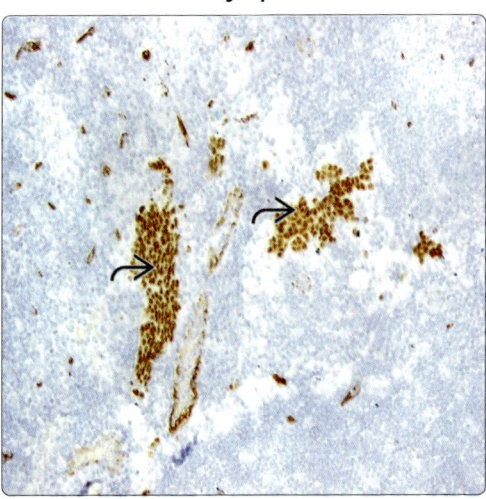

(Left) Metastasis to regional lymph nodes is an indicator of stage III Wilms tumor, and will result in local radiotherapy. Sometimes, the metastatic foci might be microscopic and difficult to visualize on initial H&E assessment. Immunohistochemical staining may be helpful in such instances. (Right) IHC staining for WT1 confirms the microscopic presence of metastasis in this case. However, one needs to be aware of the fact that all Wilms tumors are not positive for WT1.

Metastasis: Liver

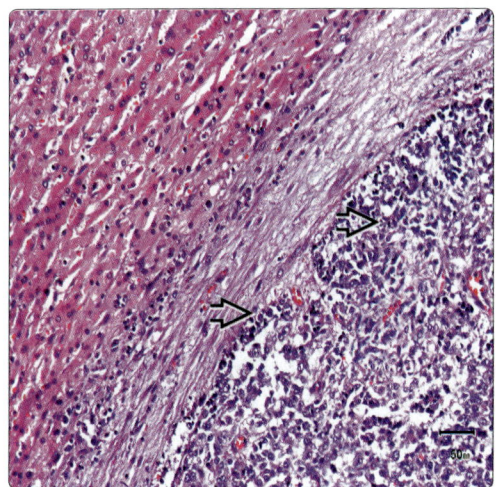

Metastasis: Lung

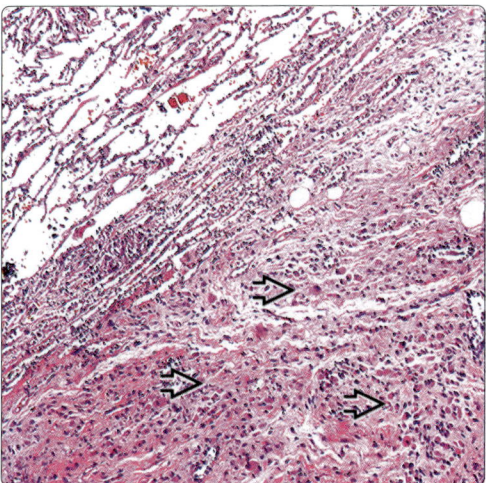

(Left) Wilms tumor mainly metastasizes to the 3 Ls: Lymph nodes, liver, and lungs. Other sites of metastasis are rare. Notice the benign hepatic parenchyma on the left side. (Right) The lung is a common site of metastasis for Wilms tumor. In spite of the basic differences in therapeutic approaches between COG and SIOP, overlaps are not uncommon. Most stage IV diseases in COG are treated by chemotherapy, and posttherapy resection specimens often show regression or differentiation, e.g., rhabdomyoblasts.

Cystic Partially Differentiated Nephroblastoma

KEY FACTS

TERMINOLOGY
- Cystic partially differentiated nephroblastoma (CPDN)
  - Entirely multilocular cystic tumor, mostly occurring before 2 years of age
  - Tumor with thin septations showing clusters of blastemal cells admixed with their derivatives
  - No expansile masses altering smooth contours of septa

CLINICAL ISSUES
- Radiologic distinction of cystic nephroma (CN), CPDN, and cystic Wilms tumor (CWT) is quite difficult
  - Definitive discrimination between 3 only possible on histologic evaluation
  - Distinction is essential for further therapy, since biologic behaviors are different
- Only 2 cases with recurrence, both with incomplete resection or spillage during surgery
  - 1 bilateral case with relapse as CWT also described

MACROSCOPIC
- No grossly apparent solid areas
- Often large (up to 18 cm), multicystic tumors

MICROSCOPIC
- Multilocular cystic tumor
- Cyst walls with blastemal clusters or their epithelial derivatives
  - Occasional mesenchymal elements also seen
- No expansile masses that alter smooth shape of septa

TOP DIFFERENTIAL DIAGNOSES
- Pediatric cystic nephroma
  - Previously regarded as related to CPDN; recently reported to be quite distinct with *DICER1* mutations
- CWT
- Cystic renal dysplasia
- Localized or segmental cystic kidney disease

Gross Features

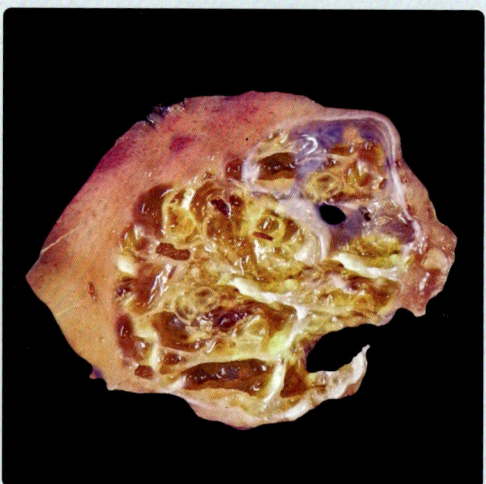

Histological Features

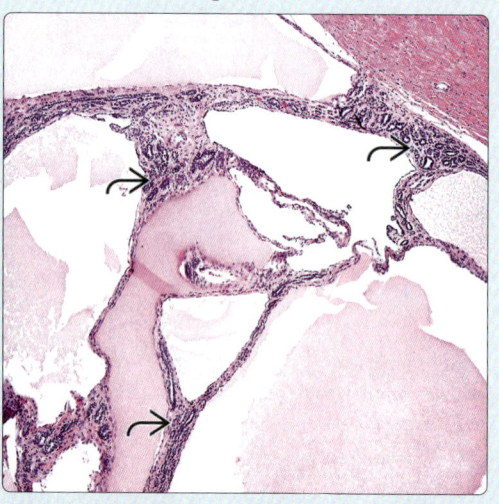

(Left) Multicystic tumor in pediatric kidneys may represent, among others, a cystic nephroma or cystic partially differentiated nephroblastoma (CPDN). Gross distinction between these entities is difficult. (Right) CPDN shows multilocular cysts with thin fibrovascular septa. Clusters of blastemal elements ⇨ are dispersed within the septa, without any distortion of the septal contours, or any expansile nodules.

Histological Features

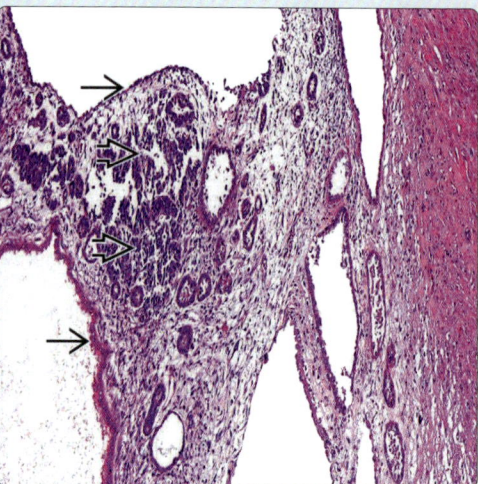

Differential Diagnosis: Cystic Wilms Tumor

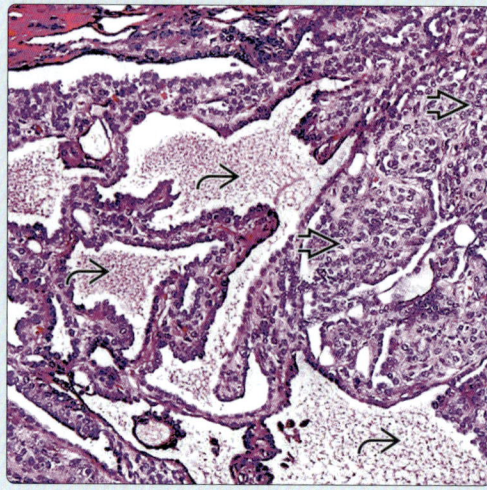

(Left) Cysts of CPDN may be lined by flat or cuboidal epithelium ⇨. Occasional cases show papillary excrescences. Immature blastemal or differentiating epithelial elements ⇨ within the septations of a multicystic tumor, without forming a nodular or mass-forming expansion, is diagnostic. (Right) This predominantly cystic ⇨ tumor shows solid areas of differentiating blastema/epithelial elements ⇨. Such expansile areas preclude its consideration as a CPDN and are characteristic of cystic Wilms tumor.

Cystic Partially Differentiated Nephroblastoma

TERMINOLOGY

Abbreviations
- Cystic partially differentiated nephroblastoma (CPDN)

Definitions
- Entirely multilocular cystic tumor, mostly occurring before 2 years of age
  - Tumor with thin septations showing clusters of blastemal cells admixed with their derivatives
  - No expansile masses altering smooth contours of septa
  - Luminal papulonodular protrusions are acceptable; such tumors classified as papulonodular type of CPDN

CLINICAL ISSUES

Histology vs. Radiologic Evaluation
- Radiologic distinction of cystic nephroma (CN), CPDN, and cystic Wilms tumor (CWT) quite difficult
  - CT shows well-defined expansile cystic masses
    - May also have variable amount of solid enhancing areas
- Definitive discrimination between 3 only possible on histologic evaluation
  - Distinction essential for further management, since biologic behaviors different
    - CN: Benign
    - CPDN: Usually nonaggressive clinical behavior; rare recurrences and relapses as CWT described
    - CWT: Malignant

Treatment
- COG recommends primary resection
  - No further therapy in stage I tumors
  - Rare stage II or higher stage tumors receive chemotherapy
- SIOP recommends therapy before resection
  - Since radiological evaluation not definitive, presurgery chemotherapy quite common in Europe
  - Recently, some experts questioned need of presurgery chemotherapy of cystic renal masses without any obvious solid components

Prognosis
- Only 2 cases with recurrence, both with incomplete resection or spillage during surgery
  - 1 bilateral case with relapse as CWT also described

MACROSCOPIC

General Features
- Often large (up to 18 cm), multicystic tumors
- No grossly apparent solid areas

MICROSCOPIC

Histologic Features
- Multilocular cystic tumor
  - Cysts usually lined by flat or cuboidal epithelium
  - Cyst walls with blastemal clusters or their epithelial derivatives
    - Occasional mesenchymal elements also seen
  - Some tumors with papillary or papulonodular excrescences protruding into cyst lumina
  - No expansile masses that alter smooth shape of septa

DIFFERENTIAL DIAGNOSIS

Pediatric Cystic Nephroma
- Tumor composed entirely of cysts and cyst septa without any blastemal, epithelial, or mesenchymal components
- Unlike cystic nephromas of adults, pediatric CN without any ovarian-type stroma
- Previously regarded as related to CPDN
  - Recently reported to be quite distinct, with *DICER1* mutations
  - These mutations not found in CPDN

Cystic Wilms Tumor
- Variably cystic tumor with solid expansile blastemal, epithelial, &/or mesenchymal elements
- Often, but not always, seen after chemotherapy

Cystic Renal Dysplasia
- Usually diffuse and bilateral
  - May be localized and segmental
- Often associated with obstruction to urinary outflow
  - Ureter and pelvicalyceal system often distorted and atretic
- Presence of primitive ducts lined by cuboidal to columnar epithelium, surrounded by cellular mesenchyme: Histologic hallmark
- Larger cysts lined by more flat epithelium, surrounded by fibrotic stroma, also common
- Small islands of cartilage and occasionally smooth muscle stroma may be present
- Ducts and cysts usually separated by fibrous stroma with scattered glomeruli, sometimes appearing immature or cystic

Localized or Segmental Cystic Kidney Disease
- Gross and microscopic appearance of cysts similar to that in autosomal dominant polycystic kidney disease
- Grossly, consists of clusters of spherical, thin-walled cysts, separated by areas of uninvolved kidney
- Cystic dilatation of Bowman capsule often present
  - Glomerulocystic change may be a predominant finding in infants

SELECTED REFERENCES

1. Doros LA et al: DICER1 mutations in childhood cystic nephroma and its relationship to DICER1-renal sarcoma. Mod Pathol. 27(9):1267-80, 2014
2. van den Hoek J et al: Cystic nephroma, cystic partially differentiated nephroblastoma and cystic Wilms' tumor in children: a spectrum with therapeutic dilemmas. Urol Int. 82(1):65-70, 2009
3. Baker JM et al: Stage III cystic partially differentiated nephroblastoma recurring after nephrectomy and chemotherapy. Pediatr Blood Cancer. 50(1):129-31, 2008
4. Rajangam K et al: Partial nephrectomy in cystic partially differentiated nephroblastoma. J Pediatr Surg. 35(3):510-2, 2000
5. Joshi VV et al: Pathologic delineation of the papillonodular type of cystic partially differentiated nephroblastoma. A review of 11 cases. Cancer. 66(7):1568-77, 1990
6. Joshi VV et al: Multilocular cyst of the kidney (cystic nephroma) and cystic, partially differentiated nephroblastoma. Terminology and criteria for diagnosis. Cancer. 64(2):466-79, 1989

Angiomyolipoma

KEY FACTS

TERMINOLOGY
- Angiomyolipoma (AML)
- Mesenchymal tumors believed to originate from so-called perivascular epithelioid cell (PEC)
- Closely related to other PEC-related group of tumors, including
  - Lymphangioleiomyomatosis, clear cell "sugar" tumors of lung, pancreas, and uterus, PEComas, and cardiac rhabdomyomas

ETIOLOGY/PATHOGENESIS
- ~ 80% patients of tuberous sclerosis with renal AML
- < 50% of AMLs in patients with tuberous sclerosis
- Associated with genetic alterations in tuberous sclerosis genes, *TSC1* (9q34) and *TSC2* (16p13.3)
  - Sporadic AMLs more often with mutations in *TSC2*; mutations in *TSC1* relatively infrequent

CLINICAL ISSUES
- Multifocality and bilaterality often associated with TSC
- Overwhelming majority with benign clinical behavior

MICROSCOPIC
- Typically contains adipose tissue, smooth muscle, and dystrophic vessels in variable proportions
- Uncommon types include predominantly lipomatous or leiomyomatous, lymphangioleiomyomatous, oncocytoma-like, sclerosing type, and AML with epithelial cysts
  - AMLs invariably positive for melanocytic markers [HMB-45, Melan-A (MART-1), MiTF, Cathepsin K]

TOP DIFFERENTIAL DIAGNOSES
- Liposarcoma
- Leiomyoma or leiomyosarcoma
- Renal oncocytoma
- Renal cell carcinoma with sarcomatoid differentiation

Gross Features

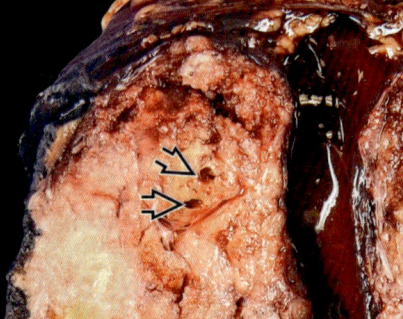

Gross Features

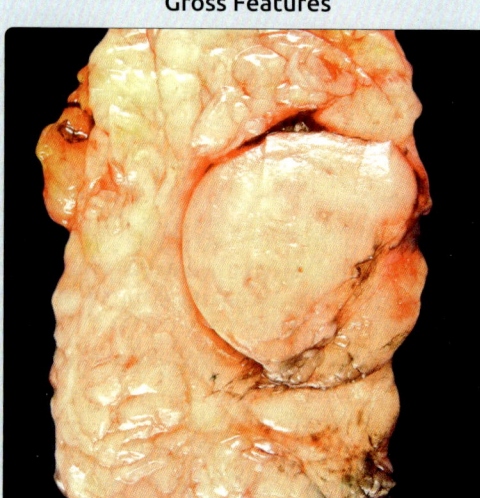

(Left) This typical angiomyolipoma (AML) with a variegated gross appearance reflects fatty ➡ and vascular ➡ areas. Some tumors, composed predominantly of smooth muscle, may have a uniform, firm, and whorled appearance, reminiscent of uterine leiomyomas. (Right) This lipomatous AML was resected with a clinical diagnosis of liposarcoma. Generous sampling is essential, and recognition of abnormal blood vessels and perivascular epithelioid cells is necessary in such tumors.

Perivascular Epithelioid Cells

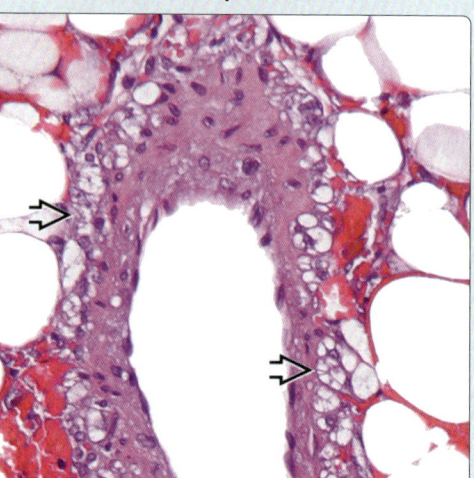

Spindle Cells

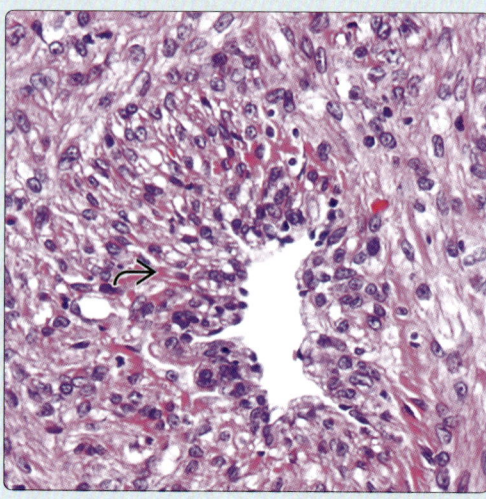

(Left) This hematoxylin and eosin section shows perivascular epithelioid cells (PEC) ➡. PEC is considered to be the cell of origin of AML and related tumors. However, no normal counterpart of PEC is known. (Right) Smooth muscle cells in AML are often seen originating and radiating out from vessel walls ➡. This typical finding helps in the accurate diagnosis in tumors with unusual histology (in lipomatous or leiomyomatous AML).

Angiomyolipoma

TERMINOLOGY

Abbreviations
- Angiomyolipoma (AML)

Definitions
- Mesenchymal tumor believed to originate from perivascular epithelioid cell (PEC)
- Closely related to other PEC-related group of tumors (e.g., lymphangioleiomyomatosis, clear cell "sugar" tumors of lung, pancreas, and uterus, PEComas, and cardiac rhabdomyomas)

ETIOLOGY/PATHOGENESIS

Tuberous Sclerosis Complex
- ~ 80% patients with tuberous sclerosis develop renal AML
- Less than 50% of patients with renal AMLs have tuberous sclerosis
- TSC associated with genetic alterations in tuberous sclerosis genes, *TSC1* (9q34) and *TSC2* (16p13.3)
  - Sporadic AMLs more often with mutations in *TSC2*; mutations in *TSC1* relatively infrequent

Mammalian Target of Rapamycin (mTOR) Pathway
- Proteins encoded by *TSC1* (hamartin) and *TSC2* genes (tuberin) function as complex to negatively regulate mammalian target of rapamycin (mTOR) signaling
  - Negative regulation done through activation of Ras homologue expressed in brain (*RHEB*)
    - *RHEB*: Specific GTPase is located downstream of tuberin
    - Altered TSC gene functions generate excessive *RHEB*-GTP
    - This leads to increased activated mTOR, activator of multiple protein synthesis pathways and possible tumorigenesis
- Activated mTOR pathway markers overexpressed in AML and related tumors

CLINICAL ISSUES

Presentation
- Most sporadic cases diagnosed incidentally by radiological investigations for other conditions
- Multifocality and bilaterality is often associated with tuberous sclerosis
  - AMLs seen in patients with tuberous sclerosis also tend to manifest at younger age
- Presence of synchronous or metachronous involvement of other sites regarded as manifestation of multicentric disease rather than metastasis
- Small tumors usually asymptomatic
  - > 75% of resected tumors in 1 recent series asymptomatic, with overall mean size of 3.5 cm
  - Larger tumors (usually > 4 cm) occasionally present with hemorrhage and shock
    - Tumor size often increases in pregnancy and may increase risk of hemorrhage
  - Extreme multifocality occasionally associated with renal failure
- Classic fat-containing tumors often easily diagnosed on radiologic evaluation
- Tumors with scant fat or other uncommon features often difficult to diagnose radiologically
  - Rarely, intratumoral hemorrhage may mask fat, hindering radiologic diagnosis

Treatment
- No treatment required in most asymptomatic, small, radiologically definite AMLs
  - Resection often delayed by surgeons until tumor attains size of 4 cm or greater

Prognosis
- Overwhelming majority with benign clinical behavior
- Retroperitoneal hemorrhage is rare complication that can be fatal
  - Large tumor size important factor in this complication
- Rare aggressive behavior, particularly those with predominant epithelioid and other atypical features

IMAGING

CT Findings
- Unenhanced CT with thin sections usually permits specific diagnosis of renal AML by demonstrating presence of intratumoral fat
  - However, intratumoral fat not detectable reportedly in ~ 5%; such tumors often difficult to diagnose both by CT or MR

MACROSCOPIC

Key Findings
- Often well circumscribed but not encapsulated
- Mean size: 6 cm (range: 0.50-25 cm)
- Cut surface variable, reflecting relative proportion of fat, smooth muscle, or vessels in tumor

MICROSCOPIC

Histologic Features
- Typically contains adipose tissue, smooth muscle, and dystrophic vessels in variable proportions
  - Areas of mature adipose tissue are present in over 90% of tumors, at least focally
  - Smooth muscle component as fascicles of spindle cells or sheets of epithelioid cells with abundant eosinophilic granular cytoplasm
    - Tumors with prominent spindled smooth muscle frequently with thin-walled vessels showing hemangiopericytoma-like architecture
    - Smooth muscle cells often appear to originate and radiate from vessel walls
  - Thickened and hyalinized vessels with eccentric lumina seen in most cases
  - Mitotic activity very rare
- Uncommon types include predominantly lipomatous or leiomyomatous, lymphangioleiomyomatous, oncocytoma-like, and sclerosing type
- Smooth muscle predominant or exclusive tumors arising from renal capsule, so-called renal capsulomas, often HMB-45(+)
  - Most believe capsulomas to be leiomyomatous AMLs
- AML with epithelial cysts (AMLEC), rare variant

Angiomyolipoma

- o Epithelial cysts lined by cuboidal to hobnailed cells
- o Layer of cellular, müllerian-like stroma with prominent admixed chronic inflammation surrounding cysts in AML
- o Cysts believed to arise from trapped renal tubules by some (supported by pax-8 positivity in these tubules); some others regard tubules as integral part of tumor
- Ultrastructural evaluation reveals
  - o Spherical structures with internal lamellations, consistent with aberrant melanosomes
  - o Rare type 2 premelanosomes; rhomboid crystals in some cases

Lymphatic/Vascular Invasion

- Vascular invasion, including that of large renal sinus vessels, renal vein, or inferior vena cava may be present
  - o No adverse influences on prognosis, if tumor otherwise typical

Lymph Nodes

- Regional lymph nodes occasionally contain AMLs
  - o Considered tumor multicentricity
  - o No such patients reported to die of disease progression

ANCILLARY TESTS

Immunohistochemistry

- Expression of melanocytic markers: HMB-45, Melan-A(MART-1), MiTF, tyrosinase, cathepsin K
  - o More common in epithelioid cells
- Expression of smooth muscle markers (actin-sm and h-caldesmon)
- Negative immunoreactivity for epithelial markers (cytokeratin, EMA/MUC1), except in epithelial cysts of AMLEC
- Periepithelial stroma in AMLEC: positive staining for ER, PR, CD10
- Immunohistochemistry useful adjunct in tumors with unusual pattern; but usually not necessary in triphasic tumors

DIFFERENTIAL DIAGNOSIS

Liposarcoma

- Mostly extrarenal, surrounding kidney
- Lack of dysmorphic vessels &/or smooth muscle component
- Negative staining for melanocytic markers [HMB-45, Melan-A (MART-1), MiTF]
  - o Caution: Immunoreactivity in fat-predominant AML usually in very few cells
- Positive immunoreactivity for mdm2 and CDK4

Leiomyoma or Leiomyosarcoma

- True primary smooth muscle tumors very rare in kidney
- No intratumoral fat or dysmorphic vessels present even after careful search for these
- Melanocytic markers negative

Renal Oncocytoma

- Cells usually arranged in nests and solid alveoli
- Uniform nuclei, with occasional foci of marked pleomorphism
- Presence of groups of smaller cells (oncoblasts)

- Epithelial markers positive; melanocytic markers negative

Renal Cell Carcinoma With Sarcomatoid Differentiation

- AML with focal epithelioid features and with prominent spindle cell component may be misinterpreted as renal cell carcinoma with sarcomatoid features
- AML may show focal dysmorphophobic vessels and lipocytes
- Immunostains and generous sampling of immense utility in difficult cases

DIAGNOSTIC CHECKLIST

Pathologic Interpretation Pearls

- Primary smooth muscle tumors of kidney are extremely rare
  - o Smooth muscle predominant AML should always be excluded before accepting such diagnosis
  - o Immunohistochemical staining for melanocytic markers of all primary smooth muscle tumors in kidney practical approach
- Lipomatous tumors lack large abnormal vessels
  - o Fat-predominant AML to be excluded even if only rare dysmorphic vessels and focal spindle cells observed
    - Staining for melanocytic markers and careful evaluation for even focal positivity imperative in such lesions

SELECTED REFERENCES

1. Martignoni G et al: PEComas of the kidney and of the genitourinary tract. Semin Diagn Pathol. 32(2):140-59, 2015
2. Kingswood JC et al: The effect of everolimus on renal angiomyolipoma in patients with tuberous sclerosis complex being treated for subependymal giant cell astrocytoma: subgroup results from the randomized, placebo-controlled, Phase 3 trial EXIST-1. Nephrol Dial Transplant. 29(6):1203-10, 2014
3. He W et al: Epithelioid angiomyolipoma of the kidney: pathological features and clinical outcome in a series of consecutively resected tumors. Mod Pathol. 26(10):1355-64, 2013
4. Lienert AR et al: Renal angiomyolipoma. BJU Int. 110 Suppl 4:25-7, 2012
5. Aydin H et al: Renal angiomyolipoma: clinicopathologic study of 194 cases with emphasis on the epithelioid histology and tuberous sclerosis association. Am J Surg Pathol. 33(2):289-97, 2009
6. Lane BR et al: Clinical correlates of renal angiomyolipoma subtypes in 209 patients: classic, fat poor, tuberous sclerosis associated and epithelioid. J Urol. 180(3):836-43, 2008
7. Pan CC et al: Constant allelic alteration on chromosome 16p (TSC2 gene) in perivascular epithelioid cell tumour (PEComa): genetic evidence for the relationship of PEComa with angiomyolipoma. J Pathol. 214(3):387-93, 2008
8. Kenerson H et al: Activation of the mTOR pathway in sporadic angiomyolipomas and other perivascular epithelioid cell neoplasms. Hum Pathol. 38(9):1361-71, 2007
9. Fine SW et al: Angiomyolipoma with epithelial cysts (AMLEC): a distinct cystic variant of angiomyolipoma. Am J Surg Pathol. 30(5):593-9, 2006
10. Martignoni G et al: Oncocytoma-like angiomyolipoma. A clinicopathologic and immunohistochemical study of 2 cases. Arch Pathol Lab Med. 126(5):610-2, 2002
11. Zamboni G et al: Clear cell "sugar" tumor of the pancreas. A novel member of the family of lesions characterized by the presence of perivascular epithelioid cells. Am J Surg Pathol. 20(6):722-30, 1996
12. Henske EP et al: Loss of heterozygosity in the tuberous sclerosis (TSC2) region of chromosome band 16p13 occurs in sporadic as well as TSC-associated renal angiomyolipomas. Genes Chromosomes Cancer. 13(4):295-8, 1995
13. Bonetti F et al: Clear cell ("sugar") tumor of the lung is a lesion strictly related to angiomyolipoma–the concept of a family of lesions characterized by the presence of the perivascular epithelioid cells (PEC). Pathology. 26(3):230-6, 1994

Angiomyolipoma

Triphasic Angiomyolipoma
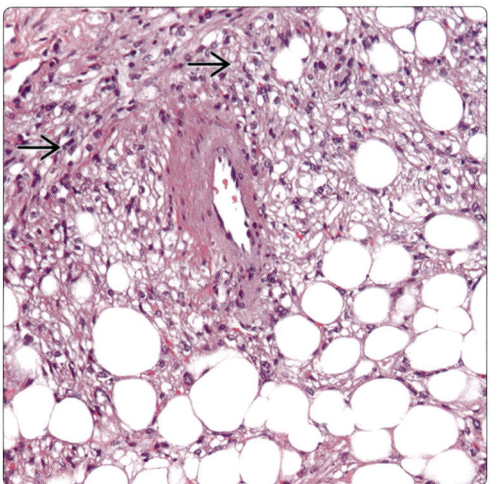

Triphasic Angiomyolipoma
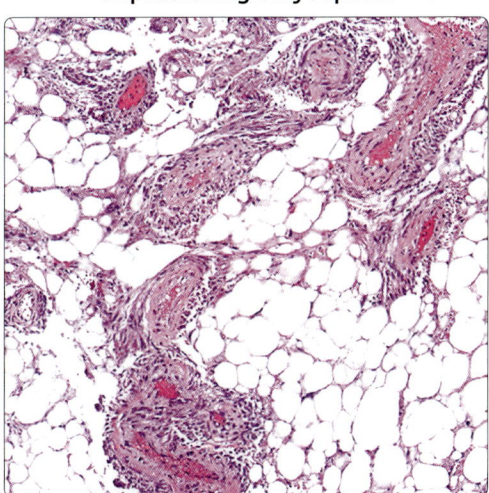

(Left) Hematoxylin and eosin stained section shows a typical triphasic AML composed of fat, spindled, smooth, muscle fascicles ➡ and a dysmorphic blood vessel. The smooth muscle cells in this image have an epithelioid appearance and emanate from the vascular wall. (Right) The vast majority of AML are triphasic. Dysmorphic vessels in these tumors often show marked variation in the thickness and disorganization of the musculature of the vessel walls.

Leiomyomatous Angiomyolipoma
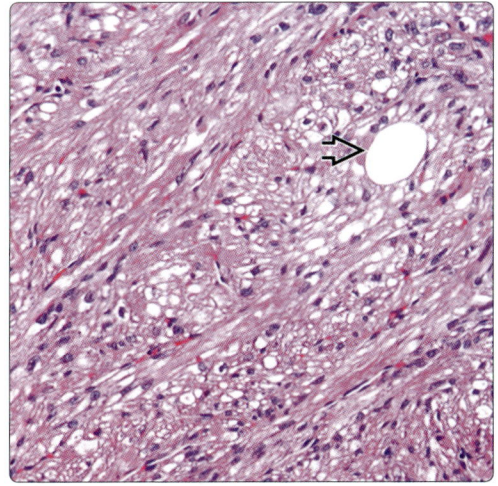

Lipomatous Angiomyolipoma
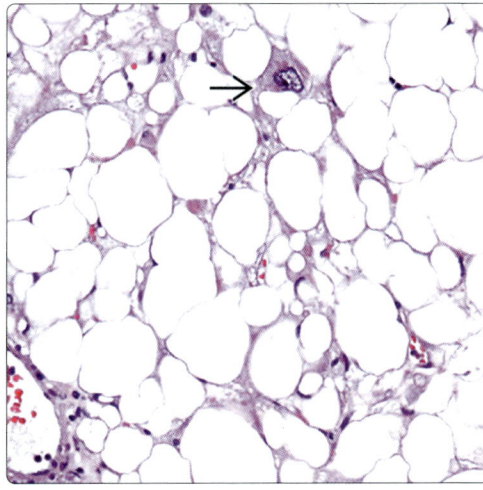

(Left) Some AMLs are predominantly leiomyomatous. Primary smooth muscle tumors of the kidney are very rare. Careful search for lipocytes ➡ and dysmorphic vessels is imperative in such tumors. (Right) Fat-predominant AML with atypical lipocytes ➡ may be mistaken for a liposarcoma. Atypical vasculature and appropriate support by immunostains for melanocytic and smooth muscle markers will help in making the correct diagnosis in both the leiomyomatous and lipomatous AML.

Focal Epithelioid Features
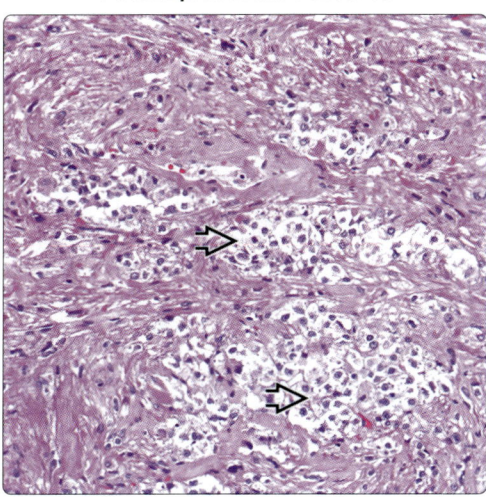

Lymphangiomyomatous Angiomyolipoma
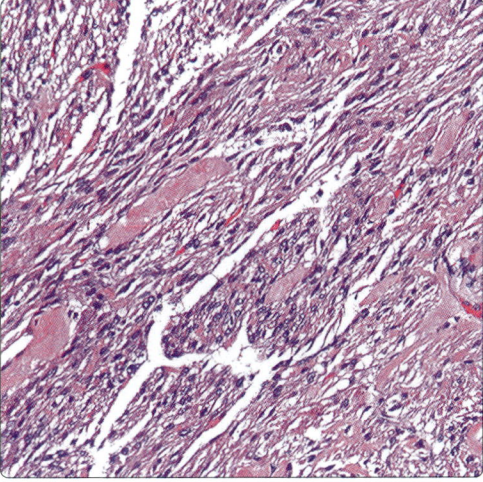

(Left) Occasionally, AMLs show foci with epithelioid features and clear cell cytology ➡. Tumors with prominence of such areas have been designated as epithelioid angiomyolipomas. These epithelioid areas are negative for cytokeratin and usually show strong expression of melanocytic markers. (Right) Smooth muscle predominant AML sometimes display a lymphangioleiomyomatous pattern. This pattern is often more conspicuous in pulmonary PEC-associated lesions in tuberous sclerosis.

Angiomyolipoma

Renal Capsuloma

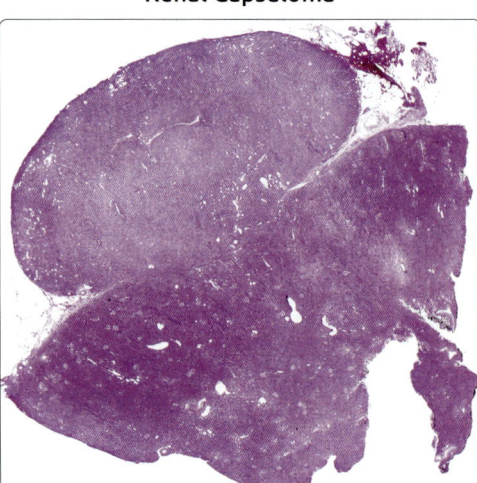

(Left) This H&E-stained section shows a whole mount of a leiomyomatous AML arising from the renal capsule. Such tumors have been called renal capsulomas by some. Immunoexpression of melanocytic markers is confirmatory of AML. (Right) Focal sclerosis is quite common in renal AML, but rare tumors may show extensive sclerosis ⟹. Such tumors have been designated as sclerosing AML. Immunohistochemistry is a useful diagnostic adjunct in AMLs with unusual histologic patterns.

Sclerosing Angiomyolipoma

Oncocytoma-Like Angiomyolipoma

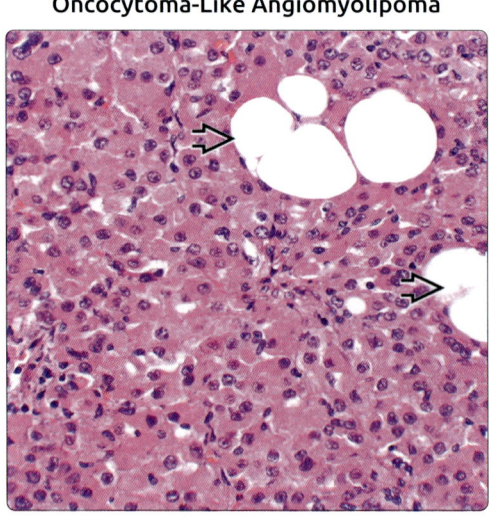

(Left) Oncocytoma-like AML is a rare variant of AML. The presence of dysmorphic vessels, sclerosing areas, adipocytes ⟹, and nuclear variability should point toward the appropriate diagnosis. These are also diffusely positive for HMB-45/Melan-A (MART-1) and negative for epithelial markers. (Right) Angiomyolipoma with epithelial cysts (AMLEC) show cysts lined by cuboidal epithelium with eosinophilic cytoplasm ⟹. Occasionally this cystic component may be conspicuous.

Angiomyolipoma With Epithelial Cysts

Vascular Invasion

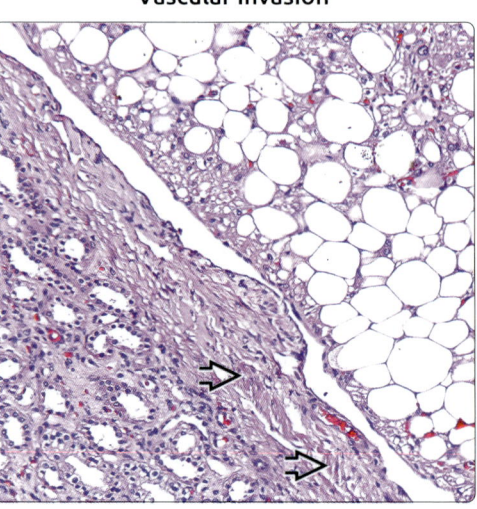

(Left) A large muscular vein ⟹ is involved by a typical triphasic neoplasm. AML may show vascular invasion, rarely even involving the renal vein or inferior vena cava. This finding is not associated with aggressive tumoral behavior. (Right) A definitive diagnosis of renal AML can be rendered on needle core biopsies. While the diagnosis is straightforward in tumors with typical triphasic morphology, immunohistochemical support is often required in tumors with mono/biphasic histology.

Angiomyolipoma in Renal Biopsy

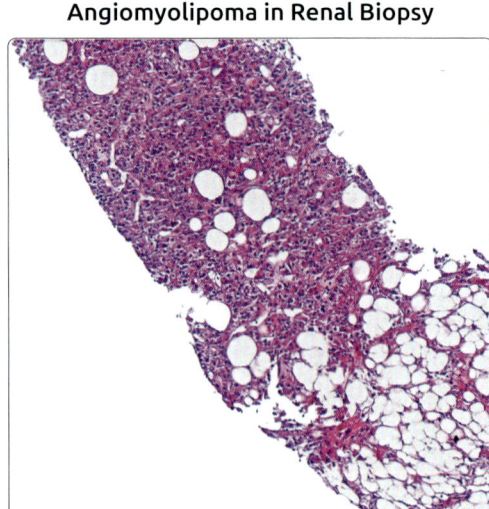

Angiomyolipoma

HMB-45
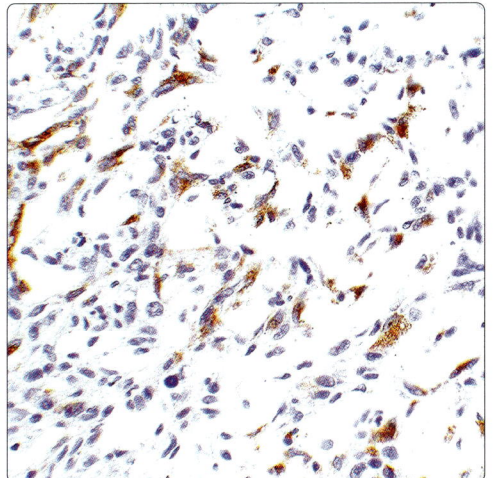

Smooth Muscle Actin
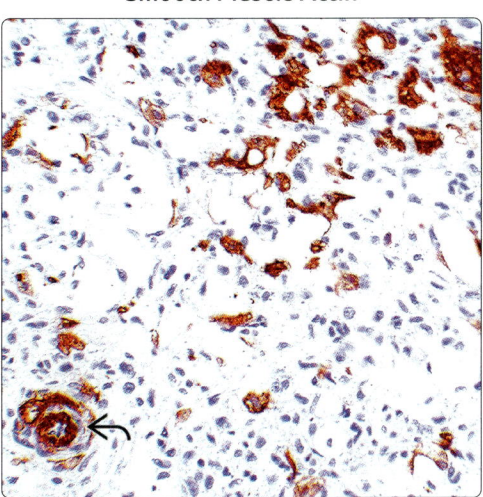

(Left) HMB-45 (seen here) &/or Melan-A (MART-1) immunostains are invariably positive in AML. The staining pattern may vary according to the cell type; positivity is often most prominent in epithelioid smooth muscle cells. (Right) Smooth muscle actin shows positivity in spindled and epithelioid smooth muscle cells. Note the positivity in a vessel wall ➔ that acts as an internal control. HMB-45 and Melan-A (MART-1) show stronger expression in epithelioid areas, while actin-sm is positive in spindled cells.

HMB-45 in Leiomyomatous Angiomyolipoma
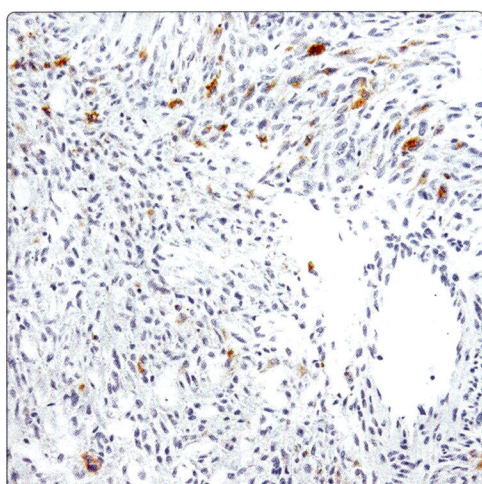

HMB-45 in Lipomatous Angiomyolipoma
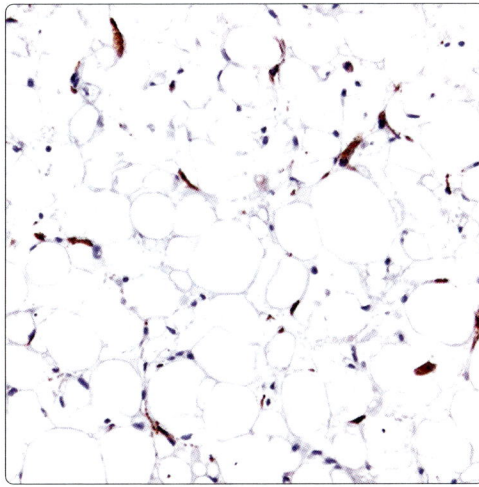

(Left) Immunohistochemical staining for HMB-45 is often only very focal in predominantly leiomyomatous or lipomatous AML. Recognition of positivity may require careful evaluation at high magnification in such tumors. (Right) HMB-45 shows positivity in a fat-predominant angiomyolipoma; the positivity is always focal in fatty areas. Nonrecognition of such focal positivity may result in misdiagnosis of a lipomatous tumor, in particular well-differentiated liposarcoma.

cathepsin-K
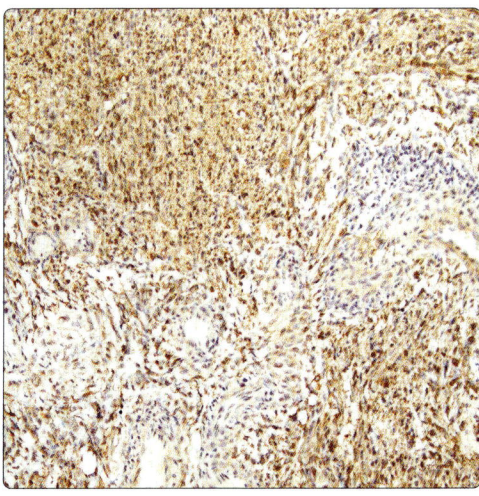

CD10 in Angiomyolipoma With Epithelial Cysts
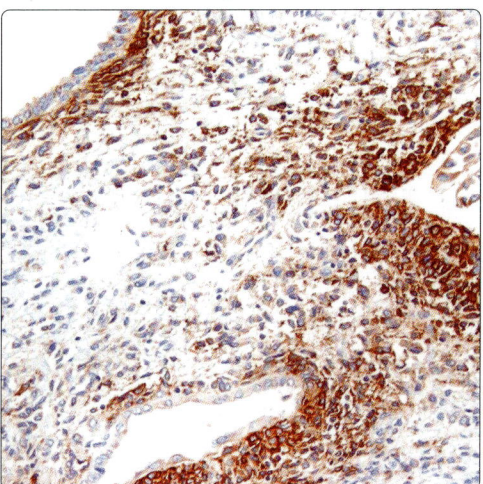

(Left) Most AMLs show strong immunoreactivity with cathepsin-K. cathepsin-K is reported to be a more sensitive marker in AML than HMB-45 and Melan-A. (Right) Spindle cells in AMLEC are usually HMB-45 and Melan-A(+), but epithelial cells lining the cysts are negative. These lining cells are often pax-8 immunoreactive. The stroma around the epithelial component is usually positive for CD10. This is in keeping with the light microscopic appearance of the spindle cells resembling cellular müllerian-like stroma.

Epithelioid Angiomyolipoma

KEY FACTS

TERMINOLOGY
- Epithelioid angiomyolipoma (E-AML)

CLINICAL ISSUES
- In one large study based on 437 consecutive resections of AML, with cut-off of ≥ 80% epithelioid cells for designation of E-AML, < 5% of all AMLs were E-AML
- Mammalian target of rapamycin (mTOR) pathway is shown to be activated in many tumors
- Many angiomyolipomas with metastases have epithelioid features and contain pleomorphic, multinucleated cells
- Overall true incidence of metastasis among all cases of E-AML likely < 5%, although higher rate has been reported

MACROSCOPIC
- Mostly solid
- Often with hemorrhagic cut surface, areas of necrosis, and cystic change

MICROSCOPIC
- Cells arranged as cohesive nests, broad alveoli, and sheets separated by thin vascular septa
- Plump spindled and epithelioid cells arranged in diffuse sheets, with less prominent vascularity
- Cells with clear or eosinophilic cytoplasm
- Pleomorphic multinucleated cells
- Tumors with ≥ 70% atypical epithelioid cells, ≥ 2 mitotic figures per 10 HPF, atypical mitotic figures, and necrosis- associated with metastasis
  - However, in primary resections, presence of these feature do not necessarily predict aggressive behavior

TOP DIFFERENTIAL DIAGNOSES
- Clear cell renal cell carcinoma
- Chromophobe renal cell carcinoma
- Metastatic malignant melanoma

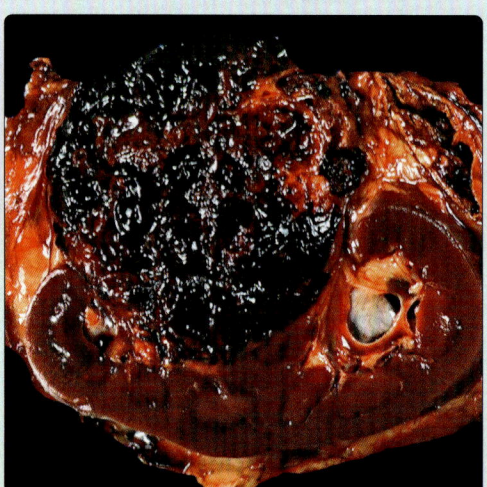

Gross Features

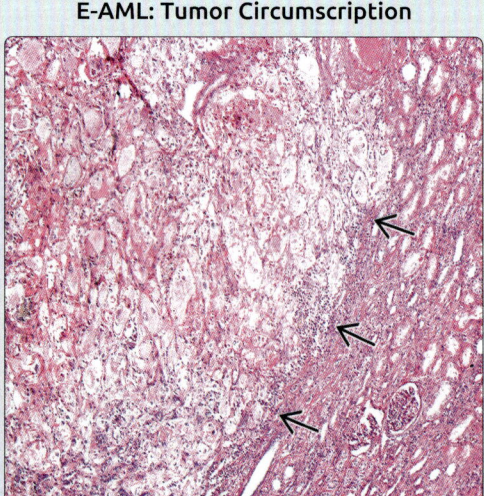

E-AML: Tumor Circumscription

(Left) Epithelioid angiomyolipomas (E-AMLs) are usually large tumors that are mostly well circumscribed, frequently with extensive hemorrhage and necrosis. Some tumors may have a more homogeneous tan cut surface. *(Right)* As often seen on gross evaluation, E-AMLs microscopically appear well circumscribed, without a discernible capsule, and in direct contact with nonneoplastic renal parenchyma ➡; however, rare tumors may show infiltrative margins.

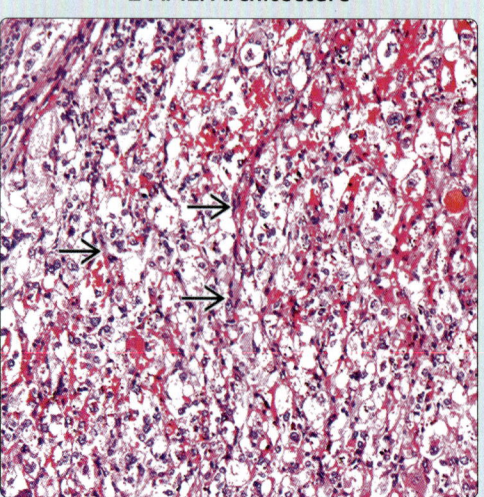

E-AML: Architecture

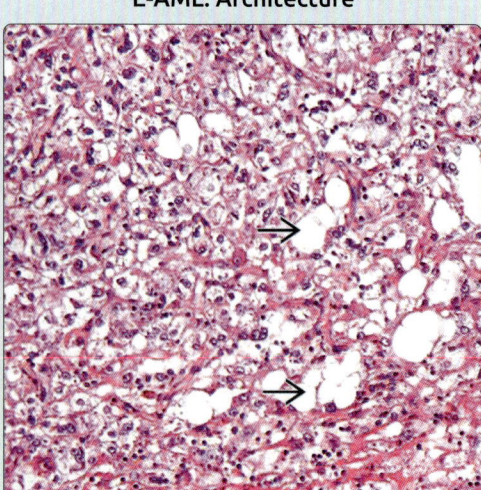

E-AML: Architecture

(Left) Microscopically, E-AMLs may show nests, alveoli, and sheets of cells separated by thin vascular septa ➡. Such architecture often leads to misdiagnosis as clear cell renal cell carcinoma. *(Right)* This E-AML shows nested growth pattern with prominent vascularity; however, the clear cells are not optically clear and show irregular cytoplasmic granularity. Many E-AMLs show the focal presence of adipocytes ➡ or dysmorphic vessels.

Epithelioid Angiomyolipoma

TERMINOLOGY

Abbreviations
- Epithelioid angiomyolipoma (E-AML)

Synonyms
- Epithelioid perivascular epithelial cell (PEC)oma (epithelioid PEComa)

Definitions
- Mesenchymal tumor believed to originate from PEC with predominant epithelioid features
  - Closely related to usual (triphasic) AML
  - Percentage of tumor with epithelioid morphology that constitutes predominant is not established
    - 2 recent large studies used cut-off of ≥ 80% and > 95% epithelioid histology
    - Others have used > 10% or > 50% epithelioid cells as cut-off
    - Based on > 110 reported cases in recent 4 largest series, all tumors developing metastases had ≥ 80% epithelioid histology
  - Some tumors are morphologically similar to PEComas of soft tissues

ETIOLOGY/PATHOGENESIS

Tuberous Sclerosis Complex and mTOR Pathway
- Like typical AML, E-AML is associated with genetic alterations in tuberous sclerosis complex (TSC) genes, *TSC1* (9q34) and *TSC2* (16p13.3)
  - *TSC2* gene involved more often than TSC1 in E-AML
- Hamartin and tuberin proteins encoded by *TSC1* and *TSC2* genes, respectively, negatively regulate mTOR signaling
  - Alterations or absence of these proteins results in increased activated mammalian target of rapamycin (mTOR), and consequential tumorigenesis
- AMLs in patients with TSC syndrome believed to more often show epithelioid features (> 25%), compared to AML in those without TSC (7%)
  - However, some more recent studies do not show such association

TP53 Mutations
- Reported in some E-AML

TFE3 Gene Fusions
- Subset of PEComas harbor *TFE3* fusions, although this event is rare among renal tumors
  - Tumors with *TFE3* fusions often do not show TSC mutations

CLINICAL ISSUES

Epidemiology
- Incidence
  - In one large study based on 437 consecutive resections of AML with cut-off of ≥ 80% epithelioid cells for designation of E-AML
    - < 5% of all AMLs as E-AML
- Age
  - Mean at presentation: 50 years (range: 14–80)

Presentation
- Mostly similar to that for usual angiomyolipoma
- Cases associated with tuberous sclerosis often present with
  - Younger age at presentation and multiple tumors including small usual angiomyolipomas
- Some tumors have metastases at presentation

Treatment
- Adjuvant therapy
  - mTOR pathway shown to be activated in many tumors
    - Targeted therapies: mTOR inhibitor sirolimus proven effective in some tumors
    - However, many tumors tend to regrow once therapy is stopped
  - EGFR inhibitor, gefitinib, has also recently been shown to be useful in rare cases

Prognosis
- E-AMLs may have metastasis or recurrence and hence are considered potentially malignant
  - Sites of metastases include
    - Liver (most common), lymph nodes, lungs, retroperitoneal organs and mesentery, bones, and other rare sites
- In spite of some studies indicating high probability of metastases, true incidence of metastasis among all cases of E-AML likely low
  - In recent largest consecutively resected E-AML series, with long mean follow-up, metastatic rate was < 5%
  - In another recent study of > 40 cases, likely influenced by referral bias, rate of metastasis as high as > 45%
- Reported pathologic indicators associated with metastatic tumors include
  - ≥ 70% atypical epithelioid cells, ≥ 2 mitotic figures per 10 HPF, atypical mitotic figures, and necrosis
    - Tumors with malignant behavior often associated with the presence of 3 or more of these features
    - Large tumors (> 5 cm), perinephric extension (Nese criteria)
- However, presence of these features in consecutively resected E-AML not necessary predictors of aggressive behavior

MACROSCOPIC

General Features
- Frequently solid
- Most are well circumscribed but some with gross extrarenal extension
- Often show hemorrhagic cut surface, frequently have necrosis and cystic change

MICROSCOPIC

Histologic Features
- Epithelioid features in tumors characterized by the following
  - Architectural patterns
    - Cells arranged as cohesive nests, broad alveoli, and sheets separated by thin vascular septa

Epithelioid Angiomyolipoma

- Plump spindled and epithelioid cells arranged in diffuse sheets, with less prominent vascularity (similar to many soft tissue PEComas)
- Occasionally, with glomus tumor-like perivascular arrangement of cells with dilated vascular spaces
  - Such tumors may also contain branching, dilated vessels with hemangiopericytomatous pattern
- Cytologic features
  - Some tumors consisting of large cells with eosinophilic cytoplasm and atypical nuclei bearing prominent nucleoli
    - Occasional eosinophilic cells with peripheral clearing; intranuclear inclusions frequent
    - Markedly pleomorphic, multinucleated giant cells also frequent
  - Others consisting of smaller, uniform epithelioid cells with clear or finely granular cytoplasm, and mostly uniform nuclei
    - Occasional tumors also show plump, spindle cells and multinucleated giant cells with uniform nuclei
  - Pleomorphic and more uniform areas may coexist in some tumors
  - Mitoses are commonly observed in E-AML
    - Most mitoses are typical; rarely atypical mitoses
    - In some cases, mitotic activity is quite brisk (> 5-8/10 HPF)
    - Mitotic activity more common and brisk in tumors with pleomorphic epithelioid and multinucleated giant cells
- Areas of tumor necrosis may be observed
- Vascular and extrarenal fat invasion, both perinephric and in renal sinus, not uncommon

ANCILLARY TESTS

Immunohistochemistry
- Epithelioid cells in E-AML usually show strong and diffuse positivity for melanocytic markers and smooth muscle markers
  - HMB-45, MITF, Melan-A (MART-1), tyrosinase: Positive; S100: Negative
  - Actin-sm frequently positive; may be focal
- Cathepsin K strongly and diffusely positive
- Epithelial markers (including EMA/MUC1 and various cytokeratins) negative
- Also reported to display positivity for CD1a, a molecule typically expressed in Langerhans cell histiocytosis

DIFFERENTIAL DIAGNOSIS

Clear Cell Renal Cell Carcinoma
- E-AML are often mistaken for clear cell renal cell carcinoma (CC-RCC) because of
  - Presence of clear cell histology
  - Eosinophilic cells with solid nested/alveolar growth pattern
  - Cells with pleomorphic lobulated nuclei (feature commonly present in high-grade CC-RCC)
- CC-RCC frequently shows
  - Intricately branching vascular septa, usually very well formed, enclosing nests of clear cells

- Careful examination of E-AML may often reveal focal presence of
  - Adipocytes &/or occasional dysmorphic vessels
- Immunostains for CA9, CD10, EMA/MUC1, and cytokeratins are usually positive in CC-RCC
  - Stains for melanocytic markers, HMB-45, Melan-A (MART-1), and MITF, Cathepsin K, and actin-sm are negative in CC-RCC

Chromophobe Renal Cell Carcinoma
- Pattern of growth is predominantly solid, separated by thin incomplete fibrovascular septa
- Most characteristic histological feature: Hyperchromatic nuclei with irregular, wrinkled outlines (raisinoid nuclei) with perinuclear halos

Metastatic Malignant Melanoma
- Melanomas show spectrum of morphologic patterns and are positive for melanocytic markers, similar to E-AML
- They are most often positive for S100, which is very uncommon in E-AML
- Adipocytes and dysmorphic vessels are not seen in malignant melanoma
- Clinical history of primary melanoma may be useful
- Metastatic malignant melanoma may be multifocal

DIAGNOSTIC CHECKLIST

Pathologic Interpretation Pearls
- Tumor with potentially aggressive biologic behavior
  - Percentage of cells with epithelioid features required to classify tumor as E-AML not finally determined
    - Almost all tumors with metastases on follow-up had ≥ 80% epithelioid cells
    - True incidence of metastatic potential < 5%
    - Most reported cases with high metastatic incidence (45-50%) primarily based on case reports or consultation cases with referral bias
- High index of suspicion for E-AML necessary before diagnosis of unclassified RCC is made
  - In needle biopsies, PAN-CK(AE1/AE3), HMB-45, Melan-A (MART-1), MITF, and cathepsin-K stain in appropriate morphological setting useful screening markers for this tumor

SELECTED REFERENCES

1. Martignoni G et al: PEComas of the kidney and of the genitourinary tract. Semin Diagn Pathol. 32(2):140-59, 2015
2. He W et al: Epithelioid angiomyolipoma of the kidney: pathological features and clinical outcome in a series of consecutively resected tumors. Mod Pathol. 26(10):1355-64, 2013
3. Martignoni G et al: Cathepsin K expression in the spectrum of perivascular epithelioid cell (PEC) lesions of the kidney. Mod Pathol. 25(1):100-11, 2012
4. Nese N et al: Pure epithelioid PEComas (so-called epithelioid angiomyolipoma) of the kidney: A clinicopathologic study of 41 cases: detailed assessment of morphology and risk stratification. Am J Surg Pathol. 35(2):161-76, 2011
5. Argani P et al: A distinctive subset of PEComas harbors TFE3 gene fusions. Am J Surg Pathol. 34(10):1395-406, 2010
6. Brimo F et al: Renal epithelioid angiomyolipoma with atypia: a series of 40 cases with emphasis on clinicopathologic prognostic indicators of malignancy. Am J Surg Pathol. 34(5):715-22, 2010
7. Krischock L et al: Sirolimus and tuberous sclerosis-associated renal angiomyolipomas. Arch Dis Child. 95(5):391-2, 2010
8. Aydin H et al: Renal angiomyolipoma: clinicopathologic study of 194 cases with emphasis on the epithelioid histology and tuberous sclerosis association. Am J Surg Pathol. 33(2):289-97, 2009

Epithelioid Angiomyolipoma

E-AML: Clear and Eosinophilic Cells

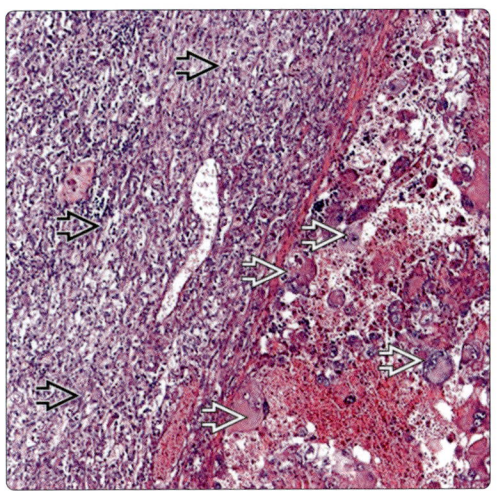

E-AML: Giant Cells

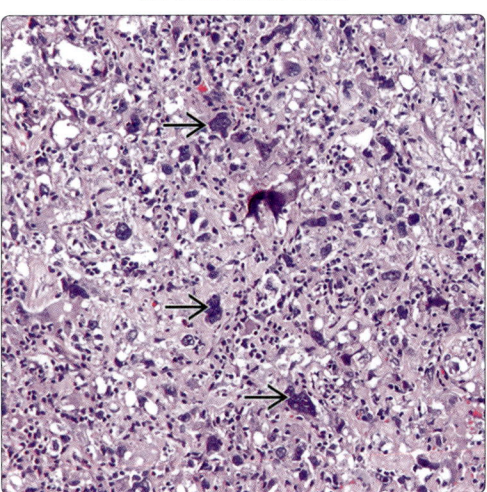

(Left) This E-AML shows a mixture of clear cell cytology ➡ with relatively low-grade nuclei and high-grade areas with eosinophilic cytoplasm and multinucleated tumor giant cells ➡. Such tumors closely mimic CC-RCC. *(Right)* It is not uncommon to see multinucleated, pleomorphic giant cells ➡ in E-AML. Presence of such giant cells in an epithelioid tumor should raise the differential diagnostic possibilities of clear cell and chromophobe RCC, in addition to E-AML. Confirmation of diagnosis needs IHC support.

E-AML: Ki-67 in Giant Cells

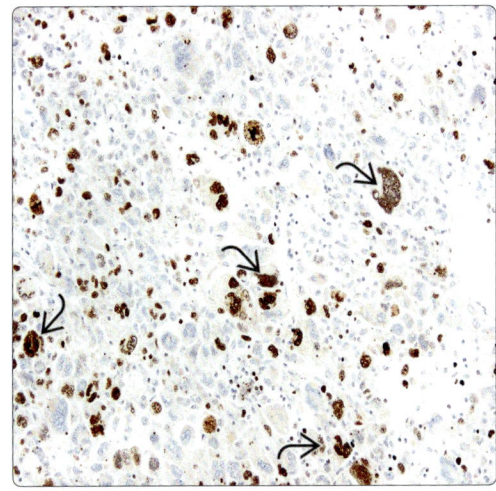

E-AML: Eosinophilic Areas

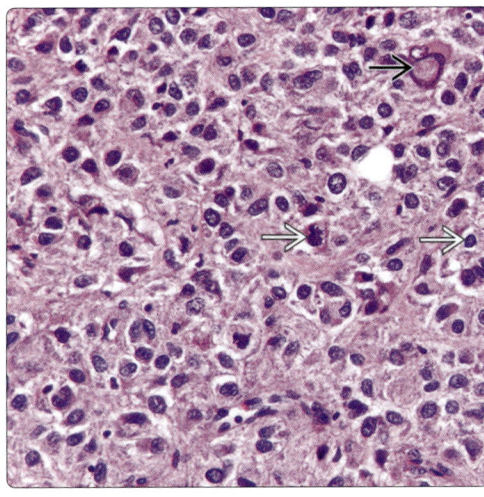

(Left) Ki-67 IHC shows that the pleomorphic giant cells in E-AML are not degenerating (as in chromophobe RCC), but an actively proliferating component of the tumor. Ki-67 shows labeling of many giant cells ➡. *(Right)* H&E shows sheet-like growth pattern of plump epithelioid cells. Note the absence of prominent vascularity in this case. Intranuclear pseudoinclusions ➡ and mitotic activity ➡ are also present; both of these features are not uncommon in E-AML.

E-AML: Clear Cells

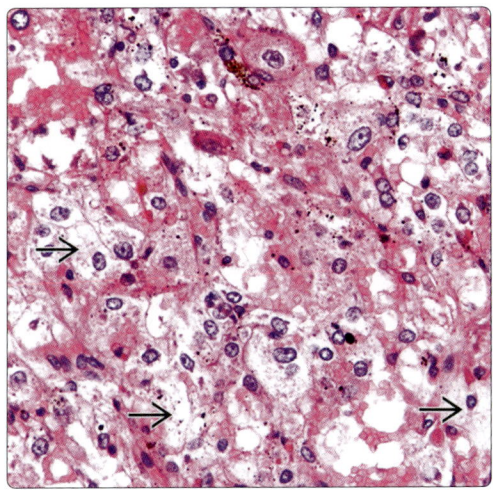

Typical AML With Epithelioid Areas

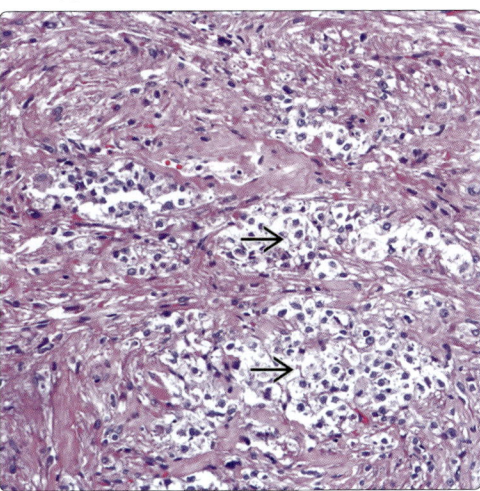

(Left) The epithelioid cells in E-AML often show clear cytoplasm. Frequently, these clear cells show irregularly dispersed intracytoplasmic granules ➡. The granularity may be perinuclear, with the periphery of the cytoplasm appearing more clear. *(Right)* A major contentious issue is when to designate an AML as E-AML. Focal epithelioid areas ➡ are often present in otherwise typical AMLs. More recent studies have used > 80% epithelioid component as the diagnostic cut-off.

Epithelioid Angiomyolipoma

E-AML: Focal Adipocytes

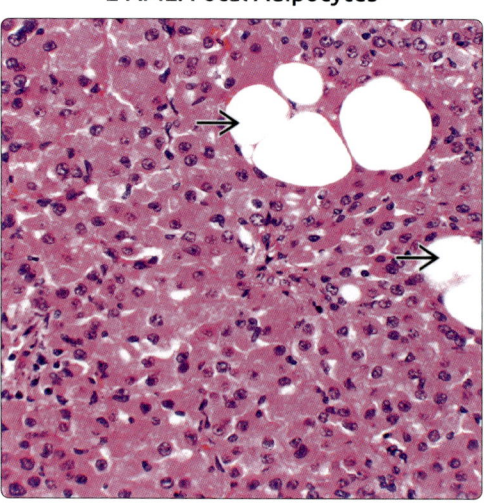

E-AML: Eosinophilic Cytoplasm

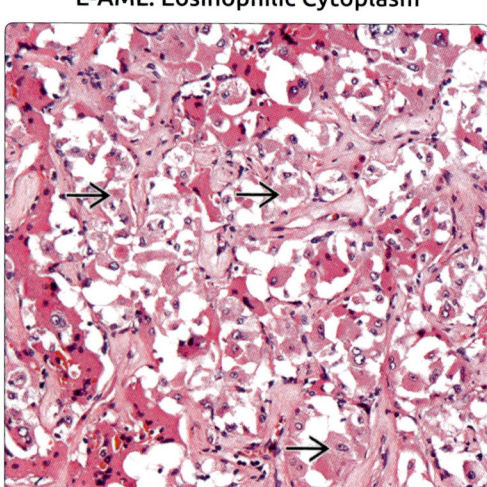

(Left) This AML with epithelioid features shows oncocytoma-like eosinophilic granularity. Careful microscopic search may lead to identification of at least focal features of typical AML, for example adipocytes ⇨, as shown here. (Right) E-AML with predominant eosinophilic cytoplasm ⇨ may superficially resemble a RCC with abundant eosinophilic cytoplasm. The diagnosis rests on exclusion of the known subtypes of RCC and appropriate immunohistochemistry.

E-AML: Necrosis

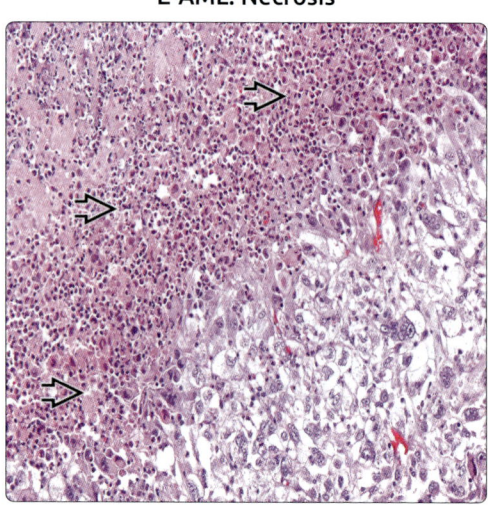

E-AML: Ganglion-Like Cells

(Left) Areas of microscopic tumor necrosis ⇨ are not infrequent in E-AML. Necrosis is mostly a feature in the tumors that show marked cytological atypia. (Right) While ≥ 70% atypical epithelioid cells, ≥ 2 mitotic figures ⇨ per 10 HPF, atypical mitotic figures, and necrosis are often present in metastatic E-AML, the presence of these features in primarily resected renal tumors does not necessarily suggest an aggressive behavior.

E-AML: Angiolymphatic Invasion

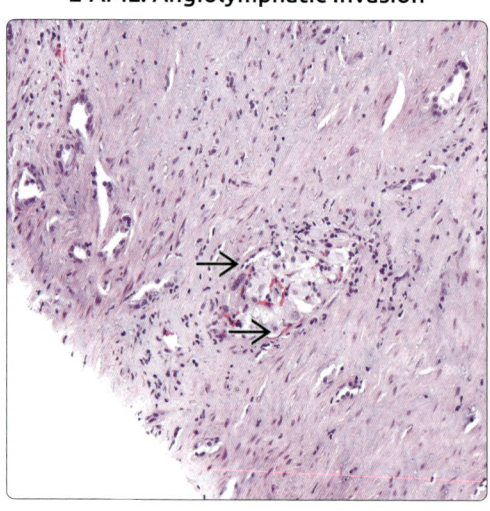

E-AML: Renal Sinus Vein Invasion

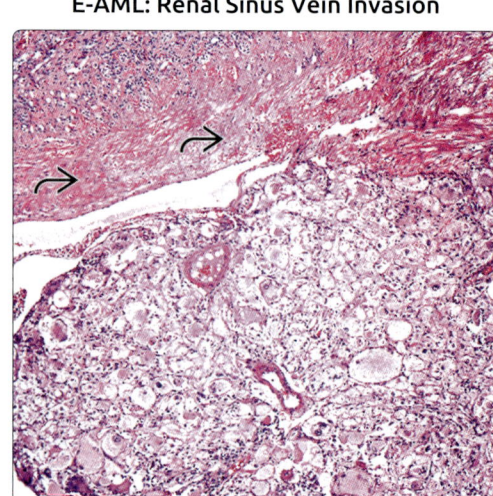

(Left) This E-AML showed angiolymphatic vascular invasion ⇨. In spite of it, and the presence of tumor necrosis, this patient showed no evidence of disease at ~ 9 years of follow-up. (Right) This epithelioid AML invades a large muscular branch of renal vein ⇨. Along with tumor necrosis, high mitotic index, perinephric involvement, and vascular invasion have been regarded as adverse markers in E-AML; however, the presence of these features should not result in the designation of a malignancy.

Epithelioid Angiomyolipoma

E-AML: Spindled and Plump Cells
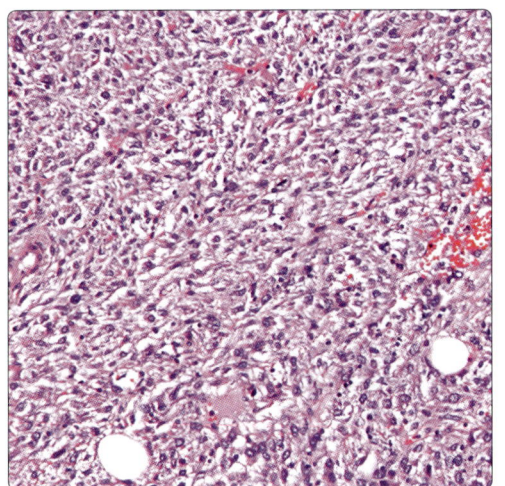

E-AML: Liver Metastasis
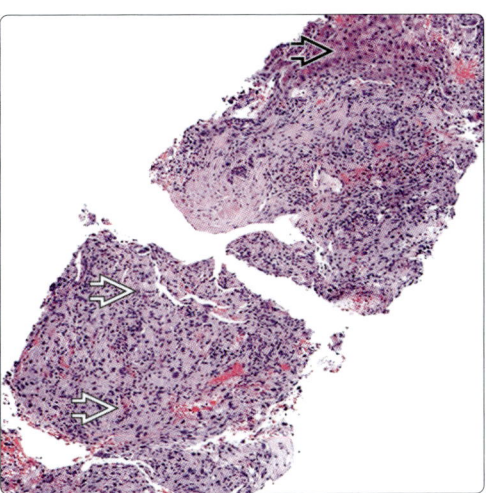

(Left) Some E-AMLs show sheets of spindled and plump epithelioid cells. Although there is noticeable vascularity in the background, the branching is irregular and does not encircle nests of tumor. **(Right)** Core needle biopsy shows an E-AML ⇨ metastatic to liver ⇨, which is the most common site for metastasis from E-AML, followed by lymph nodes and lungs.

Immunohistochemistry: HMB-45
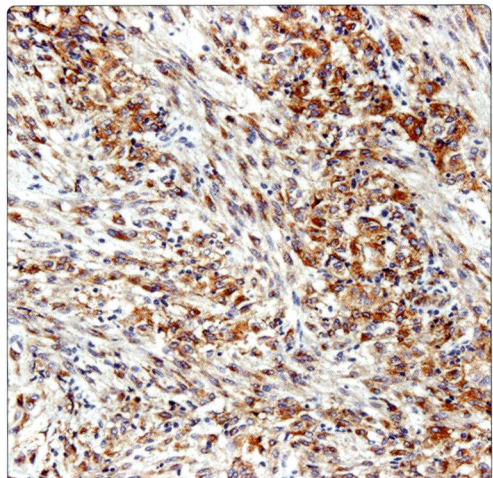

Immunohistochemistry: MITF
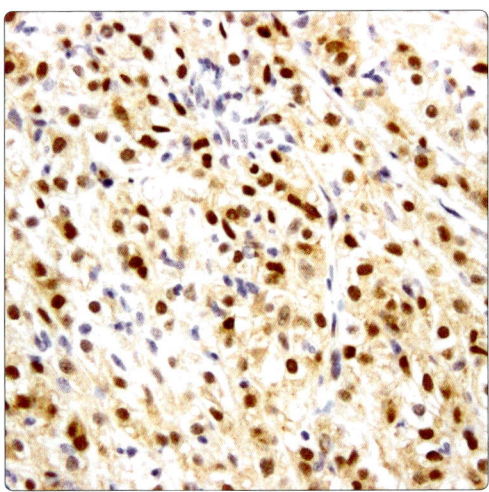

(Left) Epithelioid cells usually show diffuse and strong immunoreactivity for melanocytic markers like HMB-45 (as shown here) and Melan-A (MART-1). Besides careful attention to the histology, the tumor immunoprofile is the most distinctive feature distinguishing E-AML from RCC. **(Right)** MITF immunoreactivity is a characteristic feature of E-AML. Rarely, nuclear MITF positivity may be the only supportive melanocytic marker in E-AML.

Immunohistochemistry: cathepsin-K
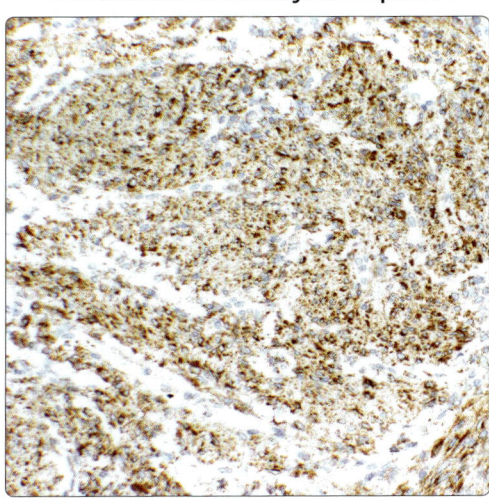

Immunohistochemistry: Phospho-S6
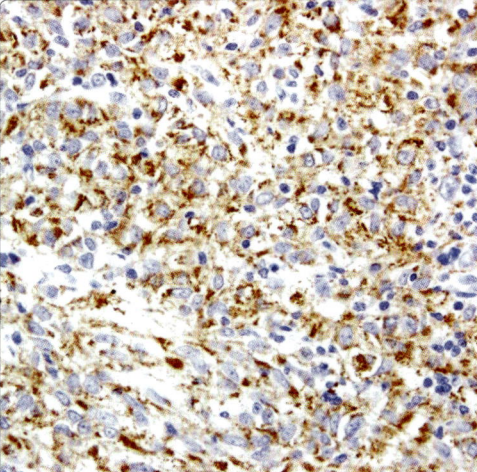

(Left) cathepsin-K has recently been found to be a highly sensitive IHC marker for AML and related tumors. It has also been shown to have higher sensitivity and greater level of expression than HMB-45 and other melanocytic markers in E-AML. **(Right)** This figure illustrates phospho-S6 positivity in an E-AML. Phospho-S6 is activated by mTOR, and overexpression of phospho-S6 is a strong indicator of an active mTOR pathway. This finding is considered a justification for using mTOR inhibitors in managing E-AML.

Congenital Mesoblastic Nephroma

KEY FACTS

TERMINOLOGY
- Congenital mesoblastic nephroma (CMN)
- Spindle cell neoplasm of kidney, composed of myofibroblasts
- Subtypes/variants: Classic, cellular, and mixed

ETIOLOGY/PATHOGENESIS
- Classic CMN typically diploid; cellular CMNs often with aneuploidy of chromosomes 11, 8, and 17
- Cellular variant has t(12;15)(p13;q25) chromosomal translocation resulting in *ETV6-NTRK3* gene fusion
  - Same translocation as seen in infantile fibrosarcoma
- Occasional association of CMN with Beckwith-Wiedemann syndrome

CLINICAL ISSUES
- Most common renal tumor of infancy
- Majority cured with surgery and have excellent outcome
- Increased risk of local recurrence with incomplete excision

MACROSCOPIC
- Solitary, unilateral; classic CMN with whorled or trabeculated, gray-white cut surface and indistinct tumor-kidney interface; cellular CMN often fleshy with circumscribed edges

MICROSCOPIC
- Classic variant (24% of cases): Intersecting bundles of spindle cells with minimal atypia and infrequent mitoses
- Cellular variant (66%): Pushing border, dense cellularity, mitoses, and sarcomatous appearance
- Mixed (10-20%): Shows combination of both histologic patterns

TOP DIFFERENTIAL DIAGNOSES
- Metanephric stromal tumor
- Clear cell sarcoma of kidney
- Wilms tumor (particularly post therapy)
- Rhabdoid tumor of kidney

Gross Features

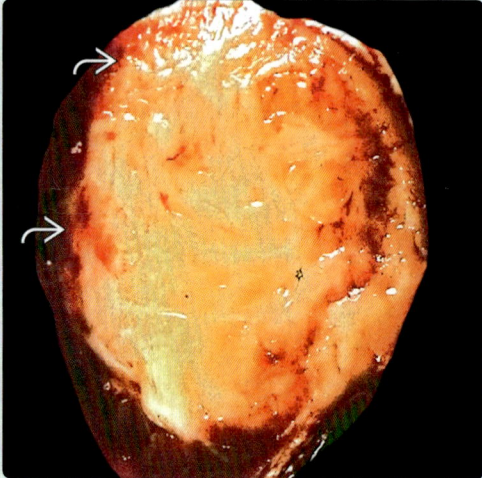

Gross Features

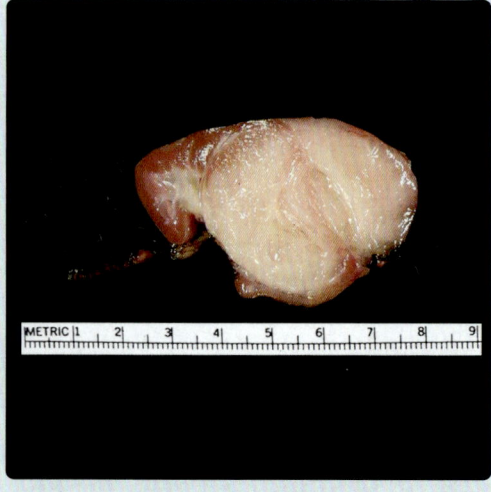

(Left) This gross picture of a classic congenital mesoblastic nephroma (CMN) shows the characteristic tan-white, fibrous, whorled, and trabeculated cut surface. The tumor-kidney interface is ill defined ⇒. (Right) Gross photograph shows another nephrectomy specimen that was resected from a 7-week-old infant. The cut surface is white-tan, resembling fibromatosis at other sites. The site of origin of this infiltrating tumor (classic variant of CMN) cannot be determined with certainty because of the size.

Classic CMN: Margins

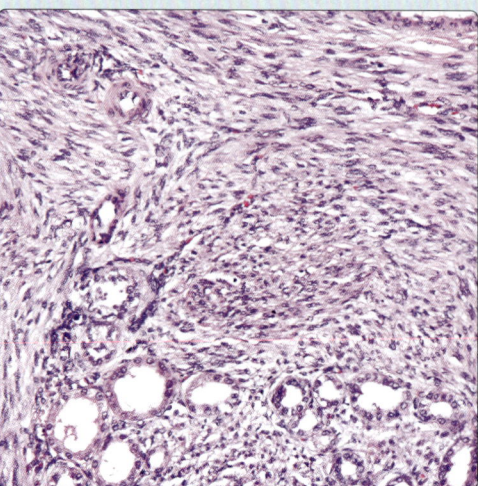

Cellular CMN: Margins

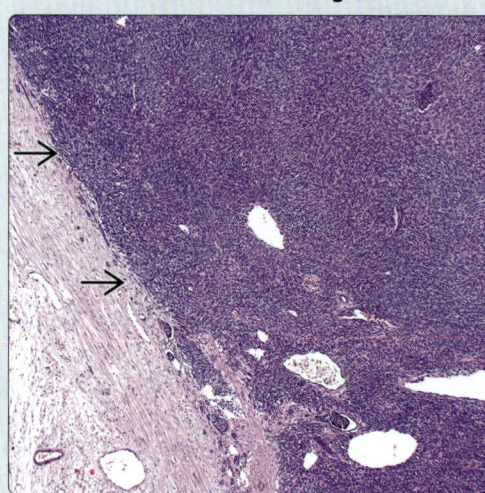

(Left) This image of CMN depicts the low-grade cytologic features seen in the classic type. With its low cellularity, minimal nuclear pleomorphism, and low mitotic activity, histologically, the classic type closely resembles fibromatosis.
(Right) The advancing edges of cellular CMN are pushing ⇒ rather than infiltrative. Cellular CMN is morphologically similar to infantile fibrosarcoma and is considered by some to be infantile fibrosarcoma centered in the renal hilum.

Congenital Mesoblastic Nephroma

TERMINOLOGY

Abbreviations
- Congenital mesoblastic nephroma (CMN)

Definitions
- Most common renal neoplasm of infancy with spindle cell features, mimicking fibromatosis or infantile fibrosarcoma

ETIOLOGY/PATHOGENESIS

Genetic Features
- Classic CMN typically diploid; cellular CMNs often with aneuploidy of chromosomes 11, 8, and 17
- Cellular variant with t(12;15)(p13;q25) chromosomal translocation resulting in *ETV6-NTRK3* gene fusion
  o Same translocation as seen in infantile fibrosarcoma; also recently reported in secretory carcinomas of breast
- No gene fusions demonstrated in mixed pattern
- Occasional association of CMN with Beckwith-Wiedemann syndrome

CLINICAL ISSUES

Presentation
- Most common renal tumor in first 3 months of life; > 90% occur in 1st year of life
- Presents as abdominal mass; may be associated with polyhydramnios, premature delivery, and nonimmune hydrops
- Hypertension (due to renin production by entrapped renal elements) may be present

Treatment
- Surgical approaches
  o Because of marked infiltrative nature of classic type, partial nephrectomy often not feasible option in many cases

Prognosis
- Majority cured with surgery with excellent outcome
  o Recurrences and metastases in ~ 5-10% of patients; risk factors for recurrence include incomplete excision, stage III or higher presentation, and involvement of intrarenal or sinus vessels

MACROSCOPIC

General Features
- Solitary, unilateral; classic CMN with whorled or trabeculated, gray-white cut surface and indistinct tumor-kidney interface; cellular CMN often fleshy with circumscribed edges
- Cysts, hemorrhage, and necrosis common, with no prognostic significance
- Tend to arise centrally within kidney and often involving renal sinus extensively

MICROSCOPIC

Histologic Features
- Classic type (24% of cases)
  o Shows intersecting bundles of spindle cells with minimal atypia and infrequent mitoses and resembles fibromatosis
  o Tumor infiltrates extensively into adjacent renal parenchyma and renal sinus structures
  o Dysplastic renal tubules and islands of cartilage are often seen trapped within tumor
- Cellular variant (66%)
  o Shows pushing borders, dense cellularity, and numerous mitoses; morphologically, similar to infantile fibrosarcoma
- Mixed (10-20%): Shows combination of both patterns

DIFFERENTIAL DIAGNOSIS

Metanephric Stromal Tumor
- May mimic classic CMN; usually does not present within 1st year of life; margins not as infiltrative as in classic CMN
- Shows dysmorphic vessels, juxtaglomerular hyperplasia, and concentric spindle cell proliferation around vessels and tubules, and usually CD34(+) stroma

Clear Cell Sarcoma of Kidney
- May mimic cellular CMN; cellular variant of CMN lacks chicken-wire vascular pattern of clear cell sarcoma of kidney (CCSK)
- Presence of other patterns of CCSK (e.g., myxoid, sclerosing, epithelioid, palisading)

Wilms Tumor
- Most difficult differential, particularly posttherapy Wilms with stromal-type residual tumor
- Wilms tumor (WT) very rare in infants, especially those < 6 months old
- Extensive necrosis, as in posttherapy WT, and rhabdomyomatous differentiation not features of CMN
- WT with compressed pseudocapsule in contrast to extensively infiltrating borders in CMN

Rhabdoid Tumor of Kidney
- Occasionally CMN may have unusually prominent nucleoli, raising suspicion of rhabdoid tumor of kidney (RTK)
  o Immunohistochemical stain for SNF5(INI1) (positive nuclear staining in CMN and absent staining in RTK) diagnostic

DIAGNOSTIC CHECKLIST

Pathologic Interpretation Pearls
- Vast majority of patients < 1 year old, at which age other pediatric renal tumors less common
- Surgical margins, especially medial margin, need careful evaluation

SELECTED REFERENCES

1. England RJ et al: Mesoblastic nephroma: a report of the United Kingdom Children's Cancer and Leukaemia Group (CCLG). Pediatr Blood Cancer. 56(5):744-8, 2011
2. Bayindir P et al: Cellular mesoblastic nephroma (infantile renal fibrosarcoma): institutional review of the clinical, diagnostic imaging, and pathologic features of a distinctive neoplasm of infancy. Pediatr Radiol. 39(10):1066-74, 2009
3. van den Heuvel-Eibrink MM et al: Characteristics and survival of 750 children diagnosed with a renal tumor in the first seven months of life: A collaborative study by the SIOP/GPOH/SFOP, NWTSG, and UKCCSG Wilms tumor study groups. Pediatr Blood Cancer. 50(6):1130-4, 2008

Congenital Mesoblastic Nephroma

(Left) Although morphologically similar to the cellular CMN, the cellular areas ⇨ in mixed CMN, interestingly, do not show the ETV6-NTRK3 gene fusion characteristic of all cellular CMN. This genetic characteristic is also absent in classic tumors and classic areas ⇨ of mixed CMN. (Right) The classic type of CMN usually shows tongue-like extensions into the surrounding renal parenchyma and soft tissues, often entrapping these elements within its advancing edges ⇨.

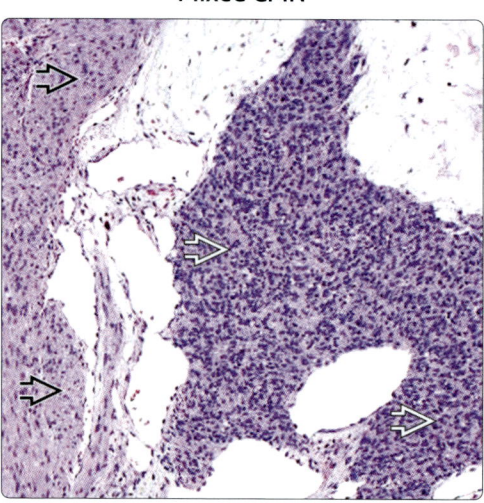
Mixed CMN

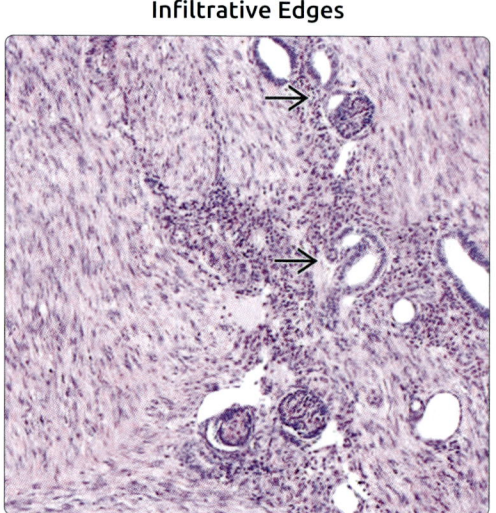
Infiltrative Edges

(Left) The infiltrativeness of classic CMN is akin to that seen in fibromatosis, with extensive infiltration in the renal sinus. These irregular infiltrating margins often make partial nephrectomy a difficult surgical option in classic CMN. (Right) Besides invading the sinus, classic CMN also extends into perinephric fat ⇨. Because of the frequent and irregular extensions into the renal sinus and perinephric fat, total or radical nephrectomy is often performed. Tumor recurrences are most commonly related to incomplete resection.

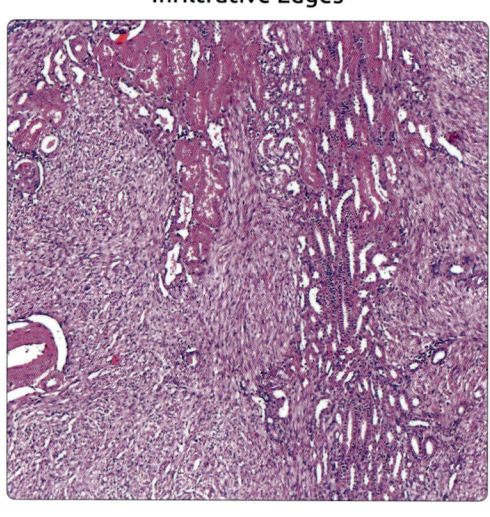
Infiltrative Edges

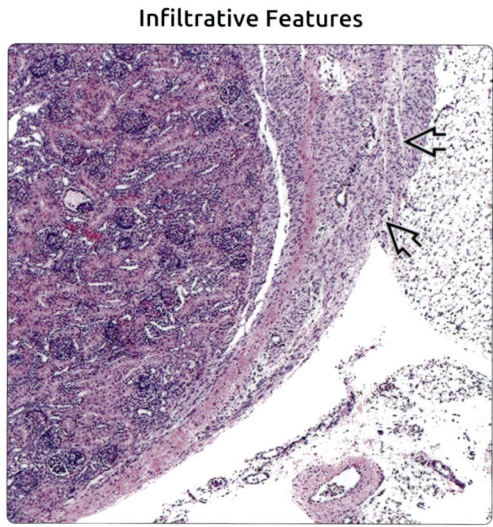
Infiltrative Features

(Left) A small but significant proportion of CMNs show mixed histologic features, with cellular ⇨ and classic ⇨ areas often present side-by-side. Cellular CMN is often mitotically active and morphologically resembles infantile fibrosarcoma. (Right) Mitotic figures ⇨ are quite frequent in cellular CMN. Recurrences and metastases occur in < 10% of patients with CMN, risk factors for which are incomplete excision, cellularity, stage III or higher tumors, and involvement of intrarenal or sinus vessels.

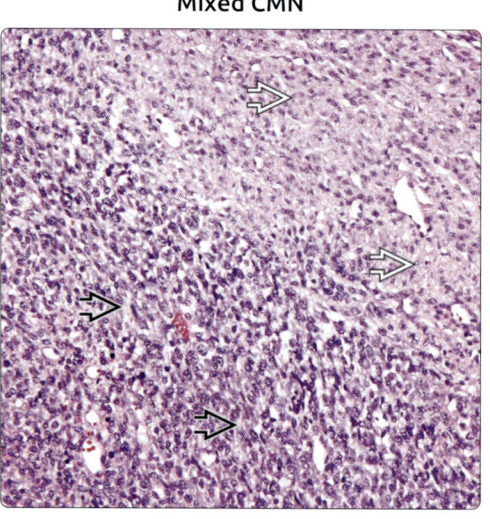
Mixed CMN

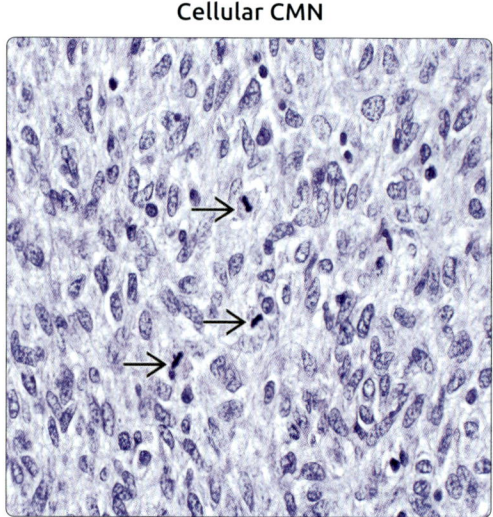
Cellular CMN

Congenital Mesoblastic Nephroma

Metaplastic Cartilage

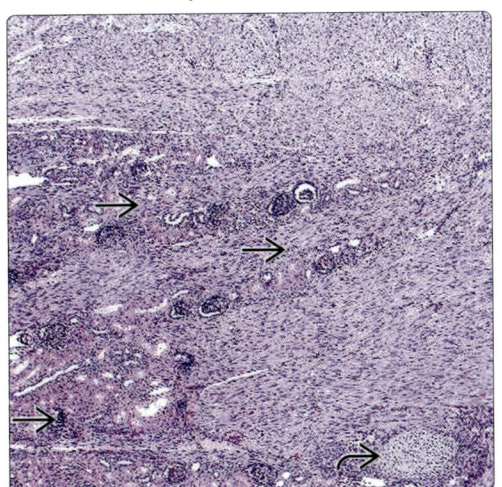

Metaplastic Cartilage

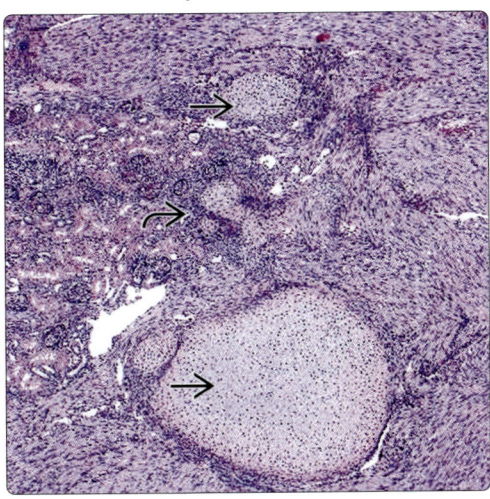

(Left) Low-power image shows a classic CMN infiltrating into adjacent renal parenchyma, forming finger-like projections ➡. Metaplastic cartilage ➡ is present at lower right. Presence of cartilaginous tissue may raise the possibility of a Wilms tumor (WT) with heterologous differentiation. (Right) The possibility of a WT with heterologous differentiation in presence of cartilage ➡ in CMN needs careful attention to the rest of the tumor. Infiltrative edges ➡, lack of blastema, and negative IHC for WT1 will favor CMN.

Differential Diagnosis: CCSK

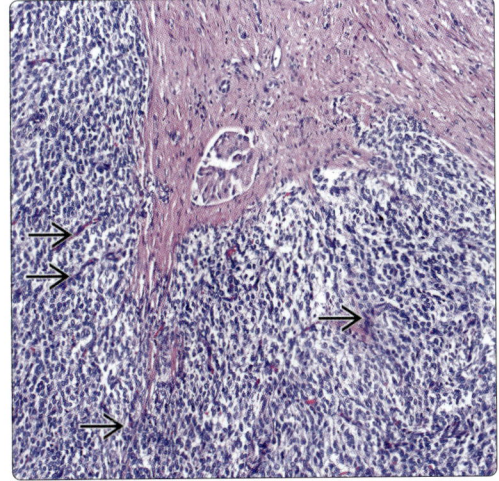

Differential Diagnosis: Spindle Cell-Predominant WT

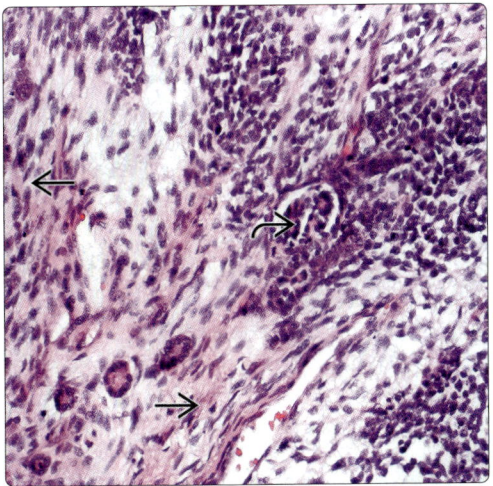

(Left) Light microscopy of this clear cell sarcoma of the kidney shows a tumor that may mimic cellular CMN. However, the classic vascular pattern ➡ is still evident evident in cellular CCSK, helping in its separation from CMN. (Right) Stromal-predominant WT ➡, particularly as seen in posttherapy setting, may be confused for CMN. Presence of even focal blastema or epithelial components ➡, as well as the usual circumscription of WT, often helps in pointing toward the correct diagnosis.

Differential Diagnosis: Rhabdoid Tumor

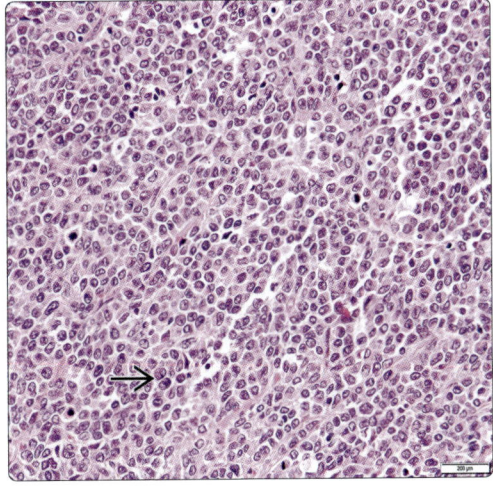

Differential Diagnosis: Metanephric Tumors

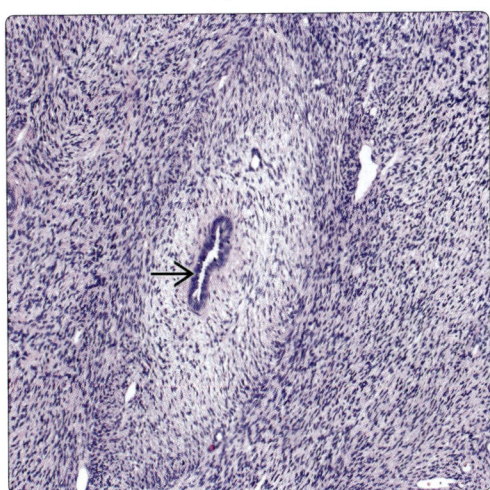

(Left) Rarely, RTK may show areas mimicking CCSK or even cellular CMN, as shown in this illustration. Presence of even focal cytoplasmic inclusions ➡, typical RTK areas, and the loss of INI1 IHC will confirm the actual diagnosis of RTK. (Right) Metanephric (M) stromal tumor and M adenofibroma can closely mimic a classic CMN. Presence of intermingled glandular elements ➡ in M adenofibroma, and other perivascular and stromal features in M stromal tumor, are very helpful in the distinction.

Clear Cell Sarcoma of Kidney

KEY FACTS

TERMINOLOGY
- Clear cell sarcoma of kidney (CCSK)
- Uncommon malignant renal neoplasm of childhood of uncertain cell of origin with aggressive clinical behavior

ETIOLOGY/PATHOGENESIS
- 2 recurrent, likely mutually exclusive, genetic aberrations recently described
  - Internal tandem duplication in *BCOR* (BCL6 corepressor) gene
  - Fusion of *YWHAE* (tyrosine 3-monooxygenase/tryptophan 5-monooxygenase activation protein, epsilon) and *NUTM2B/E* (NUT family member 2B)
- Nonrandom translocation t(10;17) and deletion 14q also described

CLINICAL ISSUES
- Treatment with doxorubicin shown to improve outcome
- Ipsilateral renal hilar lymph nodes most common site at presentation
- Bones are most common sites of recurrence
- Presence of tumor necrosis only histological prognostic variable

MICROSCOPIC
- Diagnosis primarily based on histologic criteria
- No diagnostic immunohistochemical or molecular features available at present
- Morphologic hallmark: Evenly distributed network of vascular septa, with branching chicken wire pattern

ANCILLARY TESTS
- No specific stains available for CCSK

TOP DIFFERENTIAL DIAGNOSES
- Blastema predominant Wilms tumor; mesoblastic nephroma; primitive neuroectodermal tumor; rhabdoid tumor of kidney

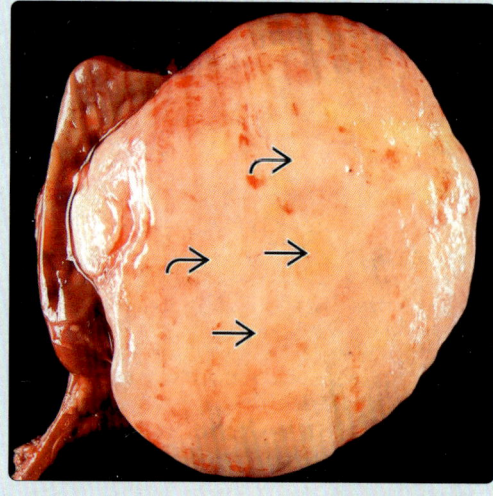

Gross Features *(Left)* Typical gross features of a clear cell sarcoma of the kidney include a large, well-circumscribed tumor ➡ with a fleshy tan, mucoid cut surface, often with variably prominent cystic areas ➡. *(Right)* Another gross example of a clear cell sarcoma of the kidney shows a predominantly pale white ➡ cut surface, alternating with somewhat myxoid areas ➡. In spite of gross well circumscription, the tumor often shows regional lymph node metastasis at the time of presentation.

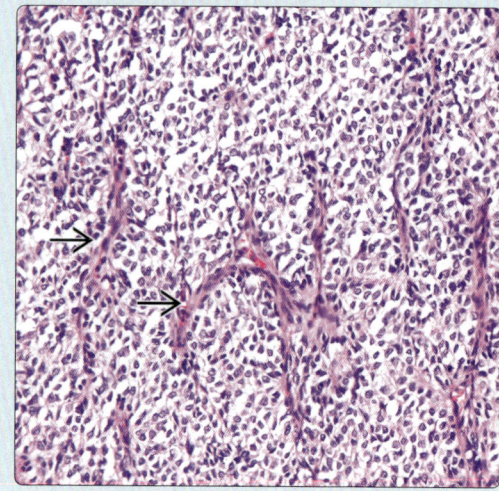

Invasive Tumor Front / "Chicken Wire" Vasculature *(Left)* Despite the well-circumscribed gross and low-power appearance, CCSK almost invariably has invasive fronts, with entrapped renal tubules ➡ and glomeruli at the periphery of the tumor. In spite of its older synonym, CCSK is more often metastatic to the local lymph nodes than bones at presentation. *(Right)* Characteristic features are seen in this classic pattern of CCSK. Cords and nests of tumor cells are separated by branching vascular septa with a chicken wire appearance ➡.

Clear Cell Sarcoma of Kidney

TERMINOLOGY

Abbreviations
- Clear cell sarcoma of kidney (CCSK)

Synonyms
- Bone-metastasizing renal tumor of childhood

Definitions
- Uncommon malignant renal neoplasm of childhood of uncertain histogenesis with aggressive clinical behavior

ETIOLOGY/PATHOGENESIS

Molecular Genetics
- 2 recurrent, likely mutually exclusive, genetic aberrations recently described
  - Internal tandem duplication in *BCOR* (BCL6 corepressor) gene; associated with epithelial-to-mesenchymal transition
  - Fusion of *YWHAE* (tyrosine 3-monooxygenase/tryptophan 5-monooxygenase activation protein, epsilon) and *NUTM2B/E* (NUT family member 2B); fusion involved in cell cycle progression
    - Fusion identical to endometrial stromal sarcoma
- Nonrandom translocation t(10;17) and deletion 14q also described
  - 17p13 is locus of *p53* gene, but *p53* alterations seen only in anaplastic CCSK

CLINICAL ISSUES

Epidemiology
- ~ 20 new cases/year in USA; comprise 3% of childhood renal tumors; M:F = 2:1
- 2 months to 14 years old; peak incidence: 2-3 years old; congenital cases and rare cases in adults reported

Presentation
- Large single renal mass, hematuria and hypertension

Treatment
- Combined therapeutic options, including nephrectomy, adjuvant chemotherapy with doxorubicin, dactinomycin, and vincristine (NWTS 4 regimen), and tumor bed radiation

Prognosis
- Aggressive clinical course; lymph nodes most common metastatic site at presentation, and bones followed by lung and retroperitoneum, most common sites of recurrence
- Independent prognostic factors for survival
  - Treatment with doxorubicin; stage 1 disease (98% overall survival); improved outcome in patients 2-4 years old; tumor necrosis (adverse factor for survival; only histological prognostic variable)

MACROSCOPIC

General Features
- Unicentric, well-circumscribed renal mass; mean diameter: 11.3 cm (range: 2.3-24 cm)
- Often homogeneous, solid, tan-gray, glistening, gelatinous cut surface; often with cystic areas and foci of hemorrhage and necrosis

MICROSCOPIC

Microscopic Features
- Diagnosis primarily based on histologic criteria; no specific immunohistochemical features available at present
- Classic pattern, present in 90% tumors at least focally
  - Almost evenly distributed network of vascular septa, with branching chicken wire pattern, similar to myxoid liposarcoma and oligodendroglioma
  - Septa divide tumor into nests and cords of polygonal cells with indistinct cell borders, nuclei showing finely granular chromatin and inconspicuous nucleoli
  - Cells often surrounded by pale, mucopolysaccharide material, often creating illusion of clear cytoplasm
  - Necrosis: Only histologic factor of adverse prognosis
  - Entrapped renal tubules along periphery
- Variant patterns (listed in order of observed frequency)
  - Myxoid, sclerosing, cellular, epithelioid trabecular, palisading/spindle cell/storiform, anaplastic (with nuclear hyperchromasia and gigantism, and atypical mitoses)
- Histologic variants do not affect prognosis

ANCILLARY TESTS

Immunohistochemistry
- IHC primarily useful for excluding other renal tumors; no specific stains available
- Vimentin and Bcl-2 (+); pax-2/pax-8 some tumors (+); epithelial markers, CD99 and WT1(-)
- p53 consistently positive in anaplastic tumors only

DIFFERENTIAL DIAGNOSIS

Blastema Predominant Wilms Tumor
- Chromatin pattern coarse with molding; WT1(+)

Primitive Neuroectodermal Tumor
- CD99 and FLI-1 (+)

Congenital Mesoblastic Nephroma, Plump Cell Pattern
- Spindled and polygonal cells, prominent nucleoli; actin (+)

Rhabdoid Tumor of Kidney
- Loss of expression for SNF5(INI1)

DIAGNOSTIC CHECKLIST

Pathologic Interpretation Pearls
- Diagnosis primarily based on histologic criteria, hallmark being evenly distributed chicken wire network of vascular septa
- Attention to overall morphology and immunohistochemical stains usually help in excluding differential diagnoses

SELECTED REFERENCES

1. Karlsson J et al: BCOR internal tandem duplication and YWHAE-NUTM2B/E fusion are mutually exclusive events in clear cell sarcoma of the kidney. Genes Chromosomes Cancer. 55(2):120-3, 2015
2. Ueno-Yokohata H et al: Consistent in-frame internal tandem duplications of BCOR characterize clear cell sarcoma of the kidney. Nat Genet. 47(8):861-3, 2015
3. Argani P et al: Clear cell sarcoma of the kidney: a review of 351 cases from the National Wilms Tumor Study Group Pathology Center. Am J Surg Pathol. 24(1):4-18, 2000

Clear Cell Sarcoma of Kidney

Architectural and Cytoplasmic Characteristics

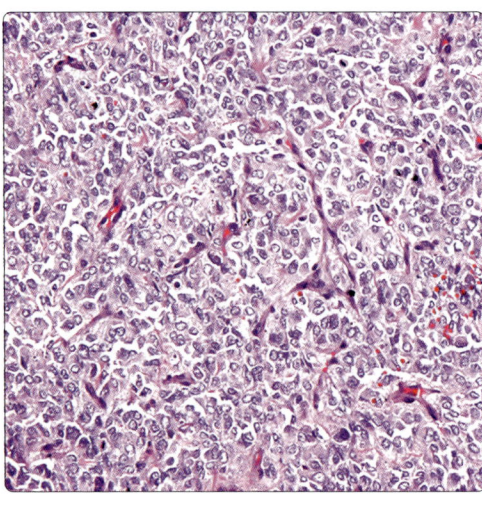

Inconspicuous Nucleoli

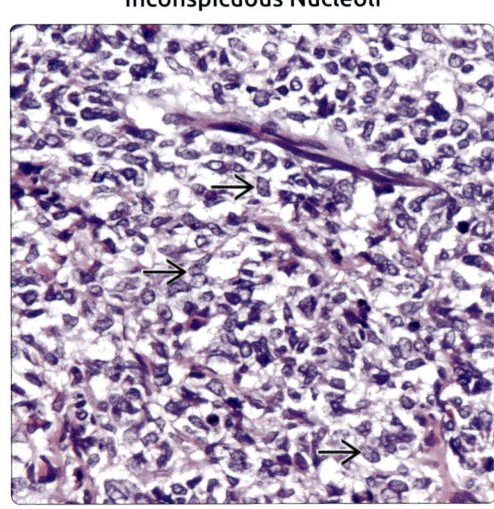

(Left) This image shows a CCSK with epithelioid features. The presence of well-defined cytoplasmic membranes and focal eosinophilic cytoplasm may raise suspicion of a rhabdoid tumor. Vesicular chromatin, lack of prominent nucleoli, and the vascular pattern point to the correct diagnosis. (Right) High magnification of classic pattern of CCSK shows tumor nuclei with vesicular, finely granular chromatin and inconspicuous nucleoli ➔. In well-fixed specimens, this chromatin pattern is the most helpful clue to the diagnosis.

Pale Intercellular Matrix

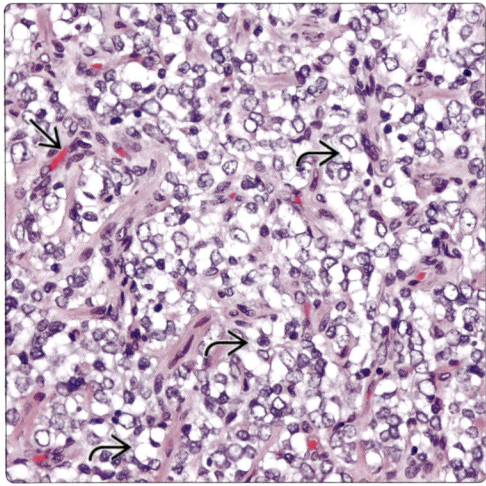

Pseudoglandular Architecture

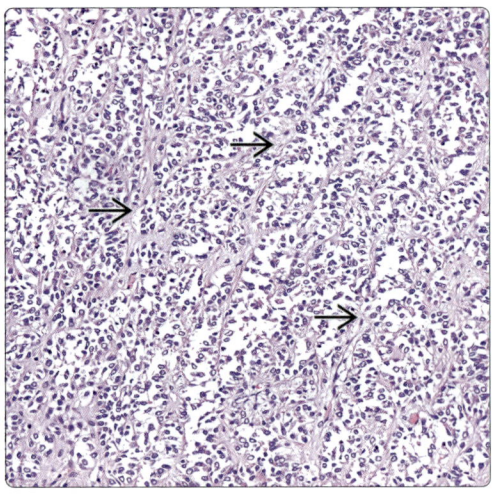

(Left) Tumor cells in CCSK show vesicular nuclei and pale cytoplasm with indistinct cell borders, separated by delicate fibrovascular septa ➔. Tumor cells are often surrounded by pale, mucopolysaccharide material ➔, creating the illusion of clear cytoplasm, as well as the pale appearance of a glass slide held against light. (Right) CCSK is shown with loosely spaced and dyscohesive cells attached to the delicate fibrovascular septa ➔. The leads to a pseudoglandular architecture in the tumor.

Variant Histology: Sclerosis

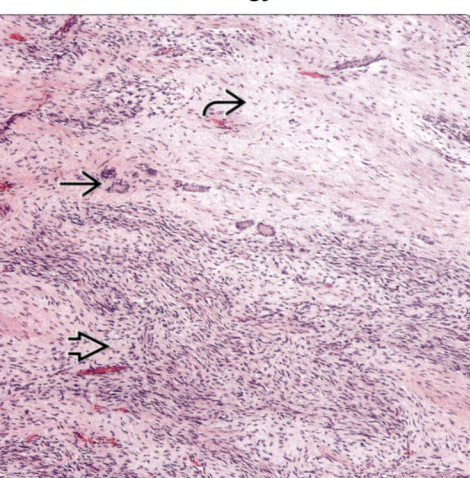

Variant Histology: Spindle Cells

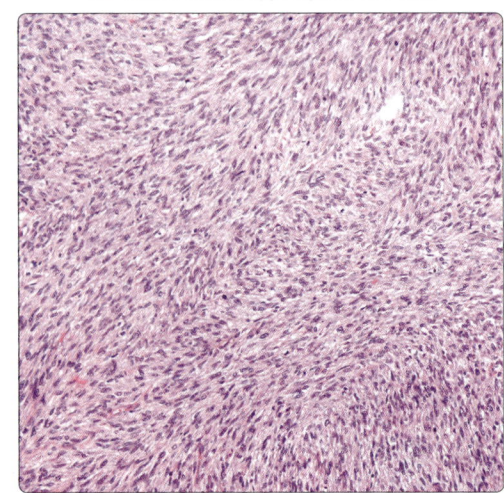

(Left) Currently, no immunohistochemical markers specific for CCSK are available. The diagnosis is primarily based on morphologic features. This medium-power view of a CCSK shows areas of hyaline sclerosis ➔ with entrapped tubules ➔, along with spindle cell patterns of growth ➔. (Right) Medium-power view of a CCSK demonstrates areas of spindle cell architecture and storiform growth pattern. Typically, adequate sampling will reveal areas of classic features in most cases.

Clear Cell Sarcoma of Kidney

Variant Histology: Palisading

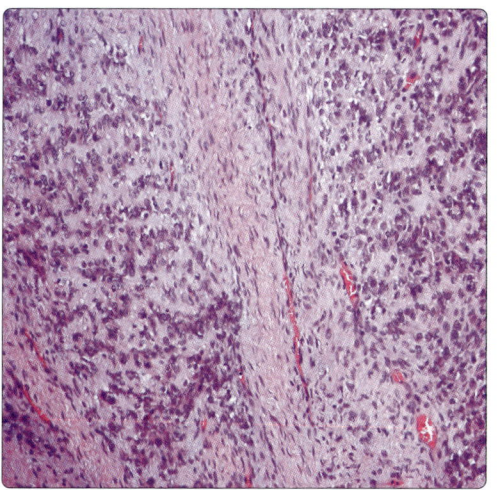

Variant Histology: High Cellularity

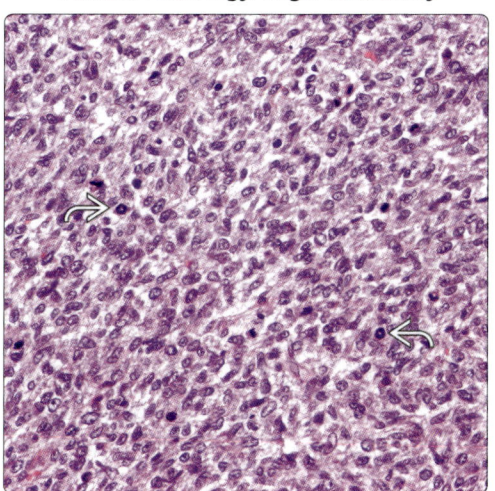

(Left) Palisading pattern may rarely be seen in CCSK and, in such areas, closely resembles schwannoma. Immunostain for S100 protein is invariably negative, excluding the possibility of a schwannoma. (Right) Some CCSK show areas of increased cellularity, nuclear hyperchromasia, mild pleomorphism, and mitotic figures ⇒. Anaplasia in CCSK is defined by nuclear hyperchromasia, nuclear gigantism, and the presence of atypical mitoses.

Embryonic-Type Metaplasia in Entrapped Tubules

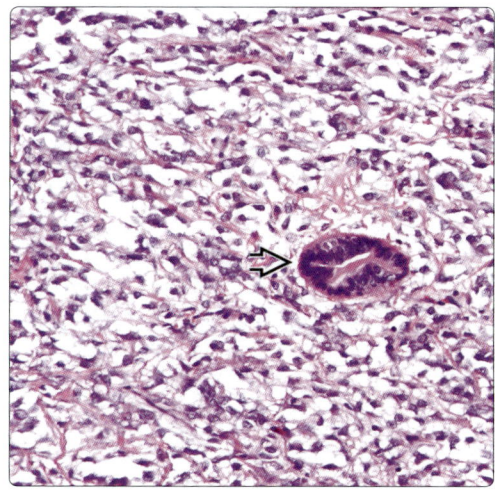

Cytoplasmic Eosinophilia

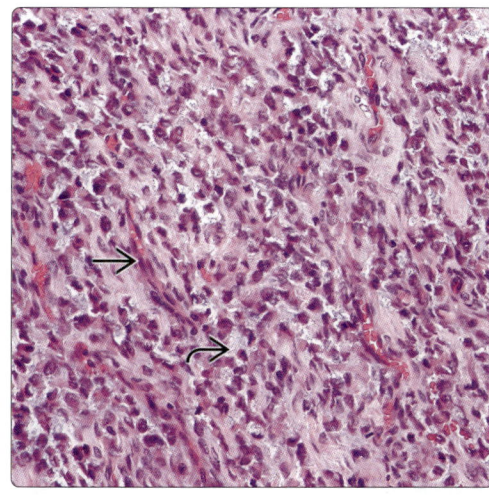

(Left) Sometimes, entrapped tubules in tumor may show embryonic-type metaplasia ⇒, raising suspicion of a Wilms tumor. The lack of blastema and presence of typical vasculature with pale nuclei in the tumor should point to the correct diagnosis. (Right) The tumor cells may show prominent eosinophilic cytoplasm reminiscent of a rhabdoid tumor of kidney. The characteristic small pools of mucin ⇒, thin fibrovascular septa ⇒, lack of high-grade nuclei, and lack of conspicuous nucleoli will help distinguish this tumor as a CCSK.

Abundant Myxoid Stroma

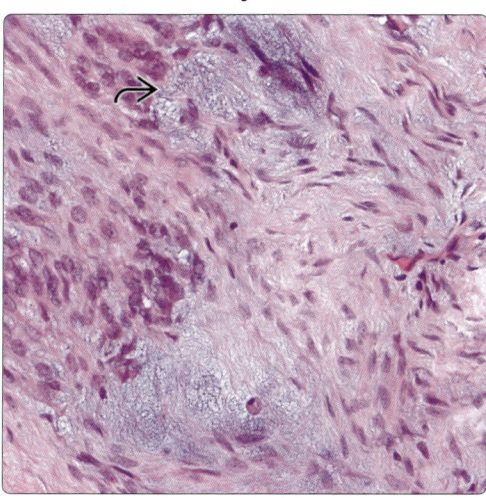

Metastasis

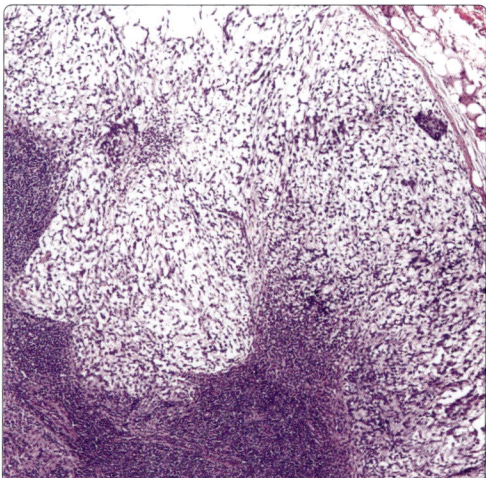

(Left) Pools of myxoid material ⇒ are seen in this CCSK at high power. Nests of round to spindle-shaped tumor cells are also present. (Right) Hematoxylin & eosin shows lymph node metastasis in a CCSK. Ipsilateral renal hilar lymph nodes are the most common site of metastasis at presentation. In contrast, osseous metastases are the most common site of recurrence, followed closely by the lungs.

Malignant Rhabdoid Tumor

KEY FACTS

TERMINOLOGY
- Malignant rhabdoid tumor of kidney (RTK)
- Highly malignant pediatric renal tumor with very poor prognosis and genetic abnormalities of *hSNF5/INI1/SMARCB1* tumor suppressor gene

ETIOLOGY/PATHOGENESIS
- Biallelic inactivation of gene, located at 22q11.2, consistent feature of RTK
- Occasional RTK with intact SMARCB1 expression harbor mutations in *SMARCA4/BRG1* gene

CLINICAL ISSUES
- Mean age of presentation: Around 1 yr old
- Predominantly affects younger children; 80% < 2 yr old, 60% < 1 yr old
- Overwhelming majority of stage IV renal tumors in 1st 7 months of life are RTK
- High tumor stage at presentation

MACROSCOPIC
- Well circumscribed and nonencapsulated
- Foci of hemorrhage and necrosis

MICROSCOPIC
- Sheets of monotonous, loosely cohesive, large ovoid-to-polygonal cells, with high nuclear grade
- Characteristic cytologic features: Vesicular chromatin, prominent eosinophilic nucleoli, and intracytoplasmic hyaline, pink inclusion, at least in some cells

ANCILLARY TESTS
- Loss of immunostaining for SNF5 (INI1) considered specific
  - Reliable surrogate marker of *hSNF5/INI1/SMARCB1* gene deletion or inactivating mutations

TOP DIFFERENTIAL DIAGNOSES
- Renal medullary carcinoma
- Cellular mesoblastic nephroma, "plump cell" variant
- Clear cell sarcoma of kidney

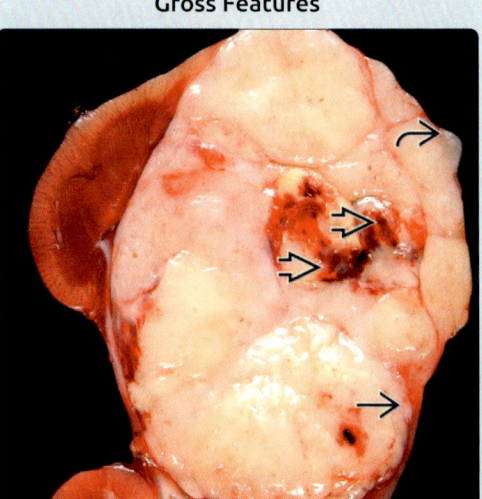

Gross Features

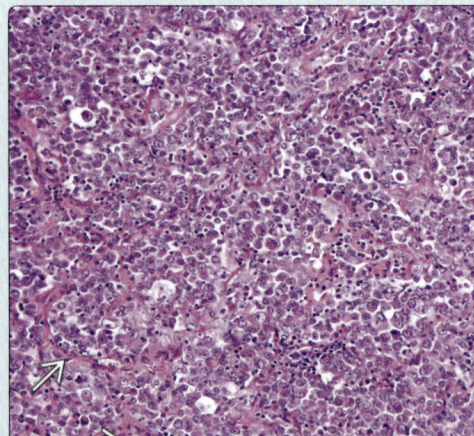

Sheet-Like Architecture

(Left) Rhabdoid tumor of kidney (RTK) is seen with necrosis ⇨, irregular invasive borders ⇨, and extension beyond renal parenchyma ⇨. Necrosis may be more extensive, and some tumors may be detected at smaller size due to presence of early disseminated metastases. (Right) Sheets of loosely cohesive tumor cells with large nuclei and abundant eosinophilic cytoplasm are typical of RTK. A delicate network of fibrovascular septa ⇨ may also be appreciated in many tumors.

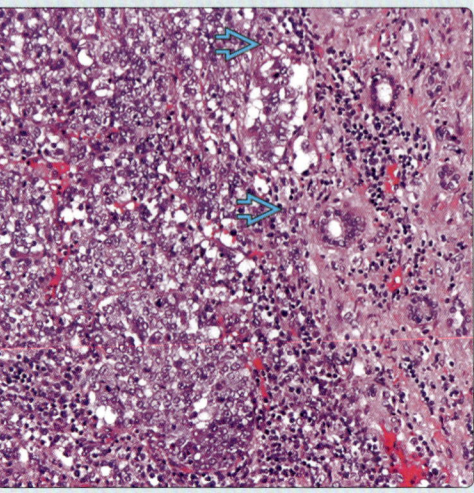

Infiltrative Borders

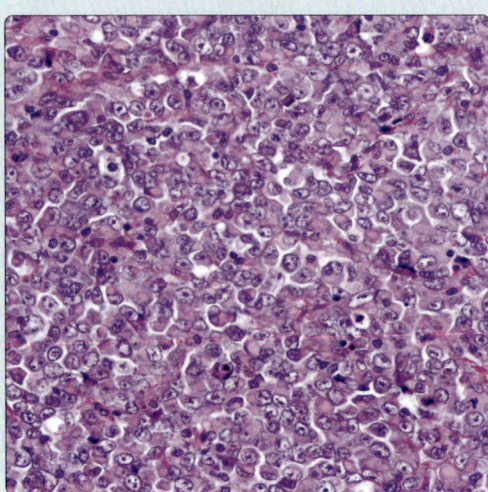

Typical Architectural and Cytological Features

(Left) Hematoxylin & eosin section shows the typical invasive border ⇨ in an RTK. No encapsulation is present in these tumors. Because of infiltrative borders, these tumors are radiologically easily differentiated from the more common Wilms tumors. (Right) Medium-power view shows sheets of loosely cohesive tumor cells with eccentric nuclei and abundant eosinophilic cytoplasm in an RTK. The nuclei show vesicular chromatin and prominent nucleoli, often easily identifiable at this magnification.

Malignant Rhabdoid Tumor

TERMINOLOGY

Abbreviations
- Rhabdoid tumor of kidney (RTK)

Definitions
- Highly malignant pediatric renal tumor with poor prognosis, and genetic abnormalities of *hSNF5/INI1/SMARCB1* tumor suppressor gene on chromosome 22

ETIOLOGY/PATHOGENESIS

HSNF5/INI1/SMARCB1 Tumor Suppressor Gene
- Biallelic inactivation of gene, located at 22q11.2 consistent feature of RTK; usually associated with deletion of 1 copy with mutation in remaining copy
  - Gene believed to be important for chromatin remodeling
- Children with concurrent RTK and atypical teratoid/rhabdoid tumor of CNS often harbor germline mutations in *HSNF5/INI1/SMARCB1* gene

SMARCA4/BRG1 Gene
- Occasional rhabdoid tumors with intact SMARCB1 expression harbor mutations in *SMARCA4/BRG1* gene

CLINICAL ISSUES

Epidemiology
- Comprise 2% of pediatric renal tumors; M:F = 1.5:1
- Mean age of presentation around 1 yr; 80% < 2 yrs old, 60% < 1 yr old; virtually nonexistent after 5 yrs of age
- RTKs constitute most stage IV renal tumors in first 7 months of life

Site
- Originally described in kidney; similar tumors later recognized in extrarenal sites, including CNS (atypical teratoid/rhabdoid tumor) and soft tissue

Presentation
- Abdominal mass most common mode of presentation; hematuria &/or fever other common symptoms; rarely hypercalcemia
  - Some tumors produce parathyroid hormone-related protein or prostaglandin E2
- > 75% present with stage III, IV, or V disease; metastases to lung, abdomen, liver, brain, and bone frequent
- Tumors in kidney, CNS, or soft tissue may occur sporadically or as part of rhabdoid tumor predisposition syndrome (1/3 of RTK cases)
  - Germline mutations of *hSNF5/INI1/SMARCB1* common in patients with apparent sporadic tumors as well as in familial rhabdoid tumor predisposition syndrome

Treatment
- Surgery, chemotherapy, radiotherapy in combination with autologous stem cell transplantation with best results

Prognosis
- Extremely poor prognosis with mortality rate > 80% within 2 yrs of diagnosis
- Predictors of poorer prognosis include: younger age, higher tumor stage, and presence of CNS lesions

MACROSCOPIC

General Features
- Typically, large tumors with ill-defined borders, often with areas of hemorrhage and necrosis in cut surface

Size
- Range, 3-17 cm in diameter (mean: 9.6 cm), sometimes replacing entire kidney

MICROSCOPIC

Histologic Features
- Sheets of monotonous loosely cohesive large, ovoid-to-polygonal cells with high nuclear grade, extensively infiltrating renal parenchyma
- Characteristic features: Vesicular chromatin; prominent eosinophilic nucleoli; cytoplasmic hyaline, pink inclusions
  - Inclusions sometimes rare; best seen around necrosis
- Brisk mitotic activity and areas of necrosis frequent, as are vascular invasion and extrarenal extension
- Variant histology present in some tumors, usually in association with typical areas, including sclerosing (most common), spindled, pseudopapillary, and cystic

ANCILLARY TESTS

Immunohistochemistry
- Among pediatric renal tumors, loss of nuclear staining for SNF5 (INI1) very sensitive and highly specific for RTK
- Nonspecific polyphenotypic patterns for other antibodies due to trapping of antibodies in hyaline inclusions

Electron Microscopy
- Ultrastructurally, hyaline inclusions correspond to whorled intermediate filaments

DIFFERENTIAL DIAGNOSIS

Renal Medullary Carcinoma
- Older age, sickle cell trait, and occasionally glandular histology; SNF5 (INI1) lost, but keratin strong (+)

Cellular Mesoblastic Nephroma, Plump Cell Variant
- Spindle cell pattern and less invasive tumor periphery

Clear Cell Sarcoma of Kidney
- Lack prominent nucleoli; retained staining for SNF5 (INI1)

DIAGNOSTIC CHECKLIST

Pathologic Interpretation Pearls
- Many renal tumors show pseudorhabdoid features, but nuclear immunoreactivity for SNF5 (INI1) is retained in all such tumors

SELECTED REFERENCES

1. Geller JI et al: Biology and treatment of rhabdoid tumor. Crit Rev Oncog. 20(3-4):199-216, 2015
2. van den Heuvel-Eibrink MM et al: Malignant rhabdoid tumours of the kidney (MRTKs), registered on recent SIOP protocols from 1993 to 2005: a report of the SIOP renal tumour study group. Pediatr Blood Cancer. 56(5):733-7, 2011
3. Weeks DA et al: Rhabdoid tumor of kidney. A report of 111 cases from the National Wilms' Tumor Study Pathology Center. Am J Surg Pathol. 13(6):439-58, 1989

Malignant Rhabdoid Tumor

Characteristic Cytological Features

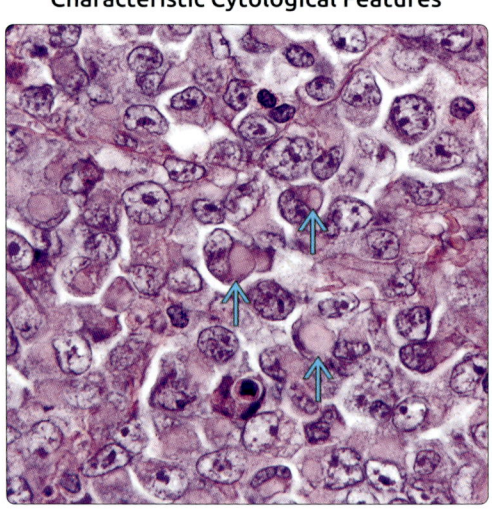

(Left) Malignant RTK typically shows mononuclear cells with pleomorphic nuclei, vesicular chromatin, conspicuous nucleoli, and intracytoplasmic eosinophilic hyaline inclusions ⇾. (Right) Besides overrunning the renal parenchyma, other features in rhabdoid tumors that indicate an aggressive phenotype include a very high mitotic index. This photomicrograph depicts a prominent mitotic activity ⇾ in an RTK.

High Mitotic Index

Trabecular/Nested Architecture

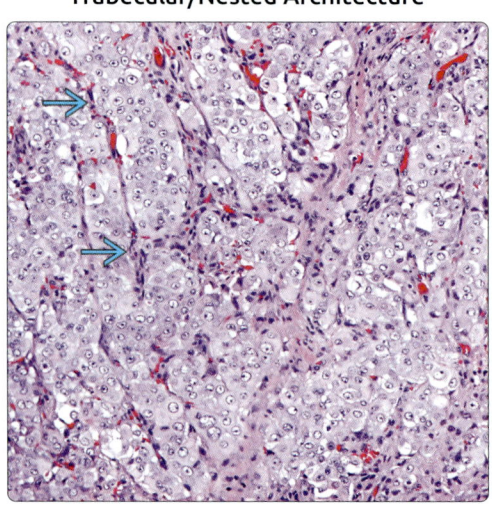

Sclerotic Variant

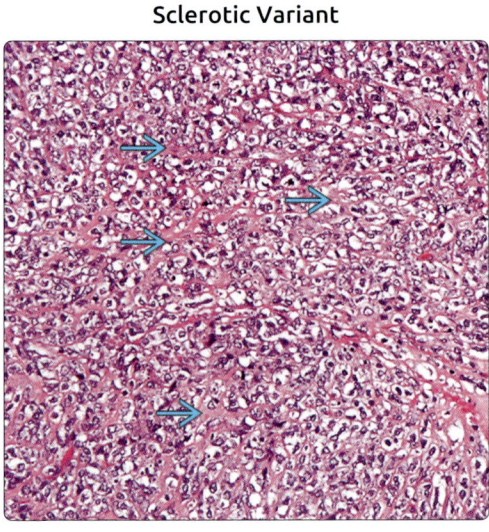

(Left) Some rhabdoid tumors show a trabecular pattern of growth. Delicate fibrovascular septations separating the tumor trabeculae ⇾ are also present here, and this may raise the suspicion of a clear cell sarcoma. The cytologic features are usually diagnostic. (Right) Some RTKs show areas with abundant sclerosis ⇾. This feature is more commonly associated with clear cell sarcoma of the kidney. Close attention to the cytologic features will help in arriving at the proper diagnosis.

Myxoid Stroma

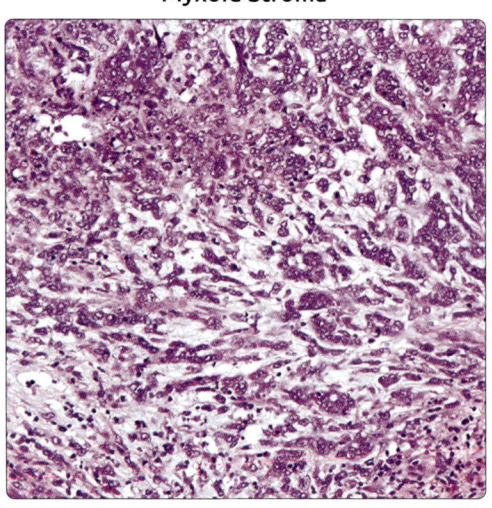

Tumor Necrosis

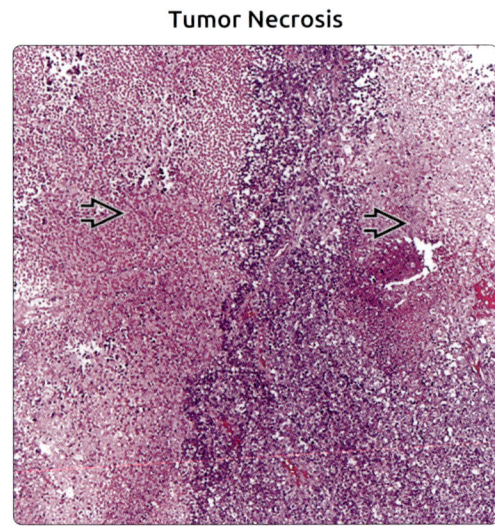

(Left) This H&E image shows marked myxoid change in the stroma of a RTK. Marked variation in the histomorphologic patterns is not infrequent in RTK, and the overall cytoarchitectural findings are essential for a proper diagnosis. (Right) H&E image shows an RTK with large areas of necrosis ⇾. Hemorrhage and necrosis are quite frequent in these tumors and support their aggressive nature. Cytoplasmic inclusions are often more abundant around the areas of necrosis.

Malignant Rhabdoid Tumor

Vascular Invasion

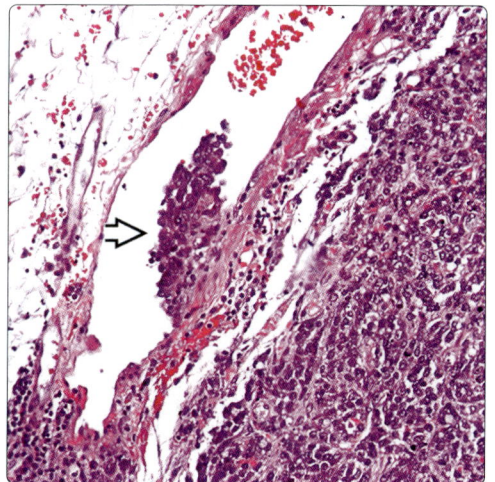

Renal Pelvis Invasion

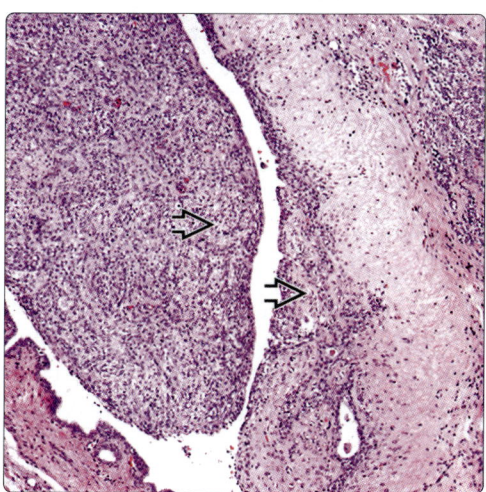

(Left) Vascular invasion ⇨ is usually extensive in malignant RTK. Many tumors show both gross and microscopic invasion of the sinus vessels, as well as the renal vein. (Right) Malignant RTKs frequently extend beyond renal parenchyma. Sinus fat or perinephric fat invasion are quite common, as is invasion of the pelvicalyceal system ⇨. Similarly, metastases involving multiple organ systems is also frequent at presentation.

Loss of Nuclear Staining for SNF5 (INI1)

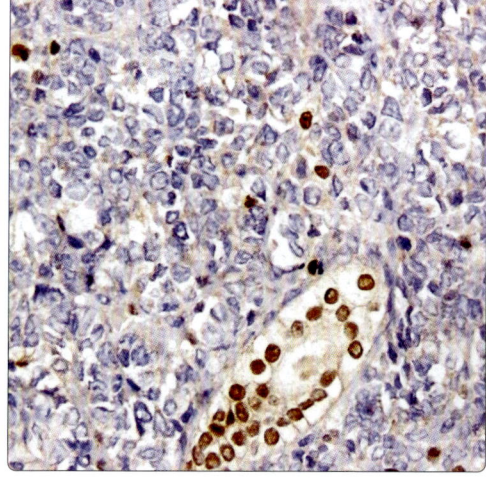

EMA

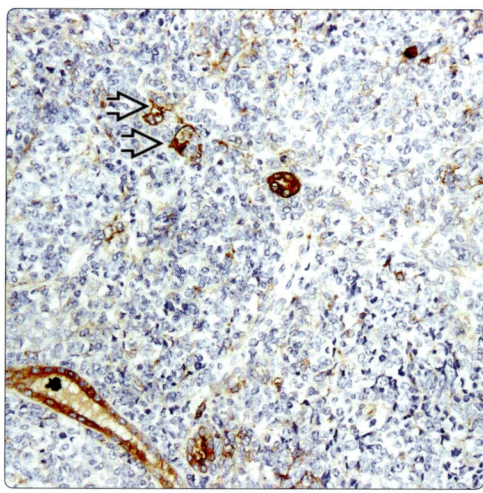

(Left) The most consistent and diagnostic immunostaining in rhabdoid and related central nervous system and soft tissue tumors is the loss of nuclear staining for SNF5. It is a reliable surrogate marker of hSNF5/INI1/SMARCB1 gene deletions or inactivating mutations. (Right) Immunostaining in RTK usually shows a polyphenotypic expression, due to nonspecific entrapment of the antibodies in the whorled structures in cytoplasmic inclusions. However, stains for EMA/MUC1 ⇨ and vimentin are often truly positive.

Differential Diagnosis: Clear Cell Sarcoma

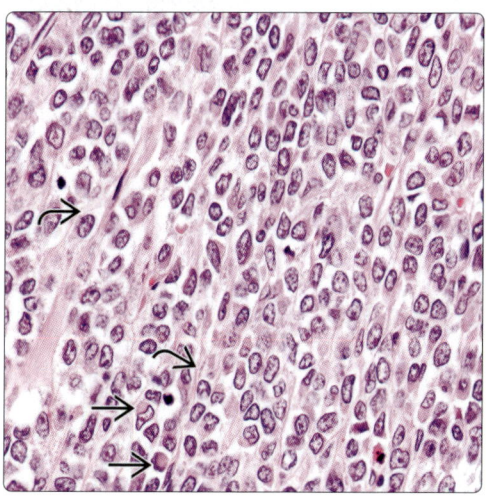

Clear Cell Sarcoma: Vimentin

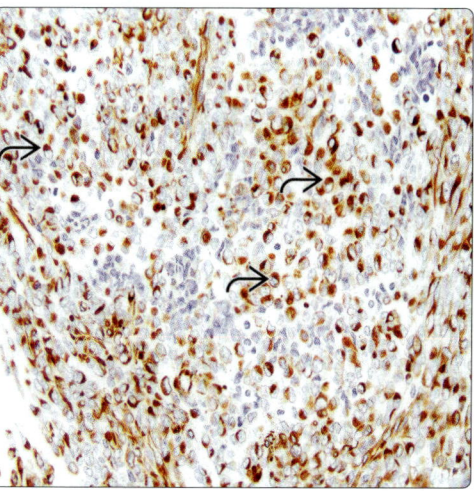

(Left) Some RTKs may show pale staining areas, and even focal vascular pattern ⇨, mimicking clear cell sarcoma. However, areas with the typical histology are often associated in such tumors. In spite of clear cell sarcoma-like histology, the characteristic cytoplasmic inclusions ⇨ are still noticeable. (Right) The tumor seen in the left frame shows the most characteristic perinuclear inclusion-like positivity ⇨ for vimentin. Such nonspecific positivity with multiple antibodies is not uncommon in RTK.

Mixed Epithelial and Stromal Tumor (MEST) Family Tumors and Pediatric Cystic Nephroma

KEY FACTS

TERMINOLOGY
- Mixed epithelial and stromal tumor (MEST) family tumors; pediatric cystic nephroma (PCN)
- MEST family of tumors show morphological spectrum ranging from variably solid to predominantly cystic (adult cystic nephroma) and contain biphasic epithelial and stromal components
- PCN (entirely distinct entity) composed purely of cysts separated by fibrous septa, sometimes containing well-differentiated tubules

ETIOLOGY/PATHOGENESIS
- Some features in MEST family tumors suggest role of steroid hormones in genesis and evolution of these tumors
- Most pediatric cystic nephromas harbor *DICER1* gene mutations

CLINICAL ISSUES
- MEST family tumors: M:F = 1:> 8; PCN: M:F = 2:1
- Incidentally detected kidney mass most common clinical presentation

MACROSCOPIC
- MEST family tumors variably solid and cystic, sometimes predominantly cystic with no apparent solid component (adult CN), or with predominant solid component
- PCN composed entirely of cysts and thin-walled septa

MICROSCOPIC
- Stroma and epithelium in both adult CN and MEST show varied histologic features
- PCN composed entirely of cysts separated by fibrous septa

TOP DIFFERENTIAL DIAGNOSES
- Multilocular cystic neoplasm of low malignant potential, tubulocystic carcinoma, cystic partially differentiated nephroblastoma (CPDN), mesoblastic nephroma (classical type), metanephric adenofibroma, renomedullary interstitial cell tumor

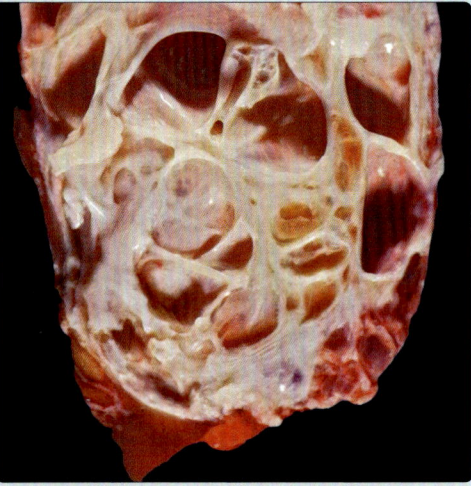

Gross Features

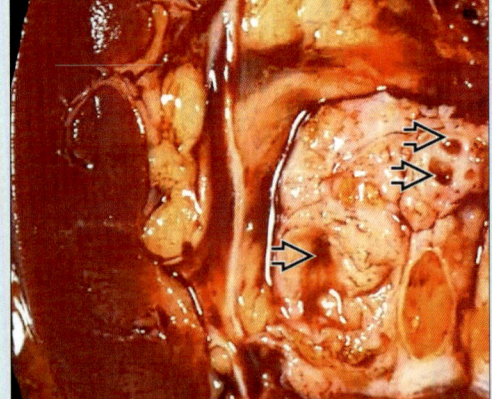

MEST: Gross Features

(Left) Gross photograph of an exclusively cystic, well-circumscribed tumor with no solid areas could represent either a pediatric cystic nephroma (PCN) or a cystic mixed epithelial and stromal (MEST) family tumor (adult cystic nephroma). Gross distinction from multilocular cystic neoplasm of low malignant potential is also not possible in such tumors. (Right) Gross appearance of this MEST shows a predominantly solid morphology. Relatively few cysts ⇨ are apparent.

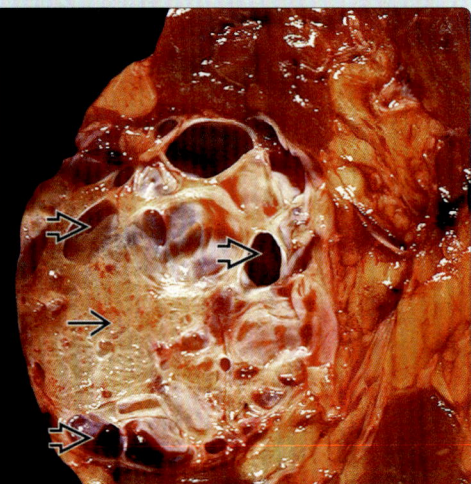

MEST: Gross Features

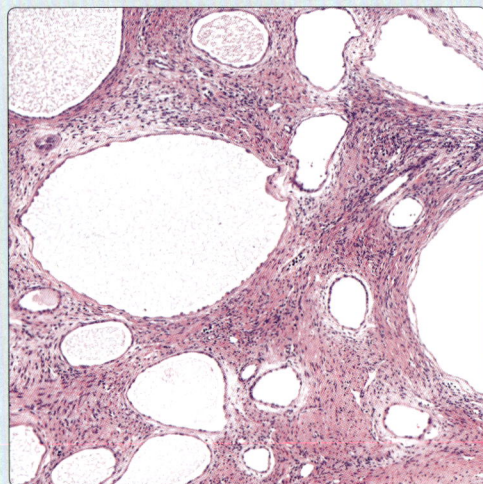

MEST: Solid Type

(Left) This tumor shows both prominent cystic areas ⇨ characteristic of adult CN and solid regions ⇨ more typical of MEST. The microscopic appearance may be influenced by variations in sampling in such a case. (Right) H&E of a MEST shows multiple variably sized tubules and cysts. Smaller cysts and complex branching glands are more common in more solid MESTs than in purely cystic MEST (adult cystic nephroma).

Mixed Epithelial and Stromal Tumor (MEST) Family Tumors and Pediatric Cystic Nephroma

TERMINOLOGY

Abbreviations
- Mixed epithelial and stromal tumor (MEST) family tumors; pediatric cystic nephroma (PCN)

Synonyms
- For MEST family tumors, renal epithelial and stromal tumor (REST); none for pediatric cystic nephroma

Definitions
- MEST family of tumors showing morphological spectrum ranging from variably solid to predominantly cystic tumors (adult cystic nephroma) containing biphasic epithelial and stromal components
- PCN (entirely distinct entity) composed purely of cysts separated by fibrous septa, sometimes containing well-differentiated tubules
  - Terminology of cystic nephroma for cystic tumors resembling PCN in adults may not be appropriate

ETIOLOGY/PATHOGENESIS

MEST Family Tumors
- Some features suggest role of steroid hormones in genesis and evolution of these tumors, including
  - Marked female predominance
  - Common history of long-term estrogen replacement in female patients
  - Frequent expression of ER and PR in tumor mesenchymal component
  - Long-term sex steroid exposure in male patients
- Gene expression profiles of mRNA demonstrate that both adult CN and MEST share similar expression profiles
  - Highest differentially expressed gene, relative to other tumors and nonneoplastic parenchyma: Insulin-like growth factor 2
  - Lowest differential expression is of carbonic anhydrase 2 gene
  - Rare case of translocation t(1;19) in MEST also reported

Pediatric Cystic Nephroma
- Most PCN harbor double-stranded RNA-specific endoribonuclease (*DICER1*) gene mutations
  - Gene located on chromosome 14q32.13 and encodes proteins belonging to RNase III family
  - Acts as endoribonuclease, cleaving double-stranded RNA
    - Required by RNA interference pathway to produce active microRNA (miRNA) and small temporal RNA (siRNA) molecules playing role in gene repression
- *DICER1* mutations not found in cystic partially differentiated nephroblastoma, suggesting that these 2 neoplasms (earlier believed to be part of continuous spectrum of disease) are in fact distinct entities
- MEST family tumors, including adult CN, do not show *DICER1* gene mutations; thus, so-called adult cystic nephromas unrelated to PCN

CLINICAL ISSUES

Epidemiology
- Age
  - MEST family tumors
    - Mean: 53 years (range: 34-78)
  - PCN
    - Mostly < 4 years
- Sex
  - MEST family tumors: M:F = 1:> 8
  - PCN: M:F = 2:1

Presentation
- MEST: Incidentally detected kidney mass most common clinical presentation; other symptoms include abdominal pain, hematuria, and urinary tract infections
- PCN: Often with pain due to tumor herniation into pelvicalyceal system

Prognosis
- All reported cases of MEST family tumors behave in benign fashion following surgical excision
  - 1 reported local recurrence 21 years after resection
- Few cases of malignant MEST reported in literature
  - Malignant phenotype observed in either epithelial or mesenchymal components
    - Spindle cell NOS, synovial sarcoma, rhabdoid, rhabdomyosarcoma, and chondrosarcoma differentiation in malignant stromal components
- PCN: Usually benign outcome; rare sarcomas (so-called DICER1 sarcomas) arising in PCN reported

MACROSCOPIC

General Features
- MEST family tumors usually solitary; very rare bilateral tumors reported
  - Most tumors well circumscribed and confined to kidney, often located close to renal hilum, but larger tumors may involve cortex
  - Variably solid and cystic, sometimes predominantly cystic with no apparent solid component (adult CN) or with predominant solid component
    - Majority of cysts contain clear serous fluid, rarely hemorrhagic or purulent material
- PCN composed entirely of cysts separated by thin-walled septa

Size
- Similar for both PCN and MEST: 1.7-21 cm (mean: 6.5 cm)

MICROSCOPIC

Histologic Features
- MEST family tumors
  - Stroma in both adult CN and MEST shows varied histologic features, including
    - Loose fibrous and edematous, dense fibrous and sclerotic, ovarian-type stroma, hypercellular spindled, NOS, or smooth muscle type
    - Ovarian-type stroma may show luteinized stromal cells
  - Prominent vasculature, more common in more solid tumors
  - Calcifications and foamy histiocytes present in both cystic and solid MEST
  - Cells in epithelial components with varied features, including

Mixed Epithelial and Stromal Tumor (MEST) Family Tumors and Pediatric Cystic Nephroma

- Flat, hobnailed, cuboidal, columnar, urothelial-like, clear cell
  - Prominent ovarian stroma, smaller cysts, complex branching glands, phyllodes gland pattern, and luteinization more common in solid MEST than adult CN
- PCN composed entirely of cysts separated by septa
  - Cysts lined by flattened, cuboidal, or hobnail epithelium, or denuded
  - Septa contain fibrous tissue with focal hypercellularity and well-differentiated tubules
    - Presence of immature nephroblastic elements indicates cystic partially differentiated nephroblastoma, and excludes diagnosis of PCN

ANCILLARY TESTS

Immunohistochemistry

- Stromal cells in MEST family tumors often positive for ER, PR, and less commonly for inhibin and calretinin (particularly in luteinized cells)

DIFFERENTIAL DIAGNOSIS

Multilocular Cystic Renal Neoplasm of Low Malignant Potential

- Differentiation required from PCN and predominantly cystic MEST
  - Multilocular cystic renal neoplasm of low malignant potential with cysts showing variable flattened lining or almost entirely larger cells with clear cytoplasm
  - Clusters or nests of clear cells always present in septa
  - No cellular or ovarian-type stroma
  - Lining cells with CA9, CD10, and often CK7 positive immunophenotype
  - No stromal immunoreactivity for ER and PR
  - PCN always seen in young children

Tubulocystic Carcinoma

- Needs to be differentiated from PCN and predominantly cystic MEST
  - Cells lining tubules and cysts in tubulocystic carcinoma have high-grade nuclei and abundant eosinophilic cytoplasm
  - Stroma usually dense fibrotic and desmoplastic
  - Septa often incomplete and free floating
  - No ER and PR positivity
  - Unlike tubulocystic carcinoma, PCN always seen in young children

Cystic Partially Differentiated Nephroblastoma

- Cystic partially differentiated nephroblastoma (CPDN) needs to be differentiated from PCN and occasionally, predominantly cystic MEST
  - Shows at least focal nephroblastematous tissue, such as blastema, immature stromal cells, and primitive epithelium in septa
  - Almost all patients < 24 months old

Mesoblastic Nephroma (Classical Type)

- Differential is with solid MEST
  - Classical mesoblastic nephroma shows finger-like extensions into surrounding renal parenchyma
  - Entrapped native tubules and glomeruli often seen in mesoblastic nephroma
    - However, seen almost entirely in periphery of tumor
  - Mesoblastic nephroma shows no ER or PR positivity

Metanephric Adenofibroma

- Metanephric adenofibroma needs to be differentiated from solid MEST
  - Epithelial component of metanephric adenofibroma typically composed of tightly packed small uniform acini
  - Epithelial component has embryonal appearance similar to metanephric adenoma
  - Stromal component in metanephric adenofibroma ER and PR negative

Renomedullary Interstitial Cell Tumor

- Almost invariably incidental finding
- Epithelial component usually with entrapped renal tubules mostly in periphery
- Stroma not ER and PR positive

DIAGNOSTIC CHECKLIST

Pathologic Interpretation Pearls

- PCN is distinct entity, separate from CPDN or completely cystic adult MEST (adult cystic nephroma)
  - Therefore, it may be prudent to use term cystic MEST for such cystic tumors in adults

SELECTED REFERENCES

1. Vanecek T et al: Mixed epithelial and stromal tumor of the kidney: mutation analysis of the DICER 1 gene in 29 cases. Appl Immunohistochem Mol Morphol. ePub, 2015
2. Doros LA et al: DICER1 mutations in childhood cystic nephroma and its relationship to DICER1-renal sarcoma. Mod Pathol. 27(9):1267-80, 2014
3. Bahubeshi A et al: Germline DICER1 mutations and familial cystic nephroma. J Med Genet. 47(12):863-6, 2010
4. Mohanty SK et al: Mixed epithelial and stromal tumors of the kidney: an overview. Arch Pathol Lab Med. 133(9):1483-6, 2009
5. Portier BP et al: Mixed epithelial and stromal tumor of the kidney. J Urol. 181(4):1879-80, 2009
6. Zhou M et al: Adult cystic nephroma and mixed epithelial and stromal tumor of the kidney are the same disease entity: molecular and histologic evidence. Am J Surg Pathol. 33(1):72-80, 2009
7. Jung SJ et al: Mixed epithelial and stromal tumor of kidney with malignant transformation: report of two cases and review of literature. Hum Pathol. 39(3):463-8, 2008
8. Kuroda N et al: Carcinosarcoma arising in mixed epithelial and stromal tumor of the kidney. APMIS. 116(11):1013-5, 2008
9. Lane BR et al: Adult cystic nephroma and mixed epithelial and stromal tumor of the kidney: clinical, radiographic, and pathologic characteristics. Urology. 71(6):1142-8, 2008
10. Montironi R et al: Cystic nephroma and mixed epithelial and stromal tumour of the kidney: opposite ends of the spectrum of the same entity? Eur Urol. 54(6):1237-46, 2008
11. Sukov WR et al: Malignant mixed epithelial and stromal tumor of the kidney with rhabdoid features: report of a case including immunohistochemical, molecular genetic studies and comparison to morphologically similar renal tumors. Hum Pathol. 38(9):1432-7, 2007
12. Turbiner J et al: Cystic nephroma and mixed epithelial and stromal tumor of kidney: a detailed clinicopathologic analysis of 34 cases and proposal for renal epithelial and stromal tumor (REST) as a unifying term. Am J Surg Pathol. 31(4):489-500, 2007
13. Antic T et al: Mixed epithelial and stromal tumor of the kidney and cystic nephroma share overlapping features: reappraisal of 15 lesions. Arch Pathol Lab Med. 130(1):80-5, 2006
14. Compérat E et al: Benign mixed epithelial and stromal tumor of the kidney (MEST) with cytogenetic alteration. Pathol Res Pract. 200(11-12):865-7, 2005
15. Michal M et al: Mixed epithelial and stromal tumors of the kidney. A report of 22 cases. Virchows Arch. 445(4):359-67, 2004

Mixed Epithelial and Stromal Tumor (MEST) Family Tumors and Pediatric Cystic Nephroma

MEST: Predominantly Cystic

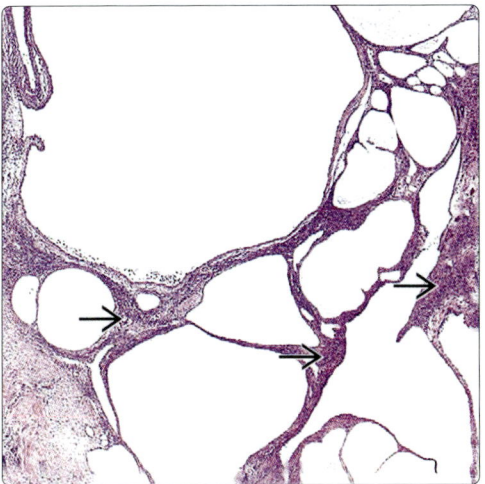

MEST: Ovarian-Type Stroma

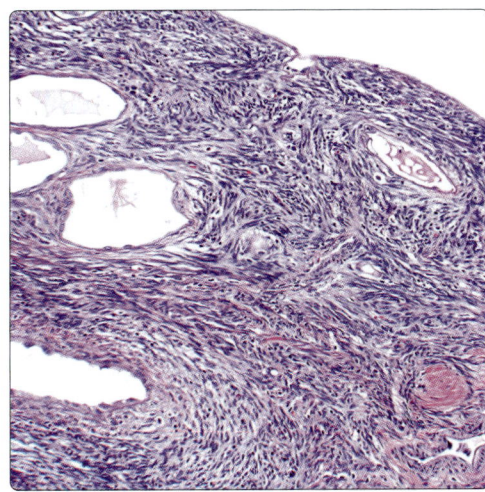

(Left) H&E shows a CN (cystic MEST) with septa composed of cellular ovarian-type stroma ➡. While such stroma may be present in cystic tumors, it is a more common finding in solid MEST. The ovarian stroma may show areas with luteinization and foam cells. (Right) Densely cellular ovarian-type stroma in MEST is shown. Predominant occurrence in females, rare tumors in males on hormone therapy, and ER/PR positivity raises the strong possibility of the role of hormones in the pathogenesis of these tumors.

MEST: Cambium-Like Stroma

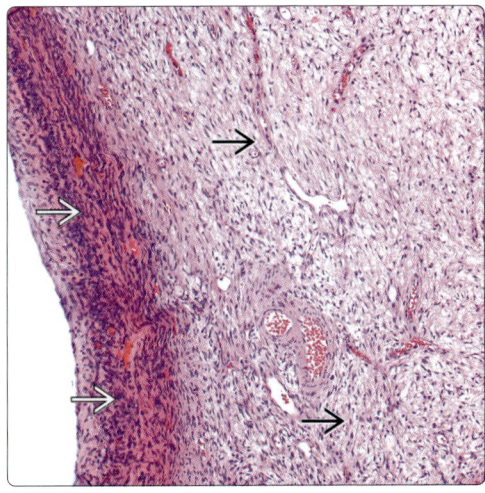

MEST: Leiomyomatous Stroma

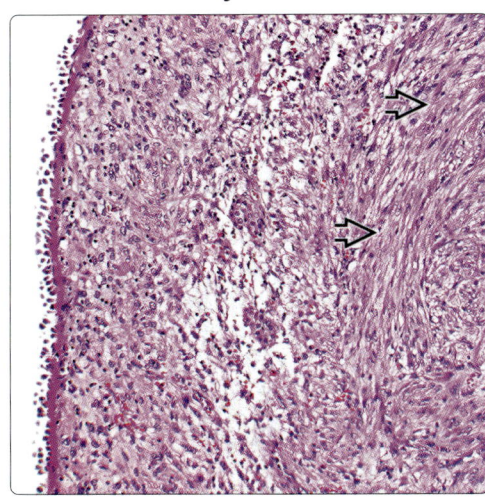

(Left) Some MESTs show a cambium-like condensed ovarian-type stroma underlying the epithelium. This image shows ovarian-type stroma ➡ under the cyst lining surrounded by more loose stroma ➡ in the rest of the tumor. ER/PR reactivity is more likely in ovarian-type stroma but may be seen in other types of stroma. (Right) Some MESTs show prominent smooth muscle differentiation ➡ of the stroma. Not unexpectedly, such areas are strongly positive for actin-sm, actin-HHF-35, and desmin.

MEST: Fatty Stroma

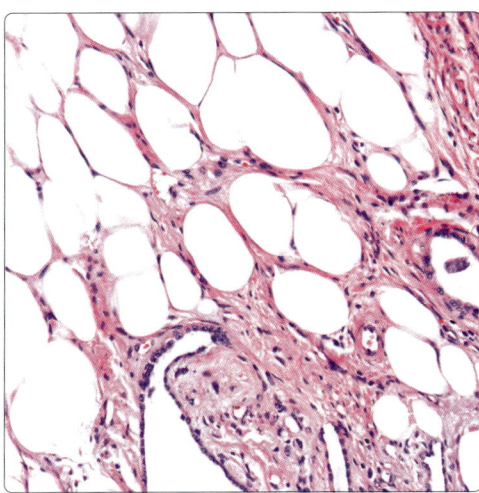

MEST: Phylloides-Like Features

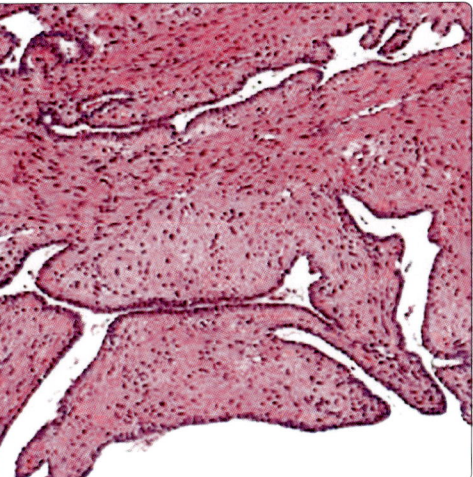

(Left) In addition to smooth muscle, the stroma in MEST may also show adipocytic differentiation. Usually, such a finding is focal, but some tumors contain a prominent fatty component. (Right) The stromal proliferation in mixed epithelial and stromal tumors may occasionally lead to leaf-like expanded (phyllodes-like) phenotype. For obvious reasons, such proliferations would not be a feature of predominantly cystic tumors.

Mixed Epithelial and Stromal Tumor (MEST) Family Tumors and Pediatric Cystic Nephroma

MEST: Corpus Albicantes-Like Focus

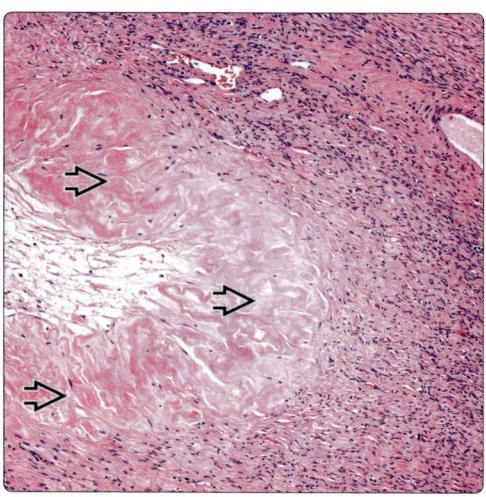

MEST: Vascular Hyalinization

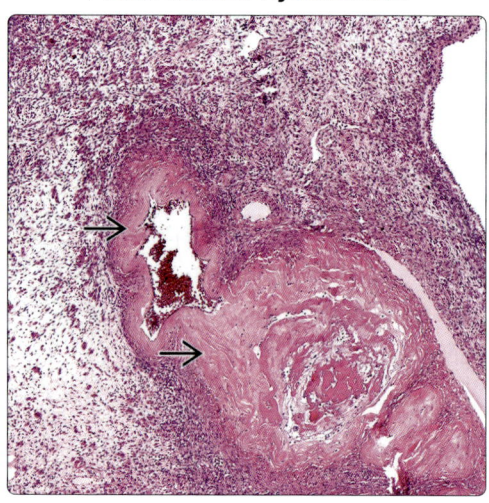

(Left) H&E shows a corpus albicantes-like structure ⇨ in a background of ovarian-type stroma. (Right) This photomicrograph depicts a large vessel with hyalinization ⇨ of the wall, supporting that the hyalinized structures are not similar to corpora albicantia of the ovary. In most cases, the pathogenesis of such structures cannot be determined, but in many cases, these seem to result from hyalinization of vessels or epithelial structures.

MEST: Cuboidal Epithelium

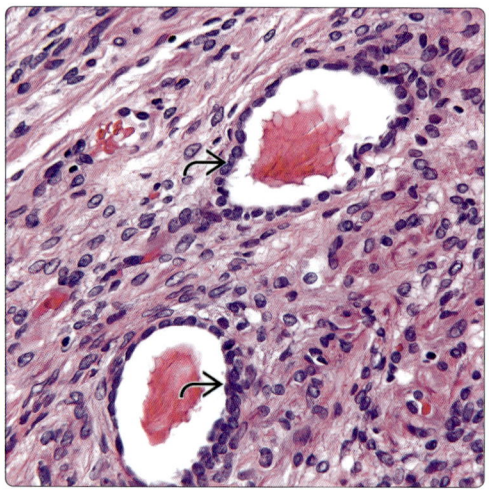

MEST: Hobnailed Epithelium

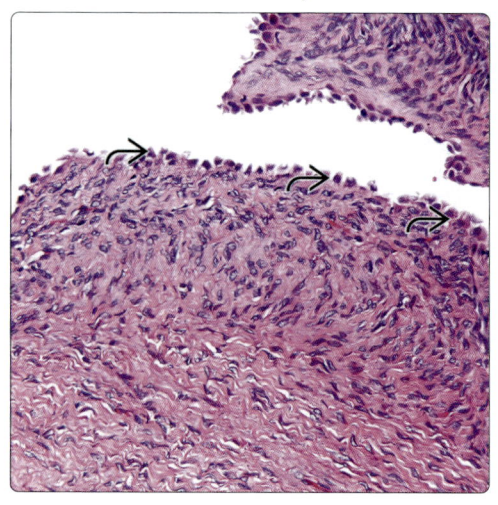

(Left) The cells in the epithelial component in mixed epithelial and stromal tumors are flat, hobnailed, cuboidal, or columnar. This image shows cuboidal epithelial lining ⇨ in small cysts of MEST. There is no nuclear atypia or nucleolar prominence. (Right) The cytological features of the cysts lining in both predominantly cystic or solid MESTs are essentially similar. This image illustrates hobnailing ⇨ of the lining epithelium in a solid MEST.

MEST: Adult Cystic Nephroma

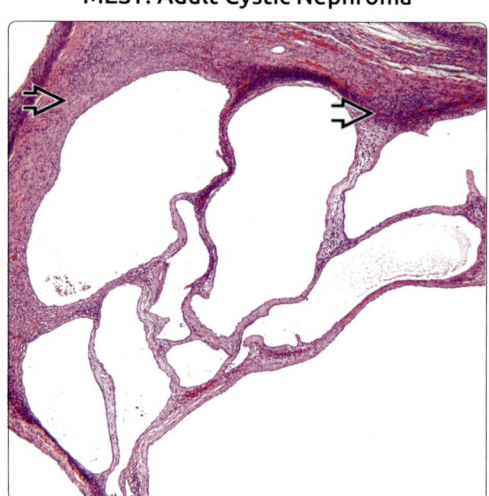

MEST: Adult Cystic Nephroma

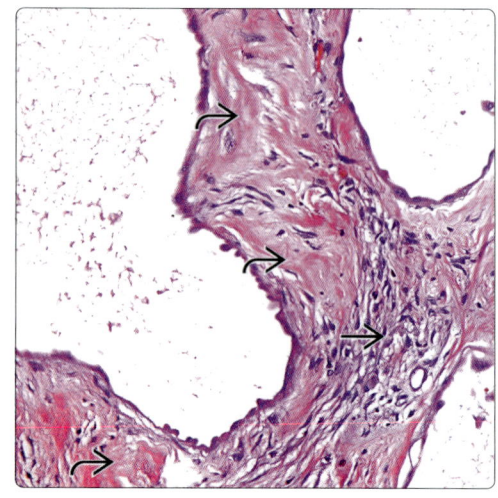

(Left) H&E shows an adult CN with slightly widened cellular septa ⇨. The lining is flattened without significant stratification. (Right) H&E of a predominantly cystic MEST (adult CN) shows a combination of sclerotic ⇨ and cellular spindle cell ⇨ stroma. Mixture of stromal patterns is common in both cystic and solid MESTs.

Mixed Epithelial and Stromal Tumor (MEST) Family Tumors and Pediatric Cystic Nephroma

MEST: Adult Cystic Nephroma

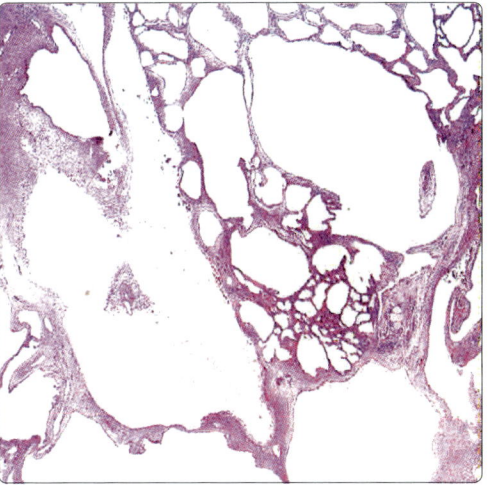

MEST: Adult Cystic Nephroma

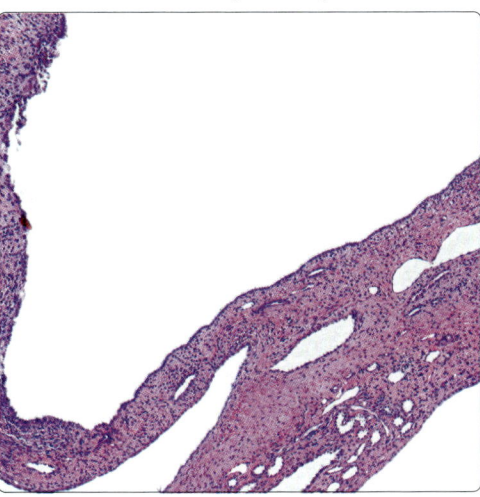

(Left) H&E of a completely cystic MEST (adult CN) shows an exclusive cystic architecture. The cysts are discrete, without any apparent interconnections. (Right) Although the separation appears to be artificial, and likely clinically irrelevant, adult CN does not show any solid areas or mural nodules. Septal thickness > 5 mm would place the tumor into the category of MEST. Even though these histologic criteria are arbitrary, these reiterate the overlap and close relationship between the two.

MEST: Clear Cell Lining

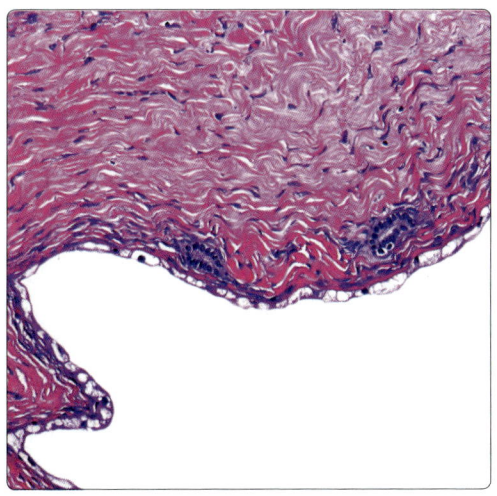

Epithelial Proliferation

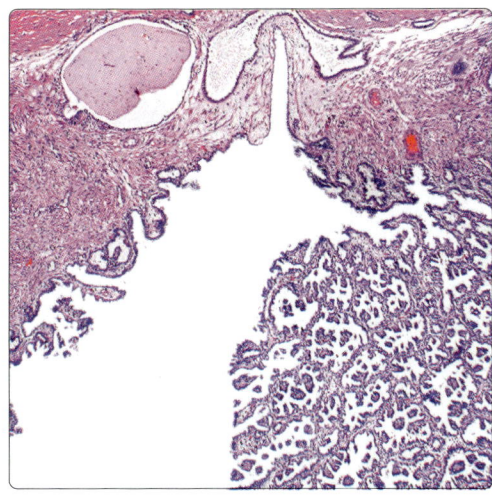

(Left) Some MESTs show variable clear cell cytology. This may raise the possibility of a multilocular cystic neoplasm of low malignant potential. However, many of these have ER/PR(+) ovarian-type stroma, and lack solid nests of clear cells in the septa. (Right) H&E shows marked epithelial proliferation in MEST. Due to lack of stromal invasion, this would qualify at least as a borderline tumor. Malignant transformation in MEST, though very rare, may occur in both epithelial and mesenchymal elements.

Malignant MEST: Sarcoma

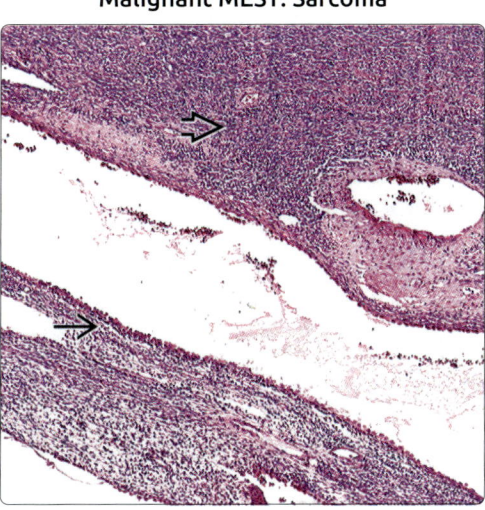

Malignant MEST: Sarcoma

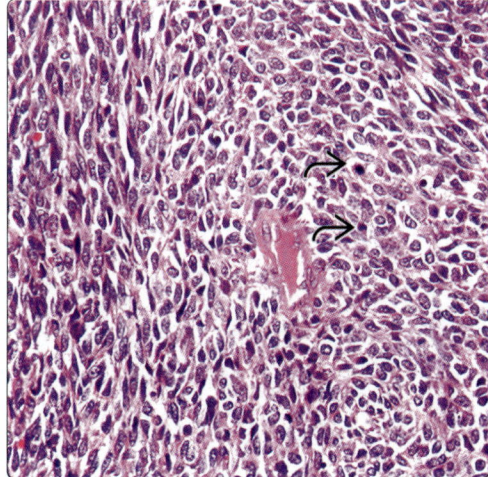

(Left) Although rare carcinomas arising in MEST are reported, most associated malignant tumors are sarcomas. This image shows a spindle cell sarcoma ⇒ arising within a MEST ⇒. (Right) Higher magnification of sarcoma arising within MEST shows marked hypercellularity, anaplastic features, and high mitotic activity ⇒ in the tumor. Synovial sarcoma, sarcomas with rhabdoid, rhabdomyo-/chondrosarcomatous differentiation have been described in mixed epithelial and stromal tumors.

Mixed Epithelial and Stromal Tumor (MEST) Family Tumors and Pediatric Cystic Nephroma

(Left) In addition to the presence of ovarian-type stroma, some mixed epithelial and stromal tumors may show dispersed luteinized cells ➔. Sometimes, these may appear in small and even focally large clusters. Such cells are often inhibin positive by immunohistochemistry. **(Right)** Lower power view depicts a minute-mixed epithelial and stromal tumor. Notice the well-circumscribed nature of the tumor, a relatively typical finding in both the cystic and solid MESTs. Interspersed within a cellular stroma are benign epithelial elements ➔.

MEST: Luteinized Cells
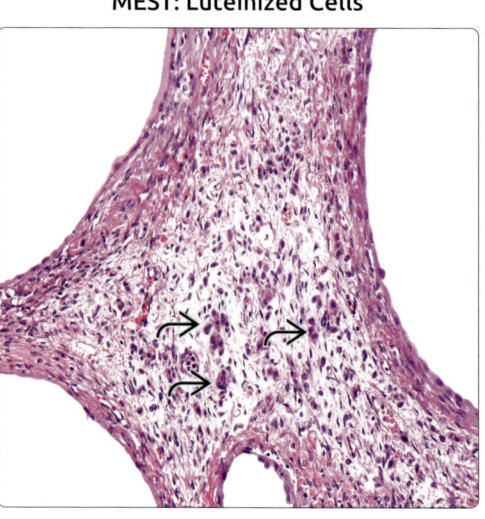

Microscopic MEST
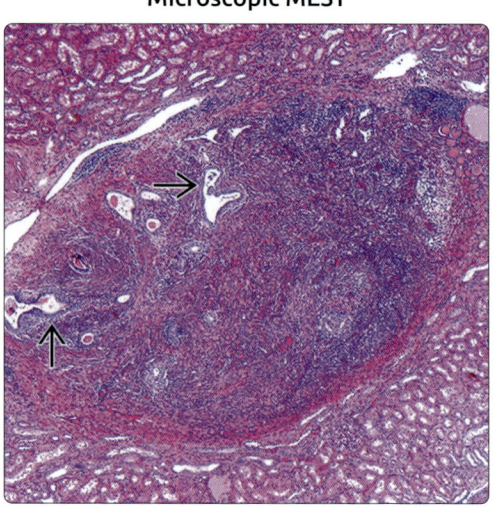

(Left) Similar to ER, PR may also be expressed in both cystic and solid MEST. While some consider such positivity as favoring specific origins for these tumors, others have shown that ER and PR immunoreactivity in renal stroma may be a metaplastic change that may be associated with obstruction and nonneoplastic cyst formation. **(Right)** In this image, CD10 positivity in the spindle cell stroma of a MEST is shown. The immunoreactivity is often concentrated around the epithelial elements ➔.

ER/PR(+) Stroma
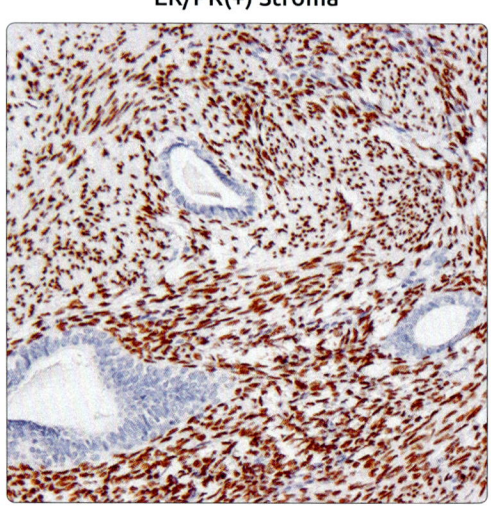

CD10
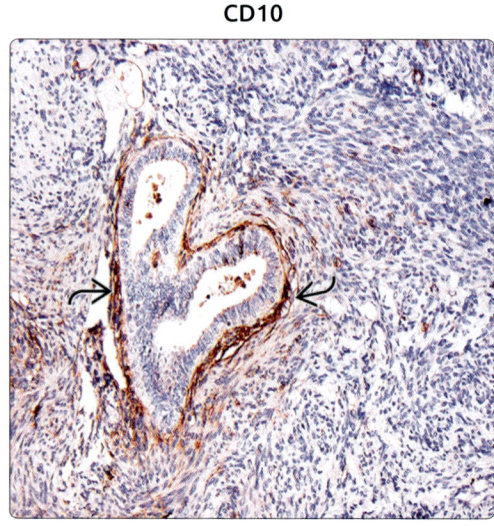

(Left) PCN is composed entirely of cysts separated by thin-walled septa. The septa contain fibrous tissue with focal, well-differentiated tubules ➔. Presence of immature nephroblastic elements indicates cystic partially differentiated nephroblastoma and excludes the diagnosis of PCN. **(Right)** In PCN, the septa contain usually paucicellular fibrous tissue. ER/PR positive stroma is absent. Notice the focal, well-differentiated tubules ➔ in the septa.

Pediatric Cystic Nephroma
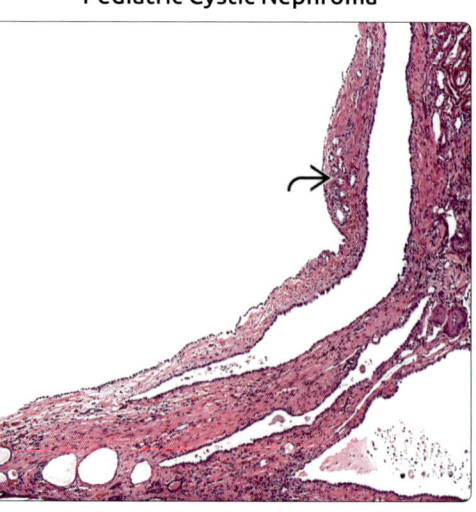

Pediatric Cystic Nephroma
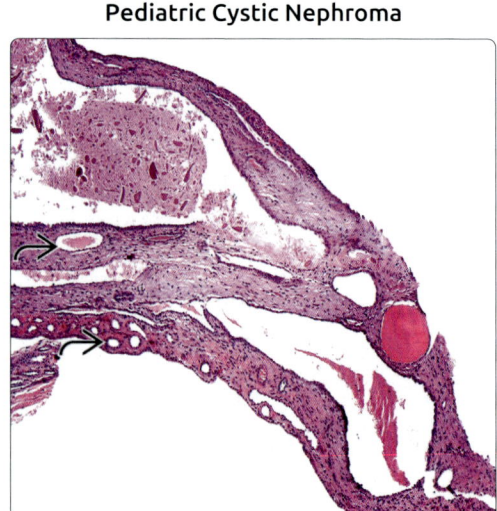

Mixed Epithelial and Stromal Tumor (MEST) Family Tumors and Pediatric Cystic Nephroma

Differential Diagnosis: CPDN

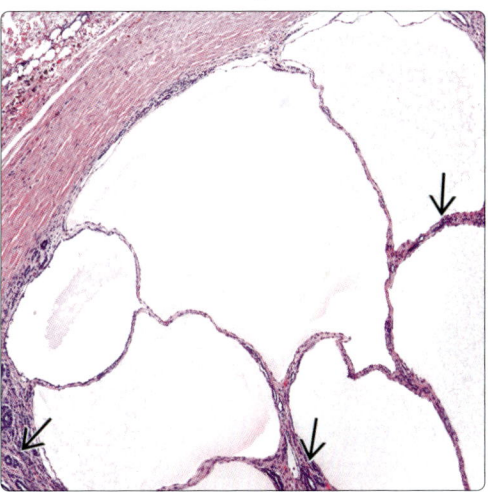

Differential Diagnosis: CPDN

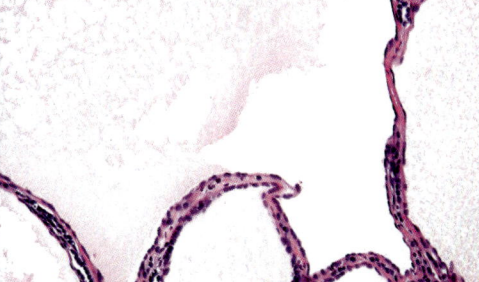
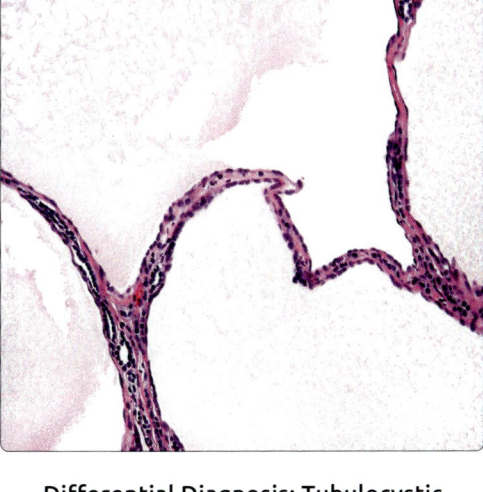

(Left) Presence of immature nephroblastic elements ⇨ in an otherwise completely cystic pediatric tumor puts it in the category of cystic partially differentiated nephroblastoma (CPDN). PCN is now regarded as a distinct entity, separate from CPDN or completely cystic adult MEST (adult CN). (Right) Most PCNs harbor DICER1 gene mutations. Such mutations have not been found in CPDN or MEST family tumors in the adults, supporting a distinct nature of CPN.

Differential Diagnosis: Tubulocystic Carcinoma

Differential Diagnosis: Tubulocystic Carcinoma

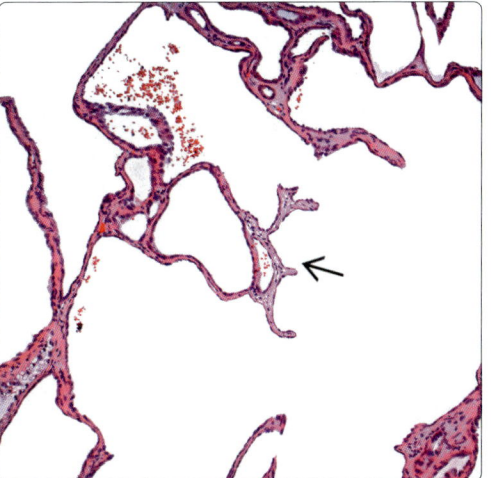
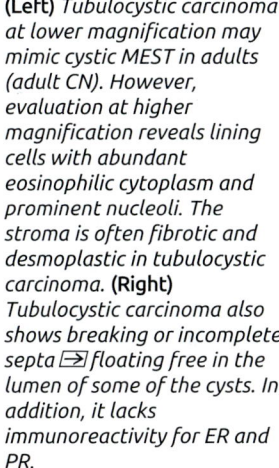

(Left) Tubulocystic carcinoma at lower magnification may mimic cystic MEST in adults (adult CN). However, evaluation at higher magnification reveals lining cells with abundant eosinophilic cytoplasm and prominent nucleoli. The stroma is often fibrotic and desmoplastic in tubulocystic carcinoma. (Right) Tubulocystic carcinoma also shows breaking or incomplete septa ⇨ floating free in the lumen of some of the cysts. In addition, it lacks immunoreactivity for ER and PR.

Differential Diagnosis: Tubulocystic Carcinoma

Differential Diagnosis: Renomedullary Interstitial Cell Tumor

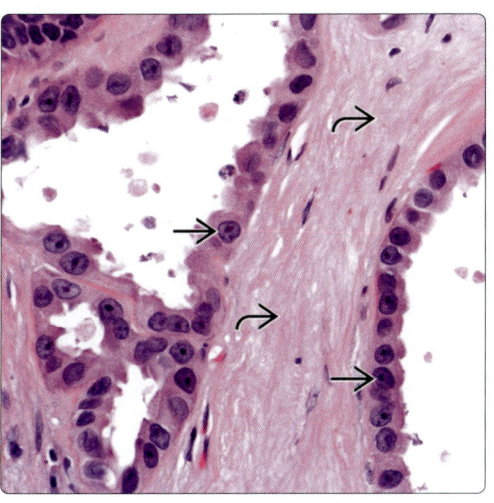
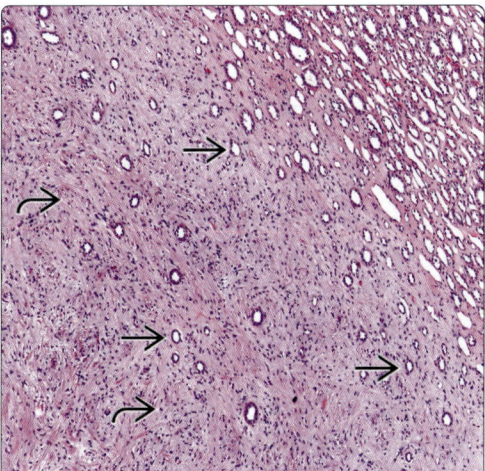

(Left) Prominence of nucleoli ⇨ in the lining cuboidal cells is a usual feature in tubulocystic carcinoma. Notice the fibrotic stromal component ⇨ as well. (Right) Unlike MEST, renomedullary interstitial cell tumor (RICT), with very rare exceptions, is an incidental finding in kidneys removed for other causes. Stroma in RICT ⇨ is not ovarian-type and is not ER and PR positive. Epithelial component usually consists of entrapped renal tubules, mostly in periphery of the lesion ⇨.

Synovial Sarcoma

KEY FACTS

TERMINOLOGY
- Synovial sarcoma (SS)
- Mesenchymal spindle cell tumor with rare epithelial differentiation and chromosomal translocation t(X;18)(p11;q11)

ETIOLOGY/PATHOGENESIS
- Primary renal SS shares characteristic *SYT-SSX* gene fusion with its more common soft tissue counterpart
- *SYT-SSX2* fusion correlates with monophasic histology in soft tissue; this may explain predominant monophasic morphology in kidney

CLINICAL ISSUES
- Rare, with ~ 80 cases described; age range: 17-78 yr (median: 36 yr); M:F = 1:1
- Aggressive with median disease-free-survival of 33 months
- Concurrent or subsequent metastases very frequent; metastatic disease with median survival of only 6 months
- Lung is most common site of metastasis; other sites include lymph nodes, liver, bones, and abdominal cavity; one of few sarcomas with lymph node metastasis

MICROSCOPIC
- Most renal SS with monophasic histology (76%)
  - Biphasic histology in 16% and poorly differentiated in 8%
- Microscopic intratumoral cysts in > 80% of tumors

ANCILLARY TESTS
- Frequently positive for Bcl-2, CD99, and vimentin; TLE1 with diffuse nuclear expression in > 90%
- FISH or reverse transcription–polymerase chain reaction (RT-PCR) for *SYT-SSX* gene fusion gold standard for diagnosis

TOP DIFFERENTIAL DIAGNOSES
- Primitive neuroectodermal tumor; blastemal Wilms tumor; cellular mesoblastic nephroma; primitive neuroectodermal tumor

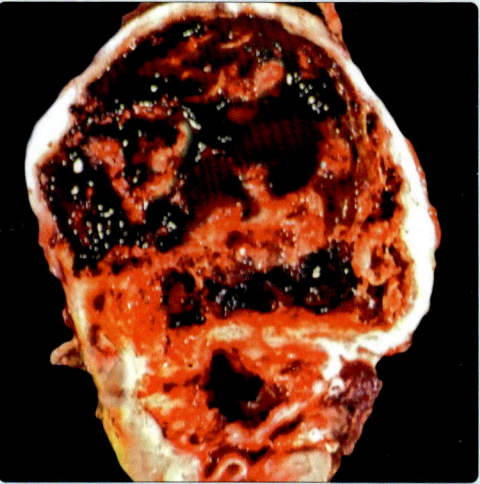

Gross Features

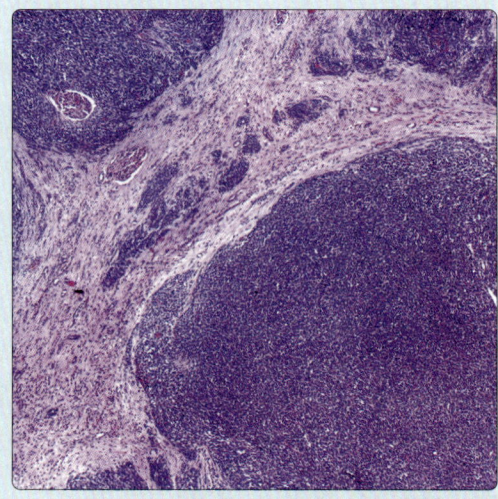

Multilobulated Architecture

(Left) This gross photograph of a primary renal synovial sarcoma (SS) shows the typical features of the tumor: Large size, extensive necrosis, cystic change, and hemorrhage. Cysts are grossly observed in 2/3 of the cases. (Right) Most renal SS show an infiltrative, multinodular growth pattern. This low-magnification view of a primary renal SS shows these typical features: Multilobulation, high cellularity, and infiltrative edges of the tumor.

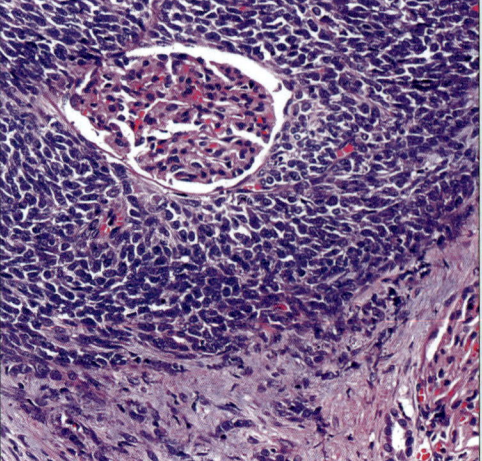

Infiltrative Borders

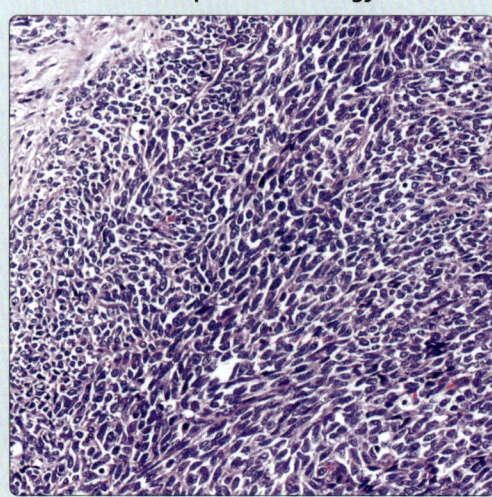

Monophasic Histology

(Left) Primary renal monophasic synovial sarcoma shows infiltrative borders, a characteristic feature of the tumor. This aggressive neoplasm often shows extrarenal extensions and vascular invasion, along with necrosis and high mitotic index. (Right) Hematoxylin & eosin shows the typical interlacing short fascicles of spindle-shaped cells in a primary renal SS. Most renal SS are of the monophasic type, with biphasic and poorly differentiated features in approximately only 1/5 of tumors.

Synovial Sarcoma

TERMINOLOGY

Abbreviations
- Synovial sarcoma (SS)

Definitions
- Mesenchymal spindle cell tumor with rare epithelial differentiation and chromosomal translocation t(X;18)(p11;q11)

ETIOLOGY/PATHOGENESIS

Molecular Features
- Primary renal SS shares characteristic *SYT-SSX* gene fusion with its soft tissue counterpart
  - Most reported renal SS with *SYT-SSX2* gene fusion
    - *SYT-SSX2* fusion correlates with monophasic histology in soft tissue; this may explain predominant monophasic morphology in kidney

CLINICAL ISSUES

Epidemiology
- Rare, with ~ 80 cases described; age range: 17-78 yr (median: 36 yr); M:F = 1:1

Presentation
- Presentation similar to that of other mass lesions; may present with symptoms related to metastases

Treatment
- Managed with combination of surgery and adjuvant chemotherapy; response rates to ifosfamide and doxorubicin-based chemotherapy ~ 24%

Prognosis
- Aggressive with median disease-free-survival of 33 months
- Concurrent or subsequent metastases very frequent; metastatic disease with median survival of only 6 months
  - Lung is most common site of metastasis; other sites include lymph nodes, liver, bones, and abdominal cavity; one of few sarcomas with lymph node metastasis

MACROSCOPIC

General Features
- Most tumors large [range,10-17 cm (mean: 11)], necrotic, and grossly cystic; gross cysts in approximately 2/3

MICROSCOPIC

Histologic Features
- Most renal SS with monophasic histology (76%)
  - Highly cellular, with plump embryonal-appearing spindle cells growing in short, intersecting fascicles
  - Cytoplasm scant and ill defined, and nuclei ovoid to fusiform with coarse chromatin, variably sized nucleoli, frequent mitoses, and extensive necrosis
  - Microscopic intratumoral cysts in > 80% of tumors
    - Cysts lined by cells with eosinophilic cytoplasm and often hobnail appearance, represent cystically dilated entrapped native tubules; such cysts led to classification as primitive sarcomas arising in cystic nephroma in past
  - Alternating hypocellular myxoid areas and prominent hemangiopericytomatous pattern common
  - Biphasic histology in 16% and poorly differentiated in 8%
  - Angiolymphatic invasion frequently present

ANCILLARY TESTS

Immunohistochemistry
- Frequently positive for Bcl-2, CD99, and vimentin; TLE1 with diffuse nuclear expression in > 90%
- CD34 and muscle markers (-); focally (+) for EMA/MUC1 and keratins (EMA/MUC1 more often than keratins) in some

Genetic Testing
- FISH or reverse transcription–polymerase chain reaction (RT-PCR) for *SYT-SSX* gene fusion gold standard for diagnosis

DIFFERENTIAL DIAGNOSIS

Primitive Neuroectodermal Tumor
- Sheets and lobules of small round cells with scant cytoplasm
- Rosette formation is useful pointer to diagnosis
- Molecular evidence of *FLI1-EWS* fusion confirmatory

Blastemal Wilms Tumor
- Wilms tumor (WT) typically seen in patients < 5 yr old; SS is tumor of older patients
- SS is usually spindle cell neoplasm, except in cases of poorly differentiated subtype
- WT1 and pax-2 is positive in WT
- Demonstration of *SYT-SSX* gene fusion is diagnostic

Cellular Mesoblastic Nephroma (CMN)
- Tumor of very young children, mostly seen in 1st year of life
- Demonstration of *SYT-SSX* gene fusion is diagnostic of SS, whereas *ETV6-NTRK3* gene fusion is characteristic of CMN

Other Monophasic Sarcomas
- Malignant peripheral nerve sheath tumor, fibrosarcoma, leiomyosarcoma, malignant solitary fibrous tumor
- Appropriate immunohistochemical panel, including S100, CD34, actin-sm, desmin

DIAGNOSTIC CHECKLIST

Pathologic Interpretation Pearls
- Monophasic spindle cell sarcoma occurring in young patient should prompt consideration for SS
  - RCC with sarcomatoid differentiation rare in this age group

SELECTED REFERENCES

1. Schoolmeester JK et al: Synovial sarcoma of the kidney: a clinicopathologic, immunohistochemical, and molecular genetic study of 16 cases. Am J Surg Pathol. 38(1):60-5, 2014
2. Iacovelli R et al: Clinical and pathological features of primary renal synovial sarcoma: analysis of 64 cases from 11 years of medical literature. BJU Int. 110(10):1449-54, 2012
3. Divetia M et al: Synovial sarcoma of the kidney. Ann Diagn Pathol. 12(5):333-9, 2008
4. Argani P et al: Primary renal synovial sarcoma: molecular and morphologic delineation of an entity previously included among embryonal sarcomas of the kidney. Am J Surg Pathol. 24(8):1087-96, 2000

Synovial Sarcoma

Cysts in Renal Synovial Sarcoma

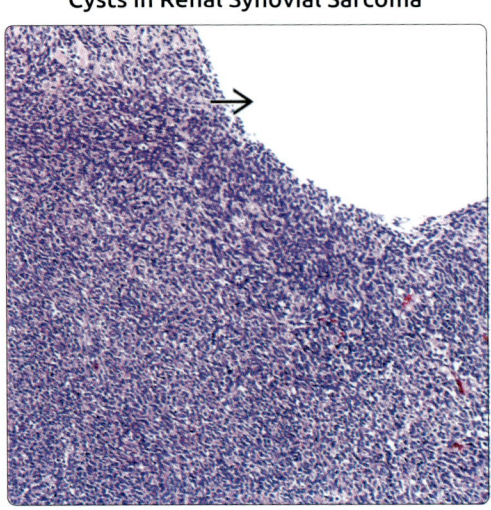

Monophasic Histology

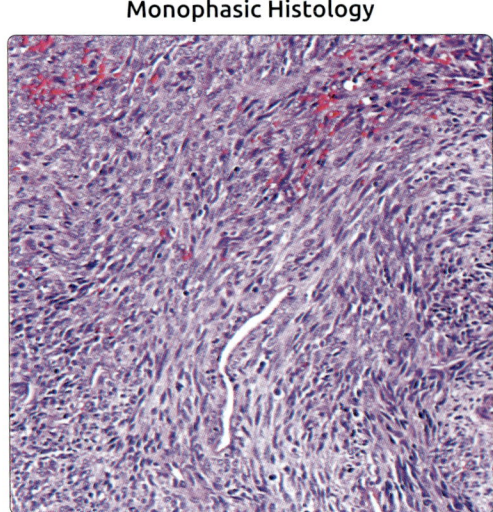

(Left) *Hematoxylin & eosin shows a cystic space ➡ surrounded by solid, highly cellular spindled tumor cells. Cysts are a characteristic feature in renal SS, being observed in > 65% of cases on gross evaluation and > 80% on light microscopy. The cysts are believed to represent entrapped and obstructed native tubules with cystic dilatation.* **(Right)** *The most prevalent spindle cell component in the tumor is histologically similar to monophasic synovial sarcoma of soft tissue.*

Prominent Mitotic Activity

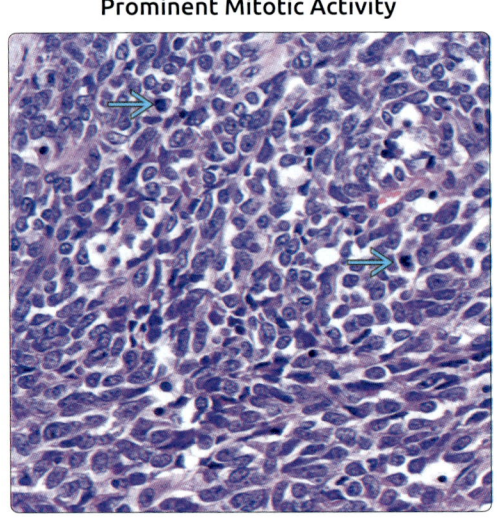

Intratumoral Cysts

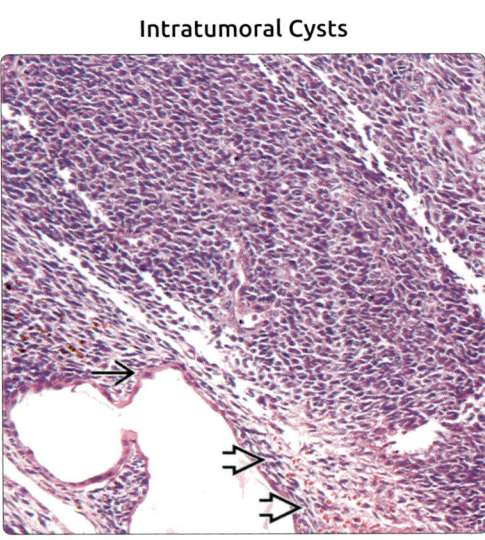

(Left) *H&E of a renal SS shows embryonal-appearing spindle cells with plump nuclei, coarse chromatin, scant cytoplasm, and indistinct cell borders. Note the prominent mitotic activity ➡ in the tumor.* **(Right)** *The cysts in renal SS are often lined by mitotically inactive, hobnailed eosinophilic cells ➡. The cysts are occasionally surrounded by ovarian-type stroma ➡, suggesting origin from cystic nephroma. However, such tumors often show the typical SYT-SSX gene fusion of SS.*

Sinus Fat Invasion

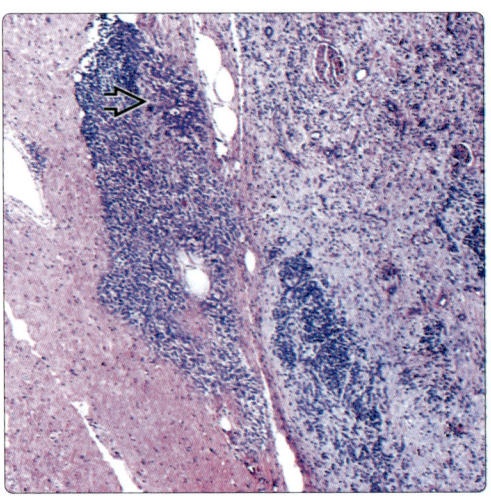

TLE1 Positivity

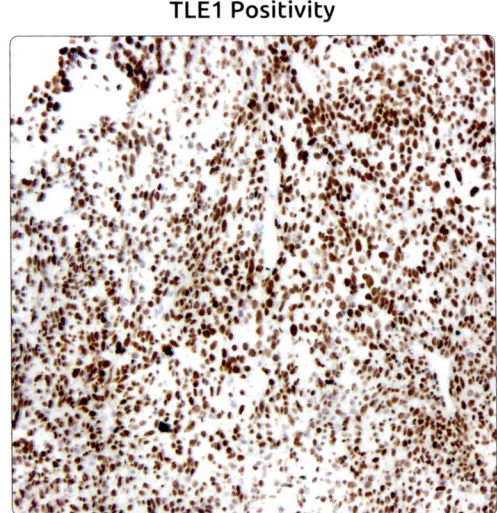

(Left) *This image shows renal sinus fat ➡ invasion by an SS. Extrarenal fat and vascular invasion are frequent in renal SS.* **(Right)** *Over 90% of synovial sarcomas show immunoreactivity for TLE1, with > 50% of the tumor cells showing nuclear positivity. While being very sensitive, TLE1 positivity is not specific, as 1/3 of other sarcomas may also show at least focal immunoreactivity for TLE1.*

Synovial Sarcoma

CD99 Positivity
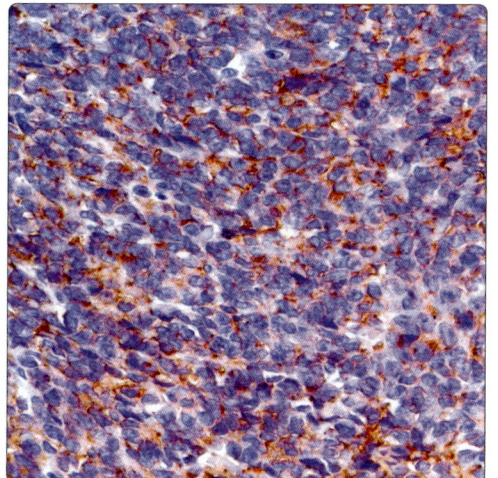

EMA/MUC1
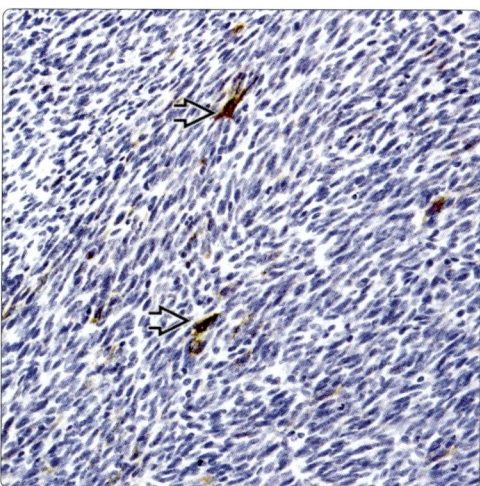

(Left) CD99 is frequently positive in renal SS, as in its extrarenal counterparts. However, unlike the diffuse, membranous positivity in renal primitive neuroectodermal tumors, the positivity is often focal and usually cytoplasmic. Bcl-2 also frequently stains synovial sarcoma. **(Right)** Epithelial markers are usually negative in the spindled cells of SS. However, focal and rare positivity may be present in some cases. EMA/MUC1 ⇨ is more sensitive antibody than pankeratin in showing this epithelial differentiation.

CD34
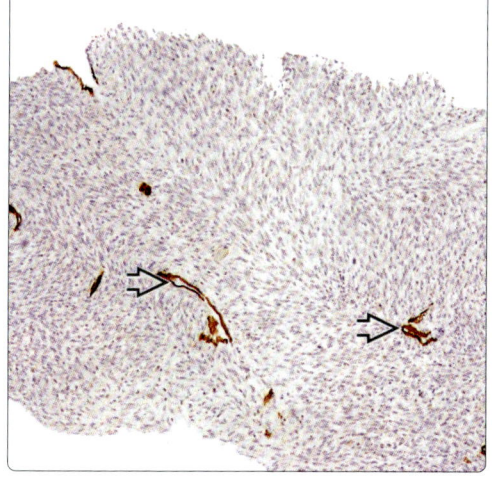

Biopsy Diagnosis
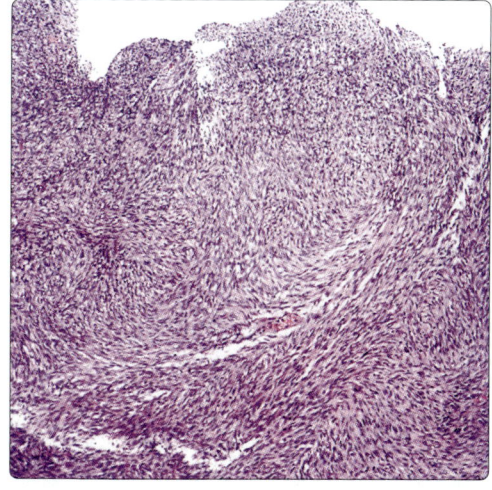

(Left) Some immunostains may suggest the diagnosis of SS but are not consistent or specific. Molecular confirmation is usually required for diagnosis. SS are consistently CD34 negative. Positive staining in the tumor vasculature ⇨ acts as internal control. **(Right)** Presence of a spindle cell sarcoma in a renal core biopsy, particularly in a young adult, should always raise the differential diagnostic possibility of renal SS, and mandates ancillary testing for appropriate classification.

Lymph Node Metastasis
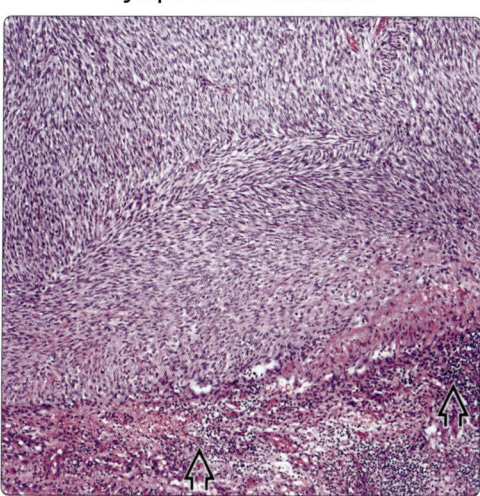

Lung Metastasis
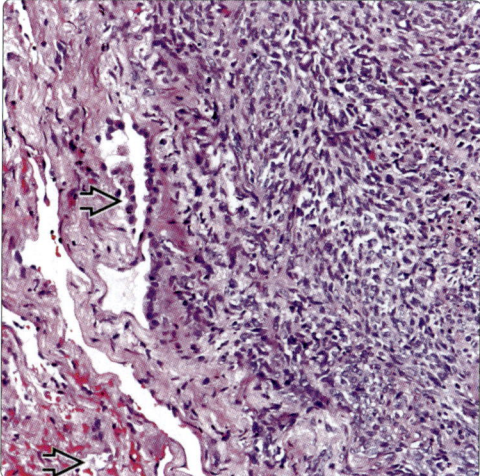

(Left) This photomicrograph shows a renal synovial sarcoma metastatic to a regional lymph node ⇨. Unlike most other sarcomas, SS, including that of renal origin, may sometimes show metastasis to the lymph nodes. However, lungs are the most common site of metastasis in renal SS. **(Right)** This image shows a renal SS metastatic to the lung ⇨. Many renal SS have lung metastasis at presentation or develop them soon after the primary diagnosis. Median survival in metastatic cases is only ~ 6 months.

Well-Differentiated Neuroendocrine Tumor (Carcinoid) and High-Grade Neuroendocrine Carcinoma

KEY FACTS

TERMINOLOGY
- Primary tumors involving renal parenchyma that demonstrate morphological &/or immunohistochemical neuroendocrine differentiation
- Tumors range from well-differentiated tumors [renal carcinoid tumor (RCT)] to high-grade neuroendocrine carcinomas [small cell neuroendocrine (SCC) and large cell neuroendocrine carcinomas (LCNEC)]

ETIOLOGY/PATHOGENESIS
- Up to 15% of primary RCT arise in horseshoe kidneys; rarely also in renal teratoma or teratoid tumors
- No predisposing genetic conditions for high-grade tumors (carcinomas)

CLINICAL ISSUES
- For RCT, most patients with metastasis show protracted clinical course; only rare reported deaths
- Patients with SCC or LCNEC: 75% dead of disease within 1 year

MICROSCOPIC
- RCT morphologically similar to carcinoid tumors at other sites; most with < 2 mitoses/10 HPF, rarely ≥ 3-4; necrosis extremely uncommon; perinephric fat invasion in > 40% cases; vascular invasion very rare
- In SCC and LCNEC, morphology similar to that in other sites, with numerous mitoses, vascular tumor emboli, and tumor necrosis; rosettes and tubules not uncommon
- RCT often with lymph node (> 1/3 of cases) metastasis; high-grade carcinomas often with systemic metastases

TOP DIFFERENTIAL DIAGNOSES
- Tumors metastatic to kidney

DIAGNOSTIC CHECKLIST
- Possibility of metastasis from other sites needs to be excluded, particularly in multifocal tumors and tumors with vascular invasion

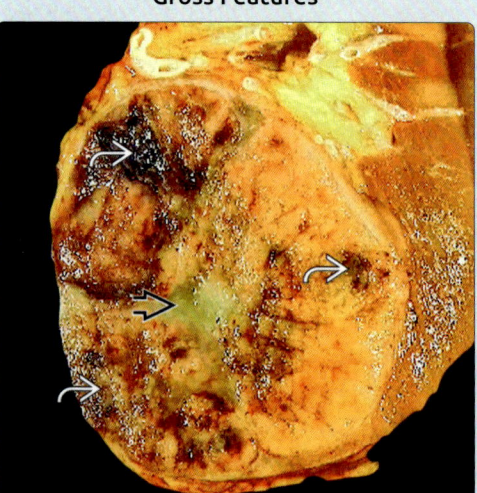

Gross Features

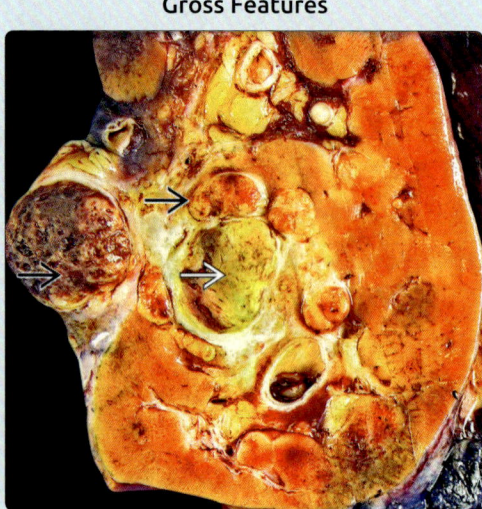

Gross Features

(Left) Primary renal carcinoid is a well-circumscribed tumor with a homogeneous cut surface. Foci of hemorrhage ⇒ are not uncommon, but necrosis is rare. A central scar ⇒ is present in this example. (Right) This gross image shows a carcinoid tumor with a multinodular growth pattern, intravascular tumor thrombi ⇒, and large area of necrosis ⇒. Such features are highly suggestive of a metastasis to the kidney and merit thorough clinical investigations for such a possibility when prior history is not known.

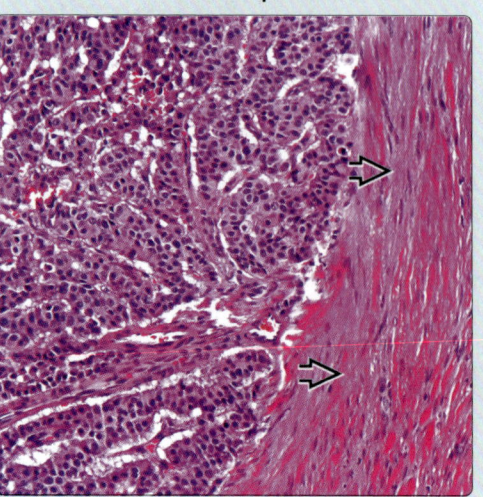

Circumscription

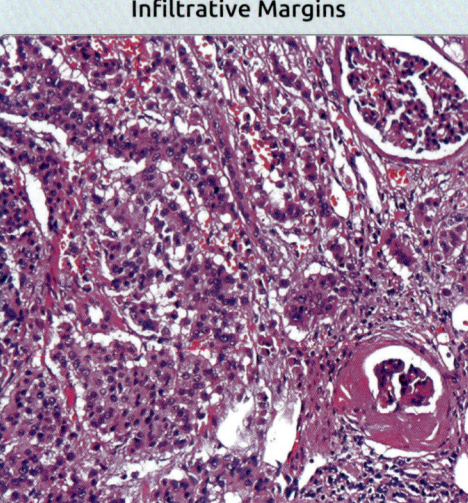

Infiltrative Margins

(Left) Most primary renal well-differentiated neuroendocrine tumors (renal carcinoids) are well circumscribed. But encapsulation is not very common. This image shows a tumor with a prominent fibrous capsule ⇒, an unusual finding that may be seen in some tumors. (Right) Rare primary renal carcinoid tumors (RCTs) may have an infiltrative margin, with irregular extensions between and surrounding the nontumorous nephrons.

Well-Differentiated Neuroendocrine Tumor (Carcinoid) and High-Grade Neuroendocrine Carcinoma

TERMINOLOGY

Abbreviations
- High-grade neuroendocrine carcinoma (HGNC)

Definitions
- Primary tumors involving renal parenchyma that demonstrate morphological &/or immunohistochemical neuroendocrine differentiation
- Tumors range from well-differentiated tumors [renal carcinoid tumor (RCT)] to high-grade neuroendocrine carcinomas [small cell neuroendocrine (SCC) and large cell neuroendocrine carcinomas (LCNEC)]

ETIOLOGY/PATHOGENESIS

Developmental Anomaly
- Up to 15% of primary RCT arise in horseshoe kidneys; rarely also in renal teratoma or teratoid tumors
- No predisposing genetic conditions for high-grade tumors (carcinomas)

CLINICAL ISSUES

Epidemiology
- Incidence
  - RCT very rare, with ~ 100 cases reported in literature; kidney 2nd most common site for genitourinary carcinoids after gonads
  - SCC and LCNEC extremely rare, mostly case reports; very few pure renal parenchymal SCC reported, most being of urothelial derivation
- Age
  - 21-87 years for RCT, with ~ 1/2 < 50 years at diagnosis; mean age for SCC: 59 years
- Sex
  - Equal distribution

Presentation
- 40% of patients with RCT present with tumor-related symptoms, including back or flank pain, hematuria, or enlarging abdominal mass; signs or symptoms of carcinoid syndrome extremely uncommon
- Most patients with high-grade NE carcinomas present with large tumors, often extending into perirenal adipose tissue
- Regional lymph node metastases and distant metastases in brain, bone, adrenal gland, and liver; very common in both

Treatment
- Nephron-sparing surgery for organ-confined RCT preferred surgical approach; for carcinomas, radical surgeries common, but often no surgeries if diagnosed on needle biopsies
- For RCT, role of adjuvant therapies uncertain; effective therapies unavailable; SCC and LCNEC often managed similar to lung tumors, platinum-based chemotherapy treatment of choice

Prognosis
- Patients with SCC or LCNEC: 75% dead of disease within 1 year
- For RCT, most patients with metastasis show protracted clinical course; only rare reported deaths
  - Reported adverse prognostic features include: ≥ 40 years of age; tumor size ≥ 4 cm; mitotic rate > 1/10 HPF; metastasis at initial diagnosis

MACROSCOPIC

General Features
- RCT usually solitary, well circumscribed, with solid homogeneous, yellow-tan, beige or red-brown cut surface, hemorrhage, calcification, or cystic change common; necrosis quite rare; size 2-17 cm (median: 6.4 cm)
- High-grade carcinomas, with soft, whitish gritty and necrotic cut surface, often extending into renal sinus adipose tissue; size: 2.5-23 cm (median: 8 cm)

MICROSCOPIC

Histologic Features
- In RCT, tumor-renal parenchymal junction sharply defined in most, with focal infiltration in occasional cases
  - Most common architectural pattern tightly packed cords and trabeculae with ribbon-like appearance; other patterns include solid sheets, solid nests, and presence of gland-like lumina
  - Cytologically similar to carcinoid tumors at other sites; most with < 2 mitoses/10 HPF, rarely ≥ 3-4; necrosis extremely uncommon; perinephric fat invasion in > 40% cases; vascular invasion very rare
- In SCC and LCNEC, morphology similar to that in other sites, with numerous mitoses, vascular tumor emboli, and tumor necrosis; rosettes and tubules not uncommon

Lymph Nodes
- RCT often with lymph node (> 1/3 of cases) metastasis; high-grade carcinomas often with lymph node and systemic metastases

DIFFERENTIAL DIAGNOSIS

Tumors Metastatic to Kidney
- Histologically similar to primary tumors, but often multiple
- Presence of multifocality and lymphovascular emboli favor metastasis

DIAGNOSTIC CHECKLIST

Pathologic Interpretation Pearls
- Possibility of metastasis from other sites needs to be excluded, particularly in multifocal tumors and tumors with vascular invasion

SELECTED REFERENCES

1. Wann C et al: Primary renal large cell neuroendocrine carcinoma in a young man. J Clin Diagn Res. 8(11):ND08-9, 2014
2. Mazzucchelli R et al: Neuroendocrine tumours of the urinary system and male genital organs: clinical significance. BJU Int. 103(11):1464-70, 2009
3. Fine SW: Neuroendocrine lesions of the genitourinary tract. Adv Anat Pathol. 14(4):286-96, 2007
4. Hansel DE et al: Renal carcinoid tumor: a clinicopathologic study of 21 cases. Am J Surg Pathol. 31(10):1539-44, 2007
5. Lane BR et al: Renal neuroendocrine tumours: a clinicopathological study. BJU Int. 100(5):1030-5, 2007
6. Yoo J et al: Primary carcinoid tumor arising in a mature teratoma of the kidney: a case report and review of the literature. Arch Pathol Lab Med. 126(8):979-81, 2002
7. Raslan WF et al: Primary carcinoid of the kidney. Immunohistochemical and ultrastructural studies of five patients. Cancer. 72(9):2660-6, 1993

Well-Differentiated Neuroendocrine Tumor (Carcinoid) and High-Grade Neuroendocrine Carcinoma

Ribbon-Like Architecture

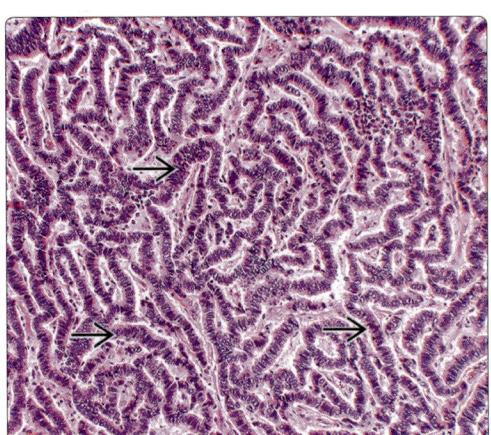

Mixed Architectural Patterns

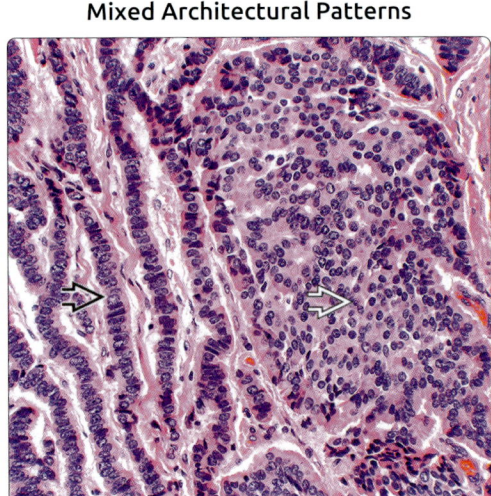

(Left) Ribbon-like ⇒ and wider cords constitute the most common architectural pattern in RCTs. This may be associated with scant or abundant, usually hyalinized stroma. **(Right)** Combination of architectural patterns is quite common in RCTs. This photomicrograph shows a tumor with mixture of cord-like ⇒ and more solid ⇒ growth patterns. Note the similarity in nuclear morphology and scant to moderate cytoplasm in both types of areas.

Cytological Features

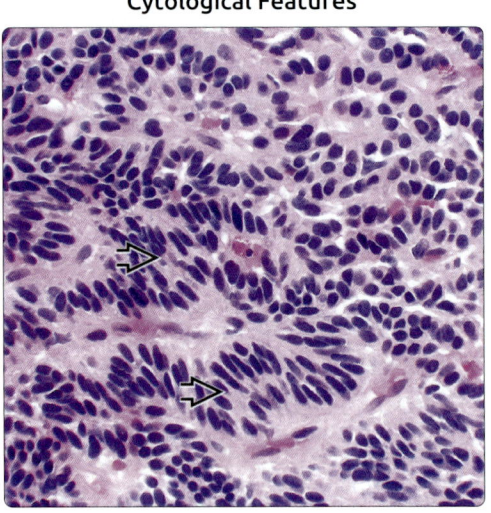

Tumor Stroma

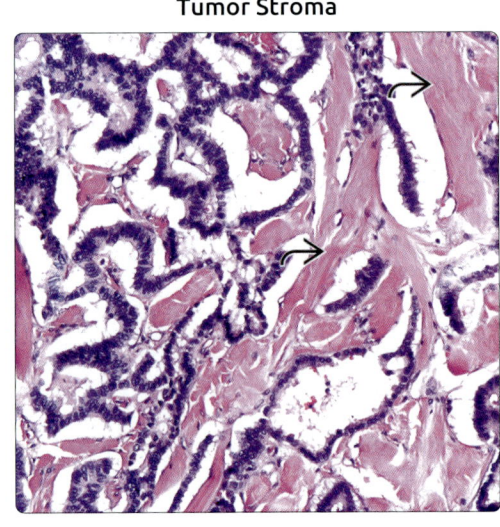

(Left) Occasionally, the nuclei may appear elongated ⇒ and oval in renal carcinoid tumors, similar to what is seen in small cell carcinomas. However, no increased mitotic activity is present. **(Right)** The intervening stroma in well-differentiated neuroendocrine tumors may range from minimal to abundant and from sclerotic to edematous. This photomicrograph demonstrates a tumor with hyalinized ⇒, abundant stroma.

Glandular Architecture

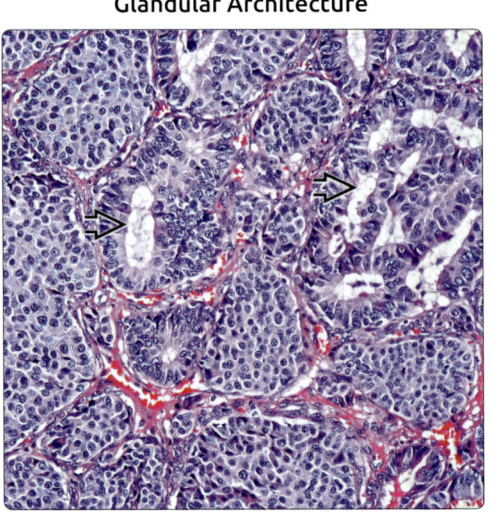

Nuclear Features

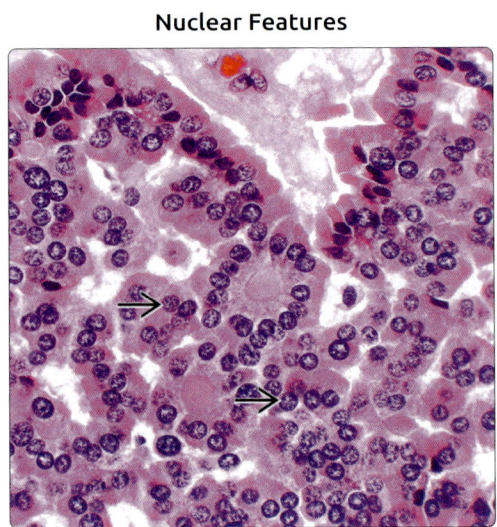

(Left) RCT, like its extrarenal counterpart, may show gland-like ⇒ features. This raises the differential diagnostic possibility of a Wilms tumor. However, the solid areas do not show the characteristics of blastema, i.e., nuclear molding and high mitotic/apoptotic index. **(Right)** As in extrarenal tumors, the nuclei in RCTs (well-differentiated neuroendocrine tumors) are relatively uniform and round. The nuclear chromatin is finely granular, showing salt and pepper appearance ⇒. Mitotic activity is usually low.

Well-Differentiated Neuroendocrine Tumor (Carcinoid) and High-Grade Neuroendocrine Carcinoma

Perirenal Invasion

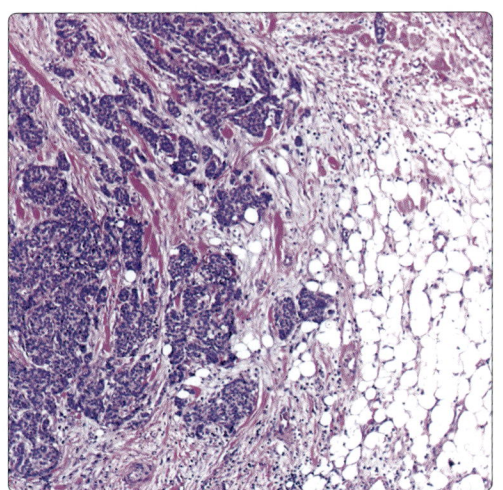

Lymph Node Metastasis

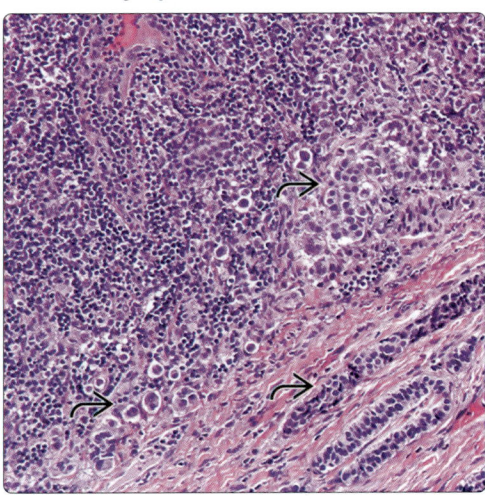

(Left) *A large proportion of renal carcinoids show invasion of the perirenal fat (stage pT3a). Some, but not all, believe this to reflect a potentially more aggressive biologic behavior.* (Right) *A large proportion of RCTs show regional node metastasis ⇨ when lymph nodes are removed at primary renal resection. However, most patients with metastasis show protracted clinical course, and only rare deaths due to disease are reported.*

Renal Teratoma With Carcinoid Tumor

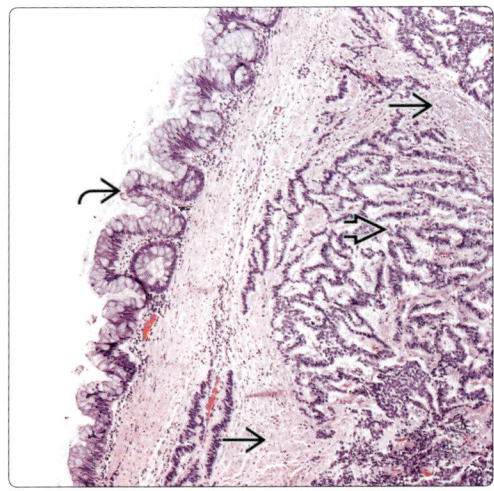

Synaptophysin

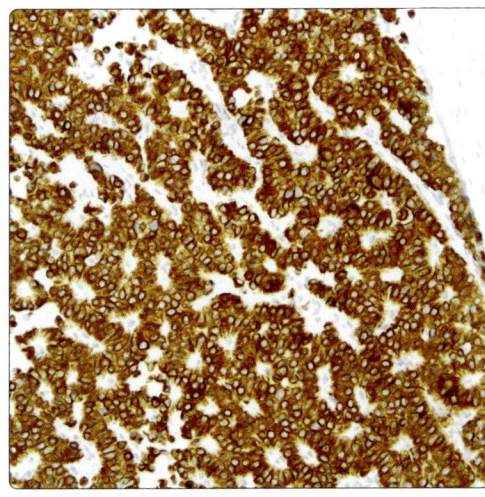

(Left) *Up to 15% of primary RCTs arise in horseshoe kidneys. Rarely, the tumors also arise in renal teratoma, an extremely uncommon tumor in kidney. This image shows one such example of teratoma, with intestinal-type lining ⇨, smooth muscle ⇨, and carcinoid tumor ⇨ present in a single field.* (Right) *This image shows diffuse immunohistochemical positivity for synaptophysin in a RCT, a relatively common finding. Chromogranin positivity may or may not be so diffuse.*

Carcinoid Tumor: Biopsy Diagnosis

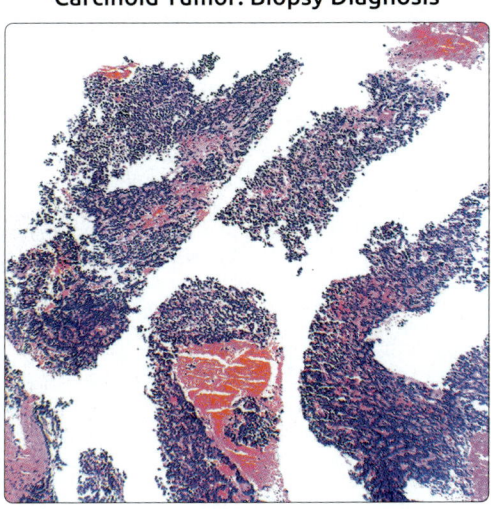

Small Cell Carcinoma: Biopsy Diagnosis

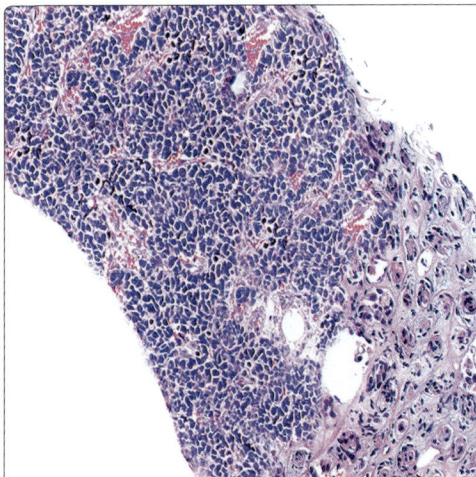

(Left) *Based on the morphological and IHC features, the diagnosis of RCT can be rendered on needle core biopsies. Exclusion of the possibility of other small blue round cell tumors requires negative staining for CD99, WT-1, muscle markers, and lymphoid markers.* (Right) *Presence of small cell carcinoma (SCC) on renal biopsies usually requires clinical exclusion of a metastatic tumor. Primary renal parenchymal SCC is very rare; most SCCs in kidney represent metastases or carcinoma of urothelial origin.*

Primitive Neuroectodermal Tumor

KEY FACTS

TERMINOLOGY
- Primitive neuroectodermal tumor (PNET)

ETIOLOGY/PATHOGENESIS
- Nontype 1 gene fusions in ES/PNET of soft tissue are associated with poor outcome
- Ewing sarcoma (ES)/PNET family of tumors characterized by fusion of *EWS* with gene from *ETS* (E-26) family of transcription factors
- In renal PNET, only 1/2 with typical type 1 fusion, other 1/2 with variant fusions that may contribute to more adverse prognosis

CLINICAL ISSUES
- Most common in young adults and adolescents
- Generally poor clinical outcome, but with current multimodal therapy-improved outcomes

MACROSCOPIC
- Usually large, with mean diameter 16 cm (range: 7-21 cm)

MICROSCOPIC
- Identical to their soft tissue counterparts
- Vaguely lobulated proliferations of primitive-appearing round cells with high nuclear:cytoplasmic ratio
- Occasionally with small amount of clear cytoplasm, and more vesicular nuclei showing small nucleoli
- Epithelial, myogenous, or cartilaginous differentiation not seen
- Frequent presence of glycogen (diastase-sensitive PAS positivity), particularly in cells with clear cytoplasm

ANCILLARY TESTS
- PNET strongly and diffusely (+) in membranous pattern for CD99; most, but not all, with FLI-1 nuclear positivity

TOP DIFFERENTIAL DIAGNOSES
- Blastemal Wilms tumor
- Other small blue round cell tumors

Gross Features

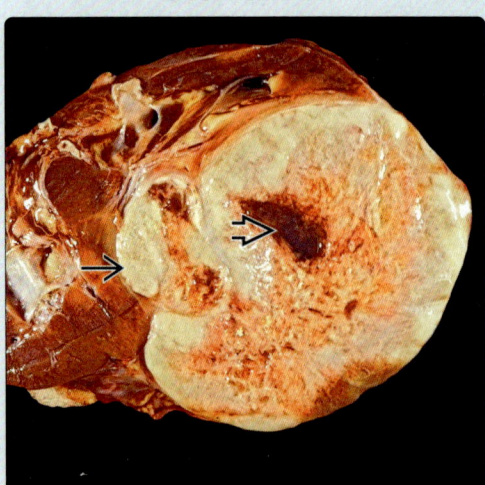

Gross Features

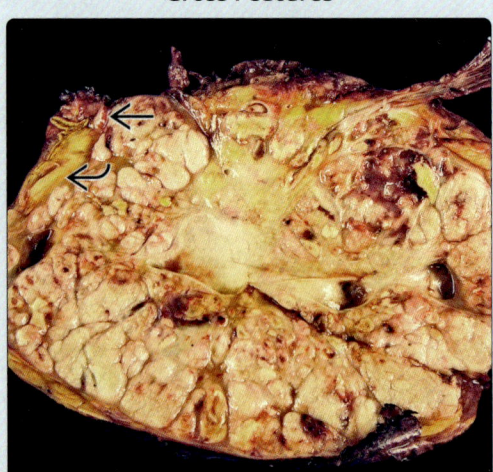

(Left) Renal primitive neuroectodermal tumors (PNET) are usually large tumors with infiltrative borders, areas of necrosis ⇨ and cystic change ⇨, multilobulated growth pattern, and tan-yellow cut surface. (Right) The typical multilobulated gross appearance is prominent in this specimen. As is common in renal PNETs, this tumor almost completely replaces the renal parenchyma. Notice the extrarenal extension into perinephric fat ⇨ close to adrenal gland ⇨.

Infiltrative Margins

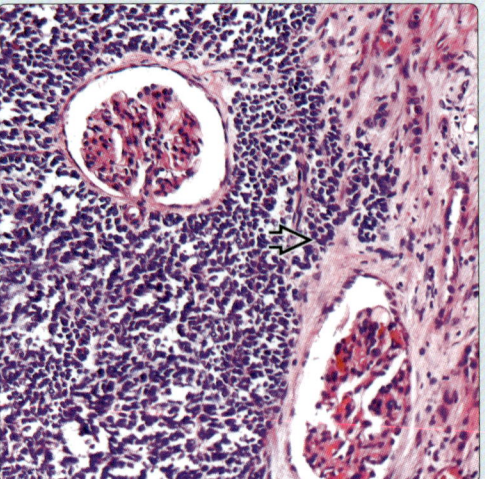

Infiltrative Margins

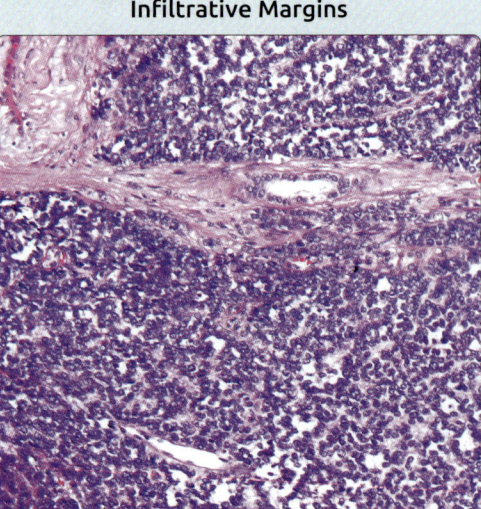

(Left) Renal PNET is morphologically similar to tumors in the bone and soft tissue and is characterized by small round blue cells. Tumor margins show irregular extensions ⇨ into surrounding kidney. (Right) Morphologically, renal PNET consists of small round/oval cells with scant cytoplasm. Because of its extreme rarity as a primary renal tumor, other rare renal round cell tumors need to be excluded before the final designation as a renal PNET.

Primitive Neuroectodermal Tumor

TERMINOLOGY

Abbreviations
- Primitive neuroectodermal tumor (PNET)

Definitions
- Aggressive blue round cell tumor with EWS and ETS (E-26) family gene fusion

ETIOLOGY/PATHOGENESIS

Molecular Features
- Similar to Ewing sarcoma (ES)/PNET of bone and soft tissue
  - Primary renal PNET also demonstrates characteristic EWS-FLI1 gene fusion resulting from translocation t(11;22)(q24;q12)
- In bone and soft tissue, 70% of EWS/FLI1 gene fusions involve fusion of EWS exon 7 and FLI1 exon 6 (so-called type 1 fusion)
  - Nontype 1 gene fusions in ES/PNET of soft tissue associated with poor outcome
  - In renal PNET, only 1/2 with type 1 fusion, other 1/2 with variant fusions that may contribute to more adverse prognosis
    - Other than FLI1, genes of ETS family that may be fused with EWS include ERG, ETV1, E1AF, FEV, and ZSG

CLINICAL ISSUES

Presentation
- Very uncommon; ~ 130 cases described; mean age: 27 years (range: 10-60)
- Presenting symptoms include abdominal pain, hematuria, palpable mass, and (rarely) night sweats
- Rarely, as 2nd tumors after therapy for leukemia, Hodgkin or non-Hodgkin lymphoma (NHL)

Prognosis
- Generally poor clinical outcome, but improved outcomes with current multimodal therapy
  - Median survival in patients with localized disease up to 60 months, compared to 15 months with regional nodal or distant metastasis

MACROSCOPIC

General Features
- Usually large tumors, mean diameter: 16 cm (range: 7-21), with tan to yellow, lobulated cut surface, often extensively replacing normal renal parenchyma
- Hemorrhage, necrosis, and cystic changes common; gross renal vein and perinephric fat invasion frequent

MICROSCOPIC

Histologic Features
- Identical to their soft tissue counterparts
- Typically infiltrates surrounding renal parenchyma in broad sheets or finger-like projections
- Vaguely lobulated proliferations of primitive-appearing round cells with high nuclear:cytoplasmic ratio
  - Occasionally with small amount of clear cytoplasm and more vesicular nuclei showing small nucleoli
- Mitotic figures and foci of necrosis common easily identified, with occasional atypical mitoses
- Rare cases with prominent Homer Wright rosettes
  - Different from early tubular differentiation of Wilms tumor that may show prominent lumina with rigid cytoplasmic luminal borders
- Epithelial/myogenous/cartilaginous differentiation absent
- Angiolymphatic invasion very common
- Frequent presence of glycogen (diastase-sensitive PAS positivity), particularly in cells with clear cytoplasm

ANCILLARY TESTS

Immunohistochemistry
- PNET strongly and diffusely (+) in membranous pattern for CD99; most, but not all, with FLI-1 nuclear positivity
- Focal positivity for cytokeratins in occasional tumors
- All tumors negative for desmin and other skeletal muscle markers, and WT1

DIFFERENTIAL DIAGNOSIS

Blastemal Wilms Tumor
- Wilms tumor (WT) typically seen in patients < 5 years old; PNET is tumor of older patients
- PNETs usually have uniform morphology/architecture throughout tumor
  - Blastemal WT often show foci of other distinctive patterns of growth in some parts of neoplasm
- Nuclei of PNET are more evenly spaced than those of blastemal WT, and nuclear chromatin of PNET less coarse than that of WT
- > 95% of PNETs demonstrate complete membranous labeling for CD99, while WT is usually negative

Other Small Round Blue Cell Tumors
- Clear cell sarcoma of the kidney (CCSK) typically occurs in patients < 5 years old, and PNET more often in young adults
- Cellular CCSK almost always shows foci of other distinctive growth patterns
- > 95% of PNETs demonstrate complete membranous labeling for CD99, while CCSK and rhabdomyosarcomas are virtually always negative
- FLI-1 nuclear positivity in PNET and negative staining for MYOD1, myogenin may also help
- Neuroblastomas with more dense chromatin, nuclear molding, and often variable neuropil
- Molecular tests diagnostic in almost all difficult cases

DIAGNOSTIC CHECKLIST

Pathologic Interpretation Pearls
- Small blue round cell tumor in young adults more likely to be PNET rather than Wilms tumor

SELECTED REFERENCES

1. Giridhar P et al: Primitive neuro-ectodermal tumour of kidney in adult: Report of four consecutive cases and review of the literature. J Egypt Natl Canc Inst. 27(4):235-8, 2015
2. Thyavihally YB et al: Primitive neuroectodermal tumor of the kidney: a single institute series of 16 patients. Urology. 71(2):292-6, 2008
3. Jimenez RE et al: Primary Ewing's sarcoma/primitive neuroectodermal tumor of the kidney: a clinicopathologic and immunohistochemical analysis of 11 cases. Am J Surg Pathol. 26(3):320-7, 2002

Primitive Neuroectodermal Tumor

(Left) *A small round blue cell tumor in the kidney may raise the possibility of a Wilms tumor, neuroblastoma, and rhabdomyosarcoma, among others. Presence of pale chromatin, lack of tubular differentiation, neuropil, or nuclear overlapping should raise the differential diagnostic possibility of PNET.* **(Right)** *The nuclear chromatin pattern in primitive neuroectodermal tumor is relatively pale and often shows small nucleoli and focal moderate amount of pale cytoplasm, unlike most other small round blue cell tumors.*

Characteristic Morphological Features
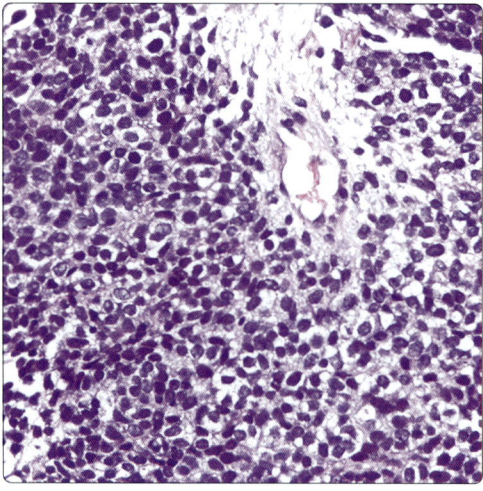

Characteristic Morphological Features
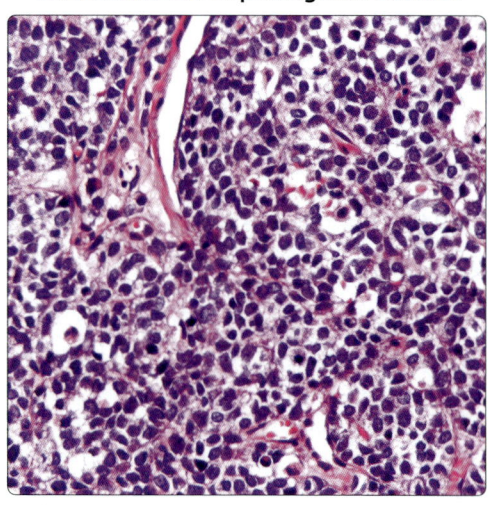

(Left) *Similar to neuroblastoma, PNET may show Homer Wright rosettes characterized by tumor cells arranged around fibrillary material ➔. However, the nuclei often show more open chromatin and lack neuropil, typical for neuroblastoma. Diffuse membranous positivity for CD99, and often FLI-1, will favor the diagnosis of PNET.* **(Right)** *Primitive neuroectodermal tumors, as at nonrenal sites, often show at least focal positivity for glycogen, as demonstrated by diastase-sensitive PAS positivity ➔.*

Characteristic Morphological Features
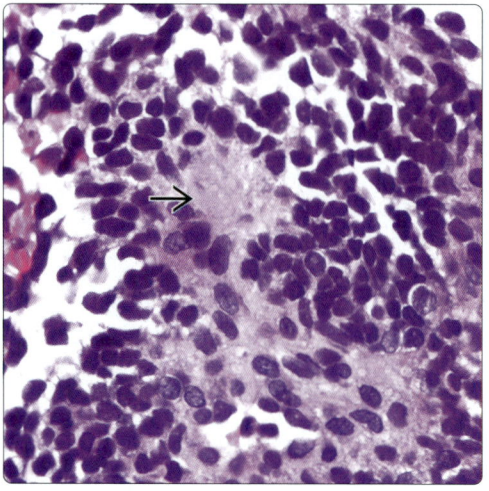

Characteristic Morphological Features
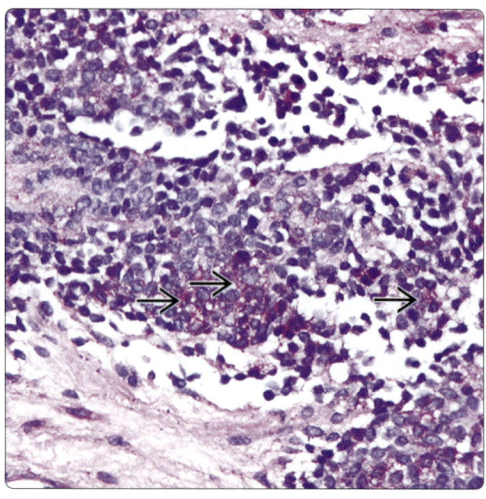

(Left) *CD99 shows diffuse membranous reactivity in PNET. Without such immunoreactivity, it may be difficult to diagnose renal PNET. At the same time, patchy CD99 positivity may be seen in other tumors, including T-lymphoblastic lymphoma, rhabdomyosarcoma, desmoplastic small round cell, and vascular tumors.* **(Right)** *FLI-1 shows strong and diffuse nuclear positivity in PNET. Positivity in isolation cannot be regarded diagnostic, as FLI-1 can also be positive in vascular and lymphoid tumors, among others.*

CD99
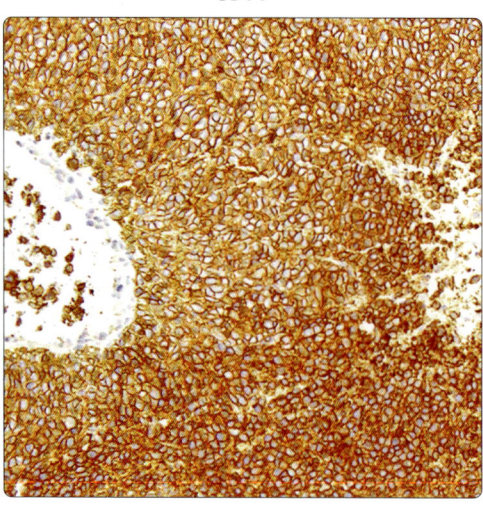

FLI-1
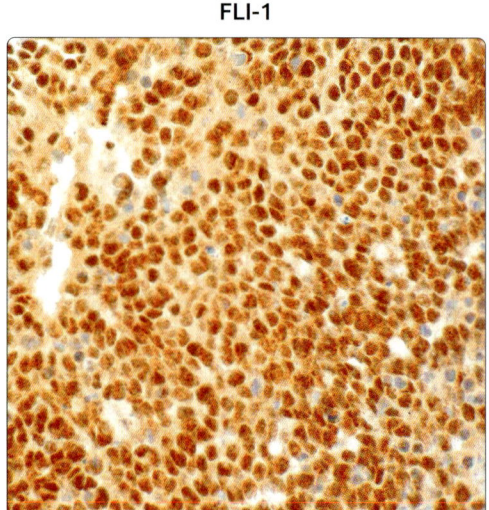

Primitive Neuroectodermal Tumor

MYOD1

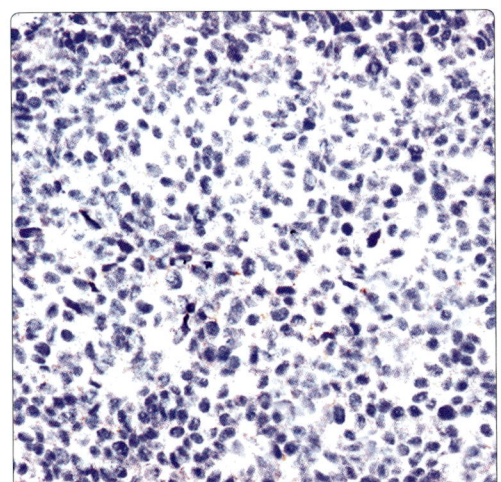

Differential Diagnosis: Neuroblastoma

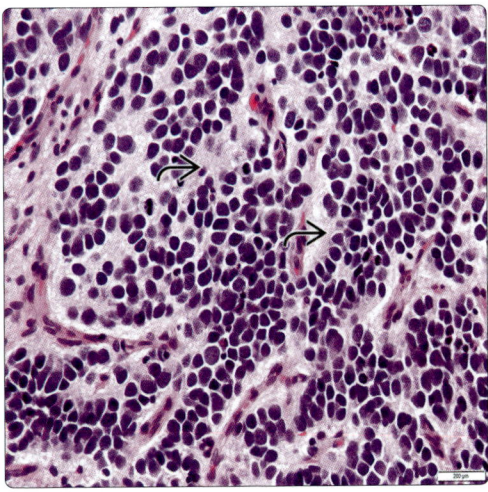

(Left) The possibility of embryonal or alveolar rhabdomyosarcoma (RMS) may arise in renal tumors with small round blue cell morphology. While CD99 is diffusely positive in PNET, it may also stain some RMS. However, MYOD1 and myogenin are always negative in PNET, as shown here. (Right) Poorly differentiated neuroblastoma (NB), as shown here, or undifferentiated NB can be a close differential diagnosis for PNET. However, presence of neuropil ⇒ is highly diagnostic of poorly differentiated neuroblastoma.

Differential Diagnosis: Alveolar Rhabdomyosarcoma

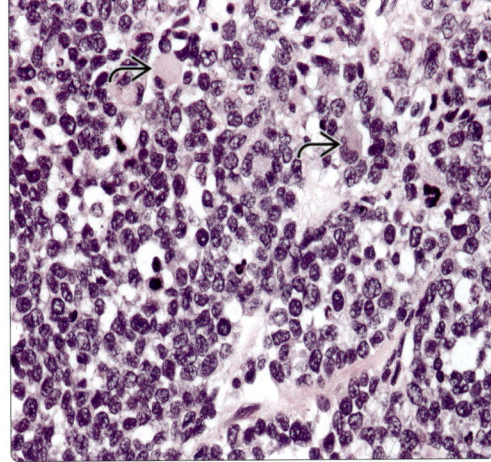

Differential Diagnosis: Epithelioid Sarcoma, Proximal Type

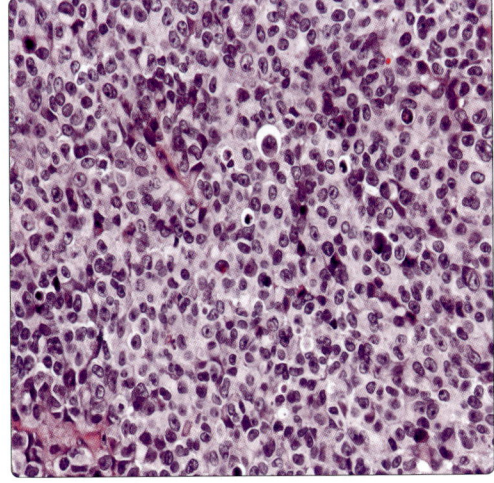

(Left) Small round blue cells in kidney may represent multiple tumors including PNET and alveolar RMS. Presence of morphological muscle differentiation ⇒, seen here, favors a rhabdomyoblastoma. (Courtesy J. Sarungbam, MD.) (Right) This small round blue cell raised the possibility of PNET and proximal-type epithelioid sarcoma, among others. Immunohistochemistry was very useful in this differentiation. (Courtesy J. Sarunbam, MD.)

INI1 in Epithelioid Sarcoma, Proximal Type

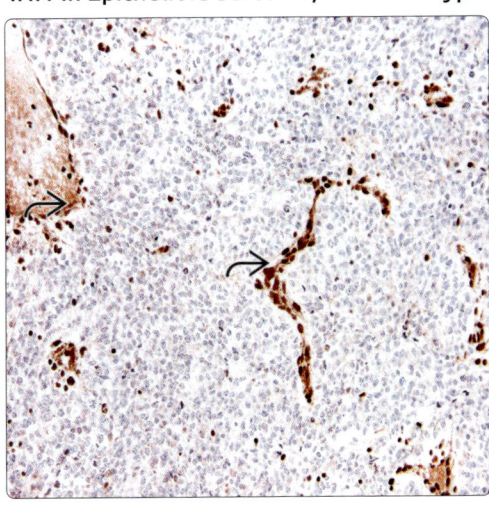

Metastatic Renal PNET

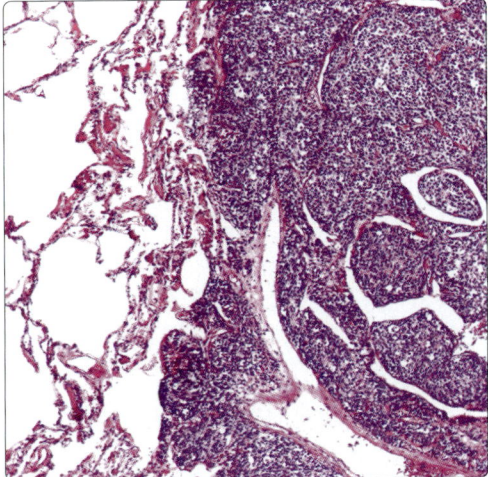

(Left) Complete loss of INI1 IHC in this small blue round cell tumor supports the diagnosis of epithelioid sarcoma. Notice the retained positivity in endothelium ⇒ and intratumoral inflammatory cells. (Courtesy J. Sarunbam, MD.) (Right) This image shows renal PNET metastatic to the lung. Among PNETs of soft tissue, gene fusions other than EWS-FLI1 are often associated with a poor clinical outcome. In renal PNET, ~ 1/2 show variant EWS fusions, and may be a factor in the poor outcome in renal PNET.

Hematopoietic Tumors

KEY FACTS

TERMINOLOGY
- Most often, kidney secondarily involved in systemic diseases but may be primary organ of involvement in very rare cases
- Tumors seen in kidney include malignant lymphoma, leukemia, plasmacytoma/myeloma, posttransplant lymphoproliferative disorders (PTLD), and very rarely intravascular lymphomas

CLINICAL ISSUES
- Lymphomas arising in urinary tract and male genital organs account for < 5% of extranodal lymphomas
- Secondary renal involvement many times more common than primary renal hematopoietic malignancies
- Prognosis for lymphomas usually not promising
- With combination of available approaches, overwhelming majority of patients with PTLD show complete long-term remission of disease

MACROSCOPIC
- 2 gross growth patterns
  - Kidney completely replaced by homogeneous gray-white tumor tissue
    - Such patterns more often seen at autopsy
  - Mass-forming lesion
    - When seen in surgical specimens, often resected under mistaken impression of renal cell carcinoma

MICROSCOPIC
- Most common growth pattern interstitial; other tumors with nodular growth pattern
- Rarely, tumor cells entirely or predominantly intravascular (intravascular lymphoma)

DIAGNOSTIC CHECKLIST
- Multifocal and bilateral renal masses should raise concern for metastasis and malignant lymphoma

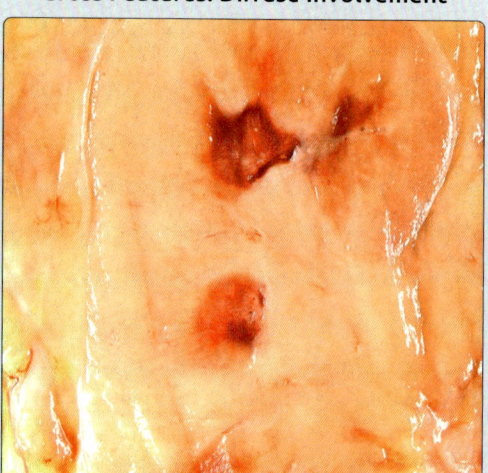

Gross Features: Diffuse Involvement

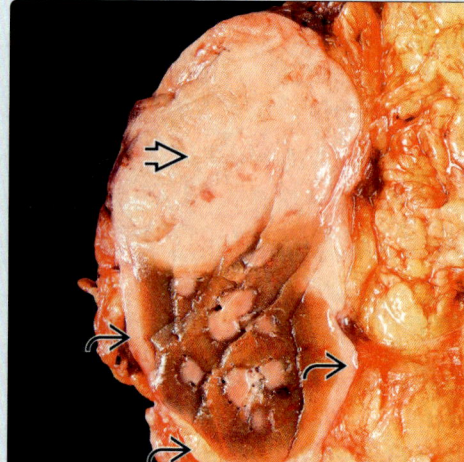

Gross Features: Mass Lesion

(Left) Gross photograph shows complete replacement of renal parenchyma by a gray-tan, fleshy tumor. Such appearance of lymphoma/leukemia involving the kidney is more often seen in autopsy specimens. (Right) Nephrectomy specimens revealing hematological malignancies usually show mass lesions ⇨. Such lesions are often clinically misdiagnosed as renal cortical tumors in which no preresection needle core biopsies have been taken. Note the sheath-like perirenal infiltration ⇨ here.

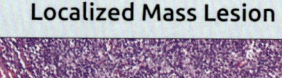

Interstitial Growth Pattern

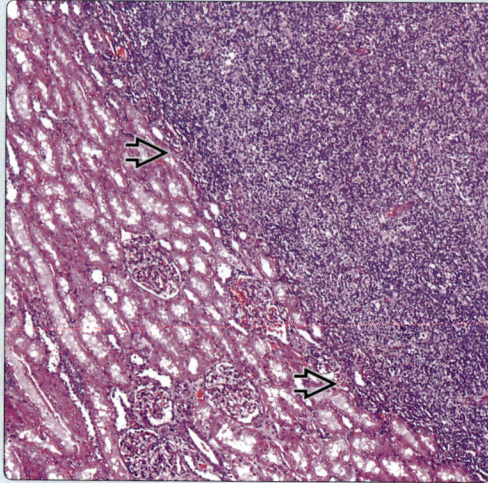

Localized Mass Lesion

(Left) The most common architectural pattern in hematopoietic tumors involving the kidney is interstitial. Sheets of tumor cells infiltrate between residual glomeruli ⇨ and tubules ⇨, although most of the nephrons are completely replaced. (Right) A less common architectural pattern is the sharply demarcated ⇨ nodular growth. Glomeruli and tubules may be entrapped within the tumor but usually only in the periphery. Such lesions are clinically difficult to differentiate from primary cortical renal cell tumors.

Hematopoietic Tumors

TERMINOLOGY

Abbreviations
- Diffuse large B-cell lymphoma (DLBCL), Burkitt lymphoma (BL), follicular lymphoma (FL), mantle cell lymphoma (MCL), mucosa-associated lymphoid tissue (MALT), intravascular lymphoma (IVL), posttransplant lymphoproliferative disorders (PTLD)

Definitions
- Lymphoid, myeloid, or other neoplastic proliferations infiltrating renal parenchyma
  - Most often, kidney is secondarily involved in systemic diseases but may be primary organ of involvement in rarer cases
  - Tumors seen in kidney include malignant lymphoma, leukemia, plasmacytoma/myeloma, and PTLD; other very rare conditions, including Langerhans cell histiocytosis, Rosai-Dorfman disease, etc.

ETIOLOGY/PATHOGENESIS

Genetic Features
- **Diffuse large B-cell lymphoma**
  - In 30-40% of DLBCL cases, translocation of *BCL6* gene (located at 3q27) with various partners present
    - Might contribute to tumorigenesis by blocking terminal lymphoid differentiation and providing resistance to apoptotic signals
  - Other alterations in some DLBCL include translocation of *BCL2* gene and translocation t(8;14) involving *MYC* gene
  - Gene expression profiling defines 3 biologically and prognostically distinct subgroups of DLBCL, 2 of which pertinent to renal lymphomas
    - Germinal center B cell-like (GCB) DLBCL, activated B cell-like DLBCL, and primary mediastinal large B-cell lymphoma
- **Burkitt lymphoma**
  - In > 80% of cases, translocation t(8;14)(q24;q32)
  - Juxtaposes *MYC* gene (located at 8q24) to immunoglobulin-heavy chain (*IGH*) locus (located at 14q32)
    - Occasionally *MYC* gene translocates to 1 of light chain loci
- **Follicular lymphoma**
  - Typically shows translocation t(14;18)(q32;q21), detected in ~ 85% of cases
  - Leads to juxtaposition of *BCL2* gene (located at 18q21) to *IGH* enhancer (located on chromosome 14)
    - Results in constitutive overexpression of *BCL2* and impaired apoptotic signaling
- **Mantle cell lymphoma**
  - Typical cytogenetic aberration, translocation t(11;14)(q13;q32), detected in almost all cases
  - Translocation leads to juxtaposition of *CCND1* gene (located at 11q13) to *IGH* enhancer
    - Results in overexpression of its gene product cyclin-D1, a key regulator of cell cycle and controller of G1/S-phase transition
- **Mucosa-associated lymphoid tissue lymphoma**
  - MALT lymphomas carry 1 of 4 known chromosomal translocations: t(11;18)(q21;q21), t(14;18)(q32;q21), t(3;14)(p14.1;q32), and t(1;14)(q22;q32)
    - Activate nuclear factor κ light chain enhancer of activated B-cells (NF-κB) pathway, which has roles in multiple cellular responses
- **Leukemias**
  - Numerous nonrandom genetic alterations reported in different forms of leukemia
  - Many of these with diagnostic, biologic, and therapeutic implications
  - Some of better known alterations include
    - t(9;22) in chronic myelogenous leukemia and ~ 20-30% of adult patients with acute lymphoblastic leukemia (ALL) → translocation between protooncogene *c-ABL* on chromosome 9 and *BCR* gene on chromosome 22
    - t(15;17) in almost all patients with acute promyelocytic leukemia; results in fusion of RARα gene on chromosome 17 with *PML* gene on chromosome 15
    - Inv(16)/t(16;16) in subgroup of patients with acute myeloid leukemia; results in fusion of *CBFβ* gene at chromosome 16q22 with *MYH11* gene at chromosome 16p13
    - t(8;21) in subgroup of patients with acute myeloid leukemia; fuses *AML1* (*RUNX1*) gene on chromosome 21 with *ETO* gene on chromosome 8
    - Most (> 95%) B-lineage ALL cases show *IG* gene rearrangements
    - *TCR* genes rearranged in most cases of T-lineage ALL

Infectious Agents
- PTLD, true Epstein-Barr virus (EBV)-driven tumors
  - Unlike malignancies occurring in immunocompetent individuals, where EBV is cofactor rather than driving influence
  - Number of factors that predispose transplant recipients to this EBV-driven PTLD include
    - Recipient EBV seronegativity and younger age at transplantation, hepatitis C infection, use of monoclonal antibodies OKT3 and antithymocyte globulin as antirejection therapy
  - Most commonly seen after solid organ but occasionally also after stem cell transplantation
- Cases of EBV-negative monomorphic T-cell PTLD involving kidneys and other organs without lymphadenopathy also reported

CLINICAL ISSUES

Epidemiology
- Incidence
  - Lymphomas arising in urinary tract and male genital organs account for < 5% of extranodal lymphomas
  - Genitourinary tract lymphomas most commonly occur in kidney, constituting 60% of all genitourinary tract lymphomas
  - Secondary renal involvement many times more common than primary renal hematopoietic malignancies

Hematopoietic Tumors

Presentation
- Because multiorgan involvement including kidneys usually clinically apparent, most secondary tumors not biopsied/sampled
- Most renal hematopoietic malignancies presented to pathologists either as multiorgan tumors on autopsy or primary tumors as mass lesions mimicking renal cell carcinoma (RCC)
- Involvement also noted incidentally in specimens resected for other causes, such as nonhematopoietic tumors or nonfunctional kidneys

Treatment
- Lymphomas and leukemias managed with type-dependent chemotherapeutic agents
- For PTLD, variety of therapeutic approaches used, including
  - Surgical resection and radiation therapy to localized disease
  - Reduction of immunosuppression, if clinically feasible, and antiviral agents, along with infusion of IL-2 activated autologous lymphocyte activated killer cells
  - Recently, humanized anti-CD20 mouse antibody, rituximab, with some promising results
  - Cytotoxic chemotherapy also often used in cases with EBV-derived lymphoma

Prognosis
- Prognosis for lymphomas usually not promising; > 35% die of disease within 2 years of presentation
- Among DLBCL, immunohistochemical algorithms (Hans algorithm) using 3 markers (CD10, Bcl-6, and MUM1) separates GCB DLBCL from non-GCB DLBCL
  - Survival significantly better for GCB subgroup than non-GCB subgroup
  - Also, based on IHC, MYC, BCL2, and Bcl-6 protein overexpression associated with adverse prognosis
- With combination of available approaches, overwhelming majority of patients with PTLD show complete long-term remission of disease, with only rare deaths due to disease
- Solitary plasmacytoma with relatively good prognosis, but local recurrence, metastasis, and progression to multiple myeloma not infrequent

MACROSCOPIC

General Features
- 2 gross growth patterns; kidney completely replaced by homogeneous gray-white tumor tissue or mass-like lesion
  - In diffuse pattern kidneys diffusely enlarged, with maintained shape, usually seen at autopsy; mass lesions grossly similar to RCC

MICROSCOPIC

Histologic Features
- Most common growth pattern interstitial; sheets of tumor cells percolating between nephrons
- Other tumors with nodular growth pattern, with few nephrons embedded at periphery
- Rarely, tumor cells entirely or predominantly intravascular (IVL)
- Number of cases diagnosed on needle core biopsy specimens in more recent past
- Subtypes of malignant lymphoma seen include DLBCL (including most of intravascular lymphomas), small cell lymphocytic lymphoma, MCL, FL, BL, MALT lymphoma
  - Other subtypes of lymphoma very rarely seen; immunophenotype similar to that in extrarenal sites
- PTLD
  - May show any of 3 histologic forms or stages of development; early hyperplastic lesion with plasma cell hyperplasia, resembling infectious mononucleosis, or atypical lymphoid hyperplasias; polymorphic PTLD, with polymorphous infiltrate; lymphomatous or monomorphic PTLD, with appearance of malignant lymphoma usually B-cell type
  - Venules often show heavy infiltration by PTLD
  - Usually accompanied by presence of irregular, serpentine areas of coagulative necrosis in surrounding renal parenchyma
  - In situ hybridization for EBER almost always positive in B-cell lymphomas developing early after transplant
  - PTLD developing after multiple years post transplant often EBV negative, and may be T-cell type
- Plasmacytoma
  - Primary plasmacytomas of kidney very rare, show proliferation of mature to atypical plasma cells; all light chain restricted, with either κ or λ phenotype on immunostaining or in situ hybridization
  - Only 24 cases primary to kidneys reported in literature
- Leukemias
  - Leukemic infiltrates often seen in autopsies on patients dying of leukemia (~ 50%)
  - Primary leukemic involvement of kidney extremely rare; designated as granulocytic sarcoma
- Other hematopoietic malignancies
  - Occasional cases of Langerhans cell histiocytosis, Rosai-Dorfman disease, and reticulum cell tumors described

DIAGNOSTIC CHECKLIST

Pathologic Interpretation Pearls
- Multifocal and bilateral renal masses should raise concern for metastasis and malignant lymphoma
- Majority of renal hematopoietic tumors are B-cell non-Hodgkin lymphoma
- Other than at autopsy, hematopoietic tumors may also be encountered by pathologists in nephrectomy specimens; often clinically misdiagnosed as parenchymal tumors

SELECTED REFERENCES
1. Hasegawa J et al: Characteristics of intravascular large B-cell lymphoma limited to the glomerular capillaries: a case report. Case Rep Nephrol Dial. 5(2):173-9, 2015
2. Hayakawa A et al: Primary pediatric stage III renal diffuse large B-cell lymphoma. Am J Case Rep. 14:34-7, 2013
3. Perry AM et al: Biological prognostic markers in diffuse large B-cell lymphoma. Cancer Control. 19(3):214-26, 2012
4. Evens AM et al: Post-transplantation lymphoproliferative disorders: diagnosis, prognosis, and current approaches to therapy. Curr Oncol Rep. 12(6):383-94, 2010
5. Kuo CC et al: Primary renal lymphoma. Br J Haematol. 144(5):628, 2009
6. Schniederjan SD et al: Lymphoid neoplasms of the urinary tract and male genital organs: a clinicopathological study of 40 cases. Mod Pathol. 22(8):1057-65, 2009
7. Haferlach T et al: Modern diagnostics in acute leukemias. Crit Rev Oncol Hematol. 56(2):223-34, 2005

Hematopoietic Tumors

Interstitial Growth Pattern

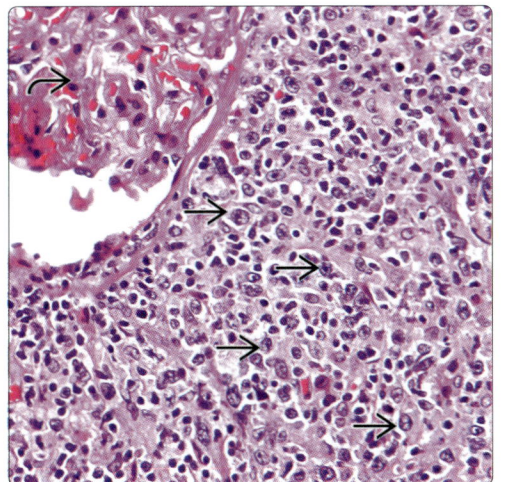

Diffuse T-Cell Lymphoma

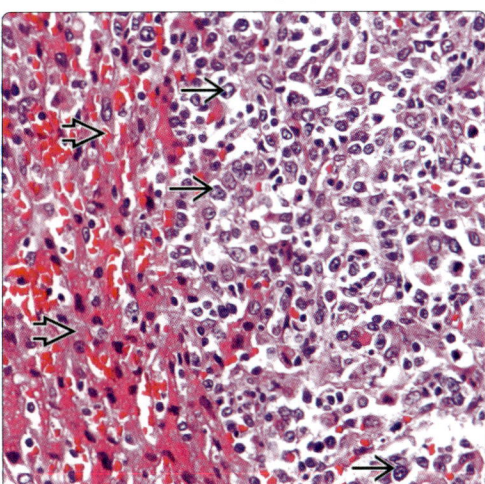

(Left) *This image from an autopsy specimen shows diffuse interstitial infiltration by large lymphoid cells ⇒ admixed with many smaller cells. Notice a glomerulus ⇒ caught within the tumor.* (Right) *This malignant lymphoid neoplasm also invaded hepatic parenchyma ⇒. Morphologically, it is composed of large ⇒ lymphoid cells with mixed cell infiltration, making specific typing difficult. This was diagnosed as diffuse T-cell/histiocyte-rich large B-cell lymphoma based on the immunophenotype.*

Follicular Lymphoma

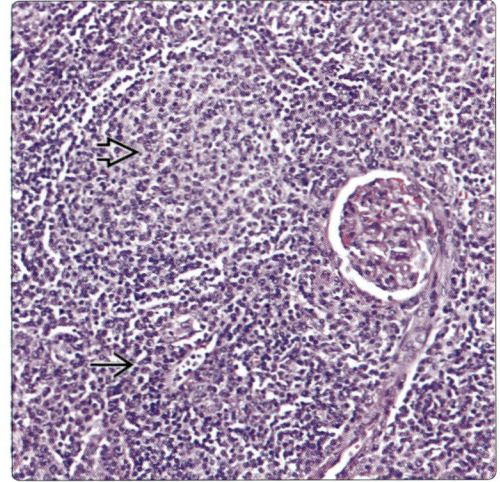

Follicular Lymphoma: CD20

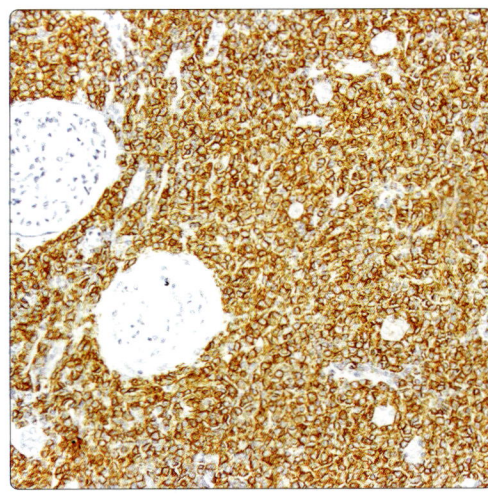

(Left) *H&E shows a lymphoid neoplastic proliferation with vague nodular ⇒ and diffuse ⇒ growth patterns. Such growth patterns suggest a follicular lymphoma. However, the possibility of a mucosa-associated lymphoid tissue lymphoma needs to be excluded, and therefore immunohistochemical confirmation is a must.* (Right) *CD20 immunostain shows diffuse positivity in this lymphoma, indicating that it is of B-cell origin. This, however, only excludes the possibility of a T-cell lymphoma.*

Follicular Lymphoma: Bcl-2

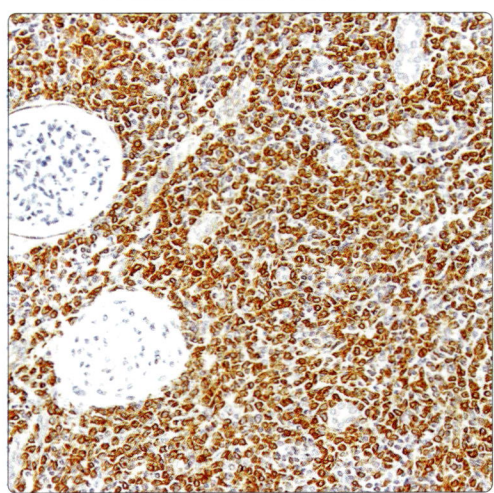

Follicular Lymphoma: CD10

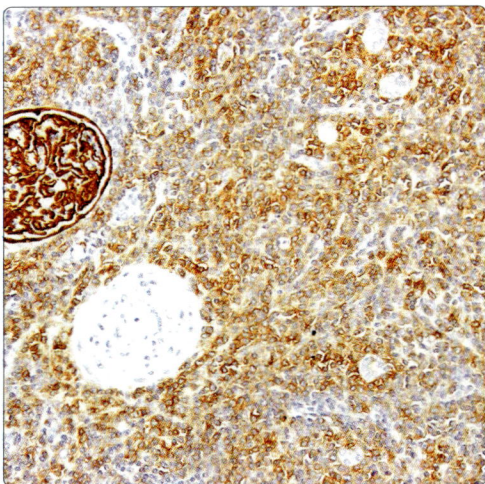

(Left) *Diffuse Bcl-2 immunoreactivity in this lymphoid tumor, along with the morphologic features, is highly suggestive of a follicular lymphoma. Diffuse large B-cell lymphomas are also often Bcl-2 positive. Therefore, morphologic as well as the expression of other immunohistochemical features are necessary for proper classification.* (Right) *Diffuse positivity for CD10, along with morphology and other immunostaining patterns, clinches the diagnosis of a follicular lymphoma in this case.*

Hematopoietic Tumors

Soft Tissue Infiltration

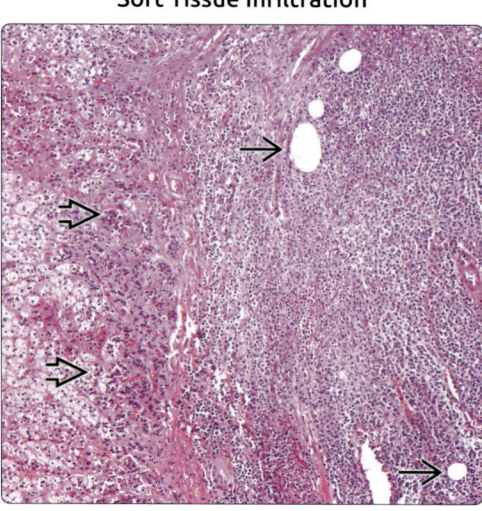

Plasmacytoma

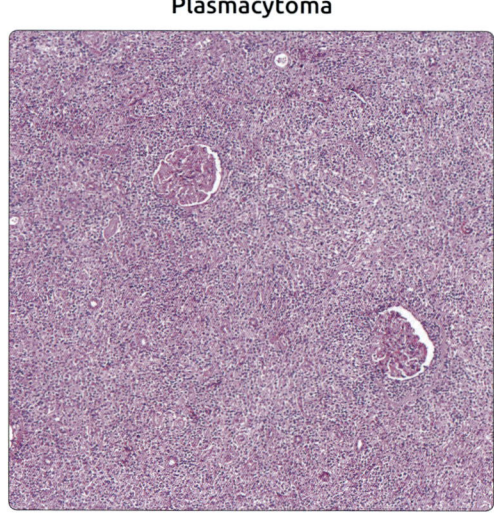

(Left) This malignant lymphoma shows diffuse infiltration of soft tissue ⇨ around the adrenal gland ⇨. Secondary malignant lymphomas of the kidneys are more often bilateral than primary renal lymphomas. They are usually also associated with extensive systemic involvement. **(Right)** Plasma cell neoplasms involving a kidney are almost always secondary. Only very rare primary renal plasmacytomas are described.

Plasmacytoma

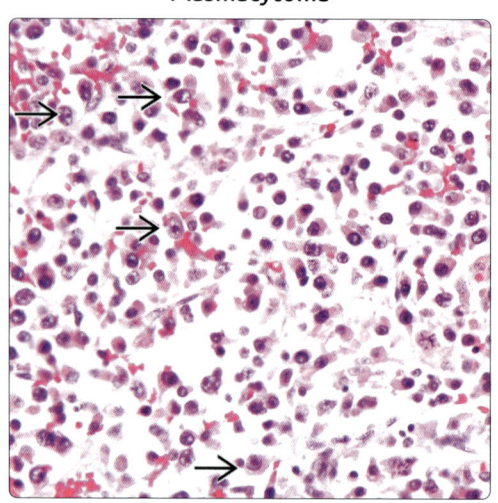

Langerhans Cell Histiocytosis

(Left) H&E shows loose sheets of neoplastic plasma cells from a case of multiple myeloma involving the kidney. Many cells are atypical, with prominent nucleoli ⇨, a common feature in plasma cell neoplasms. **(Right)** H&E shows a Langerhans cell histiocytosis ⇨ lesion, in close association with a clear cell renal cell carcinoma (RCC) ⇨. Some authors have suggested increased incidence of hematopoietic malignancies in cases with RCC, but other studies do not confirm such association.

Langerhans Cell Histiocytosis

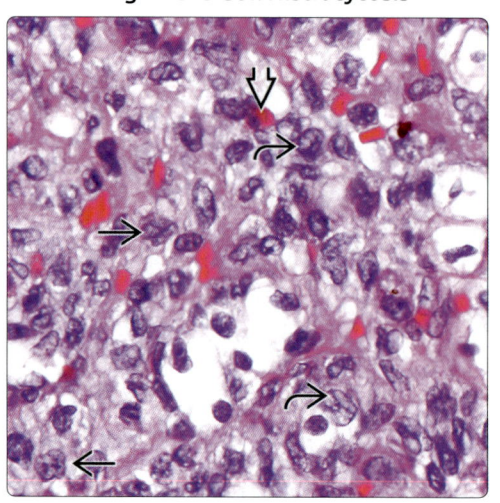

Langerhans Cell Histiocytosis: CD1a

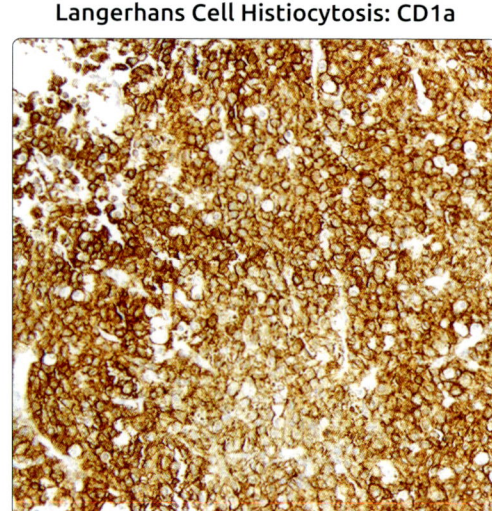

(Left) This higher magnification view depicts the typical nuclear features of Langerhans cell histiocytosis, including pale chromatin, marked nuclear angulations ⇨, and frequent grooves ⇨. A rare eosinophil is also present ⇨. **(Right)** This photomicrograph shows diffuse immunoreactivity for CD1a in a case of Langerhans cell histiocytosis involving the kidney. Such staining, along with the positivity for S100, is typical of the tumor.

Hematopoietic Tumors

Intravascular Lymphoma

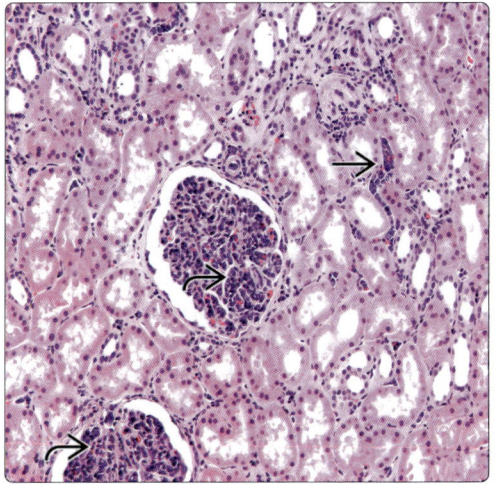

Intravascular Lymphoma: CD20

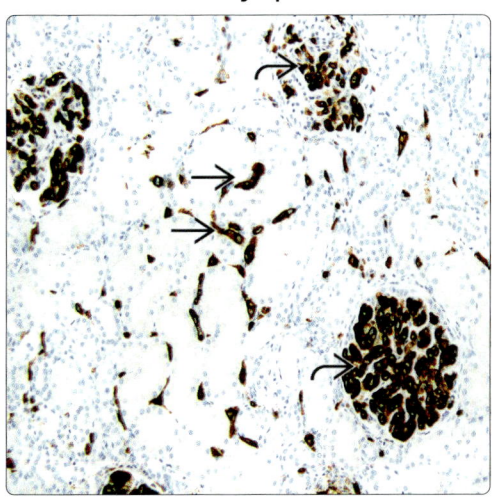

(Left) H&E depicts an intravascular lymphoma predominantly occupying the glomeruli ➡. Such lymphomas are extremely rare, and predominant involvement of glomeruli is reported. Notice the involvement of rare extraglomerular lymphatic channels ➡. (Right) CD20 immunostain confirms the presence of malignant B cells within the glomeruli ➡. Involvement of many more extraglomerular lymphovascular channels ➡ than is identified on H&E sections is highlighted on immunohistochemistry.

Posttransplant Lymphoproliferative Disorder

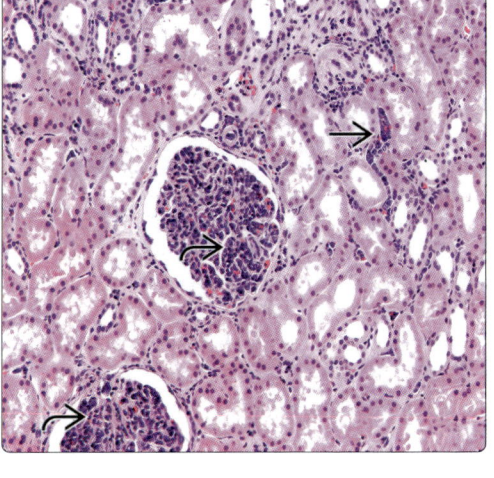

Posttransplant Lymphoproliferative Disorder

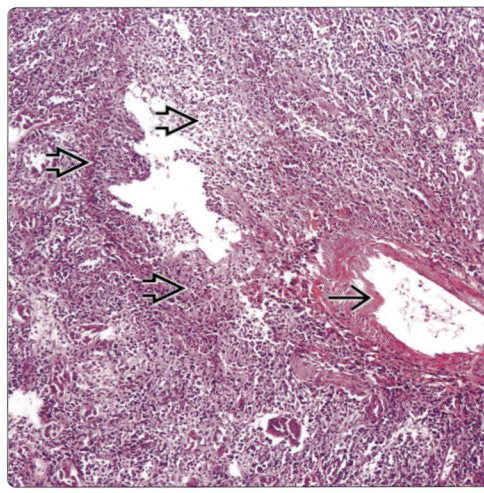

(Left) H&E shows posttransplant lymphoproliferative disorder, polymorphic type, involving the kidney. The infiltrate is polymorphous, but abundant, large atypical lymphoid cells ➡ are present. (Right) Typically, posttransplant lymphoproliferative disorder also shows venulitis ➡, within or outside the lymphoid infiltrates. The arterioles are relatively spared ➡ by the process.

Posttransplant Lymphoproliferative Disorder

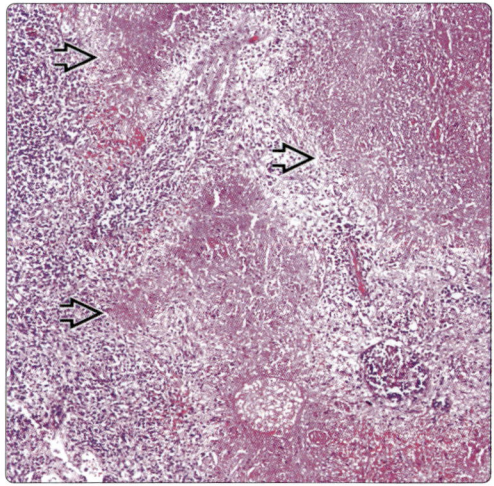

Posttransplant Lymphoproliferative Disorder

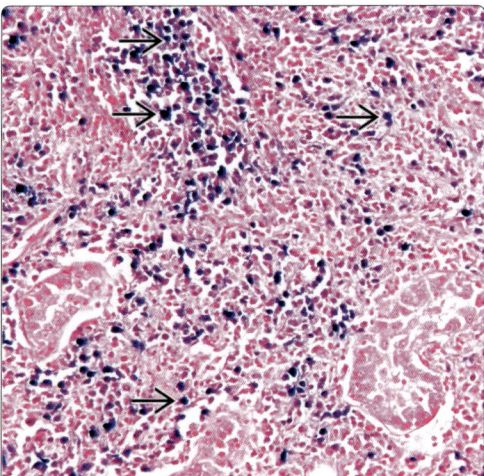

(Left) PTLD, besides the infiltrates, is characterized by serpentine, coagulative necrosis ➡ of the renal parenchyma. Presence of such necrosis on needle biopsies should alert one to the possibility of PTLD, in appropriate settings. (Right) The atypical lymphoid cells in PTLD are almost always monoclonal B cells. Only rare T or other cell type neoplasia are described. The neoplastic B cells are almost always positive for EB virus (nuclear positivity ➡ demonstrated here by in situ hybridization for EBER).

Juxtaglomerular Cell Tumor (Reninoma)

KEY FACTS

TERMINOLOGY
- Tumors derived from cells of renal juxtaglomerular apparatus, often associated with hyperreninism, hypokalemia, hyperaldosteronism, and hypertension

ETIOLOGY/PATHOGENESIS
- Loss of chromosomes 9 and 11, or LOH of same chromosomes, recurrent chromosomal abnormality

CLINICAL ISSUES
- Usually tumor of young adults
- Most present with severe hypertension showing no to minimal response to medical therapies
  - Surgical excision of tumor mostly alleviates hypertension
- Primarily, tumor with benign outcome
- Only 1 reported case with lung metastases
- All young patients with renal mass and hypertension need investigations to exclude JGCT

MACROSCOPIC
- Well-encapsulated, unilateral, solitary tumor
- Majority of tumors 2-3 cm in diameter

MICROSCOPIC
- Glomoid appearance with sheets of uniform round-to-polygonal cells with clear-to-slightly eosinophilic cytoplasm
- Numerous capillaries, branching blood vessels, and sinusoids similar to those of hemangiopericytoma
- Tumors often contain dispersed lymphoplasmacytic infiltrates
- Diffuse (+) staining with antibodies to renin, vimentin, CD34, and CD117; variable positivity for actin-sm
- Ultrastructure reveals typical membrane-bound rhomboid crystals representing renin protogranules

TOP DIFFERENTIAL DIAGNOSES
- Glomus tumor
- Solitary fibrous tumor/hemangiopericytoma

Gross Features
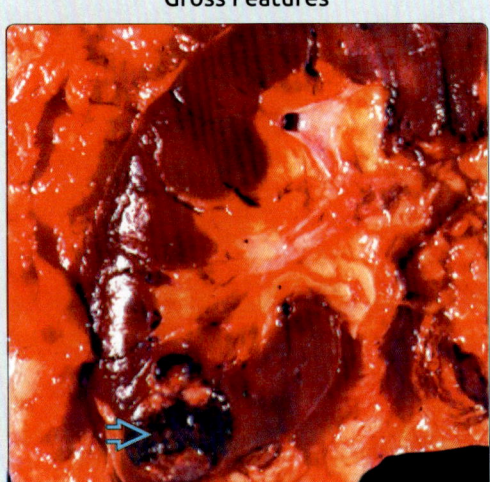

Tumor Circumscription
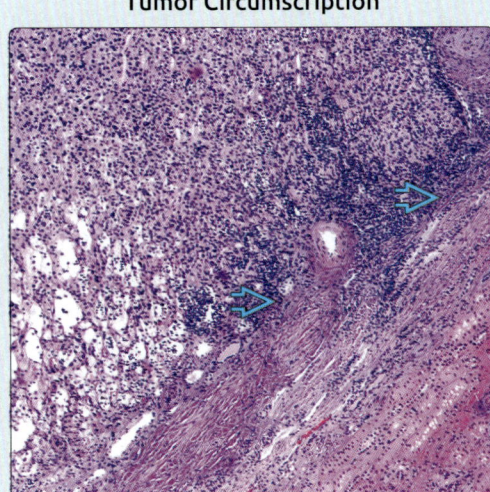

(Left) Juxtaglomerular cell tumors of the kidney are usually small, well-circumscribed tumors. Most tumors are less than 2-3 cm in size. Cut surface is usually light tan to yellow, mostly homogeneous, but may be hemorrhagic ➡ and partially cystic. (Right) Most juxtaglomerular cell tumors are well circumscribed with a well-formed, fibrous capsule. Occasionally, the capsule may show focal discontinuity ➡. Notice the marked lymphocytic infiltration in the tumor periphery in this case.

Glomus Tumor-Like Features
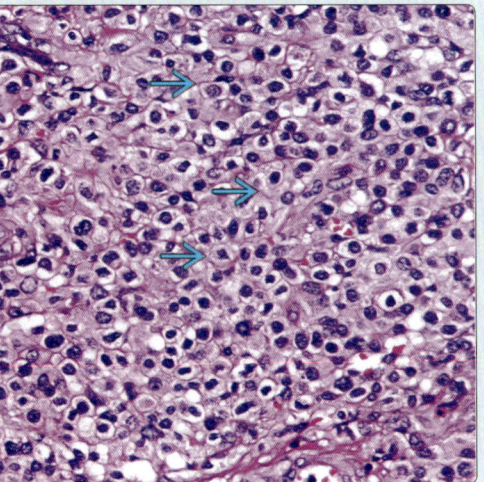

Nuclear Uniformity
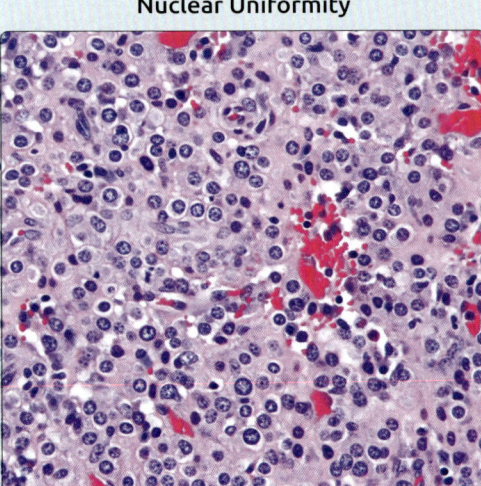

(Left) Juxtaglomerular cell tumors often show relative uniformity of nuclear size and shape. Cells often contain a moderate amount of eosinophilic cytoplasm and cell membranes are usually prominent ➡. These morphological features closely resemble those seen in glomus tumors. (Right) In addition to the frequent nuclear uniformity, most juxtaglomerular cell tumors are highly vascular, often with a hemangiopericytoma-like pattern, thus focally resembling SFT/hemangiopericytoma.

Juxtaglomerular Cell Tumor (Reninoma)

TERMINOLOGY

Abbreviations
- Juxtaglomerular cell tumor (JGCT)

Synonyms
- Reninoma

Definitions
- Tumors derived from cells of renal juxtaglomerular apparatus, often characterized by
  o Association with hyperreninism, hypokalemia, and hyperaldosteronism
  o Hypertension that usually does not respond to medical antihypertensive therapy

ETIOLOGY/PATHOGENESIS

Hyperreninemia
- With rare exceptions of nonfunctional tumors, most patients have elevated serum renin levels

Genetic Features
- Loss of chromosomes 9 and 11, or LOH of same chromosomes, recurrent chromosomal abnormality
  o Whole genome expression analysis in 2 cases with 415 up-regulated (including renin and CD117) and 325 down-regulated genes (including some protein tyrosine phosphatases)

CLINICAL ISSUES

Presentation
- Rare tumor, < 100 cases reported; more often reported in females than males (1.5:1)
- Usually tumor of young adults (2nd-3rd decade); however, age range of 6 to > 80 yr (mean: 24 yr)
- Hypertension
  o Most patients present with severe hypertension that shows no or only minimal response to medical therapies
    – Usually associated with hyperreninemia, hypokalemia, and hyperaldosteronism
  o Radiologically, no evidence of renal artery stenosis
  o All young patients with renal mass and hypertension need investigations to exclude JGCT
  o Surgical excision of tumor mostly alleviates hypertension; in rare cases, persistent hypertension after nephrectomy due to secondary hypertensive angiopathy

Treatment
- Partial or total nephrectomy

Prognosis
- Benign outcome after resection; < 10% with persistent postnephrectomy hypertension, usually less severe
- Only 1 reported case with lung metastases

IMAGING

General Features
- Radiologic studies essential to rule out other causes of hypertension
- Renal arteriography helps to exclude renal artery stenosis

MACROSCOPIC

General Features
- Well-encapsulated, unilateral, solitary tumor; tan-to-yellow cut surface, mostly solid, but occasionally with small, cysts

Size
- Majority of tumors 2-3 cm in diameter; range < 1-15 cm

MICROSCOPIC

Histologic Features
- Histologic appearance highly variable
  o Typically, glomoid appearance with sheets of uniform round-to-polygonal cells with clear-to-slightly eosinophilic cytoplasm, and distinct cell borders
  o Occasionally, sheets or irregular cords of polygonal to spindle cells with indistinct cell borders
  o Most with numerous capillaries, branching blood vessels, and sinusoids similar to those of hemangiopericytoma
  o Stroma is scanty, hyalinized, or myxoid
  o Tumors often contain dispersed lymphocytic infiltrates
  o Some tumors with entrapped tubules in periphery, sometimes hyperplastic and with papillary configuration
  o Rare cases with prominent papillary pattern; likely representing entrapped epithelium
  o Mitotic activity or necrosis uncommon

ANCILLARY TESTS

Immunohistochemistry
- Diffuse (+) staining with antibodies to renin, vimentin, CD34, and CD117; variable positivity for actin-sm
- Neuroendocrine markers and keratins (-); cytokeratins label entrapped tubules but not polygonal or spindle cells

Electron Microscopy
- Reveals typical membrane-bound rhomboid crystals representing renin protogranules

DIFFERENTIAL DIAGNOSIS

Glomus Tumor
- Marked morphologic overlap with JGCT
- JGCT most often with history of hypertension
- CD34(-) or only focally (+) in glomus tumor; laminin shows pericellular positivity, and CD117(-)
- Glomus tumor lacks typical ultrastructural crystals

Solitary Fibrous Tumor/Hemangiopericytoma
- Usually spindle cell but may have round cell areas
- SFT/hemangiopericytomas (+) for STAT-6, bcl-2 and CD99, and (-) for CD117 and renin; CD34(+) in both

SELECTED REFERENCES

1. Kuroda N et al: Juxtaglomerular cell tumor: a morphological, immunohistochemical and genetic study of six cases. Hum Pathol. 44(1):47-54, 2013
2. Kuroda N et al: Review of juxtaglomerular cell tumor with focus on pathobiological aspect. Diagn Pathol. 6:80, 2011
3. Kim HJ et al: Juxtaglomerular cell tumor of kidney with CD34 and CD117 immunoreactivity: report of 5 cases. Arch Pathol Lab Med. 130(5):707-11, 2006
4. Squires JP et al: Juxtaglomerular cell tumor of the kidney. Cancer. 53(3):516-23, 1984

Juxtaglomerular Cell Tumor (Reninoma)

(Left) A consistent feature in juxtaglomerular cell tumors is the presence of widely dispersed clusters of lymphocytic infiltrates ➡. **(Right)** The lymphocytic infiltrates in juxtaglomerular cell tumors are usually small and resemble foci of extramedullary hematopoiesis ➡. Occasionally, some mast cells may be admixed with them. Presence of mast cells in the tumor may make the interpretation of CD117 immunohistochemical stain difficult in some cases.

Lymphocytic Infiltrates

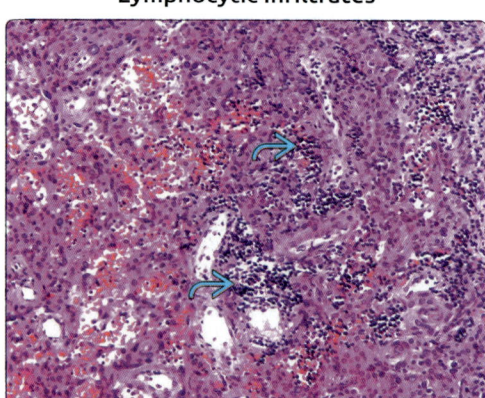

Lymphocytic Infiltrates

(Left) Overall, JGCT appears morphologically to be a low-grade neoplasm, with cytological uniformity, usual absence of mitoses, and lack of tumor necrosis. However, rare mitotic figures ➡ and indistinct cell borders ➡ may be seen in some tumors, the presence of which does not influence prognosis. **(Right)** This JGCT with polygonal cells contains scant to moderate eosinophilic cytoplasm. The cells are in small clusters and may raise the possibility of a renal epithelial neoplasm. Cytokeratin stain is typically negative.

Mitotic Activity

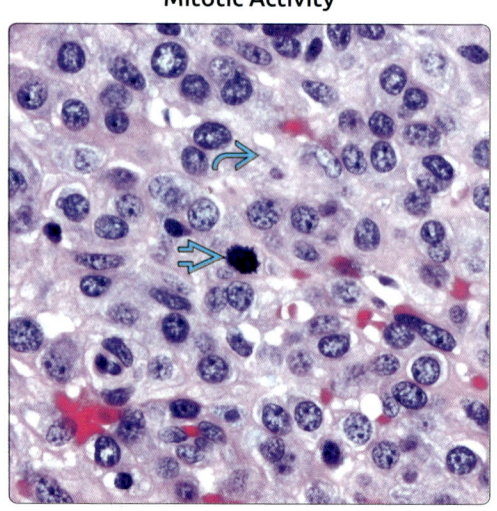

Cytoplasmic Eosinophilia

(Left) Focal, marked nuclear atypia ➡ may be present in juxtaglomerular cell tumor. The presence of such focal endocrine-like, markedly atypical, polyploid, hyperchromatic nuclei is not uncommon and has no bearing on prognosis. **(Right)** This photomicrograph shows a spindle cell phenotype in a juxtaglomerular cell tumor. This architectural feature is usually focal. The differential diagnosis with solitary fibrous tumor is resolved by immunohistochemistry, including STAT-6, Bcl-2, and CD99.

Endocrine-Like Nuclear Atypia

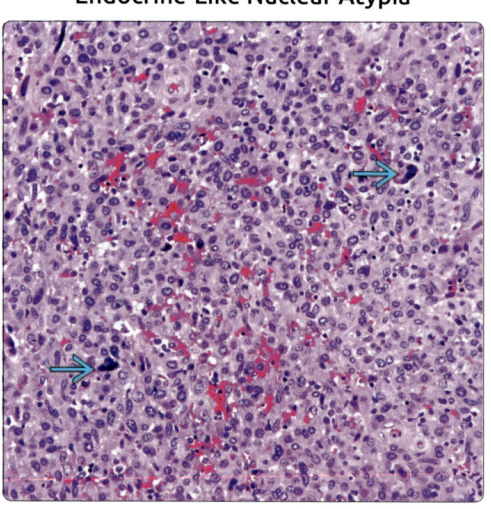

Spindle Cell Features

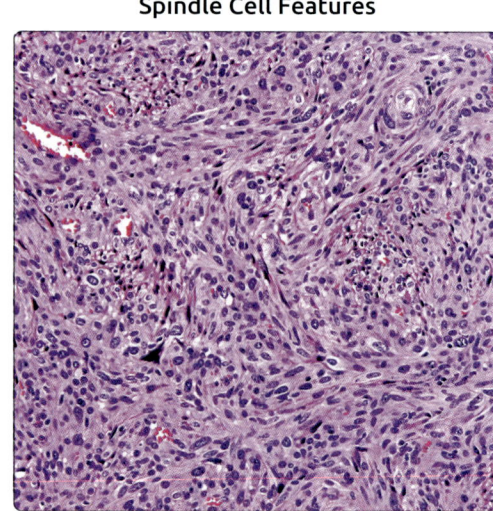

Juxtaglomerular Cell Tumor (Reninoma)

Intratumoral Edema

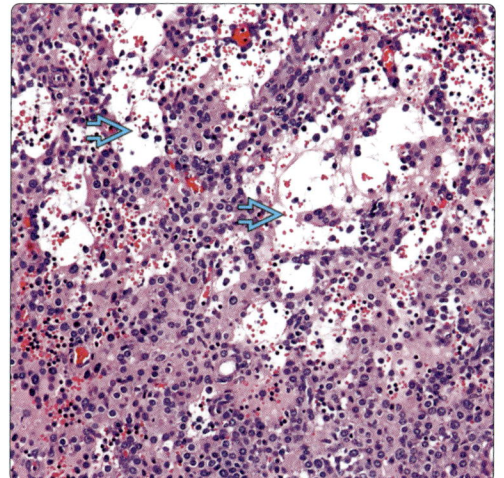

Papillary Architecture

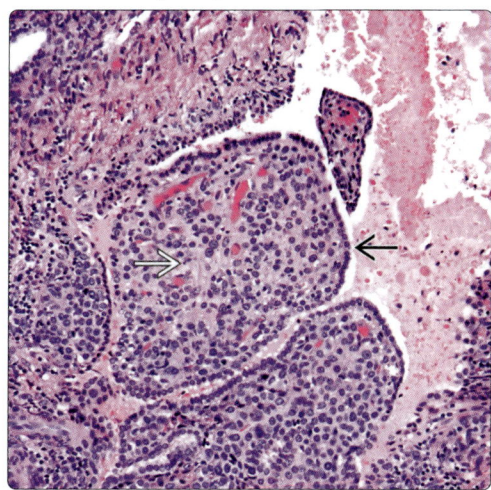

(Left) Most JGCTs are highly vascular. Some may show thin-walled edematous cystic foci ➡ as a prominent pattern in the tumor. Others may have antler-like vascularity, similar to that seen in solitary fibrous tumor/hemangiopericytoma. (Right) Juxtaglomerular cell tumors with markedly prominent papillary features have been described. In this image, a papillary configuration is seen with a number of tubular structures ➡ occupying the cores of the papillae ➡.

Immunohistochemistry: CD34

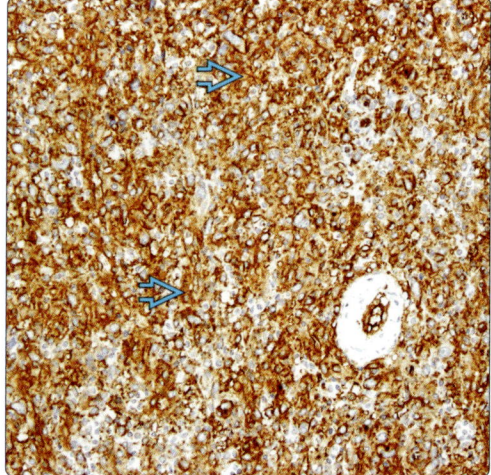

Immunohistochemistry: CD117

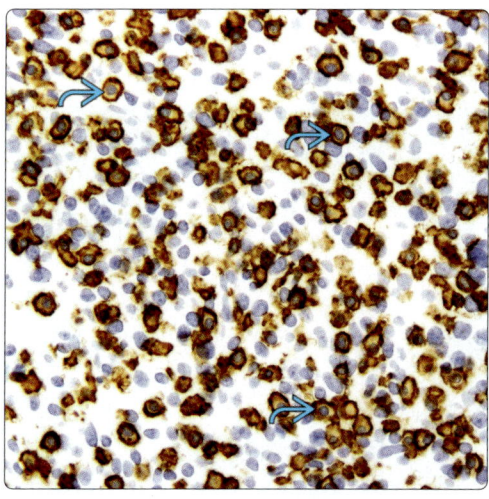

(Left) Diffuse immunohistochemical positivity for CD34 ➡ is present in most juxtaglomerular cell tumors. Such diffuse immunoreactivity is important in the distinction of JGCT from glomus tumor of the kidney. (Right) Immunoreactivity for CD117 is also present in JGCT. However, many tumors show abundant mast cell infiltration ➡, associated with lymphoplasmacytic infiltrates. Therefore, interpretation of the results with CD117 positivity requires caution.

Differential Diagnosis: Glomus Tumor

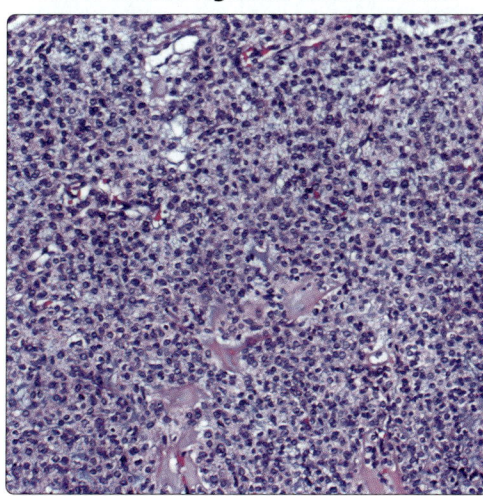

Differential Diagnosis: Solitary Fibrous Tumor

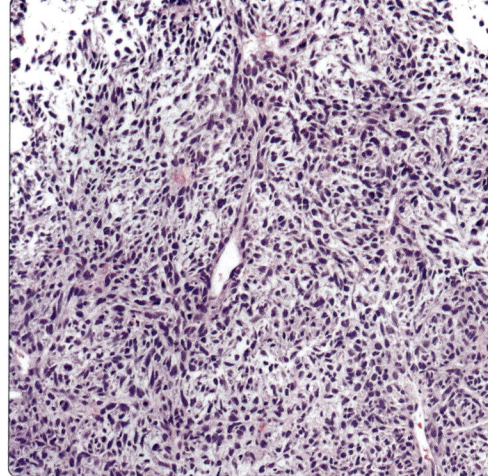

(Left) Presence of glomus tumor-like features in JGCT can make the distinction difficult. However, unlike JGCT, glomus tumor is usually CD34 and CD117 negative, stains positive for laminin, and is not associated with hypertension. (Right) Presence of spindle cell morphology in JGCT, or epithelioid/round cells in some solitary fibrous tumor, in the presence of branching vasculature, can create difficulties in the distinction between the pair. STAT-6 positivity in SFT is very helpful in their separation.

Renomedullary Interstitial Cell Tumor

KEY FACTS

TERMINOLOGY
- Benign renal medullary neoplasm arising from renomedullary interstitial cells

CLINICAL ISSUES
- Most common kidney tumor of adults
- Most often, incidental finding in nephrectomies performed for other tumors or at autopsy
- Incidence in autopsy series varies from 16-42%
- Rare mass lesions detected by radiologic imaging performed for other indications
- Very rarely, tumor may compress pelvicalyceal system, leading to hydronephrosis and urosepsis

MACROSCOPIC
- Most measure < 5 mm in greatest dimension (usually 1-10 mm)
- Very occasionally, much larger masses (≥ 5 cm) reported
  - Some of these protrude into renal pelvis and may be associated with hydronephrosis

MICROSCOPIC
- Densely collagenized tumors with sparse spindle cells
  - Keloid-like collagenous bands may be present in such tumors
- Or variably cellular tumors usually with abundant spindle to stellate cells in myxoid stroma

TOP DIFFERENTIAL DIAGNOSES
- Mixed epithelial and stromal tumor (MEST)
  - Usually larger mass lesion and primary reason for nephrectomy
  - Epithelial component in MEST distributed throughout tumor, and stroma in MEST usually ER and PR positive

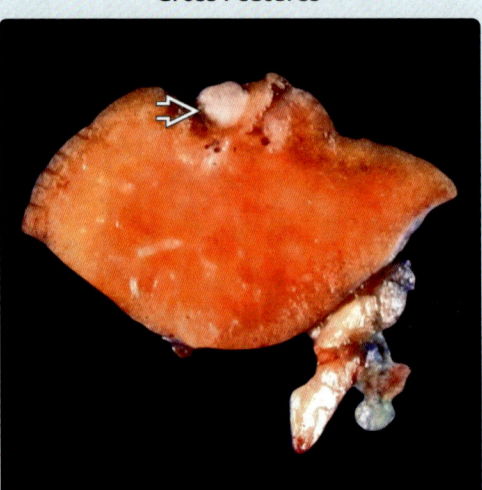

Gross Features

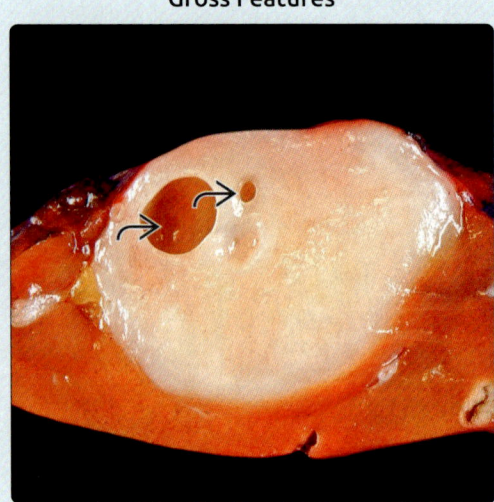

Gross Features

(Left) Renomedullary interstitial cell tumors are usually subcentimeter, white or tan nodules ⇨, mostly detected incidentally at autopsy or in nephrectomy specimens resected for other conditions. *(Right)* Very rarely, renomedullary interstitial cell tumors may be quite large and detected radiologically. This example shows some cystic areas ⇨ that on microscopy appear as cystically dilated entrapped tubules. An occasional case may compress the pelvicalyceal system and result in hydronephrosis.

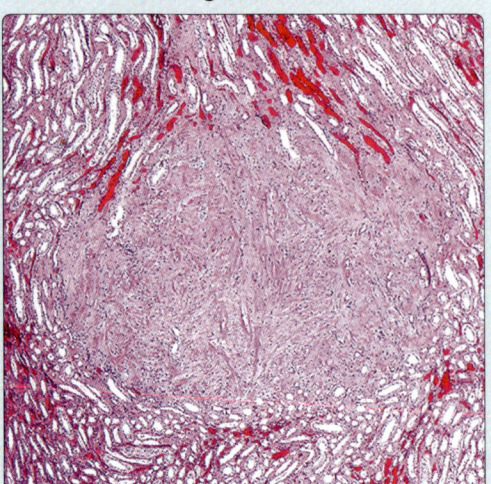

Histological Features

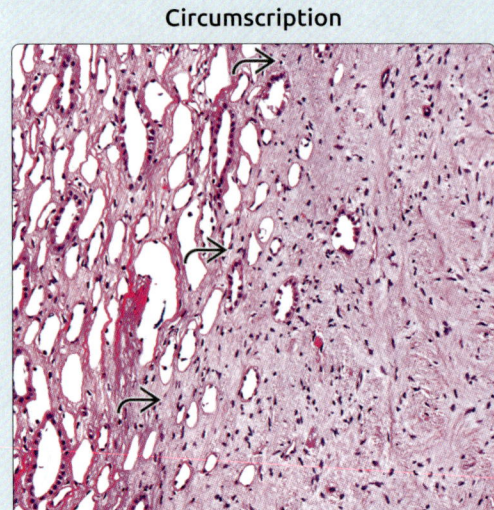

Circumscription

(Left) Renomedullary interstitial cell tumors (RMICT) are well-circumscribed nodules, almost invariably present in the renal medulla. These are the most common renal tumors, and thorough sampling of the kidneys reveals an incidence of > 40%. *(Right)* Although RMICT is almost always well circumscribed, it does not show any encapsulation. This H&E image shows a well-circumscribed renomedullary interstitial tumor imperceptibly merging with the surrounding renal medullary tissue ⇨.

Renomedullary Interstitial Cell Tumor

TERMINOLOGY

Abbreviations
- Renomedullary interstitial cell tumor (RMICT)

Synonyms
- Medullary fibroma

Definitions
- Benign renal medullary neoplasm arising from renomedullary interstitial cells

ETIOLOGY/PATHOGENESIS

Renal Medullary Interstitial Cell
- Renomedullary interstitial cells (RMIC) normally located in inner renal medulla
  - These cells express receptors for multiple vasoactive peptides, including angiotensin II
  - RMIC plays important role in renin release and regulation of sodium excretion
    - These, in turn, maintain renal blood flow and normal blood pressure
- RMIC tumors are believed by many to develop in response to systemic hypertension
  - Others have found no such relationship between these tumors and systemic hypertension
- Concomitant expression of COX-2, microsomal prostaglandin E synthase-1, and prostaglandin E2 (PGE2) receptor demonstrated in RMIC tumors
  - COX-2 activity known to provide antiapoptotic protection of interstitial cells during osmotic stress
  - RMIC tumors show constitutive activation of COX-2, resulting in increased PGE2 production and activation of PGE2 receptors
    - This activation acts in autocrine manner, leading to tumoral proliferation of interstitial medullary cells

CLINICAL ISSUES

Epidemiology
- Incidence
  - Most common kidney tumor of adults, with 16-42% incidence in autopsy series; increasing incidence with age
    - Very rare in young patients (youngest: 14 years old)

Presentation
- Mostly incidental finding in nephrectomies performed for other tumors or at autopsy
  - Rarely as mass lesions detected by radiologic imaging performed for other indications
- Occasional associations between multiple RMICTs and systemic hypertension also reported

Prognosis
- Benign tumors

MACROSCOPIC

General Features
- Well-circumscribed, tan to white nodules within renal medulla
- Most measure < 5 mm in greatest dimension (usually 1-10 mm)
- Very occasionally, much larger masses (≥ 5 cm) reported that sometimes protrude into renal pelvis and are associated with hydronephrosis

MICROSCOPIC

Histologic Features
- Stroma in RMICT either loose and myxoid, or densely collagenized, occasionally with keloid-like collagen
- Stromal cells may be scant and widely separated, or hypercellular and tightly packed
  - Stromal cells spindled or stellate with uniform chromatin, absent to minimal nuclear pleomorphism, and no mitotic activity; no necrosis
  - May show presence of lipid droplets, similar to that in nonneoplastic RMIC, as confirmed by oil red O stain
- Tumors with mixed patterns common
- Occasional tumors with amyloid deposition in stroma
- Entrapped normal tubules frequently seen, particularly at periphery of tumor, rarely with cystic dilatation

ANCILLARY TESTS

Immunohistochemistry
- Stromal cells in RMICT show some immunohistochemical features resembling myofibroblasts, but IHC rarely required in diagnostic practice
  - Stain positive for smooth muscle actin, COX-2, PGE2 and CD35; CD34 and S100 protein negative
  - Tumors have not been investigated for ER and PR

Electron Microscopy
- Ultrastructural features similar to nonneoplastic RMIC
  - Electron-dense osmiophilic droplets (lipid), cisternae, and cytoplasmic processes most consistent features

DIFFERENTIAL DIAGNOSIS

Mixed Epithelial and Stromal Tumor
- Mixed epithelial and stromal tumor (MEST) usually larger mass lesion and primary reason for nephrectomy; RMICT almost invariably incidental finding
- Epithelial component in MEST is distributed randomly and throughout tumor; RMICT usually with entrapped renal tubules only in periphery
- Stroma in MEST usually ER and PR positive
  - No reports of ER and PR positivity in RMIC tumors, although nontumorous RMICs have been reported to be ER &/or PR positive

DIAGNOSTIC CHECKLIST

Pathologic Interpretation Pearls
- Benign stromal tumor of kidney that is often incidentally detected and which is composed of bland stellate cells

SELECTED REFERENCES

1. Bazzi WM et al: Clinicopathologic features of renomedullary interstitial cell tumor presenting as the main solid renal mass. Urology. 83(5):1104-6, 2014
2. Faris G et al: Urosepsis as a presenting symptom of renomedullary interstitial cell tumor causing renal obstruction. Isr Med Assoc J. 11(8):509-10, 2009
3. Gatalica Z et al: COX-2 gene polymorphisms and protein expression in renomedullary interstitial cell tumors. Hum Pathol. 39(10):1495-504, 2008

Renomedullary Interstitial Cell Tumor

(Left) A consistent feature in renomedullary interstitial cell tumors is the presence of entrapped tubules ➔, particularly in the periphery of the tumor. Notice the adjacent renal medulla ➔, in which almost all of these tumors are located. **(Right)** Most renomedullary interstitial cell tumors are paucicellular, with dispersed spindle or stellate cells dispersed within the stroma. This image shows loose myxoid stroma in a tumor with low cellularity.

Entrapped Tubules
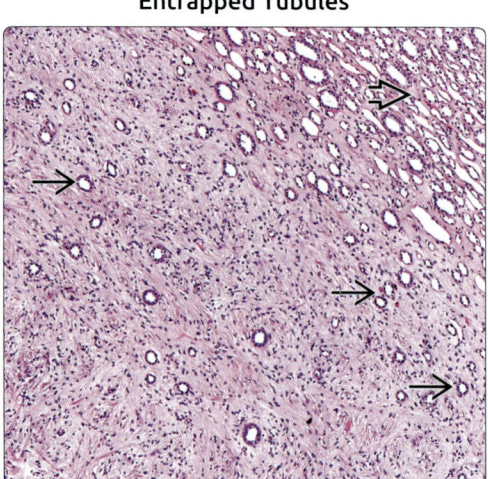

Loose Myxoid Stroma
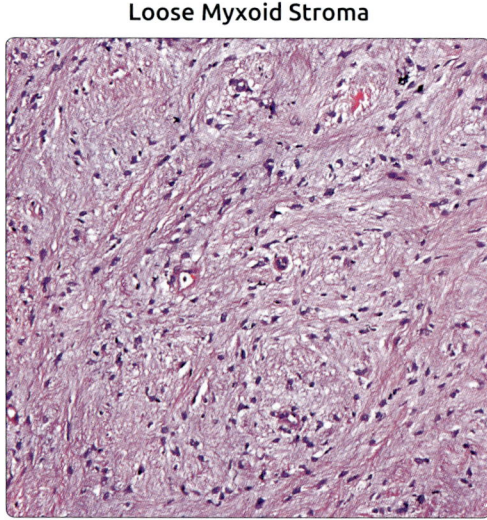

(Left) Some renomedullary interstitial cell tumors show sclerotic stroma and relatively scant spindle or stellate cells. However, the stroma is more loose ➔ and faintly basophilic, at least focally, in most cases. **(Right)** In some cases of renomedullary interstitial cell tumor, in addition to the loose myxoid and fibrotic-like stroma in variable proportions, keloid-like ➔ hyalinized bands of collagen that do not stain with Congo red may also be present. Rare cases with stromal amyloid deposition are also reported.

Sclerotic Stroma
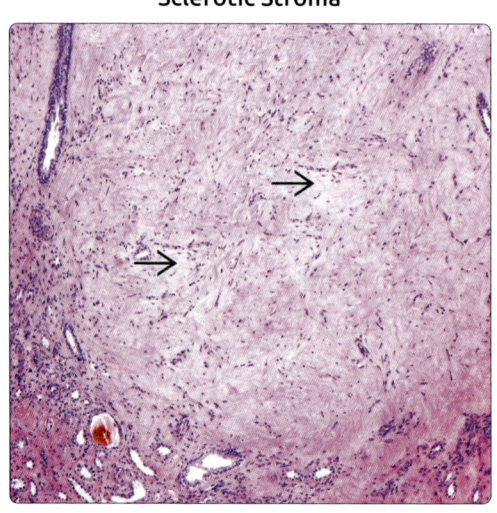

Keloid-Like Bands
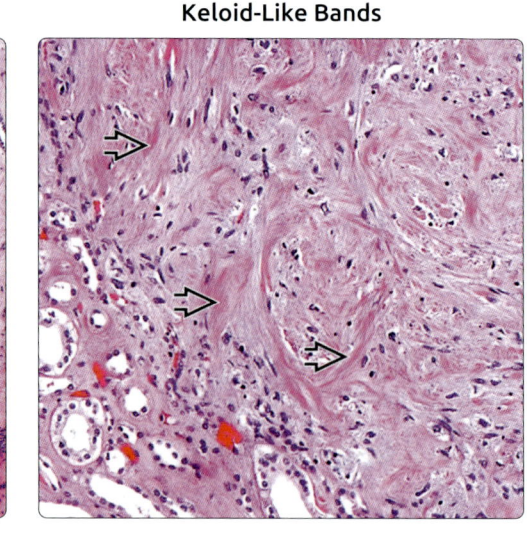

(Left) Rarely, renomedullary interstitial cell tumors may show cystic dilatation ➔ of the entrapped tubules. Notice the stromal sclerosis and keloid-like collagen ➔ in this tumor. **(Right)** The spindled or stellate cells in renomedullary interstitial cell tumors are generally loosely arranged in a myxoid or fibrotic stroma. Most of these cells are myofibroblastic in origin. However, CD35(+) dendritic cells may also be present.

Cystic Entrapped Tubules
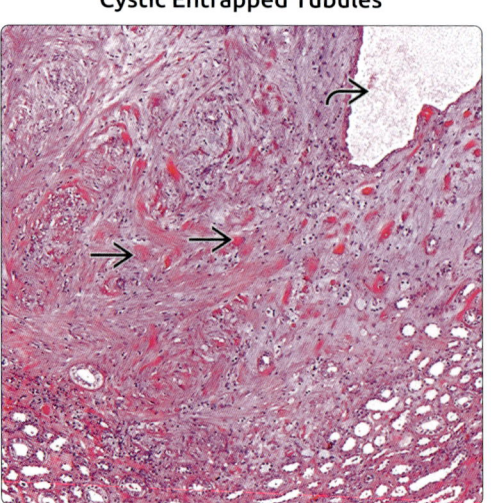

Spindle/Stellate Cells
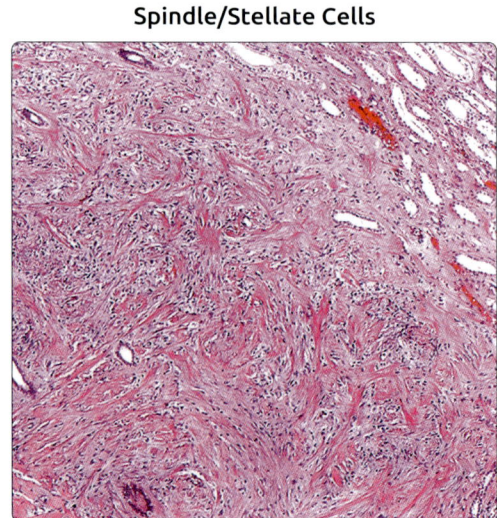

Renomedullary Interstitial Cell Tumor

Myxoid Stroma

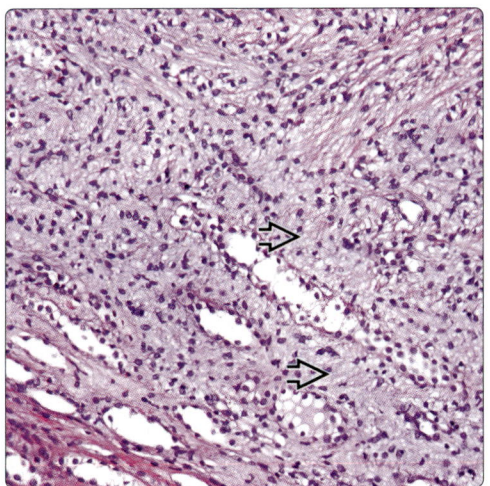

Cellular Stroma

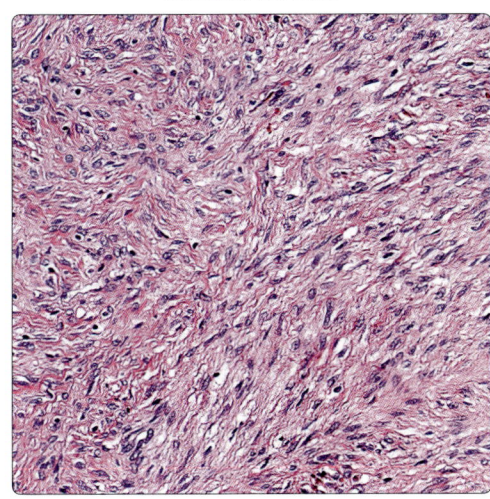

(Left) In some renomedullary interstitial tumors, the stroma may be entirely myxoid or basophilic ➡. In many tumors, however, both the sclerotic and basophilic-type stroma are present in combination, in variable proportions. (Right) Some renomedullary interstitial cell tumors may appear more cellular, and have more densely collagenized stroma. Such appearance may focally resemble fibromatosis. However, circumscription and other typical myxoid areas in the tumor exclude that possibility.

Cellular Stroma

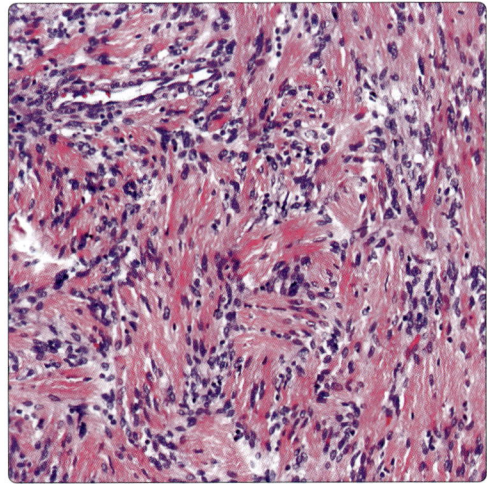

Bland Cytology

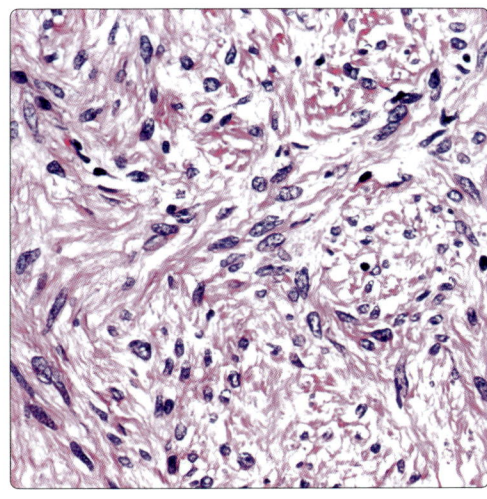

(Left) Some renomedullary interstitial cell tumors are quite cellular. This cellular tumor has a fibrotic/sclerotic stroma. These tumors are negative for CD34 and S100 (unlike solitary fibrous tumor or schwannoma), and often stain positive for smooth muscle actin. (Right) This cellular renomedullary interstitial cell tumor shows the bland nuclear features characteristic of the tumor. The nuclei depict minimal variation in shape and size, and have open chromatin. Mitotic activity is almost always nonexistent.

Bland Cytology, Open Chromatin

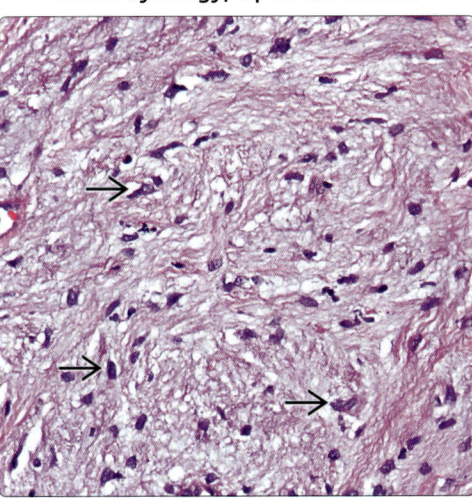

MEST: Differential Diagnosis

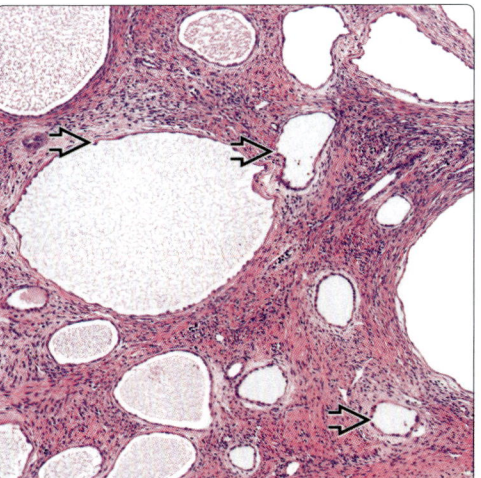

(Left) The bland spindled or stellate cells ➡ in RMICT show open chromatin and minimal atypia. Oil red O histochemical stain often reveals lipid droplets in these cells, similar to that found in nonneoplastic RMICs. (Right) Renal mixed epithelial and stromal tumors (MEST) may sometimes be difficult to distinguish from renomedullary interstitial cell tumor. Unlike RMICT, MEST is a large, radiologically identifiable tumor. The epithelial component ➡ is widely dispersed throughout the tumor, unlike RMICT.

Other Rare Tumors

TERMINOLOGY

Definitions
- Uncommon tumors that include
  - Benign and malignant mesenchymal neoplasms, neuroendocrine tumors other than carcinoid tumor, and other rare tumors

EPIDEMIOLOGY

Incidence
- Primary mesenchymal tumors of kidney constitute ≤ 1% of all renal tumors
- Among sarcomas, largest reported series of 26 cases represents 25 yr of experience at Memorial Sloan Kettering Cancer Center, New York
- After angiomyolipoma, leiomyoma is 2nd most common benign mesenchymal tumor of kidney
  - Based on older autopsy series, reported incidence is > 5%
    - However, we are now aware that most renal leiomyomatous tumors in fact represent leiomyomatous angiomyolipomas
    - Therefore, actual incidence of renal leiomyomas likely much lower than reported in literature
- Other rarer benign mesenchymal tumors described in kidneys include
  - Hemangioma, lipoma, solitary fibrous tumor, schwannoma, neurofibroma, myxoma, myopericytoma, and lymphangioma
- < 20 primary high-grade neuroendocrine carcinomas (mostly small cell carcinoma) and < 15 renal glomus tumors described in the literature
- Very few cases of renal-adrenal fusion reported
  - However, ectopic adrenal tissue is more common
  - Very occasional adrenal cortical tumor arising from renal-adrenal fusion or ectopic adrenal tissue also described

CLINICAL IMPLICATIONS

Clinical Presentation
- Most benign or low-grade tumors detected incidentally on evaluation of unrelated symptoms
  - Others may present with palpable mass or hematuria
- Sarcomas and other high-grade tumors often present with flank or abdominal pain and palpable mass, or occasionally with hematuria
  - Rare cases may present with symptoms related to metastases

Clinical Risk Factors
- Prognostic factors and risk
  - Sarcomas of kidney usually aggressive tumors with reported 5-year survival rates of < 30%
    - Tumor size and metastasis at presentation are the most significant predictors of disease-specific survival in GU, including renal, sarcomas
  - Renal high-grade neuroendocrine carcinomas are highly aggressive neoplasms, like their counterparts in other sites
    - Metastasis from another site should be ruled out before tumor is reported as primary
    - Distant metastases to brain, bone, adrenal gland, and liver frequent
    - Prognosis highly dependent on stage and complete resectability of tumor
    - Approximately 75% of patients reported to be dead of disease within 1 yr of diagnosis
    - However, with current therapies available for small cell carcinoma, prognosis may not be so dismal
  - Visceral location, size > 2 cm, nuclear atypia, significant mitotic activity, or atypical mitoses reported to predict aggressive behavior in glomus tumors
    - However, most reported renal glomus tumors have been > 2 cm, and all have had benign clinical course on relatively short follow-ups
    - Degenerative-type nuclear atypia also reported in renal glomus tumors, with no adverse influence on biologic behavior

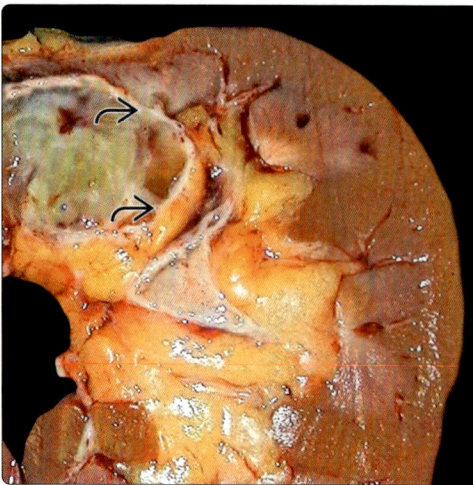

Glomus Tumor: Gross Features

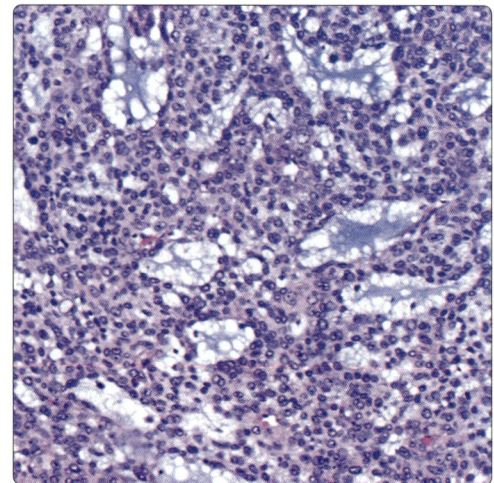

Glomus Tumor: Typical Histology

(Left) This well-circumscribed and encapsulated ⇨ tumor represents a glomus tumor. It shows a prominent myxoid cut surface. Glomus tumors of the kidney are quite rare, and at both the gross and microscopic levels need distinction from juxtaglomerular cell tumor. *(Right)* Microscopically, glomus tumors show relatively uniform cells, with smooth nuclear contours, open and speckled chromatin, moderate amount of eosinophilic to amphophilic cytoplasm, and distinct cell borders.

Other Rare Tumors

MACROSCOPIC

General Features

- Leiomyomas and lipomas: Well circumscribed, usually small; rare large tumors, including a 37 kg lipoma, also described
  - Gross appearance similar to that in soft tissue counterparts
- Hemangiomas usually small (1-2 cm), mostly localized but not well circumscribed
  - Rare tumors ≤ 8 cm in size and filling pelvicalyceal system have been also described
  - Usually hemorrhagic-appearing cut surface; rarely solid-tan appearance
- Glomus tumors well circumscribed and encapsulated
  - Cut surface may be uniform and tan, or with variegated mucoid/myxoid appearance
- Sarcomas usually large tumors
  - Mean size: 10.5 cm (range: 2.5-30 cm); tumor size closely related to biologic behavior
- Most patients with renal high-grade neuroendocrine carcinoma present with locally advanced disease and regional lymph node metastases
  - Majority of tumors located close to pelvicalyceal system
  - Size ranges from 2.5-23 cm (median: 8 cm)
    - Invasion into renal sinus adipose tissue very frequent
  - Cut surface usually soft, whitish, gritty, and necrotic

MICROSCOPIC

General Features

- Leiomyomas, lipomas, and hemangiomas: Morphologic features similar to those in soft tissue
  - Possibility of angiomyolipoma needs to be excluded in all smooth muscle and lipomatous tumors of kidney
    - Most leiomyomas recently reported to be in perimenopausal females
  - As in soft tissue, mitotic activity, nuclear atypia, necrosis, and large size in leiomyomatous tumor favor leiomyosarcoma
  - Hemangiomas usually of cavernous type; capillary hemangiomas are unusual
  - Recently described rare hemangioma variant, anastomosing hemangioma, appears unique to kidney vascular tumors
    - Shows anastomosing sinusoidal capillary-sized vessels with scattered hobnail endothelial cells
    - Morphology displays overlapping features of both sinusoidal hemangioma and hobnail hemangioma of soft tissue and skin
    - May mimic angiosarcoma
    - Also described in end-stage kidney disease
- Solitary fibrous tumor
  - Histological appearance the same as that at more common soft tissue locations
- Schwannoma
  - Histological appearance similar to that at more common locations, with palisading (Antoni A) and less cellular, loosely arranged (Antoni B) areas
- Glomus tumor: Represents group of tumors composed of glomus cells, blood vessels, and smooth muscle cells in various proportions
  - Glomus cells typically small, round-to-oval uniform cells with distinct cell borders
  - Have moderate amount of eosinophilic to amphophilic cytoplasm, and smooth nuclear contours with open and speckled chromatin
  - Areas with marked nuclear pleomorphism, likely representing symplastic/degenerative changes, may be present
  - Based on histologic features, 3 subtypes described
    - Solid glomus tumors, with sheets of glomus cells usually within background of compressed capillary framework
    - Glomangiomas that are highly vascular, with dilated vascular channels and dispersed glomus cells in stroma between vessels
    - Glomangiomyomas showing large branching and gaping vessels with spindled cells in stroma resembling smooth muscle cells
- Sarcomas: Most sarcomas involving kidney originate in retroperitoneum with invasion of kidney
  - Primary sarcomas of kidney extremely rare
    - Leiomyosarcoma most common renal sarcoma, followed by liposarcoma
    - Leiomyosarcoma involving kidney frequently arises from renal vein or its major branches
    - Some apparent leiomyosarcomas in kidney may actually be dedifferentiated liposarcomas with smooth muscle differentiation
    - Other subtypes of sarcoma exceedingly rare and include
      - Rhabdomyosarcoma
      - Osteosarcoma
      - Synovial sarcoma
    - Morphologic features similar to those in soft tissues
- High-grade neuroendocrine carcinoma: Very uncommon primary renal tumor
  - Before accepting it as primary renal neoplasm, metastasis from other more common sites needs to be excluded
  - Many of the tumors associated with nonneuroendocrine carcinomas, particularly renal pelvic urothelial carcinoma
  - Most reported cases with features of small cell carcinoma, morphologically similar to those in lung
    - Very rare large cell neuroendocrine carcinoma also described
- Renal-adrenal fusion and ectopic adrenal tissue
  - Adrenal tissue fused to kidney often lacks capsule, and in areas lacking capsule, adrenal cortical tissue shows infiltrative growth
  - Ectopic adrenal tissue always lacks medulla and is composed of cortical tissue only
  - Clear cells of adrenal cortical tissue almost always show "bubbly" cytoplasm and not transparent clear cytoplasm

DIFFERENTIAL DIAGNOSIS

Angiomyolipoma

- In all leiomyomatous and lipomatous tumors in kidney, smooth muscle or fat-predominant angiomyolipoma needs to be excluded
- Performing immunostaining for melanocytic markers prudent in all such cases

Other Rare Tumors

- Leiomyomatous angiomyolipoma may show focal adipocytes or dysmorphic vessels
- Dysmorphic vessels &/or leiomyomatous foci in lipomatous angiomyolipomas should be carefully searched for, although they are frequently absent
- Epithelioid cells cuffing small vessels may be present and point toward actual diagnosis in many of these lesions
- At least focal positivity for HMB-45, cathepsin-K, and Melan-A (MART-1) will resolve differential diagnostic issues in most cases

Extrarenal or Metastatic Tumors

- Tumors arising in retroperitoneum usually impinge on and compress/deform renal parenchyma without invading it
- Extrarenal tumors invading renal parenchyma usually show bulk of tumor in extrarenal location often with focal renal parenchymal invasion
- Clinical history of prior neuroendocrine carcinoma in lung or other organs is useful in separating primary from metastatic neuroendocrine carcinoma

Clear Cell Renal Cell Carcinoma (RCC)

- Ectopic adrenal tissue and adrenal cortical neoplasms involving kidney may be mistaken for clear cell RCC
- Adrenal cortical cells with clear cell features almost always show bubbly, and not optically clear, cytoplasm
- Adrenal cortical cells are immunoreactive for inhibin, Melan-A (MART-1), and synaptophysin, and usually negative for EMA/MUC1, cytokeratins, and CA9

Sarcomatoid Carcinoma

- Renal cell or urothelial carcinomas with predominant or exclusive sarcomatoid features may be confused with sarcoma
- Any epithelial foci need to be meticulously looked for
- Presence of urothelial carcinoma in situ also needs to be excluded
- Epithelial immunohistochemical markers may be needed
  - However, some sarcomas, particularly leiomyosarcoma, epithelioid angiosarcoma and myofibroblastic sarcoma may be focally positive
  - CA9 often shows diffuse membranous positivity in sarcomatoid areas of clear cell RCC
    - Patchy positivity may be present in sarcomas, particularly in areas of ischemia

IMMUNOHISTOCHEMISTRY

Leiomyoma and Lipomatous Tumors

- Stains for HMB-45, Melan-A (MART-1), and other melanocytic markers are completely negative
- Liposarcomas are usually Mdm2 and CDK4 positive

Glomus Tumor

- Tumors are actin-sm and common muscle actin positive
- Desmin and CD34 are usually negative, although focal positivity for CD34 may be observed
- Unlike juxtaglomerular tumor, CD117 is negative in glomus tumor

Adrenal Cortical Lesions

- These are EMA/MUC1, cytokeratin, and CA9 negative
- Stains for inhibin, Melan-A (MART-1), and synaptophysin are usually positive

Solitary Fibrous Tumor

- Usually positive for CD34, CD99, and Bcl2
- Consistent positivity for STAT6 (a consequence of recurrent *NAB2-STAT6* gene fusions in tumor)

Angiosarcoma

- Immunostains may be required in poorly differentiated or epithelioid variants
  - Tumors are CD31, CD34, ERG, and FLI-1 positive
  - Cytokeratins may show variable positivity, especially in tumors with epithelioid features

DIAGNOSTIC CHECKLIST

Diagnostic Interpretation Pearls

- Tumors with unusual morphologic features mainly require exclusion of metastases from other primary sites
- In case of mesenchymal neoplasm involving kidney, direct extension from extrarenal, retroperitoneal neoplasms needs to be excluded
- Malignant spindle cell neoplasms always need exclusion of sarcomatoid carcinoma
- Primary smooth muscle or lipomatous tumors of kidney are extremely rare
  - In all such cases, exclusion of angiomyolipoma with predominant leiomyomatous or lipomatous differentiation is imperative
    - Immunostains for melanocytic markers in all such tumors is essential

SELECTED REFERENCES

1. Patil PA et al: Renal leiomyoma: a contemporary multi-institution study of an infrequent and frequently misclassified neoplasm. Am J Surg Pathol. 39(3):349-56, 2015
2. Samaratunga H et al: Mesenchymal tumors of adult kidney. Semin Diagn Pathol. 32(2):160-71, 2015
3. Kryvenko ON et al: Haemangiomas in kidneys with end-stage renal disease: a novel clinicopathological association. Histopathology. 65(3):309-18, 2014
4. Mazzucchelli R et al: Neuroendocrine tumours of the urinary system and male genital organs: clinical significance. BJU Int. 103(11):1464-70, 2009
5. Ye H et al: Intrarenal ectopic adrenal tissue and renal-adrenal fusion: a report of nine cases. Mod Pathol. 22(2):175-81, 2009
6. Al-Ahmadie HA et al: Glomus tumor of the kidney: a report of 3 cases involving renal parenchyma and review of the literature. Am J Surg Pathol. 31(4):585-91, 2007
7. Kuroda N et al: Renal leiomyoma: an immunohistochemical, ultrastructural and comparative genomic hybridization study. Histol Histopathol. 22(8):883-8, 2007
8. Lee TY et al: Renal angiosarcoma: a case report and literature review. Can J Urol. 14(1):3471-6, 2007
9. Dotan ZA et al: Adult genitourinary sarcoma: the 25-year Memorial Sloan-Kettering experience. J Urol. 176(5):2033-8; discussion 2038-9, 2006
10. Moazzam M et al: Leiomyosarcoma presenting as a spontaneously ruptured renal tumor-case report. BMC Urol. 2:13, 2002
11. Tamboli P et al: Benign tumors and tumor-like lesions of the adult kidney. Part II: Benign mesenchymal and mixed neoplasms, and tumor-like lesions. Adv Anat Pathol. 7(1):47-66, 2000
12. Berkmen F et al: Adult genitourinary sarcomas: a report of seventeen cases and review of the literature. J Exp Clin Cancer Res. 16(1):45-8, 1997
13. Melamed J et al: Renal myxoma. A report of two cases and review of the literature. Am J Surg Pathol. 18(2):187-94, 1994
14. Dineen MK et al: Pure intrarenal lipoma–report of a case and review of the literature. J Urol. 132(1):104-7, 1984

Other Rare Tumors

Glomus Tumor: Encapsulation

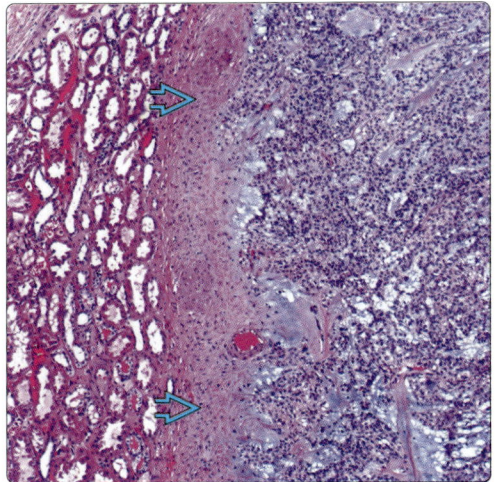

Glomus Tumor: Solid Pattern

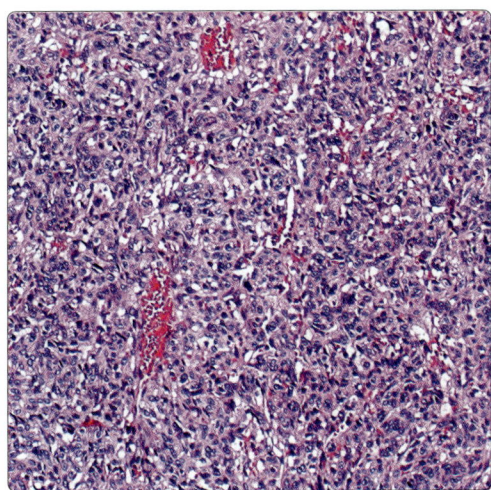

(Left) Renal glomus tumors are well circumscribed and mostly encapsulated ➡. Unlike juxtaglomerular cell tumors, which often contain glomus-like areas, glomus tumors are not associated with hypertension. (Right) Glomus tumors are composed of a mixture of glomus cells, blood vessels, and smooth muscle cells in various proportions. This example shows sheets of glomus cells within a background of compressed capillary framework. Such tumors are designated as solid glomus tumor.

Glomus Tumor: Glomangioma Pattern

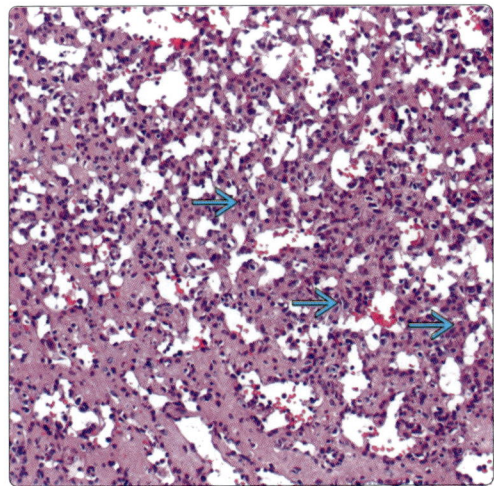

Glomus Tumor: Glomangiomyoma Pattern

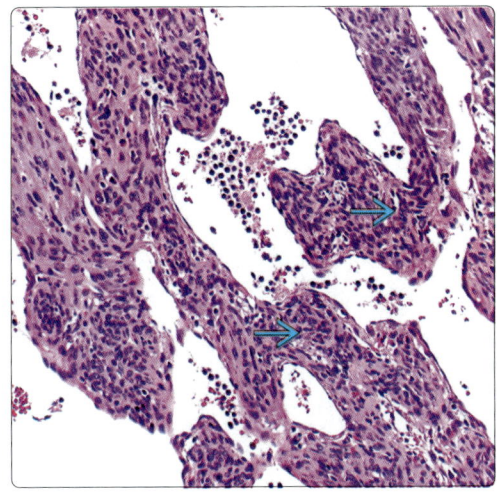

(Left) Some glomus tumors are highly vascular, with dilated vascular channels and round-to-oval glomus cells dispersed in the stroma between the vessels ➡. Such tumors have been designated as glomangiomas. (Right) Some other glomus tumors may show large branching and gaping vessels with spindled cells ➡ in the stroma resembling smooth muscle cells. Such tumors have been called glomangiomyomas. All 3 architectural patterns may sometimes be noted within the same tumor.

Actin-sm

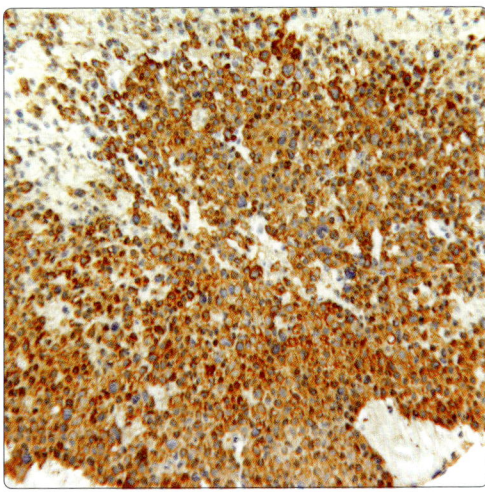

Laminin: Pericellular Staining

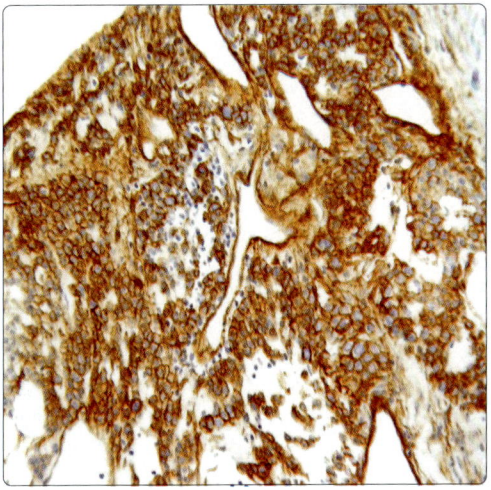

(Left) Glomus tumors show diffuse immunoreactivity for actin-sm and common muscle actin. However, staining for desmin is negative, even in tumors with glomangiomyoma features. (Right) This photomicrograph shows diffuse pericellular staining for laminin in a renal glomus tumor, a consistent and characteristic finding in the tumor. Unlike the peripheral glomus tumors, renal and other visceral glomus tumors are usually negative for CD34. However, focal reactivity has been reported in some renal tumors.

Other Rare Tumors

(Left) Other than angiomyolipoma, benign mesenchymal tumors are very rare in kidney. Leiomyoma, as depicted here, may arise within the renal parenchyma, or from the renal capsule or walls of hilar vessels. **(Right)** Leiomyomas of the kidney are very rare. Most of the previously reported renal leiomyomas, particularly those arising from the capsule, possibly represent leiomyomatous angiomyolipomas.

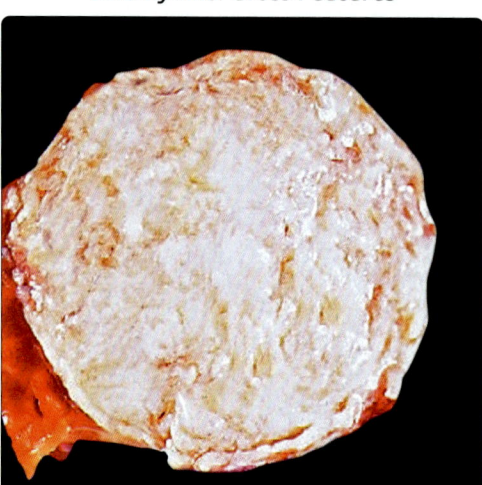
Leiomyoma: Gross Features

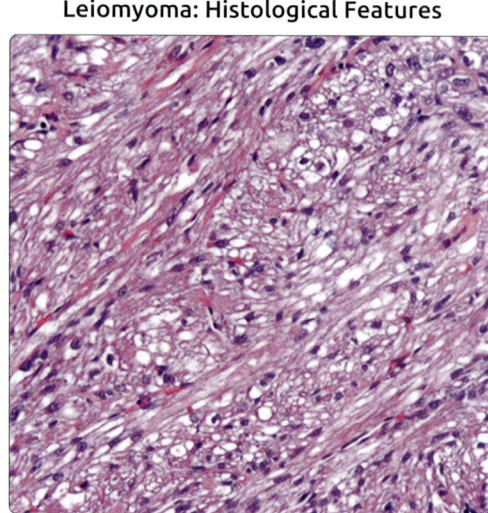
Leiomyoma: Histological Features

(Left) Diffuse positivity for actin-sm in a renal neoplasm does not differentiate between leiomyoma and smooth muscle-rich angiomyolipoma. **(Right)** Almost all renal capsular leiomyomatous tumors, which make the largest proportion of tumors in older literature, are now considered to be leiomyomatous angiomyolipomas. This image depicts HMB-45 immunoreactivity ➔ in a renal smooth muscle tumor, confirming it to be an AML, rather than a leiomyoma.

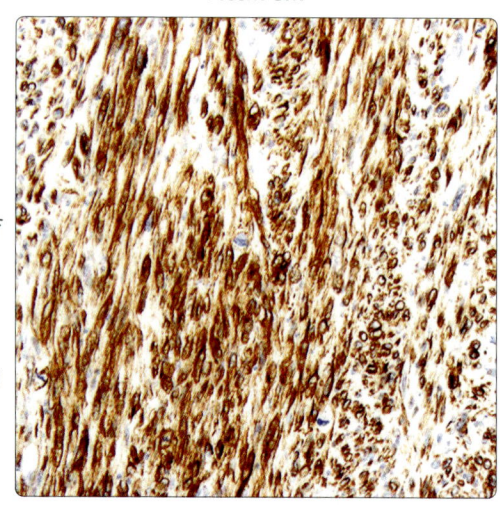
Actin-sm

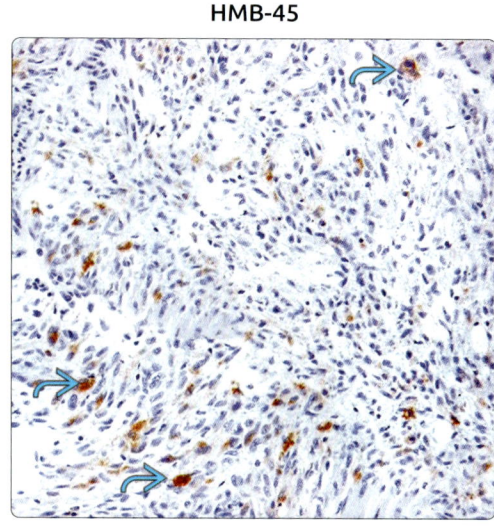
HMB-45

(Left) Leiomyosarcoma (LMS) is the most common sarcoma of the kidney. Most leiomyosarcomas involving the kidney arise in the retroperitoneal soft tissue or renal vein, and due to marked compression ➔ and distortion of the kidney, are clinically thought to arise from it. **(Right)** The morphological features of renal leiomyosarcoma are identical to those of leiomyosarcomas arising at other sites, including mitotic activity ➔, nuclear atypia ➔, necrosis, and large size.

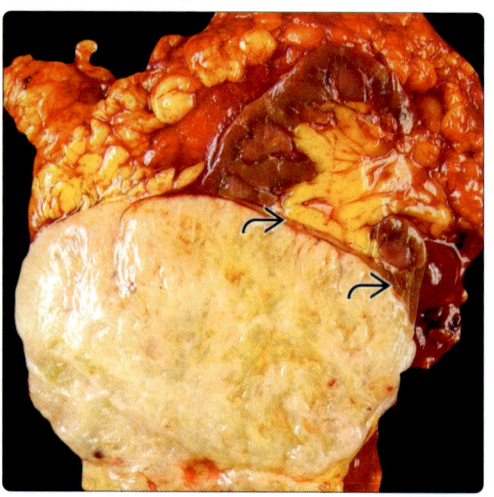
Leiomyosarcoma: Gross

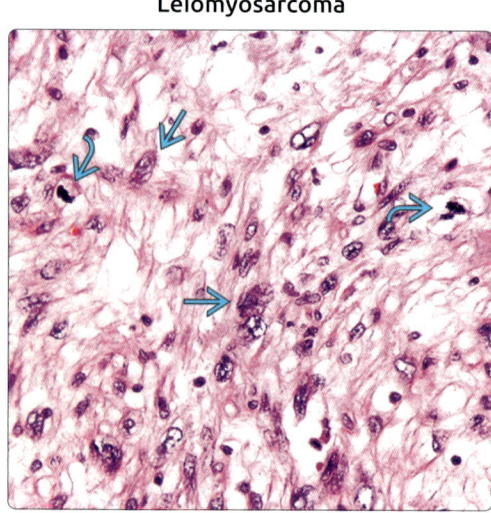
Leiomyosarcoma

Other Rare Tumors

Leiomyosarcoma: Necrosis

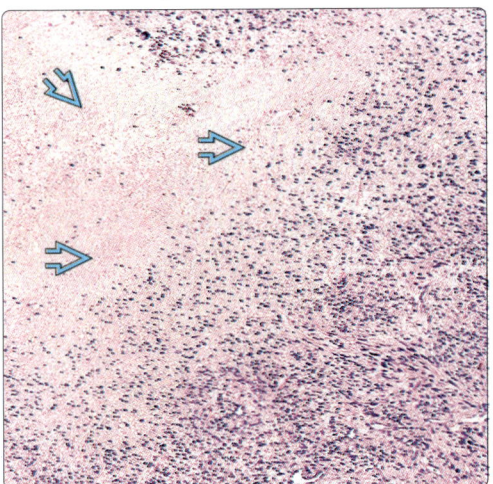

Small Cell Carcinoma

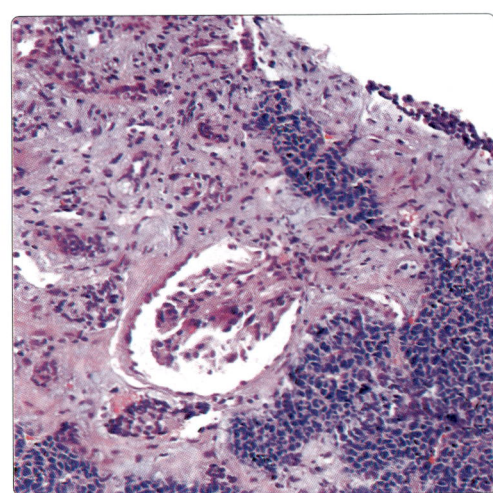

(Left) This image of a leiomyosarcoma shows a large area of tumor necrosis ⇨. Immunohistochemically, the majority of tumors are negative for cytokeratin and epithelial membrane antigen. However, a few tumors may show focal positivity for both. (Right) This tumor represents a small cell carcinoma involving the kidney. Most such tumors are metastases from other sites. However, very occasional primary small cell carcinomas of kidney are described.

Small Cell Carcinoma: Synaptophysin

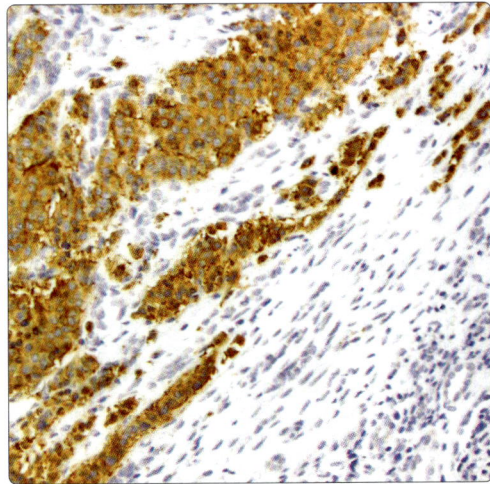

Small Cell Carcinoma: TTF-1

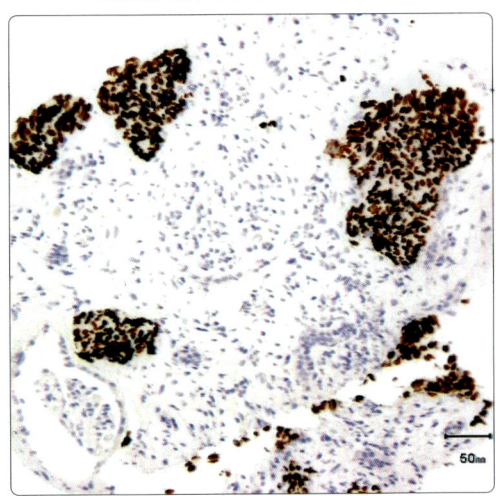

(Left) Most small blue round cell tumors in the kidney need ancillary studies, including immunostaining and molecular analysis, for proper diagnosis. This image depicts a small cell carcinoma (SCC) showing diffuse immunoreactivity for synaptophysin. (Right) TTF-1 immunostain shows diffuse and strong nuclear staining in this small, blue, round cell tumor of the kidney, supporting the diagnosis of a SCC. TTF-1 positivity may be present in SCC at any site and does not necessarily confirm origin from the lung.

Hemangioma

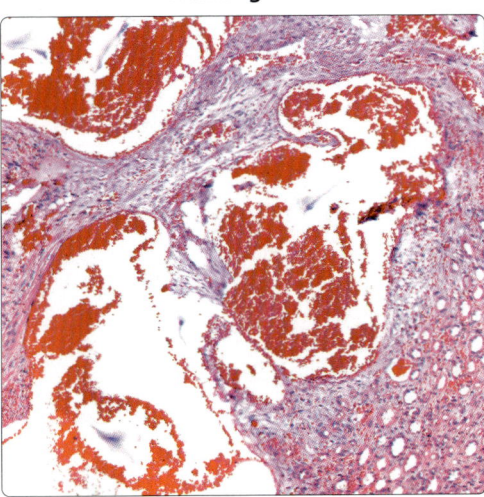

Cavernous Hemangioma

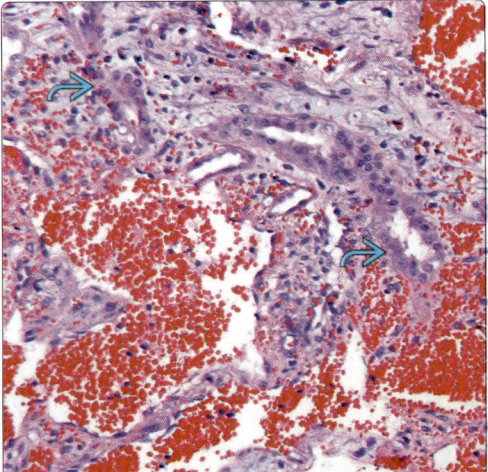

(Left) After angiomyolipoma and leiomyoma, hemangioma and lipoma are the other most frequent benign mesenchymal renal tumors, although both are extremely uncommon. This image shows a primary renal hemangioma. (Right) Renal hemangiomas usually have irregular, infiltrative-appearing borders ⇨. Both capillary and cavernous hemangiomas are described, and most described cases have been of the cavernous type, as shown here.

Other Rare Tumors

(Left) This liposarcoma shows a predominant fleshy cut surface ⇨, suggesting dedifferentiation, and smaller, yellow-tan, well-differentiated component ⇨. Most sarcomas involving the kidney originate in perirenal soft tissue. **(Right)** This high-grade spindle cell neoplasm invading the kidney was a retroperitoneal liposarcoma with dedifferentiation. The diagnosis was revealed by adequate sampling of perirenal soft tissue that showed its well-differentiated liposarcomatous component.

Liposarcoma: Gross Features

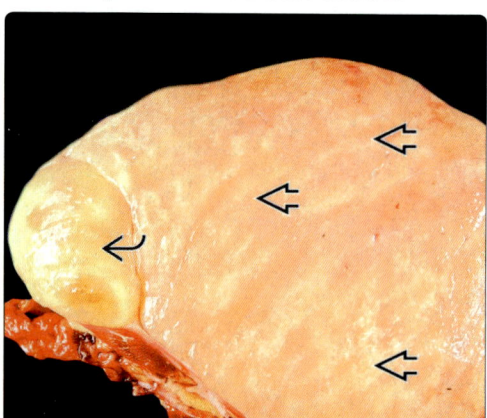

Dedifferentiated Liposarcoma

(Left) This gross image shows an extrarenal angiosarcoma (ANGS) with the typical hemorrhagic cut surface, compressing ⇨ and markedly deforming adjacent renal parenchyma. While primary ANGSs of the kidney do occur, renal involvement by ANGS arising in the retroperitoneum is more common. **(Right)** This light microscopic image from a renal angiosarcoma shows the most characteristic features of the tumor: A vasoformative neoplasm with the vascular spaces lined by high-grade tumor cells.

Angiosarcoma: Gross Features

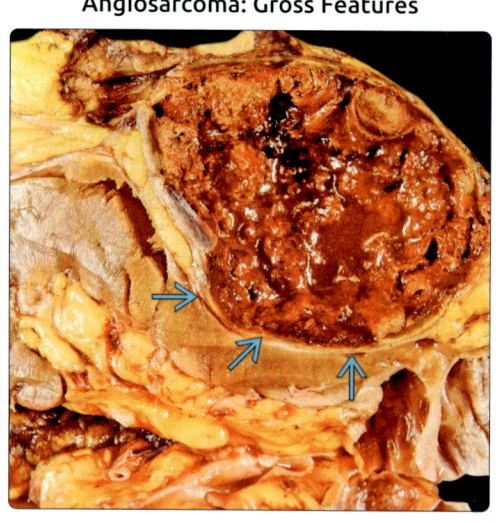

Angiosarcoma: Histological Features

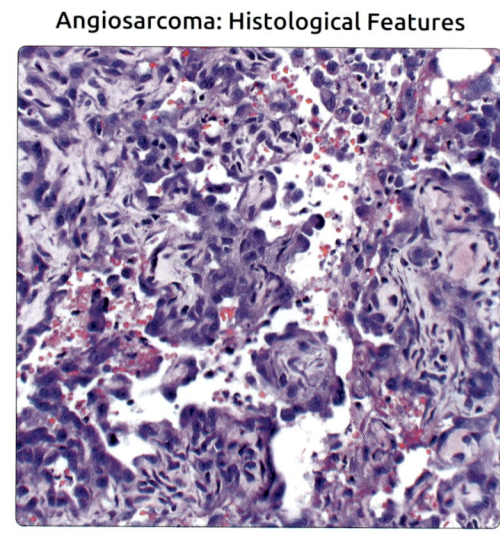

(Left) This primary angiosarcoma of the kidney shows an infiltrative tumor within the renal parenchyma. In this field, the tumor is predominantly composed of nondiagnostic pleomorphic large cells, necessitating immunostaining to confirm the diagnosis. **(Right)** This metastatic angiosarcoma in a renal hilar lymph node shows epithelioid features ⇨. Distinction from a carcinoma will require the support of immunohistochemistry for endothelial markers, such as CD31, CD34, ERG, or FLI1.

Angiosarcoma: Histological Features

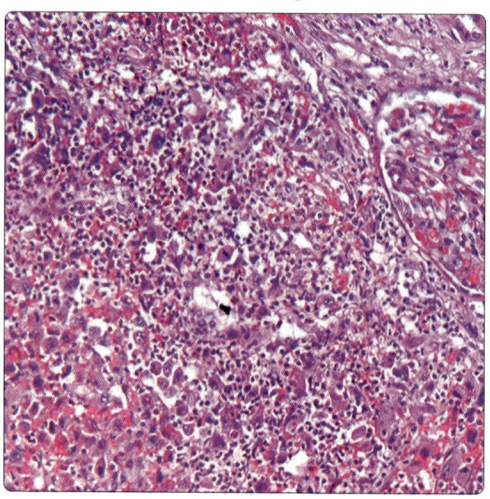

Angiosarcoma: Epithelioid Features

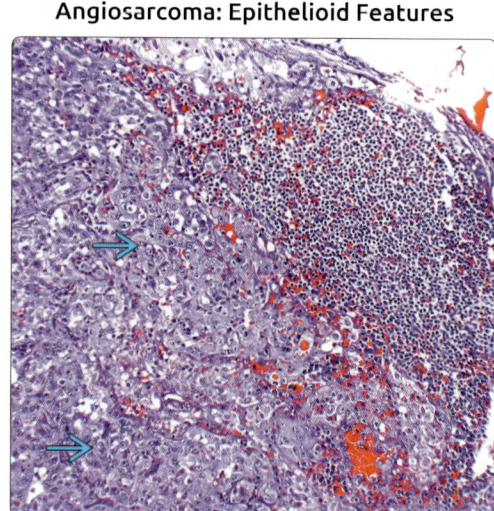

Other Rare Tumors

Angiosarcoma: CD31

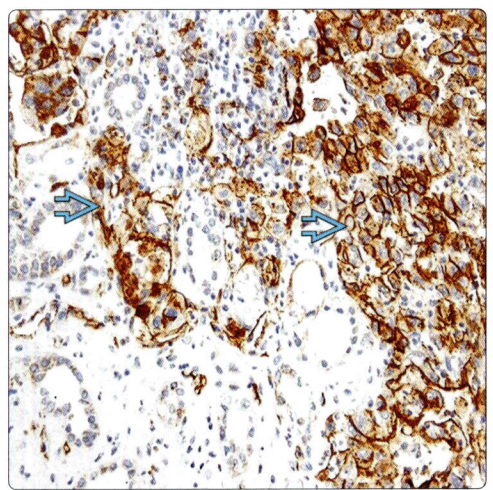

Epithelioid Angiosarcoma: CK-PAN

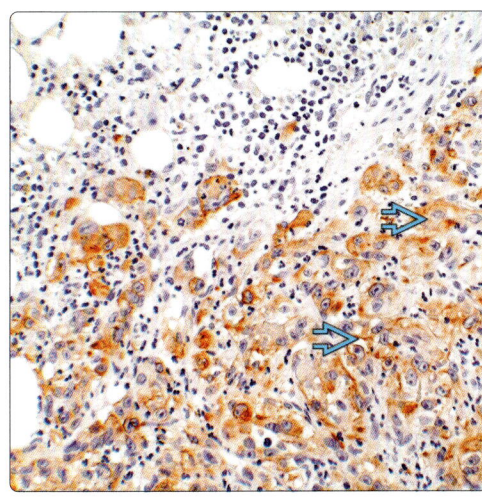

(Left) Immunostaining for CD31 is confirmatory ➡ in renal angiosarcoma, similar to that in other sites. Immunostains are particularly useful in poorly differentiated tumors. Stains for CD34, ERG, and FLI-1 may also help in the diagnosis. *(Right)* Rare angiosarcomas, particularly those with epithelioid features, may show immunoreactivity for cytokeratins like CK-PAN(AE1/AE3) ➡. If immunostaining for endothelial markers is not performed, this may lead to misdiagnosis as a carcinoma.

Malignant Spindle Cell Tumor: Sarcomatoid Carcinoma

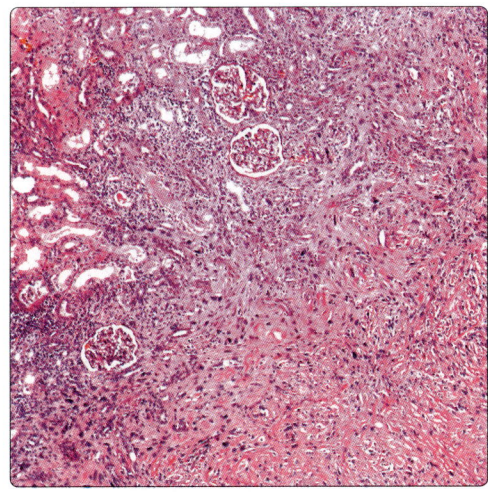

Renal-Adrenal Fusion: Gross Features

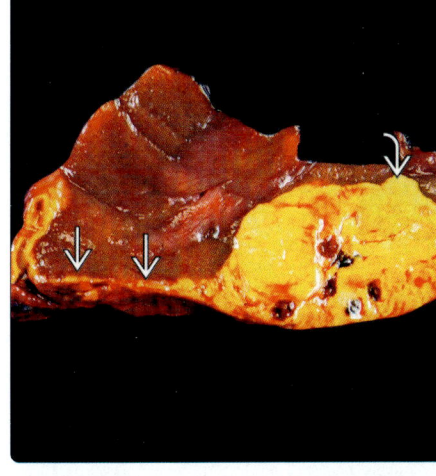

(Left) Adequate sampling and ancillary studies (e.g., immunostaining) are essential for proper classification of malignant spindle cell tumors. Most of these are sarcomatoid carcinomas, although rare cases may represent true sarcoma. *(Right)* Renal-adrenal fusion and adrenal cortical neoplasms arising therefrom are not very rare. Adrenal tissue fused to kidney often lacks a capsule ➡, and cortical nodules arising from fused adrenal may have irregular edges ➡.

Ectopic Intrarenal Adrenal Tissue

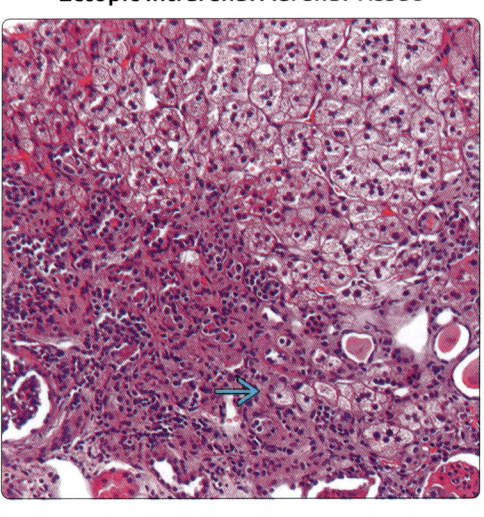

Renal-Adrenal Fusion: Partial Encapsulation

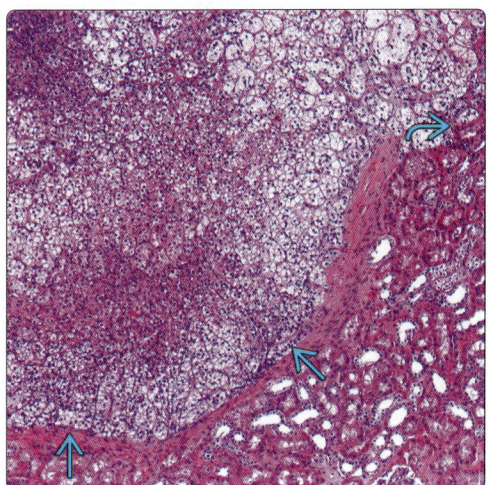

(Left) Ectopic intrarenal adrenal tissues usually show gross circumscription, but on microscopy often depict an infiltrative ➡ growth pattern. Such nodules are mostly noted in the superior pole but may be seen elsewhere in kidney. Ectopic adrenal tissue present at any site does not contain any medullary cells. *(Right)* This instance of renal-adrenal fusion shows partial encapsulation ➡ delimiting renal from adrenal tissue. In the area lacking the capsule, adrenal cortical tissue shows an infiltrative pattern of growth ➡.

Metastatic Tumors

KEY FACTS

TERMINOLOGY
- Involvement of kidney by primary tumors of other organs
- Direct extension from adjacent organs does not qualify as metastasis

CLINICAL ISSUES
- Reported to constitute up to ~ 3% of all malignant renal tumors in surgical specimens
- Kidney and ureter most common sites with metastatic tumors in urinary and male genital tract, followed closely by bladder
- Often occurs as part of widespread tumor dissemination
- In some cases, tumor may be solitary and mimic primary renal tumor
- Most common reported sources of metastasis to kidney include lung (most common), colon-rectum, stomach, pancreas, uterus, and skin (melanoma)

MICROSCOPIC
- Common histologic features in metastatic carcinoma are
  - Adenocarcinoma (30%), squamous cell carcinoma (28%), small cell carcinoma (8%), and malignant melanoma (6%)
- Often show multinodular growth pattern, even when apparently well circumscribed on gross evaluation
- Tumor emboli in vessels frequently present

TOP DIFFERENTIAL DIAGNOSES
- Collecting duct carcinoma
- Urothelial carcinoma

DIAGNOSTIC CHECKLIST
- Unusual morphologic features in renal tumor should alert one to possibility of metastatic carcinoma
- Clinical history of primary carcinoma elsewhere is often crucial in establishing diagnosis
- Immunohistochemical profile may also be useful in differential diagnosis

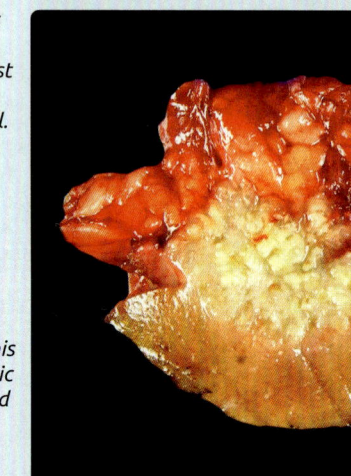

Metastatic Colonic Adenocarcinoma: Gross

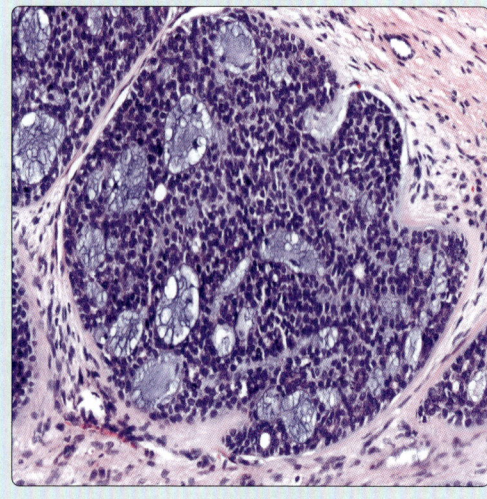

Metastatic Salivary Gland Adenoid Cystic Carcinoma

(Left) This gross image shows a colonic adenocarcinoma metastatic to the kidney. Most metastatic tumors are multifocal and often bilateral. Solitary metastasis makes such a presumption clinically difficult. (Right) While metastases to the kidney are more common from lung, breast and female genital tract, tumors from head and neck are also known to metastasize to the kidney. This image shows an adenoid cystic carcinoma from salivary gland metastatic to the kidney.

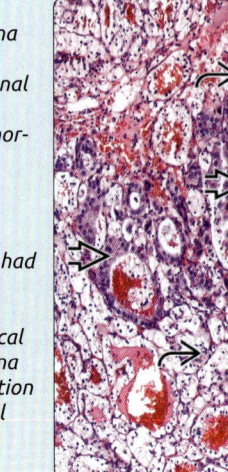

Tumor-to-Tumor Metastasis

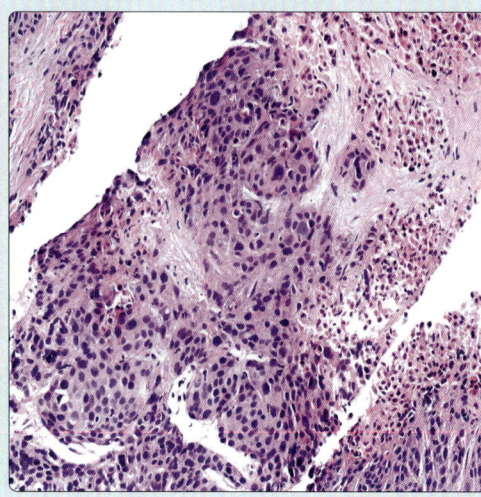

Metastatic Squamous Cell Carcinoma

(Left) This images shows metastatic breast carcinoma ➡ to a clear cell renal cell carcinoma ➡. Clear cell renal cell carcinoma is the most common recipient of a tumor-to-tumor metastasis in the kidney. (Right) Metastatic squamous cell carcinoma (SCC) is seen on this renal needle biopsy. The patient had a prior history of a cervical squamous cell carcinoma. Without the available clinical history, urothelial carcinoma with squamous differentiation would be in the differential diagnosis.

Metastatic Tumors

TERMINOLOGY

Definitions

- Involvement of kidney by primary tumors of other organs
  - Word metastasis is derived from Greek, meaning next placement or displacement
  - Almost always result of vascular or lymphatic spread from primary tumor
    - Direct extension from adjacent organs does not qualify as metastasis
    - Metastasis from contralateral kidney vs. bilateral primary tumors is extremely difficult to prove even when morphologically similar
    - Some hematopoietic malignancies involving kidney may also be considered metastatic but are not discussed here

CLINICAL ISSUES

Epidemiology

- Incidence
  - Reported to constitute up to ~ 3% of all malignant renal tumors in surgical specimens
  - Kidney and ureter most common sites with metastatic tumors in urinary and male genital tract, followed closely by bladder
  - Metastases to kidney are reported to be higher in autopsy series (range: 9-20% in patients dying of tumors)
- Sex
  - Reported male:female ratio: 2.2:1 in older series
    - Higher incidence in males believed to be due to difference in lung cancer incidences over that time period

Presentation

- Often occurs as part of widespread tumor dissemination
  - Renal involvement is frequently bilateral and multinodular in such situations
- In some cases, tumor may be solitary and mimic primary renal tumor
  - Metastatic tumors to kidney presenting in surgical specimens these days are more likely to be mimickers of primary tumor
  - History of extrarenal primary in remote past may be obtained in most such cases on careful scrutiny
- Very rarely, metastasis in kidney may be initial manifestation of primary tumor elsewhere
- Most common reported sources of metastasis to kidney include
  - Lung (most common), colon-rectum, stomach, pancreas, uterus, and skin (malignant melanoma)
  - Other, much rarer sources include breast, salivary gland, and thyroid, among others

MACROSCOPIC

General Features

- Metastatic carcinomas are often multifocal and bilateral, particularly at autopsy; concurrent metastatic involvement of other organ systems is very frequent in such scenario
- Occasionally, tumor may be unicentric, with no other clinically detectable metastatic tumors
  - In such cases, nephrectomy is usually performed with clinical impression of primary renal tumor

MICROSCOPIC

Histologic Features

- Most common primary sites of metastasis include lung, breast, head and neck, female genital tract, and colon-rectum
- Histologic features commonly that of
  - Adenocarcinoma, squamous cell carcinoma, small cell carcinoma, and malignant melanoma
  - Other rare histologic patterns, depending on primary tumor, are also seen and some of these include
    - Salivary gland-type, including adenoid cystic, myoepithelial, and epithelial-myoepithelial carcinoma
    - Thyroid type, including follicular, papillary, undifferentiated, anaplastic, and medullary carcinoma
    - Carcinoid tumor
    - Lobular or signet ring cell type, from breast or gastrointestinal tract
- Often show multinodular growth pattern, even when apparently well circumscribed on gross evaluation
- Tumor emboli in vessels frequently present
- Sometimes tumors centered on pelvicalyceal system and ureter
  - Rarely, tumor cells may replace lining urothelium, giving impression of in situ carcinoma of urothelium
- Occasionally, particularly when metastasis is clinically suspected, needle core biopsies or fine-needle aspirations may be performed
  - Morphologic features unusual for renal cell tumor, even on biopsies, should always raise suspicion of metastasis and be investigated for it
- Tumor to tumor metastasis may occur in preexisting renal cell carcinoma (RCC) or oncocytoma

DIFFERENTIAL DIAGNOSIS

Collecting Duct Carcinoma

- Stromal desmoplasia, multinodular growth pattern, usual glandular phenotype common to both metastases and collecting duct carcinoma
- Clinical history of tumor elsewhere and immunoprofile typical of primary tumor site often crucial in distinction

Urothelial Carcinoma

- Variety of morphologic phenotypes, and stromal desmoplasia may be similar to that in metastatic carcinoma
- Presence of noninvasive papillary or in situ components supports urothelial carcinoma
- Urothelial carcinomas usually CK7, CK20, GATA3, HMCK(34βE12), and p63(+); this immunophenotype is uncommon in other tumors

SELECTED REFERENCES

1. Wu AJ et al: Metastases to the kidney: a clinicopathological study of 43 cases with an emphasis on deceptive features. Histopathology. Histopathology. 66(4):587-97,2015
2. Morichetti D et al: Secondary neoplasms of the urinary system and male genital organs. BJU Int. 104(6):770-6, 2009
3. Chin-Aleong J et al: Secondary neoplasms of the kidney: a clinico-pathological review of 443 cases. J Pathol. 190[Suppl]:42A, 2000

Metastatic Tumors

Metastatic Adenocarcinoma

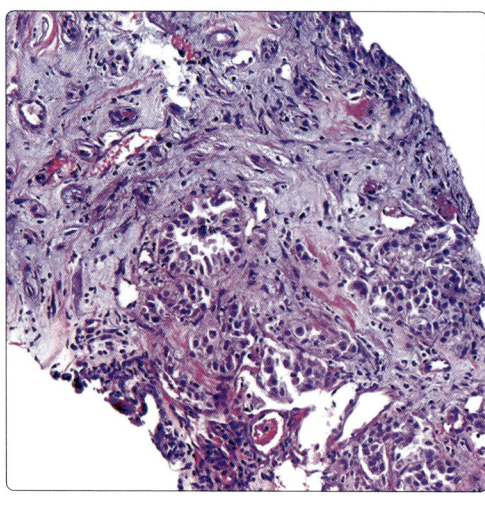

Immunohistochemistry: TTF-1

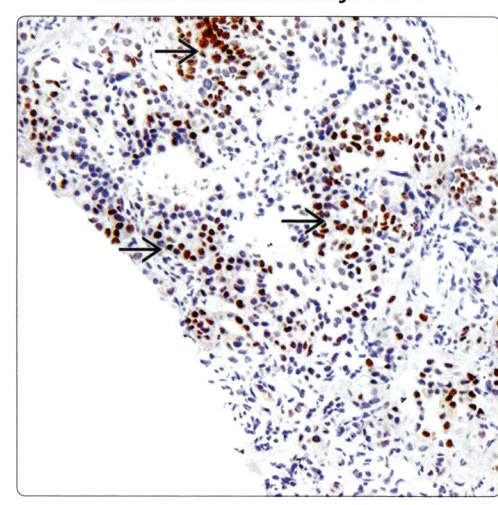

(Left) Core biopsy shows an adenocarcinoma that raises the differential of a collecting duct carcinoma. There was a history of lung adenocarcinoma, diagnosed 2 years earlier, that initiated comparison with prior material and rendering of the appropriate diagnosis of metastatic lung carcinoma. (Right) Immunohistochemical stain for TTF-1 showed diffuse nuclear positivity ⇨ in this tumor. In addition to the comparison with the patient's lung primary, IHC confirmed a metastasis from the lung.

Metastatic Squamous Cell Carcinoma From Lung

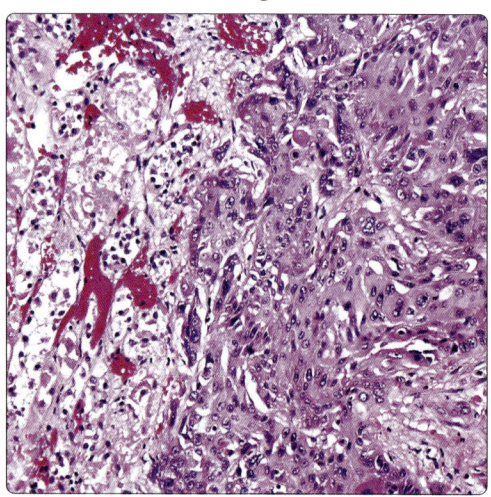

Metastatic Colorectal Adenocarcinoma

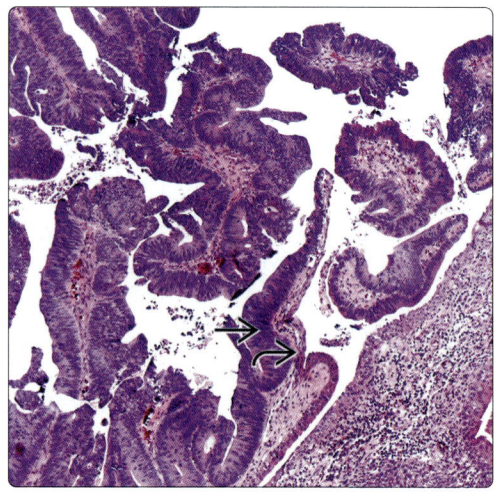

(Left) This image depicts a metastatic SCC from the lung. While a primary urothelial SCC may have similar morphologic features, this patient had bilateral cortical-based tumors with no in situ or papillary urothelial components. (Right) This metastatic colorectal adenocarcinoma, centered in the renal pelvis, completely replaces ⇨ the surface urothelial lining ⇨ in some areas. Such events are rare but raise the possibility of in situ component of a primary tumor.

Metastatic Parotid Tumor: Gross

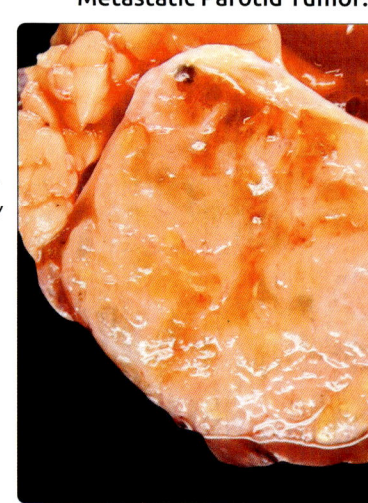

Metastatic Adenoid Cystic Carcinoma

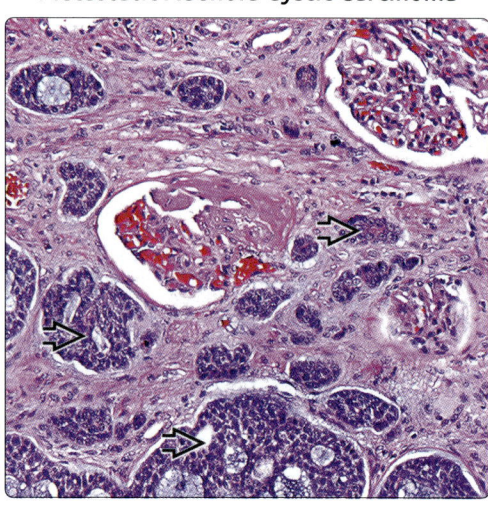

(Left) This solitary tumor in the kidney was resected with the clinical diagnosis of a primary renal tumor. History of a parotid tumor, 15 years earlier, was present. Considering the solitary tumor and very remote history, a new renal primary was clinically favored. (Right) Microscopic evaluation revealed a metastatic adenoid cystic carcinoma ⇨. Review of the slides obtained from the prior salivary gland resection showed a primary salivary gland adenoid cystic carcinoma.

Metastatic Tumors

CK-PAN
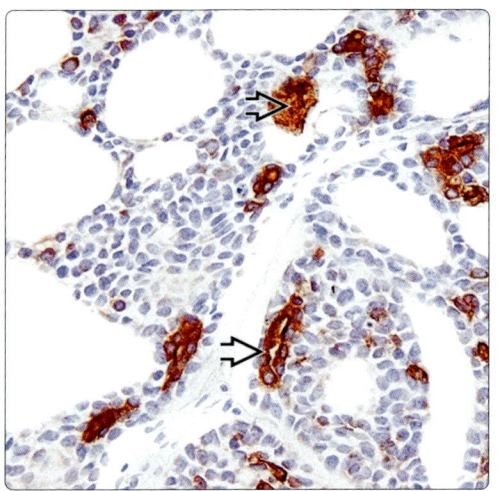

p63 Staining Pattern
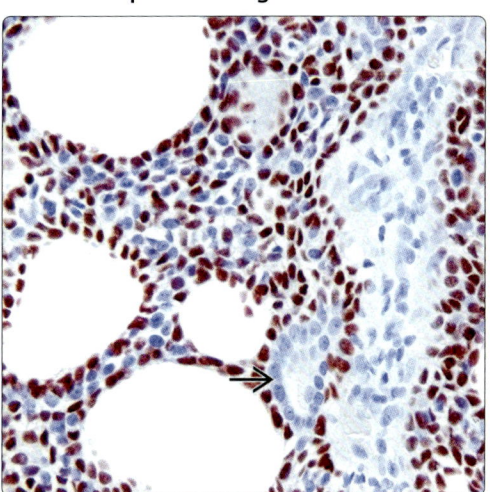

(Left) Immunostain for CK-PAN (AE1/AE3) reveals focal positivity only in the epithelial cells ⇒, while most of the myoepithelial cells of this adenoid cystic carcinoma are negative. (Right) p63 highlights the myoepithelial cells in the tumor, without staining the epithelial component ⇒. Unusual morphology in a biopsy or resection specimen requires obtaining clinical history. Metastatic tumors may mimic the morphology of primary renal tumors, leading to misdiagnoses in the absence of available clinical history.

High-Grade, Poorly Differentiated Carcinoma
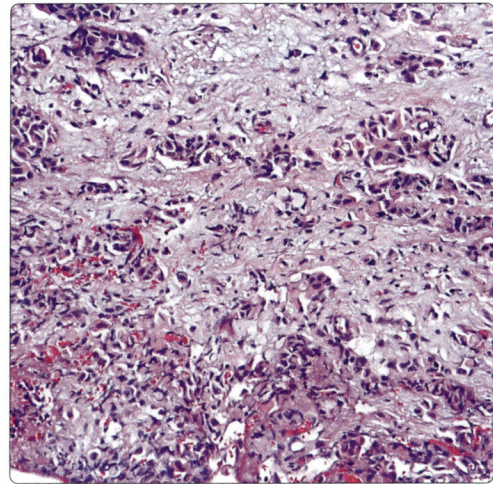

ER Immunohistochemistry
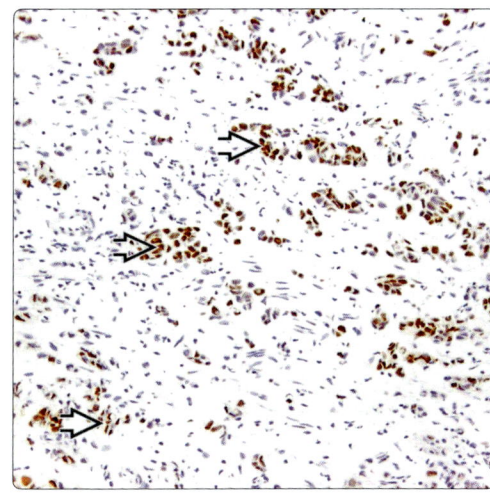

(Left) Needle core biopsy of a renal mass shows a high-grade carcinoma with differential diagnostic possibilities of a urothelial, collecting duct, or metastatic carcinoma. The known history of invasive ductal carcinoma with focal micropapillary features in this case helped in taking the proper approach, including comparison with the prior material from the breast. (Right) Like the breast primary, this renal tumor also was ER(+) ⇒, PR(-), and HER2(-).

Metastatic Adenocarcinoma
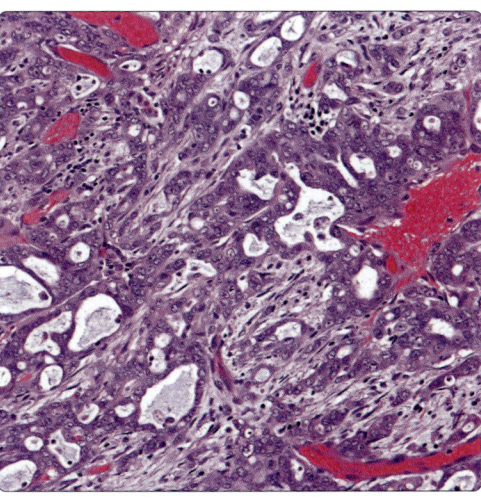

Invasive Urothelial Carcinoma
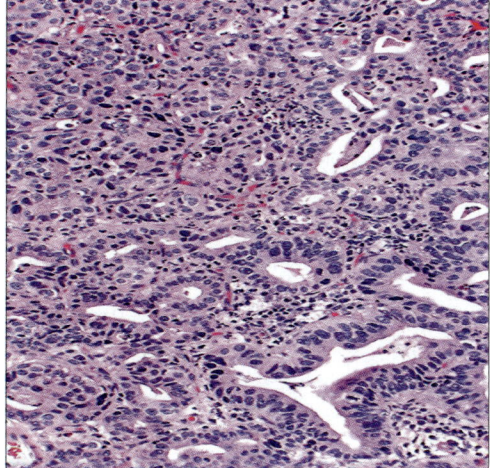

(Left) Clinical history and immunostains for HMCK (34βE12), ULEX-1, pax-2, and pax-8 may help in the distinction of metastatic adenocarcinoma and collecting duct carcinoma, but the staining patterns, especially for the first 2 antibodies, are not consistent or specific. (Right) Invasive urothelial carcinoma may also mimic metastatic carcinoma. Careful evaluation for urothelial in situ change is a must. Stains for CK7, CK20, GATA3, HMCK, and p63 may also help in most, but not all, cases.

Immunohistochemistry, Kidney

Renal Tumors With Clear-/Light-Staining Cytoplasm

Antibody	Clear Cell RCC	Chromophobe RCC, Classical	MITF/TFE Family Translocation-Associated Carcinoma	Clear Cell Papillary RCC	Epithelioid Angiomyolipoma	TCEB1-Mutated RCC
CAIX	(+) (diffuse membranous, box-like pattern)	(-) [(+) perinecrotic areas]	(-) [(+) in some cases]	(+) (diffuse membranous, cup-shaped pattern)	(-)	(+) (diffuse membranous, box-like pattern)
CK7	(-) [(+) in tumors with cystic areas]	(+) (diffuse, occasionally patchy)	(-)	(+) (diffuse, almost 100% tumor cells)	(-)	(+) (patchy)
CD10	(+) (membranous)	(-)/[rarely (+)]	(+) [but often (-) in TFEB carcinoma]	(-) (or focal, at the most)	(-)	(+) (usually focal)
Vimentin	(+)	(-)	(-/+)	(+)	(-)	ND
Ksp-cadherin	(-)	(+)	(-) (occasionally in TFEB carcinoma)	ND	(-)	ND
CD117	(-)	(+) (diffuse, often peripheral membranous accentuation)	(-)	(-)	(-)	(-)
AMACR	(-) [rarely focal (+)]	(-)	(+) (usually)	(-)	(-)	Often (+)
CK-PAN (AE1/AE3)	(+)	(+)	(-) [rarely focal (+)]	(+)	(-)	(+)
TFE3/TFEB	(-)	(-)	(+)	(-)	(-)	(-)
Melan-A (MART-1)	(-)	(-)	(+) in TFEB carcinoma, rarely (+) in TFE3	(-)	(+)	ND
HMB-45	(-)	(-)	(+) in TFEB carcinoma, rarely (+) in TFE3	(-)	(+)	ND
MiTF	(-)	(-)	(+) in TFEB carcinoma, rarely (+) in TFE3	(-)	(+)	ND
Actin-sm	(-)	(-)	(-)	(-)	(+/-)	(+) (in fibromuscular stroma)
cathepsin-K	(-)	(-)	(+) in TFEB carcinoma, + in 50% TFE3 carcinoma	(-)	(+)	ND
HMWCK (34BE12)	(-)	(-)	(-)	(+)	(-)	(-)

Renal Tumors With Papillary or Tubulopapillary Architecture

Antibody	Papillary RCC	Collecting Duct Carcinoma	Metanephric Adenoma	Mucinous Tubular and Spindle Cell Carcinoma	Clear Cell Papillary RCC	Hereditary Leiomyomatosis Renal Cell Carcinoma-Associated RCC
CK7	(+)	(+)	(-) [may be (+) in branching tubules or papillary structures]	(+)	(+) (almost 100% cells)	(-) [rarely focal (+)]
CD10	(+) (often luminal pattern)	(-)	(-)	(-/+) (focal)	(-) [rarely (+), focal]	(+)
AMACR	(+)	(-)	(-/+)	(+)	(-)	(+)
WT1	(-)	(-)	(+)	(-)	(-)	(-)
HMCK (34βE12)	(-)	(+/-)	(-)	(-/+)	(+)	(-)
INI1	(+)	(+) (lost in renal medullary carcinoma)	(+)	(+)	(+)	(+)

Immunohistochemistry, Kidney

Renal Tumors With Papillary or Tubulopapillary Architecture (Continued)

Antibody	Papillary RCC	Collecting Duct Carcinoma	Metanephric Adenoma	Mucinous Tubular and Spindle Cell Carcinoma	Clear Cell Papillary RCC	Hereditary Leiomyomatosis Renal Cell Carcinoma-Associated RCC
Ulex-1	(-)	(+)	(-)	(-)	ND	ND
CAIX	(-) [(+) perinecrotic areas and papillary tips]	(-/+) (perinecrotic area)	ND	ND	(+) (diffuse membranous, cup-shaped pattern)	(-)
Fumarate hydratase	(+)	(+)	(+)	(+)	(+)	Completely lost in tumor cells
BRAF (V600E)	(-) [rarely focal (+)]	(-)	(+)	(-)	ND	ND

Renal Tumors With Granular/Eosinophilic Cytoplasm

Antibody	Clear Cell RCC, Eosinophilic	Chromophobe RCC, Eosinophilic	Oncocytoma	MiTF/TFE Family Translocation-Associated Carcinoma	Epithelioid Angiomyolipoma	SDHB-Deficient RCC
Vimentin	(+/-)	(-) [rarely (+)]	(-)	(-/+)	(+)	(+/-)
CD117	(-)	(+)	(+)	(-)	(-)	(-) (highlights intratumoral mast cells)
pax-2/pax-8	(+)	(-) [rarely (+)]	(+)	V	(-)	(+)
CK7	(-)	(+/-)	(-)	(-)	(-)	(-)
CD10	(+)	(-/+)	(+)	(+) in TFE3 carcinoma, often (-) in TFEB	(-)	(-)
TFE3/TFEB	(-)	(-)	(-)	(+)	(-)	(-)
HMB-45/Melan-A (MART-1)/MITF	(-)	(-)	(-)	(+) in TFEB carcinoma, rarely (+) in TFE3	(+)	(-)
cathepsin-K	(-)	(-)	(-)	(+) in TFEB carcinoma, (+) in 50% TFE3 carcinoma	(+)	(-)
Actin-sm	(-)	(-)	(-)	(-)	(+/-)	(-)
HMCK (34βE12)	(-)	(-) [rarely focal (+)]	(-)	(-) [occasionally focal (+)]	(-)	(-)
CAIX	(+)	(-)	(-)	(-) [(+) in some cases]	(-)	(-)
S100A	(+/-)	(-) [rarely (+)]	(+)	(-)	(-)	(-)
SDHB	(+)	(+)	(+)	(+)	(+)	Completely lost in tumor cells

Tumors With Spindle Cell Morphology

Antibody	Spindle Cells in Sarcomatoid RCC	Mucinous Tubular and Spindle Cell Carcinoma	Sarcoma	Angiomyolipoma
CK-PAN (AE1/AE3)	(+) (may be focal/rare cells)	(+) (usually diffuse)	(-) [may be focal (+) in leiomyosarcoma]	(-)
Cam5.2	(+) (may be focal/rare cells)	(+)	(-) [may be focal (+) in leiomyosarcoma]	(-)
EMA/MUC1	(+) (may be focal/rare cells)	(+)	(-) [may be focal (+) in leiomyosarcoma]	(-)
Desmin	(-) [may occasionally be (+)]	(-)	(+) in myosarcomas, occasionally in others	(+)

Immunohistochemistry, Kidney

Tumors With Spindle Cell Morphology (Continued)

Antibody	Spindle Cells in Sarcomatoid RCC	Mucinous Tubular and Spindle Cell Carcinoma	Sarcoma	Angiomyolipoma
Actin-sm	(-) [may occasionally be (+)]	(-)	(+) in myosarcomas, occasionally in others	(+)
CD99	(-)	(-)	(+) in synovial sarcoma	V
S100	(-)	(-)	V	V
HMB-45/Melan-A (MART-1)/MITF	(-)	(-)	(-)	(+)
cathepsin-K	(-)	(-)	V	(+)
HMCK (34βE12)	(-)/[rarely focal (+)]	(-/+)	(-)	(-)
CK7	(-)/[rarely focal (+)]	(+)	(-)	(-)
CAIX	(+/-) [often (+) in sarcomatoid clear cell RCC]	(-)	(-) [(+) in perinecrotic areas]	(-)
cathepsin-K	(-)	(-)	V	(+)

Poorly Differentiated Carcinomas

Antibody	RCC, Unclassified	Collecting Duct Carcinoma	Urothelial Carcinoma
CK7	(-/+)	(+)	(+)
CK20	(-)	(-) [rarely focal (+)]	(+/-)
p63	(-)	(-/+)	(+)
HMCK (34βE12)	(-/+)	(+/-)	(+)
Thrombomodulin	(-)	(-)	(+/-)
uroplakin-3/uroplakin-2	(-)	(-)	(+/-)
CD10	(+/-)	(-)	(-/+)
CK5/6	(-)	(-)	(+/-)
INI1	(+)	(+) (lost in renal medullary carcinoma)	(+)
Ulex-1	(-)	(+)	(-/+)
Fumarate hydratase	(+) (retained)	(+) (retained)	(+) (retained)

Small Blue Round Cell Tumors of Kidney

Antibody	Wilms Tumor	Ewing Sarcoma/PNET	Small Cell Carcinoma	Lymphoma	Desmoplastic Small Round Cell Tumor	Synovial Sarcoma, Poorly Differentiated
WT1	(+)	(-)	(-)	(-)	(+)	(-)
S100	(-)	(-)	(-)	(-)	V	(-/+)
FLI-1	(-)	(+)	(-)	(-)	(-)	(-)
CD99	(+/-)	(+)	(-)	(+/-)	(-/+)	(-/+)
HMCK (34βE12)	(-)	(-/+)	(+) (often dot-like)	(-)	(-)	(-/+)
EMA/MUC1	(-/+)	(-)	(-/+)	(-)	(-)	(-/+)
CD45 (LCA)	(-)	(-)	(-)	(+)	(-)	(-)
Chromogranin	(-)	(-)	(+)	(-)	(-)	(-)
Desmin	(-)	(-)	(-)	(-)	(+)	(-)
pax-2/pax-8	(+)	ND	ND	ND	ND	ND
CK-PAN (AE1/AE3)	(+) (in tubules)	(+/-) (focal)	(+) (often dot-like)	(-)	(+)	(-/+)

V = variable; ND = no data.

Immunohistochemistry, Kidney

Carbonic Anhydrase IX in Clear Cell RCC

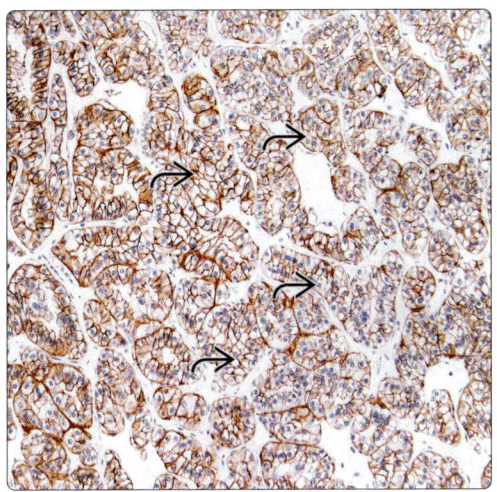

Carbonic Anhydrase IX in Clear Cell Papillary RCC

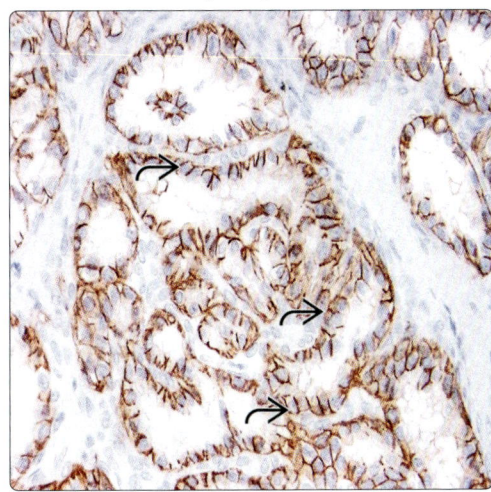

(Left) Carbonic anhydrase IX is one of the most useful immunohistochemical markers of clear cell RCC. It shows diffuse, membranous positivity in > 90% of the tumors, highlighting all the cell membranes (box-like pattern) ⮕. (Right) While CA9 shows diffuse, membranous immunoreactivity in clear cell papillary renal cell carcinoma as well, it generally does not stain the luminal aspects of the cells, resulting in a characteristic cup-shaped staining pattern ⮕. Tumors not showing this pattern likely do not represent CC-PRCC.

Carbonic Anhydrase IX in *TCEB1*-Mutated RCC

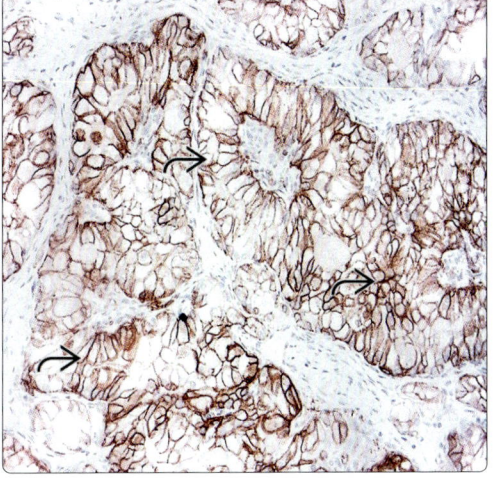

Carbonic Anhydrase IX in Clear Cell RCC

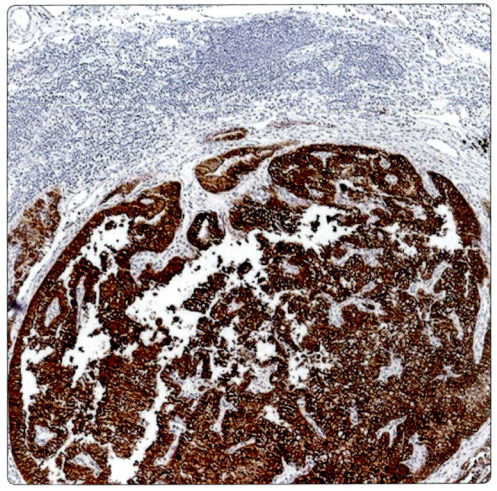

(Left) Many tumors with CCP-like areas show box-like CA9 staining pattern unlike CCP-RCC. This example of TCEB1-mutated RCC is diffusely positive for CA9, but the box-like ⮕ staining pattern goes against the diagnosis of CCP-RCC. (Right) Diffuse, membranous box-like positivity for CA9 may be helpful in determining the origin of tumors at metastatic sites, as in this lymph node metastasis. This staining pattern is retained at most of the metastatic sites, and > 2/3 of CC-RCC with sarcomatoid differentiation.

CK7 in Papillary RCC

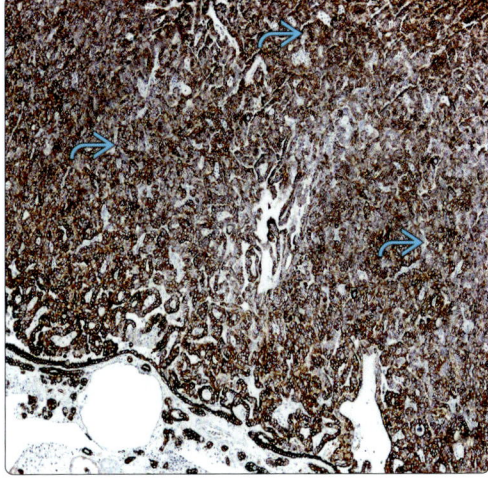

CK7 in Clear Cell Papillary RCC

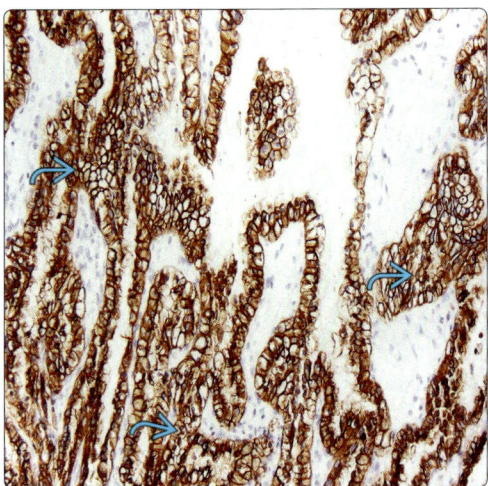

(Left) CK7 is a useful stain in the differentiation of renal cell tumors. Diffuse positivity is very common in type 1 papillary RCC ⮕. However, positivity may be absent or very focal in type 2 tumors. (Right) CCP-RCC is one of the few renal tumors consistently showing CK7 positivity in almost 100% tumor cells, as seen here ⮕. Lack of such positivity in tumors resembling CCP-RCC is not compatible with the diagnosis of CCP-RCC. Diffuse CK7 staining may also be seen in multilocular cystic renal neoplasms of low malignant potential.

Immunohistochemistry, Kidney

(Left) CK7 usually shows patchy to diffuse membrane-predominant immunoreactivity in classical chromophobe RCC. Reactivity is generally more focal in the eosinophilic variants of chromophobe RCC. (Right) AMACR immunostain shows diffuse, granular cytoplasmic reactivity ➡ in papillary RCCs, but similar diffuse staining may also be seen in many other renal tumors with or ± papillary architecture. In the absence of reactivity for CK7 and AMACR, alternative diagnostic possibilities should be considered.

CK7 in Chromophobe RCC
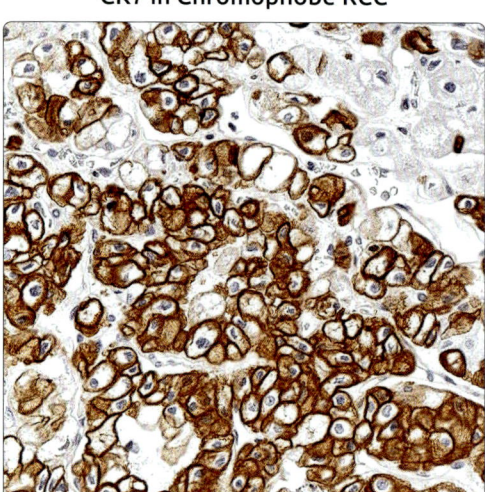

AMACR in Papillary RCC
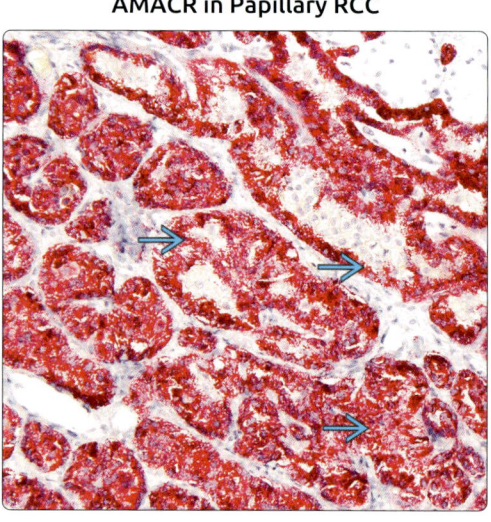

(Left) Diffuse AMACR positivity is also typical of ACD-associated RCC. In spite of some tumors with predominant papillary architecture, overall morphological features and usual CK7 negativity should point to the diagnosis of other than PRCC. (Right) Renal tumors with spindle cell features raise a multitude of possibilities. The morphological features and HMB-45 staining are usually necessary to make the diagnosis of AML, particularly in tumors with predominant spindle cell features.

AMACR in ACD-Associated RCC
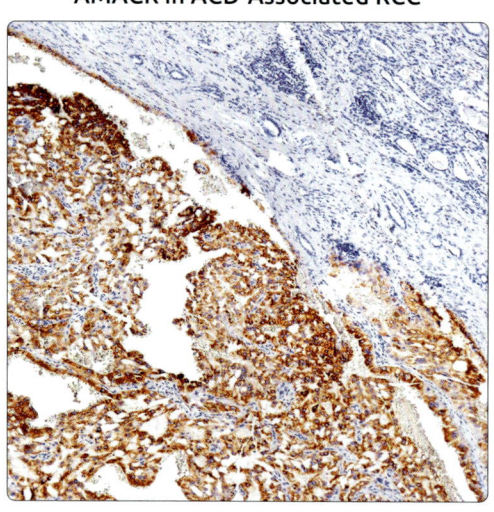

Angiomyolipoma: HMB-45
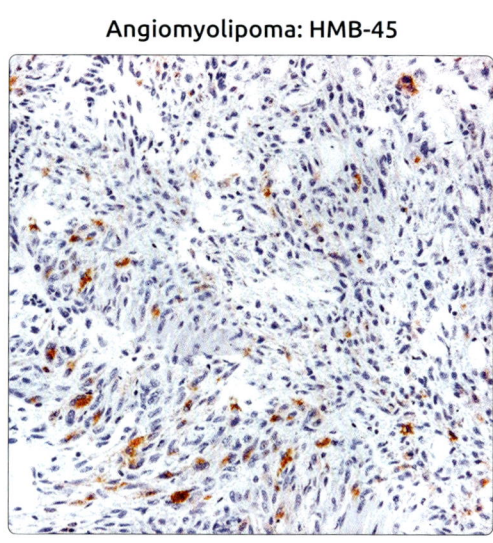

(Left) Cathepsin-K is reported to be more sensitive for all variants of AML, compared to the more traditional IHC markers. Diffuse cytoplasmic staining is shown here in a predominantly leiomyomatous tumor ➡. (Right) Immunostaining for WT1 may be needed in the distinction of small, blue round cell tumors. WT1 usually shows diffuse nuclear immunoreactivity in the blastemal and epithelial components of Wilms tumor. Positivity may also be observed in desmoplastic small round cell tumor and metanephric adenomas.

Cathepsin-K in Angiomyolipoma
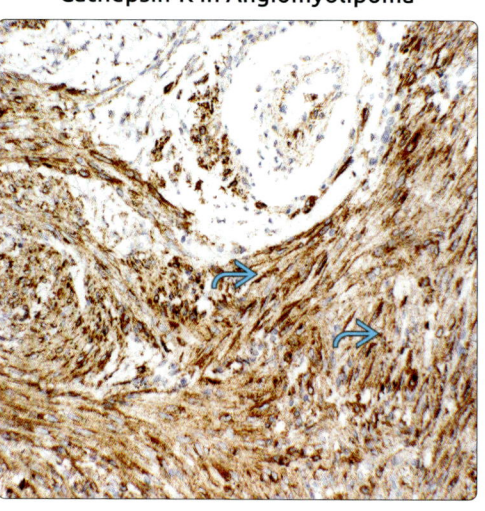

WT1
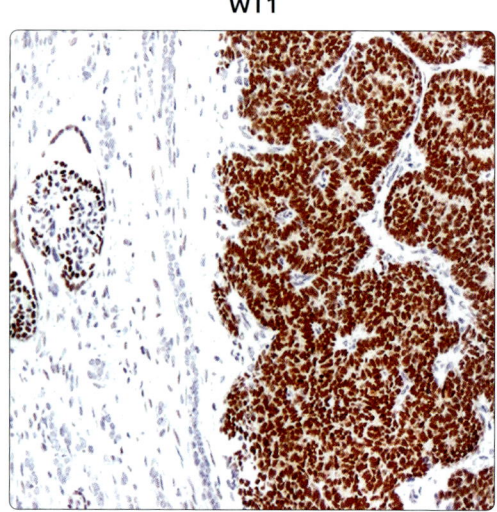

Immunohistochemistry, Kidney

WT1 in Metanephric Adenoma

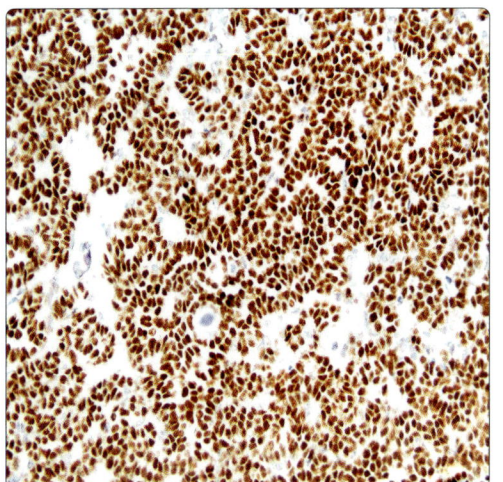

BRAF (V600E) in Metanephric Adenoma

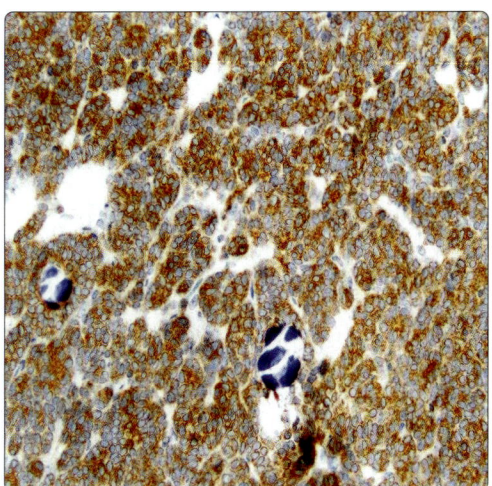

(Left) Metanephric adenomas, like most Wilms tumors, often show diffuse nuclear staining for WT1. This often helps in differentiation from purely tubular papillary RCC. (Right) More than 90% of metanephric adenomas show mutations in BRAF, and immunohistochemistry for V600E BRAF is invariably positive in such tumors. Metanephric adenoma is one of the rare benign tumors with this mutation and immunohistochemical immunoreactivity. Most other BRAF-mutated tumors are malignant.

Fumarate Hydratase in HLRCC

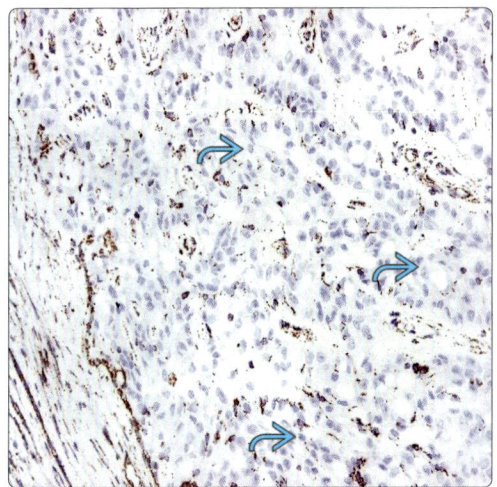

SDHB-Deficient RCC

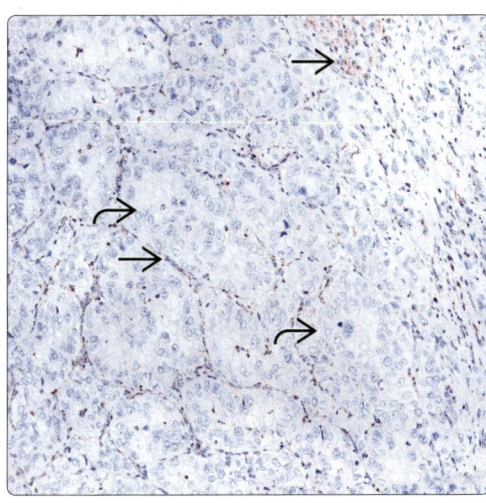

(Left) A number of renal tumors have characteristic and diagnostic absence of normally present IHC markers. Complete fumarate hydratase absence in tumor cells ➡ compared to retained staining in vascular endothelium and inflammatory cells is highly suggestive of HLRCC-associated RCC. (Right) SDHB-deficient RCC usually shows low-grade oncocytic features with characteristic cytoplasmic vacuoles. IHC for SDHB is completely negative in tumor cells ➡, with positive staining in the internal controls ➡.

SNF5/Baf47 Loss in Renal Medullary Carcinoma

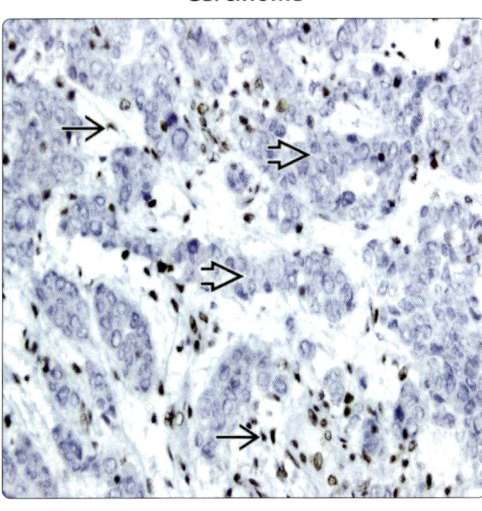

TFE3 Carcinoma

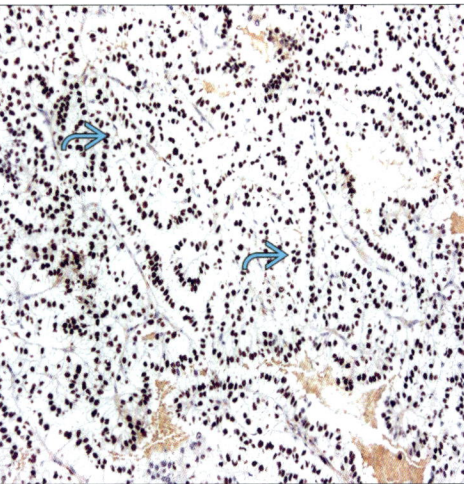

(Left) SNF5/Baf 47 immunostain shows complete loss of nuclear expression in renal medullary carcinoma ➡. Rhabdoid tumor of the kidney also shows complete loss of the stain. The background stromal cells and lymphocytes retain positivity ➡. (Right) Diffuse and strong TFE3 ➡ or TFEB IHC staining is highly characteristic of MiTF/TFE family carcinomas. However, weak and even diffuse staining requires FISH confirmation, because of the nonspecific nature of immunohistochemistry.

SECTION 2
Urinary Bladder

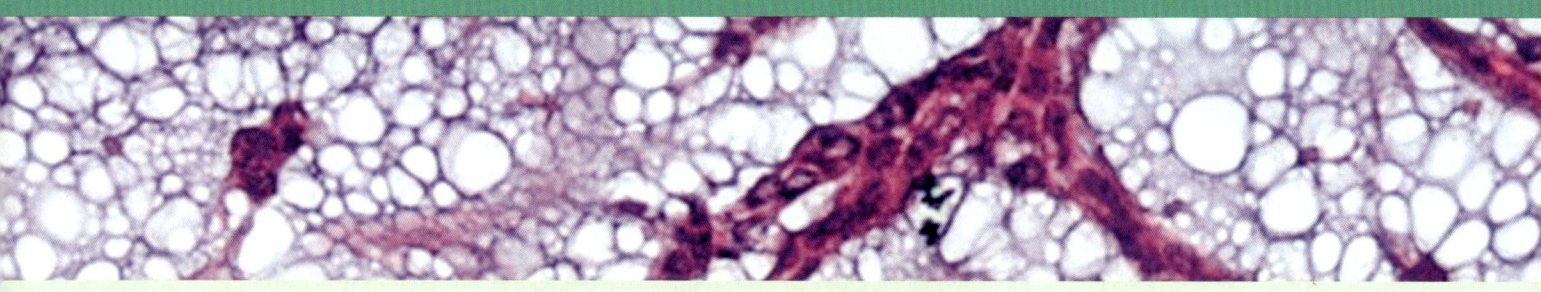

Introduction and Overview
Classification of Bladder Tumors and Tumor-Like
  Lesions   250

Microscopic Anatomy
Microscopic Anatomy of Urinary Bladder   252
Microscopic Anatomy of Urethra   256
Microscopic Anatomy of Ureter   260
Microscopic Anatomy of Renal Pelvis   262

Nonneoplastic Lesions of Urinary Tract
Overview of Cystitis   266
Papillary-Polypoid Cystitis   272
Malakoplakia   280
Schistosomiasis   286
von Brunn Nests   288
Nephrogenic Adenoma (Metaplasia)   294
Fibroepithelial Polyp   302
Prostatic-Type Polyp (Ectopic Prostate)   306
Amyloidosis   312
Müllerian Lesions   314
Pseudocarcinomatous Hyperplasia   318
Hamartoma   326

Urothelial Neoplasms, General
Overview of Urinary Bladder Neoplasms   328

Flat Urothelial Lesions
Urothelial Carcinoma In Situ   332
Flat Urothelial Lesions Other Than Carcinoma In Situ   340

Urothelial Neoplasms, Noninvasive
Urothelial Papilloma   344
Papillary Urothelial Neoplasm of Low Malignant
  Potential   350
Low-Grade Papillary Urothelial Carcinoma   354

High-Grade Papillary Urothelial Carcinoma   358
Inverted Urothelial Neoplasia   364

Urothelial Neoplasms, Invasive
Invasive Urothelial Carcinoma   374
Overview of Invasive Carcinoma Subtypes   382

Glandular Lesions
Cystitis Cystica and Glandularis   404
Villous Adenoma   408
Invasive Adenocarcinoma   410
Clear Cell Adenocarcinoma   416

Squamous Lesions
Squamous Proliferations Other Than Carcinoma   422
Invasive Squamous Cell Carcinoma   426

Mesenchymal Lesions
Myofibroblastic Proliferations   432
Smooth Muscle Tumors   440
Skeletal Muscle Tumors   448
Other Mesenchymal Tumors   454

Other Tumors of Urinary Bladder
Paraganglioma   462
Metastatic and Secondary Carcinomas   470

Diverticula of Urinary Tract
Diverticula   478
Diverticular-Associated Neoplasia   482

Urethra
Inflammatory Lesions of Urethra   486
Carcinoma of Urethra   490
Other Tumors and Tumor-Like Lesions of Urethra   494

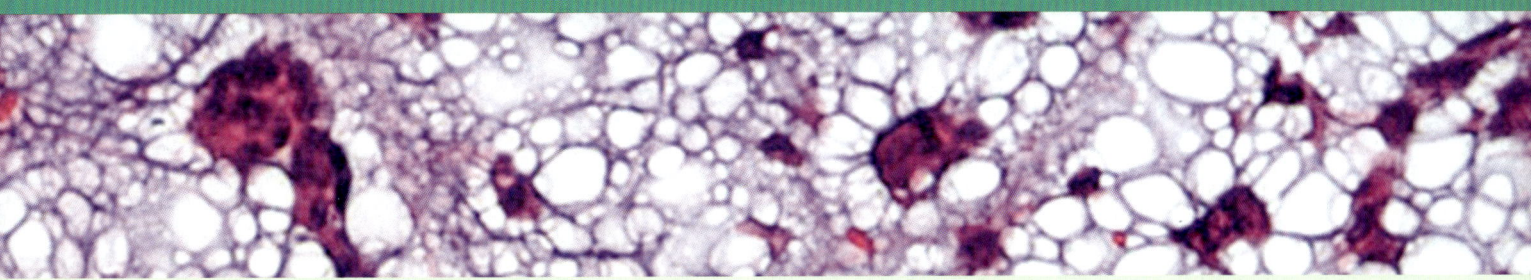

Ureter
Urothelial Carcinoma of Ureter	**498**
Other Tumors and Tumor-Like Lesions of Ureter	**502**

Renal Pelvis
Urothelial Carcinoma of Renal Pelvis	**506**
Other Tumors and Tumor-Like Lesions of Renal Pelvis	**514**

Urachus
Urachal Remnants	**520**
Tumors of Urachus	**522**

Immunohistochemical Profiles for Tumors Involving Urinary Bladder
Immunohistochemistry, Urinary Tract	**528**

Classification of Bladder Tumors and Tumor-Like Lesions

NONNEOPLASTIC LESIONS

Tumor-Like Lesions

- Amyloidosis
- Cystitis
  - Emphysematous
  - Encrusted
  - Eosinophilic
  - Follicular
  - Gangrenous
  - Giant cell
  - Granulomatous
  - Hemorrhagic
  - Infectious
  - Interstitial
  - Radiation
- Cystitis cystica and glandularis
  - ± intestinal metaplasia
  - ± mucin extravasation
- Fibroepithelial polyp
- Hamartoma
- Malakoplakia
- Müllerian lesions
- Nephrogenic adenoma
- Papillary-polypoid cystitis
- Postoperative lesions
  - Granulomas
  - Spindle cell nodule
- Prostatic-type polyps
- Pseudocarcinomatous hyperplasia
- Schistosomiasis
- Squamous lesions
  - Squamous metaplasia (keratinizing and nonkeratinizing)
  - Squamous hyperplasia, papillary and flat
- von Brunn nests

NEOPLASMS

Flat Urothelial Lesions

- Flat urothelial lesions with atypia
  - Flat urothelial hyperplasia
  - Reactive urothelial atypia
  - Urothelial atypia of unknown significance
  - Dysplasia
  - Urothelial carcinoma in situ

Noninvasive Inverted (Endophytic) Urothelial Neoplasms

- Benign
  - Inverted urothelial papilloma
  - Inverted urothelial neoplasm of low malignant potential
- Malignant
  - Low-grade inverted urothelial carcinoma
  - High-grade inverted urothelial carcinoma

Noninvasive Papillary Urothelial Neoplasms

- Benign
  - Urothelial papilloma
  - Papillary urothelial neoplasm of low malignant potential
- Malignant
  - Low-grade papillary urothelial carcinoma
  - High-grade papillary urothelial carcinoma
    - Glanadular/villoglandular differentiation
    - Squamous differentiation
    - Micropapillary

Invasive Neoplasms

- Microinvasive urothelial carcinoma
- Invasive urothelial carcinoma
  - Typical
  - Urothelial carcinoma with divergent differentiation
    - Squamous differentiation
    - Glandular differentiation
    - Trophoblastic differentiation
  - Deceptively benign features
    - Nested
    - Large nested
    - Small tubular
    - Microcystic
    - Inverted
  - Unusual cytoplasmic features
    - Clear cell (glycogen rich)
    - Plasmacytoid
    - Rhabdoid
    - Lipoid (lipid cell) features
  - Unusual stromal reactions
    - Pseudosarcomatous stroma
    - Stromal osseous or cartilaginous metaplasia
    - Osteoclast-type giant cells
    - With prominent lymphoid infiltrate
    - With myxoid stroma/chordoid
  - Micropapillary
  - Lymphoepithelioma-like
  - Small cell carcinoma
  - Sarcomatoid carcinoma
  - Large cell undifferentiated carcinoma

Glandular Lesions

- Villous adenoma
- Invasive adenocarcinoma
  - Adenocarcinoma, not otherwise specified
  - Enteric
  - Mucinous/colloid
  - Signet ring
  - Hepatoid
  - Mixed
- Clear cell adenocarcinoma
- Urachal neoplasia
  - Low-grade mucinous neoplasm
  - Adenocarcinoma

Squamous Lesions

- Squamous papilloma
- Condyloma
- Squamous dysplasia
- Squamous cell carcinoma

Smooth Muscle Tumors

- Leiomyoma
- Leiomyosarcoma

Classification of Bladder Tumors and Tumor-Like Lesions

Skeletal Muscle Tumors
- Rhabdomyosarcoma (embryonal, alveolar)

Other Mesenchymal Neoplasms
- Undifferentiated pleomorphic sarcoma
- Myofibroblastic proliferations
  - Inflammatory myofibroblastic tumor/pseudosarcomatous myofibroblastic proliferation
- Solitary fibrous tumor
- PEComa
- Neurofibroma
- Granular cell tumor
- Hemangioma/vascular malformation
- Angiosarcoma
- Postradiation sarcoma

Other Tumors, Including Hematopoietic Tumors
- Carcinoid
- Paraganglioma
- Melanoma
- Lymphoma
- Plasmacytoma

Metastatic Tumors
- Prostatic adenocarcinoma
- Colonic adenocarcinoma
- Other (rectum, cervix, endometrium, breast, ovary)

Microscopic Anatomy of Urinary Bladder

MACROSCOPIC

Anatomic Features

- Urinary bladder: Epithelial-lined muscular viscus in which urine is collected prior to micturition
  - Pelvic organ, situated anteriorly in pelvis minor, inferior to peritoneum when empty
    - Full and distended bladder extends into abdomen and may reach level of umbilicus
- In infants and children, until puberty, it is located in part within abdomen
- Posterior surface (base of bladder) faces posteriorly and inferiorly; separated from rectum by uterine cervix and proximal portions of vagina in females and by seminal vesicles and parts of vasa deferentia in males
- Anterior and lateral to bladder, boundaries include pubic bones and internal obturator and levator ani muscles
- Superior surface is partially covered by pelvic peritoneum
- Bladder lies relatively freely within fibrofatty tissues of pelvis
  - In area of bladder neck, it is firmly secured by pubovesical ligaments in females and puboprostatic ligaments in males
- Apex of bladder (dome) is most anterosuperior point of bladder and is site of insertion of median umbilical ligament where urachal remnant may be present
- Trigone is located at base of bladder and extends to posterior bladder neck
  - Ureteral orifices are located at proximal and lateral aspects of trigone
- Bladder neck is most distal portion of bladder and opens into urethra
  - In male bladder, bladder neck merges with prostate gland
  - Occasional prostatic ducts may be present in this area
- Internal sphincter of urethra, composed of smooth muscle derived predominantly from middle circular layer of detrusor muscle at junction of urethra with urinary bladder, is located in this general area

MICROSCOPIC

General Features

- Urinary bladder consists of 4 layers: **Urothelium, lamina propria, muscularis propria, and adventitia** (partial serosal layer present at dome/anterior wall)
  - These anatomic landmarks are important for tumor staging
- **Urothelium**, formerly referred to as "transitional epithelium," is multilayered epithelium with variable thickness depending on degree of bladder distension (ranging 2-7 cells thick)
- 3 cell types generally recognized (superficial, intermediate, and basal)
  - Superficial (umbrella) cells in contact with urinary space
    - Large, elliptical cells, may be binucleated and have abundant eosinophilic cytoplasm
    - In distended bladder, they become flattened and barely discernible
    - May become detached, or may overlie frank carcinoma in situ
  - Intermediate cells: May be up to 5 cells thick in contracted bladder, but may become inconspicuous or only 1 cell thick and flattened in distended bladder
    - Oriented with long axis perpendicular to basement membrane
    - Contain oval nuclei, nuclear grooves, finely stippled chromatin, absent or indistinct nucleoli
    - Ample cytoplasm, distinct cytoplasmic membranes
  - Basal cells: Lie on thin and continuous basement membrane
    - Composed of cuboidal cells, which are evident only in contracted bladder
  - Common urothelial variants include formation of Brunn nests (invaginations of surface urothelium into underlying lamina propria), cystitis cystica, and cystitis glandularis

Normal Urothelial Mucosa

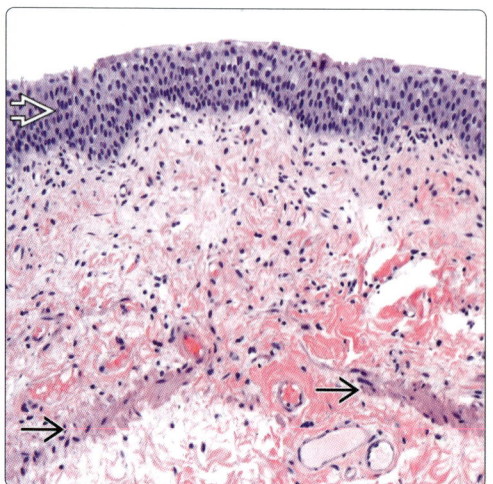

Normal Urothelium

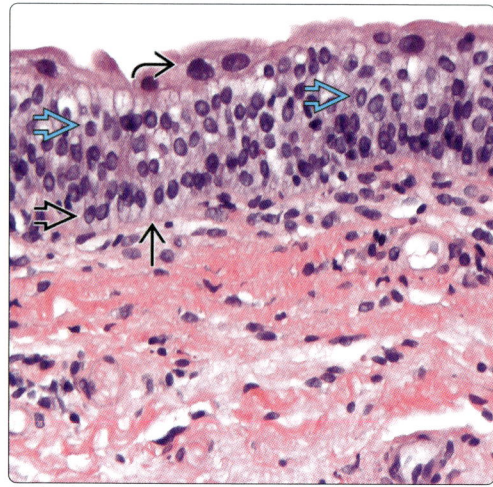

(Left) Normal urothelial mucosa consists of an orderly, multilayered lining ➡. The lamina propria contains loose connective tissue and thin bundles of smooth muscle that form the muscularis mucosae ➡. (Right) Normal urothelium is shown. The superficial cells ➡ are characterized by abundant eosinophilic cytoplasm and large, occasionally multinucleated nuclei. The intermediate cells ➡ have relatively uniform, oval nuclei. The basal cells ➡ have small nuclei and lie immediately above the basement membrane ➡.

Microscopic Anatomy of Urinary Bladder

- Urothelium frequently undergoes metaplastic changes (squamous or glandular), most commonly as response to chronic inflammatory stimuli such as urinary tract infection, calculi, diverticula, or frequent catheterization
- **Lamina propria** lies between mucosal basement membrane and muscularis propria
  - Composed of dense connective tissue containing rich vascular network, lymphatic channels, sensory nerve endings, and a few elastic fibers
  - Thickness of lamina propria varies with degree of bladder distention
    - Generally thinner in areas of trigone and bladder neck (may contain muscularis propria directly beneath mucosa with lamina propria being virtually indiscernible)
  - In midportion of lamina propria of bladder lie intermediate-sized arteries and veins
  - Wisps of smooth muscle are commonly found in lamina propria, usually associated with these vessels
    - These fascicles of smooth muscle are not connected to muscularis propria and appear as isolated bundles but may form discontinuous thin layer of muscle
    - Anatomic relationship of these fibers to overlying urothelium can be severely disrupted by inflammation or prior therapeutic intervention when they may be seen juxtaposed to basement membrane
    - Uncommonly, these muscle fibers may present as continuous layer of muscle within lamina propria, thus forming true muscularis mucosae (important distinction form muscularis propria)
  - Muscularis mucosae muscle bundles may be hyperplastic (seen frequently in dome) or nonhyperplastic
    - Hyperplastic muscularis mucosae muscle bundles may be arranged in 2 patterns: Haphazard (loose muscle bundles with jagged outlines) or compact regular pattern (small muscle bundles similar to muscularis propria)
  - Distribution of muscularis mucosa muscle bundles is variable and ranges from being absent, isolated, or scattered and nondispersed (forming recognizable layer)
    - Muscularis mucosa can be present as near-continuous linear layer or as variably discontinuous/interrupted layer
  - Adipose tissue may be encountered within lamina propria and muscularis propria (should not be misinterpreted as evidence of perivesical fat in transurethral resection specimens)
    - Typically situated in deeper aspect of lamina propria near superficial border of muscularis propria and rarely seen in superficial lamina propria abutting mucosa or in trigone
- **Muscularis propria** is generally regarded to consist of 3 smooth muscle coats, inner and outer longitudinal layers, and central circular layer
  - For practical purposes, longitudinal and circular layers mix freely and have no definite orientation
  - In contracted bladder, fascicles of muscle fibers are arranged in relatively coarse bundles, separated by moderate to abundant connective tissue containing blood vessels, lymphatics, and nerves
  - Typically arranged in groups or bundles both horizontally and vertically, forming layers with distinct round thick compact muscle bundles with smooth contours
  - Mature adipose tissue may also be present between groups of muscle bundles
  - Very infrequently, nests of paraganglia may be identified, usually associated to neural or vascular structures
  - For staging purposes, muscularis propria has been divided into 2 segments: Superficial and deep (T2a and T2b, respectively)
  - No anatomical landmarks can be used to make this distinction (must be done by direct visualization on light microscopy)
  - Prior transurethral resection will alter anatomy of site and mask normal landmarks, making proper staging difficult, if not impossible
- **Adventitia** is outermost connective tissue covering of bladder
  - At dome/anterior wall, a serosal surface is present, representing part of abdominal peritoneum
  - In other regions of bladder, adventitia connects to perivesical adipose tissue
  - Boundary between muscularis propria and perivesical fat is not always well demarcated, occasionally presenting difficulties in assigning proper stage for invasive tumors

SELECTED REFERENCES

1. Ananthanarayanan V et al: Influence of histologic criteria and confounding factors in staging equivocal cases for microscopic perivesical tissue invasion (pT3a): an interobserver study among genitourinary pathologists. Am J Surg Pathol. 38(2):167-75, 2014
2. Paner GP et al: Further characterization of the muscle layers and lamina propria of the urinary bladder by systematic histologic mapping: implications for pathologic staging of invasive urothelial carcinoma. Am J Surg Pathol. 31(9):1420-9, 2007
3. Philip AT et al: Intravesical adipose tissue: a quantitative study of its presence and location with implications for therapy and prognosis. Am J Surg Pathol. 24(9):1286-90, 2000
4. Engel P et al: The muscularis mucosae of the human urinary bladder. Implications for tumor staging on biopsies. Scand J Urol Nephrol. 26(3):249-52, 1992
5. Ro JY et al: Muscularis mucosa of urinary bladder. Importance for staging and treatment. Am J Surg Pathol. 11(9):668-73, 1987
6. Dixon JS et al: Histology and fine structure of the muscularis mucosae of the human urinary bladder. J Anat. 136(Pt 2):265-71, 1983
7. Paner GP et al: Diagnostic utility of antibody to smoothelin in the distinction of muscularis propria from muscularis mucosae of the urinary bladder: a potential ancillary tool in the pathologic staging of invasive urothelial carcinoma. Am J Surg Pathol. 33(1):91-8, 2009
8. Paner GP et al: Diagnostic use of antibody to smoothelin in the recognition of muscularis propria in transurethral resection of urinary bladder tumor (TURBT) specimens. Am J Surg Pathol. 34(6):792-9, 2010

Microscopic Anatomy of Urinary Bladder

(Left) Bladder wall shows urothelium ➡, muscularis mucosae ➡, medium-sized vessels of the lamina propria ➡, and muscularis propria ➡. The muscularis mucosae in this case is conspicuous but discontinuous in nature. **(Right)** H&E shows bladder wall with surface urothelium and lamina propria without appreciable muscularis mucosae. Muscle bundles of muscularis propria are present ➡. Adipose tissue is present in the lamina propria; when present in here, it is frequently more deeply situated ➡.

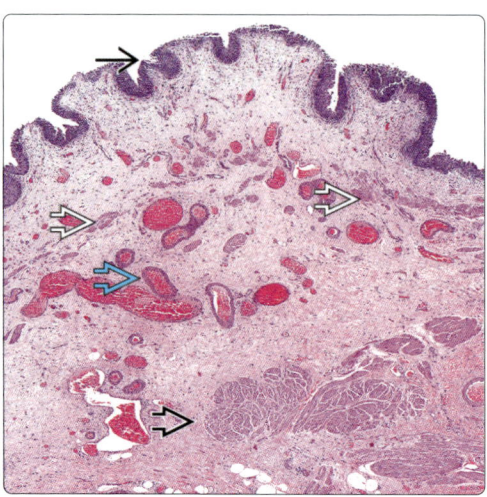
Bladder Wall

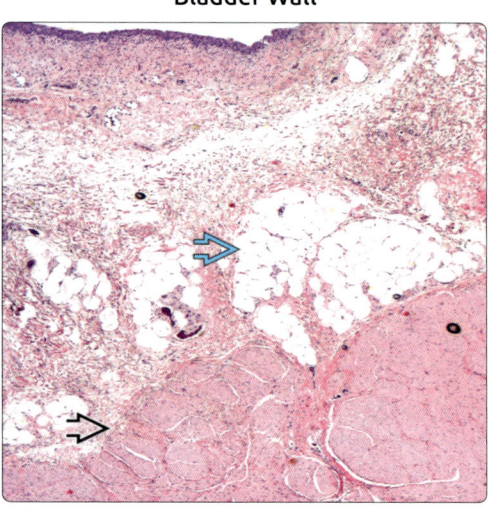
Bladder Wall

(Left) In this low-magnification image, the lamina propria contains a nonhyperplastic, continuous layer of muscularis mucosae ➡ and loose connective tissue abutting the muscularis propria in the deeper aspect. **(Right)** H&E shows bladder wall at the trigone. Note the near absence of lamina propria elements and the close proximity of small bundles of muscularis propria to the surface urothelium. The muscularis propria muscle bundles tend to become smaller in caliber as they reach the surface in this location.

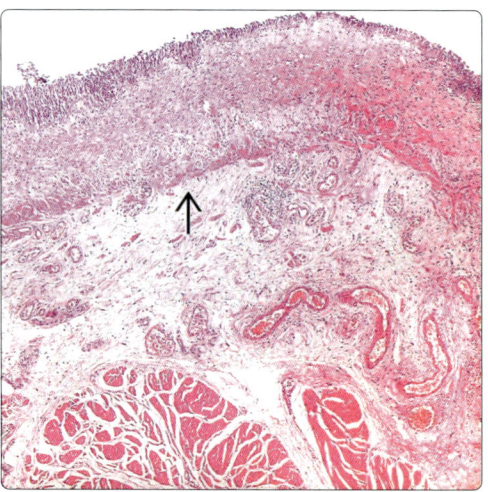
Muscularis Mucosae

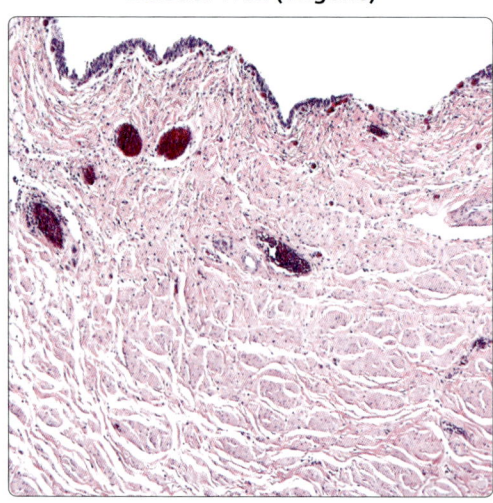
Bladder Wall (Trigone)

(Left) Hypertrophic bundles of muscularis mucosae (MM) are shown with haphazard orientation and jagged outlines. This feature serves to distinguish MM from the rounded, smooth contours of muscularis propria (MP) in TURBT specimens. **(Right)** Hypertrophic MM resembling muscularis propria is shown, posing a diagnostic challenge in TURBT specimens. If round fascicles of muscle are associated with other fascicles oriented both vertically and horizontally in compact bundles, MP is favored. Muscle location is also important.

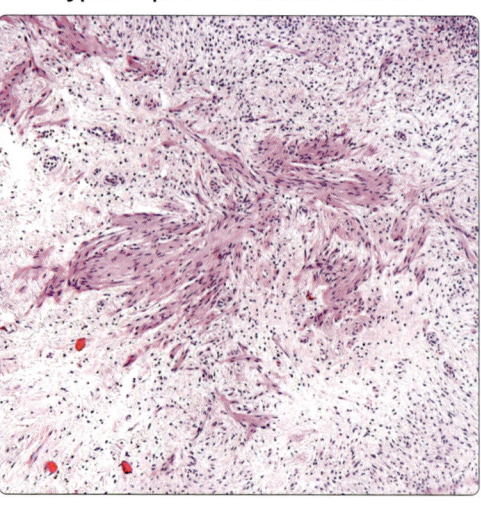
Hypertrophic Muscularis Mucosae

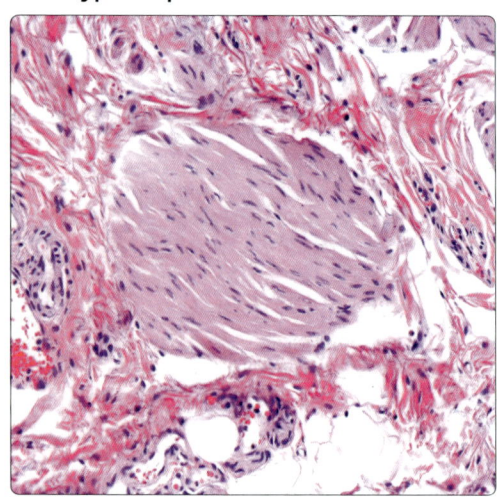
Hypertrophic Muscularis Mucosae

Microscopic Anatomy of Urinary Bladder

Histology of Muscularis Propria

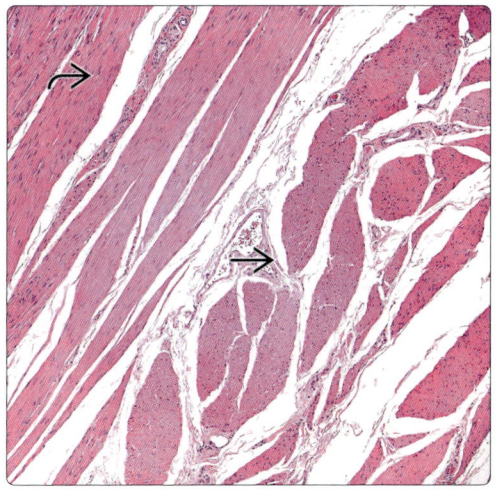

Muscularis Propria With Adipose Tissue

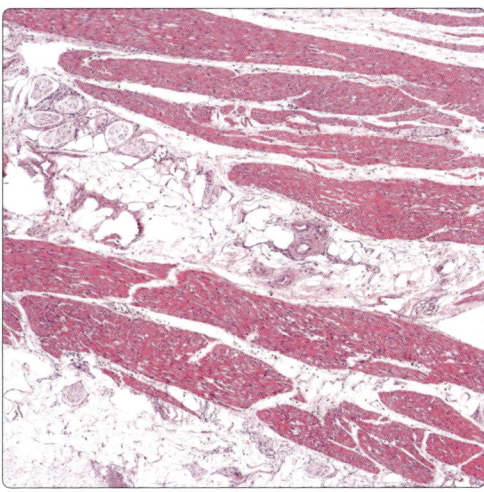

(Left) Longitudinal ➡ and circular ➡ muscle layers comprise the muscularis propria (MP) of the urinary bladder wall. Horizontal and vertical orientation of the muscle fascicles with rounded, smooth contours and arranged in bundles serves as a useful feature in the recognition of MP. (Right) Adipose tissue is frequently present between the layers of MP in the bladder wall. It is important to note this feature in the context of interpreting TURBT specimens containing adipose tissue for staging of bladder tumors.

Bladder Wall (Muscularis Propria and Perivesical Fat)

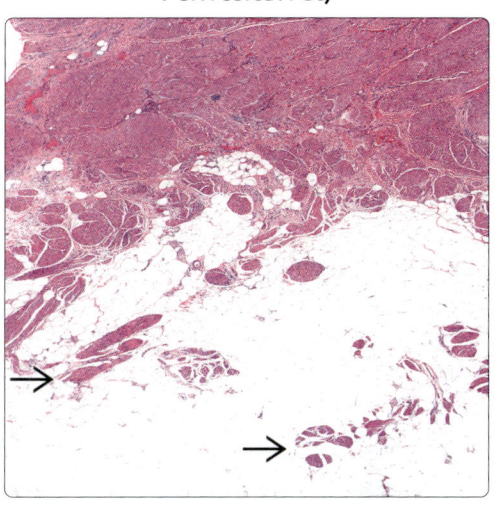

Bladder Wall (Muscularis Propria)

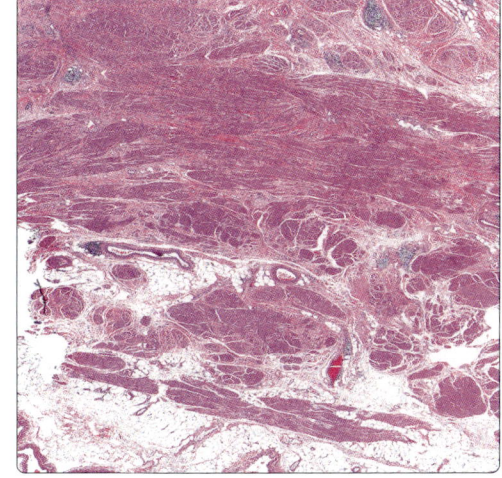

(Left) Interface of the muscularis propria ➡ and perivesical fat (PVF) shows irregular boundaries between MP and PVF, a staging dilemma. (Right) Bladder wall shows different layers of the muscularis propria. The muscularis propria muscle fascicles tend to be arranged in bundles separated by loose fibroconnective tissue or adipose tissue. Each group contains muscle bundle layers stacked horizontally and vertically. These are useful features to bear in mind when interpreting muscle in TURBT specimens.

SMA Staining in Bladder Wall

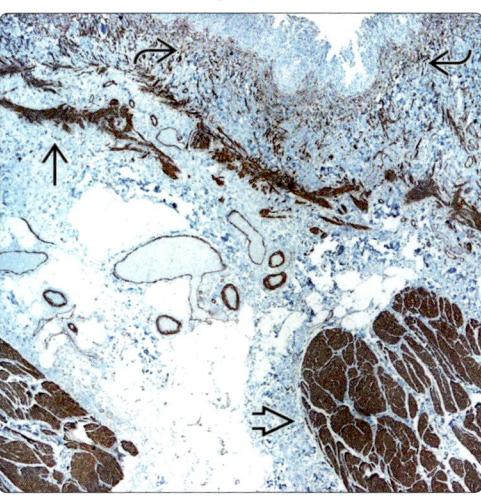

Smoothelin Staining in Bladder Wall

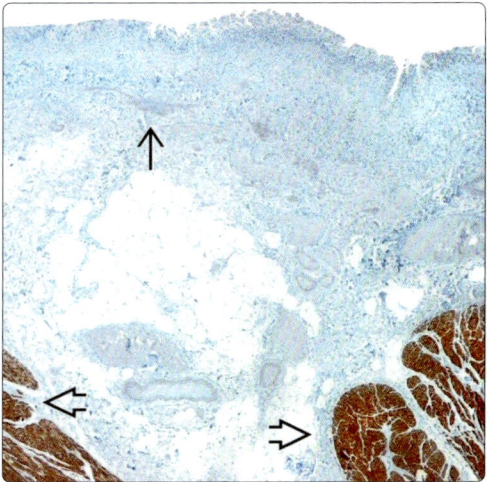

(Left) Smooth muscle actin immunohistochemical stain demonstrates diffuse and strong positivity in both the muscularis mucosae ➡ and muscularis propria ➡. A band of subintimal myofibroblasts also stains positively with smooth muscle actin ➡. (Right) Smoothelin immunostaining demonstrates striking differential immunoreactivity and aids in distinguishing between muscularis propria (strong and diffuse staining ➡) and muscularis mucosae (negative staining ➡).

Microscopic Anatomy of Urethra

MACROSCOPIC

General Features

- Tubal structure connecting urinary bladder to external urethra orifice (meatus of glans penis)
- Transports urine from bladder to exterior through urethral meatus
- In males, also serves as conduit for semen
- Urethral lining epithelium derived from endodermal urogenital sinus
  - Epithelial lining of fossa navicularis in males is of ectodermal origin
  - Urogenital sinus separated from anorectal canal at ~ 4th week gestation
  - Penile urethra formed from urethral groove under influence of dihydrotestosterone
- Male urethra
  - 15-20 cm in length
  - Divided into 3 anatomic segments based on structures that invest it
  - Prostatic urethra
    - Extends from bladder neck (apex of trigone) to prostatic apex
    - 3-4 cm long
    - Forms gentle anterior 45° curve as it descends through prostate
    - Supported by urogenital diaphragm and perineal membrane inferiorly
    - Merges with membranous urethra at urogenital diaphragm
    - One of key landmarks for microanatomic division of prostate (McNeal model)
    - Contains urethral crest
      - Intraluminal longitudinal ridge from posterior aspect of urethral wall
    - Verumontanum (colliculus seminalis) located in central part of prostatic urethra
      - Most prominent part of urethral crest

Prostatic Urethra at Verumontanum

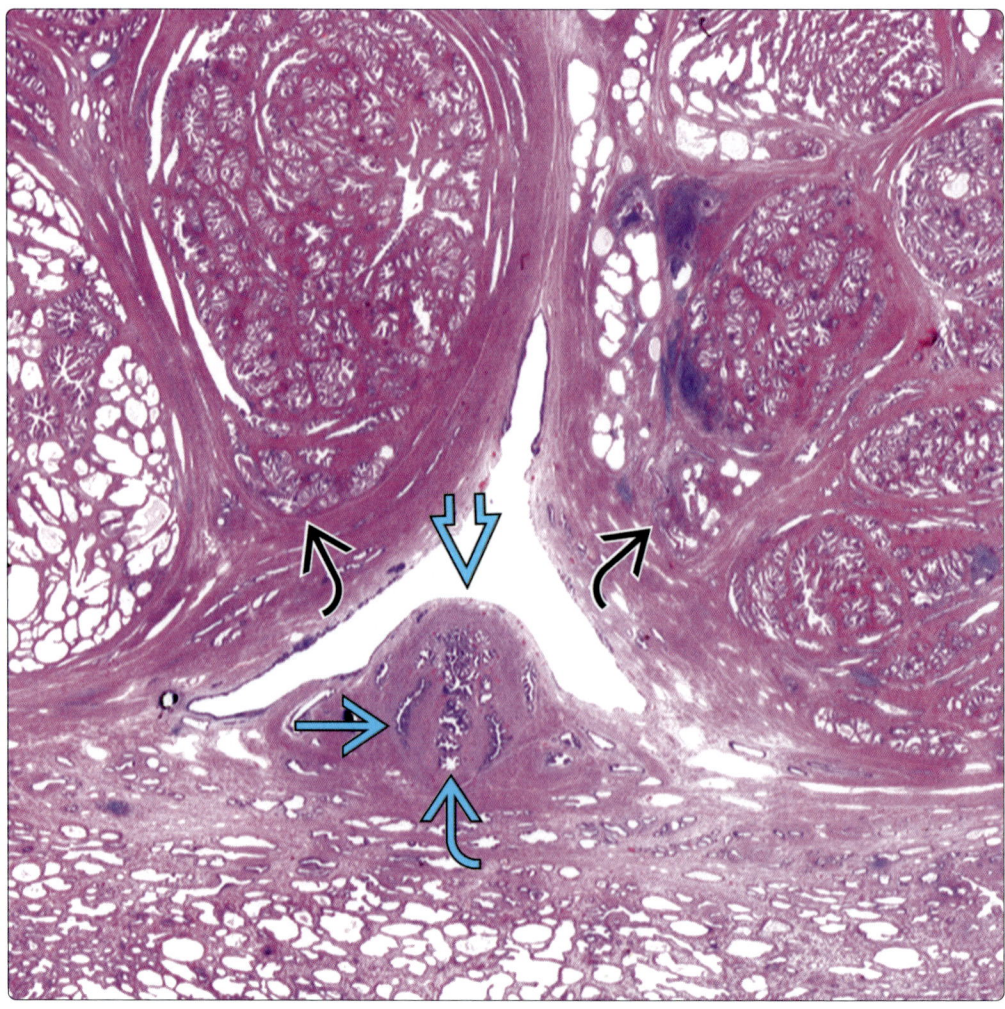

Verumontanum ➡ is a prominence at the mid-urethra where the ejaculatory ducts ➡ (bilateral) exit. Prostatic utricle ➡ is a diverticulum situated at the center of verumontanum in between the 2 ejaculatory ducts. The verumontanum bulges into the urethral lumen from the posterior wall and serves as a landmark in urethroscopy and for orientation histologically (points to anterior of prostate). In this prostate, the urethra is compressed by nodular hyperplasia of transition zone ➡. The peripheral zone with its stream of ducts and acini is seen subjacent to verumontanum.

Microscopic Anatomy of Urethra

- □ No physiologic significance but a key landmark in urethroscopy, transurethral resection, and pathological examination of prostate
- – Contains prostatic utricle
  - □ Midline epithelial-lined blind sac at verumontanum representing müllerian vestige
  - □ Opens into verumontanum
- – Ejaculatory duct empty into urethra on either side of prostatic utricle at verumontanum
- – Most prostatic ducts open along posterior and lateral walls of prostatic urethra
  - □ Proximal prostatic ducts lined by urothelium, which transitions to prostatic acinar and basal cells distally
  - □ Theoretically, urothelial carcinoma may arise primarily within prostate from proximal urethral ducts urothelium
  - □ Urothelial carcinoma from urethra may spread through ducts
- o Bulbo-membranous urethra
  - – Membranous urethra
    - □ Shortest segment of urethra (~ 1.0-2.5 cm)
    - □ Least distensible portion of urethra
    - □ Extends from prostatic apex to bulb of penis
    - □ Traverses urethral sphincter and urogenital diaphragm and is surrounded by muscle fibers
    - □ Extends to posterior margin of penile bulb
  - – Cowper (bulbourethral) glands
    - □ Located adjacent to membranous urethra bilaterally within skeletal muscle of urogenital diaphragm
    - □ Their ducts empty into posterior aspect of bulbomembranous urethra
    - □ Male homologue of Bartholin gland
  - – Bulbous urethra
    - □ Begins immediately distal to urogenital diaphragm at root of penis
    - □ 3-4 cm in length
    - □ Relatively larger caliber than membranous and prostatic segments
- o Penile (spongy) urethra
  - – Longest segment of urethra, 10-15 cm
  - – Extends from urogenital diaphragm to fossa navicularis, where it opens into external urethral meatus
    - □ Meatus is slightly ventral at glans tip with slit-like opening oriented sagittally
  - – Surrounded by corpus spongiosum, below paired corpora cavernosa
    - □ Corpora are spongy structures consisting of irregular sinus spaces lined by endothelial cells
    - □ Sinuses separated by trabeculae containing collagenous, elastic, and smooth muscle fibers and nerves
    - □ Important landmark for staging penile carcinoma
  - – Opens externally at tip of glans penis as external urethral meatus
  - – Scattered mucus-secreting glands (Littré glands), except anteriorly
- o Alternative division of male urethra
  - – **Proximal/posterior urethra** represents prostatic and membranous segments
  - – **Distal/anterior urethra** represents penile segment
  - o Preprostatic urethra (bladder neck) can also be considered distinct part
- Female urethra
  - o Short (~ 4 cm in length)
  - o Periurethral glands (Skene glands) near external orifice
- Lymphatic drainage
  - o Lymphatics of prostatic and bulbo-membranous urethra drain to external iliac and obturator lymph nodes
  - o Lymphatics of penile urethra drain to superficial inguinal lymph nodes
- Vascular supply
  - o Inferior vesical artery supplies prostatic urethra
  - o Bulbourethral artery supplies bulbo-membranous urethra
  - o Venous counterparts drain similar urethral segments

MICROSCOPIC

Mucosal Epithelium in Male Urethra

- Prostatic urethra
  - o Generally lined by urothelium, but could have columnar lining
  - o Verumontanum normally composed of closely apposed small glands, often containing eosinophilic to brown concretions
  - o Periurethral prostatic glands comprised of short ducts and acini usually present along proximal segment of prostatic urethra
- Membranous urethra
  - o Lined by pseudostratified columnar epithelium
  - o Has rich, vascular mucosa
- Penile urethra
  - o Lined by pseudostratified columnar epithelium, except at fossa navicularis, which is lined by nonkeratinized squamous epithelium
  - o Mucosa has several small recesses called lacunae of Morgagni, which extend deeper into mucin-secreting glands of Littré
  - o Largest recesses at fossa navicularis called lacuna magna

Mucosal Epithelium in Female Urethra

- Urothelium lines proximal 1/3
- Nonkeratinized squamous epithelium lines distal 2/3

Lamina Propria

- Composed of loose fibroconnective tissue with numerous elastic bundles
- Contains scattered smooth muscle fascicles, which are predominantly longitudinally oriented, as well as circular smooth muscle bundles in outer layers
- Membranous urethra surrounded by striated muscle of urogenital diaphragm

SELECTED REFERENCES

1. Pradidarcheep W et al: Anatomy and histology of the lower urinary tract. Handb Exp Pharmacol. 202:117-48, 2011
2. Carroll PR et al: Surgical anatomy of the male and female urethra. Urol Clin North Am. 19(2):339-46, 1992

Microscopic Anatomy of Urethra

Prostatic Urethra

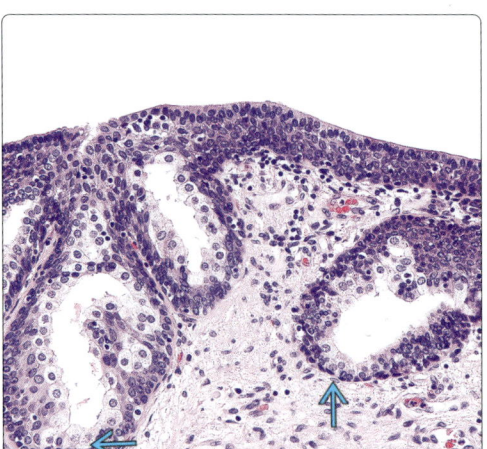

Prostatic Urethra

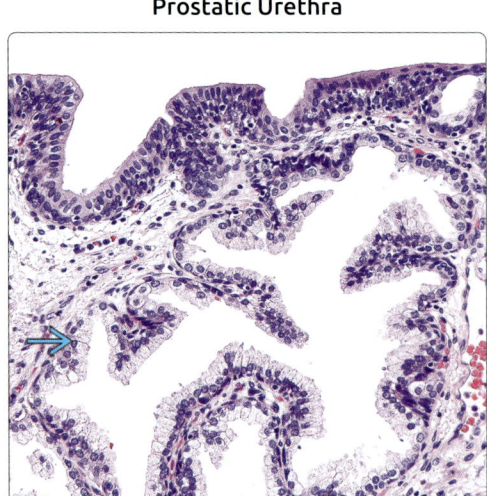

(Left) This segment of prostatic urethra shows the urothelial lining and periurethral glands. These glands are often abortive and commonly lined by prostatic-type cells ➡. **(Right)** This segment of prostatic urethra shows a periurethral gland ➡ lined by secretory and basal cells. These glands are phenotypically similar to those deep within the prostate parenchyma, including positivity for PSA and basal cell markers. The periurethral glandular region may be considered a distinct zone of the prostate.

Prostatic Ducts

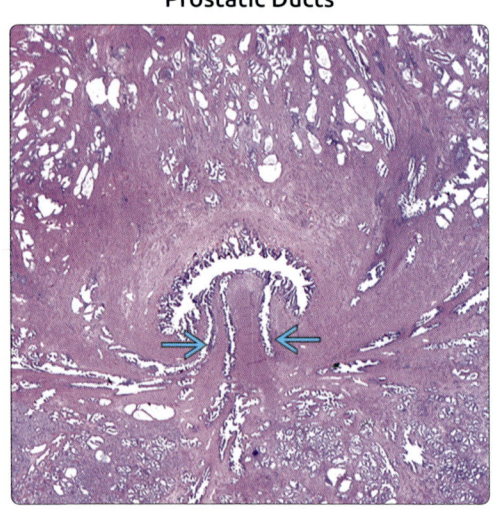

Prostatic Ducts

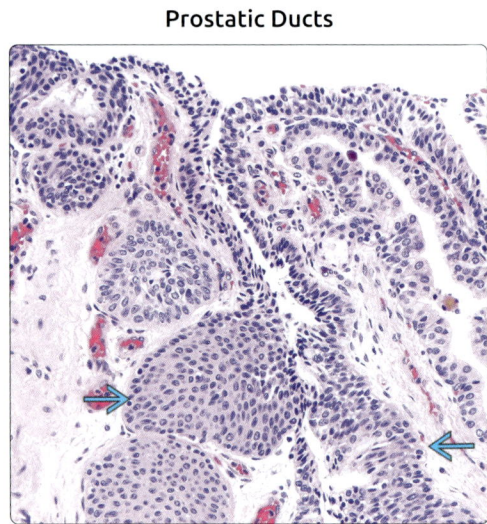

(Left) Low-power view shows prostatic ducts opening into the urethra ➡. The prostatic ducts can be seen either extending posteriorly or curving anteriorly. Prostate carcinoma (PCa) may spread within these ducts (intraductal carcinoma) and extend and protrude into the urethra. **(Right)** Proximal portion of prostatic ducts may contain a urothelial lining ➡. Urothelial carcinoma may spread via these ducts and may extend into the prostate. Urothelial carcinoma confined within these ducts is still considered an in situ disease.

Verumontanum Glands

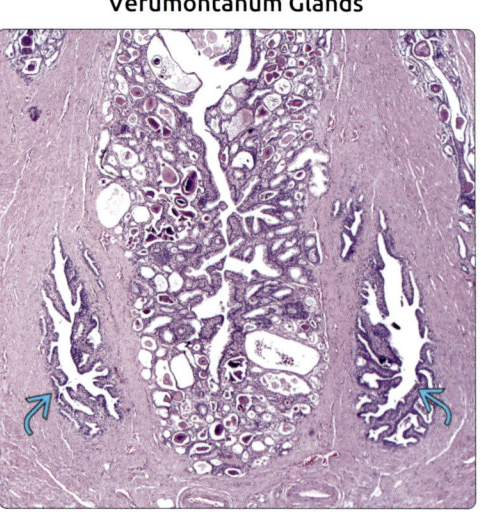

Prostatic Utricle

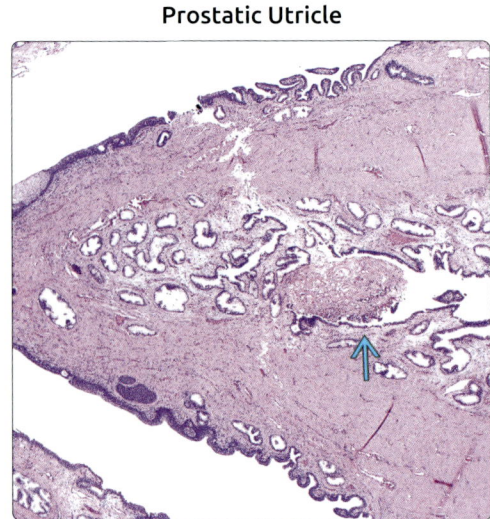

(Left) Note the well-circumscribed small glandular proliferation with eosinophilic concretions in the verumontanum between bilateral ejaculatory ducts ➡. These closely packed and often anastomosing hyperplastic glands should not be mistaken for PCa. **(Right)** Prostatic utricle ➡ is a small epithelium-lined diverticulum of prostatic urethra located between the openings of ejaculatory ducts. It is composed of glandular units lined by columnar epithelium and surrounded by fibroconnective tissue.

Microscopic Anatomy of Urethra

Verumontanum Glands

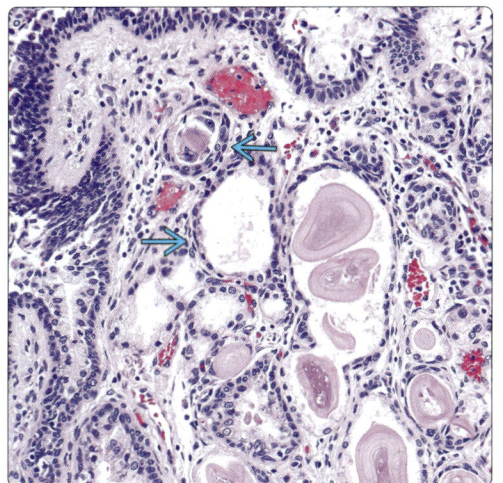

Cowper Gland

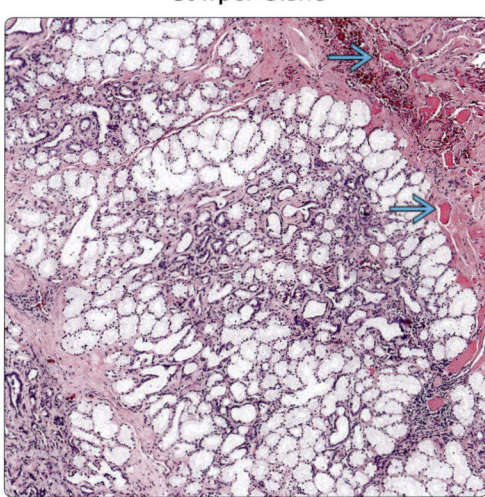

(Left) Verumontanum mucosal glands usually contain corpora amylacea. These glands may become hyperplastic and may mimic PCa. Unlike PCa, verumontanum glands lack nuclear atypia, and the double layer of cells is usually discernible ➡ on H&E stain. (Right) Low-power view shows Cowper glands composed of circumscribed lobules of small, compact tubuloalveolar glands that resemble minor salivary glands admixed with excretory ducts/ductules. Cowper gland is usually associated with skeletal muscles ➡.

Cowper Gland

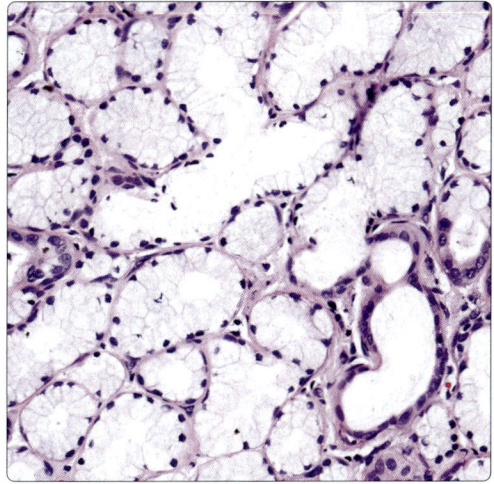

Penile Urethra

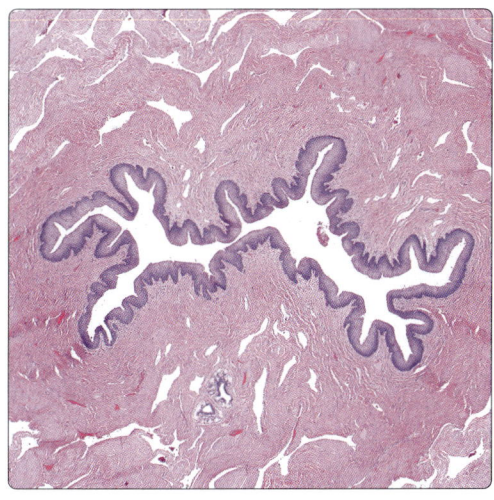

(Left) Cowper gland shows tubuloalveolar acini with cuboidal cells containing pale-staining mucinous cytoplasm and small, bland, basally located nuclei. The basal cell layer may not be readily apparent on H&E stain, and these glands may be confused with PCa, particularly foamy gland PCa, in needle core biopsies. (Right) Low-power magnification shows lumen of penile urethra with recesses. This urethral segment is lined by squamous epithelium. The sinus spaces of corpus spongiosum are seen surrounding the urethra.

Penile Urethra

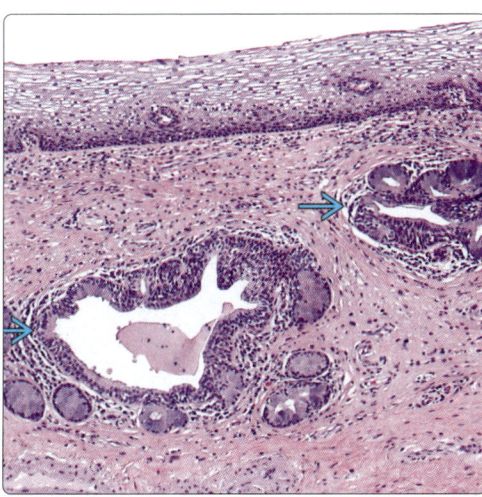

Penile Urethra

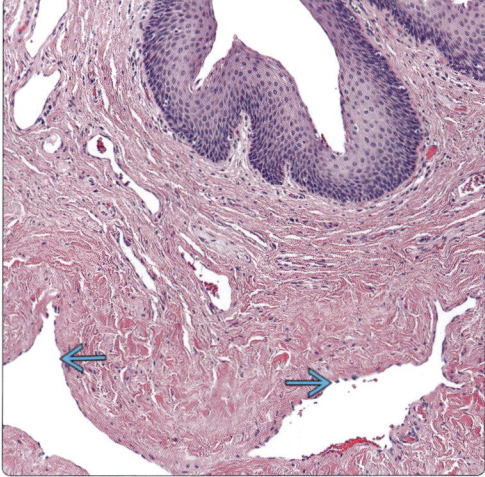

(Left) This segment of urethra is lined by squamous epithelium, and mucus-secreting glands (Littré glands) ➡ are seen. These tubuloacinar glands are in close relation with erectile tissue. Inflammation of Littré glands can clinically simulate a tumor. (Right) Low-power view shows nonkeratinized squamous epithelium of penile urethra. Around this urethral segment is the corpus spongiosum, composed of dilated sinus spaces lined by endothelial cells ➡, which is a landmark in staging penile carcinoma (pT2 disease).

Microscopic Anatomy of Ureter

MACROSCOPIC

Gross Anatomy

- Ureter is tubular viscus that enables active, peristaltic transport of urine from kidney to urinary bladder
  - 20-30 cm in length in adults; 1/2 abdominal and 1/2 pelvic
- Ureter begins within or immediately outside renal hilum, distal to ureteropelvic junction
  - Emerges posterior to renal artery and vein
- Ureter descends caudally, anterior to psoas muscle, with gonadal vessels crossing it anteriorly
- Ureter enters pelvis, anterior to sacroiliac joint, then descends to cross anterior to iliac vessels, usually at their bifurcation
- Ureter then courses downward along lateral pelvic sidewall, turning anteromedially to enter posterolateral wall of urinary bladder
  - Courses within wall of bladder 1-2 cm before ending at luminal ureteral orifice
    - Waldeyer sheath of fibromuscular tissue envelops most distal/intravesical portion

Segmental Anatomy

- Upper ureter: Upper 1/3, extending from ureteropelvic junction to upper border of sacrum
- Middle ureter: Middle 1/3, extending from upper to lower border of sacrum
- Lower ureter (distal or pelvic ureter): Lower 1/3, extending from lower border of sacrum to bladder

MICROSCOPIC

General Features

- Ureter is lined by **urothelium**; previously called transitional epithelium
- This stratified epithelium is generally 5-7 cell layers thick; may be hyperplastic in reactive setting
- Urothelium shows **basal cells**, which are cuboidal, small, and attenuated, scattered along basement membrane
- **Intermediate cells** are variable in number, slightly more plump with more cytoplasm, make up most of epithelium
  - Small, oval nuclei with even chromatin and no more than micronucleoli
- **Umbrella cells** are largest and most superficial and form lining directly juxtaposed to luminal contents
- Similar to bladder and other sites, ureteral **lamina propria** represents connective tissue that lies directly under thin, subepithelial basement membrane
  - Variably collagenized connective tissue with microvasculature, lymphatics, and chronic inflammation
  - Looser lamina propria in ureter with elastic fibers enables mucosal folding when lumen is physiologically variably distended
- Ureter has **no muscularis mucosae**, smaller wispy bundles of smooth muscle in lamina propria seen in bladder
- In proximal ureter, **muscularis propria** (also called muscularis), or definitive muscular coat, is often seen as single layer with smooth muscle fibers of admixed orientation
  - More distally, 2 distinct layers tend to develop
    - Longitudinal oriented smooth muscle bundles of innermost layer
    - Circular orientation of smooth muscle bundles of outer layer
- Beyond muscularis propria is adventitia, adipose connective tissue with rich anastomotic plexus of arteries, veins, and lymphatics

SELECTED REFERENCES

1. Gupta R et al: Neoplasms of the upper urinary tract: a review with focus on urothelial carcinoma of the pelvicalyceal system and aspects related to its diagnosis and reporting. Adv Anat Pathol. 15(3):127-39, 2008
2. Delahunt B et al: Pathology of the renal pelvis and ureter. In Amin MB et al: Urological Pathology. Philadelphia: Wolters Kluwer Health/Lippincott Williams & Wilkins, 2014
3. Reuter V et al: Urinary bladder, ureter, and pelvis. In Mills SE et al: Histology for Pathologists. 4th ed. Philadelphia: LWW, 2012
4. Anderson JK et al: Surgical anatomy of the retroperitoneum, adrenals, kidneys, and ureters. In Wein AJ et al: Campbell-Walsh Urology. 10th ed. London: Elsevier Health Sciences, 2011

(Left) The ureter emerges posterior to the renal vessels and courses inferiorly along the anterior psoas muscle, crossing the iliac vessels at their bifurcation, posterolaterally along the pelvic sidewall, and then anteromedially into the posterolateral bladder wall. (Right) The upper ureter extends from renal hilum ⇒ to the upper border of the sacrum ⇒, the middle ureter between upper ⇒ and lower ⇒ borders of the sacrum, and the lower ureter from lower border of the sacrum ⇒ to its orifice in the bladder ⇒.

Course of Ureter

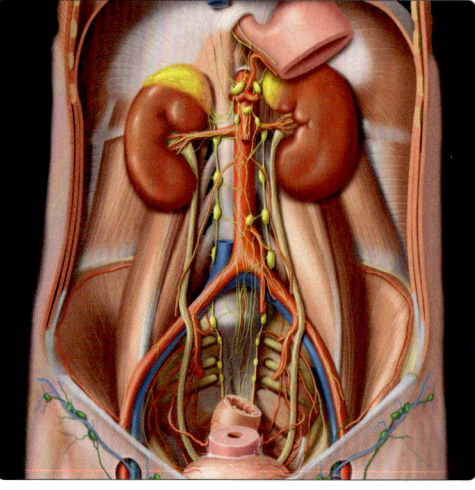

Segmental Anatomy of Ureter

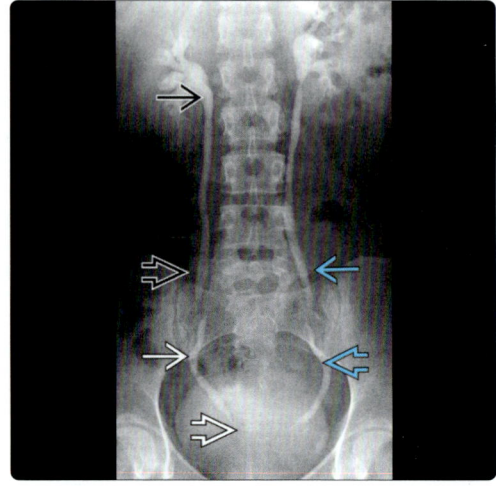

Microscopic Anatomy of Ureter

Cross Section at Mid Ureter

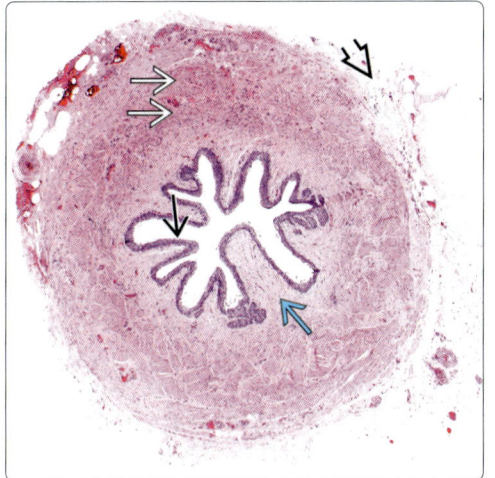

Urothelium and Lamina Propria

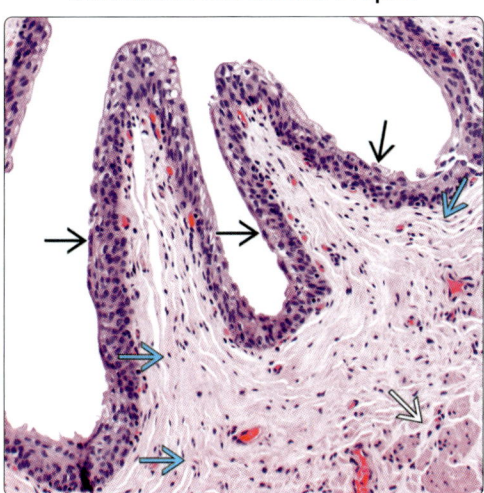

(Left) Innermost is the luminal urothelial-lined mucosa ➡, then the folded, underlying, loosely collagenized lamina propria ➡, then the smooth muscle layer of the muscularis propria ➡, and then the outer fibroadipose adventitia ➡. (Right) Here, the urothelium, 3-5 cell layers thick with well-demonstrated luminal umbrella cells ➡, lines the loosely fibrovascular, underlying lamina propria ➡. No muscularis mucosae is present here; the smooth muscle seen in the lower right is the inner longitudinal bands of the muscularis propria ➡.

Muscularis Propria of Ureter

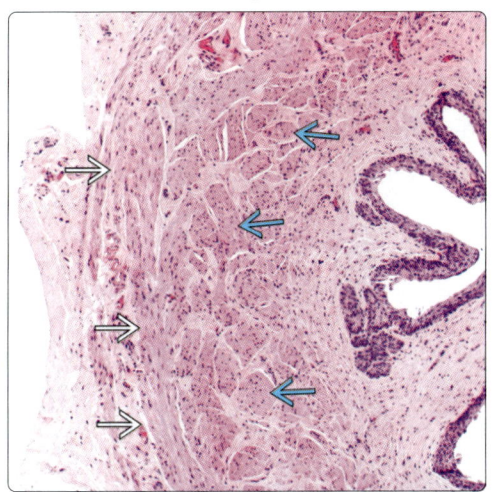

Ureteral Adventitia

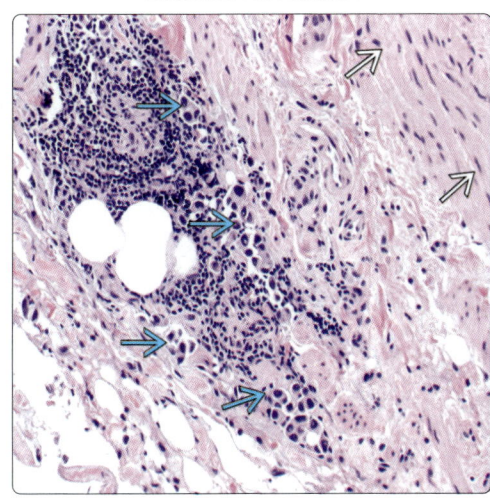

(Left) While often discussed physiologically as a 2-layered, inner longitudinal ➡, and outer circular ➡ layer, the muscularis propria of the ureter often shows admixture of fibers oriented both longitudinally and circularly. (Right) The adventitia of the ureter is a rich vascular plexus seen peripherally beyond the outermost, circularly oriented bundles of muscularis propria (upper right ➡). Here, metastatic urothelial carcinoma with lymphangitic spread highlights the rich lymphatic plexus in this area ➡.

Distal Ureter

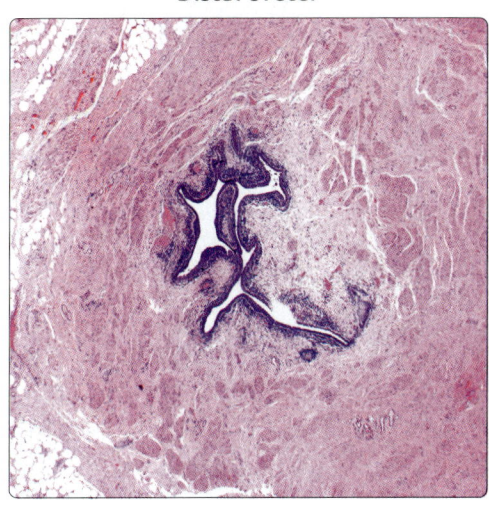

Papillary/Polypoid Ureteritis

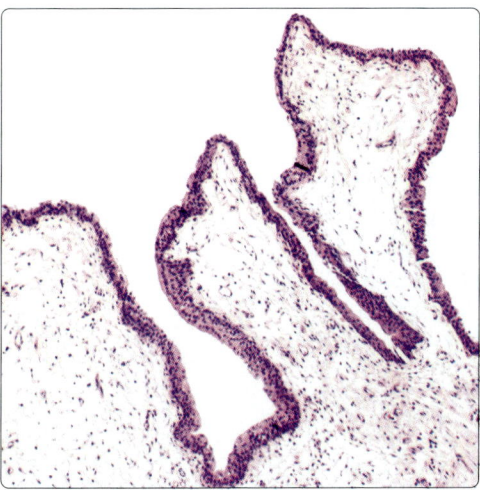

(Left) In this section taken in the plane of the ureterovesical junction, the distal part of the lower ureter is seen entering the lateral wall of the bladder. The muscularis propria of the ureter is seen blending into the muscularis propria of the bladder. Brisk chronic inflammation is apparent in the superficial lamina propria, associated with prior stenting. (Right) In this section taken from a dilated hydroureter, confluent lamina propria edema has rendered the folds of the ureteral mucosa polypoid, simulating a papillary lesion.

Microscopic Anatomy of Renal Pelvis

MACROSCOPIC

Gross Anatomy

- Renal parenchyma shows three histoanatomic and functional components: **Cortex**, **medulla**, and **pelvicalyceal system**
- **Cortex** is outer tubular parenchyma, with glomeruli, proximal, and distal tubules, containing nephrons
- **Medulla** is zone of kidney composed of loops of Henle and converging **collecting tubules** of collecting system
  - Medulla is conical in shape, often also called pyramids
    - Usually, medulla appears darker grossly
- Centrally, within kidney but deep to cortex and medulla, is **renal sinus**
  - **Renal sinus** contains **renal calyces**, more proximal part of the **renal pelvis**, vessels, nerves and adipose tissue
- More distal portion of pelvicalyceal system or proximal ureter exits kidney at **renal hilum**
  - **Renal hilum** is recessed area, between upper and lower poles, and medial to sinus
  - Renal artery, vein, distal portion of renal pelvis, and proximal ureter course through this area
  - Occasionally lymph nodes are located here

Functional Anatomy: Pelvicalyceal System

- Medulla contains converging collecting ducts of many nephrons, which together empty at **papilla** (tip) into minor calyx
- Papillae, thus, provide dividing mark between pelvicalyceal system and most distal renal parenchyma
  - Important distinction for staging of pelvicalyceal urothelial carcinomas
- Renal papillae are quite variable in number (4-18), usually 7-10 per kidney, and are aligned in rows, anterior and posterior
  - Anterior row of papillae have tips that point medially
  - Posterior row of papillae point anteriorly
- **Minor calyces** surround and collect effluent urine of each papilla, may be single or compound

Renal Pelvis and Calyces

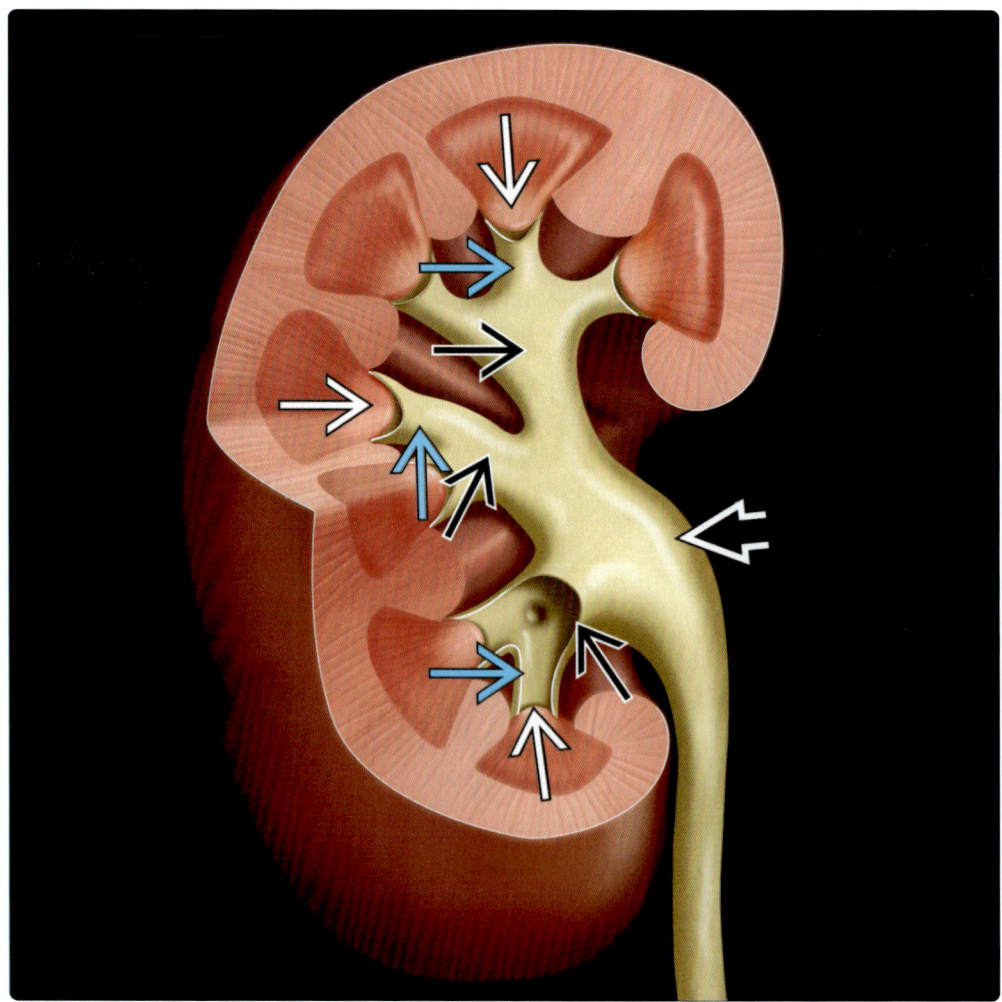

In the kidney, 7-10 renomedullary pyramids ➡ empty at their papillae into urothelial-lined minor calyces ➡, which pass through infundibula to collect into 2-3 major calyces ➡, which converge into the renal pelvis ➡.

Microscopic Anatomy of Renal Pelvis

- o Particularly at upper and lower poles, 2 or more papillae may share compound minor calyx
- Each minor calyx then progresses through variable area of narrowing called **infundibulum**
  - o 2 or more minor calyceal infundibula converge to form **major calyx**
  - o Usually 2-3 major calyces total arise in superior, interpolar, and inferior kidney
- From confluence of these calyces arises variably sized renal pelvis
  - o Some pelves are small structures, contained entirely within renal sinus adipose tissue
  - o Some pelves are quite large, protruding beyond renal hilum into retroperitoneal adipose
- High degree of structural anatomic variation, such that functional studies are often needed to prove pathologic dysfunction
  - o Gross examination should be circumspect regarding assessment of disease on anatomic grounds alone
- Pelvis then usually narrows at ureteropelvic junction to give rise to ureter
- Blood supply for renal pelvis is derived from branches of renal arteries
- Venous drainage is via renal vein
- Lymphatic drainage is to renal sinus lymph nodes, highlighting importance of gross dissection to identify any lymph node candidates in cancer cases

MICROSCOPIC

Urothelium

- Mucosa of renal pelvis shares many features with that of urinary bladder, ureter, and proximal urethra
- Pelvicalyceal mucosa is lined by **urothelium**, previously called transitional epithelium
- This stratified epithelium varies from 5-7 cell layers thick in well-formed areas, such as deeper in pelvis (or bladder), to quite thin and attenuated
  - o Often only 2-3 cells thick in minor calyces or at tips of papillae
- Urothelium shows **basal cells**, which are cuboidal, small, and attenuated, scattered along basement membrane
- **Intermediate cells** are variable in number, slightly more plump with more cytoplasm, make up most of epithelium
  - o Small, oval nuclei with even chromatin and no more than micronucleoli
- **Umbrella cells** are largest and most superficial and form lining directly juxtaposed to luminal contents
  - o Express proteins called **uroplakins**, which are involved in membrane-cytoplasmic cycling vesicles that expand luminal surface when distended by urine
    - Uroplakins 2 and 3 may be used as highly specific markers of urothelial differentiation
  - o Umbrella cells may be multinucleate or show degenerative-type atypia

Lamina Propria

- Similar to other sites of urinary tract, renal pelvic **lamina propria** represents connective tissue that lies directly under thin subepithelial basement membrane
- Variably collagenized connective tissue with microvasculature, lymphatics, and chronic inflammation

- In renal papillae, lamina propria is absent, in favor of denser basement membrane material surrounding distal collecting ducts
- Lamina propria may be quite thin in proximal parts of minor calyces
- In areas of renal pelvis, lamina propria is more loosely collagenized to allow rugations and mucosal folding when it is not distended
  - o Scattered elastic fibers facilitate folding when not distended by urine
- No muscularis mucosae is present in pelvicalyceal system or ureter
  - o These smaller wispy bundles of smooth muscle in lamina propria are only apparent in urinary bladder

Muscularis Propria

- In renal pelvis, muscularis propria is usually present as single layer
  - o Contrasting 2-layered (inner longitudinal, outer circular) muscularis propria developing more distally in ureter
- In more proximal pelvicalyceal system, muscularis propria of minor calyxes is even more attenuated: Single layer that may be discontinuous
- Within renal sinus, muscularis propria is surrounded by renal sinus fat
- More distally in renal hilum, renal pelvis is again surrounded by peripelvic adipose tissue and vascular and lymphatic spaces in adventitia
  - o Peripelvic fat includes vascular and lymphatic spaces, which merge distally into adventitia of ureter

SELECTED REFERENCES

1. Delahunt B et al: Pathology of the renal pelvis and ureter. In Amin M et al: Urological Pathology. 1st ed. Philadelphia: Lippincott Williams & Wilkins. 261-94, 2014
2. Anderson JK et al: Surgical anatomy of the retroperitoneum, adrenals, kidneys, and ureters. In McDougal W et al: Campbell-Walsh Urology. 10th ed. Philadelphia: Elsevier Saunders. 2-9, 2012
3. Reuter V et al: Urinary bladder, ureter, and pelvis. In Mills S: Histology for Pathologists. 4th ed. Philadelphia: Lippincott Williams & Wilkins. 971-86, 2012
4. Gupta R et al: Neoplasms of the upper urinary tract: a review with focus on urothelial carcinoma of the pelvicalyceal system and aspects related to its diagnosis and reporting. Adv Anat Pathol. 15(3):127-39, 2008
5. Olgac S et al: Urothelial carcinoma of the renal pelvis: a clinicopathologic study of 130 cases. Am J Surg Pathol. 28(12):1545-52, 2004

Microscopic Anatomy of Renal Pelvis

Papilla and Minor Calyx

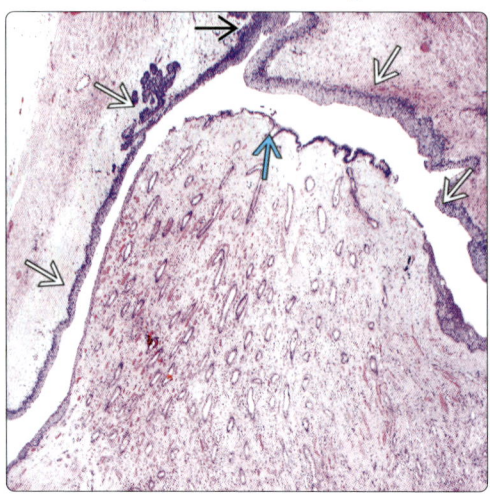

Papilla and Minor Calyx: Smooth Muscle Actin

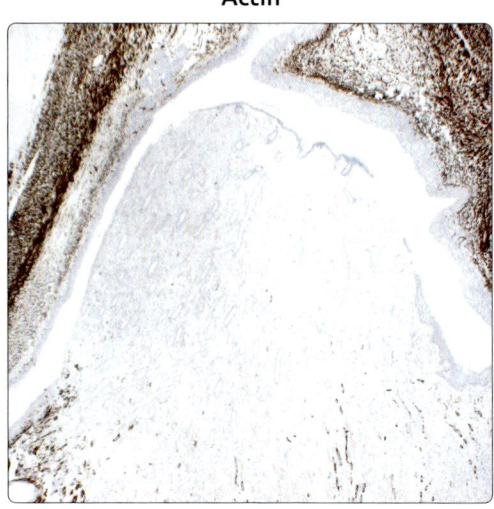

(Left) The papilla, or distal tip ➡, of the renal medullary collecting system protrudes into its surrounding minor calyx ➡. Distally, the infundibulum of the minor calyx is apparent as a narrowing ➡ before joining an adjacent minor calyx to form a major calyx. (Right) Smooth muscle actin (SMA) immunostain demonstrates the conspicuous lack of SMA(+) lamina propria fibroblasts in the papilla, which contain basement membrane only between collecting ducts and beneath the overlying urothelium.

Urothelium of the Minor Calyx

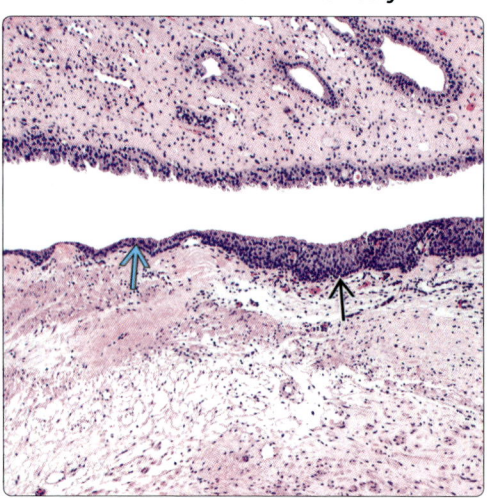

Urothelium of the Papilla

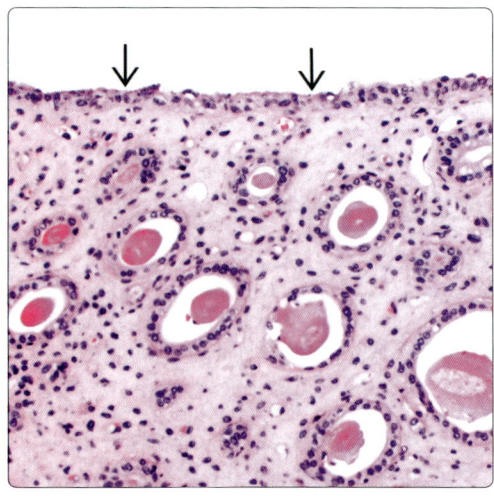

(Left) Here the tip of a papilla (upper) is juxtaposed to the wall of the minor calyx (lower). The urothelium, reactive-appearing and lining the minor calyx, ranges from more normal thickness ➡ to quite attenuated ➡. (Right) The urothelial lining of the tip of the papilla is quite attenuated, in some areas comprising only 2-3 cell layers ➡. No lamina propria is present such that the tubular basement membrane of the collecting ducts directly underlies the urothelium, with important consequences for staging carcinomas.

Lamina Propria and Smooth Muscle

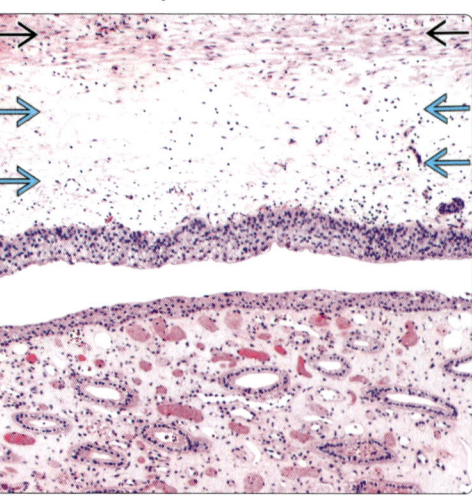

Lamina Propria and Smooth Muscle: Smooth Muscle Actin

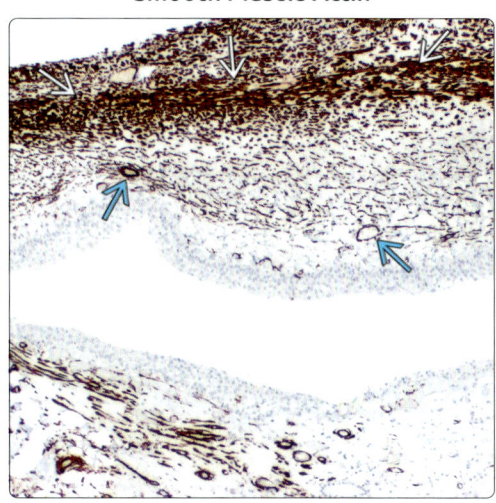

(Left) The lamina propria of the minor calyx is a loosely collagenized layer of fibroblasts and lymphovascular tissue ➡. A variable smooth muscle layer lies deep to the lamina propria ➡, but is less developed in the minor calyx than major calyces and renal pelvis. (Right) SMA stain highlights lamina propria myofibroblasts and the walls of scattered arterioles ➡; denser staining is apparent in the attenuated muscularis in this area ➡.

Microscopic Anatomy of Renal Pelvis

Muscularis Propria: Variability
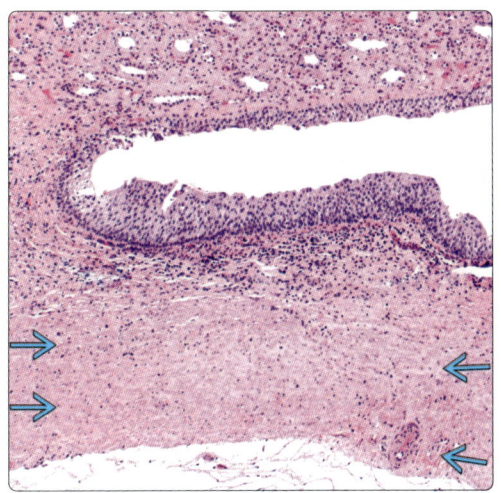

Muscularis Propria: Variability
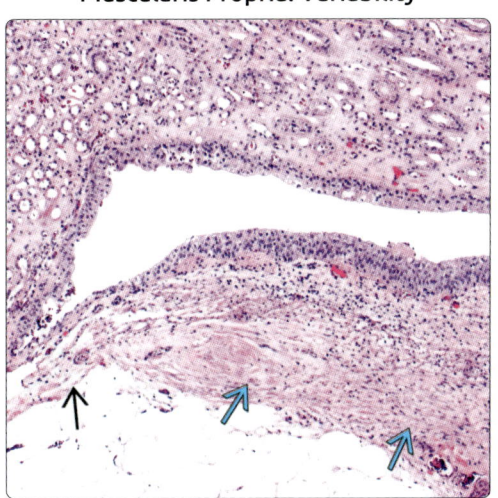

(Left) In the minor calyces, the smooth muscle layer of the muscularis propria is markedly variable, providing challenges in staging when there is involvement by a urothelial carcinoma. In this example, the muscularis is well developed ➡. (Right) Contrasting the case at left, the wall of this example of the minor calyx demonstrates a a wispy, attenuated muscularis ➡ that is focally absent, with lamina propria overlying renal sinus adipose ➡.

Renal Pelvis
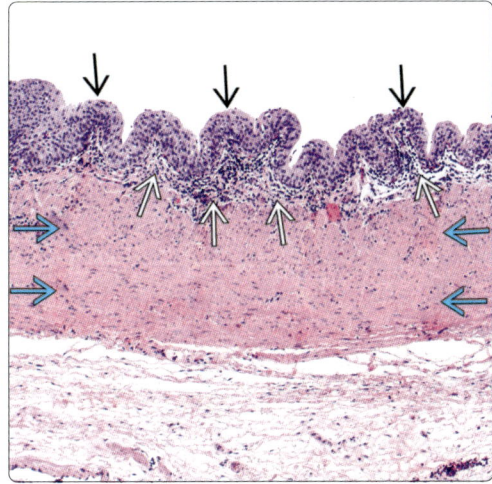

Proliferative Pyelitis
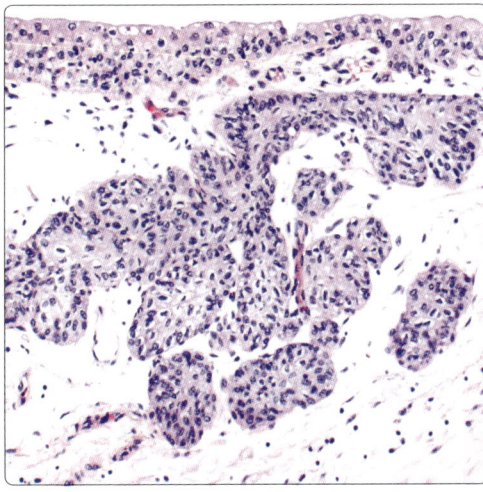

(Left) The renal pelvis shows a urothelial lining of the mucosa ➡, folded over the underlying lamina propria in the non-distended state ➡, with a well-formed, continuous underlying muscularis ➡. (Right) Similar to the urothelium of the ureter and bladder, the pelvicalyceal urothelium may show proliferation of nests of von Brunn. Cases of florid proliferative pyelitis may raise consideration of inverted urothelial papilloma.

Renal Sinus Soft Tissue
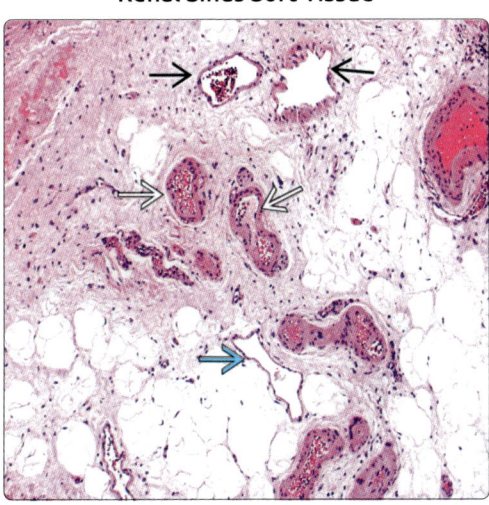

Renal Sinus Soft Tissue: Paraganglia
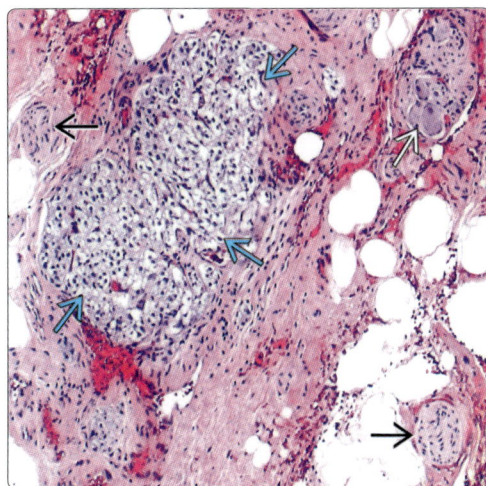

(Left) Interspersed between the renal calyces and the pelvis is the soft tissue of the renal sinus, a rich, variably fibrous and adipose connective tissue milieu with arteries ➡, veins ➡, and lymphatics ➡ representing favored sites for vascular invasion by both pelvicalyceal urothelial carcinomas and renal cell carcinomas. (Right) Here, incidental paraganglia ➡ are encountered closely juxtaposed to nerve branches ➡ and ganglia ➡. Paraganglia should not be mistaken for invasive urothelial or renal carcinoma.

Overview of Cystitis

TERMINOLOGY

Abbreviations
- Bacillus Calmette-Guérin (BCG)

Definitions
- Spectrum of nonneoplastic inflammatory conditions may involve urinary bladder

CYSTITIS SUBTYPES

Granulomatous Cystitis
- BCG effect following intravesical therapy for bladder carcinoma
  - Caseating or noncaseating granulomatous inflammation
  - Overlying urothelium may show reactive atypia or ulceration
  - Ziehl Neelsen stain may reveal acid-fast bacilli
    - Not generally performed
- Postsurgical granuloma (postsurgical necrobiotic granuloma)
  - Develops after transurethral resection of bladder
  - Traumatic granulomatous process
    - Linear or serpiginous contours with central fibrinoid necrosis
    - Rimmed by palisading histiocytes, some multinucleated
    - May resemble rheumatoid nodule
    - Surrounding inflammation comprised of lymphocytes and plasma cells
    - Eosinophils prominent following post excision to biopsy interval of < 1 month
    - Necrotic outlines of surrounding vessels may be seen
  - Tuberculous cystitis
    - Usually caseating granulomas with central necrosis surrounded by histiocytes and multinucleated giant cells
    - Early lesions generally in region of ureteral orifice
    - Systemic or localized tuberculosis infection
    - Most commonly caused by *Mycobacterium tuberculosis*
    - *Mycobacterium bovis* may rarely be causative agent
    - Acid-fast bacilli may be seen on Ziehl Neelsen stain
    - Typically no history of prior transurethral procedure or intravesical therapy
    - Urine or tissue cultures may be needed for diagnosis
  - Other rare noninfectious causes
    - Sarcoidosis
    - Crohn disease
    - Rheumatoid arthritis (rheumatoid nodule)

Follicular Cystitis
- Nonspecific pattern of inflammation
  - Lymphoid follicles with germinal center formation in lamina propria
  - Associated with bladder cancer, treatment or urinary tract infection
  - More prevalent in children but spans all ages
- Differential diagnosis
  - Low-grade lymphoma, such as follicular lymphoma
  - Readily distinguished by immunohistochemistry as in other sites

Eosinophilic Cystitis
- Descriptive term applied to mixed inflammatory infiltrates of lamina propria rich in eosinophils
  - Not a single diagnostic entity
- Often has polypoid appearance
  - May mimic polypoid cystitis or urothelial carcinoma in adults or rhabdomyosarcoma in children
- 4 clinical settings
  - Nonspecific localized process
    - Pattern of injury associated with a variety of etiologies
    - Prostatic hyperplasia, bladder carcinoma, or prior transurethral biopsy
  - Allergy associated
    - In children, seen in association with allergic gastroenteritis, asthma, or other allergic disorders
    - May rarely be drug induced
    - Peripheral blood eosinophilia may seen
  - Rarely, may be secondary to parasitic infection
  - Also seen in chronic granulomatous disease of childhood

BCG Granuloma

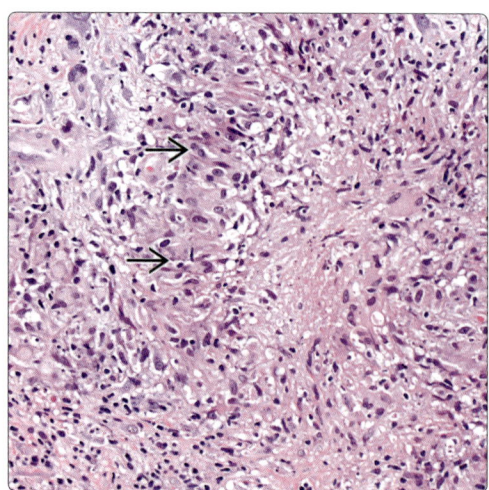

Eosinophilic Cystitis

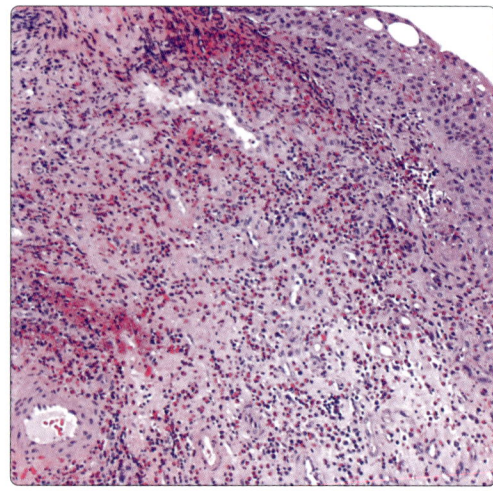

(Left) The palisading histiocytes ➡ forming this granuloma are secondary to intravesical bacillus Calmette-Guérin (BCG) therapy that was administered for urothelial carcinoma. (Right) In this example of eosinophilic cystitis, the eosinophilic infiltrate is striking. This may rarely be seen with allergic conditions in children. In adults, parasitic infection or association with an adjacent carcinoma or prior biopsy may be seen.

Overview of Cystitis

Emphysematous Cystitis
- Presence of gas-filled vesicles in bladder that are visible by cystoscopy or gross examination
- More common in women
- Clinical associations
  - Adults
    - Most commonly associated with diabetes mellitus/hyperglycemia
  - Children
    - Most commonly seen as complication of necrotizing enterocolitis
- By histology, multiple blebs (empty cavities) within lamina propria
  - Histiocytes, often multinucleate, or thin fibrous tissue surround clear spaces
- Caused by gas-forming bacteria
  - *Aerobacter aerogenes*
  - *Escherichia coli*
  - *Clostridium perfringens*

Interstitial Cystitis
- Chronic inflammatory process of unknown etiology
- Occurs almost exclusively in middle-aged and older women
- Some research has suggested possibility of autoimmune disorder
- Clinical symptoms
  - Urinary frequency, urgency, suprapubic pressure, and pain with either bladder distention or voiding
- Cystoscopy
  - Early nonulcer type
    - Small submucosal hemorrhagic foci (glomerulations) and linear cracks under hydrodistention
  - Classic ulcer type (Hunner ulcer)
    - Multiple reddened foci with small vessels radiating toward central scar or ulcer with fibrin accumulation
    - Increasing hydrodistention causes mucosal rupture at ulcer with oozing of blood
    - Bullous edema also common after distention
- Clinical diagnosis of exclusion
  - Urodynamic studies typically reveal decreased bladder-filling capacity
  - Urine cultures are negative, by definition
  - Prior therapies with known bladder irritants, concomitant urothelial neoplasia, and infections exclude interstitial cystitis
- Histologic features
  - No pathognomonic features
    - Important role for pathologists is exclusion of urothelial carcinoma in situ or specific form of cystitis
  - Common findings
    - Ulceration with variably admixed fibrin, erythrocytes, and inflammatory cells, especially neutrophils
    - Associated granulation tissue and perineural lymphocytic infiltrates are common
    - Urothelial denudation is frequent
    - Ulcers typically extend deep into lamina propria with surrounding edema and congestion
    - Without ulcers, morphologic changes may be subtle: Suburothelial hemorrhage, edema, and mucosal tears
    - Fibrosis of muscularis propria in longstanding disease
- Considerable debate regarding utility of mast cell counts in distinction from other inflammatory processes
  - Specificity in distinction from other inflammatory processes is questionable
  - Reports of increased intravesical mast cell infiltrates in patients with interstitial cystitis are cited
- Final diagnosis of interstitial cystitis requires close clinical (i.e., history, cystoscopy, and voiding studies) and pathologic correlation

Infectious Cystitis
- Not typically histologic diagnosis
  - Culture and serum tests are usually used for diagnosis
- Bacterial
  - Sexually active women (20-40 years old)
  - Dysuria, frequency, urgency, voiding small quantity
  - Common etiologies
    - *E. coli*, *Staphylococcus*, *Klebsiella*, *Proteus*, *Enterococci*
  - Tissue biopsy plays little role in diagnosis
    - Diagnosis by urine culture, urinalysis, and clinical symptoms
- Viral
  - Human papillomavirus
    - Associated with condyloma
  - Adenovirus
    - Important cause of hemorrhagic cystitis in children, particularly types 11 and 21
    - May occur after bone marrow or solid organ transplantation in any age group or in otherwise healthy children
  - Polyoma (BK) virus
    - Infection of immunocompromised (such as renal transplant) patients
    - Results in large nuclear inclusions in urothelial cells, so-called decoy cells, which may mimic carcinoma in situ
      - May be difficult to recognize in paraffin embedded sections
      - More easily seen in cytology preparations
  - Other viral causes of hemorrhagic cystitis
    - Polyomavirus and herpes simplex type 2
  - Herpes zoster may be associated with reversible voiding dysfunction
  - Cytomegalovirus may rarely involve bladder in immunocompromised patients
- Fungal
  - Fungal cystitis is uncommon
  - Debilitated patients on antibiotics or diabetics
  - *Candida albicans* most common; rarely *Aspergillus*
    - Secondary to ascending urethral infection or hematogenous spread
  - Cystoscopically
    - Small white mucosal plaques, but large fungal balls may rarely be seen
  - Histology
    - Ulceration and inflammation in lamina propria
    - Fungal hyphae may be visible on routine stains
    - Pseudohyphae and yeast forms in tissue section with PAS and silver stain

Overview of Cystitis

Giant Cell Cystitis
- Similar cells may be seen in patients treated with chemotherapeutic agents and radiation
- Not a clinical entity
  - Normal histologic finding
    - Commonly seen in bladder biopsy specimen without apparent pathology
  - Presence of atypical stromal cells in lamina propria of bladder
    - Enlarged, hyperchromatic, multilobated nuclei
    - Degenerative atypia
    - Mitoses absent or rare
- Differential diagnosis
  - Radiation atypia
    - More pronounced atypia with nucleoli
  - Sarcoma
    - Bladder sarcomas are almost always more cellular

Hemorrhagic Cystitis
- Severe hematuria shortly after exposure to inciting agent
  - Chemotherapeutic agents
    - Cyclophosphamide
    - Busulfan and thiotepa
  - Industrial exposure
    - Aniline and toluidine derivatives used in dyes and insecticides
  - Viral etiologies also well described
    - Adenovirus, types 11 and 21
    - Polyomavirus
      - Increasingly recognized after allogeneic hematopoietic stem cell transplantation for hematopoietic malignancy
    - Herpes simplex type 2
- Morphology
  - Extensive hemorrhage into lamina propria with vascular congestion and edema
  - Overlying epithelium with ulceration, necrosis, and nuclear atypia
    - Similar to radiation or intravesical chemotherapy-associated changes

Encrusted Cystitis
- Deposition of inorganic salts in bladder mucosa
- Caused by urea-splitting bacteria that alkalinize urine
- Most common in women
- Presenting symptoms are similar to other urinary tract infections
- Cystoscopically
  - Diffuse gritty appearance
- Morphologically
  - Fibrinous exudate with admixed calcified, necrotic debris, and inflammatory infiltrates
- Differential diagnosis
  - Carcinoma may have overlying calcification
    - Correlation with cystoscopic impression is important

Radiation Cystitis
- Urothelium may show striking cytologic atypia
  - Cytoplasmic and nuclear vacuolation with normal nuclear/cytoplasmic ratio
  - Karyorrhexis
- Stromal changes also seen
  - Atypical mesenchymal cells similar to those seen in giant cell cystitis in lamina propria
    - Usually have more pronounced atypia with nucleoli
  - Marked stromal edema or fibrosis
  - Prominent telangiectatic vessels with hyalinization and thrombosis
- Pseudocarcinomatous hyperplasia of epithelium may be seen
  - 75% are associated with pelvic radiation
  - Close mimic of invasive carcinoma
  - Epithelium closely associated with vessels and fibrin
- Differential diagnosis
  - Urothelial carcinoma in situ
    - Lack cytoplasmic vacuolization
    - More uniform nucleomegaly and hyperchromasia
    - Diffuse cytoplasmic cytokeratin 20 immunoreactivity throughout urothelium

Gangrenous Cystitis
- Necrosis generally begins in mucosa and may progress to involve entire wall to serosa
- Most commonly complication of infection
- Other causes
  - Systemic disorders
    - Severe diabetes mellitus
    - Sepsis
    - Vascular disease
  - Corrosive chemical injury

SELECTED REFERENCES

1. Amano M et al: Emphysematous cystitis: a review of the literature. Intern Med. 53(2):79-82, 2014
2. Gilis L et al: High burden of BK virus-associated hemorrhagic cystitis in patients undergoing allogeneic hematopoietic stem cell transplantation. Bone Marrow Transplant. 49(5):664-70, 2014
3. Kauffman CA: Diagnosis and management of fungal urinary tract infection. Infect Dis Clin North Am. 28(1):61-74, 2014
4. Kryvenko ON et al: Pseudocarcinomatous urothelial hyperplasia of the bladder: clinical findings and followup of 70 patients. J Urol. 189(6):2083-6, 2013
5. Kulchavenya E: Best practice in the diagnosis and management of urogenital tuberculosis. Ther Adv Urol. 5(3):143-51, 2013
6. Hinev A et al: Gangrenous cystitis: report of a case and review of the literature. Urol Int. 85(4):479-81, 2010
7. Kim MS et al: Eosinophilic cystitis associated with eosinophilic enterocolitis: case reports and review of the literature. Br J Radiol. 83(990):e122-5, 2010
8. Meria P et al: Encrusted cystitis and pyelitis. J Urol. 160(1):3-9, 1998
9. White MD et al: Gangrenous cystitis in the elderly: pathogenesis and management options. Br J Urol. 82(2):297-9, 1998
10. Bauer SB et al: Vesical manifestations of chronic granulomatous disease in children. Its relation to eosinophilic cystitis. Urology. 37(5):463-6, 1991
11. Eble JN et al: Post-surgical necrobiotic granulomas of urinary bladder. Urology. 35(5):454-7, 1990
12. Hansson S et al: Follicular cystitis in girls with untreated asymptomatic or covert bacteriuria. J Urol. 143(2):330-2, 1990
13. Gillenwater JY et al: Summary of the National Institute of Arthritis, Diabetes, Digestive and Kidney Diseases Workshop on Interstitial Cystitis, National Institutes of Health, Bethesda, Maryland, August 28-29, 1987. J Urol. 140(1):203-6, 1988
14. Hellstrom HR et al: Eosinophilic cystitis. A study of 16 cases. Am J Clin Pathol. 72(5):777-84, 1979
15. Fajardo LF et al: Radiation injury in surgical pathology. Part I. Am J Surg Pathol. 2(2):159-99, 1978
16. Rubin JS et al: Cyclophosphamide hemorrhagic cystitis. J Urol. 96(3):313-6, 1966

Overview of Cystitis

Hemorrhagic Cystitis

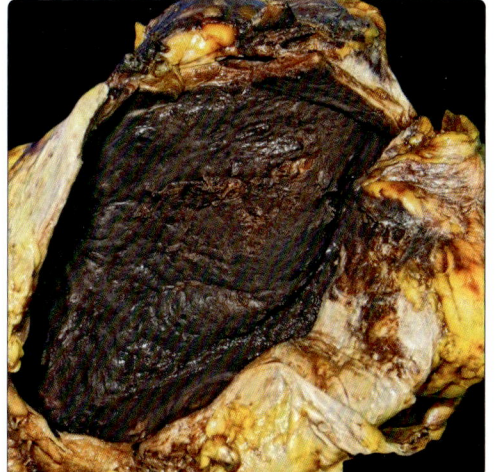

Follicular Cystitis

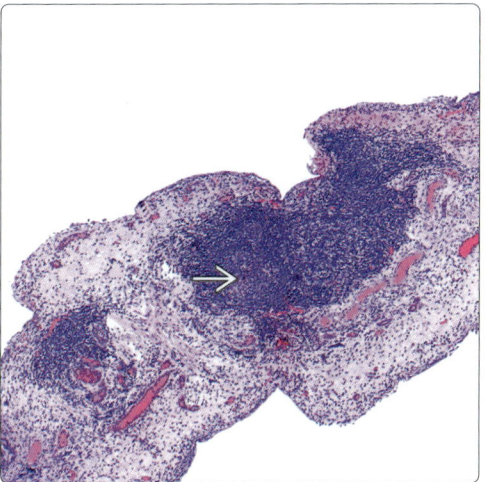

(Left) This urinary bladder specimen from a patient with hemorrhagic cystitis shows diffuse mucosal hemorrhage. Tissue biopsies are rarely performed in such patients. (Courtesy D. Regula, MD.) (Right) Follicular cystitis shows a dense lymphocytic inflammatory infiltrate in the lamina propria with central germinal center formation ➡. This pattern of inflammation is nonspecific but is most commonly associated with urinary tract infection.

Nonspecific Inflammation

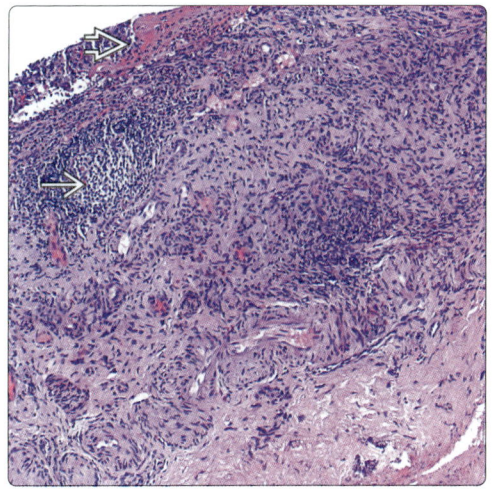

Nonspecific Inflammation

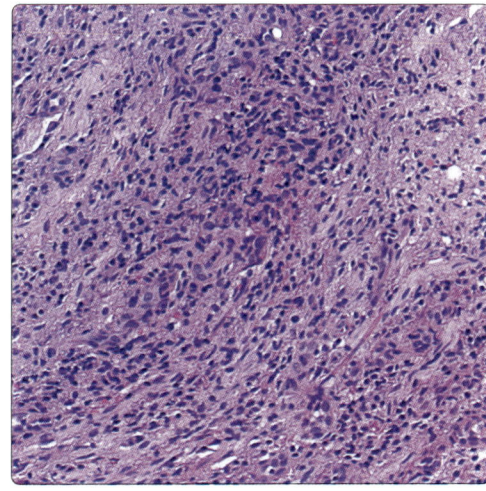

(Left) This bladder biopsy specimen shows evidence of ulceration ➡ and a mixed inflammatory infiltrate filling the lamina propria with rare lymphoid follicles ➡. This pattern is nonspecific and in some cases an etiology is not known. Such cases are best diagnosed descriptively. (Right) Occasionally, reactive lymphoid infiltrates of the bladder, as in this case of unknown etiology, may mimic lymphoma. B- and T-cell immunohistochemical markers show a mixed population in reactive lesions.

Normal Multinucleated Stromal Cells

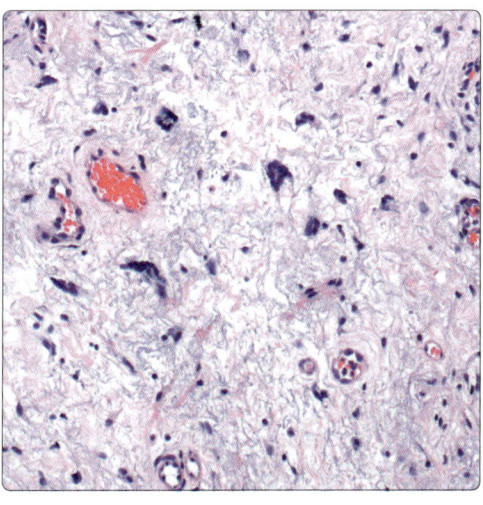

BCG Granuloma

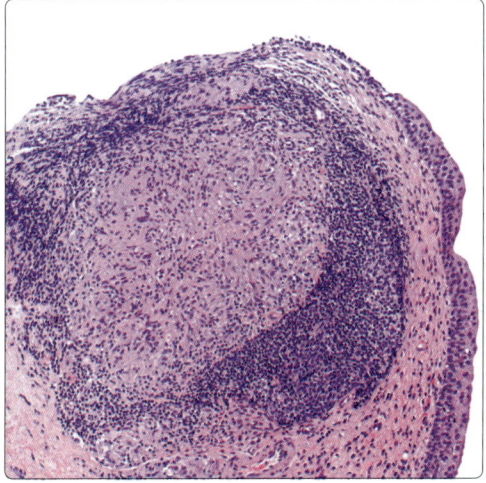

(Left) Multinucleated stromal cells within the lamina propria are a normal histologic feature, but have been referred to as giant cell cystitis when prominent. it is important to distinguish this from sarcomas or sarcomatoid carcinomas, which are much more cellular and mitotically active. (Right) This tightly formed, noncaseating granuloma with a cuff of lymphocytes was associated with prior bacillus Calmette-Guérin therapy. In the appropriate clinical context, stains for infectious organisms are not required.

Overview of Cystitis

Interstitial Cystitis

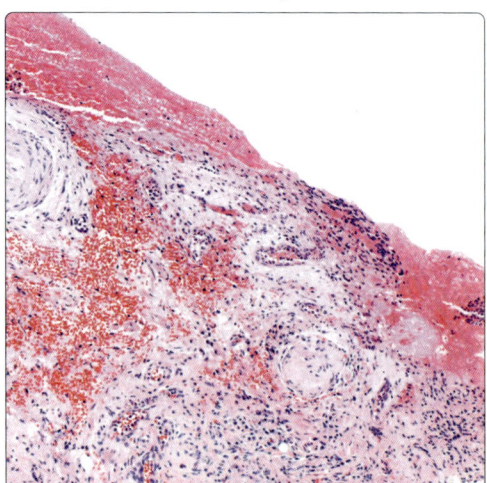

(Left) Many of the histologic changes seen in interstitial cystitis are nonspecific, such as ulceration, hemorrhage, and a mixed inflammatory infiltrate. Biopsy is important to exclude other causes, such as urothelial carcinoma in situ.

Interstitial Cystitis

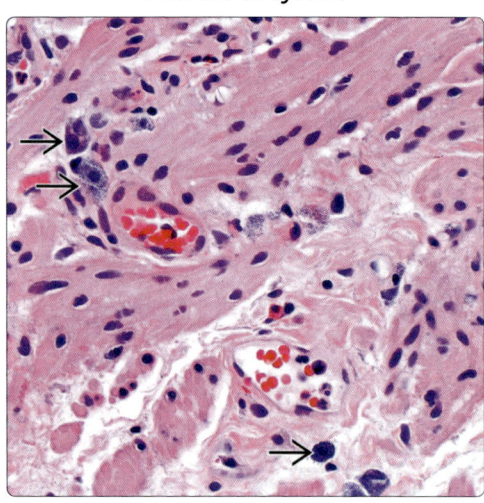

(Right) Increased numbers of mast cells ➡ may be seen within the muscularis propria in interstitial cystitis. The significance of mast cell counts to diagnose interstitial cystitis is controversial.

Interstitial Cystitis

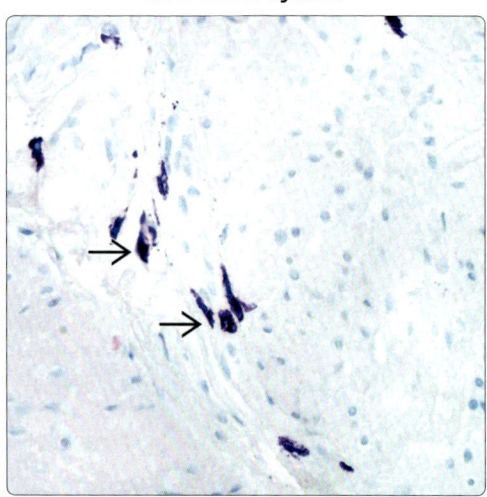

(Left) A pinacyanol erythrosinate stain highlights mast cells ➡ within the muscularis propria in interstitial cystitis. CD117 immunohistochemistry may also be used. The specificity of this finding for interstitial cystitis is controversial. Ultimately, the diagnosis of interstitial cystitis requires close correlation with voiding studies and cystoscopic findings.

Eosinophilic Cystitis

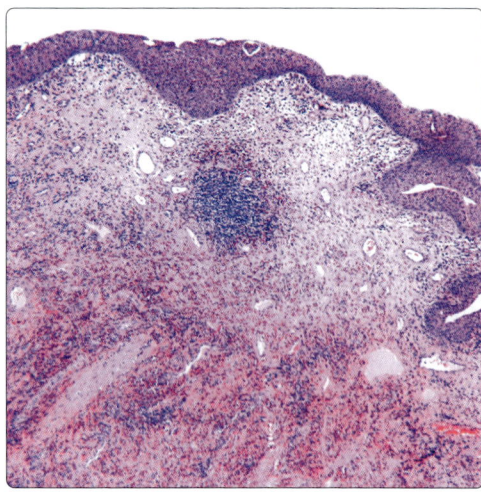

(Right) Eosinophilic cystitis is a nonspecific inflammatory infiltrate that is rich in eosinophils, which may form a radiographic mass lesion.

Encrusted Cystitis

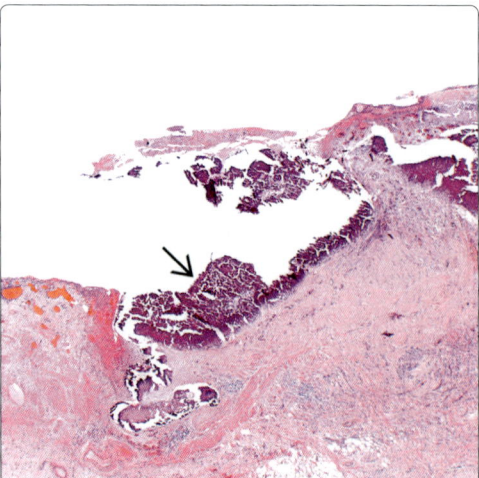

(Left) Occasionally, urea-splitting bacteria may alkalinize the urine and cause precipitation of inorganic salts. Morphologically, this results in calcified debris ➡ in the bladder mucosa, often with associated inflammatory infiltrates.

Encrusted Cystitis

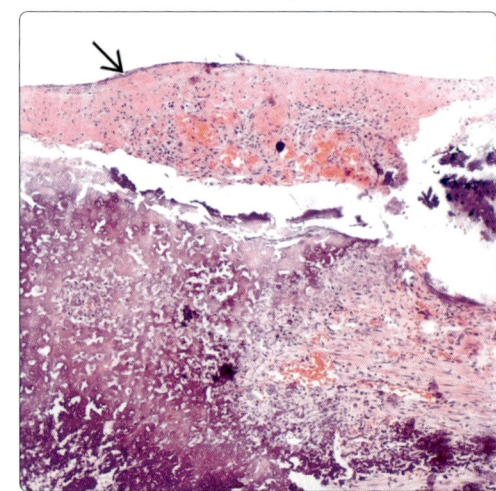

(Right) Calcified debris is associated with fibrin deposition ➡ in this encrusted cystitis. This may also be seen in other conditions that cause necrosis. Calcification overlying a necrotic carcinoma is the major differential consideration.

Overview of Cystitis

Radiation Cystitis
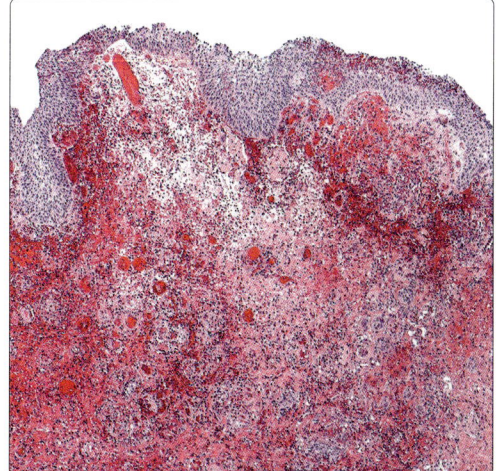

Radiation Cystitis
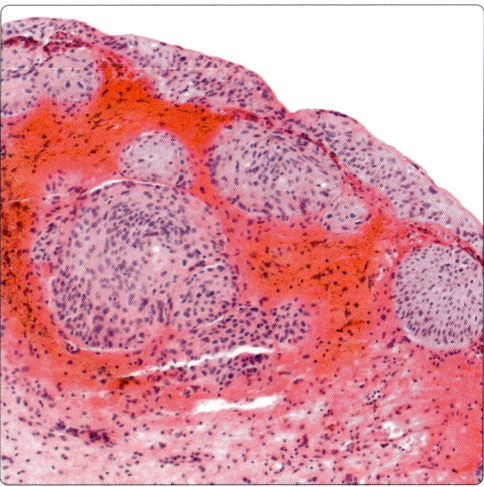

(Left) The first histologic clue to radiation cystitis is typically extensive hemorrhage into the lamina propria, typically with abnormal blood vessels and fibrin. (Right) Radiation may induce a variety of histologic changes, such as stromal hemorrhage, as seen in this example. Displaced nests of benign urothelium are also common. Radiation therapy for prostate and gynecologic tract cancers is the most common association.

Radiation Cystitis
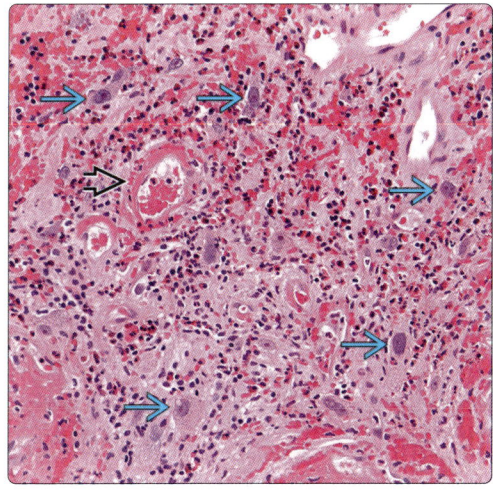

Radiation Cystitis: Pseudocarcinomatous Hyperplasia
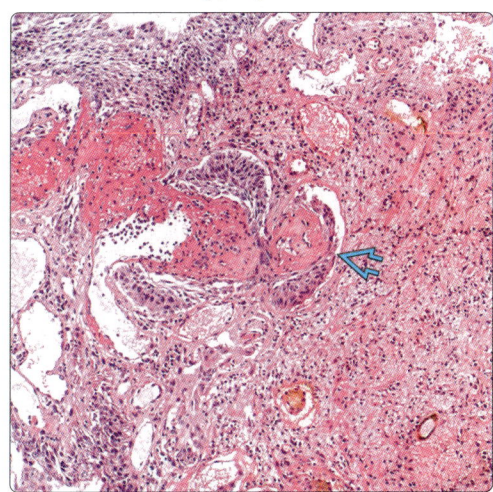

(Left) In addition to hemorrhage, radiation cystitis is also commonly characterized by the presence of large atypical stromal cells ➡. Abnormal vessels with fibrinoid change are also common and are present in this example ➡. (Right) Rare cases of radiation cystitis have areas showing urothelial nests deep in the lamina propria with associated fibrin and hemorrhage ➡. This pattern of injury may closely mimic carcinoma. Fibrin within vessels and associated atypical stromal cells are useful in correct identification.

Biopsy-Related Granuloma
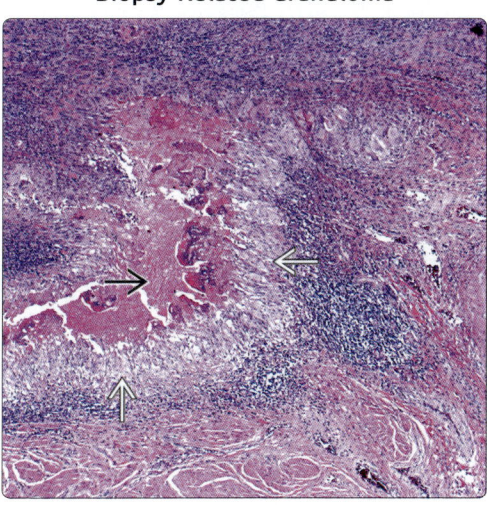

Biopsy-Related Changes
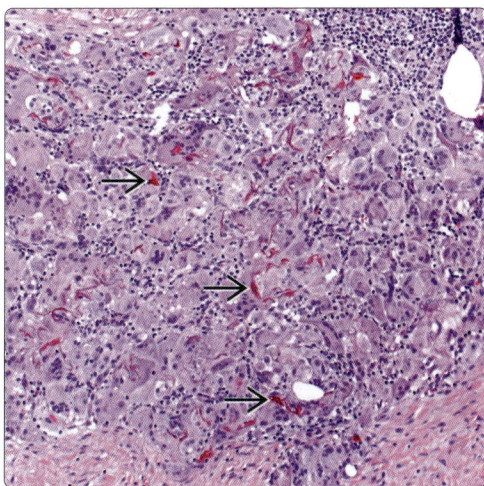

(Left) This granuloma is associated with a prior transurethral resection for a noninvasive papillary urothelial carcinoma. These granulomas commonly have linear or serpiginous contours with central fibrinoid necrosis ➡ and a rim of palisading histiocytes ➡, some multinucleated. (Right) Postbiopsy granulomas may also be associated with pigment deposition ➡ from hemorrhage and subsequent red cell breakdown products.

Papillary-Polypoid Cystitis

KEY FACTS

TERMINOLOGY
- Papillary-polypoid cystitis is nonneoplastic inflammatory lesion of urinary bladder
- Characterized by edema of lamina propria and exophytic polypoid or papillary projections

ETIOLOGY/PATHOGENESIS
- Many cases are related to indwelling catheter or vesical fistula

CLINICAL ISSUES
- May affect any age group
- Hematuria
- Irritative bladder symptoms from underlying cause
- No excision required if appropriately identified as nonneoplastic

MICROSCOPIC
- Characterized by variable exophytic projections of urothelium secondary to lamina propria edema
- Papillae lack complex branching typical of papillary urothelial neoplasia
- Stromal cores are composed of edema and fibrosis, not typical fibrovascular cores of papillary urothelial neoplasia
- Stromal cores are characteristically broader at base and taper to point distally
- Reactive urothelial atypia may be prominent

TOP DIFFERENTIAL DIAGNOSES
- Papillary urothelial neoplasia
  - Papilloma and papillary urothelial neoplasm of low malignant potential most commonly considered
  - With marked reactive urothelial atypia, carcinomas may also be considered
- Exophytic prostatic adenocarcinoma of prostatic urethra
  - May be very subtle lesion with bland adenomatous appearance
- Papillary nephrogenic adenoma
  - Single cuboidal layer of lining epithelium

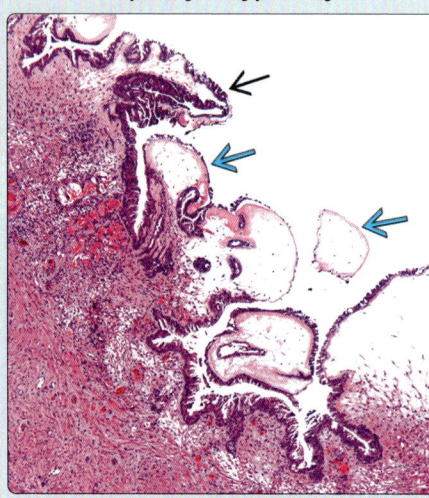

Papillary-Polypoid Cystitis

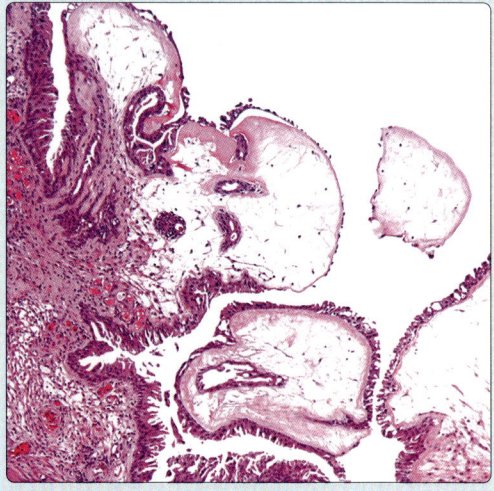

Papillary-Polypoid Cystitis

(Left) This architecture, best seen at low magnification, is characterized by broad, bulbous excrescences of the urothelium ➡ and is typical of papillary-polypoid cystitis. Occasional slender papillary excrescences ➡ are also seen in this example. (Right) Marked stromal edema is striking within the exophytic polypoid excrescences in this example of papillary-polypoid cystitis. There are associated urothelial changes, including extensive denudation. Where present, the urothelium is unremarkable or shows reactive atypia.

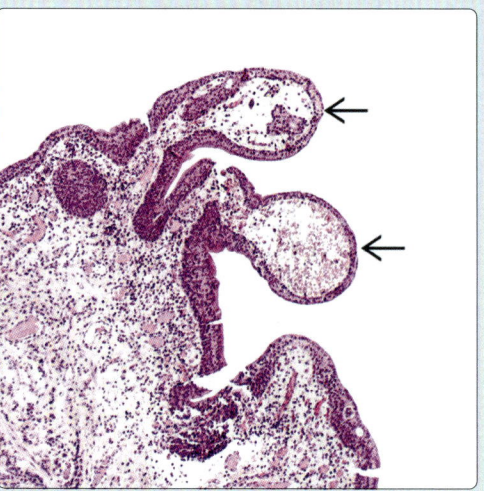

Papillary-Polypoid Cystitis

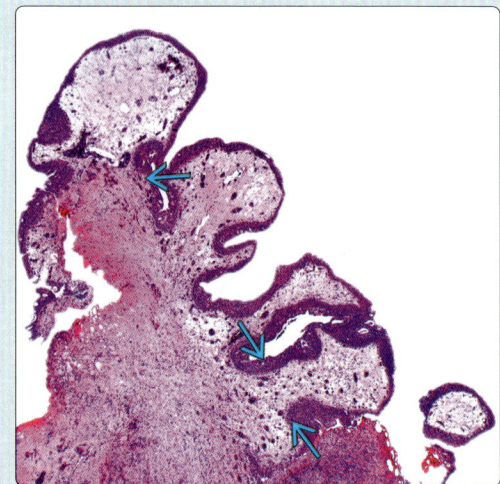

Papillary-Polypoid Cystitis

(Left) The bulbous tips ➡ of these simple papillae are characteristic of papillary-polypoid cystitis. This expansion is secondary to edema within the stalk and lamina propria. (Right) The broad-based connections of the polypoid excrescences to the underlying bladder ➡ are a key diagnostic feature of papillary-polypoid cystitis. The excrescences do not have significant branching.

Papillary-Polypoid Cystitis

TERMINOLOGY

Synonyms
- Papillary cystitis
- Polypoid cystitis
- Bullous cystitis
- Catheter-induced pseudopolyps

Definitions
- Nonneoplastic inflammatory lesion of urinary bladder
  - Exophytic polypoid or papillary projections
  - Characterized by edema and fibrosis of lamina propria

ETIOLOGY/PATHOGENESIS

Instrumentation
- Indwelling catheter

Inflammatory Conditions
- Vesical fistula

Radiation Therapy
- May follow regional radiation therapy
  - Gynecologic, prostatic, or bladder cancer most common

Tumor Association
- May be seen in association with urothelial carcinoma

CLINICAL ISSUES

Epidemiology
- Age
  - May affect any age group
- Sex
  - Equal gender distribution

Presentation
- Hematuria
- Irritative bladder symptoms from underlying cause
- Often seen incidentally in pathology specimens sent for other lesions
  - Also found in urethra, ureter, and renal pelvis

Endoscopic Findings
- Multifocal
- Appears as friable mucosal irregularity
  - Edematous broad or elongated, thin papillae adjacent to inflamed area
- Generalized edema common

Treatment
- No excision needed if appropriately clinically recognized as nonneoplastic
- Removal of inciting inflammatory factors required

Prognosis
- Benign lesion with no risk of evolving into carcinoma

MACROSCOPIC

Size
- Usually small lesions (up to 5 mm)

MICROSCOPIC

Histologic Features
- Variable exophytic projections of urothelium secondary to lamina propria edema
- Papillae lack complex secondary or tertiary branching typical of papillary urothelial neoplasia
- Stromal cores are composed of edema and fibrosis
  - Characteristically broader at base and taper to point toward lumen
  - Not typical fibrovascular cores of papillary urothelial neoplasia
  - Edema is more pronounced in early lesions with resultant broader papillae
  - Papillae become thin with more fibrotic stroma over time
- Acute and chronic inflammation may be seen in underlying lamina propria
- Hyperplastic urothelium may be seen
- Reactive urothelial atypia may be prominent
  - May add to morphologic overlap with papillary urothelial neoplasia
    - Potential for significant overdiagnosis as carcinoma
- Occasional areas may show foci indistinguishable from papillary urothelial neoplasia
  - In such cases, important to assess lesion in its entirety
  - If background lamina propria and other papillae are edematous and inflamed, diagnosis of papillary-polypoid cystitis is likely

Cytologic Features
- Reactive

Predominant Pattern/Injury Type
- Papillary
- Interstitial edema
- Fibrosis

Predominant Cell/Compartment Type
- Epithelial, urothelial

Bullous Cystitis
- Elevations are broad; width greater than height
- Extensive edema

Polypoid Cystitis
- Broad-based thick papillae

Papillary Cystitis
- Well-developed, slender, finger-like papillae with associated lamina propria fibrosis

DIFFERENTIAL DIAGNOSIS

Papillary Urothelial Neoplasia
- Urothelial papilloma and papillary urothelial neoplasm of low malignant potential are closest mimics
- Papillary cores are typically thin and delicate in lower grade papillary urothelial neoplasms
  - Compared to broad and edematous in papillary-polypoid cystitis

Papillary-Polypoid Cystitis

- Detached distal papillary fronds of papillary cystitis without underlying lamina propria may closely mimic papillary urothelial neoplasia
- Papillary urothelial neoplasms generally branch into smaller papillae
  - Complex anastomosis or secondary/tertiary branching favors carcinoma
- Low-grade and high-grade papillary urothelial carcinomas have greater degree of cytologic atypia
  - Must be distinguished from reactive atypia common to papillary-polypoid cystitis

Papillary Nephrogenic Adenoma
- May have admixed architectural patterns
  - Papillary
  - Tubular/tubulocystic
  - Solid/diffuse
    - Recognition of solid or tubular patterns excludes papillary/polypoid cystitis
- Lined by single layer of cytologically bland cuboidal epithelium
  - In contrast to stratified layer of urothelial cells in papillary urothelial lesions
- Epithelial cells show strong nuclear pax-8 expression by immunohistochemistry
- May also have variable intralesional GATA3 staining

Fibroepithelial Polyp
- More common in ureter and renal pelvis
- Large bulbous polypoid lesion covered by urothelium
  - Stroma more fibrous
    - More cellular and may contain atypical stromal cells or rarely myxoid matrix
- Some authors have suggested it may represent late phase of papillary-polypoid cystitis
  - Distinction in difficult cases has little clinical significance

Hamartoma
- Typically has more cellular stroma
- Invaginated epithelium may resemble cystitis glandularis

Prostatic-Type Polyp (Ectopic Prostate)
- Similar architecture
- Contains prostatic secretory and basal epithelium admixed with urothelium
  - Immunoreactivity for PSA, PAP, PSMA, and NKX-3.1

Tamm-Horsfall Polyp
- Very rare lesion
- Contain waxy eosinophilic material

Collagen Polyp
- Incidental finding after collagen injection utilized during surgical procedures
  - Often for urinary incontinence
- Contains very dense, homogeneous collagen

Amyloid
- Rarely, amyloid may present as polypoid mass
- May be confirmed by adjunctive testing to distinguish from collagen
  - Congo red stain
  - Thioflavin S fluorescence

Prostatic Adenocarcinoma
- Ductal type adenocarcinoma more commonly presents as urethral polyp
  - May be histologically subtle lesion
    - Often cytologically bland adenomatous appearance
    - Pseudostratified columnar lining common
    - More architecturally complex prostatic epithelium
      - Cribriform foci with acinar formation is feature of carcinoma
- Rare prostatic acinar adenocarcinomas have papillary or pseudopapillary architecture
- PSA, PAP, PSMA, and NKX-3.1 immunoreactivity in epithelium
- Once prostatic adenocarcinoma is suspected, basal cell layer markers are important to be performed; absence of expression confirms carcinoma

DIAGNOSTIC CHECKLIST

Clinically Relevant Pathologic Features
- Gross appearance
  - May be cystoscopically similar to papillary neoplasm
  - Edema and inflammatory changes are common
- Urologist often has endoscopic impression of nonneoplastic inflammatory process

Pathologic Interpretation Pearls
- Papillary-polypoid cystitis must be considered in differential of papillary urothelial neoplasms
  - Architecture as evaluated at screening magnification is critical to recognition
- Urothelial neoplasms should be diagnosed with caution in patients with indwelling catheters or vesical fistulas
- Great caution should be exercised in small ureter or renal pelvic biopsies
  - More difficult distinction due to smaller samples obtained
  - Superficial biopsies of only papillary tips may be impossible to diagnose correctly

SELECTED REFERENCES

1. Gordetsky J et al: Pseudopapillary features in prostatic adenocarcinoma mimicking urothelial carcinoma: a diagnostic pitfall. Am J Surg Pathol. 38(7):941-5, 2014
2. Aydin H et al: Ductal adenocarcinoma of the prostate diagnosed on transurethral biopsy or resection is not always indicative of aggressive disease: implications for clinical management. BJU Int. 105(4):476-80, 2010
3. Lane Z et al: Polypoid/papillary cystitis: a series of 41 cases misdiagnosed as papillary urothelial neoplasia. Am J Surg Pathol. 32(5):758-64, 2008
4. Kiliç S et al: Polypoid cystitis unrelated to indwelling catheters: a report of eight patients. Int Urol Nephrol. 34(3):293-7, 2002
5. Norlén LJ et al: Effects of indwelling catheters on the urethral mucosa (polypoid urethritis). Scand J Urol Nephrol. 22(2):81-6, 1988
6. Young RH: Papillary and polypoid cystitis. A report of eight cases. Am J Surg Pathol. 12(7):542-6, 1988
7. Milles G: Catheter-induced hemorrhagic pseudopolyps of the urinary bladder. JAMA. 193:968-9, 1965

Papillary-Polypoid Cystitis

Polypoid Cystitis
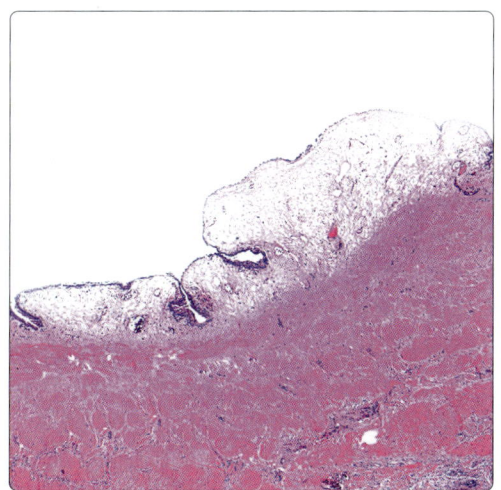

Polypoid Cystitis
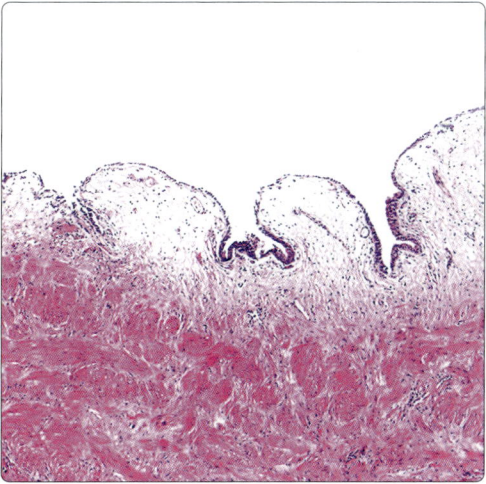

(Left) *In this example, the excrescences are much broader than they are tall. Even at low magnification, there is an edematous appearance to the lamina propria. This feature represents the earliest form of papillary-polypoid cystitis and is seen very commonly in the renal pelvis.* **(Right)** *As papillary-polypoid cystitis develops, the bulbous processes become more elongated, but the base remains much broader than typical of papillary urothelial neoplasia.*

Polypoid Cystitis/Urethritis
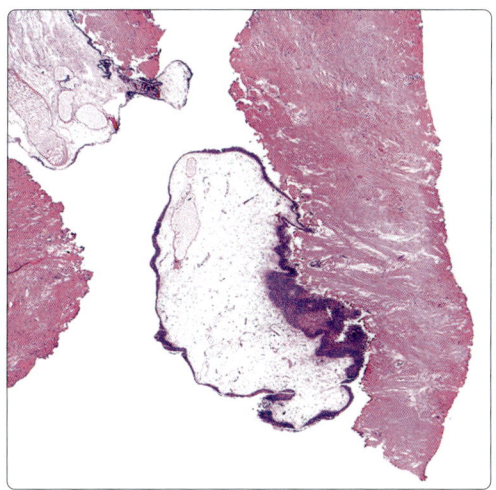

Polypoid Cystitis
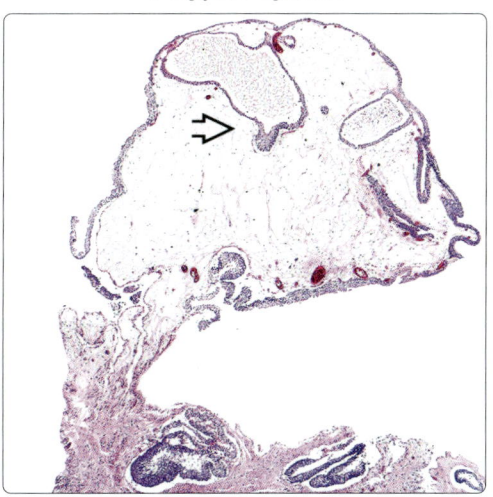

(Left) *In this transurethral resection specimen performed for benign prostatic hyperplasia, foci of polypoid urethritis were present. As in other locations, it is characterized by broad bulbous excrescences with central edema. The connection with the the surface urothelium may not be seen in unoriented fragments.* **(Right)** *Occasional examples of polypoid cystitis may have entrapped urothelium (cystitis cystica) ➔. The bulbous architecture and prominent edema are distinctive.*

Papillary-Polypoid Cystitis
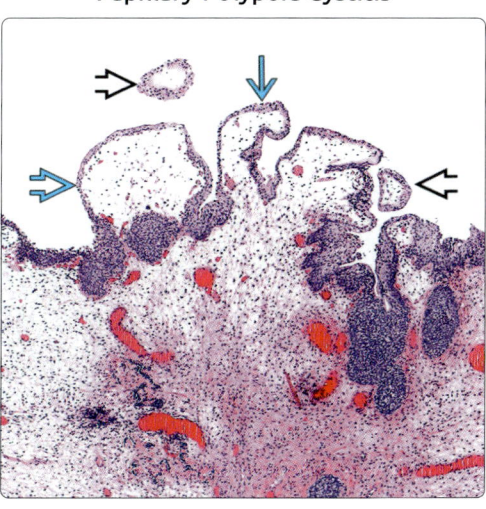

Papillary Cystitis Mimicking Urothelial Carcinoma
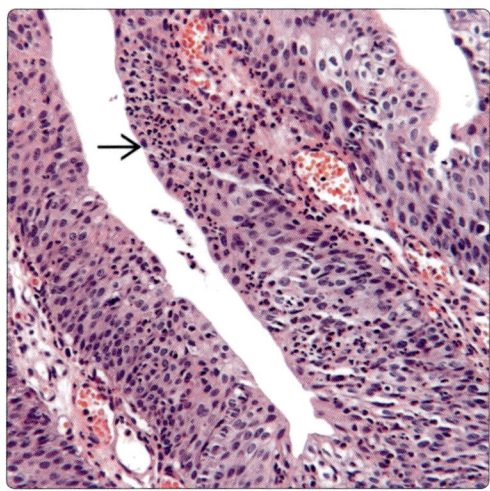

(Left) *This example of papillary-polypoid cystitis shows an admixture of bulbous ➔ and more slender ➔ excrescences. Out of context, the tips of the excrescences ➔ may be indistinguishable from papillary neoplasia.* **(Right)** *Out of context, this area in a urothelial proliferation mimics urothelial carcinoma. The prominent neutrophilic infiltrate ➔ is helpful in recognizing the inflammatory nature of this lesion as the background lesion had typical histology of papillary-polypoid cystitis.*

Papillary-Polypoid Cystitis

(Left) As papillary-polypoid cystitis progresses, the papillary cores often become more fibrotic and the excrescences may become more elongated. In contrast to urothelial neoplasms, complex hierarchical branching is absent. **(Right)** The larger bulbous excrescence in this example of papillary-polypoid cystitis is more fibrotic ➡ than edematous and is becoming somewhat more elongated. The attachment at the base remains relatively broad ➡.

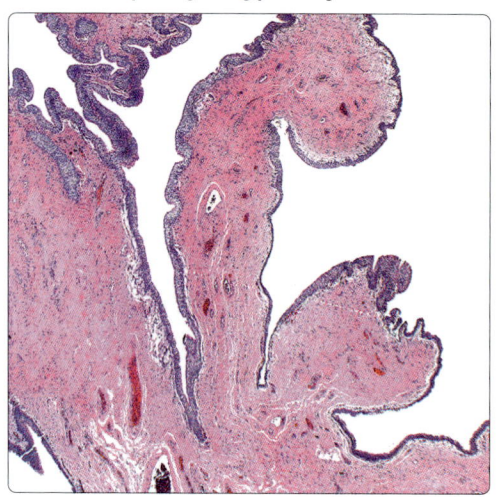
Papillary-Polypoid Cystitis

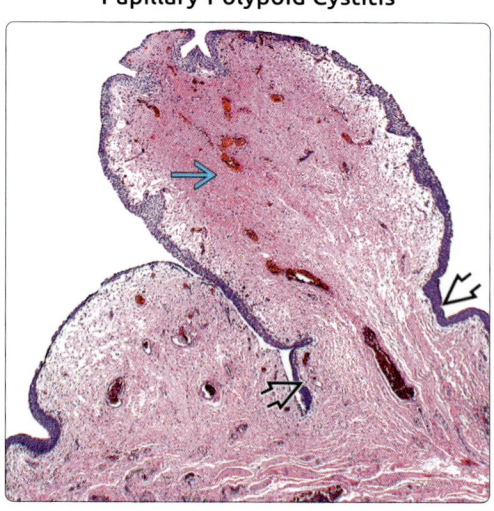
Papillary-Polypoid Cystitis

(Left) If the tips of the excrescences are cut tangentially ➡ such that some are not connected to the underlying bladder, the architecture may appear somewhat more complex than typical. The lack of secondary and tertiary branching and the broad connection at the base are characteristic of papillary-polypoid cystitis. **(Right)** This example of papillary-polypoid cystitis shows a typical bulbous excrescence with a broad base ➡. Simple branching with more slender papillae may be seen ➡.

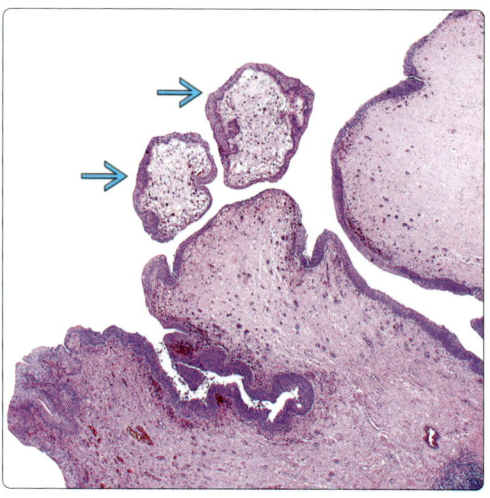
Papillary-Polypoid Cystitis

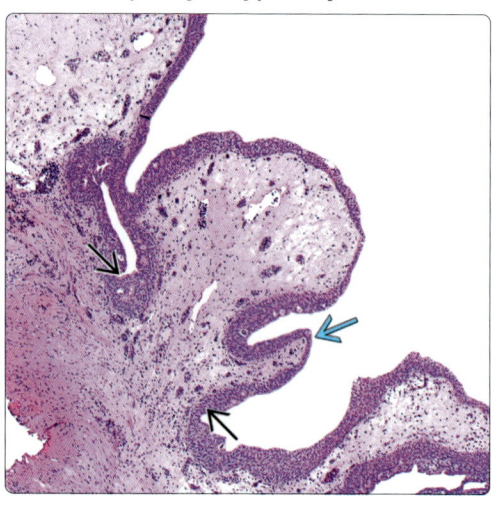
Papillary-Polypoid Cystitis

(Left) Focal areas within papillary-polypoid cystitis may be practically indistinguishable from a small papillary urothelial neoplasm ➡, but the broad-based bulbous excrescence is diagnostic ➡. It is important to evaluate the context of the entire lesion. **(Right)** In late phases of papillary-polypoid cystitis ➡, the exophytic processes may lack the prototypical bulbous edema; however, the absence of secondary and tertiary branching should aid in the recognition as papillary cystitis.

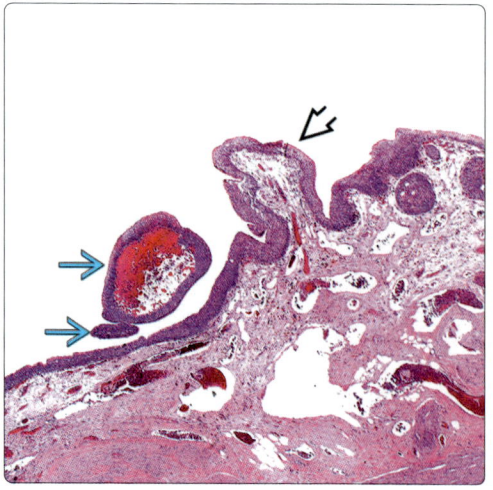
Papillary-Polypoid Cystitis

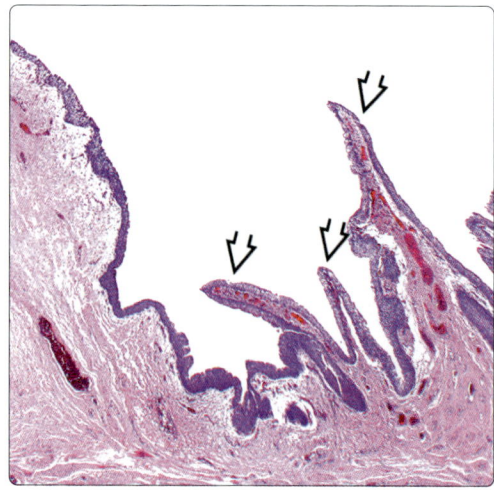
Papillary-Polypoid Cystitis

Papillary-Polypoid Cystitis

Papillary-Polypoid Cystitis

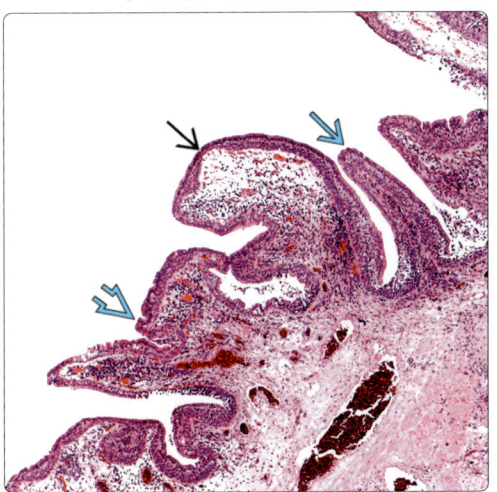

Papillary-Polypoid Cystitis

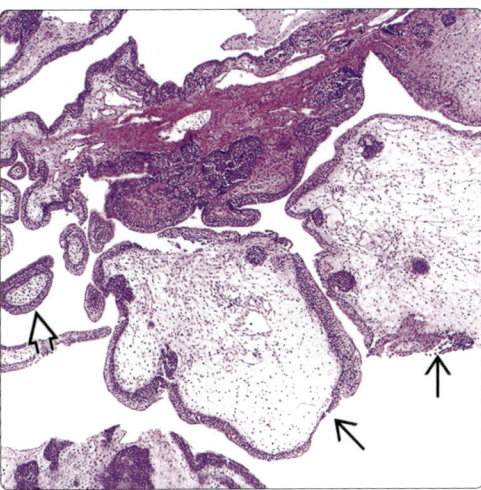

(Left) This example of papillary-polypoid cystitis shows a heterogeneous group of both slender ⇨ and bulbous ⇨ excrescences. Some excrescences have a simple branching architecture ⇨. **(Right)** Admixed large edematous papillae ⇨ are diagnostic of papillary-polypoid cystitis. Smaller papillae ⇨ may cause diagnostic confusion.

Papillary-Polypoid Cystitis

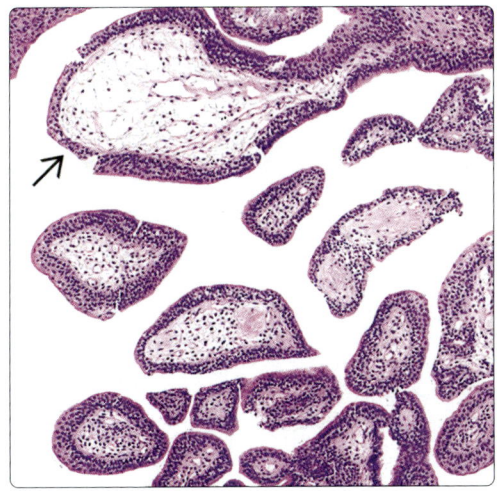

Papillary Urothelial Neoplasm

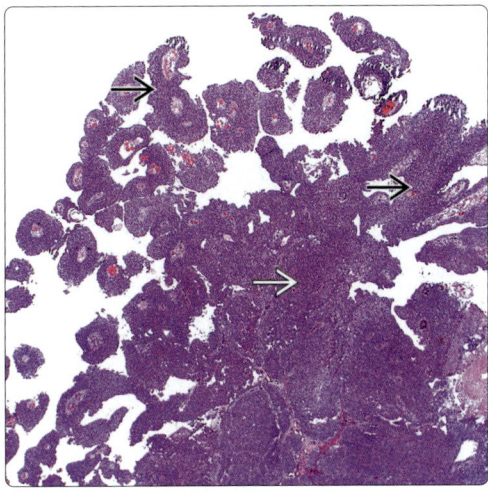

(Left) When the distal tips of papillary-polypoid cystitis are biopsied, there may be significant overlap with a papillary urothelial neoplasm. Recognition of the more broad papillae toward the base, scattered edematous cores ⇨, and the absence of complex anastomosing or hierarchical branching aids in recognition as papillary cystitis. **(Right)** This degree of epithelial confluence ⇨ and the areas of solid growth ⇨ are diagnostic of a papillary urothelial neoplasm and would preclude a diagnosis of papillary cystitis.

Urothelial Papilloma

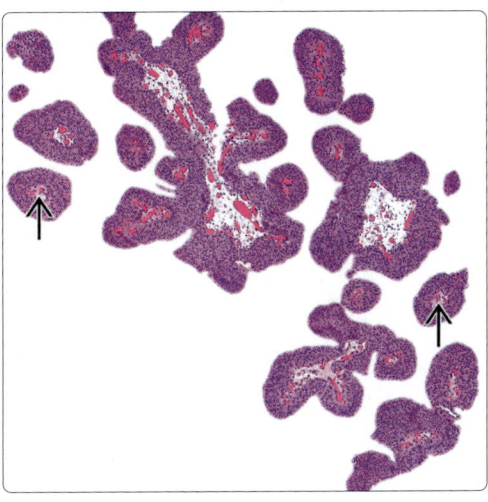

Urothelial Papilloma

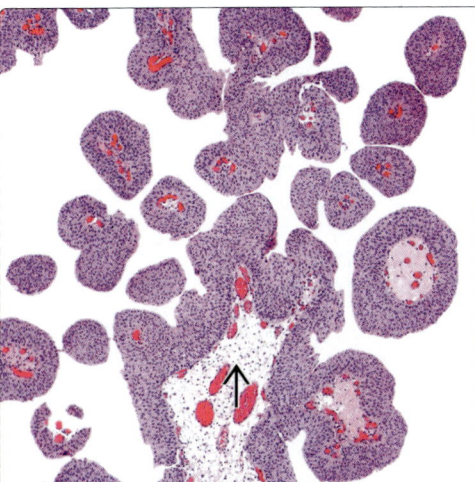

(Left) Very thin fibrovascular cores ⇨, as seen in this example of urothelial papilloma, are typical of papillary urothelial neoplasms. The papillae of papillary-polypoid cystitis generally have a greater amount of stroma with prominent edema. **(Right)** This urothelial papilloma has prominent secondary branching from a central fibrovascular core ⇨, a feature typical of papillary urothelial neoplasms.

Papillary-Polypoid Cystitis

(Left) Urothelial papilloma may have some unique architectural patterns within the cores. This example highlights an unusual gland-in-gland pattern ⇨ and dilated lymphatics with prominent fluid within the core ⇨, features not typical of papillary-polypoid cystitis. **(Right)** The central lymphatic fluid ⇨ seen in this example is a histologic feature that is more common in urothelial papilloma.

Urothelial Papilloma
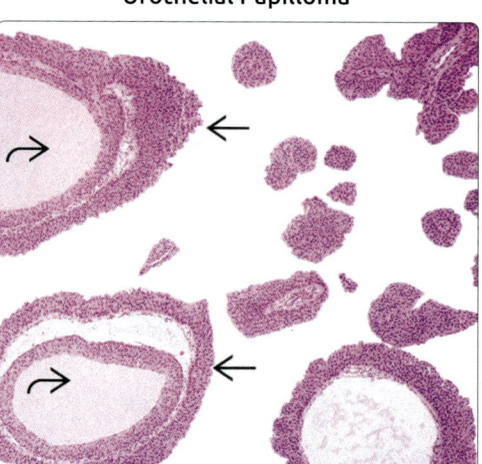

Urothelial Papilloma
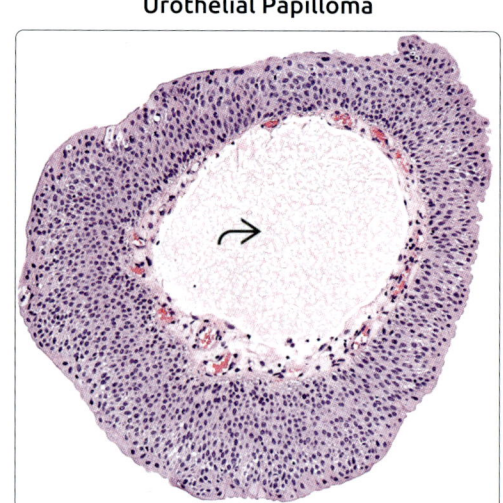

(Left) Urothelial papilloma has more complex papillary architecture and often has a very prominent layer of vacuolated umbrella cells ⇨. Thin fibrovascular cores are helpful to exclude papillary cystitis. **(Right)** Papillary nephrogenic adenoma is shown with variably sized papillae lined by a single cuboidal epithelial layer. Associated edema is not prominent. Admixed glandular/tubular patterns may also be seen ⇨, aiding in the diagnosis. Reactive atypia of the lining cells mimics glandular neoplasia.

Urothelial Papilloma
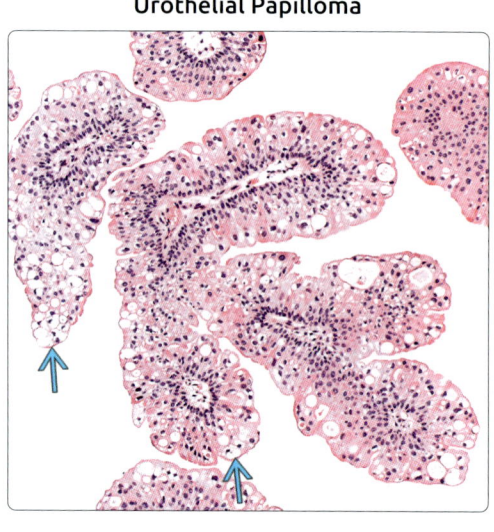

Nephrogenic Adenoma
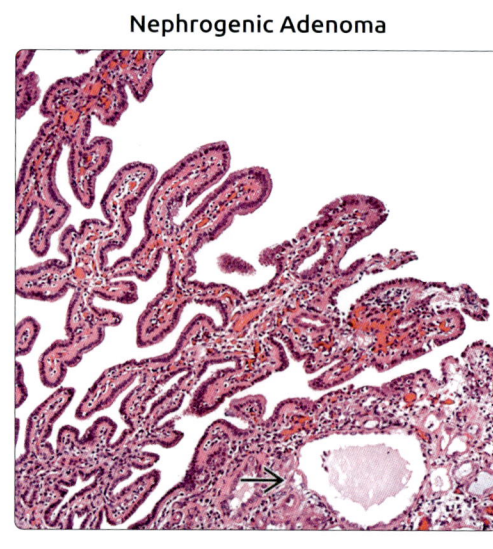

(Left) Papillary nephrogenic adenoma is characteristically lined by a single cuboidal layer of epithelium with bland cytologic figures. In contrast, papillary cystitis has larger and thicker papillae with a stratified urothelial layer. **(Right)** On high magnification, the single cuboidal layer of epithelium lining the papillary cores is highlighted. This feature is characteristic of nephrogenic adenoma. Background inflammation and neovascularity may be prominent.

Nephrogenic Adenoma
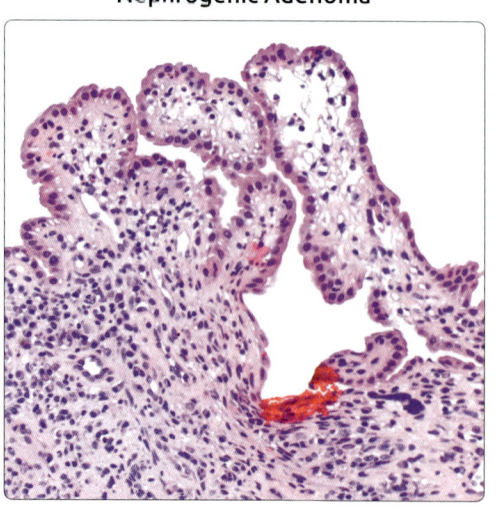

Nephrogenic Adenoma
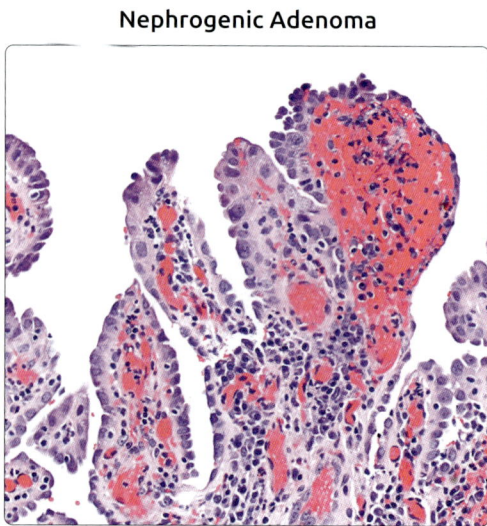

Papillary-Polypoid Cystitis

Prostatic Ductal Carcinoma

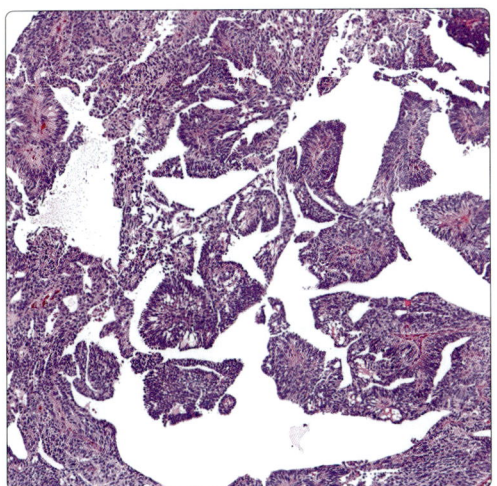

Prostatic Ductal Carcinoma

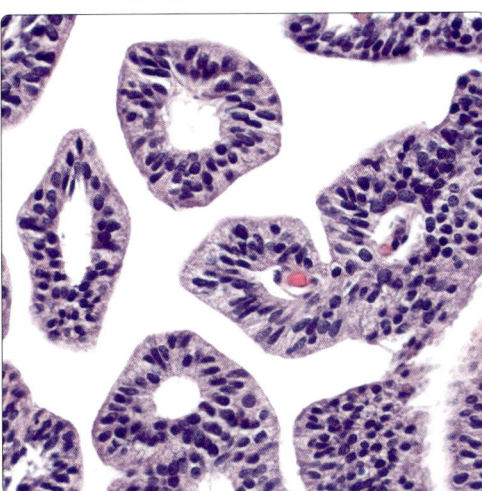

(Left) Prostatic ductal adenocarcinoma often has a papillary architecture and may present as a primary urethral lesion. The papillae may have variable architecture, but the complexity and the cytologic features are distinctive. This combination has a distinctive adenomatous appearance. **(Right)** *On high-power magnification, prostatic ductal adenocarcinoma may appear cytologically bland and the pseudostratified columnar arrangement may be subtle and difficult to appreciate in some foci.*

Prostatic Ductal Carcinoma

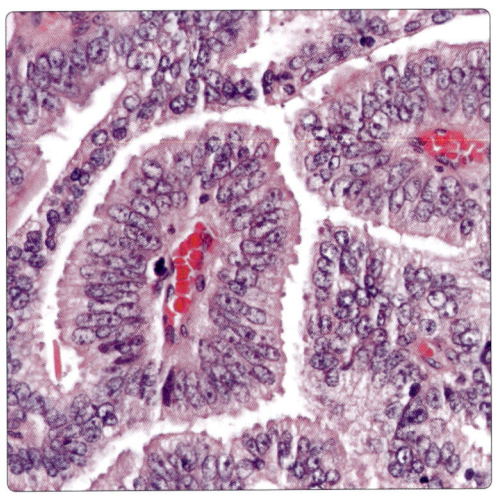

Prostatic Ductal Carcinoma

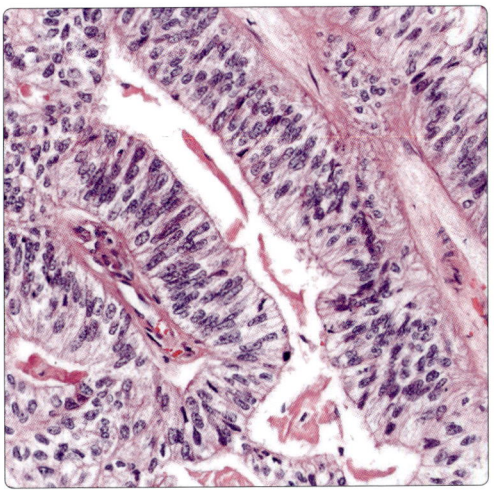

(Left) In this example of prostatic ductal adenocarcinoma, the cytologic features should suggest prostatic adenocarcinoma given the monomorphic cells with nucleomegaly and prominent nucleoli. **(Right)** *Prostatic ductal adenocarcinoma is shown with well-developed pseudostratified columnar epithelium, a very characteristic feature that should aid in distinction from reactive or benign papillary lesions. Enteric lesions of bladder occur in background of intestinal metaplasia.*

Prostatic Adenocarcinoma: Papillary Pattern

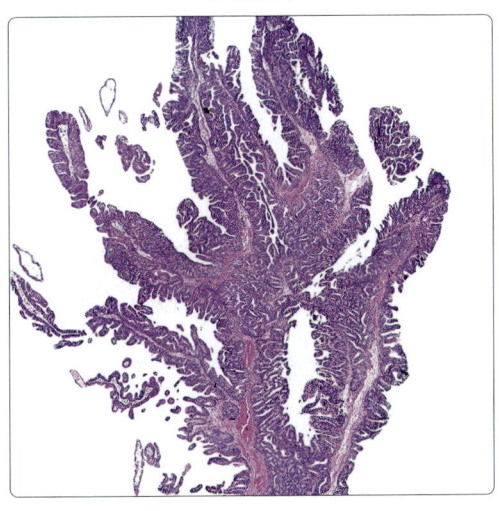

Prostatic Adenocarcinoma: Papillary Pattern

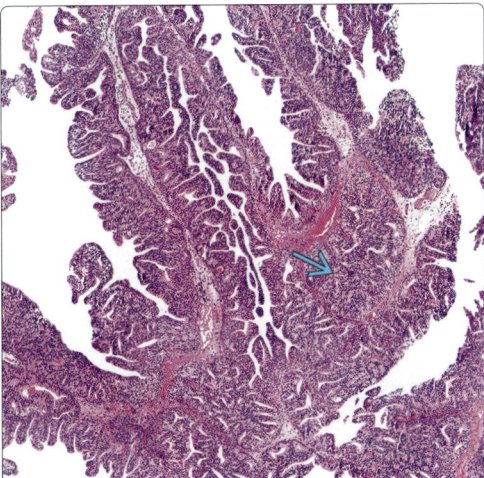

(Left) Rare cases of prostatic adenocarcinoma may have a papillary appearance that closely mimics a variety of urothelial lesions. **(Right)** *The degree of architectural complexity in this unusual exophytic example of prostatic adenocarcinoma, characterized by extensive secondary tufting and solid areas ➡, precludes the diagnosis of a reactive nonneoplastic process.*

Malakoplakia

KEY FACTS

TERMINOLOGY
- Mass-forming histiocytic & fibroinflammatory infiltrate with characteristic cytoplasmic inclusions (may be very focal)

ETIOLOGY/PATHOGENESIS
- *Escherichia coli* and other gram-negative coliform bacilli
- Secondary to defective phagolysosomal activity

CLINICAL ISSUES
- Typically polypoid bladder mass covered with intact mucosa
- Treated by eradicating infection

MICROSCOPIC
- Sheets of round histiocytes with abundant eosinophilic granular cytoplasm (von Hansemann cells)
  - Round nuclei with variable nucleoli
  - Rounded concentric basophilic intracytoplasmic inclusions (Michaelis-Guttman bodies)
  - Admixed acute and chronic inflammation common
  - May have obscuring abscess formation
  - May occasionally be fibroblastic with spindle cell predominant pattern
- Overlying urothelium may show reactive atypia

ANCILLARY TESTS
- PAS, von Kossa, and iron stains highlight intracytoplasmic inclusions
- Histiocytic markers (CD68 and CD163) show diffuse cytoplasmic immunoreactivity
- Cytokeratins are nonreactive in lesional cells

TOP DIFFERENTIAL DIAGNOSES
- Atypical mycobacterial spindle cell pseudotumor
- Extranodal Rosai-Dorfman disease
- Urothelial carcinoma
- Xanthogranulomatous inflammation

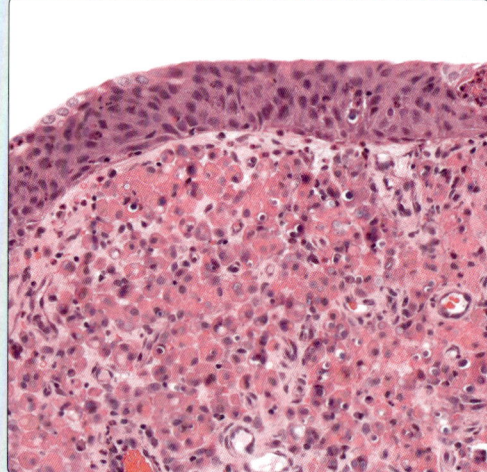

Malakoplakia: Typical Pattern

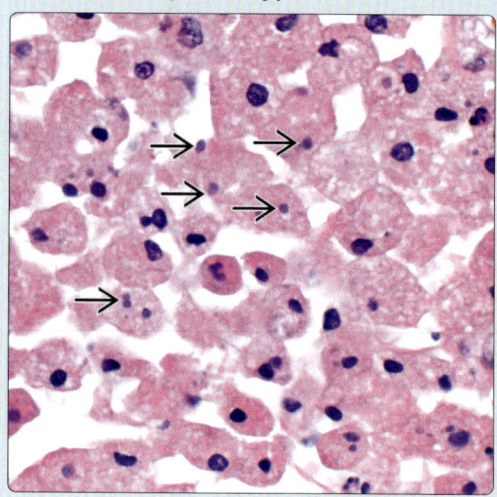

Malakoplakia: Typical Pattern

(Left) This bladder biopsy shows a superficial collection of sheets of round histiocytes with rather homogeneous eosinophilic cytoplasm. The overlying urothelium may be inflamed and may show reactive urothelial atypia, as in this specific case. (Right) The histiocytes of malakoplakia have abundant eosinophilic cytoplasm and intracytoplasmic inclusions (Michaelis-Guttman bodies) ➡. Inclusions aid in the distinction from other histiocytic lesions.

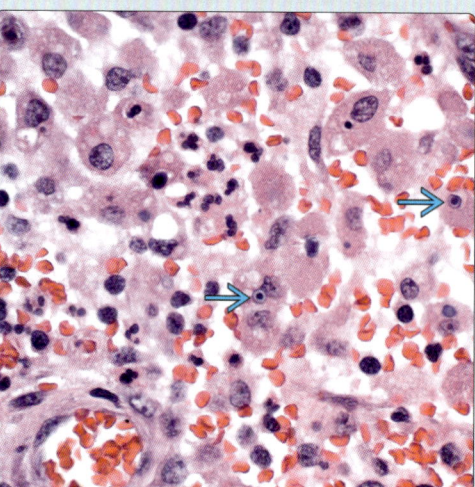

Malakoplakia: Typical Pattern

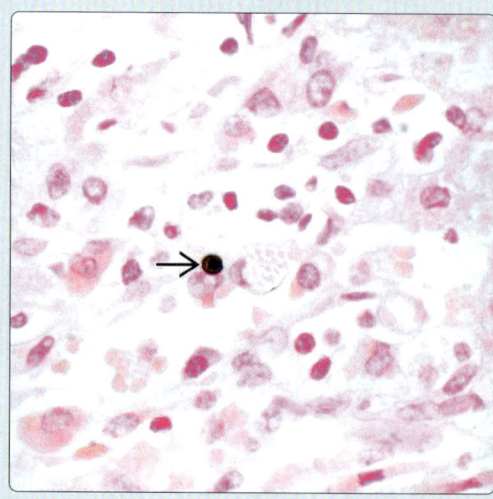

Malakoplakia: von Kossa Stain

(Left) The characteristic histiocytes of malakoplakia (von Hansemann cells) have eosinophilic cytoplasm and round nuclei. The distinct, sometimes targetoid intracytoplasmic inclusions (Michaelis-Guttman bodies) are prominent in this case ➡. (Right) In this von Kossa stain, there is a large Michaelis-Guttman body ➡ that confirms the diagnosis of malakoplakia. Histiocytic markers may be useful if carcinoma is in the differential diagnosis.

Malakoplakia

TERMINOLOGY

Synonyms
- Malacoplakia

Definitions
- Fibrohistiocytic infiltrate with unique cytoplasmic inclusions

ETIOLOGY/PATHOGENESIS

Infectious Agents
- *Escherichia coli* and other gram-negative coliform bacilli
  - Defective phagocytosis by macrophages

CLINICAL ISSUES

Epidemiology
- Age
  - Wide range from children to adults
- Sex
  - More common in females

Site
- Throughout genitourinary tract (most common in bladder trigone)

Presentation
- Bladder irritability and hematuria

Endoscopic Findings
- Polypoid mass covered usually by intact mucosa

Treatment
- Antibacterial agents with good intracellular concentration, anticholinergic agents, and ascorbic acid

MACROSCOPIC

General Features
- Single or multiple, soft yellow or yellow-brown plaques on mucosal surface
- May appear nodular or polypoid with central umbilication or ulceration

MICROSCOPIC

Histologic Features
- Collection of histiocytes with granular eosinophilic cytoplasm (von Hansemann cells)
  - Scattered histiocytes contain Michaelis-Guttman bodies
    - Rounded concentric basophilic intracytoplasmic inclusions
    - In early lesions, may be small dot with surrounding halo
- Variable inflammatory infiltrate: Neutrophils, lymphocytes, plasma cells, and eosinophils
  - Abscess formation or granulation tissue may obscure typical findings
- Stromal reaction may be variable with fibroblastic proliferation or fibrosis

Predominant Pattern/Injury Type
- Diffuse

Predominant Cell/Compartment Type
- Histiocyte/macrophage

ANCILLARY TESTS

Histochemistry
- von Kossa, iron stain, and periodic acid-Schiff
  - Highlight intracytoplasmic inclusions
  - PAS may be only positive stain in early lesions
    - Mineralization occurs later in disease, so calcium and iron stains are negative

Immunohistochemistry
- Cytokeratins are nonreactive in lesional cells
- CD68 and CD163 show diffuse cytoplasmic reactivity

DIFFERENTIAL DIAGNOSIS

Urothelial Carcinoma
- Undifferentiated or plasmacytoid carcinoma may be considered
- Cytokeratin stains should resolve difficult cases

Prostatic Adenocarcinoma
- Express cytokeratin, NKX3.1, PSA, and PAP

Xanthogranulomatous Inflammation
- Morphologically and pathogenetically similar to malakoplakia
- Lack Michaelis-Guttman bodies

Extranodal Rosai-Dorfman Disease
- Histiocytes with emperipolesis
- Cells are immunoreactive for S100 protein

Atypical Mycobacterial Spindle Cell Pseudotumor
- Acid-fast bacilli present by special stains
- Intracytoplasmic inclusions typical of malakoplakia not seen

Histiocytic Sarcoma
- Larger cells with more prominent cytoplasm and more nuclear variability
- Michaelis-Guttman bodies absent

Myeloid Leukemia
- May have mass-forming disease outside bone marrow
- Larger nuclei with greater cytologic atypia and express myeloid/granulocytic/monocytic markers

DIAGNOSTIC CHECKLIST

Pathologic Interpretation Pearls
- Michaelis-Guttman bodies may be difficult to visualize on H&E in early disease process
  - von Kossa (calcium), Perls stain (iron), and periodic acid-Schiff highlight inclusions

SELECTED REFERENCES

1. Long JP Jr et al: Malacoplakia: a 25-year experience with a review of the literature. J Urol. 141(6):1328-31, 1989
2. Lou TY et al: Malakoplakia: pathogenesis and ultrastructural morphogenesis. A problem of altered macrophage (phagolysosomal) response. Hum Pathol. 5(2):191-207, 1974

Malakoplakia

Malakoplakia: Typical Pattern

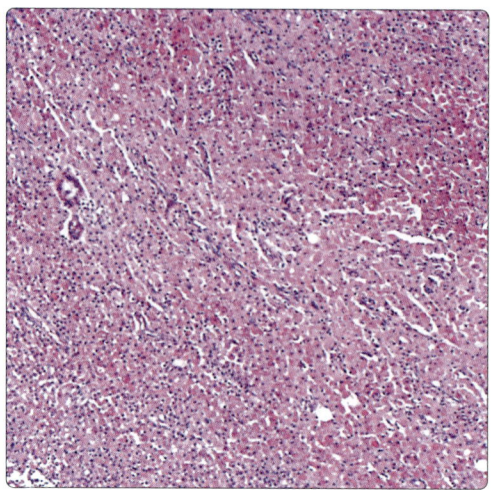

Malakoplakia: Typical Pattern

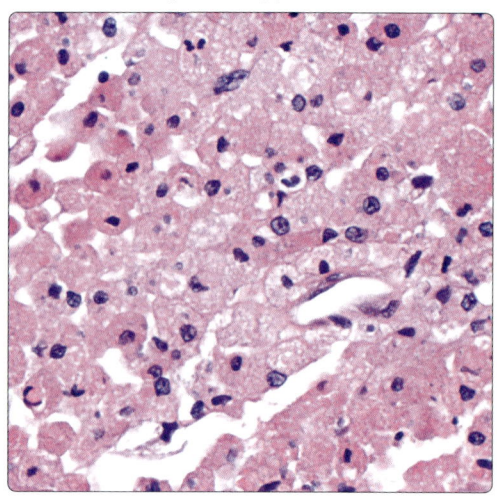

(Left) *Malakoplakia is characterized by sheets of histiocytes with abundant eosinophilic cytoplasm. This sheet-like growth may mimic a variety of malignant neoplasms.* (Right) *Sheets of histiocytes with abundant eosinophilic cytoplasm are characteristic of malakoplakia. This pattern may suggest a diffuse type carcinoma, such as from gastric or breast origin. Immunoreactivity for histiocytic, but not epithelial, markers will resolve most difficult cases.*

Malakoplakia: Typical Pattern

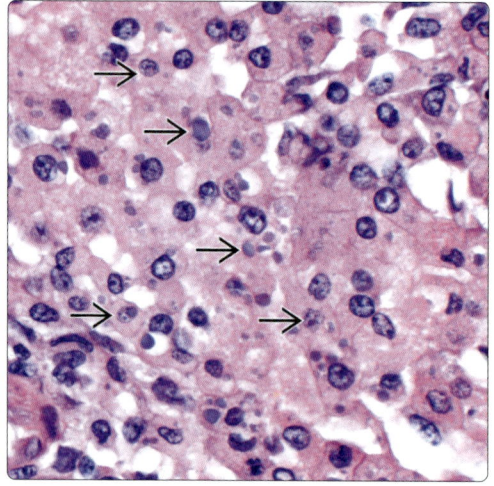

Malakoplakia: Typical Pattern

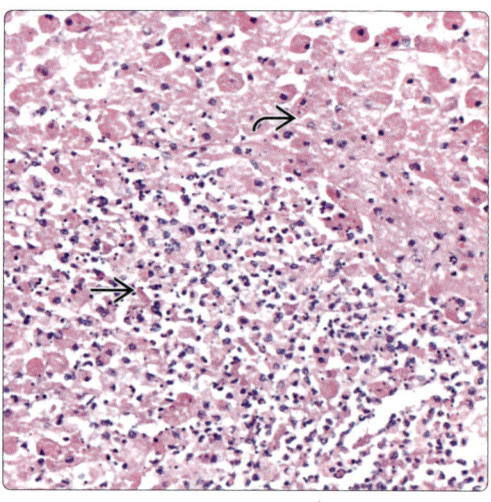

(Left) *Numerous intracytoplasmic inclusions (Michaelis-Guttman bodies) ➔ are present within the eosinophilic histiocytes of malakoplakia. Identification of these characteristic inclusions help to exclude the possibility of other histiocytic infiltrates.* (Right) *The histiocytes of malakoplakia ➔ are often admixed with acute inflammation ➔. This may cause consideration of tuberculosis or fungal-associated granulomas. The nature and extent of inflammatory reaction varies between lesions.*

Malakoplakia: Typical Pattern

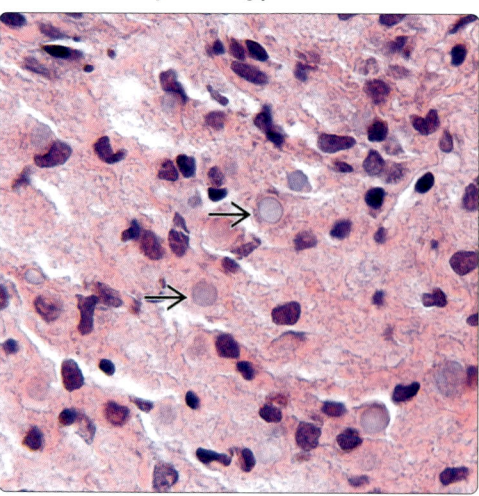

Malakoplakia: von Kossa Stain

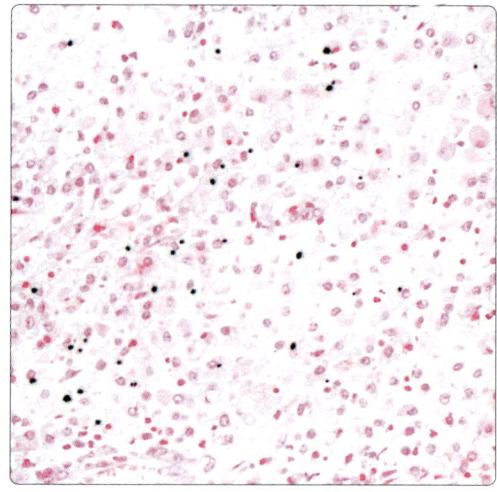

(Left) *Under high-power examination with oil immersion, the lamellated nature of the intracytoplasmic Michaelis-Guttman bodies is evident ➔. These inclusions are sufficient for a diagnosis of malakoplakia.* (Right) *A von Kossa stain highlights innumerable intracytoplasmic inclusions (black dots) in this example of malakoplakia. In early lesions, prior to mineralization, von Kossa stains may be negative. PAS stains may be more useful in that setting.*

Malakoplakia

Malakoplakia: Spindled Pattern

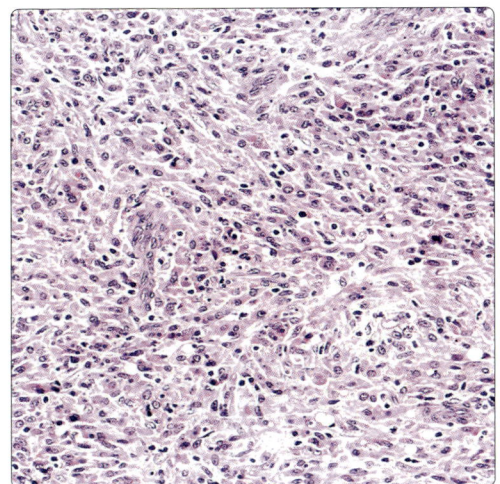

Malakoplakia: Spindled Pattern

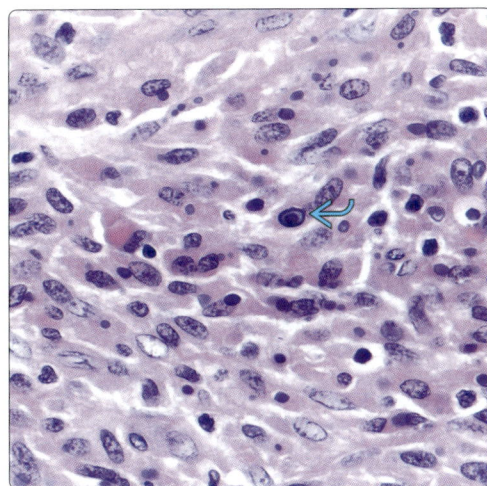

(Left) This example of malakoplakia has a more prominent spindled appearance and scant inflammatory infiltrate. Because the histiocytes appear spindled, lesions such as reactive stromal proliferations or spindle cell neoplasms may be considered in the differential diagnosis. (Right) This high-power view of malakoplakia shows histiocytes with a more elongated shape imparting a spindled appearance. A typical MG body ⇨ is present.

Extranodal Rosai-Dorfman

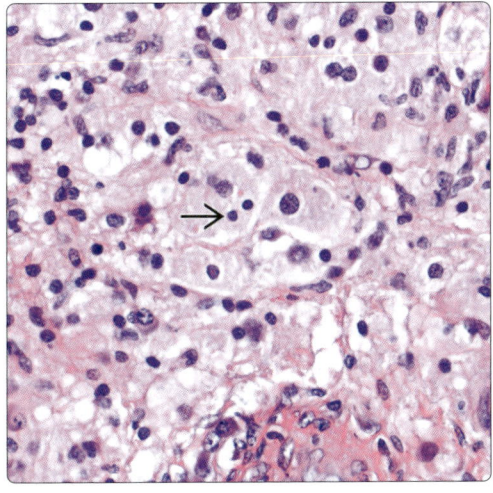

Extranodal Rosai-Dorfman

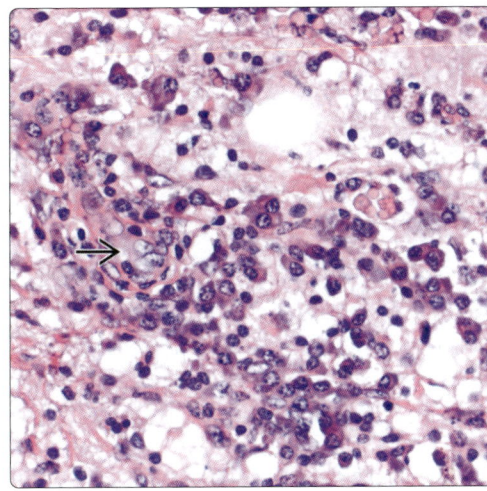

(Left) Extranodal Rosai-Dorfman disease is well documented in the genitourinary tract and may closely resemble other histiocytic infiltrates, such as malakoplakia. The histiocytes of Rosai-Dorfman disease often contain more voluminous cytoplasm and emperipolesis may be present ⇨. Emperipolesis may potentially mimic inclusions. (Right) Perivascular plasma cells (endothelial cells highlighted ⇨) are also characteristic of Rosai-Dorfman disease.

Extranodal Rosai-Dorfman: S100 Protein

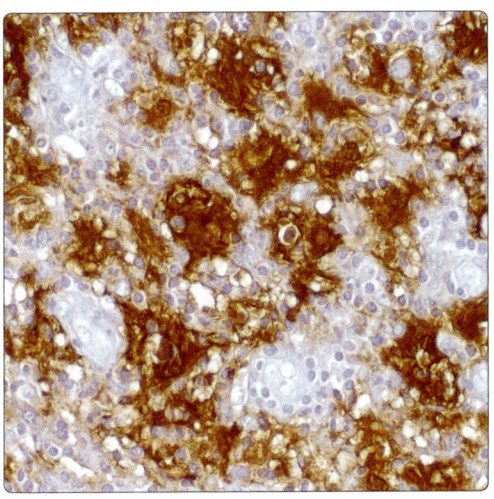

Granulomatous Inflammation: Fungal

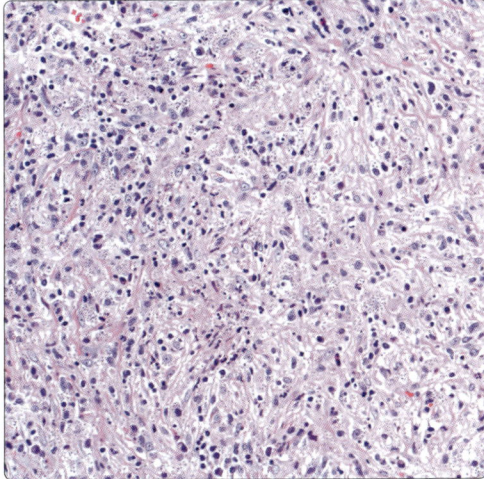

(Left) The histiocytes of Rosai-Dorfman disease, unlike malakoplakia, show diffuse cytoplasmic and nuclear reactivity for S100 protein. (Right) This histiocytic infiltrate represents granulomatous inflammation due to a fungal infection. The sheet-like appearance of histiocytes in a fibrotic background with mixed inflammatory cells mimics malakoplakia. The spindled histiocytes in this case also resemble a spindle cell neoplasm.

Malakoplakia

Granulomatous Inflammation: Fungal
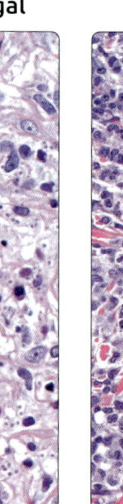

Leukemia in Bladder
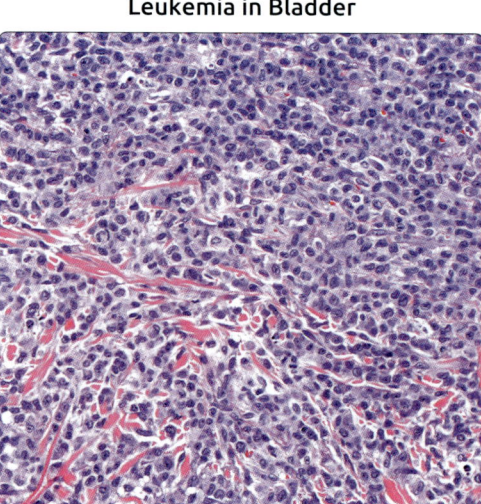

(Left) *Note the fungal organisms ➡ in this high-power image of granulomatous inflammation mimicking malakoplakia. The background contains a mixed inflammatory infiltrate and plump histiocytes.* **(Right)** *Myeloid sarcoma, especially those with histiocytic or megakaryocytic differentiation, may present in parenchymal organs. The sheets of cells with amphophilic cytoplasm may provoke a differential that includes malakoplakia, especially since histiocytic markers may be positive.*

Prostatic Adenocarcinoma
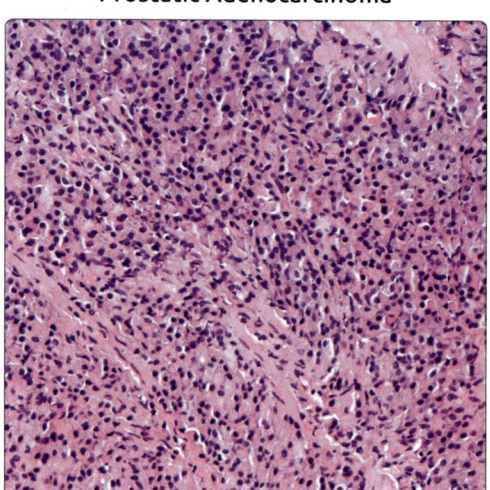

Prostatic Adenocarcinoma
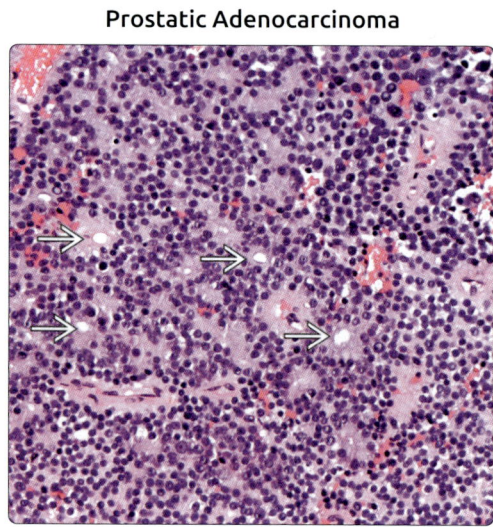

(Left) *This example of Gleason pattern 5 prostatic adenocarcinoma involving the bladder has eosinophilic cytoplasm that may prompt consideration of malakoplakia. Immunohistochemistry is helpful in difficult cases. Prostatic adenocarcinoma should express cytokeratin and PSA/PAP or NKX3.1.* **(Right)** *The identification of foci with luminal differentiation in this neoplasm greatly aids in recognizing prostatic adenocarcinoma ➡.*

Urothelial Carcinoma
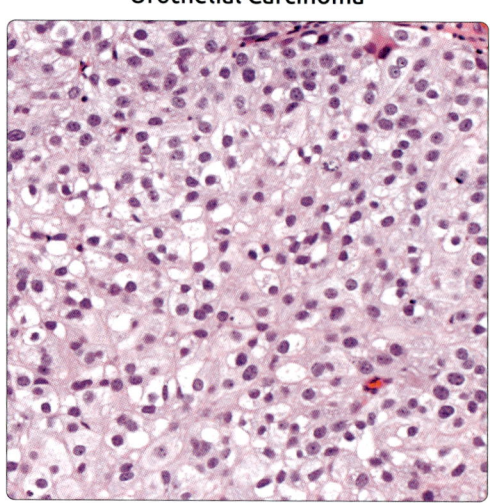

Urothelial Carcinoma
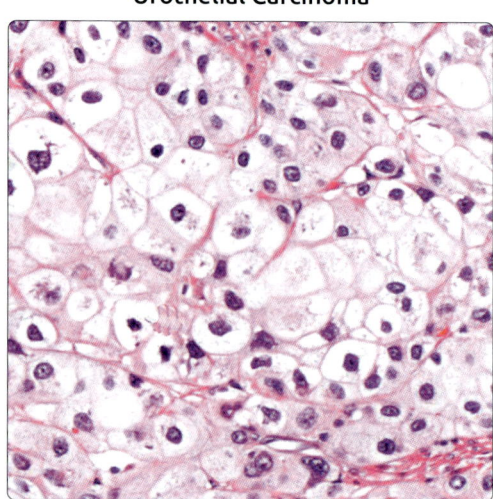

(Left) *In this example of invasive urothelial carcinoma, the sheet-like growth is associated with more abundant frothy and lightly eosinophilic cytoplasm. These cells are more uniformly cohesive than typically expected in a histiocytic infiltrate, such as malakoplakia.* **(Right)** *At high-power evaluation of this invasive urothelial carcinoma, the abundant lightly eosinophilic cytoplasm with a frothy appearance and the relatively round nuclei may suggest histiocytes.*

Malakoplakia

Urothelial Carcinoma
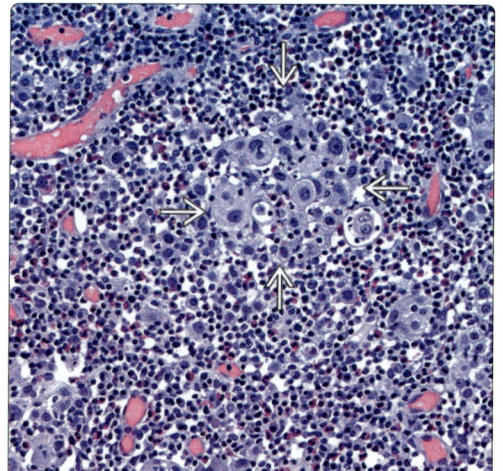

Urothelial Carcinoma
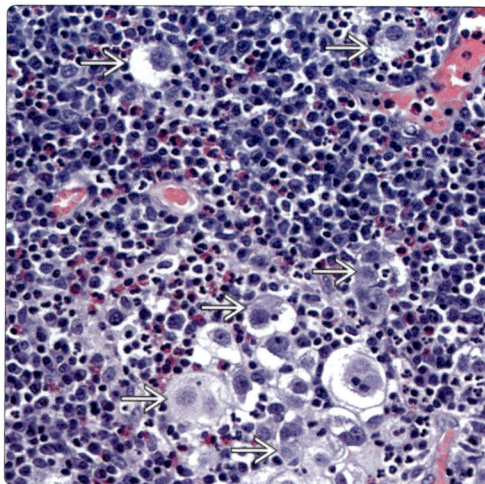

(Left) This example of invasive urothelial carcinoma with an associated mixed inflammatory infiltrate has a morphology with striking resemblance to histiocytes ➡. (Right) On high-power evaluation, the neoplastic cells ➡ of this invasive urothelial carcinoma have abundant "frothy" cytoplasm that has marked overlap with histiocytes. Demonstration of cytokeratin reactivity with a broad spectrum keratin is important in difficult cases.

Mycobacterial Spindle Cell Pseudotumor
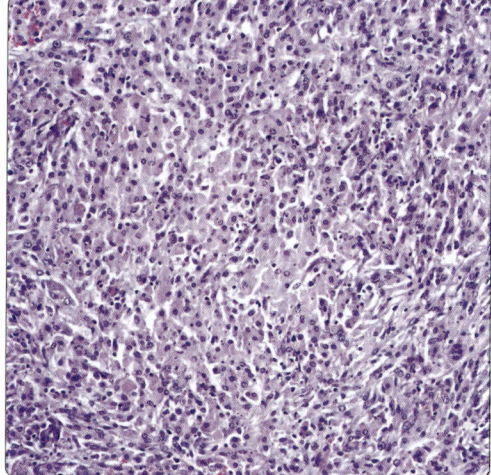

Mycobacterial Spindle Cell Pseudotumor: Acid-Fast Stain
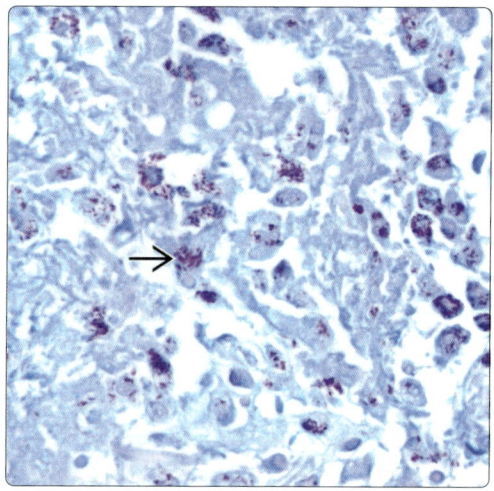

(Left) Mycobacterial spindle cell pseudotumor has overlapping morphologic features with malakoplakia. Note the sheet-like aggregates of spindled histiocytes with an inflammatory infiltrate. (Right) An AFB stain demonstrates numerous clusters of intracytoplasmic acid-fast bacilli ➡ in this example of mycobacterial spindle cell pseudotumor. AFB stains are important when considering the possibility of this diagnosis.

Primary Signet Ring Cell Adenocarcinoma
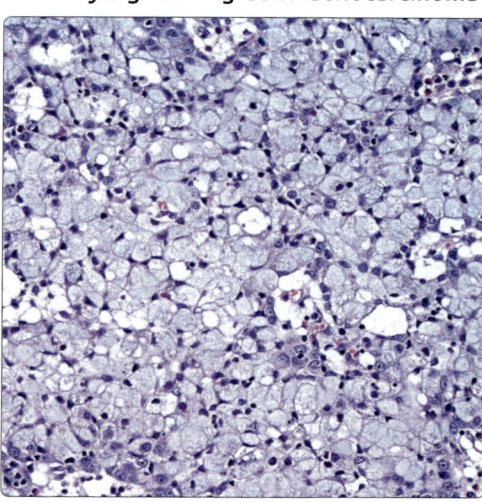

Plasmacytoid Urothelial Carcinoma
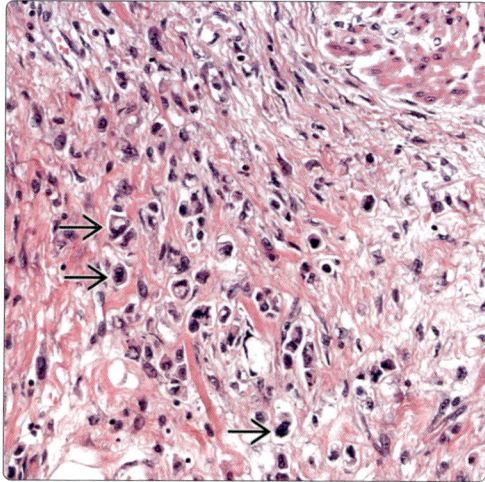

(Left) Primary signet ring cell adenocarcinoma of the urinary bladder, as in other anatomic sites, may have morphologic overlap with histiocytes. The peripheral nuclei and intracytoplasmic mucin are distinctive features. The nuclei are often indented by the cytoplasmic contents. (Right) In this invasive plasmacytoid urothelial carcinoma, the neoplastic cells infiltrate separately, which may suggest inflammatory cells, but the peripheral nuclei are larger and more atypical ➡ than seen in histiocytes.

Schistosomiasis

KEY FACTS

TERMINOLOGY
- Urinary bladder infection by *Schistosoma*
- a.k.a. bilharziasis or Katayama fever

ETIOLOGY/PATHOGENESIS
- Water-borne trematode infection
  - Initially enters host through skin within water
  - *Schistosoma haematobium* infects bladder
- Endemic in eastern Mediterranean and sub-Saharan Africa
  - Large percentage of population affected, although incidence is decreasing

CLINICAL ISSUES
- Hematuria most common presentation
  - Due to egg deposition in established phase
- Morbidity and mortality is determined by parasitic burden, risk of reinfection, and chronicity
  - Untreated chronic infection has serious morbidity
    - Hydronephrosis
    - Pyelonephritis
    - Renal failure
    - Bacterial coinfection
    - Squamous cell carcinoma (most common type)
    - Urothelial carcinoma or adenocarcinoma

MICROSCOPIC
- Numerous ova
  - Become calcified over time
- Inflammatory response
  - Acute and chronic inglammation
  - Granulomatous response
- Epithelial changes
  - Keratinizing squamous metaplasia and dysplasia
  - Intestinal metaplasia

TOP DIFFERENTIAL DIAGNOSES
- Encrusted cystitis
- Selective internal radiation therapy (SIRT) microspheres

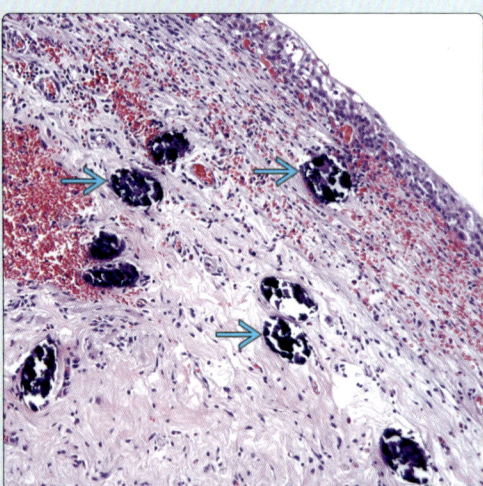

Schistosomiasis

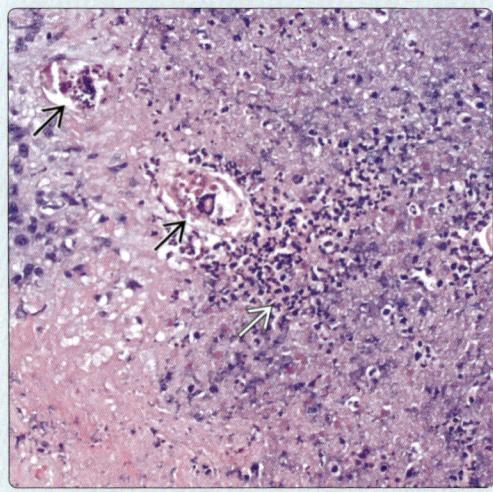

Schistosomiasis

(Left) Numerous calcified ova of Schistosoma haematobium ⇒ are present in the lamina propria of the urinary bladder in this superficial biopsy. Surrounding fibrosis is common in the late phases. The lining mucosa here is urothelial in nature, although most frequently, it is keratinizing squamous epithelium. (Right) Noncalcified Schistosoma haematobium eggs ⇒ associated with necrosis and an acute inflammatory infiltrate ⇒. Metaplastic changes and calcifications are associated with chronicity.

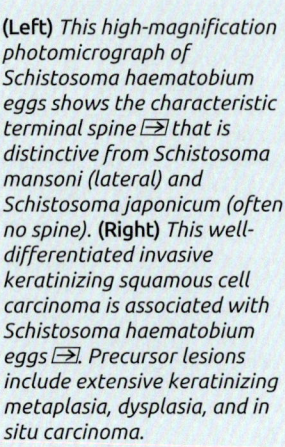

Schistosomiasis

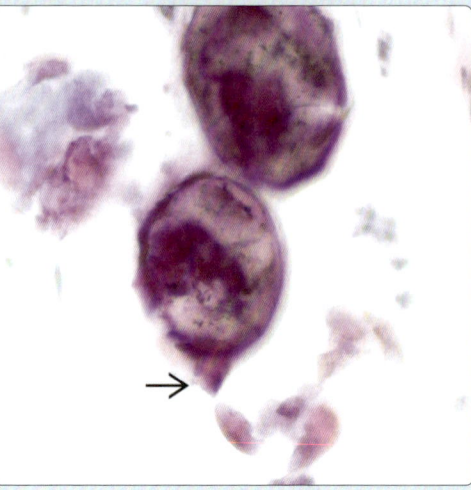

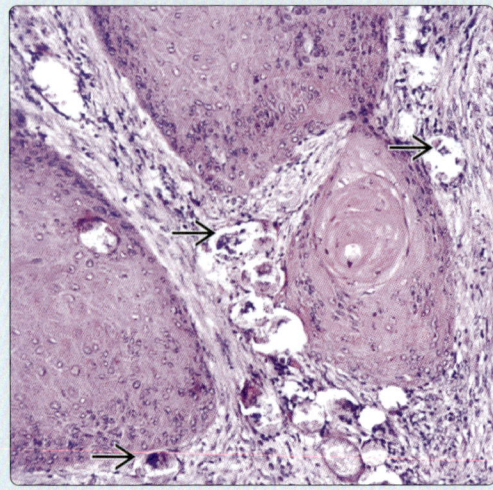

Schistosomiasis With Associated Carcinoma

(Left) This high-magnification photomicrograph of Schistosoma haematobium eggs shows the characteristic terminal spine ⇒ that is distinctive from Schistosoma mansoni (lateral) and Schistosoma japonicum (often no spine). (Right) This well-differentiated invasive keratinizing squamous cell carcinoma is associated with Schistosoma haematobium eggs ⇒. Precursor lesions include extensive keratinizing metaplasia, dysplasia, and in situ carcinoma.

Schistosomiasis

TERMINOLOGY

Synonyms
- Bilharziasis

Definitions
- Urinary bladder infection by *Schistosoma*

ETIOLOGY/PATHOGENESIS

Infectious Agents
- Water-borne trematode infection
  - *Schistosoma haematobium* infects bladder
  - *Schistosoma mansoni* and *Schistosoma japonicum* are typically intestinal infections
- Acquired by exposure to infected water
  - Eggs enter fresh water through urine or feces contamination
  - Larval stages develop in water
    - Freshwater snails are intermediate host
  - Infection of humans by penetration through skin within water source

CLINICAL ISSUES

Epidemiology
- Incidence
  - Endemic areas
    - Mediterranean and sub-Saharan Africa

Presentation
- Hematuria most common

Laboratory Tests
- Diagnosed by identifying eggs in urine
- Newer serologic tests
  - ELISA specific for *Schistosoma* antigens

Natural History
- Ova are deposited in veins of muscularis propria of bladder where they become permeable
  - Infiltrates bladder tissues and incites inflammatory reaction

Treatment
- Drugs
  - Medications with antischistosomal effect

Prognosis
- Morbidity and mortality is determined by parasitic burden, risk of reinfection, and chronicity
  - Untreated chronic infection has serious morbidity
    - Hydronephrosis, pyelonephritis, or renal failure
- Predisposing factor for bladder carcinoma
  - Primary squamous cell carcinoma
    - Arises through squamous metaplasia-dysplasia-carcinoma sequence
  - Urothelial carcinoma or adenocarcinoma
    - Arises through urothelial dysplasia-carcinoma sequence and glandular metaplasia-dysplasia-carcinoma sequence

MACROSCOPIC

General Features
- Rough granular mucosal surface
  - "Sandy patches"
- Sharp ulcerations and transverse fissures
- Polyps less common

MICROSCOPIC

Histologic Features
- Numerous ova are present with surrounding inflammatory response
  - Granulomas with acute and chronic inflammation
  - Hemorrhage and ulceration
- In chronic infection, bladder wall may show extensive fibrosis
- Eggs calcify over time
- Associated keratinizing squamous metaplasia and dysplasia may be seen
- *Schistosoma haematobium* vs. *Schistosoma mansoni*/*Schistosoma japonicum*
  - Terminal spines seen in *S. haematobium*
    - *S. mansoni* has lateral spine
    - *S. japonicum* has no spine or small inconspicuous subterminal spine
  - *S. mansoni* and *S. japonicum* infection typically based in intestines

DIFFERENTIAL DIAGNOSIS

Encrusted Cystitis
- Irregular calcified aggregates distinct from rounded/oval calcified eggs
- Associated with bladder infections or overlying carcinoma
  - Usually in areas of necrosis

Selective Internal Radiation Therapy (SIRT) Microspheres
- Round microspheres may resemble *Schistosoma* ova
  - Greater awareness of this potential therapy effect reduces possibility of misidentification
    - More spherical than *Schistosoma* eggs
- Seen mostly in stomach and duodenum following intrahepatic treatment of metastatic colorectal adenocarcinoma
  - Other clinical uses may be emerging

DIAGNOSTIC CHECKLIST

Pathologic Interpretation Pearls
- Occasionally, infection is 1st diagnosed on bladder biopsy

SELECTED REFERENCES

1. Obeng BB et al: Application of a circulating-cathodic-antigen (CCA) strip test and real-time PCR, in comparison with microscopy, for the detection of Schistosoma haematobium in urine samples from Ghana. Ann Trop Med Parasitol. 102(7):625-33, 2008
2. Ghoneim MA: Bilharziasis of the genitourinary tract. BJU Int. 89 Suppl 1:22-30, 2002
3. El-Bolkainy MN et al: The impact of schistosomiasis on the pathology of bladder carcinoma. Cancer. 48(12):2643-8, 1981
4. Zahran MM et al: Bilharziasis of urinary bladder and ureter: comparative histopathologic study. Urology. 8(1):73-9, 1976

von Brunn Nests

KEY FACTS

TERMINOLOGY
- Invaginated nests of cytologically benign urothelial cells in lamina propria

ETIOLOGY/PATHOGENESIS
- Variant of normal urothelial histology
- May occur as result of local inflammation

CLINICAL ISSUES
- Common finding in 85-95% of bladders
- Usually incidental microscopic finding
- Entirely benign

MICROSCOPIC
- Solid nests of urothelial cells in superficial lamina propria
- Nests have smooth, round contours
- Evenly spaced nests with lobular configuration
- Sharp linear border at deep junction with lamina propria
- Urothelial cells do not have dysplastic features

TOP DIFFERENTIAL DIAGNOSES
- Nested variant of urothelial carcinoma
  - More extensive epithelium and irregular distribution
- Inverted papilloma
  - Often cord-like, anastomosing growth
- Carcinoid tumor
  - More architecturally complex epithelium (cribriforming)
- Paraganglioma and normal paraganglionic cells
  - May have deep location; cytokeratin negative
- Pseudocarcinomatous hyperplasia
  - Nests juxtaposed to vessels containing fibrin thrombi

DIAGNOSTIC CHECKLIST
- In superficial biopsies, may have significant morphologic overlap with nested urothelial carcinoma
  - Architectural distribution of nests at low magnification is critical

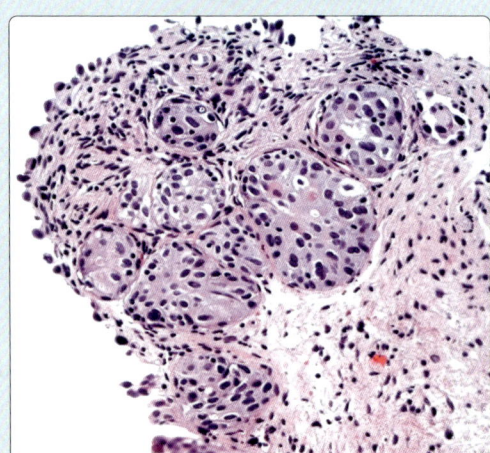

von Brunn Nests

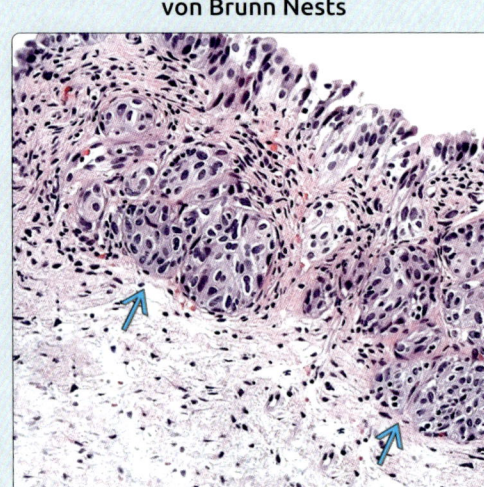

von Brunn Nests

(Left) von Brunn nests are characterized by aggregated individual urothelial nests with a lobular arrangement. There is typically a sharp linear border at the junction with the lamina propria. (Right) The sharp linear border at the base of the lesion ➡ is characteristic of von Brunn nests and aids in the distinction from subtle variants of carcinoma, such as nested variant or microcystic variant.

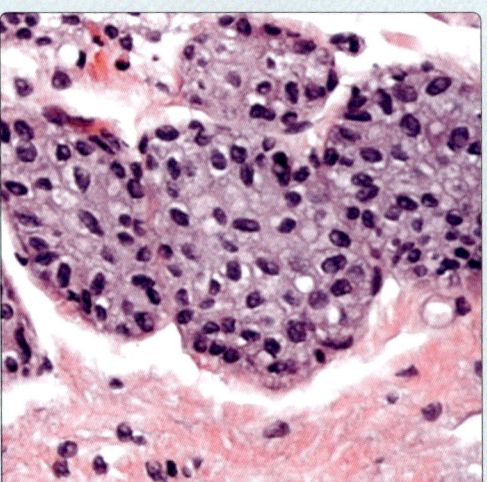

von Brunn Nests

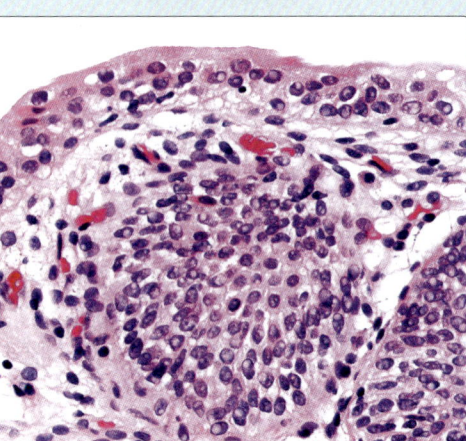

von Brunn Nests

(Left) von Brunn nests have small nuclei and bland cytologic features. Some nested carcinomas share similar features; hence, appreciation of the architecture is important to distinguish von Brunn nests from subtle patterns of carcinoma. (Right) The cytologic features of the urothelial cells in von Brunn nests are similar to the overlying normal urothelium. The nests have smooth round contours.

von Brunn Nests

TERMINOLOGY

Synonyms
- Proliferative cystitis

Definitions
- Invaginated nests of cytologically benign urothelial cells in lamina propria

ETIOLOGY/PATHOGENESIS

Etiology
- Variant of normal urothelial histology
- May occur as result of local inflammation

CLINICAL ISSUES

Epidemiology
- Incidence
  - Common finding (85-95% of bladders)
- Age
  - Frequency increases with age

Site
- Bladder trigone, renal pelvis, and ureter

Presentation
- Usually incidental microscopic finding

Prognosis
- Benign (not neoplastic precursor lesion)

MACROSCOPIC

General Features
- Typically < 5 mm in diameter
- Most are not grossly visible
  - May be cystoscopically visible when prominent
  - May appear as mucosal blebs

MICROSCOPIC

Histologic Features
- Solid nests of urothelial cells in superficial lamina propria; variable continuity with surface urothelium
  - Nests typically have smooth, round contours
    - Some have minor branching and some minimal confluence
  - Clustered individual nests have orderly arrangement
    - Evenly spaced with lobular configuration
  - Sharp epithelial-stromal interface at deep aspect
  - Normal cytology similar to overlying surface urothelium
- May be associated with other florid conditions, including cystitis cystica and cystitis glandularis
- Stromal reaction is absent

Cytologic Features
- Identical to normal urothelium

Predominant Pattern/Injury Type
- Nests

DIFFERENTIAL DIAGNOSIS

Nested Variant of Urothelial Carcinoma
- Typically larger lesion
- In very superficial biopsies, may be histologically indistinguishable from von Brunn nests
- Has more disorganized arrangement of nests
  - Nonlobular, random distribution often into deep lamina propria
  - Nests often have greater confluence at least focally
  - Invasion of muscularis propria is diagnostic of carcinoma

Inverted Papilloma
- More numerous and crowded urothelial nests
- Peripheral basal palisading of neoplastic cells is common
- Trabecular architecture are also common
- Spindling of cells within nests may be seen
- Distinction of florid von Brunn nests from inverted papilloma may be arbitrary in some cases
  - Size of lesion and presence of cystoscopic lesion are helpful in diagnosis of lesion
  - Greater epithelial to stromal ratio in papilloma

Carcinoid Tumor (Low-Grade Neuroendocrine Neoplasm)
- Mixed nested and trabecular architecture common
  - More complex anastomosing growth
- Neoplastic cells with stippled nuclear chromatin
- Expresses neuroendocrine markers

Paraganglioma and Normal Paraganglionic Cells
- Nests usually more numerous and crowded
- Vascular septa may be prominent
- Not confined to superficial location

Pseudocarcinomatous Hyperplasia
- Urothelial nests in lamina propria closely associated with blood vessels containing fibrin
- Nests show atypia in range of reactive etiology

DIAGNOSTIC CHECKLIST

Pathologic Interpretation Pearls
- Significant morphologic overlap with nested urothelial carcinoma
- Clinical presentation should be carefully reviewed in superficial biopsies thought to represent mass lesion
  - Consider nested carcinoma in cases with any aggressive clinical findings (large mass or ureteral obstruction)
  - Caution in making this diagnosis in renal pelvis or ureteral biopsy

SELECTED REFERENCES

1. Volmar KE et al: Florid von Brunn nests mimicking urothelial carcinoma: a morphologic and immunohistochemical comparison to the nested variant of urothelial carcinoma. Am J Surg Pathol. 27(9):1243-52, 2003
2. Wiener DP et al: The prevalence and significance of Brunn's nests, cystitis cystica and squamous metaplasia in normal bladders. J Urol. 122(3):317-21, 1979

von Brunn Nests

(Left) von Brunn nests are cytologically benign invaginations of urothelium into the lamina propria. These nests are very common and represent a variant of normal histology. **(Right)** This relatively superficial collection of urothelial nests with a rounded, lobular configuration is typical of von Brunn nests.

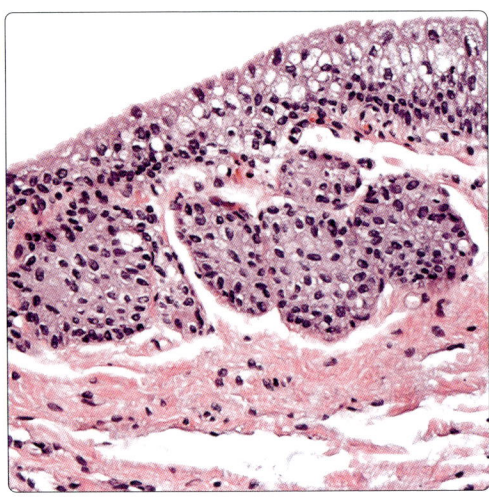
von Brunn Nests

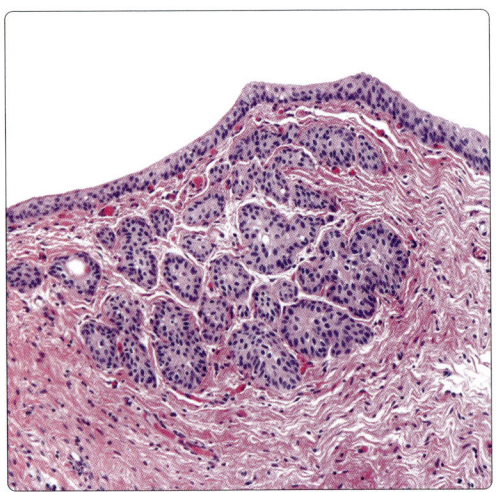
von Brunn Nests: Lobular Pattern

(Left) Note the characteristic superficial location of von Brunn nests ➡. There is a sharp border at the base of the urothelial nests, a feature that is key to the distinction from carcinoma. There is a close relationship, or sometimes a connection with the overlying surface. **(Right)** These von Brunn nests have the typical rounded contours and are aggregated into tight superficial clusters. Carcinomas typically have a more random distribution and deeper extension into the lamina propria (or muscularis propria).

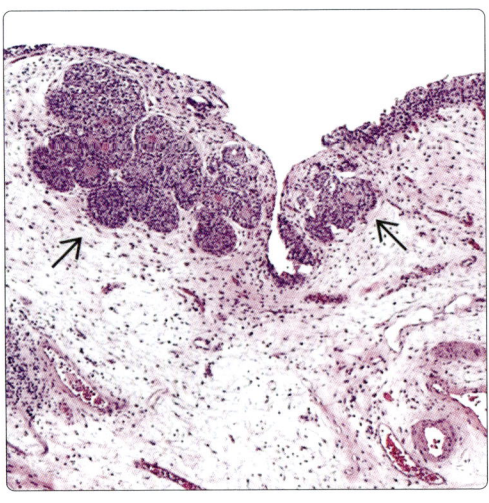
von Brunn Nests: Sharp Base

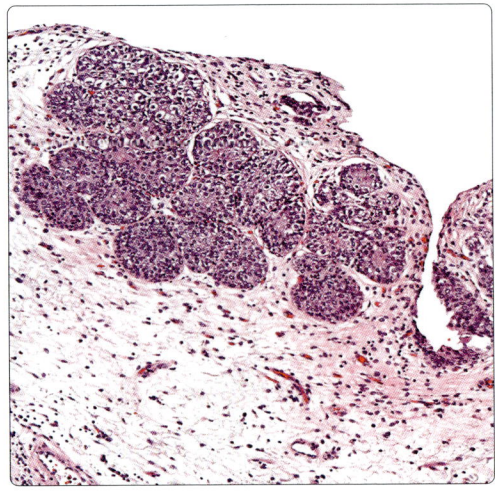
von Brunn Nests: Lobular Configuration

(Left) Although not needed, in some examples of von Brunn nests, a residual connection to the surface urothelium may be seen ➡. **(Right)** This example of von Brunn nests is characterized by multiple groups of clustered urothelial nests with a superficial location and sharp border ➡ at the lower junction with the lamina propria.

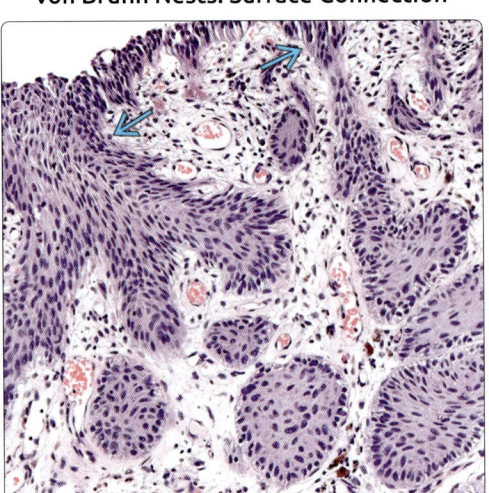
von Brunn Nests: Surface Connection

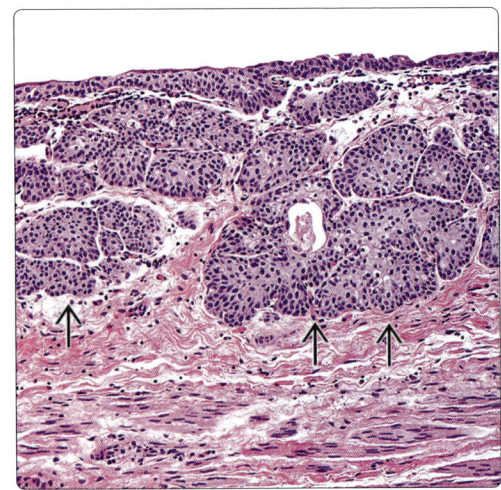
von Brunn Nests: Regular Nests, Sharp Base

von Brunn Nests

von Brunn Nests: Ureter
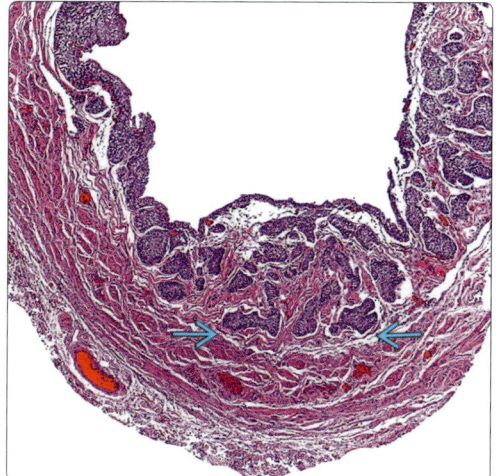

von Brunn Nests: Ureter
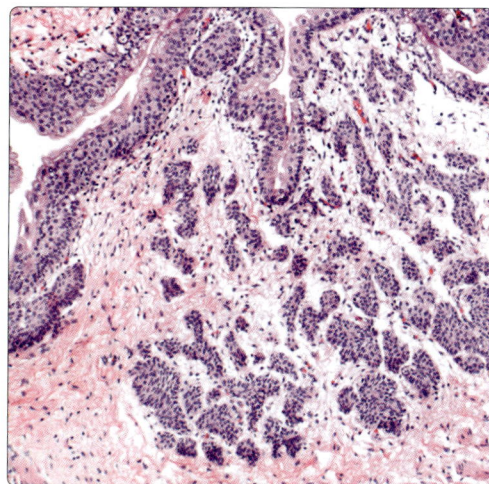

(Left) In the ureter, von Brunn nests are often smaller and have a more complex branching pattern; however, they still extend to a uniform level at the base of the lesion ➡. **(Right)** On a small superficial biopsy from the ureter that does not include the base of the lesion, these nests could present a difficult diagnostic challenge. A low-power lobular configuration is the most helpful feature. One should be very hesitant to make a diagnosis of nested urothelial carcinoma in ureter or pelvicalyceal system unless there is a mass lesion.

von Brunn Nests: Irregular Outline
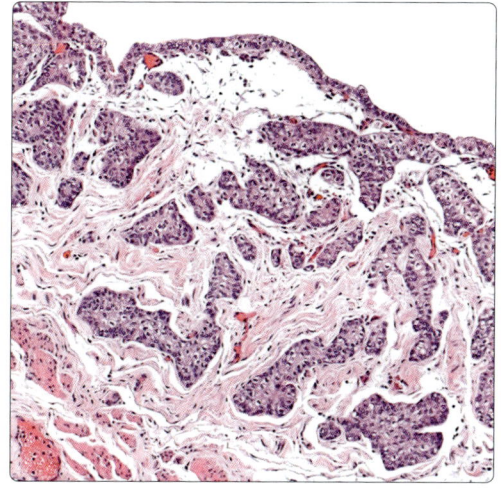

von Brunn Nests: Maintain Lobularity
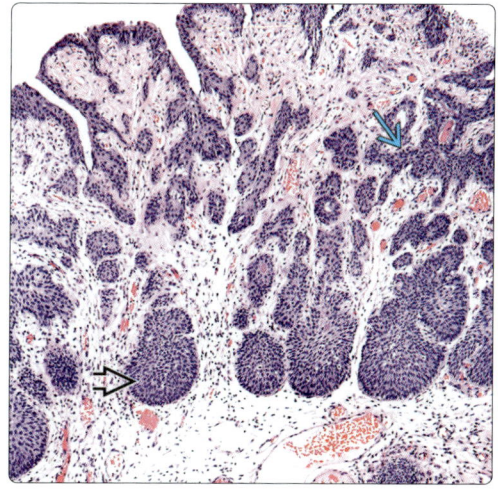

(Left) This example demonstrates the degree of epithelial nest elongation and branching that is more commonly seen in von Brunn nests of the ureter. **(Right)** Despite the larger nests at the base ➡ and the presence of some epithelial branching ➡, the sharply delineated border at the base of this lesion is characteristic of von Brunn nests. This example also shows some connection to the surface.

von Brunn Nests
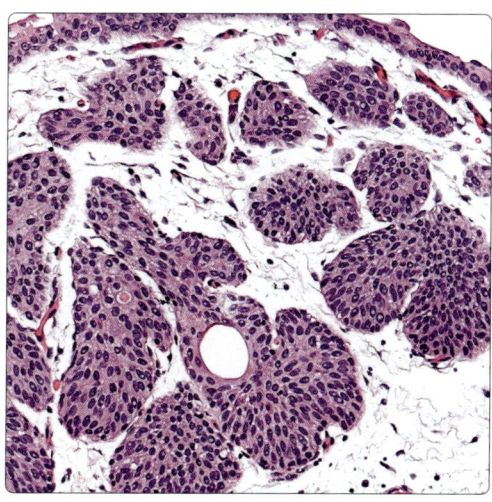

von Brunn Nests: Clear Cell Change
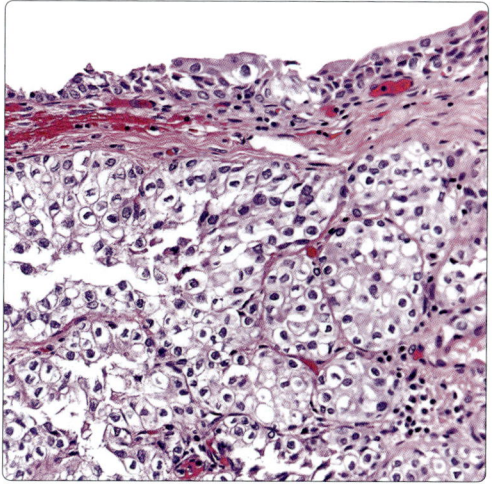

(Left) The urothelial aggregates of von Brunn nests may have some degree of branching, as in this example. The overall organized architecture argues for a benign diagnosis. **(Right)** Some examples of von Brunn nests have clear cytoplasm, which may occasionally suggest the possibility of renal cell carcinoma. The superficial location of the nests and well-delineated/lobular architecture, as well as the clinical history, should help in this distinction.

von Brunn Nests

Nested Urothelial Carcinoma
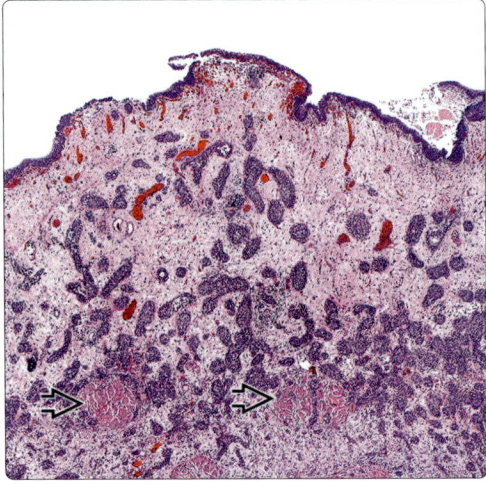

Nested Urothelial Carcinoma
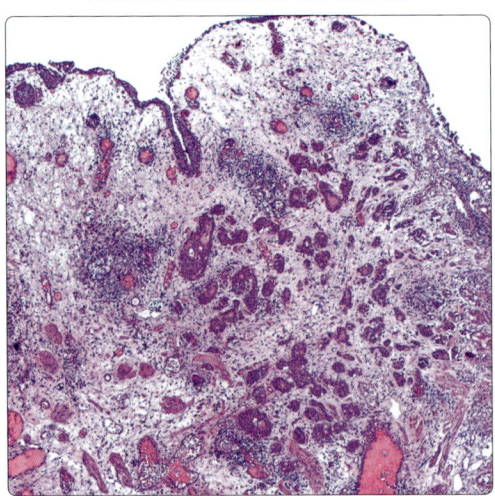

(Left) Evaluation of the architectural distribution of the urothelial nests at relatively low magnification is most important to the recognition of nested carcinoma. Invasion of the muscularis propria is diagnostic ⇒. (Right) This photomicrograph highlights the deep, irregular invasion of the lamina propria by nested urothelial carcinoma. The nests lack the aggregated, lobular arrangement typical of von Brunn nests, which are more superficial with a sharp linear border at the base.

Nested Urothelial Carcinoma
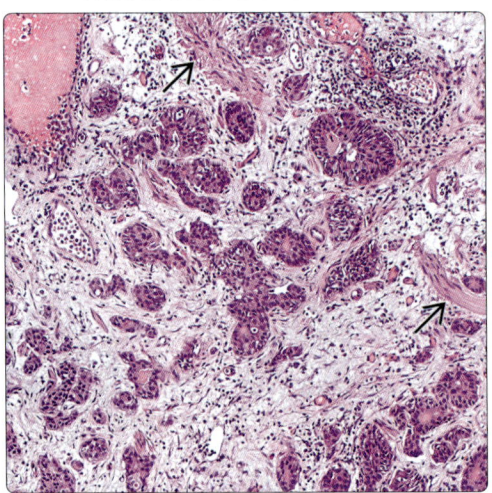

Nested Urothelial Carcinoma
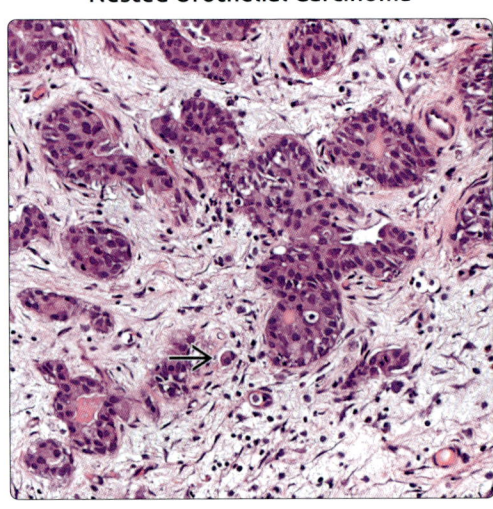

(Left) Nested urothelial carcinomas show deeper invasion into the lamina propria with involvement of the muscularis mucosae ⇒. Deep involvement is not seen with von Brunn nests and is diagnostic of neoplasia. (Right) Clues to the diagnosis of nested carcinoma include more variation in size and shape of urothelial nests and small clusters with retraction ⇒. The cytology of the malignant cells is extremely bland, which adds to the degree of histologic overlap with von Brunn nests.

Pseudocarcinomatous Hyperplasia
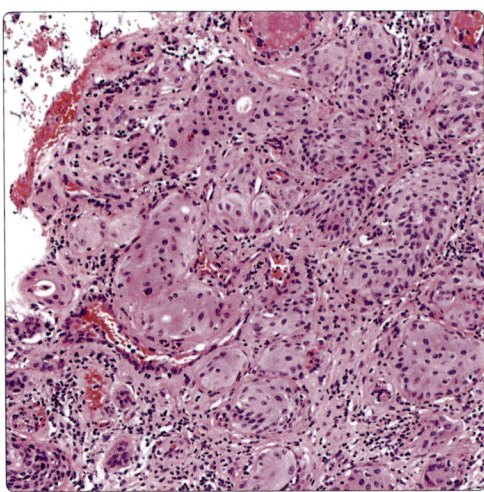

Pseudocarcinomatous Hyperplasia
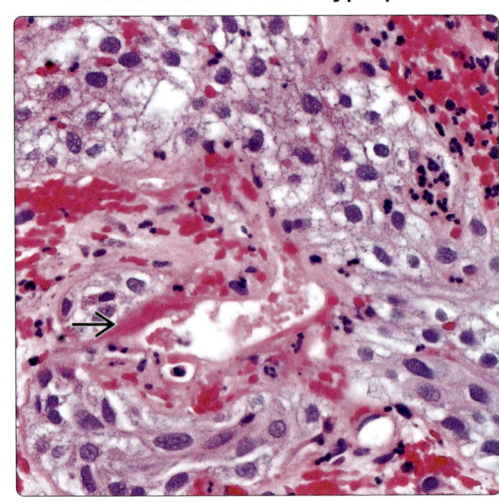

(Left) This florid reactive urothelial proliferation is from a patient who underwent radiation therapy for prostate cancer. Despite the back-to-back nests, the cytology of the urothelial cells is bland, and at most is in the range of reactive atypia. (Right) This blood vessel has fibrin within the wall ⇒, is encircled by cytologically bland urothelium, and has associated extravasated red blood cells and acute inflammation. These features are typical of pseudocarcinomatous hyperplasia.

von Brunn Nests

Inverted Papilloma

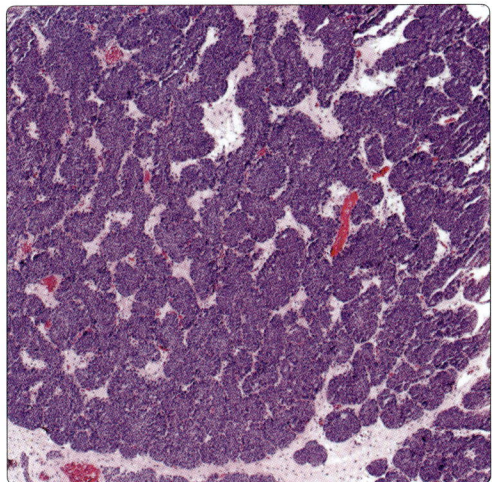

Inverted Papilloma

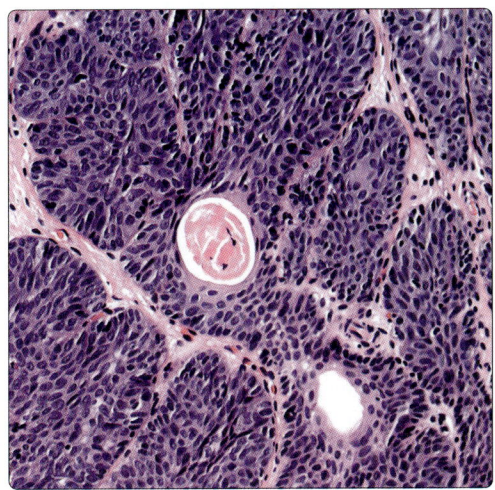

(Left) Inverted papillomas also have an endophytic growth but they typically show a more trabecular, anastomosing growth pattern. The distinction in small lesions may be arbitrary, although more established architecture and expansile growth favors inverted papilloma. (Right) Inverted papillomas may have areas with a cystitis cystica-like pattern. In the context of the appropriate architecture as evaluated at low magnification, this feature should not alter the diagnosis.

Carcinoid Tumor (Low-Grade Neuroendocrine Neoplasm)

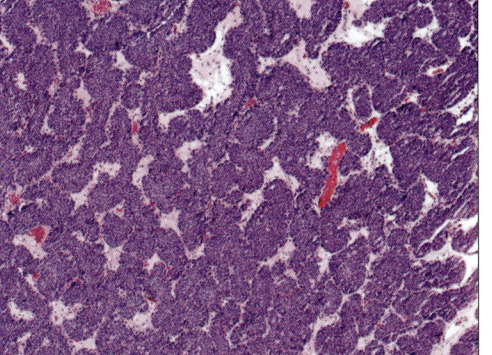

Carcinoid Tumor (Low-Grade Neuroendocrine Neoplasm)

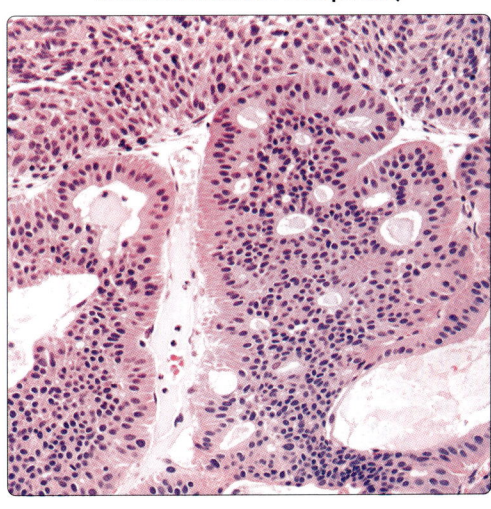

(Left) When seen on a superficial biopsy, the typical monomorphic cytology may cause consideration of a benign lesion. The complex cribriforming ➡ or ribbon-like growth should alert one to the possibility of a carcinoid tumor. (Right) Despite the bland cytologic features, this degree of architectural complexity with cribriform growth should lead to consideration of a neoplastic process such as carcinoid tumor. Expression of synaptophysin would be helpful.

Paraganglia

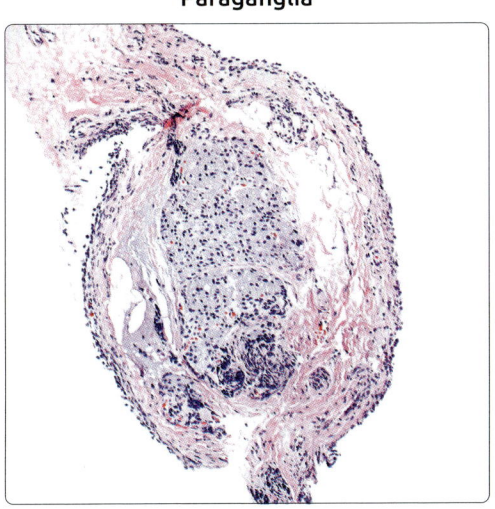

Paraganglia

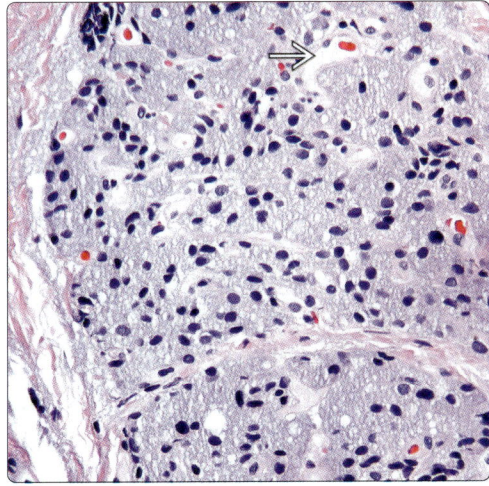

(Left) Paraganglionic tissue in a biopsy specimen shows the lesion is well demarcated and unrelated to urothelium. Paraganglia are present in the lamina propria, rarely in muscularis propria or deeper. Accurate distinction from von Brunn nests is not that clinically significant. (Right) In this paraganglionic tissue, note nested architecture with abundant amphophilic cytoplasm and fine blood vessels (sinusoidal pattern) ➡ between nests. In small biopsy specimens, distinction from a paraganglioma may not be possible.

Nephrogenic Adenoma (Metaplasia)

KEY FACTS

ETIOLOGY/PATHOGENESIS
- Many are secondary to urothelial injury

CLINICAL ISSUES
- Usually incidental microscopic findings
  - May have irritative symptoms from underlying inflammatory process
  - Common in diverticuli

MACROSCOPIC
- May appear as papillary-polypoid mass or irregular flat velvety lesion

MICROSCOPIC
- Papillary and glandular patterns most common
- Papillary cores lined by single cuboidal epithelial layer
- Tubular pattern with hobnail appearance of epithelial cells
- Rare cases have myxoid stroma and cording or spindling of cells (fibromyxoid pattern)
- Rare cases have diffuse sheet-like growth
- Thick basement membrane/hyalinized sheath may underlie epithelium
- Degenerative-type atypia may be present

ANCILLARY TESTS
- Express cytokeratins, pax-2, and pax-8
- May express PSA, PAP (rare and usually focal), and AMACR
- GATA3 expression is variable

TOP DIFFERENTIAL DIAGNOSES
- Clear cell adenocarcinoma of bladder
  - More atypia and mitotic activity
- Prostatic adenocarcinoma
  - May closely mimic tubular nephrogenic adenoma
- Urothelial carcinoma with glandular differentiation
- Nested or tubular variant of urothelial carcinoma
- Papillary urothelial neoplasia

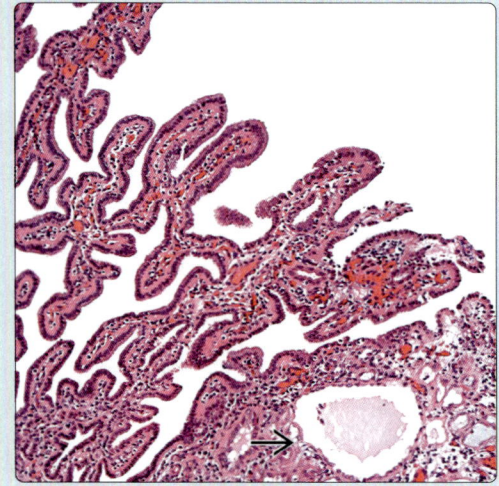

Nephrogenic Adenoma: Papillary Predominant

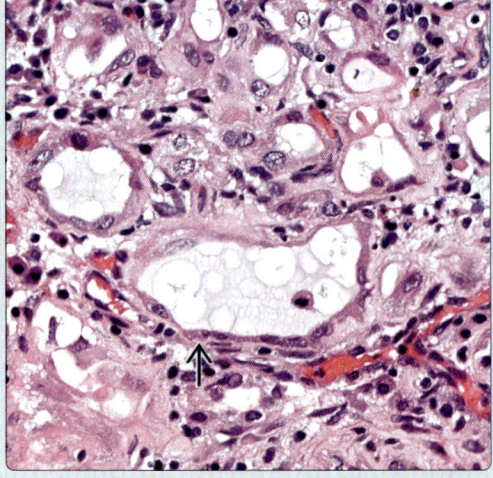

Nephrogenic Adenoma: Tubular

(Left) Mixed exophytic papillary (filiform), cystic, and tubular patterns ➡ of nephrogenic adenoma are common. The papillary cores are characteristically lined by a single layer of cuboidal epithelial cells. (Right) Nephrogenic adenoma commonly shows a tubular pattern in the lamina propria with variably sized lumina lined by flattened atrophic or hobnailed epithelium ➡. Intraluminal mucinous material is also common.

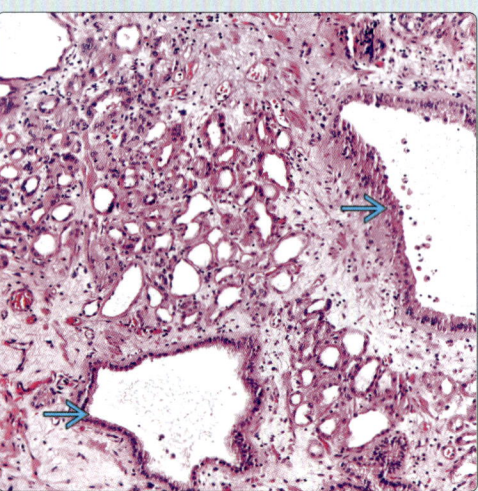

Nephrogenic Adenoma: Tubular and Cystic

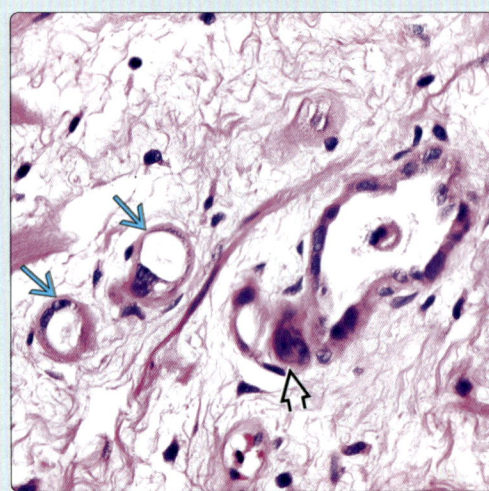

Nephrogenic Adenoma: Tubular With Nucleoli

(Left) This crowded glandular/tubular pattern of nephrogenic adenoma is common. The tubules are often located very superficially beneath the urothelium. Not uncommonly, other patterns are admixed, such as the cystic pattern seen in this example ➡. (Right) Some tubules of nephrogenic adenoma with very small lumina closely resemble vascular spaces ➡. In addition, some of the cells may show nuclear enlargement and nucleoli ➡. The basement membrane is thickened, a helpful feature.

Nephrogenic Adenoma (Metaplasia)

TERMINOLOGY

Abbreviations
- Nephrogenic adenoma (NA)

Synonyms
- Nephrogenic metaplasia

Definitions
- Benign epithelial lesion of urinary tract characterized by tubular, glandular, &/or papillary growth pattern that commonly occurs secondary to injury of urothelium or renal seeding, e.g., post transplantation

ETIOLOGY/PATHOGENESIS

Injury of Urothelium
- Many are secondary to urothelial injury
  - Infections, calculi, instrumentation, intravesical BCG therapy, and surgery
  - May be seen in association with carcinoma
- Also commonly seen within diverticuli
- Combination of renal tubular cell seeding and metaplasia possibly linked to etiopathogenesis

Renal Transplant
- Frequent in renal transplant patients
  - Supports proposed renal tubular origin

CLINICAL ISSUES

Presentation
- Usually incidental microscopic finding
  - Difficult to attribute irritative voiding symptoms to NA given other associated inflammatory findings
- Most commonly in adults but also described in pediatric patients
- Lesions in renal transplant patients may be large

Treatment
- Simple curetting for larger lesions

Prognosis
- Completely benign, but recurrence is described

MACROSCOPIC

General Features
- May appear as papillary-polypoid mass or irregular, flat, velvety lesion

MICROSCOPIC

Histologic Features
- Broad spectrum of architectural patterns (often admixed)
  - Tubular/glandular pattern
    - Most common
    - Low-power architecture may appear pseudoinfiltrative
    - Lining cells may have hobnail appearance
    - Single cells with minute lumen may closely mimic blood vessels or signet ring cells
      - May contain basophilic or eosinophilic intraluminal secretions
    - Thick basement membrane/hyalinized sheath may surround glands
  - Papillary pattern
    - Exophytic papillary cores of variable complexity
      - Broad edematous papillae most common
      - Thin filiform papillae also seen
    - Lined by single layer of cuboidal epithelium
  - Cystic pattern
    - Dilated tubules lined by variably atrophic epithelium
  - Fibromyxoid pattern
    - Rare cases have predominance of myxoid or collagenized stroma
    - Subtle minor population of epithelial cells
      - Most commonly contains spindled epithelial cells
      - Rarely admixed epithelial cords and tubules
  - Diffuse pattern
    - Rare cases have diffuse sheet-like growth
    - Typically with clear cytoplasm
    - Resembles clear cell renal cell carcinoma
  - Flat pattern
    - Single layer of bland cuboidal cells on surface; rarely tangentional sectioning may result in multilayered appearance
    - Resembles denuded urothelium with intact basal layer
- Cytologic features
  - Cytologically bland, cuboidal cells
  - Cytoplasm varies from eosinophilic to clear
  - Nucleoli may be present; in range of reactive atypia
  - Degenerative-type atypia may be present
- Microscopic distribution
  - Located in superficial lamina propria
  - Typically does not show diffuse infiltration of muscularis propria
  - In perirenal region, rare cases show involvement of adipose tissue

Predominant Pattern/Injury Type
- Glandular

Predominant Cell/Compartment Type
- Epithelial

ANCILLARY TESTS

Immunohistochemistry
- Express cytokeratins and EMA
  - Pan keratin
  - CK7
  - High molecular weight cytokeratin
- Express nuclear pax-2 and pax-8
- May express cytoplasmic markers associated with prostatic epithelial origin
  - PSA (rare, focal)
  - PAP (rare, focal)
  - AMACR/racemase/P504S
    - Not biotin artifact
- May express patchy to rarely diffuse GATA3 (40%)
- Multiplex (cocktail) immunostains with AMACR + basal cell markers
  - Staining is extremely variable

Nephrogenic Adenoma (Metaplasia)

- Expression of high molecular weight cytokeratin is seen in most cases
- p63 expression is rare (AMACR + p63 is less useful)
- Often excludes prostatic adenocarcinoma
- Small foci may rarely have identical immunophenotype to prostatic adenocarcinoma
- S100-A1 immunoreactivity is also reported in NA

DIFFERENTIAL DIAGNOSIS

Clear Cell Adenocarcinoma of Urinary Bladder
- Often mixed papillary and cystic tubular patterns
  - Histologic overlap with NA may be striking
  - May have associated densely hyalinized stroma in papillary cores
- Variable nuclear pleomorphism
- Appreciation of cytologic atypia is key
- Mitotically active
  - May show high proliferation rate by Ki-67
- May express p53 and CA125
- Also express nuclear pax-8 and pax-2

Prostatic Adenocarcinoma
- Prostatic adenocarcinoma involving urinary bladder is typically high Gleason grade
  - Solid or cribriform architecture common
- Does not express CK7, pax-2, and pax-8
- Typically more homogeneous glands
  - Cystic and atrophic patterns, as seen in NA, are uncommon
  - Periglandular sheaths of basement membrane-like material are not seen in prostate cancer
- Often has elevated serum PSA
- Immunostains with common prostatic epithelial markers may compound overlapping histologic features
- None or extremely rare immunoreactivity with S100-A1

Urothelial Carcinoma With Glandular Differentiation
- Admixed typical urothelial carcinoma may be present
  - Papillary, in situ, or invasive
- Subset express Uroplakin-2 and GATA3
  - GATA3 may also be expressed in NA
- Typically deeply invasive
- More cytologic atypia than NA

Nested or Tubular or Microcystic Pattern Variant of Urothelial Carcinoma
- Admixed typical urothelial carcinoma may be present
  - Papillary, in situ, or invasive
- More irregular nests of urothelium
- Cytology often very bland
- Deep, irregular infiltration of lamina propria or muscularis propria
- Stromal clefting around invasive foci is common
- Usually express p63

Papillary Urothelial Carcinoma
- Lined by stratified layer of urothelium
- Admixed tubular/glandular pattern in stalks or underlying lamina propria is uncommon
- Frequently express urothelial markers
  - Uroplakin-2, GATA3, p63, and CK20
  - May also express pax-8 and pax-2

Urothelial Carcinoma In Situ
- Flat NA may cause consideration of denuding carcinoma in situ
- Urothelial carcinoma in situ has more atypia
  - Larger nuclei
  - Coarse nuclear chromatin
  - Frequent mitotic activity
  - Occasional pagetoid spread into adjacent urothelium

Other Secondary Adenocarcinomas
- Greater cytologic atypia and destructive invasion
- Most commonly colorectal with enteric features
- Endocervical adenocarcinomas may be deceptively bland

DIAGNOSTIC CHECKLIST

Clinically Relevant Pathologic Features
- Frequently misinterpreted as low-grade prostatic adenocarcinoma or urothelial papilloma

Pathologic Interpretation Pearls
- Knowledge of wide spectrum of morphologic patterns, which commonly occur in various combinations, is essential
- NA may express immunohistochemical markers expected in prostate cancer, especially AMACR
- NA should be considered in superficial urethral biopsies
  - Especially if low-grade prostatic adenocarcinoma is considered

SELECTED REFERENCES

1. McDaniel AS et al: Immunohistochemical staining characteristics of nephrogenic adenoma using the PIN-4 cocktail (p63, AMACR, and CK903) and GATA-3. Am J Surg Pathol. 38(12):1664-71, 2014
2. Diolombi M et al: Nephrogenic adenoma: a report of 3 unusual cases infiltrating into perinephric adipose tissue. Am J Surg Pathol. 37(4):532-8, 2013
3. Kao CS et al: Nephrogenic adenomas in pediatric patients: a morphologic and immunohistochemical study of 21 cases. Pediatr Dev Pathol. 16(2):80-5, 2013
4. López JI et al: Nephrogenic adenoma of the urinary tract: clinical, histological, and immunohistochemical characteristics. Virchows Arch. 463(6):819-25, 2013
5. Piña-Oviedo S et al: Flat pattern of nephrogenic adenoma: previously unrecognized pattern unveiled using PAX2 and PAX8 immunohistochemistry. Mod Pathol. 26(6):792-8, 2013
6. Rahemtullah A et al: Nephrogenic adenoma: an update on an innocuous but troublesome entity. Adv Anat Pathol. 13(5):247-55, 2006
7. Tong GX et al: PAX2: a reliable marker for nephrogenic adenoma. Mod Pathol. 19(3):356-63, 2006
8. Skinnider BF et al: Expression of alpha-methylacyl-CoA racemase (P504S) in nephrogenic adenoma: a significant immunohistochemical pitfall compounding the differential diagnosis with prostatic adenocarcinoma. Am J Surg Pathol. 28(6):701-5, 2004

Nephrogenic Adenoma (Metaplasia)

Nephrogenic Adenoma: Cystic
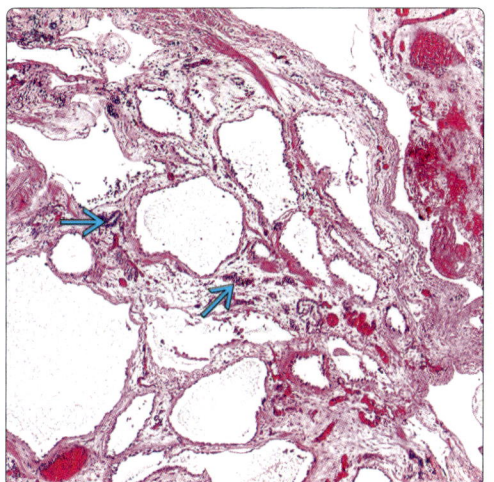

Nephrogenic Adenoma: Tubular
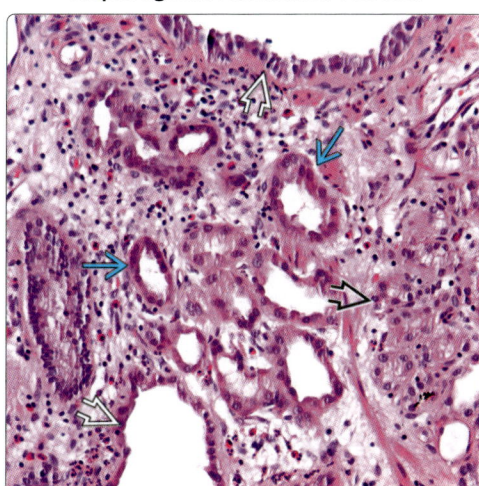

(Left) Large dilated cysts are sometimes the predominant pattern of nephrogenic adenoma. They are usually lined by eosinophilic cells with an atrophic or hobnail arrangement. Smaller tubules are often intermixed ➡ but may be obscured. (Right) This is the prototypical tubular pattern of nephrogenic adenoma resembling renal tubules ➡. Other adjacent patterns include cystic glands ➡ and solid nests/cords ➡. The stroma is edematous.

Nephrogenic Adenoma: Solid Cords
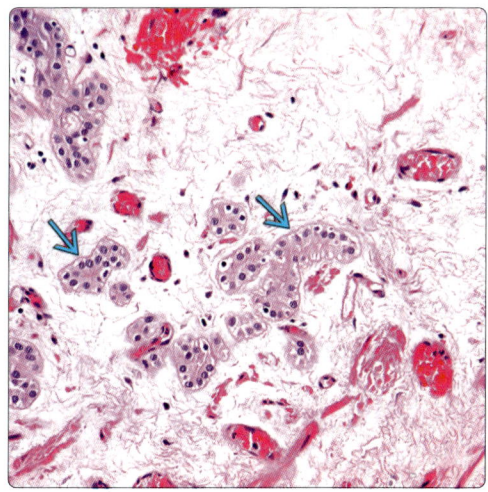

Nephrogenic Adenoma: Papillary
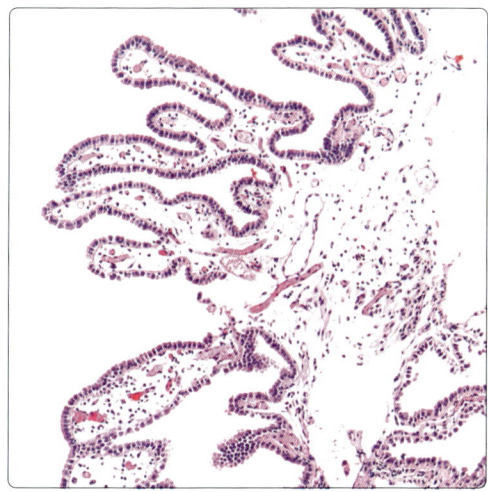

(Left) Small tubules of nephrogenic adenoma may have a pseudoinfiltrative appearance that closely mimics prostatic adenocarcinoma. Although not always seen, the thin rim of basement membrane-like material ➡ is characteristic. (Right) The papillary pattern of nephrogenic adenoma may have variable filiform or larger edematous papillae. Unlike papillary urothelial neoplasia, the papillae are lined by a single layer of cytologically bland cuboidal epithelial cells.

Nephrogenic Adenoma: Flat
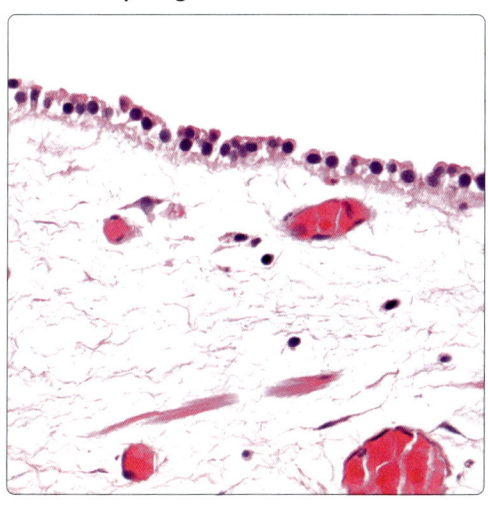

Nephrogenic Adenoma: Solid Nests
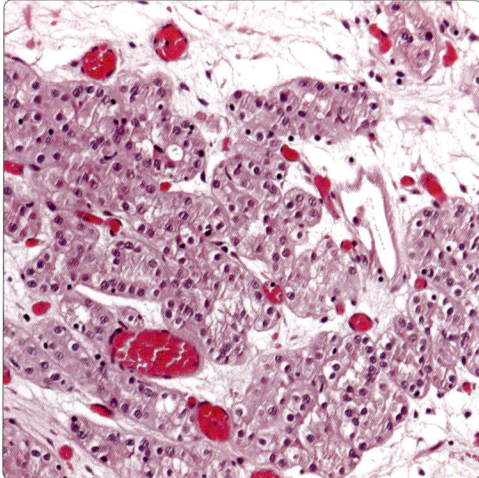

(Left) The recently described flat pattern of nephrogenic adenoma is difficult to distinguish from denuded urothelium with residual basal cells but is usually seen adjacent to other patterns. Bland cytology is distinct from urothelial carcinoma in situ. IHC may be helpful. (Right) The tubules of nephrogenic adenoma may occasionally have a solid or cord-like pattern. This histologic appearance may closely mimic prostatic adenocarcinoma due to the monomorphic nuclei. When seen back to back, a diffuse pattern is created.

Nephrogenic Adenoma (Metaplasia)

Nephrogenic Adenoma: Signet Ring-Like
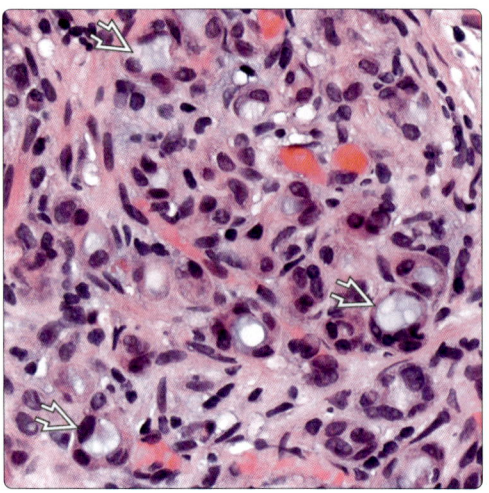

Nephrogenic Adenoma: Fibromyxoid
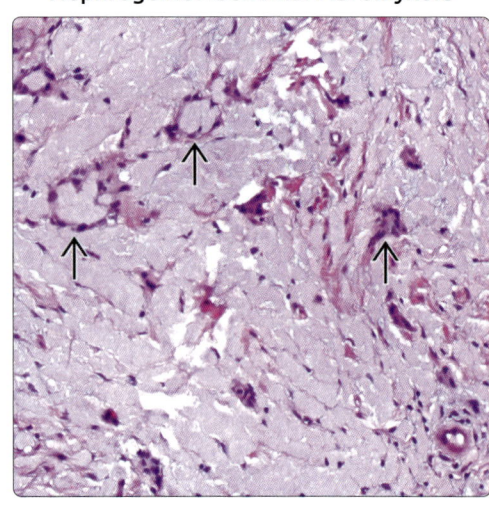

(Left) Small tubules of nephrogenic adenoma may contain intraluminal basophilic material that closely mimics a signet ring cell adenocarcinoma ➡. Other more typical patterns of nephrogenic adenoma are almost always present to aid in diagnosis. (Right) The fibromyxoid pattern of nephrogenic adenoma is characterized by prominent myxoid stroma and scattered irregular cords of epithelium ➡. Awareness of this rare pattern is important because it may possibly mimic myxoid mesenchymal neoplasms.

Nephrogenic Adenoma: Diffuse
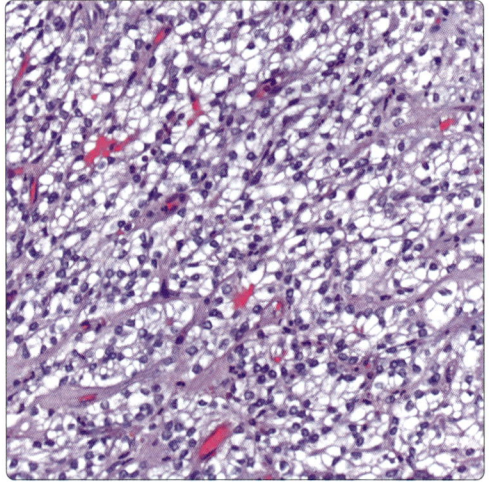

Nephrogenic Adenoma: Pseudoinfiltrative
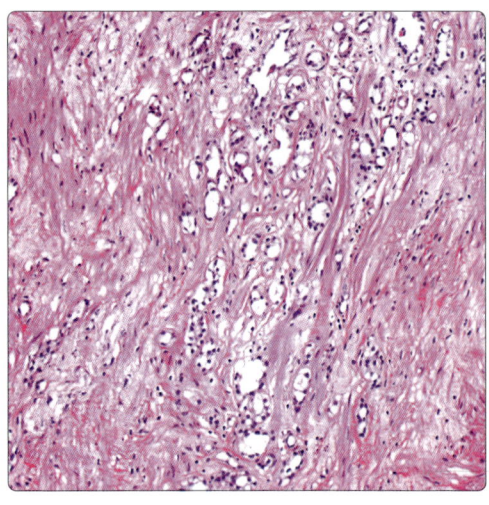

(Left) Solid growth in nephrogenic adenoma has been described as the diffuse pattern, and it resembles renal cell carcinoma. (Right) The tubular pattern of nephrogenic adenoma may appear pseudoinfiltrative, another feature that may be confused with prostatic carcinoma. It is important to carefully consider nephrogenic adenoma in bladder and urethral biopsies. The immunohistochemical overlap further compounds the problem.

Nephrogenic Adenoma: Compressed Tubules
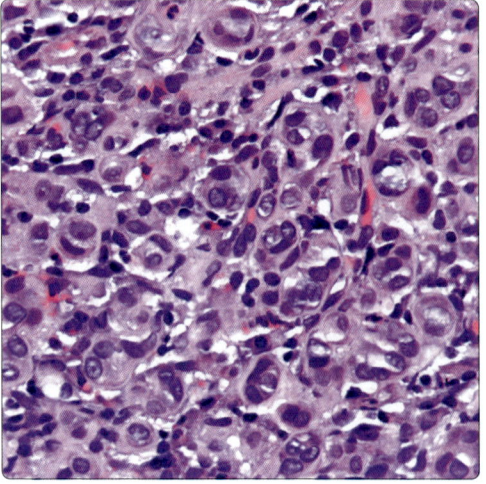

Nephrogenic Adenoma: Tubular/Cystic
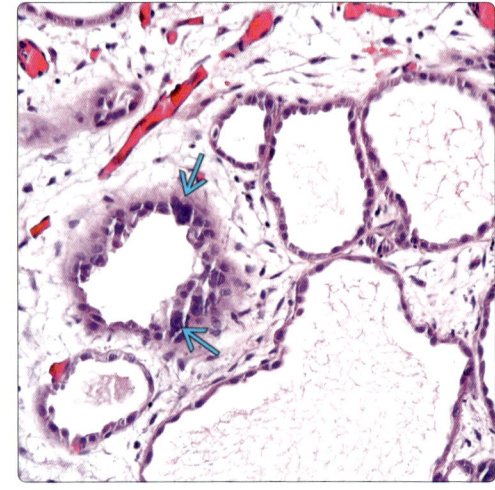

(Left) Tightly packed tubules of nephrogenic adenoma may create a solid appearance simulating a carcinoma or paraganglioma. This architectural pattern may be difficult to recognize, but multiple patterns are often intermixed to aid in the differential diagnosis. (Right) These cystically dilated tubules of nephrogenic adenoma show a focus with atypical epithelial cells ➡. They are not mitotically active. This finding is not uncommon and should not alter the diagnosis.

Nephrogenic Adenoma (Metaplasia)

Nephrogenic Adenoma: pax-8
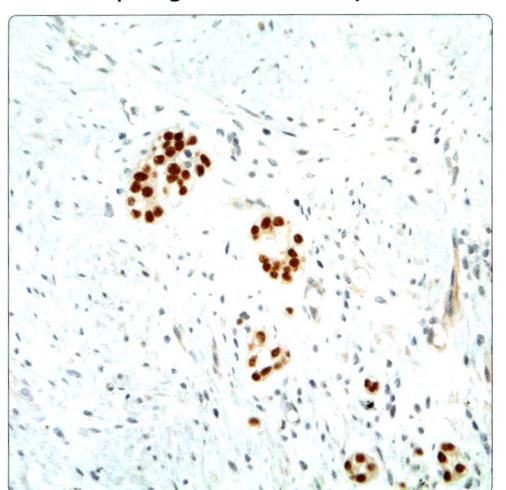

Nephrogenic Adenoma: pax-2
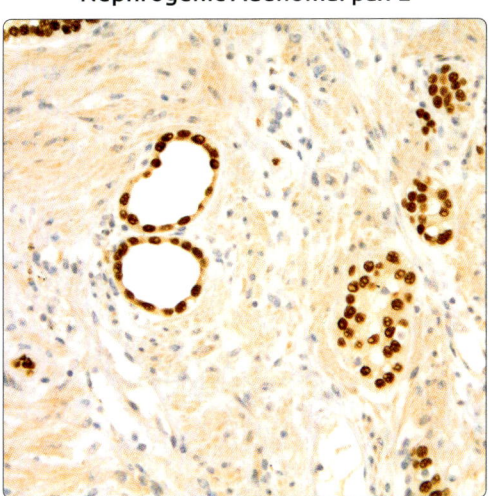

(Left) Strong nuclear staining for pax-8 is typical of nephrogenic adenoma. To date, prostatic adenocarcinomas have been uniformly negative for pax-8. Urothelium may express pax-8, including urothelial carcinomas (especially in the upper tract). A combination of markers employed depending on the histology including racemase and low Ki-67 are helpful. (Right) Nuclear pax-2 staining is also expected in nephrogenic adenoma. Clear cell adenocarcinoma, which is in the differential, may also express pax-2 or pax-8.

Nephrogenic Adenoma: CK7
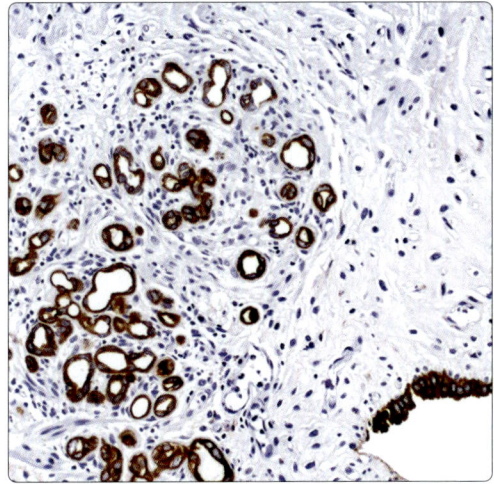

Nephrogenic Adenoma: GATA3
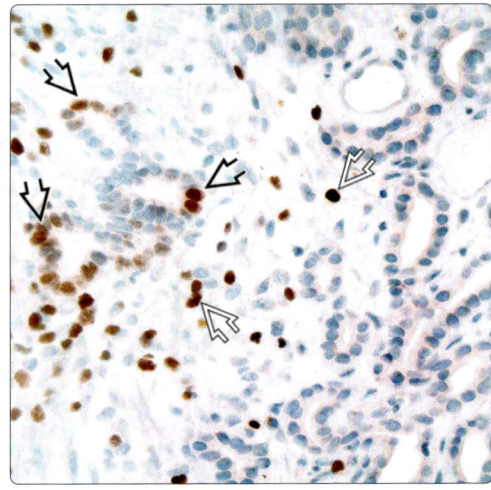

(Left) Strong cytoplasmic immunoreactivity for CK7 is typical of nephrogenic adenoma, whereas prostatic adenocarcinoma is typically negative. (Right) Patchy nuclear GATA3 staining is seen in up to 40% of nephrogenic adenomas ⇒, as in this example; therefore, it is not useful in distinction from urothelial tumors. A subset of background lymphocytes are typically positive for GATA3 as well ⇒.

Nephrogenic Adenoma: AMACR + p63
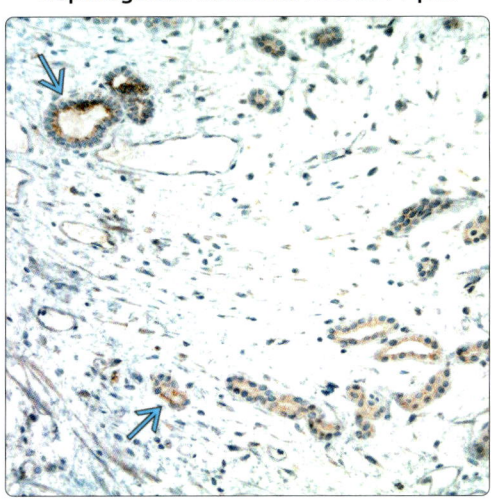

Nephrogenic Adenoma: PSA
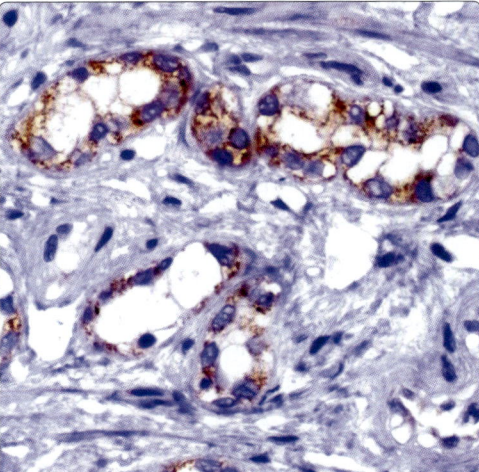

(Left) This multiplex AMACR and p63 immunostain highlights the potential pitfall in the distinction from a low-grade prostate cancer. p63 immunoreactivity is almost always absent, whereas luminal AMACR staining ⇒ is common. High molecular weight cytokeratin is a more useful marker in this combination setting. (Right) Strong cytoplasmic immunoreactivity for PSA may be seen in nephrogenic adenoma. This finding represents a major diagnostic pitfall in the distinction from prostatic adenocarcinoma.

Nephrogenic Adenoma (Metaplasia)

Urothelial Papillary Neoplasia

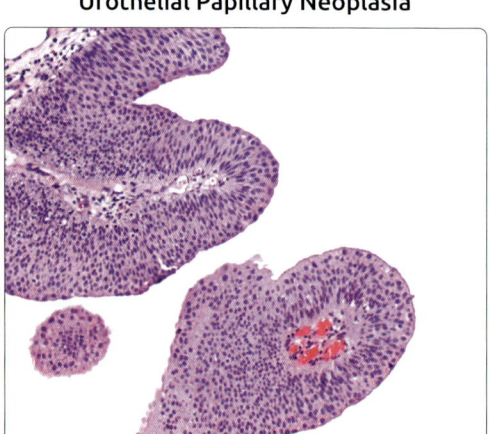

Urothelial Papillary Neoplasia

(Left) *In contrast to papillary nephrogenic adenoma that is characterized by a single cuboidal layer of epithelium lining the papillary cores, papillary urothelial neoplasms have a stratified layer of epithelium. An accompanying endophytic component is unusual in urothelial neoplasms, whereas it is typical in nephrogenic adenoma.* (Right) *Papillary urothelial carcinoma is distinct from the papillary component of nephrogenic adenoma because of the stratified layer of epithelium.*

Prostatic Adenocarcinoma

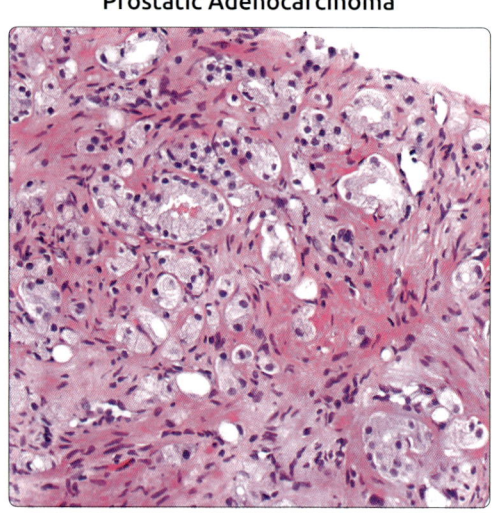

Prostatic Adenocarcinoma

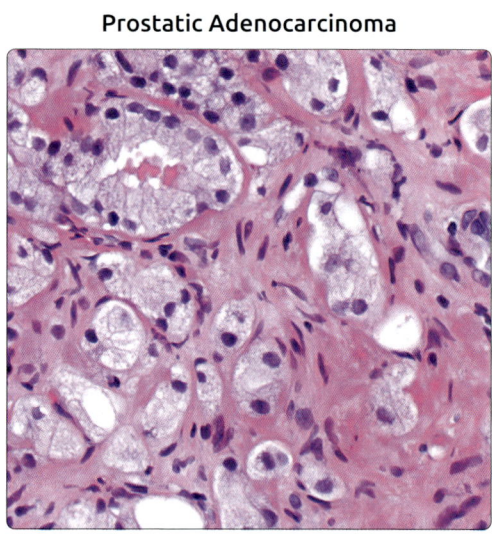

(Left) *When involving the urinary bladder, prostatic carcinoma is typically of higher grade.* (Right) *This prostatic carcinoma shows the potential morphologic overlap with nephrogenic adenoma. In difficult cases, pax-2/pax-8 immunohistochemistry may be useful, as it is positive in nephrogenic adenoma. Strong PSA/PAP suggests a diagnosis of prostate cancer, but staining may be seen in nephrogenic adenoma as well. NKX3, PSMA, and P501S more useful to confirm prostatic carcinoma.*

Urothelial Carcinoma: Microcystic

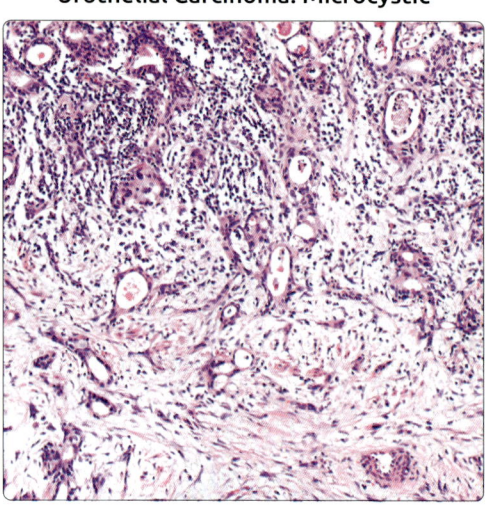

Urothelial Carcinoma: Small Tubules

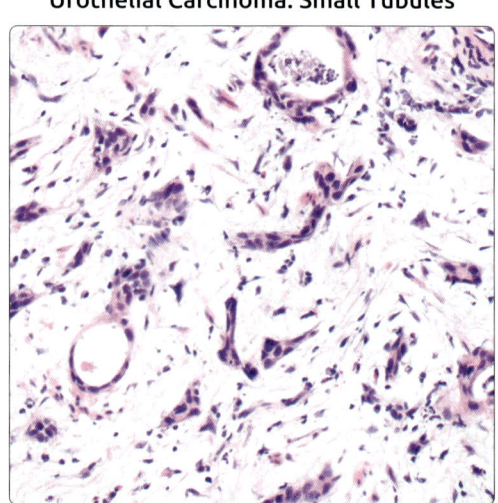

(Left) *This example of invasive urothelial carcinoma with a microcystic pattern may also mimic nephrogenic adenoma. The stromal reaction and typically deep irregular invasion help in the distinction from nephrogenic adenoma.* (Right) *The individual neoplastic cells in urothelial carcinoma with small tubules may be deceptively bland. The haphazard architectural distribution and stromal reaction are important features in the distinction from nephrogenic adenoma.*

Nephrogenic Adenoma (Metaplasia)

Urothelial Carcinoma: Chordoid/Myxoid

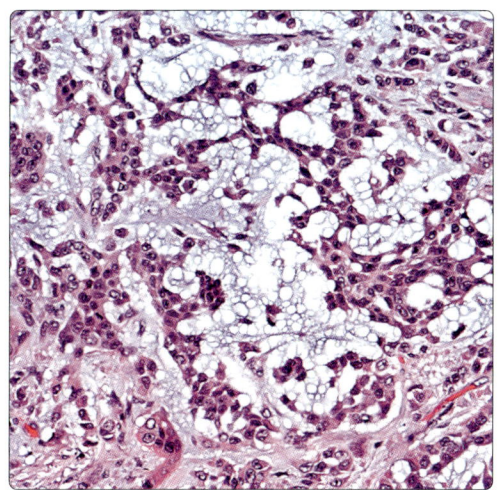

Urothelial Carcinoma: Glandular Differentiation

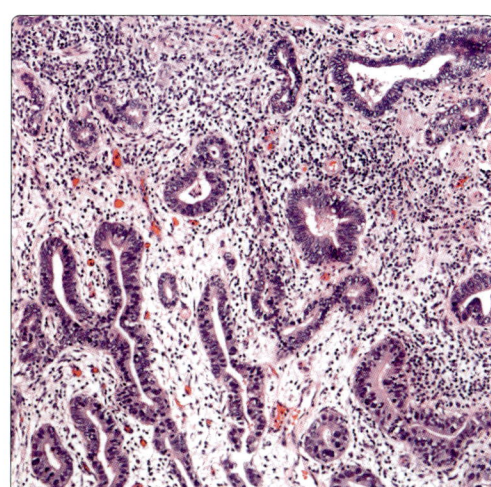

(Left) *Invasive urothelial carcinoma with myxoid stroma may mimic fibromyxoid nephrogenic adenoma, especially in small biopsy specimens. Carcinomas have more prominent epithelium, and other typical patterns of urothelial carcinoma are commonly present.* (Right) *This urothelial carcinoma had extensive glandular differentiation. The degree and extent of cytologic atypia is beyond that seen in nephrogenic adenoma. In addition, these tumors are typically diffusely invasive into muscularis propria.*

Clear Cell Adenocarcinoma

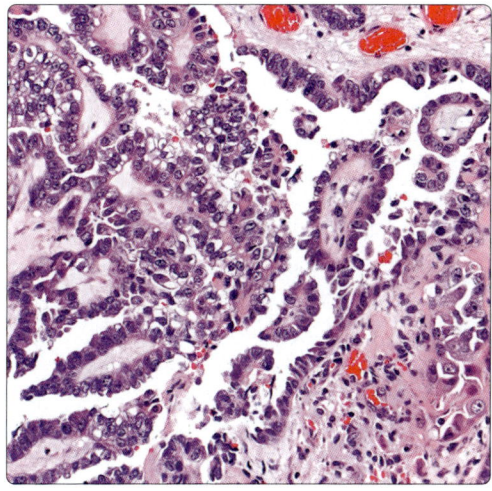

Clear Cell Adenocarcinoma

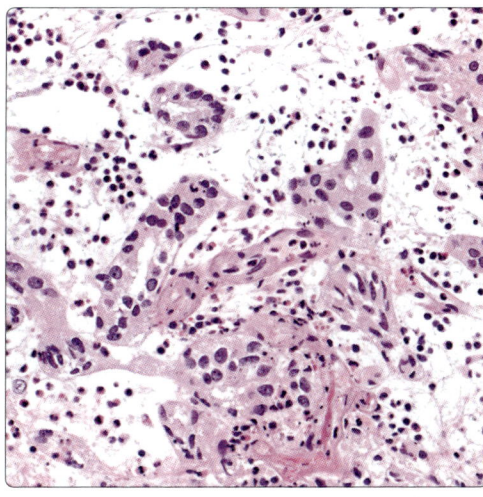

(Left) *Clear cell adenocarcinoma of the bladder may have a papillary growth pattern with a single cuboidal lining. In contrast to papillary NA, clear cell adenocarcinoma has a greater degree of nuclear atypia and may have areas of epithelial stratification and tufting.* (Right) *Tubular/glandular pattern of clear cell adenocarcinoma has significant morphologic overlap with NA, but subtle variations in nuclear size and shape need consideration of malignancy.*

Clear Cell Adenocarcinoma

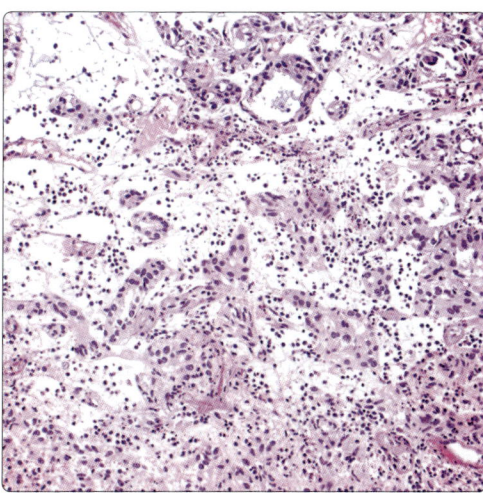

Clear Cell Adenocarcinoma

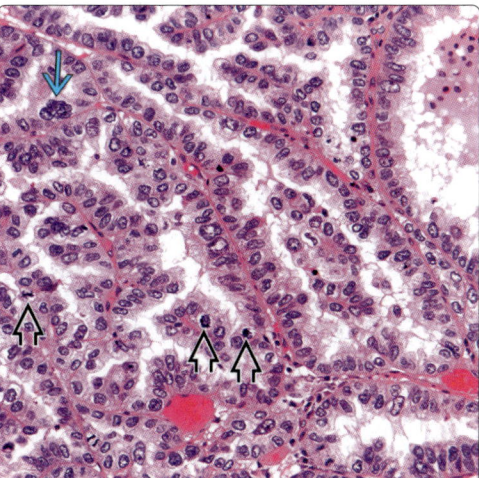

(Left) *Clear cell adenocarcinoma of the urinary bladder with a tubular/glandular pattern may closely mimic nephrogenic adenoma, especially on low-power histologic evaluation.* (Right) *In contrast to nephrogenic adenoma, clear cell adenocarcinoma typically has morphologic features of malignancy that include more coarse nuclear chromatin, obvious nuclear pleomorphism ➡, and easily identified mitotic activity ➡.*

Fibroepithelial Polyp

KEY FACTS

TERMINOLOGY
- Nonneoplastic polyp of bladder

CLINICAL ISSUES
- Usually reported in children and adolescents
- Almost exclusively in males
- More commonly occurs in urethra and ureter
- Treatment is conservative transurethral resection
- Nonrecurring lesion

MICROSCOPIC
- Polypoid excrescence with variably bulbous to elongated papillae
- Cloverleaf-like or club-like projections of mucosa
- Florid cystitis glandularis of nonintestinal type in stalk
- Urothelial lining typical or reactive; rarely hyperplastic
- Typically fibrous stroma
- Scattered atypical stromal cells may be present
- Stroma may rarely show myofibroblastic or smooth muscle features

TOP DIFFERENTIAL DIAGNOSES
- Botryoid rhabdomyosarcoma
  - Often has similar polypoid architecture
  - Cambium layer is often well-developed
  - Rhabdomyoblasts may be seen
  - Immunoreactivity for myogenin is diagnostic
- Prostatic type polyp
  - Contains admixed prostatic secretory epithelium
  - Immunoreactivity for prostatic markers
    - PSA
    - Other: PSMA, NKX 3.1, PAP
- Inverted papilloma
  - Epithelial predominant
  - More confluent and anastomosing urothelial architecture

Fibroepithelial Polyp: Macroscopic Features

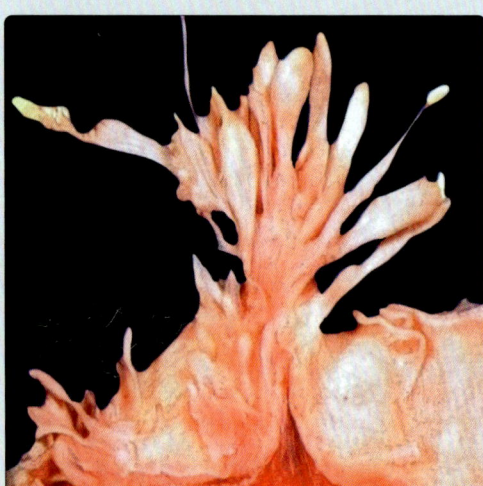

Fibroepithelial Polyp: Cystitis Glandularis-Like

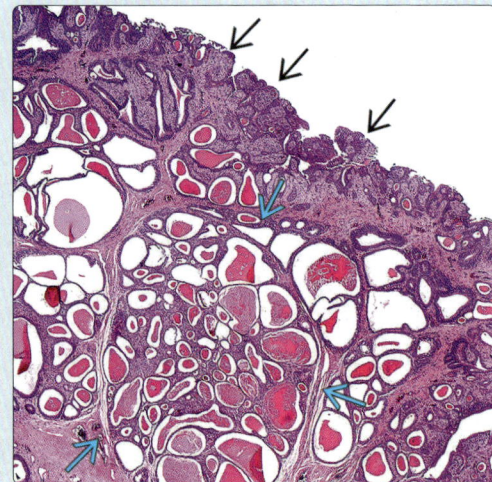

(Left) Fibroepithelial polyp with polypoid and papillary projections is shown. In contrast to papillary tumors, each papillary structure is more distinct due to a more prominent fibrous component, and there is less complex branching. **(Right)** The surface of this fibroepithelial polyp shows the typical club-like projections ➡. Deeper in the stalk, there are crowded collections of benign glands identical to florid cystitis glandularis ➡.

Fibroepithelial Polyp: Benign Urothelium

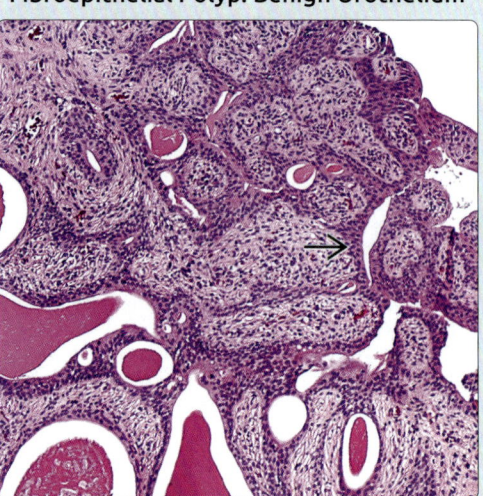

Fibroepithelial Polyp: Benign Urothelium

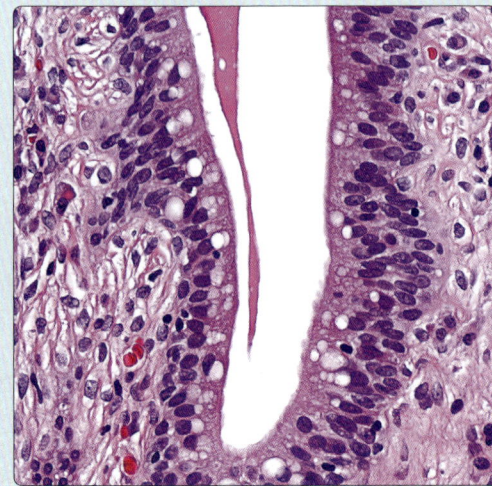

(Left) The lining of a fibroepithelial polyp is typically urothelial ➡. The rest of the epithelial component varies from resembling florid von Brunn nests to cystitis cystica or glandularis. **(Right)** High-power magnification of fibroepithelial polyp shows the bland cytology of the epithelium that is identical to that of cystitis glandularis.

Fibroepithelial Polyp

TERMINOLOGY

Abbreviations
- Fibroepithelial polyp (FEP)

Synonyms
- Congenital posterior urethral polyp
- Botryoid fibroepithelial polyp

Definitions
- Nonneoplastic polyp of bladder
  - May be hamartomatous process

CLINICAL ISSUES

Epidemiology
- Incidence
  - Rare lesion
    - ~ 180 reported
- Age
  - Usually reported in children and adolescents
  - In adults, median age: 44 years old
- Sex
  - Almost exclusively in males

Site
- Usually near verumontanum or bladder neck
- More commonly occurs in urethra and ureter

Presentation
- Acute urinary retention with bladder outlet obstruction
- Hematuria

Treatment
- Conservative transurethral resection

Prognosis
- Benign
  - Nonrecurring, if completely excised

MACROSCOPIC

General Features
- Papillary or polypoid lesion
  - Usually 1-2 cm

MICROSCOPIC

Histologic Features
- Polypoid excrescence with variably bulbous to elongated papillae
  - Cloverleaf-like projections of lining urothelium
    - Reminiscent of adenofibromas of gynecologic tract
  - Florid cystitis glandularis of nonintestinal type in stalk
  - Urothelial lining typical, reactive or hyperplastic
  - Secondary papillae with elongated, finger-like projections may be seen
  - Typically fibrous stroma
    - Scattered atypical stromal cells may be present
    - Myofibroblastic proliferation has also been described

DIFFERENTIAL DIAGNOSIS

Embryonal Rhabdomyosarcoma
- Polypoid, botryoid growth pattern of fibroepithelial polyp may closely resemble embryonal rhabdomyosarcoma
- Usually more cellular stroma
  - Cambium layer is typically present
  - May have obvious rhabdomyoblasts
- Coexpression of cytoplasmic desmin with nuclear myogenin &/or MYOD1 is diagnostic of rhabdomyosarcoma

Florid Cystitis Cystica/Glandularis
- Endophytic nests in fibroepithelial polyp are identical to cystitis cystica/glandularis
- No exophytic papillary component

Papillary-Polypoid Cystitis
- More edematous stroma with admixed chronic inflammation
- More simple papillary architecture
- Cystitis cystica/glandularis component not prominent feature
- Some reported fibroepithelial polyps may represent papillary-polypoid cystitis
  - Fibroepithelial polyp may be end stage of papillary-polypoid cystitis

Urothelial Papilloma
- More slender papillae with secondary branching
  - Less bulbous appearance
- Prominent umbrella cells are common
  - May have extensive vacuolization

Inverted Papilloma
- Endophytic growth with thin anastomosing cords
- More epithelial predominant lesion

Bladder Hamartoma
- Extremely rare lesion
- More extensive epithelial nests distributed haphazardly within stalk
- Squamous metaplasia may be present

Prostatic-Type Polyp
- Contains admixed prostatic secretory cells and urothelium
  - Express PSA and PAP by immunohistochemistry

DIAGNOSTIC CHECKLIST

Pathologic Interpretation Pearls
- In children, botryoid rhabdomyosarcoma must be excluded
  - Some embryonal rhabdomyosarcomas are deceptively bland
  - Immunohistochemistry with myogenin may be useful

SELECTED REFERENCES

1. Tsuzuki T et al: Fibroepithelial polyp of the lower urinary tract in adults. Am J Surg Pathol. 29(4):460-6, 2005
2. Musselman P et al: The spectrum of urinary tract fibroepithelial polyps in children. J Urol. 136(2):476-7, 1986
3. Young RH: Fibroepithelial polyp of the bladder with atypical stromal cells. Arch Pathol Lab Med. 110(3):241-2, 1986

Fibroepithelial Polyp

Fibroepithelial Polyp: Architecture

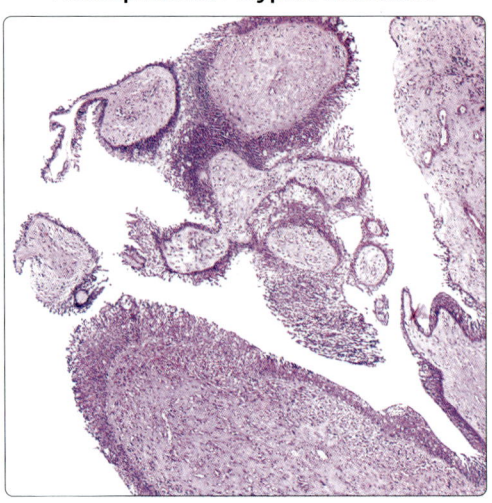

Fibroepithelial Polyp: Architecture

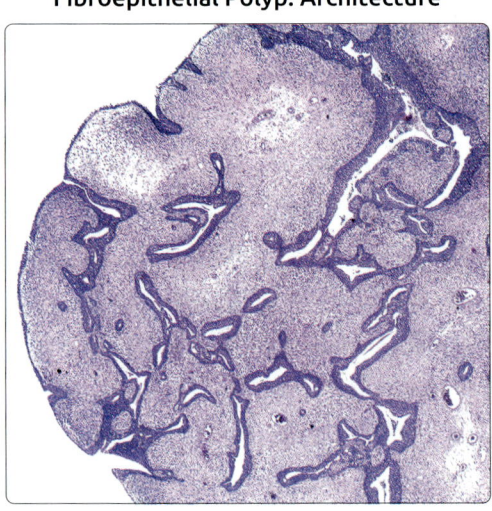

(Left) The surface of fibroepithelial polyps often has a bulbous, polypoid architecture that may mimic a urothelial neoplasm or papillary-polypoid cystitis. The stroma is typically more cellular than that seen in papillary-polypoid cystitis. (Right) Fibroepithelial polyps may have a relatively complex mixed stromal-epithelial architecture, as in this example. The epithelium is not as prominent nor as complex as that seen in inverted urothelial papilloma.

Fibroepithelial Polyp: Architecture

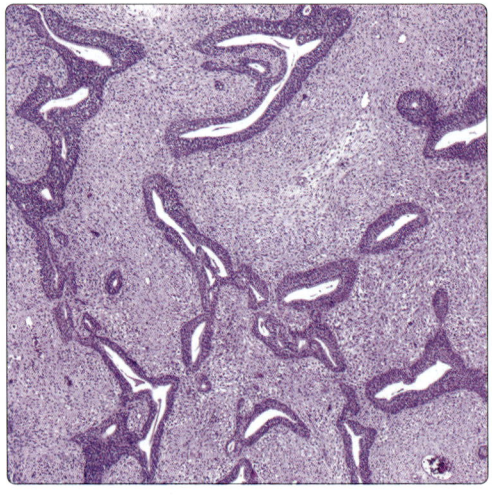

Fibroepithelial Polyp: Epithelium

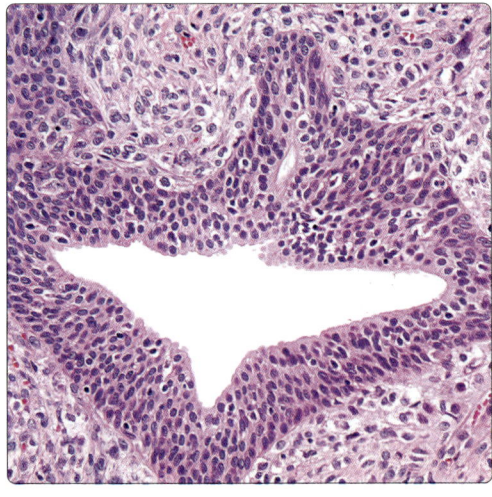

(Left) In this example, the invaginated epithelium has a branching architecture and consists of urothelium with normal cytologic features. Invasive urothelial carcinoma or adenocarcinoma typically shows a greater degree of cytologic atypia. The typical fibrotic stroma contrasts with a desmoplastic stromal response of carcinoma. (Right) The invaginated epithelium has an appearance of cytologically normal urothelium with a central luminal space.

Fibroepithelial Polyp: Architecture

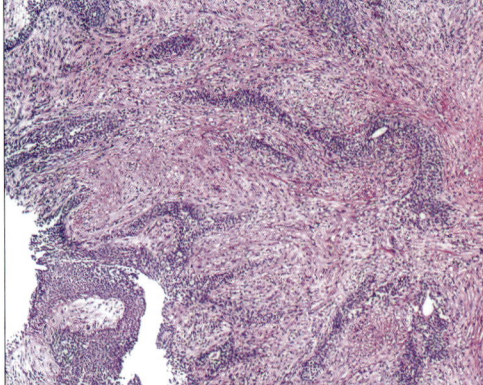

Fibroepithelial Polyp: Epithelium

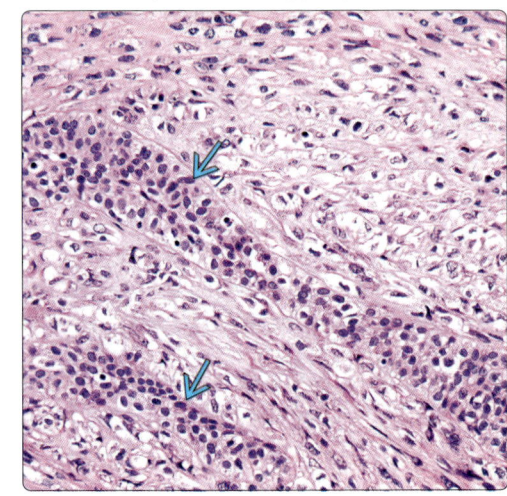

(Left) In this fibroepithelial polyp, there are invaginated cords of urothelium. This pattern may closely mimic inverted urothelial papilloma. Inverted urothelial papilloma shows greater epithelial predominance and complexity. (Right) This invaginated epithelium in a fibroepithelial polyp ⇒ does not have the complex anastomosing growth or the peripheral palisading typical of inverted urothelial papilloma.

Fibroepithelial Polyp

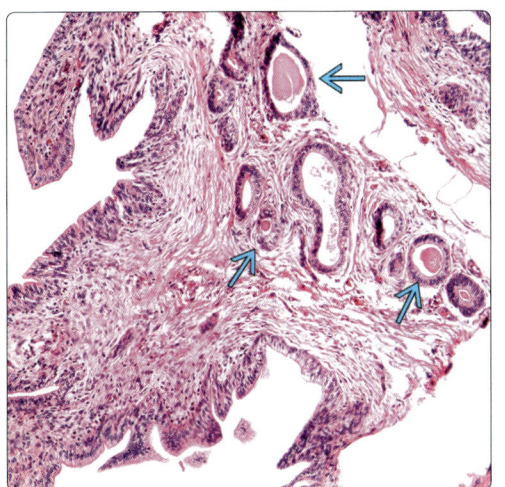

Fibroepithelial Polyp: Epithelium

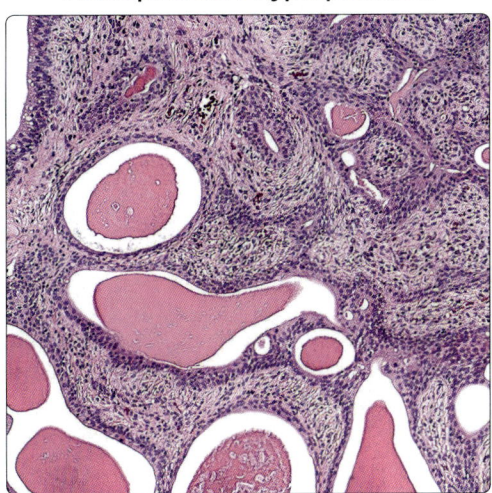

Fibroepithelial Polyp: Epithelium

(Left) The glands within the stalk of a fibroepithelial polyp ➡ may have an intraluminal secretion and often resemble florid cystitis cystica or cystitis glandularis, which do not share the polypoid, club-like architecture or more cellular stroma. (Right) The stalks of fibroepithelial polyps commonly contain crowded benign dilate von Brunn nests or glands reminiscent of cystitis cystica or cystitis glandularis. The central lumina may be filled with thick eosinophilic secretions.

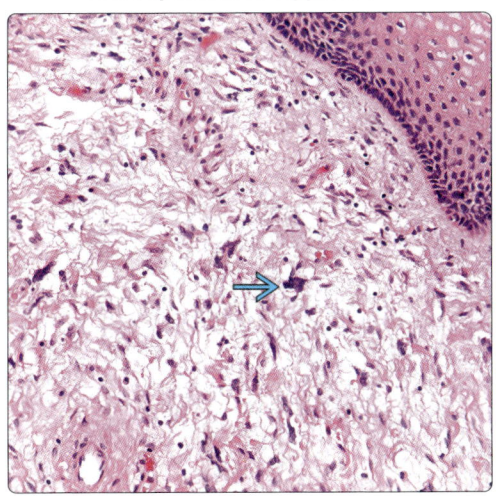

Fibroepithelial Polyp: Stroma

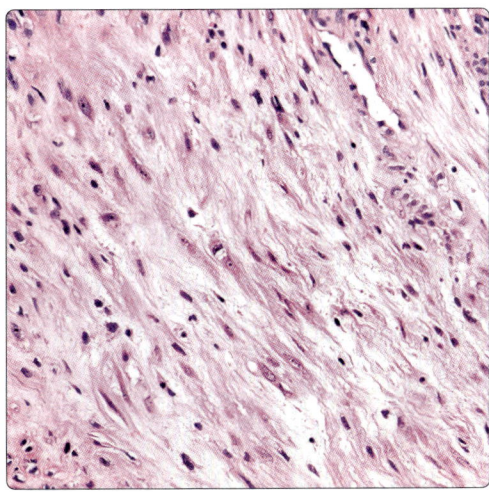

Fibroepithelial Polyp: Stroma

(Left) Fibroepithelial polyps may contain atypical stromal cells with multilobated nuclei ➡. This finding does not change the expected benign behavior. In addition, the subepithelial stroma may occasionally resemble the cambium layer of rhabdomyosarcoma. (Right) The stroma may have cellular foci with a myofibroblastic appearance, similar to inflammatory myofibroblastic tumor, characterized by elongated cytoplasmic processes, elongated nuclei with fine chromatin, and variable nucleoli.

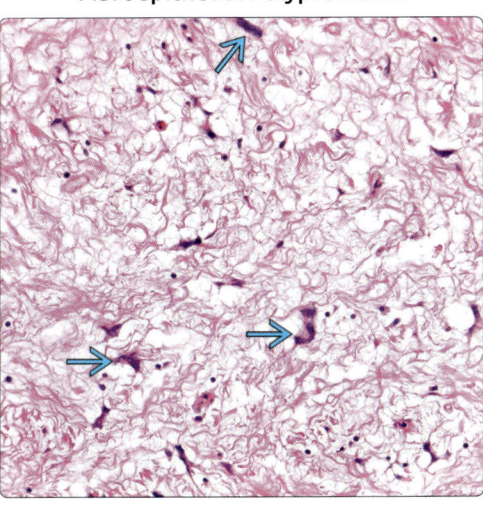

Fibroepithelial Polyp: Stroma

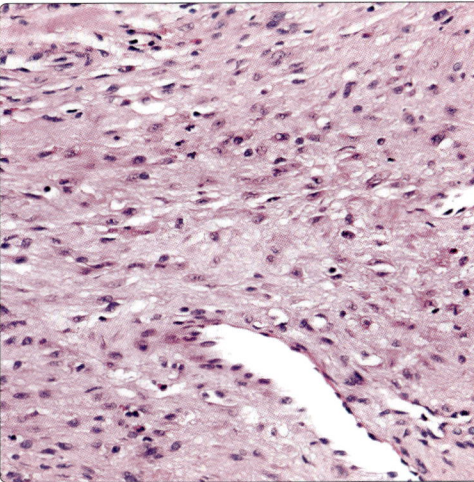

Fibroepithelial Polyp: Stroma

(Left) The stromal cells in fibroepithelial polyps may show "degenerate atypia" ➡ as described in other anatomic sites. These cells often show eccentric, multilobated nuclei identical to those historically described as "giant cell cystitis." (Right) Some foci may show a cellular fibroblastic stroma. This stromal component is one of the main distinguishing features form papillary-polypoid cystitis.

Prostatic-Type Polyp (Ectopic Prostate)

KEY FACTS

ETIOLOGY/PATHOGENESIS
- Multiple theories proposed
  - Metaplastic, ectopia, developmental anomaly, or prolapse

CLINICAL ISSUES
- Broad range: 19-89 years
- Trigone is most common site in bladder
- Most common in prostatic urethra
- Hematuria, hematospermia
- Polypoid mass with variable exophytic fronds

MICROSCOPIC
- Polypoid or papillary/filiform exophytic process
- Stroma contains benign prostatic-type secretory glandular epithelium and admixed urothelium
- Excrescences lined by cytologically benign prostatic secretory cells &/or urothelium
- Long, finger-like projections are rarely seen

ANCILLARY TESTS
- Immunoreaction for PSA and PAP in prostatic secretory cells

TOP DIFFERENTIAL DIAGNOSES
- Prostatic ductal adenocarcinoma
- Papillary urothelial neoplasm
- Benign prostatic hyperplasia
- Nephrogenic adenoma
- Papillary-polypoid cystitis
- Cystitis cystica/glandularis

DIAGNOSTIC CHECKLIST
- Prostatic ductal carcinoma must be carefully considered and excluded by morphology
  - Has subtle, often cytologically bland stratified columnar lining with adenomatous appearance
  - Corpora amylacea and 2 cell-type lining are useful in recognizing as benign

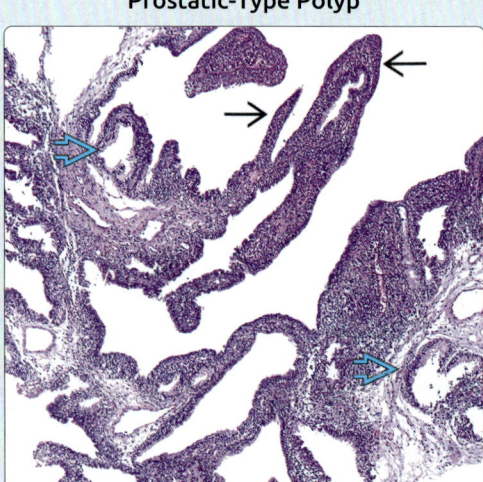

Prostatic-Type Polyp

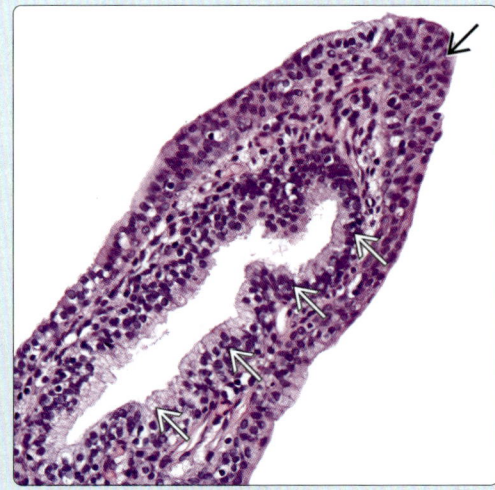

Prostatic-Type Polyp

(Left) *Prostatic-type polyps range from polypoid to villiform ➡, as seen in this example. The key diagnostic feature is the presence of prostatic secretory glands within the stroma ➡.* (Right) *On high-power examination of this prostatic-type polyp, the contrast between the lining urothelial cells ➡ and the prostatic secretory epithelium ➡ is highlighted.*

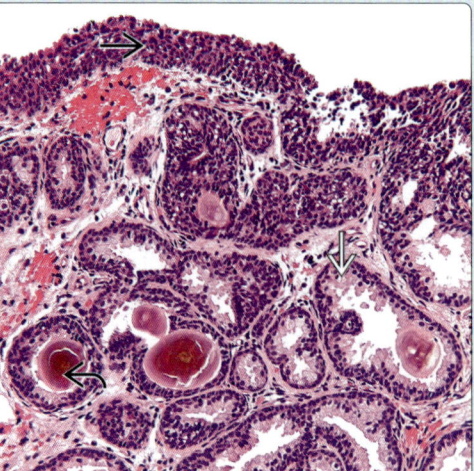

Prostatic-Type Polyp

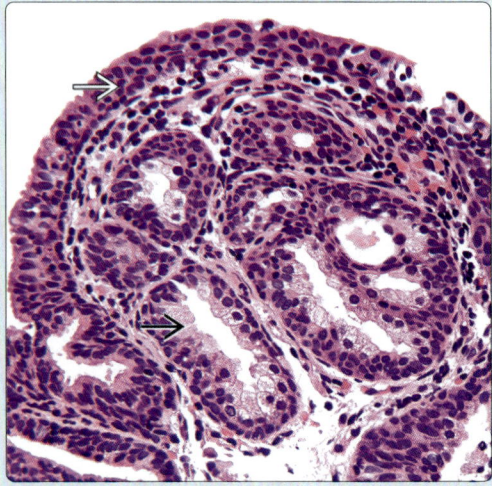

Prostatic-Type Polyp

(Left) *Prostatic-type polyps may have a polypoid growth pattern. Prostatic glands ➡ are present in the stroma underlying the urothelium ➡. The presence of corpora amylacea ➡ is helpful.* (Right) *The lightly eosinophilic frothy cytoplasm of the prostatic glands ➡ is distinct from the stratified urothelium that lines the surface of the polyp ➡. This admixture of cell types is characteristic of a prostatic-type polyp (ectopic prostate).*

Prostatic-Type Polyp (Ectopic Prostate)

TERMINOLOGY

Synonyms
- Ectopic prostate
- Benign prostatic epithelial polyp

Definitions
- Urothelial tract polyp comprised of benign prostatic glands and stroma

ETIOLOGY/PATHOGENESIS

Controversial, Unproven Etiology
- Metaplastic process, prostate gland ectopia, developmental anomaly, or prolapse proposed

CLINICAL ISSUES

Epidemiology
- Age
  - Broad range: 19-89 years

Site
- Most common in prostatic urethra
- Trigone most common in bladder

Presentation
- Gross or microscopic hematuria
- Hematospermia

Endoscopic Findings
- Polypoid mass with variable exophytic fronds

Treatment
- Simple excision often curative of symptoms

Prognosis
- Benign

MACROSCOPIC

General Features
- Papillary or polypoid, sometimes multiple

MICROSCOPIC

Histologic Features
- Polypoid or papillary/filiform exophytic process
  - Contains benign prostatic-type secretory glandular epithelium
    - Prostatic glands vary greatly in number and may contain corpora
    - Light, faintly eosinophilic cytoplasm
    - Round nuclei without prominent nucleoli
    - Both secretory and basal cell layer lining present
  - Admixed urothelium, often with cystitis glandularis

Predominant Cell/Compartment Type
- Epithelial, glandular

ANCILLARY TESTS

Immunohistochemistry
- Immunoreactivity for PSA and PAP in prostatic secretory cells
- GATA-3 reactivity in admixed urothelium

DIFFERENTIAL DIAGNOSIS

Prostatic Ductal Adenocarcinoma
- Most important differential consideration
  - Aggressive malignancy that occurs in prostatic urethra
  - Potential morphologic overlap with prostatic-type polyp on small superficial biopsies
- Typical cellular features
  - Pseudostratified columnar cells lining glands
  - Nucleoli prominent
- More complex architectural growth patterns than prostatic-type polyp
  - Cribriform &/or anastomosing cords
- Shares PSA and PAP reactivity with prostatic-type polyp

Papillary Urothelial Neoplasm
- More complex papillary architecture with secondary or tertiary branching
- Absence of prostatic secretory cells is distinctive

Benign Prostatic Hyperplasia
- May protrude into bladder lumen, forming polypoid mass
- Admixture of benign prostatic glands and spindled cells

Nephrogenic Adenoma
- Mixed papillary and tubular pattern is common
  - Tubules often smaller and more atrophic
  - Papillae lined by single cuboidal layer of epithelial cells
- Express nuclear pax-2 and pax-8 by immunohistochemistry
- May occasionally show weak immunoreactivity for PSA &/or PAP

Papillary-Polypoid Cystitis
- Architectural features may be identical to prostatic-type polyp
- No admixed prostatic secretory cells

Cystitis Cystica/Cystitis Glandularis
- Glands are of varying size and shape without basal cell layer
  - Accentuated luminal cytoplasm may closely mimic prostatic secretory epithelium
- Corpora amylacea are absent, and PSA is negative

Urothelial Carcinoma With Glandular Differentiation
- Greater degree of cytologic atypia
- More architectural complexity

DIAGNOSTIC CHECKLIST

Pathologic Interpretation Pearls
- Prostatic ductal carcinoma must be considered and excluded by morphology

SELECTED REFERENCES

1. Anjum MI et al: Benign polyps with prostatic-type epithelium of the urethra and the urinary bladder. Int Urol Nephrol. 29(3):313-7, 1997
2. Chan JK et al: Prostatic-type polyps of the lower urinary tract: three histogenetic types? Histopathology. 11(8):789-801, 1987
3. Remick DG Jr et al: Benign polyps with prostatic-type epithelium of the urethra and the urinary bladder. A suggestion of histogenesis based on histologic and immunohistochemical studies. Am J Surg Pathol. 8(11):833-9, 1984

Prostatic-Type Polyp (Ectopic Prostate)

Prostatic-Type Polyp

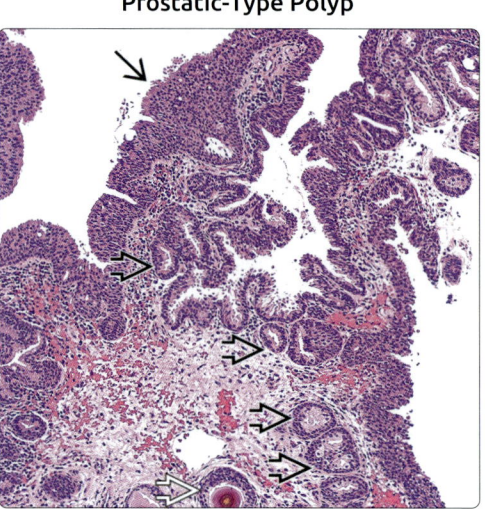

Prostatic-Type Polyp

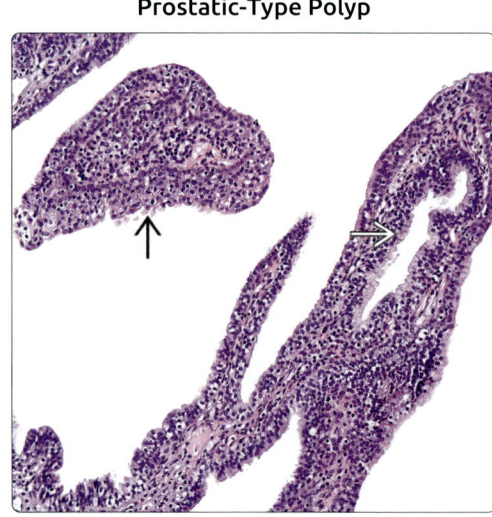

(Left) This prostatic-type polyp has urothelial-lined papillae ➡ mimicking a papillary urothelial neoplasm, but prostatic glands are present throughout the underlying stroma ➡. Corpora amylacea may occasionally be seen in the prostate glands ➡. (Right) Villiform prostatic-type polyps may mimic papillary urothelial neoplasms because the tips of the papillae may be morphologically indistinguishable ➡. The benign prostate glands ➡ are diagnostic of a prostatic-type polyp.

Prostatic-Type Polyp

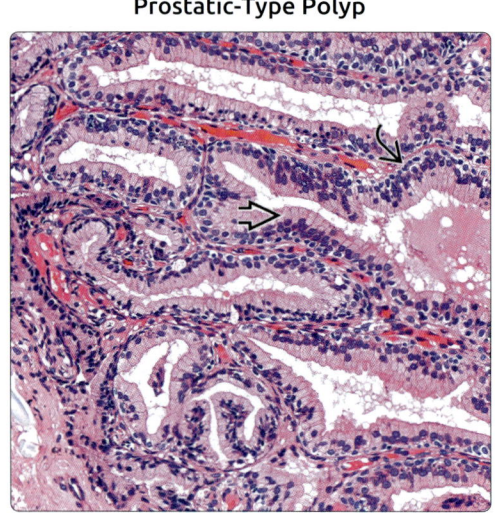

Prostatic-Type Polyp

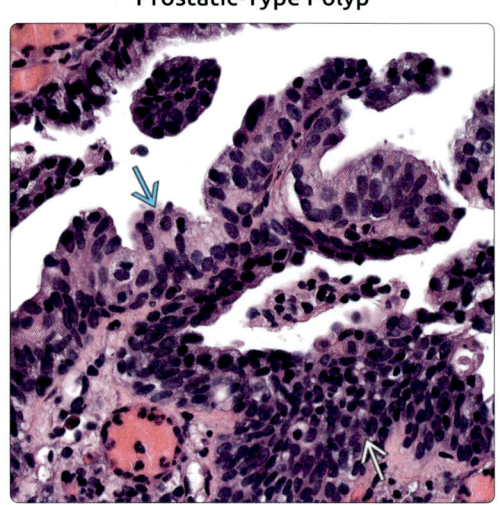

(Left) In some prostatic-type polyps, the prostate glands may predominate. The characteristic bland cytologic features and the presence of 2 cell types (secretory ➡ and basal cells ➡) point to a benign diagnosis. (Right) This high-magnification photomicrograph shows the abrupt transition from prostatic secretory epithelium ➡ to urothelium ➡ that may be seen in prostatic-type polyps of the urinary tract.

Prostatic-Type Polyp

Prostatic-Type Polyp: PSA

(Left) The more frothy eosinophilic cytoplasm of the cells forming the underlying glands is typical of prostatic secretory epithelium ➡, which is diagnostic of a prostatic-type polyp. (Right) Strong PSA positivity helps confirm the diagnosis. Cystitis cystica/glandularis may be in the differential diagnosis. Although PSA positivity confirms prostatic origin, the difference between benign and malignant is identified with light microscopy.

Prostatic-Type Polyp (Ectopic Prostate)

Prostatic Adenocarcinoma: Ductal

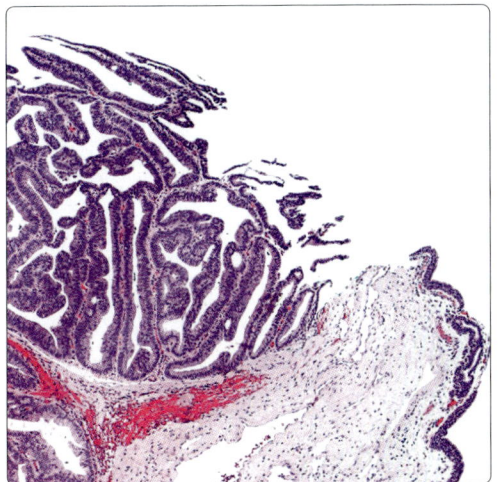

Prostatic Adenocarcinoma: Ductal

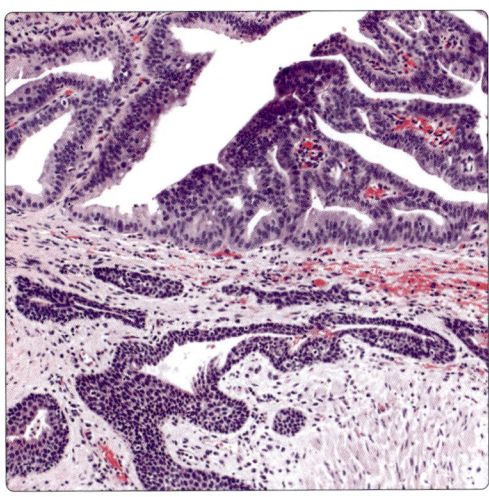

(Left) *Prostatic ductal carcinoma may extend intraluminally within the prostatic urethra to involve the urinary bladder. In small biopsies, these carcinomas may potentially have morphologic overlap with a prostatic-type polyp due to the low-grade nuclear features.* (Right) *The admixture of prostatic epithelium and urothelium may suggest a prostatic-type polyp (ectopic prostate), but the degree of architectural complexity would strongly suggest a carcinoma in this example.*

Prostatic Adenocarcinoma: Ductal

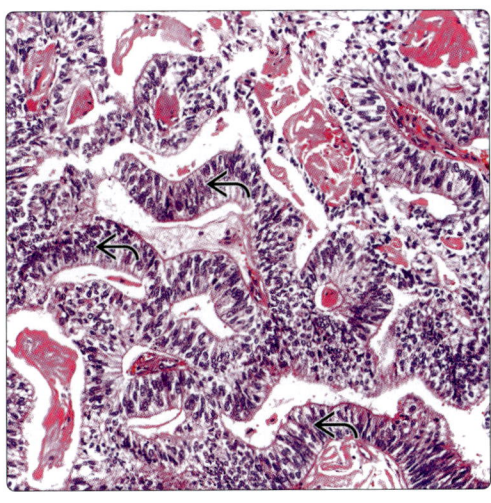

Prostatic Adenocarcinoma: Unusual Papillary Pattern

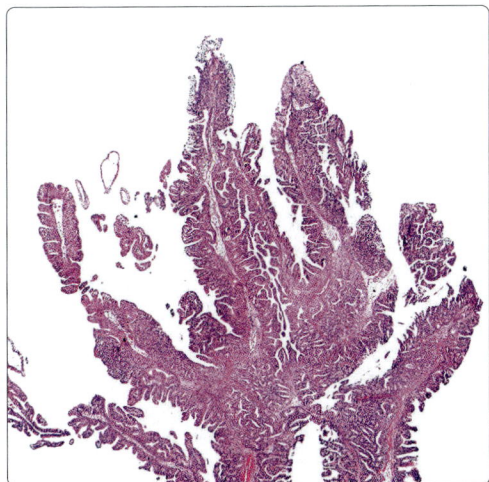

(Left) *The pseudostratified columnar lining epithelial cells ➡ are characteristic of prostatic ductal adenocarcinoma. The degree of glandular complexity is beyond what would be seen in a prostatic-type polyp.* (Right) *Prostatic adenocarcinomas may rarely involve the urinary tract as exophytic polypoid or even papillary mass lesions. High index of suspicion and confirmation by immunohistochemistry are necessary.*

Prostatic Adenocarcinoma: Unusual Papillary Pattern

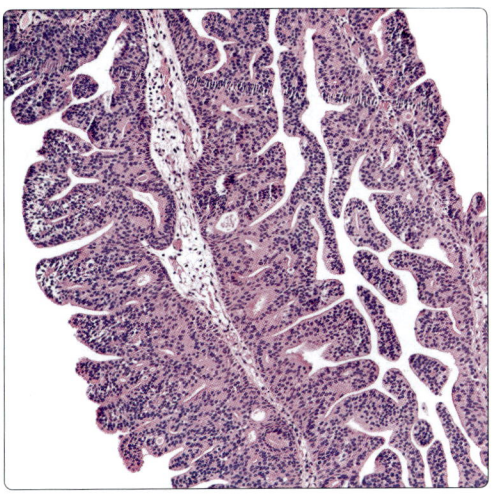

Prostatic Adenocarcinoma: Unusual Papillary Pattern

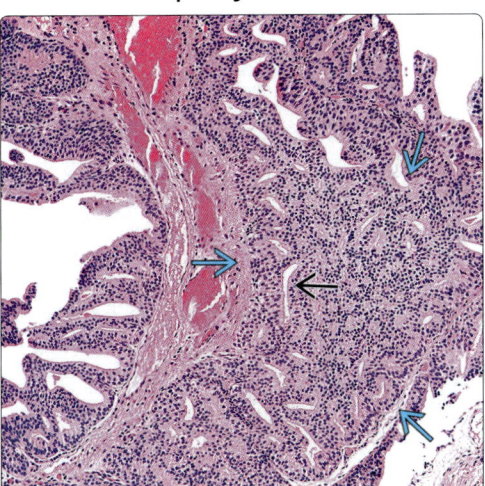

(Left) *The complexity of the epithelium in this very unusual example of an exophytic prostatic adenocarcinoma is well beyond the architecturally simple glands that are characteristic of prostatic-type polyps.* (Right) *Areas of epithelial confluence ➡ with formation of acinar spaces ➡ are a feature of prostatic adenocarcinoma and would argue against a benign prostatic-type polyp.*

Prostatic-Type Polyp (Ectopic Prostate)

Noninvasive Papillary Urothelial Neoplasm

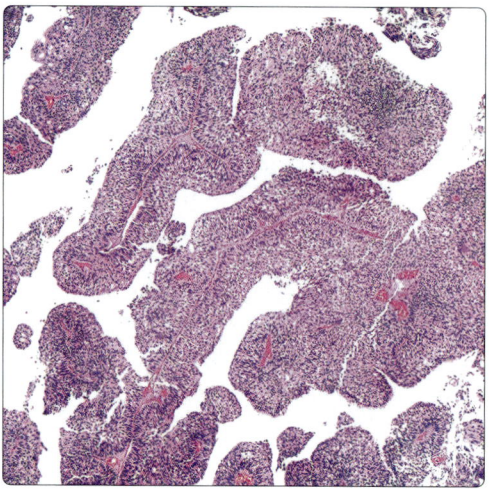

Noninvasive Papillary Urothelial Neoplasm: Gland-Like Spaces

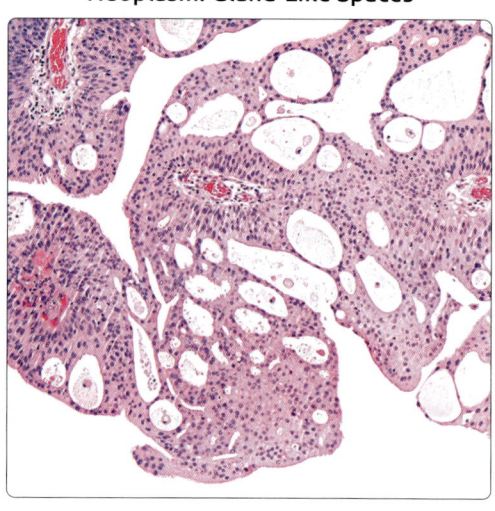

(Left) The degree of epithelial stratification in this exophytic papillary mass in the urinary bladder is characteristic of a noninvasive papillary urothelial neoplasm. In addition, no glandular component is present. (Right) Some papillary urothelial neoplasms may have intraepithelial spaces that can contain intraluminal necrotic &/or apoptotic debris. This should not be mistaken for an associated glandular component.

Papillary Urothelial Carcinoma: Glandular Differentiation

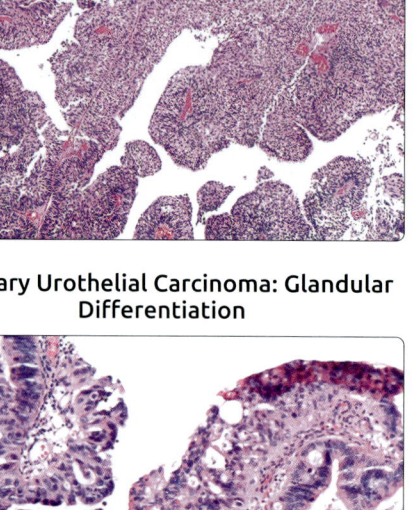

Papillary Urothelial Carcinoma: Glandular Differentiation

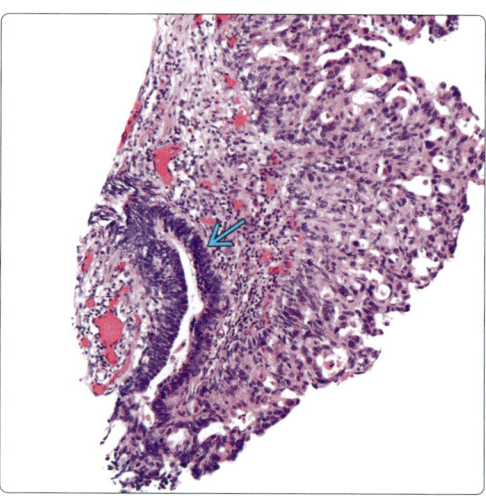

(Left) The high-grade cytology of the urothelial cells ➡ and the atypical glandular component should allow quick distinction of urothelial carcinoma with glandular differentiation from a prostatic-type polyp. (Right) In urothelial carcinomas showing glandular differentiation, the glands are lined by cytologically atypical epithelium that is often pseudostratified with an adenomatous appearance ➡.

Papillary Urothelial Carcinoma: Glandular Differentiation

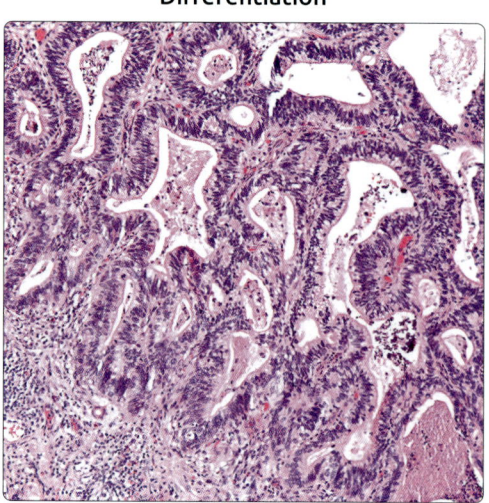

Papillary Urothelial Carcinoma: Glandular Differentiation

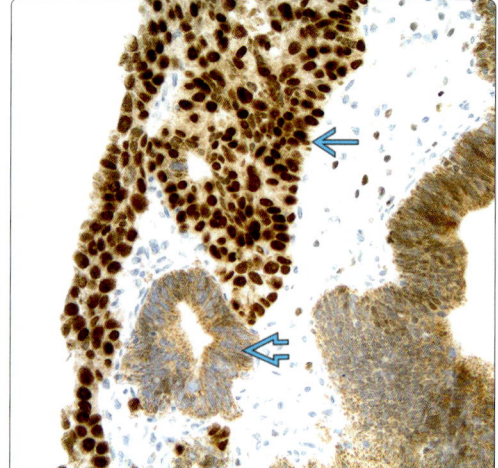

(Left) In this example of urothelial carcinoma with extensive glandular differentiation, the glands are lined by a pseudostratified columnar epithelium with an enteric appearance, which is distinct from prostatic secretory glands. (Right) GATA3 shows strong nuclear immunoreactivity in the urothelial component ➡, but not in the areas of glandular differentiation ➡. This would also be seen in a prostatic-type polyp. The cytologic atypia in both components of urothelial carcinoma is distinctive.

Prostatic-Type Polyp (Ectopic Prostate)

Nephrogenic Adenoma

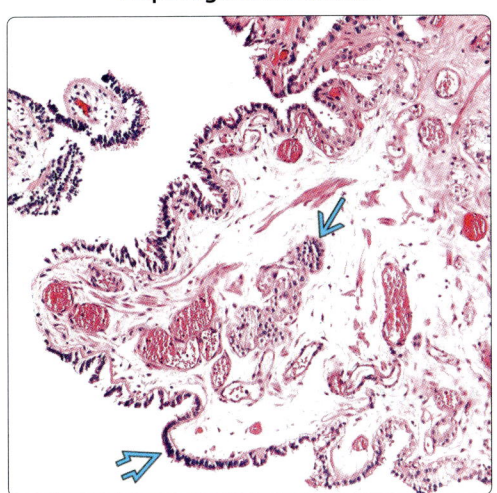

Nephrogenic Adenoma

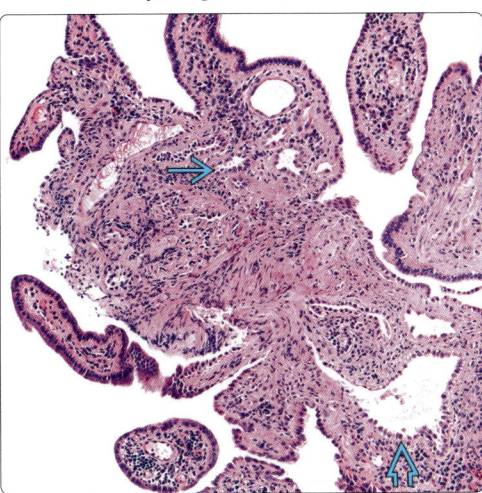

(Left) Nephrogenic adenoma may have a mixed papillary-polypoid pattern ⇒ with tubules in the underlying stroma ⇒. These tubules may closely resemble prostatic secretory glands. In addition, prostatic secretory markers may be expressed in nephrogenic adenoma epithelium. (Right) The underlying tubules in nephrogenic adenoma may be small ⇒ or cystically dilated ⇒. Secretions are usually "colloid" type in nature.

Cystitis Cystica

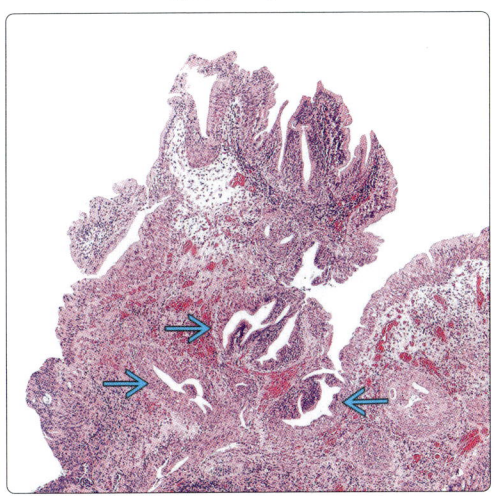

Cystitis Glandularis

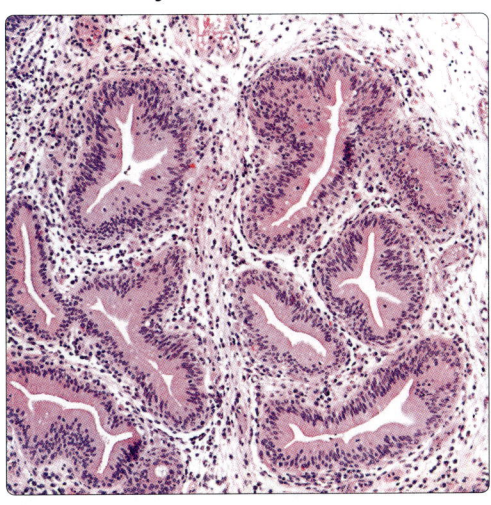

(Left) Florid cystitis cystica may have a polypoid appearance that closely mimics a prostatic-type polyp. In contrast, the underlying gland-like structures of cystitis cystica are lined by urothelium ⇒. (Right) Cystis glandularis of the bladder has greater variation of glandular size and shape without corpora amylacea. The PSA stain is negative. Cystis glandularis and prostatic-type polyp are both benign lesions; hence, distinction between them is not as critical as with prostatic ductal carcinoma.

Benign Prostatic Hyperplasia

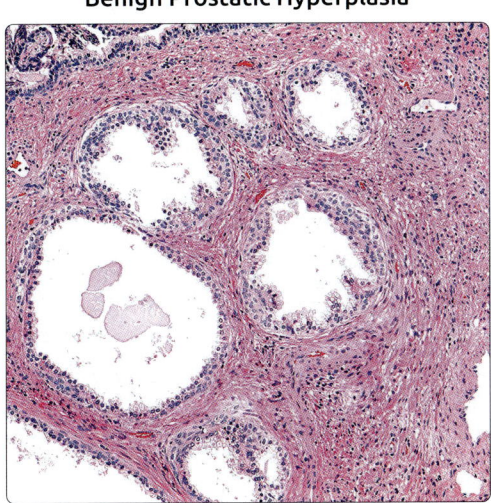

Papillary-Polypoid Cystitis

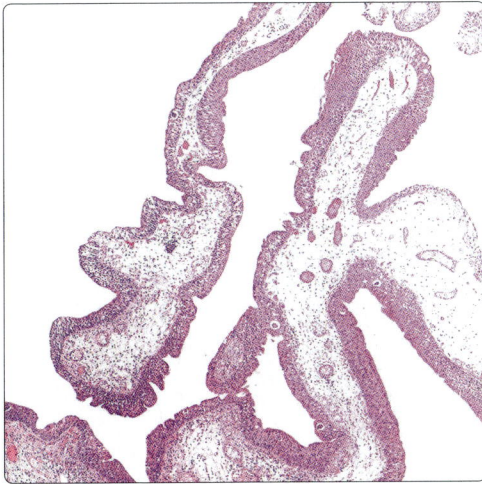

(Left) Benign prostatic hyperplasia may produce a polypoid mass that bulges into the urinary bladder near the bladder neck (clinically called median lobe hypertrophy). The associated stroma and clinical scenario should aid in its distinction from prostatic-type polyp. (Right) The exophytic simple papillary or polypoid architecture of papillary-polypoid cystitis may be very similar to a prostatic-type polyp; however, there are no associated prostatic secretory glands.

Amyloidosis

KEY FACTS

TERMINOLOGY
- Deposition of amyloid protein in urinary bladder
- 2 types
  - Localized process
    - Unknown etiology
    - Most commonly AL type
      - Comprised of immunoglobulin light chains
  - Systemic amyloidosis
    - Primary
      - Typically AL-type amyloid
    - Secondary
      - Often associated with chronic inflammatory conditions
      - Commonly AA-type amyloid
    - Familial
      - Transthyretin mutation
      - Other proteins are extremely rare

MICROSCOPIC
- Deposition of eosinophilic amorphous material in lamina propria and superficial muscularis propria
- May be associated with histiocytic and giant cell reaction

ANCILLARY TESTS
- "Apple green" birefringence on Congo red under polarized light
- Thioflavin T fluorescence is seen
- Randomly arranged, rigid, nonbranching, 8- to 10-nm fibrils by electron microscopy
- Amyloid subtyping now commonly performed by mass spectrometry on paraffin embedded tissue

TOP DIFFERENTIAL DIAGNOSES
- Fibrosis/collagenization
  - Highlighted by trichrome stain
  - No green birefringence on Congo red stain
  - No thioflavin T fluorescence

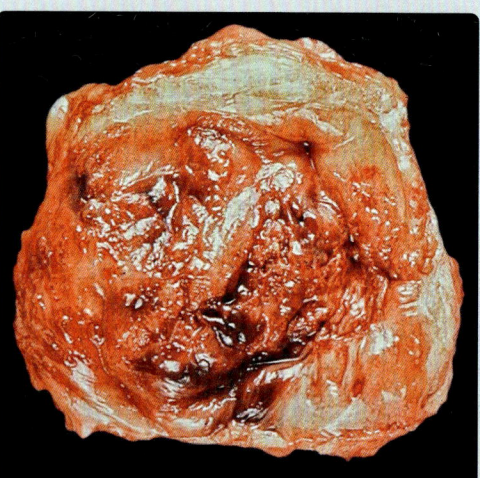

Amyloid: Macroscopic

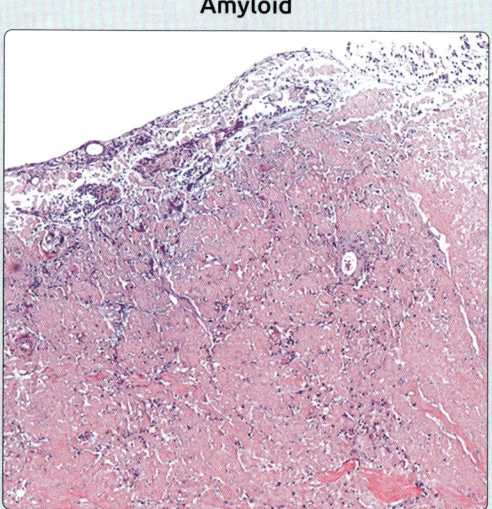

Amyloid

(Left) Partial cystectomy shows "tumor" forming amyloidosis (amyloidoma). Large lesions may ulcerate the overlying mucosa due to a large submucosal and mural mass. Surgery is often restricted to cases with uncontrolled bleeding. (Right) At scanning magnification, the lamina propria of the urinary bladder is filled by dense eosinophilic material. Deposition in the vessel wall is less common in bladder lesions and is more commonly associated with systemic amyloidosis. Muscularis propria may be rarely involved.

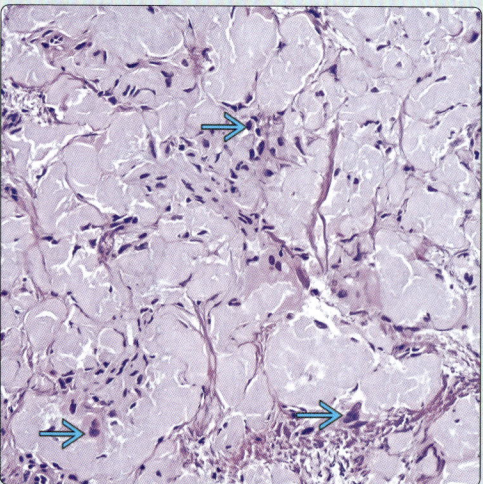

Amyloid

Amyloid: Congo Red

(Left) Amorphous eosinophilic material is characteristic of amyloid, as in other anatomic sites. Congo red is useful in the distinction from collagen. Associated histiocytic ➔ and giant cell infiltrates are commonly seen. (Right) With Congo red stain, amyloid deposits produce characteristic "apple green" birefringence under polarized light ➔.

Amyloidosis

TERMINOLOGY

Synonyms
- Amyloid tumor (if localized)

Definitions
- Deposition of amyloid protein in urinary bladder
  - Primary localized or systemic process

ETIOLOGY/PATHOGENESIS

Systemic
- Primary
  - AL-type amyloid
- Secondary
  - Associated with chronic inflammatory conditions
    - Autoimmune causes, such as rheumatoid arthritis and ankylosing spondylitis
    - Infectious causes, such as tuberculosis and osteomyelitis
  - AA-type amyloid
- Familial
  - Transthyretin mutations most common
  - Other proteins are extremely rare

Localized Type
- Unknown etiology
- Most commonly AL type

CLINICAL ISSUES

Epidemiology
- Incidence
  - Rarely bladder is primary site of disease
- Age
  - After 5th decade

Site
- Posterior and posterolateral walls most common

Presentation
- Painless hematuria

Treatment
- Surgical approaches
  - Local excision or laser ablation for localized amyloid
  - Partial cystectomy occasionally required for bleeding

Prognosis
- Local recurrence of primary amyloid is not uncommon
- Secondary amyloid depends on primary cause

MACROSCOPIC

General Features
- Diffuse amyloidosis
  - Mucosal erythema, sometimes petechial hemorrhage and necrosis
- Localized amyloidosis
  - On cystoscopy, may be polypoid mass lesion

MICROSCOPIC

Histologic Features
- Deposition of eosinophilic afibrillar material in lamina propria and superficial muscularis propria
  - Deposition in vessel wall is less common and usually seen in systemic form
- Florid histiocytic and foreign body type giant cell reaction may be seen

ANCILLARY TESTS

Histochemistry
- Congo red
  - Afibrillar material has dense orange "congophilia" under light microscopy
  - "Apple green" birefringence under polarized light

Immunohistochemistry
- Amyloid panel of κ light chain, λ light chain, prealbumin, β-2 microglobulin, and SAA1 may be helpful

Immunofluorescence
- Fluorescence with Thioflavin T stain is seen

Electron Microscopy
- Randomly arranged, rigid, nonbranching, 8-10 nm fibrils

Mass Spectrometry
- Increasingly used for amyloid subtyping in paraffin

DIFFERENTIAL DIAGNOSIS

Fibrosis/Collagenization
- Collagen deposition may appear similar to amyloid
  - Highlighted by trichrome stain
  - No green birefringence on Congo red stain
  - No thioflavin T fluorescence

Hematopoietic Neoplasms
- Occasionally associated with dense fibrosis that may closely mimic amyloid

DIAGNOSTIC CHECKLIST

Clinically Relevant Pathologic Features
- May be interpreted as neoplasm on cystoscopy
- Determination of amyloid type may aid clinical work-up of patient

Pathologic Interpretation Pearls
- Because of rarity, may be overlooked as organizing fibrosis
- Does not necessarily indicate systemic process

SELECTED REFERENCES

1. Zhou F et al: Primary localized amyloidosis of the urinary tract frequently mimics neoplasia: a clinicopathologic analysis of 11 cases. Am J Clin Exp Urol. 2(1):71-5, 2014
2. Merrimen JL et al: Localized amyloidosis of the urinary tract: case series of nine patients. Urology. 67(5):904-9, 2006
3. Tirzaman O et al: Primary localized amyloidosis of the urinary bladder: a case series of 31 patients. Mayo Clin Proc. 75(12):1264-8, 2000

Müllerian Lesions

KEY FACTS

TERMINOLOGY
- Ectopic benign müllerian tissue within wall of urinary bladder

CLINICAL ISSUES
- Typically reproductive age women

MICROSCOPIC
- Cytologically benign glands of müllerian type within bladder wall
  o Endometriosis
    – Endometrial type glands and stroma
  o Endocervicosis
    – Columnar cells with abundant pale cytoplasm
  o Endosalpingiosis
    – Tubal type epithelium
      □ Ciliated cells often prominent
  o Müllerianosis
    – Admixture of different types of müllerian epithelium

TOP DIFFERENTIAL DIAGNOSES
- Invasive adenocarcinoma
  o More pronounced cytologic atypia
  o Enteric appearance common
  o Associated desmoplasia may be seen
- Urothelial carcinoma with glandular differentiation
  o Overlying component of intermixed typical urothelial carcinoma common
    – Noninvasive papillary carcinoma, carcinoma in situ, or invasive carcinoma
- Microcystic urothelial carcinoma
  o Typically more microcystic structures with flattened or columnar lining with irregular distribution and infiltration
  o More typical component of urothelial carcinoma may be seen
- Secondary involvement by adenocarcinoma
  o Colorectal adenocarcinoma most common

Endometriosis
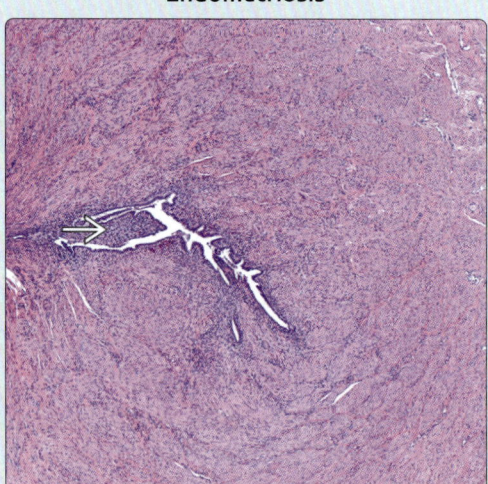

Endometriosis
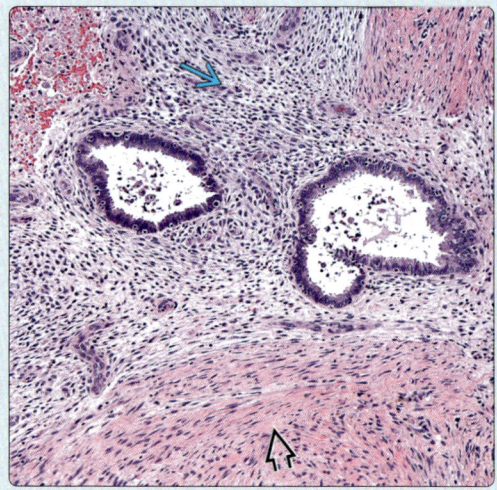

(Left) The presence of large branching glands and the associated endometrial stroma ➡ are characteristic features of endometriosis. As seen in this case, the glands may be deep within the muscularis propria of the urinary bladder. (Right) In endometriosis of the urinary bladder (as in other locations), the glands are lined by benign tubal-type cells and are surrounded by endometrial-type stroma ➡. Compared to the endometriotic stroma, the surrounding muscularis propria has more eosinophilic cytoplasm ➡.

Endosalpingiosis
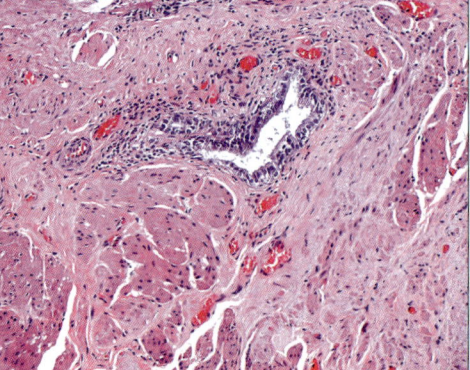

Endocervicosis
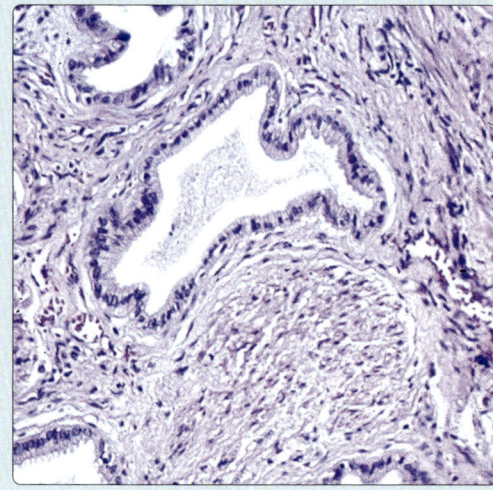

(Left) In this example of endosalpingiosis, the benign glandular structure is admixed with the thick smooth muscle bundles of the muscularis propria with some surrounding fibrosis. (Right) The bland cytologic features and pale mucinous cytoplasm of these glands within the muscularis propria of the urinary bladder are characteristic of endocervicosis. Nuclei are often basally located.

Müllerian Lesions

TERMINOLOGY

Definitions
- Ectopic müllerian tissue within wall of urinary bladder
  - Endometriosis
    - Cytologically benign endometrial glands and stroma
  - Endocervicosis
    - Cytologically benign endocervical-type glands
  - Endosalpingiosis
    - Cytologically benign glands with tubal-type epithelium
  - Müllerianosis
    - Admixture of different types of benign müllerian epithelium
- Müllerian duct cyst/remnant
  - Benign müllerian-type glands between bladder and rectum of men
    - ± involvement of posterior bladder wall
- Paramesonephric (müllerian) sinus of urinary bladder
  - Sinus tract lined by müllerian-type epithelium
  - Connects posterolateral wall of the bladder to broad ligament in women

ETIOLOGY/PATHOGENESIS

Predisposing Factors
- Müllerianosis spectrum
  - 50% of cases have history of previous surgery
    - Most commonly cesarean section

CLINICAL ISSUES

Epidemiology
- Incidence
  - Endometriosis
    - Involvement of urinary tract in < 2% of patients with endometriosis
    - Bladder most common genitourinary site
  - Endocervicosis, endosalpingiosis, and müllerianosis are rare
  - Both müllerian duct cyst/remnant and paramesonephric (müllerian) sinus of urinary bladder are very rare
- Age
  - Müllerianosis spectrum
    - Typically reproductive age
    - Rarely postmenopausal if receiving hormones
  - Müllerian duct cyst/remnant
    - Peak age range is 20-40 years
- Sex
  - Müllerianosis spectrum
    - Female
    - Rare cases reported in males receiving estrogen therapy
  - Müllerian duct cyst/remnant
    - Men
  - Paramesonephric (müllerian) sinus of urinary bladder
    - Women

Presentation
- Müllerianosis spectrum
  - Dysuria
    - Urinary urgency, frequency, suprapubic pain
  - Hematuria, mucosuria
  - > 50% of patients have no vesical symptoms
  - Endometriosis may produce pain with menstrual cycle
  - Mass lesion in some cases
- Müllerian duct cyst/remnant
  - Hematospermia
  - Azoospermia
  - Hematuria
- Paramesonephric (müllerian) sinus of urinary bladder
  - Irritative voiding symptoms

Endoscopic Findings
- Müllerianosis spectrum
  - Cystoscopic findings not entirely specific
    - Appear as congested, edematous mucosal elevations overlying cysts
    - May show hemorrhagic or blue-tinged mucosa
    - Rarely, polypoid mass lesion

Treatment
- Surgical approaches
  - Definitive surgery for women beyond reproductive age
  - Müllerian duct cyst/remnants may be managed conservatively in some cases
- Drugs
  - Conservative surgery and hormonal therapy in women who desire fertility

Prognosis
- Benign
  - Treatment for symptoms
- Malignant transformation of endometriosis in bladder has been reported (rare)
  - Carcinoma of müllerian type
    - Clear cell adenocarcinoma
    - Endometrioid adenocarcinoma
  - Endometrial stromal sarcoma
  - Adenosarcoma

IMAGING

General Features
- Location
  - Endometriosis most common on serosal surface near vesicouterine pouch
    - May extend into muscularis propria to produce mass lesion
    - Rarely, submucosal nodule
  - Müllerian duct cyst/remnant
    - Midline, between bladder and rectum
  - Paramesonephric (müllerian) sinus of urinary bladder
    - Posterolateral wall of bladder to broad ligament

MACROSCOPIC

General Features
- Müllerianosis spectrum
  - Palpable suprapubic mass in almost 50% of cases
  - Hemorrhagic ill-defined mass may project into bladder lumen
- Müllerian duct cyst/remnant
  - Often unilocular or multilocular cysts

Müllerian Lesions

- Paramesonephric (müllerian) sinus of urinary bladder
  - Sinus tract

MICROSCOPIC

Histologic Features

- Cytologically benign glands of müllerian type within bladder wall
  - Endometriosis
    - Resemble endometriosis at other sites
    - Intimate admixture of endometrial-type glands with surrounding endometrial stroma
  - Endocervicosis
    - Benign glands resembling endocervix
      - Epithelium lining glands consists of single layer of columnar cells with abundant pale cytoplasm
      - Ciliated cells are often interspersed among mucinous cells
      - When glands are dilated, epithelium is cuboidal or flattened
  - Endosalpingiosis
    - Tubal-type glands
      - Lined by ciliated, intercalated, and peg cells
  - Müllerianosis
    - Admixture of tubal, endocervical, &/or endometrial-type glands
- Fibrosis and hyperplastic muscle around lesional glands may thicken bladder wall
- Most involve muscularis propria, but mucosa and adventitia also may be involved
- Müllerian duct cysts and remnants are also lined by benign müllerian-type epithelium
  - Denudation of cysts is common
- Paramesonephric (müllerian) sinus of urinary bladder
  - Branching tubular structures without surrounding smooth muscle
  - Lined by single columnar to cuboidal epithelium
    - Mucinous cytoplasm with scattered ciliated cells

ANCILLARY TESTS

Immunohistochemistry

- Typically not needed for evaluation

DIFFERENTIAL DIAGNOSIS

Primary Invasive Adenocarcinoma of Urinary Bladder

- Obvious cytologic atypia
- Glands may show more architectural complexity
  - Cribriforming with comedonecrosis
  - Destructive, angulated glands
- Stromal desmoplastic reaction common

Microcystic Urothelial Carcinoma

- May have bland cytologic features
- Lumina may contain mucinous material
- May have admixed areas of more typical urothelial carcinoma
  - Often with nested features
- More glandular structures with irregular invasion
  - Including irregular distribution in lamina propria

Urothelial Carcinoma With Glandular Differentiation

- Intermixed typical urothelial component is diagnostic
  - Noninvasive papillary urothelial carcinoma
  - Urothelial carcinoma in situ
  - Invasive urothelial carcinoma
- Prior history of urothelial carcinoma also suggestive

Secondary Involvement by Adenocarcinoma

- Carcinomas from other sites may involve urinary bladder, often by direct extension
  - Colorectal adenocarcinoma most common
  - Urethral adenocarcinoma
  - Direct extension from gynecologic tract
    - Endocervical or endometrial adenocarcinoma
    - Rarely ovarian carcinomas

Mixed Epithelial Stromal Neoplasm of Seminal Vesicle

- Spindled stromal component surrounds benign glands
  - May have stromal invaginations into gland lumina creating phyllodes-like pattern
  - Malignant stroma may be seen in rare cases
- Glands have features of seminal vesicle epithelium
  - Nuclear pleomorphism; inclusions
  - Intracytoplasmic lipofuscin pigment may be seen

Urachal Cysts

- Deep location, midline, dome, deep in muscularis propria
- Lining varies from urothelium, glandular NOS, mucinous ± intestinal metaplasia

DIAGNOSTIC CHECKLIST

Pathologic Interpretation Pearls

- Some features should raise possibility of müllerianosis over invasive carcinoma
  - Bland-appearing, well-formed glandular structures deep in bladder wall
  - Admixed ciliated cells

SELECTED REFERENCES

1. Furuya R et al: New classification of midline cysts of the prostate in adults via a transrectal ultrasonography-guided opacification and dye-injection study. BJU Int. 102(4):475-8, 2008
2. Comiter CV: Endometriosis of the urinary tract. Urol Clin North Am. 29(3):625-35, 2002
3. Edmondson JD et al: Endosalpingiosis of bladder. J Urol. 167(3):1401-2, 2002
4. Oliva E et al: Clear cell carcinoma of the urinary bladder: a report and comparison of four tumors of mullerian origin and nine of probable urothelial origin with discussion of histogenesis and diagnostic problems. Am J Surg Pathol. 26(2):190-7, 2002
5. Young RH et al: Müllerianosis of the urinary bladder. Mod Pathol. 9(7):731-7, 1996
6. Clement PB et al: Endocervicosis of the urinary bladder. A report of six cases of a benign müllerian lesion that may mimic adenocarcinoma. Am J Surg Pathol. 16(6):533-42, 1992
7. Ritchey ML et al: Management of müllerian duct remnants in the male patient. J Urol. 140(4):795-9, 1988
8. Felderman T et al: Müllerian duct cysts: conservative management. Urology. 29(1):31-4, 1987

Müllerian Lesions

Endometriosis With Endocervicosis-Like Foci

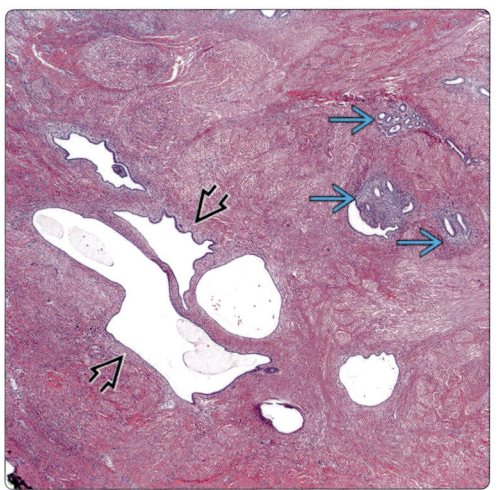

Müllerianosis

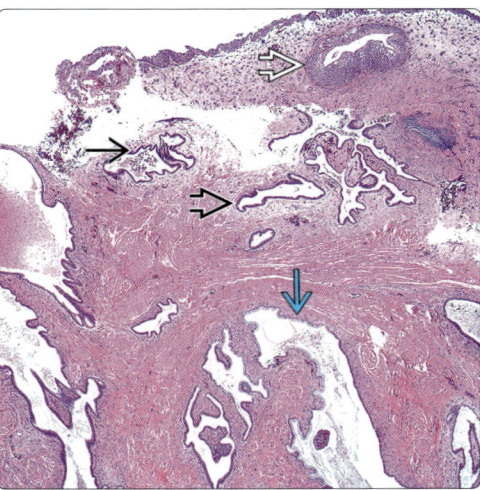

(Left) Endometriosis ➡ of the urinary bladder may be admixed with foci that have the morphology of endocervicosis ➡. This has led to the suggestion that they may be related. (Right) In this section of the urinary bladder wall, there is an admixture of benign tubal-type ➡ and benign endocervical-type ➡ glands. The glands may extend to involve the lamina propria ➡. The superficial areas show surface urothelium and von Brunn nests ➡.

Endosalpingiosis

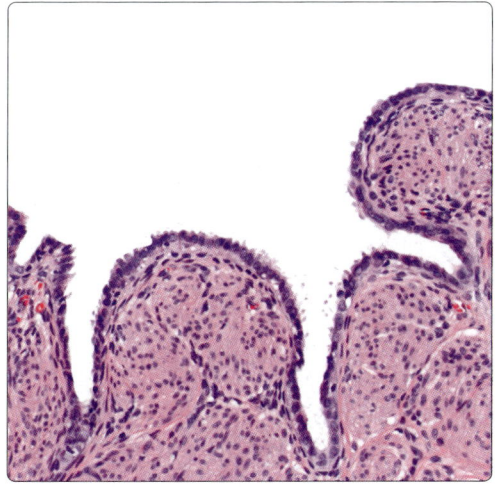

Müllerianosis

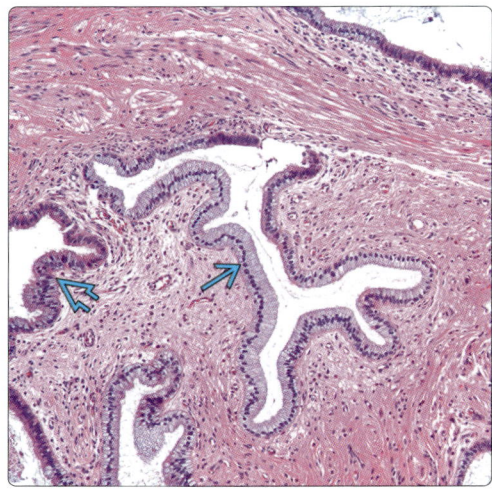

(Left) An endosalpingiotic gland with tubal-type lining epithelium (without surrounding endometrial stroma) is shown in this example of endosalpingiosis. Lesions in which the glands have a combination of endometrial-type, endocervical-type, or endosalpingiotic epithelium are referred to as müllerianosis. (Right) In this example of müllerianosis, benign glands are lined by an admixture of mucinous endocervical-type ➡ and ciliated tubal-type ➡ epithelium.

Müllerianosis

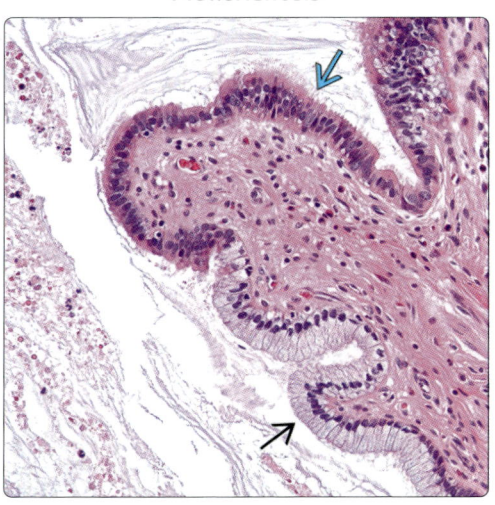

Endometriosis

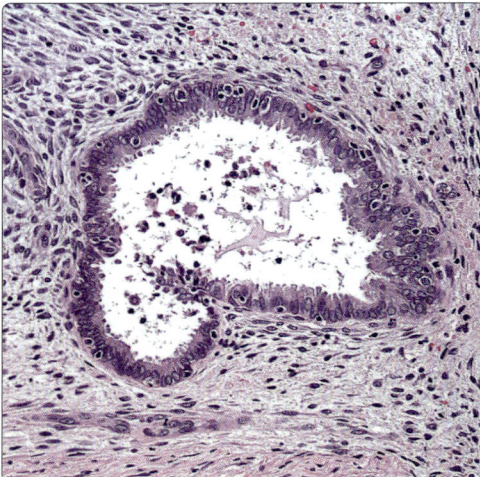

(Left) At high-power magnification, the benign ciliated epithelium (tubal or salpingitic-type) ➡ is admixed with benign endocervical-type epithelium ➡. This admixture of cell types is the characteristic histologic feature of müllerianosis. (Right) This benign tubal-type epithelium is surrounded by endometrial stroma, a histologic feature diagnostic of endometriosis.

Pseudocarcinomatous Hyperplasia

KEY FACTS

ETIOLOGY/PATHOGENESIS
- Described in association with chemotherapy &/or radiation therapy
- Subset of cases with no prior therapy
  - Have other ischemia-inducing conditions or factors

CLINICAL ISSUES
- Symptoms of radiation/chemotherapy cystitis
- Most appear polypoid

MICROSCOPIC
- Small urothelial nests with rounded or irregular, jagged borders
- Prominent cytoplasmic eosinophilia imparting "squamoid" appearance
- Some have frankly squamous differentiation
- Epithelium characteristically encircles vessels and fibrin aggregates
- Mitotic figures usually absent
- Stromal hemorrhage and hemosiderin deposition
- Vascular ectasia
- Stromal &/or intravascular fibrin deposition
- Associated ulceration common
- Stromal fibrosis
- Typical radiation-induced epithelial changes
- Atypical fibroblasts

TOP DIFFERENTIAL DIAGNOSES
- Invasive urothelial carcinoma
- Nested variant of urothelial carcinoma
- Florid von Brunn nests
- Invasive squamous cell carcinoma
- Inverted urothelial neoplasia
- Verrucous carcinoma

DIAGNOSTIC CHECKLIST
- Attention to associated background ischemic/radiation changes is crucial to avoid misdiagnosis

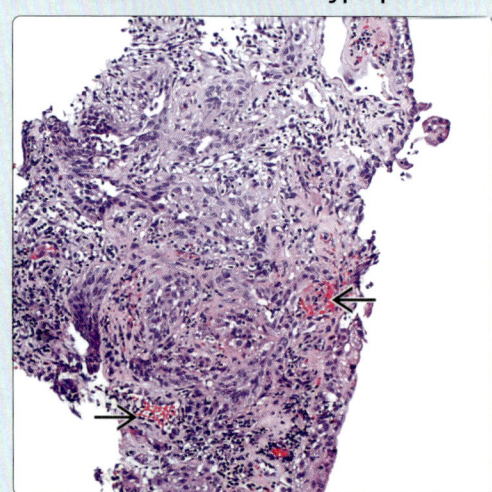

Pseudocarcinomatous Hyperplasia

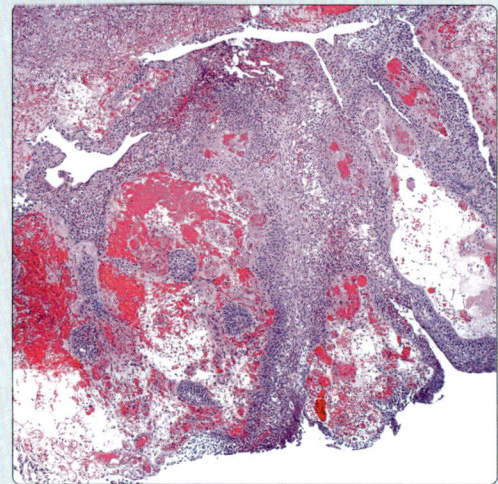

Pseudocarcinomatous Hyperplasia

(Left) This example of pseudocarcinomatous hyperplasia is secondary to radiation therapy for cervical cancer, and shows nests of urothelium with associated blood vessels ⇥ and collagen. (Right) Extensive hemorrhage and fibrin deposition is typically associated with the invaginated urothelium in pseudocarcinomatous hyperplasia. The process is typically more endophytic than exophytic.

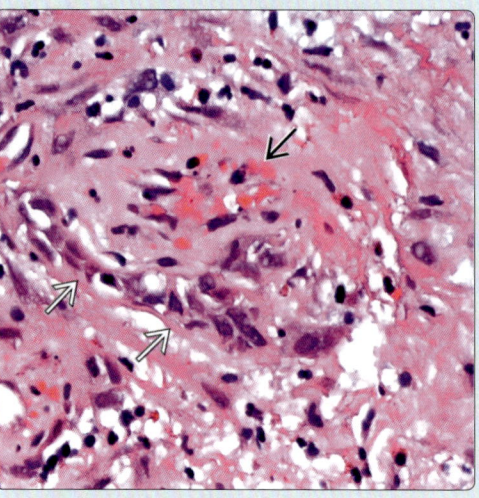

Pseudocarcinomatous Hyperplasia

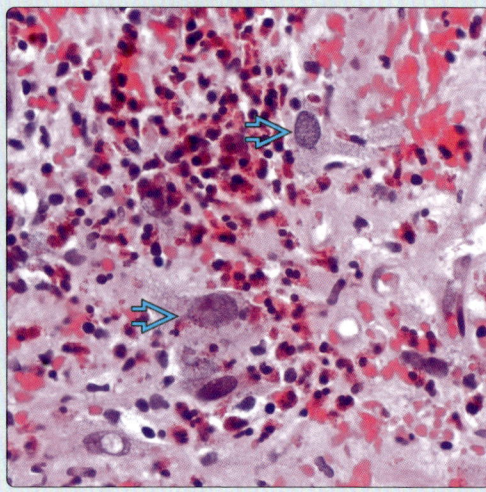

Radiation Atypia

(Left) This is the typical epithelial-stromal relationship of pseudocarcinomatous hyperplasia, which is characterized by epithelial nests encircling an abnormal blood vessel with dense hyalinization ⇥. The urothelial nest in this example is irregular and jagged, a feature that closely mimics invasive carcinoma ⇥. (Right) This high-power photomicrograph of atypical stromal cells ⇥ is from a patient with a history of radiation therapy for prostate cancer.

Pseudocarcinomatous Hyperplasia

TERMINOLOGY

Synonyms
- Radiation/chemotherapy cystitis
- Radiation-induced pseudocarcinomatous hyperplasia
- Postchemotherapy pseudocarcinomatous hyperplasia
- Pseudocarcinomatous proliferation

Definitions
- Florid benign urothelial proliferation with pseudoinfiltrative growth pattern mimicking invasive carcinoma
  - Most commonly in patients with prior radiation &/or chemotherapy

ETIOLOGY/PATHOGENESIS

Environmental Exposure
- Thought to be caused by urinary bladder ischemia of varying etiology
- Most commonly associated with prior pelvic radiation therapy (75% of cases)
  - In males, most commonly for prostatic carcinoma
  - In females, most commonly for gynecologic malignancy
    - Cervical or endometrial carcinoma most common
- Less commonly associated with prior systemic or intravesical chemotherapy
  - Thiotepa
  - Mitomycin
  - Cyclophosphamide
  - BCG therapy
- Subset of cases with no prior radiation or chemotherapy
  - Other rare associations suggest underlying ischemic etiology
    - Peripheral vascular disease
    - Atrial fibrillation
    - Diabetes
    - Indwelling Foley catheter
    - Prior local surgery
      - Radical prostatectomy
    - Sickle cell disease
    - Vascular malformation
- Rare cases have no known cause identified

CLINICAL ISSUES

Epidemiology
- Incidence
  - Rare
- Age
  - Mean: 67 years
  - Range: 33-85 years
- Sex
  - Most commonly reported in males (M:F = 6:1)

Site
- Urinary bladder

Presentation
- Symptoms of radiation/chemotherapy cystitis
  - Hematuria

Endoscopic Findings
- Most appear erythematous
- May be polypoid mass lesion
- Other rare findings
  - Bullous edema
  - Trabeculations
  - Bleeding ulcers

Natural History
- Average time from radiation to radiation cystitis is 55 months; wide time range
- Morphologic features of radiation cystitis may persist for years

Treatment
- Options, risks, complications
  - Symptomatic care and follow-up
  - Remove inciting factors if possible
- Surgical approaches
  - None required

Prognosis
- Benign, reactive condition
- Bleeding may rarely necessitate therapy

MACROSCOPIC

General Features
- Small polypoid lesion

MICROSCOPIC

Histologic Features
- Urothelial proliferation
  - Small to intermediate-sized urothelial nests with rounded or irregular, jagged borders
  - Prominent cytoplasmic eosinophilia imparting "squamoid" appearance
  - Some have frankly squamous differentiation
  - Epithelium characteristically encircles or wraps around blood vessels and fibrin aggregates
  - Extent of lamina propria involvement varies (> 50% in some cases)
  - Variation in nuclear size and shape
  - Mitotic figures usually absent
- More typical radiation-induced epithelial changes may be present in adjacent urothelium
  - Cytoplasmic ballooning and nuclear multilobation
  - Smudged chromatin
  - Nuclear and cytoplasmic vacuoles
  - Karyorrhectic cellular debris
- Other associated stromal changes
  - Vascular ectasia and edema
  - Stromal hemorrhage and hemosiderin deposition
  - Stromal &/or intravascular fibrin deposition
  - Markedly atypical fibroblasts common
  - Stromal fibrosis
  - Variable acute and chronic inflammation
  - Atherosis
  - Frank tissue necrosis
- Other associated nonneoplastic reactive changes
  - Reactive urothelial atypia common

Pseudocarcinomatous Hyperplasia

- May have denudation with residual clinging reactive urothelial cells
  - Deep ulceration with necrosis and fibroinflammatory reaction
  - Associated papillary-polypoid cystitis

Predominant Pattern/Injury Type
- Hyperplasia

Predominant Cell/Compartment Type
- Urothelial

DIFFERENTIAL DIAGNOSIS

Typical Invasive Urothelial Carcinoma
- May have associated papillary or in situ component
- More pronounced cytologic atypia in epithelium
- Mitotic activity may be seen
- Invasion of muscularis propria diagnostic
- Lacks epithelial cells encircling blood vessels with fibrin deposition
- Background radiation cystitis typically less pronounced in postradiation setting
  - Pools of blood and fibrin uncommon

Nested Variant of Urothelial Carcinoma
- Nests and cords of cytologically bland urothelial cells within lamina propria
  - More epithelial predominant
  - More architecturally complex growth pattern
- Invasion of muscularis propria is most definitive feature
- Lacks epithelial cells encircling blood vessels with fibrin deposition
- Background radiation cystitis typically less pronounced (if postradiation setting)
  - Pools of blood and fibrin uncommon

Florid von Brunn Nests
- More uniformly rounded nests of urothelium in lamina propria
  - Lobular configuration of nests
  - Sharp line of demarcation with underlying lamina propria
  - Typically lack squamoid appearance
- May have admixed cystitis cystica or glandularis
- Background hemorrhage and vascular changes absent
- Distinction not clinically relevant

Invasive Squamous Cell Carcinoma
- More cytologic atypia in epithelium
- Mitotic activity may be seen
- Associated stromal myofibroblastic proliferation not uncommon
- Invasion of muscularis propria is most definitive feature
- Other associated squamous lesions may be present
  - May have adjacent keratinizing squamous metaplasia &/or squamous dysplasia
  - Squamous dysplasia or carcinoma in situ may also be seen
- Typically lacks background hemorrhage and fibrin
- Often have history of chronic inflammatory process

Inverted Urothelial Neoplasia
- Epithelial predominant lesion
  - Interconnecting, anastomosing cords of noninvasive urothelium with rounded contours within lamina propria
- May have associated typical invasive carcinoma component to aid diagnosis
- Inverted papilloma may have additional unique features
  - Peripheral nuclear palisading in urothelial nests
  - Central epithelial spindling in nests
- Typically lacks background stromal changes or hemorrhage

Fibromyxoid Pattern of Nephrogenic Adenoma
- Stromal predominant lesion
- Sclerotic background with entrapped epithelium
- May have myxoid component
- Epithelium more corded or spindled
- Epithelium expresses pax-8
- May be admixed with more typical patterns of nephrogenic adenoma

Verrucous Carcinoma
- Has deep, cytologically bland squamous nests
- More confluent epithelium with sharply delineated base
- Has surface verrucous/papillary component
- Absence of typical background radiation changes

DIAGNOSTIC CHECKLIST

Clinically Relevant Pathologic Features
- Very close histologic mimic of invasive carcinoma
  - Cystoscopic impression may suggest radiation injury
- No treatment typically necessary

Pathologic Interpretation Pearls
- Knowledge of this specific pattern of injury is key to avoiding misdiagnosis as malignancy
- Attention to associated background ischemic/radiation changes is crucial to avoid misdiagnosis
  - Pools of hemorrhage and fibrin are first clue at scanning magnification
  - Vascular and stromal changes due to radiation are present in postradiation cases
  - History of radiation therapy rarely given
  - Radiation therapy may be very remote
- Epithelial nests wrapping around abnormal blood vessels is characteristic
  - Specific diagnostic feature of this hyperplastic process

SELECTED REFERENCES
1. Kryvenko ON et al: Pseudocarcinomatous urothelial hyperplasia of the bladder: clinical findings and followup of 70 patients. J Urol. 189(6):2083-6, 2013
2. Lane Z et al: Pseudocarcinomatous epithelial hyperplasia in the bladder unassociated with prior irradiation or chemotherapy. Am J Surg Pathol. 32(1):92-7, 2008
3. Chan TY et al: Radiation or chemotherapy cystitis with "pseudocarcinomatous" features. Am J Surg Pathol. 28(7):909-13, 2004
4. Baker PM et al: Radiation-induced pseudocarcinomatous proliferations of the urinary bladder: a report of 4 cases. Hum Pathol. 31(6):678-83, 2000
5. Suresh UR et al: Radiation disease of the urinary tract: histological features of 18 cases. J Clin Pathol. 46(3):228-31, 1993

Pseudocarcinomatous Hyperplasia

Pseudocarcinomatous Hyperplasia
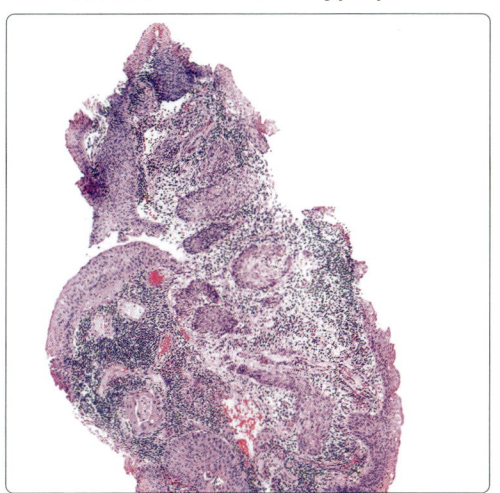

Pseudocarcinomatous Hyperplasia
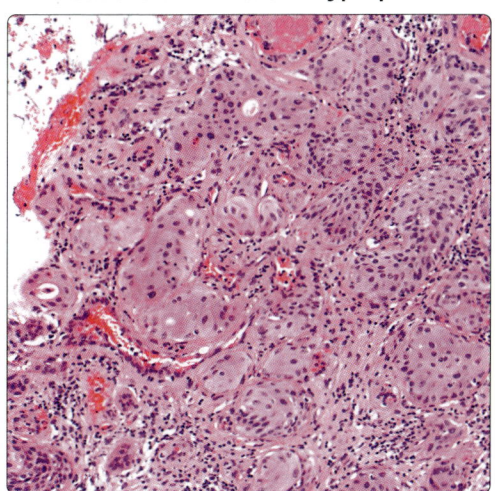

(Left) *This low-power photomicrograph shows an epithelial proliferation that could easily be mistaken for an invasive urothelial (or squamous cell) carcinoma.* **(Right)** *This florid reactive urothelial proliferation is from a patient who underwent radiation therapy for prostate cancer. Despite the back-to-back nests, the cytology of the urothelial cells is bland and at best is the range of reactive atypia.*

Pseudocarcinomatous Hyperplasia
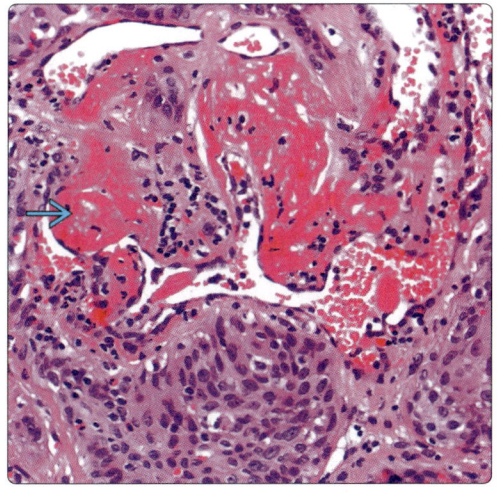

Pseudocarcinomatous Hyperplasia
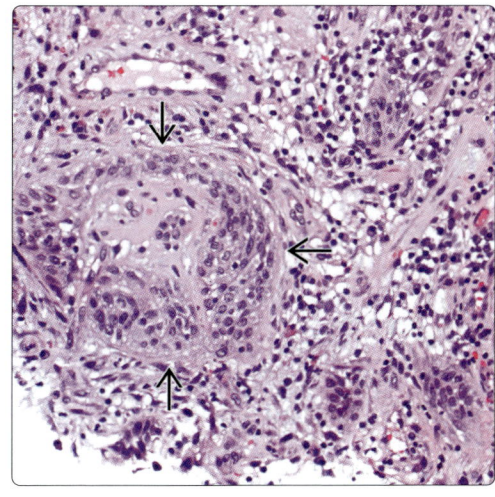

(Left) *The association between the urothelial nests and intravascular and stromal fibrin ➡ is characteristic of this florid reactive process known as pseudocarcinomatous hyperplasia.* **(Right)** *These nests of urothelium can be seen encircling dense collagen ➡ or fibrin in this hyperplastic lesion. This is one of the most important histologic features for distinguishing pseudocarcinomatous hyperplasia from carcinoma.*

Pseudocarcinomatous Hyperplasia
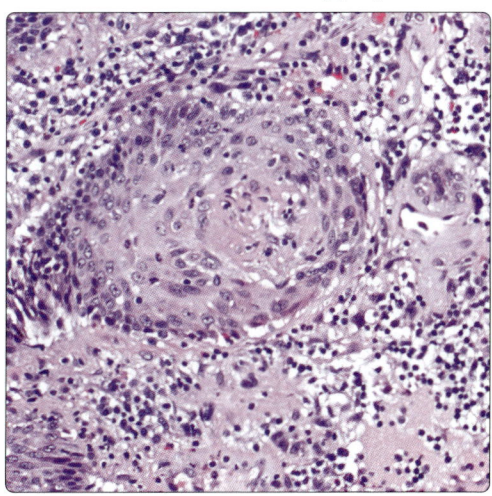

Pseudocarcinomatous Hyperplasia
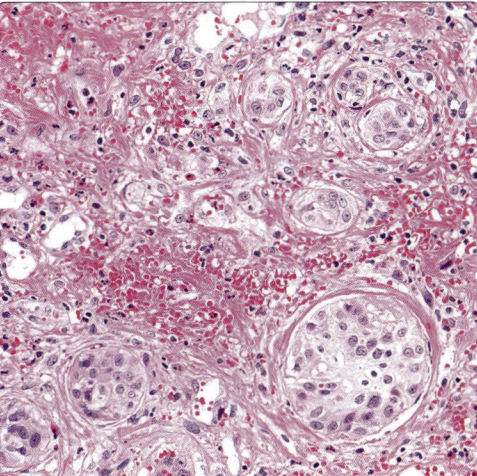

(Left) *The epithelial nests in pseudocarcinomatous hyperplasia often have a "squamoid" appearance. The nuclear features remain bland, in contrast to urothelial carcinoma with squamous differentiation.* **(Right)** *Nests of urothelium present deep within the lamina propria are a common finding in pseudocarcinomatous hyperplasia. The surrounding extravasated red blood cells would be unusual in an invasive urothelial carcinoma.*

Pseudocarcinomatous Hyperplasia

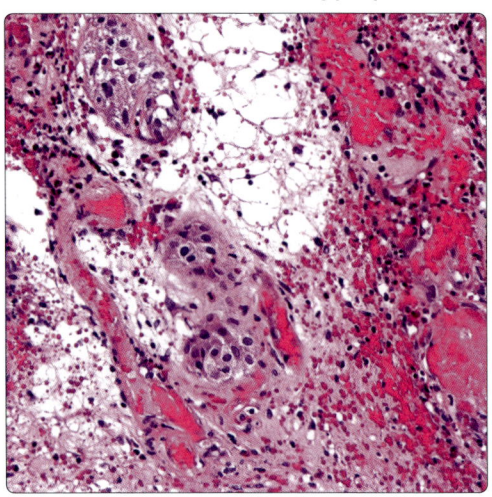

Pseudocarcinomatous Hyperplasia

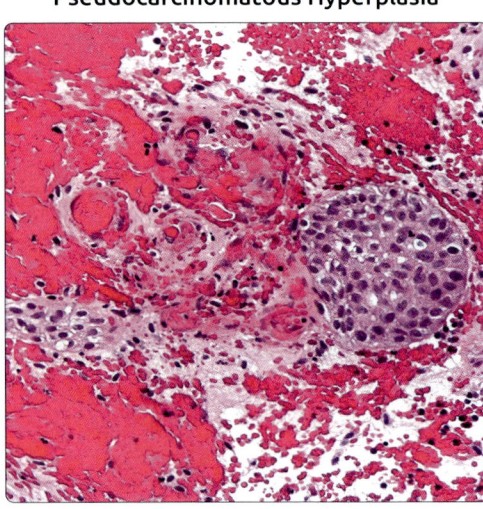

Pseudocarcinomatous Hyperplasia

(Left) The nests of urothelium are present deep in the lamina propria with associated stromal hemorrhage and intravascular fibrin accumulation. The urothelial nests have bland cytologic features. (Right) The extensive hemorrhage is a strong clue to the diagnosis of a pseudocarcinomatous hyperplasia, especially when associated with fibrin. The epithelial nests may be more dispersed in some examples, which makes the diagnosis somewhat easier.

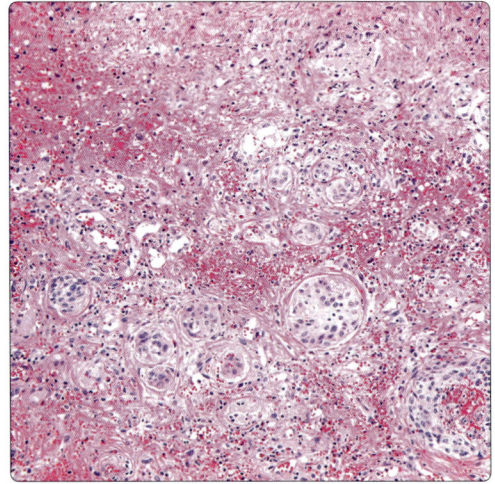

Pseudocarcinomatous Hyperplasia

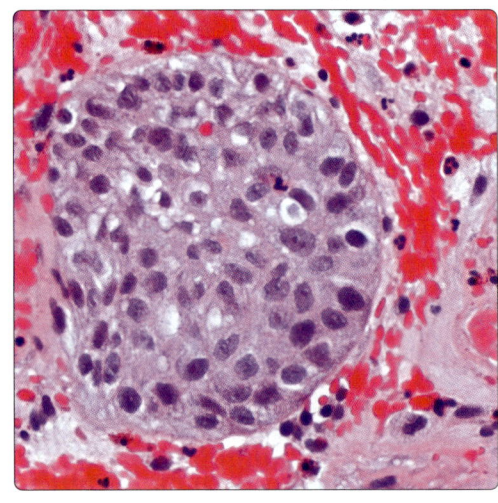

Pseudocarcinomatous Hyperplasia

(Left) The presence of nests of urothelium associated with extravasated blood and fibrin is characteristic of this radiation-induced reparative process. An initial assessment at low-power magnification is very important. (Right) This high-power photomicrograph shows minimal variation in the size of the nuclei and variably prominent pinpoint nucleoli in the urothelial nests.

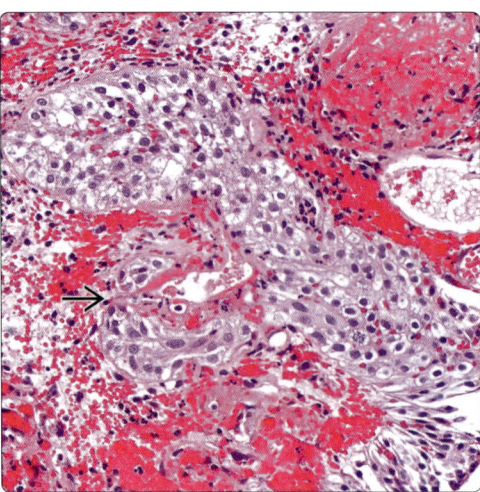

Pseudocarcinomatous Hyperplasia

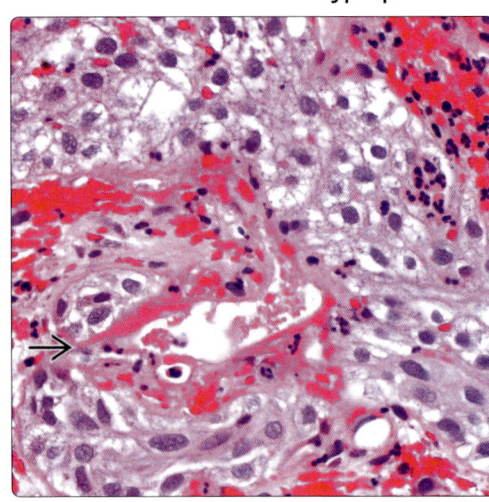

Pseudocarcinomatous Hyperplasia

(Left) This example of pseudocarcinomatous hyperplasia shows the characteristic "wrapping" of urothelium around abnormal blood vessels ⇨ with hyalinization &/or intravascular fibrin. (Right) This blood vessel has fibrin within the wall ⇨, is encircled by cytologically bland urothelium, and has associated extravasated red blood cells and acute inflammation. These features are typical of pseudocarcinomatous hyperplasia.

Pseudocarcinomatous Hyperplasia

Other Radiation-Associated Changes

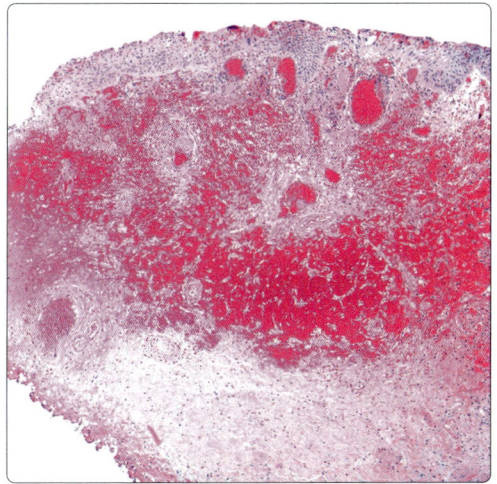

Other Radiation-Associated Changes

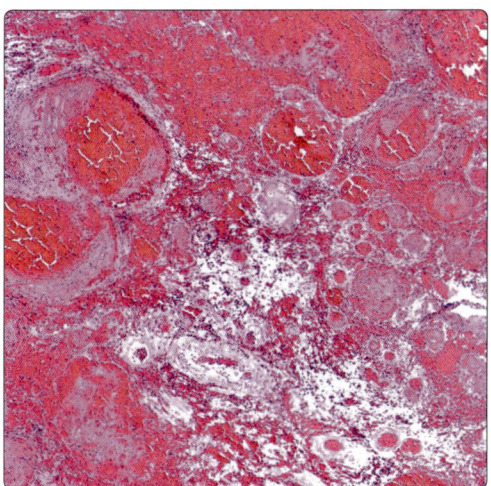

(Left) On low-power evaluation, extensive hemorrhage in the lamina propria (while not entirely specific) should alert one to the possibility of radiation. (Right) This is a florid example of vascular ectasia with both extensive intravascular and stromal fibrin. This feature in the tissue surrounding an epithelial proliferation should prompt strong consideration of a nonneoplastic process, possibly related to prior therapy.

Other Radiation-Associated Changes

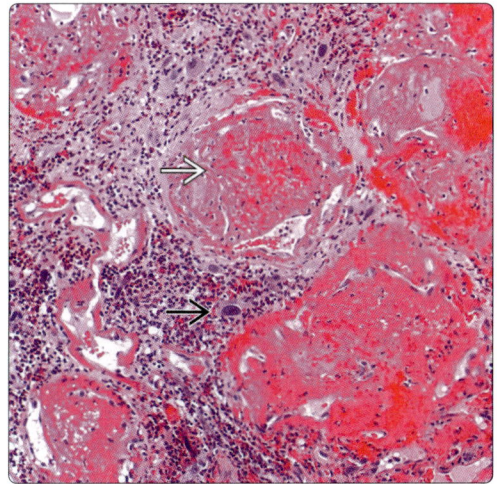

Other Radiation-Associated Changes

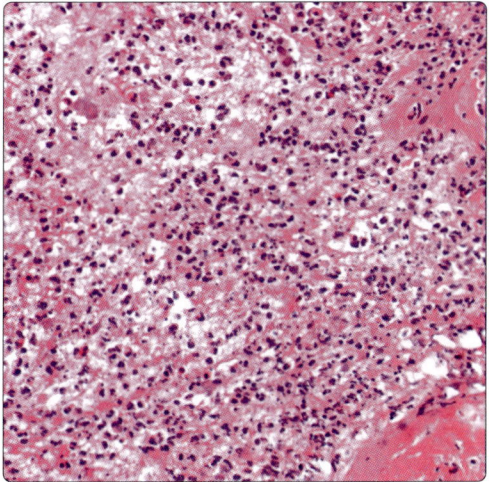

(Left) Prominent vascular ectasia with intravascular fibrin ➡ is present in this example with an associated history of radiation therapy. Scattered atypical fibroblasts are present in the background stroma ➡ as well. (Right) Admixed acute and chronic inflammation is a common finding because of tissue ischemia and may obscure the fibrin deposition. Areas of frank tissue necrosis may be seen.

Other Radiation-Associated Changes

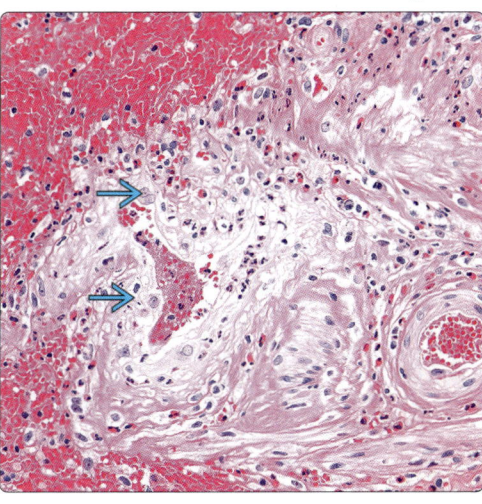

Other Radiation-Associated Changes

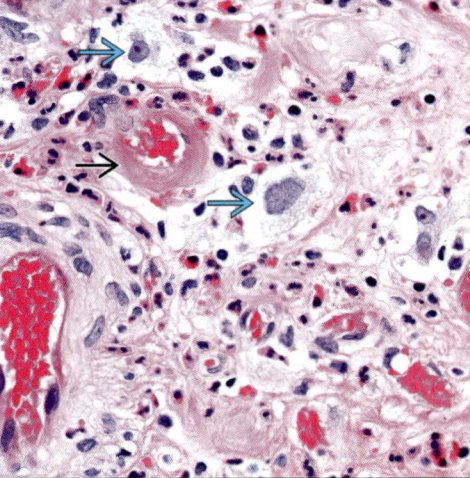

(Left) Abnormal blood vessels are another sign of prior radiation therapy. In this example, there are mildly atypical cells within the vessel wall ➡ as well as inflammatory cells. (Right) The presence of large, individual atypical cells ➡ (beyond what is usually seen in lamina propria stromal cells), is also a feature that should suggest prior radiation. This example also shows fibrinoid necrosis of a small blood vessel wall ➡.

Pseudocarcinomatous Hyperplasia

Papillary-Polypoid Cystitis
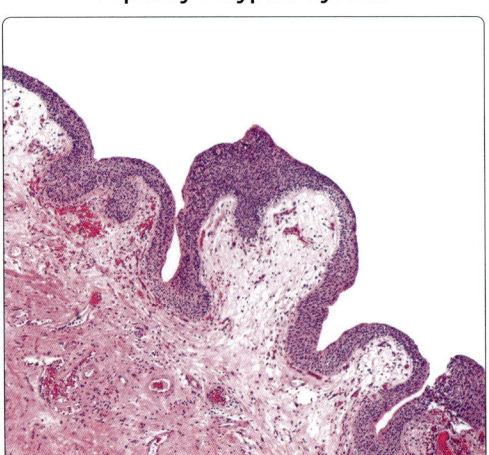

Reactive Urothelial Atypia
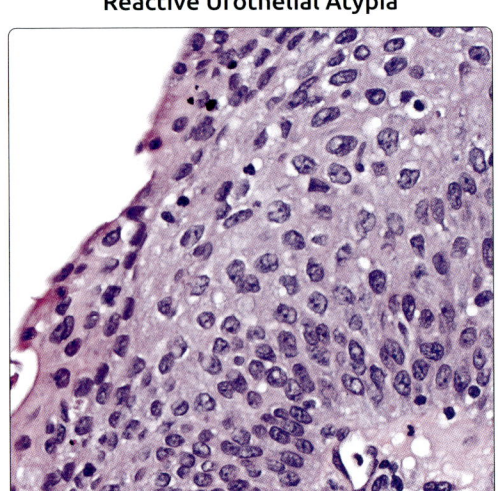

(Left) Adjacent urothelium may show nonspecific reactive changes, including papillary-polypoid cystitis. This may mimic a noninvasive papillary urothelial neoplasm. (Right) The overlying surface urothelium in pseudocarcinomatous hyperplasia shows reactive urothelial changes characterized by mild nucleomegaly, fine nuclear chromatin, and pinpoint nucleoli. The absence of associated urothelial carcinoma in situ or papillary urothelial neoplasia is important.

Radiation Atypia in Urothelium
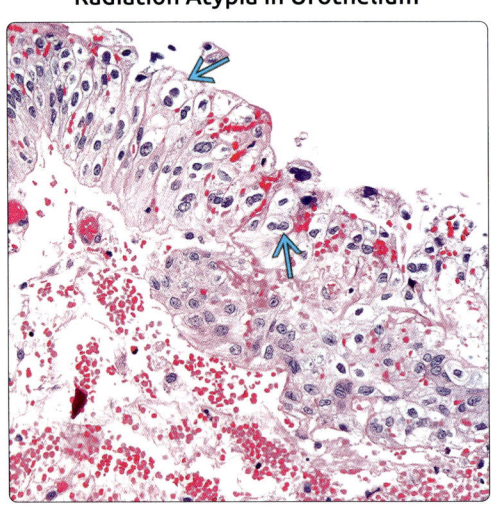

Radiation Atypia in Urothelium
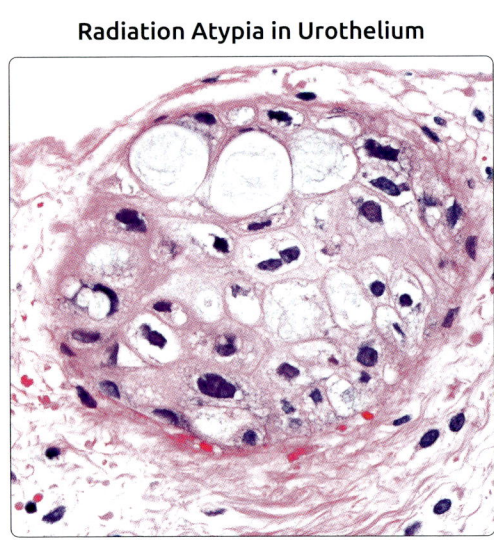

(Left) Urothelium may show radiation-induced changes, which often include cytoplasmic vacuolization and binucleation ➡, in addition to some nuclear enlargement and small nucleoli. (Right) This high-power photomicrograph better highlights common radiation-induced changes, characterized in this example by very prominent cytoplasmic vacuolization and some binucleation.

Urothelial Denudation
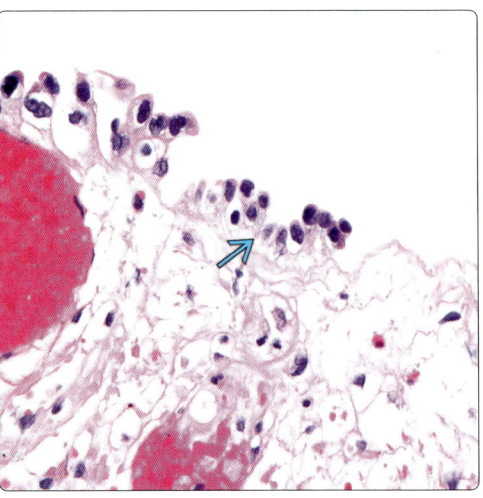

Surface Ulceration
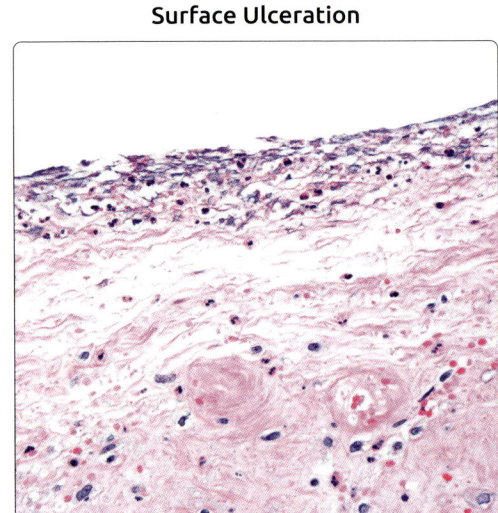

(Left) Urothelial denudation may be seen, similar to other reactive/inflammatory conditions. The individual clinging reactive urothelial cells ➡ do not show the degree of nucleomegaly or nuclear hyperchromasia seen in urothelial carcinoma in situ. (Right) Complete surface ulceration with underlying acute inflammation (and sometimes necrosis) may be seen in association with radiation. All of these changes may be variably present in a patchy distribution. Note obliterative changes in the blood vessels.

Pseudocarcinomatous Hyperplasia

Invasive Urothelial Carcinoma

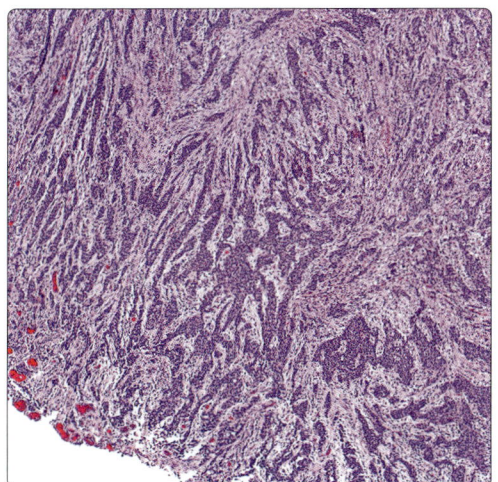

Invasive Urothelial Carcinoma

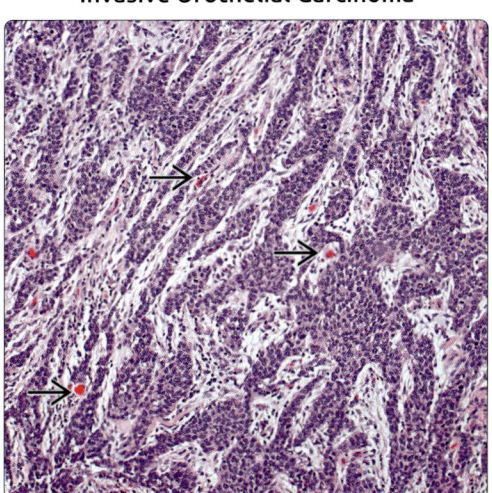

(Left) This is an example of invasive urothelial carcinoma in a patient with a history of radiation therapy. The nests of urothelium are more complex and interanastomosing than typically seen in pseudocarcinomatous hyperplasia. (Right) This degree of epithelial confluence should suggest the diagnosis of carcinoma in this case. The associated blood vessels are not associated with fibrin and are not hyalinized ⇒.

Invasive Urothelial Carcinoma

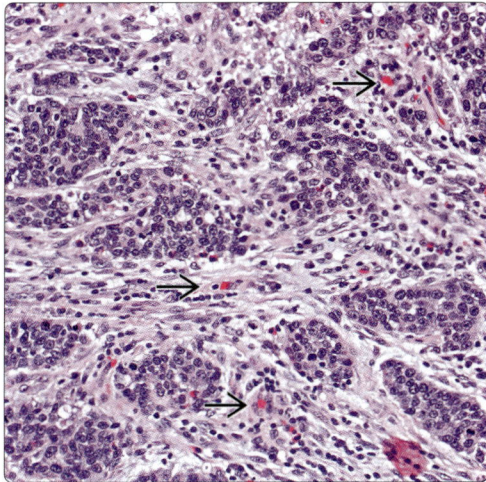

Invasive Urothelial Carcinoma

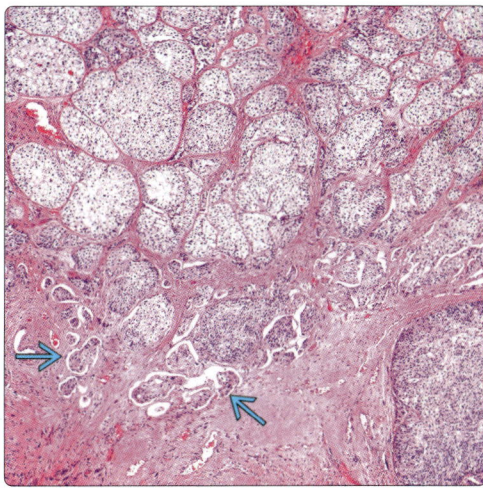

(Left) This invasive urothelial carcinoma, although monomorphic, has a higher nuclear:cytoplasmic ratio and larger nucleoli compared to pseudocarcinomatous hyperplasia. In addition, the small capillary-sized blood vessels appear normal ⇒. (Right) Cytologically bland invasive carcinomas with areas of nested morphology may mimic pseudocarcinomatous hyperplasia. The absence of background radiation changes and the foci with stromal retraction ⇒ are clues to the diagnosis of carcinoma.

Invasive Urothelial Carcinoma

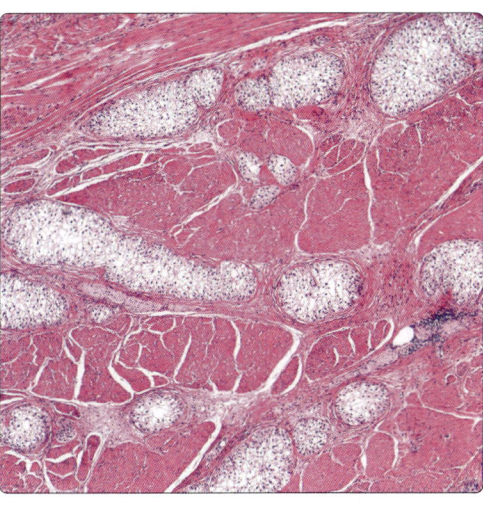

Verrucous Carcinoma

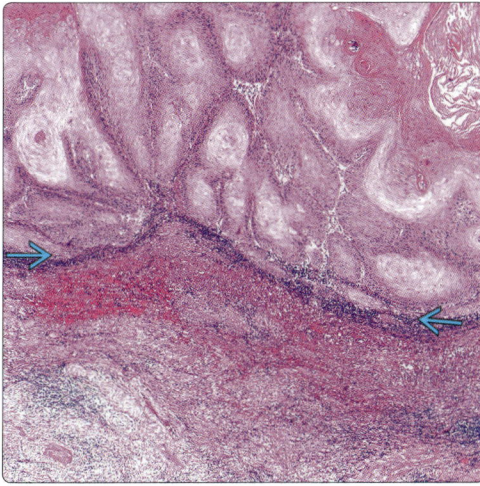

(Left) Definitive invasion of underlying muscularis propria is one of the most useful features of invasive carcinoma, as seen in this example with bland cytologic features and glycogen-rich cytoplasm. (Right) Verrucous carcinoma has a pushing broad front of nondestructive invasion. The squamous epithelium is more confluent with a sharp, rounded border at the interface with the lamina propria ⇒. In addition, a surface verrucous component is invariably present.

Hamartoma

KEY FACTS

TERMINOLOGY
- Rare polypoid bladder mass comprised of benign urothelium resembling cystitis glandularis and variable stroma

CLINICAL ISSUES
- Symptoms
  - Hematuria
  - Urinary voiding symptoms
- Treatment
  - Conservative excision
- Age
  - May occur in children, but varies

MICROSCOPIC
- Resemble spectrum of invaginated urothelial nests
  - Cystitis cystica/glandularis ± intestinal metaplasia
- More pronounced and irregularly distributed epithelium than cystitis cystica spectrum

- Variable stromal component
  - Cellular spindled foci common
  - May be smooth muscle, fibrous, or edematous

TOP DIFFERENTIAL DIAGNOSES
- Embryonal rhabdomyosarcoma
  - May have similar biphasic appearance with periglandular stroma
  - Expresses markers of skeletal muscle differentiation
    - Such as myogenin
- Cystitis glandularis
  - Superficial location of nests favors cystitis cystica
  - Absence of distinct stromal component

DIAGNOSTIC CHECKLIST
- Botryoid rhabdomyosarcoma must be carefully considered in younger patients

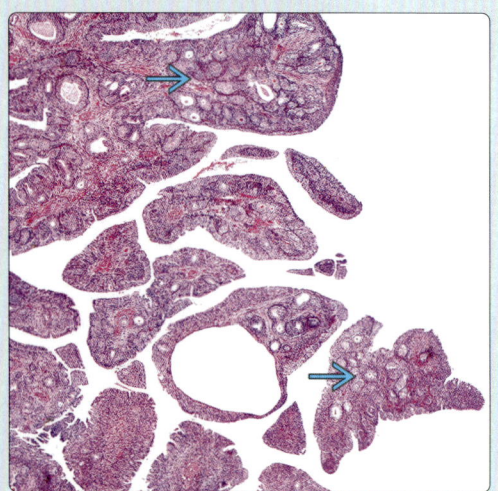

Bladder Hamartoma

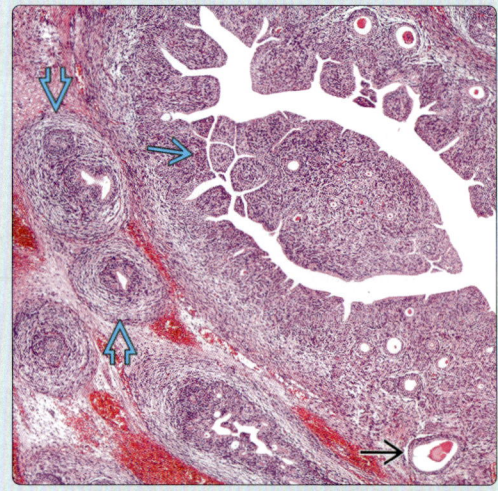

Bladder Hamartoma

(Left) This bladder hamartoma has a papillary and polypoid architecture with a lining of benign urothelium and crowded invaginations of epithelium resembling the spectrum of cystitis cystica ➡. (Right) Bladder hamartoma may have a phyllodes-type architecture ➡ and cellular periglandular stroma may be prominent ➡. The epithelial glands have a morphology identical to cystitis cystica ➡. This appearance may closely mimic rhabdomyosarcoma.

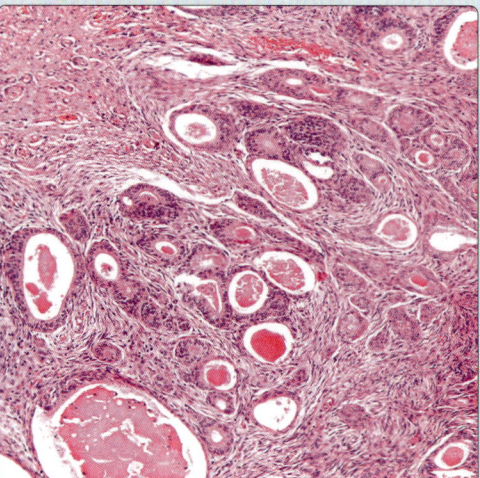

Bladder Hamartoma

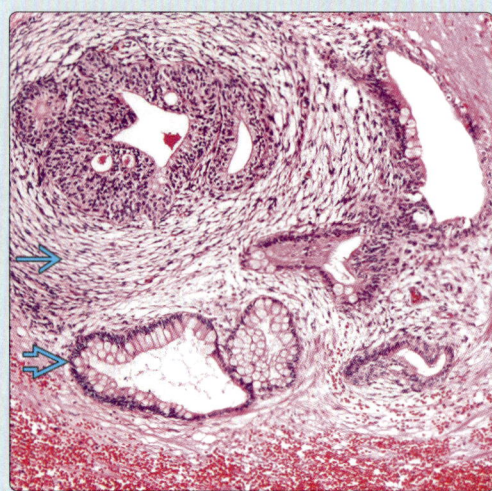

Bladder Hamartoma

(Left) The polyps of bladder hamartoma are filled with crowded collections of epithelium resembling von Brunn nests, cystitis cystica, and cystitis glandularis. The surrounding spindled stroma is also characteristic. (Right) Bladder hamartoma may have glands with intestinal metaplasia ➡, similar to cystitis glandularis of intestinal type. The background cystitis, cystica-like component shows the characteristic surrounding spindled stroma ➡.

Hamartoma

TERMINOLOGY

Synonyms
- Lesions reported as hamartoma have varied
  - Similar lesions have been described as adenoma
  - First reported case of nephrogenic adenoma called hamartoma

Definitions
- Extremely rare polypoid bladder mass
  - Comprised of benign urothelium resembling cystitis glandularis spectrum with variable stromal component

ETIOLOGY/PATHOGENESIS

Genetic
- Occurrence in siblings suggests genetic component in some cases

CLINICAL ISSUES

Presentation
- Hematuria
- Urinary voiding symptoms

Treatment
- Conservative excision

Prognosis
- Benign
  - Nonrecurring

Age
- May occur in children, but varies

IMAGING

Cystoscopy
- Polypoid mass in bladder lumen
- May fill entire bladder

MACROSCOPIC

General Features
- Exophytic polypoid mass of varying size

MICROSCOPIC

Histologic Features
- Papillary/polypoid lesion
- Benign urothelial nests
  - Resemble spectrum of invaginated urothelial nests
    - von Brunn nests
    - Cystitis cystica
    - Cystitis glandularis
      - Intestinal metaplasia may be seen
  - More pronounced and irregularly distributed than cystitis cystica spectrum
- Variable stromal component
  - Varies in histologic appearance
    - Fibrous
    - Muscular
    - Edematous
    - Cellular spindled foci
  - Often encircles urothelial nests

Cytologic Features
- Bland cytologic features of epithelial and stromal components

ANCILLARY TESTS

Immunohistochemistry
- Not helpful except to exclude differential diagnostic considerations

DIFFERENTIAL DIAGNOSIS

Embryonal Rhabdomyosarcoma
- Cellular spindled stroma around glands often suggests botryoid rhabdomyosarcoma
- Rhabdomyosarcoma does not generally have as much of epithelial component
- Expression of skeletal muscle markers may aid in difficult cases
  - Myogenin and MyoD1

Cystitis Glandularis
- May be polypoid
- Some small lesions have been reported as hamartoma
  - Might be better regarded as florid examples of cystitis cystica spectrum
- Superficial location of nests would favor cystitis cystica
  - Cystitis cystica typically has sharp interface at epithelial-stromal junction
- Absence of distinct stromal component would favor cystitis cystica

Exstrophy Polyp
- By definition, arise in association with bladder exstrophy
- Have morphologic overlap with hamartoma
  - Deep cystitis, cystica-like epithelium
  - Onion-skin fibrosis around glands
- Greater degree of inflammation
- Squamous metaplasia frequent

DIAGNOSTIC CHECKLIST

Clinically Relevant Pathologic Features
- Botryoid rhabdomyosarcoma must be considered in younger patients

Pathologic Interpretation Pearls
- Disorganized collection of glands and stroma in polypoid mass of the bladder suggest hamartoma
  - Extent is beyond what is typically seen in cystitis cystica

SELECTED REFERENCES

1. Fan R et al: Exstrophy polyp is a unique pathology entity. Pediatr Dev Pathol. 15(6):471-7, 2012
2. Keating MA et al: Hamartoma of the bladder in a 4-year-old girl with hamartomatous polyps of the gastrointestinal tract. J Urol. 138(2):366-9, 1987
3. Billis A et al: Adenoma of bladder in siblings with renal dysplasia. Urology. 16(3):299-302, 1980

Overview of Urinary Bladder Neoplasms

EPIDEMIOLOGY

Incidence

- 9th most common cancer worldwide
  - 260,000 new cases each year in men
  - 76,000 new cases each year in women
- In USA, 4th most common cancer in men, with estimated 74,000 new cases in 2014
  - > 90% are urothelial in origin
  - Pure squamous cell carcinoma and adenocarcinoma represent < 5%
- In regions of endemic schistosomiasis, squamous cell carcinoma is most common

Ethnicity and Geographic Relationship

- Highest incidence in Western Europe, North America, and Australia
- Incidence in developed countries is 6x higher than nondeveloped countries
- 2x more common in American white males than African American males, particularly in superficial tumors; similar risk in invasive disease

Gender

- ~ 3-4x more common in males than females

Natural History

- ~ 70-80% of newly diagnosed bladder cancer patients present with noninvasive or early invasive disease (stages Ta, Tis, or T1)
  - These tumors typically show frequent recurrences but low progression rate
- For noninvasive tumors, recurrence and progression rates depend on grade
  - Urothelial papilloma
    - Recurrence: 0-8%
    - Grade or stage progression: 0%
  - Papillary urothelial neoplasm of low malignant potential (LMP)
    - Recurrence: 25-47%
    - Grade or stage progression: 8%
  - Low-grade carcinoma
    - Recurrence: 48-71%
    - Progression and death due to disease: < 5%
  - High-grade carcinoma
    - Almost all disease-related deaths are in patients with high-grade tumors
    - 40-45% of newly diagnosed bladder cancer is high grade
    - Stage progression: 20% progress to invasion and 12% die of disease
- For invasive tumors, outcome depends on stage
  - Lamina propria invasion (pT1)
    - For some patients, conservative surgical management is sufficient in addition to intravesical therapy
    - Subset will progress to pT2 disease and require cystectomy
  - Invasion of muscularis propria and beyond (greater than pT2)
    - 50% of patients with pT2 or greater disease have occult metastases at diagnosis
    - Most of these develop overt signs of metastasis within 1 year
  - Distant metastasis
    - Very poor prognosis
    - Poor response to adjuvant therapy

Age Range

- Typically seen in adults
  - More common after 60 years of age (median age: 65-70 years) but wide range of age distribution including children
- In children and adolescents, urothelial papilloma and papillary urothelial neoplasm of LMP may be seen
  - Urothelial carcinoma is very rare in young patients
  - Congenital bladder exstrophy is associated with increased risk of developing adenocarcinoma, squamous cell carcinoma, or urothelial carcinoma in bladder remnant, even following early treatment with reconstructive surgery

Classification of Papillary Urothelial Neoplasms

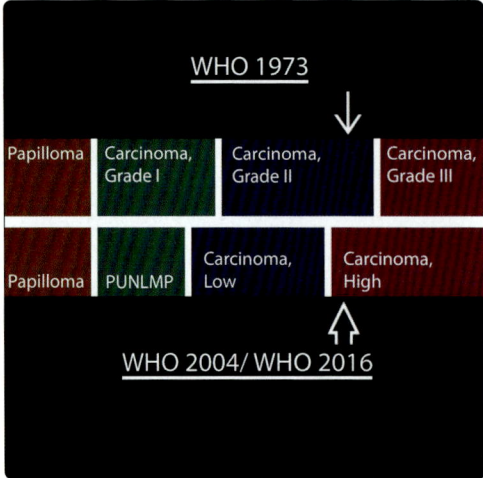

Pathogenesis of Urothelial Neoplasia

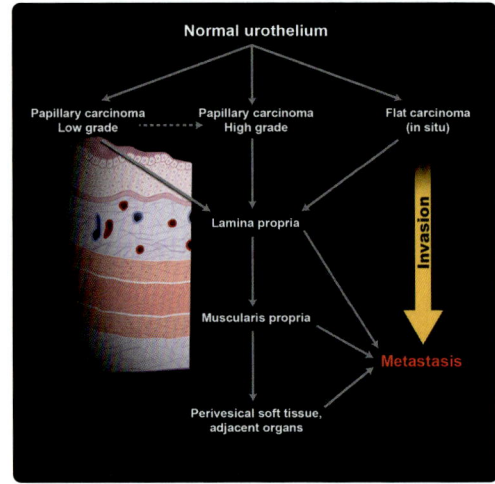

(Left) The threshold for high grade was lowered in WHO 2004/2016 system. A subset of cases classified as grade II ⇒ would now be classified as high grade ⇒. This is important for treatment, because some grade II tumors may now receive intravesical therapy. Urologists should understand that grade II does not equal low grade in all cases. (Right) Graphic shows the proposed pathways for carcinogenesis developing along the papillary and flat pathways. High-grade lesions are more likely to develop invasion & metastases.

Overview of Urinary Bladder Neoplasms

Environmental Factors

- Tobacco smoking
  - Major established risk factor for bladder cancer
    - 2.6x increased risk in smokers; ~ 50% of bladder cancer in men and 23% in women may be attributed to smoking
    - Risk correlates with duration and intensity of smoking (pack years); cessation may gradually decrease risk of bladder cancer with time
- Occupational exposure
  - Aniline dye, aromatic amines (benzidine, 2-naphthylamine; also linked to cigarette smoking)
  - Increased arsenic levels in drinking water and soil in certain parts of world is environmental risk factor
- Chronic inflammation
  - Chronic urinary tract infection and calculi proposed as risk factors
- Other drugs
  - Chronic abuse of analgesics that include phenacetin
  - Cyclophosphamide for cancer therapy
  - Chlornaphazine
  - Pelvic radiation

Infectious Etiology

- Schistosomiasis (particularly *Schistosoma haematobium*) is associated with increased risk for squamous cell carcinoma but also for urothelial carcinoma and adenocarcinoma
- Human papillomavirus (HPV) is rare etiology for bladder cancer but may increase risk for condyloma and rarely squamous cell carcinoma

CLINICAL IMPLICATIONS

Grading Issues

- Multiple grading schemes have been used, but WHO/International Society of Urological Pathology (ISUP) 2004/2016 is now widely accepted
  - Adopted by American Joint Committee on Cancer, 7th Edition and American Urologic Association
  - Papillary urothelial carcinoma is divided into low-grade and high-grade categories; 2-tier system that increases interobserver reproducibility and improves risk stratification
  - Recent consensus statement by International Consortium on Urologic Diseases and European Association of Urology has endorsed WHO/ISUP system and have provided nomenclature for inverted lesions
  - Overall similar approach and analogy in grading of flat, papillary, and endophytic urothelial lesions
- WHO/ISUP classification of papillary neoplasia
  - Urothelial papilloma
  - Papillary urothelial neoplasm of LMP
  - Papillary urothelial carcinoma, low grade
  - Papillary urothelial carcinoma, high grade
- WHO/ISUP classification of flat lesions with atypia
  - Reactive urothelial atypia
  - Urothelial atypia of uncertain significance
  - Urothelial dysplasia
  - Urothelial carcinoma in situ
- Endophytic neoplasia
  - Inverted papilloma
  - Endophytic urothelial neoplasm of LMP
  - Endophytic urothelial carcinoma, low grade
  - Endophytic urothelial carcinoma, high grade, noninvasive
  - Endophytic urothelial carcinoma, high grade, invasive
- Invasive carcinoma
  - No consensus grading scheme
  - Evidence suggests grade of invasive component is not prognostic
    - In United States, most experts consider all invasive carcinomas as high grade despite lower grade cytology in rare cases, such as nested variant
    - In Europe, invasive tumors are frequently graded as grades 2 and 3; this grading schema may be required by some institutions and for eligibility in clinical trials in Europe
    - Prognosis is dependent on depth of invasion rather than grade
    - Grading schema are developed for flat lesions, exophytic papillary and endophytic lesions
      - Criteria for lesions in these categories are similar and can be extrapolated

Management

- "Superficial" bladder cancer (pTcis, pTa, pT1 disease)
  - Urothelial carcinoma in situ, high-grade papillary, and invasive urothelial carcinoma involving lamina propria
    - Usually treated with intravesical therapy, such as Bacillus Calmette-Guérin
    - Cystectomy for tumors refractory to conservative management
  - Low-grade carcinoma and papillary urothelial neoplasm of LMP
    - Usually treated by transurethral resection and surveillance
    - Urine cytology screening
    - Adjunctive molecular screening
- Urothelial carcinoma invasive into muscularis propria
  - Generally warrants radical cystectomy; radiation therapy offered in many countries
  - Use of neoadjuvant/adjuvant therapy is common, but its use varies among institutions
- New role for molecular based therapies, limited applications, primarily in advanced/metastatic disease

Prognostic Factors

- **Noninvasive papillary tumors**
  - Histologic grade most important prognostic factor for recurrence and progression
    - Urothelial papilloma and papillary urothelial neoplasm of LMP: Minimal risk for progression; LMP lesions often recur
    - All carcinomas (low or high grade) frequently recur
    - Low-grade and high-grade papillary carcinoma: Increased risk of progression; more in high grade than in low grade
  - Size of tumor
    - Large tumors (often > 3 cm) increased risk of recurrence and progression
  - Multifocality
    - Multifocal tumors (in bladder or in ureters and urethra) increase risk of recurrence and progression

Overview of Urinary Bladder Neoplasms

Analogy for Application of WHO/ISUP System to Inverted Neoplasia

Degree of Atypia	Exophytic Papillary Lesions	Flat Lesions	Endophytic/Inverted Papillary Lesions
None	Papilloma	Normal urothelium	Inverted papilloma
Minimal	Papillary urothelial neoplasm of low malignant potential (PUNLMP)	Urothelial hyperplasia	Inverted PUNLMP
Distinct, mild-moderate	Papillary urothelial carcinoma, low grade, noninvasive	Urothelial dysplasia	Inverted papillary urothelial carcinoma, low grade, noninvasive
Moderate-severe; severe	Papillary urothelial carcinoma, high grade, noninvasive	Urothelial carcinoma in situ	Inverted papillary urothelial carcinoma, high grade, noninvasive
Severe	Papillary urothelial carcinoma, high grade, invasive	Not applicable	Inverted papillary urothelial carcinoma, high grade, invasive

- Presence of urothelial carcinoma in situ in adjacent nonpapillary mucosa generally associated with increased risk of recurrence and progression; may represent increased urothelial instability
- **Urothelial carcinoma in situ**
  - Worse outcome associated with presentation with high-grade papillary carcinoma, multifocal disease, involvement of prostatic urethra and failure to respond to intravesical therapy
- **Invasive urothelial carcinoma**
  - Depth of invasion in bladder wall determines stage and prognosis
  - Lymph node and distant metastasis portend poor prognosis
  - Involvement of prostatic gland and seminal vesicles- poor prognosis
  - Some variant histologic types may portend worse prognosis or have therapeutic implications
    - Small cell carcinoma
    - Micropapillary carcinoma
    - Nested variant urothelial carcinoma (limited experience)
    - Sarcomatoid carcinoma
    - Carcinoma with rhabdoid features
    - Plasmacytoid carcinoma
    - Lymphoepithelioma-like carcinoma
    - Undifferentiated carcinoma
  - Lymphovascular invasion
    - Controversial prognostic factor
    - Utilized for management decisions in some centers
    - Because of frequent retraction artifact in invasive carcinoma, reproducibility of lymphovascular invasion diagnosis is problematic
    - Strict morphologic criteria should be used in recognition
    - Immunohistochemistry with endothelial markers may rarely be required; not routinely recommended
  - Multifocal disease and the presence of urothelial carcinoma in situ of urethra and ureter may portend worse outcome
  - Surgical margin involvement by invasive carcinoma adverse risk factor primarily for local recurrence
  - Histologic grade less important in invasive disease

Intraoperative (Frozen Section) Evaluation

- General intraoperative issues
  - Frozen section artifact may induce or exaggerate atypical features in urothelium
  - Using stromal lymphocytes as gauge of nuclear size is useful
  - Establishing minimal threshold for carcinoma in situ is key on frozen section analysis of flat lesions
  - Variant invasive patterns, as plasmacytoid, mimic inflammatory cells, but more commonly have subtle spread along perivesical and periureteral soft tissue
  - Frozen section usually performed for urothelial margin evaluation
    - Ureters
      - Should generally be sectioned en face
      - En face sections should include entire wall (urothelium, muscularis, and adventitia)
      - Examination usually to rule out carcinoma in situ; invasive carcinoma may rarely be seen in soft tissue around ureter
      - von Brunn nests are common and should be distinguished from tumor
    - Urethra
      - Examination usually to rule out carcinoma in situ; its presence may effect type of urinary diversion post cystectomy
      - Carcinoma in situ may be subtle and pagetoid in histology
  - Ureteral and urethral mucosa retracts more than muscle and soft tissue; important to ensure its presence in sections prepared for frozen section

SELECTED REFERENCES

1. Amin MB et al: Update for the practicing pathologist: The International Consultation On Urologic Disease-European association of urology consultation on bladder cancer. Mod Pathol. 28(5):612-630, 2015
2. Ferlay J et al: Cancer incidence and mortality worldwide: sources, methods and major patterns in GLOBOCAN 2012. Int J Cancer. 136(5):E359-86, 2015
3. American Joint Committee on Cancer: AJCC Cancer Staging Manual. 7th ed. New York: Springer, 2009
4. Eble et al: Tumors of the urinary system. In: World Health Organization Classification of Tumors. Pathology & Genetics. Tumors of the Urinary System and Male Genital Organs. Lyon: IARC Press. 89-149, 2004
5. Epstein JI et al: The World Health Organization/International Society of Urological Pathology consensus classification of urothelial (transitional cell) neoplasms of the urinary bladder. Bladder Consensus Conference Committee. Am J Surg Pathol. 22(12):1435-48, 1998

Overview of Urinary Bladder Neoplasms

Invasive Urothelial Carcinoma (Muscularis Propria)

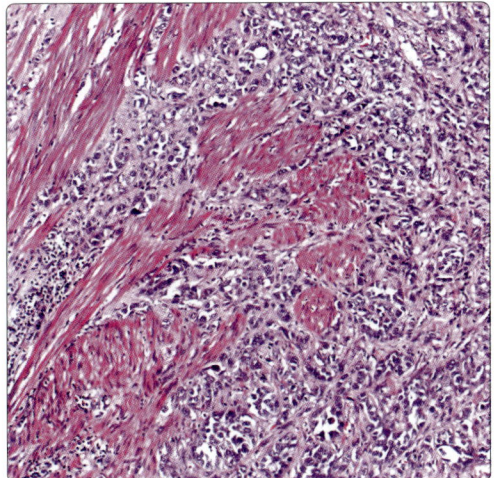

Prostatic Involvement by Urothelial Carcinoma

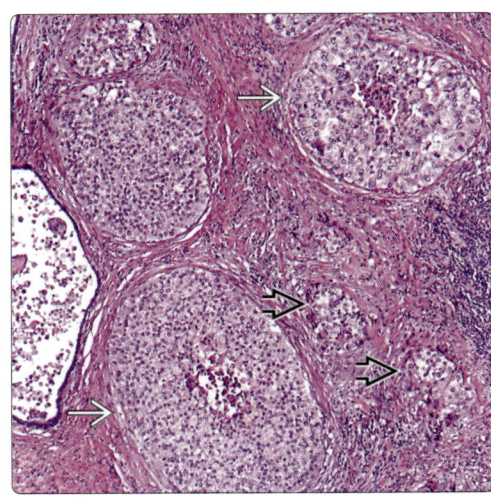

(Left) Urothelial carcinoma is shown invading into thick muscle bundles, representative of muscularis propria. This is an important stage-determining histologic parameter with implication on subsequent radical therapy (e.g., cystectomy). (Right) Urothelial carcinoma extensively involving prostatic ducts ➡ and invading the prostatic stroma ➡ is shown. The latter finding is particularly important (and may require extensive sampling of the prostate) because it is associated with adverse outcome.

Urothelial Carcinoma With Lymphovascular Invasion

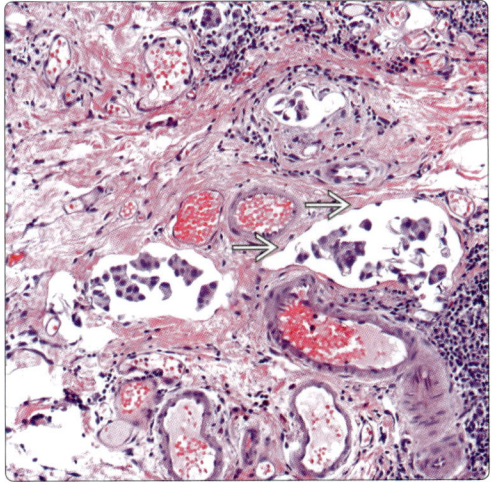

Invasive Urothelial Carcinoma With Stromal Retraction

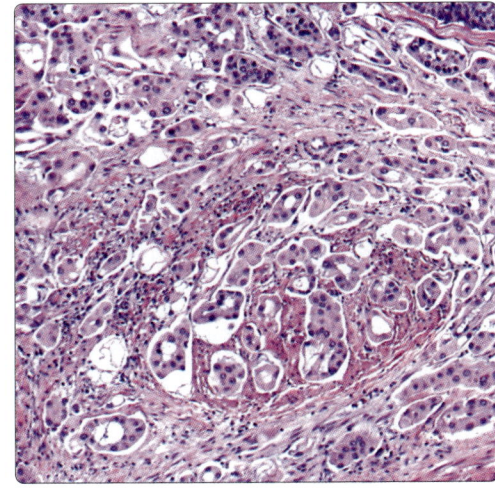

(Left) This invasive urothelial carcinoma has invaded vascular spaces. The distribution of tumor and the presence of readily identifiable endothelial cells lining the clear spaces ➡ is characteristic. This finding was was further confirmed by immunostain D2-40. (Right) In contrast, this invasive urothelial carcinoma exhibits marked stromal retraction, mimicking lymphovascular invasion. Immunostains with endothelial markers failed to identify endothelial cells surrounding any of the tumor clusters.

Frozen Section of Peritoneal Soft Tissue (Plasmacytoid Carcinoma)

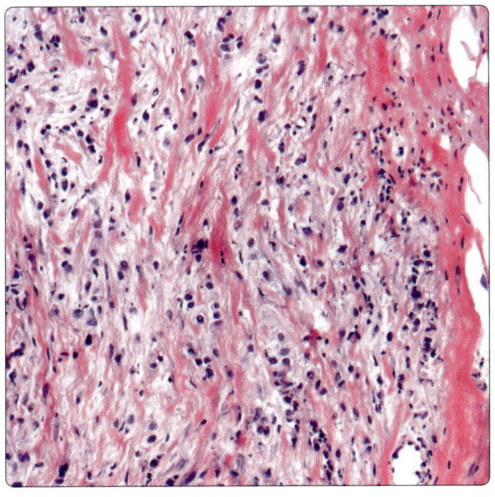

Ureter Margin Frozen Section

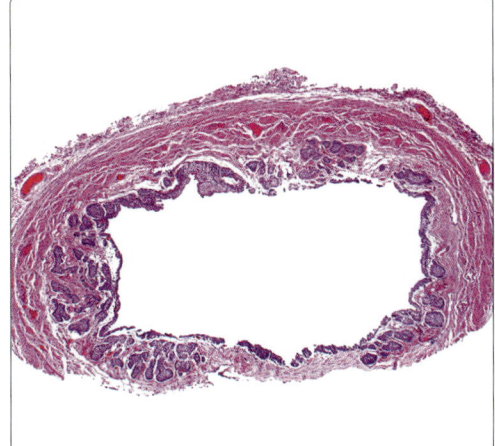

(Left) Subtle case on frozen section of a peritoneal biopsy from a patient with plasmacytoid carcinoma of the bladder is shown. Note the dyscohesive infiltrative nature of the tumor cells. Radical cystectomy was aborted upon reporting the presence of tumor. (Right) Suboptimal ureteral margin submitted for evaluation by frozen section is shown. Although complete urothelium is seen, the entire muscularis and adjacent soft tissue is not visualized.

Urothelial Carcinoma In Situ

KEY FACTS

TERMINOLOGY
- Malignant flat urothelial lesion comprised of cytologically high-grade cells

ETIOLOGY/PATHOGENESIS
- Multiple predisposing environmental factors are known

CLINICAL ISSUES
- Most common in men, 6th-7th decades
- Multifocality common, including upper urinary tract involvement
- May progress to invasive carcinoma

MICROSCOPIC
- Unequivocal high-grade cytologic atypia may involve either full or partial thickness of urothelium
- Marked nucleomegaly is typical
- Nuclear hyperchromasia with coarse condensed chromatin is typical
- Spectrum of atypia and growth patterns exist
- Loss of polarity to basement membrane is common

ANCILLARY TESTS
- CK20, CD44, and p53 immunohistochemistry may be useful in distinction from nonneoplastic reactive atypia
  - Diffuse cytoplasmic staining for CK20 in atypical cells is common in carcinoma in situ (CIS)
  - Membranous CD44 staining in atypical cells more common in benign reactive lesions

TOP DIFFERENTIAL DIAGNOSES
- Urothelial dysplasia and flat atypia of uncertain significance
- Reactive atypia (including therapy effect)

DIAGNOSTIC CHECKLIST
- Key to interpreting flat lesions is developing appropriate minimal threshold for CIS
- Intraurothelial inflammation should prompt consideration of reactive atypia

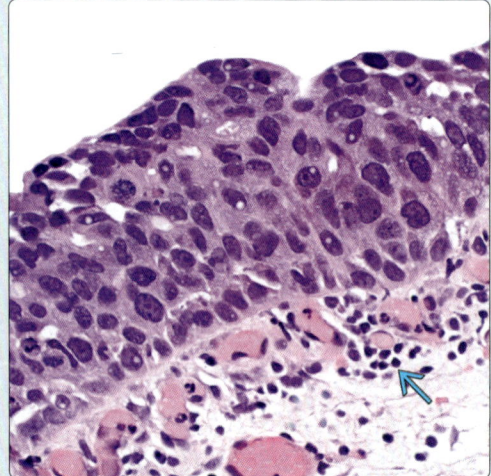

Urothelial Carcinoma In Situ: Nuclear Size

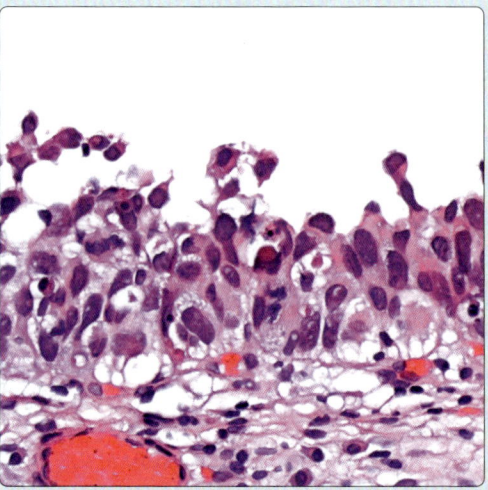

Urothelial Carcinoma In Situ: Pleomorphism

(Left) *Marked nucleomegaly is a very useful diagnostic feature of carcinoma in situ (CIS) and involves the full thickness seen in this example. In this case, the neoplastic nuclei are approximately 5-6x the size of the underlying lymphocytes ⇨, a useful gauge of nucleomegaly.* (Right) *CIS is characterized by cellular disorder, pronounced nucleomegaly, and variable pleomorphism. There may be cellular dyscohesion, as seen here toward the surface. The thickness of the mucosa involved by CIS varies considerably.*

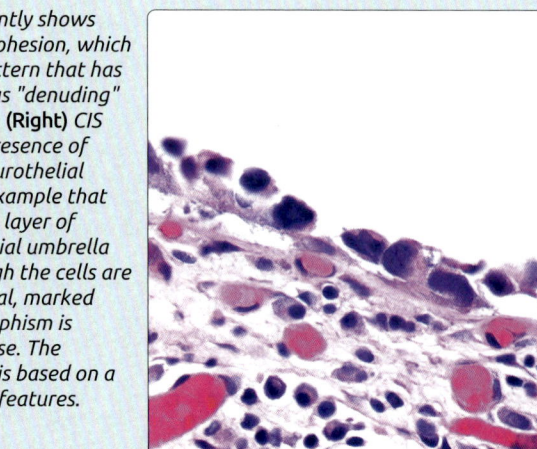

Urothelial Carcinoma In Situ: Denudation

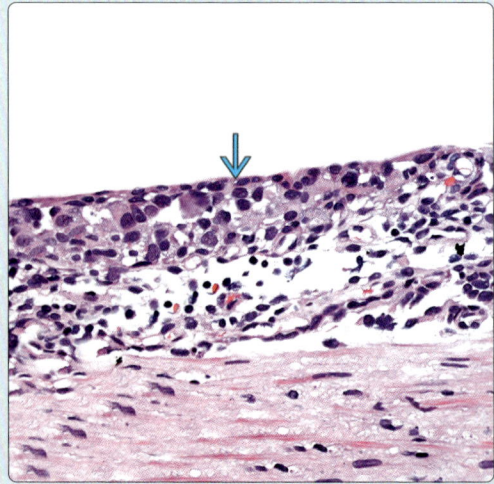

Urothelial Carcinoma In Situ: Preserved Umbrella Layer

(Left) *CIS frequently shows loss of cellular cohesion, which can lead to a pattern that has been described as "denuding" or "clinging" CIS.* (Right) *CIS may show the presence of residual benign urothelial cells, as in this example that has a subtle thin layer of residual superficial umbrella cells ⇨. Although the cells are large and atypical, marked nuclear pleomorphism is absent in this case. The diagnosis of CIS is based on a constellation of features.*

Urothelial Carcinoma In Situ

TERMINOLOGY

Abbreviations
- Urothelial carcinoma in situ (CIS)
- Bacillus Calmette-Guérin (BCG)

Synonyms
- Urothelial carcinoma in situ is only appropriate term for this lesion under WHO 2004/ISUP classification system

Definitions
- Flat urothelial lesion comprised of cytologically malignant cells, which may involve either full or partial thickness of urothelium

ETIOLOGY/PATHOGENESIS

Environmental Exposure
- Tobacco smoking, analgesic abuse, and arylamine compounds are known predisposing factors

Molecular Pathogenesis
- Molecular data have identified several genetic changes associated with CIS
  - Amplification/mutation of *p53* gene
  - Aneuploidy common

CLINICAL ISSUES

Epidemiology
- Incidence
  - Primary (de novo) CIS is rare (< 3% of all urothelial neoplasms)
  - CIS is commonly detected with high-grade papillary and invasive urothelial carcinoma
- Age
  - Most typically seen in men in 6th or 7th decade

Presentation
- Asymptomatic, or may present with dysuria, nocturia, urgency, or frequency of micturition
- Hematuria, if present, is typically microscopic

Treatment
- Different forms of intravesical therapy
  - BCG is standard treatment
- Cystectomy is common treatment for patients refractory to intravesical therapy

Prognosis
- Behavior of CIS is somewhat unpredictable
  - ~ 50% of patients develop invasive carcinoma within 5 years
  - Primary (de novo) CIS seems to have lower progression rate than secondary or concomitant CIS

MACROSCOPIC

General Features
- Cystoscopic appearance may range from normal to erythematous, edematous, or erosive
- Multifocality is common
  - Either within urinary bladder &/or including upper urinary tract

MICROSCOPIC

Histologic Features
- Unequivocal high-grade cytologic atypia may involve either full or partial thickness of urothelium
  - Nuclear anaplasia may be obvious
  - Spectrum of cytologic atypia exists
    - Marked nucleomegaly is typical (3-6x size of normal lymphocyte nucleus)
    - Coarse, condensed nuclear chromatin is typical
    - Prominent nucleoli, multiple nucleoli, nucleolar pleomorphism
    - Mitoses are variable, but atypical forms may be present, even toward surface
    - Loss of cellular cohesion may be prominent
    - Loss of polarity and crowding is common
    - Some examples have abundant eosinophilic cytoplasm
      - High nuclear:cytoplasmic ratio is not sensitive finding
- Urothelial thickness varies greatly in CIS
  - Varies from denuded (with only single cell layer) to normal to hyperplastic
- Different morphologic patterns are described
  - Pleomorphic
    - Very recognizable, given degree of nuclear anaplasia
  - Nonpleomorphic
    - More monomorphic population of cells
    - Still have degree of nucleomegaly and hyperchromasia required for diagnosis
    - May have abundant cytoplasm
    - Prominent nucleoli or consistent chromatin irregularity
  - Small cell
    - Neoplastic cells have little to no cytoplasm
    - Descriptive term that does not denote neuroendocrine differentiation
  - Pagetoid
    - Individual neoplastic cells colonize normal urothelium
    - Highly variable number of malignant cells are present
  - "Clinging" (dyscohesive)
    - Few remaining epithelial cells attached to mucosa, but with features of CIS
    - In cases with complete denudation, correlation with cytology is important
  - Undermining (or overriding)
    - Rare cases show growth underneath adjacent normal urothelium
    - Spread above adjacent normal urothelium is very rare
- CIS may be associated with microinvasion

ANCILLARY TESTS

Immunohistochemistry
- CK20 and CD44 may be useful in distinction of reactive atypia from CIS
- Normal urothelium and reactive atypia
  - CK20 expressed (cytoplasmic) in superficial umbrella cells only
  - CD44 stains only basal and parabasal cell layer with increased membranous staining in reactive atypia

Urothelial Carcinoma In Situ

- In contrast, CIS has distinct immunophenotype
  - Full thickness cytoplasmic staining for CK20
  - CD44 is absent or confined to residual basal cells only
- Some authors have suggested diagnostic utility for other markers
  - HER2/neu
    - Strong membranous staining in CIS
  - CK5/6
    - Cytoplasmic expression in reactive atypia, but not CIS
      - Similar cellular staining to CD44
    - Diagnostic pitfall in lesions with squamous differentiation
      - Strong and diffuse cytoplasmic staining in squamous cell CIS
  - p16
    - Strong cytoplasmic staining in CIS
  - AMACR
    - Strong cytoplasmic staining in CIS (50-78%)
  - p53
    - Strong, diffuse nuclear reactivity in CIS
    - Variable weak or patchy staining in normal or reactive urothelium
    - p53 staining varies between immunohistochemical laboratories
      - If utilized, strict adherence to requirement for strong and diffuse nuclear reactivity must be maintained

DIFFERENTIAL DIAGNOSIS

Urothelial Dysplasia and Flat Atypia of Uncertain Significance
- Dysplasia has unequivocal nuclear atypia (beyond reactive urothelial changes) that falls short of threshold for CIS
  - This lesion has significant problems related to intraobserver reproducibility
  - Many genitourinary pathologists use term flat urothelial atypia for lesions that fall short of CIS yet are not unequivocally nonneoplastic
- Most important to have appropriate minimal diagnostic threshold for CIS

Reactive Urothelial Atypia
- Intraepithelial inflammation is usually prominent
- Although there is nuclear enlargement, it is usually uniform
  - Usually < 3x size of normal lymphocyte nucleus
- Nucleoli are common
- Chromatin remains relatively evenly dispersed
- Mitotic figures may be increased and may extend into upper levels of urothelium, but are not atypical

Radiation/Chemotherapy Effect
- May induce full-thickness nuclear atypia
- Cells often have intracytoplasmic and nuclear vacuolization
- Cells may have multinucleation
- Associated radiation-induced changes in underlying tissue
  - Stromal hemorrhage
  - Atypical fibroblasts
  - Damaged blood vessels

BK Viral Cytopathic Effect
- Nucleomegaly with dark, smudgy nuclear chromatin
- More easily identified in cytologic preparations

Intravesical BCG or Mitomycin-Associated Changes
- Urothelial denudation and associated inflammation are common
- Nuclear enlargement and nucleoli are common
- Prominent eosinophilic cytoplasm may be seen

DIAGNOSTIC CHECKLIST

Clinically Relevant Pathologic Features
- Multifocality and microinvasion

Pathologic Interpretation Pearls
- Key to interpreting flat lesions is developing appropriate minimal threshold for urothelial CIS
  - Definite nucleomegaly with nuclear hyperchromasia/irregular chromatin is required
    - Lymphocytes are useful internal control for nuclear size
    - Comparison to adjacent normal urothelium is also helpful
  - Elevated mitotic rates and prominent nucleoli alone are not sufficient, as they may be seen in reactive lesions
  - Intraurothelial inflammation should prompt careful consideration of other diagnoses
    - Reactive urothelial atypia
    - Urothelial atypia of uncertain significance
- While certain immunohistochemical profiles correlate with different diagnostic categories of urothelial atypia, routine morphology remains gold standard for diagnosis
- Important to look for invasion or microinvasion when CIS is present

SELECTED REFERENCES

1. Amin MB et al: Best practices recommendations in the application of immunohistochemistry in urologic pathology: report from the International Society of Urological Pathology consensus conference. Am J Surg Pathol. 38(8):1017-22, 2014
2. Amin MB et al: Best practices recommendations in the application of immunohistochemistry in the bladder lesions: report from the International Society of Urologic Pathology consensus conference. Am J Surg Pathol. 38(8):e20-34, 2014
3. Jung S et al: The role of immunohistochemistry in the diagnosis of flat urothelial lesions: a study using CK20, CK5/6, P53, Cd138, and Her2/Neu. Ann Diagn Pathol. 18(1):27-32, 2014
4. Aron M et al: Utility of a triple antibody cocktail intraurothelial neoplasm-3 (IUN-3-CK20/CD44s/p53) and α-methylacyl-CoA racemase (AMACR) in the distinction of urothelial carcinoma in situ (CIS) and reactive urothelial atypia. Am J Surg Pathol. 37(12):1815-23, 2013
5. Oliva E et al: Immunohistochemistry as an adjunct in the differential diagnosis of radiation-induced atypia versus urothelial carcinoma in situ of the bladder: a study of 45 cases. Hum Pathol. 44(5):860-6, 2013
6. Murata S et al: Molecular and immunohistologic analyses cannot reliably solve diagnostic variation of flat intraepithelial lesions of the urinary bladder. Am J Clin Pathol. 134(6):862-72, 2010
7. Sesterhenn IA: Urothelial carcinoma in situ. In Eble JN et al: World Health Organization Classification of Tumours. Pathology & Genetics. Tumours of the Urinary System and Male Genital Organs. Lyon: IARC Press, 2004
8. McKenney JK et al: Discriminatory immunohistochemical staining of urothelial carcinoma in situ and non-neoplastic urothelium: an analysis of cytokeratin 20, p53, and CD44 antigens. Am J Surg Pathol. 25(8):1074-8, 2001
9. McKenney JK et al: Morphologic expressions of urothelial carcinoma in situ: a detailed evaluation of its histologic patterns with emphasis on carcinoma in situ with microinvasion. Am J Surg Pathol. 25(3):356-62, 2001
10. Epstein JI et al: The World Health Organization/International Society of Urological Pathology consensus classification of urothelial (transitional cell) neoplasms of the urinary bladder. Bladder Consensus Conference Committee. Am J Surg Pathol. 22(12):1435-48, 1998

Urothelial Carcinoma In Situ

Urothelial Carcinoma In Situ: Nuclear Size

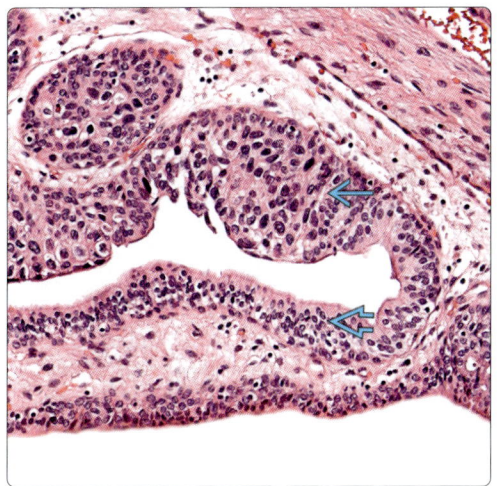

Urothelial Carcinoma In Situ: Nuclear Size

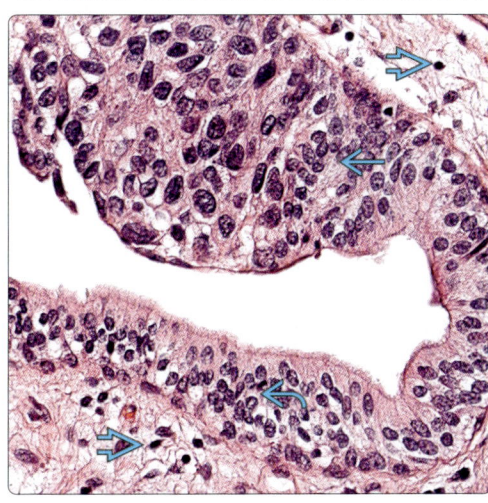

(Left) The degree of nucleomegaly of the CIS ⇨ is obvious when compared to the normal urothelium below ⇨. The diagnosis of CIS is made on the basis of the overall constellation of nuclear abnormalities. (Right) CIS ⇨ in this example is characterized by marked nucleomegaly, nuclear hyperchromasia, and some degree of pleomorphism. The nuclei of the normal urothelium ⇨ are only 1-2x the size of a stromal lymphocyte ⇨, in contrast to at least 4x in this CIS.

Urothelial Carcinoma In Situ: Comparison to Normal

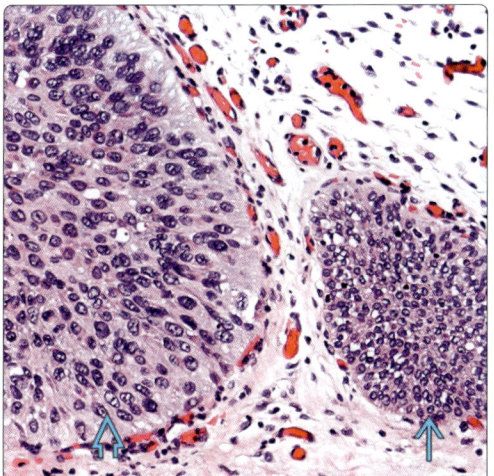

Urothelial Carcinoma In Situ: Pleomorphism

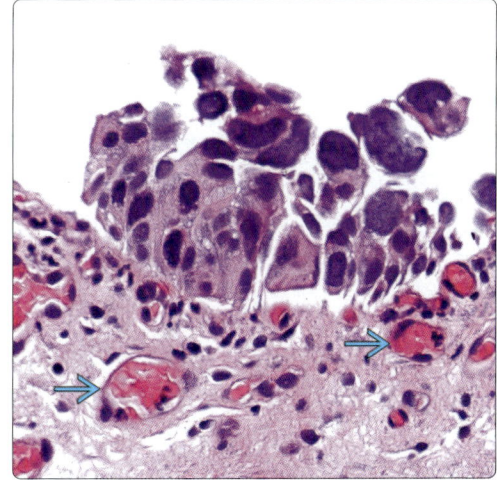

(Left) Cells of urothelial CIS colonizing a von Brunn nest on the left ⇨ show obvious marked nucleomegaly and coarse chromatin compared to the von Brunn nest with normal urothelial cells on the right ⇨. (Right) This CIS has marked nuclear pleomorphism. Loss of cellular cohesion, as also seen in this example, is common. Frequently, there is neovascularization in the superficial lamina propria ⇨.

Urothelial Carcinoma In Situ: Variation in Thickness

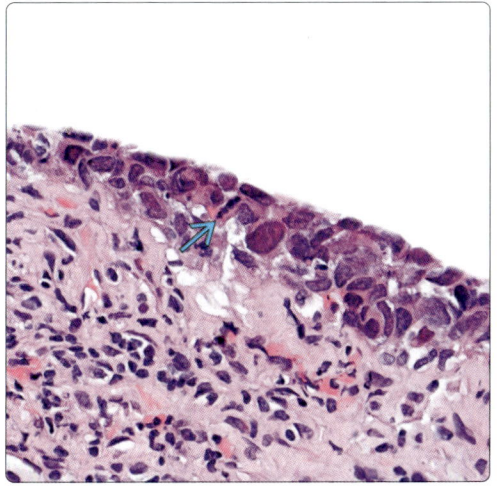

Urothelial Carcinoma In Situ: Less Than Full-Thickness Involvement

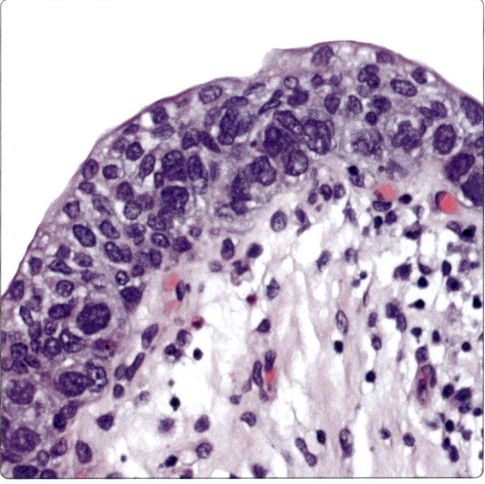

(Left) CIS may occasionally consist of a very thin urothelium. The urothelial cells are markedly enlarged with irregular coarse chromatin and obvious mitotic figures ⇨, features useful in the diagnosis of CIS. (Right) In CIS, the neoplastic cells may not show full-thickness involvement. In this example, they are confined to the lower 2/3 of the urothelium. In contrast to precursor lesions in some other anatomic sites, the presence of markedly atypical cells at any level is sufficient for the diagnosis as CIS.

Urothelial Carcinoma In Situ

Urothelial Carcinoma In Situ: Pleomorphic Pattern

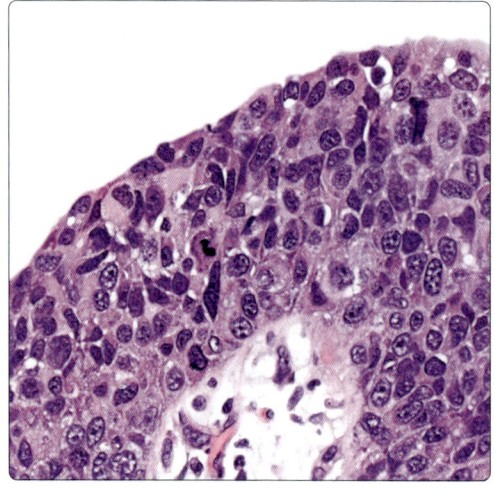

Urothelial Carcinoma In Situ: So-Called "Small Cell" Pattern

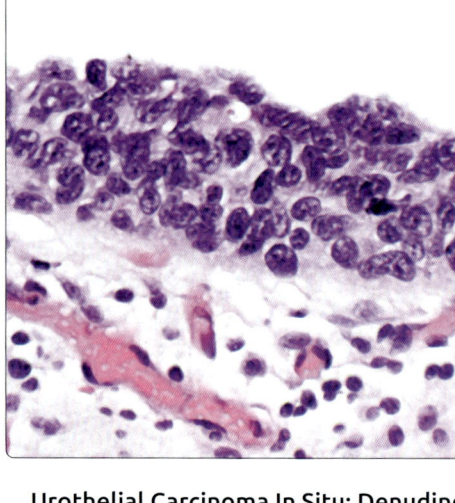

(Left) CIS shows a range of histologic diversity, with unequivocal high-grade nuclear atypia, which may include pleomorphism, prominent nucleoli, and atypical mitoses toward the surface. (Right) So-called small cell CIS has a high nuclear to cytoplasmic ratio. This term does not imply neuroendocrine differentiation or relation to small cell carcinoma.

Urothelial Carcinoma In Situ: Nonpleomorphic Pattern

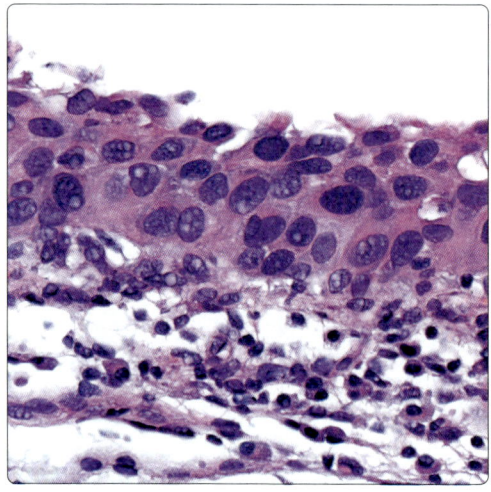

Urothelial Carcinoma In Situ: Denuding Pattern

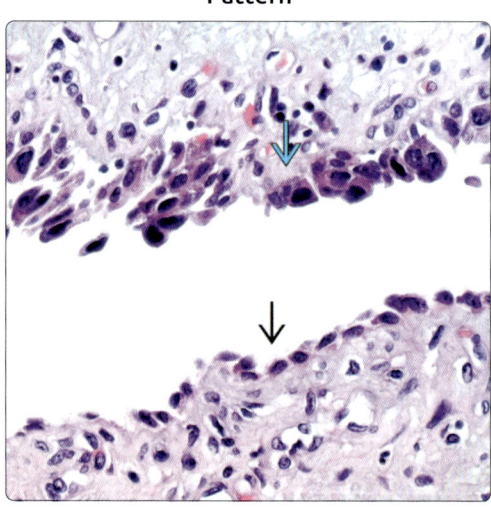

(Left) Some examples of CIS referred to as nonpleomorphic large cell CIS have less significant pleomorphism and may have more abundant eosinophilic cytoplasm. The degree of nucleomegaly and coarse nuclear chromatin, however, are diagnostic of CIS. (Right) "Clinging" urothelial CIS is characterized by individual residual carcinoma cells ➡ attached to the basement membrane. The nucleomegaly and nuclear hyperchromasia of this "clinging" CIS are contrasted to the normal residual basal cells below ➡.

Urothelial Carcinoma In Situ: Pagetoid Pattern

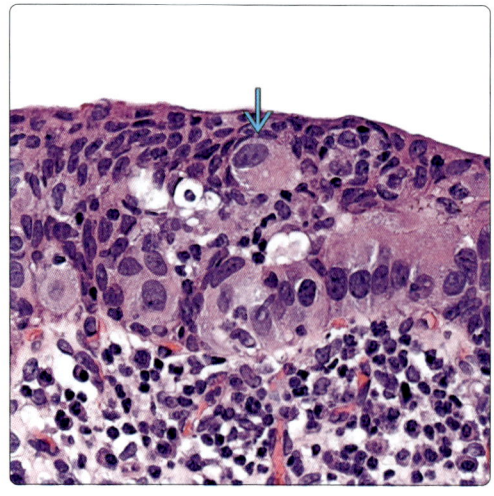

Urothelial Carcinoma In Situ: Undermining Pattern

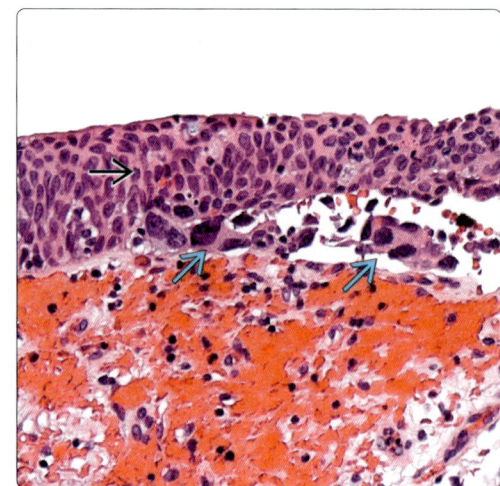

(Left) Pagetoid urothelial CIS is characterized by clusters or individual carcinoma cells ➡ that colonize normal urothelium in a pattern similar to mammary Paget disease. (Right) Undermining urothelial CIS is characterized by extension of carcinoma cells ➡ underneath adjacent normal urothelium ➡. The difference in nuclear size between the 2 populations is striking.

Urothelial Carcinoma In Situ

Urothelial Carcinoma In Situ: Comparison to Normal

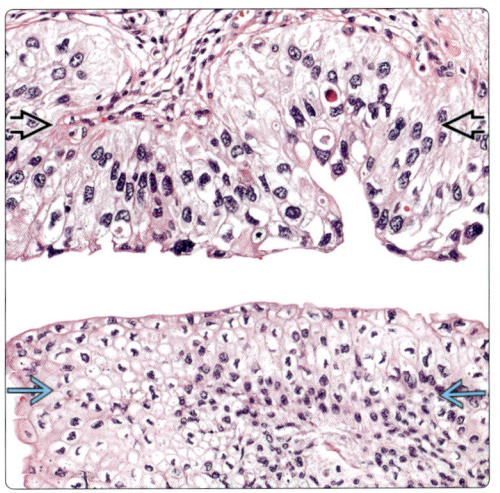

Urothelial Carcinoma In Situ: Mitoses

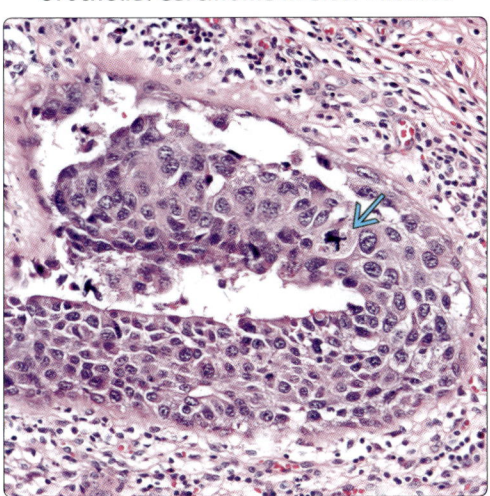

(Left) Identification of adjacent normal urothelium ⇨ is valuable in assessing flat urothelial lesions with atypia. The markedly enlarged nuclei with nuclear hyperchromasia are sufficient for diagnosis of CIS ⇨. (Right) Mitotic figures may be seen in reactive urothelial atypia, but the presence of atypical mitotic figures ⇨ should prompt careful consideration of CIS. In this example, the degree of nuclear enlargement and hyperchromasia are well beyond the threshold for CIS.

Urothelial CIS Colonizing von Brunn Nests

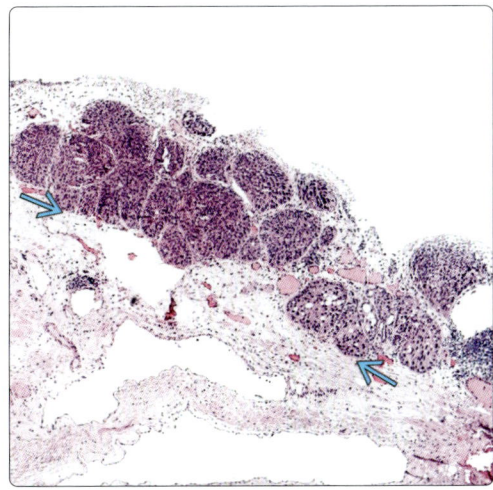

Urothelial CIS Colonizing von Brunn Nests

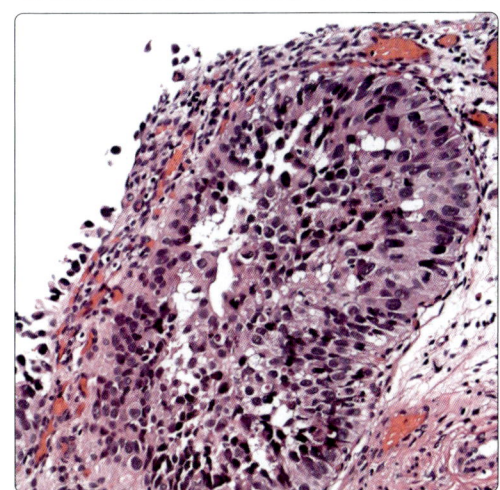

(Left) These von Brunn nests are colonized by urothelial CIS. The sharp linear border at the underlying junction with the lamina propria ⇨ and the rounded borders of the nests help in the distinction from invasive urothelial carcinoma of the nested type. (Right) The sharp round contour of this large epithelial aggregate is characteristic of a von Brunn nest colonized by urothelial carcinoma in situ.

Urothelial CIS With Microinvasion

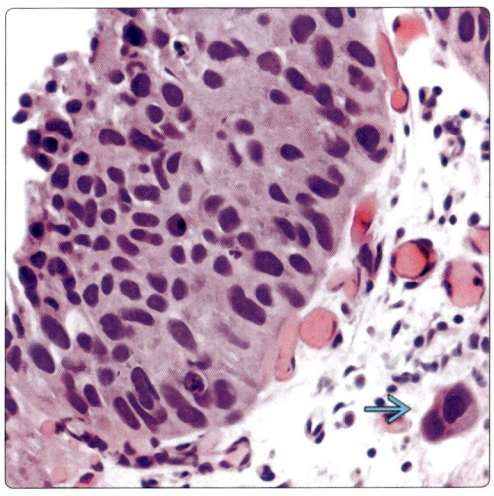

Urothelial CIS With Underlying Invasion

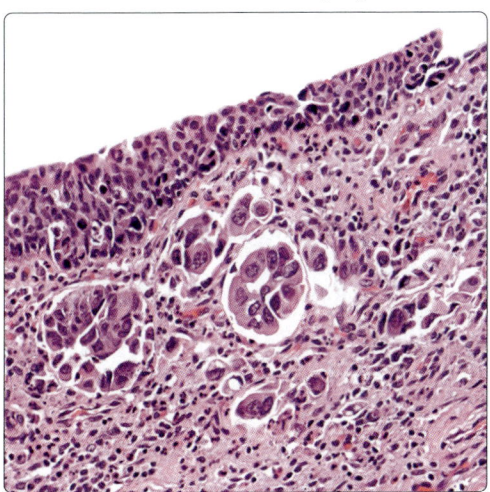

(Left) The small cluster of neoplastic cells ⇨ underlying the CIS indicates focal invasion into the lamina propria (i.e., pT1 disease). (Right) These neoplastic cells in the superficial lamina propria, which are characterized by individual cells and clusters of cells with eosinophilic cytoplasm and surrounding retraction spaces, represent lamina propria invasion. Stromal clefts are characteristic of invasion and exclude the possibility of von Brunn nests colonized by CIS.

Urothelial Carcinoma In Situ

CK20: Urothelial Carcinoma In Situ

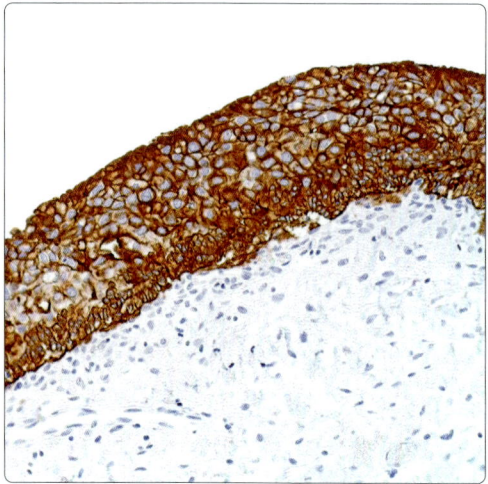

CK20: Urothelial Carcinoma In Situ

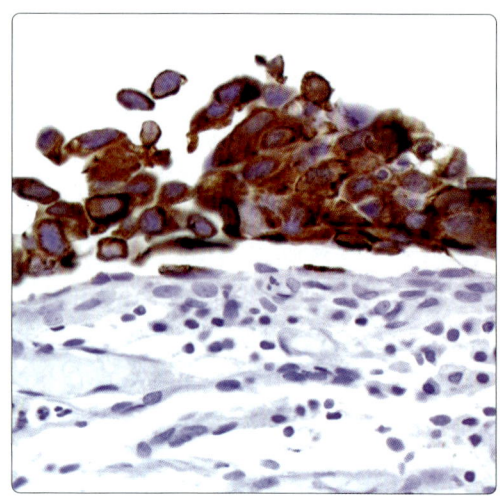

(Left) *Diffuse cytoplasmic reactivity for CK20 is commonly seen in urothelial CIS. In normal and reactive urothelium, CK20 staining is confined to the superficial umbrella cell layer; staining may be completely negative if these cells are not present.* (Right) *Denuding urothelial CIS commonly shows diffuse strong cytoplasmic reactivity for CK20. Normal basal and parabasal cells do not typically express CK20, even in cases with significant reactive atypia.*

CD44: Negative in Pagetoid Urothelial CIS

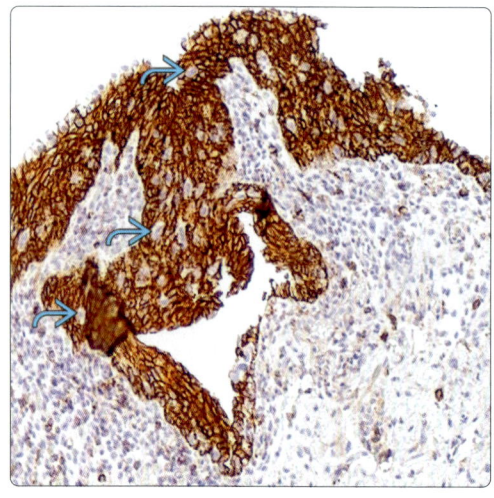

p53: Positive in Pagetoid Urothelial CIS

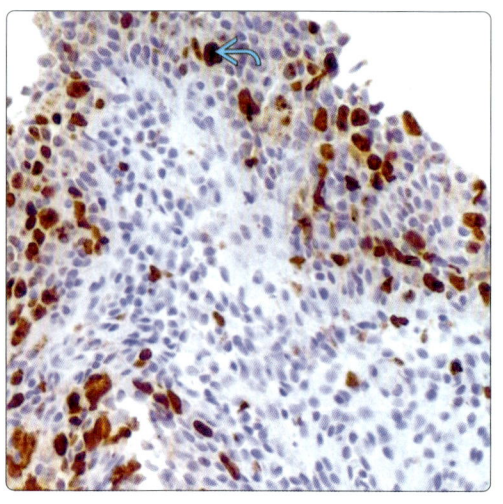

(Left) *In this cystectomy specimen with pagetoid urothelial CIS, immunohistochemistry for CD44 standard isoform shows strong membranous reactivity in the normal reactive urothelial cell population, as expected. The scattered negative cells represent CIS ⇨.* (Right) *Scattered neoplastic cells of pagetoid CIS ⇨ are highlighted by nuclear immunoreactivity for p53, which is less sensitive than CK20.*

CD44: Reactive Urothelial Atypia

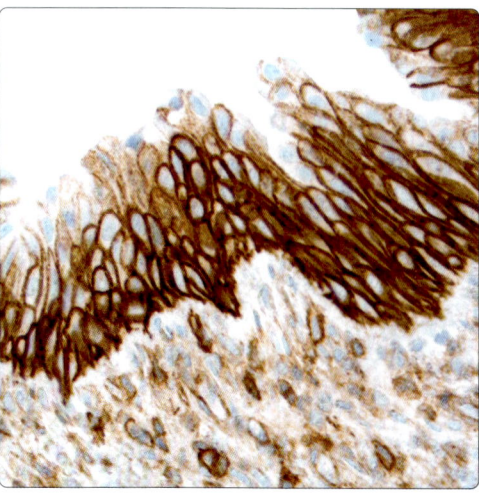

CK20, CD44, p53 Cocktail Immunostain: Pagetoid Urothelial CIS

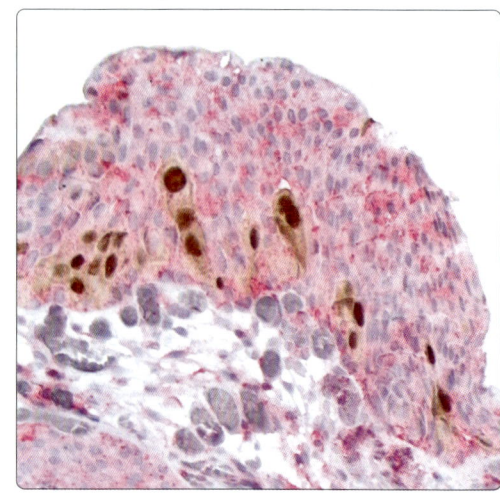

(Left) *This pattern of CD44 immunoreactivity in the basal and upper layers (with membranous accentuation) is commonly seen in reactive urothelial atypia. In contrast, urothelial CIS typically shows a loss of staining in the atypical cell population.* (Right) *This triple antibody cocktail consists of CK20 (brown cytoplasmic), CD44 (red membranous), and p53 (brown nuclear). The CK20 and p53 highlight the carcinoma cells, while CD44 is expressed in the background nonneoplastic cells.*

Urothelial Carcinoma In Situ

Reactive Urothelial Atypia
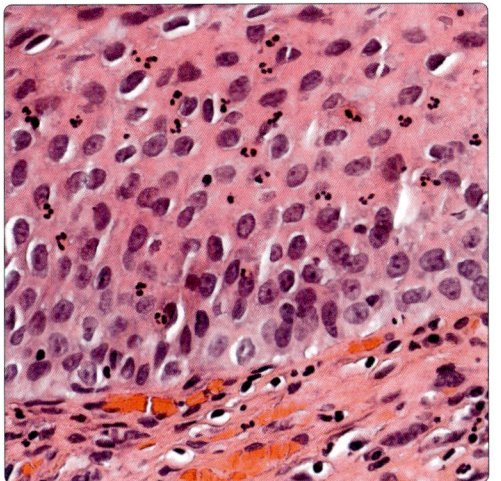

Reactive Urothelial Atypia
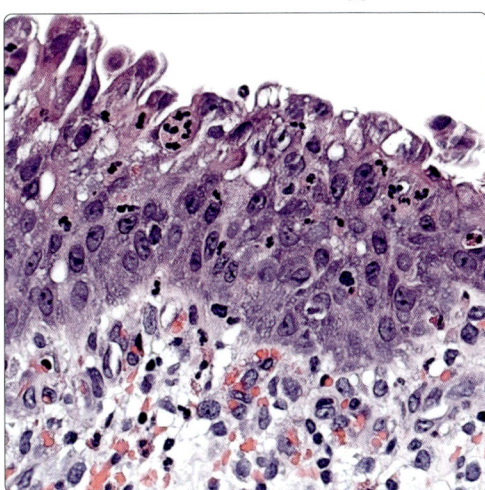

(Left) In this example of reactive atypia, the nuclei are more rounded, but maintain fine nuclear chromatin and show small nucleoli. The homogeneously even chromatin and associated intraurothelial neutrophils support a designation as a reactive lesion. (Right) This florid example of reactive atypia in a young patient is associated with an indwelling catheter. Despite the enlarged nucleoli, the relatively fine chromatin and intraurothelial neutrophils support a reactive diagnosis.

Benign Urothelium
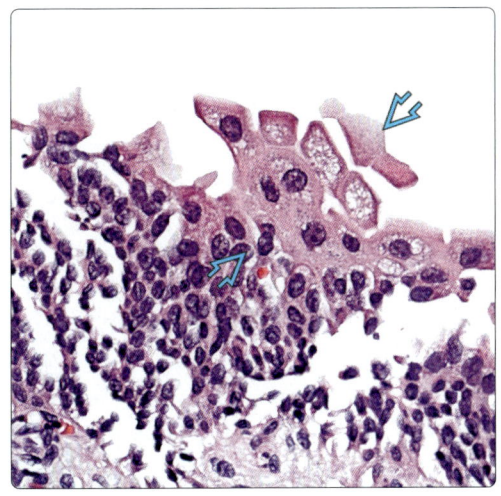

Benign Urothelium
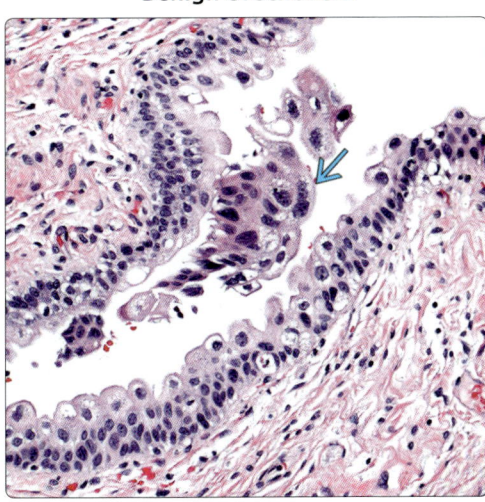

(Left) Normal superficial umbrella cells ⇨ may show some level of cytologic atypia with nucleomegaly and multinucleation that may potentially mimic urothelial CIS, especially if sectioned somewhat tangentially. (Right) This example of tangentially sectioned umbrella cells ⇨ demonstrates the degree of urothelial atypia that may be seen in these superficial benign cells.

Urothelial Atypia of Unknown Significance
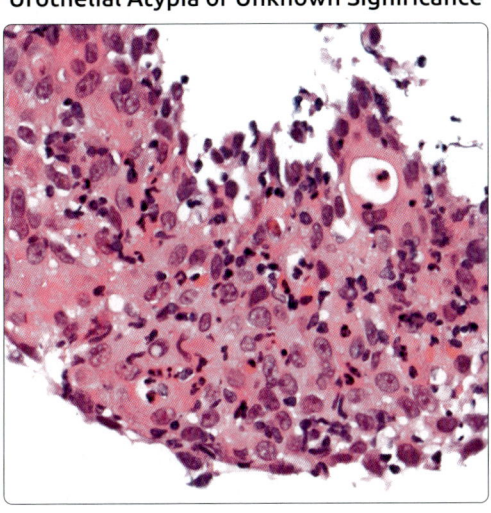

Urothelial Atypia
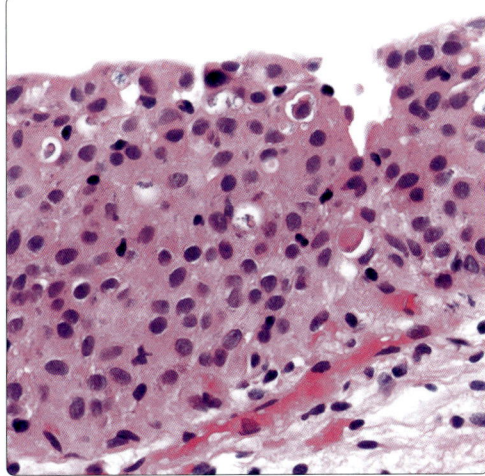

(Left) These urothelial cells show macronucleoli, variation in size and shape, and cellular disorder. Given the amount of associated inflammation, this example would be designated as urothelial atypia of unknown significance. (Right) This lesion has nuclear rounding and loss of cellular order, but does not show the degree of nucleomegaly and nuclear hyperchromasia to meet the minimal diagnostic threshold for urothelial CIS. This might be designated as dysplasia or urothelial atypia of unknown significance.

Flat Urothelial Lesions Other Than Carcinoma In Situ

KEY FACTS

TERMINOLOGY

- Reactive urothelial atypia
  - Benign reactive or regenerative epithelial changes, secondary to infection, prior therapy, or intravesical catheter
  - Typically associated with intraurothelial inflammatory infiltrate or inflammation in lamina propria
  - Mild nucleomegaly, fine chromatin, and prominent nucleoli
  - No pleomorphism
- Urothelial atypia of unknown significance
  - Subtle but definite alterations that are not categorically either reactive or dysplastic
  - Descriptive diagnosis to ensure clinical follow-up in difficult to classify cases
- Urothelial dysplasia
  - Controversial category with poor reproducibility and poorly understood significance
  - Unequivocal cytologic and architectural changes felt to be preneoplastic but below threshold for urothelial carcinoma in situ
  - Mild nucleomegaly
  - Subtle loss of polarity
  - Minimal irregularity of nuclear contours
  - Increased cytoplasmic eosinophilia

CLINICAL ISSUES

- Reactive atypia
  - Treated by alleviating underlying etiology
- Urothelial atypia of unknown significance/urothelial dysplasia
  - Requires clinical follow-up with urine cytology/cystoscopy

TOP DIFFERENTIAL DIAGNOSES

- Urothelial carcinoma in situ

Reactive Urothelial Atypia
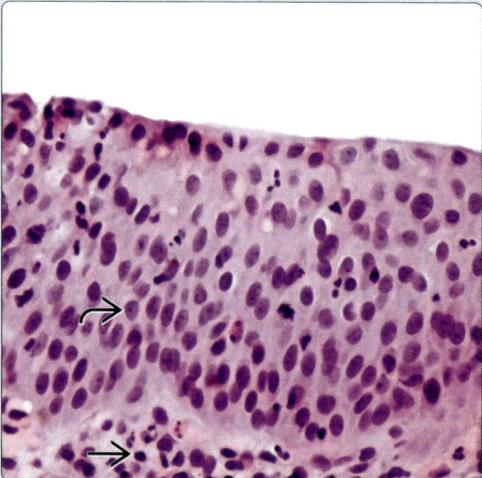

Reactive Urothelial Atypia
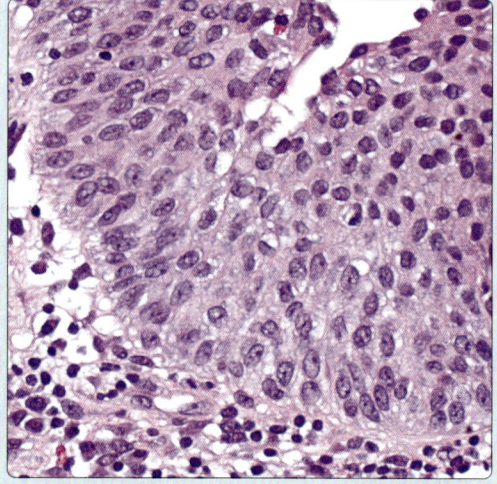

(Left) In this example of reactive urothelial atypia, numerous intraurothelial neutrophils are present. The nuclei of the urothelial cells ⇨ are only 2-3x the size of a stromal lymphocyte ⇨, as expected, and the chromatin remains evenly dispersed with small nucleoli. (Right) In reactive atypia, prominent nucleoli are obvious, but the nuclear chromatin is evenly dispersed. There is overall maintained polarity and monotony of nuclei. Inflammation is variable in reactive atypia.

Radiation Atypia
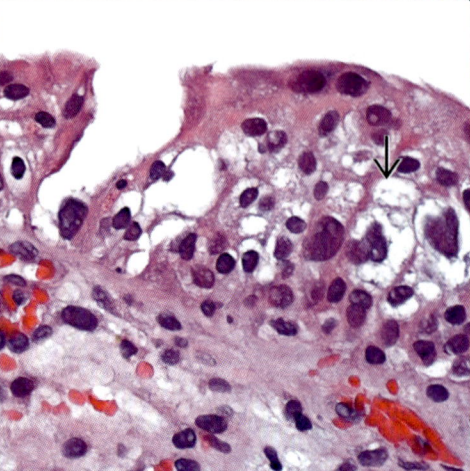

Urothelial Atypia of Unknown Significance
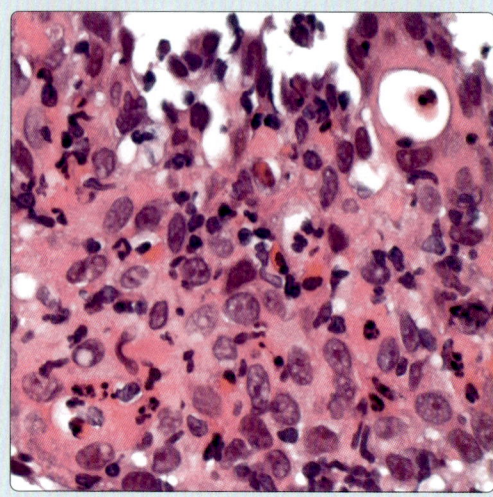

(Left) This example of reactive urothelial atypia secondary to radiation therapy shows characteristic radiation changes that include large nuclei with "smudgy" chromatin and cytoplasmic vacuolization ⇨. (Right) Nuclear rounding, mild variation in nuclear size and shape, and macronuclei are present. With this degree of intraurothelial inflammation, the suggested diagnosis would be "atypia of unknown significance," as the possibility of an underlying neoplasia cannot be entirely ruled out.

Flat Urothelial Lesions Other Than Carcinoma In Situ

TERMINOLOGY

Abbreviations
- Carcinoma in situ (CIS)

Definitions
- Reactive urothelial atypia
  - Benign reactive or regenerative epithelial changes
- Urothelial atypia of unknown significance
  - Flat lesions with subtle but definite alterations that are not categorically either reactive or neoplastic
  - Descriptive diagnosis to ensure clinical follow-up in difficult to classify cases
- Urothelial dysplasia
  - Lesions with unequivocal cytologic and architectural changes felt to be preneoplastic but that fall below threshold for diagnosis of urothelial CIS
    - Controversial category with poor reproducibility

CLINICAL ISSUES

Presentation
- Irritative bladder symptoms

Treatment
- Reactive urothelial atypia
  - Treatment should be based on alleviating underlying cause
- Urothelial atypia of unknown significance
  - Requires clinical follow-up with urine cytology/cystoscopy
- Urothelial dysplasia
  - Requires clinical follow-up with urine cytology/cystoscopy

Prognosis
- Reactive atypia
  - Benign
- Urothelial atypia of unknown significance
  - Not fully known
- Urothelial dysplasia
  - In rare series diagnosed as dysplasia, progression to bladder neoplasia (including CIS), seen in 5-19% of cases

MACROSCOPIC

General Features
- May have hyperemic mucosa at cystoscopy

MICROSCOPIC

Reactive Urothelial Atypia
- Nucleomegaly with prominent nucleoli
  - Usually 2-3x size of lymphocyte nucleus
  - Nucleoli usually pin-point but may be larger
- Nuclear chromatin fine and evenly dispersed
- Cells maintain polarity perpendicular to basement membrane
- Intraurothelial acute or chronic inflammation
- Increased mitotic activity (not atypical forms) may be present, even in upper layers
- Ulceration or inflammation in lamina propria

Urothelial Atypia of Unknown Significance
- Used as diagnostic category in cases with inflammation in which severity of atypia appears to be out of proportion to extent of inflammation
  - Preneoplastic lesion cannot be confidently excluded

Urothelial Dysplasia
- Some genitourinary pathologists diagnose such lesions as urothelial atypia of unknown significance
  - Controversial category with poor reproducibility
  - Poorly understood clinical significance
  - No known treatment implication
- Clear-cut nuclear atypia is evident but is not severe enough to merit diagnosis of CIS
  - Mild nucleomegaly with subtle loss of polarity
    - Nuclear crowding and rounded to polygonal cells
  - Minimal irregularity of nuclear contours and chromatin distribution

DIFFERENTIAL DIAGNOSIS

Urothelial Carcinoma In Situ
- Marked nucleomegaly (often ≥ 4x size of lymphocyte nucleus)
- Nuclear pleomorphism and hyperchromasia
- Loss of normal polarity and presence of nuclear crowding common
- Immunohistochemistry may have utility in distinction from reactive atypia
  - CIS commonly has full-thickness cytoplasmic expression of CK20
    - Normal or reactive urothelium shows CK20 only in umbrella cell layer
    - Reactive atypia often has CD44 membranous reactivity in atypical cells

Normal Urothelium
- Flat lesions with benign cytology and minimal disorder should be considered within spectrum of normal

DIAGNOSTIC CHECKLIST

Pathologic Interpretation Pearls
- Developing appropriate threshold for urothelial CIS is critical in diagnosing flat lesions
  - Nuclear size and chromatin character are critical morphologic features
- Great caution should be exercised before lesion is diagnosed as de novo dysplasia (i.e., with no prior history of urothelial neoplasia)
  - Designating these cases as atypia of unknown significance is recommended

SELECTED REFERENCES

1. Eble JN et al: World Health Organization Classification of Tumour. Pathology & Genetics. Tumour of the Urinary System and Male Genital Organs. Lyon: IARC Press. 111-12, 2004
2. Epstein JI et al: The World Health Organization/International Society of Urological Pathology consensus classification of urothelial (transitional cell) neoplasms of the urinary bladder. Bladder Consensus Conference Committee. Am J Surg Pathol. 22(12):1435-48, 1998

Flat Urothelial Lesions Other Than Carcinoma In Situ

Reactive Urothelial Atypia

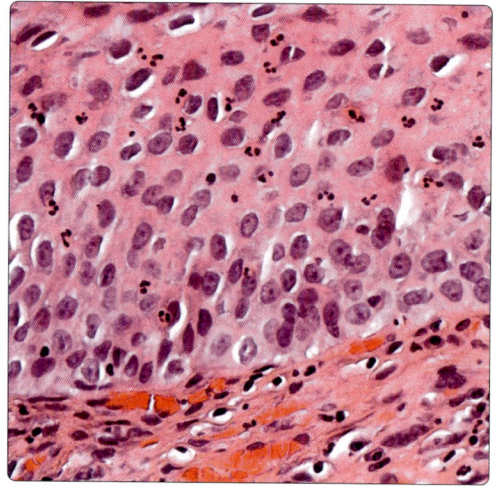

(Left) In this reactive urothelial atypia, there is marked intraurothelial acute inflammation. As typical, the chromatin is fine and nucleoli are prominent. (Right) Florid reactive urothelial atypia may have brisk mitotic activity ➔ that extends into the upper urothelial layers, as seen in this case. The fine nuclear chromatin, small pin-point nucleoli, and normal polarity (upward streaming of the urothelial cells) all support a reactive diagnosis.

Reactive Urothelial Atypia

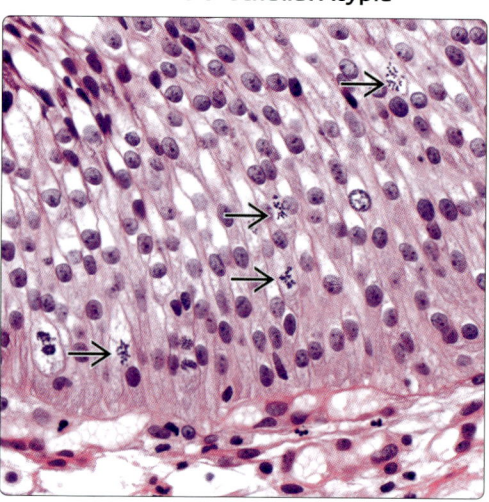

Reactive Urothelial Atypia

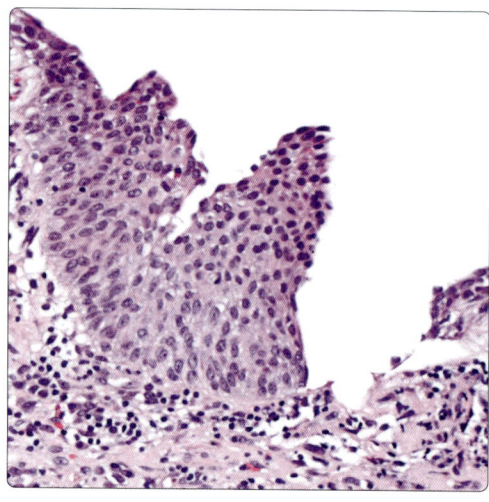

(Left) In this example of reactive urothelial atypia, the nuclei of the urothelial cells are only slightly enlarged with small and rarely prominent nucleoli. There is nuclear monotony. (Right) In this example of florid reactive urothelial atypia associated with intravesical catheterization, intraurothelial inflammation may be present with associated nuclear enlargement and 1 or more prominent nucleoli.

Reactive Urothelial Atypia

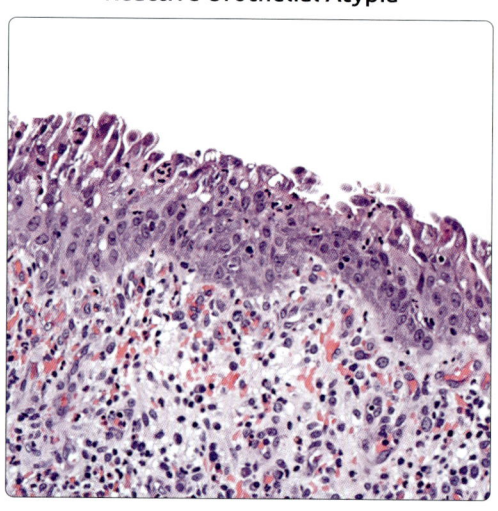

CK20: Reactive Urothelial Atypia

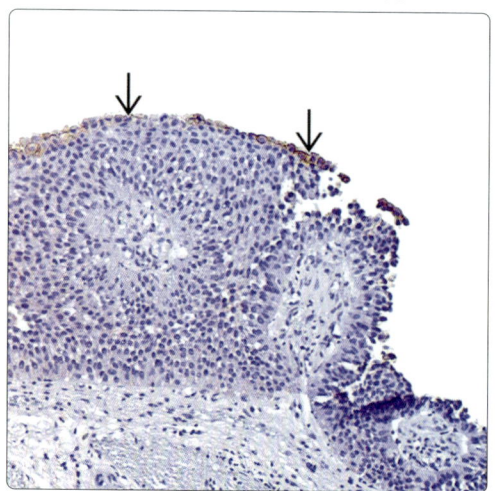

(Left) Immunohistochemistry is useful in the distinction of carcinoma in situ from reactive atypia. CK20 stains only umbrella cells in normal or reactive urothelium ➔. Diffuse full-thickness staining is common in carcinoma in situ. (Right) Membranous immunoreactivity with CD44 extending into the intermediate/upper levels of the urothelium is characteristic of reactive atypia. Carcinoma in situ has absent CD44 expression or staining only in residual basal cells.

CD44: Reactive Urothelial Atypia

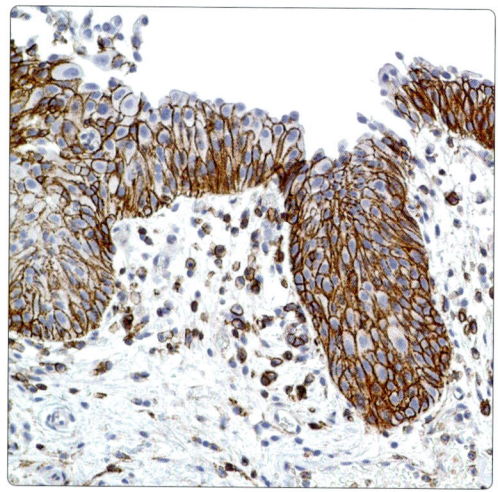

Flat Urothelial Lesions Other Than Carcinoma In Situ

Polyomavirus

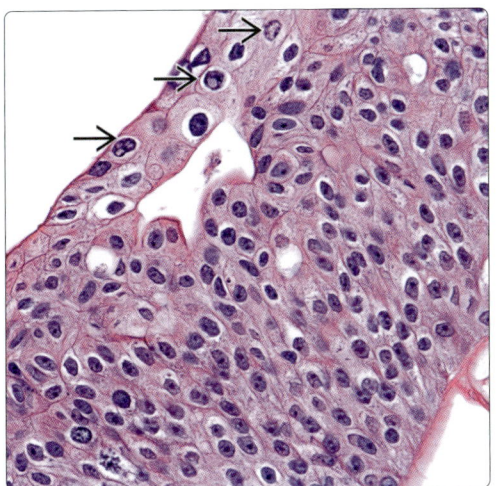

Polyomavirus

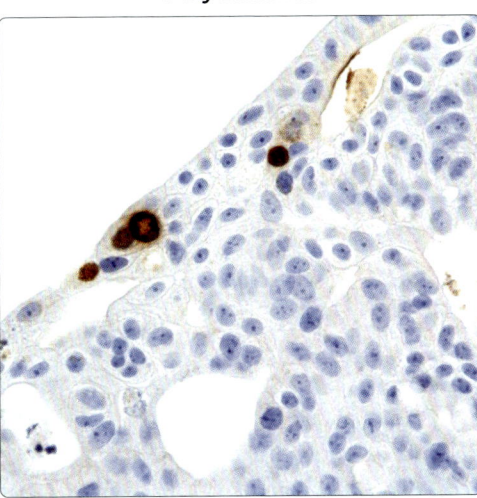

(Left) *Specific forms of reactive nonneoplastic urothelial changes, such as this example of polyomavirus infection, may also mimic urothelial neoplasia. In this example, there is "smudgy" nuclear chromatin and intranuclear inclusions ⇒ in scattered superficial urothelial cells. The urothelium in the lower levels has a typical reactive appearance.* (Right) *Strong nuclear reactivity for polyomavirus, which is typically superficial, is diagnostic of infection.*

Radiation Atypia

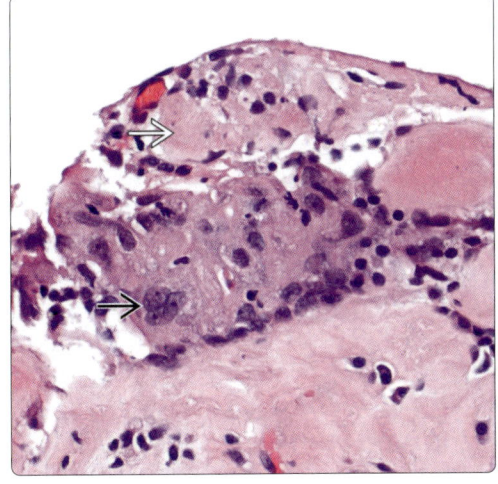

Urothelial Atypia

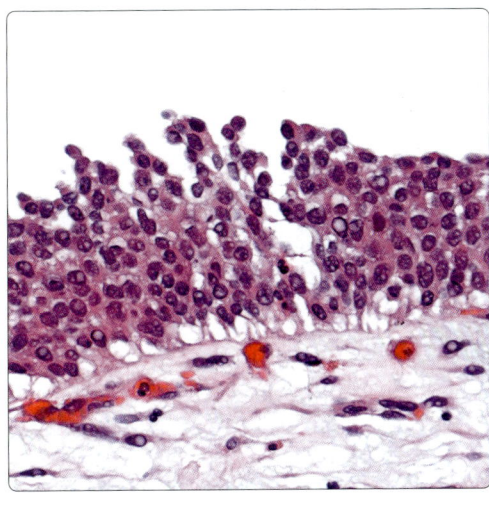

(Left) *Multinucleation ⇒ and fibrin aggregates ⇒ are commonly seen in radiation-associated atypia. Other features associated with radiation injury, such as stromal hemorrhage and vascular changes, may be seen in the lamina propria.* (Right) *This lesion has round nuclei with mild enlargement, some polarity loss, and no significant chromatin abnormality. We would classify this lesion as atypia of unknown significance, but some might regard such lesions as urothelial dysplasia.*

Urothelial Atypia

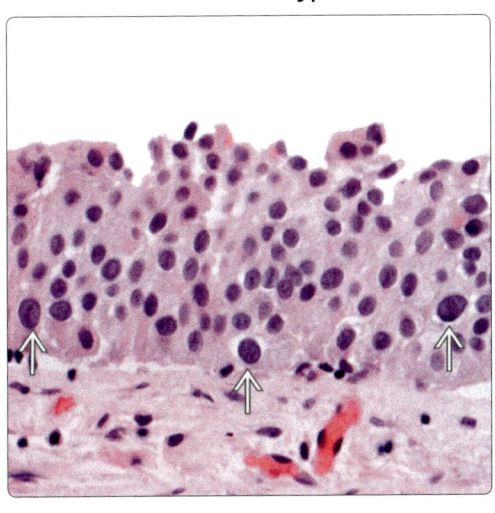

Urothelial Carcinoma In Situ

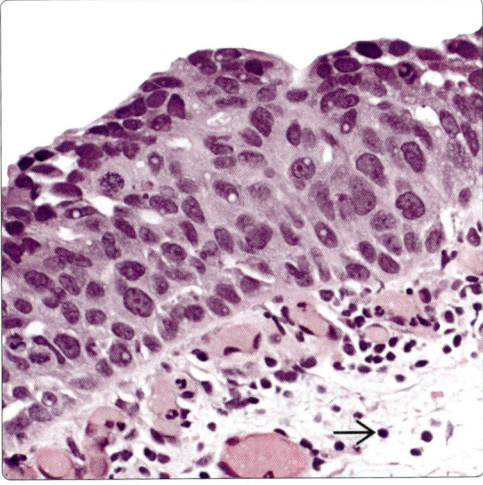

(Left) *Occasional cells are enlarged with mild chromatin alteration ⇒, and there is some crowding and nuclear rounding. This atypia falls short of CIS. Some experts might regard this lesion as urothelial dysplasia.* (Right) *Although nucleoli are prominent, the degree of nucleomegaly (> 5x the size of lymphocyte nuclei ⇒ in some cells), marked variation in nuclear size and shape, loss of polarity, and nuclear membrane irregularity all support a diagnosis of urothelial carcinoma in situ in this case.*

Urothelial Papilloma

KEY FACTS

CLINICAL ISSUES
- Very uncommon urothelial lesion (~ 1% of papillary urothelial neoplasms)
- Typically occur in younger adult patients; may be seen in children
- Gross or microscopic hematuria
- Recurrence is rare (0-8%)
- Posterior or lateral walls of bladder, close to ureteral orifices
- Urethra is another common site of occurrence
- Lesions often very small in size

MICROSCOPIC
- Exophytic papillary neoplasm lined by normal-appearing urothelium
- No significant cytologic atypia
- Slender, minimally branching papillary architecture
- Superficial umbrella cells often prominent
- Prominent vacuolization of umbrella cells is common
- Umbrella cells may be enlarged and multinucleated

ANCILLARY TESTS
- CK20 expression typically confined to umbrella cells, as in normal urothelium
- Alteration of p53 expression is not seen

TOP DIFFERENTIAL DIAGNOSES
- Papillary urothelial neoplasm of low malignant potential
  - Thicker urothelial lining with increased cell density
- Papillary-polypoid cystitis
  - Broad base with nonhierarchical branching
  - May have reactive urothelial atypia
- Papillary nephrogenic adenoma
  - Single layer of lining cuboidal epithelium

DIAGNOSTIC CHECKLIST
- More common in younger patients
- Important not to interpret umbrella cells in assessment of degree of atypia

Urothelial Papilloma
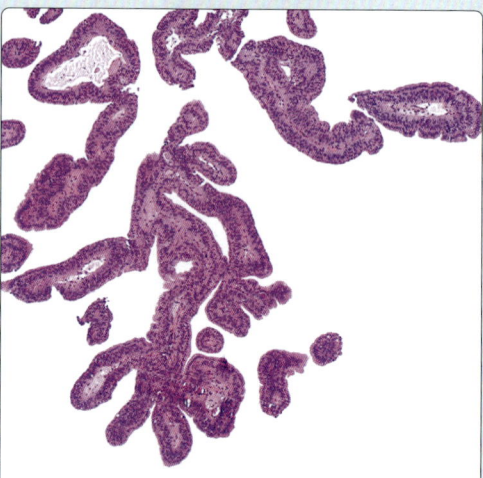

Urothelial Papilloma
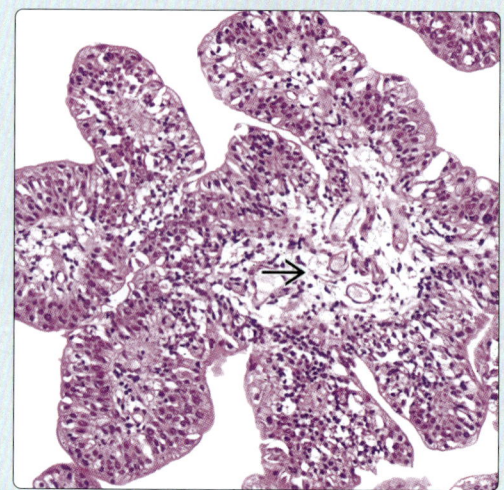

(Left) Characteristic elongated slender papillae are seen in this urothelial papilloma. The normal thickness of the urothelium distinguishes papilloma from a papillary urothelial neoplasm of low malignant potential. (Right) This urothelial papilloma shows slender papillae branching from a larger central core ➡. There is normal cytology and nuclear polarity, features that allow classification as papilloma.

Urothelial Papilloma
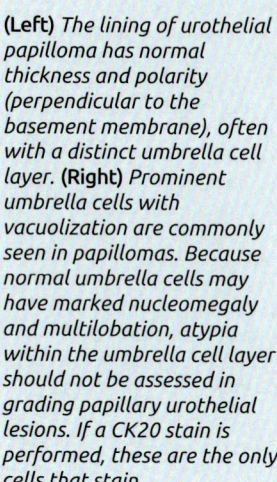

Urothelial Papilloma
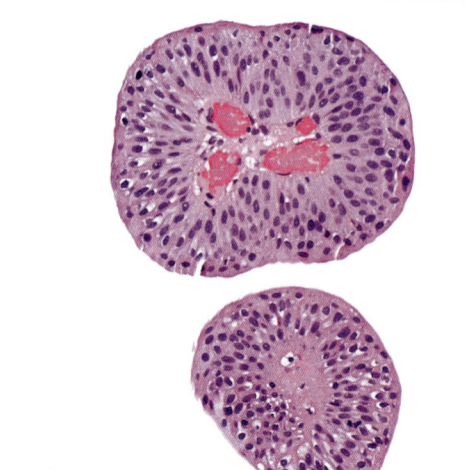
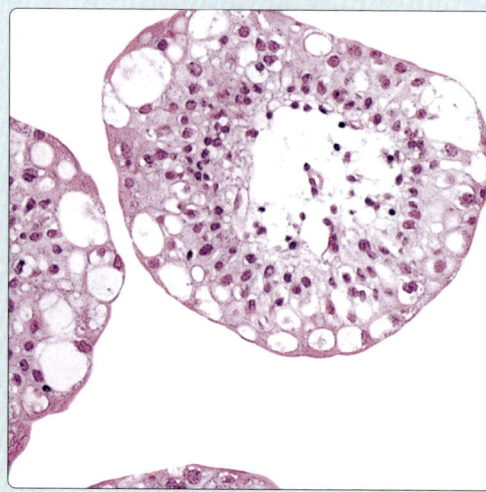

(Left) The lining of urothelial papilloma has normal thickness and polarity (perpendicular to the basement membrane), often with a distinct umbrella cell layer. (Right) Prominent umbrella cells with vacuolization are commonly seen in papillomas. Because normal umbrella cells may have marked nucleomegaly and multilobation, atypia within the umbrella cell layer should not be assessed in grading papillary urothelial lesions. If a CK20 stain is performed, these are the only cells that stain.

Urothelial Papilloma

TERMINOLOGY

Synonyms
- Transitional cell papilloma

Definitions
- Exophytic papillary urothelial neoplasm
  - Fibrovascular cores lined by histologically normal urothelium

CLINICAL ISSUES

Epidemiology
- Incidence
  - ~ 1% of papillary urothelial neoplasms
- Age
  - Tends to occur in younger adult patients
  - May be seen in children
- Sex
  - M:F = 1.9:1

Site
- Posterior or lateral walls of bladder
- Urethra is also common site of occurrence

Presentation
- Gross or microscopic hematuria
- Frequently present de novo (in patients without history of bladder neoplasia)
- May occur in patients with prior or simultaneous papillary bladder neoplasms
  - Including higher grade lesions

Endoscopic Findings
- Cystoscopic features identical to other low-grade papillary urothelial neoplasms; lesions often smaller

Treatment
- Surgical approaches
  - Complete transurethral resection

Prognosis
- Clinical course is benign
- Recurrence is rare (0-8%)

MACROSCOPIC

General Features
- Most are solitary

MICROSCOPIC

Histologic Features
- Exophytic papillary neoplasm lined by normal-appearing urothelium
  - No significant cytologic atypia
  - Slender, minimally branching papillary architecture
  - Cores may contain prominent dilated lymphatics
  - Cores occasionally show gland-in-gland pattern
- Superficial umbrella cells often prominent
  - Prominent vacuolization of umbrella cells common
  - May be enlarged and multinucleated
- Mitoses are typically absent
- Concomitant inverted pattern may be seen

Predominant Pattern/Injury Type
- Papillary

Predominant Cell/Compartment Type
- Epithelial

ANCILLARY TESTS

Immunohistochemistry
- Alteration of p53 is not seen
- CK20 expression typically confined to umbrella cells, as in normal urothelium

DIFFERENTIAL DIAGNOSIS

Papillary Urothelial Neoplasm of Low Malignant Potential
- Urothelium that is thicker than papilloma
- Cell density appears to be increased compared to normal

Papillary Urothelial Carcinoma, Low Grade
- Subtle variation in nuclear polarity, size, shape, outlines, or chromatin distribution

Papillary-Polypoid Cystitis
- Broader papillary bases that taper toward tips
- Nonhierarchical branching

Nephrogenic Adenoma
- Pure papillary forms may mimic papilloma
- Single layer of cuboidal epithelial cells
- Express pax-8 by immunohistochemistry

Papillary Clear Cell Adenocarcinoma
- More atypical areas are almost always present
- Lined by single layer of cuboidal epithelium

Prostatic-Type Polyp
- Admixed prostatic secretory cells

Prostatic Ductal Carcinoma
- Columnar pseudostratified PSA positive lining cells

DIAGNOSTIC CHECKLIST

Clinically Relevant Pathologic Features
- More common in younger patients
  - Urothelial carcinoma would be rare in children, adolescents, and young adults

Pathologic Interpretation Pearls
- Important not to interpret umbrella cells in assessment of atypia
- Papilloma should be considered in children

SELECTED REFERENCES

1. Magi-Galluzzi C et al: Urothelial papilloma of the bladder: a review of 34 de novo cases. Am J Surg Pathol. 28(12):1615-20, 2004
2. McKenney JK et al: Urothelial (transitional cell) papilloma of the urinary bladder: a clinicopathologic study of 26 cases. Mod Pathol. 16(7):623-9, 2003
3. Cheng L et al: Urothelial papilloma of the bladder. Clinical and biologic implications. Cancer. 86(10):2098-101, 1999

Urothelial Papilloma

(Left) At low magnification, this urothelial papilloma has the typical slender papillae with minimal branching. Significant anastomosing or confluent sheet-like epithelial growth, which is more common in higher grade lesions, is not seen. **(Right)** Urothelial papilloma typically has a simple, minimally branching papillary architecture without confluent epithelial aggregates and has a urothelial lining of normal thickness that is usually 3-6 layers.

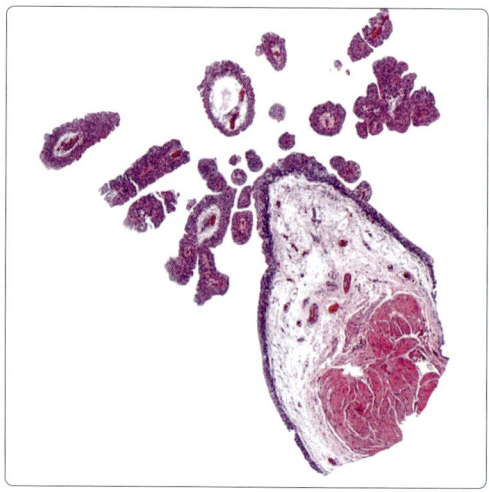
Urothelial Papilloma

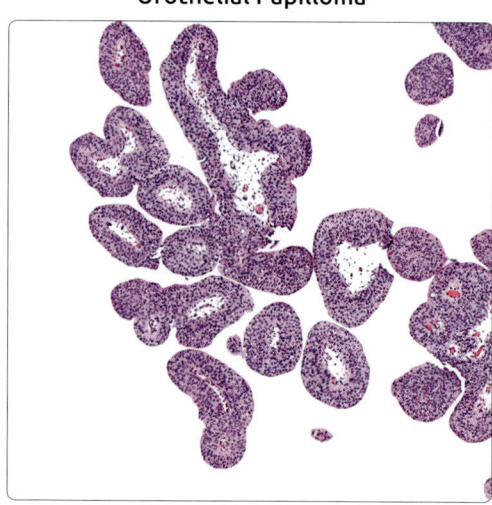
Urothelial Papilloma

(Left) This typical urothelial papilloma is characterized by a simple branching architecture and an urothelium of normal thickness. The homogeneous thin papillae help distinguish papilloma from papillary cystitis, which would have more broad bulbous papillae toward the base. **(Right)** Urothelial papillomas may show dilated lymphatics in the papillary cores ⇨ and occasionally a unique gland-in-gland pattern ⇨. The urothelium is of normal thickness, as required for a diagnosis of papilloma.

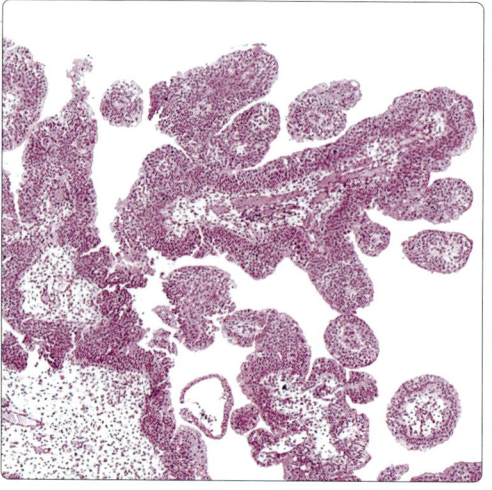
Urothelial Papilloma

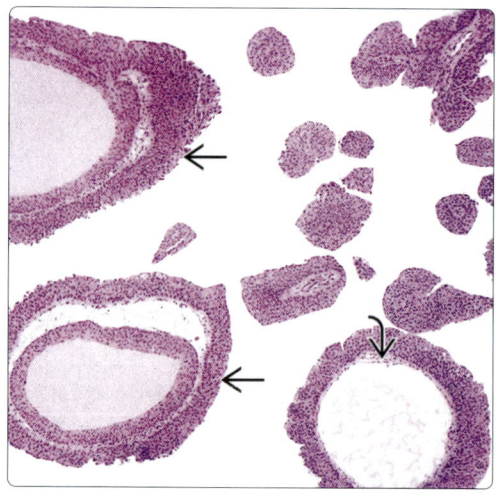
Urothelial Papilloma

(Left) In urothelial papilloma, the simple papillary architecture may be very similar to papillary urothelial neoplasm of low malignant potential. The urothelium in this example is of normal thickness, consistent with papilloma. **(Right)** Dilated lymphatics within the papillary cores are sometimes prominent in urothelial papilloma. This feature is not commonly seen in other reactive or neoplastic papillary urothelial lesions.

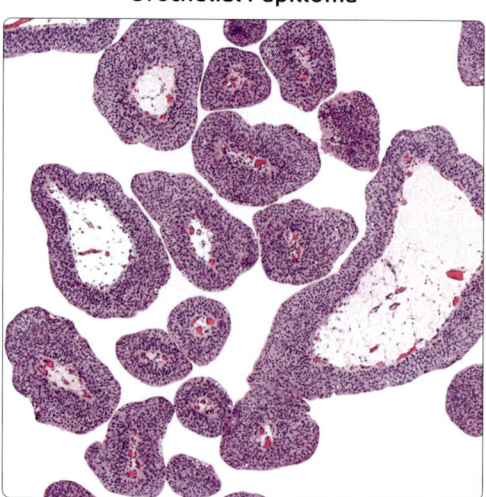
Urothelial Papilloma

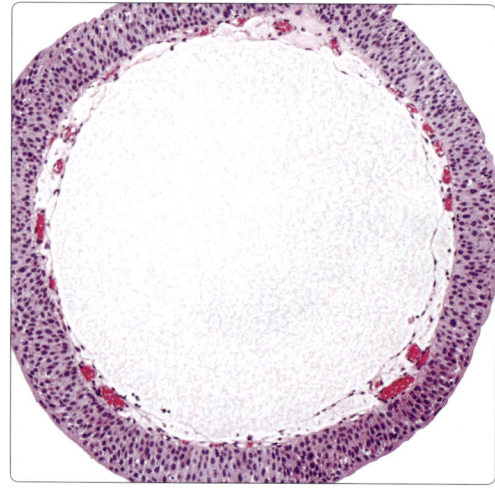
Urothelial Papilloma

Urothelial Papilloma

Urothelial Papilloma

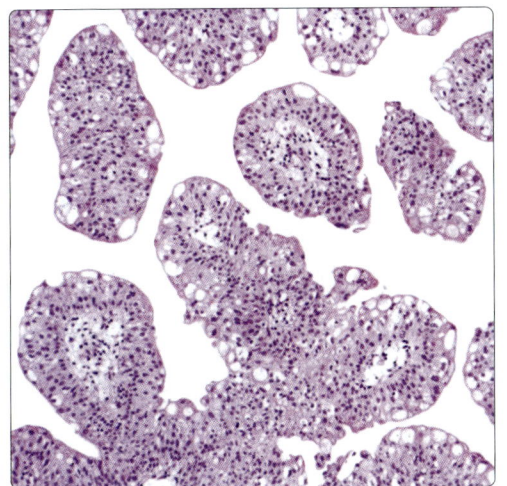

Urothelial Papilloma

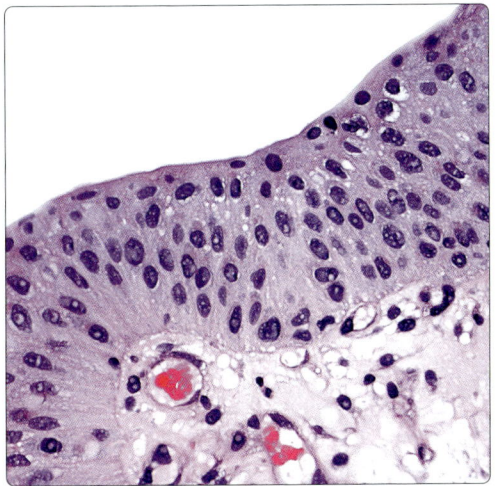

(Left) *Urothelial papillomas often have a prominent umbrella cell layer, which may show extensive cytoplasmic vacuolization.* (Right) *This high-power photomicrograph of the surface lining demonstrates the characteristic normal urothelium of urothelial papilloma. The nuclei are small with fine chromatin and stream upward from the basement membrane.*

Mixed Features With PUNLMP

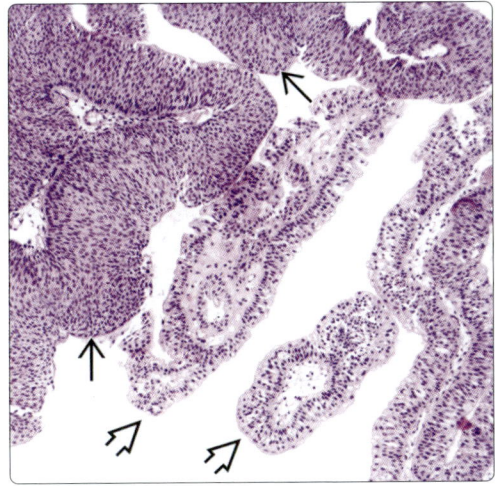

Mixed Features With PUNLMP

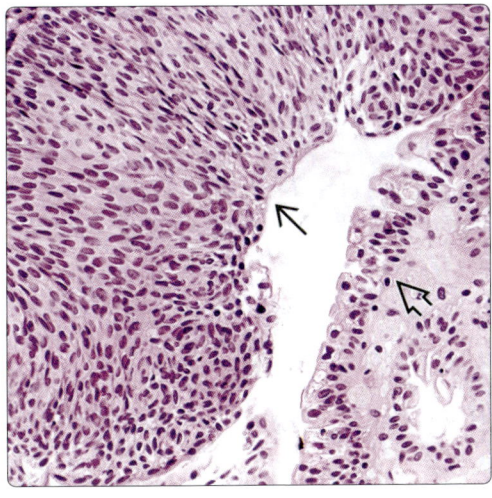

(Left) *Papillary urothelial neoplasm with mixed features contrasts foci with a morphology of urothelial papilloma on the right ➡ and papillary urothelial neoplasm of low malignant potential (PUNLMP) on the left ➡.* (Right) *Increased thickness of the urothelium and increased cell density in PUNLMP ➡ is compared to the papilloma-like component ➡. It would be classified by its highest grade focus as a PUNLMP, but this example contrasts the difference in thickness.*

PUNLMP

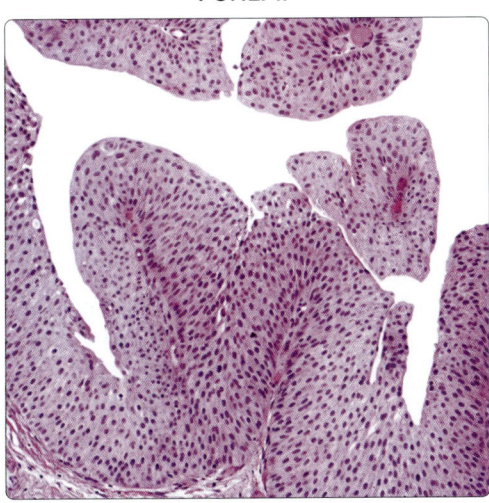

PUNLMP

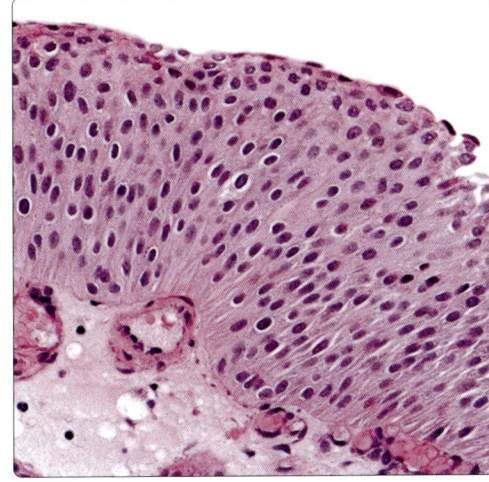

(Left) *PUNLMP has a hyperplastic urothelial lining, in contrast to the urothelium of normal thickness seen in papilloma.* (Right) *On high-power examination of this papillary neoplasm, the urothelium has bland cytology and normal perpendicular orientation to the basement membrane. Despite this normal cytology, the hyperplastic urothelium warrants designation as PUNLMP over papilloma.*

Urothelial Papilloma

Urothelial Carcinoma

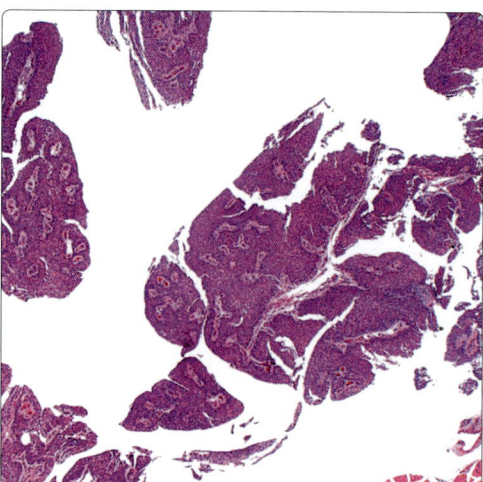

Urothelial Carcinoma

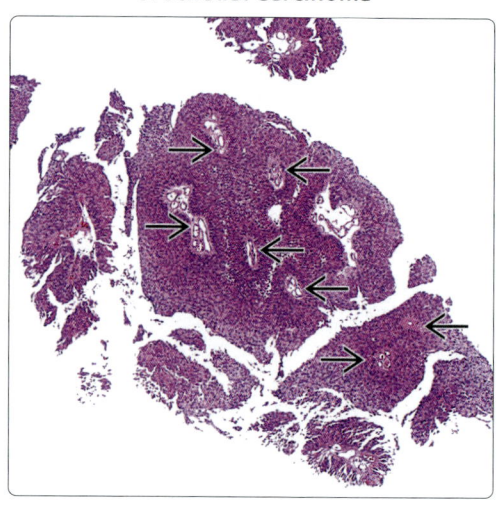

(Left) On low-power examination, this papillary urothelial carcinoma has more epithelial confluence than urothelial papilloma, which would maintain simple discrete papillae. The degree of hyperchromasia is also unusual for papilloma. **(Right)** This example of papillary urothelial carcinoma shows complex epithelial growth that encases multiple different papillary cores ⇨. This degree of epithelial confluence would preclude classification as urothelial papilloma. The degree of hyperchromasia is also unusual for papilloma.

Urothelial Carcinoma

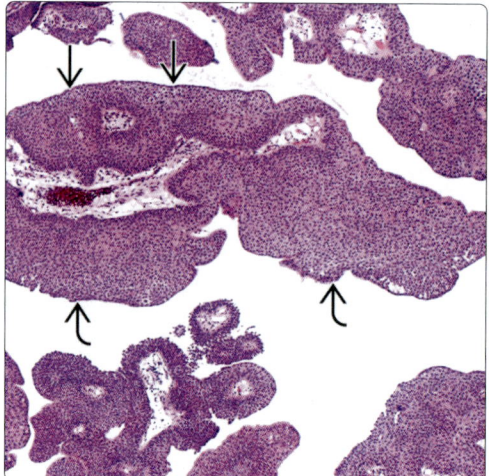

Urothelial Carcinoma

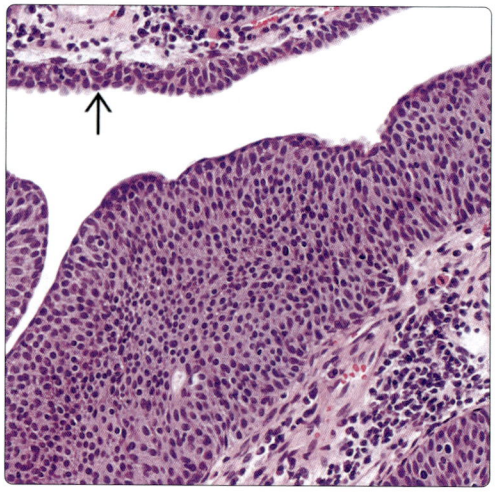

(Left) This papillary urothelial carcinoma has foci with obviously thickened urothelium (hyperplasia) ⇨ and more epithelial confluence ⇨ than seen in urothelial papilloma. **(Right)** On high-power examination, the disordered urothelium (loss of polarity) with increased thickness warrants classification as low-grade carcinoma. The adjacent normal urothelium ⇨ allows comparison with normal thickness.

Nephrogenic Adenoma

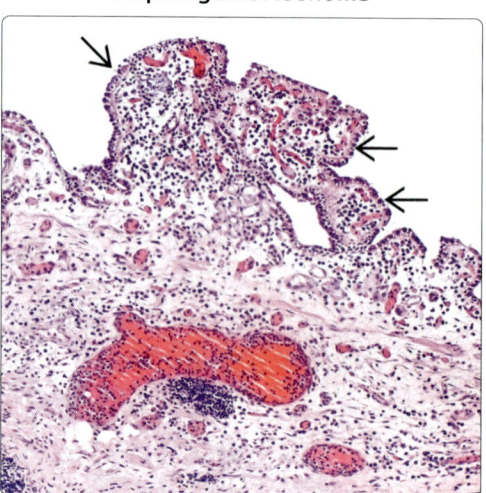

Nephrogenic Adenoma

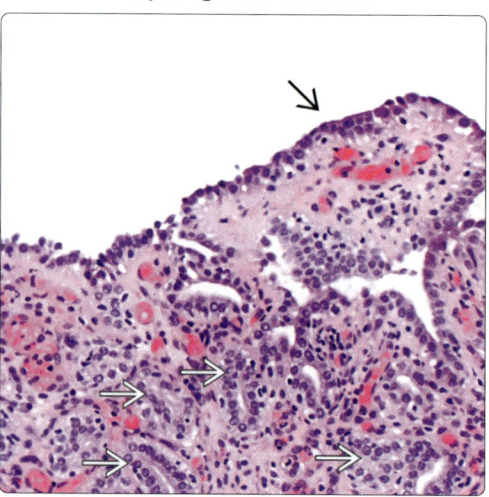

(Left) Papillary nephrogenic adenoma is distinguished from urothelial papilloma by the single cuboidal layer of lining epithelium ⇨. **(Right)** The admixed tubular component in the lamina propria ⇨ is a distinctive feature of nephrogenic adenoma. In addition, the papillae are lined by a single cuboidal layer of epithelium ⇨. In contrast, urothelial papilloma is lined by multilayered urothelium.

Urothelial Papilloma

Prostatic-Type Polyp

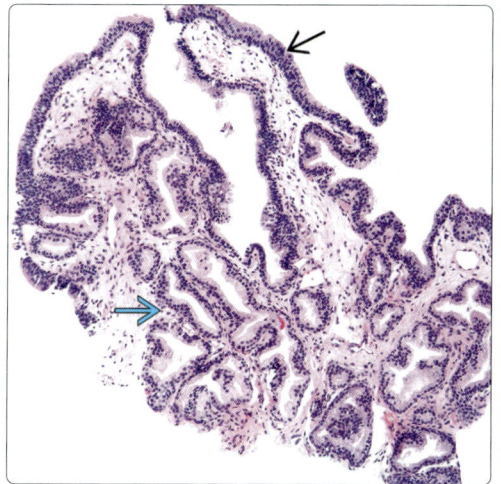

Prostatic-Type Polyp

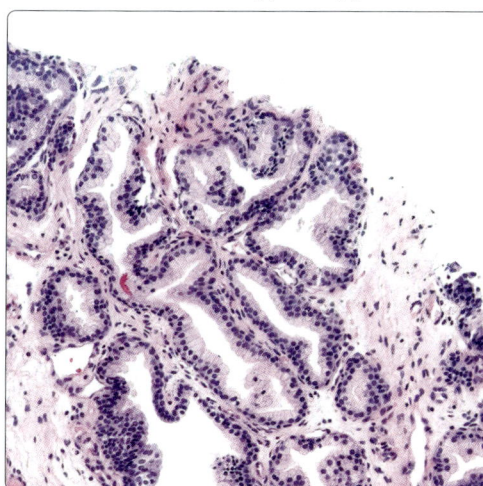

(Left) In this example of a prostatic-type polyp, the surface of the papillary excrescences is lined by urothelium ➡, while the cores contain prostatic secretory type glands ➡. *(Right)* The presence of prostatic secretory glands in the stalk is characteristic of a prostatic-type polyp. Although not typically necessary for diagnostic purposes, the glands would express positivity for PSA by IHC.

Papillary-Polypoid Cystitis

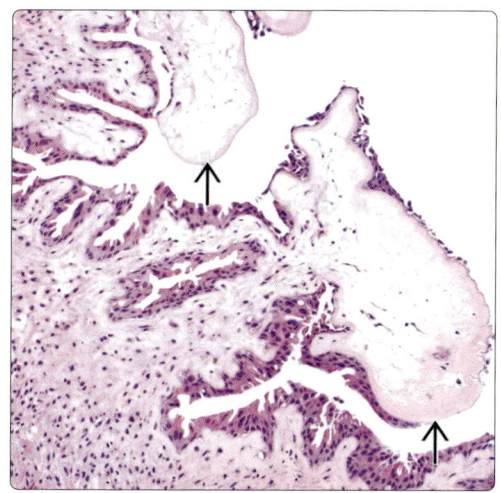

Papillary-Polypoid Cystitis

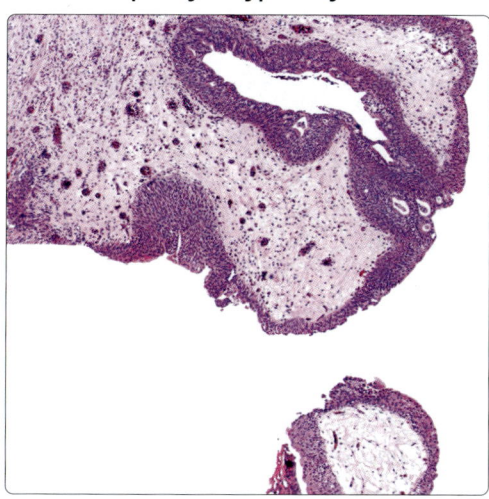

(Left) This example of papillary-polypoid cystitis shows the typical bulbous tips ➡ of the papillary excrescences. *(Right)* Papillary-polypoid cystitis is a reactive lesion that may closely mimic urothelial papilloma. In contrast to the thin papillae of urothelial papilloma, papillary-polypoid cystitis is characterized by broad bulbous excrescences with stromal edema. The lining varies from being normal to hyperplastic to reactive.

Clear Cell Adenocarcinoma

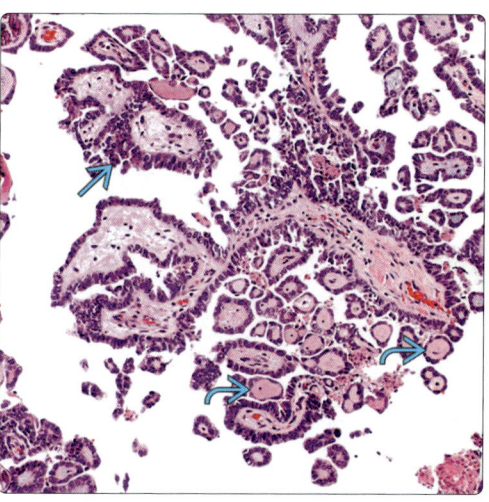

Clear Cell Adenocarcinoma

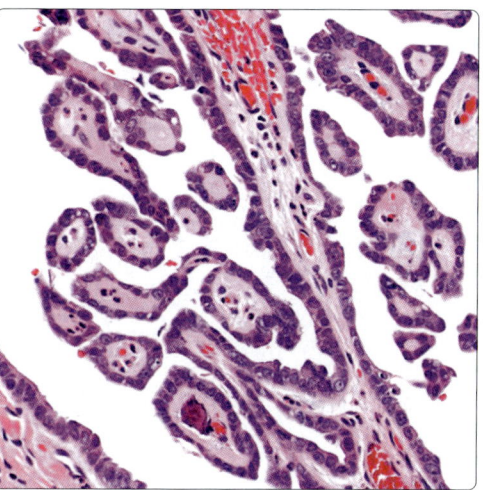

(Left) Papillary foci of clear cell adenocarcinoma may also potentially mimic a benign lesion, such as papilloma. Although there is some stratification ➡, most of the papillae are lined by a single epithelial lining. The papillae are smaller than typically seen in papilloma, and some have a hyalinized core ➡. *(Right)* As seen here, papillary clear cell adenocarcinomas may have deceptively bland foci, but other areas with typical levels of cytologic atypia are usually present. These lesions typically form larger masses.

Papillary Urothelial Neoplasm of Low Malignant Potential

KEY FACTS

CLASSIFICATION
- Rare papillary urothelial neoplasm when strictly defined

CLINICAL ISSUES
- Incidence is 3/100,000 individuals per year
- Wide age range that includes children and adolescents
- Male predominance (M:F = 3-5:1)
- Gross or microscopic hematuria
- Recurrence rate: 25-47%
- Progression rate to higher grade: 8%

MACROSCOPIC
- Typically 1-2 cm exophytic papillary tumor

MICROSCOPIC
- Papillae of papillary urothelial neoplasm of low malignant potential (PUNLMP) are typically discrete and slender
- Lined by hyperplastic, cellular urothelium
- Minimal to absent cytologic atypia and normal architecture
- Cells are monotonous with normal size, shape, and chromatin distribution
- Cells stream upward, perpendicular to basement membrane (polarity is preserved)
- Mitoses are extremely rare and, if present, have basal location
- Endophytic pattern may also be seen but rare

TOP DIFFERENTIAL DIAGNOSES
- Urothelial papilloma
  - Thinner, less cellular urothelial lining
- Low-grade papillary urothelial carcinoma
  - More cellular disorder and more cytologic atypia
- Papillary-polypoid cystitis
  - Less complex excrescences with broad base and edematous inflamed lamina propria
- Papillary nephrogenic adenoma
  - Lined by single cuboidal epithelial layer
  - Other admixed patterns common (tubular or cystic)

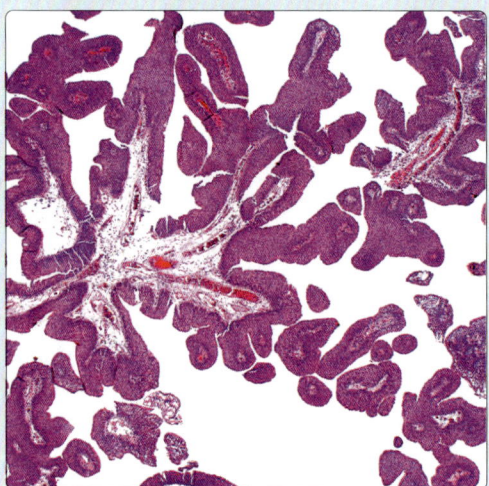

PUNLMP: Low-Power Architecture

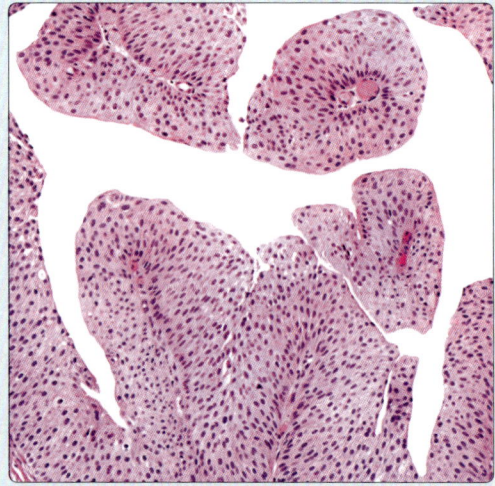

PUNLMP: Urothelial Thickness

(Left) The simple papillary architecture of this papillary urothelial neoplasm of low malignant potential (PUNLMP) with minimal branching may also be seen in urothelial papilloma, but the hyperplastic urothelial lining at low power is typical of PUNLMP. *(Right)* PUNLMP shows a hyperplastic urothelial lining with increased cell density; however, the polarity of the urothelial cells and the bland cytology are maintained.

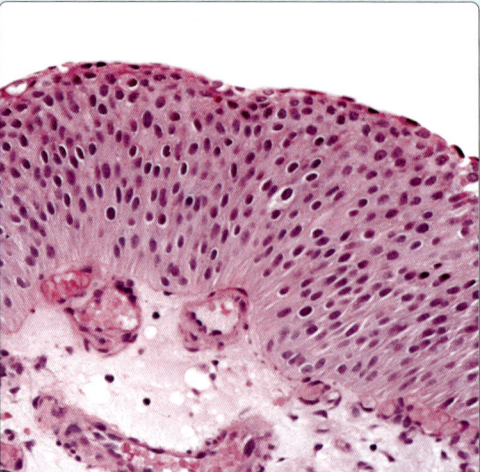

PUNLMP: Cytologic Features

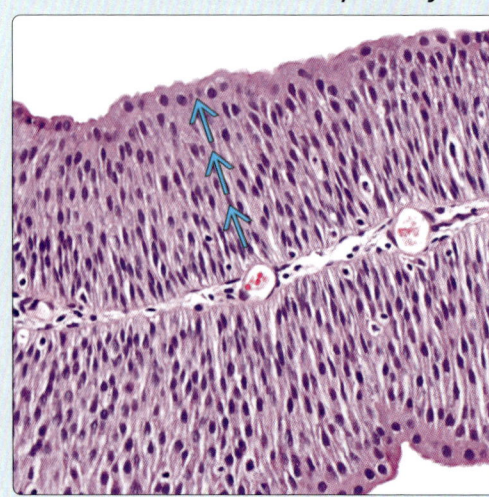

PUNLMP: Cellular Order/Polarity

(Left) This high-power photomicrograph of a PUNLMP demonstrates the required bland cytologic features of the neoplastic urothelial cells and their preserved order. *(Right)* PUNLMP is characterized by papillae lined by a thickened urothelium with normal cytologic features and preserved cellular order (i.e., streaming of the neoplastic urothelial cells ➡ perpendicular to the basement membrane).

Papillary Urothelial Neoplasm of Low Malignant Potential

TERMINOLOGY

Abbreviations
- Papillary urothelial neoplasm of low malignant potential (PUNLMP)

Synonyms
- Represents subset of tumors previously classified as transitional cell carcinoma, grade 1 (WHO 1973)

Definitions
- Papillary urothelial tumor, which resembles exophytic urothelial papilloma, but with increased thickness &/or cell density of lining urothelium
  - Cytologic features of normal urothelium

CLINICAL ISSUES

Epidemiology
- Incidence
  - Rare bladder lesion: ~ 3/100,000 individuals per year
- Age
  - Wide range
    - May occur in children and adolescents
- Sex
  - Male predominance (M:F = 3-5:1)

Presentation
- Gross or microscopic hematuria
- Urine cytology is usually negative

Treatment
- Surgical approaches
  - Complete transurethral resection

Prognosis
- Recurrence rate: 25-47%
- Progression rate to higher grade is ~ 8%
- Stage progression is very rare

MACROSCOPIC

General Features
- Typically, 1- to 2-cm exophytic papillary tumor

MICROSCOPIC

Histologic Features
- Papillae of PUNLMP are typically discrete and slender
  - Lined by hyperplastic urothelium (increased cell layers or increased cell density)
  - Minimal to absent cytologic atypia and normal architecture (should be evaluated in well-oriented section)
    - Cells are monotonous with normal size, shape, and chromatin distribution
    - Cells stream upward, perpendicular to basement membrane (polarity is preserved)
    - Umbrella cell layer is often preserved
    - Mitoses are extremely rare and, if present, have basal location
    - Basal layer may show palisading
  - Loss of polarity is minimal to absent and distinct nuclear atypia is not allowed

Predominant Pattern/Injury Type
- Papillary

DIFFERENTIAL DIAGNOSIS

Urothelial Papilloma
- Papillae are lined by urothelium of normal thickness
  - Key distinction from PUNLMP, which is hyperplastic and cellular
- Cytology may be identical to PUNLMP

Low-Grade Papillary Urothelial Carcinoma
- Papillary architecture is similar to PUNLMP but may have more confluence/complexity
- Lining urothelial cells show obvious loss of orientation to basement membrane (i.e., disorder/loss of polarity)
- Mild but distinct cytologic atypia
  - Subtle variation in nuclear size and shape or chromatin abnormality

Papillary-Polypoid Cystitis
- Exophytic papillary-polypoid structures on low power
  - Edematous or fibrotic papillary cores
    - No significant branching architecture or epithelial confluence
    - Broad base of excrescences may taper to slender papillae toward lumen

Nephrogenic Adenoma
- Papillae lined by single layer of cuboidal epithelium
- May have other associated endophytic growth patterns, including glandular and tubulocystic

DIAGNOSTIC CHECKLIST

Clinically Relevant Pathologic Features
- Clinical follow-up for PUNLMP similar to low-grade carcinoma

Pathologic Interpretation Pearls
- Strict criteria for PUNLMP must be applied
  - Little morphologic heterogeneity allowed under WHO/International Society of Urological Pathology (ISUP) criteria
    - Relatively uncommon but preserves prognostic distinction from low-grade papillary urothelial carcinoma

SELECTED REFERENCES

1. Fine SW et al: Urothelial neoplasms in patients 20 years or younger: a clinicopathological analysis using the world health organization 2004 bladder consensus classification. J Urol. 174(5):1976-80, 2005
2. Campbell PA et al: Papillary urothelial neoplasm of low malignant potential: reliability of diagnosis and outcome. BJU Int. 93(9):1228-31, 2004
3. Johansson SL et al: Papillary urothelial neoplasm of low malignant potential. In Eble JN et al: World Health Organization Classification of Tumours. Pathology & Genetics. Tumours of the Urinary System and Male Genital Organs. Lyon: IARC Press, 2004
4. Yin H et al: Histologic grading of noninvasive papillary urothelial tumors: validation of the 1998 WHO/ISUP system by immunophenotyping and follow-up. Am J Clin Pathol. 121(5):679-87, 2004
5. Fujii Y et al: Long-term outcome of bladder papillary urothelial neoplasms of low malignant potential. BJU Int. 92(6):559-62, 2003

Papillary Urothelial Neoplasm of Low Malignant Potential

PUNLMP: Urothelial Thickness

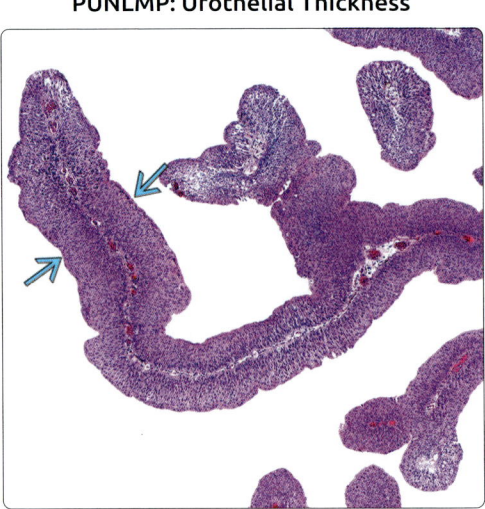

PUNLMP: Cytology

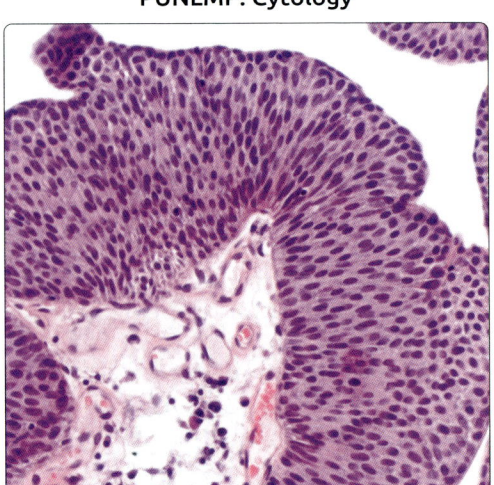

(Left) This papillary urothelial neoplasm is lined by a thickened urothelium ⇒, a feature that would raise a differential of PUNLMP vs. low-grade carcinoma. High-power examination of the cytology and cellular orientation are needed for distinction. (Right) The cells of the hyperplastic urothelium lining the papillae of PUNLMP have uniform cytology, usually with an elongated fusiform shape. They stream perpendicularly between the basement membrane and bladder lumen.

PUNLMP: Polarity

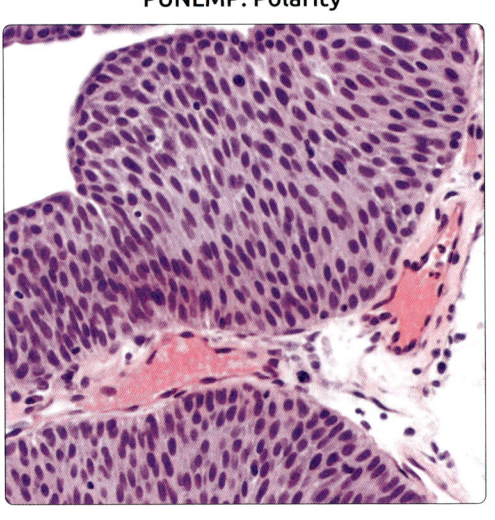

PUNLMP: Umbrella Cell Layer

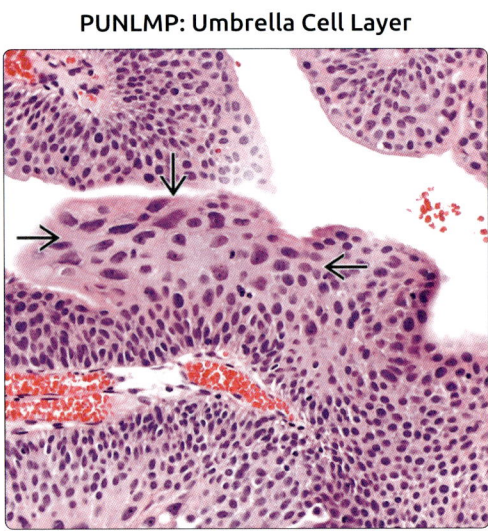

(Left) The normal polarity of the lining neoplastic urothelium in this papillary urothelial neoplasm is characteristic of PUNLMP; there is no crowding. (Right) Tangentially sectioned superficial (umbrella) cells ⇒ may occasionally be seen in a PUNLMP. The normal degree of nucleomegaly and the occasional multilobation of umbrella cells should be discounted and not prompt designation as a higher grade lesion. It is also important to evaluate well-oriented sections in the evaluation of polarity.

Urothelial Papilloma

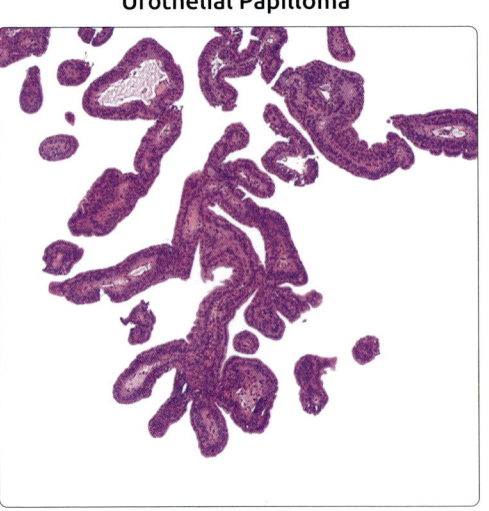

Urothelial Papilloma

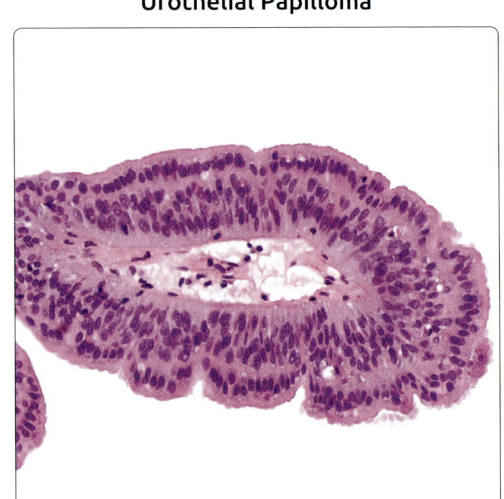

(Left) The thin, simple branching in this urothelial papilloma is similar to that seen in PUNLMP. In contrast to PUNLMP, the lining urothelium is of normal thickness. (Right) The prominent umbrella cell layer and the normal cytology and polarity are all features that may be seen in urothelial papilloma and PUNLMP. The thin (normal) lining urothelium warrants classification of this tumor as urothelial papilloma. The normal urothelium and that of papilloma is typically 3-6 layers.

Papillary Urothelial Neoplasm of Low Malignant Potential

Urothelial Papilloma

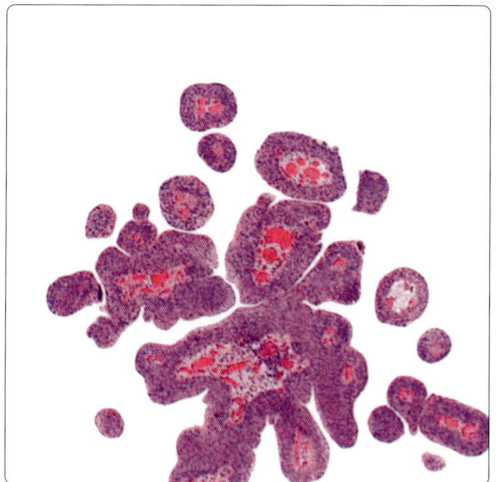

Urothelial Papilloma

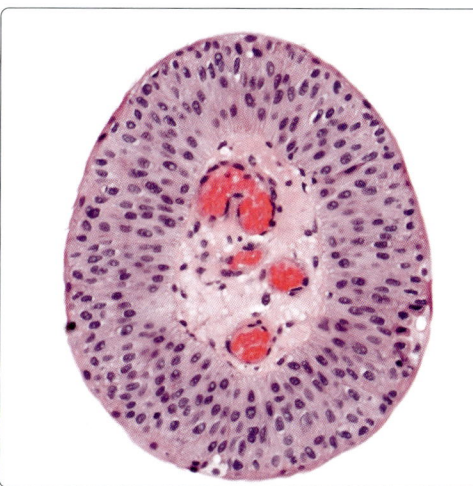

(Left) Urothelial papilloma shares a relatively simple papillary architecture with PUNLMP at low-power magnification. In general, significant fusion between adjacent papillae is not prominent. *(Right)* On high-power magnification, the urothelial lining of papilloma is of normal thickness, normal cytology, and normal orientation. The absence of hyperplasia is the most distinctive feature compared to PUNLMP.

Papillary/Polypoid Cystitis

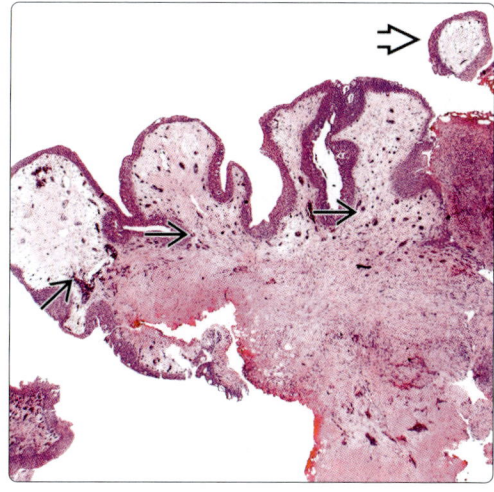

Low-Grade Carcinoma

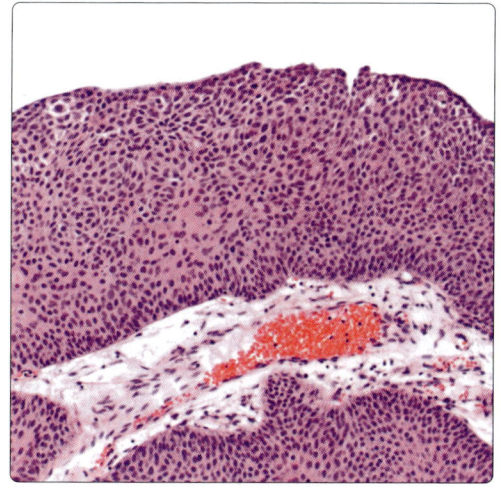

(Left) The edematous polypoid stalks with a broad base ⇨ are characteristic of papillary-polypoid cystitis. The sectioned ends of the papillae ⇨ may mimic a PUNLMP, which typically has more slender papillae with at least some degree of simple branching. *(Right)* Although the lining urothelium of this papillary tumor is thickened, the cells do not have the orderly arrangement of PUNLMP. This architectural disorder is sufficient for classification as low-grade papillary urothelial carcinoma.

Low-Grade Carcinoma

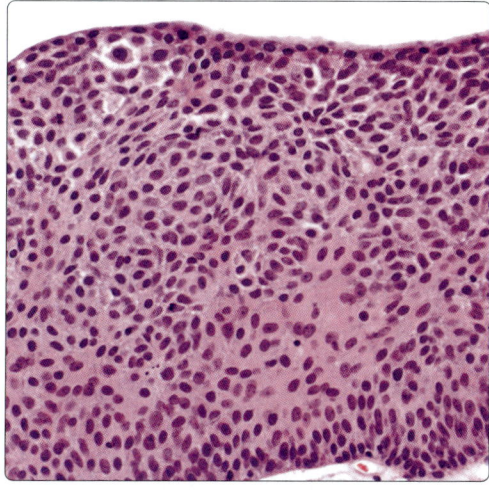

Low-Grade Carcinoma

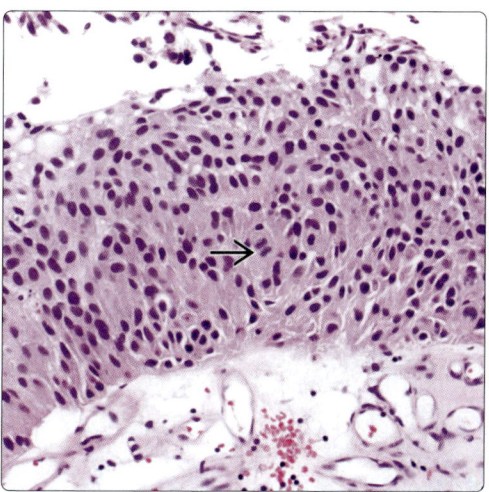

(Left) In this low-grade papillary urothelial carcinoma, the nuclei are small and the chromatin is evenly dispersed; however, there is loss of orientation to the basement membrane, which precludes a diagnosis of PUNLMP. *(Right)* This low-grade carcinoma has too much architectural disorder to qualify as PUNLMP and is probably a closer mimic of high-grade carcinoma. In addition, rare mitotic figures are seen ⇨, a feature that should prompt careful consideration of carcinoma over PUNLMP.

Low-Grade Papillary Urothelial Carcinoma

KEY FACTS

TERMINOLOGY

- Definitions
  - Papillary urothelial neoplasm with some degree of cytoarchitectural disorder and distinct but low-grade cytologic abnormality
  - No high-grade cytologic features (pleomorphism, mitoses toward surface and nucleoli throughout)

CLINICAL ISSUES

- Mean age: 70 years
- Male predilection
  - M:F = 3:1
- Gross or microscopic hematuria common
- Progression and death from disease is rare (< 5% of patients) but recurrence/new occurrence is common (48-71%)

MICROSCOPIC

- Cells are relatively uniform in size without significant nuclear pleomorphism or nucleomegaly
- Subtle variation in nuclear size may be present
- Relatively fine nuclear chromatin
- Loss of cellular polarity
  - Random distribution of cells in urothelium
  - Loss of linear perpendicular orientation to basement membrane
- Mitotic figures are rare and distributed randomly
  - Generally mitoses restricted to lower 1/2 of urothelium

TOP DIFFERENTIAL DIAGNOSES

- Papillary urothelial neoplasm of low malignant potential (PUNLMP)
- High-grade papillary urothelial carcinoma
- Papillary-polypoid cystitis

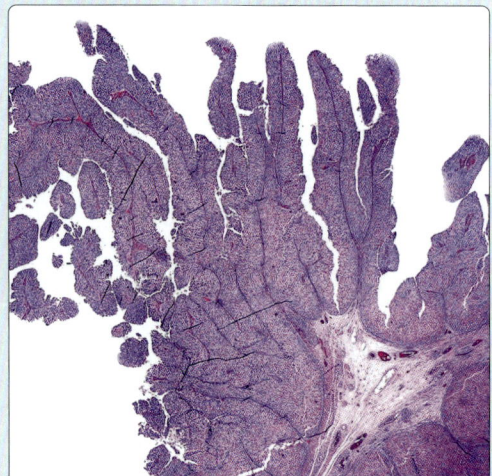

Low-Grade Papillary Urothelial Carcinoma: Long Branching Papillae

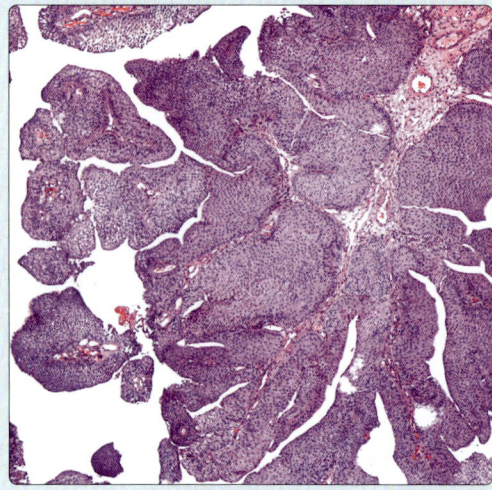

Low-Grade Papillary Urothelial Carcinoma: Papillary Thickening and Fusion

(Left) Low-magnification view shows a low-grade papillary urothelial carcinoma. Multiple long, slender, and branching papillary fronds are present. *(Right)* Low-grade papillary urothelial carcinoma has well-formed papillae with minimal papillary fusion or branching. The urothelium is thickened but the level of cytoarchitectural disorder is minimal.

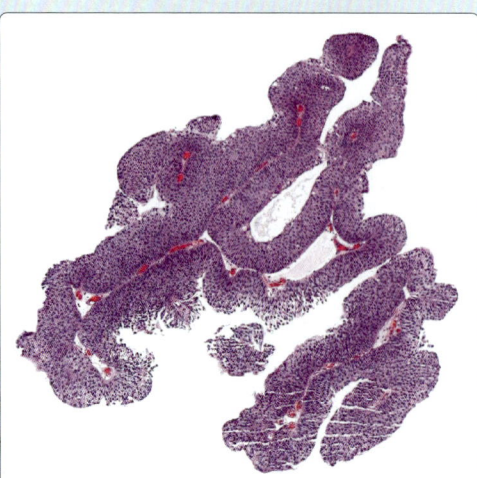

Low-Grade Papillary Urothelial Carcinoma: Mild Architectural Disorder

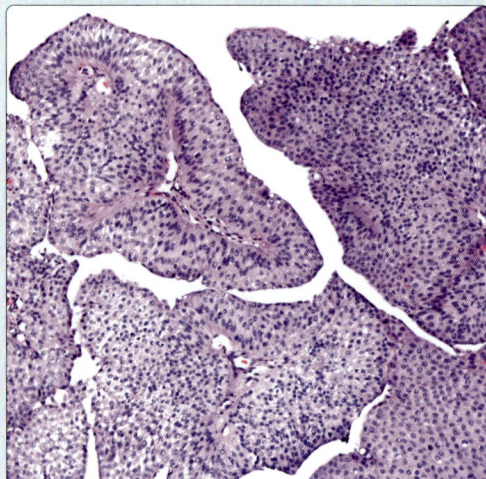

Low-Grade Papillary Urothelial Carcinoma: Loss of Order

(Left) Intermediate magnification shows a low-grade papillary urothelial carcinoma from a transurethral resection specimen. Mild architectural disorder is appreciated at this magnification. *(Right)* Low-grade papillary urothelial carcinoma with minimal epithelial fusion and loss of order is shown at low power; no obvious nuclear pleomorphism or hyperchromasia is seen.

Low-Grade Papillary Urothelial Carcinoma

TERMINOLOGY

Definitions
- Papillary urothelial neoplasm with some degree of cytoarchitectural disorder and distinct but low-grade cytologic abnormality
  - Exhibits minimal architectural and cytologic variability but overall orderly appearance (recognized at scanning magnification)
    - Low-grade papillary urothelial carcinoma is not synonymous with WHO 1973 grade 1

CLINICAL ISSUES

Epidemiology
- Incidence
  - 5 per 100,000 individuals per year
- Age
  - Mean: 70 years
- Sex
  - Male predilection (M:F = 3:1)

Site
- Most commonly on posterior bladder wall

Presentation
- Gross or microscopic hematuria common
- Cytology of urine may show cellular clusters/papillae suspicious for carcinoma

Treatment
- Surgical approaches
  - Complete transurethral resection
- Adjuvant therapy
  - Intravesical therapies not generally used for low-grade carcinomas; may be used for large or recurrent tumors

Prognosis
- Recurrence/new occurrence is common (48-71%)
- Progression and death from disease rare (< 5%)

MACROSCOPIC

General Features
- Cystoscopy shows exophytic fronds of tumor, solitary or multiple lesions, wide range of lesion size

MICROSCOPIC

Histologic Features
- Cells are relatively uniform in size without significant nuclear pleomorphism or nucleomegaly
  - Subtle variation in nuclear size may be present
- Variable loss of cellular polarity, random distribution of cells in urothelium
  - Loss of linear perpendicular orientation to basement membrane
- Nuclei are often rounded with occasional irregularities of nuclear contour
- Relatively fine to slightly abnormal chromatin distribution
- Mitotic figures are rare and distributed randomly, but usually limited to low half of urothelium
- Nucleoli may be present, but inconspicuous

ANCILLARY TESTS

Immunohistochemistry
- Not routinely used for classifying papillary urothelial neoplasms

DIFFERENTIAL DIAGNOSIS

Papillary Urothelial Neoplasm of Low Malignant Potential (PUNLMP)
- Similar to low-grade papillary urothelial carcinoma at low and intermediate magnification
- Lacks distinct nuclear abnormalities or architectural disorder (no variation in nuclear shape or size, maintains normal polarity/order)

High-Grade Papillary Urothelial Carcinoma
- Wide morphologic spectrum; high-grade features may be diffuse, focal, or patchy
- Marked nucleomegaly and variation in size and shape of nuclei
- Irregular nuclear membranes and clumped nuclear chromatin; dyscohesion on surface
- Mitotic figures readily identifiable
- May be associated with invasive carcinoma

Papillary-Polypoid Cystitis
- Exophytic papillary excrescences associated with edematous or fibrotic papillary cores, no significant branching architecture and no anastomosing epithelial growth
  - Broad base of excrescences may taper to slender papillae toward lumen
- May have associated reactive atypia of lining

DIAGNOSTIC CHECKLIST

Pathologic Interpretation Pearls
- Distinction between low- and high-grade noninvasive papillary urothelial carcinoma is often therapeutic threshold for intravesical therapy
  - Establishing morphologic threshold for high-grade carcinoma is important
    - Well-oriented longitudinal sections of papillae should be chosen for evaluation to avoid artifactual crowding from tangential sectioning
    - Atypia in superficial umbrella cells should be discounted while grading, as these may have inherent atypia

SELECTED REFERENCES

1. Montironi R et al: The 2004 WHO classification of bladder tumors: a summary and commentary. Int J Surg Pathol. 13(2):143-53, 2005
2. Johansson SL et al: Non-invasive Papillary Urothelial Carcinoma, Low Grade. In Eble JN et al: World Health Organization Classification of Tumours. Pathology & Genetics. Tumours of the Urinary System and Male Genital Organs. Lyon: IARC Press, 2004
3. Yin H et al: Histologic grading of noninvasive papillary urothelial tumors: validation of the 1998 WHO/ISUP system by immunophenotyping and follow-up. Am J Clin Pathol. 121(5):679-87, 2004
4. Epstein JI et al: The World Health Organization/International Society of Urological Pathology consensus classification of urothelial (transitional cell) neoplasms of the urinary bladder. Bladder Consensus Conference Committee. Am J Surg Pathol. 22(12):1435-48, 1998

Low-Grade Papillary Urothelial Carcinoma

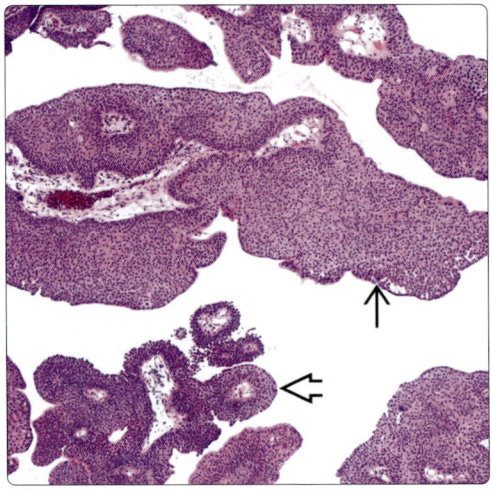

Low-Grade Papillary Urothelial Carcinoma: Thick and Thin Papillae

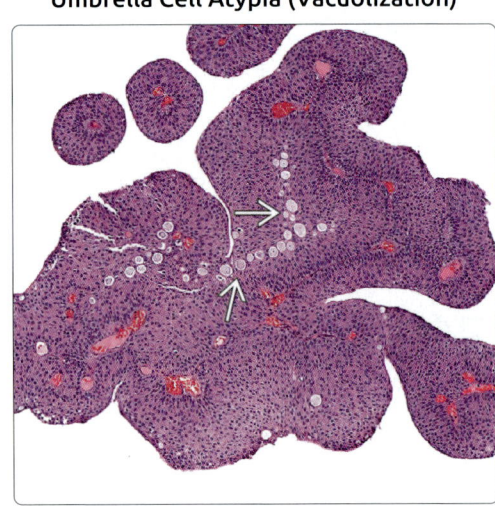

Low-Grade Papillary Urothelial Carcinoma: Umbrella Cell Atypia (Vacuolization)

(Left) Low-grade papillary urothelial carcinoma is shown with heterogeneous architectural patterns of complex markedly thickened urothelium ➡ and simple papillae with a thin urothelial lining ➡. **(Right)** Low-grade papillary urothelial carcinoma exhibits cytoarchitectural disorder. Note the atypia and vacuoles associated with the umbrella cells ➡.

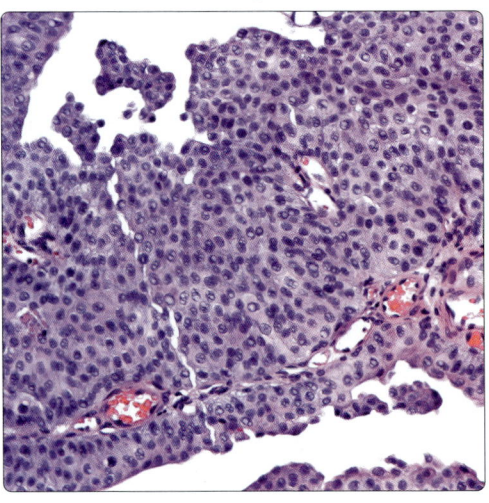

Low-Grade Papillary Urothelial Carcinoma: Nuclear Rounding and Disorder

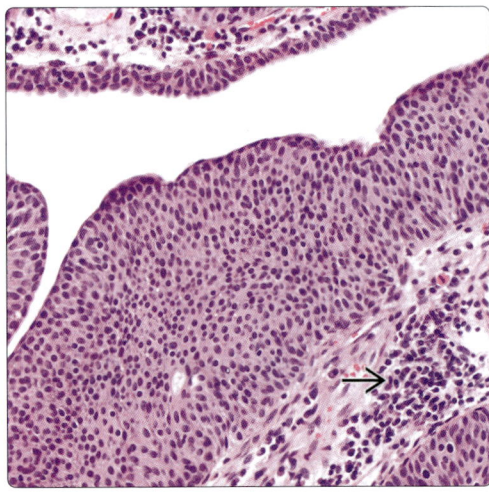

Low-Grade Papillary Urothelial Carcinoma: Nuclear Uniformity

(Left) There is thickened urothelium, marked nuclear rounding, and disorder in this low-grade papillary urothelial carcinoma. **(Right)** Low-grade papillary urothelial carcinoma shows cellular disorder, but no pleomorphism. The small size of the neoplastic cells is seen by comparison to the stromal inflammatory cells ➡. Pleomorphism, lack of prominent nucleoli throughout, and lack of surface mitoses argue against high-grade lesion.

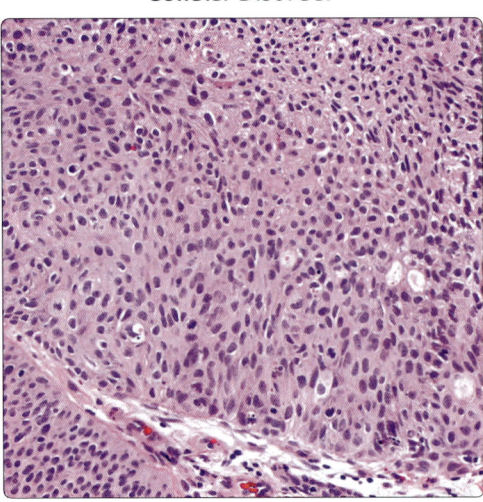

Low-Grade Papillary Urothelial Carcinoma: Cellular Disorder

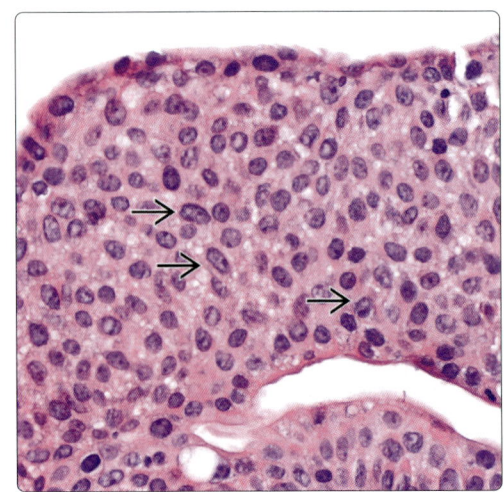

Low-Grade Papillary Urothelial Carcinoma: Minimal Size Variation

(Left) Low-grade papillary urothelial carcinoma is shown with areas of cellular disorder but no significant nucleomegaly, pleomorphism, or hyperchromasia present, excluding a high-grade carcinoma. **(Right)** High-magnification view shows low-grade papillary urothelial carcinoma with minimal variation in nuclear size and chromatin quality. The nuclei occasionally have irregular nuclear contours ➡. These features are consistent with the classification of low-grade over high-grade papillary urothelial carcinoma.

Low-Grade Papillary Urothelial Carcinoma

Low-Grade Papillary Urothelial Carcinoma: Inverted Growth

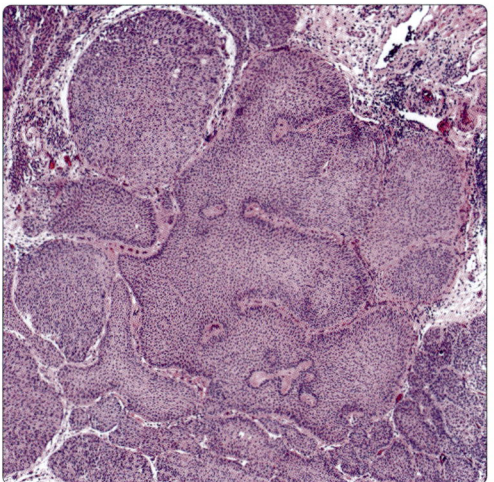

Low-Grade Papillary Urothelial Carcinoma: Endophytic Growth

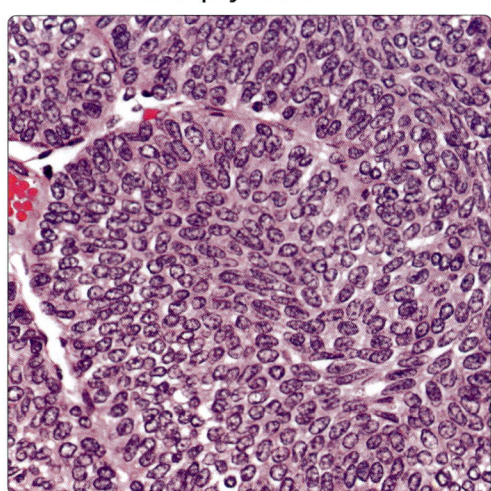

(Left) Low-grade carcinomas may have an endophytic growth pattern that may potentially mimic an inverted papilloma. *(Right)* High magnification shows an endophytic urothelial neoplasm. The cells have only mild variation in nuclear size and shape with mild disorder, slightly enlarged nuclei, and indistinct nucleoli. These features are consistent with the classification of low-grade urothelial carcinoma.

High-Grade Papillary Urothelial Carcinoma

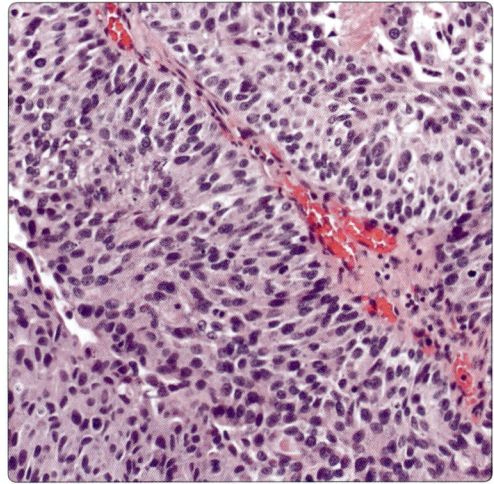

High-Grade Papillary Urothelial Carcinoma

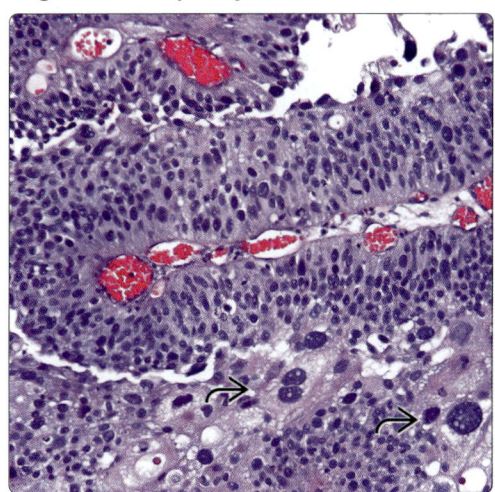

(Left) This high-grade papillary urothelial carcinoma does not show marked pleomorphism, but the hyperchromatic nuclei with irregular, clumped chromatin warrants a high-grade designation. *(Right)* Despite the noticeable atypia in the umbrella cells ⇨, this papillary urothelial neoplasm exhibits more pronounced nuclear pleomorphism and hyperchromasia, consistent with high-grade papillary urothelial carcinoma.

Invasive Urothelial Carcinoma: Deceptively Bland Histology

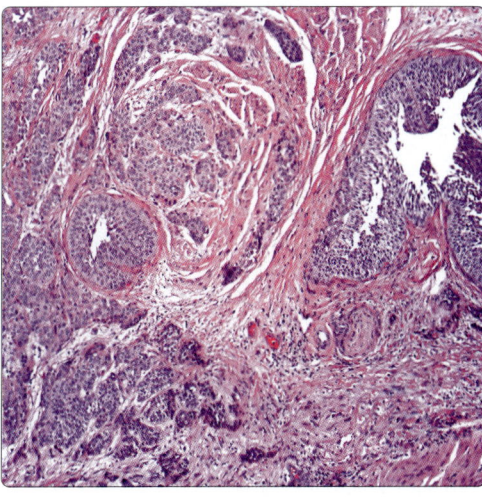

Low-Grade Papillary Urothelial Carcinoma: Superficial Invasion

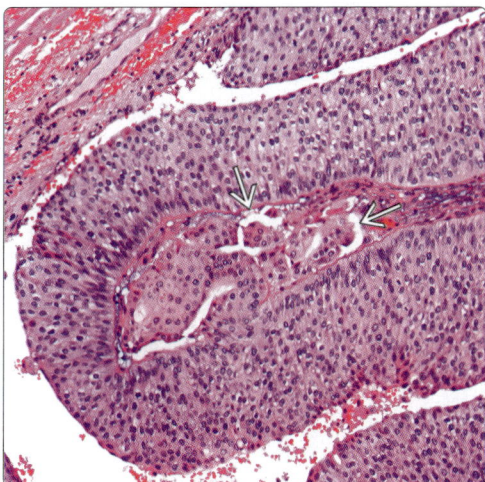

(Left) This invasive urothelial carcinoma shows deceptively bland features with nested features. Appreciation that the architecture is haphazard, as well as widespread infiltrating pattern is important to recognize the lesion as carcinoma. *(Right)* In this low-grade urothelial carcinoma, the advancing edge of the tumor was not invasive, but invasive small and irregular tumor nests were identified in the stalks of papillary fronds. Note the presence of retraction artifact associated with invasive foci ⇨.

High-Grade Papillary Urothelial Carcinoma

KEY FACTS

TERMINOLOGY
- Papillary urothelial neoplasm with moderate to marked nuclear atypia and architectural disorder

CLINICAL ISSUES
- Most occur in 6th decade or later
- Strong male predominance (M:F = 6-8:1)
- Gross or microscopic hematuria is common
- High rate of progression to invasive disease
- Patients may have prior, concurrent or future high- or low-grade carcinoma

MICROSCOPIC
- Often have complex papillary architecture (solid to fused) on low-power examination
- Level of nuclear atypia is variable
- Some have obvious nuclear pleomorphism
- Other tumors have more monomorphic nuclei
- Nucleomegaly is consistently present
- Irregular clumped nuclear chromatin is typical
- Neoplastic cells are often crowded and overlapping
- Cells lose linear orientation perpendicular to basement membrane
- Mitotic activity may be brisk, atypical mitoses and toward surface
- Cellular dyscohesion is common
- May be associated with low-grade component
- Important to rule out invasion

ANCILLARY TESTS
- Not required for diagnosis

TOP DIFFERENTIAL DIAGNOSES
- Low-grade urothelial carcinoma
- Papillary-polypoid cystitis
- Papillary nephrogenic adenoma
- Prostatic-type polyp
- Prostatic ductal carcinoma

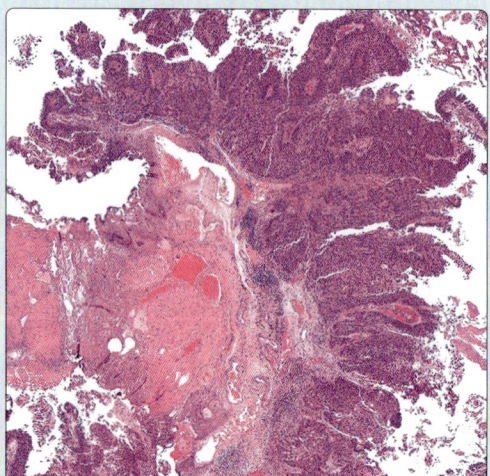

High-Grade Papillary Urothelial Carcinoma: Complex Architecture

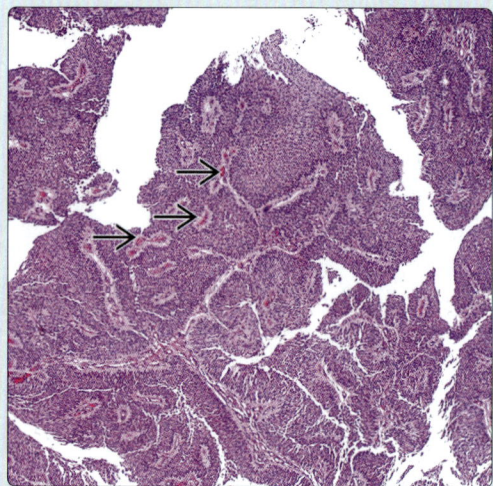

High-Grade Papillary Urothelial Carcinoma: Confluent Growth

(Left) Marked nuclear atypia and architectural disorder are evident on this low-power magnification. There is complex architecture characterized by fusion and confluence of papillae. There is dyscohesion toward the surface. (Right) High-grade papillary urothelial carcinoma shows confluent urothelial growth entrapping multiple fibrovascular cores ➡. This degree of architectural complexity and fusion between papillae is more common in higher grade lesions.

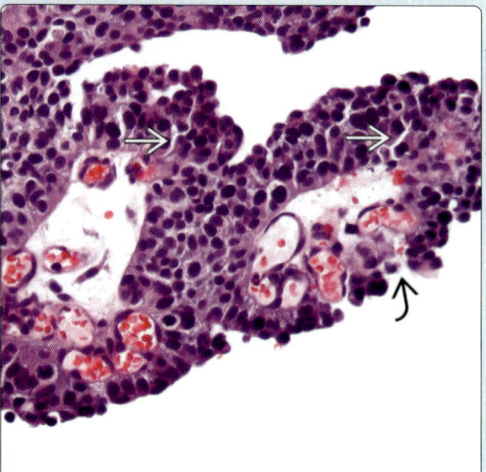

High-Grade Papillary Urothelial Carcinoma: Nuclear Atypia and Hyperchromasia

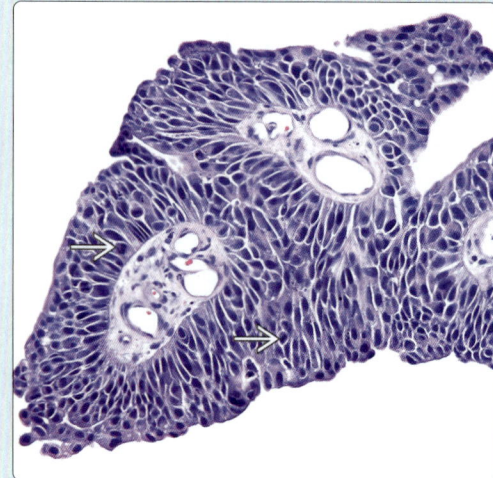

High-Grade Papillary Urothelial Carcinoma: Mitoses

(Left) In this example, marked nuclear hyperchromasia, as well as tumor cell dyscohesion ➡ and partial denudation ➡, are present. Although quite monotonous, there is no polarity, features arguing for the high-grade nature of this tumor. (Right) In this high-power view, there is pronounced nuclear atypia (hyperchromatic nuclei) and increased nuclear:cytoplasmic ratio. Mitotic figures are readily identified ➡.

High-Grade Papillary Urothelial Carcinoma

TERMINOLOGY

Definitions
- Papillary urothelial carcinoma with distinct nuclear abnormalities, including presence of moderate to marked nuclear atypia, nucleoli, and pleomorphism

CLINICAL ISSUES

Epidemiology
- Most occur in 6th decade or later
- Strong male predominance (M:F = 6-8:1)

Presentation
- Gross or microscopic hematuria is common
- Urine cytology often shows carcinoma

Treatment
- Surgical approaches
  - Transurethral resection and fulguration of visible tumor
- Adjuvant therapy
  - Intravesical immunotherapy with bacillus Calmette-Guérin
  - Intravesical chemotherapy with thiotepa or mitomycin-C

Prognosis
- High rate of progression to invasive disease

MACROSCOPIC

General Features
- Exophytic papillary growth

MICROSCOPIC

Histologic Features
- Often have complex papillary architecture on low-power examination
  - Anastomosis of papillae and confluence, cellular dyscohesion and denudation
- Range of nuclear atypia is included in this category
  - Some have obvious nuclear pleomorphism (subset shows marked nuclear anaplasia)
  - Other common features: Nucleomegaly with irregular clumped nuclear chromatin; nuclear rounding; irregular nuclear contour, prominent nucleoli, multiple nucleoli, and nucleolar pleomorphism
- Neoplastic cells are often crowded and overlapping (urothelial disorder: Cells typically lose linear orientation perpendicular to basement membrane)
- Mitotic activity may be brisk, including on surface
- May be admixed with lower grade foci of carcinoma

ANCILLARY TESTS

Immunohistochemistry
- Not required for diagnosis (expression of CK20 and p53 more frequent in high-grade carcinoma)

DIFFERENTIAL DIAGNOSIS

Low-Grade Urothelial Carcinoma
- Nuclear features and urothelial disorder less atypical than in high-grade carcinoma
- Cells are more uniform in size and evenly distributed at low-power magnification (order of architecture)
- Nuclei may be rounded, have more evenly distributed chromatin and occasional nucleoli
- Mitoses are variable but not in upper 3rds
- Cellular dyscohesion less common
- Prominent umbrella cells are occasionally seen

Papillary-Polypoid Cystitis
- Broad papillae with stromal edema
- Do not have complex secondary or tertiary branching typical of papillary urothelial neoplasia
- May have reactive urothelial atypia (nucleoli, finely speckled chromatin)
  - Mitotic activity is common
- Clinical impression is usually reactive

Papillary Nephrogenic Adenoma
- Papillae lined by single cuboidal layer and prominent basement membrane
- May have other admixed morphologic patterns (tubular/tubulocystic, diffuse/solid)
  - May mimic invasion
- Immunoreactivity for pax-2 and pax-8 characteristic

Prostatic-Type Polyp
- Papillae lined by admixed prostatic and urothelial cells
- Express PSA and PAP in secretory cell component

Prostatic Ductal Carcinoma
- Papillary neoplasm that may extend into bladder from prostatic urethra
- Papillae typically lined by monomorphic columnar cells
- PSA and PAP positive by immunohistochemistry

DIAGNOSTIC CHECKLIST

Clinically Relevant Pathologic Features
- High-grade designation is clinical threshold for adjuvant intravesical therapy
- Nonpapillary urothelium may show carcinoma in situ

Pathologic Interpretation Pearls
- WHO 2004/International Society of Urological Pathology (ISUP) has lowered threshold for diagnosis as high grade
  - High-grade category includes subset of tumors previously considered grade 2 by WHO 1973
    - Therefore, grades cannot be simply translated
  - Invasion must be meticulously excluded

SELECTED REFERENCES

1. Reuter VE. Non-invasive papillary urothelial carcinoma, high grade. In Eble JN et al: World Health Organization Classification of Tumours. Pathology & Genetics. Tumours of the Urinary System and Male Genital Organs. Lyon: IARC Press, 2004
2. Amin MB et al: Update for the practicing pathologist: The International Consultation On Urologic Disease-European association of urology consultation on bladder cancer. Mod Pathol. 28(5):612-630, 2015
3. Babjuk M et al: EAU guidelines on non-muscle-invasive urothelial carcinoma of the bladder: update 2013. Eur Urol. 64(4):639-53, 2013
4. Epstein JI et al: The World Health Organization/International Society of Urological Pathology consensus classification of urothelial (transitional cell) neoplasms of the urinary bladder. Bladder Consensus Conference Committee. Am J Surg Pathol. 22(12):1435-48, 1998

High-Grade Papillary Urothelial Carcinoma

(Left) High-grade urothelial carcinoma shows nuclear rounding (in contrast to normal fusiform to spindled shape of tumor cells), pleomorphism, hyperchromasia, cellular disorganization, and loss of polarity. **(Right)** The urothelial nests have obvious nuclear pleomorphism and hyperchromasia, features diagnostic of high-grade urothelial carcinoma. Assessment of invasion is better performed on low-power view, and grading of the tumor is best assessed on a higher power view.

High-Grade Papillary Urothelial Carcinoma: Cellular Disorganization and Loss of Polarity

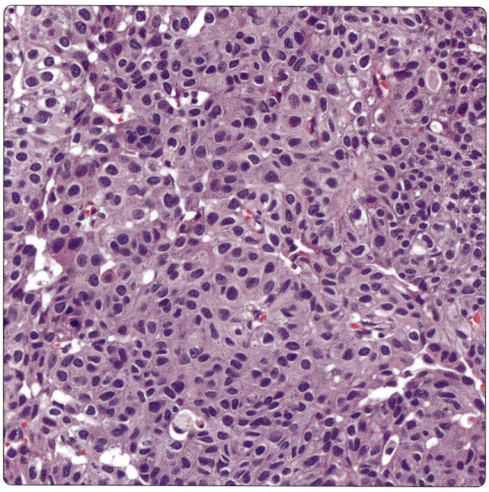

High-Grade Papillary Urothelial Carcinoma: Marked Nuclear Atypia and Hyperchromasia

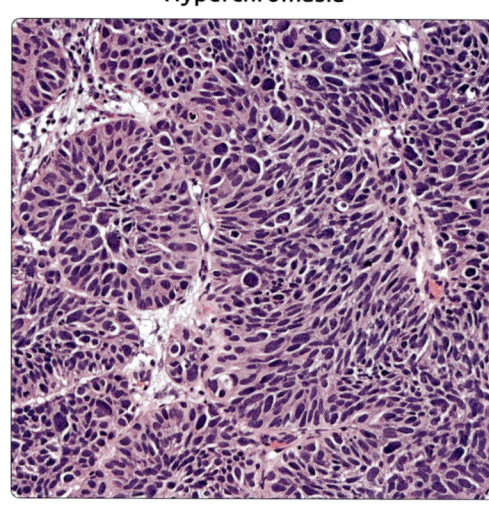

(Left) High-grade carcinoma with marked disorder and many atypical cells exhibits prominent pleomorphic nuclei and anaplastic features. Other cellular and architectural features typical of high-grade disease are also evident. **(Right)** Anaplastic nuclei can be focal, as seen in this example ➡ that otherwise exhibits recognizable features of high-grade carcinoma. These changes represent the extreme end of the spectrum of atypia but are not prerequisite for the diagnosis of high-grade disease.

High-Grade Papillary Urothelial Carcinoma: Architectural Disorder and Anaplasia

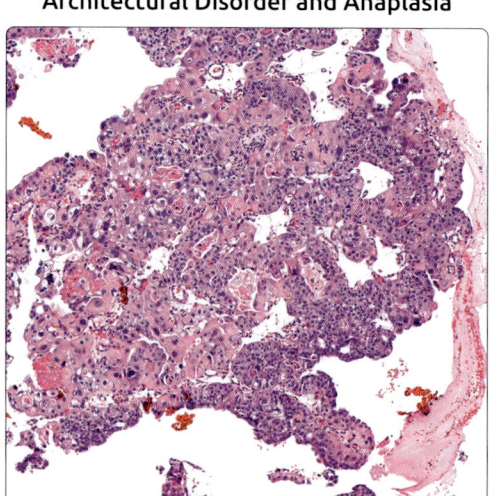

High-Grade Papillary Urothelial Carcinoma: Giant Nuclei

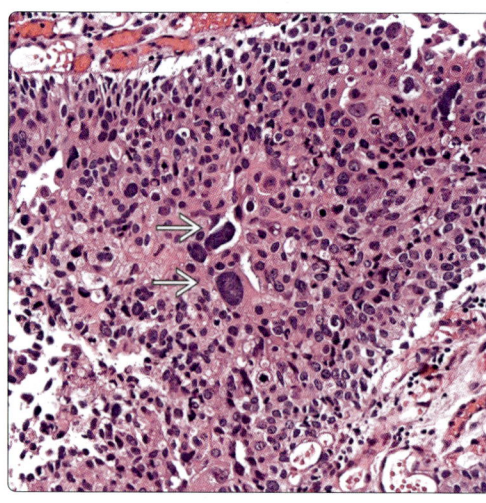

(Left) High-grade urothelial carcinoma commonly has irregular nuclear contours, obvious pleomorphism, mitotic activity/apoptotic debris, and loss of normal perpendicular alignment to the basement membrane. **(Right)** This high-grade carcinoma is more monomorphic without prominent loss of order. The nuclear chromatin is irregular and clumped, creating marked hyperchromasia. This tumor might have been classified as grade 2 in the WHO 1973 classification system, it is high grade by the current WHO/ISUP classification.

High-Grade Papillary Urothelial Carcinoma: Apoptotic Changes and Nuclear Pleomorphism

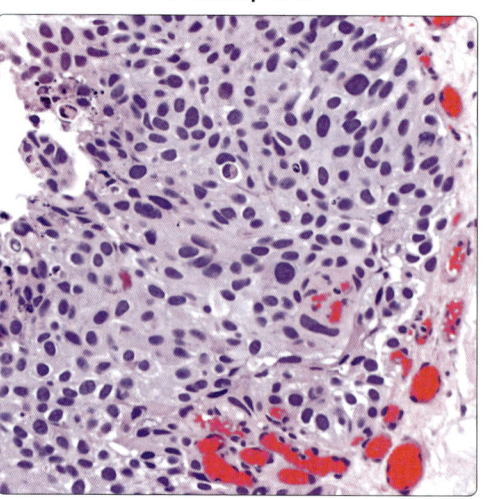

High-Grade Papillary Urothelial Carcinoma: Nuclear Monotony

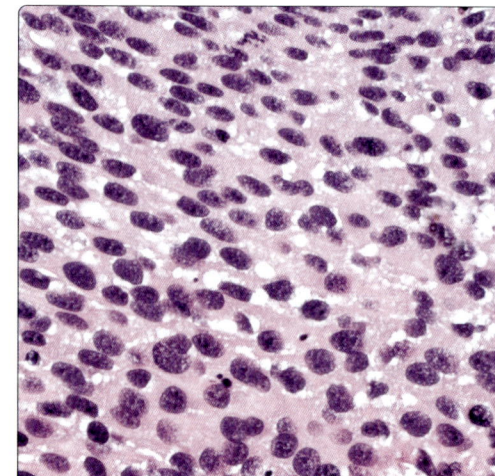

High-Grade Papillary Urothelial Carcinoma

High-Grade Papillary Urothelial Carcinoma: Micropapillary (Noninvasive)

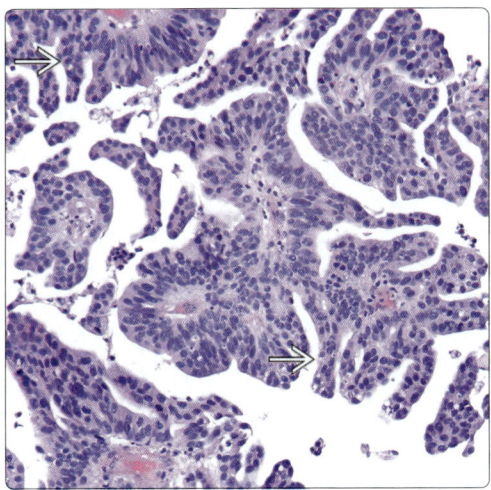

High-Grade Papillary Urothelial Carcinoma: Microcystic and Micropapillary

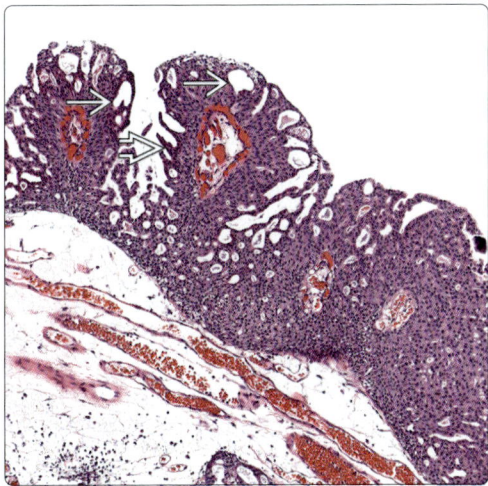

(Left) This is another example of architectural complexity in the form of secondary branching and formation of micropapillary structures ➡. The high-grade nuclear and architectural features are also evident. *(Right)* Another example of high-grade papillary urothelial carcinoma shows complex architecture forming microcystic ➡ and micropapillary structures ➡, in addition to the overall high-grade papillary configuration. Some areas are solid.

High-Grade Papillary Urothelial Carcinoma: Adjacent Flat Carcinoma In Situ

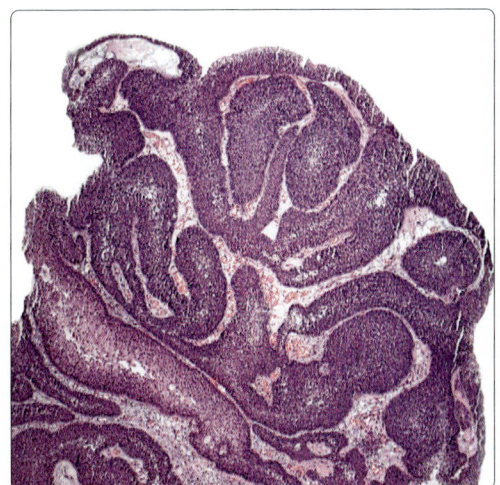

High-Grade Papillary Urothelial Carcinoma: Endophytic Growth

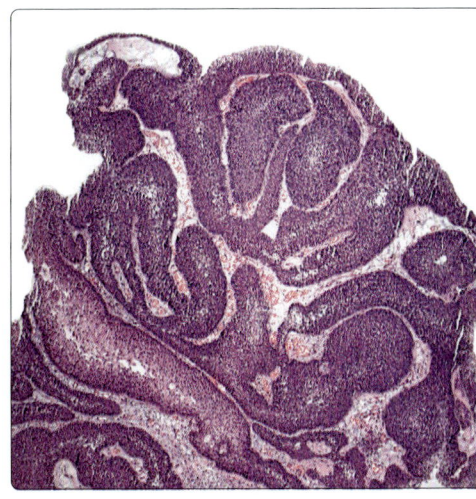

(Left) In addition to the high-grade papillary component ➡, this tumor exhibits unequivocal flat disease (urothelial carcinoma in situ) at the shoulder of the tumor ➡ adjacent to the papillary component. This observation is not uncommonly encountered in this disease. *(Right)* This represents an uncommon noninvasive endophytic pattern of high-grade urothelial carcinoma. The trabecular growth is reminiscent of inverted papilloma, but the individual cords are broader and more expansile in carcinomas.

High-Grade Papillary Urothelial Carcinoma: Superficial Invasion

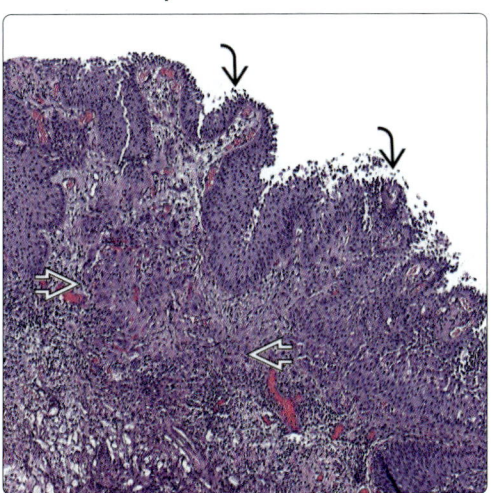

High-Grade Papillary Urothelial Carcinoma: Marked Denudation

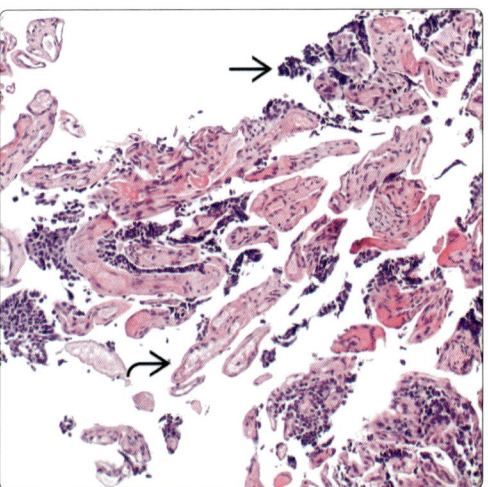

(Left) Obvious papillary carcinoma with readily recognizable high-grade features ➡ is shown. Upon careful inspection, there is a microscopic focus of invasive carcinoma in the superficial lamina propria ➡. High-grade tumors have higher chances of invasion and should be carefully evaluated for this finding. *(Right)* The papillae in high-grade papillary urothelial carcinoma may show extensive denudation ➡ and dyscohesion ➡. Denudation is uncommon in low-grade tumors unless cautery is utilized.

High-Grade Papillary Urothelial Carcinoma

(Left) Low-grade papillary urothelial carcinoma shows tangentially cut umbrella cells exhibiting significant nucleomegaly, atypia, and disorder ⇥. This may be mistaken for the possibility of focal high-grade cytology in low-grade urothelial neoplasms. **(Right)** While areas of this tumor may resemble low-grade carcinoma (left side of the image), there is unequivocal pleomorphism and disorder to warrant a more accurate diagnosis of high-grade carcinoma ⇥.

Low-Grade Papillary Urothelial Carcinoma

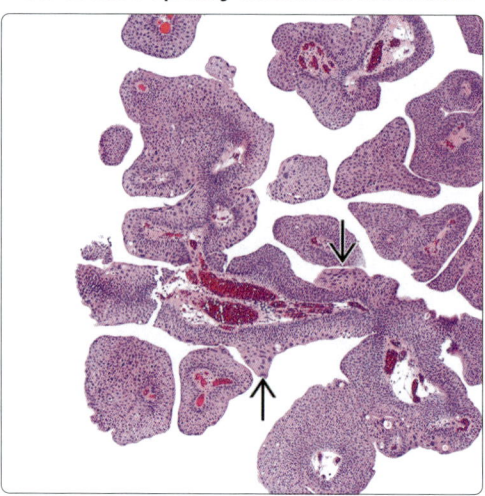

High-Grade Papillary Urothelial Carcinoma: Areas of Low-Grade Morphology

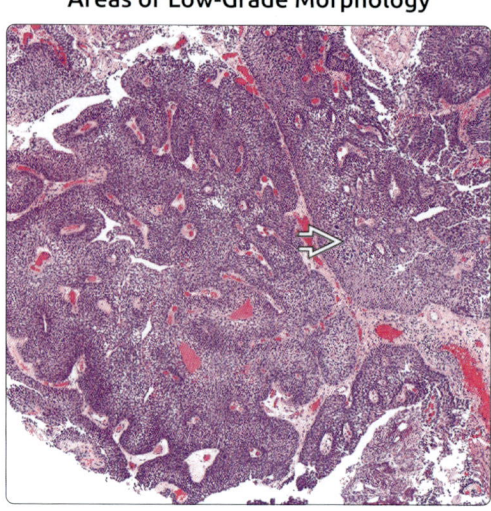

(Left) Polypid cystitis exhibits broad papillary formation and stromal edema but no complex secondary or tertiary branching. The overlying urothelial cells may also exhibit reactive atypia. **(Right)** Papillary nephrogenic adenoma has a single layer of low cuboidal lining cells. The possibility of denudation in a high-grade carcinoma might be considered, but the cellular uniformity, presence of inflammation, and prominent basement membrane are important features to correctly identify this entity.

Polypoid Cystitis

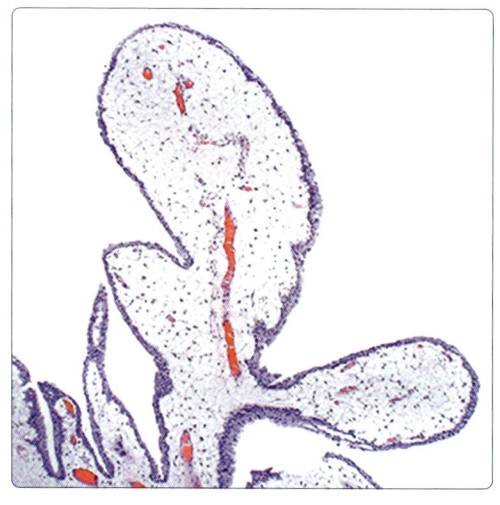

Nephrogenic Adenoma

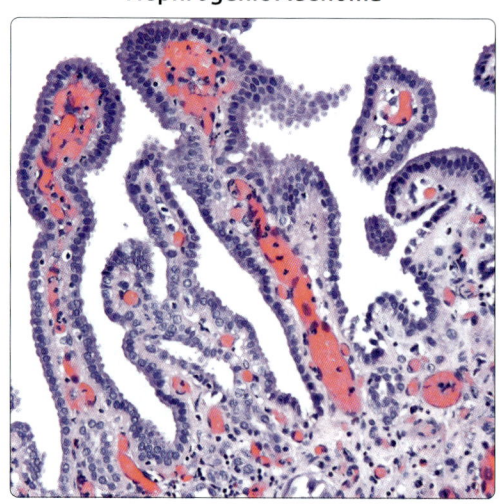

(Left) Nephrogenic adenoma exhibits complex papillary architecture. The bland histology, inflammation, and columnar appearance of a single layer of cells are important microscopic clues to the right diagnosis. **(Right)** This is the superficial component of an adenocarcinoma of the bladder, which may be mistaken for high-grade papillary urothelial carcinoma. The presence of typical features of adenocarcinoma elsewhere in the tumor enabled the correct diagnosis to be made.

Nephrogenic Adenoma

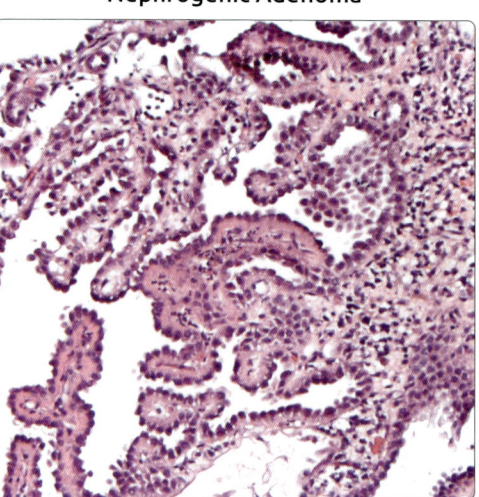

Adenocarcinoma of Bladder

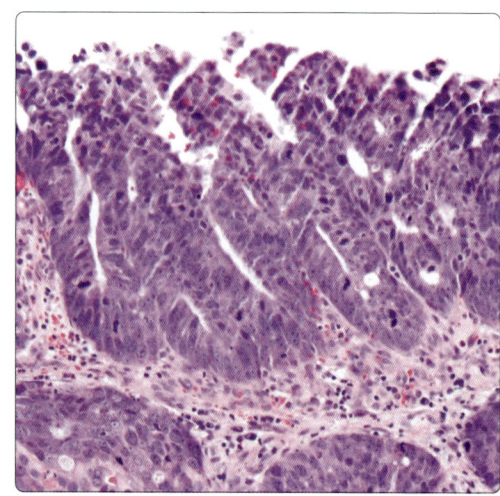

High-Grade Papillary Urothelial Carcinoma

Prostatic-Type Polyp

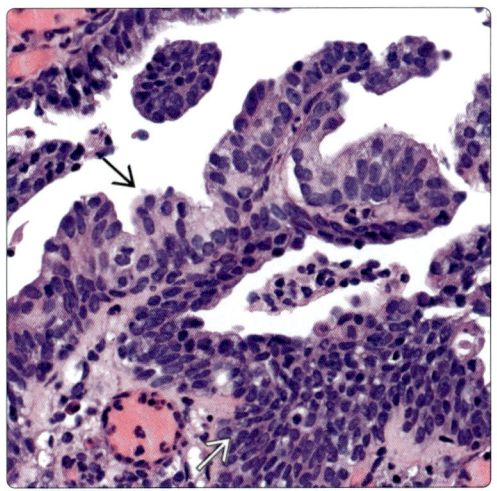

Prostatic-Type Polyp

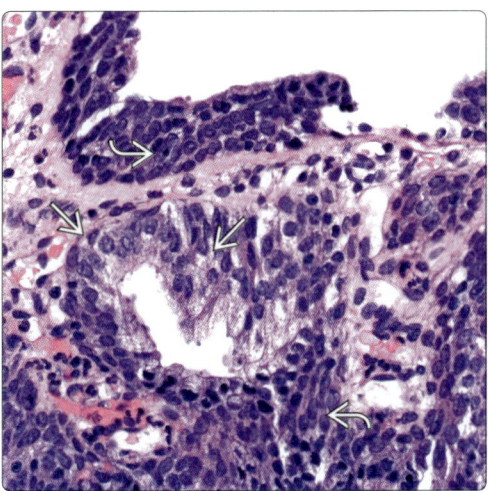

(Left) *Prostatic-type polyps are comprised of both prostatic secretory ⇒ and urothelial ⇒ cells. The urothelial cells are cytologically bland and have normal perpendicular streaming from the basement membrane.* (Right) *Prostatic secretory cells have a more "frothy" cytoplasm ⇒ and can be highlighted by PSA immunostains in difficult cases. Admixed urothelial cells are also present in this case ⇒. The underlying lamina propria often shows benign-appearing prostatic acini.*

Prostatic Adenocarcinoma Involving Bladder

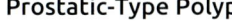

Prostatic Adenocarcinoma Involving Bladder

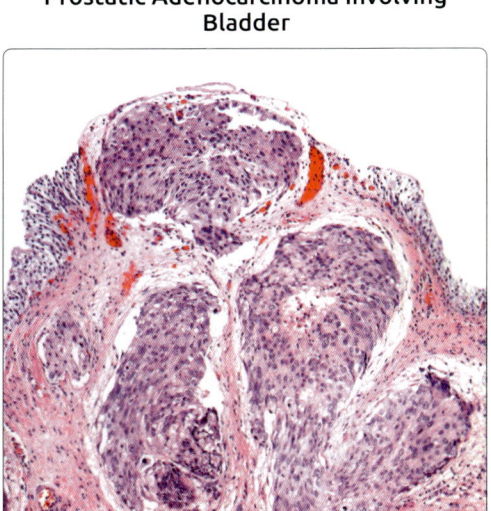

(Left) *This tumor exhibits papillary architecture and high nuclear grade. The presence of relatively uniform nuclei and prominent nuclei is helpful in suggesting a prostatic origin of this tumor. Accurate diagnosis can be achieved by proper immunostains of prostatic differentiation.* (Right) *In this example, prostatic adenocarcinoma invades the bladder wall as irregular nodules with occasional central necrosis. The clinical history of prostate cancer prompted the performance of immunostains that confirmed the diagnosis.*

Prostatic Adenocarcinoma Ductal Pattern

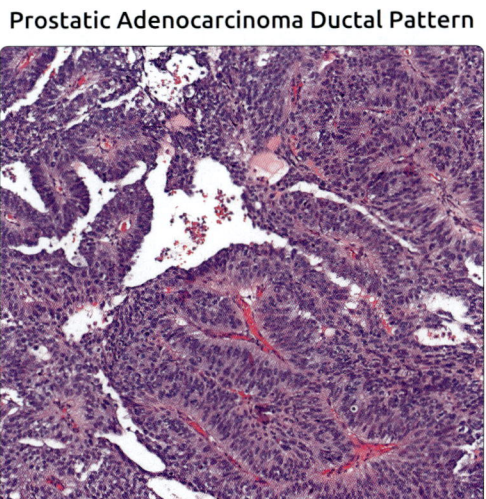

Prostatic Adenocarcinoma Involving Bladder With Surface Involvement

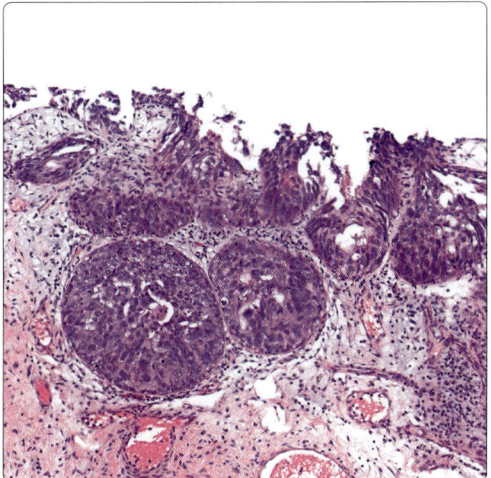

(Left) *Prostate cancer presenting as a bladder tumor is shown. There is extensive papillary formation and nuclear hyperchromasia. Applying relevant immunostains is critical to establish the diagnosis.* (Right) *Prostate cancer is shown involving the bladder as both invasive growth as well as colonization of the urothelial surface, strongly mimicking urothelial carcinoma. Awareness of such presentation is important in the work-up of such tumors.*

Inverted Urothelial Neoplasia

KEY FACTS

TERMINOLOGY
- Noninvasive pattern of urothelial neoplasia with predominantly endophytic growth pattern

CLINICAL ISSUES
- Inverted papilloma
  - Very uncommon urothelial lesion (1% of urothelial neoplasms)
  - Most common in trigone and bladder neck region
  - Recurrence rate: < 1%
- Other inverted urothelial neoplasms
  - More common with recurrence/progression rates similar to papillary counterparts

MICROSCOPIC
- Inverted papilloma
  - Urothelium invaginates into lamina propria
  - Forms thin interconnecting cords/trabeculae
  - Periphery of cords typically show palisading of basal cells
  - Central areas of cords may be spindled
  - Lesion has smooth pushing contour
  - Rare tumors have mixed inverted and exophytic patterns of urothelial papilloma
  - Scattered cells with "degenerative" atypia may be seen
  - Surface urothelium is normal
- Other inverted urothelial neoplasms
  - Urothelium invaginates into lamina propria
  - Forms interconnecting cords/trabeculae with areas of expansile growth or prominent thickening
  - Marked cytologic atypia would warrant classification as carcinoma regardless of architecture

TOP DIFFERENTIAL DIAGNOSES
- Nested urothelial carcinoma
- Large nested carcinoma
- Paraganglioma
- Florid von Brunn nests/cystitis cystica
- Carcinoid tumor

Inverted Papilloma

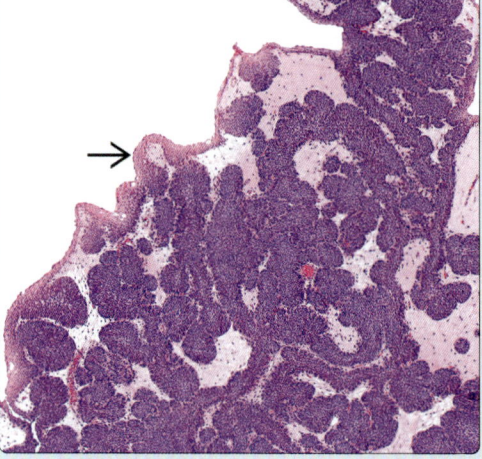

Inverted Papilloma

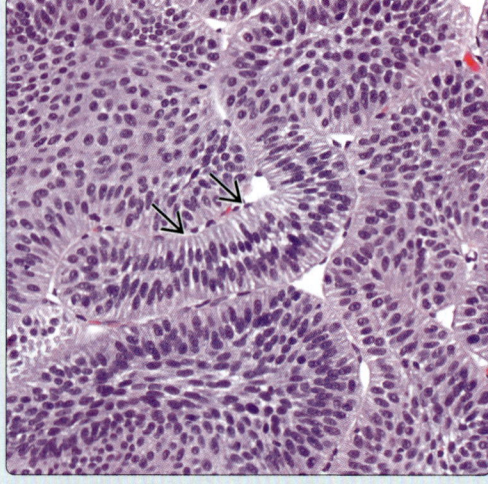

(Left) *Inverted urothelial papilloma is characterized by endophytic growth into the lamina propria with anastomosing thin trabecular architecture. The overlying urothelium is normal ➡. Unlike inverted carcinomas, the cords are thin, without expansile foci.* (Right) *In this high-power field showing inverted urothelial papilloma, there is striking basal palisading that is accentuated by a reverse polarity ➡, reminiscent of ameloblastoma. This feature is more typically seen in papillomas.*

Inverted PUNLMP

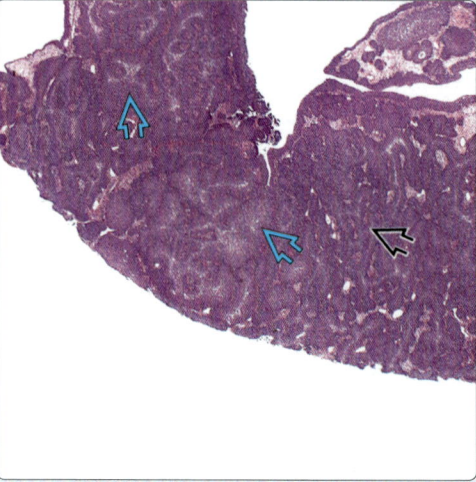

Inverted PUNLMP

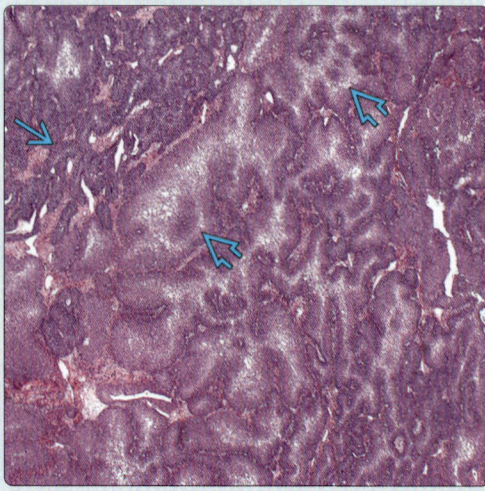

(Left) *In contrast to inverted papilloma, other noninvasive urothelial neoplasms with an inverted/endophytic pattern are 1st detected at low-power magnification by identifying areas where the cords of cells become expanded ➡. In other foci, the cords are identical to inverted papilloma ➡.* (Right) *In this noninvasive PUNLMP with an endophytic growth pattern, the nests and cords are too large ➡ to consider inverted papilloma. Some foci have cords with a caliber allowable in inverted papilloma ➡.*

Inverted Urothelial Neoplasia

TERMINOLOGY

Abbreviations
- Papillary urothelial neoplasm of low malignant potential (PUNLMP)

Synonyms
- Endophytic urothelial lesions

Definitions
- Inverted papilloma
  o Benign urothelial neoplasm with predominantly endophytic growth pattern
    - Involves lamina propria
- Other inverted urothelial neoplasms
  o Noninvasive endophytic pattern of urothelial neoplasia (of any grade) that pushes downward into lamina propria

CLINICAL ISSUES

Epidemiology
- Incidence
  o Inverted papilloma
    - Very uncommon urothelial lesion (1% of urothelial neoplasms)
  o Other inverted urothelial neoplasms
    - Underreported histologic pattern of urothelial neoplasia
    - Admixture with papillary urothelial neoplasia is common
- Age
  o Inverted papilloma
    - 1st to 8th decade
  o Other inverted urothelial neoplasms
    - More common over 50 years of age
- Sex
  o Male predominance (similar to papillary urothelial neoplasia)

Site
- Occurs anywhere along urothelial tract
  o Most common in trigone

Presentation
- Gross or microscopic hematuria

Endoscopic Findings
- Smooth or nodular polypoid structures
  o May be sessile or contain short stalk
- May have concomitant papillary component

Treatment
- Surgical approaches
  o Complete transurethral resection
- Adjuvant therapy
  o Intravesical therapy for high-grade carcinomas
    - Similar to high-grade papillary urothelial carcinoma

Prognosis
- Inverted papilloma
  o Recurrence rate: < 1%
- Other inverted urothelial neoplasms
  o Reported outcome for predominant or pure endophytic neoplasms is limited
  o Assumed similar recurrence and progression potential to papillary counterpart
    - Some have suggested higher recurrence rate

MACROSCOPIC

General Features
- Polypoid with smooth mucosal surface

Size
- Inverted papilloma
  o Most are < 3 cm
  o Rare tumors may be up to 8 cm or more
    - Larger tumors require extensive or complete sampling
- Other inverted urothelial neoplasms
  o Varies widely

MICROSCOPIC

Histologic Features
- Inverted papilloma
  o Urothelium invaginates into lamina propria
    - Forms thin interconnecting cords/trabeculae
  o Surface epithelium is normal
    - Presence of more than occasional exophytic papillae argues for mixed inverted and exophytic patterns of urothelial papilloma
  o Periphery of cords typically show palisading of basal cell nuclei
    - Mitotic figures are rarely seen at basal layer
    - Should be very few in papilloma
  o Lesion has smooth pushing contours
    - Central areas of cords may show cellular spindling
    - Distinct from irregular small nests of invasive carcinoma
    - No stromal reaction
    - Retraction artifact uncommon
  o Epithelial nests may become centrally cystic with cuboidal epithelial lining
    - Cystitis cystica or cystitis glandularis-like patterns
  o Bland cytologic features
    - Scattered cells with "degenerative" atypia or nuclear multilobation may be seen
  o Rare cases may contain foamy or vacuolated cytoplasm
  o Nonkeratinizing squamous metaplasia may also be present
- Inverted PUNLMP
  o Areas of expansive growth
    - Cords become thicker than in inverted papilloma
    - Expanded foci have bland nuclear features and ordered arrangement
      □ Central areas of expanded nests may have stellate reticulum-like appearance, similar to papilloma
      □ Basal palisading may be preserved
  o May be admixed with areas identical to inverted papilloma
- Inverted low-grade carcinoma
  o Areas of expansile growth

Inverted Urothelial Neoplasia

- Cords become thicker to nodular than in inverted papilloma
- Urothelial cells in expanded foci have architectural disorder
  - Cytologic atypia below threshold for high-grade designation
- Inverted high-grade carcinoma
  - Areas of expansile growth
    - Cords become thicker to nodular than in inverted papilloma
  - Defined by presence of high-grade cytology
  - Associated invasion should be assessed more closely in high-grade carcinoma

Predominant Pattern/Injury Type
- Inverted trabeculae/cord

Predominant Cell/Compartment Type
- Epithelial, urothelial

DIFFERENTIAL DIAGNOSIS

Invasive Urothelial Carcinoma, Typical Type
- Smaller, more irregular angulated nests of invasion
  - May or may not show stromal reaction
- More cytoplasmic eosinophilia common (i.e., "paradoxical maturation")
- Surrounding retraction artifact also common

Nested Urothelial Carcinoma
- More irregular distribution of urothelial nests
- Trabecular growth pattern not predominant
- More expansile nests may be present
- Irregular invasion of lamina propria/muscularis propria is common
- Surrounding retraction spaces may be seen
- Admixed microcystic pattern of carcinoma not uncommon

Large Nested Carcinoma
- Similar features to more common nested carcinoma
- Larger size of invasive nests closely mimics noninvasive endophytic pattern
- Low-power architecture critical to recognition
  - Less corded growth
  - Irregular distribution throughout lamina propria
  - Involvement of muscularis propria is diagnostic

Paraganglioma
- Nested (zellballen) pattern
- Sclerotic stromal pattern may create less of nested architecture
- Often show marked variation in nuclear size (i.e., "endocrine anaplasia")
- Immunoreactivity for synaptophysin and chromogranin
  - S-100 protein positive sustentacular cells
  - Cytokeratin negative in most cases
- Immunohistochemical pitfall
  - Characteristically has nuclear GATA3 expression
    - Overlap with urothelial cells

Florid von Brunn Nests/Cystitis Cystica
- Rounded nests of urothelium
  - Often lobular distribution
  - Lacks trabecular or cord-like pattern
  - Nests are more architecturally complex in ureter and renal pelvis
- Distinction from cystitis cystica-like pattern of inverted papilloma may be arbitrary in some cases

Carcinoid Tumor
- May have similar trabecular/nested architecture
  - Often more complex architecture with acinar or cribriform component
- Neuroendocrine type nuclear features
  - Stippled chromatin
- Immunoreactivity for synaptophysin &/or chromogranin

DIAGNOSTIC CHECKLIST

Clinically Relevant Pathologic Features
- Inverted papilloma
  - May be cystoscopically similar to other bladder neoplasms
  - Clinically benign despite unusual morphologic patterns (e.g., spindling)
- Inverted urothelial neoplasia should be distinguished from invasive carcinoma

Pathologic Interpretation Pearls
- Urothelial carcinoma with endophytic growth pattern must be considered when diagnosing inverted papilloma
  - Contain more expansile trabeculae or solid areas
  - Greater degree of cytologic atypia often present
- Inverted papilloma-like areas may be present in other endophytic lesions of higher grade/stage
- As with papillary neoplasms (particularly high-grade subset), careful evaluation for stromal invasion is critical

SELECTED REFERENCES

1. Maxwell JP et al: Long-term outcome of primary Papillary Urothelial Neoplasm of Low Malignant Potential (PUNLMP) including PUNLMP with inverted growth. Diagn Pathol. 10:3, 2015
2. Chen YB et al: Primary carcinoid tumors of the urinary bladder and prostatic urethra: a clinicopathologic study of 6 cases. Am J Surg Pathol. 35(3):442-6, 2011
3. Hodges KB et al: Urothelial lesions with inverted growth patterns: histogenesis, molecular genetic findings, differential diagnosis and clinical management. BJU Int. 107(4):532-7, 2011
4. Albores-Saavedra J et al: Inverted urothelial papilloma of the urinary bladder with focal papillary pattern: a previously undescribed feature. Ann Diagn Pathol. 13(3):158-61, 2009
5. Jones TD et al: Urothelial carcinoma with an inverted growth pattern can be distinguished from inverted papilloma by fluorescence in situ hybridization, immunohistochemistry, and morphologic analysis. Am J Surg Pathol. 31(12):1861-7, 2007
6. Fine SW et al: Inverted urothelial papillomas with foamy or vacuolated cytoplasm. Hum Pathol. 37(12):1577-82, 2006
7. Sung MT et al: Natural history of urothelial inverted papilloma. Cancer. 107(11):2622-7, 2006
8. Broussard JN et al: Atypia in inverted urothelial papillomas: pathology and prognostic significance. Hum Pathol. 35(12):1499-504, 2004
9. Amin MB et al: Urothelial transitional cell carcinoma with endophytic growth patterns: a discussion of patterns of invasion and problems associated with assessment of invasion in 18 cases. Am J Surg Pathol. 21(9):1057-68, 1997

Inverted Urothelial Neoplasia

Inverted Papilloma: Anastomosing Cords

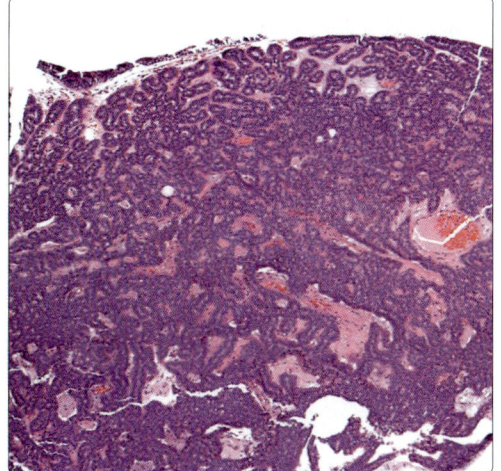

Inverted Papilloma: Basal Palisading

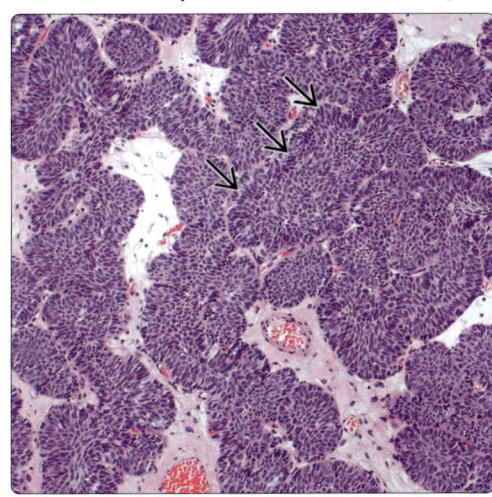

(Left) At scanning magnification, the endophytic growth of thin, anastomosing urothelial cords/trabeculae may be appreciated in this example of inverted urothelial papilloma. (Right) This typical inverted urothelial papilloma of the urinary bladder shows the usual endophytic growth into the lamina propria, distinct trabecular architecture, and nuclear palisading ➡ at the periphery of the cords/nests. Lesions appear alarmingly hyperchromatic at low power due to scant cytoplasm.

Inverted Papilloma: Anastomosing Cords

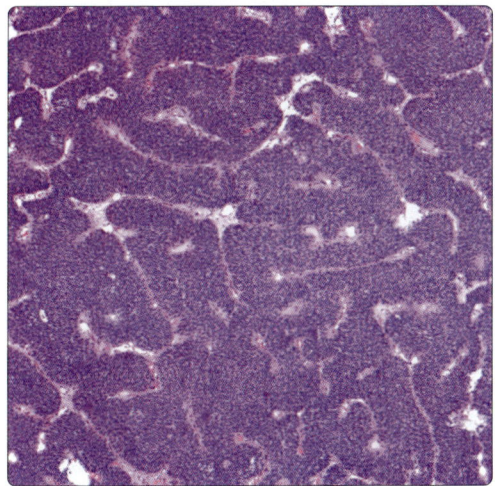

Inverted Papilloma: Trabecular Growth and Palisading

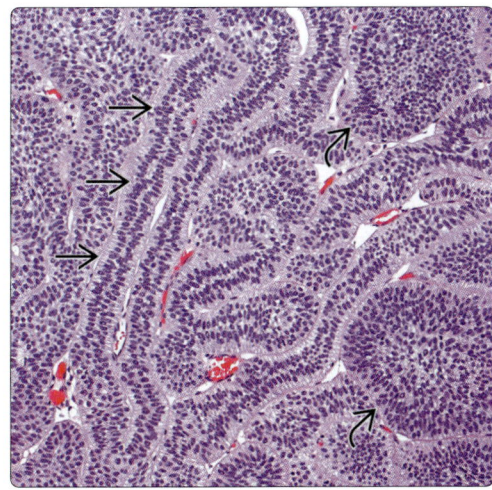

(Left) Inverted urothelial papilloma commonly displays well-formed invaginated epithelial trabeculae/cords that create an anastomosing network. The relatively thin cords aid in the distinction from endophytic urothelial neoplasm of low malignant potential or carcinoma. (Right) This example of inverted urothelial papilloma has a striking trabecular architecture with prominent basal palisading ➡, a feature typical of inverted papilloma. In addition, there is an admixture of more rounded nests ➡.

Inverted Papilloma: Central Spindling

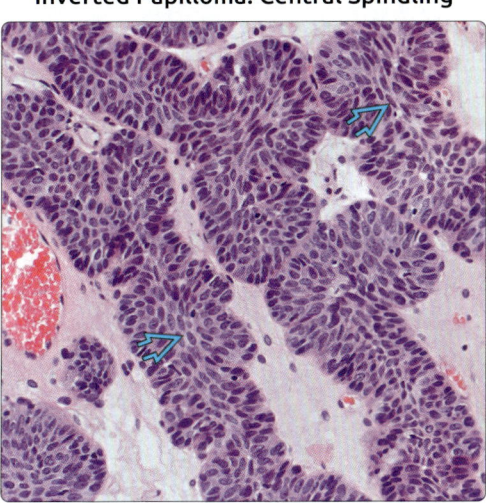

Inverted Papilloma: Bland Cytology

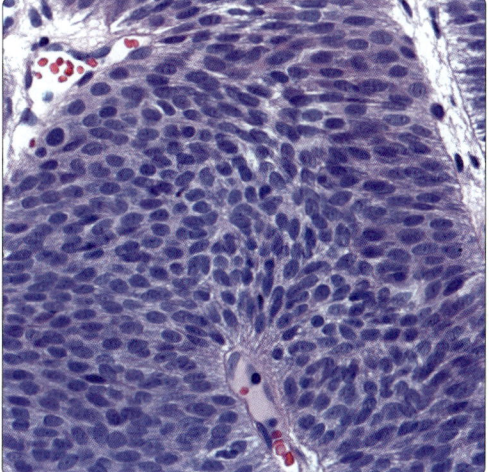

(Left) On high-power examination of this inverted urothelial papilloma, the bland cytologic features of the urothelial cells within the thin trabeculae are evident. In addition, the central cells have subtle early spindling ➡. (Right) This inverted urothelial papilloma demonstrates the characteristic bland monomorphic nuclear features at high-power examination. Mitotic figures and apoptotic debris are typically absent, in contrast to urothelial carcinoma.

Inverted Urothelial Neoplasia

Inverted Papilloma: Central Spindling

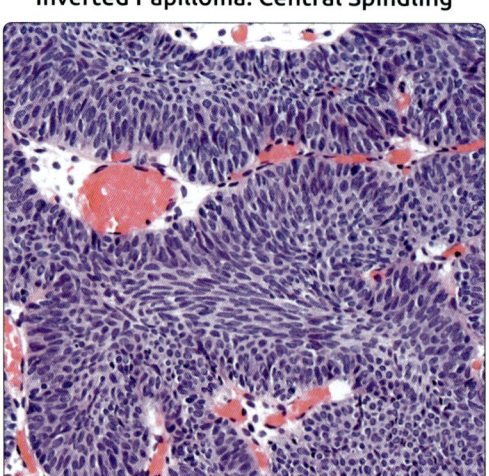

(Left) This inverted urothelial papilloma has characteristic trabecular growth and also demonstrates prominent basal palisading and central spindling of the neoplastic cells, features that are commonly seen. (Right) This high-power photomicrograph highlights the basal palisading and central streaming/spindling of the neoplastic urothelial cells, features that are characteristic of inverted urothelial papilloma.

Inverted Papilloma: Cystitis Cystica/Glandularis Pattern

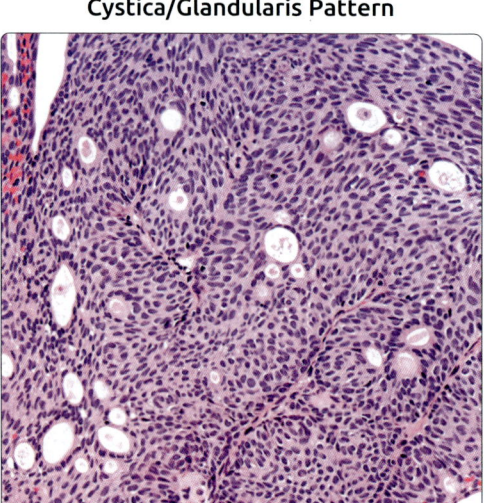

(Left) Inverted urothelial papillomas may have areas with luminal formation that are reminiscent of cystitis glandularis or cystitis cystica. (Right) This high-power photomicrograph of an inverted urothelial papilloma highlights scattered lumina with surrounding neoplastic cells containing apical cytoplasm. This cystitis glandularis-like pattern is well described in a subset of inverted papillomas.

Inverted Papilloma: Stellate Reticulum Appearance

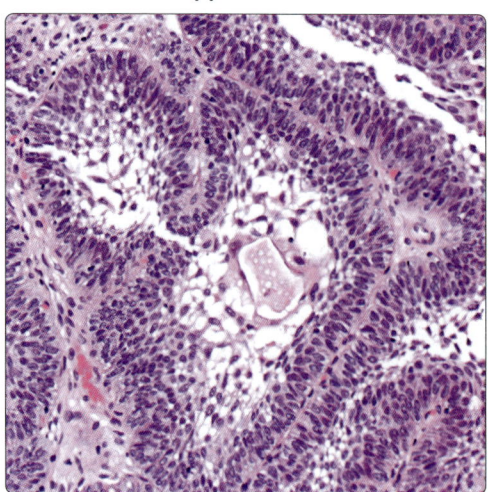

Inverted Papilloma: Degenerative Atypia

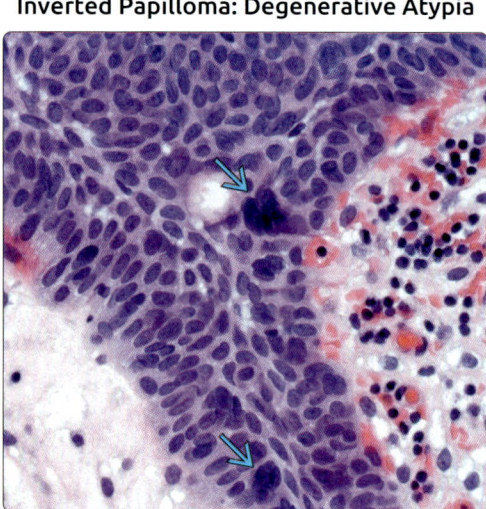

(Left) Rare examples of inverted urothelial papilloma, as seen in this H&E, have endophytic nests with central edema creating a stellate reticulum-like appearance. In this example, the basal palisading is also prominent. (Right) Inverted urothelial papillomas occasionally have scattered, enlarged multilobated cells with a degenerative appearance ➡. This feature should not be regarded as high-grade cytologic atypia; therefore, it should not warrant a diagnosis of carcinoma.

Inverted Urothelial Neoplasia

Inverted PUNLMP: Expanded Endophytic Nests

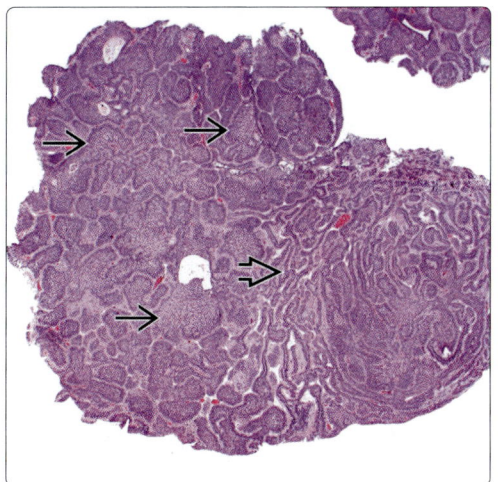

Inverted PUNLMP: Expanded Endophytic Cords

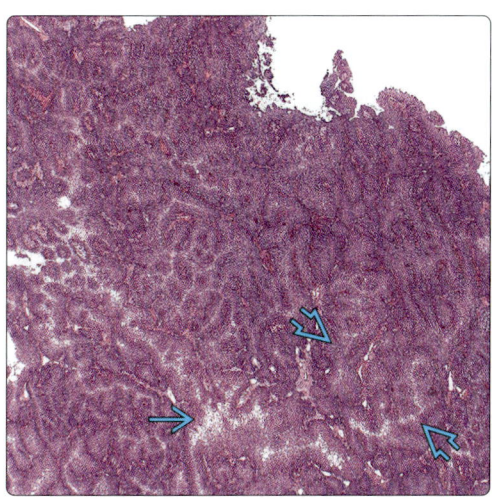

(Left) In this inverted PUNLMP, tissue fragments appear polypoid, but the endophytic and corded growth is distinct from a papillary tumor. Expansile areas ➡ with loss of thin cord-like growth ➡ are distinct from inverted papilloma. (Right) In this example of inverted PUNLMP, areas of epithelial expansion are identified ➡ that would preclude a diagnosis of inverted papilloma. In some foci, central clearing within the expanded areas correspond to a stellate-reticulum-like pattern ➡.

Inverted PUNLMP: Retained Palisading

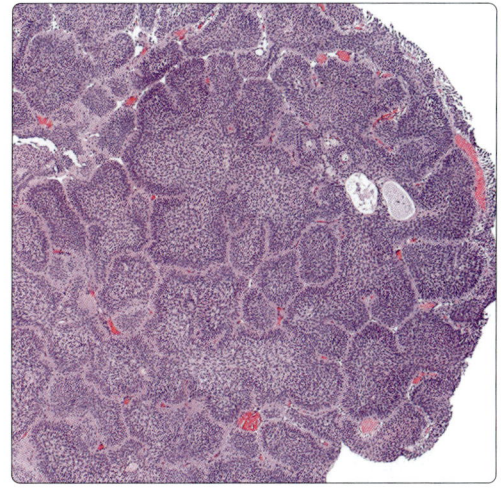

Inverted PUNLMP: Bland Cytology

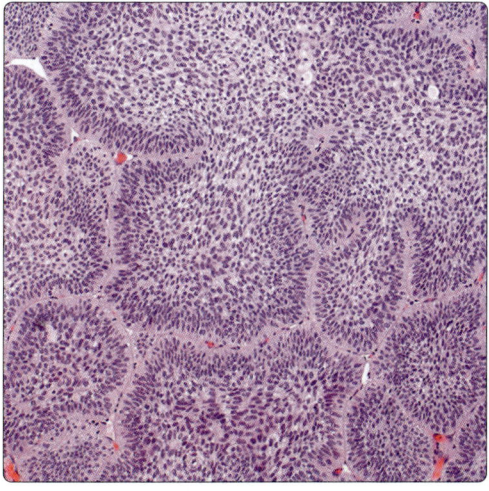

(Left) The endophytic epithelium in this polypoid bladder neoplasm does not have the thin cords characteristic of inverted papilloma. The urothelial nests are expanded, but there is retained nuclear palisading and the central areas have bland cytology and an ordered arrangement. (Right) On high-power magnification, these expanded nests show a level of nuclear cytology and cellular organization that are acceptable for a diagnosis as inverted/endophytic PUNLMP.

Inverted PUNLMP: Expanded Cords

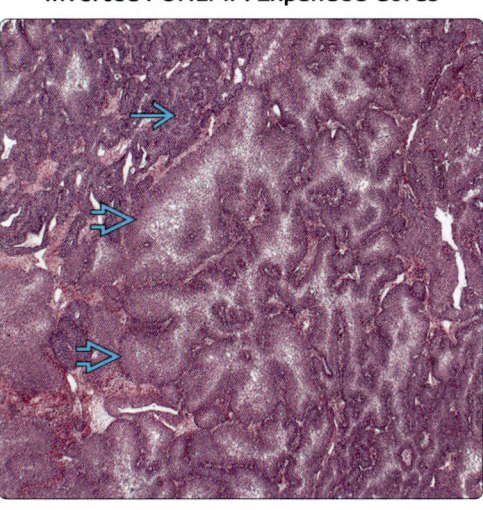

Inverted PUNLMP: Expanded Edematous Foci

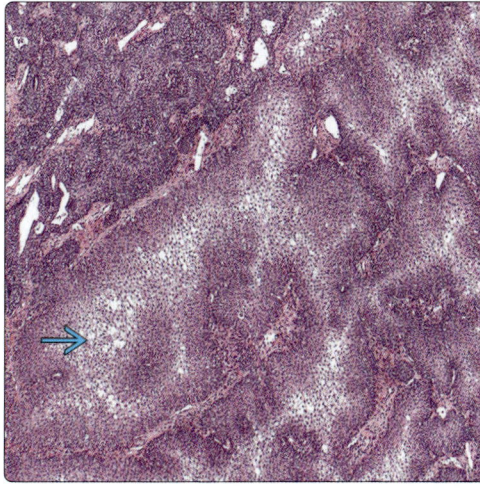

(Left) This degree of bulbous expansion of the cords/trabeculae ➡ of urothelium would preclude consideration of inverted papilloma. There are focal inverted papilloma-like areas ➡. (Right) The expanded nests have central clearing as the cells become less tightly arranged with an edematous appearance ➡, a feature not uncommon in inverted PUNLMP. The cords are too expanded for a papilloma diagnosis. Absence of cytologic atypia argues against a carcinoma diagnosis.

Inverted Urothelial Neoplasia

Inverted Low-Grade Carcinoma: Expanded Cords

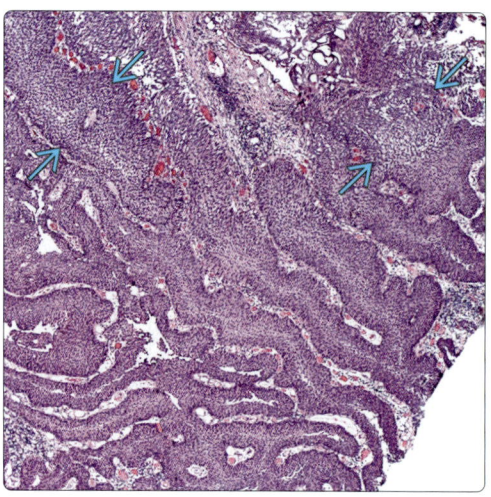

Inverted Low-Grade Carcinoma: Markedly Expanded Endophytic Nests

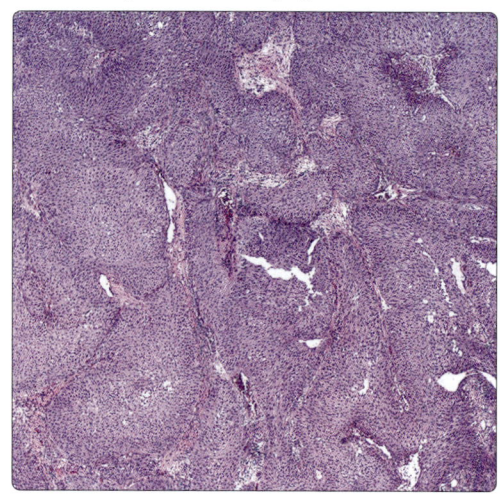

(Left) This endophytic urothelial carcinoma displays prominent trabecular growth that has significant morphologic overlap with inverted papilloma; however, it shows a greater expansion (width) of the cords ➡ than is typically seen in inverted papilloma. (Right) Inverted papilloma would not be considered here because the cords are not thin. Differential diagnosis would include large nested carcinoma, which would be distinguished by assessing the lower power epithelial distribution and interface with the stroma.

Inverted Low-Grade Carcinoma: Markedly Expanded Endophytic Nests

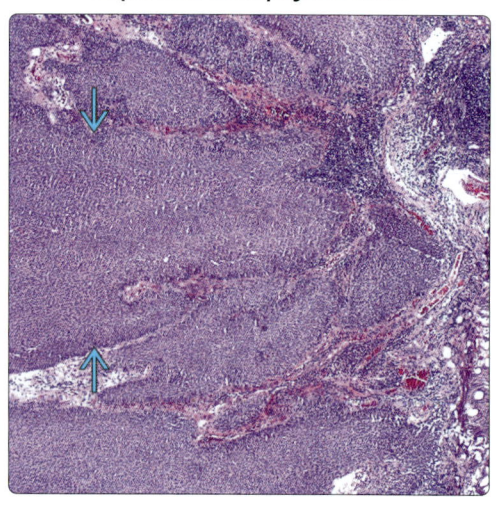

Inverted Low-Grade Carcinoma: Cellular Disorder

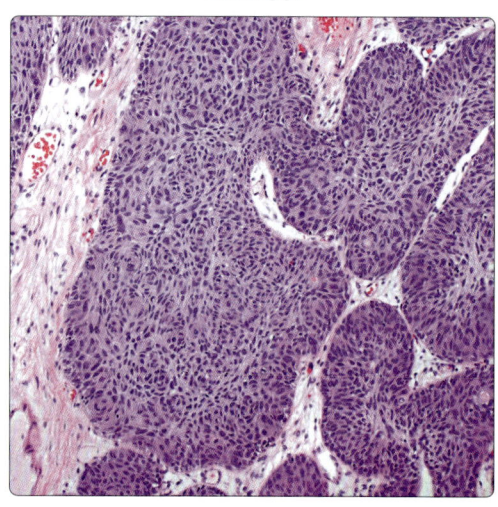

(Left) Despite the endophytic architecture of this neoplasm, the degree of expansile and solid growth ➡ is diagnostic of endophytic urothelial carcinoma. (Right) This endophytic low-grade urothelial carcinoma shows expansion of trabeculae and has a very disordered urothelium with loss of polarization to the surrounding basement membrane. The overall smooth contours of the urothelial proliferation argue for endophytic growth rather than destructive invasion.

Inverted Low-Grade Carcinoma: Subtle Cellular Disorder

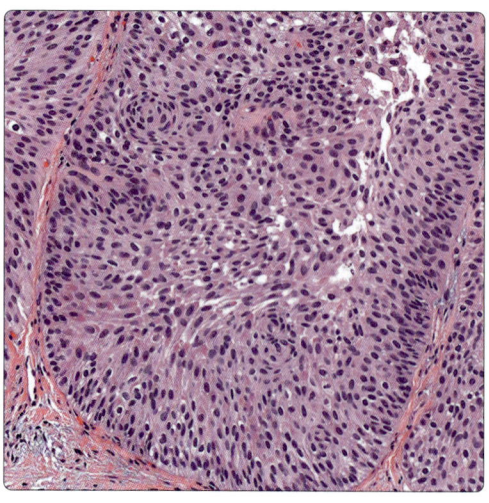

Inverted Carcinoma: Low-Grade Cytology

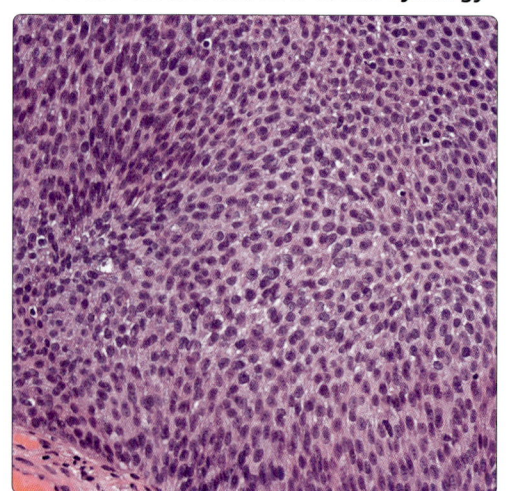

(Left) While inverted PUNLMP might be considered, this case exceeds the threshold for cellular disorder with random distribution of the cells. This case would be classified as noninvasive endophytic urothelial carcinoma, low grade. (Right) On high-power magnification, these nuclei are rather monomorphic. This degree of cytologic atypia based on nuclear size, nuclear chromatin distribution, and nuclear variability does not meet the threshold for a high-grade designation.

Inverted Urothelial Neoplasia

Inverted High-Grade Carcinoma: Expanded Endophytic Cords

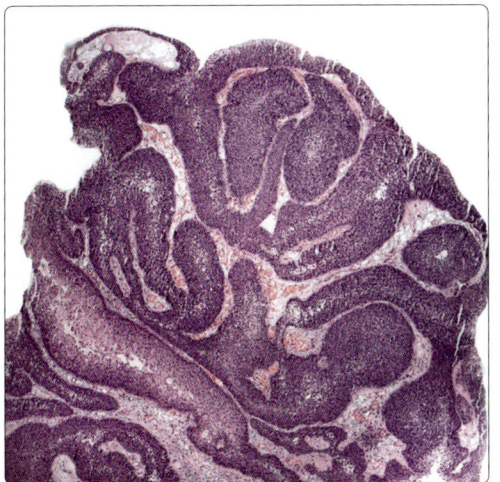

Inverted High-Grade Carcinoma: Expanded Endophytic Nests

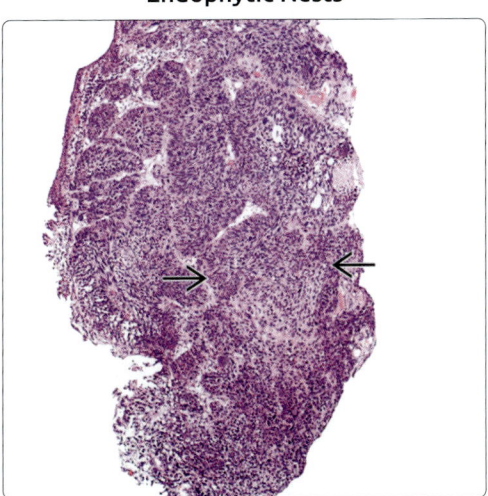

(Left) The anastomosing cords of urothelium with rounded edges are characteristic of a noninvasive endophytic pattern of urothelial neoplasia. The expansion of the cords would preclude a diagnosis of inverted papilloma. *(Right)* In this endophytic urothelial neoplasm identified in a transurethral resection specimen there is some expansile solid growth ➡, which should prompt consideration of a carcinoma. Cytologic features of malignancy were present at higher power.

Inverted Carcinoma: High-Grade Cytology

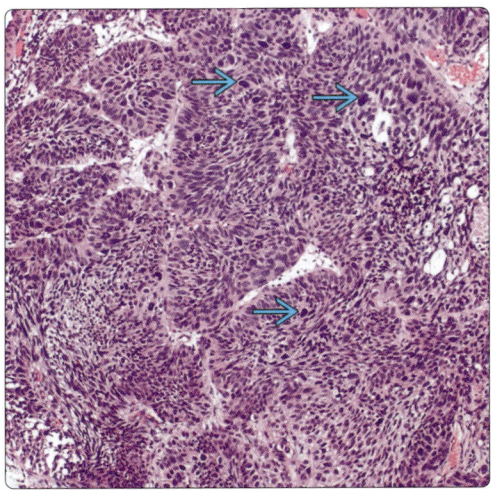

Inverted Carcinoma: High-Grade Cytology

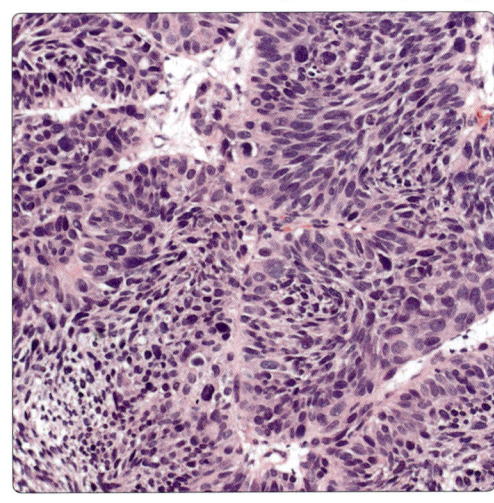

(Left) Even at low-power examination, scattered nuclear pleomorphism ➡ may be appreciable in high-grade endophytic urothelial carcinomas. The nests and cords are more expansile than typical of inverted urothelial papilloma. *(Right)* On high-power magnification the neoplastic cells show marked nucleomegaly, nuclear hyperchromasia, and some degree of pleomorphism. These features are diagnostic of a high-grade carcinoma. The atypia is not degenerate in nature.

Inverted Carcinoma: High-Grade Cytology

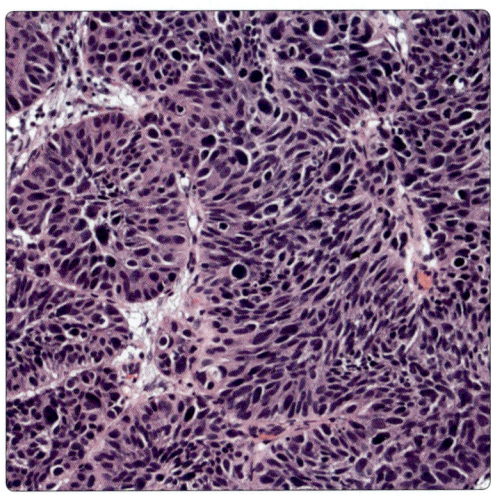

Inverted Carcinoma: High-Grade Cytology

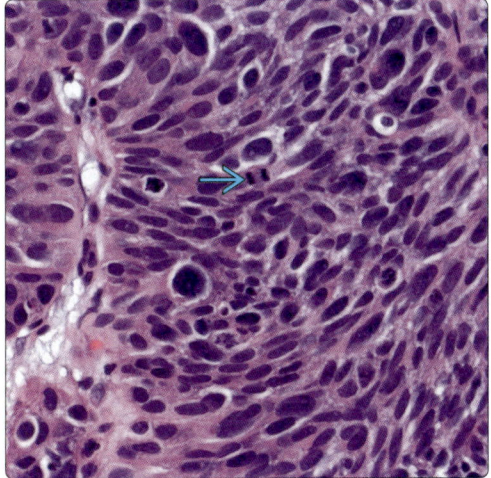

(Left) While this neoplasm had a "basaloid" appearance at low-power magnification, the degree of nucleomegaly and the marked variation in nuclear size and shape are well beyond the threshold for classification as high-grade carcinoma. *(Right)* On higher power examination, significant nuclear pleomorphism is evident in this high-grade endophytic urothelial carcinoma. In addition, there is loss of polarity with disorganization of the neoplastic cells within the nests and mitotic activity ➡.

Inverted Urothelial Neoplasia

(Left) When faced with a noninvasive endophytic/inverted urothelial carcinoma (especially if high grade), a careful assessment for areas of stromal invasion should be performed. (Right) As in other flat or papillary urothelial carcinomas, invasion is often characterized by small nests of tumor cells within retraction spaces ⇨. As seen in this example, these are often identifiable at low-power screening evaluation.

Noninvasive Carcinoma With Endophytic/Inverted Pattern

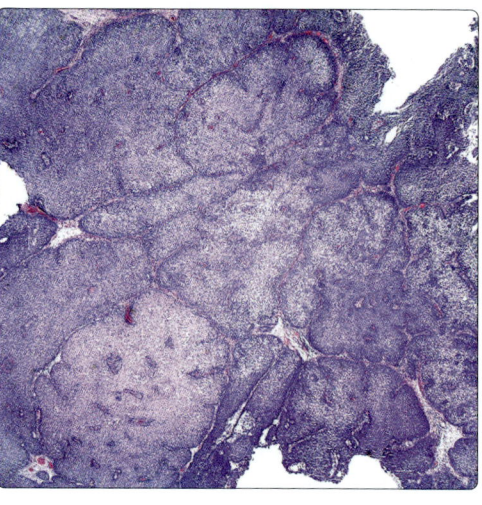

Stromal Invasion

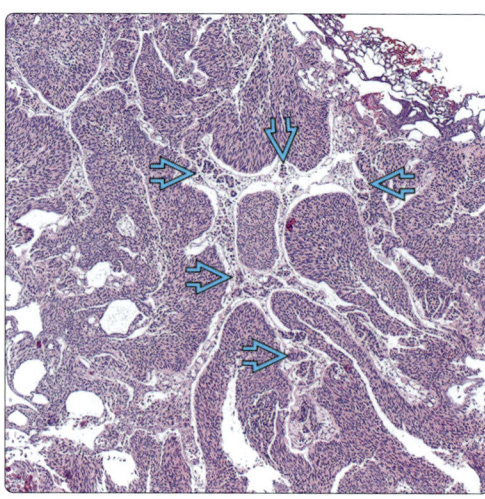

(Left) These nests and clusters of urothelial cells ⇨, some within retraction spaces, are diagnostic of stromal invasion (lamina propria invasion in this example). The large rounded aggregates of carcinoma cells ⇨ represent the noninvasive endophytic component. (Right) This focus of detached clusters/nests of urothelial carcinoma with associated cleft-like retraction spaces ⇨ is characteristic of focal invasion.

Stromal Invasion Admixed With Noninvasive Component

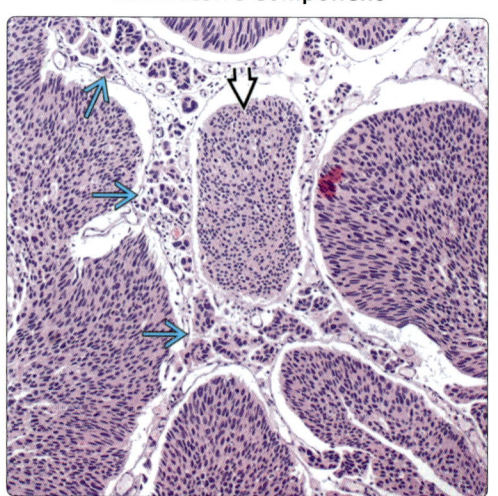

Stromal Invasion: Retraction

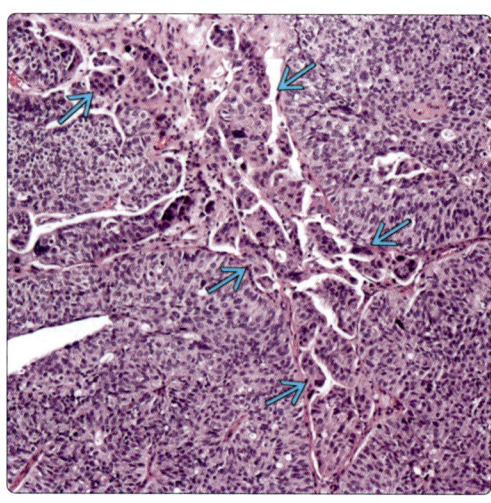

(Left) In contrast to the noninvasive endophytic component ⇨, the small irregular clusters ⇨ with a subtle degree of cytoplasmic eosinophilia represent a small focus of stromal (lamina propria) invasion. (Right) The contours of the small cords of urothelial carcinoma cells are too irregular for a noninvasive focus ⇨. In addition, there are admixed detached clusters of cells with cytoplasmic eosinophilia that should strongly suggest invasion. The noninvasive component shows larger, more rounded aggregates ⇨.

Stromal Invasion: Cytoplasmic Eosinophilia

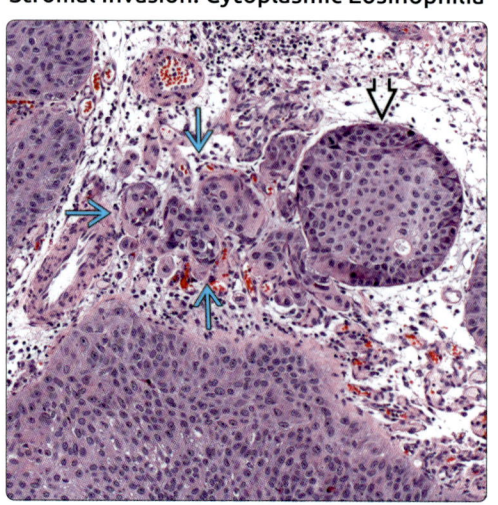

Stromal Invasion: Irregular Contours

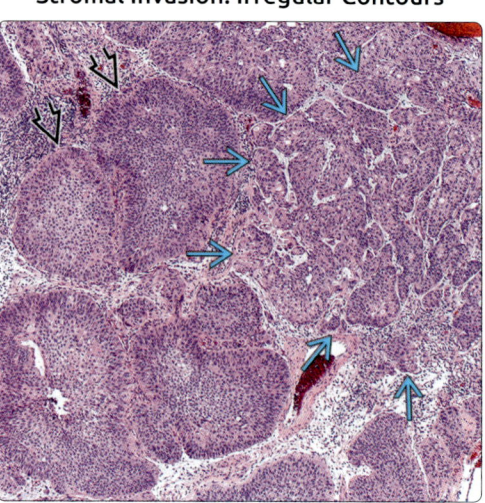

Inverted Urothelial Neoplasia

von Brunn Nests vs. Inverted Papilloma

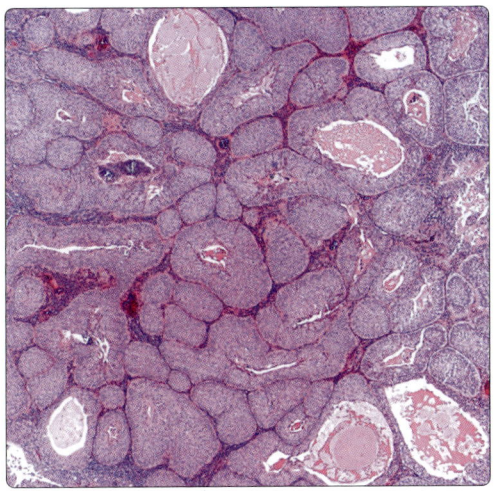

Paraganglioma

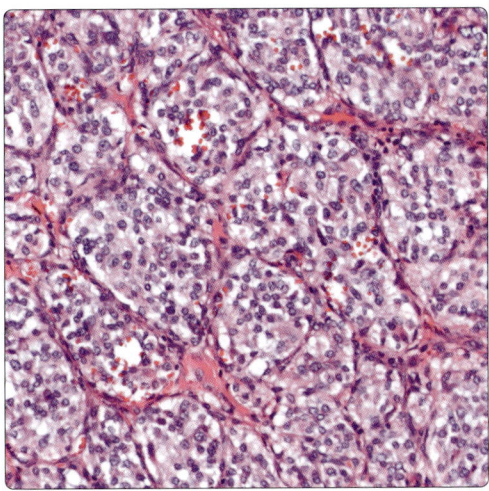

(Left) As seen in this example, the distinction between inverted papilloma with a cystitis cystica-like pattern and florid von Brunn nests/cystitis cystica may be arbitrary and suffers from interobserver variability. (Right) Paraganglioma is characterized by neoplastic cells randomly distributed within nests; inverted papilloma would be expected to show a distinctly palisaded basal layer. A sinusoidal architecture and synaptophysin reactivity is confirmatory.

Carcinoid Tumor

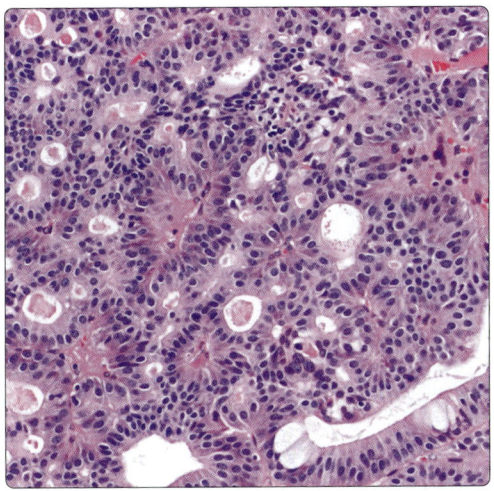

Synaptophysin: Carcinoid Tumor

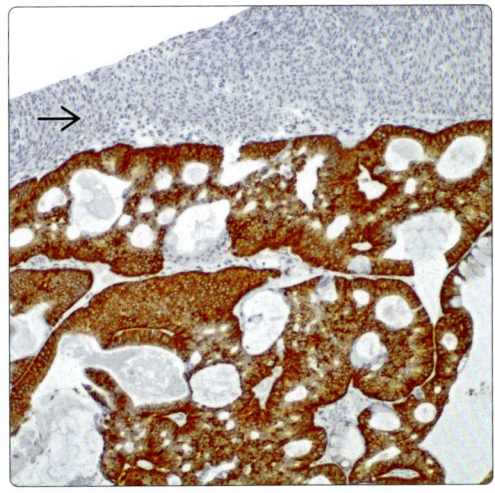

(Left) This trabecular and cystitis cystica-like growth pattern in a rare carcinoid tumor of the urinary bladder may suggest the diagnostic possibility of inverted papilloma with cystitis cystica-like pattern. (Right) Strong, diffuse synaptophysin reactivity is seen in this carcinoid tumor, but negative in the overlying urothelium ⇒. Neuroendocrine immunohistochemical markers may be very useful in diagnostically challenging superficial biopsies.

Invasive Nested Urothelial Carcinoma

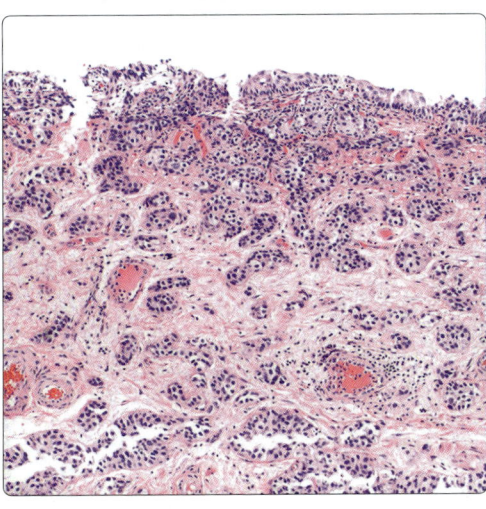

Invasive Nested Urothelial Carcinoma

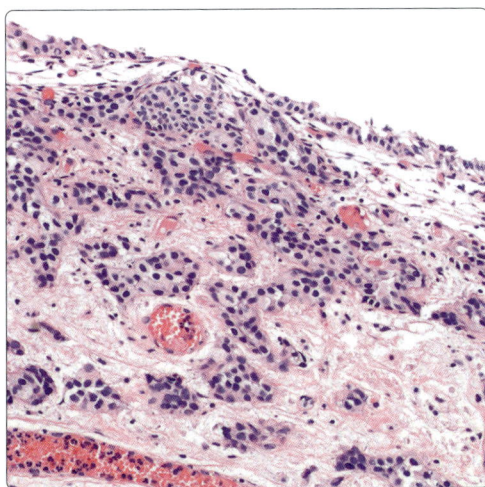

(Left) These urothelial nests do not have the anastomosing cord-like arrangement that is typical of a noninvasive endophytic urothelial neoplasm. The random distribution with abundant intervening stroma strongly suggests the nested variant of invasive urothelial carcinoma. (Right) On high-power magnification, the cytologic features of invasive nested urothelial carcinoma are deceptively bland. The stromal response seen here is not typical of invasive urothelial carcinoma.

Invasive Urothelial Carcinoma

KEY FACTS

TERMINOLOGY
- Urothelial carcinoma that invades beyond basement membrane

CLINICAL ISSUES
- Invasion into lamina propria usually managed with intravesical therapy
- Invasion into muscularis propria usually managed by radical cystectomy; radiation therapy in some centers
- Neoadjuvant or adjuvant chemotherapy may be offered

MICROSCOPIC
- Small nests, clusters, &/or single cells within lamina propria
- Surrounding retraction artifact is common
- Other stromal reactions include desmoplasia, sclerosis, myxoid change and inflammation
- May have irregular, jagged tongues of epithelium in continuity with overlying noninvasive component

TOP DIFFERENTIAL DIAGNOSES
- Prostatic adenocarcinoma involving bladder
- Gynecologic carcinomas involving bladder
- Paraganglioma
- Inverted patterns of noninvasive urothelial neoplasia
- Nephrogenic adenoma
- Pseudocarcinomatous hyperplasia

DIAGNOSTIC CHECKLIST
- Important to state depth of invasion by clearly reporting invasion of lamina propria or muscularis propria
- Recognizing heterogeneity of urinary bladder microanatomy is important to avoid overstaging
- Several variant forms or aberrant squamous or glandular differentiation may exist

Invasive Urothelial Carcinoma
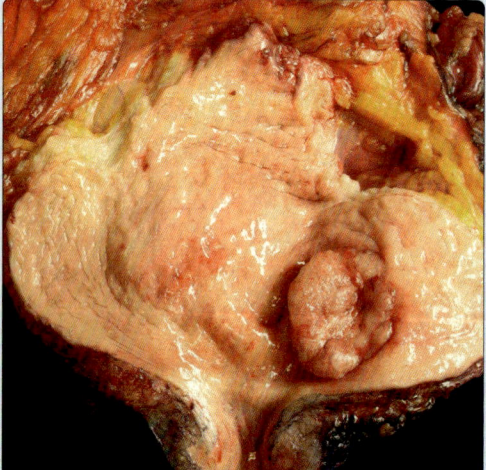

Invasive Urothelial Carcinoma
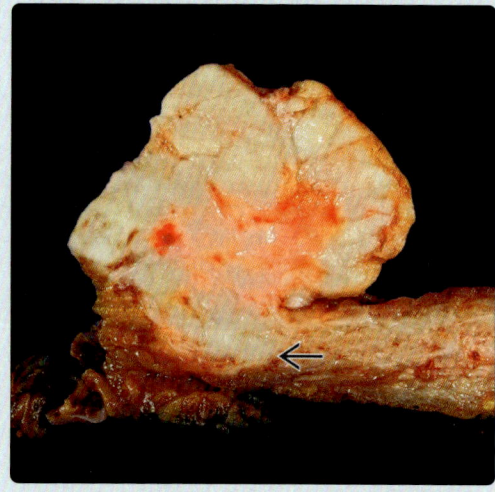

(Left) Invasive urothelial carcinoma presents as a solitary tumor on the side wall of the bladder adjacent to the left ureteral opening. The remainder of the urothelial mucosa is mildly erythematous but otherwise largely unremarkable. *(Right)* Cut section of the bladder wall from a pelvic exenteration specimen is shown. Note the presence of a large tumor with yellow-tan fleshy cut surface protruding into the bladder cavity. Note the deeply invasive border of the tumor into the outer half of the bladder wall ➡.

Papillary Urothelial Carcinoma
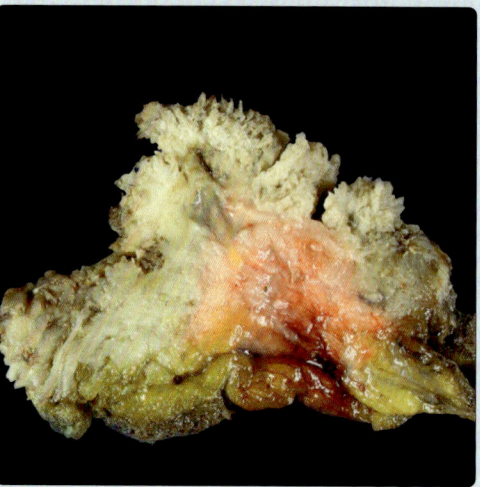

Multifocal Urothelial Carcinoma
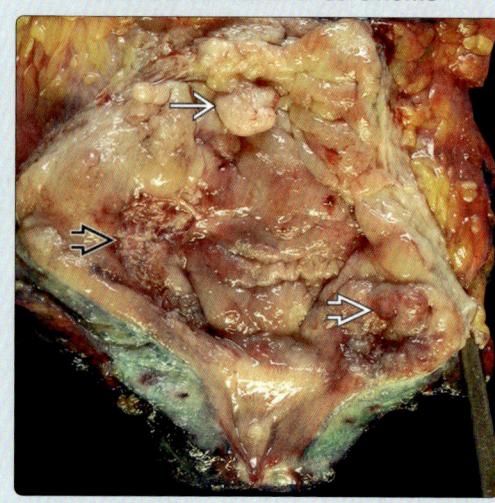

(Left) Cross section shows a bulky papillary tumor covering much of the bladder mucosal surface and filling the bladder cavity. Although this tumor was not deeply invasive, the large size could only be managed by radical cystectomy. *(Right)* In this cystoprostatectomy specimen, there are multiple invasive urothelial carcinomas with exophytic ➡, endophytic ➡, and ulcerated ➡ appearances. There were other smaller tumors identified microscopically that were not recognized grossly.

Invasive Urothelial Carcinoma

TERMINOLOGY

Synonyms
- Invasive transitional cell carcinoma

Definitions
- Urothelial carcinoma that invades beyond basement membrane

CLINICAL ISSUES

Treatment
- Surgical approaches
  - Transurethral resection of visible tumor
    - Also required for accurate assessment of presence and extent of invasion
  - Invasion into lamina propria usually managed conservatively with intravesical therapy
    - Bacillus Calmette-Guérin
    - Mitomycin and other intravesical therapies
    - Radical cystectomy in select patients with high-risk features (large size, recurrent or refractory disease, tumor multifocality, extensive CIS, etc.)
  - Invasion into muscularis propria usually managed by radical cystectomy ± chemotherapy (adjuvant or neoadjuvant)
    - Radiation therapy consideration in certain situations (palliative or bladder preservation strategies)

Prognosis
- Stage dependent
  - Deeply invasive tumors (pT2 or greater/muscularis propria and beyond); poor prognosis
  - Superficially invasive tumors (pT1/lamina propria); may have excellent prognosis

MACROSCOPIC

General Features
- May be papillary, polypoid, nodular, solid, or ulcerated
- Background urothelium may be normal or erythematous
- Solitary or multifocal

MICROSCOPIC

Key Descriptors
- Predominant cell/compartment type: Epithelial, urothelial

Patterns of Invasion
- Small nests or clusters/single cells within lamina propria
  - Surrounding retraction artifact is common
  - Other stromal reactions include desmoplasia, sclerosis, myxoid change and inflammation
  - Microinvasion: Focal invasion of single cells or small clusters, < 2 mm in depth
- May have more abundant eosinophilic cytoplasm than adjacent noninvasive component
  - Paradoxical maturation/differentiation
- May have irregular, jagged tongues of epithelium in continuity with overlying noninvasive component
- Most invasive urothelial carcinomas are high grade
  - Exceptions are nested and tubular variants
- Grade of invasive component does not affect prognosis as all have recurring and metastatic potential

ANCILLARY TESTS

Immunohistochemistry
- General comments
  - Usually immunoreactive for p63, CK7, CK20, thrombomodulin and HMCK(34βE12)
    - Low specificity
  - Uroplakin-2, uroplakin-3, GATA3, and S100p are more specific markers of urothelial lineage
    - Relatively low sensitivity (except GATA3)
  - Smoothelin immunostains may be helpful in distinguishing muscularis mucosae from muscularis propria
    - Weak, patchy staining in muscularis mucosae
    - Strong, diffuse reactivity in muscularis propria
      - May be useful when tumor obliterates muscularis propria and only scant residual muscle is seen
  - Cytokeratin stains may be useful in identifying subtle foci of invasive carcinoma
    - Should not be confused with cytokeratin positive myofibroblasts
      - Spindled cells with tapered cytoplasmic processes
      - Also coexpress actin-sm

DIFFERENTIAL DIAGNOSIS

Other Nonurothelial Neoplasms
- Prostatic adenocarcinoma involving bladder
  - Monomorphic round cells with prominent nucleoli
  - May have gland/acinar formation
  - Immunoreactive for PSA &/or PAP
  - Usually negative for p63 and HMCK(34βE12)
  - CK7/CK20 immunophenotype is highly variable in high-grade prostatic adenocarcinomas
- Gynecologic carcinomas involving bladder
  - Cervical squamous cell carcinomas may mimic urothelial carcinoma with squamous differentiation
  - High-grade uterine carcinomas may mimic poorly differentiated urothelial carcinoma or urothelial carcinoma with glandular differentiation
    - Often express ER &/or WT1
  - Clinical/radiographic correlation is critical
- Paraganglioma
  - Nested aggregates of epithelioid cells
    - Often have closely associated surrounding vascular network
  - Sclerotic/hyalinized examples may be pseudoinfiltrative
    - Closely mimics invasive carcinoma
  - May have scattered pleomorphic cells
    - Endocrine anaplasia
  - Immunophenotype is distinctive
    - Positive for synaptophysin but not cytokeratins
    - S100(+) sustentacular cells may be seen
- Inverted patterns of noninvasive urothelial neoplasia
  - Crowded endophytic nests or trabeculae of urothelium with sharp, rounded contours
    - Range from inverted papilloma to inverted high-grade carcinoma, based on cytologic features

Invasive Urothelial Carcinoma

- No surrounding retraction or other stromal changes
- No jagged nests

Benign Mimics
- Nephrogenic adenoma, generally mimicker of glandular lesions
  - Small tubules in lamina propria, often with thick basement membrane, lined by flattened or hobnail cells
  - Rare diffuse or solid pattern may closely mimic malignancy
  - Diffuse nuclear pax-2/pax-8 immunoreactivity
  - May also stain with AMACR (P504s)
- Pseudocarcinomatous hyperplasia
  - Often associated with prior radiation or chemotherapy
  - Rare cases have no prior therapy
  - Squamoid epithelial nests in lamina propria may be jagged but are associated with fibrin and blood vessels
    - Epithelial aggregates characteristically envelop blood vessels that are obliterated by fibrin
  - Lamina propria is often hemorrhagic with extravasated fibrin
  - Other radiation-associated changes may be seen such as stromal cell atypia
- Cystitis cystica/glandularis
  - Invaginated urothelial nests with superficial location in lamina propria
    - Rounded contours of nests
    - May have lobular architecture
  - Sharp border with lamina propria at base
  - No stromal reaction
  - Intestinal type may have associated mucin extravasation
    - May closely mimic malignancy clinically

DIAGNOSTIC CHECKLIST

Clinically Relevant Pathologic Features
- Hypertrophied patterns of muscularis mucosae are not restricted to men with prostatic hyperplasia

Pathologic Interpretation Pearls
- Recognizing heterogeneity of urinary bladder microanatomy is important to avoid overstaging
  - Morphology of muscularis mucosae is more variable than originally reported
- Stromal retraction should not be overinterpreted as vascular invasion
  - In some centers, presence of vascular invasion may affect clinical management (controversial)

STAGING

Difficult Staging Distinctions
- Noninvasive urothelial carcinoma involving prostatic glands
  - Rounded contours of epithelial nests
    - May be expansile
    - No irregular jagged nests or small nests with surrounding retraction
    - No stromal response
  - May have residual basal cells or adjacent normal prostatic glands
  - Because of thick fibromuscular stroma in this location, may mimic muscularis propria invasion
- Muscularis mucosae invasion vs. muscularis propria
  - Nonclassic patterns of muscularis mucosa may be difficult
    - Individual small rounded aggregates of thick smooth muscle separated by stroma
    - In contrast, muscularis propria has large confluent aggregates of thick muscle
  - In some bladders, junction of muscularis propria and lamina propria is not well defined
    - Dispersed thick muscle extending luminally toward lamina propria particularly in trigone
- Invasion of perivesical tissue (pT3 disease)
  - Cannot be diagnosed on biopsy
    - Adipose tissue is present throughout normal bladder wall, including lamina propria and muscularis propria, and cannot be used to determine depth of invasion

REPORTING

Issues in Transurethral Biopsy
- Important to state depth of invasion by clearly reporting invasion of lamina propria or muscularis propria
  - Reporting muscle invasion without further specification is inappropriate
    - Does not distinguish between muscularis mucosae (pT1) and propria (at least pT2)
- Diagnosis of invasive urothelial carcinoma involving muscle of indeterminant type is warranted in some cases
  - Carcinoma involving smooth muscle (difficulty in determining mucosae vs. propria)
    - Requires restaging biopsies

SELECTED REFERENCES

1. Council L et al: Differential expression of immunohistochemical markers in bladder smooth muscle and myofibroblasts, and the potential utility of desmin, smoothelin, and vimentin in staging of bladder carcinoma. Mod Pathol. 22(5):639-50, 2009
2. Paner GP et al: Diagnostic utility of antibody to smoothelin in the distinction of muscularis propria from muscularis mucosae of the urinary bladder: a potential ancillary tool in the pathologic staging of invasive urothelial carcinoma. Am J Surg Pathol. 33(1):91-8, 2009
3. Paner GP et al: Further characterization of the muscle layers and lamina propria of the urinary bladder by systematic histologic mapping: implications for pathologic staging of invasive urothelial carcinoma. Am J Surg Pathol. 31(9):1420-9, 2007
4. Vakar-Lopez F et al: Muscularis mucosae of the urinary bladder revisited with emphasis on its hyperplastic patterns: a study of a large series of cystectomy specimens. Ann Diagn Pathol. 11(6):395-401, 2007
5. Jimenez RE et al: pT1 urothelial carcinoma of the bladder: criteria for diagnosis, pitfalls, and clinical implications. Adv Anat Pathol. 7(1):13-25, 2000
6. Philip AT et al: Intravesical adipose tissue: a quantitative study of its presence and location with implications for therapy and prognosis. Am J Surg Pathol. 24(9):1286-90, 2000
7. Ro JY et al: Muscularis mucosa of urinary bladder. Importance for staging and treatment. Am J Surg Pathol. 11(9):668-73, 1987

Invasive Urothelial Carcinoma

Invasive Urothelial Carcinoma, Large Tumor

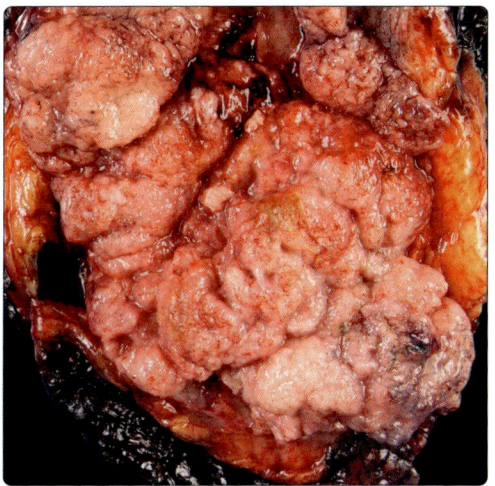

Bladder Wall Microanatomy (Muscularis Mucosae)

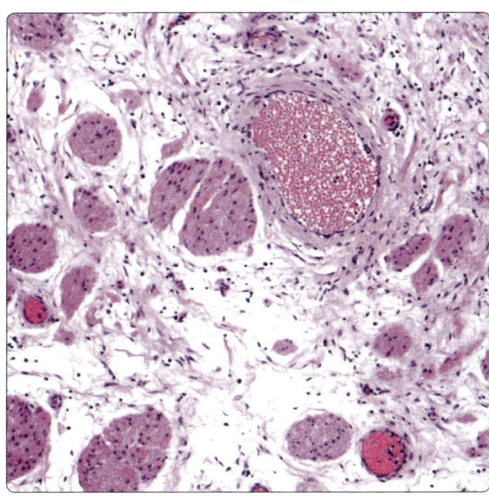

(Left) This radical cystectomy specimen with urothelial carcinoma contains a fungating and ulcerated mass that involves the entire mucosal surface of the bladder. There are areas of hemorrhage and necrosis. **(Right)** Section of muscularis mucosae consists of individual rounded bundles of smooth muscle separated by loose stroma. In contrast, muscularis propria consists of confluent, tightly packed, large smooth muscle aggregates.

Bladder Wall Microanatomy (Muscularis Mucosae)

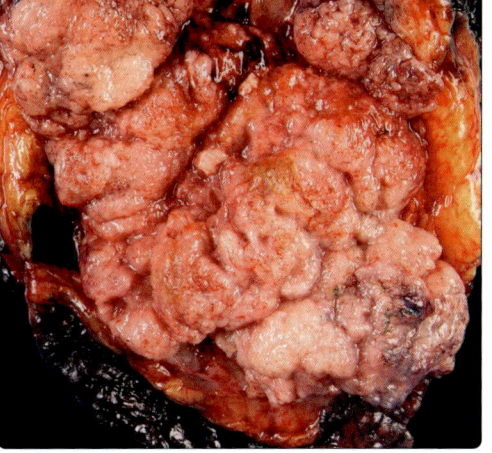

Bladder Wall Microanatomy (Muscularis Propria)

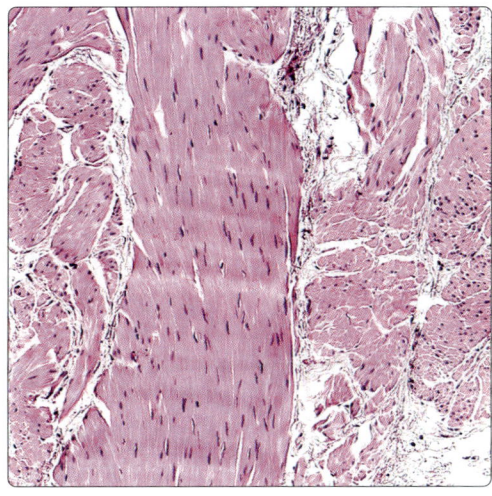

(Left) Disorganized, thin, wispy bundles of smooth muscle are characteristic of muscularis mucosae. Their location varies from superficial to deep in the lamina propria. The term "muscle invasion" should not be used in reports as it does not distinguish muscularis mucosae from muscularis propria. **(Right)** The large size of these smooth muscle bundles, which are arranged in a fascicular pattern, is diagnostic of muscularis propria. The presence of muscularis propria in a TUR specimen is important for sample adequacy.

Bladder Wall Microanatomy (Lamina Propria)

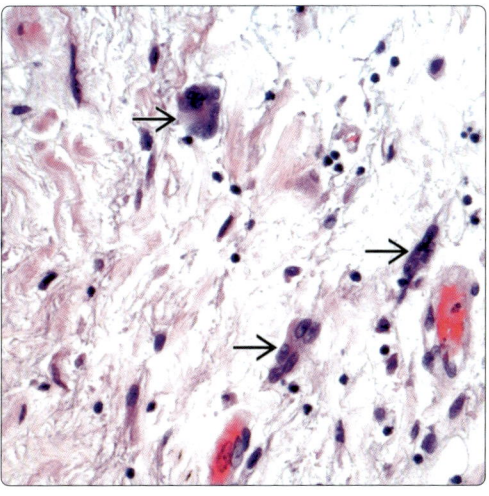

Bladder Wall Microanatomy (Lamina Propria)

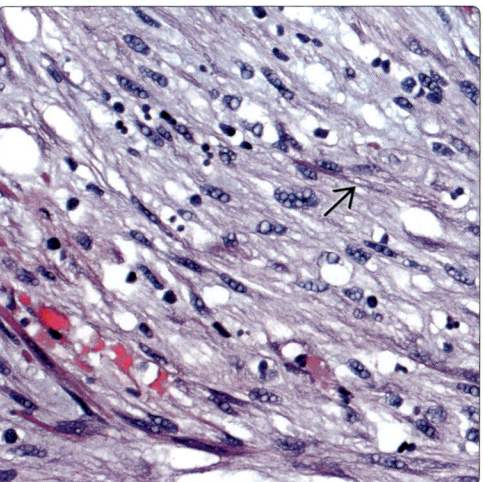

(Left) These stromal cells of the lamina propria have multilobated nuclei and dark smudgy chromatin ➡. This may represent a normal variation in the stroma, even in the absence of prior radiation, and should not be confused with a malignant spindle cell neoplasm. **(Right)** Elongated cytoplasmic processes ➡ and fine nuclear chromatin are typical features of myofibroblasts. Such reactive lesions often lack the eosinophilia of smooth muscle.

Invasive Urothelial Carcinoma

Invasive Urothelial Carcinoma

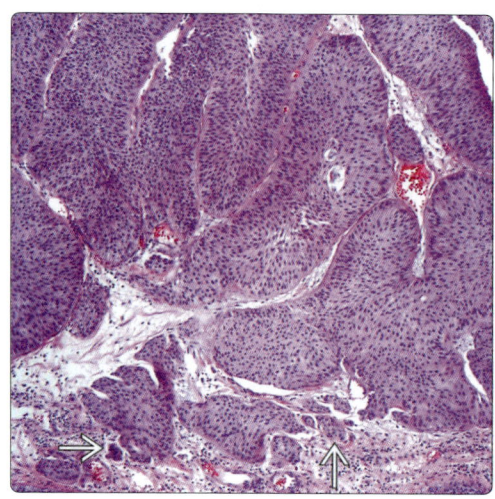

Invasive Urothelial Carcinoma

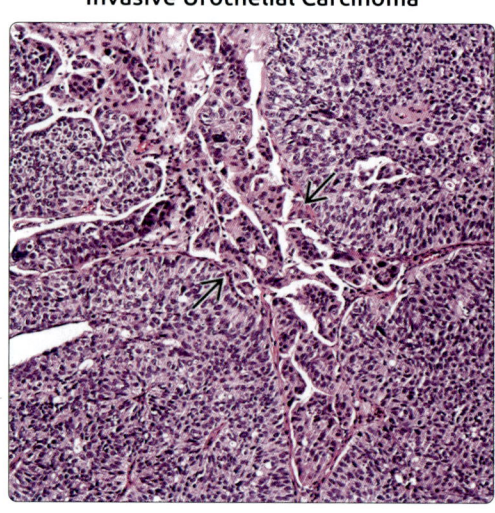

(Left) Irregular tumor nests invade the superficial lamina propria ➡ associated with myxoid stroma. The invasive component loses the normal contours seen at the base of the noninvasive component. (Right) Invasion into the stalk of a papillary urothelial carcinoma is often characterized by small aggregates and nests of urothelium with surrounding retraction artifact ➡. This would be designated as lamina propria invasion and staged as pT1.

Early Invasion: Paradoxical Differentiation

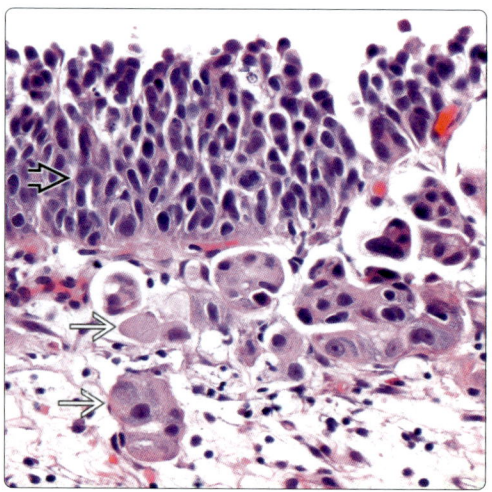

Desmoplastic Response

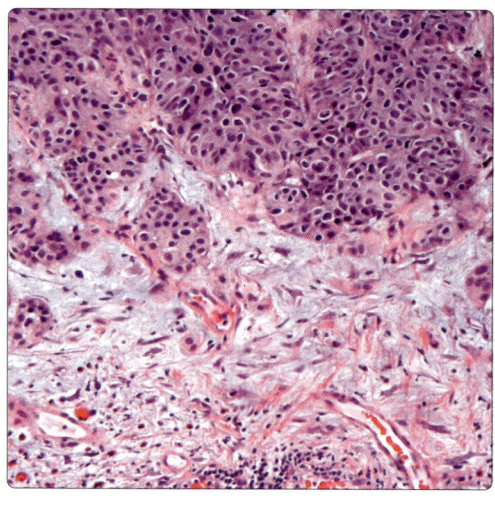

(Left) Invasion of the superficial lamina propria is shown. There are irregular nests of tumor cells with increased amount of eosinophilic cytoplasm (paradoxical differentiation) ➡ compared to those of the noninvasive carcinoma ➡. Stromal retraction is also present associated with the invasive tumor. (Right) Invasive urothelial carcinoma into superficial lamina propria is shown. Irregular nests and individual cells of invasive tumor are present within desmoplastic bluish stroma.

Lamina Propria Invasion

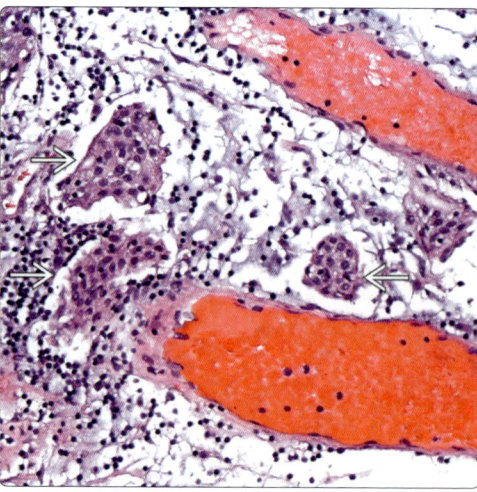

Individual and Scattered Cells of Invasion

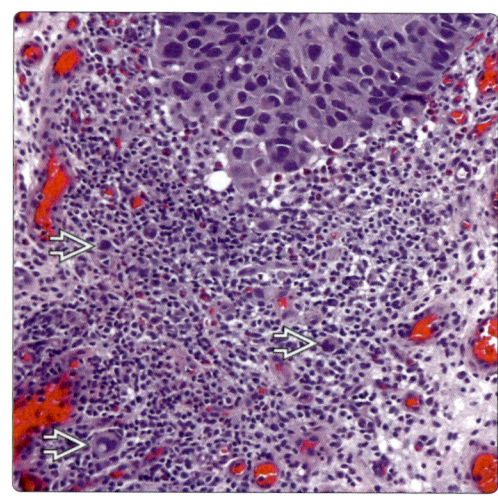

(Left) These rounded aggregates of invasive urothelial carcinoma with surrounding retraction ➡ and inflammation were present in the deep lamina propria. The edematous stroma and blood vessels are characteristic findings of the lamina propria. (Right) Invasive urothelial carcinoma into superficial lamina propria is present as individual tumor cells ➡ admixed with an intense mixed inflammatory infiltrate. Immunostains for epithelial markers may help to identify the presence and extent of the invasive disease.

Invasive Urothelial Carcinoma

Invasion of Muscularis Mucosae

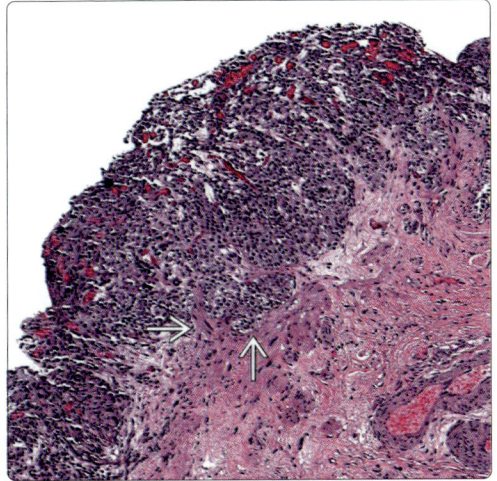

Lamina Propria Invasion

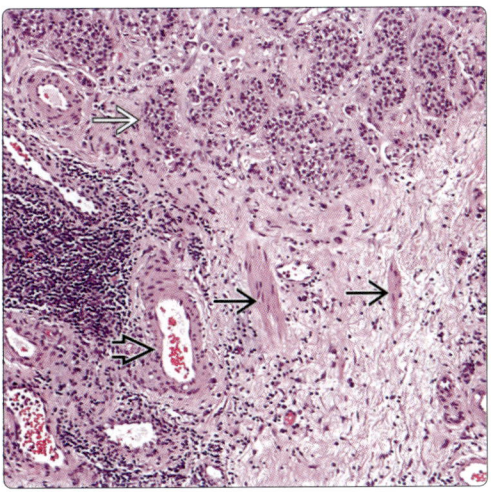

(Left) Urothelial carcinoma is shown invading muscle fibers that are characteristic of muscularis mucosae ➡. These thin and superficial bundles of smooth muscle should not be mistaken for muscularis propria. (Right) The irregular nests of this invasive urothelial carcinoma ➡ invade the lamina propria. Typical features of lamina propria (variably sized blood vessels ➡ and wispy fascicles of the muscularis mucosae ➡) are seen.

Diagnostic Stromal Invasion: Desmoplasia

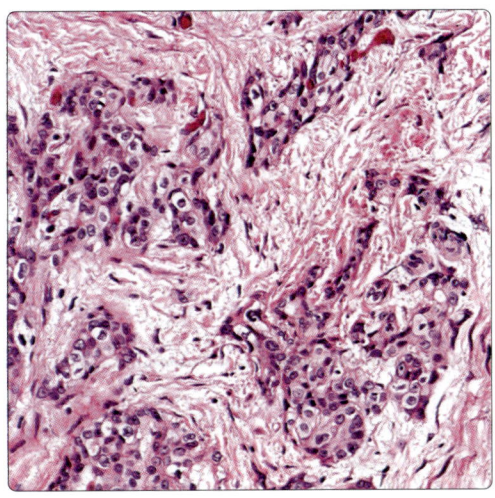

Pseudosarcomatous Myofibroblastic Reaction to Invasion

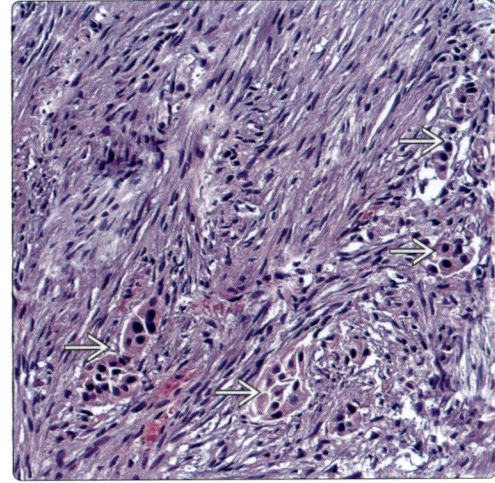

(Left) The irregular, jagged nests of urothelium present in this example of urothelial carcinoma are diagnostic of stromal invasion into the lamina propria. No muscularis propria is seen. (Right) This pseudosarcomatous myofibroblastic proliferation is associated with invasive urothelial carcinoma ➡. The cytologically bland tapered spindled cells with a blue hue are typical of myofibroblasts. This may potentially be confused with muscle invasion or sarcomatoid carcinoma.

Extensive Invasion Between Muscle Fibers

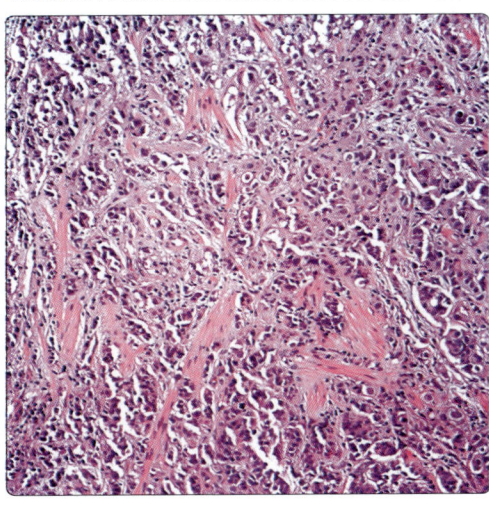

Supporting Muscularis Propria Invasion (Smoothelin Stain)

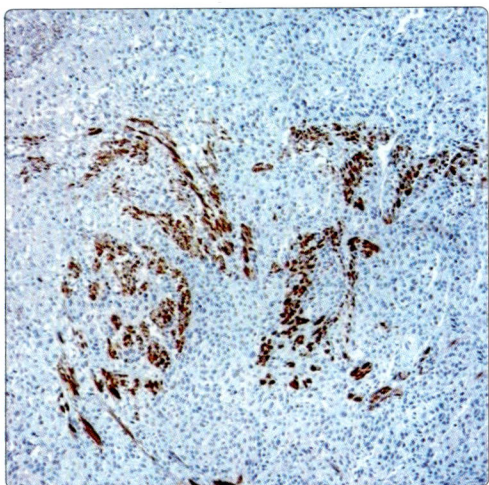

(Left) This invasive urothelial carcinoma involves scattered fragmented smooth muscle aggregates. The differential diagnosis includes muscularis mucosae invasion or destructive permeation of muscularis propria. The presence of such muscle throughout an entire tissue fragment is strongly suggestive of muscularis propria. (Right) Strong and diffuse immunoreactivity for smoothelin in the entrapped smooth muscle cells supports the diagnosis of muscularis propria invasion.

Invasive Urothelial Carcinoma

Invasive Urothelial Carcinoma

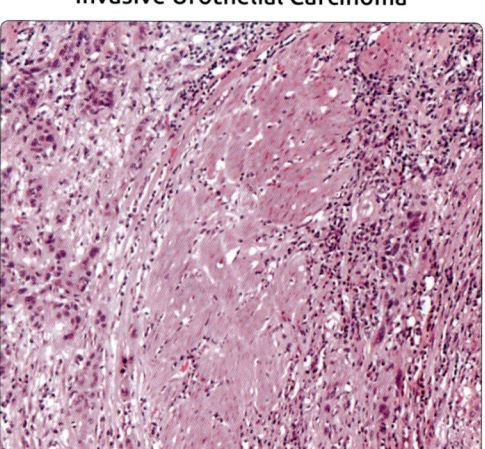

(Left) This example of invasive urothelial carcinoma shows prototypical invasion of the muscularis propria, which is characterized by infiltrating tumor cells that surround large confluent aggregates of compact smooth muscle. (Right) Invasive urothelial carcinoma dissects between confluent bundles of smooth muscle, a finding diagnostic of muscularis propria invasion (at least pT2 disease in transurethral resections). There is thermal artifact ➡ that, if severe, may preclude recognition of the carcinoma.

Invasive Urothelial Carcinoma (Thermal Artifact)   Invasive Urothelial Carcinoma (Keratin Stain)

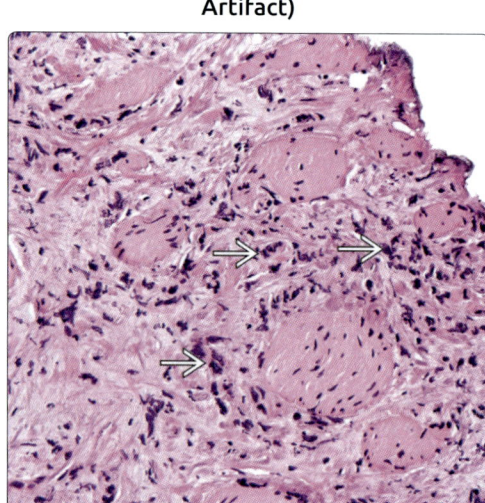 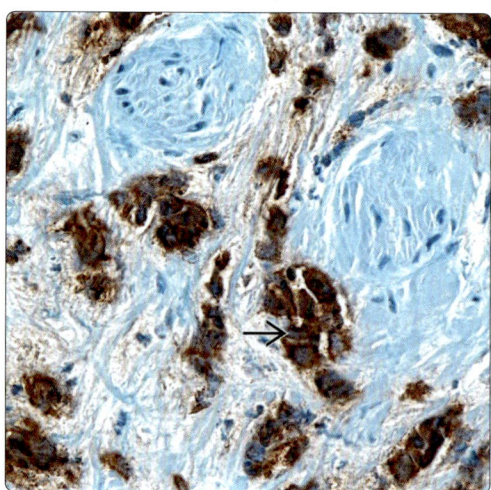

(Left) Invasive urothelial carcinomas ➡ may be masked by thermal artifact. Cytokeratin may be required to highlight infiltrating tumor cells in cases of such severe artifact. (Right) This CK-PAN (AE1/AE3) immunostain highlights the invasive carcinoma cells ➡ that are masked by crush artifact. Cytokeratin may also stain reactive myofibroblasts; therefore, careful correlation with the morphology is essential.

Invasive Urothelial Carcinoma   Invasive Urothelial Carcinoma

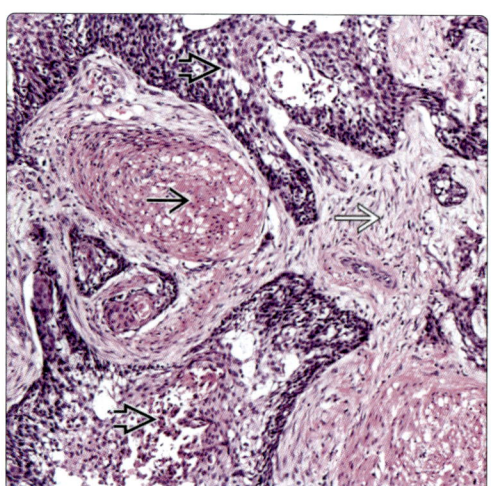 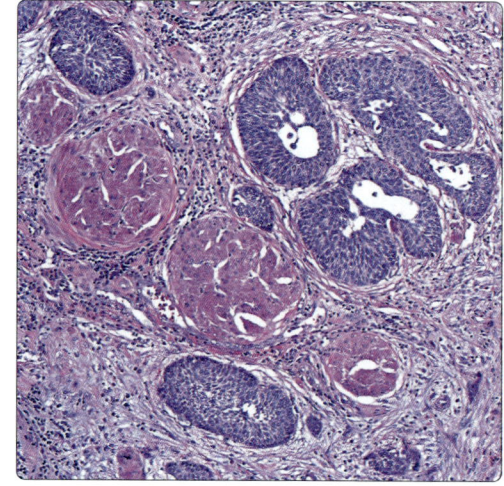

(Left) This invasive urothelial carcinoma ➡ contrasts the eosinophilic muscle bundles of the muscularis propria ➡ with the more myxoid and spindled reactive myofibroblastic proliferation ➡. (Right) Medium-sized nests of urothelium with bland histology surrounded by mild stromal reaction and inflammatory infiltrate are shown. Their presence deep at the level of muscularis propria is diagnostic of invasive carcinoma despite the bland cellular features.

Invasive Urothelial Carcinoma

Prostatic Adenocarcinoma Involving Bladder

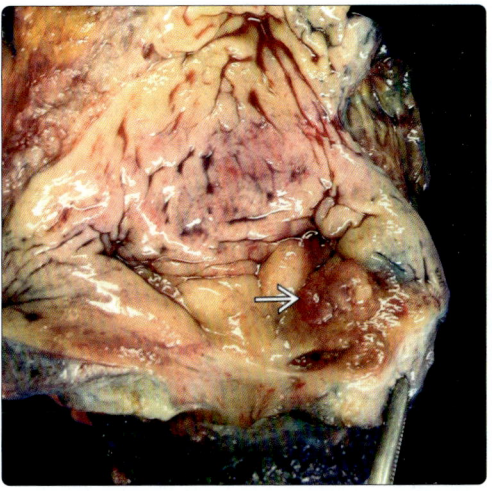

Prostatic Adenocarcinoma Involving Bladder

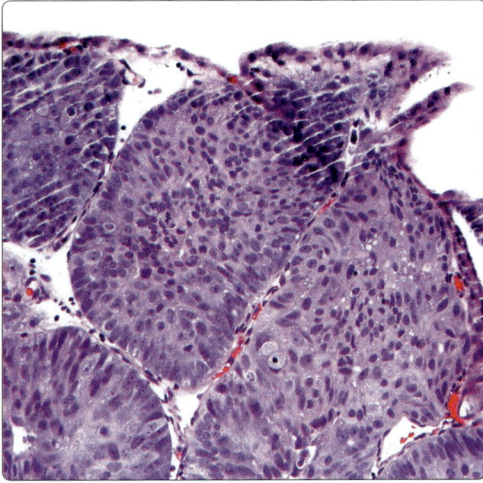

(Left) This is a locally advanced prostate cancer refractory to hormone deprivation therapy. The tumor extensively involved the prostate and extended to the wall of the bladder, mimicking a primary bladder cancer ➡. **(Right)** A bladder mass was discovered in a patient who presented with hematuria. Prostatic adenocarcinoma was the diagnosis and confirmed by immunostains PSA and PSMA. The relative uniformity of tumor nuclei and occasional nucleoli are helpful features to consider prostatic origin for this tumor.

Prostatic Adenocarcinoma Involving Bladder

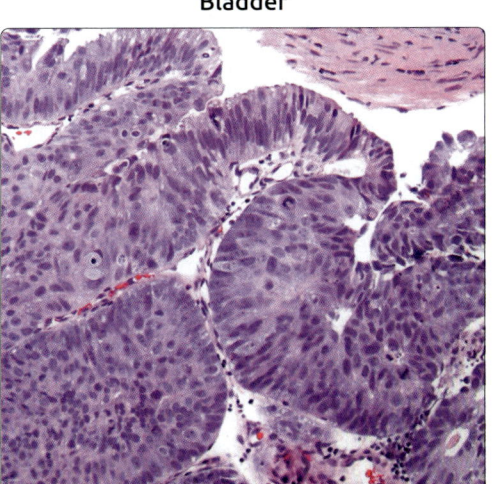

Prostatic Adenocarcinoma Involving Bladder

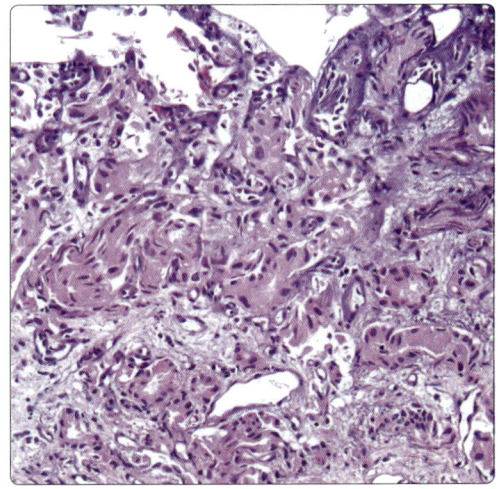

(Left) This prostatic adenocarcinoma is colonizing the surface urothelium, superficially resembling a noninvasive papillary urothelial carcinoma. These areas were immunoreactive with PSA and PSMA, confirming the prostatic origin of this tumor. **(Right)** This TUR specimen contains tumor tissue with thermal artifact, which masked the glandular differentiation and complicated the proper identification of the prostatic origin of the tumor.

Metastatic Serous Carcinoma to Bladder

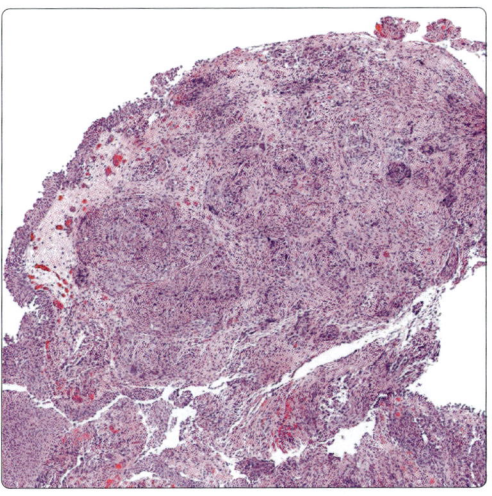

Metastatic Breast Cancer to Bladder

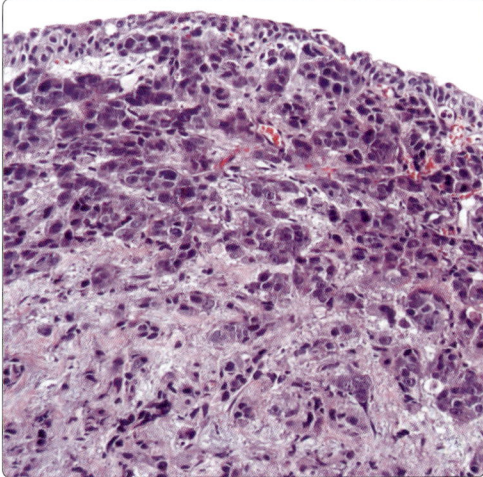

(Left) This poorly differentiated carcinoma discovered in bladder biopsy morphologically resembled a primary urothelial carcinoma. A prior history of high-grade serous carcinoma of the uterus in this patient was crucial in establishing the metastatic origin of this tumor, which was further confirmed by immunostains. **(Right)** Another poorly differentiated carcinoma discovered in the bladder represents metastasis from breast cancer, 13 years post mastectomy. The clinical history is very important for this diagnostic consideration.

Overview of Invasive Carcinoma Subtypes

TERMINOLOGY

Definitions

- Invasive urothelial carcinoma (UC) with morphology distinct from the usual or typical pattern

CLINICAL IMPLICATIONS

Gender

- Variants are most common in older men
  - Similar to urothelial carcinoma in general

Clinical Presentation

- Hematuria most common

Treatment

- Urothelial carcinoma variants are treated similarly to conventional urothelial carcinoma with some exceptions
  - Small cell carcinoma treated by separate chemotherapy regimen
  - Pure lymphoepithelioma-like carcinoma may be more responsive to chemotherapy
  - Micropapillary carcinoma may be treated by radical surgery at low stage (pT1) in some centers
  - Urothelial carcinoma with squamous differentiation is less responsive to adjuvant therapy

Prognosis

- Variant invasive urothelial carcinomas have poor prognosis
  - Generally present at high stage
  - Uncertain whether prognosis is worse than urothelial carcinoma of similar stage in some variants

MACROSCOPIC

General Features

- Typically large infiltrative mass lesion

UC WITH ALTERNATIVE/ABERRANT DIFFERENTIATION

Microscopic Features

- By definition, contains component of typical papillary, in situ, or invasive urothelial carcinoma at least focally
  - Squamous differentiation
    - Keratinization and intracellular bridges
    - May be focal or extensive
  - Glandular differentiation
    - Glandular component identical to adenocarcinoma
  - Trophoblastic differentiation
    - Scattered syncytiotrophoblasts within high-grade urothelial carcinoma
    - Rarely choriocarcinomatous differentiation

NESTED CARCINOMA

Microscopic Features

- Nests of infiltrative tumor cells with relatively bland cytologic appearance
  - Irregular infiltrating border with lamina propria is characteristic
  - Muscularis propria is commonly involved
  - Tumor nests often have some degree of complex anastomosis at least focally
  - Invasion with surrounding retraction may be present focally
  - Generally show increasing levels of atypia toward deeper portions of tumor
  - May be admixed with urothelial carcinoma with small tubules or microcystic patterns

Differential Diagnosis

- von Brunn nests
  - More rounded urothelial nests
  - Lobular configuration
  - Superficial location with sharp border at deep interface with lamina propria
- Cystitis cystica/glandularis

Urothelial Carcinoma With Squamous Differentiation

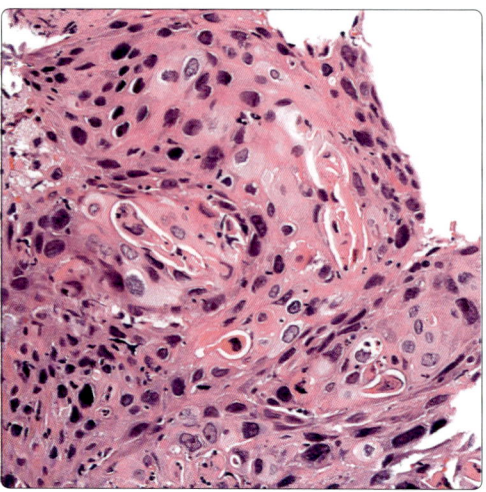

Nested Carcinoma

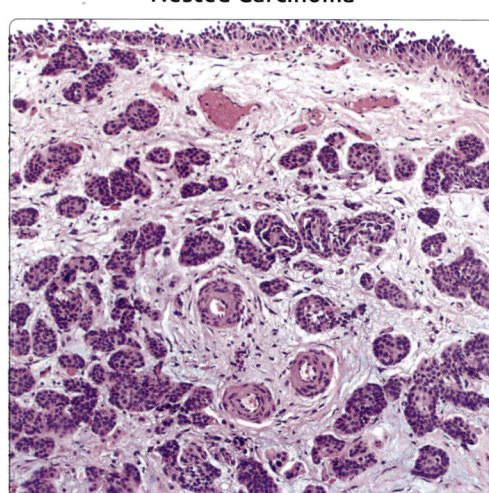

(Left) Urothelial carcinomas, not uncommonly, show areas of squamous differentiation that are histologically indistinguishable from squamous cell carcinoma. Identification of a urothelial component is key to the distinction. (Right) The nested variant of urothelial carcinoma is cytologically bland, but the presence of irregularly distributed nests throughout the lamina propria and the complex epithelial growth is diagnostic.

Overview of Invasive Carcinoma Subtypes

- o More superficially located
- o Also has sharp border at interface with lamina propria
- Nephrogenic adenoma
  - o More tubular appearance
  - o Prominent basement membranes may surround tubules
  - o Lining epithelium may have hobnail appearance
  - o Other admixed patterns may be present: Papillary, solid/diffuse, cystic

LARGE NESTED CARCINOMA

Microscopic Features

- Very large nests of urothelial cells with relatively bland cytologic features
  - o Numerous and irregularly distributed throughout the lamina propria
  - o May have central cystic change
  - o Rare areas with stromal reaction may be seen
  - o Invasion of muscularis propria is diagnostic

Differential Diagnosis

- Noninvasive endophytic low-grade urothelial carcinoma (or PUNLMP)
  - o More anastomosing cord-like architecture
  - o Sharp rounded interface with underlying tissue

UC WITH SMALL TUBULES

Microscopic Features

- Invasive carcinoma with small gland-like spaces lined by urothelial cells
  - o No intracellular mucin
  - o No columnar lining
- May be admixed with nested variant
  - o Same differential considerations as nested variant

MICROCYSTIC CARCINOMA

Microscopic Features

- Dilated microcysts in invasive component
  - o Microcysts may reach 1-2 mm in diameter
  - o Urothelial lining
- May be associated with nested variant

Differential Diagnosis

- Urothelial carcinoma with glandular differentiation
  - o Glandular component lined by columnar cells or has abundant intracytoplasmic mucin
- Nephrogenic adenoma
  - o More superficial location
  - o No destructive invasion
- Cystitis cystica/glandularis
  - o Sharp linear base at junction with lamina propria
- Müllerianosis
  - o Endocervical, tubal, or endometrial-type glands
  - o Bland cytologic features

PLASMACYTOID CARCINOMA

Microscopic Features

- Poorly to undifferentiated malignant cells closely resemble plasma cells set in myxoid or loose edematous stroma
  - o Eccentric nuclei
  - o Abundant glassy eosinophilic cytoplasm
- Clusters of neoplastic cells may be surrounded by retraction spaces
- Concomitant conventional urothelial carcinoma may be admixed
- Signet ring-like cells are not uncommon
- More extensive spread in abdominal cavity than other variants of urothelial carcinoma
  - o May recur with malignant effusions or peritoneal carcinomatosis

Differential Diagnosis

- Plasmacytoma and lymphoma
  - o Plasmacytoid carcinoma may express CD138
  - o Strong cytokeratin reactivity supports carcinoma
  - o Evaluation of κ and λ ratio may be helpful
- Signet ring adenocarcinoma
  - o Diagnosis restricted to cases with extracellular mucin

MICROPAPILLARY CARCINOMA

Microscopic Features

- Small nests and papillae with surrounding retraction spaces
  - o Resembles ovarian serous carcinoma
  - o Confluent retraction spaces are characteristic
  - o Multiple nests in same retraction space is common
- Although nuclear grade is typically high, may also have relatively low-grade appearance
- Most are muscle invasive with vascular invasion
  - o CD31, CD34, and Podoplanin (D2-40) may help to distinguish true lymphatic invasion from retraction artifact
- Immunohistochemically, tumor is reactive for EMA/MUC1, CK7, CK20
  - o Immunoreactivity for HER2 and CA125 may also be seen

Differential Diagnosis

- Ovarian serous carcinoma
  - o Clinical/radiographic correlation is needed
  - o Immunohistochemical expression of ER and WT1 is common in ovarian primary
- Typical invasive urothelial carcinoma with stromal retraction
  - o Larger nests
  - o Does not typically show multiple small nests in same retraction space
  - o Significant immunophenotypic overlap with micropapillary carcinoma: May also express EMA/MUC1, CA125, and HER2
  - o In some cases, distinction may be very difficult

LYMPHOEPITHELIOMA-LIKE CARCINOMA

Microscopic Features

- Resembles undifferentiated carcinomas of nasopharynx
  - o Individual neoplastic cells arranged in syncytia with obscuring chronic inflammation
    - Cytoplasmic borders are most often indistinct
    - Inflammation consists of a mixture of polyclonal B and T lymphocytes, histiocytes, eosinophils, and plasma cells
- Pure forms are reportedly more responsive to chemotherapy

Overview of Invasive Carcinoma Subtypes

- o Percentage of lymphoepithelioma-like areas should be reported

Differential Diagnosis

- Lymphoma or chronic inflammation
  - o CD45(LCA) reactivity in neoplastic cells
  - o No cytokeratin-positive population
- Small cell carcinoma
  - o Neuroendocrine chromatin features
  - o Cellular molding
  - o High mitotic and apoptotic index
  - o Coexpress cytokeratin and synaptophysin
- Urothelial carcinoma with prominent lymphoid stroma
  - o Lacks syncytia of cells
  - o Poorly differentiated urothelial carcinoma histology

SMALL CELL CARCINOMA

Microscopic Features

- Sheets and occasionally nests of cells with scant cytoplasm and high nuclear:cytoplasmic ratio
  - o Chromatin is finely stippled, and nucleoli are inconspicuous
  - o Geographic areas of necrosis, high mitotic rate, and areas of crush artifact are also frequent
- Other subtypes of primary bladder carcinoma may be admixed
  - o Urothelial carcinoma in situ, invasive urothelial carcinoma, squamous cell carcinoma, adenocarcinoma, or sarcomatoid carcinoma
  - o Identical pattern of allelic loss in small cell carcinoma and adjacent conventional urothelial carcinoma suggest shared lineage
- Highly aggressive clinical behavior
- Even focal small cell component should be reported

Differential Diagnosis

- Metastatic small cell carcinoma
  - o Histologically and immunophenotypically indistinguishable unless conventional urothelial carcinoma is present
  - o CK7(+)/CK20(-) phenotype common
  - o Both metastases and primary tumors may express TTF-1
- Lymphoma
  - o Express hematopoietic markers
  - o Cytokeratin negative
- Poorly differentiated urothelial carcinoma
  - o Does not express synaptophysin or chromogranin
- Rhabdomyosarcoma
  - o May express synaptophysin
  - o Nuclear myogenin reactivity diagnostic of skeletal muscle differentiation

SARCOMATOID UC

Microscopic Features

- Neoplasms containing both epithelial and mesenchymal differentiation by morphology or immunohistochemistry
  - o Epithelial component may be any subtype of bladder carcinoma
    - Urothelial carcinoma in situ, invasive urothelial carcinoma, squamous cell carcinoma, or adenocarcinoma
  - o Mesenchymal component usually has high-grade spindle cell morphology
  - o Heterologous elements may be present
    - Osteosarcoma, chondrosarcoma, and rhabdomyosarcoma
- Immunohistochemical expression of HMCK(34βE12), CK5/6 and p63 in both epithelial and spindled component

Differential Diagnosis

- Pseudosarcomatous myofibroblastic proliferation
  - o Fine nuclear chromatin
  - o Actin expression common
  - o In contrast to carcinoma, cytokeratin expression limited to low molecular weight forms
  - o Does not express p63
  - o Subset expresses ALK1 by immunohistochemistry
- Urothelial carcinoma with pseudoangiosarcomatous
  - o Bladder cancer with prominent dyscohesion of cells resembling angiosarcoma
- Primary leiomyosarcoma
  - o Expresses desmin and actin
  - o In contrast to carcinoma, cytokeratin expression limited to low molecular weight forms
  - o Up to 23% express p63
- Other primary vesical sarcoma
  - o No carcinomatous component or recent history of urothelial carcinoma
  - o Nonepithelial immunophenotype

UC WITH OSTEOCLAST-LIKE GIANT CELLS

Microscopic Features

- Prominent osteoclast-type giant cells are seen in rare undifferentiated carcinomas
  - o Giant cells are histiocytic in origin
- Background spindled and mononuclear cells are cytokeratin positive

UC WITH RHABDOID FEATURES

Microscopic Features

- Very rare morphologic subtype
- Neoplastic cells with large vesicular nuclei, prominent nucleoli, and eosinophilic cytoplasmic inclusions
  - o Resembles malignant extrarenal rhabdoid tumor
  - o Does not have deletion of *INI1* at 22q11
  - o Usually adult tumor, unlike malignant extrarenal rhabdoid tumor
- Very aggressive clinical course

UC WITH MYXOID STROMA (INCLUDING CHORDOID)

Microscopic Features

- Typical urothelial carcinoma almost always present
- Prominent myxoid stroma
  - o Proportion of tumor highly variable
- Neoplastic cells may "float" in myxoid matrix in aggregates or chains

Overview of Invasive Carcinoma Subtypes

- Small round cells with eosinophilic cytoplasm are common

Differential Diagnosis
- Myxoid sarcoma
  - Urothelial carcinomas with myxoid stroma maintain epithelial immunophenotype
- Chordoma
  - Nuclear brachyury expression

UC WITH CLEAR CYTOPLASM (GLYCOGEN RICH)

Microscopic Features
- Abundant clear cytoplasm secondary to glycogen accumulation
- Typically focal pattern in otherwise typical urothelial carcinoma

Differential Diagnosis
- Renal cell carcinoma
  - Obvious renal mass present
  - Expression of pax-8/pax-2 may be seen
- Clear cell adenocarcinoma, primary or gynecologic
  - Distinct mixed tubulocystic and papillary pattern with hobnail cells typical

UC WITH LIPOID FEATURES (LIPID RICH/LIPID CELL)

Microscopic Features
- Rare urothelial carcinomas have foci with intracellular lipid
  - Closely resemble lipoblasts
- Most admixed with typical urothelial carcinoma
- Maintain cytokeratin immunoreactivity, even in lipid-rich cells

Differential Diagnosis
- Primary liposarcoma
  - Lack component of typical urothelial carcinoma
  - Epithelioid variant of pleomorphic liposarcoma is close mimic that may express keratin
- Sarcomatoid urothelial carcinoma with heterologous liposarcoma
  - Usually has pleomorphic spindled component
  - Lipoblasts do not express cytokeratin
  - Other heterologous components may be admixed
- Signet ring cell adenocarcinoma
  - Smaller cells with single intracytoplasmic vacuoles
  - Often infiltrate as individual cells

POORLY DIFFERENTIATED UROTHELIAL CARCINOMA

Microscopic Features
- Poorly differentiated pleomorphic carcinoma without histologic features typical of urothelial carcinoma (also called large cell undifferentiated)

Differential Diagnosis
- Lymphoma
  - Expresses hematopoietic markers
- Secondary carcinoma from another anatomic site
  - Requires clinical correlation
- Melanoma
  - Expresses S-100 protein

DIFFERENTIAL DIAGNOSIS

Secondary Carcinomas From Nonbladder Sites
- Variant morphologic patterns of urothelial carcinoma may suggest nonbladder primary
- Most urothelial carcinoma variants maintain urothelial immunophenotype
  - CK7 and CK20 coexpression common
  - Express HMCK(34βE12)
  - Nuclear p63 reactivity
  - Uroplakin 2
  - GATA3

DIAGNOSTIC CHECKLIST

Pathologic Interpretation Pearls
- Variant morphology carcinoma: Primary carcinoma involving bladder and not conforming to morphology of typical urothelial carcinoma
- Variant histology must be documented, including percentage, if not pure in histology
  - Variant histology may present at metastatic site; facilitates association with bladder primary
- Variant histology may have diagnostic, prognostic, or therapeutic significance
- Metastatic carcinoma or carcinoma secondarily involving bladder must be ruled out in all cases

SELECTED REFERENCES

1. Paner GP et al: Pseudoangiosarcomatous urothelial carcinoma of the urinary bladder. Am J Surg Pathol. 38(9):1251-9, 2014
2. Cox R et al: Large nested variant of urothelial carcinoma: 23 cases mimicking von Brunn nests and inverted growth pattern of noninvasive papillary urothelial carcinoma. Am J Surg Pathol. 35(9):1337-42, 2011
3. Williamson SR et al: Lymphoepithelioma-like carcinoma of the urinary bladder: clinicopathologic, immunohistochemical, and molecular features. Am J Surg Pathol. 35(4):474-83, 2011
4. Lopez-Beltran A et al: Urothelial carcinoma of the bladder, lipid cell variant: clinicopathologic findings and LOH analysis. Am J Surg Pathol. 34(3):371-6, 2010
5. Lopez-Beltran A et al: Large cell undifferentiated carcinoma of the urinary bladder. Pathology. 42(4):364-8, 2010
6. Sangoi AR et al: Interobserver reproducibility in the diagnosis of invasive micropapillary carcinoma of the urinary tract among urologic pathologists. Am J Surg Pathol. 34(9):1367-76, 2010
7. Amin MB: Histological variants of urothelial carcinoma: diagnostic, therapeutic and prognostic implications. Mod Pathol. 22 Suppl 2:S96-S118, 2009
8. Cox RM et al: Invasive urothelial carcinoma with chordoid features: a report of 12 distinct cases characterized by prominent myxoid stroma and cordlike epithelial architecture. Am J Surg Pathol. 33(8):1213-9, 2009
9. Nigwekar P et al: Plasmacytoid urothelial carcinoma: detailed analysis of morphology with clinicopathologic correlation in 17 cases. Am J Surg Pathol. 33(3):417-24, 2009
10. Baydar D et al: Osteoclast-rich undifferentiated carcinomas of the urinary tract. Mod Pathol. 19(2):161-71, 2006
11. Cheng L et al: Small cell carcinoma of the urinary bladder: a clinicopathologic analysis of 64 patients. Cancer. 101(5):957-62, 2004
12. Lopez-Beltran A et al: Carcinosarcoma and sarcomatoid carcinoma of the bladder: clinicopathological study of 41 cases. J Urol. 159(5):1497-503, 1998
13. Drew PA et al: The nested variant of transitional cell carcinoma: an aggressive neoplasm with innocuous histology. Mod Pathol. 9(10):989-94, 1996
14. Amin MB et al: Micropapillary variant of transitional cell carcinoma of the urinary bladder. Histologic pattern resembling ovarian papillary serous carcinoma. Am J Surg Pathol. 18(12):1224-32, 1994

Overview of Invasive Carcinoma Subtypes

Urothelial Carcinoma With Squamous Differentiation

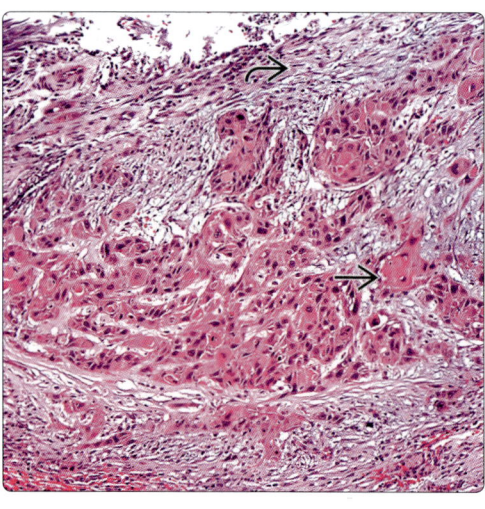

Urothelial Carcinoma With Squamous Differentiation

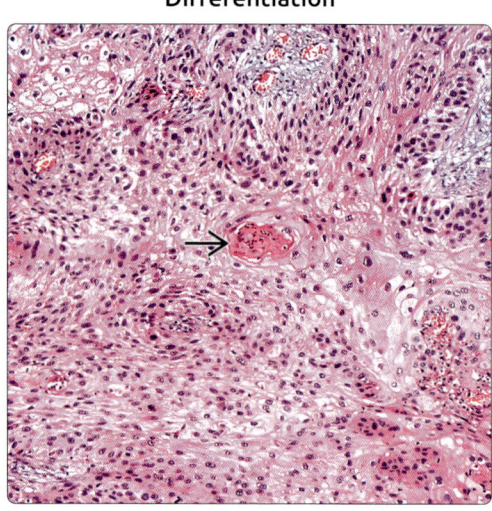

(Left) *Invasive urothelial carcinomas may show squamous differentiation. The cytoplasm is more eosinophilic than typical urothelial carcinoma, and keratin formation ➔ is seen. These carcinomas are frequently associated with a florid stromal myofibroblastic proliferation ➔. The presence of typical urothelial carcinoma precludes a diagnosis of primary squamous cell carcinoma.* (Right) *Squamous differentiation with keratin formation ➔ may also be seen in the noninvasive component.*

Urothelial Carcinoma With Squamous Differentiation

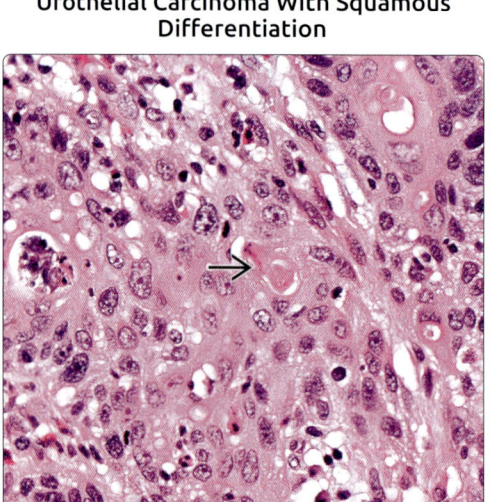

Urothelial Carcinoma With Squamous Differentiation

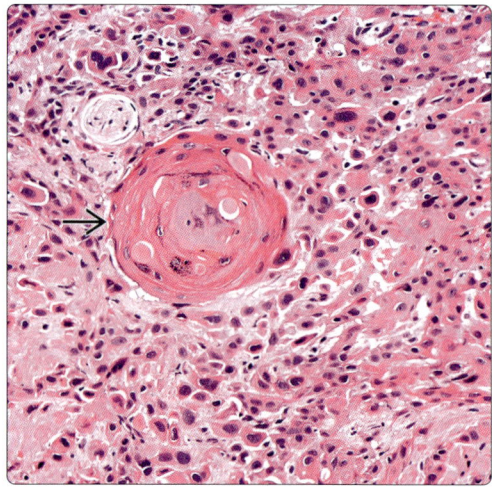

(Left) *Focal keratin formation ➔ is seen in this example of urothelial carcinoma with squamous differentiation.* (Right) *Keratin pearl formation ➔ is the prototypical feature of squamous differentiation. In contrast to primary squamous cell carcinoma, urothelial carcinoma with squamous differentiation has areas of conventional papillary, invasive, or in situ urothelial carcinoma. In addition, primary squamous cell carcinoma arises in a background of squamous metaplasia/dysplasia.*

Urothelial Carcinoma With Glandular Differentiation

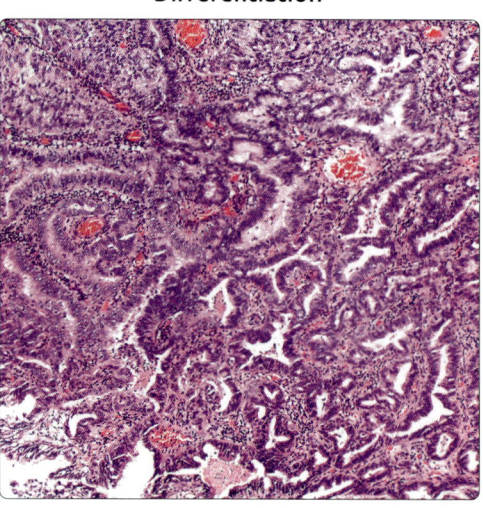

Concomitant Urothelial Carcinoma In Situ

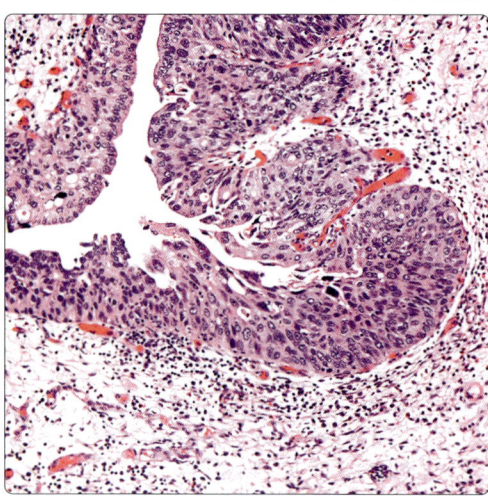

(Left) *Invasive urothelial carcinoma may show glandular differentiation that is morphologically identical to adenocarcinoma. The presence of a component of conventional urothelial carcinoma is distinctive.* (Right) *The presence of associated urothelial carcinoma in situ, as seen here, is diagnostic of urothelial carcinoma when alternative differentiation is present. Typical noninvasive papillary or invasive urothelial carcinoma is also sufficient.*

Overview of Invasive Carcinoma Subtypes

Urothelial Carcinoma With Syncytiotrophoblasts

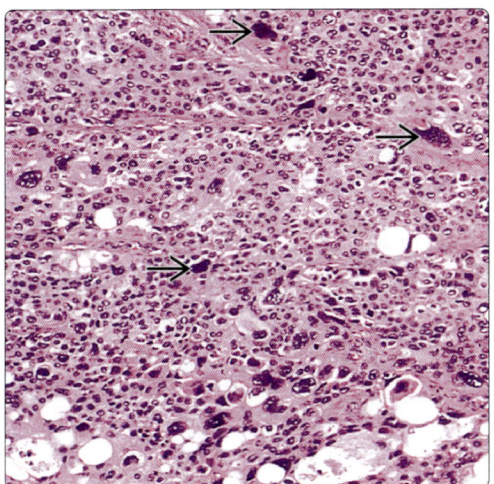

Urothelial Carcinoma With Syncytiotrophoblasts

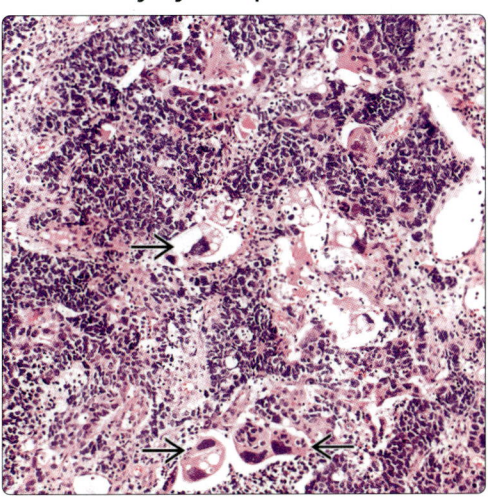

(Left) Multinucleated cells with dense nuclear chromatin ➡, characteristic of syncytiotrophoblasts, are present amidst this high-grade invasive urothelial carcinoma. This is distinct from choriocarcinoma, which would also contain central nests of cytotrophoblasts. (Right) This example of poorly differentiated urothelial carcinoma of the urinary bladder had both small cell differentiation and numerous scattered syncytiotrophoblasts ➡.

Urothelial Carcinoma With Syncytiotrophoblasts

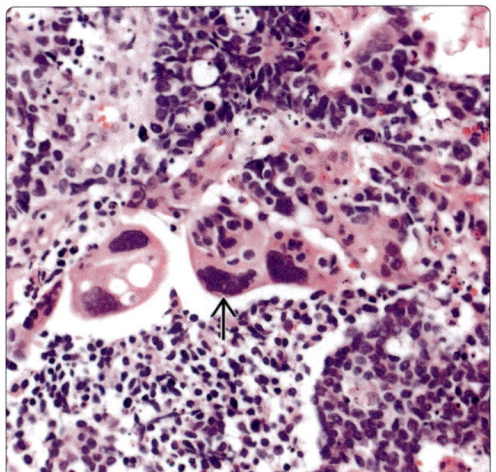

Urothelial Carcinoma With Choriocarcinoma

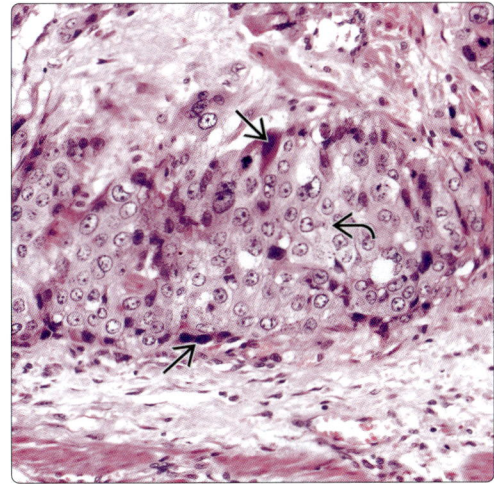

(Left) This photomicrograph shows the characteristic multinucleation of syncytiotrophoblasts ➡ and small cell carcinoma. (Right) To diagnose urothelial carcinoma with choriocarcinomatous differentiation, the classic biphasic architecture of choriocarcinoma must be seen: Nests of mononuclear cytotrophoblasts ➡ enveloped by syncytiotrophoblasts ➡. Scattered syncytiotrophoblasts are not sufficient for a diagnosis of choriocarcinoma.

Urothelial Carcinoma With Choriocarcinoma

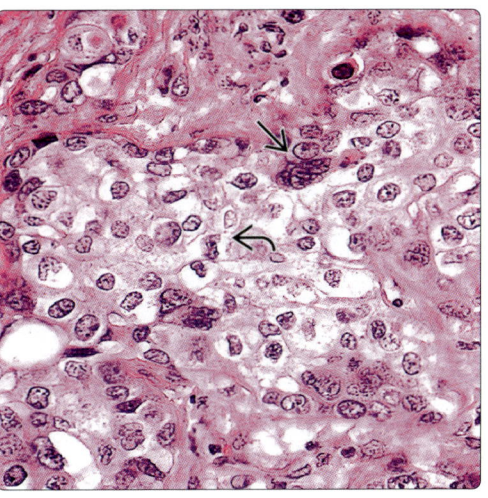

β-HCG: Urothelial Carcinoma With Choriocarcinoma

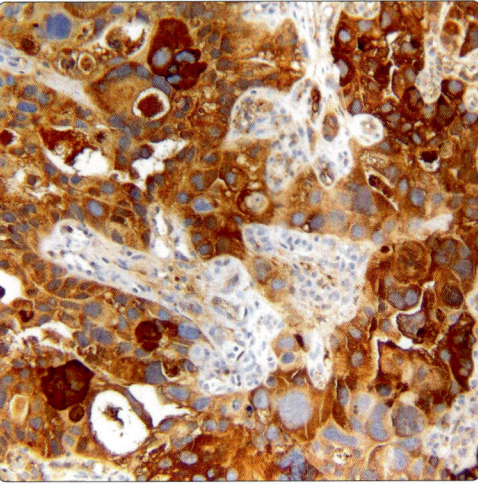

(Left) In this case of urothelial carcinoma with choriocarcinomatous differentiation, multinucleated syncytiotrophoblasts ➡ are seen wrapping around mononuclear cytotrophoblasts ➡. (Right) As in this example with choriocarcinomatous differentiation, β-HCG reactivity is typically strong; however, β-HCG reactivity may also be seen in poorly differentiated urothelial carcinoma without trophoblasts. Morphologic context is critical.

Overview of Invasive Carcinoma Subtypes

(Left) On low-power examination, nested urothelial carcinoma has more epithelial nests present deeper in the lamina propria and areas with more complex architecture than seen in benign mimics, such as florid von Brunn nests and cystitis cystica. (Right) Nested variant is a histologically subtle form of malignancy that has relatively bland cytologic features. The haphazard distribution of the nests, seen here at low power, is helpful in recognizing this variant of bladder cancer.

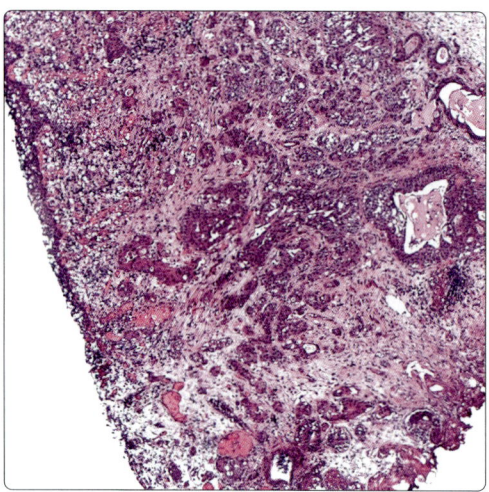
Nested Carcinoma: Architectural Distribution

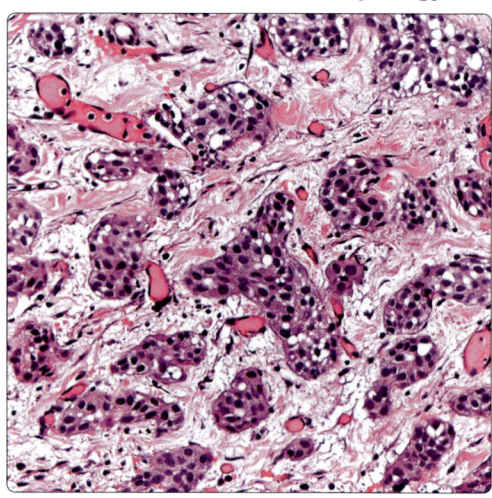
Nested Carcinoma: Bland Cytology

(Left) This nested urothelial carcinoma highlights the bland cytologic features of the neoplastic cells ⇨ compared to the normal overlying urothelium ⇨. (Right) The neoplastic cells of nested urothelial carcinoma have a subtle increase in the nuclear/cytoplasmic ratio. A mitotic figure ⇨ is also seen in this nest. It is difficult to recognize this form of carcinoma only by cytology. In small superficial bladder biopsy specimens, a definitive diagnosis may sometimes be impossible.

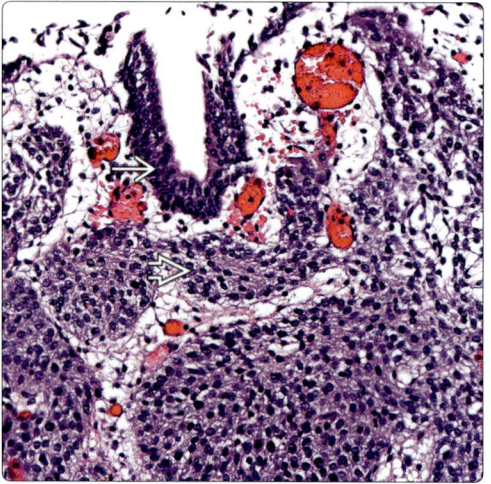
Nested Carcinoma: Bland Cytology

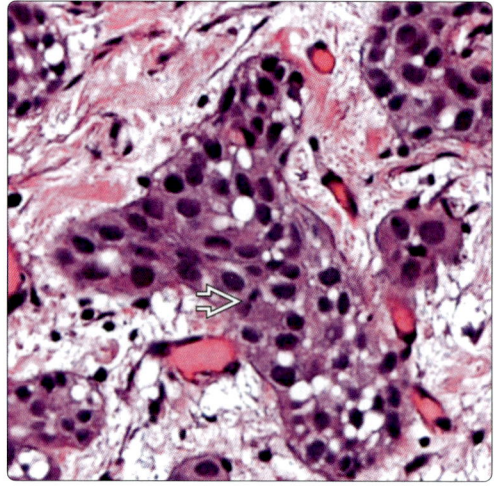
Nested Carcinoma: Subtle Features

(Left) Invasion of the muscularis propria is diagnostic of carcinoma. In some cases, rebiopsy may be necessary to document invasion. Even in the deeply invasive areas, the bland cytology may be retained, as in this example. (Right) Lymph node metastases ⇨ are not uncommon in nested carcinoma, as seen in this photomicrograph. The nested architecture and bland cytology are retained. These tumors should be treated similar to conventional high-grade invasive urothelial carcinoma.

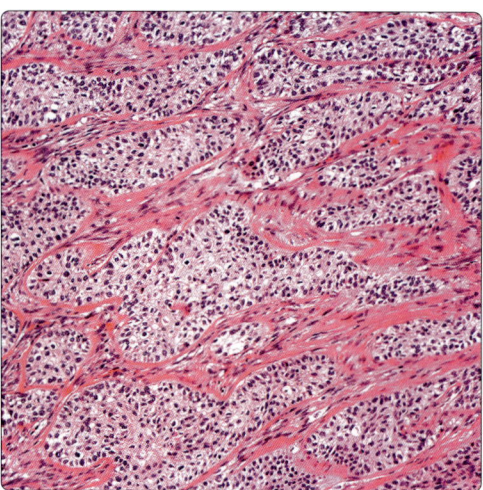
Nested Carcinoma: Deep Invasion

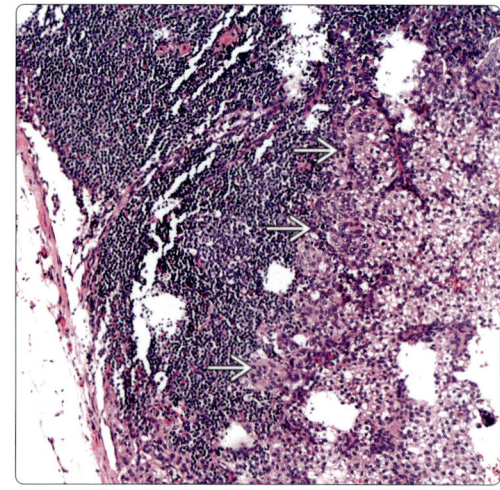
Nested Carcinoma: Lymph Node Metastasis

Overview of Invasive Carcinoma Subtypes

Large Nested Carcinoma: Low-Power Architectural Distribution

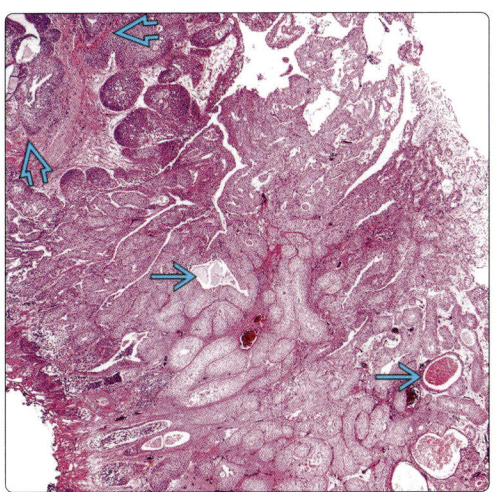

Large Nested Carcinoma: Subtle Features

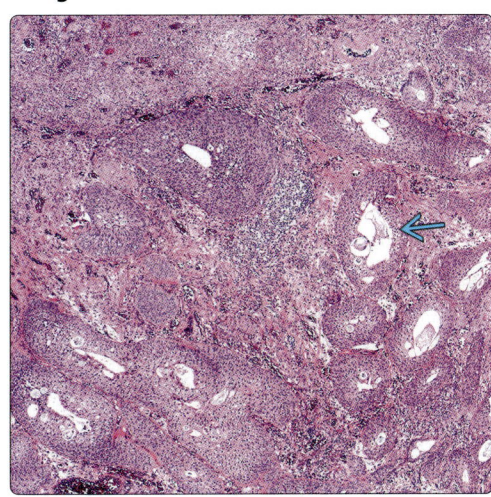

(Left) This amount of epithelium seen at low-power magnification should prompt consideration of large nested carcinoma. Central cystic areas ➡ are a subtle clue, but the irregular border ➡ is most diagnostic in the distinction from a noninvasive nested pattern. (Right) Central lumina with inspissated material ➡ may also be seen in cystitis glandularis, but these nests are irregularly distributed throughout the lamina propria and filled most of the submitted tissue fragments.

Large Nested Carcinoma: Necrosis

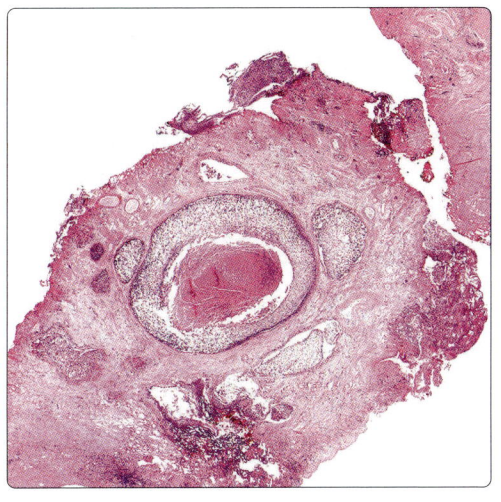

Large Nested Carcinoma: Architectural Distribution

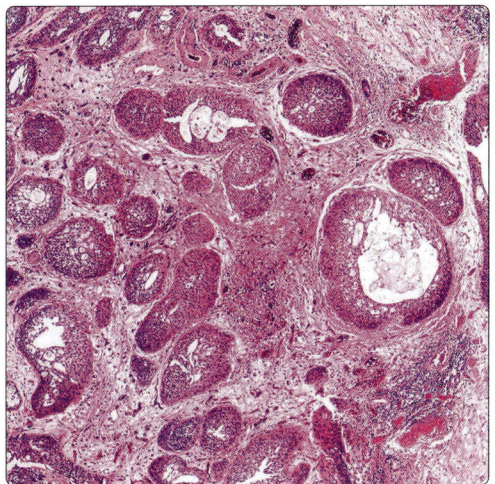

(Left) Areas of central necrosis may be seen in large nested carcinoma, a feature that should prompt consideration of malignancy. The size and the irregular distribution of the urothelial nests also suggest the possibility of large nested carcinoma. (Right) The irregular, random distribution of the urothelial nests in the lamina propria argues against the benign mimics of large nested carcinoma such as cystitis cystica and cystitis glandularis.

Large Nested Carcinoma: Focal Stromal Response

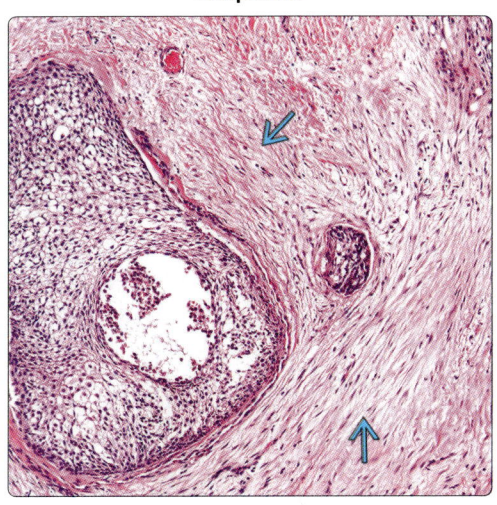

Large Nested Carcinoma: Deep Invasion

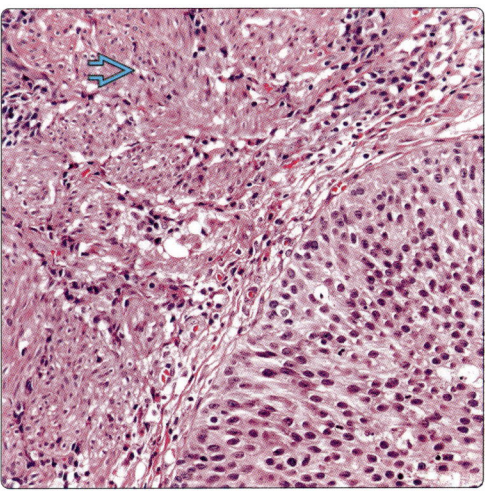

(Left) In rare foci, large nested carcinoma may be associated with a subtle degree of stromal reaction, characterized by a rim of elongated myofibroblasts ➡, as seen in this example. (Right) Identification of invasion into muscularis propria ➡ is diagnostic of invasive carcinoma. This high-power photomicrograph demonstrates the relatively bland cytologic features of large nested carcinoma.

Overview of Invasive Carcinoma Subtypes

(Left) This invasive urothelial carcinoma has an admixture of nests ⇨ and tubules ⇨. The distribution in the lamina propria is more irregularly dispersed than in benign mimics. (Right) On high-power examination, this invasive urothelial carcinoma is comprised of elongated nests ⇨ with occasional tubule formation ⇨. The reactive stromal changes and the irregular, randomly distributed nests are features that should suggest a diagnosis of carcinoma.

Urothelial Carcinoma With Small Tubules

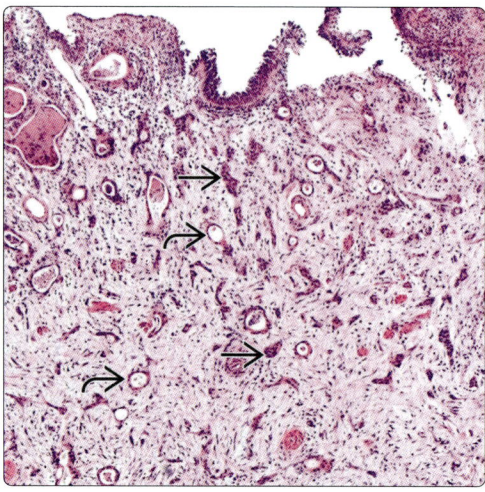

Urothelial Carcinoma With Small Tubules

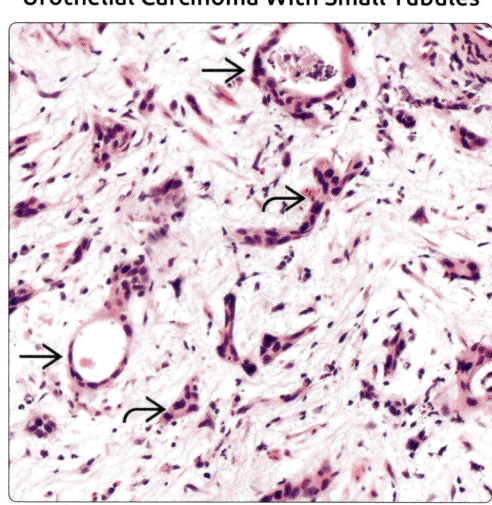

(Left) This deeply invasive carcinoma has a deceptively bland appearance with small luminal structures that mimic blood vessels on low-power evaluation ⇨. The associated stromal reaction ⇨ should suggest a neoplastic process. (Right) Microcystic urothelial carcinoma shows deceptively bland features mimicking cystitis glandularis. The irregular and haphazard nature of the proliferation, as well as widespread involvement of lamina propria, aid in recognition as carcinoma.

Microcystic Carcinoma

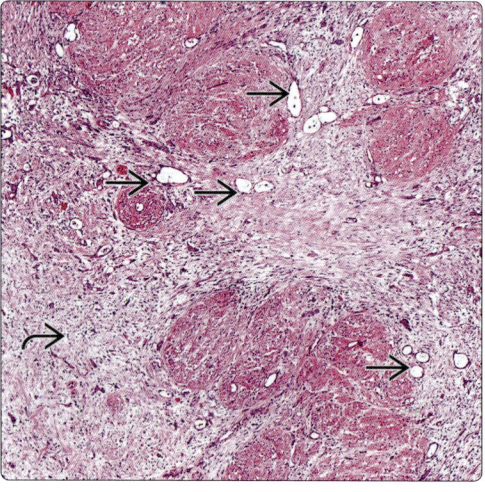

Microcystic Carcinoma

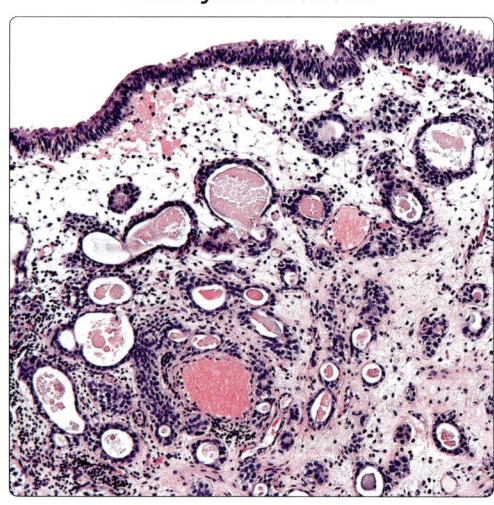

(Left) Microcystic urothelial carcinoma is shown with innocuous nuclear features. The variably sized and shaped cysts are lined by flattened to columnar epithelium or multilayered urothelium. (Right) The extremely bland cytology of the neoplastic cells in this microcystic carcinoma is appreciated. In contrast to the typical pseudostratified columnar lining cells of adenocarcinoma, these neoplastic cells are flattened. Expression of urothelial markers is common.

Microcystic Carcinoma

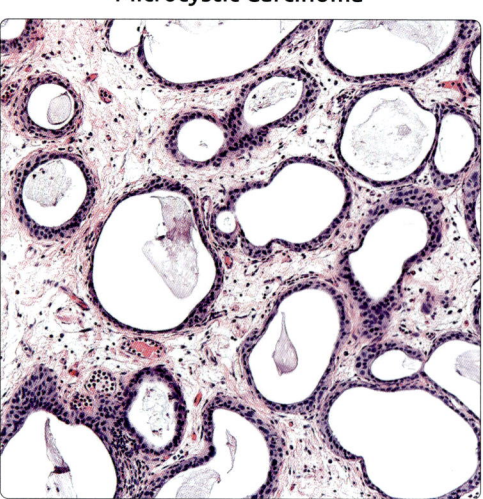

Microcystic Carcinoma

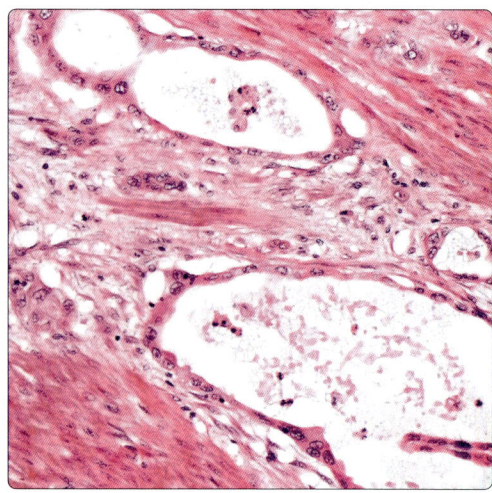

Overview of Invasive Carcinoma Subtypes

Plasmacytoid Carcinoma
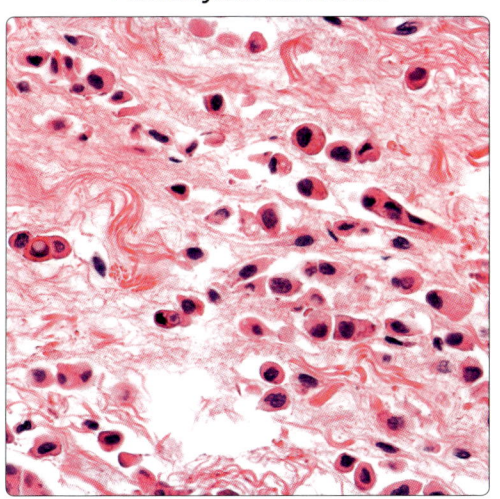

Plasmacytoid Carcinoma
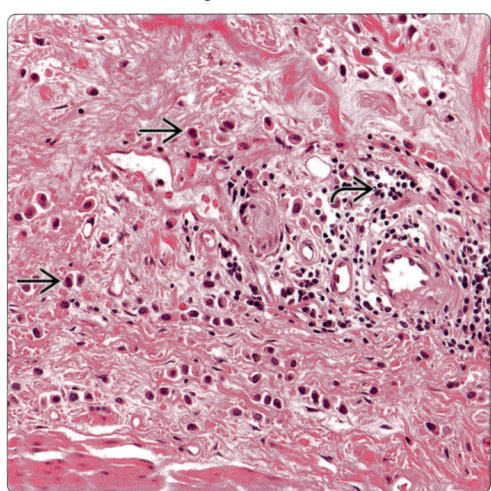

(Left) Plasmacytoid urothelial carcinoma is characterized by individual round neoplastic cells with eccentric nuclei and deep eosinophilic cytoplasm. They often infiltrate in a pattern similar to signet ring adenocarcinoma. **(Right)** This low-power image shows the subtle morphology of plasmacytoid urothelial carcinoma ➡ adjacent to an inflammatory infiltrate ➡. The neoplastic cells are easily confused with plasma cells or histiocytes at this magnification.

Plasmacytoid Carcinoma
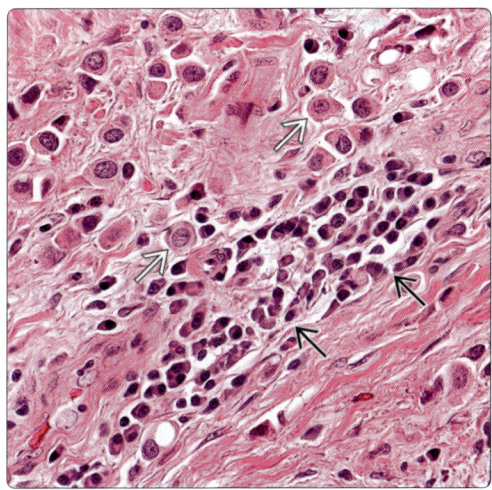

Plasmacytoid Carcinoma
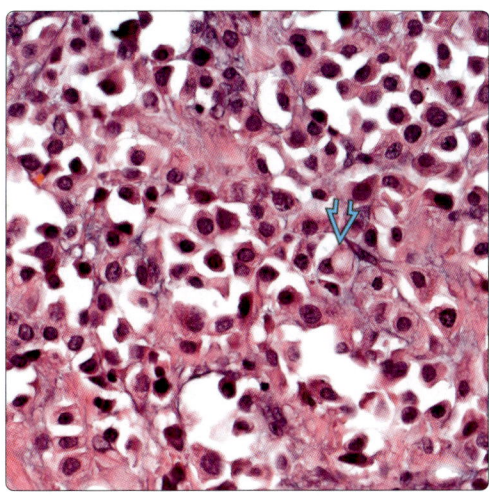

(Left) The large size of the neoplastic plasmacytoid carcinoma cells ➡ can be compared to the smaller adjacent normal plasma cells ➡. This pattern may be very difficult to recognize on intraoperative frozen section evaluation of margins. **(Right)** The presence of multiple dyscohesive neoplastic cells within retraction spaces is typical of the plasmacytoid variant of urothelial carcinoma. It is not uncommon for admixed signet ring-like cells ➡ to be present, and should not change the diagnosis.

Plasmacytoid Carcinoma
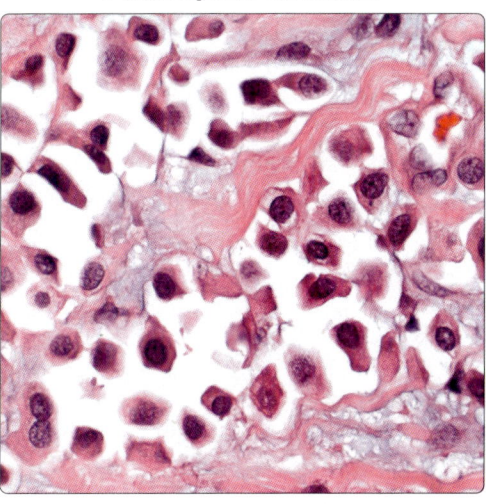

Cytokeratin: Plasmacytoid Carcinoma
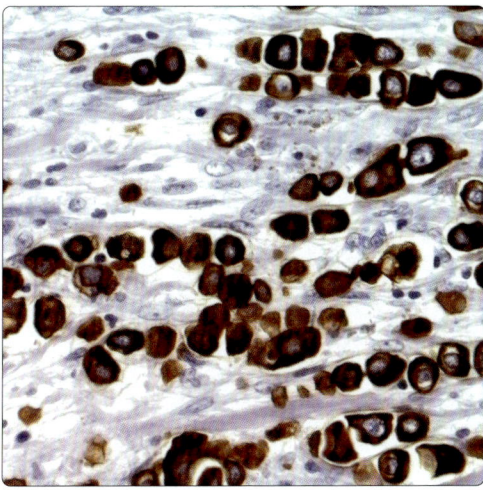

(Left) The round eccentric nuclei and the eosinophilic cytoplasm are characteristic of plasmacytoid urothelial carcinoma. In difficult cases, immunohistochemistry may aid in the distinction from inflammatory cells. **(Right)** Diffuse cytoplasmic immunoreactivity for broad spectrum cytokeratin is very helpful in establishing the diagnosis of carcinoma in difficult cases. It is important to realize that these carcinomas may also express CD138, further mimicking a plasma cell infiltrate.

Overview of Invasive Carcinoma Subtypes

Plasmacytoid Carcinoma in Seminal Vesicle

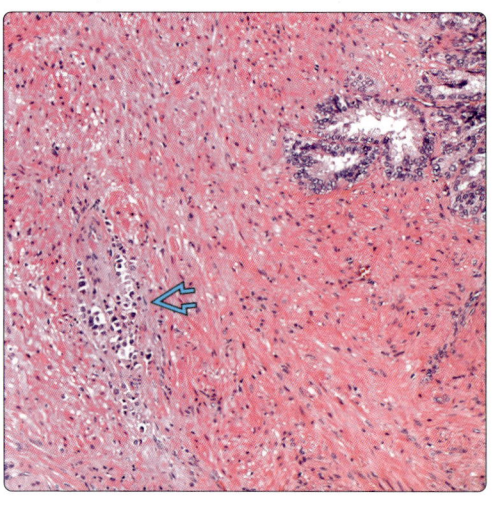

Plasmacytoid Carcinoma in Fallopian Tube

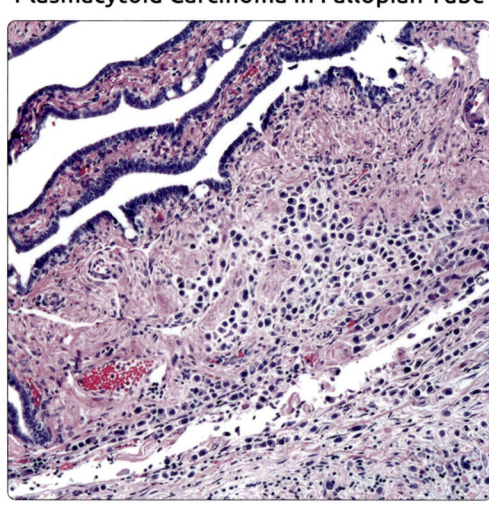

(Left) *Plasmacytoid carcinoma has a propensity for high stage, disseminated disease. In this example, the carcinoma involves the wall of the seminal vesicle ➡ where it could be mistaken for inflammatory cells.* (Right) *This plasmacytoid carcinoma involves the fallopian tube. The plasmacytoid variant of urothelial carcinoma has an unusual, but characteristic, pattern of spread to peritoneal surfaces. The behavior is similar to diffuse gastric cancer and lobular breast carcinoma.*

Plasmacytoid Carcinoma in Periureteral Tissue

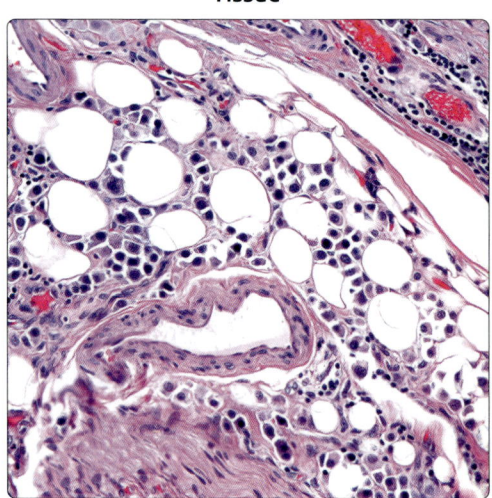

Plasmacytoid Carcinoma in Lymph Node

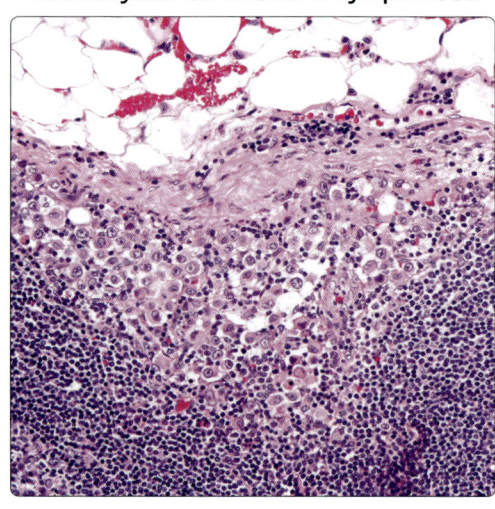

(Left) *When involving soft tissues (e.g., periureteral or perivesical), the neoplastic cells permeate adipose and fibrous tissue in an individual cell pattern that may closely mimic inflammatory cells. Prior knowledge of a plasmacytoid carcinoma diagnosis is helpful.* (Right) *When metastatic to lymph nodes, the plasmacytoid variant of urothelial carcinoma may closely mimic sinus histiocytes or other intranodal inflammatory cells.*

Plasmacytoid Carcinoma in Lymph Node

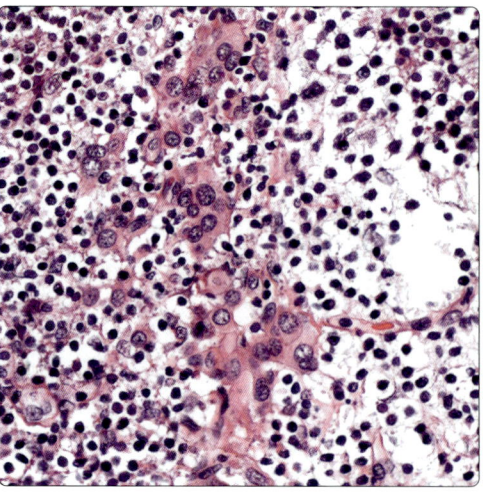

Cytokeratin: Plasmacytoid Carcinoma

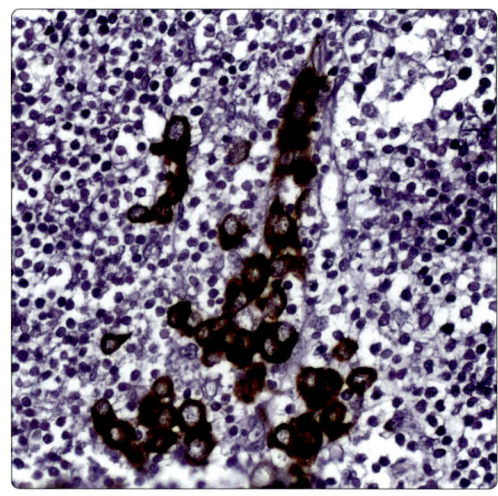

(Left) *Metastatic plasmacytoid urothelial carcinoma in a lymph node may be deceptively bland, where it closely mimics sinus histiocytes or intranodal plasma cells.* (Right) *Cytokeratin immunostains may be helpful in difficult cases, as they highlight the subtle population of metastatic plasmacytoid carcinoma cells. It is very helpful to know that a plasmacytoid morphology is present when screening excised lymph nodes.*

Overview of Invasive Carcinoma Subtypes

Noninvasive Papillary Urothelial Carcinoma

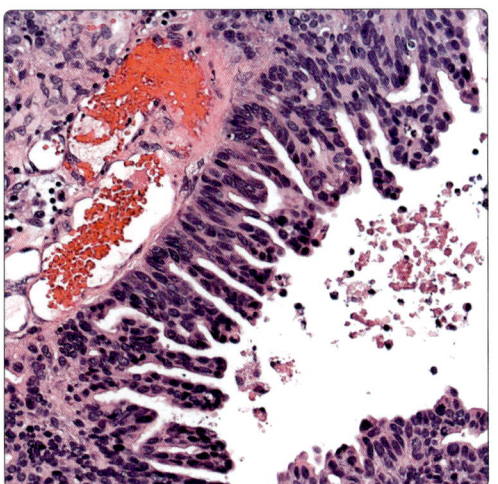

Noninvasive Papillary Urothelial Carcinoma

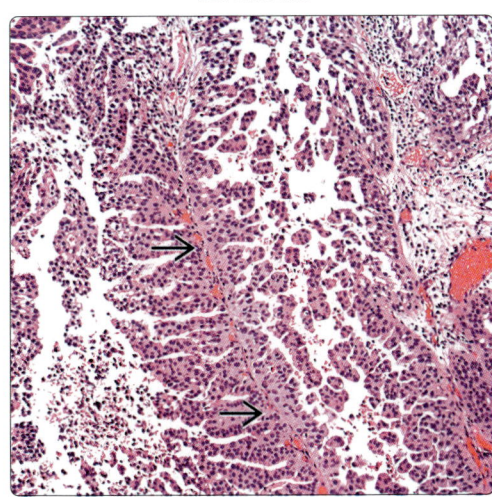

(Left) Noninvasive papillary urothelial carcinomas may also have a micropapillary architecture characterized by thin elongated micropapillae that have a greater length than width. This should not be diagnosed as micropapillary carcinoma. (Right) This noninvasive urothelial carcinoma also has micropapillary architecture characterized by elongated filiform papillae arising from the main papillary core ➡. This should not be diagnosed as micropapillary carcinoma as the clinical implications are not the same.

Micropapillary Carcinoma

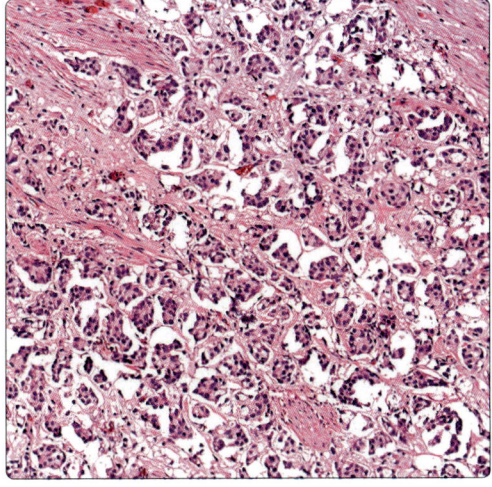

Micropapillary Carcinoma

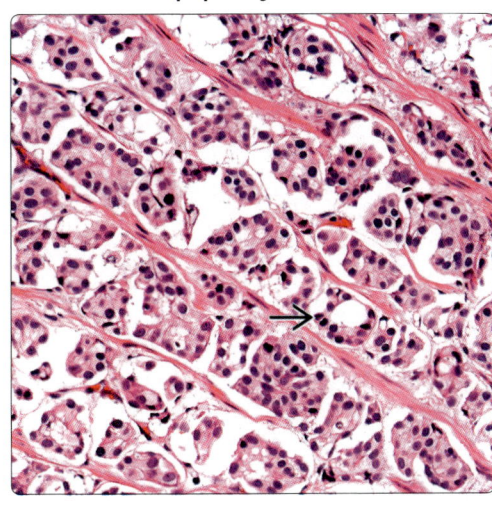

(Left) Invasive micropapillary carcinoma is characterized by back-to-back lacunar spaces containing small nests of carcinoma, as seen in this example. (Right) Nests and ring forms ➡ within back-to-back lacunar spaces are characteristic of invasive micropapillary carcinoma. The cytology of the neoplastic cells may be rather bland, despite the deeply invasive growth and the common presentation with metastases. Vascular invasion is typically present in this variant.

Micropapillary Carcinoma

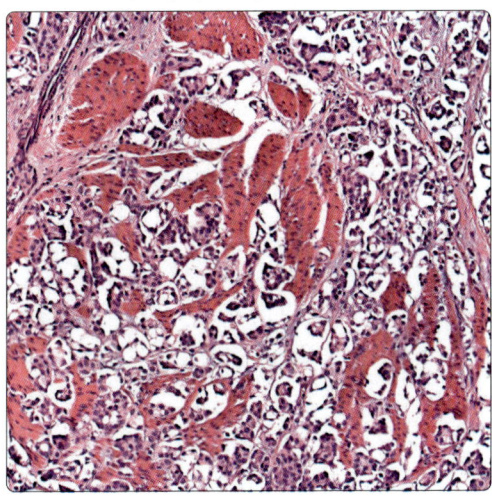

Micropapillary Carcinoma

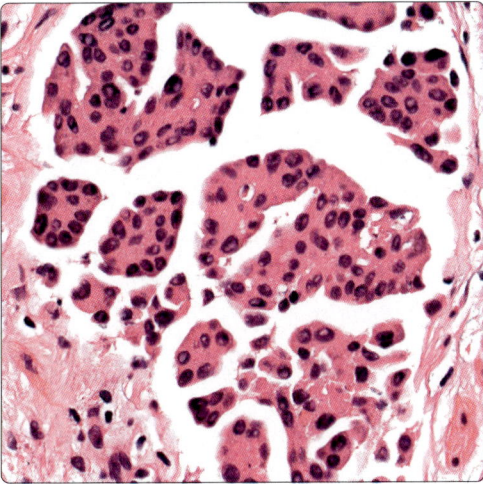

(Left) Micropapillary carcinoma commonly presents at high stage. This example shows extensive involvement of the muscularis propria. The tumor maintains characteristic features such as back-to-back lacunar spaces, multiple nests in a single retraction space, and ring forms. (Right) Micropapillary carcinoma may have a striking resemblance to ovarian serous carcinoma. Micropapillary carcinoma of the urinary bladder maintains a urothelial phenotype and typically lacks a true fibrovascular core.

Overview of Invasive Carcinoma Subtypes

Micropapillary Carcinoma

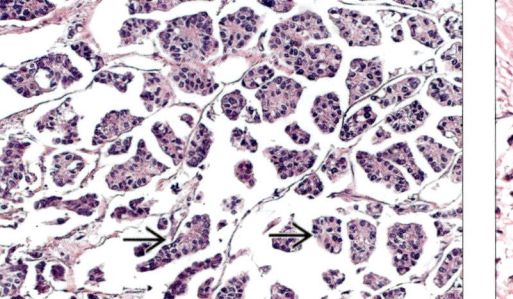

Micropapillary Carcinoma

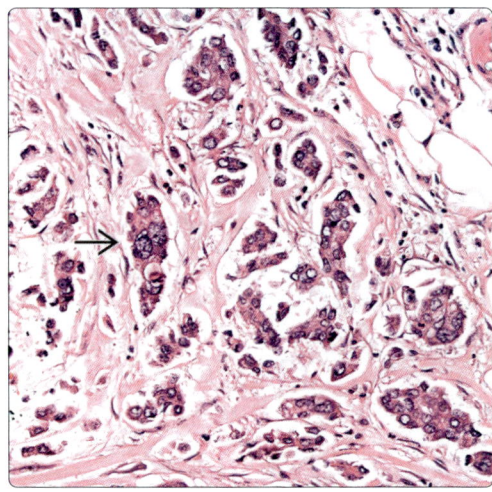

(Left) Although not present in all cases, the peripheral orientation of the nuclei in these nests ➡ is another feature that may be seen in micropapillary carcinoma. The back-to-back lacunar spaces and the presence of multiple nests in a single lacunar space are other characteristic features. (Right) There is a broad spectrum of cytologic atypia in micropapillary carcinoma. This example shows more nuclear pleomorphism ➡ than typically seen in micropapillary carcinoma.

Micropapillary Carcinoma: Mixed Pattern

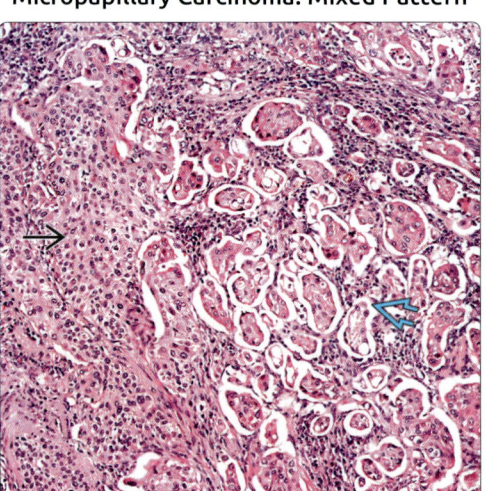

Micropapillary Carcinoma in Lymph Node

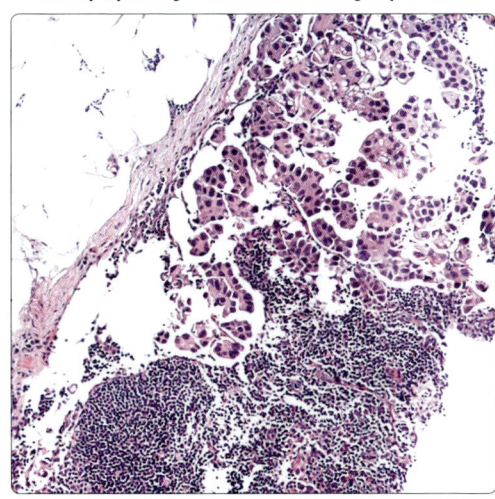

(Left) In this example of a urothelial carcinoma with mixed histologic patterns, sheets of conventional urothelial carcinoma ➡ are adjacent to the small epithelial nests within lacunar spaces ➡ that are characteristic of micropapillary carcinoma. (Right) Metastatic sites of spread, as highlighted by this lymph node metastasis, commonly retain the micropapillary histologic features of the primary tumor.

Typical Urothelial Carcinoma With Retraction Spaces

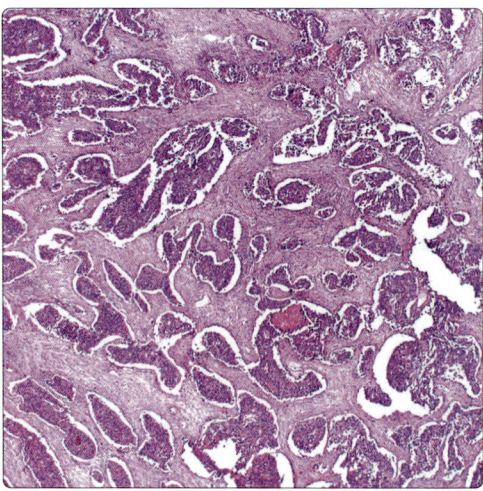

Typical Urothelial Carcinoma With Retraction Spaces

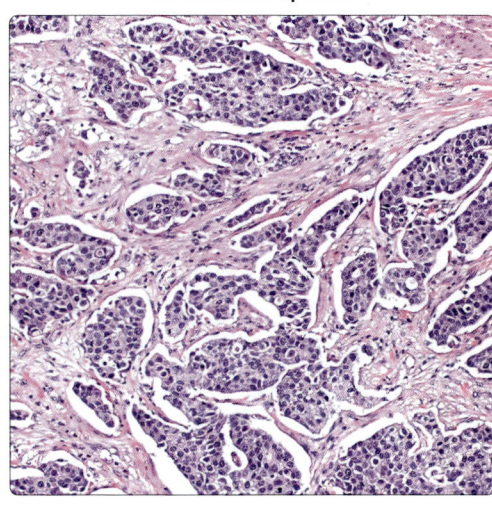

(Left) Despite the prominent retraction spaces, this should be regarded as typical invasive urothelial carcinoma. The epithelial nests are much larger than those seen in micropapillary carcinoma. (Right) On higher power evaluation, this typical invasive urothelial carcinoma has larger nests and more confluent, branching epithelium than micropapillary carcinoma. These urothelial carcinomas with extensive retraction may have an identical immunophenotype to micropapillary carcinoma.

Overview of Invasive Carcinoma Subtypes

Lymphoepithelioma-Like Carcinoma

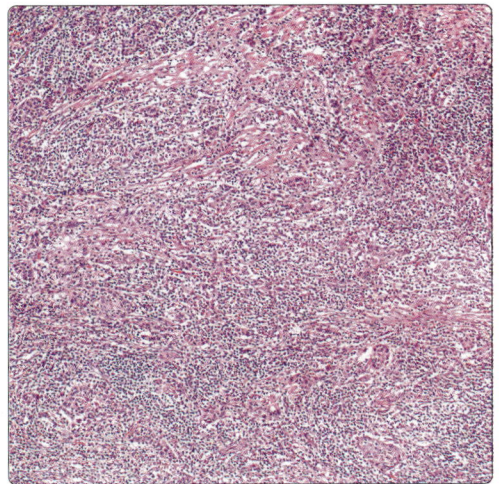

Lymphoepithelioma-Like Carcinoma

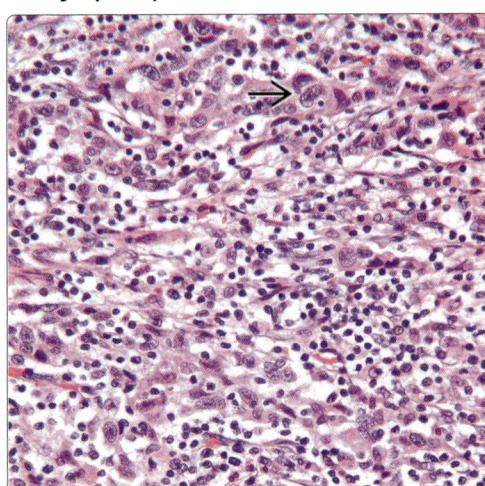

(Left) At low-power evaluation, lymphoepithelioma-like carcinoma closely mimics an inflammatory infiltrate or lymphoma. Recognition as carcinoma depends on identification of the carcinomatous component at high magnification. *(Right)* At high-power evaluation, there is a dense inflammatory infiltrate, but a 2nd subtle population of cells is also seen ➡. This 2nd population is the carcinomatous component and may be highlighted by cytokeratin immunostains.

Lymphoepithelioma-Like Carcinoma

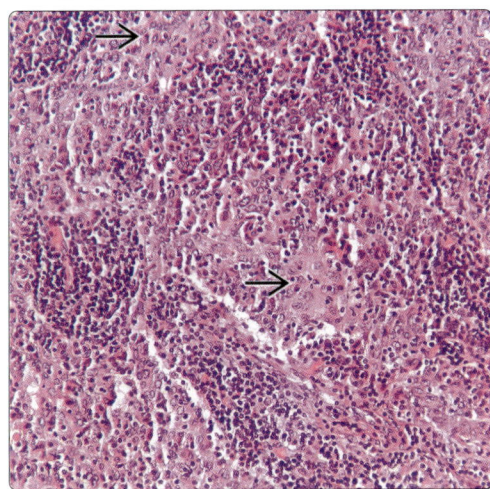

Lymphoepithelioma-Like Carcinoma

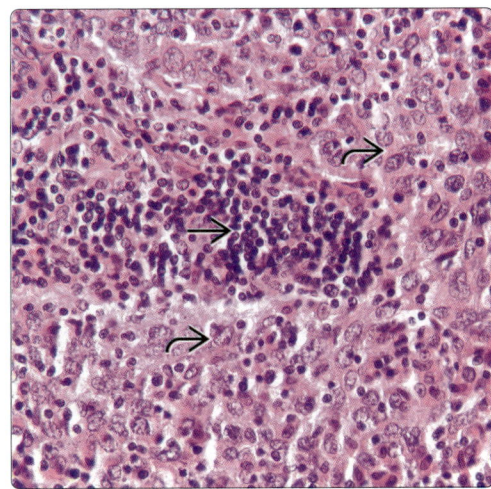

(Left) This example of lymphoepithelioma-like carcinoma in the urinary bladder has a more pronounced epithelial component ➡, even at low-power magnification. *(Right)* On high power, the larger size of the cells in the carcinomatous component ➡ are contrasted with the lymphocytes ➡. Bladder lymphoepithelioma-like carcinoma is not associated with EBV infection. Lymphoepithelioma-like carcinomas may be pure, predominant, or a focal finding.

Lymphoepithelioma-Like Carcinoma

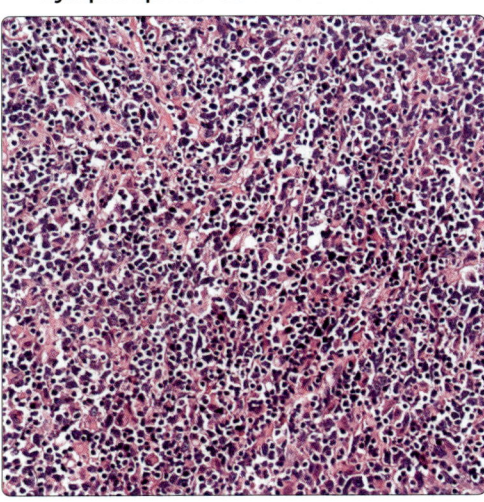

Cytokeratin: Lymphoepithelioma-Like Carcinoma

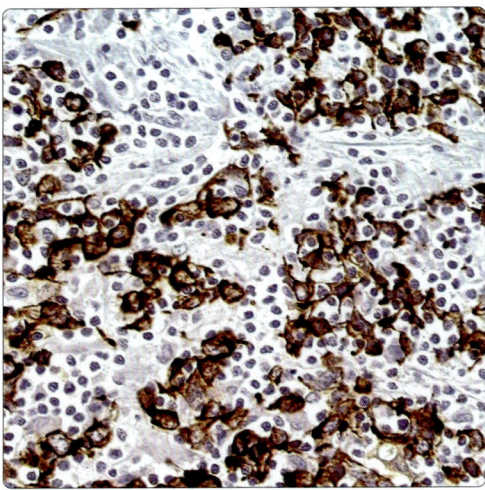

(Left) This lymphoepithelioma-like carcinoma has an absence of epithelial aggregates and closely mimics a lymphomatous process. Immunohistochemical evaluation is important in such cases. *(Right)* This lymphoepithelioma-like carcinoma is highlighted by CK-PAN (AE1/AE3) immunostains. A broad spectrum cytokeratin stain is helpful in excluding other diagnoses, such as lymphoma, that would not show an admixed population of epithelial cells.

Overview of Invasive Carcinoma Subtypes

Small Cell Carcinoma
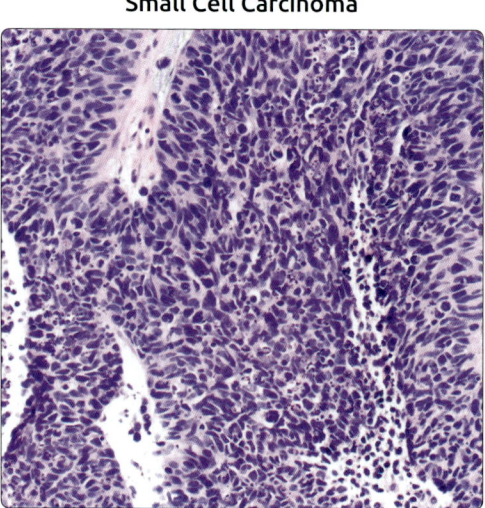

Small Cell Carcinoma
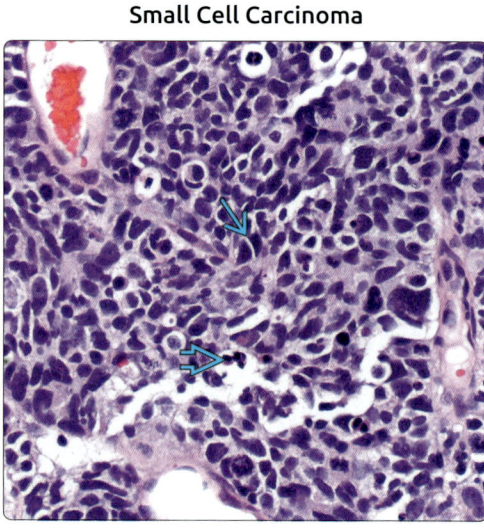

(Left) Small cell carcinoma of the urinary bladder is morphologically similar to pulmonary primaries with high nuclear:cytoplasmic ratio, nuclear molding, and high mitotic rate. In the urinary bladder, this pattern is often interpreted as poorly differentiated urothelial carcinoma, but recognition as small cell carcinoma is important because it requires a different chemotherapeutic regimen. **(Right)** Small cell carcinoma often has high nuclear:cytoplasmic ratio, nuclear molding ➡, and frequent apoptotic bodies ➡.

Small Cell Carcinoma
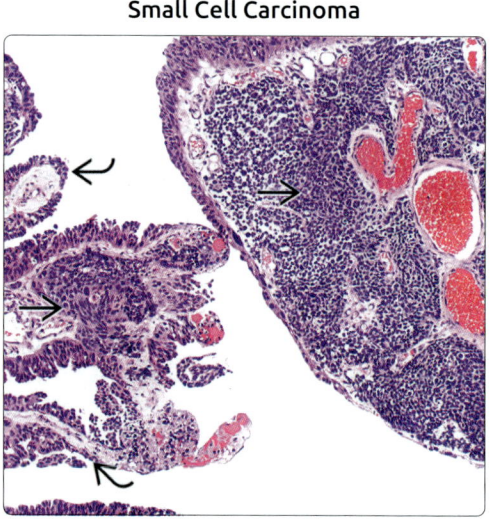

Synaptophysin: Small Cell Carcinoma
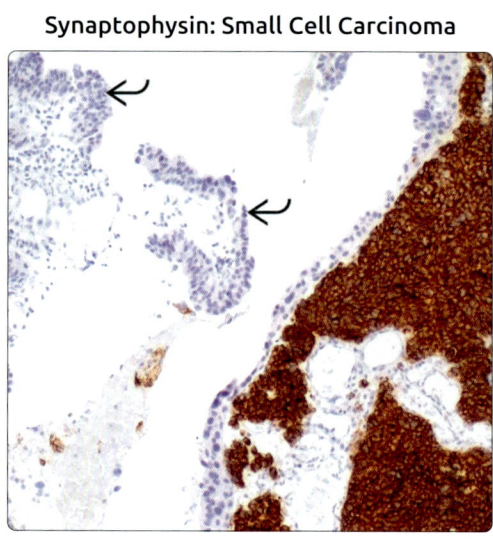

(Left) Small cell carcinoma component ➡ adjacent to a conventional papillary urothelial carcinoma ➡. **(Right)** Strong diffuse synaptophysin reactivity is seen in the small cell carcinoma, but not in the adjacent conventional papillary urothelial carcinoma ➡. Synaptophysin stains must be carefully interpreted in the context of the morphology, as prostatic adenocarcinoma and alveolar rhabdomyosarcoma involving the bladder often express synaptophysin.

Glycogen-Rich Urothelial Carcinoma
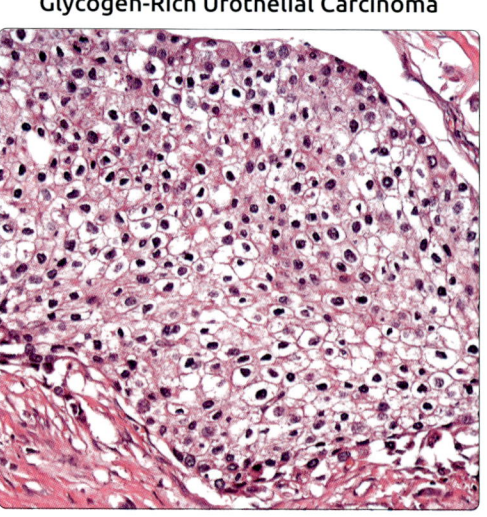

Glycogen-Rich Urothelial Carcinoma
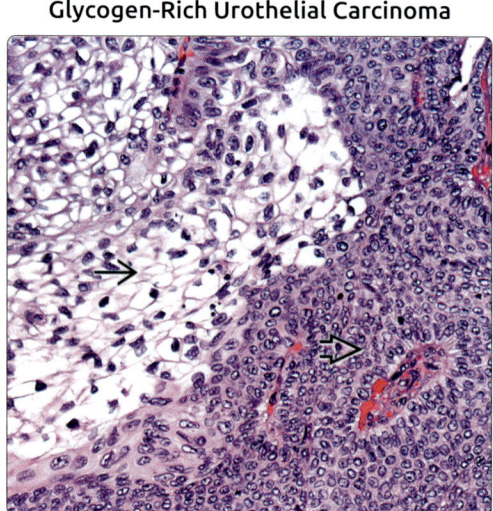

(Left) Rare urothelial carcinomas have abundant clear cytoplasm secondary to intracytoplasmic glycogen accumulation. This feature is typically present only focally in an otherwise typical urothelial carcinoma, which allows distinction from other clear tumors, such as renal cell carcinoma. **(Right)** This urothelial carcinoma of the urinary bladder has a component with intracytoplasmic glycogen ➡ adjacent to a more typical urothelial carcinoma ➡.

Overview of Invasive Carcinoma Subtypes

Poorly Differentiated Urothelial Carcinoma

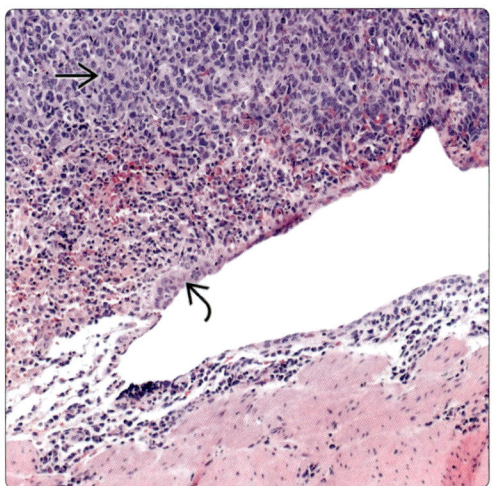

Poorly Differentiated Urothelial Carcinoma

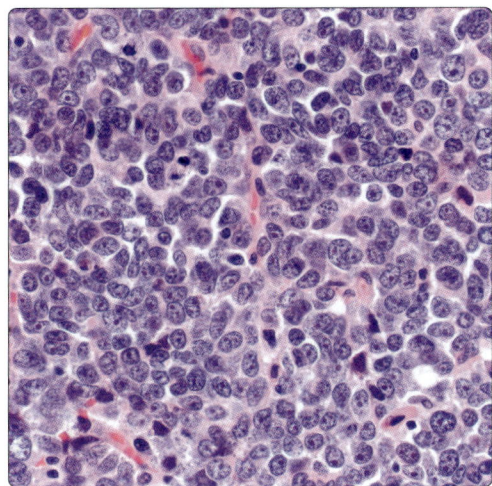

(Left) A poorly differentiated round cell malignancy ⇒ is present underlying the urothelium ⇒. Immunohistochemistry would be needed to confirm urothelial differentiation. **(Right)** On high-power examination of a bladder resection specimen, this poorly differentiated urothelial carcinoma has a morphology that overlaps with lymphoma, rhabdomyosarcoma, small cell carcinoma, and other round cell malignancies. A broad panel of immunohistochemical stains is critical in evaluating such cases.

HMCK (34βE12): Poorly Differentiated Urothelial Carcinoma

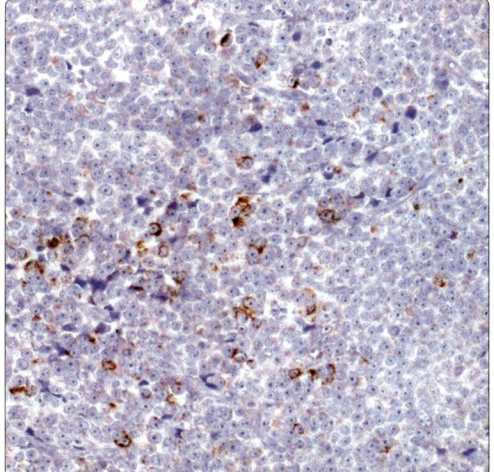

p63: Poorly Differentiated Urothelial Carcinoma

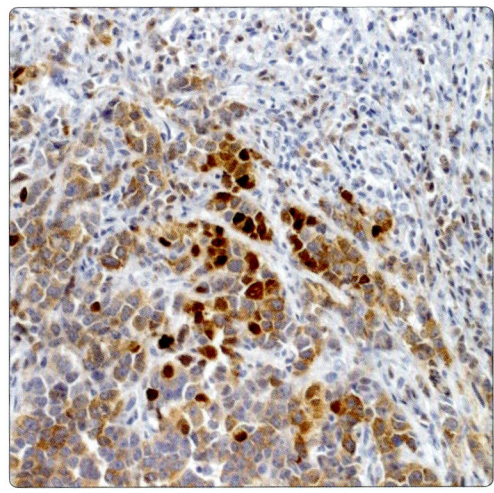

(Left) Patchy cytoplasmic immunoreactivity for HMCK (34βE12) is seen in this poorly differentiated urothelial carcinoma. Hematopoietic [CD45 (LCA) and CD43], skeletal muscle (desmin and myogenin), and neuroendocrine markers (synaptophysin) were all negative. **(Right)** Patchy nuclear p63 immunoreactivity is also seen in this poorly differentiated neoplasm, supporting classification as poorly differentiated urothelial carcinoma. GATA3 and uroplakin-2 are also useful stains.

Urothelial Carcinoma With Osteoclast-Type Giant Cells

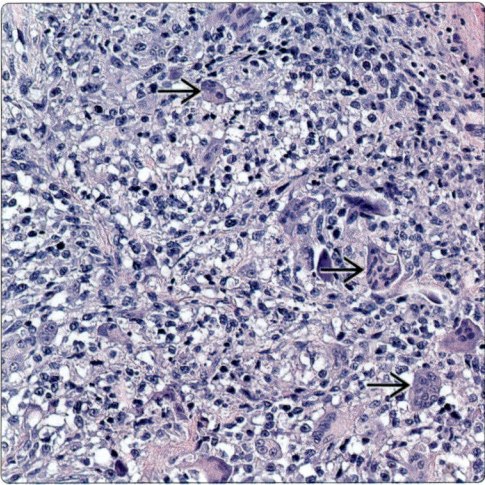

Urothelial Carcinoma With Osteoclast-Type Giant Cells

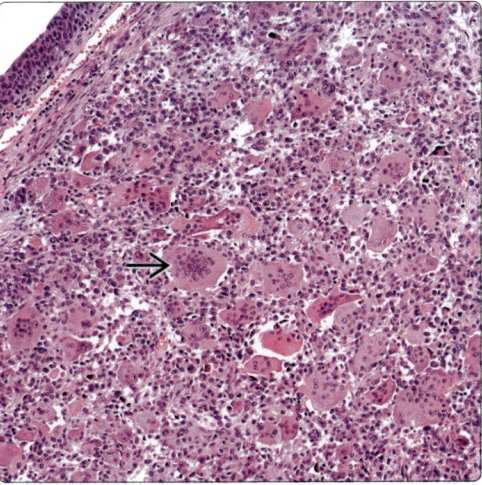

(Left) Urothelial carcinomas may have admixed osteoclast-like giant cells ⇒. This population of multinucleated giant cells stains with histiocytic markers but not cytokeratin. **(Right)** Rare urothelial carcinomas have abundant osteoclast-like giant cells ⇒ that create a morphologic appearance similar to giant cell tumor of bone or soft tissue. The background mononuclear cells express cytokeratin, confirming an epithelial lineage.

Overview of Invasive Carcinoma Subtypes

(Left) The presence of infiltrating urothelial carcinoma ⇒ adjacent to a malignant spindle cell neoplasm ⇒ is diagnostic of sarcomatoid urothelial carcinoma. When a carcinomatous component is not present, immunohistochemistry may be needed. (Right) This sarcomatoid carcinoma has a degree of nuclear chromatin irregularity diagnostic of malignancy. Cytology is the most useful feature in the distinction from a myofibroblastic proliferation.

Sarcomatoid Urothelial Carcinoma: Carcinomatous Component

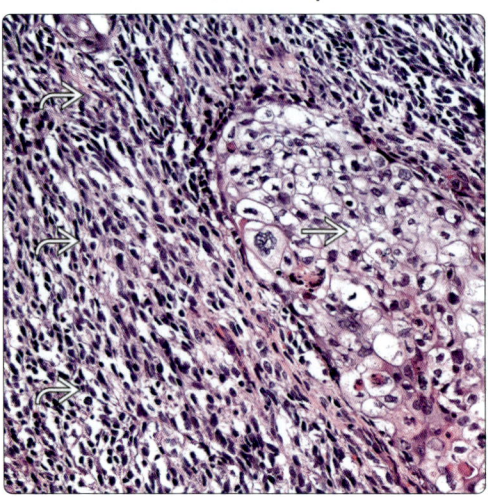

Sarcomatoid Urothelial Carcinoma

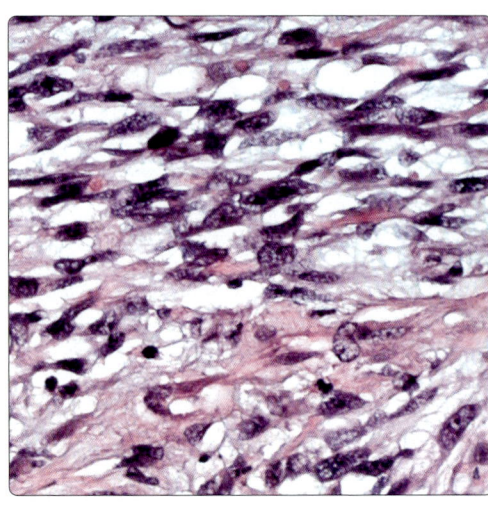

(Left) Spindled sarcomatoid carcinoma may be indistinguishable from a variety of soft tissue sarcomas. Expression of epithelial markers, such as HMCK(34βE12) and p63, are helpful; myofibroblastic and smooth muscle tumors only express low molecular weight keratin. (Right) Pure spindled sarcomatoid carcinomas may be deceptively bland with only subtle nuclear chromatin changes. Evaluation of the entire tumor usually reveals areas with more pronounced atypia.

Sarcomatoid Urothelial Carcinoma

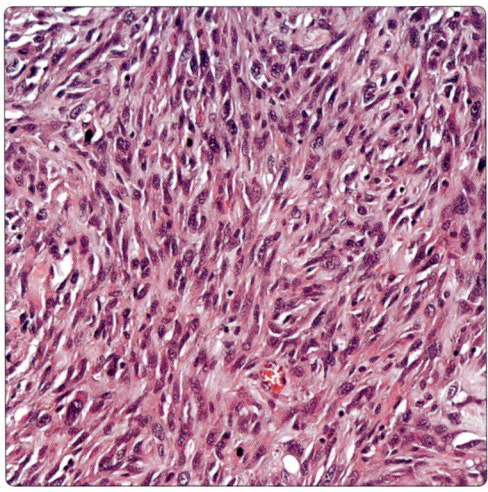

Sarcomatoid Urothelial Carcinoma

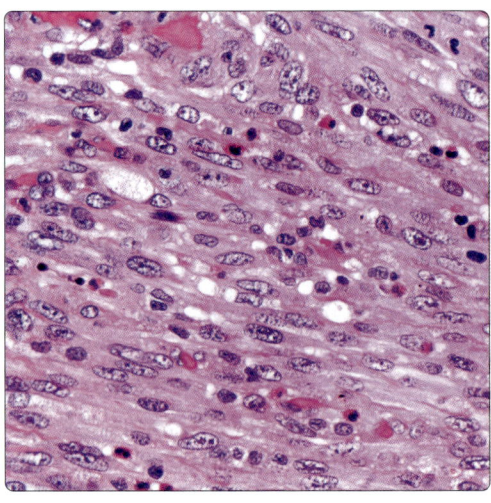

(Left) This example of sarcomatoid urothelial carcinoma shows areas with obvious nuclear pleomorphism and nuclear chromatin abnormalities that are beyond that seen in myofibroblastic lesions. If a carcinomatous component is not seen, leiomyosarcoma should still be excluded immunohistochemically. (Right) The presence of foci with a more epithelioid morphology should prompt careful consideration of a carcinoma and appropriate immunohistochemical evaluation.

Sarcomatoid Urothelial Carcinoma

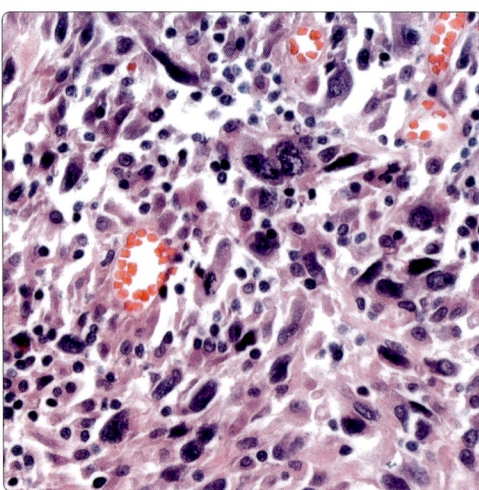

Sarcomatoid Urothelial Carcinoma: Epithelioid Focus

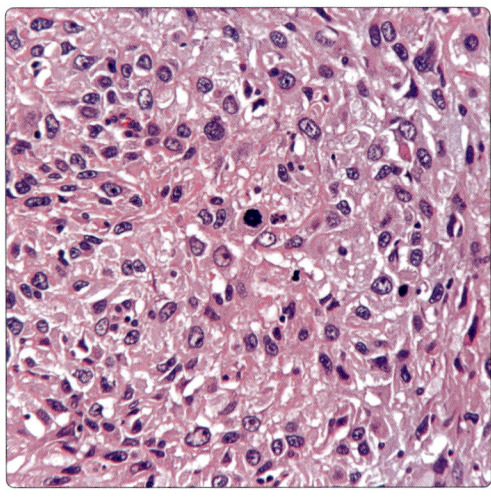

Overview of Invasive Carcinoma Subtypes

Sarcomatoid Urothelial Carcinoma

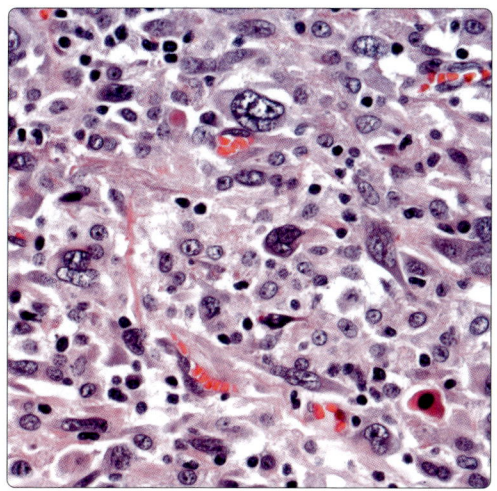

Sarcomatoid Urothelial Carcinoma: Myxoid Pattern

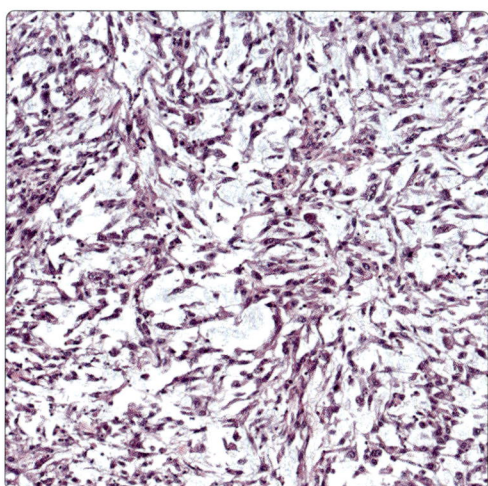

(Left) Some sarcomatoid urothelial carcinomas have pleomorphic undifferentiated foci. This neoplasm also had areas of both typical urothelial carcinoma and spindle cell morphology. (Right) Myxoid and spindle cell patterns of sarcomatoid urothelial carcinoma may closely mimic myxoid leiomyosarcoma or a myofibroblastic proliferation. IHC analysis may be critical in such cases. Myofibroblastic proliferations and urothelial neoplasia may coexist. Distinction between the two is based on cytologic features.

Sarcomatoid Urothelial Carcinoma: Myxoid Pattern

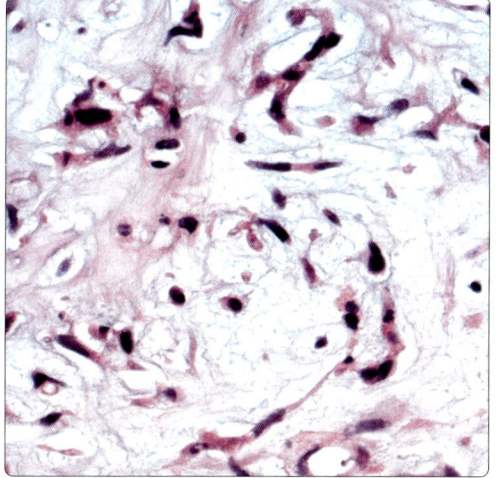

Sarcomatoid Urothelial Carcinoma: Heterologous Rhabdomyosarcoma

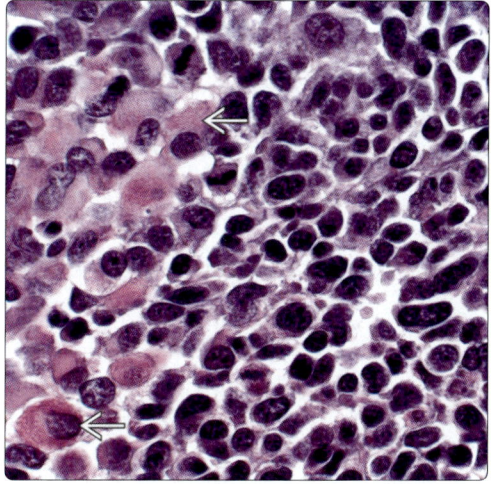

(Left) A subset of sarcomatoid carcinomas have prominent myxoid stroma. Although this may cause confusion with myofibroblastic lesions, the degree of nuclear chromatin changes is more than that seen in myofibroblastic lesions. In this case, conventional urothelial carcinoma was present elsewhere. (Right) This sarcomatoid urothelial carcinoma shows a focus of heterologous rhabdomyosarcoma. Numerous rhabdomyoblasts are seen ⇒.

Sarcomatoid Urothelial Carcinoma

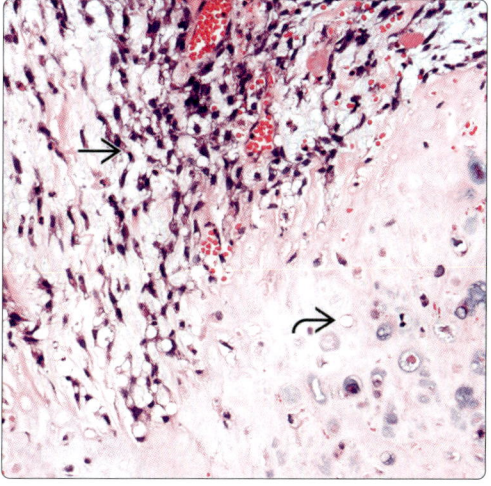

Sarcomatoid Urothelial Carcinoma: Heterologous Osteosarcoma

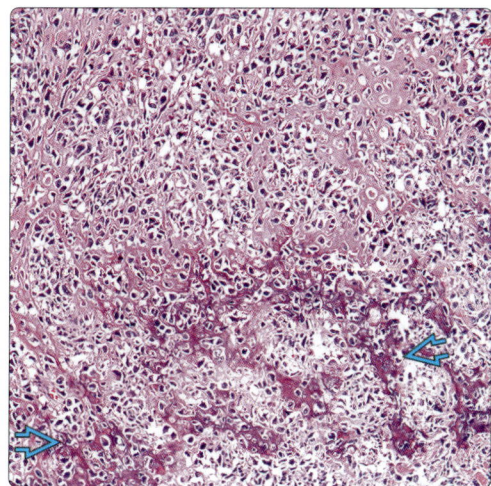

(Left) The malignant spindle cell component ⇒ merges with a focus of heterologous chondrosarcoma ⇒. Osteosarcoma and chondrosarcoma are rare and, when present, should prompt a search for a carcinomatous component. (Right) Sarcomatoid carcinomas may have heterologous differentiation. This example shows osteosarcoma, but chondrosarcoma and rhabdomyosarcoma may also be seen. While collagen may mimic osteoid, matrix calcification ⇒ is a more specific feature.

Overview of Invasive Carcinoma Subtypes

(Left) *Sarcomatoid urothelial carcinomas are very heterogeneous neoplasms. This example shows a region mimicking a myxoid spindle cell sarcoma ⇨, while other foci show poorly differentiated carcinoma ⇨.* (Right) *Heterologous osteosarcoma in a sarcomatoid urothelial carcinoma may also have admixed osteoclast-type giant cells. Osteoid was seen in other areas of the tumor.*

Sarcomatoid Urothelial Carcinoma

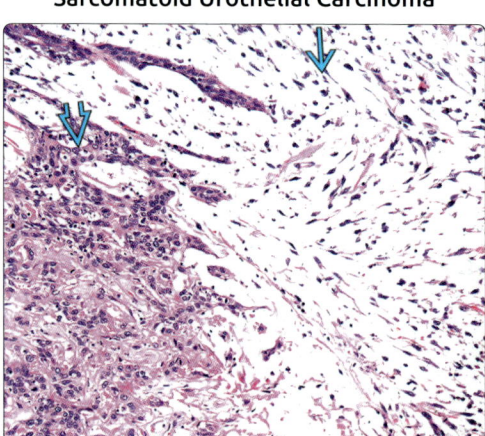

Sarcomatoid Urothelial Carcinoma: Heterologous Osteosarcoma

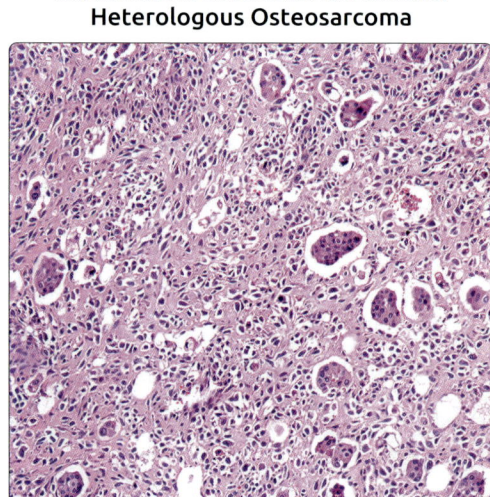

(Left) *The presence of a component of urothelial carcinoma, such as the micropapillary carcinoma in this case ⇨, strongly supports a diagnosis as sarcomatoid urothelial carcinoma.* (Right) *Sarcomatoid urothelial carcinomas may have a concomitant component of typical urothelial carcinoma, as the urothelial carcinoma in situ in this case. This feature would make the diagnosis more straightforward.*

Sarcomatoid Urothelial Carcinoma

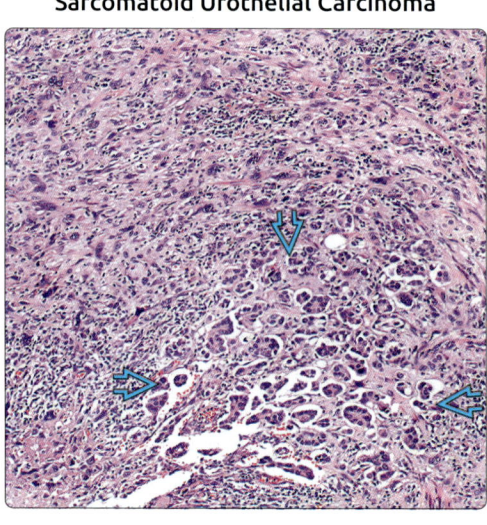

Sarcomatoid Urothelial Carcinoma

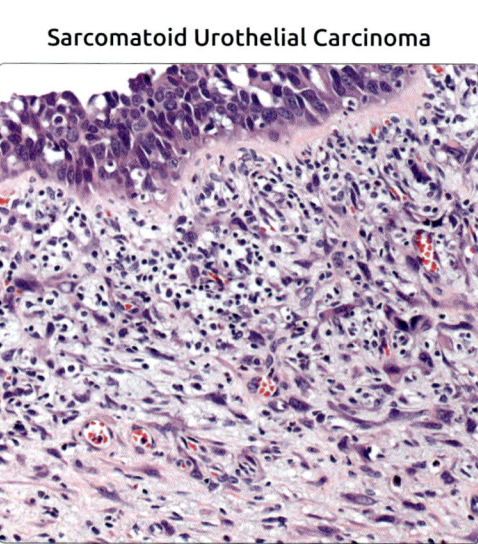

(Left) *Rare sarcomatoid urothelial carcinomas have areas of acantholysis that create pseudovascular spaces ⇨, mimicking angiosarcoma.* (Right) *Lymph node metastases from sarcomatoid urothelial carcinomas with a pseudoangiosarcomatous pattern may mimic both benign and malignant lesions including: angiosarcoma, normal sinuses, or vascular transformation of sinuses. Occasionally the cells may be more epithelioid or of poorly differentiated urothelial carcinoma.*

Sarcomatoid Urothelial Carcinoma: Pseudoangiosarcomatous

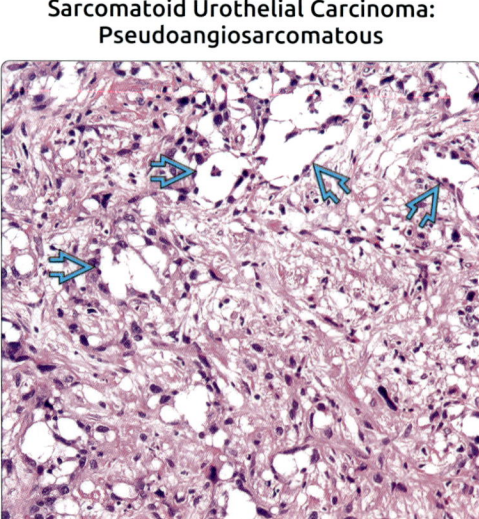

Sarcomatoid Urothelial Carcinoma: Pseudoangiosarcomatous

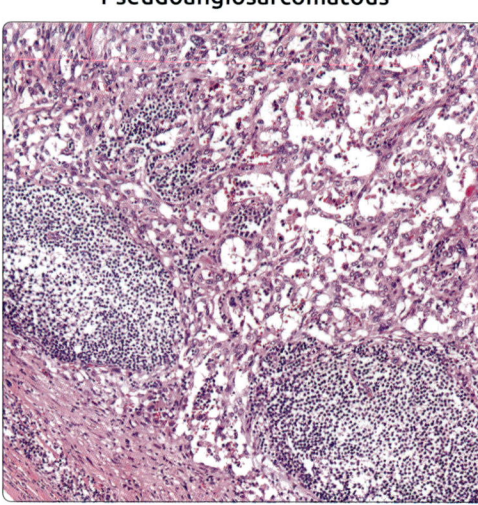

Overview of Invasive Carcinoma Subtypes

Cytokeratin: Sarcomatoid Urothelial Carcinoma

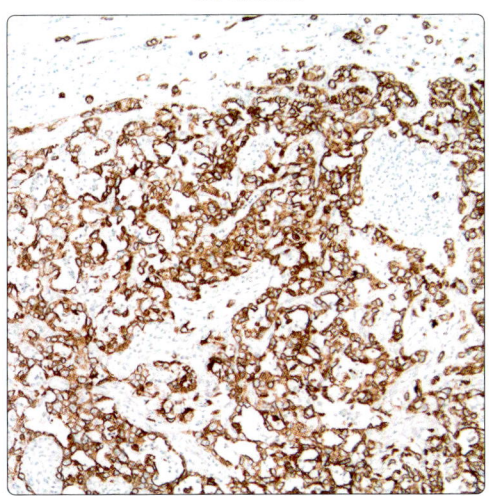

CAM5.2: Sarcomatoid Urothelial Carcinoma

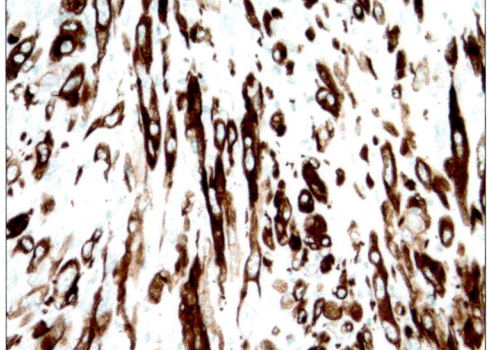

(Left) While "pan" keratins may be used as immunohistochemical screens for documenting sarcomatoid carcinoma, they are not entirely specific. Both smooth muscle and myofibroblastic lesions may also express "pan" keratins. (Right) Low molecular weight forms of cytokeratin may be positive in sarcomatoid urothelial carcinomas, but are also commonly expressed in myofibroblastic proliferations, and (less commonly) in smooth muscle tumors.

HMWCK: Sarcomatoid Urothelial Carcinoma

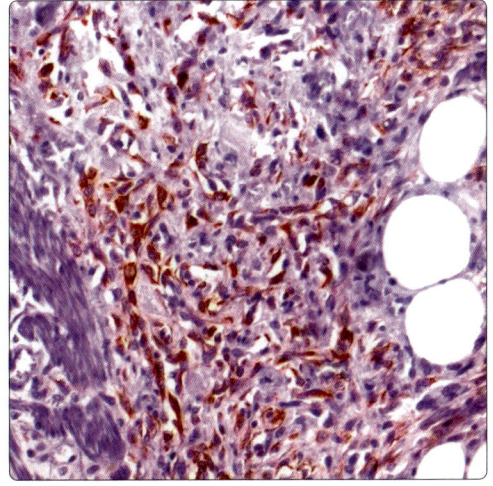

p63: Sarcomatoid Urothelial Carcinoma

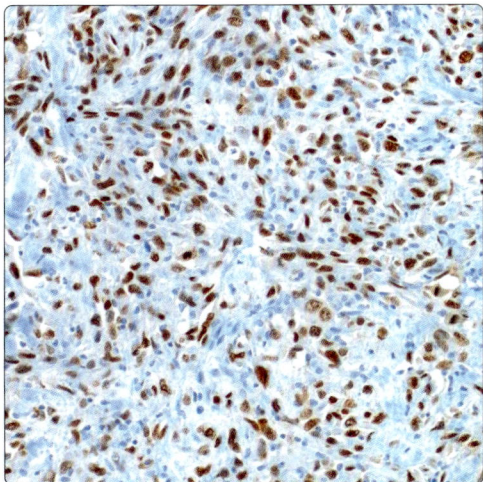

(Left) Sarcomatoid urothelial carcinoma typically expresses HMCK(34βE12). In contrast, when keratin expression is present, myofibroblastic proliferations and leiomyosarcomas only show immunoreactivity with low molecular weight cytokeratin. (Right) Nuclear p63 immunoreactivity is characteristic of sarcomatoid urothelial carcinoma. Other spindle cell mimics, such as florid myofibroblastic proliferations, do not show p63 expression. Leiomyosarcoma may occasionally be p63 positive.

GATA3: Sarcomatoid Urothelial Carcinoma

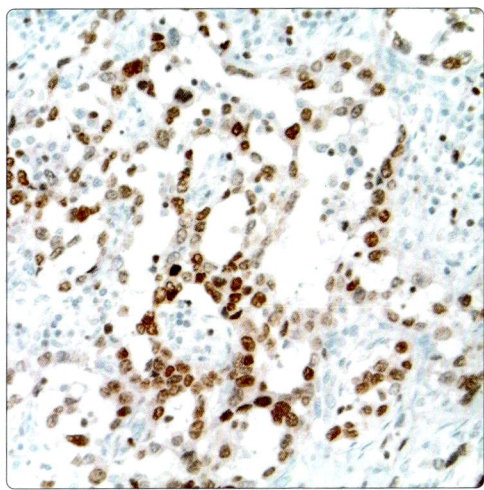

ERG: Sarcomatoid Carcinoma

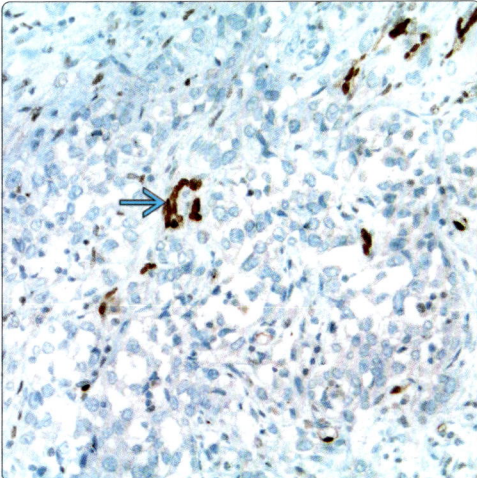

(Left) Nuclear GATA3 immunoreactivity may be retained in sarcomatoid urothelial carcinoma. (Right) A "pseudoangiosarcomatous" pattern of sarcomatoid urothelial carcinoma does not show immunophenotypic evidence of true endothelial differentiation. This ERG immunostain is negative in the neoplastic cells (with strong nuclear internal controls in benign blood vessels ➡).

Overview of Invasive Carcinoma Subtypes

(Left) Rare examples of invasive urothelial carcinoma are associated with abundant myxoid stroma that may mimic an adenocarcinoma or a spectrum of mesenchymal neoplasms, raising the possibility of sarcomatoid urothelial carcinoma. **(Right)** In the early phases, the neoplastic cells within the epithelial aggregates of these urothelial carcinomas become separated by gradual accumulation of myxoid matrix. More developed neoplasms are hypocellular with a predominance of myxoid stroma.

Urothelial Carcinoma With Chordoid Features

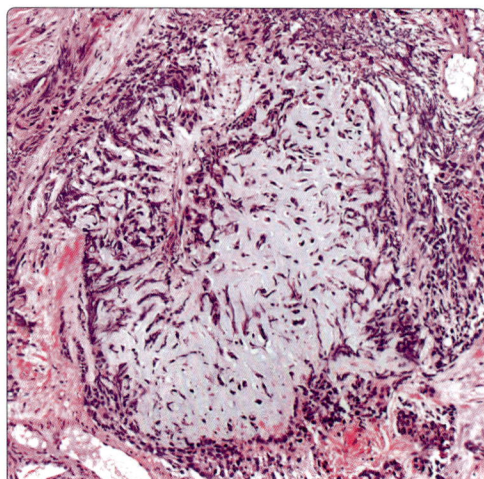

Urothelial Carcinoma With Chordoid Features

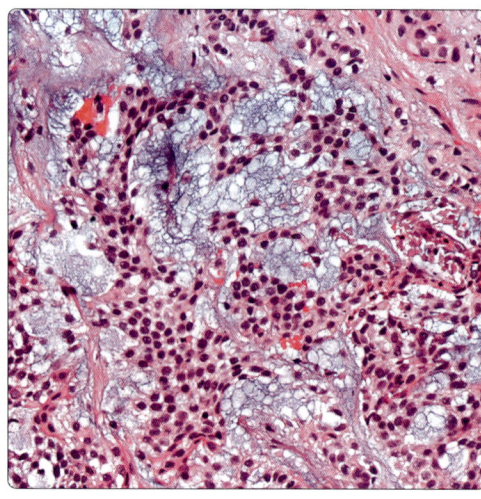

(Left) Invasive urothelial carcinomas with myxoid stroma may have a single file cord-like epithelial architecture. This pattern of carcinoma may mimic a variety of myxoid mesenchymal neoplasms, especially if seen in metastatic lesions. **(Right)** Invasive urothelial carcinomas with myxoid stroma may have a complex cord-like epithelial architecture. This pattern of carcinoma may closely mimic chordoma or extraskeletal myxoid chondrosarcoma.

Urothelial Carcinoma With Chordoid Features

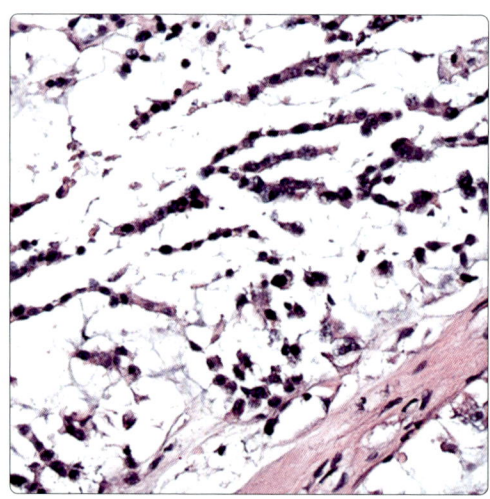

Urothelial Carcinoma With Chordoid Features

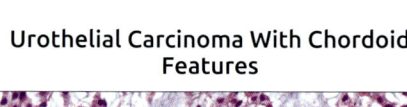

(Left) Diffuse cytoplasmic HMCK(34βE12) immunoreactivity is generally retained in these urothelial carcinomas despite the unusual morphologic features. **(Right)** p63 is maintained in urothelial carcinomas with myxoid stroma, a finding that supports epithelial lineage. The expression of any or all of HMCK(34βE12), p63, CK20, CK5/6, and GATA3 help confirm urothelial differentiation in the appropriate clinical context. Uroplakin-2 is specific but not sensitive.

HMCK(34βE12): Urothelial Carcinoma With Chordoid Features

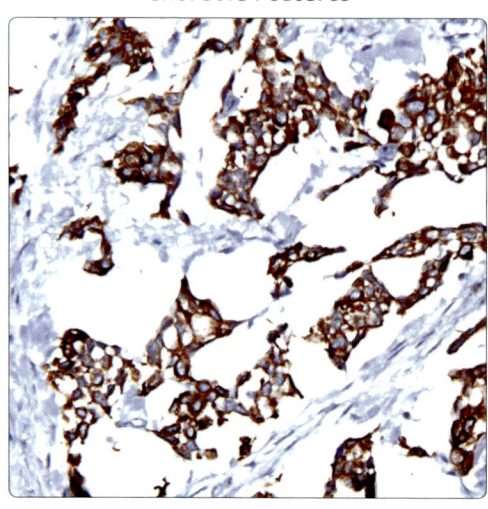

p63: Urothelial Carcinoma With Chordoid Features

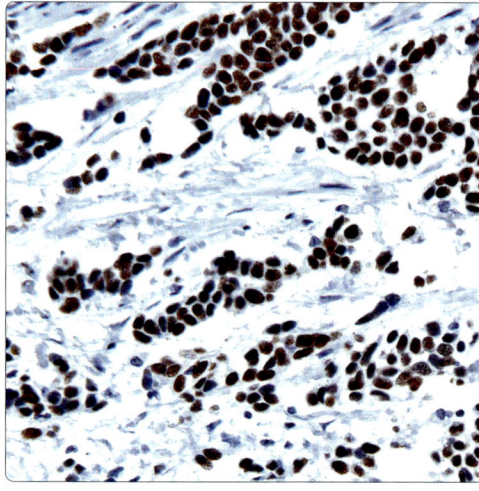

Overview of Invasive Carcinoma Subtypes

Urothelial Carcinoma With Rhabdoid Features

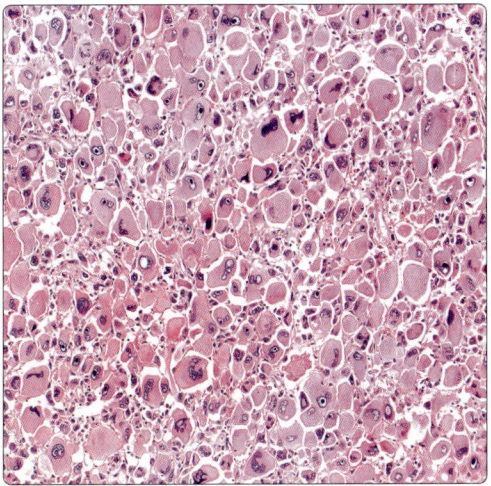

Urothelial Carcinoma With Rhabdoid Features

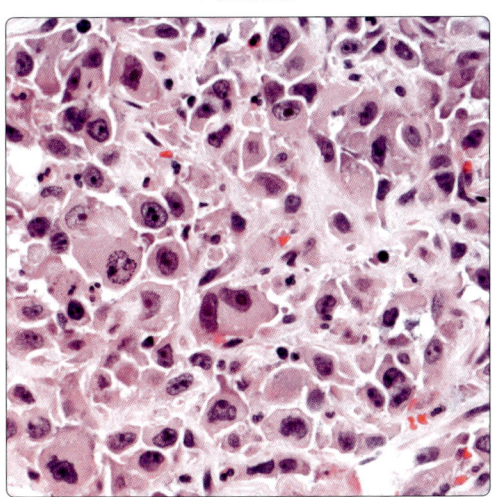

(Left) Invasive urothelial carcinoma with rhabdoid features is characterized by sheets of neoplastic cells showing abundant eosinophilic cytoplasm and eccentric nuclei with vesicular chromatin. These tumors resemble malignant extrarenal rhabdoid tumors but do not have chromosome 22 deletion or INI1 mutation. *(Right)* Urothelial carcinoma with rhabdoid features has obvious features of malignancy, with marked nucleomegaly and prominent macronucleoli.

Lipid-Rich (Lipoid) Urothelial Carcinoma

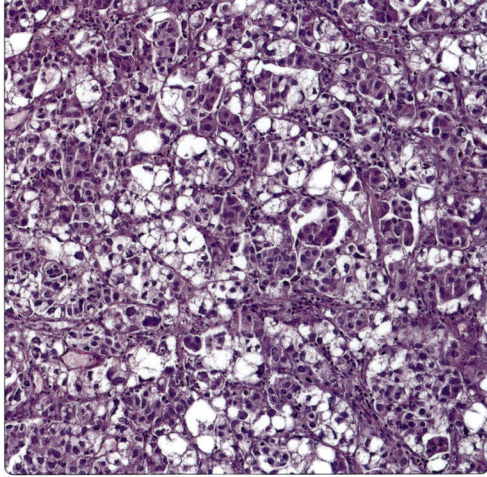

Lipid-Rich (Lipoid) Urothelial Carcinoma

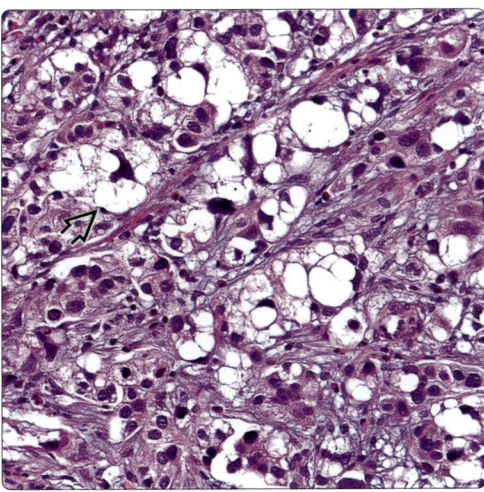

(Left) On low-power examination of this invasive lipid-rich urothelial carcinoma, there are scattered neoplastic cells with clear multivacuolated cytoplasm admixed with more conventional urothelial carcinoma. *(Right)* These rare high-grade carcinomas contain scattered neoplastic cells with intracytoplasmic lipid ➽ that resemble pleomorphic lipoblasts. This may closely mimic pleomorphic liposarcoma, but obvious typical urothelial carcinoma is usually admixed.

Lipid-Rich (Lipoid) Urothelial Carcinoma

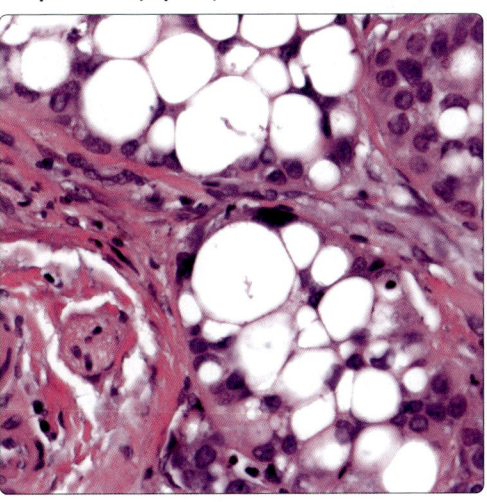

Cytokeratin: Lipid-Rich (Lipoid) Urothelial Carcinoma

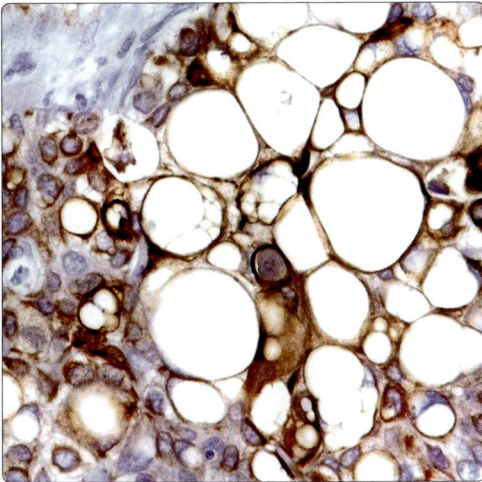

(Left) The neoplastic urothelial cells are distended by lipid droplets with thin septations. These features are typical of the "lipoid" or lipid-rich variant of urothelial carcinoma, but out-of-context may mimic heterologous liposarcoma. *(Right)* CK-PAN(AE1/AE3) immunohistochemistry shows strong cytoplasmic staining in the neoplastic cells, even in the scant peripheral cytoplasm of the population with intracytoplasmic lipid. S100 stain is negative. These findings should aid in the distinction from primary or heterologous liposarcoma.

Cystitis Cystica and Glandularis

KEY FACTS

TERMINOLOGY

- Invaginated urothelial nests in superficial lamina propria with cystic dilatation forming luminal space
- Cystitis glandularis has luminal cuboidal or columnar lining cells
- Cystitis glandularis of intestinal type contains goblet cells
- Cystitis cystica and glandularis with mucin extravasation

ETIOLOGY/PATHOGENESIS

- May be normal variant or secondary to localized inflammatory response

CLINICAL ISSUES

- Usually incidental finding
- When florid, may have polypoid appearance clinically
- No convincing evidence that this lesion represents neoplastic precursor condition

MICROSCOPIC

- Cystitis cystica has superficial nests of urothelium with central cysts
- Glandular cells (columnar or cuboidal cells) line central lumen in cystitis glandularis
- Cystitis glandularis with intestinal metaplasia contains goblet cells; rarely Paneth cells may be present
- Rare cases have extensive mucin extravasation

TOP DIFFERENTIAL DIAGNOSES

- Invasive adenocarcinoma
- Noninvasive urothelial carcinoma with glandular differentiation (adenocarcinoma in situ)
- Nested urothelial carcinoma with associated tubules
- Inverted papilloma with glandular features
- Bladder hamartoma

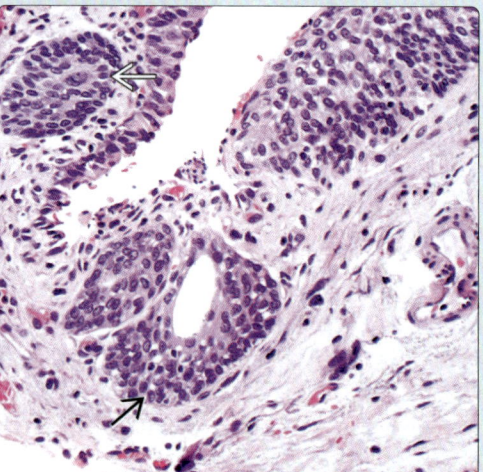

von Brunn Nests With Cystitis Cystica

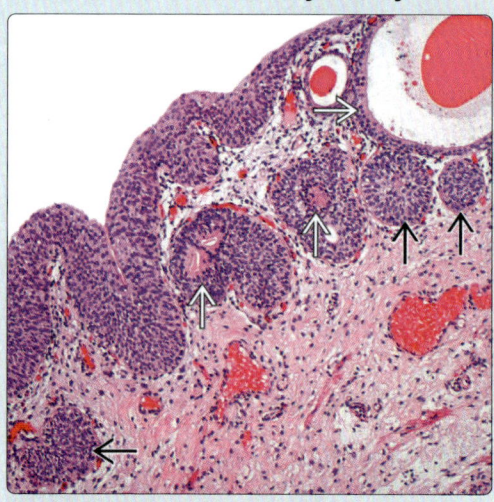

von Brunn Nests With Cystitis Cystica

(Left) von Brunn nests ➡ with cystitis cystica ➡ show a lumen with flattened urothelial lining but without luminally oriented cytoplasm. No columnar cells/glandular epithelia is present to support a cystitis glandularis designation. (Right) H&E shows von Brunn nests ➡ interspersed with cystitis glandularis ➡, a frequent combination. The superficial location and sharp linear border at the base help in the distinction from invasive mimics, such as nested urothelial carcinoma.

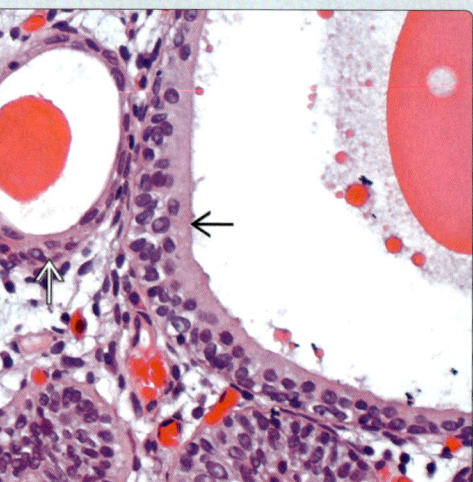

Cystitis Cystica and Glandularis

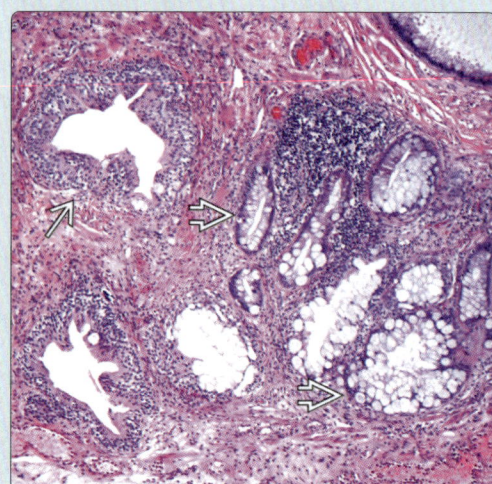

Cystitis Cystica and Glandularis With Intestinal Metaplasia

(Left) The luminally oriented cytoplasm of cystitis glandularis ➡ contrasts with the flattened urothelial lining in cystitis cystica ➡. These 2 patterns may occur together along with florid von Brunn nests. (Right) A section of urothelial mucosa with cystitis cystica and glandularis is shown. Cystically dilated von Brunn nests ➡ adjacent to glands are lined by enteric-type cells ➡. There is chronic inflammation in the background.

Cystitis Cystica and Glandularis

TERMINOLOGY

Definitions
- Cystitis cystica
  - Invaginated urothelial nests in superficial lamina propria with cystic dilatation forming luminal space
  - No cuboidal or columnar luminal cells are present
- Cystitis glandularis
  - Cystitis cystica with luminal cuboidal or columnar lining cells
- Cystitis glandularis with intestinal metaplasia (intestinal type)
  - Cystitis glandularis with at least focal intestinal-type goblet cells
- Cystitis cystica and glandularis with mucin extravasation

ETIOLOGY/PATHOGENESIS

Environmental Exposure
- May be secondary to localized inflammatory response

CLINICAL ISSUES

Presentation
- Usually incidental finding
- When florid, small raised lesion with intact urothelium may be seen
- Rare cases with intestinal metaplasia and extensive mucin extravasation may form large mass lesion that can mimic malignancy

Prognosis
- No convincing evidence that cystitis cystica or glandularis represents neoplastic precursor lesion

MACROSCOPIC

General Features
- May form polypoid mass in some florid examples
  - Intact overlying mucosa with variable translucent appearance
- Usually < 1 cm; rarely large-sized

MICROSCOPIC

Histologic Features
- Cystitis cystica
  - Superficial nests of invaginated urothelium in lamina propria
    - Connection to surface urothelium is variable
    - May have lobular configuration
    - In contrast to von Brunn nests, this lesion has cystically dilated lumina
    - No glandular-lining cells are present
    - Often admixed with von Brunn nests
- Cystitis glandularis
  - Identical to cystitis cystica, except glandular cells line central lumen
    - Cuboidal or columnar cells with luminally oriented cytoplasm
- Cystitis glandularis with intestinal metaplasia
  - Identical to cystitis glandularis with at least scattered intestinal-type goblet cells or, rarely, Paneth cells
- Rare cases may have extensive mucin extravasation
  - No significant cytologic atypia
  - No irregular epithelial aggregates
  - No destructive invasion of muscularis propria
  - Intact glands floating in mucin is helpful feature to distinguish from carcinoma

DIFFERENTIAL DIAGNOSIS

Invasive Adenocarcinoma
- Usually high stage with destructive invasion into muscularis propria
- Greater degree of nuclear atypia with free-floating single cells and small clusters
- In mucinous (colloid) variant, epithelium forms irregular aggregates within stromal mucin
  - Distinctive feature from cystitis glandularis with mucin extravasation

Nested Urothelial Carcinoma With Associated Tubules
- Individual nests may have significant overlap with cystitis cystica or glandularis on superficial biopsy
  - Generally have more infiltrating borders and stacking of tumor nests
- Typically extends deeply into lamina or muscularis propria

Prostatic-Type Polyp
- Glands within stroma have prostatic secretory phenotype
  - Lightly eosinophilic, frothy cytoplasm
  - Round nuclei
  - PSA and PAP positive

Inverted Urothelial Papilloma With Glandular Features
- May have cystitis cystica-like pattern
- Endophytic thin anastomosing cords are typical
  - More complex architecture compared to separate individual nests/glands of cystitis glandularis
- Basal nuclear palisading around nests is typical

Bladder Hamartoma
- More irregularly distributed epithelium with variable stromal component

DIAGNOSTIC CHECKLIST

Clinically Relevant Pathologic Features
- Extensive cystitis glandularis with intestinal metaplasia and mucin extravasation may closely mimic bladder cancer on cystoscopy

Pathologic Interpretation Pearls
- Low-power architectural evaluation is very helpful in distinction from carcinomas
  - Superficial location with sharp base at junction with lamina propria

SELECTED REFERENCES

1. Smith AK et al: Role of cystitis cystica et glandularis and intestinal metaplasia in development of bladder carcinoma. Urology. 71(5):915-8, 2008
2. Corica FA et al: Intestinal metaplasia is not a strong risk factor for bladder cancer: study of 53 cases with long-term follow-up. Urology. 50(3):427-31, 1997

Cystitis Cystica and Glandularis

(Left) Section of urothelial mucosa shows dilated von Brunn nests ⮕ consistent with cystitis cystica. Note the presence of mild inflammation and edema in the background. **(Right)** On high-power examination, the glandular epithelium within the lamina propria has abundant luminally oriented cytoplasm, a feature that distinguishes cystitis glandularis from cystitis cystica.

von Brunn Nest and Cystitis Cystica
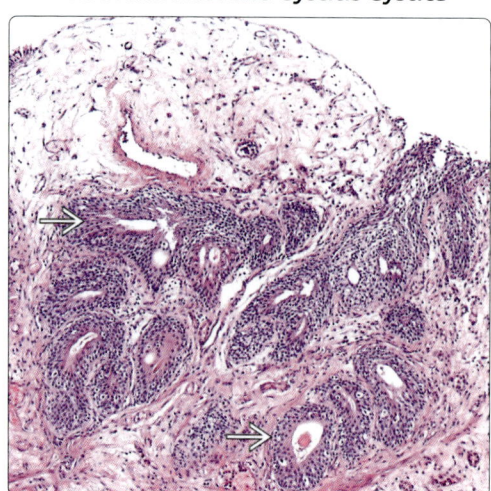

Cystitis Cystica and Glandularis
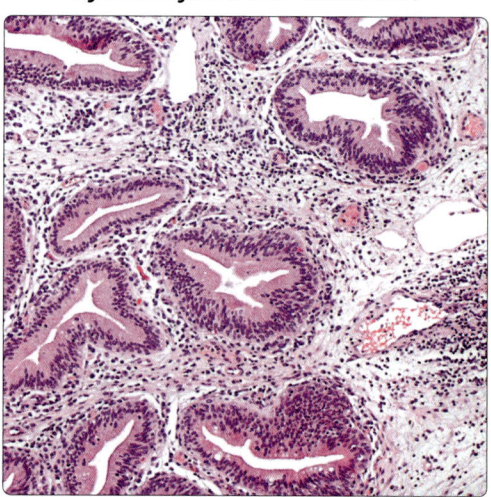

(Left) Superficial collection of tightly packed aggregate of urothelial nests with central lumina and columnar epithelium is characteristic of florid cystitis glandularis. These florid examples may form a cystoscopic lesion. **(Right)** Florid cystitis glandularis has the characteristic well-developed, luminally oriented cytoplasm ⮕. The lesional cells lack the degree of cytologic atypia expected in adenocarcinoma. Overall low-power features of organization are key to recognize the lesion as benign.

von Brunn Nest and Cystitis Cystica
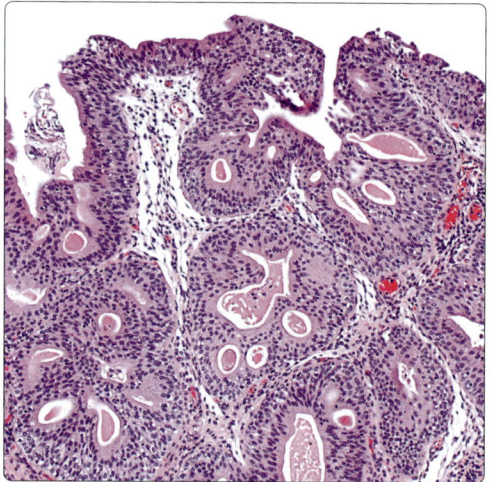

von Brunn Nest and Cystitis Cystica
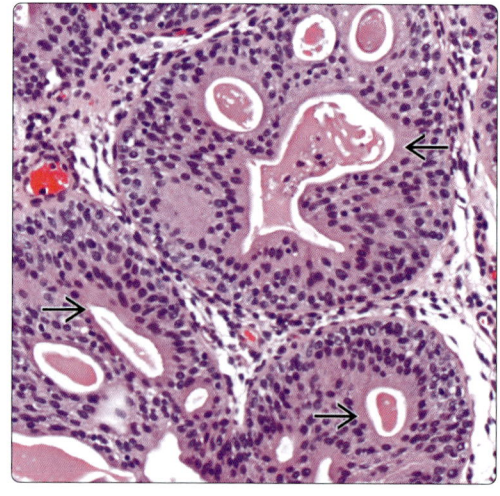

(Left) This example shows an admixture of cystitis glandularis without intestinal metaplasia ⮕ next to an area of almost complete intestinal metaplasia ⮕. Inflammation may vary between cases and may not be conspicuous. **(Right)** Some cases of cystitis glandularis with intestinal metaplasia show extensive mucin extravasation ⮕. The intact glands and absence of epithelial aggregates in the mucin distinguish this lesion from mucinous adenocarcinoma, which may have a similar appearance during cystoscopy.

Cystitis Cystica and Glandularis With Intestinal Metaplasia
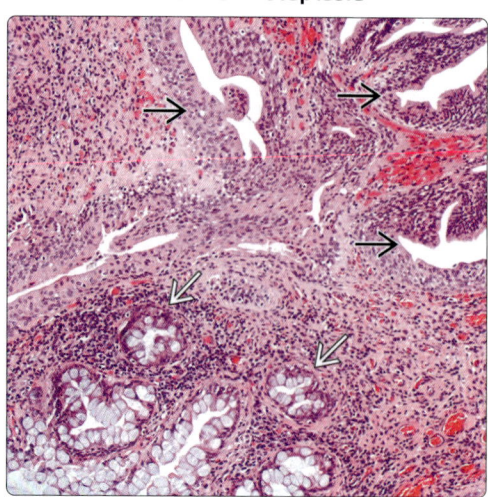

Cystitis Cystica and Glandularis With Mucin Extravasation
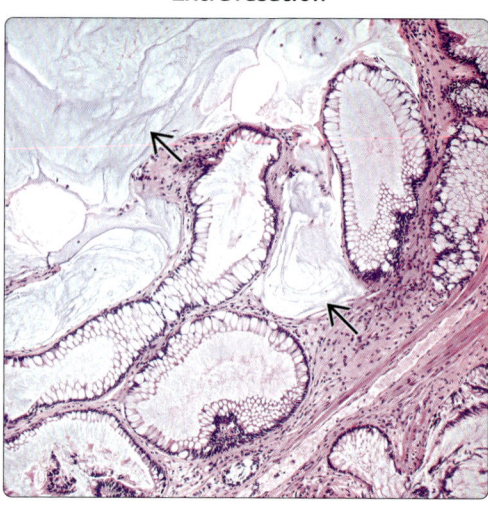

Cystitis Cystica and Glandularis

Cystitis Glandularis
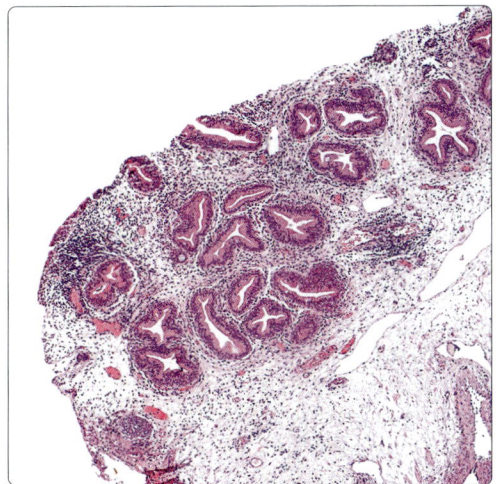

Nested Urothelial Carcinoma
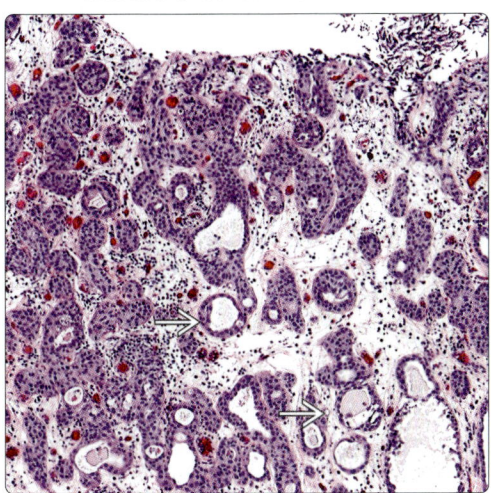

(Left) This collection of glandular structures within the superficial lamina propria has overall lobularity and a sharp linear border at the base, features typical of cystitis glandularis. (Right) Nested variant of urothelial carcinoma shows occasional microcysts ➡. Unlike cystitis cystica, there are too many haphazardly arranged nests to be acceptable as a benign process. In addition, the tumor spanned the entire lamina propria and invaded beyond it into the bladder wall.

Nested Urothelial Carcinoma
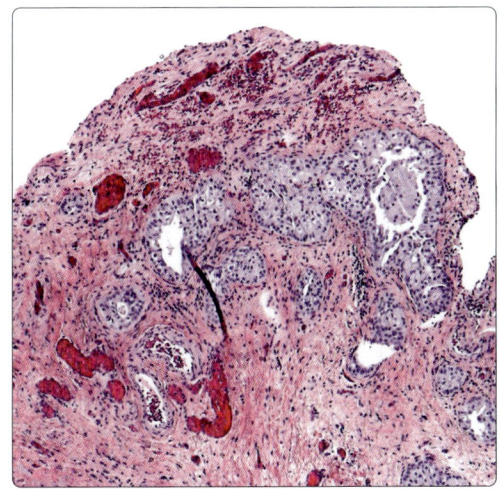

Nested Urothelial Carcinoma
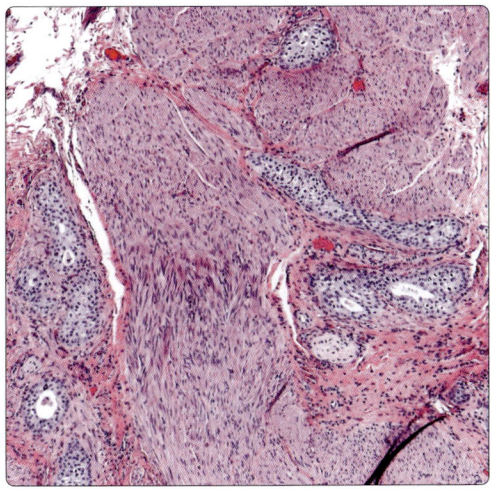

(Left) Nested variant of urothelial carcinoma is shown. In this superficial biopsy, there is striking resemblance to cystitis cystica with the presence of the cystically dilated nests and bland cytologic features. (Right) Nested variant of urothelial carcinoma infiltrates deep into the muscularis propria. Note the bland histologic features of the infiltrating nests. The presence of urothelial nests within muscularis propria should trigger concern for an invasive urothelial process.

Adenocarcinoma In Situ
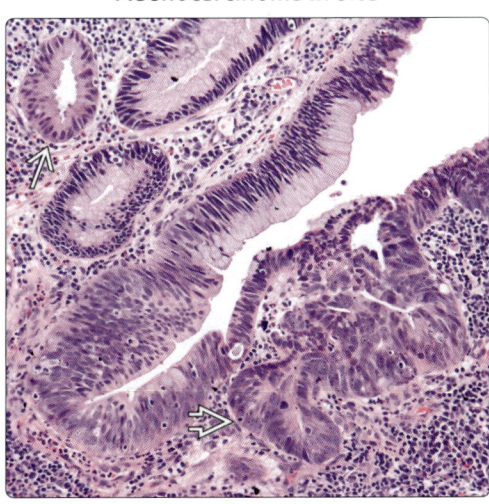

Inverted Papilloma With Colloid Cysts
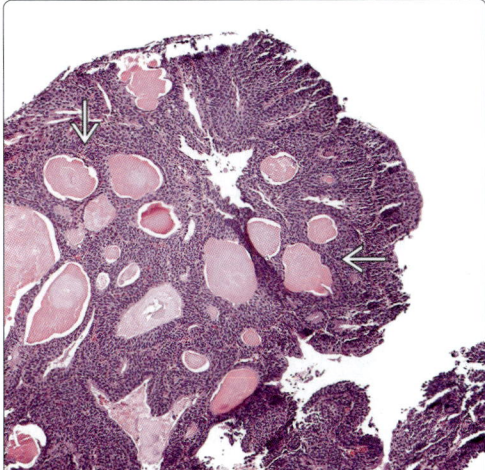

(Left) Adenocarcinoma in situ of the bladder with suspicion for early invasion is shown. Despite the presence of bland-appearing glands ➡, there is clear evidence of a true malignant glandular process (i.e., adenocarcinoma) ➡ in this section. (Right) Inverted papilloma comprised of anastomosing cords of tumor cells with interspersed colloid cysts ➡ demonstrates central cystic change. When prominent, this pattern may be readily mistaken for cystitis cystica.

Villous Adenoma

KEY FACTS

TERMINOLOGY
- Benign glandular neoplasm arising from urothelium

CLINICAL ISSUES
- Presenting symptoms
  - Hematuria
  - Irritative urinary symptoms
  - Rarely, mucosuria can be seen
- Therapy: Complete transurethral resection
- Excellent prognosis for
  - Villous adenoma with no invasive component
  - Villous adenoma completely resected

MICROSCOPIC
- Villoglandular architecture
  - Fibrovascular cores lined by pseudostratified columnar epithelium
  - Complex architecture (cribriform growth), marked nuclear atypia: Indicate high-grade dysplasia, criteria similar to enteric villous adenoma
- Invasive adenocarcinoma of enteric type may arise from villous adenoma

TOP DIFFERENTIAL DIAGNOSES
- Invasive adenocarcinoma of urinary bladder
- Papillary urothelial carcinoma with glandular differentiation

DIAGNOSTIC CHECKLIST
- All tissue should be submitted for histologic evaluation to exclude invasive component
- All efforts made to distinguish it from metaplastic lesion
  - Association with inflammation and granulation tissue
  - History of chronic irritation (stones, catheter, fistula, etc.)
- No histologic features of high-grade dysplasia/intraepithelial carcinoma
- No histologic features of frank malignancy (i.e., adenocarcinoma)

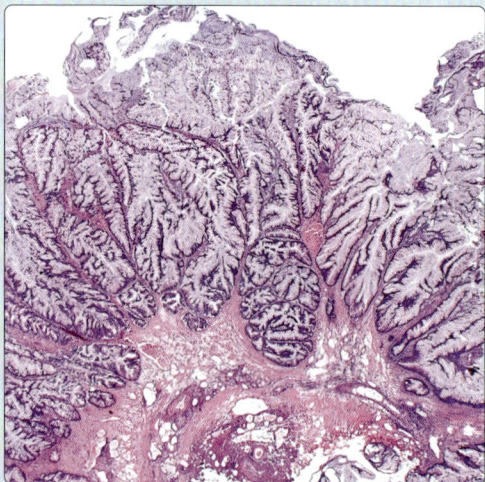

Villous Adenoma: Complex Branching Papillary Architecture

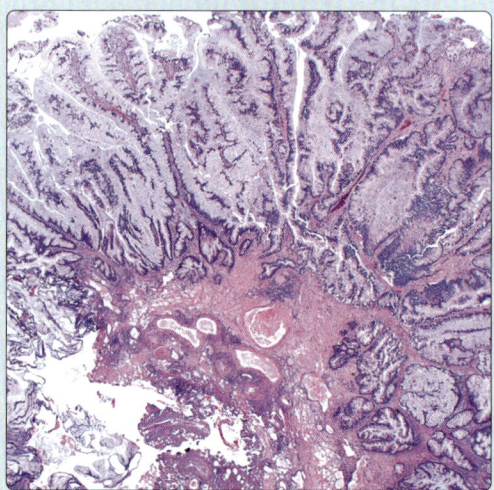

Villous Adenoma: Abundant Mucin Production

(Left) Villous adenoma of the urinary bladder has an identical morphology to its more common colorectal counterpart with variable papillary architecture and obvious intracellular mucin. (Right) This low-power photomicrograph shows the typical exophytic papillary appearance of villous adenoma. There is typically abundant mucin production within the tumor cells. All visible tissue must be resected and histologically examined before a diagnosis of villous adenoma is made.

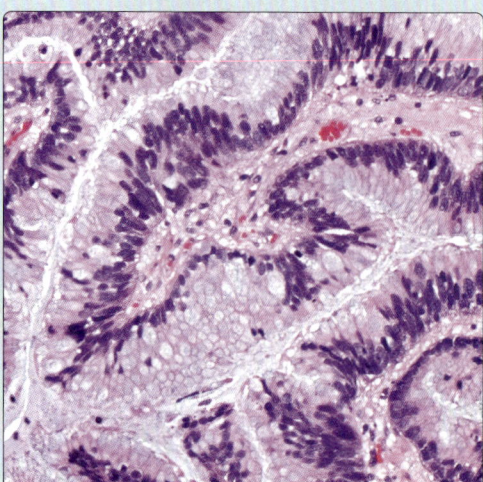

Villous Adenoma: Nuclear Pseudostratification

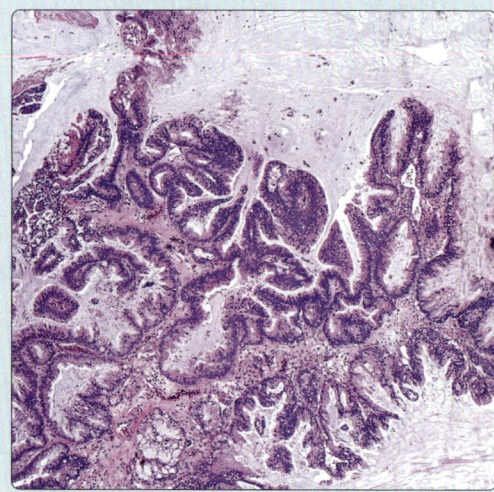

Villous Adenoma: Extracellular Mucin

(Left) On high-power examination, villous adenoma is characterized by pseudostratified columnar epithelium showing nuclear crowding and hyperchromasia. Typically, many tumor cells contain abundant mucinous material. (Right) Hematoxylin and eosin section shows the typical exophytic, papillary appearance of villous adenoma. There are areas of nuclear stratification typically seen in these lesions and evidence of extracellular mucin.

Villous Adenoma

TERMINOLOGY

Definitions
- Benign glandular neoplasm of urinary bladder
  - Histologically identical to colorectal adenomas

CLINICAL ISSUES

Epidemiology
- Incidence
  - Rare primary bladder neoplasm
- Age
  - Wide age range
    - Mean: 65 years
- Sex
  - M > F

Site
- Common sites include bladder dome and trigone
- May also occur in urachus

Presentation
- Hematuria
- Irritative bladder symptoms
- Rarely, mucosuria can be seen

Natural History
- Rare cases may progress to invasive adenocarcinoma

Treatment
- Complete transurethral resection

Prognosis
- Excellent for villous adenoma with no invasive component and complete resection
- Prognosis for invasive lesions depends on stage of disease

MACROSCOPIC

General Features
- Exophytic papillary/villiform tumor
  - May be identical to papillary urothelial neoplasm on cystoscopy

MICROSCOPIC

Histologic Features
- Papillary architecture
  - Central fibrovascular cores lined by pseudostratified columnar epithelium with mucin depletion
    - Stratification
    - Crowding
    - Nuclear hyperchromasia
- May have high-grade dysplasia/adenocarcinoma in situ
- Invasive adenocarcinoma of enteric type may arise from villous adenoma

Predominant Pattern/Injury Type
- Papillary

Predominant Cell/Compartment Type
- Epithelial, glandular

ANCILLARY TESTS

Immunohistochemistry
- Enteric immunophenotype
  - Immunoreactivity for CK20, CDX2, and CEA

DIFFERENTIAL DIAGNOSIS

Invasive Adenocarcinoma of Urinary Bladder
- Irregular gland contours with stromal reaction
  - May have complex gland formation, such as cribriforming
- Typically deeply invasive into muscularis propria

Papillary Urothelial Carcinoma With Glandular Differentiation
- Obvious urothelial component typically present
  - Invasive, papillary, or in situ
- More heterogeneous glandular component
  - Intracytoplasmic mucin is rare pattern

Secondary Involvement by Adenocarcinoma
- Colonic adenocarcinoma
  - Superficial biopsies may appear deceptively bland and may simulate surface lesion
  - Invasion should be obvious on adequate biopsies
    - Deep involvement of bladder wall
- Endometrial adenocarcinoma
  - Endometrioid type may appear enteric
  - Typically express PR &/or ER by immunohistochemistry

Cystitis Cystica/Glandularis With Intestinal Metaplasia and Mucin Extravasation
- May form conspicuous mass lesion
- Associated with pools of mucin containing intact glands with enteric-type epithelium
  - In large lesions, mucin extravasation may be extensive
- Lining epithelium may be bland or occasionally reactive

DIAGNOSTIC CHECKLIST

Pathologic Interpretation Pearls
- All tissue should be submitted for histologic evaluation
  - Invasive component must be excluded
- Secondary involvement by adenocarcinoma may have surface villous component mimicking primary

SELECTED REFERENCES

1. Pal DK: Villous adenoma of the urinary bladder. J Cancer Res Ther. 11(3):665, 2015
2. Nakamura Y et al: A case of villous adenoma of the urinary bladder with tubulovillous architecture: characterization by immunohistochemical analysis. Pol J Pathol. 62(3):179-82, 2011
3. Lane Z et al: Immunohistochemical expression of prostatic antigens in adenocarcinoma and villous adenoma of the urinary bladder. Am J Surg Pathol. 32(9):1322-6, 2008
4. Sung W et al: Villous adenoma of the urinary bladder. Int J Urol. 15(6):551-3, 2008
5. Tamboli P et al: Villous adenoma of urinary tract: a common tumor in an uncommon location. Adv Anat Pathol. 7(2):79-84, 2000
6. Cheng L et al: Villous adenoma of the urinary tract: a report of 23 cases, including 8 with coexistent adenocarcinoma. Am J Surg Pathol. 23(7):764-71, 1999
7. Trotter SE et al: Villous adenoma of the bladder. Histopathology. 24(5):491-3, 1994

Invasive Adenocarcinoma

KEY FACTS

ETIOLOGY/PATHOGENESIS
- Predisposing factors
  - Associated with bladder exstrophy
  - Nonfunctioning bladder, chronic inflammation, schistosomiasis (rare)

CLINICAL ISSUES
- Rare primary bladder neoplasm (< 2% of bladder malignancies)
- Peak incidence in 6th decade
- Most common presentation is hematuria
- Poor prognosis (5-yr survival rate varies from 18-47%) secondary to high stage at presentation

MICROSCOPIC
- Nearly pure glandular differentiation
- Associated adenocarcinoma in situ may be seen
- Indistinguishable from adenocarcinomas of other organs

ANCILLARY TESTS
- CK20(+), CK7(-)
- May express villin and CDX-2
- Does not express nuclear β-catenin
- PAP reactivity is reported, but PSA is typically negative

TOP DIFFERENTIAL DIAGNOSES
- Direct invasion by prostatic adenocarcinoma
- Direct invasion or metastatic colorectal adenocarcinoma
- Other metastatic adenocarcinoma
- Cystitis glandularis
- Invasive urothelial carcinoma with glandular differentiation or small tubules
- Müllerianosis
- Urachal adenocarcinoma

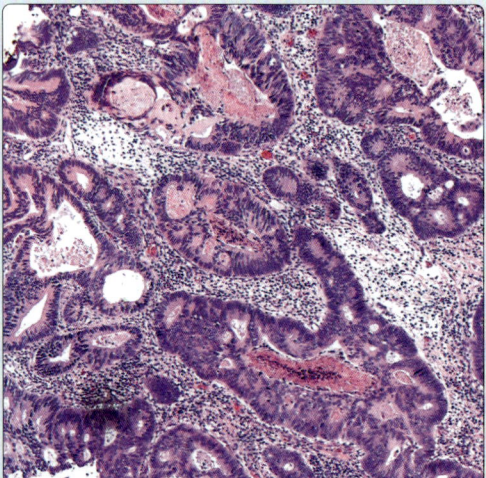

Adenocarcinoma of Bladder

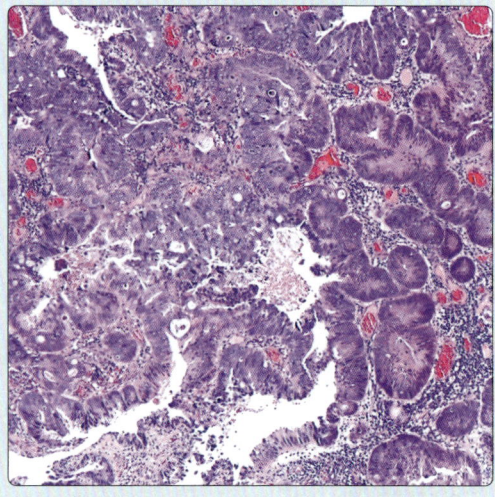

Adenocarcinoma of Bladder

(Left) This is a primary adenocarcinoma of the bladder with enteric morphology, identical to colorectal adenocarcinoma. The possibility of metastasis or direct extension from a primary adenocarcinoma of the GI tract must always be considered. (Right) This is another example of an adenocarcinoma primary in the bladder with morphologic features indistinguishable from colorectal adenocarcinoma.

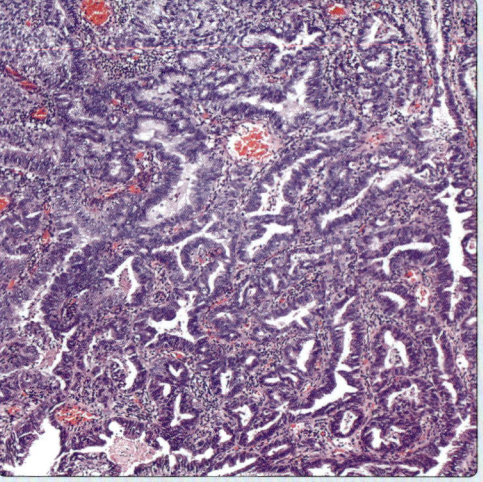

Adenocarcinoma of Bladder

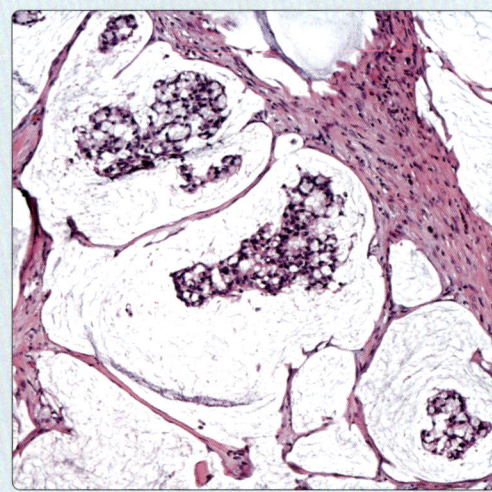

Adenocarcinoma of Bladder

(Left) In this gland-forming carcinoma of the bladder with no associated component of urothelial carcinoma, a primary adenocarcinoma should be considered. Metastatic carcinoma is always a consideration when dealing with these tumors. (Right) In this primary mucinous adenocarcinoma of the urinary bladder, irregular clusters of epithelial nests are seen floating in mucin. The associated atypia is beyond what is acceptable for a benign or reactive process such as cystitis cystica with mucin extravasation.

Invasive Adenocarcinoma

TERMINOLOGY

Definitions
- Primary gland-forming carcinoma of urinary bladder not associated with urothelial or squamous carcinoma component
- Specific form may occur within urachal remnant or cyst

ETIOLOGY/PATHOGENESIS

Developmental Anomaly
- Associated with bladder exstrophy (~ 4-7% risk)

Chronic Irritation
- Nonfunctioning bladder, obstruction, schistosomiasis

CLINICAL ISSUES

Epidemiology
- Incidence
  - Rare primary bladder neoplasm (< 2% of bladder malignancies)
- Age
  - Peak incidence in 6th decade
- Sex
  - M:F = 2.6:1.0

Site
- Bladder base is most common

Presentation
- Hematuria, dysuria, mucosuria

Treatment
- Radical cystectomy; adjuvant radiation &/or chemotherapy

Prognosis
- Poor prognosis (5-year survival rate varies from 18-47%) due to high stage at presentation

MACROSCOPIC

General Features
- Exophytic, papillary, sessile, or infiltrating mass

MICROSCOPIC

Histologic Features
- Nearly pure glandular differentiation with varying morphologic patterns: Enteric, adenocarcinoma, not otherwise specified, mucinous/colloid, signet ring cell, hepatoid, mixed, clear cell carcinoma
- May be associated with intestinal metaplasia
- May be associated with noninvasive component (adenocarcinoma in situ)

ANCILLARY TESTS

Immunohistochemistry
- Enteric adenocarcinoma may have significant overlap with colonic adenocarcinoma
  - Typically expresses CK20; may express villin and CDX-2
  - CK7 expression is variable, usually negative
  - Does not express nuclear β-catenin

DIFFERENTIAL DIAGNOSIS

Direct Invasion by Prostatic Adenocarcinoma
- More common than primary adenocarcinoma
- Monomorphic round nuclei with prominent nucleoli suggest prostate origin
- Ductal adenocarcinoma of prostate has significant morphologic overlap with enteric adenocarcinoma
- Often expresses PSA, PAP, PSMA, NK3.1, P501S (prostein) and PSMA
  - Note that rare primary bladder adenocarcinoma may focally express PAP, PSMA and prostein

Direct Extension or Metastatic Colorectal Adenocarcinoma
- Morphologically indistinguishable from bladder primary
- Frequently expresses nuclear β-catenin (caveat, not all primary colorectal carcinomas express nuclear β-catenin)
- Colonoscopy is often required for distinction
- May have surface component mimicking in situ change

Other Metastatic Adenocarcinoma
- Gastric signet ring cell and ovarian serous and clear cell carcinomas may be indistinguishable morphologically
- May have surface component mimicking in situ change

Extensive Cystitis Glandularis
- Superficial location and bland nuclear cytology
- Sharp linear border with underlying lamina propria
- Rare cases have mucin extravasation, mimicking mucinous adenocarcinoma (but no irregular epithelial aggregates)

Invasive Urothelial Carcinoma With Glandular Differentiation or Small Tubules
- Identifiable component of papillary, in situ, or invasive urothelial carcinoma

Müllerianosis
- Endocervical, tubal, or endometrial-type glands
- May be present deeply in muscularis propria or adventitia
  - Distinction: Bland nuclear cytology, no stromal response

Urachal Adenocarcinoma
- Distinguished by anatomic location in urachus/dome

DIAGNOSTIC CHECKLIST

Pathologic Interpretation Pearls
- Primary adenocarcinoma of bladder is extremely rare
  - Possibility of origin from distant or contiguous anatomic site should be carefully considered before diagnosis is rendered

SELECTED REFERENCES

1. Zaghloul MS et al: Long-term results of primary adenocarcinoma of the urinary bladder: a report on 192 patients. Urol Oncol. 24(1):13-20, 2006
2. Suh N et al: Value of CDX2, villin, and alpha-methylacyl coenzyme A racemase immunostains in the distinction between primary adenocarcinoma of the bladder and secondary colorectal adenocarcinoma. Mod Pathol. 18(9):1217-22, 2005
3. Wang HL et al: Immunohistochemical distinction between primary adenocarcinoma of the bladder and secondary colorectal adenocarcinoma. Am J Surg Pathol. 25(11):1380-7, 2001
4. Grignon DJ et al: Primary adenocarcinoma of the urinary bladder. A clinicopathologic analysis of 72 cases. Cancer. 67(8):2165-72, 1991

Invasive Adenocarcinoma

Invasive Adenocarcinoma

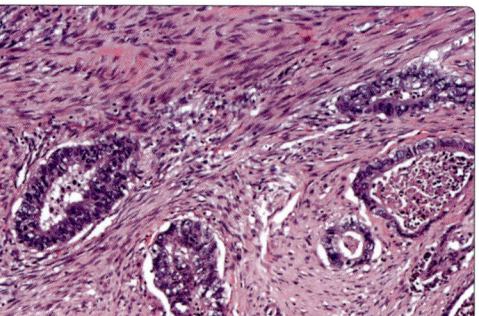

Enteric Features

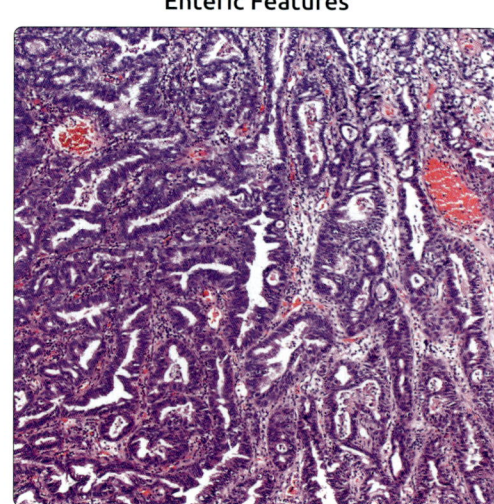

(Left) Primary adenocarcinoma with invasion into muscularis propria may be morphologically indistinguishable from colorectal adenocarcinoma. Clinical history is of paramount importance. **(Right)** This invasive bladder adenocarcinoma has a well-formed glandular pattern and a minimal desmoplastic stromal response. This degree of low-power complexity helps in the distinction from benign mimics, such as florid cystitis glandularis.

Mimicking Colorectal Carcinoma

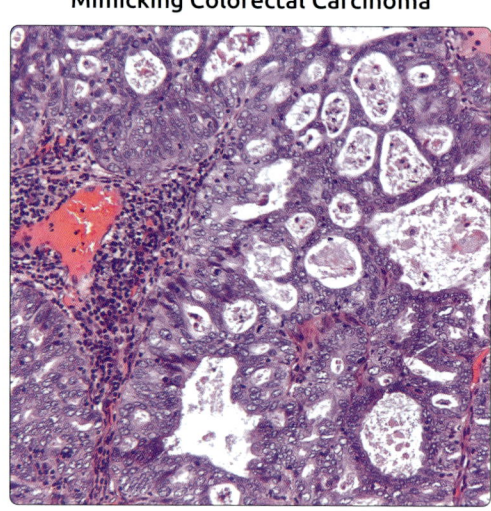

Cytologic Atypia

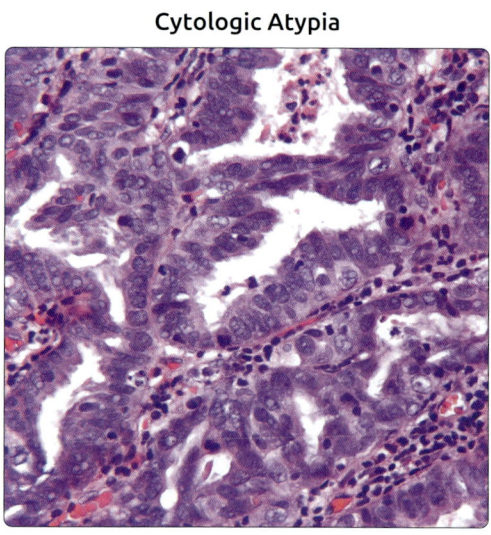

(Left) Complex cribriform architecture with dirty necrosis is present in this primary bladder adenocarcinoma that closely resembles colorectal carcinoma. Because colorectal carcinoma may directly invade into the bladder, this diagnostic possibility must be carefully considered prior to diagnosing a bladder primary. **(Right)** On high power, this primary vesical adenocarcinoma, enteric morphology, has a high nuclear:cytoplasmic ratio, elongated nuclei, and nuclear membrane irregularities.

Comedonecrosis

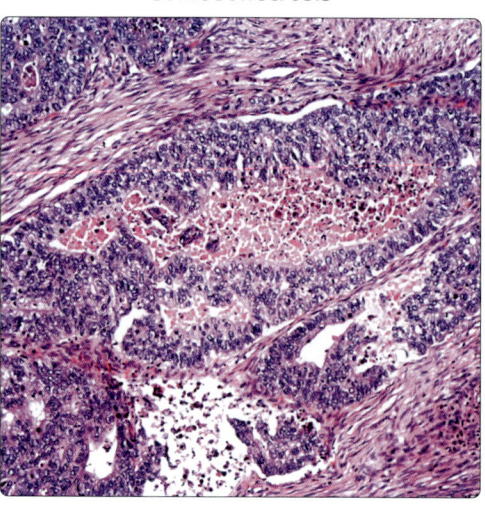

Exophytic and Invasive Histology

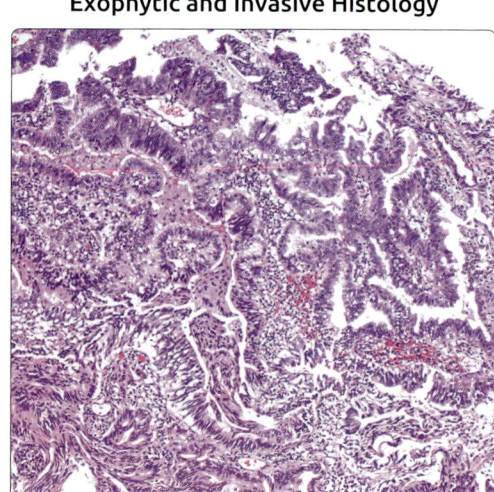

(Left) Enteric-type adenocarcinoma with comedonecrosis may be morphologically indistinguishable from colon cancer. Clinical correlation is essential in this setting, and colonoscopy is often useful if there is no prior diagnosis. **(Right)** A primary bladder adenocarcinoma with both the exophytic and invasive components is shown. The exophytic areas also have a glandular phenotype. In contrast, urothelial carcinoma with glandular differentiation has a urothelial morphology in some areas.

Invasive Adenocarcinoma

Adenocarcinoma of Bladder

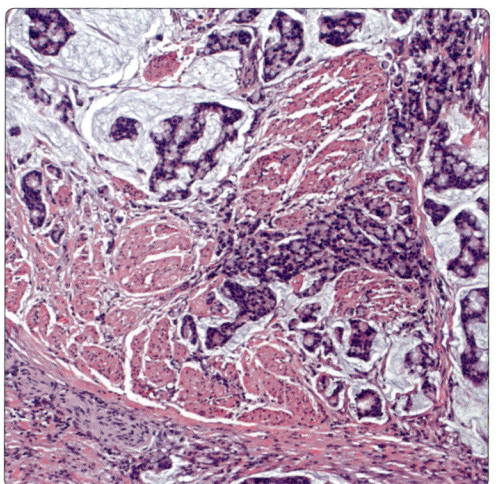

Adenocarcinoma of Bladder

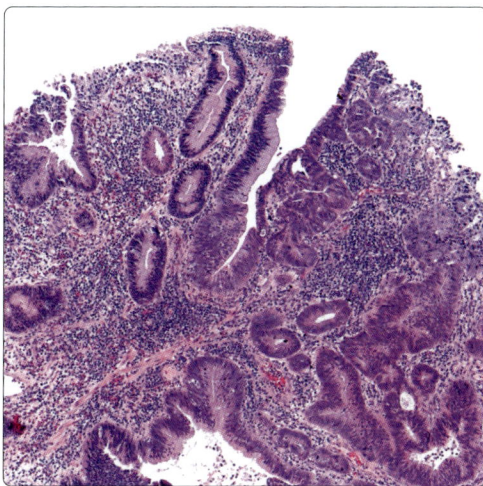

(Left) Primary vesical adenocarcinoma (enteric and colloid type) is typically high stage and shows obvious destructive invasion of the muscularis propria. This feature is very useful in the distinction from cystitis glandularis with mucin extravasation. Observation of partial & poorly formed glands is also useful. **(Right)** This is the superficial component of otherwise invasive enteric-type adenocarcinoma of the bladder. Note the adenomatous changes that are similar to what is generally encountered in the GI tract.

Adenocarcinoma of Bladder

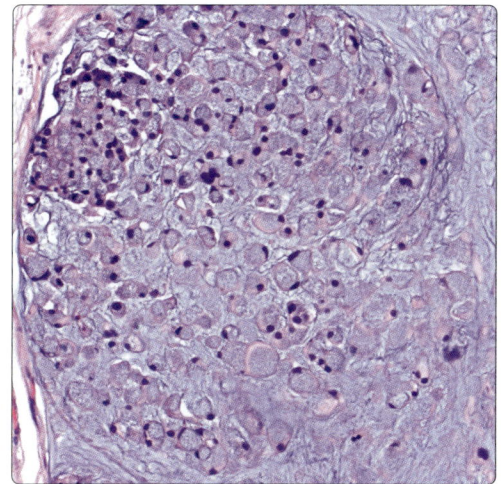

Adenocarcinoma of Bladder

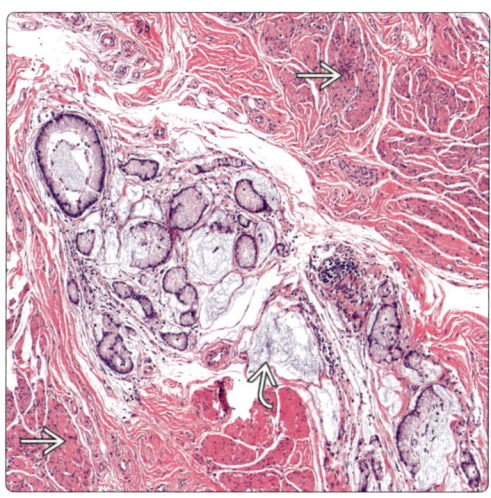

(Left) Signet ring cell adenocarcinoma of the urinary bladder is rare but is morphologically indistinguishable from metastatic gastric signet ring cell adenocarcinoma. Mixed patterns of adenocarcinoma are common in the bladder. **(Right)** Despite the bland look of some of the glands in this tumor, the infiltrating nature (note the presence of muscularis propria ➡ on either side of the tumor) is strong evidence of its malignant nature. Note the presence of mucinous material next to the tumor ➡.

Adenocarcinoma of Bladder: Immunohistochemistry (CK20)

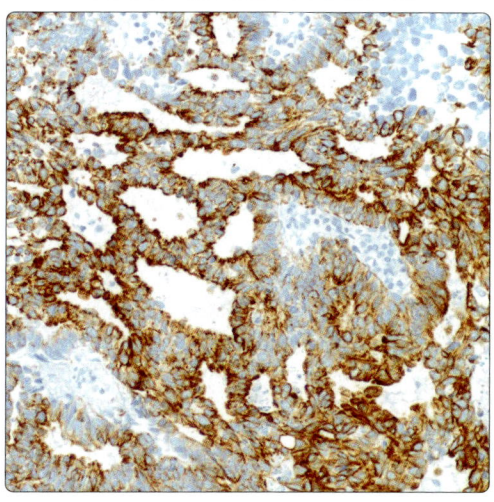

Adenocarcinoma of Bladder: Immunohistochemistry (CDX-2)

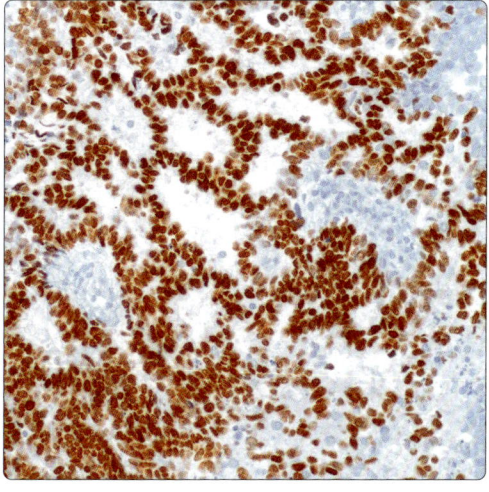

(Left) Primary adenocarcinoma of the urinary bladder may have a complete enteric immunophenotype with strong and diffuse CK20 expression. CK7 reactivity is more variable. **(Right)** Nuclear immunoreactivity for CDX-2 may be seen in primary bladder adenocarcinoma but is not present as frequently as in colorectal adenocarcinoma. There may be complete immunophenotypic overlap between these 2 lesions and adenocarcinomas arising in the urachus.

Invasive Adenocarcinoma

(Left) Urachal adenocarcinoma may be morphologically identical to adenocarcinomas developing elsewhere in the bladder. Location in the dome is the strongest clue to the diagnosis of urachal carcinoma. **(Right)** Urachal adenocarcinoma is seen with enteric morphologic appearance. The entire range of primary mucosal-based vesical adenocarcinoma histology may also be seen in urachal adenocarcinomas.

Urachal Adenocarcinoma

Urachal Adenocarcinoma

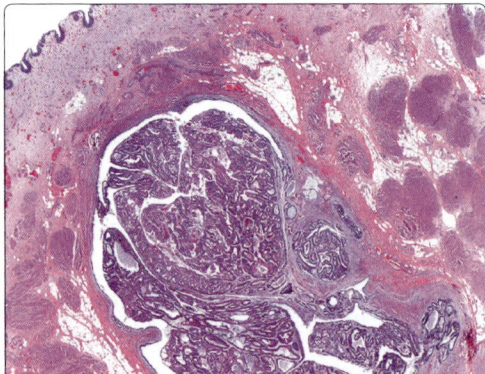

(Left) Urachal adenocarcinomas are indistinguishable from primary vesical adenocarcinoma. The presence of a muscularis propria-based tumor in the dome and absence of surface lesions favor a urachal primary. **(Right)** This is a bladder tumor in a patient with a known history of primary colonic adenocarcinoma, which was morphologically similar to the tumor in the bladder. Note the intact surface urothelium overlying the metastatic tumor.

Urachal Adenocarcinoma

Metastatic Colonic Adenocarcinoma to Bladder

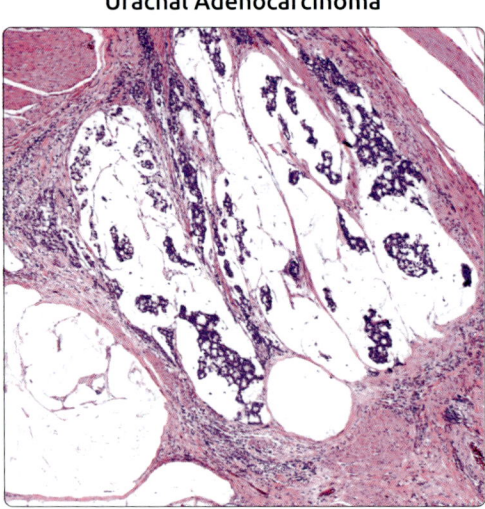

(Left) Lesions in the spectrum of müllerianosis may also enter the differential diagnosis of adenocarcinoma because of the presence of glands deep within the bladder wall, including the muscularis propria ⇨. **(Right)** Endocervicosis contains glands comprised of cytologically bland cuboidal cells ⇨. Invasive adenocarcinomas have a greater degree of cytologic atypia with nucleomegaly and irregular nuclear chromatin, and they are typically associated with a stromal reaction.

Müllerianosis of Bladder

Müllerianosis of Bladder

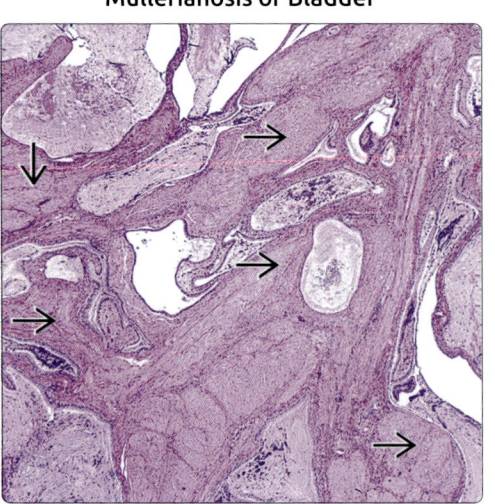 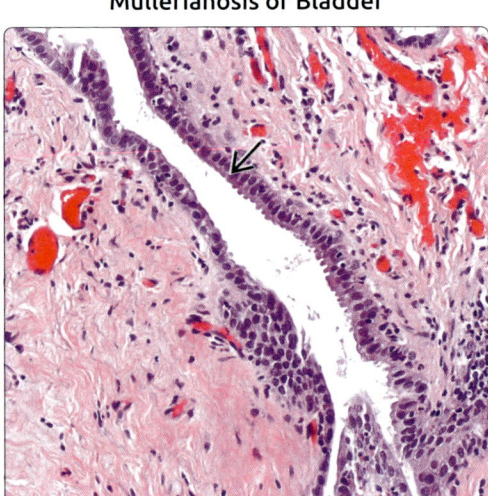

Invasive Adenocarcinoma

Prostatic Adenocarcinoma

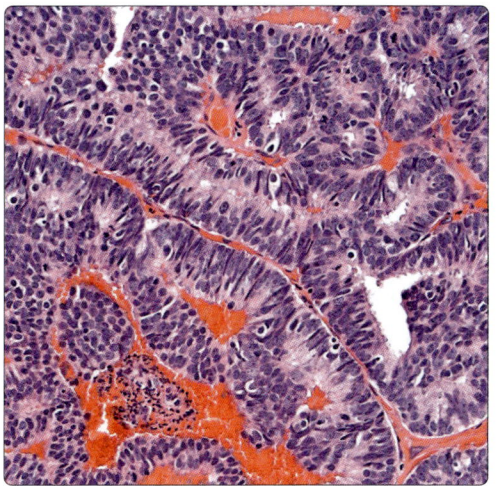

Prostatic Adenocarcinoma

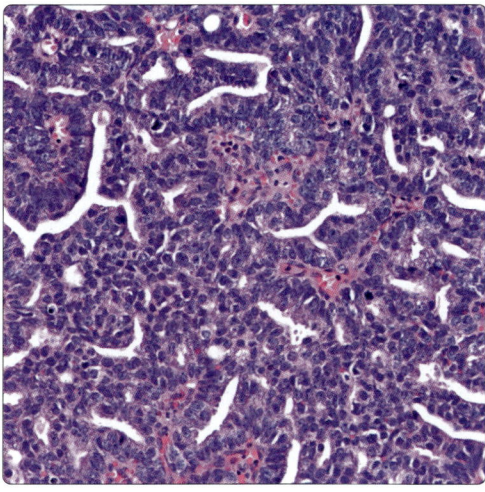

(Left) *Prostatic adenocarcinoma may involve the lumina of the prostatic urethra and may extend superiorly to involve the bladder. The columnar cells of ductal carcinoma more closely mimic enteric-type vesical adenocarcinoma.* (Right) *Prostatic adenocarcinoma with secondary involvement of the bladder may have a gland-forming pattern that mimics a primary adenocarcinoma. In comparison to vesical adenocarcinomas, prostatic carcinoma has more rounded monomorphic nuclei.*

Prostatic Adenocarcinoma: Immunohistochemistry (PSA)

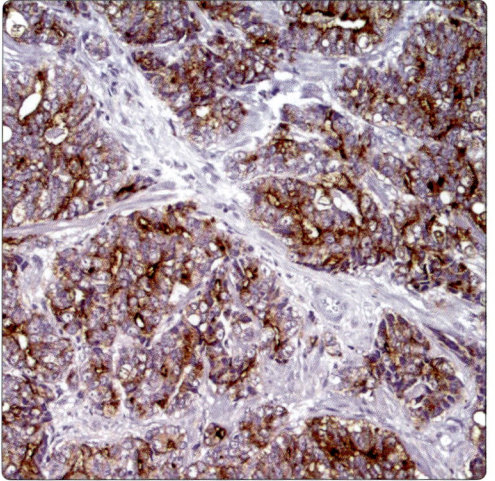

Urothelial Carcinoma With Tubular Morphology

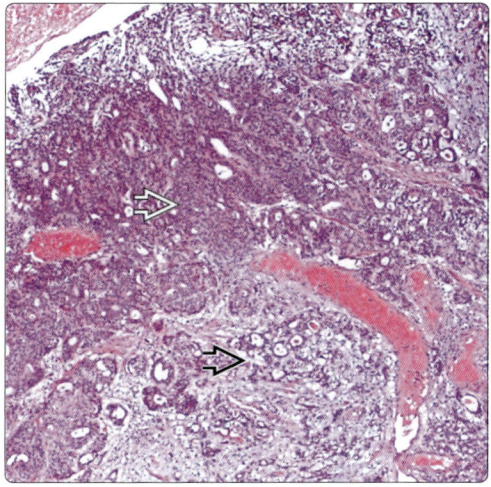

(Left) *Immunoreactivity for PSA (and other prostatic markers) is useful in the distinction of prostatic adenocarcinoma with secondary involvement of the bladder from a primary vesical adenocarcinoma. For primary vesical adenocarcinomas, there is no specific marker that indicates origin from the bladder.* (Right) *This example of invasive urothelial carcinoma with small tubular differentiation highlights the dimorphic appearance with an admixture of both typical urothelial carcinoma ⇒ and distinct tubules ⇒.*

Urothelial Carcinoma With Tubular Features

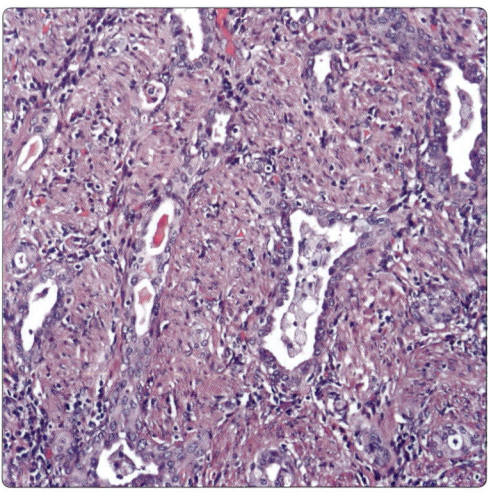

Cystitis Glandularis With Intestinal Metaplasia

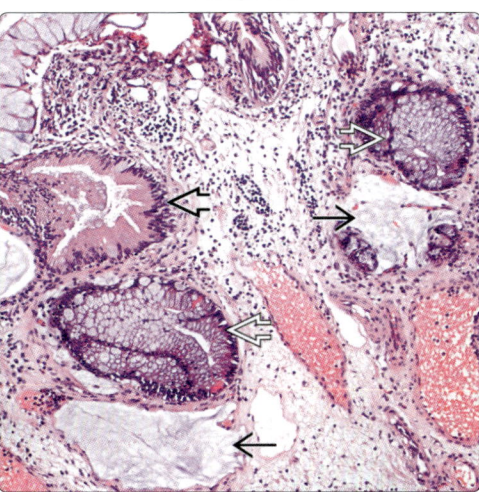

(Left) *In this field, the bland-looking tubular structures invade deeply into the bladder wall and represent a tubular component of otherwise classic urothelial carcinoma elsewhere in the tumor, effectively ruling out the diagnosis of adenocarcinoma.* (Right) *Cystitis glandularis with intestinal metaplasia may mimic adenocarcinoma in some cases. Some glands have prominent luminal cytoplasm ⇒, and others show extensive goblet cell metaplasia ⇒. Mucin extravasation may be present and is occasionally extensive ⇒.*

Clear Cell Adenocarcinoma

KEY FACTS

ETIOLOGY/PATHOGENESIS
- Subset of clear cell adenocarcinoma (CCC) in female patients arises in association with endometriosis or ectopic müllerian glands
- Some cases arise in background of typical urothelial carcinoma

CLINICAL ISSUES
- Extremely rare
- Female predominance
- Hematuria and dysuria
- Deeply invasive CCC is highly aggressive

MICROSCOPIC
- Mixed tubulocystic, papillary, and solid/diffuse patterns
- Tumor cells typically range from flat to cuboidal
- Hobnail pattern of cells commonly seen
- Mixed clear and eosinophilic cytoplasm
- Papillae may have densely hyalinized cores
- Cytologic atypia usually moderate to severe, but areas with low-grade features may be present
- Mitotic figures are frequent
- Tumor invasion readily identified but may be difficult to assess in small or superficial biopsies

ANCILLARY TESTS
- Positive for CK7, CEA, and CA125; occasionally for CK20
- Also express pax-8, pax-2, and AMACR
- MIB-1 proliferation index is high

TOP DIFFERENTIAL DIAGNOSES
- Nephrogenic adenoma
- Secondary involvement (direct extension) from gynecologic tract CCC
- Urothelial carcinoma with clear cytoplasm
- Urothelial carcinoma with glandular differentiation
- Renal cell carcinoma

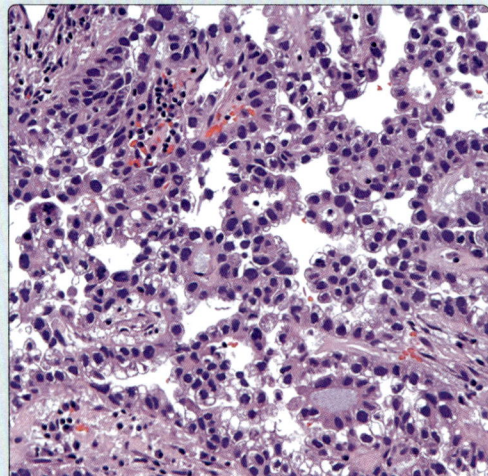

Clear Cell Adenocarcinoma of Bladder: Predominant Papillary Architecture

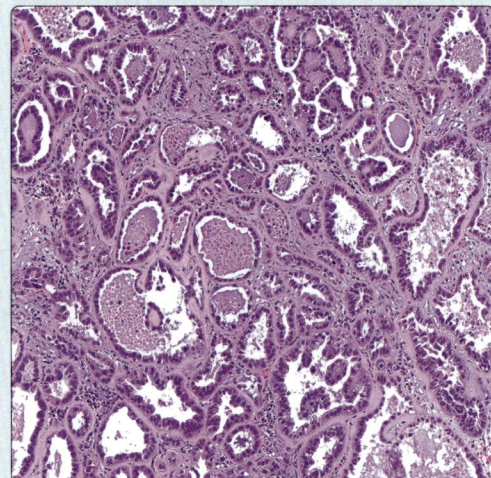

Clear Cell Adenocarcinoma of Bladder: Tubulocystic Architecture

(Left) Clear cell adenocarcinoma of the bladder usually exhibits papillary architecture with cuboidal cells containing clear to eosinophilic cytoplasm and multiple areas with a hobnail appearance. (Right) The tumor may also exhibit tubular arrangement of variable sizes and shapes with readily appreciated infiltration and stromal reaction. Architectural diversity is the rule rather than an exception in clear cell adenocarcinoma.

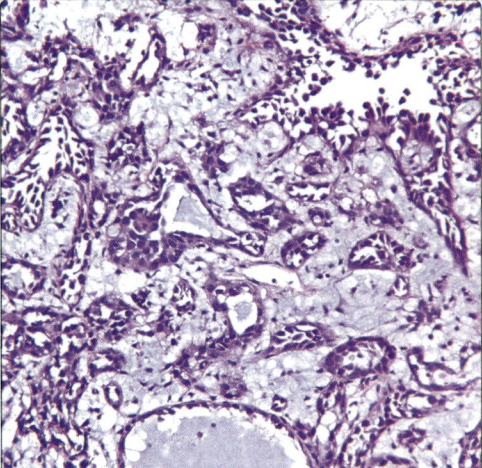

Clear Cell Adenocarcinoma of Bladder: Invasion and Myxoid Stromal Reaction

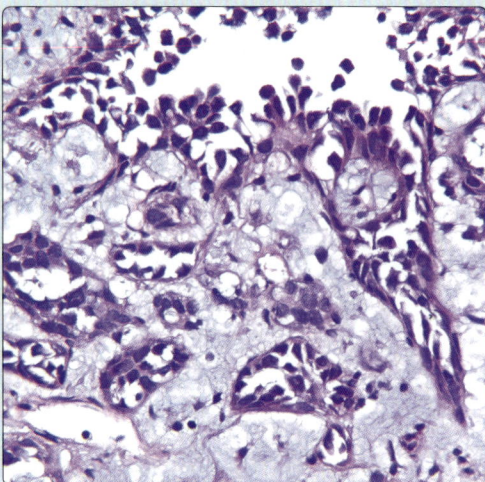

Clear Cell Adenocarcinoma of Bladder: Nuclear Pleomorphism and Hyperchromasia

(Left) A low-power photomicrograph shows clear cell adenocarcinoma with a classic tubulocystic pattern. The lining neoplastic cells have a striking hobnail appearance in this example. There is also associated myxoid stroma, which is a common finding. (Right) This high-power photomicrograph of the tubulocystic growth pattern highlights this typical hobnail appearance of the neoplastic cells in clear cell adenocarcinoma.

Clear Cell Adenocarcinoma

TERMINOLOGY

Abbreviations
- Clear cell adenocarcinoma (CCC)

Synonyms
- Mesonephric adenocarcinoma

Definitions
- Distinct morphologic variant of bladder adenocarcinoma
  - Identical to müllerian-type CCC of female genital tract

ETIOLOGY/PATHOGENESIS

Urothelial Origin
- Some cases arise in background of typical urothelial carcinoma (as divergent differentiation)

Müllerian Origin
- Subset of CCC in female patients arises in association with endometriosis or ectopic müllerian glands

Unknown
- In many cases, origin cannot be determined
  - No immunohistochemical stains are diagnostic

CLINICAL ISSUES

Epidemiology
- Incidence
  - Extremely rare
- Age
  - Wide age range (22-83 years)
- Sex
  - Female predominance

Presentation
- Hematuria and dysuria

Prognosis
- Stage dependent
  - Deeply invasive CCC is highly aggressive

MACROSCOPIC

General Features
- Papillary, polypoid mass, may be ulcerative

MICROSCOPIC

Histologic Features
- Mixed tubulocystic, papillary, and solid/diffuse patterns
- Tumor cells typically range from flat to cuboidal, with clear to eosinophilic cytoplasm
- Papillae may have densely hyalinized cores
- Hobnail pattern of cells may be seen
- Cytologic atypia is usually moderate to severe
  - Level of cytologic atypia may be heterogeneous
- Mitotic figures are frequent (correlates with high MIB-1 positivity)
- Typically have obvious invasion
- Associated myxoid stroma is also common

ANCILLARY TESTS

Immunohistochemistry
- Usually positive for CK7, CEA, and CA125
  - Occasionally positive for CK20
- No immunoreactivity for PSA, ER, or PR
- Also expresses pax-2, pax-8, and AMACR
- Frequently shows nuclear p53 expression

DIFFERENTIAL DIAGNOSIS

Nephrogenic Adenoma
- Low-power architecture may be identical to CCC
  - Generally, mixed tubulocystic and papillary but rarely solid and diffuse pattern
- Lacks significant nuclear pleomorphism, but nucleoli may be present; mitosis rare
- Noninvasive or limited "invasion" associated with inflammation
- Also expresses pax-2 and pax-8

Secondary Involvement (Direct Extension) From Gynecologic Tract Clear Cell Adenocarcinoma
- Morphologically identical to bladder CCC
- In female patients, gynecologic origin must be excluded clinically/radiologically

Urothelial Carcinoma With Clear Cytoplasm
- Cytoplasmic clearing typically focal
  - Usually adjacent typical urothelial carcinoma present
- Contains cytoplasmic glycogen

Urothelial Carcinoma With Glandular Differentiation
- Tubulopapillary architecture may mimic CCC, but neoplastic cells are columnar

Renal Cell Carcinoma
- Associated renal mass (clinical history important)
- Typically lack mixed clear cell and papillary pattern
- Expression of pax-8/pax-2 in both renal cell carcinoma and CCC may be pitfall

DIAGNOSTIC CHECKLIST

Clinically Relevant Pathologic Features
- Extent of invasion is key prognostic feature

Pathologic Interpretation Pearls
- CCC should be considered when considering large nephrogenic adenoma or those with marked atypia
  - Significant morphologic overlap
  - Metastasis should be ruled out

SELECTED REFERENCES

1. Tong GX et al: Expression of PAX8 in nephrogenic adenoma and clear cell adenocarcinoma of the lower urinary tract: evidence of related histogenesis?. Am J Surg Pathol. 32(9):1380-7, 2008
2. Oliva E et al: Clear cell carcinoma of the urinary bladder: a report and comparison of four tumors of mullerian origin and nine of probable urothelial origin with discussion of histogenesis and diagnostic problems. Am J Surg Pathol. 26(2):190-7, 2002
3. Gilcrease MZ et al: Clear cell adenocarcinoma and nephrogenic adenoma of the urethra and urinary bladder: a histopathologic and immunohistochemical comparison. Hum Pathol. 29(12):1451-6, 1998

Clear Cell Adenocarcinoma

Clear Cell Adenocarcinoma of Bladder: Papillary Morphology Without Stratification

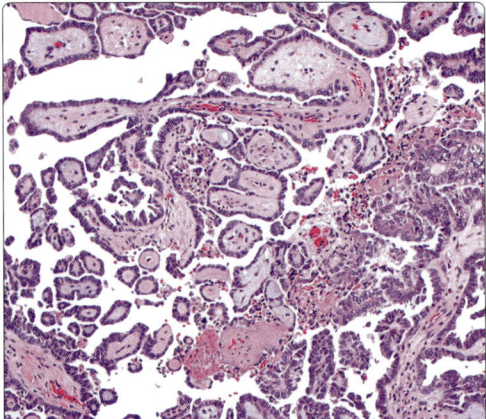

Clear Cell Adenocarcinoma of Bladder: Papillary Tufting and Stromal Invasion

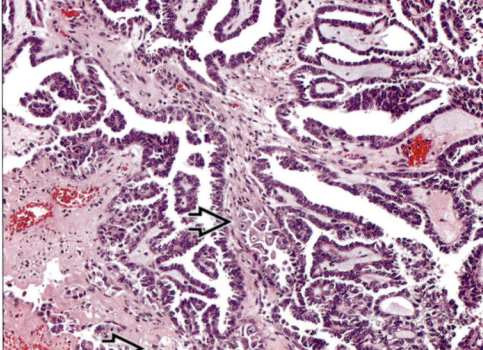

(Left) Some examples of clear cell adenocarcinoma have a predominant exophytic papillary appearance. The papillae are lined by a single layer of cuboidal cells, a feature distinct from typical papillary urothelial carcinoma. *(Right)* This example of clear cell adenocarcinoma with a papillary growth pattern shows prominent epithelial tufting. There is subtle stalk invasion ⇨ that, with haphazard growth when present, is diagnostic of adenocarcinoma.

Clear Cell Adenocarcinoma of Bladder: Bland Morphologic Features

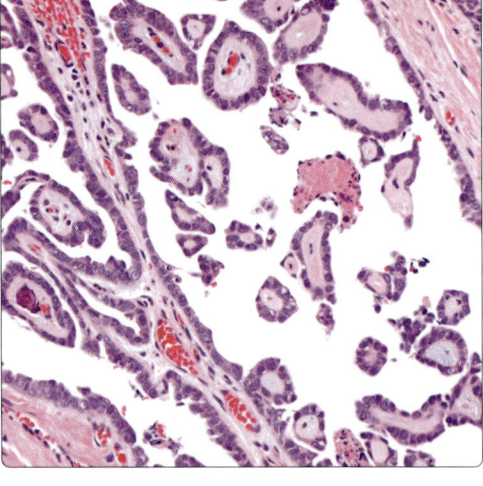

Clear Cell Adenocarcinoma of Bladder: Nuclear Atypia and Prominent Nucleoli

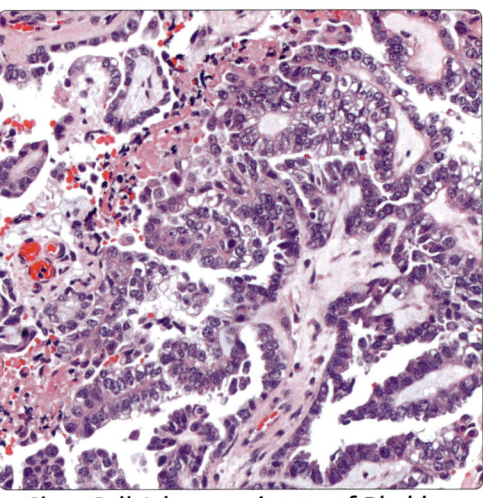

(Left) The degree of cytologic atypia may be variable within a given clear cell adenocarcinoma. This papillary focus is relatively bland, which may lead to confusion with nephrogenic adenoma. Areas with more typical cytologic features of carcinoma should be sought and are generally identified. *(Right)* High-power examination of this clear cell adenocarcinoma shows the typical degree of marked nuclear atypia with nucleomegaly, nuclear pleomorphism, and prominent macronucleoli.

Clear Cell Adenocarcinoma of Bladder: Heterogeneous Tumor Patterns

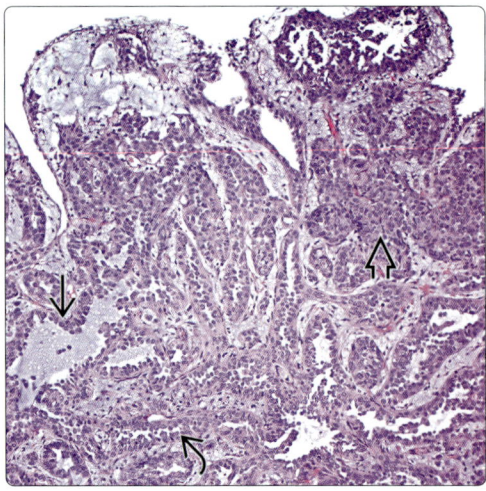

Clear Cell Adenocarcinoma of Bladder: Marked Eosinophilic Cytoplasm and Myxoid Stroma

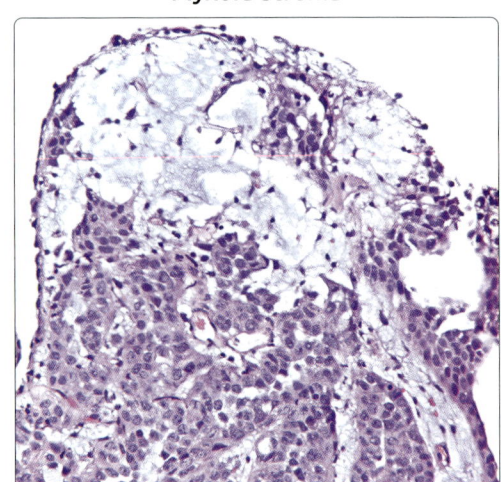

(Left) Multiple admixed architectural growth patterns are common in clear cell adenocarcinoma of the bladder. On this low-power field, there are cystic ⇨, tubular ⇨, and solid ⇨ components. *(Right)* Clear cell adenocarcinoma may show a tubular pattern with solid intraluminal growth. The neoplastic cells have a more eosinophilic cytoplasm, which may be very striking in some cases.

Clear Cell Adenocarcinoma

Clear Cell Adenocarcinoma of Bladder: High-Power View, Solid Growth

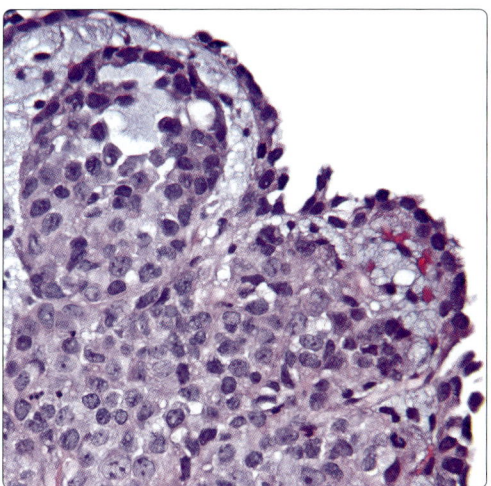

Clear Cell Adenocarcinoma of Bladder: Round Uniform Cuboidal Cells

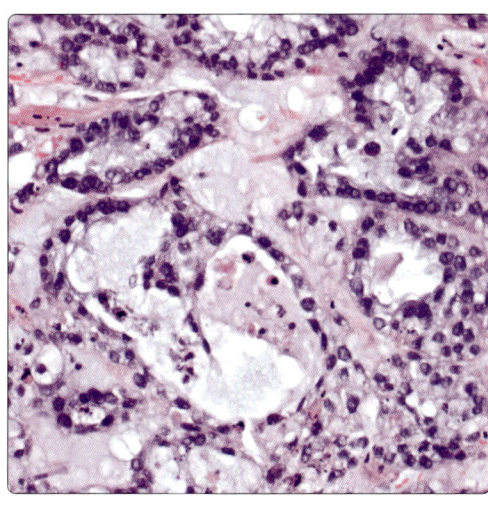

(Left) The foci of solid intratubular growth may mimic a poorly differentiated urothelial carcinoma, especially if the cytoplasm is more eosinophilic, as in this example. Identification of more characteristic patterns of clear cell adenocarcinoma is helpful. GATA3 and uroplakin-2 should be negative. *(Right)* The round nuclear contours are typical of clear cell adenocarcinoma and contrast with the columnar cells present in many other adenocarcinomas.

Clear Cell Adenocarcinoma of Bladder: Short Papillae and Nuclear Hobnailing

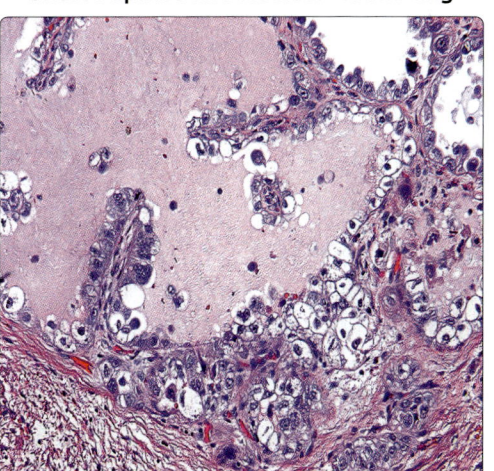

Clear Cell Adenocarcinoma of Bladder: Invasive With Minimal Stromal Reaction

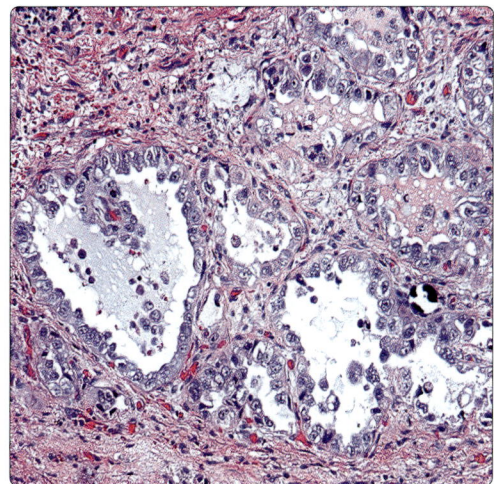

(Left) Clear cell adenocarcinoma with small papillary projections is shown. Tumor cells contain clear to eosinophilic cytoplasm with an occasional hobnail appearance. *(Right)* In this tumor with predominant tubular arrangement, there is minimal stromal reaction, but the nuclear features are indicative of a high-grade malignant process. A focus of calcification is noted. Nephrogenic adenoma and metastatic carcinoma are important differentials.

Clear Cell Adenocarcinoma of Bladder: Bland Features, Cystic and Flattened Tumor Nuclei

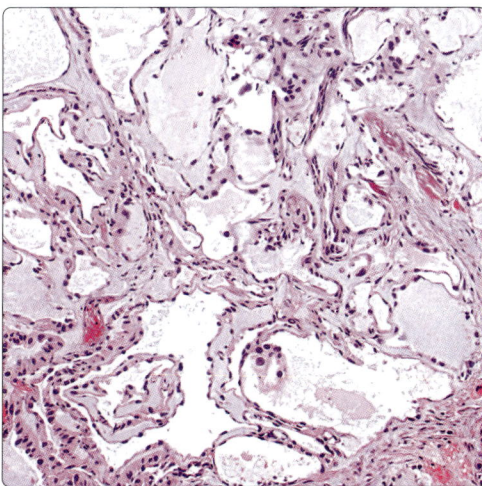

Clear Cell Adenocarcinoma of Bladder: Tumor Heterogeneity, Cystic and Papillary Patterns

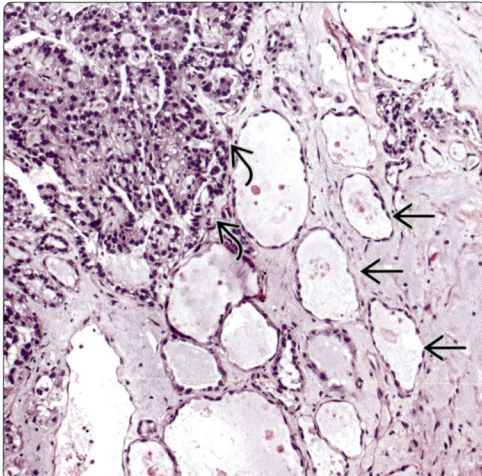

(Left) This example of clear cell adenocarcinoma has dilated tubulocystic foci with very bland cytologic features. This pattern could cause diagnostic confusion with a cystic nephrogenic adenoma or other benign glandular lesions. *(Right)* In this example of clear cell adenocarcinoma, a morphologically subtle tubulocystic pattern in the lower right ➡ merges into a more obviously malignant pattern in the upper left ➡. This degree of intratumoral heterogeneity is not uncommon in clear cell adenocarcinoma.

Clear Cell Adenocarcinoma

Clear Cell Adenocarcinoma of Bladder: Nuclear Pleomorphism, Hyperchromasia and Hobnail Appearance

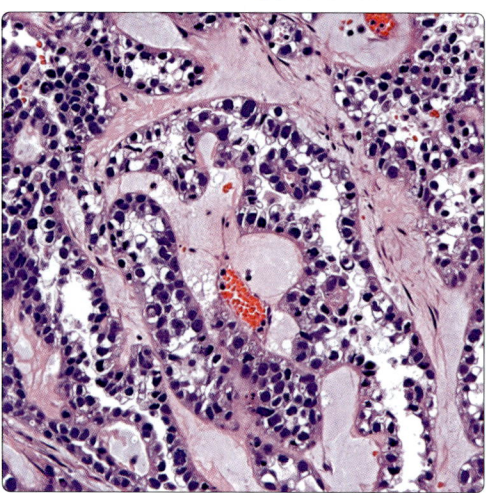

Clear Cell Adenocarcinoma of Bladder: Morphologic Similarity to Gynecologic Tract Tumors

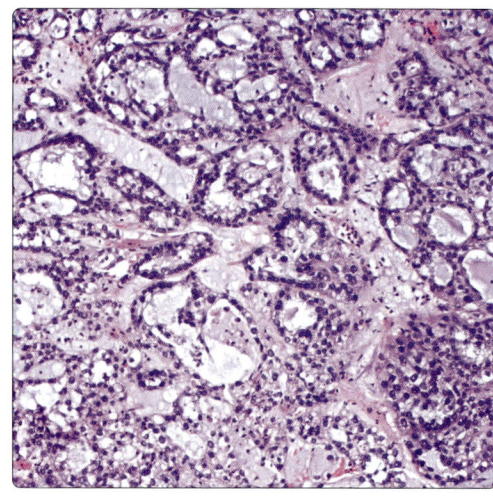

(Left) This example of clear cell adenocarcinoma has interconnecting tubules lined by neoplastic cells with a hobnail appearance. There is a subtle yet distinct variation in nuclear size and shape and chromatin characteristics to render a malignant diagnosis. **(Right)** Tubulocystic patterns of clear cell adenocarcinoma may mimic direct extension or metastasis from another primary site. Clinical correlation is necessary, as immunostaining is not always reliable.

Clear Cell Adenocarcinoma of Bladder: Solid Growth and Clear Cytoplasm

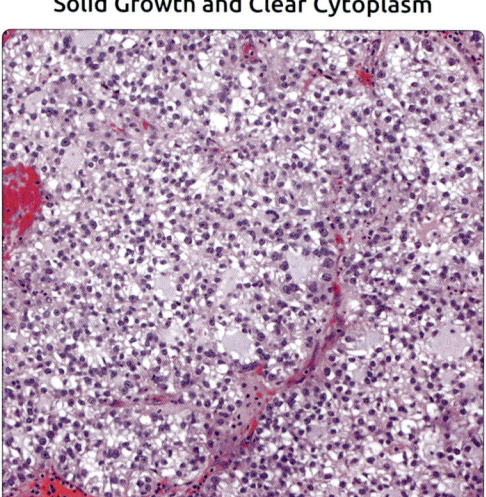

Clear Cell Adenocarcinoma of Bladder: Clear Cytoplasm and Prominent Nucleoli

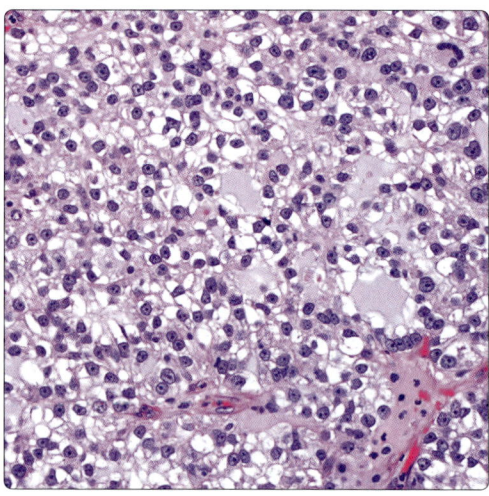

(Left) Solid growth may also be seen in clear cell adenocarcinoma of the urinary bladder, which may mimic other poorly differentiated carcinomas, including renal cell carcinoma. **(Right)** This field shows areas of solid growth in clear cell adenocarcinoma of the urinary bladder. The small rim of clear cytoplasm, the rounded nuclei, and the prominent nucleoli are typical features of this tumor.

Clear Cell Adenocarcinoma of Bladder: Clear Cytoplasm and Stromal Hyalinization

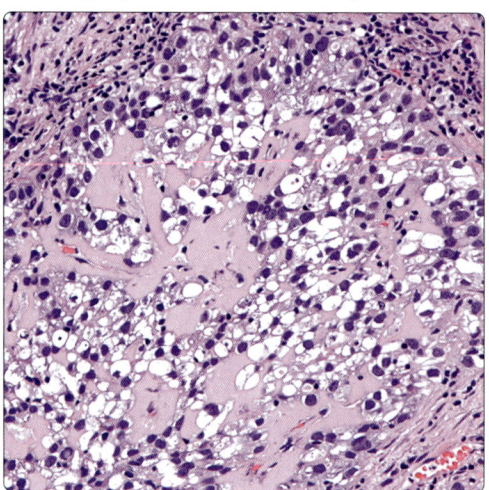

Clear Cell Adenocarcinoma of Bladder: Nuclear Pleomorphism and Mitotic Figures

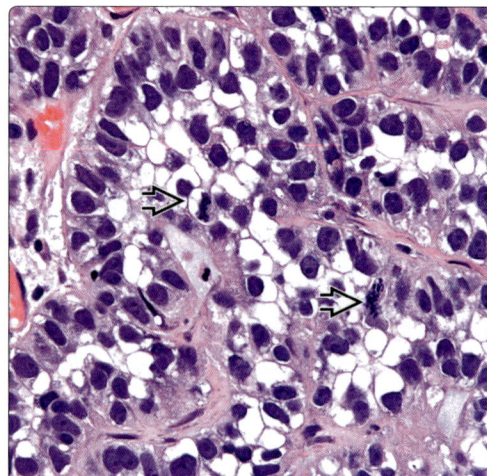

(Left) Dense stromal hyalinization, admixed with nests and individual tumor cells, and the abundant clear cytoplasm are typical features of clear cell adenocarcinoma but may not be always present in all cells. **(Right)** Mitotic figures ⇒ are variable in clear cell adenocarcinoma but should be easily identifiable. Such a finding, along with the more atypical cytologic features (nuclear pleomorphism, hyperchromasia, and markedly prominent nucleoli), is also helpful in the distinction from nephrogenic adenoma.

Clear Cell Adenocarcinoma

Nephrogenic Adenoma

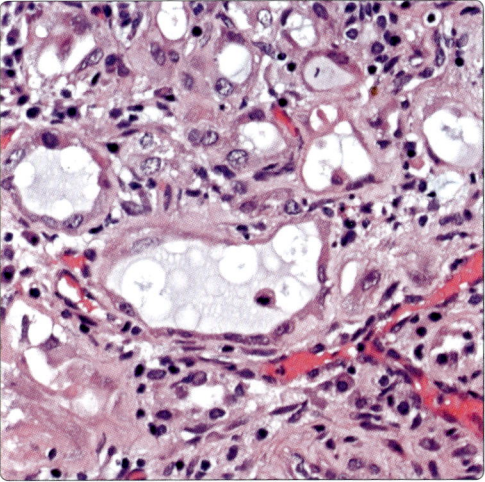

Nephrogenic Adenoma

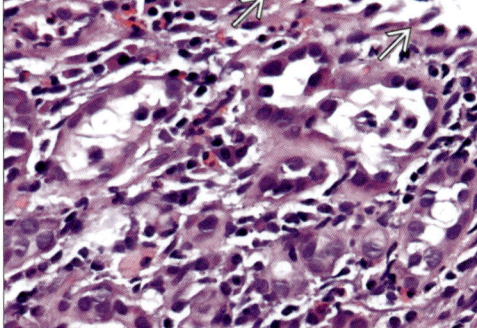

(Left) Nephrogenic adenoma, shown here, may cause diagnostic confusion with clear cell adenocarcinoma. The lack of significant cytologic atypia and the flattened lining epithelium are characteristic of nephrogenic adenoma. (Right) Some examples of nephrogenic adenoma may have a hobnail pattern ➡, as this example shows. Other patterns of more typical nephrogenic adenoma are usually present, and mitotic figures are usually absent.

Clear Cell Adenocarcinoma of Bladder: Superficial Biopsy Mimicking Nephrogenic Adenoma

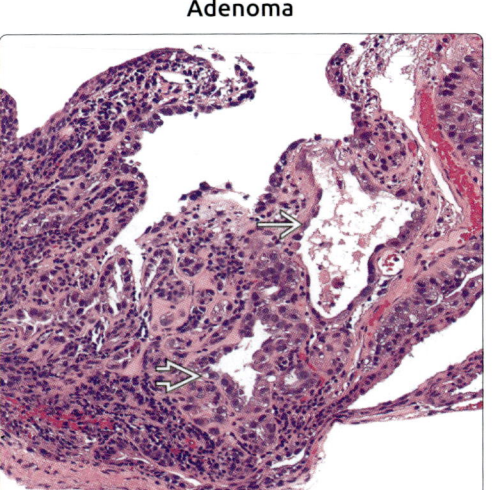

Urothelial Carcinoma With Clear Cell Features

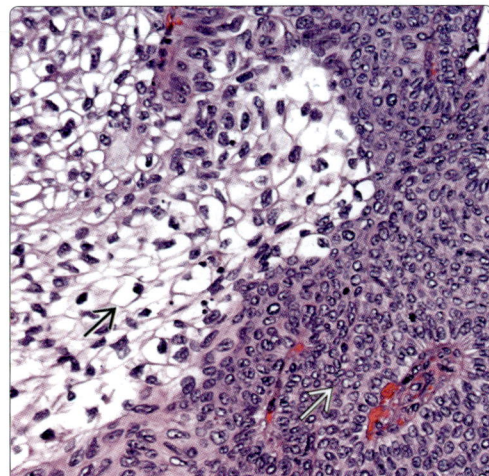

(Left) Superficial biopsy of a clear cell adenocarcinoma of the bladder resembles nephrogenic adenoma, in particular the inflammatory background and focally flattened cells ➡. More atypical features, however, were also present in this field ➡ and elsewhere in the tumor. (Right) This urothelial carcinoma shows an abrupt transition from typical morphology ➡ to areas with prominent clear cytoplasm ➡. The focality of this glycogen-rich appearance is typical and is distinct from clear cell carcinoma.

Urothelial Carcinoma With Large Vacuolated Clear Cells

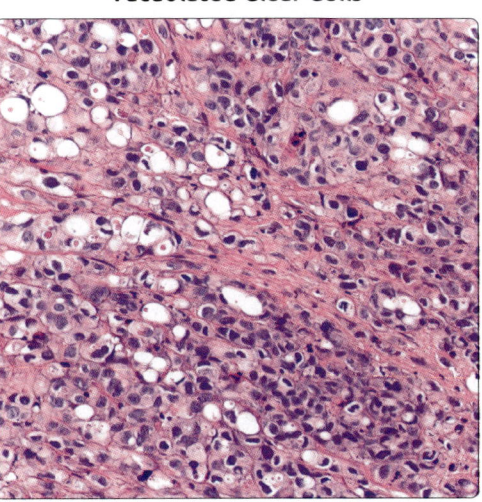

Urothelial Carcinoma With Papillary Architecture

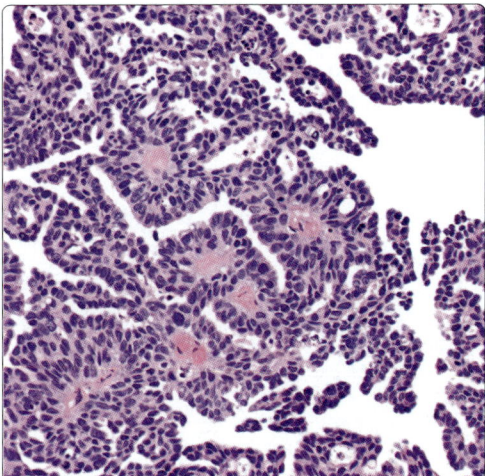

(Left) This is another example of high-grade urothelial carcinoma with clear cells due to large cytoplasmic vacuoles. The presence of otherwise typical areas of urothelial carcinoma is helpful in establishing the diagnosis. (Right) This is a papillary neoplasm with features suggestive of clear cell adenocarcinoma. The presence of complex micropapillary structures and multilayering of the urothelial lining should correctly place this tumor into urothelial carcinoma diagnosis (urothelial carcinoma with villoglandular features).

Squamous Proliferations Other Than Carcinoma

KEY FACTS

ETIOLOGY/PATHOGENESIS

- Keratinizing squamous metaplasia
  - May be associated with chronic irritation
  - Catheters, stones, or parasitic infection
  - Neurogenic bladder
- Condyloma of bladder
  - Contains human papillomavirus (HPV) DNA

CLINICAL ISSUES

- Squamous papilloma
  - Elderly women
- Condyloma
  - Young, sexually active population

MICROSCOPIC

- Nonkeratinizing glycogenated squamous mucosa
  - Very common in trigone of women
  - Normal variation in histology
- Keratinizing squamous metaplasia
  - Hyperkeratotic squamous epithelium lining bladder lumen
- Condyloma
  - Resembles condyloma at other sites
  - Koilocytotic cytologic features
- Squamous papilloma
  - Papillary cores lined by cytologically benign squamous epithelium
  - No viral cytopathic effect is seen

TOP DIFFERENTIAL DIAGNOSES

- Squamous dysplasia
- Urothelial carcinoma in situ
- Noninvasive papillary urothelial carcinoma
- Verrucous carcinoma

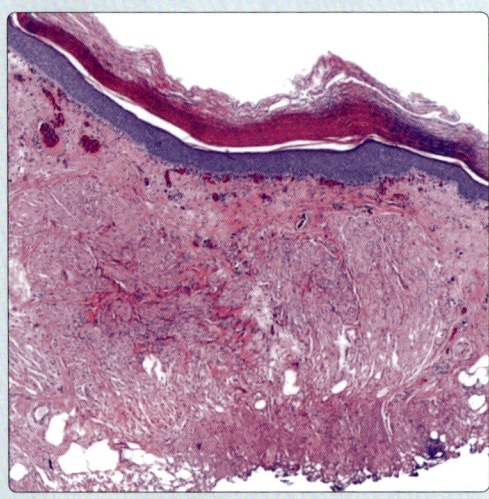
Keratinizing Squamous Metaplasia

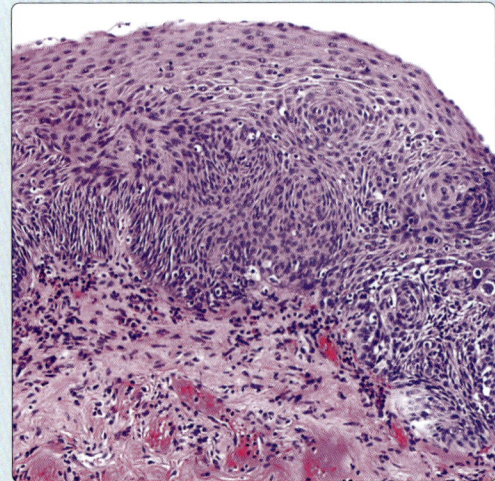
Squamous Metaplasia

(Left) Keratinizing squamous metaplasia is characterized by hyperkeratosis and parakeratosis without dysplasia. When this is extensive, sampling of multiple areas is important to explore the possibility of an associated in situ neoplasia. (Right) This hyperplastic squamous mucosa shows reactive changes associated with inflammation. Higher-power evaluation of cytologic features is necessary to rule out in situ neoplasia.

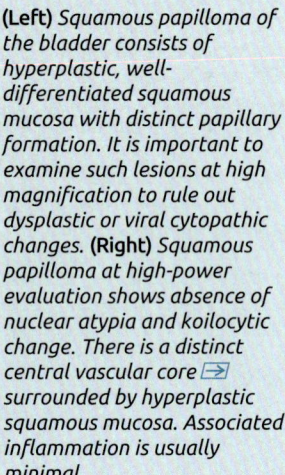
Squamous Papilloma

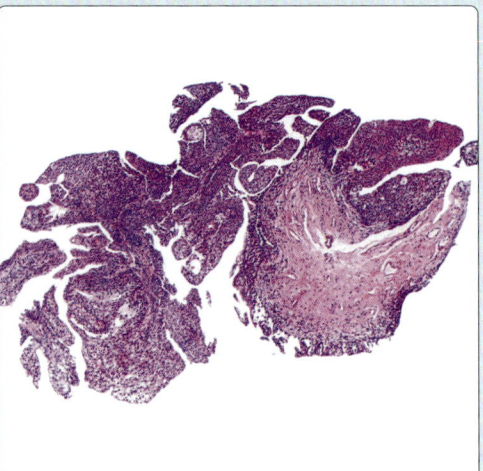

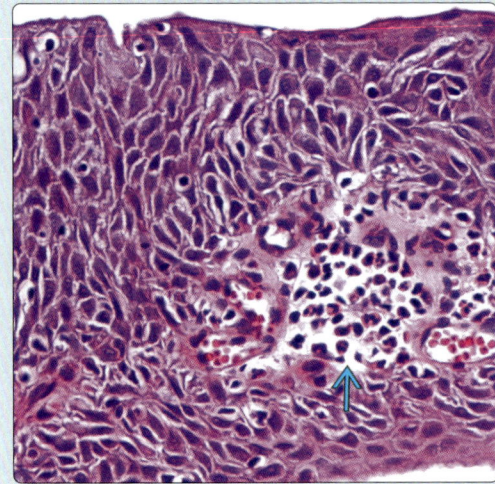
Squamous Papilloma

(Left) Squamous papilloma of the bladder consists of hyperplastic, well-differentiated squamous mucosa with distinct papillary formation. It is important to examine such lesions at high magnification to rule out dysplastic or viral cytopathic changes. (Right) Squamous papilloma at high-power evaluation shows absence of nuclear atypia and koilocytic change. There is a distinct central vascular core ⇒ surrounded by hyperplastic squamous mucosa. Associated inflammation is usually minimal.

Squamous Proliferations Other Than Carcinoma

TERMINOLOGY

Definitions
- Squamous metaplasia
  - Urothelium replaced by stratified squamous epithelium (nonkeratinized or keratinized)
- Squamous papilloma
  - Rare benign exophytic papillary squamous neoplasm
    - Unrelated to human papillomavirus (HPV) infection
- Condyloma
  - Exophytic squamous proliferation with HPV viral cytopathic effect
- Squamous hyperplasia, papillary and flat
  - Multiple layers of cytologically bland metaplastic squamous epithelium with flat or papillary architecture

ETIOLOGY/PATHOGENESIS

Environmental Exposure
- Keratinizing squamous metaplasia: Chronic irritation, catheters, stones, parasitic infection

Infectious Agents
- Condyloma of bladder: Contains HPV DNA

CLINICAL ISSUES

Epidemiology
- Incidence
  - Isolated urinary tract involvement by condyloma is rare (usually also involves urethra, vulva, vagina, or anus)
- Age
  - Squamous papilloma: Elderly women
  - Condyloma: Young, sexually active population

Endoscopic Findings
- Squamous metaplasia: Pale gray-white patches with irregular borders, often surrounded by erythema
- Condyloma and squamous papilloma: Exophytic, polypoid

Prognosis
- Keratinizing squamous metaplasia and condyloma: Risk of malignant transformation (squamous dysplasia/carcinoma)
- Squamous papilloma: Benign clinical course

MICROSCOPIC

Squamous Metaplasia
- Nonkeratinizing glycogenated squamous metaplasia, nontrigonal location
  - In trigone, it is normal variation and not metaplasia
- Keratinizing squamous metaplasia
  - Hyperkeratotic squamous epithelium lining bladder

Condyloma Acuminatum
- Rarely involves bladder, usually by direct extension from genital lesions
- Resembles condyloma at other sites
  - Papillary fronds, hyperplastic squamous epithelium, koilocytosis, hyperchromatic wrinkled nuclei; parakeratosis, hyperkeratosis, and granular layer

Squamous Papilloma
- Papillary fronds with cytologically benign squamous epithelium; no viral cytopathic effect

Squamous Hyperplasia
- Metaplastic squamous mucosa with increased cell thickness and normal cytology; reactive changes may be present

ANCILLARY TESTS

In Situ Hybridization
- Condyloma is positive for HPV

DIFFERENTIAL DIAGNOSIS

Squamous Dysplasia and Carcinoma In Situ
- Condyloma may progress to frank squamous dysplasia (lack of maturation, high N:C ratio, increased mitoses)

Urothelial Carcinoma In Situ
- Lacks features of squamous epithelium (no keratinization or intercellular bridges) or condyloma

Noninvasive Papillary Urothelial Carcinoma
- Papillary urothelial carcinoma has distinct papillary architecture from condyloma
  - Fine papillary cores and long, branching papillae
  - Occasional squamous metaplasia (no koilocytes, no HPV by adjunctive studies)

Verrucous Carcinoma
- Generally larger mass, verrucoid architecture, bland cytology without koilocytic changes

Radiation Atypia
- Squamoid appearance with multinucleation and cytoplasmic vacuolization may mimic koilocytes
- No history of HPV-related lesions elsewhere
  - Most bladder condylomas have other lesions
- Clinical history of prior radiation therapy

Polyomavirus
- Nuclear inclusions in superficial urothelium, smooth nuclear membranes, reactivity with polyomavirus antibodies

DIAGNOSTIC CHECKLIST

Pathologic Interpretation Pearls
- Presence and extent of keratinizing squamous metaplasia should be reported
- Nonkeratinizing glycogenated squamous epithelium is normal in trigone and bladder neck in women
  - Should not be diagnosed as squamous metaplasia

SELECTED REFERENCES

1. Ahmad I et al: Keratinizing squamous metaplasia of the bladder: a review. Urol Int. 81(3):247-51, 2008
2. Guo CC et al: Noninvasive squamous lesions in the urinary bladder: a clinicopathologic analysis of 29 cases. Am J Surg Pathol. 30(7):883-91, 2006
3. Khan MS et al: Keratinising squamous metaplasia of the bladder: natural history and rationalization of management based on review of 54 years experience. Eur Urol. 42(5):469-74, 2002
4. Cheng L et al: Squamous papilloma of the urinary tract is unrelated to condyloma acuminata. Cancer. 88(7):1679-86, 2000
5. Iwasawa A et al: Presence of human papillomavirus 6/11 DNA in condyloma acuminatum of the urinary bladder. Urol Int. 48(2):235-8, 1992

Squamous Proliferations Other Than Carcinoma

Nonkeratinizing Squamous Mucosa

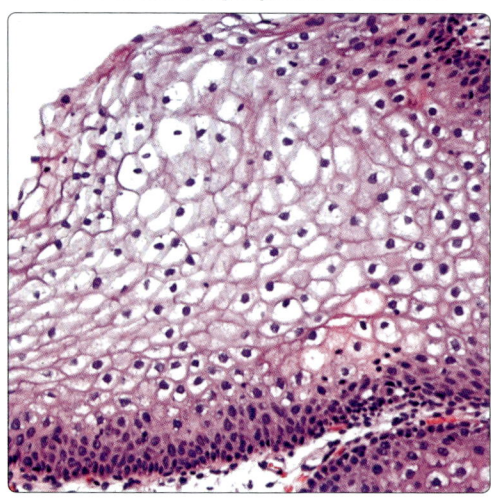

Squamous Metaplasia

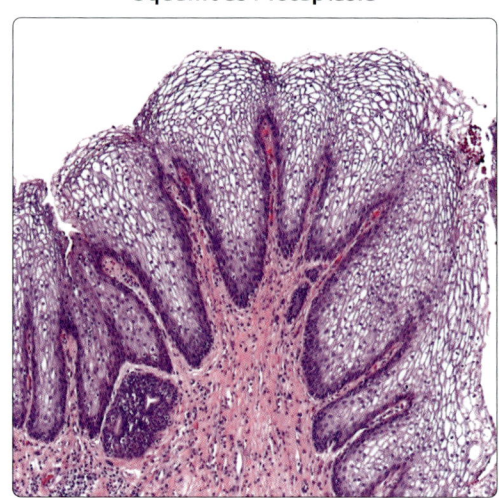

(Left) Glycogenated nonkeratinizing squamous mucosa commonly occurs in the trigone and bladder neck of women. This is a normal finding and does not have any pathologic risk for progression to neoplasia. (Right) This section shows extensive squamous metaplasia of the bladder in a patient with neurogenic bladder that required repeated catheterization. Additional sampling revealed the presence of squamous cell carcinoma elsewhere in the bladder.

Squamous Metaplasia

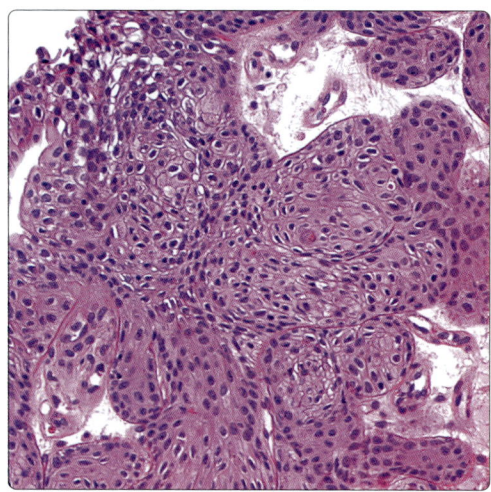

Keratinizing Squamous Metaplasia

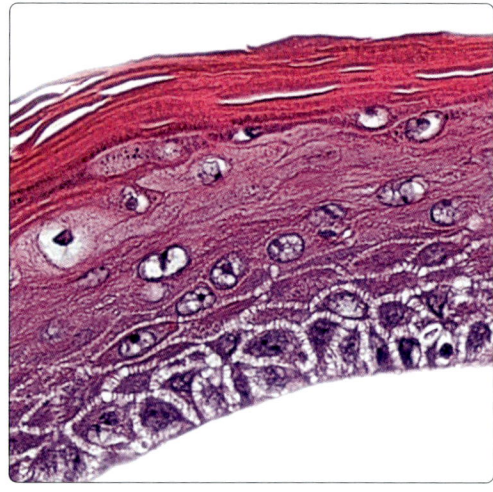

(Left) This focus shows metaplastic squamous changes involving von Brunn nests with focal aberrant keratinization but bland cytology. When extensive and associated with inflammation, the superimposed reactive changes may raise concern for neoplasia. (Right) Keratinizing squamous metaplasia may be seen in longstanding inflammatory conditions. This finding should be reported as, when extensive and widespread, it may be associated with risk of obstruction or progression to neoplasia.

Condyloma

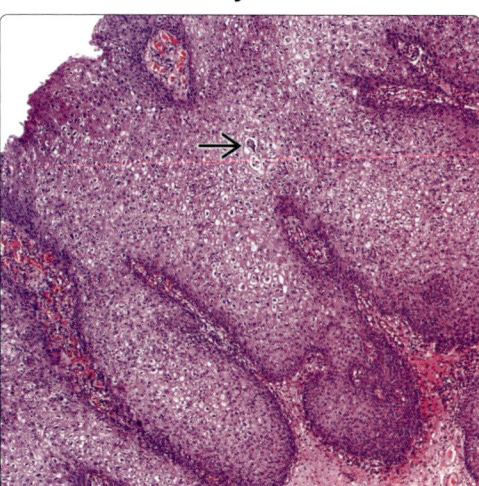

Squamous Cell Carcinoma

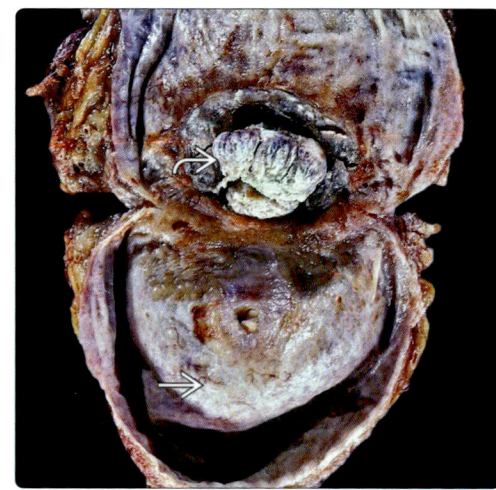

(Left) Evidence of enlarged koilocytes may be seen ➡, even at low-power magnification. Condylomas of the urinary bladder are typically associated with other human papillomavirus (HPV)-associated lesions, such as perineal squamous dysplasia or urethral condylomas. (Right) This cystectomy specimen shows a white, exophytic squamous cell carcinoma ➡ arising in a background of widespread plaque-like keratinizing squamous metaplasia ➡ and keratinizing dysplasia.

Squamous Proliferations Other Than Carcinoma

Condyloma

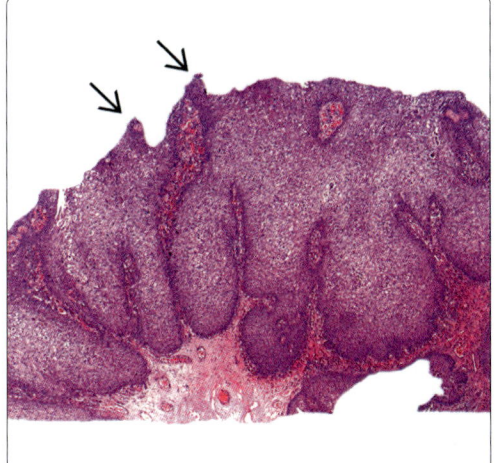

Urinary Bladder Condyloma: Marked Cellular Atypia

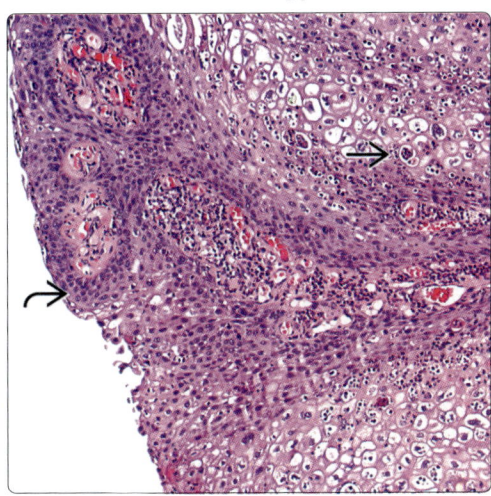

(Left) At low-power evaluation, condyloma of the urinary bladder, as in other anatomic sites, is characterized by hyperplastic squamous epithelium exhibiting a papillomatous architecture ➡. **(Right)** The degree of viral cytopathic effect in condyloma may vary greatly. In some foci, the perinuclear clearing, nuclear hyperchromasia and membrane irregularity are striking ➡. Other foci in the same lesion do not show these nuclear changes ➡.

Condyloma

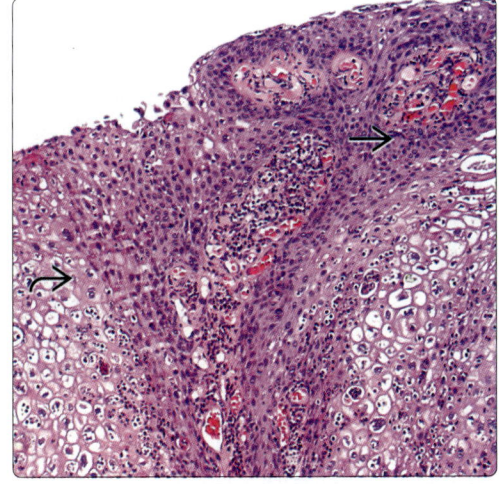

Condyloma

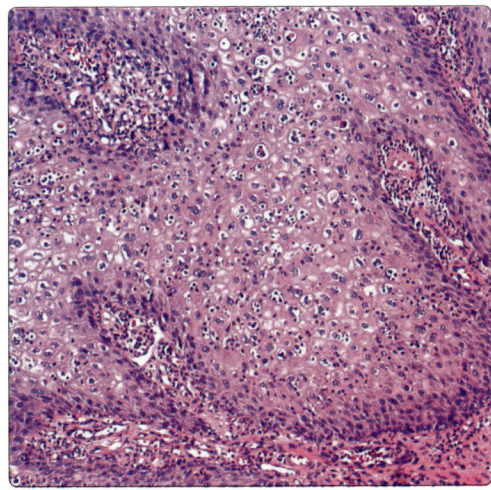

(Left) Variable degree of viral cytopathic effects in condyloma may vary greatly, ranging from foci with virtually no changes ➡ to areas with prominent perinuclear clearing, nuclear hyperchromasia, and nuclear membrane irregularity ➡. **(Right)** In some cases of condyloma, extensive acute inflammation may make interpretation difficult by masking the viral cytopathic effects.

Condyloma

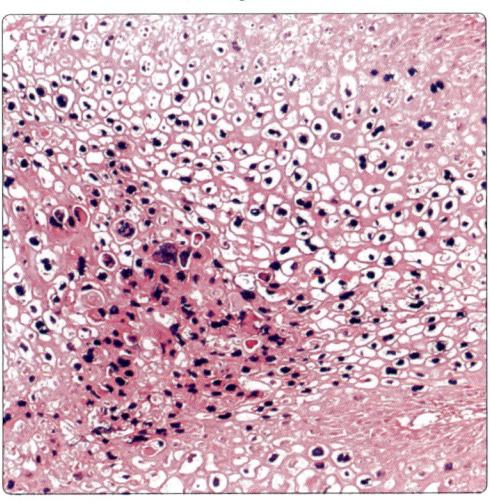

Verrucous Carcinoma of Bladder

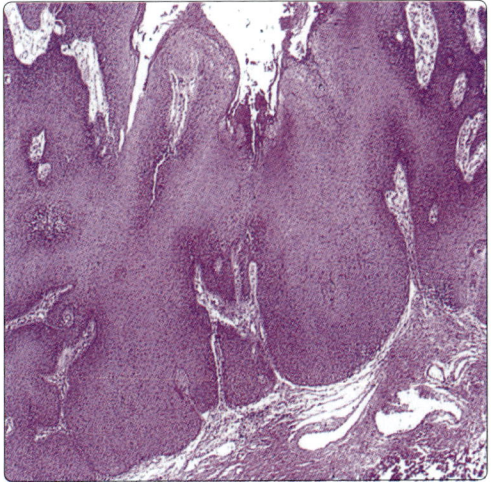

(Left) In situ hybridization studies for HPV show diffuse nuclear positivity. This is not usually needed to render a diagnosis of condyloma but demonstrates the viral etiology. This study is typically negative in a squamous papilloma. **(Right)** Verrucous carcinoma involving the bladder may be confused with squamous papilloma or squamous hyperplasia. The typical large size and the rounded contours at the base of the proliferation, which extend/push into the lamina propria, aid in this distinction.

Invasive Squamous Cell Carcinoma

KEY FACTS

TERMINOLOGY
- Malignant epithelial neoplasm of bladder with pure squamous cell phenotype

ETIOLOGY/PATHOGENESIS
- Smoking
- Chronic inflammatory conditions with squamous metaplasia
- Strongly associated with *Schistosoma* infection

CLINICAL ISSUES
- Varies with geographic region (incidence higher in areas of endemic schistosomiasis)
- Hematuria
- Dysuria
- May be large bulky tumors
- Radical cystectomy with or without adjuvant chemotherapy or radiation therapy

MICROSCOPIC
- Typical/classic squamous cell carcinoma
  - Irregular jagged invasive aggregates of tumor cells
  - Evidence of keratin production: Squamous pearls, intercellular bridges, etc.
  - By definition, no component of urothelial carcinoma or glandular component
- Verrucous carcinoma
  - Verrucous fronds of well-differentiated, acanthotic squamous epithelium with hyperkeratosis
  - Sharp rounded "pushing" base
  - Minimal cytologic atypia
  - Frequently associated with *Schistosoma* infection

TOP DIFFERENTIAL DIAGNOSES
- Invasive urothelial carcinoma with squamous differentiation
- Metastatic or secondary squamous cell carcinoma

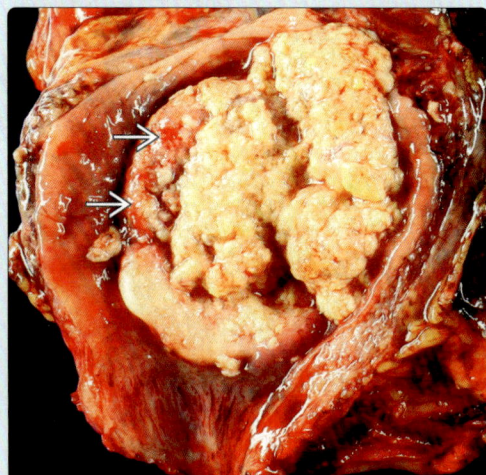

Squamous Cell Carcinoma of Bladder

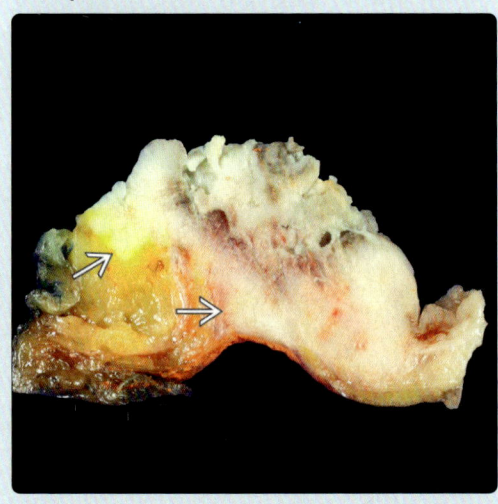

Squamous Cell Carcinoma of Bladder

(Left) This is a large tumor occupying the majority of the posterior wall of the bladder and compressing the ureteral openings. Note the yellowish-white color of the tumor and the presence of ulceration ➡. (Right) In this longitudinal section of a urinary bladder with squamous cell carcinoma, the tumor is deeply invasive. Note the extensive involvement of bladder wall and the deep invasion into perivesical fat ➡.

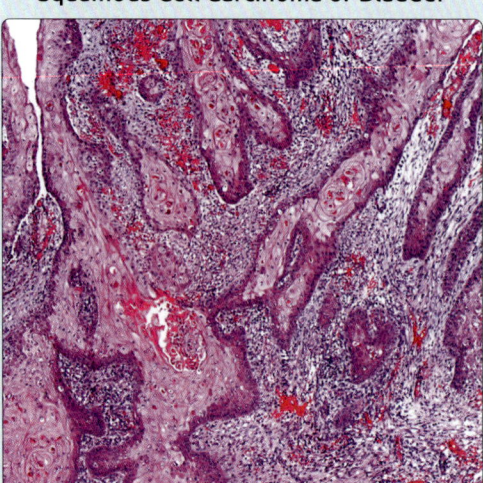

Squamous Cell Carcinoma of Bladder

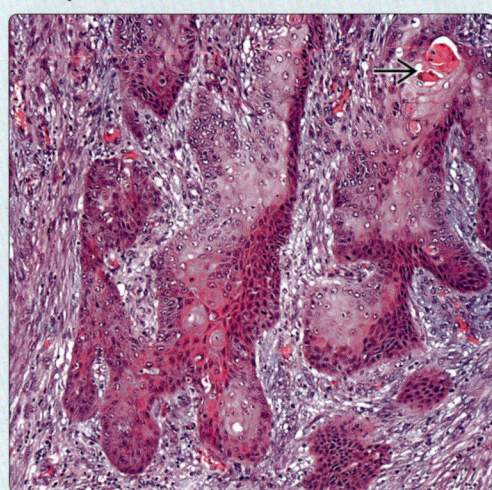

Squamous Cell Carcinoma of Bladder

(Left) On low-power evaluation, the jagged outlines of epithelial tongues and associated stromal reaction are diagnostic of invasion in this primary squamous cell carcinoma of the urinary bladder. (Right) Irregular jagged nests of epithelium with eosinophilic cytoplasm and keratinization ➡ are features of typical/classic invasive squamous cell carcinoma in the urinary bladder.

Invasive Squamous Cell Carcinoma

TERMINOLOGY

Abbreviations
- Squamous cell carcinoma (SCC)

Definitions
- Malignant epithelial neoplasm of bladder with pure squamous cell phenotype

ETIOLOGY/PATHOGENESIS

Developmental Anomaly
- Bladder exstrophy

Environmental Exposure
- Tobacco smoking (5x ↑ risk over nonsmokers)
- Chronic inflammatory conditions with squamous metaplasia are risk factors
  - Bladder stones, chronic indwelling catheters, neurogenic bladder, prolonged cyclophosphamide treatment

Infectious Agents
- Strongly associated with schistosomal infection
  - Includes *S. haematobium* and *S. mansoni* (common in Egypt and other parts of Africa)
  - Verrucous carcinoma is more in this setting
- HPV association is very rare
  - May be seen in cases associated with condyloma or in association with chronic injury

CLINICAL ISSUES

Epidemiology
- Incidence
  - Varies by geographic region
    - 5% of bladder tumors in USA
    - 75% in Egypt/Sudan (endemic schistosomiasis)
  - Verrucous carcinoma of urinary bladder very rare in USA
- Age
  - Most common in 6th decade
- Sex
  - Male predominance, but lower than in urothelial carcinoma

Presentation
- Hematuria, dysuria

Endoscopic Findings
- Large white exophytic mass
- Surface of bladder may show white, plaque-like thickening

Treatment
- Surgical approaches
  - Radical cystectomy is standard therapy
- Adjuvant therapy
  - Often have neoadjuvant or adjuvant radiation
  - Adjuvant chemotherapy is less standardized

Prognosis
- Poor prognosis (nonverrucous SCC)
  - High-stage disease at presentation is common
  - Reported 5-year survival = 7-50% (in pT3 disease = 13%)
- Pure verrucous carcinoma has favorable prognosis with no metastatic risk

MACROSCOPIC

General Features
- Fungating, tan-white mass
  - Typically large and deeply invasive, often ulcerated

MICROSCOPIC

Invasive Squamous Cell Carcinoma, Typical/Classic Type
- Irregular jagged invasive aggregates of malignant squamous cells distributed randomly
  - Stromal myofibroblastic proliferation common
- Displays wide range of differentiation
- No component of urothelial carcinoma (invasive and noninvasive) or adenocarcinoma
- Often associated with surface keratinizing metaplasia and squamous dysplasia

Pure Verrucous Squamous Cell Carcinoma
- Verrucous fronds of well-differentiated, acanthotic squamous epithelium with hyperkeratosis
- Rounded "pushing" base
  - Admixed lymphocytic infiltrate common at base
  - No jagged, irregularly invasive nests
- Minimal cytologic atypia
- Diagnosis is made only in completely resected tumor.
- In partial sample: Well-differentiated SCC with verrucous carcinoma histology

DIFFERENTIAL DIAGNOSIS

Invasive Urothelial Carcinoma With Squamous Differentiation
- Associated component of urothelial carcinoma

Keratinizing Squamous Metaplasia
- May mimic verrucous carcinoma
  - No deep extension into lamina propria

Condyloma Acuminatum
- Koilocytic atypia and no deep extension into lamina propria

Metastatic or Secondary Squamous Cell Carcinoma
- May be morphologically identical to primary vesical SCC
- Requires close clinical and radiographic correlation
- Background squamous dysplasia argues for primary process

DIAGNOSTIC CHECKLIST

Pathologic Interpretation Pearls
- Carcinoma must be of pure squamous histology and primary without elsewhere to classify as primary SCC

SELECTED REFERENCES

1. Lagwinski N et al: Squamous cell carcinoma of the bladder: a clinicopathologic analysis of 45 cases. Am J Surg Pathol. 31(12):1777-87, 2007
2. Rundle JS et al: Squamous cell carcinoma of bladder. A review of 114 patients. Br J Urol. 54(5):522-6, 1982

Invasive Squamous Cell Carcinoma

(Left) *Irregularly formed, jagged tongues of neoplastic squamous epithelium extend into the deep lamina propria with associated stromal inflammatory changes in this biopsy specimen of primary bladder squamous cell carcinoma.* (Right) *Obvious keratinization, often with dyskeratosis ⇨, is commonly seen in primary invasive squamous cell carcinoma. These carcinomas are indistinguishable from squamous carcinomas arising in other anatomic sites.*

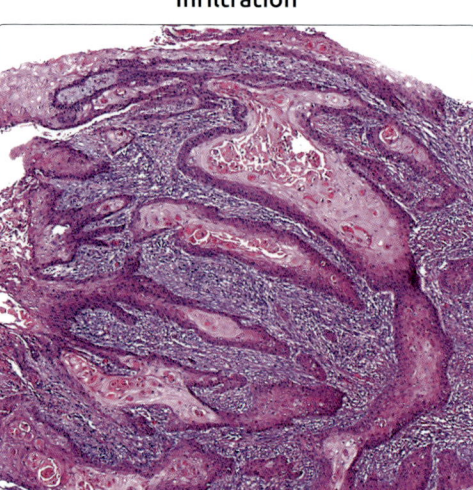
Infiltration

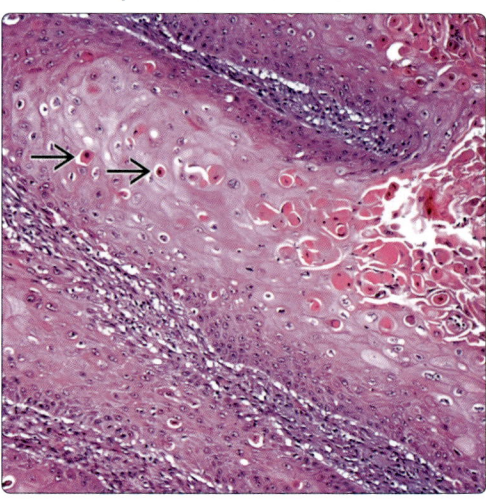
Squamous Differentiation

(Left) *Keratinization is usually obvious in invasive squamous cell carcinoma. By definition, no component of papillary, invasive, or in situ urothelial carcinoma or glandular component is present.* (Right) *This primary vesical invasive squamous cell carcinoma has typical features, including irregular nests, stromal reaction, keratin pearl formation ⇨, and dyskeratosis. These features distinguish typical/classic squamous cell carcinoma from verrucous carcinoma.*

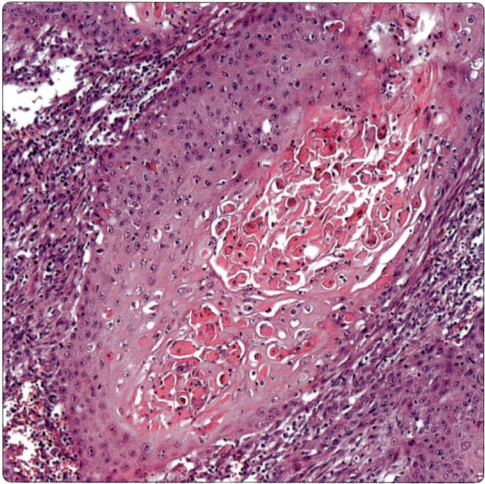
Prominent Keratinization

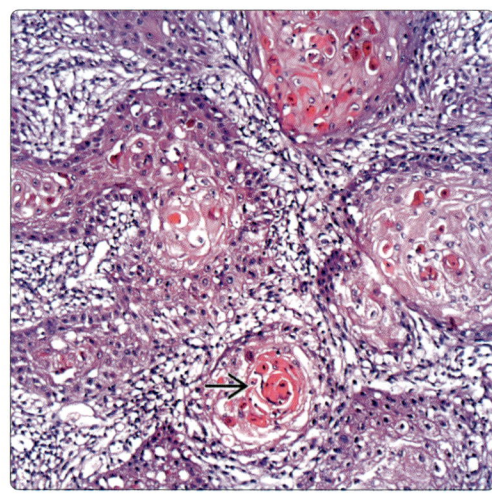
Destructive Invasion

(Left) *The jagged irregular nests of invasive SCC are commonly associated with a myofibroblastic proliferation, which, if prominent, may raise the diagnostic possibility of sarcomatoid carcinoma.* (Right) *The spindle cells associated with this squamous cell carcinoma are cytologically bland with elongated cytoplasmic processes, features typical of myofibroblasts. In contrast, the spindle cell component of sarcomatoid carcinoma usually has marked nuclear hyperchromasia and obvious pleomorphism.*

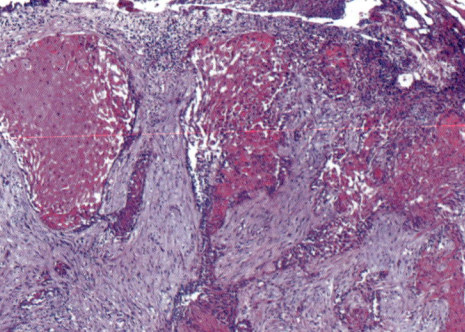
With Pseudosarcomatous Reaction

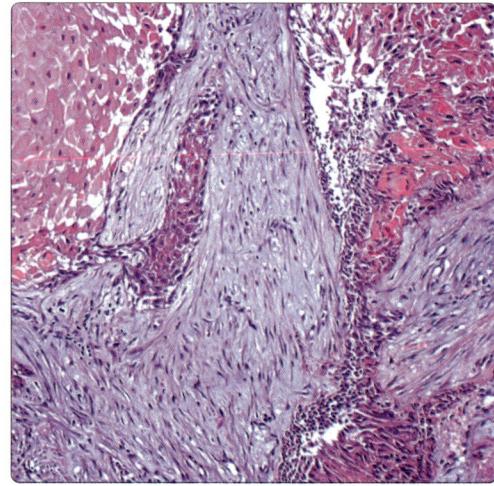
With Pseudosarcomatous Reaction

Invasive Squamous Cell Carcinoma

Squamous Cell Carcinoma of Bladder

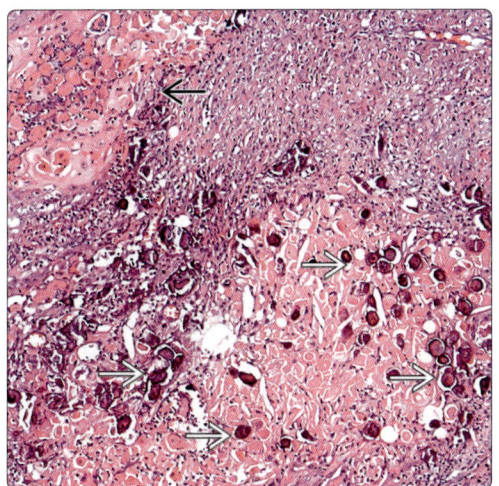

Schistosomiasis

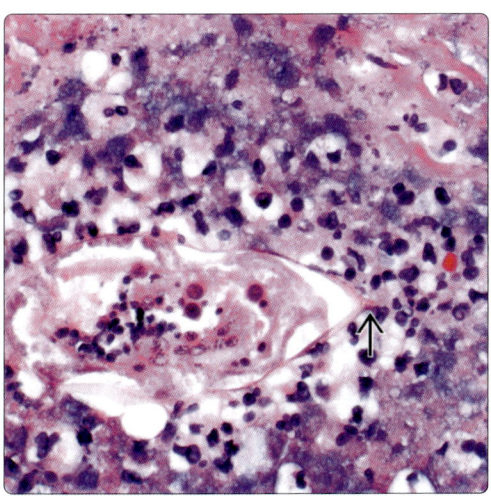

(Left) This squamous cell carcinoma ➡ arose in association with schistosomal infection. Numerous calcified eggs ➡ are present in the adjacent tissue. A spectrum of bladder tumors, including urothelial carcinoma, occurs with schistosomiasis. (Right) Noncalcified Schistosoma haematobium eggs with characteristic terminal spines ➡ may be identified in the urinary bladder of infected patients. Note the presence of multiple organelles within the egg.

Verrucous Carcinoma of Bladder

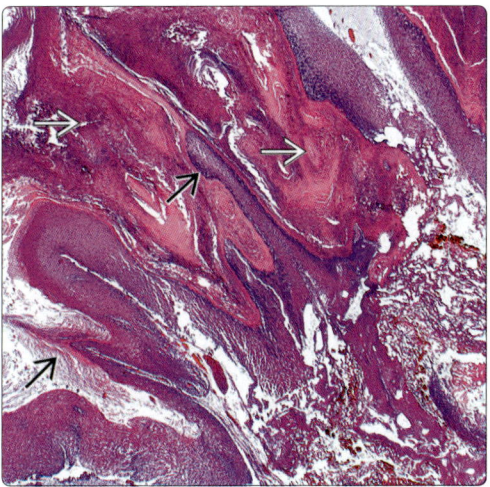

Verrucous Carcinoma of Bladder

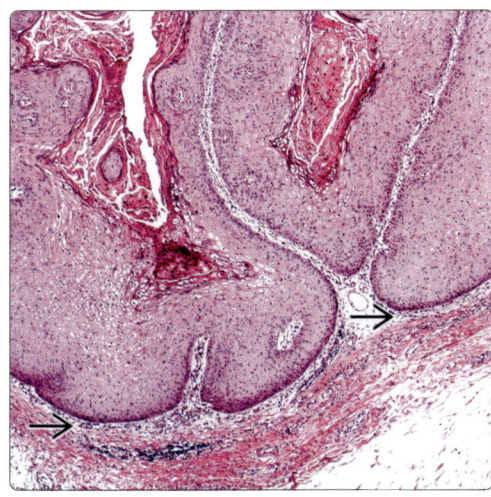

(Left) Long exophytic papillary processes ➡ are typical of verrucous carcinoma and may produce a warty appearance. Marked hyperkeratosis may also be seen ➡. (Right) The round "pushing" base at the deep aspect ➡ is characteristic of the invasion pattern of verrucous carcinoma. Typical invasive squamous cell carcinoma has more irregular nests at the base of the tumor.

Verrucous Carcinoma of Bladder

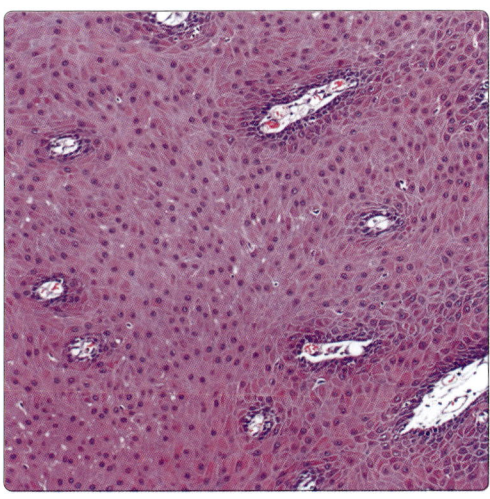

Squamous Cell Carcinoma of Bladder

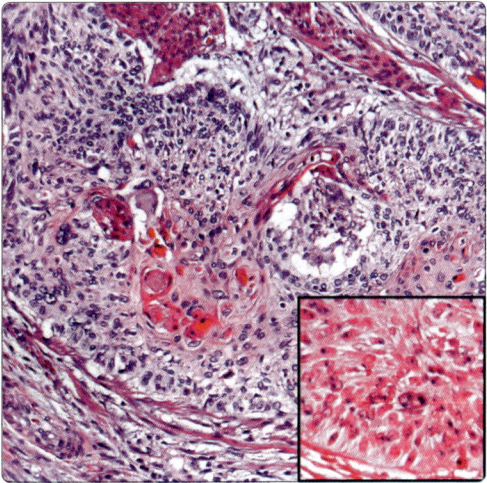

(Left) Unlike typical invasive SCC, verrucous carcinoma lacks significant nuclear pleomorphism. If the entire lesion is not sampled, diagnostic terms, such as "well-differentiated SCC with verrucous carcinoma histology," may be used. (Right) Squamous cell carcinoma developing in a neurogenic bladder associated with HPV infection (inset, HPV in situ hybridization) is shown. The patient was self catheterizing multiple times per day and the bladder had extensive squamous metaplasia.

Invasive Squamous Cell Carcinoma

(Left) *Keratinizing squamous metaplasia is commonly seen in the bladder mucosa surrounding squamous cell carcinoma.* **(Right)** *The background mucosa in squamous cell carcinoma may show a spectrum from low-grade dysplasia to squamous carcinoma in situ. Dysplastic changes, including nucleomegaly and hyperchromasia, are seen here. Severe dysplasia and in situ carcinoma are synonymous in bladder squamous lesions.*

Keratinizing Squamous Metaplasia
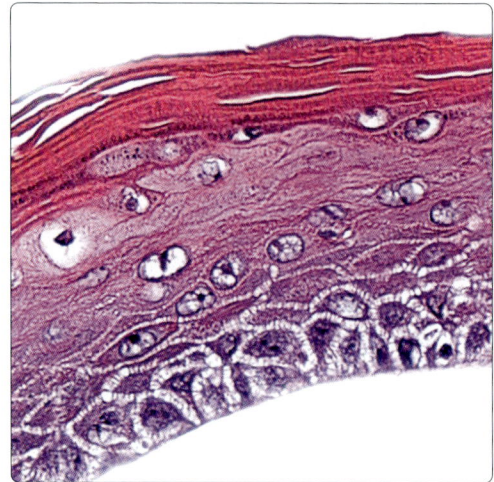

Severe Squamous Dysplasia
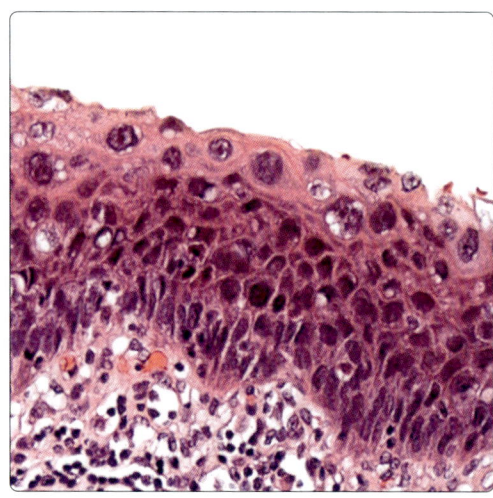

(Left) *Squamous dysplasia may show a subtle differentiated type without full-thickness involvement by basaloid cells with high nuclear:cytoplasmic ratio. Note the presence of nucleomegaly, hyperchromasia, and mitoses at the base ➡.* **(Right)** *The presence of calcification and keratin debris should suggest the possibility of an unsampled SCC or squamous dysplasia. Secondary infection, ulceration, and necrosis are not uncommon with SCC, and may be seen in superficial biopsy specimens.*

Severe Squamous Dysplasia
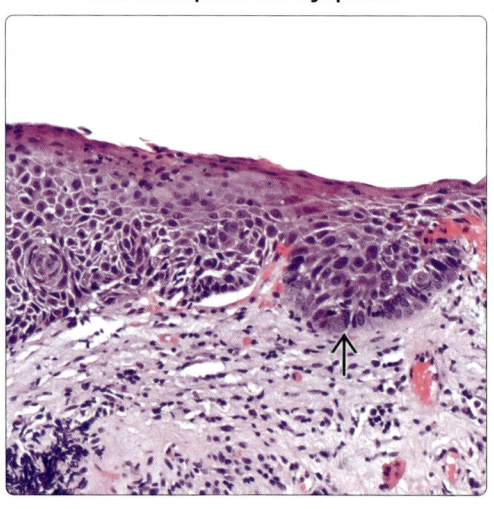

Keratinous Debris and Calcification
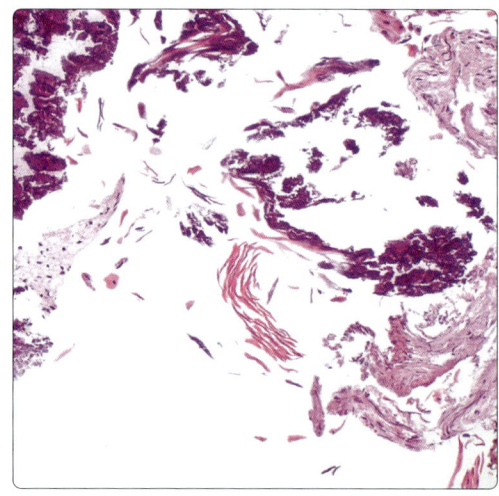

(Left) *Not all schistosomal infestation of the bladder are associated with squamous cell carcinoma. Calcified schistosomal eggs with associated inflammation might be seen in specimens sampled for hematuria or irritative symptoms.* **(Right)** *The terminal spine of Schistosoma haematobium eggs ➡ may also be identified in completely calcified forms. Identification of associated Schistosoma eggs provides strong evidence of a primary bladder squamous cell carcinoma over secondary spread.*

Schistosomal Infection
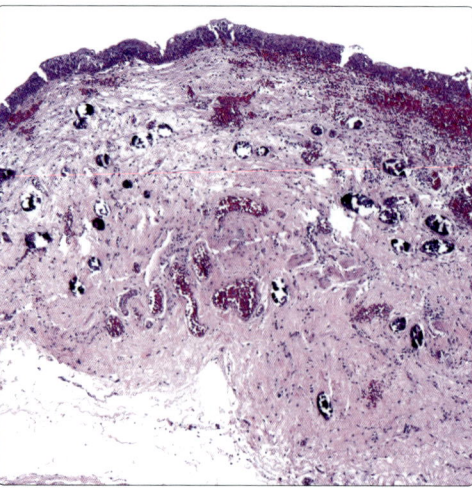

Schistosomal Eggs
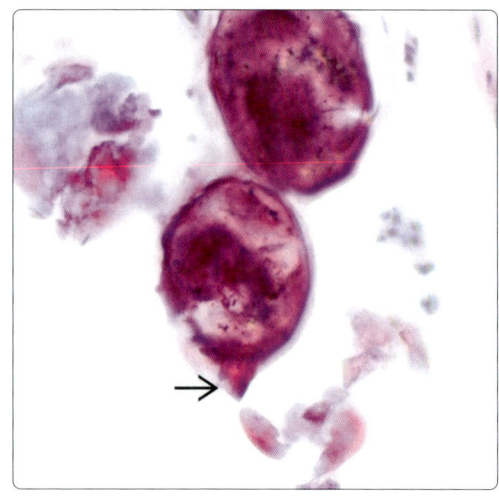

Invasive Squamous Cell Carcinoma

Secondary Squamous Cell Carcinoma of Bladder

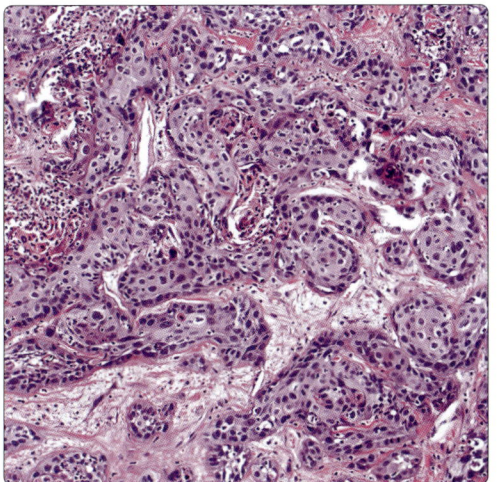

Secondary Squamous Cell Carcinoma of Bladder

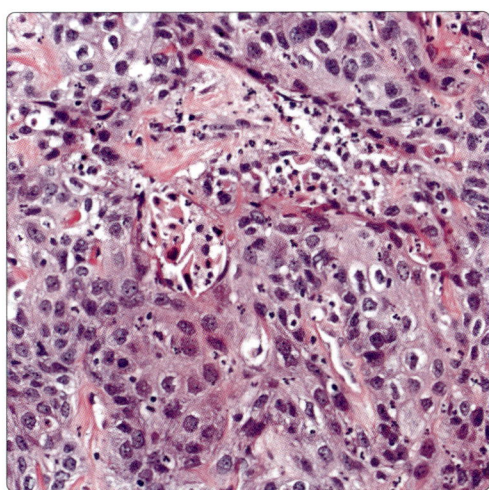

(Left) Invasive squamous cell carcinoma from adjacent anatomic regions may involve the urinary bladder by direct extension, as seen in this example of cervical squamous cell carcinoma in a transurethral biopsy specimen of the bladder. **(Right)** This cervical squamous cell carcinoma in a bladder biopsy specimen is indistinguishable from a primary bladder squamous carcinoma. Very close clinical and imaging correlation is essential in this differential diagnostic setting.

Secondary Squamous Cell Carcinoma of Bladder (p16)

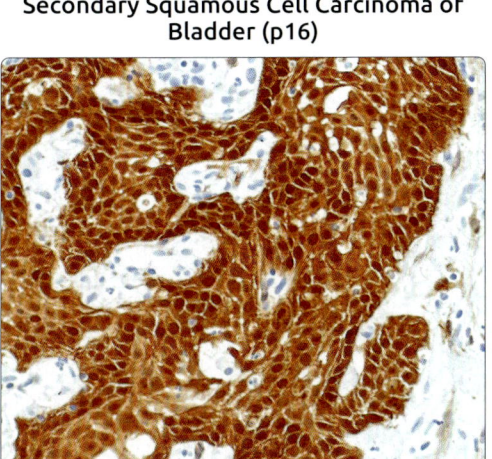

Squamous Metaplasia

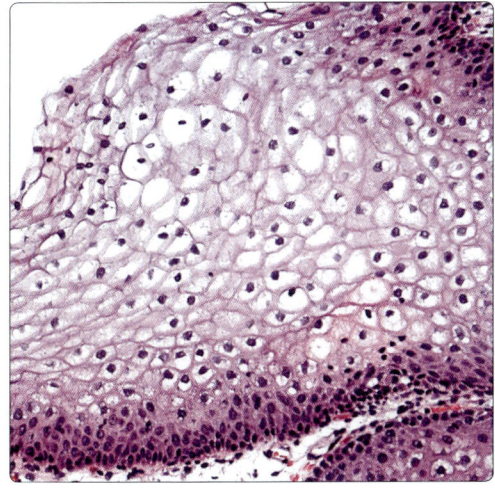

(Left) Diffuse cytoplasmic and nuclear p16 immunoreactivity is seen in this cervical squamous cell carcinoma that secondarily involved the urinary bladder by direct extension. Although p16 is a surrogate marker for HPV, it is not very specific, as it may occasionally be seen in bladder cancers that are not HPV related. **(Right)** Glycogenated squamous metaplasia is a common finding in the trigone of premenopausal women and should not be used as evidence in support of diagnosis of primary urinary bladder squamous cell carcinoma.

Urothelial Carcinoma With Squamous Differentiation

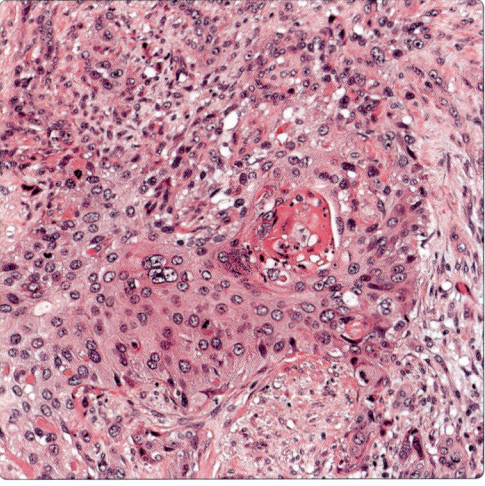

Secondary Squamous Cell Carcinoma of Bladder

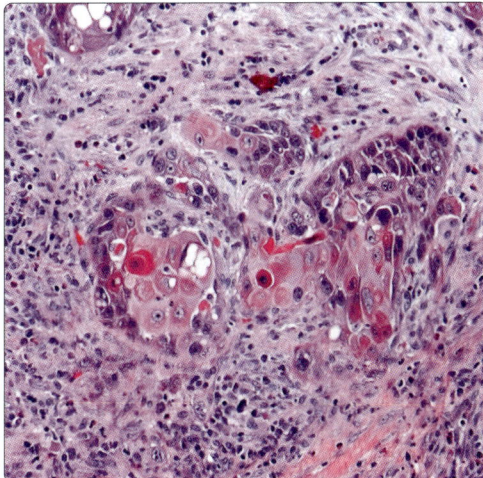

(Left) Urothelial carcinoma with squamous differentiation may be indistinguishable from primary squamous cell carcinoma. The identification of any urothelial component warrants classification as urothelial carcinoma. **(Right)** Squamous cell carcinoma histology is shown in the bladder of a patient with known history of prostatic adenocarcinoma status post radiation therapy. Squamous differentiation was extensive in this case, but a minor component of prostatic adenocarcinoma was identified.

Myofibroblastic Proliferations

KEY FACTS

TERMINOLOGY
- Different names have been used for identical, cytologically benign myofibroblastic proliferations
  - Pseudosarcomatous myofibroblastic proliferation
  - Inflammatory myofibroblastic tumor

CLINICAL ISSUES
- Rare
- 10% local recurrence rate; no metastases reported

MICROSCOPIC
- Loose fascicular architecture
- Individual cells tapered with elongated cytoplasmic processes
- Chromatin fine and evenly distributed
- Scattered nuclei enlarged with macronucleoli
- Invasion of muscularis propria does not denote malignancy
- Cellularity variable with loose and edematous, or myxoid stroma
- Mitotic activity may be brisk
- Admixed inflammatory cells present, including eosinophils and plasma cells
- Necrosis may be present

ANCILLARY TESTS
- Commonly coexpress smooth muscle actin and cytokeratin (low molecular weight forms)
- ALK1 expression by immunohistochemistry varies widely

TOP DIFFERENTIAL DIAGNOSES
- Rhabdomyosarcoma
  - Must be carefully considered in children
- Sarcomatoid carcinoma
  - Nuclear features important; coexistent carcinoma
- Leiomyosarcoma
  - May be difficult distinction
  - Nuclear hyperchromasia in sarcoma

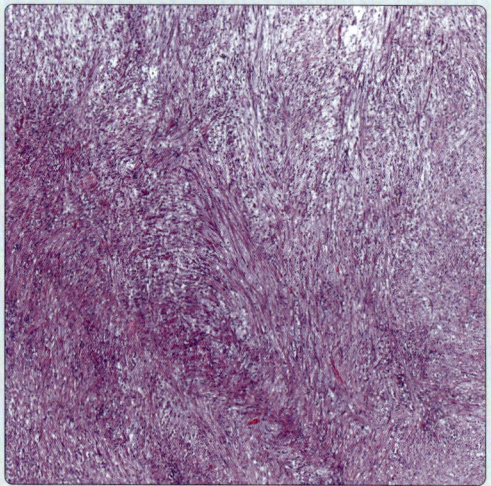

Myofibroblastic Proliferation: Cellular Spindle Cell Population

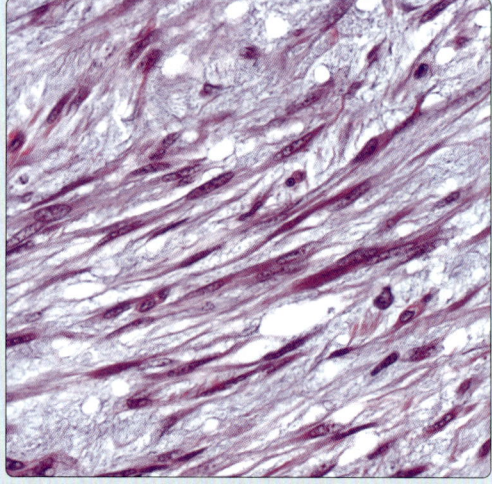

Myofibroblastic Proliferation: Tapered Cells and Myxoid Stroma

(Left) *Urinary bladder pseudosarcomatous myofibroblastic proliferations (inflammatory myofibroblastic tumors) are typically characterized by spindle cells with a loose fascicular architecture and variable cellularity, often with myxoid stroma.* (Right) *These cells are typical myofibroblasts with elongated tapered cytoplasmic processes, fine nuclear chromatin, and pinpoint nucleoli. Individual cells are commonly separated by myxoid stroma.*

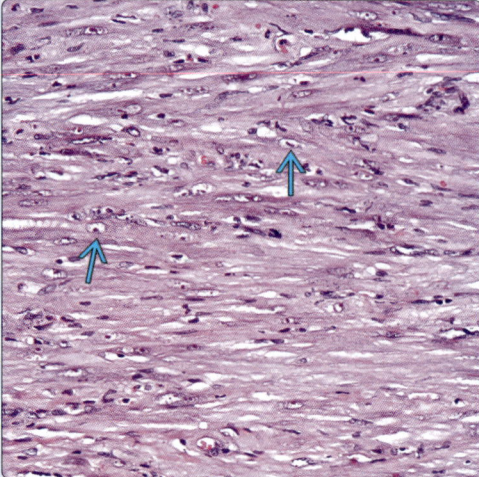

Myofibroblastic Proliferation: Prominent Nucleoli

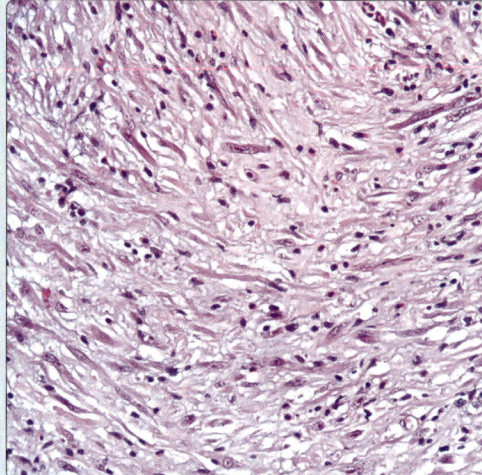

Myofibroblastic Proliferation: Admixed Inflammation

(Left) *The lesional cells composing myofibroblastic proliferations in the urinary bladder may have variability in nuclear size and shape, but the nuclear chromatin is relatively open. Nucleoli ➔ of varying sizes are also common.* (Right) *As in this example of a myofibroblastic proliferation in the urinary bladder, admixed inflammatory cells are relatively common. Cellularity and amount of stroma varies within and between lesions.*

Myofibroblastic Proliferations

TERMINOLOGY

Synonyms
- Pseudosarcomatous myofibroblastic proliferation
- Pseudosarcomatous fibromyxoid tumor
- Inflammatory myofibroblastic tumor (IMT)
- Postoperative spindle-cell nodule
- Inflammatory pseudotumor
  - Not recommended

Definitions
- Cytologically benign myofibroblastic proliferation of urinary bladder
- Different names have been used for identical lesions

ETIOLOGY/PATHOGENESIS

Infectious Agents
- No known inflammatory or infectious etiology

Associations
- May have history of trauma/prior instrumentation
  - Often referred to as "postoperative spindle-cell nodule"
- Some invasive urothelial carcinomas have an associated florid myofibroblastic proliferation
  - Invasive urothelial carcinoma with pseudosarcomatous stroma
- De novo lesions without predisposing factors also seen, but various names applied
  - Pseudosarcomatous myofibroblastic proliferation
  - Inflammatory myofibroblastic tumor (IMT)

Systemic Disease
- Evidence argues strongly against relationship with systemic IgG4 sclerosing disease

CLINICAL ISSUES

Epidemiology
- Incidence
  - Rare
- Age
  - Typically in 2nd to 4th decade
  - Also in children

Site
- Urinary bladder most common site in genitourinary tract

Presentation
- Gross hematuria, abdominal pain, irritative or obstructive voiding symptoms

Treatment
- Transurethral resection common
- Partial cystectomy for larger lesions

Prognosis
- 10% local recurrence rate
- No metastases reported
- Major risk is obstructive symptoms

MACROSCOPIC

General Features
- Polypoid or submucosal nodule
- Cut surface is often pale, firm, and gelatinous

Size
- 1.5-13 cm

MICROSCOPIC

Histologic Features
- Proliferation of spindle cells
  - Loose fascicular architecture
  - Elongated cytoplasmic processes
  - Chromatin fine and evenly distributed
  - Scattered nuclei enlarged with macronucleoli
  - Cellularity variable with edematous or myxoid stroma
  - Mitotic activity may be brisk, but not atypical mitoses
- Zonation common
  - Hypocellularity common superficially with higher cellularity deeper
- Granulation tissue-type vascularity
- Invasion of muscularis propria is not uncommon and does not denote malignancy
- Necrosis may be seen
- Admixed inflammatory cells often present

Predominant Cell/Compartment Type
- Myofibroblast

ANCILLARY TESTS

Immunohistochemistry
- Commonly express smooth muscle actin
- Cytokeratin immunoreactivity is very common
  - Low molecular weight forms
- Typically nonreactive for high molecular weight keratins
  - CK34βE12 and CK5/6
- ALK1 expression by immunohistochemistry varies widely in literature (8-89%)
  - Due to varying antibodies and staining conditions
- Desmin reactivity is variable
- Rare cases reported to have GATA3 expression
- No increase in IgG4 positive plasma cell ratio
- Typically negative for smoothelin
  - Unlike true smooth muscle tumors

In Situ Hybridization
- Subset shows *ALK* rearrangements by FISH
  - ~ 70% by current methods

DIFFERENTIAL DIAGNOSIS

Sarcomatoid Urothelial Carcinoma
- Myxoid and sclerosing pattern may closely mimic myofibroblastic process
- Nuclear pleomorphism and hyperchromasia is key feature of malignancy
- Heterologous elements may be seen
  - Chondrosarcoma
  - Osteosarcoma

Myofibroblastic Proliferations

- Rhabdomyosarcoma
- May have component of conventional urothelial carcinoma or history of urothelial carcinoma, papillary or flat in situ disease
    - More typical invasive urothelial carcinoma (or variant pattern)
        - May also have associated myofibroblasts
- Expression of p63, CK5/6, and HMCK(34βE12) in carcinoma is distinctive
- GATA3 nuclear staining may be retained
- Smooth muscle actin expression is not uncommon
    - Desmin expression unexpected, but may be seen with heterologous skeletal muscle differentiation

Leiomyosarcoma

- Morphologically heterogeneous
    - Cellular form with tight intersecting fascicles
        - More pronounced cytoplasmic eosinophilia
    - Myxoid pattern may closely mimic myofibroblastic process
- Nuclear pleomorphism and hyperchromasia
- Commonly express desmin and smooth muscle actin
    - Aberrant low molecular weight keratin expression also common; p63 and HMCK are negative

Rhabdomyosarcoma

- Embryonal subtype may be cytologically bland in some foci
    - Cambium layer (subepithelial condensation) is often present
    - More cellular foci with nuclear hyperchromasia
    - Scattered rhabdomyoblasts may be seen
- Must be carefully considered in children
    - Immunohistochemical confirmation important in small samples
        - Express cytoplasmic desmin and nuclear myogenin

Fibromyxoid Nephrogenic Adenoma

- Prominent myxoid or collagenized background stroma
- Scattered corded or spindled epithelial cells
    - Express typical markers of nephrogenic adenoma
        - Cytokeratin, pax-2, and pax-8
- Other concurrent patterns of nephrogenic adenoma often seen in adjacent tissue
    - Tubular, papillary, or cystic most common
- May be seen adjacent to carcinoma

Urothelial Carcinoma With Myxoid Stroma

- Prominent myxoid stroma
- Often has cord-like growth of epithelial cells
- Immunoprofile typical of urothelial carcinoma
    - p63, HMWCK, and GATA3 expression

Other Primary Sarcomas of Urinary Bladder

- Undifferentiated pleomorphic sarcoma
    - May have focal myxoid component
    - Nuclear pleomorphism and hyperchromasia are characteristic

Iatrogenic Soft Tissue Filler

- Soft tissue fillers may be used during stress incontinence procedures
- Localized accumulation may clinically present as mass lesion
- Prior urologic procedure often not given in history
- Different types of soft tissue fillers
    - Some have myxoid appearance by histology
        - Particularly polyacrylamide
    - May have histiocytic or associated giant cell reaction
    - Some may elicit granulomatous response

Neurofibroma

- Bland spindle cell proliferation
- Scattered degenerative-type nuclear atypia may be seen
- Express S100 protein and SOX10 by immunohistochemistry

DIAGNOSTIC CHECKLIST

Clinically Relevant Pathologic Features

- Nuclear features are key to distinguish myofibroblasts from a malignant process
    - Clinical management differences after pre and post resection

Pathologic Interpretation Pearls

- Close morphologic overlap between myofibroblasts and malignant spindle cell neoplasms
    - Some foci may be indistinguishable
    - Nuclear chromatin distinguishes myofibroblastic proliferations from malignancy
        - Malignant neoplasms have at least some foci with irregular, coarse nuclear chromatin
        - Chromatin is fine and evenly dispersed in myofibroblasts, but macronucleoli may be present
    - Deep invasion is not a sign of clinical malignancy
    - Myofibroblastic proliferations may be associated with urothelial carcinoma

SELECTED REFERENCES

1. Choi E et al: Inflammatory myofibroblastic tumor of the urinary bladder: the role of IgG4 and the comparison of two immunohistochemical antibodies and fluorescence in situ hybridization for the detection of ALK Alterations. Histopathology. 67(1):20-38, 2014
2. Teoh JY et al: Inflammatory myofibroblastic tumors of the urinary bladder: a systematic review. Urology. 84(3):503-8, 2014
3. Council L et al: Differential expression of immunohistochemical markers in bladder smooth muscle and myofibroblasts, and the potential utility of desmin, smoothelin, and vimentin in staging of bladder carcinoma. Mod Pathol. 22(5):639-50, 2009
4. Westfall DE et al: Utility of a comprehensive immunohistochemical panel in the differential diagnosis of spindle cell lesions of the urinary bladder. Am J Surg Pathol. 33(1):99-105, 2009
5. Christensen L: Normal and pathologic tissue reactions to soft tissue gel fillers. Dermatol Surg. 33 Suppl 2:S168-75, 2007
6. Sukov WR et al: Utility of ALK-1 protein expression and ALK rearrangements in distinguishing inflammatory myofibroblastic tumor from malignant spindle cell lesions of the urinary bladder. Mod Pathol. 20(5):592-603, 2007
7. Harik LR et al: Pseudosarcomatous myofibroblastic proliferations of the bladder: a clinicopathologic study of 42 cases. Am J Surg Pathol. 30(7):787-94, 2006
8. Montgomery EA et al: Inflammatory myofibroblastic tumors of the urinary tract: a clinicopathologic study of 46 cases, including a malignant example inflammatory fibrosarcoma and a subset associated with high-grade urothelial carcinoma. Am J Surg Pathol. 30(12):1502-12, 2006
9. Freeman A et al: Anaplastic lymphoma kinase (ALK 1) staining and molecular analysis in inflammatory myofibroblastic tumours of the bladder: a preliminary clinicopathological study of nine cases and review of the literature. Mod Pathol. 17(7):765-71, 2004
10. Tsuzuki T et al: ALK-1 expression in inflammatory myofibroblastic tumor of the urinary bladder. Am J Surg Pathol. 28(12):1609-14, 2004

Myofibroblastic Proliferations

Myofibroblastic Proliferation: Loose Fascicles

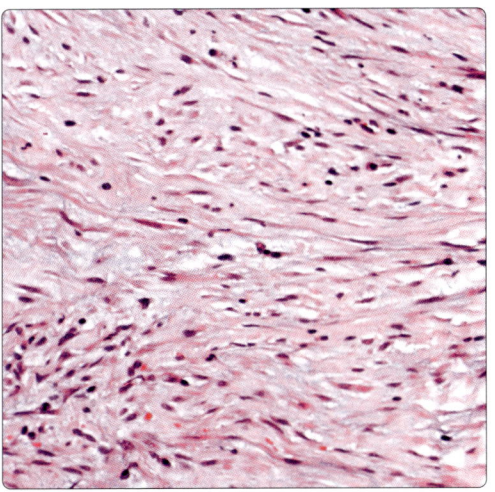

Myofibroblastic Proliferation: Tapered Cytoplasmic Processes

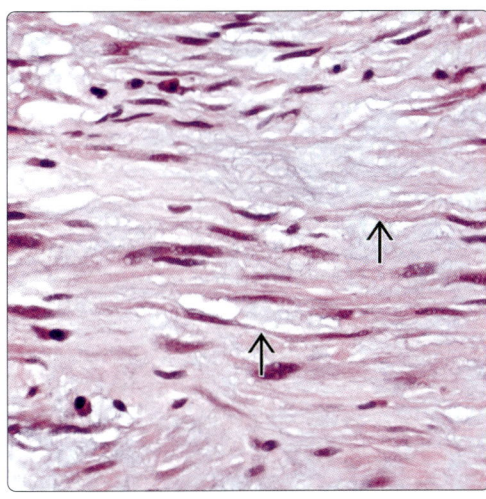

(Left) Spindled myofibroblasts, as seen in pseudosarcomatous myofibroblastic proliferation, are typically arranged into loose, poorly formed fascicles and are commonly associated with myxoid stroma. (Right) These typical myofibroblasts highlight the characteristic tapered nuclei and thin elongated cytoplasmic processes ➡. The fine nuclear chromatin distinguishes myofibroblasts from malignant lesions, such as leiomyosarcoma (LMS) and sarcomatoid carcinoma.

Myofibroblastic Proliferation: Prominent Myxoid Stroma and Epithelioid Cells

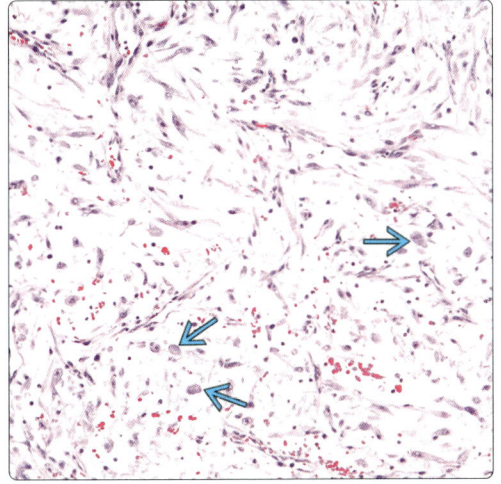

Myofibroblastic Proliferation: Myometrial Invasion

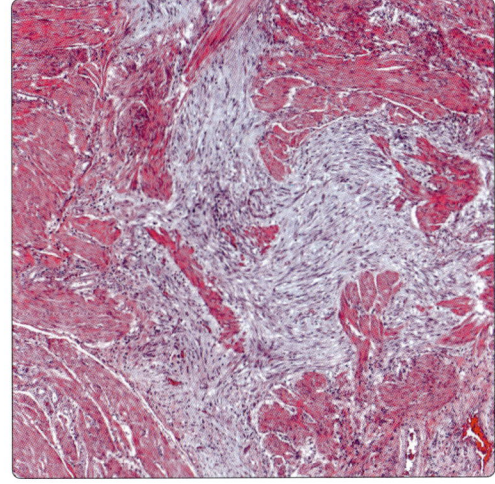

(Left) This myofibroblastic proliferation of the urinary bladder is associated with abundant myxoid stroma and contains some scattered neoplastic cells with a more epithelioid appearance ➡, another histologic feature that may be seen. (Right) Involvement of the muscularis propria by these florid myofibroblastic proliferations is common and may be extensive. This infiltrative growth does not denote malignancy.

Myofibroblastic Proliferation: Fine Nuclear Chromatin

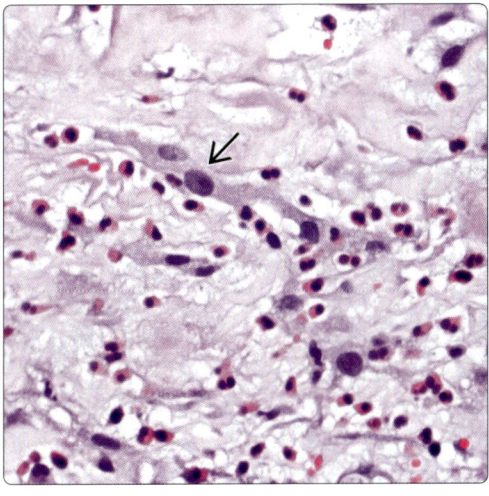

Myofibroblastic Proliferation: Cell Variation

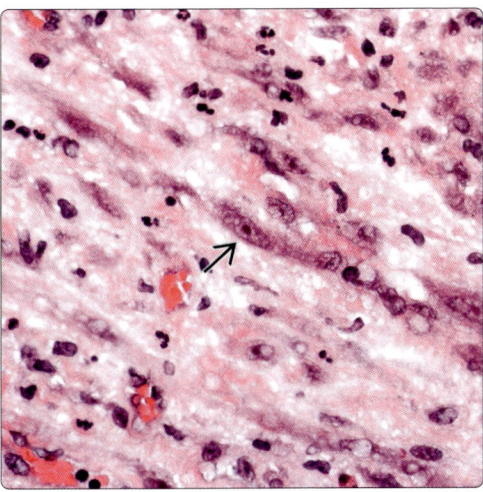

(Left) Myofibroblasts may show variation in nuclear size and may have prominent nucleoli ➡. Despite these features, the chromatin is fine and evenly dispersed. Malignant spindle cell lesions typically show coarse nuclear chromatin. (Right) This myofibroblastic proliferation shows the spectrum of nuclear size and shape that may be seen. This variation in cell size and the presence of prominent nucleoli ➡ are common and should not prompt a diagnosis of malignancy. Inflammatory cells and extravasated red cells are common.

Myofibroblastic Proliferations

Myofibroblastic Proliferation

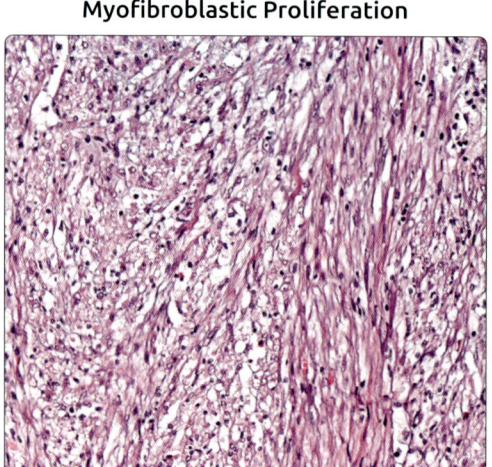

Myofibroblastic Proliferation

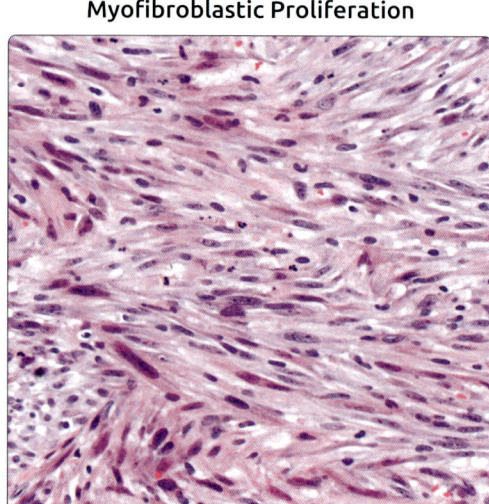

(Left) Some myofibroblastic proliferations are more cellular and eosinophilic, closely mimicking a smooth muscle neoplasm. This example arose 1 month following a transurethral biopsy (postoperative spindle cell nodule). (Right) This cellular myofibroblastic proliferation is arranged into a distinct fascicular architecture and has admixed inflammatory cells, a feature that is common. More cellular lesions may closely mimic a true smooth muscle tumor.

Actin: Myofibroblastic Proliferation

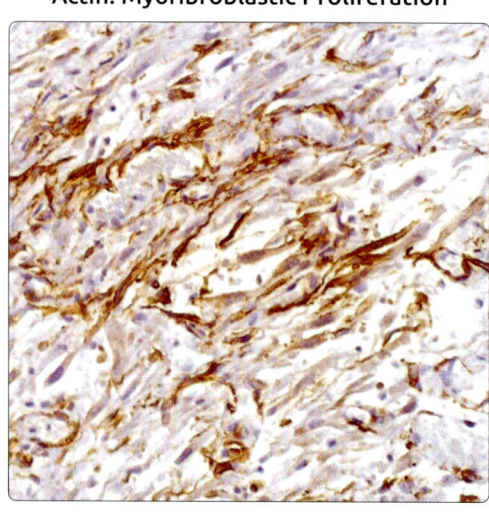

ALK1: Myofibroblastic Proliferation

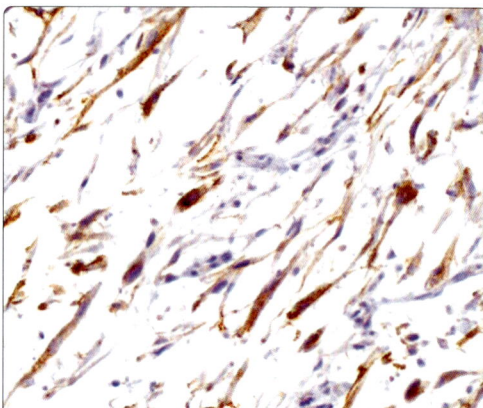

(Left) Diffuse immunoreactivity for smooth muscle actin is typical of myofibroblasts. Myofibroblasts do not commonly coexpress desmin, a distinguishing feature from smooth muscle. (Right) Strong cytoplasmic immunohistochemical staining with ALK1 may be seen in these myofibroblastic proliferations, but this finding varies widely in the literature. This feature has suggested a relationship to inflammatory myofibroblastic tumor.

Cytokeratin AE1/3: Myofibroblastic Proliferation

Cytokeratin CAM5.2: Myofibroblastic Proliferation

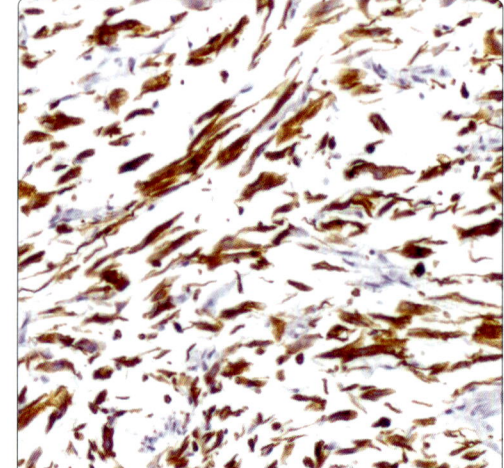

(Left) Cytoplasmic reactivity to CK AE1/3 may cause diagnostic confusion with sarcomatoid carcinoma, but low molecular weight CK staining is fairly common in these myofibroblastic proliferations. (Right) Keratin subtyping reveals that the myofibroblastic cells express only low molecular weight CK. In contrast, sarcomatoid carcinoma expresses HMCK as well as nuclear p63. Strong CK staining in the right context favors myofibroblastic proliferation.

Myofibroblastic Proliferations

Myofibroblastic Proliferation Associated With Urothelial Carcinoma

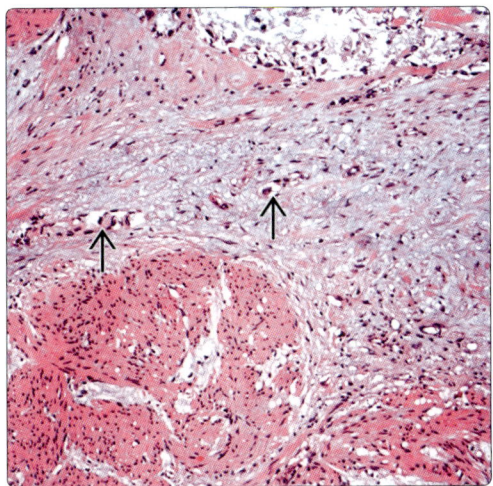

Myofibroblastic Proliferation Associated With Urothelial Carcinoma

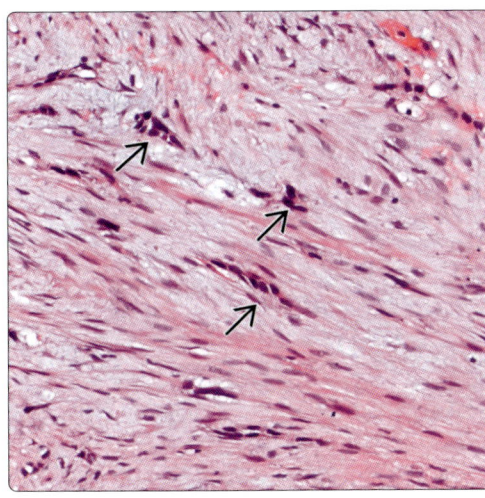

(Left) Invasive urothelial carcinoma ➡ may be associated with a florid myofibroblastic proliferation that may mimic a primary myofibroblastic process. (Right) This example has a florid myofibroblastic proliferation that is associated with scant, subtle aggregates of invasive carcinoma ➡. The individual myofibroblasts are identical to those seen in other myofibroblastic lesions. It is important to exclude the possibility of a morphologically subtle carcinoma in this setting.

Myofibroblastic Proliferation Associated With Urothelial Carcinoma

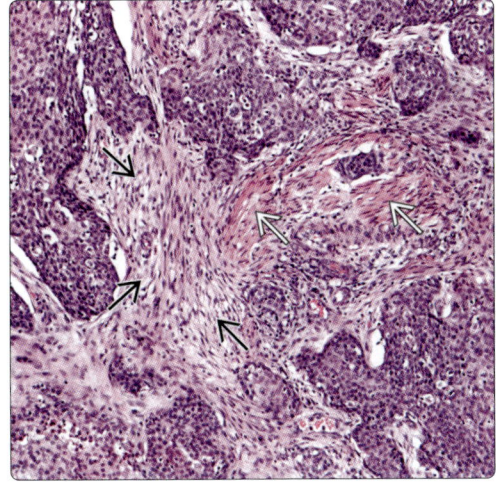

Myofibroblastic Proliferation Associated With Urothelial Carcinoma

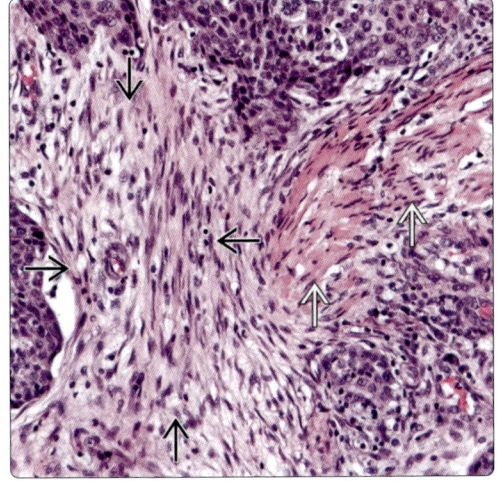

(Left) This invasive urothelial carcinoma involves the muscularis propria ➡ and is also associated with a myofibroblastic proliferation ➡. (Right) The myofibroblastic proliferation ➡ that is associated with carcinoma has less eosinophilic cytoplasm than the adjacent smooth muscle of the muscularis propria ➡. The myofibroblasts are cytologically bland, which aids in distinction from sarcomatoid carcinoma.

Myofibroblastic Proliferation Associated With Urothelial Carcinoma

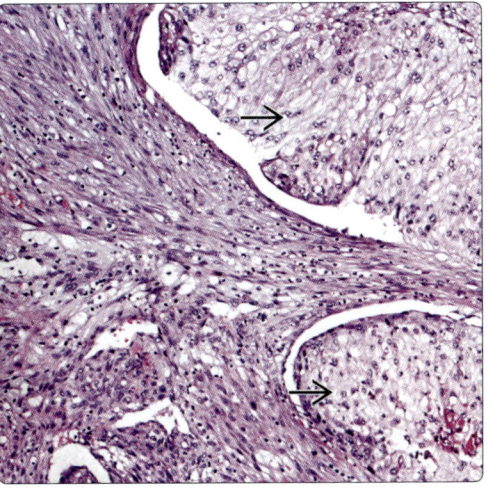

Myofibroblastic Proliferation Associated With Urothelial Carcinoma

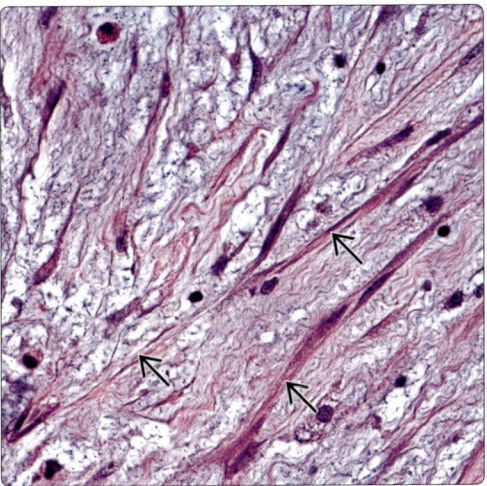

(Left) Invasive urothelial carcinoma with associated "pseudosarcomatous" stroma may suggest sarcomatoid carcinoma when the carcinomatous component ➡ is prominent. These myofibroblasts are associated with an inflammatory infiltrate similar to primary myofibroblastic proliferations. (Right) On high-power examination, these spindle cells that were associated with carcinoma in other fields show the long cytoplasmic processes ➡ and fine nuclear chromatin, typical of myofibroblasts.

Myofibroblastic Proliferations

Leiomyosarcoma

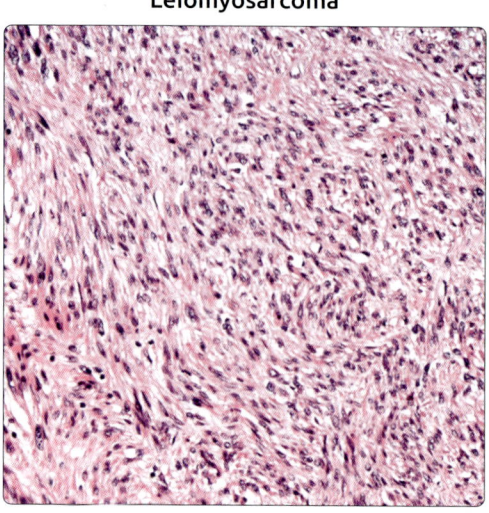

(Left) True smooth muscle tumors of the urinary bladder, as in this example of LMS, typically have more eosinophilic cytoplasm compared to myofibroblasts and have more cellular and better developed fascicular growth. (Right) The degree of cytologic atypia in this smooth muscle tumor, which was desmin and smooth muscle actin positive, is diagnostic of malignancy (i.e., LMS).

Leiomyosarcoma

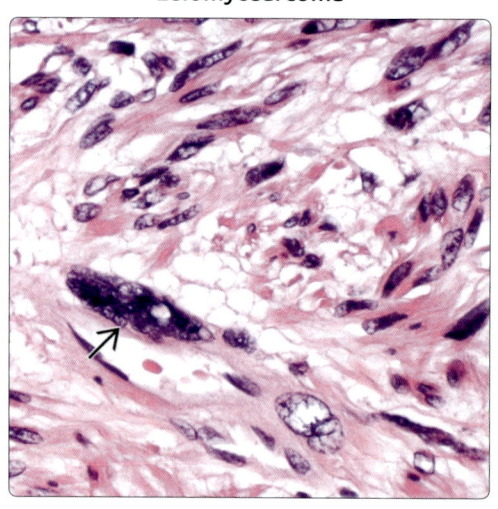
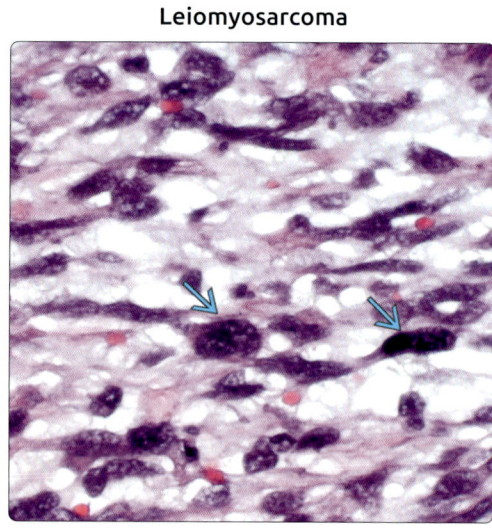

(Left) This example of LMS shows individual neoplastic cells with marked nuclear pleomorphism and nuclear hyperchromasia ⇒, features that are most useful in the distinction from myofibroblasts. (Right) The degree of nuclear hyperchromasia/irregular clumped chromatin ⇒ in this sarcomatoid urothelial carcinoma is diagnostic of malignancy and should exclude the diagnosis of a benign myofibroblastic process.

Leiomyosarcoma **Myxoid Leiomyosarcoma**

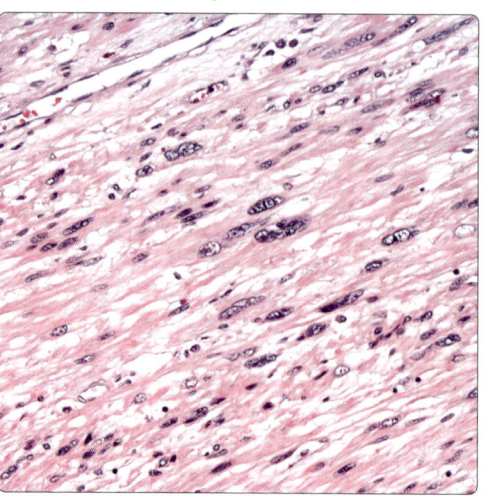
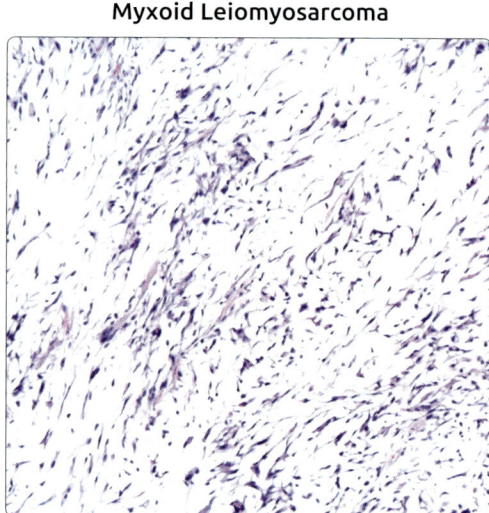

(Left) The degree of pleomorphism and hyperchromasia in this LMS is beyond what is acceptable in a myofibroblastic proliferation of the bladder. (Right) LMS in the bladder may be associated with myxoid stroma. In more monomorphic regions, this may cause diagnostic confusion with myofibroblasts. Careful evaluation of nuclear cytology is critical. CK is typically negative and only rarely focally positive. Desmin is more commonly expressed in LMS over myofibroblastic proliferations.

Myofibroblastic Proliferations

Rhabdomyosarcoma
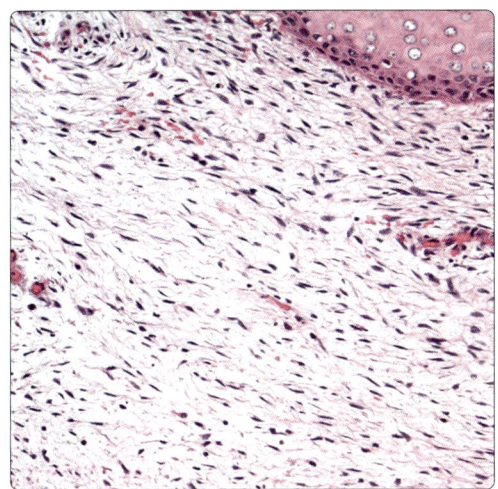

Rhabdomyosarcoma
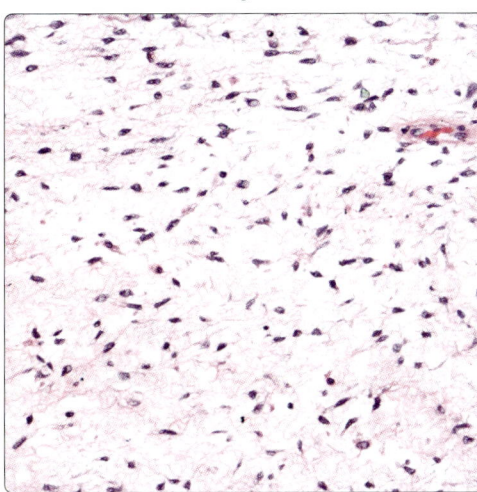

(Left) Particularly in children, the possibility of rhabdomyosarcoma should be considered when faced with a spindle cell proliferation. Some foci in embryonal rhabdomyosarcoma may be deceptively bland. (Right) On high-power magnification, there is a subtle degree of nuclear hyperchromasia; however, in some hypocellular foci, morphologic overlap with myofibroblasts may be striking. Myogenin immunostains can be useful in this setting.

Sarcomatoid Urothelial Carcinoma
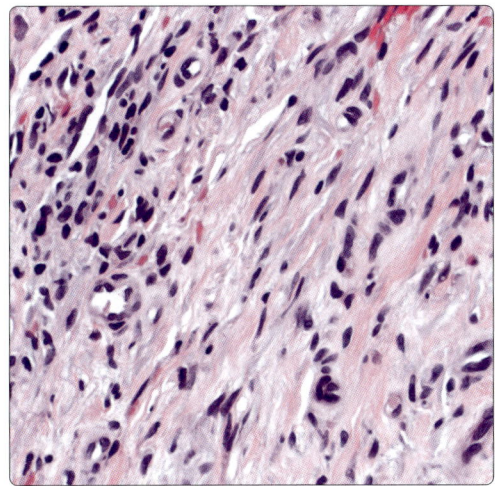

Sarcomatoid Urothelial Carcinoma
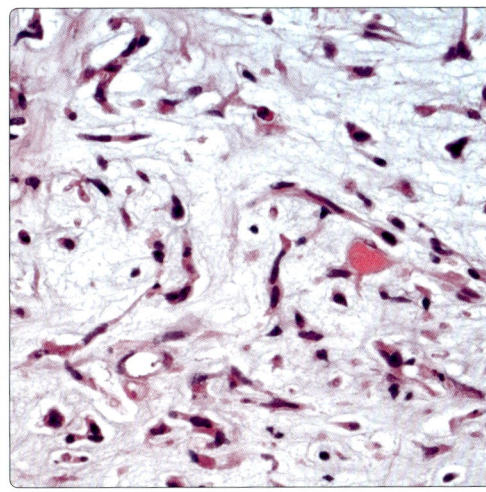

(Left) Focal areas in malignant tumors may have significant overlap with pseudosarcomatous myofibroblastic proliferation. This example of sarcomatoid urothelial carcinoma had more striking nuclear atypia in other areas of the tumor. (Right) Sarcomatoid urothelial carcinoma may also be associated with myxoid stroma. This morphologic pattern may very closely mimic a myofibroblastic proliferation. More conventional areas with definitive malignant cytology should be sought.

Fibromyxoid Nephrogenic Adenoma
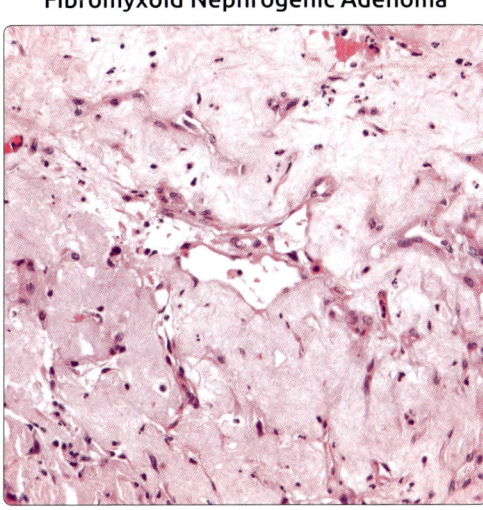

Soft Tissue Filler
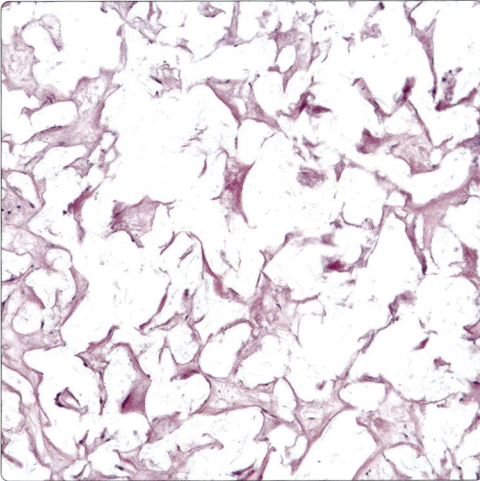

(Left) Rare nephrogenic adenomas are associated with myxoid or collagenized stroma that may mimic a mesenchymal lesion. Identification of classic patterns of nephrogenic adenoma or cytokeratin &/or pax-8 immunoreactivity may aid in recognition. (Right) With surgeries for urinary incontinence utilizing soft tissue fillers, unusual patterns of myxoid/mucinous and collagenized appearing material may cause diagnostic consideration of a myxoid neoplasm if presenting as a mass lesion.

Smooth Muscle Tumors

KEY FACTS

CLINICAL ISSUES
- Leiomyosarcoma is rare but most common primary vesical sarcoma
- Complete excision is curative for leiomyoma
- Leiomyosarcoma has high recurrent and metastatic rate

MICROSCOPIC
- Leiomyoma
  - Interlacing fascicles of spindle cells with prominent eosinophilic cytoplasm
  - Low cellularity is typical
  - No nuclear pleomorphism and fine nuclear chromatin
- Leiomyosarcoma
  - Fascicles of spindle cells with variable eosinophilic cytoplasm
  - Scattered pleomorphic, hyperchromatic cells are common
  - Rarely, marked nuclear anaplasia is seen
  - Mitotic figures are usually easily identified

ANCILLARY TESTS
- Express smooth muscle actin, caldesmon, and desmin
- Focal expression of cytokeratin may be seen
  - Typically low molecular weight forms
- No expression of skeletal muscle markers

TOP DIFFERENTIAL DIAGNOSES
- Sarcomatoid urothelial carcinoma
  - Must be excluded before accepting primary vesical sarcoma diagnosis
- Pseudosarcomatous myofibroblastic proliferation (inflammatory myofibroblastic tumor)
- Perivascular epithelioid cell neoplasm (PEComa)

DIAGNOSTIC CHECKLIST
- Nuclear cytology is key feature in distinguishing leiomyosarcoma from benign mimics

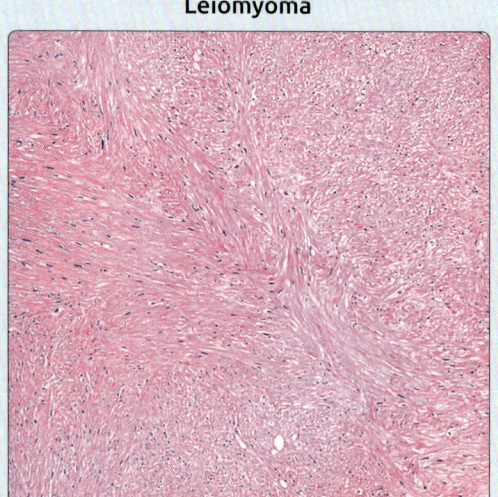
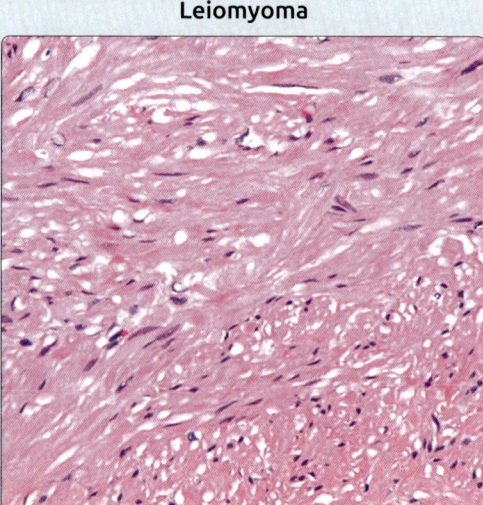

Leiomyoma (Left) Benign leiomyomas are characterized by well-developed fascicles of cytologically bland spindle cells with prominent eosinophilic cytoplasm. These histologic features are reminiscent of normal smooth muscle. **(Right)** The neoplastic cells of leiomyomas have abundant eosinophilic cytoplasm, an elongated spindled morphology, and bland cytologic features, as seen in this example.

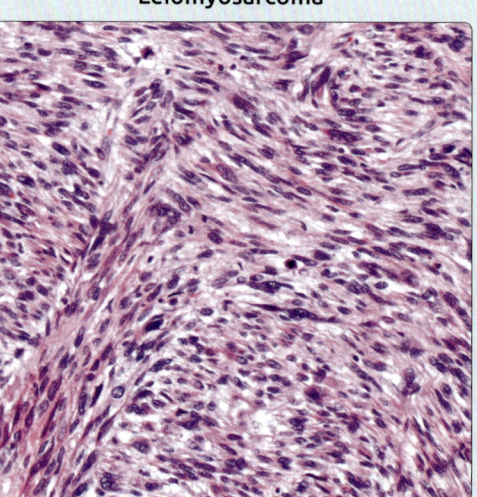
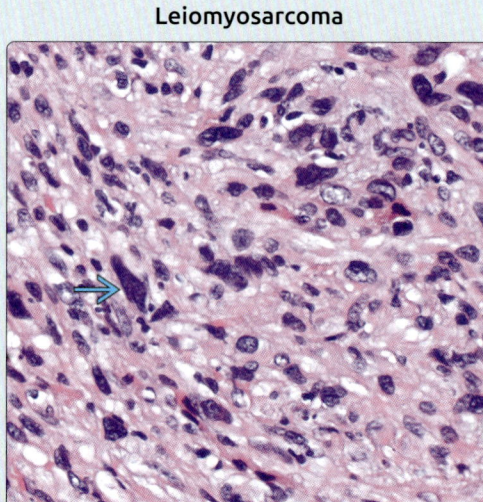

Leiomyosarcoma (Left) Intersecting fascicular growth and variable eosinophilic cytoplasm are characteristic of smooth muscle tumors. Tumors with this cellularity should be carefully examined for features of leiomyosarcoma. **(Right)** Scattered neoplastic cells with nucleomegaly and nuclear hyperchromasia are typically found in leiomyosarcoma ➡. This degree of atypia would not be seen in leiomyoma or pseudosarcomatous myofibroblastic proliferation (inflammatory myofibroblastic tumor).

Smooth Muscle Tumors

TERMINOLOGY

Definitions
- Leiomyoma
  - Benign mesenchymal neoplasm showing smooth muscle differentiation
- Leiomyosarcoma
  - Morphologically and clinically malignant mesenchymal neoplasm with smooth muscle differentiation

ETIOLOGY/PATHOGENESIS

Iatrogenic
- History of chemotherapy reported in some cases of leiomyosarcoma

CLINICAL ISSUES

Epidemiology
- Incidence
  - Leiomyoma is most common benign mesenchymal neoplasm of bladder
  - Leiomyosarcoma is rare but most common primary vesical sarcoma in adults
    - < 1% of all bladder malignancies
- Age
  - Wide range for both leiomyoma and leiomyosarcoma
- Sex
  - Female predilection for leiomyoma
  - Male predominance in leiomyosarcoma (M:F = 2:1)

Presentation
- Urinary symptoms
  - Obstruction
  - Irritative symptoms
  - Hematuria

Treatment
- Leiomyoma
  - Transurethral resection or open resection
- Leiomyosarcoma
  - Radical surgical resection

Prognosis
- Leiomyoma
  - Complete excision is curative
- Leiomyosarcoma
  - High recurrence/metastatic rate (~ 70%)

MACROSCOPIC

Leiomyoma
- Typically small, circumscribed mass lesion within bladder wall
- Mean size: < 2 cm
- Rare leiomyomas up to 25 cm are reported
- Usually lack necrosis
  - Infarction may be present in large tumors

Leiomyosarcoma
- Typically large, solid, infiltrating intramural mass
- Mean size: 7 cm
- Foci of geographic necrosis are common

MICROSCOPIC

Histologic Features
- Leiomyoma
  - Interlacing fascicles of spindle cells with prominent eosinophilic cytoplasm
    - Lacks compact round bundles of smooth muscle typical of normal muscularis propria
  - Low cellularity and circumscription is typical
  - No nuclear pleomorphism and fine nuclear chromatin
  - Mitotic figures are rare or absent
  - No areas of coagulative tumor cell necrosis
- Leiomyosarcoma
  - Interlacing fascicles of spindle cells with prominent eosinophilic cytoplasm
  - Wide range of cytologic atypia, infiltrative growth pattern
    - Scattered pleomorphic, hyperchromatic cells are common
    - Rarely, marked nuclear anaplasia is seen
  - Coagulative tumor cell necrosis may be present
  - Mitotic figures are usually easily identified
  - Myxoid stroma may be dominant feature in subset of cases
  - Rare cases have epithelioid morphology
- Atypical (symplastic) leiomyoma
  - Rare descriptions of smooth muscle neoplasms with scattered cytologic atypia, but no mitotic activity and no necrosis
  - Controversial diagnostic entity in bladder
    - No long-term clinical outcome studies

Leiomyosarcoma Grading Scheme
- Low grade
  - Mitoses < 5 per 10 HPF
  - Usually mild to moderate cytologic atypia
- High grade
  - Mitoses > 5 per 10 HPF
  - Marked nuclear pleomorphism and hyperchromasia
  - Necrosis common

ANCILLARY TESTS

Immunohistochemistry
- Diffuse cytoplasmic reactivity for muscle markers
  - Smooth muscle actin
  - Caldesmon
  - Desmin
- Stronger staining more common in leiomyoma
- Focal expression of cytokeratin may be seen
  - Typically found with low molecular weight subtypes
- ALK1, p63, or HMCK(34βE12) are typically negative
- No expression of skeletal muscle markers
  - Myogenin
  - MYOD1

DIFFERENTIAL DIAGNOSIS

Sarcomatoid Urothelial Carcinoma
- Should be excluded for any malignant spindle cell neoplasm in bladder

Smooth Muscle Tumors

- Spindled component may be histologically indistinguishable from leiomyosarcoma
- Some features add strong diagnostic support without immunohistochemistry
  - Associated papillary, in situ, or invasive urothelial carcinoma
  - Prior history of urothelial carcinoma at same site
- Immunoreactivity for epithelial markers
  - p63
  - HMCK(34βE12)
  - Subset may retain nuclear GATA3 expression
- May have heterologous differentiation
  - Skeletal muscle and cartilage most common
  - Osteosarcoma may also be seen
- Diagnostic pitfall
  - May express smooth muscle markers

Pseudosarcomatous Myofibroblastic Proliferation (Inflammatory Myofibroblastic Tumor)

- Distinguished from leiomyosarcoma by cytologic features
  - Enlarged nuclei with nucleoli and fine nuclear chromatin
- Myxoid stroma and granulation tissue type vascularity are common
- Commonly express smooth muscle actin, but desmin staining is variable
- ALK1 immunoreactivity is identified in subset of cases
- Diagnostic pitfall
  - May be associated with invasive urothelial carcinoma

Benign Nerve Sheath Tumor

- Cellular fascicular areas may closely mimic smooth muscle in some cases
- May have degenerative atypia (ancient change) that mimics malignancy
- Diffuse cytoplasmic and nuclear immunoreactivity for S100 protein is diagnostic
- Also express SOX10
- Does not express smooth muscle markers

Perivascular Epithelioid Cell Neoplasm (PEComa)

- May closely mimic smooth muscle neoplasia
  - Fascicular growth with eosinophilic cytoplasm
  - Less commonly epithelioid
- May be more nested
- Cytoplasmic clearing common
- Neoplastic cells are frequently associated with walls of intratumoral blood vessels
- Commonly expresses smooth muscle actin, less commonly desmin
- Expresses melanocytic markers
  - HMB45, melan-A, cathepsin-K
- Rare subset have TFE3 fusion

Solitary Fibrous Tumor

- Some examples previously called hemangiopericytoma in literature
- No pronounced cytoplasmic eosinophilia
- Generally less organized into fascicles
- Often more collagenized stroma or, less commonly, myxoid
- Associated hemangiopericytic blood vessels common
- Express CD34
- Characterized by *NAB2-STAT6* fusion
  - Nuclear *STAT6* expression by immunohistochemistry may be used as surrogate for diagnosis

Rhabdomyosarcoma

- More common in children
- Typically not as uniformly eosinophilic-appearing
- Some examples could mimic leiomyosarcoma with myxoid stroma or cellular fascicles
- Nuclear myogenin expression is diagnostic

Gastrointestinal Stromal Tumor (Secondary Involvement)

- May involve peritoneal surface over bladder
- Histologically mimics smooth muscle tumors
  - May be spindle cell or epithelioid
- Express c-kit (CD117) and DOG1

Other High-Grade Sarcomas (Rarely Described)

- Angiosarcoma
  - Commonly vasoformative
  - Pure epithelioid angiosarcomas do occur
  - Express endothelial markers
    - CD31 and CD34
    - ERG (nuclear)
- Undifferentiated pleomorphic sarcoma
  - No histologic or immunophenotypic evidence of specific line of differentiation
  - Absence of smooth muscle differentiation
- Liposarcoma
  - Dedifferentiated liposarcoma mimics other high-grade sarcomas
  - Has MDM2 amplification by FISH

DIAGNOSTIC CHECKLIST

Pathologic Interpretation Pearls

- Nuclear cytology is key feature in distinguishing leiomyosarcoma from benign mimics
- Primary vesical sarcoma is diagnosis of exclusion
  - For high-grade tumors, immunohistochemistry is commonly required to exclude sarcomatoid urothelial carcinoma

SELECTED REFERENCES

1. Rodríguez D et al: Clinical features of leiomyosarcoma of the urinary bladder: analysis of 183 cases. Urol Oncol. 32(7):958-65, 2014
2. Lee TK et al: Smooth muscle neoplasms of the urinary bladder: a clinicopathologic study of 51 cases. Am J Surg Pathol. 34(4):502-9, 2010
3. Lindberg MR et al: Leiomyosarcoma of the urinary bladder: a clinicopathological study of 34 cases. J Clin Pathol. 63(8):708-13, 2010
4. Westfall DE et al: Utility of a comprehensive immunohistochemical panel in the differential diagnosis of spindle cell lesions of the urinary bladder. Am J Surg Pathol. 33(1):99-105, 2009
5. Martin SA et al: Smooth muscle neoplasms of the urinary bladder: a clinicopathologic comparison of leiomyoma and leiomyosarcoma. Am J Surg Pathol. 26(3):292-300, 2002
6. Goluboff ET et al: Leiomyoma of bladder: report of case and review of literature. Urology. 43(2):238-41, 1994
7. Mills SE et al: Leiomyosarcoma of the urinary bladder. A clinicopathologic and immunohistochemical study of 15 cases. Am J Surg Pathol. 13(6):480-9, 1989

Smooth Muscle Tumors

Leiomyoma
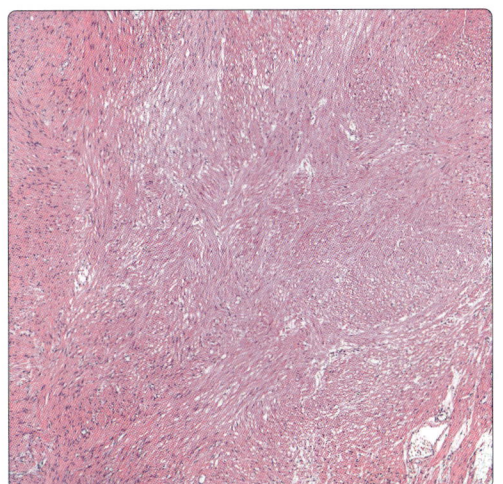

Leiomyoma
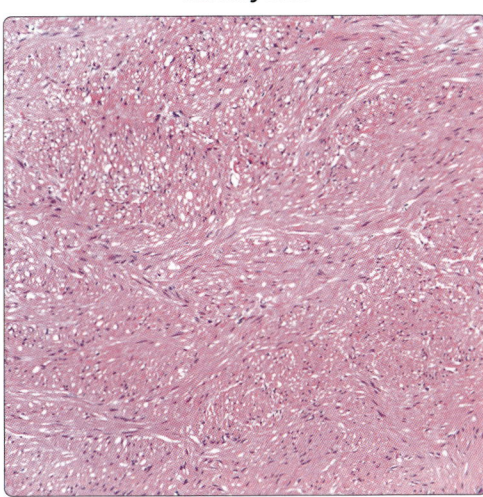

(Left) At low-power magnification, the well-developed fascicular architecture and the prominent cytoplasmic eosinophilia are characteristic features of leiomyoma. (Right) In this bladder leiomyoma, the neoplastic cells are evenly spaced and the nuclei are cytologically bland with fine chromatin and no pleomorphism. These features are similar to the more common uterine leiomyomas.

Leiomyoma
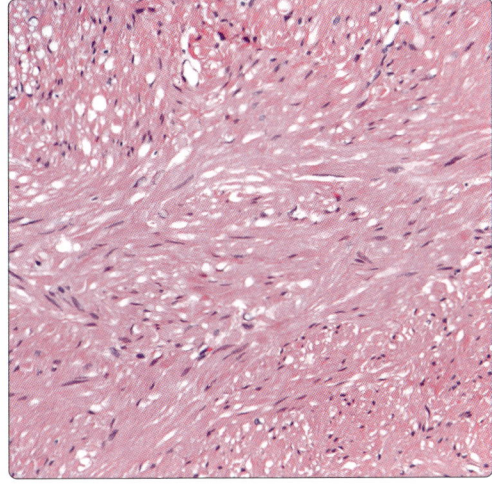

Leiomyoma
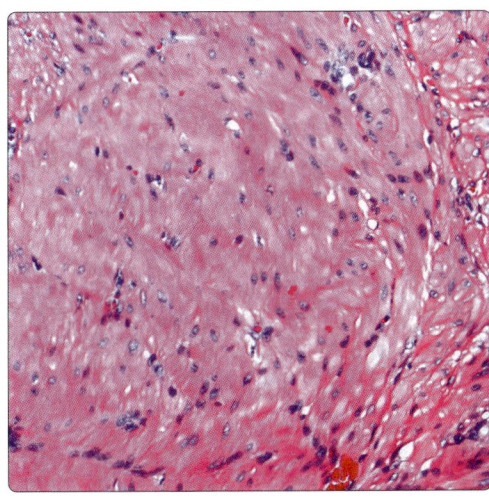

(Left) On high-power magnification, the absence of significant cytologic atypia or mitotic activity in leiomyomas may be appreciated. (Right) The small, monotonous smooth muscle cells in this leiomyoma have a very bland cytology with fine nuclear chromatin. The tumor is very hypocellular, a feature typical of benign leiomyomas. The cytologic features in smooth muscle tumors are the key in distinguishing benign from malignant tumors.

Leiomyosarcoma
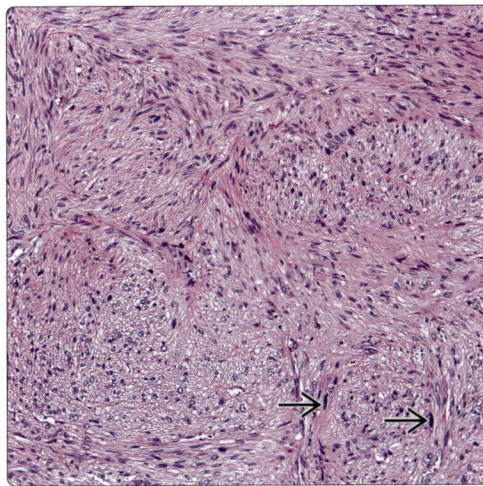

Leiomyosarcoma
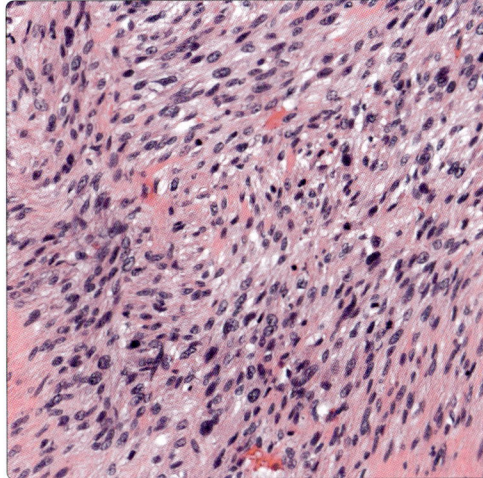

(Left) In contrast to leiomyoma, this leiomyosarcoma has scattered hyperchromatic cells ➡ visible at low-power magnification. Such findings should prompt careful consideration of malignancy. (Right) Leiomyosarcomas have a wide spectrum of atypia. This example does not show significant nuclear pleomorphism, but there is nuclear membrane irregularity and clumped chromatin imparting a hyperchromatic appearance.

Smooth Muscle Tumors

(Left) This spindle cell neoplasm had evidence of smooth muscle differentiation by immunohistochemistry (diffuse desmin reactivity). The variation in nuclear size, nuclear hyperchromasia ➔, and mitotic activity ➔ all support a diagnosis of leiomyosarcoma. (Right) This degree of nuclear pleomorphism ➔ and hyperchromasia is diagnostic of malignancy and supports a diagnosis of leiomyosarcoma if sarcomatoid urothelial carcinoma is excluded.

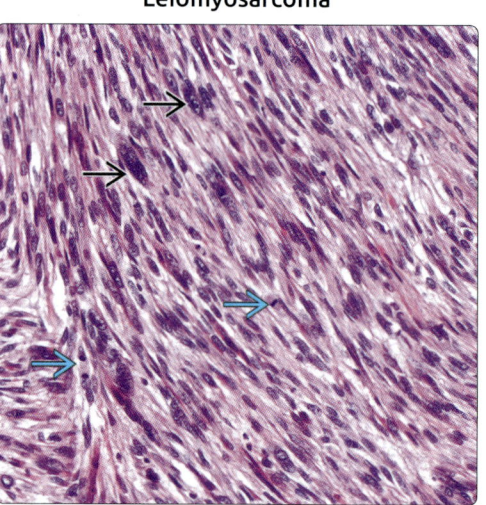
Leiomyosarcoma

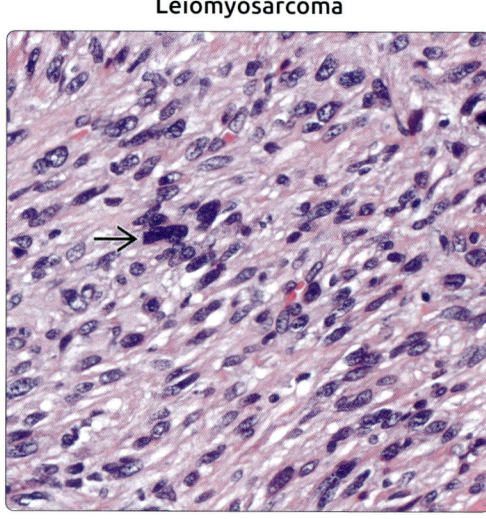
Leiomyosarcoma

(Left) This leiomyosarcoma contains scattered cells with obvious nuclear pleomorphism. Most of these tumors have easily identifiable mitotic figures at higher power examination. (Right) The clumped, irregular nuclear chromatin of leiomyosarcoma ➔ is a key feature in the morphologic distinction of leiomyosarcomas from pseudosarcomatous myofibroblastic proliferations (inflammatory myofibroblastic tumors).

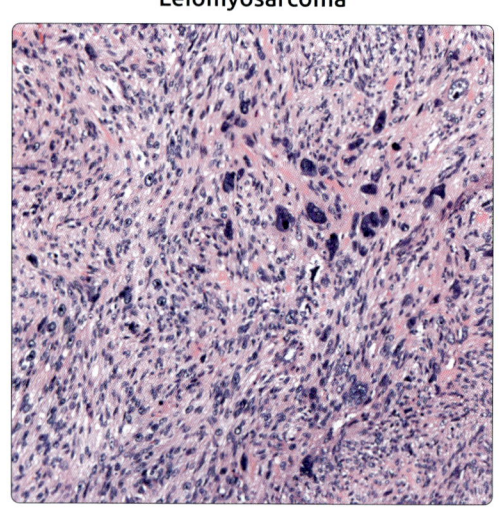
Leiomyosarcoma

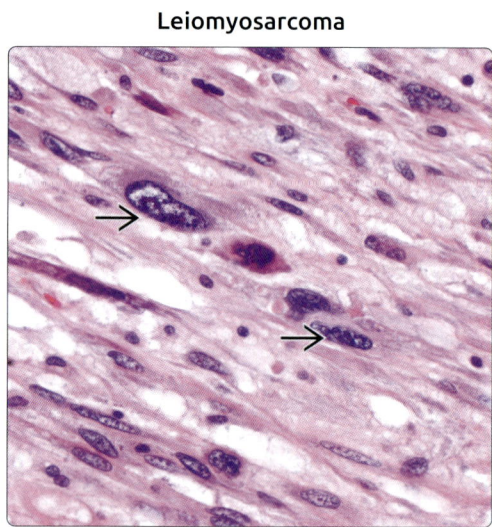
Leiomyosarcoma

(Left) On high-power magnification, the neoplastic cells of this leiomyosarcoma show nucleomegaly and nuclear hyperchromasia ➔. (Right) Immunohistochemistry is very useful in establishing the lineage of spindle cell neoplasms in the urinary bladder. Diffuse cytoplasmic desmin reactivity, as seen here, is strong evidence for a smooth muscle phenotype. It should be remembered that smooth muscle tumors may have aberrant cytokeratin expression, but this is typically seen only with low molecular weight keratins.

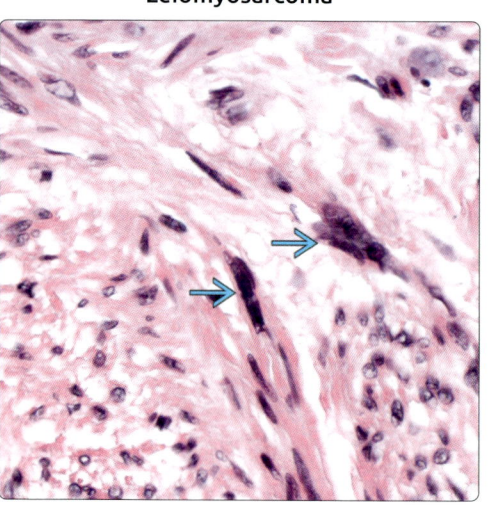
Leiomyosarcoma

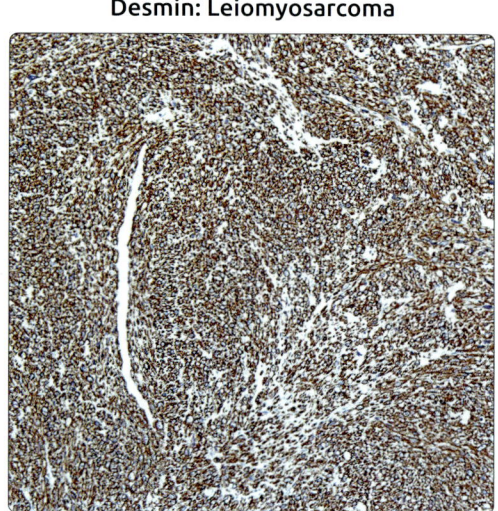
Desmin: Leiomyosarcoma

Smooth Muscle Tumors

Sarcomatoid Carcinoma
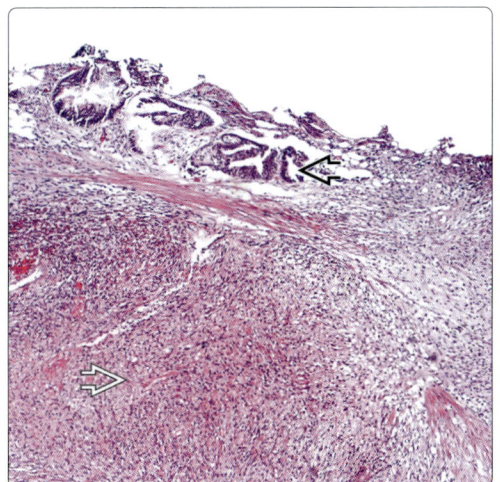

Sarcomatoid Carcinoma
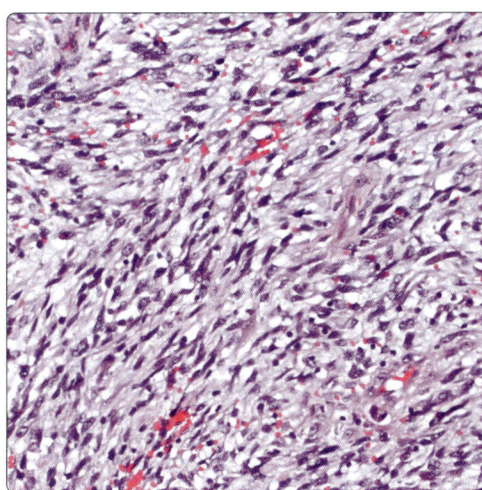

(Left) This biphasic sarcomatoid carcinoma has an adenocarcinoma component ⇨ adjacent to the malignant spindle cell component ⇨. This biphasic morphology is diagnostic of sarcomatoid carcinoma. (Right) This myxoid and sclerosing sarcomatoid carcinoma mimics a leiomyosarcoma or pseudosarcomatous myofibroblastic proliferation. The cellularity and nuclear hyperchromasia are diagnostic of malignancy, but a smooth muscle lineage should be excluded by immunohistochemistry.

Sarcomatoid Carcinoma
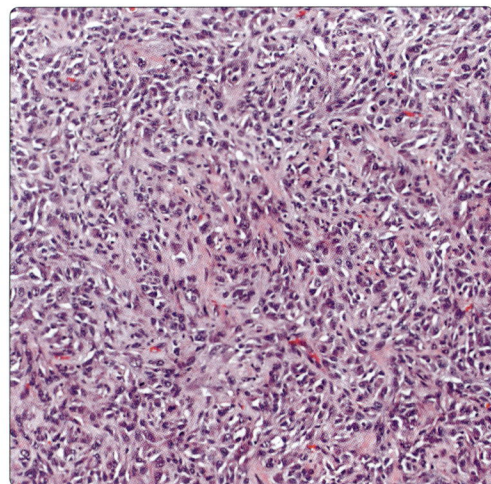

Sarcomatoid Carcinoma
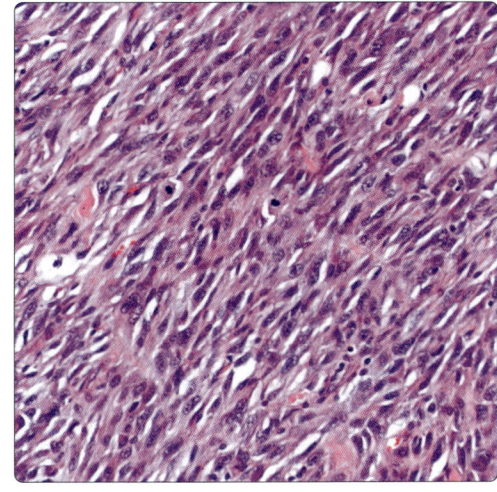

(Left) A mixed spindled and epithelioid appearance should suggest the possibility of a sarcomatoid urothelial carcinoma. If a typical component of in situ, papillary, or invasive urothelial carcinoma is not present, then immunohistochemistry is typically required. History of prior urothelial carcinoma in the bladder is usually sufficient evidence for a carcinoma diagnosis. (Right) Pure spindled sarcomatoid carcinomas may closely mimic a primary vesical sarcoma, such as leiomyosarcoma.

p63: Sarcomatoid Carcinoma
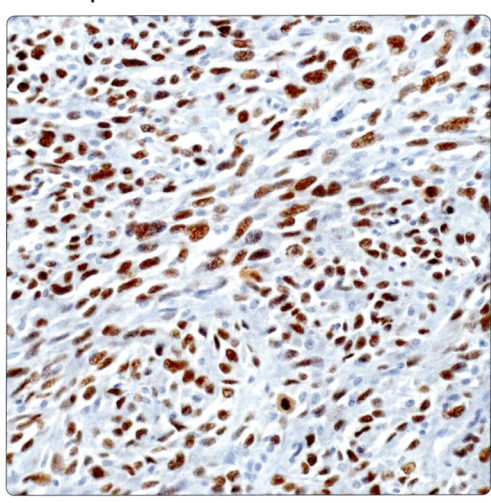

HMWCK: Sarcomatoid Carcinoma
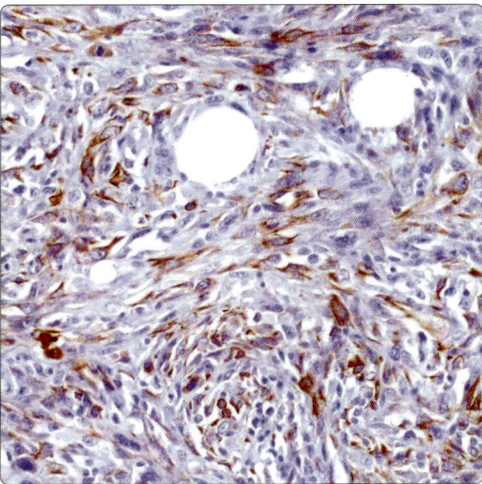

(Left) Nuclear p63 immunoreactivity provides strong evidence of an epithelial origin and is maintained in the spindle cell components. (Right) Cytoplasmic reactivity for HMWCK(34βE12) is a feature of epithelial lineage. Keratin expression in smooth muscle cells and myofibroblasts is typically only found with low molecular weight cytokeratins. Due to the marked overlap in morphology and immunohistochemistry, a broad panel of markers is necessary.

Smooth Muscle Tumors

(Left) Invasion of muscularis propria ⇨ is common in pseudosarcomatous myofibroblastic proliferations. This finding should not be regarded as a feature of malignancy. **(Right)** This pseudosarcomatous myofibroblastic proliferation (inflammatory myofibroblastic tumor) has a fascicular growth pattern that closely resembles a smooth muscle tumor. Cytologic features are most important in the distinction from a malignant tumor.

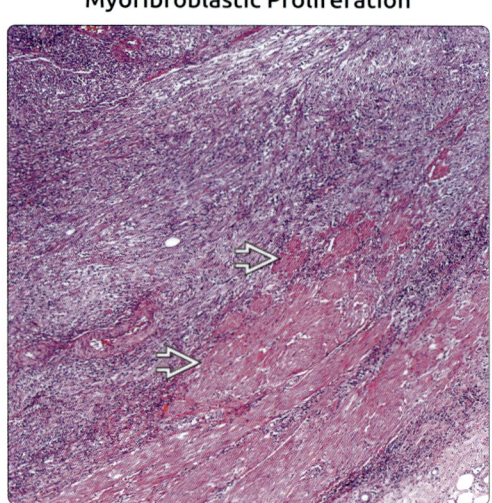

Myofibroblastic Proliferation | Myofibroblastic Proliferation

(Left) Myofibroblastic proliferations of the urinary bladder often have an associated myxoid stroma. These changes may mimic a myxoid leiomyosarcoma, but the nuclear cytology is distinct in myofibroblasts with an absence of nuclear hyperchromasia. **(Right)** Cytoplasmic ALK1 reactivity is seen in a subset of pseudosarcomatous myofibroblastic proliferations, but it is not typically seen in sarcomatoid carcinoma or leiomyosarcoma.

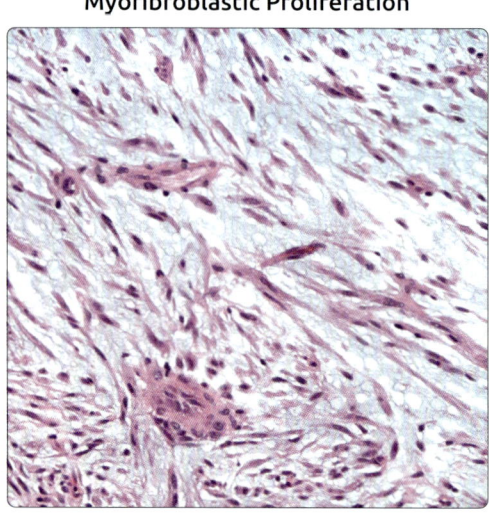
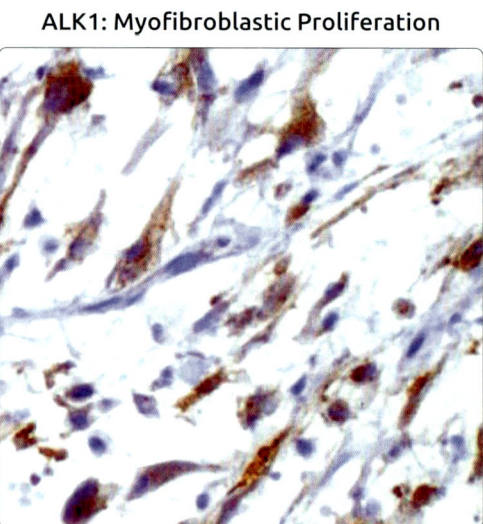

Myofibroblastic Proliferation | ALK1: Myofibroblastic Proliferation

(Left) Solitary fibrous tumor (some examples of which were previously called hemangiopericytoma) has less organization without well-developed fascicles. The stroma may be myxoid or collagenized. **(Right)** Solitary fibrous tumors harbor a distinct recurring fusion involving NAB2 and STAT6. Nuclear expression of STAT6 by immunohistochemistry is a very specific surrogate for the fusion and may be used to confirm the diagnosis.

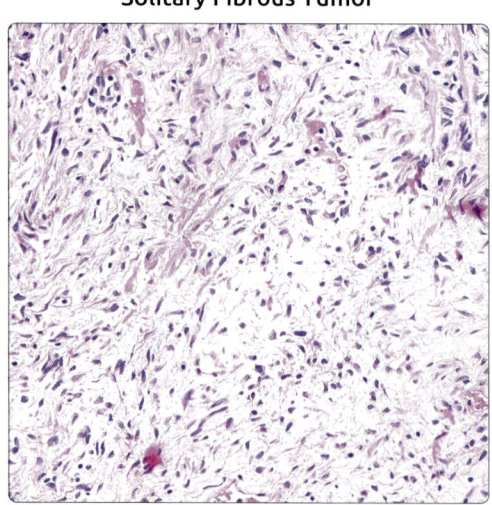
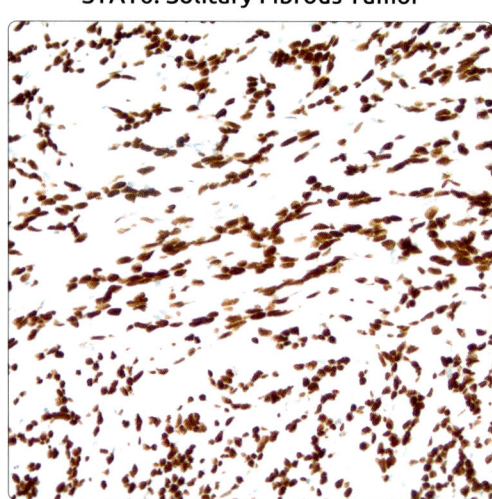

Solitary Fibrous Tumor | STAT6: Solitary Fibrous Tumor

Smooth Muscle Tumors

Cellular Schwannoma
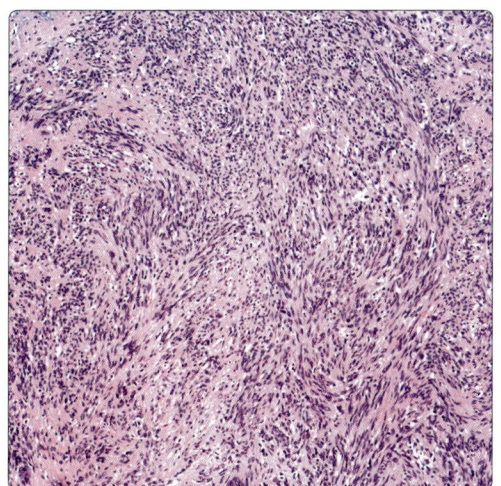

Cellular Schwannoma
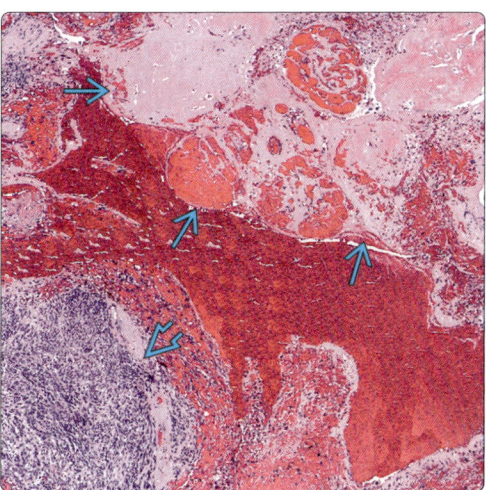

(Left) Cellular foci of a schwannoma often have organized cellular fascicles that may create an appearance that closely mimics a smooth muscle tumor. (Right) In some foci, schwannomas commonly have large, dilated blood vessels with associated fibrin ⇒. When associated with a cellular spindle cell neoplasm ⇒, these changes should at least suggest the possibility of a schwannoma.

Schwannoma With Ancient Change
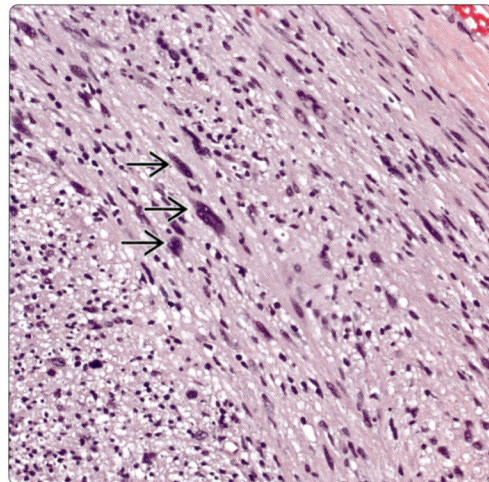

S100 Protein: Schwannoma
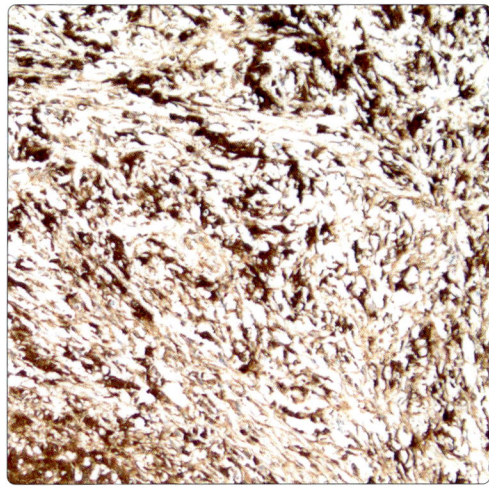

(Left) This benign nerve sheath tumor (schwannoma) shows scattered cells with degenerative-type atypia ⇒ that may mimic malignancy. Demonstration of diffuse immunoreactivity for S100 protein is an important diagnostic feature in this distinction. (Right) Diffuse cytoplasmic and nuclear immunoreactivity for S100 protein is a characteristic feature of benign nerve sheath tumors.

PEComa
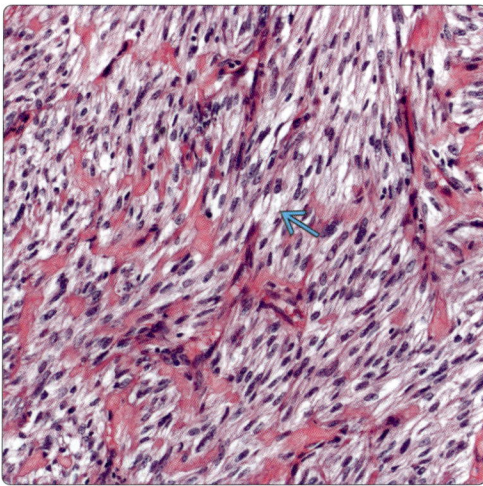

HMB45: PEComa
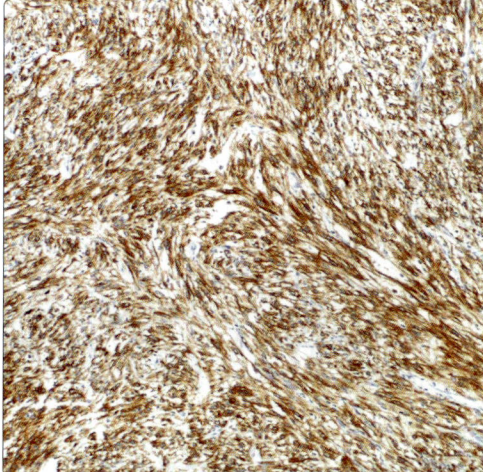

(Left) PEComa, which rarely occurs in the urinary bladder, may very closely mimic a smooth muscle neoplasm. They commonly have areas with subtle cytoplasmic clearing ⇒ &/or a nested growth. (Right) PEComas show coexpression of both smooth muscle (smooth muscle actin) and melanocytic markers (HMB45, melan-A, tyrosinase, cathepsin-K) by immunohistochemistry. HMB45 staining may be relatively focal, but is rather diffuse in this example.

Skeletal Muscle Tumors

KEY FACTS

CLINICAL ISSUES
- Most common bladder tumor of childhood
- Extraordinarily rare in adults
- Current therapies have greatly improved survival in pediatric group

MICROSCOPIC
- Embryonal RMS is heterogeneous
  - Spindle cells and more fusiform cells common
  - Loose myxoid stroma common
  - Rhabdomyoblasts variably present
- Classic alveolar RMS has back-to-back "round cells" with high nuclear:cytoplasmic ratio
  - May have classic alveolar arrangement with fibrous septa
  - May be solid pattern
- Vesical RMS in adults often have alveolar or unclassifiable RMS histology with anaplasia

ANCILLARY TESTS
- Desmin and smooth muscle actin are typically strongly positive
- Nuclear myogenin and MYOD1 expression characteristic
- Alveolar RMS may have *FKHR* (*FOXO1a*) rearrangements

TOP DIFFERENTIAL DIAGNOSES
- Inflammatory myofibroblastic tumor
- Fibroepithelial polyp
- Small cell carcinoma in adults
- Sarcomatoid urothelial carcinoma in adults
  - May have rhabdomyoblastic differentiation
- Lymphoma

DIAGNOSTIC CHECKLIST
- Embryonal RMS should be carefully ruled out when considering vesical inflammatory myofibroblastic tumor in a child

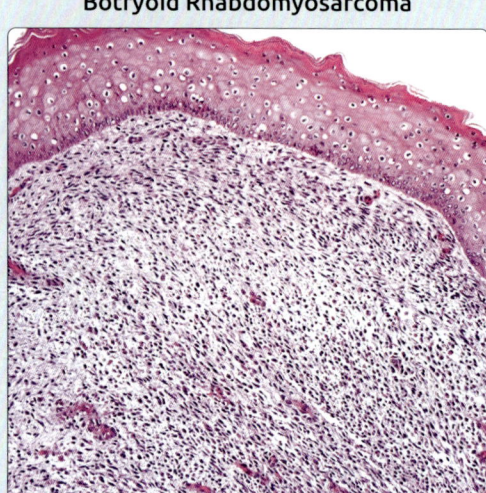

Botryoid Rhabdomyosarcoma

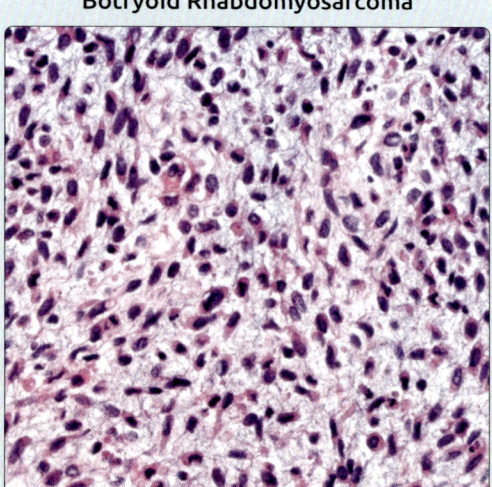

Botryoid Rhabdomyosarcoma

(Left) A subepithelial proliferation of spindle cells is characteristic of the botryoid variant of embryonal rhabdomyosarcoma, the most common type of rhabdomyosarcoma in the urinary bladder. *(Right)* Spindled to round or fusiform neoplastic cells with a variable rim of eosinophilic cytoplasm is typical of embryonal rhabdomyosarcoma. The associated myxoid stroma is also commonly seen in embryonal types of rhabdomyosarcoma.

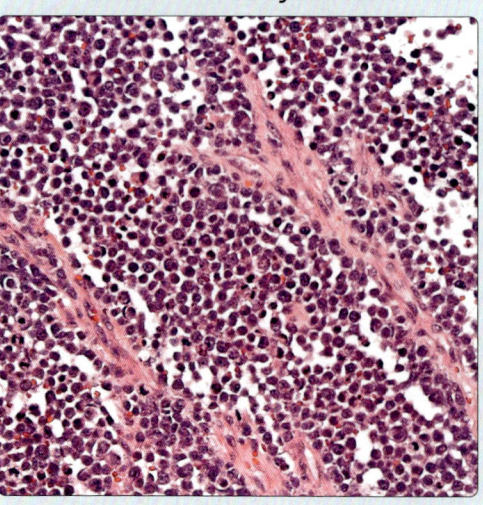

Alveolar Rhabdomyosarcoma

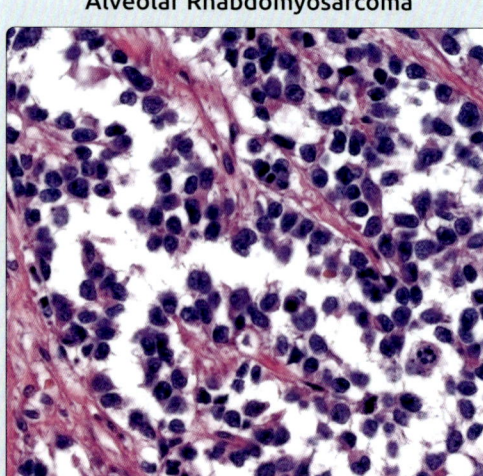

Alveolar Rhabdomyosarcoma

(Left) This is a classic example of alveolar rhabdomyosarcoma with fibrovascular septa creating the prototypical alveolar architecture. The neoplastic cells typically appear dyscohesive and have a "malignant small round blue cell" morphology. *(Right)* The neoplastic small round cells of alveolar rhabdomyosarcoma cling to the fibrous septa in a hobnail pattern. The alveolar subtype is extremely rare in the urinary bladder. It may occur in adults where it mimics small cell carcinoma.

Skeletal Muscle Tumors

TERMINOLOGY

Abbreviations
- Rhabdomyosarcoma (RMS)

Definitions
- Malignant neoplasm recapitulating morphologic and molecular features of skeletal muscle

CLINICAL ISSUES

Epidemiology
- Incidence
  - Most common urinary bladder tumor in childhood and adolescence
  - Extraordinarily rare in adults
- Age
  - Mean at diagnosis is 4 years
- Sex
  - Male predominance (M:F = 3:2)

Presentation
- Gross hematuria is most common initial symptom

Treatment
- Combined surgery and chemotherapy have greatly improved survival in pediatric group

Prognosis
- Excellent in children with newer chemotherapy regimens
- Extremely poor in adults

MACROSCOPIC

General Features
- Typically polypoid (botryoid)

MICROSCOPIC

Histologic Features
- Embryonal RMS is composed of proliferation of spindled tumor cells with variable cellularity
  - Botryoid subtype has condensation of tumor cells (cambium layer) beneath surface epithelium
  - Marked variability with fusiform, spindled, and rounded neoplastic cells may be seen
  - May have scattered rhabdomyoblasts ("strap cells")
  - Foci may be markedly hypocellular with bland cytology
  - Myxoid stroma is common
- Classic alveolar RMS
  - Characterized by back-to-back "round cells" with high nuclear:cytoplasmic ratio
  - Neoplastic cells have nuclear morphology reminiscent of lymphoma
  - May have fibrous septa or may grow in solid pattern
- Vesical RMS in adults
  - Often have alveolar or unclassifiable RMS histology
  - Areas of nuclear anaplasia are common

Predominant Pattern/Injury Type
- Spindled

Predominant Cell/Compartment Type
- Skeletal muscle

ANCILLARY TESTS

Immunohistochemistry
- Desmin is typically strongly positive
- Nuclear myogenin and MYOD1 expression define skeletal muscle phenotype
  - MYOD1 commonly has nonspecific cytoplasmic staining, which is nondiagnostic

In Situ Hybridization
- Alveolar RMS may have rearrangements involving *FKHR (FOX01a)* and either *PAX3* or *PAX7*

DIFFERENTIAL DIAGNOSIS

Inflammatory Myofibroblastic Tumor
- Spindle cells with elongated, eosinophilic cytoplasmic processes
- Myxoid stromal matrix is common
- Admixed inflammatory cells
- Typically coexpress smooth muscle actin and cytokeratin
- No nuclear myogenin or MYOD1 expression

Small Cell Carcinoma in Adults
- May be morphologically indistinguishable from alveolar RMS
- Typical urothelial carcinoma may also be present
- Immunohistochemistry for synaptophysin and chromogranin are positive
  - Synaptophysin may also be positive in RMS
- Express cytokeratin in dot-like pattern
- No nuclear myogenin or MYOD1 expression

Fibroepithelial Polyp
- Polypoid exophytic growth may clinically simulate botryoid RMS; microscopic reactive stromal cells raise possibility of neoplasm
- No cambium layer or myogenin expression

Sarcomatoid Urothelial Carcinoma in Adults
- Component of urothelial carcinoma
- RMS is common heterologous element in carcinosarcoma

Lymphoma
- Lymphomas may have identical cytology to alveolar RMS
- Immunohistochemistry helps exclude hematopoietic lineage

DIAGNOSTIC CHECKLIST

Pathologic Interpretation Pearls
- Embryonal RMS should be ruled out if considering vesical inflammatory myofibroblastic tumor in children
- RMS and small cell carcinoma may be morphologically indistinguishable in adults

SELECTED REFERENCES

1. Paner GP et al: Rhabdomyosarcoma of the urinary bladder in adults: predilection for alveolar morphology with anaplasia and significant morphologic overlap with small cell carcinoma. Am J Surg Pathol. 32(7):1022-8, 2008
2. Leuschner I et al: Rhabdomyosarcoma of the urinary bladder and vagina: a clinicopathologic study with emphasis on recurrent disease: a report from the Kiel Pediatric Tumor Registry and the German CWS Study. Am J Surg Pathol. 25(7):856-64, 2001

Skeletal Muscle Tumors

(Left) The cambium layer (subepithelial condensation of the neoplastic cells) is typical of the botryoid variant of embryonal rhabdomyosarcoma. In children, the clinical presentation of an exophytic bladder mass should strongly suggest this diagnosis. (Right) There is a broad morphologic spectrum for rhabdomyosarcoma. This embryonal type has a cellular fascicular pattern of growth with scant myxoid stroma. The patient's age is important in arriving at the appropriate diagnosis.

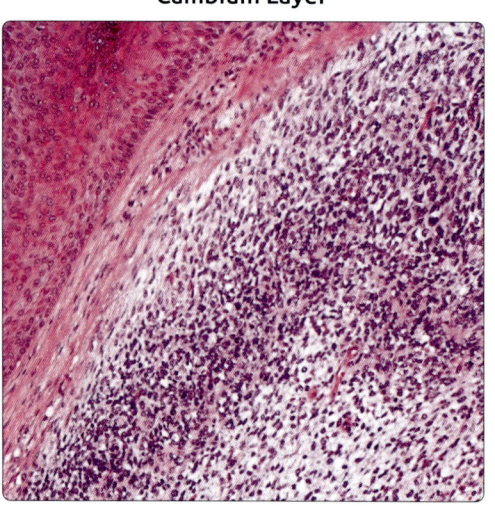

Cambium Layer

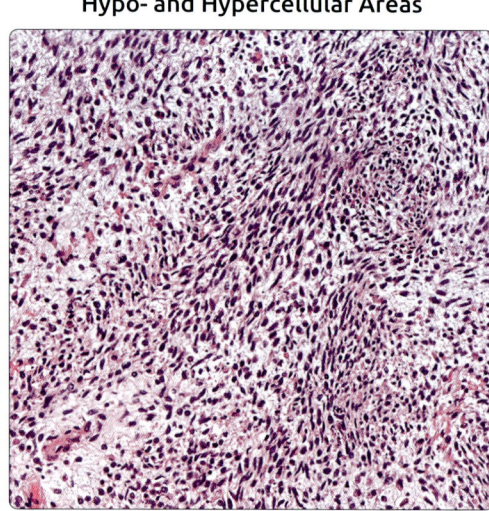

Hypo- and Hypercellular Areas

(Left) Myxoid stroma is common in embryonal rhabdomyosarcoma. In the urinary bladder, this may cause diagnostic consideration of a myofibroblastic proliferation, which may also occur in children. (Right) Some foci in embryonal rhabdomyosarcoma may have very bland nuclear cytology that may closely mimic a benign process. In children, the index of suspicion for rhabdomyosarcoma should be high and prompt an immunohistochemical work-up.

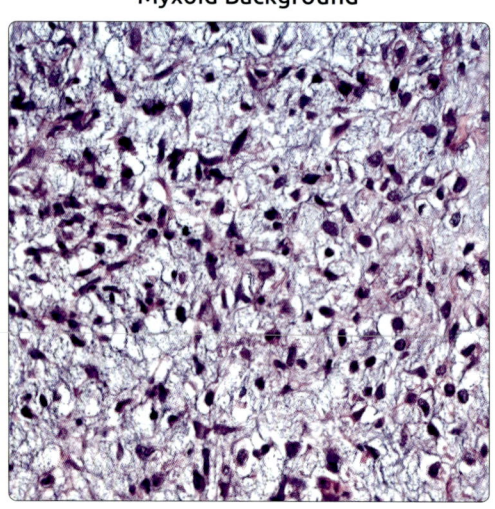

Myxoid Background

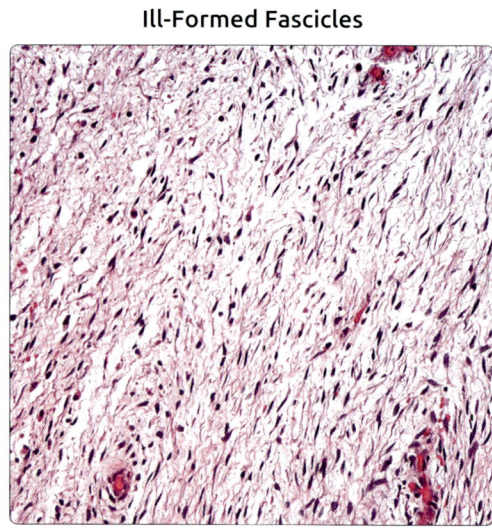

Ill-Formed Fascicles

(Left) Classic rhabdomyoblasts or "strap cells" with cross striations may be identified ➡. These are diagnostic of rhabdomyoblastic differentiation. (Right) Focal cartilaginous differentiation is well described in rhabdomyosarcoma of the gynecologic and genitourinary tracts. This may cause diagnostic confusion with a sarcomatoid carcinoma. The presence of cartilage does not alter the favorable prognosis for a patient with a childhood bladder rhabdomyosarcoma.

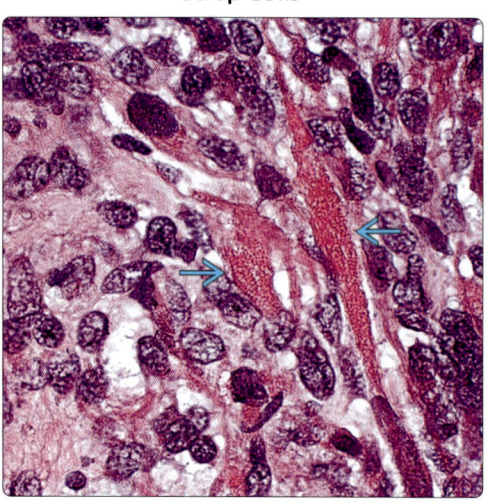

Strap Cells

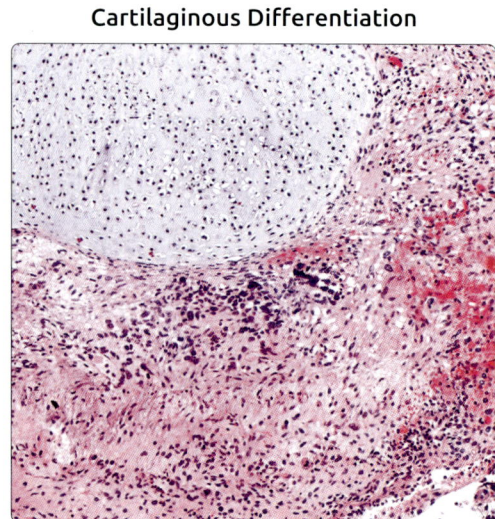

Cartilaginous Differentiation

Skeletal Muscle Tumors

Cellular Foci in Embryonal Rhabdomyosarcoma

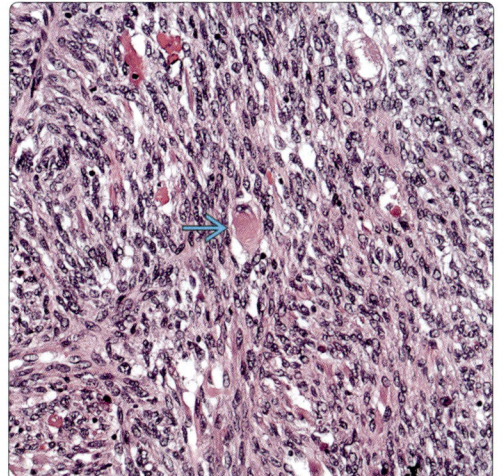

Cellular Foci in Embryonal Rhabdomyosarcoma

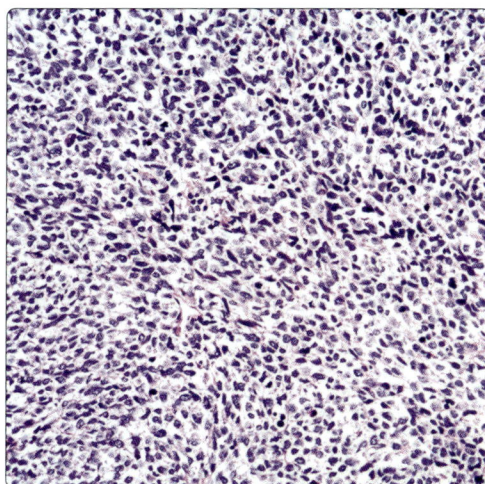

(Left) Some embryonal rhabdomyosarcomas may have very cellular foci. The spindled morphology and easily identified rhabdomyoblasts ➡ suggest an embryonal subtype. (Right) When cellular foci of embryonal rhabdomyosarcoma have more fusiform cells, there is a greater degree of histologic overlap with the alveolar subtype. The myogenin staining pattern and adjunctive FISH testing may help in difficult cases.

Alveolar Rhabdomyosarcoma

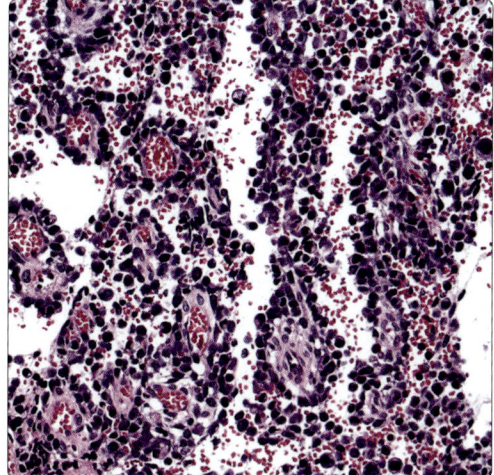

Alveolar Rhabdomyosarcoma

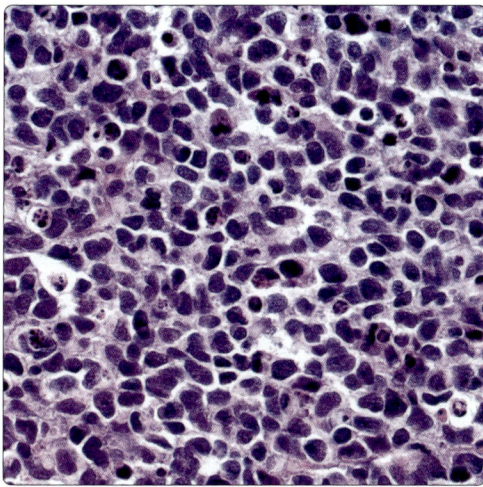

(Left) The cellular dyscohesion seen in alveolar rhabdomyosarcoma may occasionally produce a pseudo-papillary pattern, as seen in this example. (Right) This alveolar rhabdomyosarcoma has a solid pattern that lacks fibrous septa. The alveolar subtype commonly shows cytologic features that are reminiscent of a high grade lymphoma, as in this example.

Pleomorphic Rhabdomyosarcoma

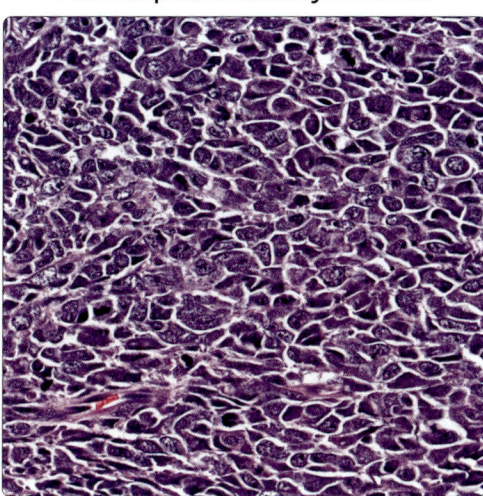

Alveolar Rhabdomyosarcoma With Anaplasia

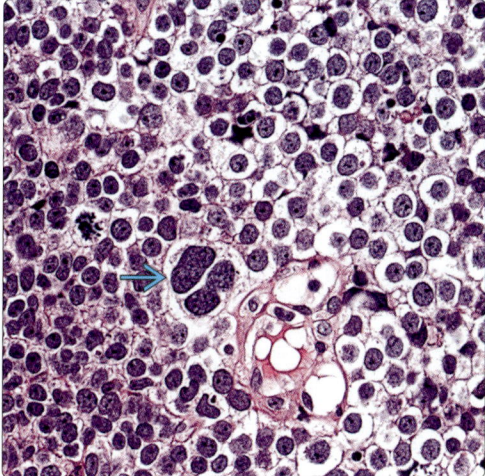

(Left) This example of rhabdomyosarcoma in an adult has a greater degree of pleomorphism than typically seen in childhood forms. This suggests the possibility of a carcinoma or an aggressive high-grade lymphoma. (Right) Adult rhabdomyosarcoma commonly has an alveolar morphology, as well as scattered neoplastic cells with marked nuclear anaplasia ➡. In adults, this should be distinguished from sarcomatoid carcinoma with rhabdomyoblastic differentiation.

Skeletal Muscle Tumors

Rhabdomyosarcoma: Myogenin

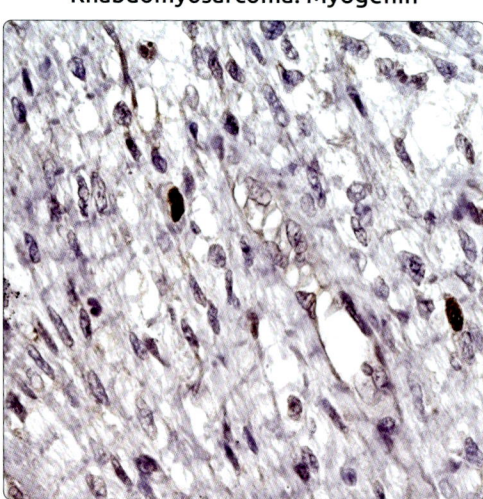

Rhabdomyosarcoma: Myogenin

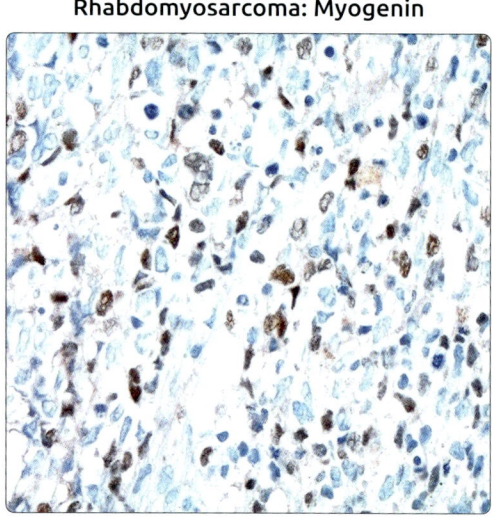

(Left) As in this example of embryonal rhabdomyosarcoma with bland cytologic features, nuclear myogenin immunoreactivity may be very patchy. In contrast, diffuse immunoreactivity (greater than 80% of neoplastic cells positive) is typical of alveolar rhabdomyosarcoma. (Right) In more cellular foci of embryonal rhabdomyosarcoma, this degree of nuclear myogenin immunoreactivity is more easily identified and more typical.

Rhabdomyosarcoma: Myogenin

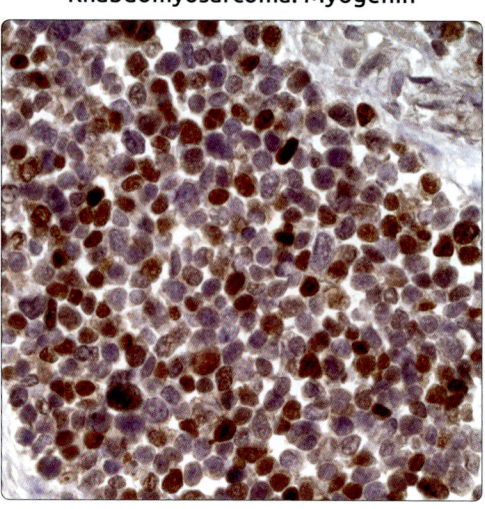

Nonspecific MYOD1 Staining

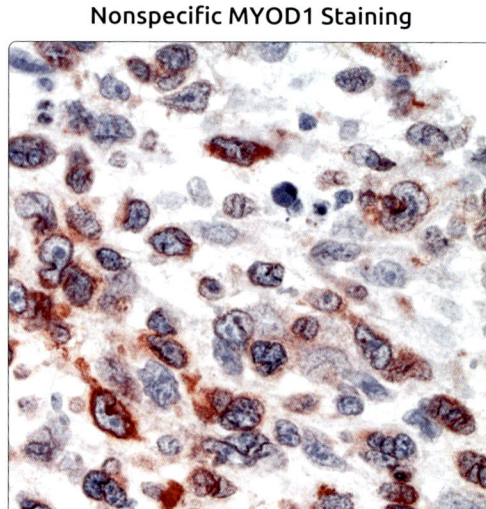

(Left) Strong and diffuse myogenin reactivity is characteristic of alveolar rhabdomyosarcoma. The percentage of cells expressing myogenin is typically much less in embryonal rhabdomyosarcoma. (Right) Careful attention to the pattern of staining is important in the interpretation of skeletal muscle markers. As in this example, nonspecific cytoplasmic staining for MYOD1 (a nuclear marker) is common but does not indicate skeletal muscle differentiation.

Rhabdomyosarcoma: Desmin

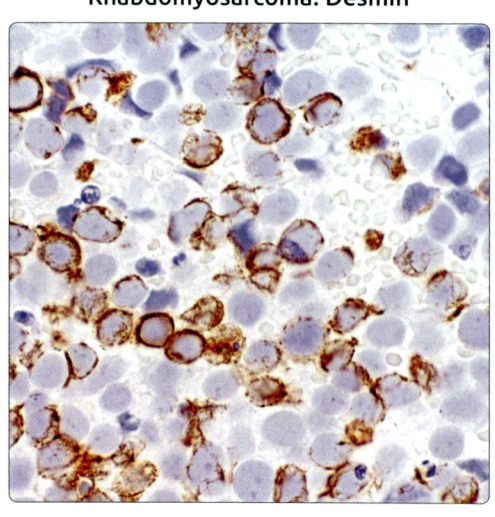

Rhabdomyosarcoma: Synaptophysin

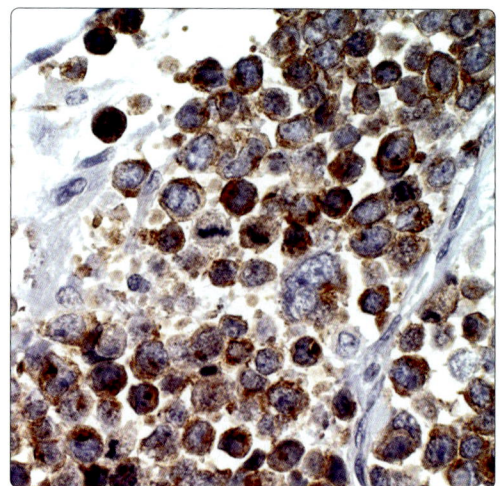

(Left) Strong cytoplasmic desmin reactivity is typical of rhabdomyosarcoma. Desmin immunoreactivity is not entirely specific for skeletal muscle, so other markers, such as myogenin and MYOD1, are often utilized. (Right) This rhabdomyosarcoma shows "aberrant" synaptophysin reactivity. It is not uncommon for RMS at any site to be positive for synaptophysin. In adults, this finding may result in further diagnostic confusion with small cell carcinoma. Cytokeratin staining is helpful to confirm a small cell carcinoma diagnosis.

Skeletal Muscle Tumors

Urothelial Carcinoma
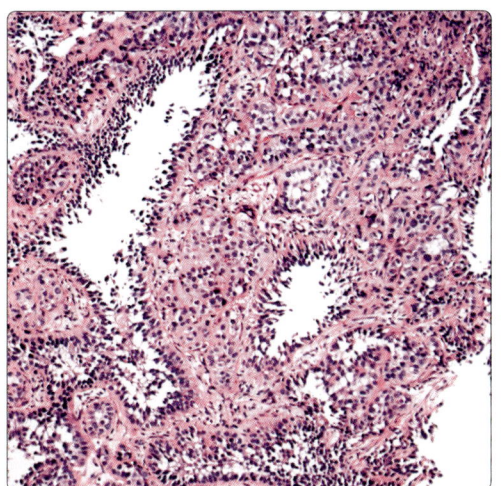

Urothelial Carcinoma
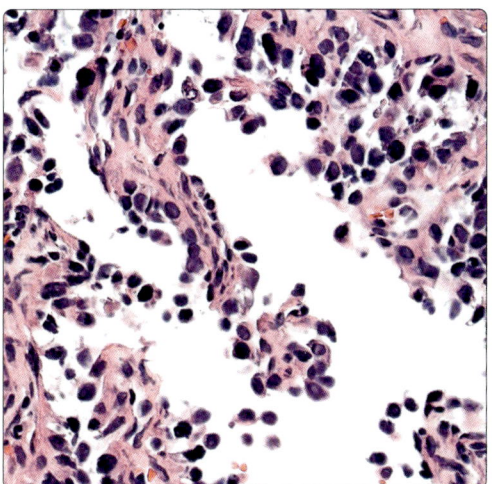

(Left) Morphologically subtle patterns of invasive urothelial carcinoma (e.g., nested or microcystic) may occasionally have cystic change with dyscohesion that may suggest an alveolar morphology on biopsy. *(Right)* Focal areas of this urothelial carcinoma have cellular dyscohesion that may suggest an alveolar rhabdomyosarcoma on a small biopsy specimen. Other foci of more typical urothelial carcinoma are usually present. Immunohistochemistry may be necessary in biopsy specimens. Cautery and crush artifact contribute to this dilemma.

Small Cell Carcinoma
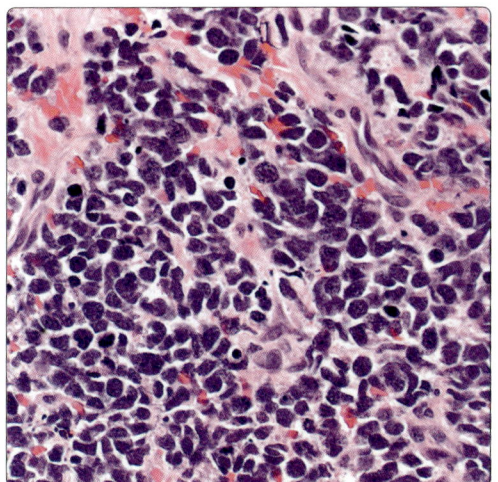

Small Cell Carcinoma
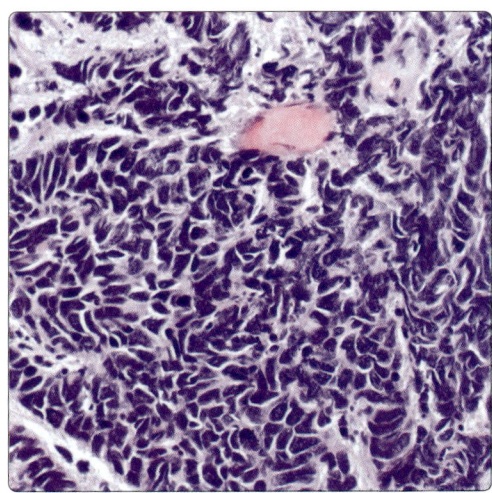

(Left) A small cell carcinoma of the urinary bladder in an adult may mimic any small round cell tumor, such as rhabdomyosarcoma, lymphoma, or malignant melanoma. *(Right)* Small cell carcinoma often has high nuclear:cytoplasmic ratio, nuclear molding, apoptotic bodies, and high mitotic index. It is negative for myogenin and MYOD1 but expresses cytokeratin, synaptophysin, and in some cases TTF-1. It is not uncommon for small cell carcinoma to have an associated urothelial carcinoma.

Myofibroblastic Proliferation
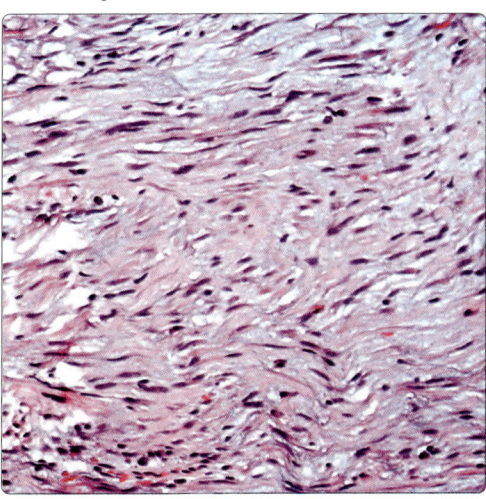

Lymphoepithelioma-Like Carcinoma
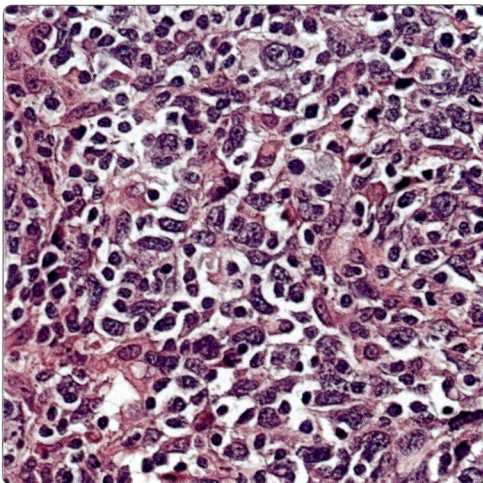

(Left) Myofibroblastic proliferations, as in this example, may closely resemble bland foci of embryonal rhabdomyosarcoma. In a child, the possibility of rhabdomyosarcoma should be carefully considered and excluded when a cytologically bland spindle cell proliferation is encountered on a biopsy specimen. *(Right)* A lymphoepithelioma-like carcinoma of the urinary bladder may also closely mimic a round cell tumor. Cytokeratin reactivity is useful in confirming an epithelial lineage.

Other Mesenchymal Tumors

KEY FACTS

CLINICAL ISSUES
- Extraordinarily rare
- Hematuria

MICROSCOPIC
- Neurofibroma
  - Proliferation of spindled cells with small tapered nuclei
  - Randomly distributed collagen bundles common
  - May mimic myofibroblastic proliferation in cellular cases
  - S100 protein positive
- Solitary fibrous tumor
  - Spindle cells arranged in haphazard pattern
  - Angulated "hemangiopericytic" blood vessels
  - Deposition of intercellular collagen
  - Neoplastic cells are positive with CD34
  - STAT6 immunohistochemistry useful as surrogate for diagnostic gene fusion
- Hemangioma/vascular malformation
  - Benign lesion comprised of aggregated blood vessels
  - No destructive invasive growth or significant cytologic atypia
- Postradiation sarcoma
  - Pleomorphic undifferentiated appearance most common
  - Distinction from sarcomatoid carcinoma may be difficult
- Other tumors
  - Angiosarcoma
    - May express cytokeratin
  - Pleomorphic undifferentiated sarcoma (malignant fibrous histiocytoma)
    - Must exclude sarcomatoid carcinoma
  - Granular cell tumor
    - Sheets of large S100 protein positive cells with granular eosinophilic cytoplasm
  - PEComa
    - Nested appearance with clear to lightly eosinophilic cells
  - Endometrial stromal sarcoma

Solitary Fibrous Tumor
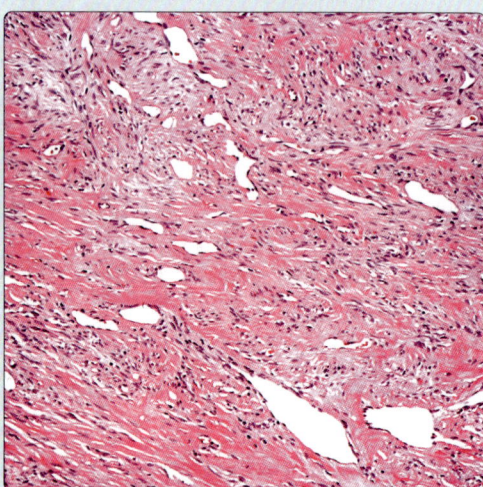

Angiosarcoma
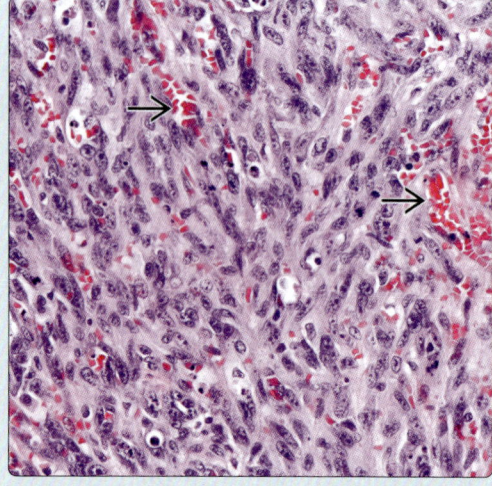

(Left) Although not common, solitary fibrous tumors are also well described in the urinary bladder. Angulated (hemangiopericytic) blood vessels and collagenization are both typical features. (Right) Vasoformation 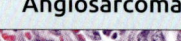 and extravasated red blood cells should suggest angiosarcoma. Spindled areas may mimic leiomyosarcoma or sarcomatoid urothelial carcinoma, which are more common than angiosarcoma. Urothelial carcinoma may have pseudoangiosarcomatous pattern.

Granular Cell Tumor
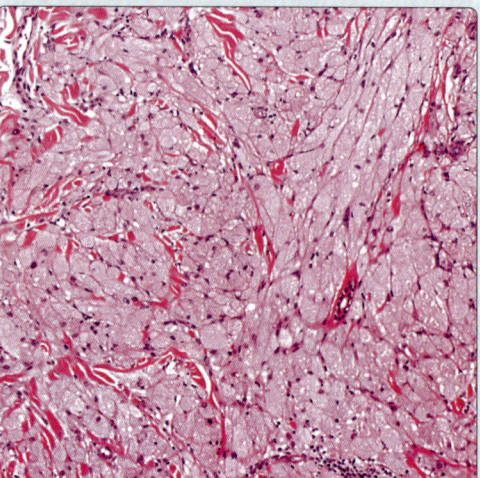

Endometrial Stromal Sarcoma
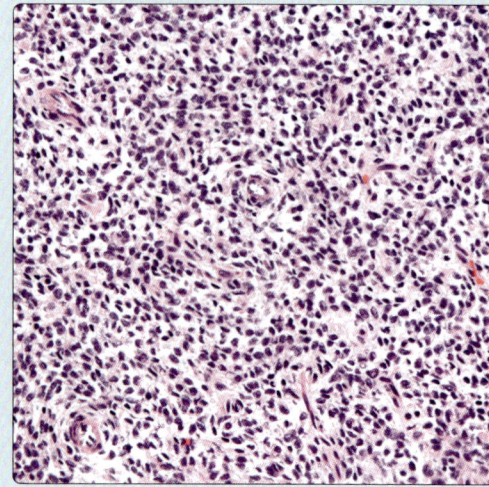

(Left) Granular cell tumors of the genitourinary tract are similar to those in other sites with a sheet-like growth pattern and abundant granular eosinophilic cytoplasm. The neoplastic cells show diffuse expression of S100 protein. (Right) Endometrial stromal sarcoma may rarely involve the bladder, either as a metastasis (usually from the uterus) or rarely as sarcomatous progression of endometriosis.

Other Mesenchymal Tumors

TERMINOLOGY

Definitions
- Mesenchymal neoplasms other than muscle and myofibroblastic lineage may occur in urinary bladder

CLINICAL ISSUES

Epidemiology
- Incidence
  - Extraordinarily rare
    - Often present in literature as single case reports

Presentation
- Hematuria
- Obstruction
- Pelvic pain

Treatment
- Surgical approaches
  - Simple transurethral resection for small benign lesions
  - Large benign lesions may need more extensive resection
  - Sarcomas generally require radical cystectomy and consideration of adjuvant therapy

MICROSCOPIC

Neurofibroma
- Proliferation of spindled cells with small tapered or wavy nuclei
- Randomly distributed individual bundles of "shredded carrot" collagen are common
- Lack of significant cytologic atypia or mitotic figures
  - Scattered degenerative atypia may be seen
- Neoplastic cells show cytoplasmic and nuclear immunoreactivity with S100 protein

Solitary Fibrous Tumor
- Most behave in benign fashion when completely resected
  - Large size, nuclear pleomorphism, and mitotic activity may predict malignant potential
- Spindle cells arranged in haphazard pattern
- Cellularity and intercellular collagen varies greatly
- Neoplastic cells are positive with CD34
- Characteristic NAB2-STAT6 gene fusion
  - Immunohistochemical expression of STAT6 (nuclear) is very sensitive and specific surrogate for fusion

Hemangioma/Vascular Malformation
- Benign lesion composed of blood vessels
  - Cytologically bland endothelial cells
  - Surrounding smooth muscle cells often seen
- Most lesions reported as hemangioma are designated as vascular malformation under recent classification systems

Postradiation Sarcoma
- Pleomorphic undifferentiated appearance most common
  - Distinction from sarcomatoid carcinoma may be very difficult
    - Especially if history of genitourinary tract carcinoma
- Commonly arises 8-10 years after radiation therapy
  - Many occur after treatment of prostatic or uterine primaries

Other Mesenchymal Neoplasia Subtypes
- Angiosarcoma
  - Vasoformative or epithelioid with sheet-like growth
    - Commonly express CD34 and CD31
      - CD31 often highlights intratumoral histiocytes and may cause confusion
    - Nuclear expression of ERG
    - May show aberrant cytokeratin expression, especially if epithelioid
      - Immunoreactivity for low molecular weight forms of keratin
      - Do not express high molecular weight keratin
- Osteosarcoma
  - Trabeculae of neoplastic bone associated with malignant cells
    - Most tumors with osteoid production represent sarcomatoid carcinoma
- Pleomorphic undifferentiated sarcoma (malignant fibrous histiocytoma)
  - Pleomorphic spindled malignant neoplasm without evidence of specific line of differentiation
- Granular cell tumor
  - Round cellular infiltrate with abundant granular eosinophilic cytoplasm
  - Express S100 protein
- PEComa
  - Variable histologic features
    - Spindled cells
      - Fascicular growth pattern
      - Clear to lightly eosinophilic cytoplasm
      - Relatively uniform nuclei
    - Epithelioid cells
      - Abundant eosinophilic cytoplasm with eccentric nucleus
      - Variable cytologic atypia
    - Nested growth pattern common
    - Neoplastic cells typically present within walls of blood vessels at least focally
    - May have intracytoplasmic lipid
    - May have an associated network of endothelial lined spaces
    - May be malignant
      - Assessed by size, nuclear atypia, and mitotic rate
  - Coexpress smooth muscle and melanocytic markers
    - Smooth muscle actin positive
    - HMB45, Melan-A, and MiTF positive
    - Cathepsin K positive
- Endometrial stromal sarcoma
  - May rarely occur in bladder
  - May be associated with endometriosis or primary uterine tumor
  - Typically express CD10 and estrogen receptor
  - Different molecular subtypes
    - Distinct low-grade and high-grade patterns
- Lipoma
  - Well-delineated collection of mature adipose tissue

Other Mesenchymal Tumors

DIFFERENTIAL DIAGNOSIS

Neurofibroma
- Low-grade malignant peripheral nerve sheath tumor
  - Better developed fascicular growth with mitotic activity
  - More heterogeneous cellularity
- Embryonal rhabdomyosarcoma
  - May have morphologically bland areas with close resemblance to neurofibroma
  - Cytoplasmic desmin and nuclear myogenin &/or MYOD1 immunoreactivity diagnostic
- Leiomyoma
  - Usually more cellular without collagen bundles
  - Express smooth muscle actin and desmin, but not S100 protein
- Myofibroblastic proliferation
  - Usually have associated mixed inflammatory infiltrate
  - Express smooth muscle actin, but not S100 protein

Solitary Fibrous Tumor
- Sarcomatoid carcinoma
  - Usually more cytologic atypia and carcinomatous component may be identified
  - Typically expresses HMCK(34βE12) and p63
- Neurofibroma
  - Diffuse S100 protein immunoreactivity
- Synovial sarcoma
  - Typically more cellular, tightly organized fascicles
  - Does not express CD34
  - Has characteristic (X;18) translocation

Hemangioma/Vascular Malformation
- Angiosarcoma has infiltrative growth and cytologic atypia
- Kaposi sarcoma typically has cellular fascicles of monomorphic spindle cells
- Granulation tissue contains tightly aggregated small vessels with associated inflammation

Postradiation Sarcoma
- Sarcomatoid urothelial carcinoma
  - Carcinomatous component may be seen
  - Carcinoma expresses high molecular weight cytokeratin and p63 (focally)
  - Very difficult distinction is some cases because many have history of prior carcinoma

Angiosarcoma
- Kaposi sarcoma
  - Predominantly spindled and expresses HHV8
- Hemangioma
  - Lobulated architecture without infiltration or significant atypia
- Sarcomatoid carcinoma with pseudoangiosarcomatous pattern
- Papillary endothelial hyperplasia (Masson lesion)

Pleomorphic Undifferentiated Sarcoma (Malignant Fibrous Histiocytoma)
- Sarcomatoid urothelial carcinoma
  - Prior history of urothelial carcinoma is helpful
  - Component of typical carcinoma or expresses epithelial markers

PEComa
- Melanoma
  - Share immunophenotypic expression of melanocytic markers
  - Diffuse S100 protein immunoreactivity
- Clear cell sarcoma
  - May have admixed multinucleated giant cells
  - Also share immunophenotypic expression of melanocytic markers
  - Diffuse S100 protein immunoreactivity
  - Characteristic EWSR1-ATF1 fusion [t(12;22)]
- Smooth muscle neoplasms
  - More homogeneously eosinophilic
  - Typically do not express melanocytic markers
- TFE3-associated renal cell carcinoma
  - pax-8 nuclear expression
  - TFE3 rearrangement
    - Fusion partner variable
    - PEComa may also have a TFE3 rearrangement in rare subset of cases
  - May have some expression of melanocytic markers
  - Cytokeratin expression may be focal or absent
- TFEB-associated renal cell carcinoma TFEB
  - pax-8 nuclear expression
  - TFEB rearrangement
  - May have some expression of melanocytic markers
  - Cytokeratin expression may be focal or absent

Endometrial Stromal Sarcoma
- Large nested carcinoma
  - Cytokeratin staining distinctive
- Paraganglioma
  - More nested architecture
- Poorly differentiated synovial sarcoma
  - Has characteristic (X;18) translocation

Mesenchymal Neoplasm With Myxoid Features
- Soft tissue filler from stress incontinence procedure
  - May contain histiocytes and giant cells

SELECTED REFERENCES

1. Tian W et al: Endometrial stromal sarcoma involving the urinary bladder: a study of 6 cases. Am J Surg Pathol. 38(7):982-9, 2014
2. Williamson SR et al: Malignant perivascular epithelioid cell neoplasm (PEComa) of the urinary bladder with TFE3 gene rearrangement: clinicopathologic, immunohistochemical, and molecular features. Am J Surg Pathol. 37(10):1619-26, 2013
3. Kang HW et al: Granular cell tumor of the urinary bladder. Korean J Urol. 51(4):291-3, 2010
4. Sukov WR et al: Perivascular Epithelioid Cell Tumor (PEComa) of the Urinary Bladder: Report of 3 Cases and Review of the Literature. Am J Surg Pathol.
5. Tavora F et al: A series of vascular tumors and tumorlike lesions of the bladder. Am J Surg Pathol. 32(8):1213-9, 2008
6. Wang W et al: Benign nerve sheath tumors on urinary bladder biopsy. Am J Surg Pathol. 32(6):907-12, 2008
7. Westra WH et al: Solitary fibrous tumor of the lower urogenital tract: a report of five cases involving the seminal vesicles, urinary bladder, and prostate. Hum Pathol. 31(1):63-8, 2000

Other Mesenchymal Tumors

Neurofibroma: Classic

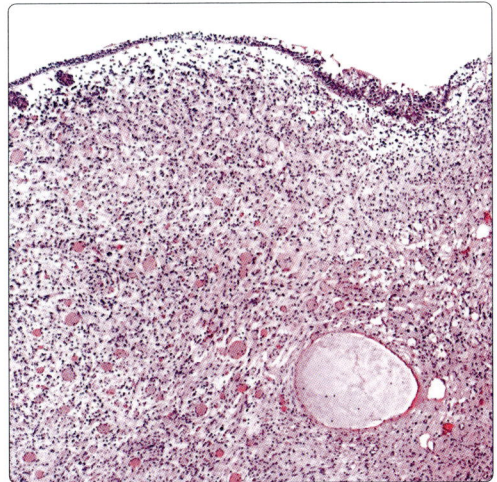

Neurofibroma: Classic

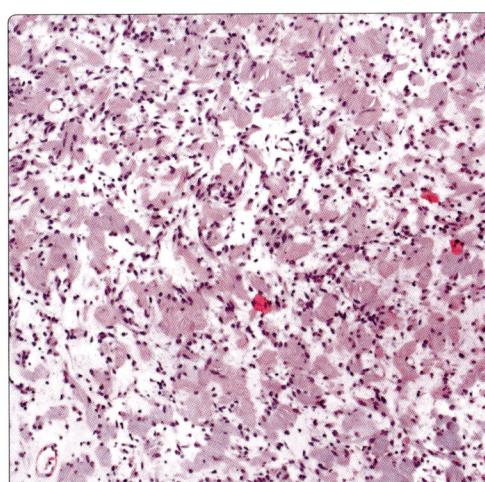

(Left) This neurofibroma is seen underlying the surface urothelium of the urinary bladder. On low-power evaluation, neural tumors may mimic a myofibroblastic or other spindle cell process. (Right) The randomly scattered collagen bundles ("shredded carrot" collagen) are characteristic of neurofibroma at any site. The neoplastic cells are usually cytologically bland, but scattered cells with degenerative atypia may be seen.

Neurofibroma: Cellular

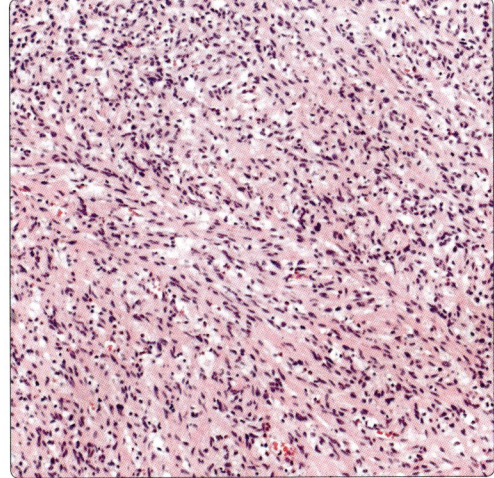

Neurofibroma: Myxoid

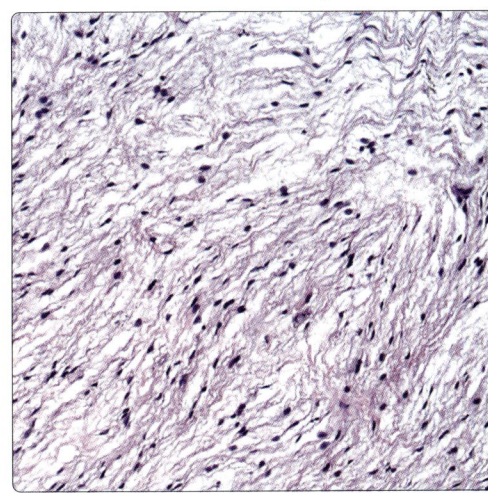

(Left) More cellular neurofibromas, such as this example, may closely mimic a myofibroblastic proliferation of the urinary bladder. Demonstration of diffuse cytoplasmic and nuclear S100 immunoreactivity is helpful in this diagnostic setting. (Right) This example of neurofibroma has a more myxoid appearance. The long cellular processes that can be seen also suggest the possibility of perineurioma, but S100 protein reactivity excludes that possibility.

Neurofibroma: Atypia

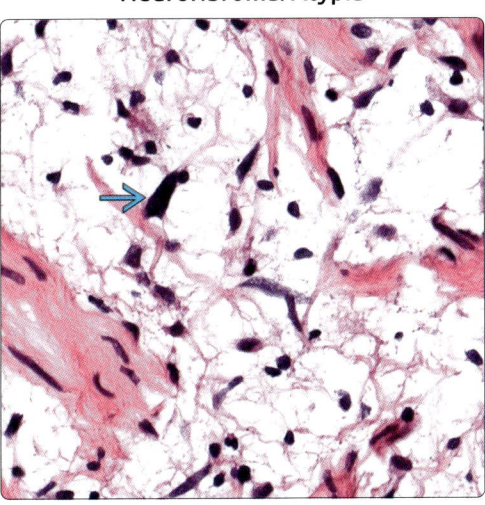

Neurofibroma: S100 Protein

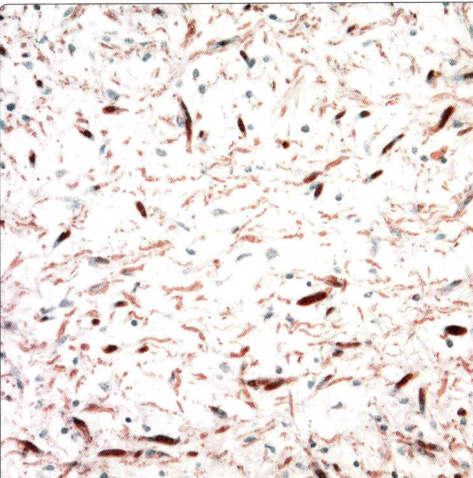

(Left) Neurofibromas may contain scattered enlarged cells ➡. In the absence of increased cellularity with fascicular growth &/or mitotic activity, this feature should not change the benign designation. (Right) Nuclear and cytoplasmic expression for S100 protein adds adjunctive support to the diagnosis of a nerve sheath tumor. In general, malignant peripheral nerve sheath tumors show more focal expression for S100 protein.

Other Mesenchymal Tumors

(Left) *In superficial biopsies, such as this example, the diagnostic consideration of a solitary fibrous tumor over other more common spindle cell lesions (such as myofibroblastic) may not be be apparent.* **(Right)** *Some examples of solitary fibrous tumor are more cellular and have also been called hemangiopericytoma in the older literature. The angulated blood vessels with hyalinization ➡ are typical of solitary fibrous tumor.*

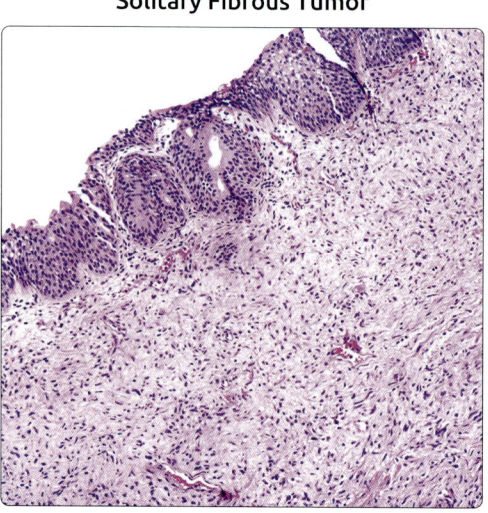
Solitary Fibrous Tumor

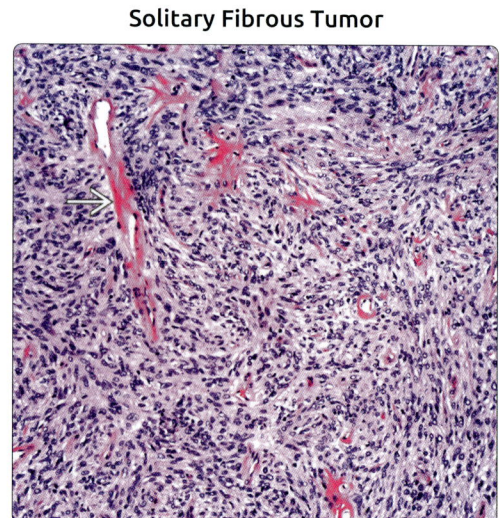
Solitary Fibrous Tumor

(Left) *The hypocellular proliferation of fibroblasts without a distinct architectural growth (so-called "patternless" pattern), the dense collagenization, and the angulated hemangiopericytic blood vessels ➡ all support a diagnosis of solitary fibrous tumor.* **(Right)** *Diffuse cytoplasmic immunoreactivity with CD34 is characteristic of solitary fibrous tumor, which would typically be negative for cytokeratin staining. Smooth muscle actin may occasionally show immunoreactivity.*

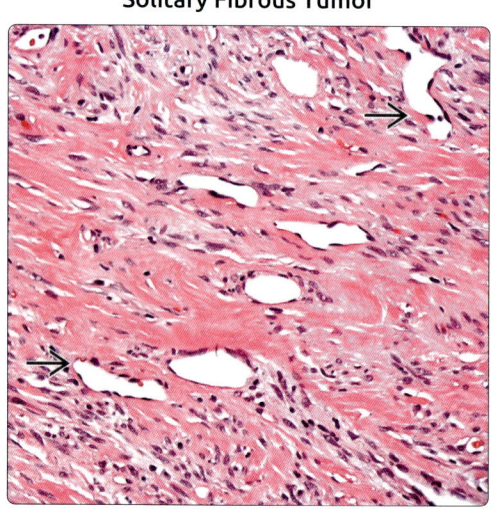
Solitary Fibrous Tumor

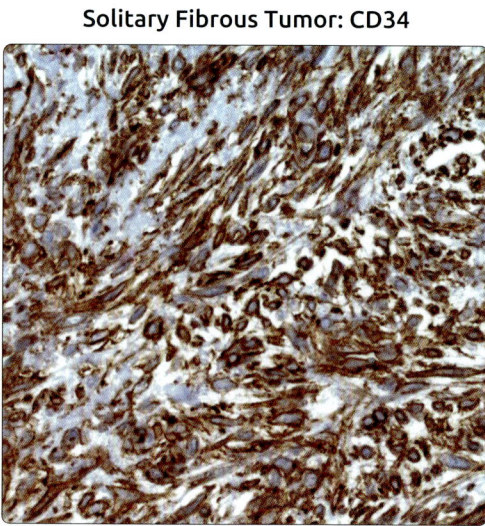
Solitary Fibrous Tumor: CD34

(Left) *Strong nuclear expression of STAT6 is a very specific feature of solitary fibrous tumor, as it provides evidence for the underlying gene fusion. Only rarely do other tumors show expression of STAT6 (e.g., dedifferentiated liposarcoma).* **(Right)** *Lipoma of the urinary bladder is extraordinarily rare. As in other anatomic sites, it consists of a sheet-like mass lesion formed by mature adipose tissue.*

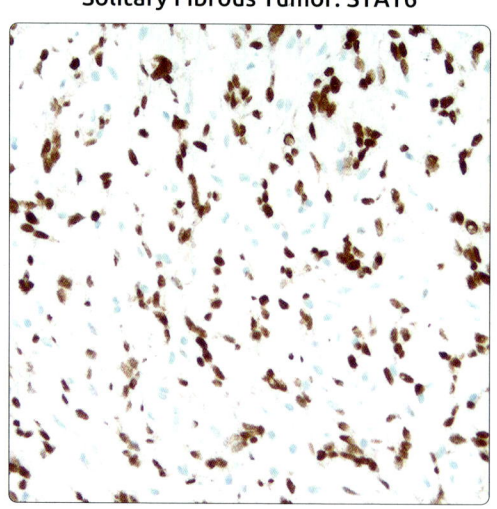
Solitary Fibrous Tumor: STAT6

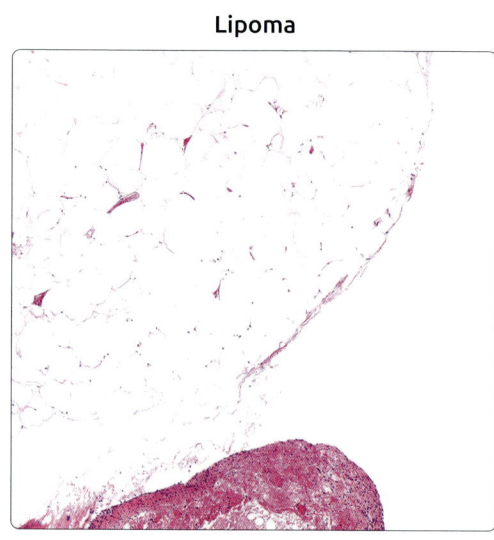
Lipoma

Other Mesenchymal Tumors

Vascular Malformation/Hemangioma

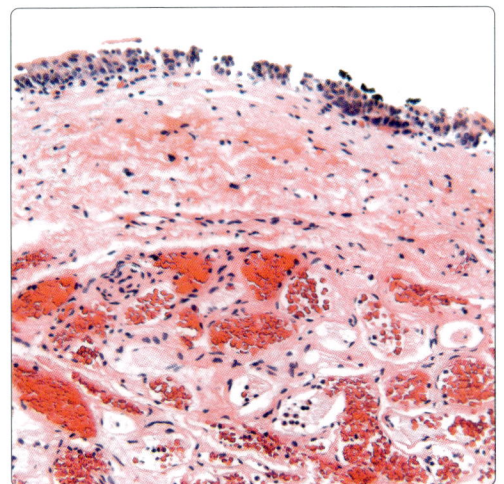

Vascular Malformation/Hemangioma

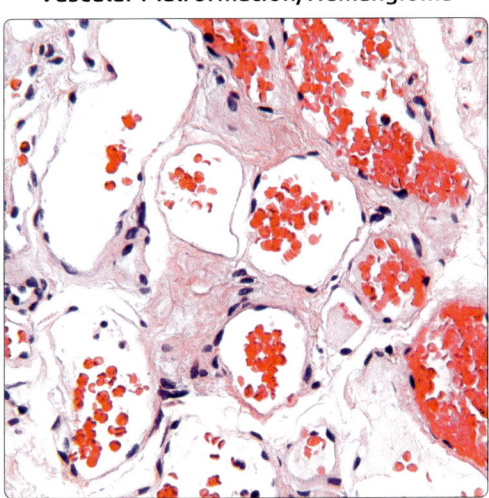

(Left) This collection of small blood vessels in the lamina propria of the bladder is sharply circumscribed, a characteristic feature of a benign vascular lesion such as hemangioma. (Right) In benign vascular lesions, the individual endothelial cells are cytologically bland. Permeation and destructive invasion of normal structures, such as muscularis propria, is not seen.

Epithelioid Angiosarcoma

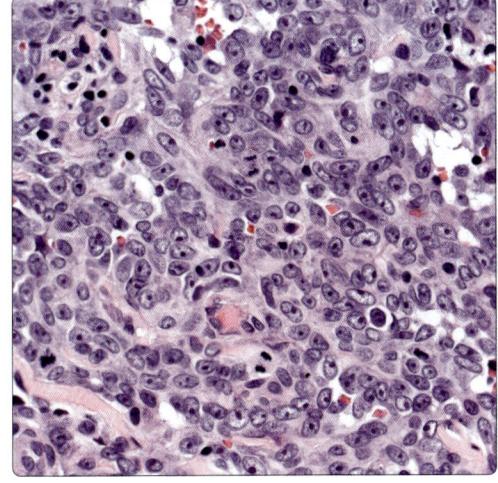

Epithelioid Angiosarcoma: ERG

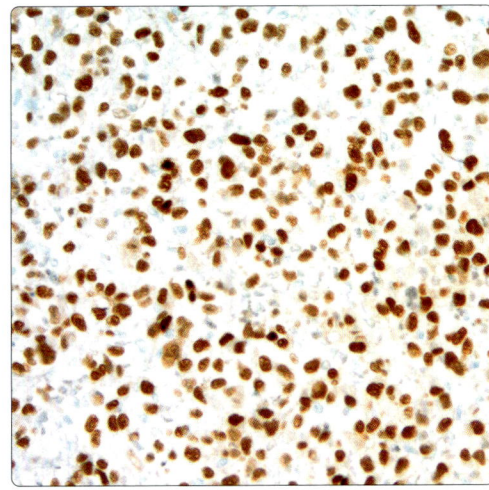

(Left) Epithelioid foci in angiosarcoma may closely mimic poorly differentiated urothelial carcinoma, especially given the frequent immunoreactivity with cytokeratin. CD31, FLI-1, and CD34 immunostains may be helpful. (Right) Strong nuclear immunoreactivity for ERG adds strong support for endothelial lineage. We typically pair this with a CD31 immunostain for added specificity. Some urothelial carcinomas may have pseudoangiosarcomatous pattern.

Undifferentiated Pleomorphic Sarcoma

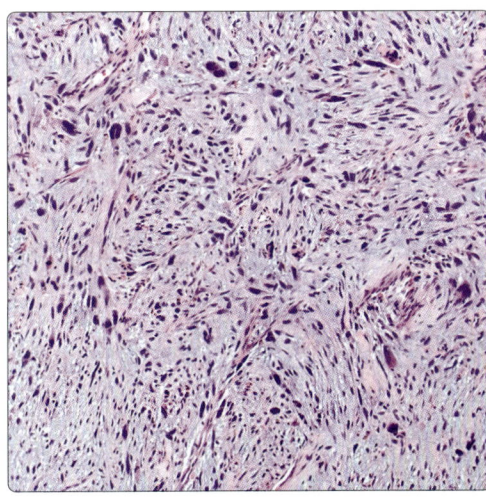

Granular Cell Tumor

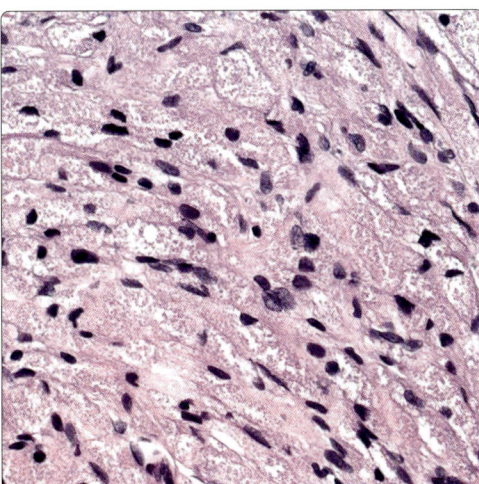

(Left) Pleomorphic undifferentiated sarcoma may look identical to a high-grade leiomyosarcoma or sarcomatoid carcinoma; however, no immunoreactivity with smooth muscle or epithelial immunohistochemical markers is demonstrable. (Right) Granular cell tumor is characterized by sheets of cells with voluminous eosinophilic cytoplasm. The cytoplasm has a striking granular appearance that correlates with lysosomes ultrastructurally.

Other Mesenchymal Tumors

PEComa

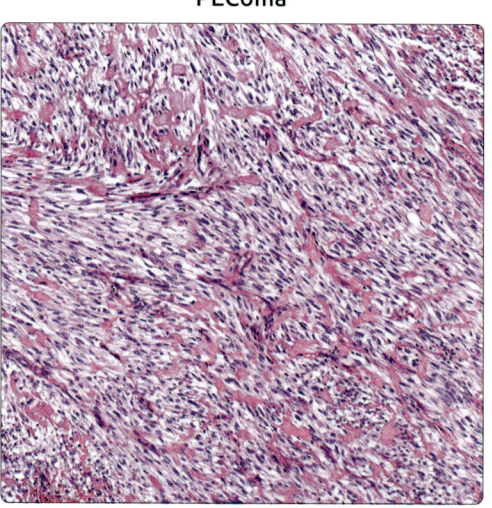

PEComa

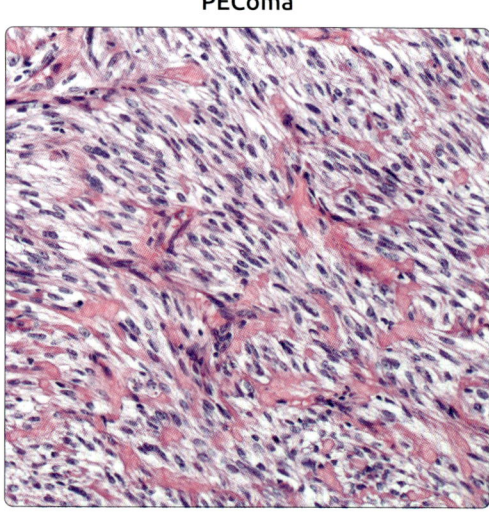

(Left) PEComas often have a spindle cell or epithelioid morphology with nested or grouped arrangement. The nests consist of short fascicles in this example. The cytoplasm characteristically appears clear or eosinophilic with a flocculent appearance. **(Right)** The neoplastic cells of PEComa often have relatively uniform nuclei. The cytoplasm is often clear with some wispy eosinophilia. Even on higher magnification, the nested architecture is apparent. cathepsin-K is a recently described useful marker.

PEComa: Smooth Muscle Actin

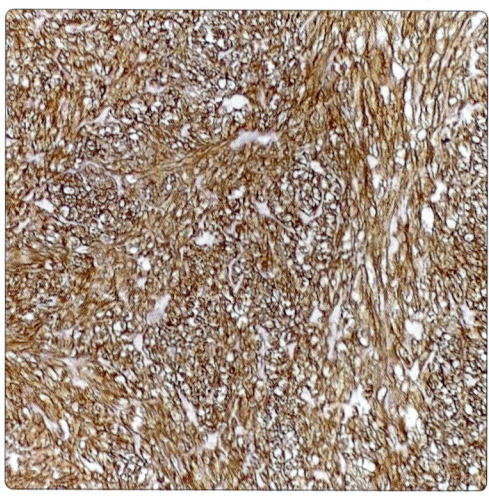

PEComa: HMB-45

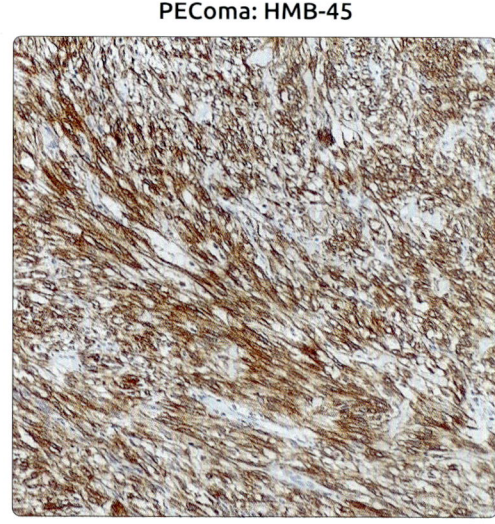

(Left) Smooth muscle actin is often reported as the most sensitive immunohistochemical marker of PEComa. In this example, there is diffuse cytoplasmic reactivity. The main differential diagnosis would be a smooth muscle neoplasm. **(Right)** PEComas often coexpress melanocytic markers (e.g., HMB-45, Melan A, MiTF, or tyrosinase), which are useful diagnostic adjuncts. This example demonstrated diffuse cytoplasmic HMB-45 reactivity. Expression may be more focal than seen in this case.

Epithelioid PEComa

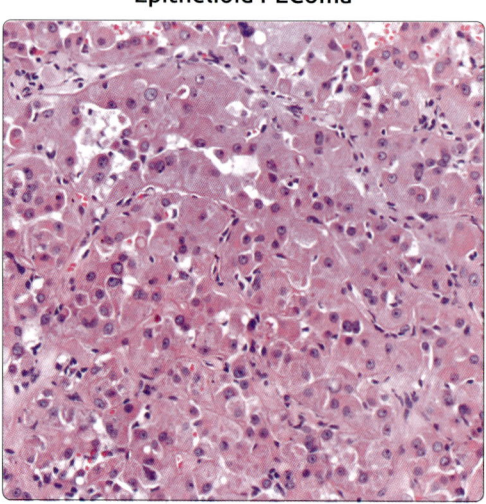

Epithelioid PEComa: Malignant

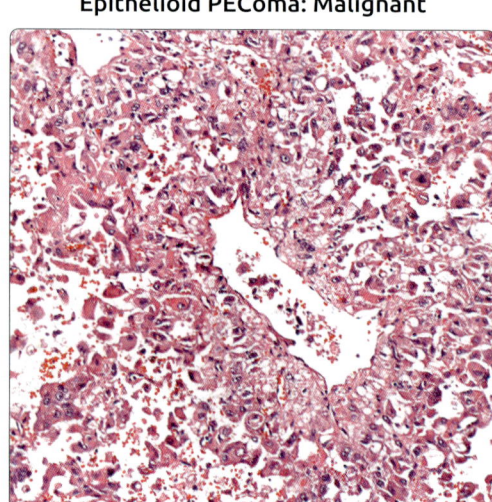

(Left) PEComa may show a predominant epithelioid morphology. This feature may suggest a carcinoma. The absence of CK expression and consideration of PEComa with appropriate markers would be needed in these more difficult cases. **(Right)** Epithelioid PEComas may also have nuclear atypia and may show signs of malignant behavior. The arrangement of the neoplastic cells within the wall of this blood vessel is a very characteristic feature that should suggest the possibility of PEComa. IHC confirmation is mandatory.

Other Mesenchymal Tumors

Endometrial Stromal Sarcoma
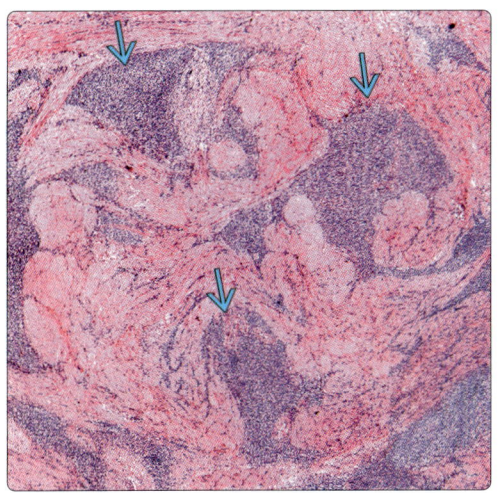

Endometrial Stromal Sarcoma
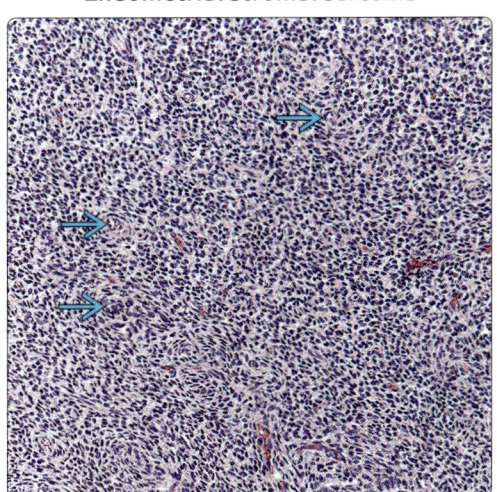

(Left) Endometrial stromal sarcoma may rarely involve the urinary bladder, either as metastatic disease or neoplastic progression from endometriosis. The infiltration of the bladder wall in large, separate irregular tongues ➡ (as also seen in the uterus) is a characteristic feature. (Right) The neoplastic cells of low-grade endometrial stromal sarcoma are typically very uniform with oval to fusiform shaped cells containing very little cytoplasm. The typical network of arterioles may be subtle ➡, particularly at low magnification.

Endometrial Stromal Sarcoma
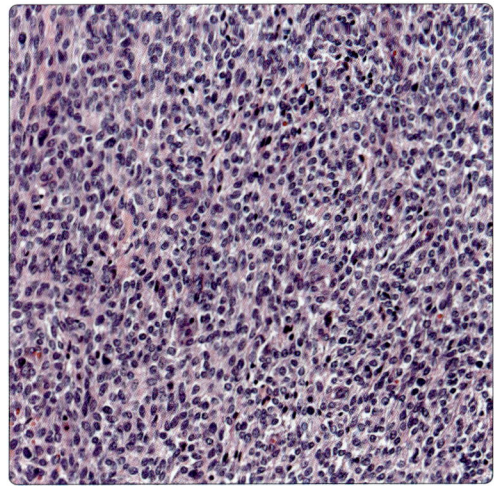

Endometrial Stromal Sarcoma
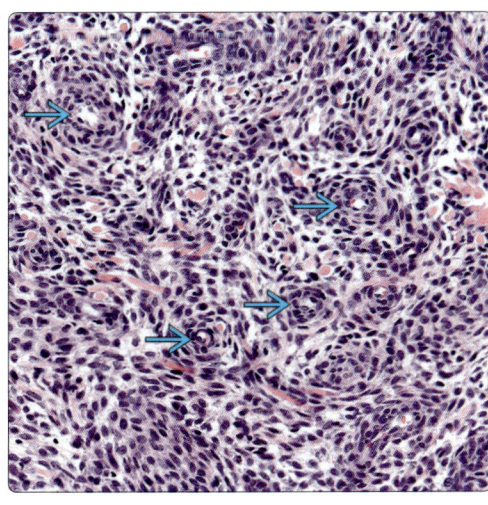

(Left) The monomorphic oval to fusiform cells with fine nuclear chromatin are demonstrated in this example of low-grade endometrial stromal sarcoma. This pattern may mimic other monomorphic sarcoma subtypes (e.g., synovial sarcoma). (Right) On higher magnification, the characteristic arteriole network of low-grade endometrial stromal sarcoma is seen ➡. The neoplastic cells may have a subtle whorled appearance around the blood vessels.

Soft Tissue Filler
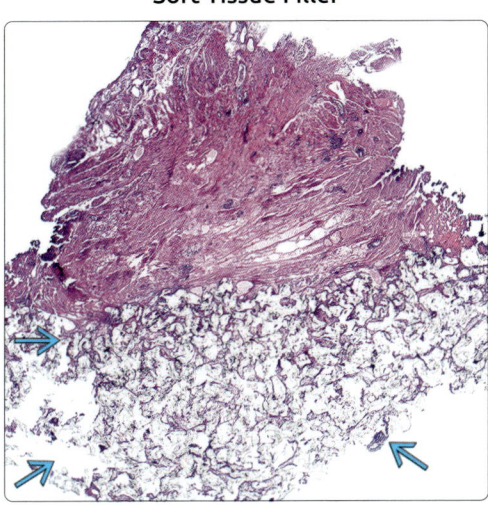

Soft Tissue Filler
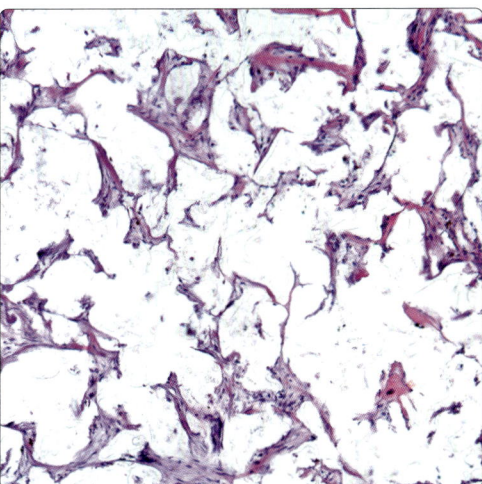

(Left) Soft tissue fillers may be utilized in surgical procedures for urinary stress incontinence. Out of context, these aggregates of soft tissue fillers may mimic a neoplastic mass ➡, both clinically and pathologically. (Right) Postsurgical aggregates of soft tissue fillers used during prior operative procedures, as for urinary stress incontinence, may later cause a mass lesion. Histologically, they often mimic a myxoid mesenchymal neoplasm. Although histiocytes and giant cells may be admixed, they lack a population of spindle cells.

Paraganglioma

KEY FACTS

CLINICAL ISSUES
- < 0.05% of bladder tumors
- Patients frequently present with hematuria
- Other systemic paraganglioma symptoms in up to 15% of cases
- Elevated levels of catecholamines in serum and urine
- Frequent association with hereditary neoplasia syndromes
  - Frequently germline *SDHB* mutation
    - More commonly have malignant behavior
  - Less commonly von Hippel Lindau disease

MACROSCOPIC
- Commonly intramural nodules on lateral wall

MICROSCOPIC
- Most have classic zellballen pattern
- Rarely, more diffuse &/or sclerosing pattern of growth
- Scattered pleomorphic cells are often present (i.e., endocrine anaplasia)

ANCILLARY TESTS
- Express neuroendocrine markers by immunohistochemistry (e.g., synaptophysin, chromogranin A, and CD56)
- Sustentacular cells highlighted by S100 protein (not always present)
- Neoplastic cells are typically negative for cytokeratin
- Also express nuclear GATA3
- Testing for *SDHB* loss by immunohistochemistry is recommended
  - High rate of associated SDH germline mutations

TOP DIFFERENTIAL DIAGNOSES
- Invasive urothelial carcinoma
- High-grade prostatic adenocarcinoma
- Metastatic renal cell carcinoma
- Malignant melanoma
- Other endocrine neoplasms

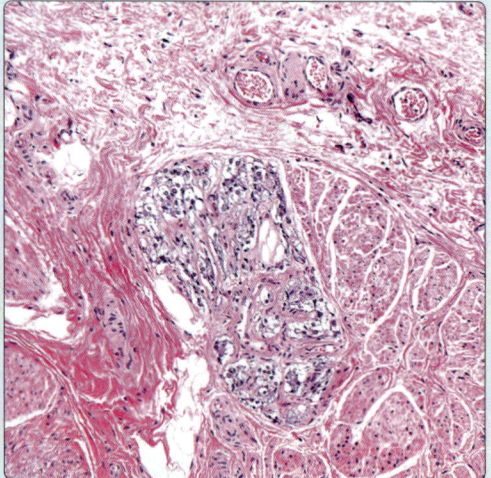
Normal Paraganglia Cells in Bladder

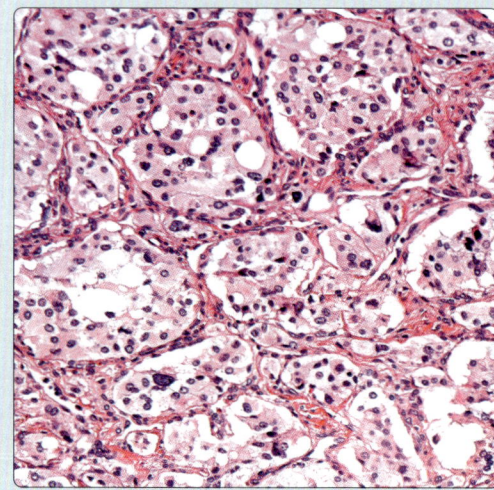
Paraganglioma Architecture

(Left) Normal collections of paraganglia cells are incidentally encountered in random histologic sections from cystectomy specimens. These cells represent the origin of the rare paraganglioma of the urinary bladder. (Right) The classic nested or zellballen architecture of paraganglioma may mimic an invasive urothelial carcinoma with a nested growth pattern. An awareness of paraganglioma is important and should be in the differential diagnosis of an unusual urothelial carcinoma with solid architecture.

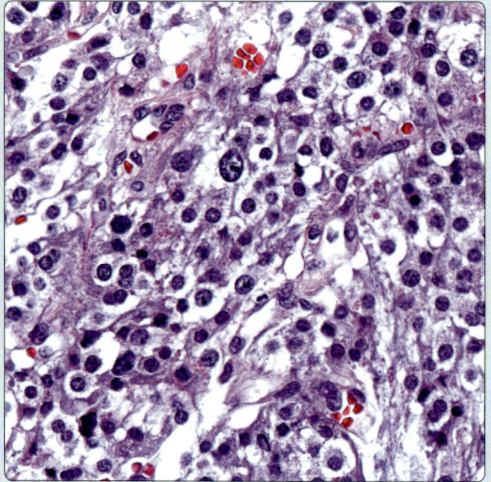
Paraganglioma Cytology

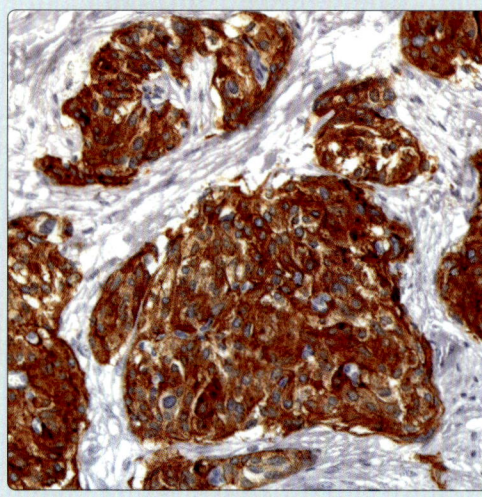
Synaptophysin in Paraganglioma

(Left) The nuclear contours of paraganglioma are typically round and sharp, but scattered individual enlarged cells may be present. This monotonous nuclear morphology may suggest prostatic adenocarcinoma, but nucleoli are not typically prominent in paraganglioma. (Right) Diffuse cytoplasmic synaptophysin immunoreactivity is a helpful ancillary finding to aid in the differential diagnosis of urothelial carcinoma. The absence of cytokeratin staining is also helpful.

Paraganglioma

TERMINOLOGY

Synonyms
- Pheochromocytoma of bladder

Definitions
- Neoplasm derived from paraganglia cells in bladder wall in which sole criterion for malignancy is metastasis

ETIOLOGY/PATHOGENESIS

Hereditary Etiology
- Paragangliomas in urinary bladder are often associated with hereditary syndrome
  - Associated with germline mutations in SDH genes
    - *SDHB* (1p35-p36.1) most common
    - *SDHA* (5p15)
    - *SDHC* (1q21)
    - *SDHD* (11q23)
  - Present at younger age
  - May have association with other neoplasms
    - Other paragangliomas
    - Unique SDH-deficient renal cell carcinomas
    - Unique gastrointestinal stromal tumors of stomach
    - Pituitary neoplasia
- Less commonly associated with von Hippel Lindau disease
  - 11% of cases from hereditary neoplasia referral center
- Rare case reports of association with neurofibromatosis

CLINICAL ISSUES

Epidemiology
- Incidence
  - Majority described in case reports
  - < 0.05% of bladder tumors
- Age
  - 10-90 years
    - Younger ages more commonly SDH deficient

Site
- Urinary bladder
  - Most frequent extraadrenal site of urinary tract

Presentation
- Hematuria
  - Most common presentation
- Other symptoms (15-30%)
  - Headache, palpitations, and sweating during micturition
  - Hypertension

Laboratory Tests
- Elevated serum and urine catecholamines are common

Natural History
- Most are clinically benign

Treatment
- Surgical approaches
  - Complete excision

Prognosis
- Local recurrence with incomplete excision
- 10% demonstrate malignant behavior (i.e., metastasis)
- Subset with *SDHB* loss is more commonly malignant

MACROSCOPIC

General Features
- Intramural nodules
  - Lateral wall common

Size
- Most < 5 cm

MICROSCOPIC

Histologic Features
- Typically well circumscribed
- Classic zellballen (or nested) arrangement of tumor cells
  - Surrounding vascular network
- Diffuse pattern of growth in subset of cases
- Sclerosing pattern may mimic invasive growth
  - Dense hyalinized collagen between nests of tumor cells
- Neoplastic cells are round to polygonal
  - Abundant eosinophilic granular to clear cytoplasm
  - Cytoplasm may occasionally be basophilic
- Central nucleus with vesicular chromatin
  - Nuclear inclusions may be present
- Mitoses can be present
- Scattered pleomorphic cells are often present (i.e., endocrine atypia)
- Rare cases may have calcification
- Surface urothelium is intact and normal
- Artifactual changes in transurethral resection of bladder specimens may create even more diagnostic difficulty
  - Cautery-induced cell spindling may closely mimic sarcoma
  - Mechanical biopsy-related trauma may create pseudopapillary architecture
  - Stromal retraction may also be present around tumor cell nests
- Very rare examples are described with features of composite paraganglioma-ganglioneuroma
- Tumors may infiltrate muscularis propria and have vascular-lymphatic invasion
- Metastasis is only reliable criterion for malignancy

Predominant Pattern/Injury Type
- Neoplastic

Predominant Cell/Compartment Type
- Neuroendocrine

ANCILLARY TESTS

Immunohistochemistry
- Express neuroendocrine markers
  - Synaptophysin, chromogranin A, and CD56
- Sustentacular cells highlighted by S100 protein (but not always present)
- Paraganglioma cells are negative for epithelial markers
  - Cytokeratin, EMA, and p63
- Nuclear expression of GATA3 is typical
  - Major diagnostic pitfall given overlap with urothelial carcinoma

Paraganglioma

- Loss of SDHB staining is not uncommon (~ 1/3 of urinary bladder paragangliomas)
  - Strongly correlates with germline SDH mutation of any type
  - SDHB-deficient cases are more commonly malignant

DIFFERENTIAL DIAGNOSIS

Invasive Urothelial Carcinoma (Nested, Large Nested, or Typical Types)

- May or may not be associated with papillary or in situ urothelial carcinoma
- Endophytic (inverted) patterns may have significant architectural overlap with paraganglioma
- Varying shapes of infiltrating nests
  - Present diffusely within lamina propria
  - Stromal reaction variable
    - Surrounding retraction spaces common
  - Nested (or large nested) variant may mimic zellballen architecture
- Immunoreactive for cytokeratin and p63
  - Key immunohistochemical distinction from paraganglioma
- May show immunoreactivity for urothelial-specific markers
  - Uroplakin-2 and -3 are reportedly specific for urothelial origin
  - GATA3 staining not useful
    - Also stains nuclei of paraganglioma

Granular Cell Tumor

- Lack fine vascular network
- Abundant eosinophilic granular cytoplasm
- Diffuse S100 protein immunoreactivity

Large Cell Neuroendocrine Carcinoma

- Necrosis, abundant mitotic activity, and cellular anaplasia common
- Positive for cytokeratin in addition to neuroendocrine markers
- Negative for S100 protein

Malignant Melanoma

- Anaplasia and prominent nucleoli
- Admixed nested and spindled components are common
- S100 protein is best screening marker
  - Strong and diffuse staining in melanoma
    - In contrast to rare, scattered sustentacular cell pattern of paraganglioma
- Also expresses SOX10
- May also express markers of melanocytic differentiation
  - HMB-45, Melan-A, MITF, and cathepsin-K
- Lack of prior history not uncommon

Metastatic Renal Cell Carcinoma

- Delicate vascular septa may mimic zellballen pattern
- Clear or eosinophilic cytoplasm
- Variable immunoreactivity for renal epithelial markers
  - pax-8, pax-2, RCCma

High-Grade Prostatic Adenocarcinoma

- More prominent nucleoli
- Less nuclear variability
- At least focal luminal differentiation typical
- Immunoreactive for PSA, PAP, and NKX3
  - May also express neuroendocrine markers
- Serum PSA often markedly elevated

Alveolar Soft Part Sarcoma

- Organoid (nested) arrangement with surrounding sinusoidal vascular channels
  - Center of tumor nests often shows loss of cellular cohesion
- Abundant granular eosinophilic cytoplasm
- Intracellular crystalline material by PAS stain
- Unbalanced t(X;17)(p11.2q25) is diagnostic
  - Results in *TFE3-ASPSCR1* fusion

DIAGNOSTIC CHECKLIST

Clinically Relevant Pathologic Features

- No reliable morphologic features for predicting malignant behavior
- Subset are associated with SDH mutation
  - Screening with *SDHB* immunohistochemistry is recommended
    - Will identify protein loss due to mutation in any of SDH genes
      - *SDHA*, *SDHB*, *SDHC*, or *SDHD*
- Rarely associated with von Hippel Lindau disease

Pathologic Interpretation Pearls

- Awareness and consideration of paraganglioma in bladder is key to its distinction from other tumors
- Paraganglioma should be considered in younger patients, in female patients, and with nested architecture and endocrine type atypia
- GATA3 cannot be used as screening marker for urothelial carcinoma in this setting
  - Cytokeratin must be included in testing panel

SELECTED REFERENCES

1. Martucci VL et al: Association of urinary bladder paragangliomas with germline mutations in the SDHB and VHL genes. Urol Oncol. 33(4):167.e13-20, 2015
2. Pai R et al: Usefulness of Succinate dehydrogenase B (SDHB) immunohistochemistry in guiding mutational screening among patients with pheochromocytoma-paraganglioma syndromes. APMIS. 122(11):1130-5, 2014
3. Mason EF et al: Identification of succinate dehydrogenase-deficient bladder paragangliomas. Am J Surg Pathol. 37(10):1612-8, 2013
4. So JS et al: GATA3 expression in paragangliomas: a pitfall potentially leading to misdiagnosis of urothelial carcinoma. Mod Pathol. 26(10):1365-70, 2013
5. Gill AJ et al: Immunohistochemistry for SDHB triages genetic testing of SDHB, SDHC, and SDHD in paraganglioma-pheochromocytoma syndromes. Hum Pathol. 41(6):805-14, 2010
6. Plaza JA et al: Sclerosing paraganglioma: report of 19 cases of an unusual variant of neuroendocrine tumor that may be mistaken for an aggressive malignant neoplasm. Am J Surg Pathol. 30(1):7-12, 2006
7. Kovacs K et al: Malignant paraganglioma of the urinary bladder: Immunohistochemical study of prognostic indicators. Endocr Pathol. 16(4):363-9, 2005
8. Zhou M et al: Paraganglioma of the urinary bladder: a lesion that may be misdiagnosed as urothelial carcinoma in transurethral resection specimens. Am J Surg Pathol. 28(1):94-100, 2004
9. Cheng L et al: Paraganglioma of the urinary bladder: can biologic potential be predicted? Cancer. 88(4):844-52, 2000
10. Moyana TN et al: Urinary bladder paragangliomas. An immunohistochemical study. Arch Pathol Lab Med. 112(1):70-2, 1988

Paraganglioma

Small, Incidental Paraganglioma

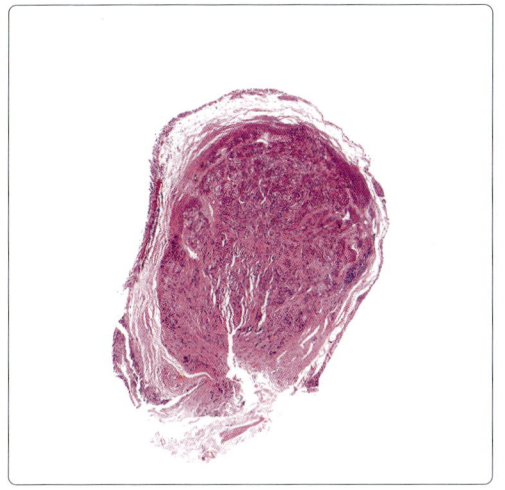

Paraganglioma (Classic Zellballen)

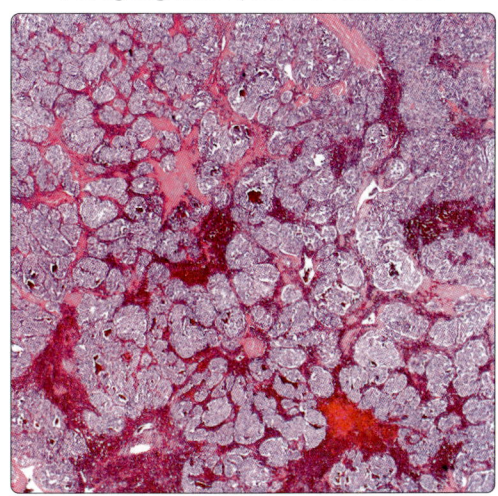

(Left) This small, incidental paraganglioma was removed during a cystoscopy performed for a resection of a papillary urothelial neoplasm. This example is more superficially located than typically seen. (Right) This low-power photomicrograph shows an example of a paraganglioma with striking nested architecture. This is the prototypical zellballen pattern that is characteristic of paraganglioma. The presence of intervening extravasated red blood cells is not uncommon.

Paraganglioma: Fibrovascular Septa

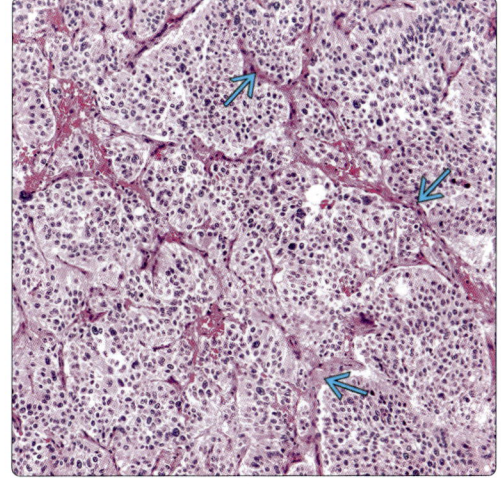

Paraganglioma: Round Nuclei

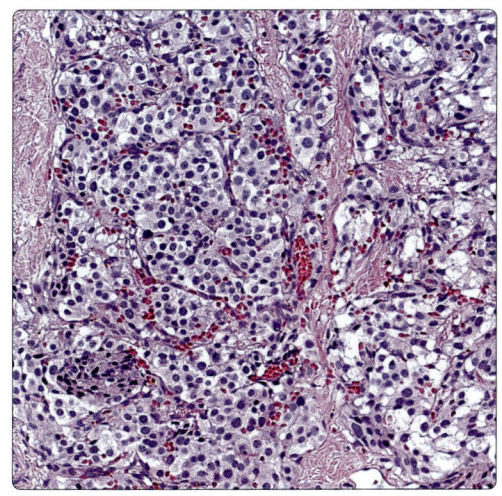

(Left) This example of paraganglioma in the urinary bladder has larger nests that appear more complex and serpiginous. Distinct vascular septa are seen between the tumor cell nests ➡. (Right) The nests of tumor cells in paraganglioma are encircled by fine vascular septa. The neoplastic cells are round and monomorphic. This pattern may suggest the possibility of an invasive urothelial carcinoma with a nested pattern or possibly a high-grade prostatic adenocarcinoma.

Paraganglioma With Basophilia

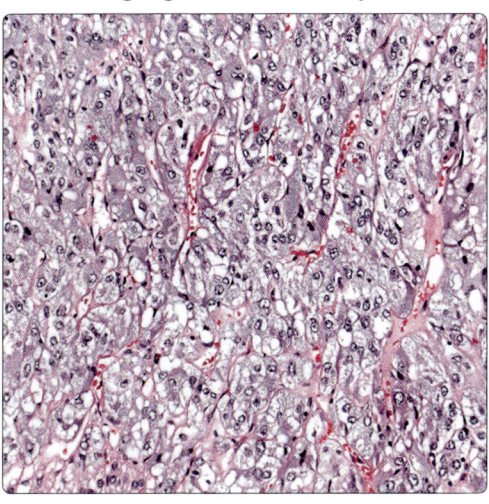

Paraganglioma With Nuclear Inclusions

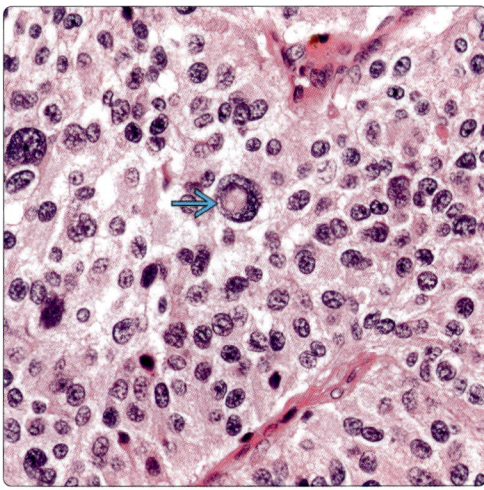

(Left) This paraganglioma has a more basophilic (or amphophilic) cytoplasm. This histologic appearance is identical to that of prototypical adrenal pheochromocytoma. In this example, the nested architecture is more subtle. (Right) In addition to the presence of scattered pleomorphic tumor cells, paragangliomas may have distinct intranuclear inclusions ➡, as seen in this example.

Paraganglioma

Paraganglioma With Endocrine Atypia
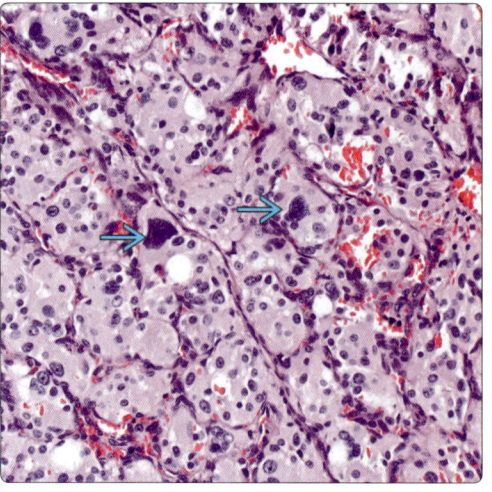

Paraganglioma With Nuclear Atypia
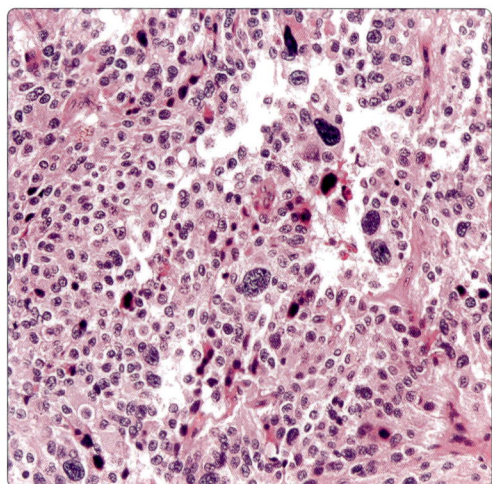

(Left) Scattered neoplastic cells with marked variation in size and shape (i.e., endocrine anaplasia) are common in paraganglioma and do not denote malignancy ⇒. This is a helpful diagnostic feature that should suggest a neuroendocrine tumor. (Right) This example of paraganglioma shows more striking nuclear atypia with pleomorphism and nuclear hyperchromasia. The majority of the background neoplastic cells show more typical monophonic round nuclei.

Paraganglioma With Less-Pronounced Nests
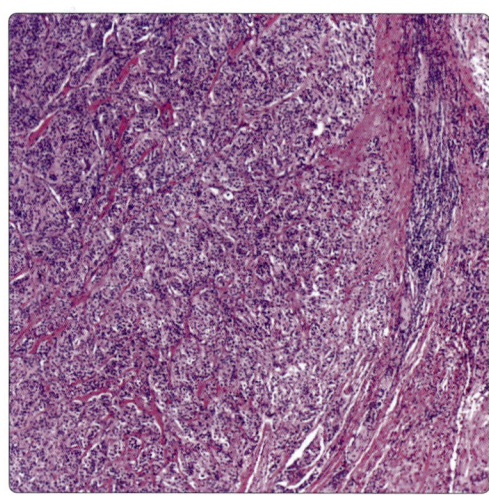

Paraganglioma With Typical Circumscription
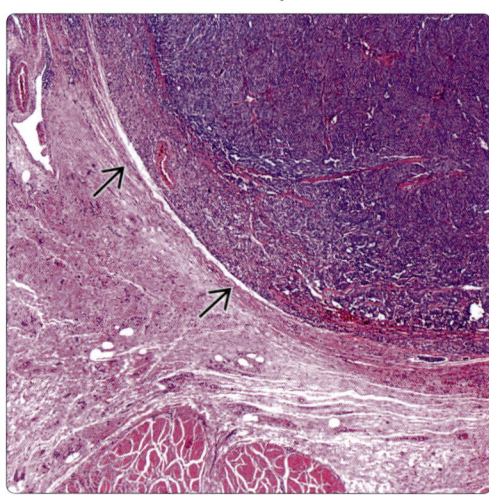

(Left) On low-power examination, this paraganglioma has a more vaguely nested growth pattern. Considering the possibility of paraganglioma at this site is important to its recognition. The correct diagnosis has prognostic and therapeutic implications. (Right) The interface of paraganglioma with the surrounding bladder soft tissues is usually well delineated ⇒. In carcinomas, a more irregular, infiltrative border is typically seen at scanning magnification.

Associated Normal Urothelium
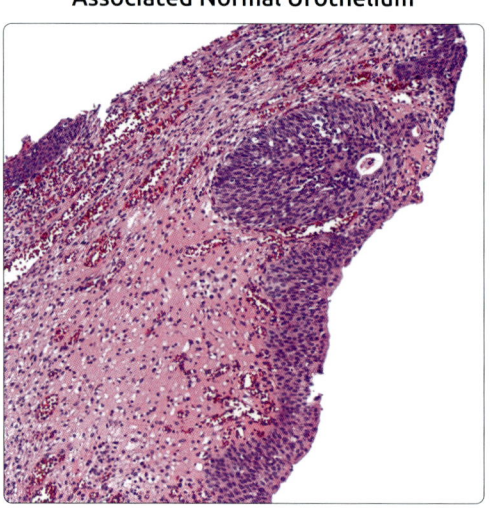

Confounding Prior Biopsy Site Changes
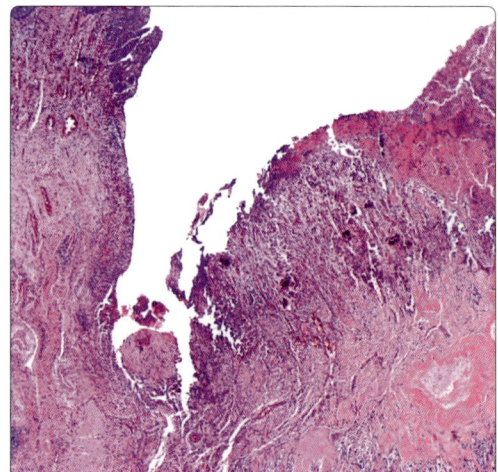

(Left) Other morphologic clues may be helpful in recognizing paraganglioma. A normal surface urothelium is typically seen overlying paragangliomas of the urinary bladder. (Right) Surface ulceration due to prior transurethral resection may distort the tissue or impart an artifactual papillary appearance in subsequent excision specimens. These changes may cause additional confusion with urothelial carcinoma.

Paraganglioma

Sclerosing Paraganglioma

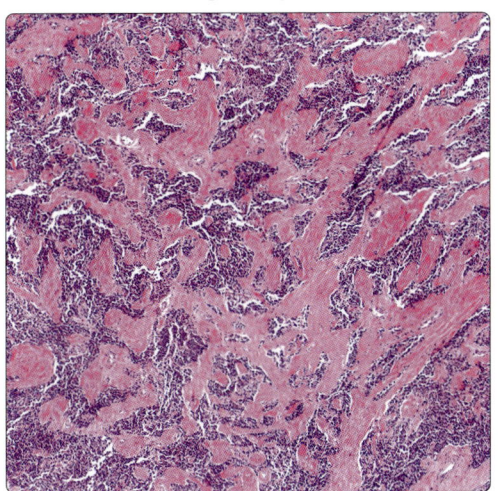

Sclerosing Paraganglioma

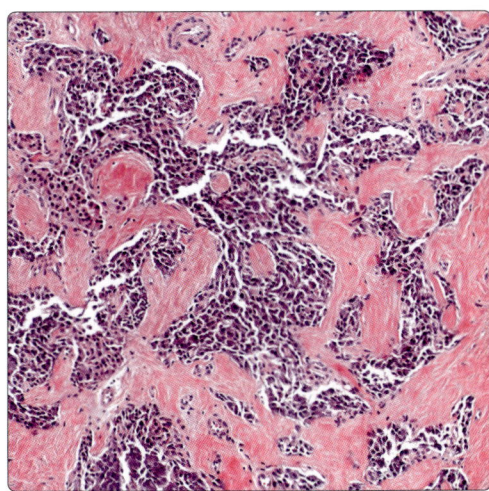

(Left) Paragangliomas may have a striking component of hyalinized collagen that distorts the typical architecture and more closely mimics invasive carcinoma. This example shows an irregular, tongue-like, anastomosing architectural growth pattern that closely mimics destructive tissue invasion. *(Right)* Because of this significant degree of morphologic overlap with invasive urothelial carcinoma, awareness of this sclerosing pattern of paraganglioma is important.

Sclerosing Paraganglioma

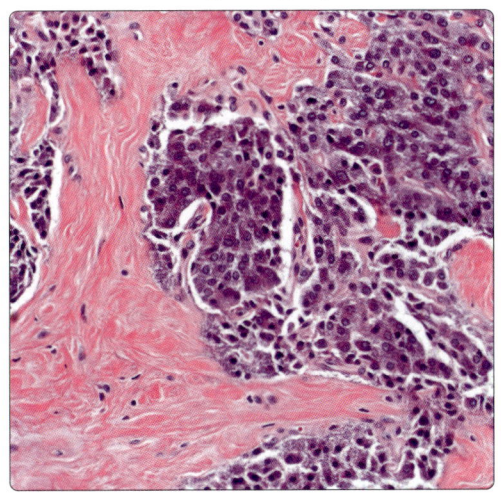

Sclerosing Paraganglioma

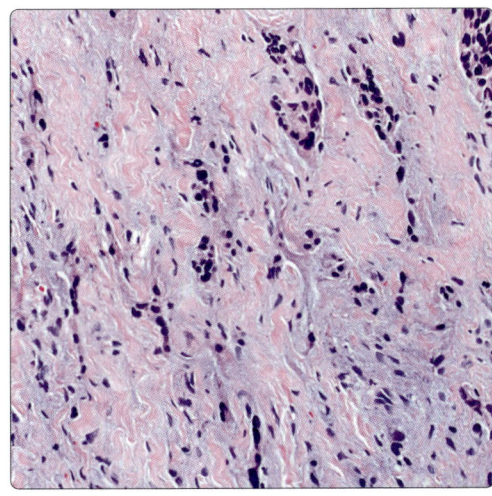

(Left) The classic individual cell nests (zellballen pattern) are often not apparent in some paragangliomas with a more sclerosing morphology. On higher magnification, the tumor cells have the typical round nuclear contours and granular cytoplasm. *(Right)* In rare examples of sclerosing paraganglioma, the fibrotic tissue may comprise the majority of the lesion. Immunohistochemical confirmation with cytokeratin (-) and synaptophysin (+) may be essential in such cases.

Sclerosing Paraganglioma

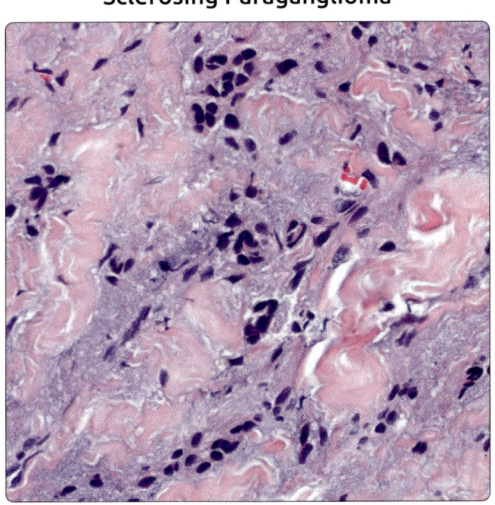

Sclerosing Paraganglioma

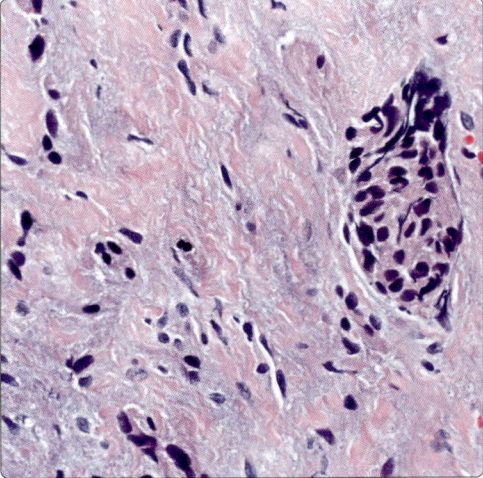

(Left) In this paraganglioma, a poorly differentiated invasive urothelial carcinoma is a strong consideration given the extensive degree of sclerosis and cord-like architectural growth. *(Right)* Recognition of rare scattered nests and a high index of suspicion for paraganglioma is essential to recognize these morphologically difficult cases. Confirmatory immunostains for synaptophysin and keratin are critical to properly classifying such cases.

Paraganglioma

Paraganglioma With Stromal Retraction
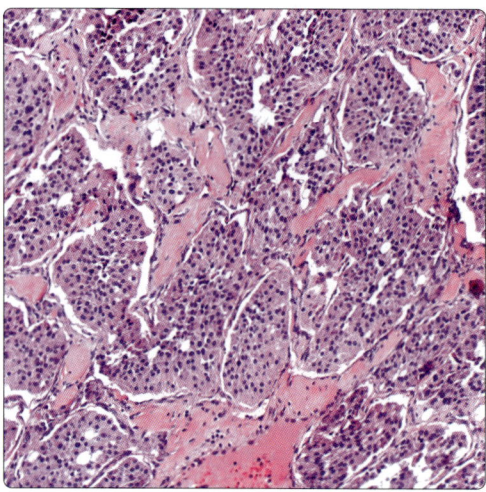

Paraganglioma With Biopsy Artifact
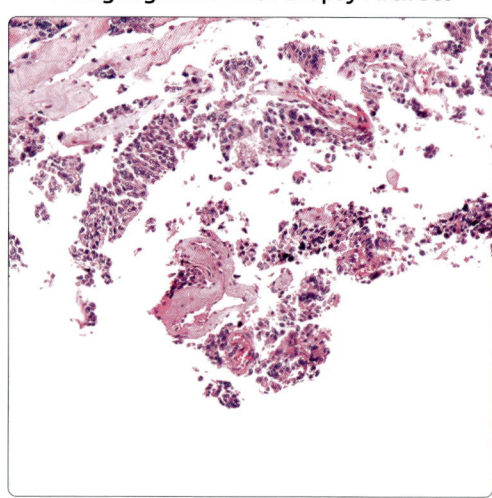

(Left) Retraction artifact, as seen in this example of paraganglioma, may closely mimic invasive urothelial carcinoma. An immunohistochemical work-up is useful in such cases. *(Right)* Mechanical biopsy artifact may lead to marked tissue disruption and can produce artifactual patterns that may potentially mimic a papillary architecture with dyscohesive tumor cells surrounding vessels.

Paraganglioma With Cautery Artifact
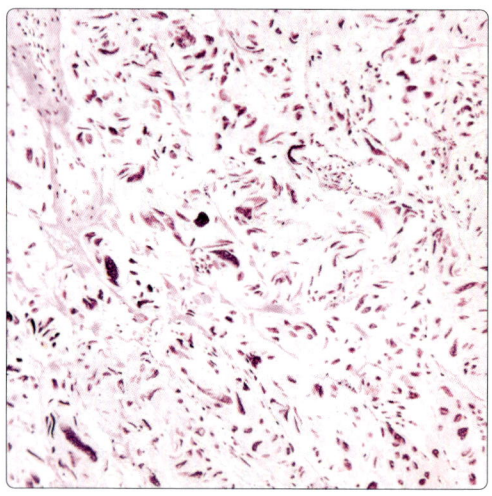

Paraganglioma With Vascular Invasion
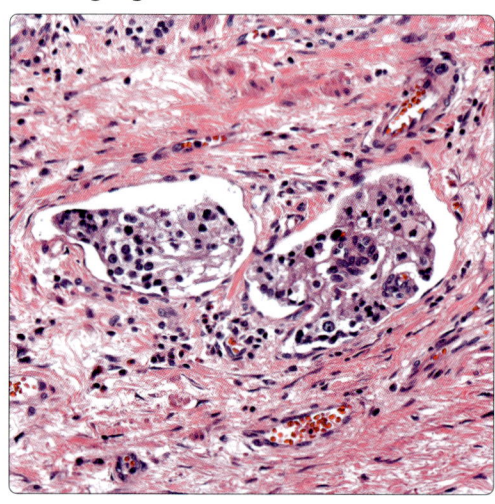

(Left) Cautery artifact due to a transurethral resection of bladder procedure may induce an appearance of cellular spindling. When seen together with nuclear pleomorphism, this may lead to confusion with a vesical sarcoma or sarcomatoid carcinoma. *(Right)* Definitive lymphovascular invasion was identified in this example of a clinically malignant paraganglioma. Malignant potential may be impossible to predict by morphologic examination.

Metastatic Paraganglioma to Lymph Node
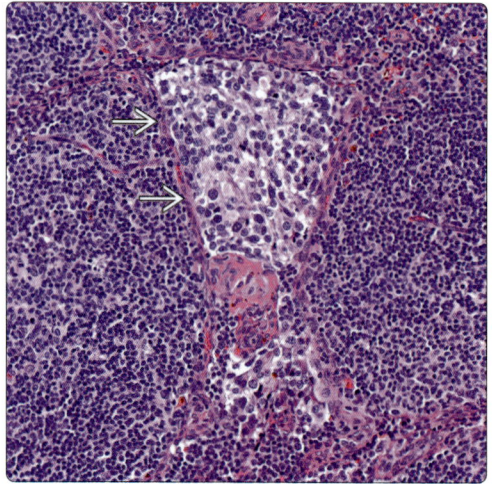

Synaptophysin in Metastatic Paraganglioma
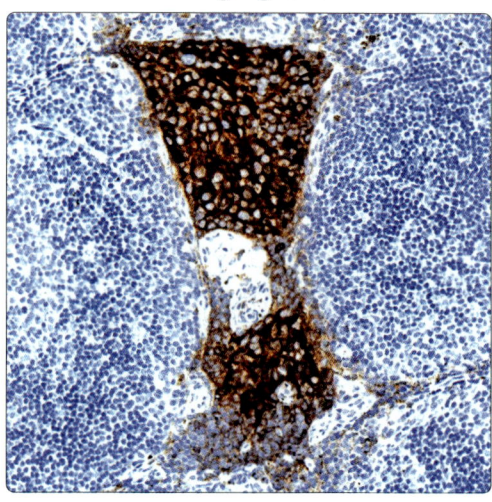

(Left) Metastatic paraganglioma may be identified in regional lymph nodes ➡. Histologic features do not adequately predict malignancy in paraganglioma, which is defined by the presence of metastasis. *(Right)* Strong cytoplasmic immunoreactivity with chromogranin highlights the metastatic paraganglioma in this lymph node. Expression of endocrine markers, in the absence of keratin expression, is characteristic of paraganglioma.

Paraganglioma

Synaptophysin in Paraganglioma
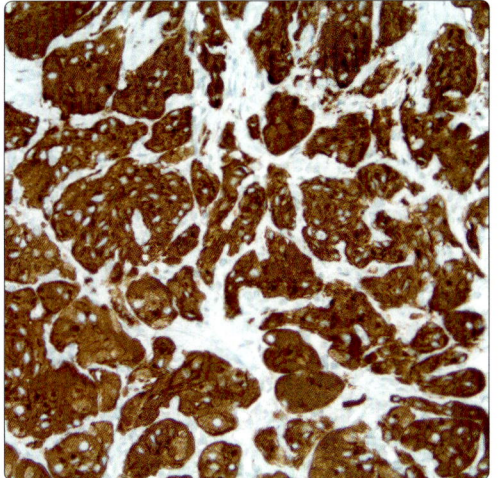

Chromogranin in Paraganglioma
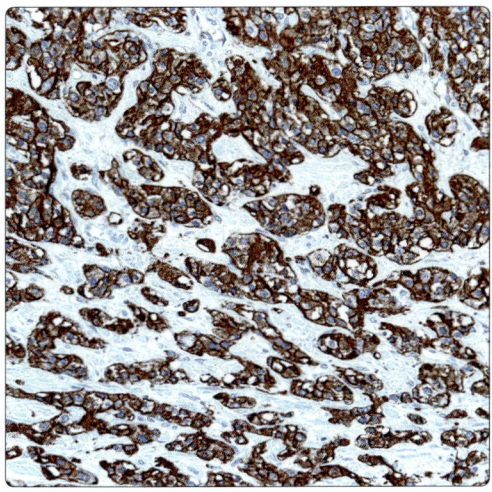

(Left) Strong and diffuse cytoplasmic reactivity with synaptophysin is characteristic of paraganglioma. In the differential diagnostic distinction with urothelial carcinoma, this finding (together with an absence of keratin expression) strongly supports a paraganglioma diagnosis. (Right) Strong cytoplasmic positivity with chromogranin A is also typical of paraganglioma.

S100 Protein in Paraganglioma
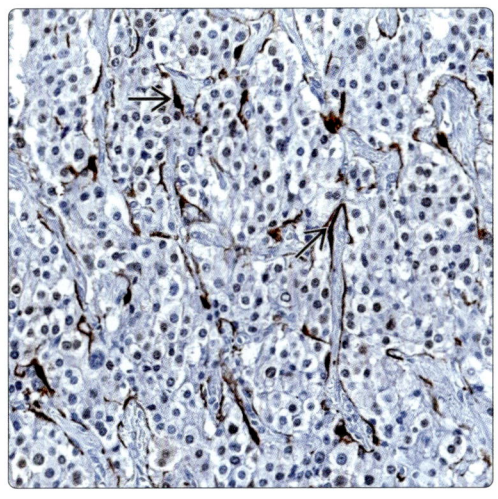

p63 in Paraganglioma
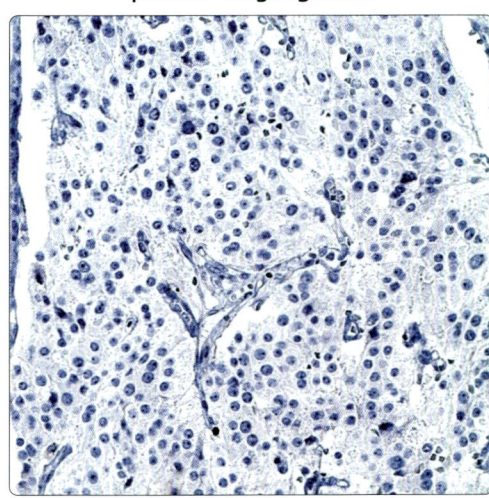

(Left) S100 protein immunohistochemistry highlights obvious sustentacular cells ➡ in this paraganglioma. These sustentacular cells may not always be readily apparent, even after immunohistochemical evaluation. Synaptophysin is, therefore, the most sensitive marker for paraganglioma. (Right) As typical, this paraganglioma does not show nuclear immunoreactivity for p63. In contrast, urothelial carcinoma commonly expresses p63.

GATA3 in Paraganglioma
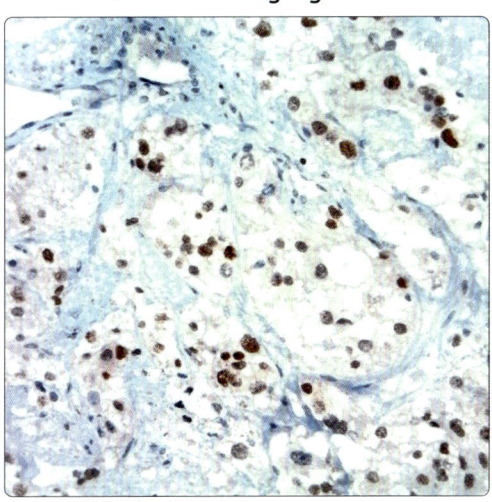

SDHB Loss in Paraganglioma
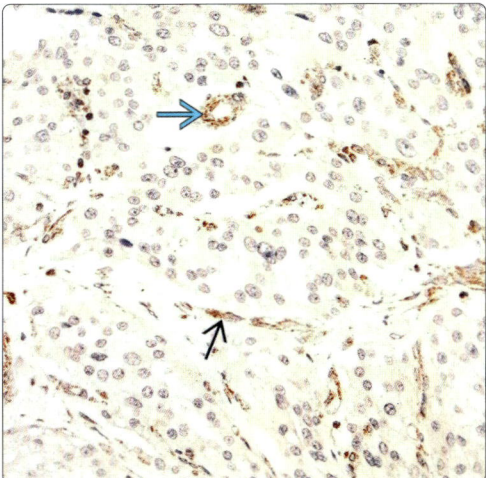

(Left) GATA3 typically shows nuclear reactivity in paragangliomas; therefore, it cannot be used in the distinction from urothelial carcinoma. (Right) In an SDH-deficient paraganglioma, there is loss of granular cytoplasmic staining in the neoplastic cells, while very good internal control staining is present in intratumoral endothelial cells ➡ and pericytes ➡. This loss has a strong correlation with an underlying germline SDH mutation.

Metastatic and Secondary Carcinomas

KEY FACTS

TERMINOLOGY
- Urinary bladder may be involved secondarily by direct extension of tumors from adjacent sites or by metastases from distant sites

CLINICAL ISSUES
- Comprise 2-15% of malignant bladder tumors
  - Prostate
  - Colorectal
  - Gynecologic tract

MACROSCOPIC
- Generally, multiple mass lesions with intramural location

MICROSCOPIC
- Metastases may have pagetoid growth

ANCILLARY TESTS
- Immunoreactivity dependent on primary site of origin
  - Colorectal adenocarcinoma and primary bladder adenocarcinoma may have identical phenotype
    - Nuclear β-catenin may be specific for colonic origin
  - Breast carcinoma may maintain GATA3, ER, GCDFP-15, and mammaglobin reactivity
- Absence of specific urothelial carcinoma markers (Uroplakin II has some potential)

TOP DIFFERENTIAL DIAGNOSES
- Primary adenocarcinoma of urinary bladder
- Urothelial carcinoma with glandular differentiation
- Urothelial carcinoma with squamous differentiation
- Primary squamous cell carcinoma of bladder
- Müllerianosis/endometriosis
- Specific variants of urothelial carcinoma
  - Plasmacytoid
  - Micropapillary
  - Glycogen-rich

Prostatic Adenocarcinoma
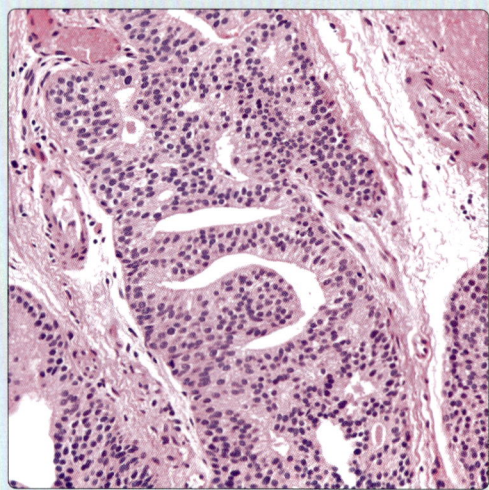

Cervical Squamous Cell Carcinoma
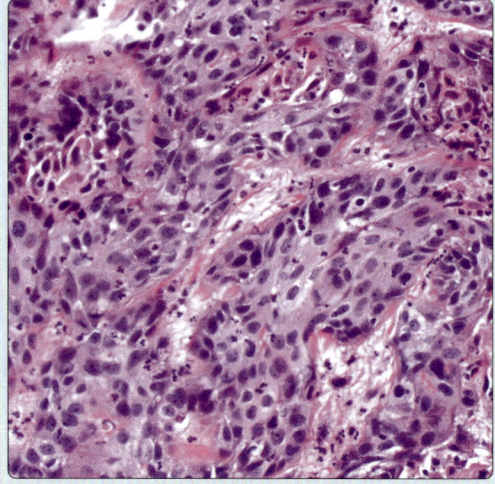

(Left) High grade prostatic adenocarcinomas, typically with solid and cribriform growth patterns, may involve the urinary bladder and can closely mimic urothelial carcinoma. (Right) Invasion of the urinary bladder from an adjacent cervical squamous cell carcinoma, as seen in this example, presents a diagnostic challenge, since squamous differentiation is not uncommon in urothelial carcinomas. Clinical/imaging correlation is essential.

Endometrioid Adenocarcinoma of Uterus
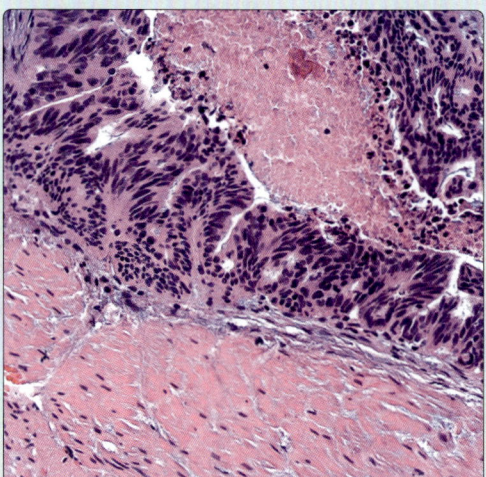

Metastatic Adenocarcinoma of Breast
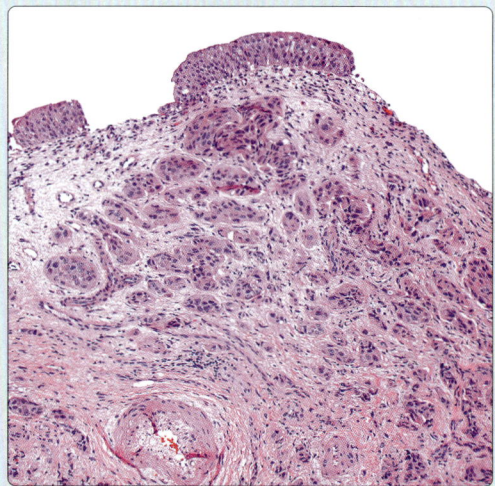

(Left) Other gynecologic tract carcinomas, such as this example of endometrioid adenocarcinoma of the uterine corpus, may involve the urinary bladder by direct extension. (Right) Rarely, distant metastases may involve the urinary bladder. These may be more difficult to diagnose because of the absence of a radiographically detectable mass in an adjacent organ.

Metastatic and Secondary Carcinomas

TERMINOLOGY

Definitions
- Urinary bladder may be involved secondarily by carcinomas
  - Direct extension from adjacent anatomic sites
  - Metastases from distant anatomic sites

CLINICAL ISSUES

Epidemiology
- Incidence
  - Comprise 2-15% of malignant tumors in the urinary bladder
  - Some common primary sites include
    - Colon (21%)
    - Prostate (19%)
    - Rectum (12%)
    - Uterine cervix (11%)
    - Melanoma, ovary, gastric, and breast (rare)

Site
- Bladder neck and trigone

Presentation
- Hematuria

Treatment
- Dependent on primary site and tumor subtype
- Resection may be required to stop hemorrhage

Prognosis
- Poor prognosis secondary to high-stage malignancy

MACROSCOPIC

General Features
- Polypoid bladder mass
  - May be multiple and often intramural

MICROSCOPIC

Histologic Features
- General features of metastatic carcinoma
  - Multiple foci of nodular aggregates of tumors cells
  - Absence of surface mucosal abnormalities
    - No urothelial carcinoma in situ
    - May create pagetoid spread or intramucosal growth
    - No papillary urothelial carcinoma
  - Tumor may show only muscularis propria involvement
  - Extensive or exclusive angiolymphatic involvement suggests metastasis
  - Unusual morphologies may suggest metastasis
- Colorectal adenocarcinoma
  - Enteric-type adenocarcinoma
    - Gland formation with pseudostratified columnar epithelium
    - May be histologically identical to primary bladder adenocarcinoma
    - Surface villous component may be misleading
  - Commonly expresses nuclear β-catenin by immunohistochemistry
    - Bladder adenocarcinomas show membranous and cytoplasmic staining
  - CK7, CK20, and CDX-2 immunophenotype may be identical to primary bladder adenocarcinoma
- Prostatic adenocarcinoma
  - May have sheet-like growth with occasional acinar formation
  - Monomorphic nuclei with round nuclear contours
  - Expresses PSA and PAP by immunohistochemistry
  - Nuclear NKX3.1 expression is very specific for prostate origin
    - Retained staining in high grade carcinomas
- Gynecologic carcinomas
  - Uterine cervical squamous cell carcinoma
    - Identical to primary bladder squamous cell carcinoma or urothelial carcinoma with squamous differentiation
    - Clinical and radiographic correlation is essential
    - Identification of high risk HPV (by PCR or CISH) is a useful adjunctive finding for cervical origin
    - p16 IHC has limited role
  - Ovarian and endometrial carcinoma
    - Clear cell adenocarcinoma
      □ Morphologically and immunophenotypically identical to clear cell adenocarcinoma of urinary tract
      □ Requires clinical and radiographic correlation
    - Serous carcinoma
      □ May mimic poorly differentiated or micropapillary urothelial carcinoma
    - Endometrioid carcinoma
      □ Mimics primary adenocarcinoma or Müllerianosis
- Breast carcinoma
  - Ductal carcinoma may closely mimic typical invasive urothelial carcinoma
  - Lobular carcinoma closely mimics plasmacytoid carcinoma of bladder
  - Expresses GATA3 with nuclear pattern (similar pattern to urothelial)
  - Absence of uroplakin II and positive ER, mammaglobin, &/or GCDFP15 staining may be helpful for confirming breast origin

ANCILLARY TESTS

Immunohistochemistry
- Immunoreactivity dependent on primary site of origin
- Absence of entirely specific urothelial carcinoma markers
  - Uroplakin II, uroplakin III, and S100p have lower sensitivity in urothelial carcinoma
  - GATA3 is sensitive, but is expressed in other carcinomas
  - Non-urothelial carcinomas may express HMWCK(34βE12) and p63; these markers are most useful if prostate adenocarcinoma is in differential

DIFFERENTIAL DIAGNOSIS

Primary Adenocarcinoma of Urinary Bladder
- May have associated precursor lesion
  - Adenocarcinoma in situ or villous adenoma
- Absence of nuclear β-catenin expression
- May have enteric immunophenotype: CK20 and CDX-2 expression

Metastatic and Secondary Carcinomas

- Colonoscopy may be needed in difficult cases to exclude colonic primary
- GATA3 immunoreactivity is rare
- Rare primary mucinous adenocarcinoma of bladder have signet ring cell features
  - May be difficult to distinguish from gastric or colorectal primary

Urothelial Carcinoma With Glandular Differentiation

- Admixed typical urothelial carcinoma component
  - Invasive, papillary, or urothelial carcinoma in situ may be seen
- Absence of nuclear β-catenin expression
- Non-glandular component often expresses more typical urothelial markers

Urothelial Carcinoma With Squamous Differentiation

- May be histologically indistinguishable from cervical primary
- p16 may be expressed in both urothelial and cervical primaries
- Testing for high risk HPV by PCR or CISH methodology is often helpful
  - Generally negative in urothelial carcinoma

Primary Squamous Cell Carcinoma of Bladder

- Often arises in chronic inflammatory conditions
- May have associated keratinizing metaplasia or dysplasia
- In some countries, associated schistosomiasis may be identified
- As in urothelial carcinoma with squamous differentiation, HPV testing may be helpful
  - HPV-related squamous cell carcinoma is exceedingly rare in the bladder
    - Generally have history of precursor HPV lesions in genital region with colonization of urinary tract

Müllerianosis/Endometriosis

- Müllerian-type glands present within bladder wall
  - Tubal or endometrial-type epithelium may be seen
    - Cytologically bland with no destructive invasion

Specific Variants of Invasive Urothelial Carcinoma

- Plasmacytoid carcinoma
  - May mimic a variety of non-urothelial neoplasms
    - Diffuse type gastric carcinoma
    - Lobular breast carcinoma
    - Plasmacytoma/myeloma
    - Lymphoma
  - Strong cytokeratin reactivity, but may also express CD138
    - p63 staining is variable
      - Other screening epithelial markers are more useful
  - Negative for CD45(LCA), ER, GCDFP-15, mammaglobin, and MUM-1
- Micropapillary carcinoma
  - Closely resembles carcinomas with micropapillary features in other sites
    - Breast
    - Ovary: High grade or low grade serous carcinoma
  - ER, pax-8, mammaglobin, and TTF-1 are negative in urothelial primaries
- Glycogen-rich carcinoma
  - May mimic renal cell carcinoma
    - Metastatic renal cell carcinoma to the bladder is quite rare
  - Maintains urothelial immunophenotype
    - Renal cell carcinoma and urothelial carcinoma may both coexpress pax-8 and GATA3
- Poorly differentiated urothelial carcinoma with syncytiotrophoblasts
  - May mimic high grade serous carcinoma with nuclear anaplasia
  - Maintains urothelial immunophenotype

Normal Histologic Variants and Nonneoplastic Changes

- Prominent von Brunn nests with clear cytoplasm may mimic renal cell carcinoma
  - More common in ureter
- Pseudocarcinomatous hyperplasia may mimic squamous cell carcinoma
  - Especially if associated with prior radiation therapy for known cervical carcinoma
  - Other radiation associated changes usually present
- Florid cystitis glandularis with mucin extravasation could mimic secondary mucinous adenocarcinoma

DIAGNOSTIC CHECKLIST

Pathologic Interpretation Pearls

- Non-bladder primaries must be considered before accepting a diagnosis of primary vesical adenocarcinoma
  - Careful radiographic correlation and colonoscopy are often essential
- Multifocality, vascular-lymphatic invasion, and normal surface mucosa should strongly raise possibility of metastasis
- Tumors with only muscularis propria involvement and those with unusual morphologies should strongly raise possibility of non-urothelial origin

SELECTED REFERENCES

1. Tian W et al: Utility of uroplakin II expression as a marker of urothelial carcinoma. Hum Pathol. 46(1):58-64, 2015
2. Gordetsky J et al: Pseudopapillary features in prostatic adenocarcinoma mimicking urothelial carcinoma: a diagnostic pitfall. Am J Surg Pathol. 38(7):941-5, 2014
3. Mohanty SK et al: Evaluation of contemporary prostate and urothelial lineage biomarkers in a consecutive cohort of poorly differentiated bladder neck carcinomas. Am J Clin Pathol. 142(2):173-83, 2014
4. Ellis CL et al: GATA-3 immunohistochemistry in the differential diagnosis of adenocarcinoma of the urinary bladder. Am J Surg Pathol. 37(11):1756-60, 2013
5. Rao Q et al: Distinguishing primary adenocarcinoma of the urinary bladder from secondary involvement by colorectal adenocarcinoma: extended immunohistochemical profiles emphasizing novel markers. Mod Pathol. 26(5):725-32, 2013
6. Bates AW et al: The significance of secondary neoplasms of the urinary and male genital tract. Virchows Arch. 440(6):640-7, 2002
7. Wang HL et al: Immunohistochemical distinction between primary adenocarcinoma of the bladder and secondary colorectal adenocarcinoma. Am J Surg Pathol. 25(11):1380-7, 2001
8. Bates AW et al: Secondary neoplasms of the bladder are histological mimics of nontransitional cell primary tumours: clinicopathological and histological features of 282 cases. Histopathology. 36(1):32-40, 2000

Metastatic and Secondary Carcinomas

Monotonous Appearance

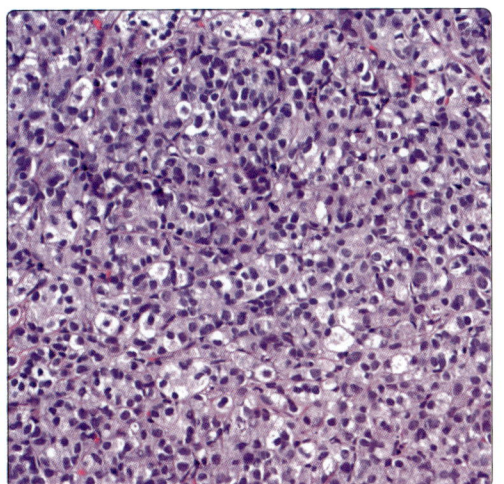

Cribriform/Acinar Pattern

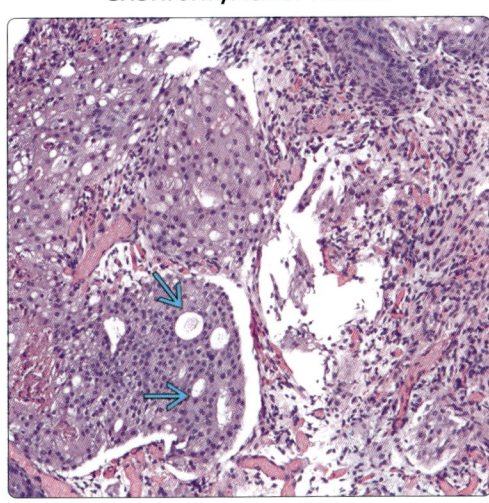

(Left) *Prostatic adenocarcinoma may extend to the bladder. The monotonous appearance of cells with relatively round nuclei and prominent nucleoli is characteristic of prostatic primaries. Immunohistochemistry for PSA(+), NKX3.1(+), and GATA3(-) often help establish prostatic origin.* **(Right)** *The presence of acinar formation with sharply rounded lumina ⇨ is a histologic feature that should strongly suggest prostatic adenocarcinoma.*

Cribriform Pattern

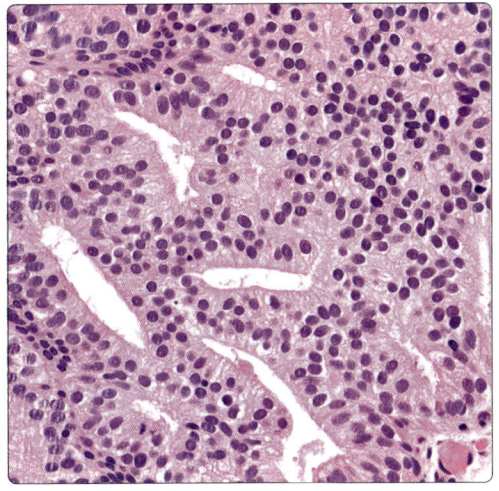

Papillary Pattern

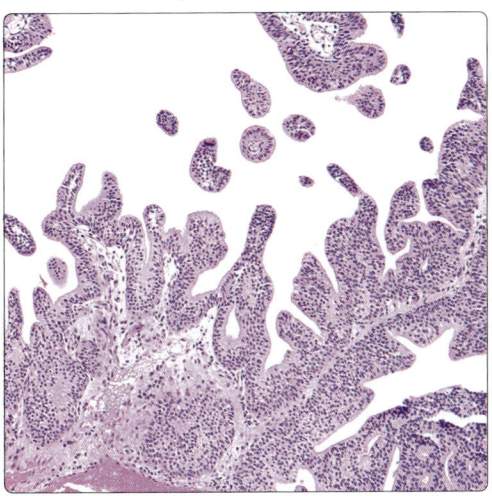

(Left) *The monomorphic appearance with round nuclear contours and acinar formation should strongly suggest the possibility of prostatic epithelial origin. This appearance is almost diagnostic. Nucleoli are not always prominent.* **(Right)** *Unusual histologic features, such as the papillary tufting in this example of prostatic adenocarcinoma involving the urinary bladder, may very closely mimic a papillary urothelial neoplasm.*

Pseudopapillary Pattern

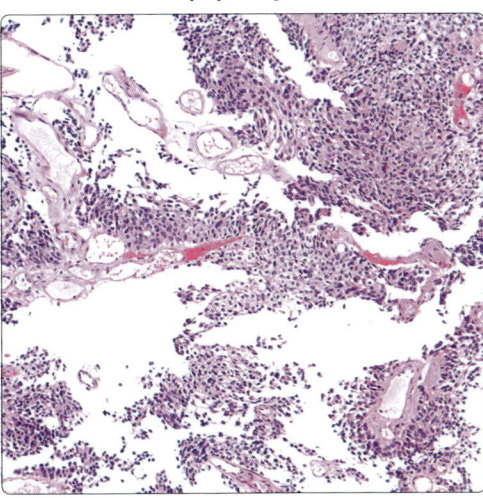

Solid Pattern

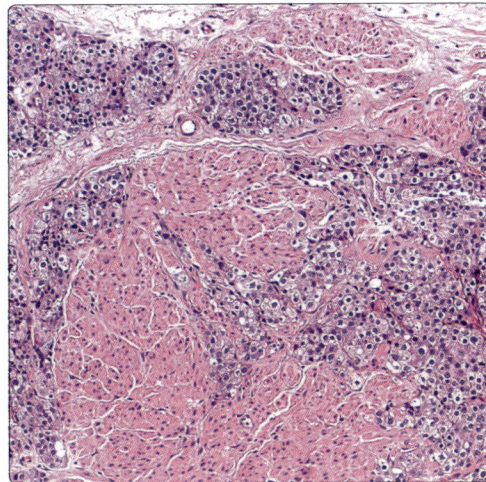

(Left) *Rarely, biopsy artifact may induce a pseudopapillary architecture in prostatic adenocarcinoma. This may cause diagnostic confusion with a noninvasive high-grade papillary urothelial carcinoma.* **(Right)** *This prostatic adenocarcinoma that secondarily involves the urinary bladder shows invasion of the muscularis propria. Out of context, this may very closely mimic primary urothelial carcinoma. Paraganglioma of bladder is also in the differential.*

Metastatic and Secondary Carcinomas

PSA: Prostatic Adenocarcinoma in Bladder

PSMA: Prostatic Adenocarcinoma in Bladder

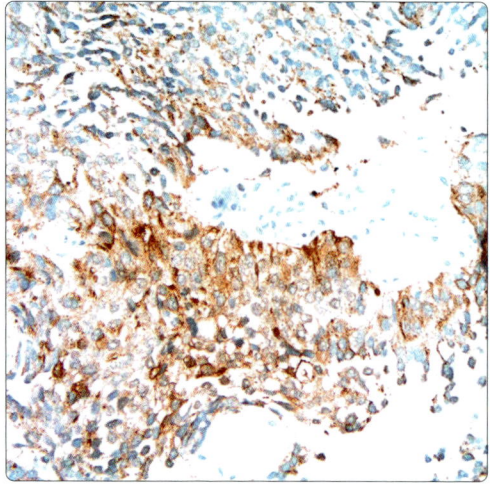
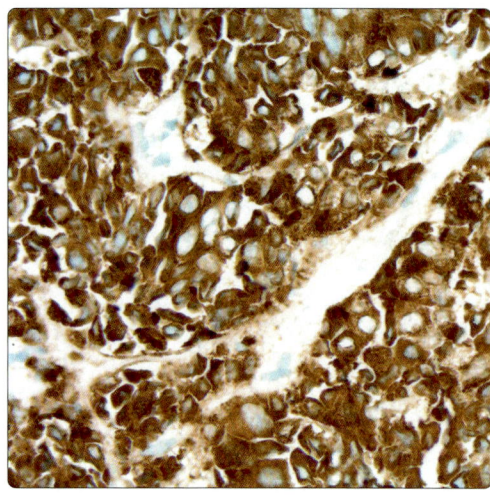

(Left) This example of PSA immunoreactivity in a prostatic adenocarcinoma involving the urinary bladder is relatively strong compared to many high grade carcinomas. Not uncommonly, the PSA staining is more patchy and weak, and may be confined to focal areas with acinar formation. **(Right)** Cytoplasmic PSMA staining in prostatic adenocarcinoma, as seen in this example that involved the urinary bladder, is often more diffuse and more intense compared to PSA.

p63: Prostatic Adenocarcinoma in Bladder

34bE12: Prostatic Adenocarcinoma in Bladder

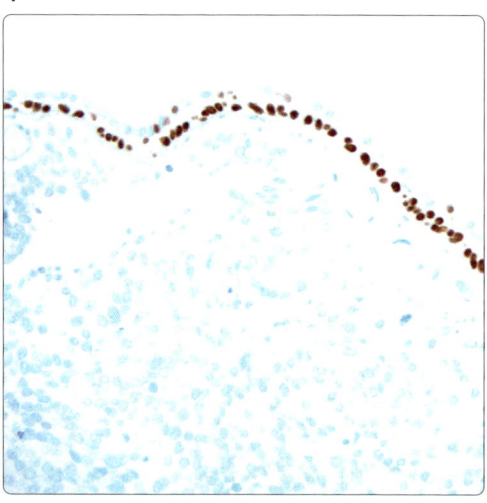

(Left) p63 is typically negative in high grade prostatic adenocarcinoma, while positive in urothelial carcinoma (or in benign urothelial cells as seen in the internal normal control tissue). The rare prostatic adenocarcinomas with p63 expression often have an unusual atrophic pattern. The staining pattern is nuclear. **(Right)** Most prostatic adenocarcinomas do not express high molecular weight cytokeratins such as 34bE12 (or cytokeratin 5/6). The staining pattern is cytoplasmic.

NKX3.1: Prostatic Adenocarcinoma in Bladder

GATA3: Prostatic Adenocarcinoma in Bladder

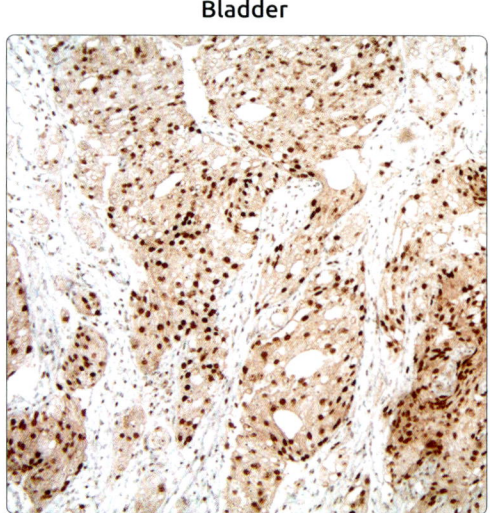
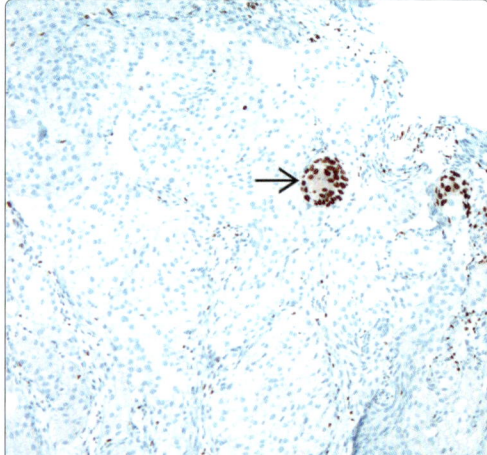

(Left) NKX3.1 is a very specific nuclear marker of prostate epithelial origin when used in the differential diagnostic distinction from urothelial carcinoma. NKX3.1 expression is often maintained in high grade carcinomas. NKX3.1, PSMA and Prostein (P501S) are useful markers to confirm prostate origin. **(Right)** GATA3, which is typically paired with NKX3.1 in this diagnostic setting, has not been reported to show reactivity in prostatic adenocarcinoma. The entrapped urothelium shows strong nuclear reactivity ➡.

Metastatic and Secondary Carcinomas

Metastatic Esophageal Adenocarcinoma

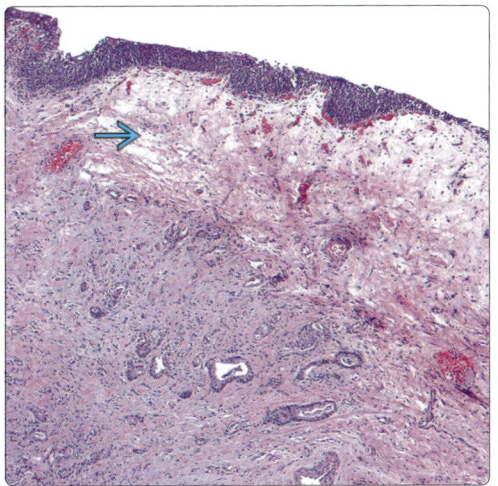

Metastatic Diffuse Gastric Carcinoma

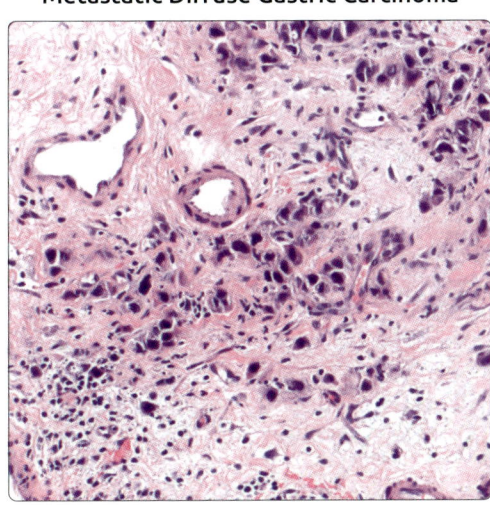

(Left) The presence of a normal surface urothelium and a zone of uninvolved lamina propria ⇨ should suggest the possibility of metastatic adenocarcinoma, as in this example of a metastasis from the distal esophagus. *(Right)* Metastatic diffuse-type gastric adenocarcinoma may be morphologically and immunophenotypically indistinguishable from the plasmacytoid variant of urothelial carcinoma. Both may also show loss of membranous e-cadherin expression.

Secondary Involvement by Colorectal Adenocarcinoma

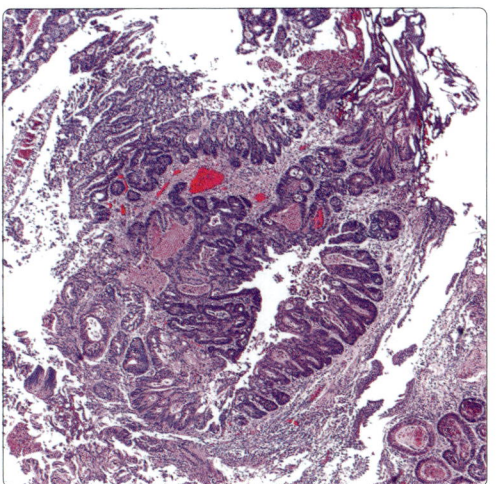

Metastatic Colorectal Adenocarcinoma

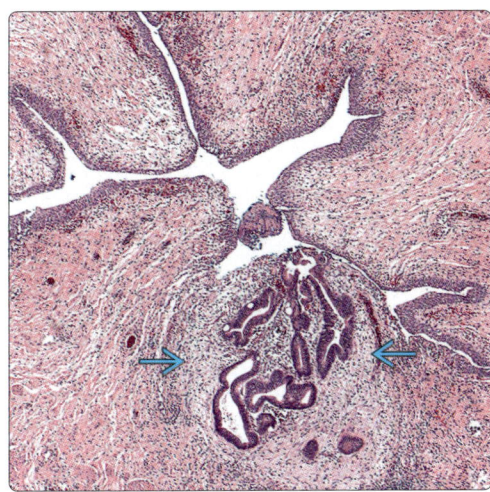

(Left) Direct invasion from gastrointestinal tract adenocarcinomas may be indistinguishable from primary bladder adenocarcinoma. Close imaging correlation and colonoscopy are often needed to aid in this distinction. *(Right)* This example of metastatic adenocarcinoma from the colon ⇨ demonstrates how well-differentiated the metastatic lesions may appear.

CK20: Colorectal Adenocarcinoma

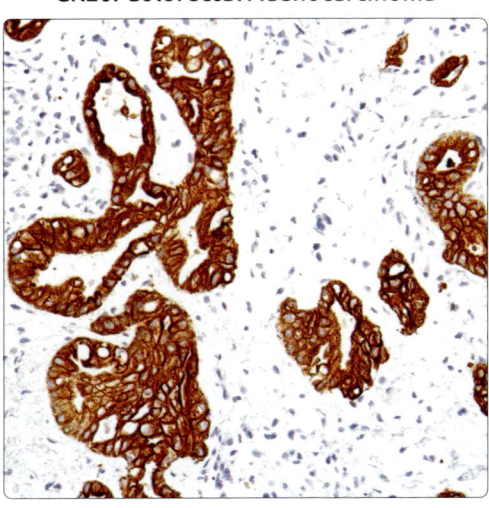

CDX2: Colorectal Adenocarcinoma

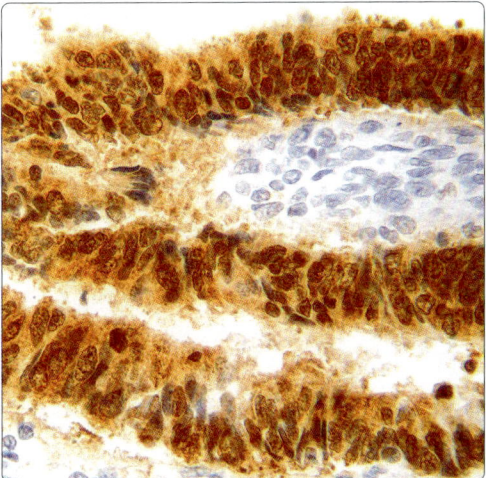

(Left) Colorectal adenocarcinoma involving the bladder shows strong cytoplasmic immunoreactivity for CK20, as in this case. CK20 expression may also be seen in enteric-type adenocarcinomas of urinary bladder origin, which often have an identical enteric immunophenotype. *(Right)* Nuclear expression of CDX2 in colorectal adenocarcinoma is seen involving the urinary bladder. Clinical history and comparison with the primary are often more useful than immunostains.

Metastatic and Secondary Carcinomas

Cervical Squamous Cell Carcinoma in Urinary Bladder

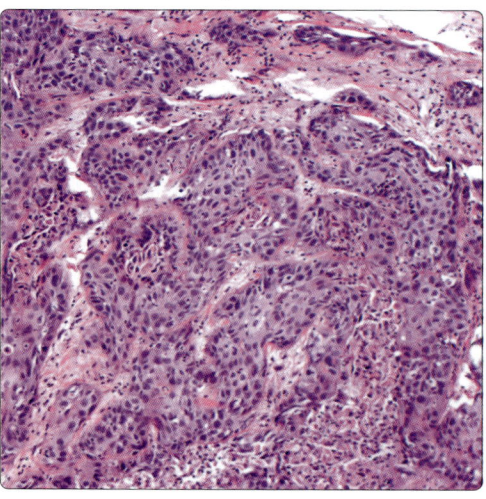

p16: Cervical Squamous Cell Carcinoma

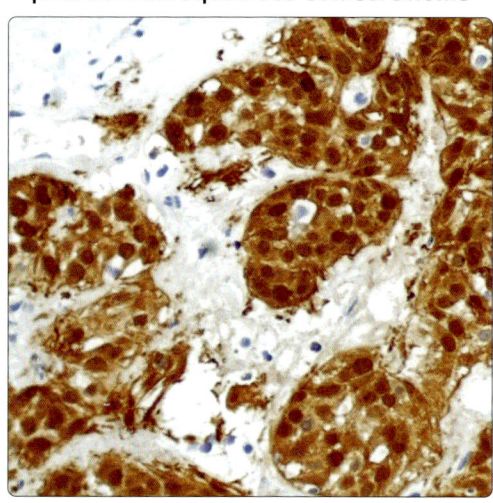

(Left) Primary squamous cell carcinoma of the uterine cervix or vagina may invade the urinary bladder by direct extension. In this setting, morphologic distinction may be impossible. **(Right)** Strong nuclear and cytoplasmic immunoreactivity for p16 is seen in this cervical squamous cell carcinoma in the bladder. p16 staining is used as an HPV surrogate, but is not specific and may be expressed in urothelial carcinoma. PCR- and CISH-based high-risk HPV testing are more specific methods.

Metastatic Papillary Serous Carcinoma

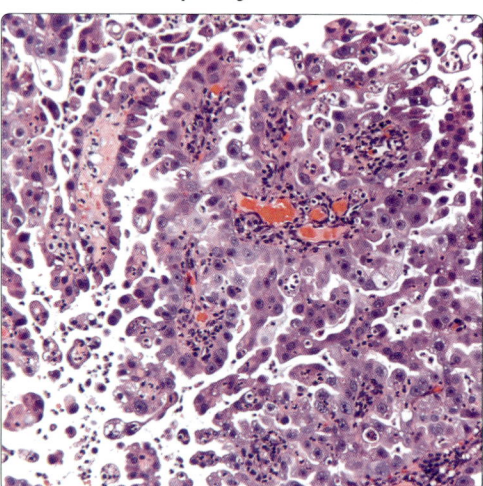

pax-8: Metastatic Papillary Serous Carcinoma

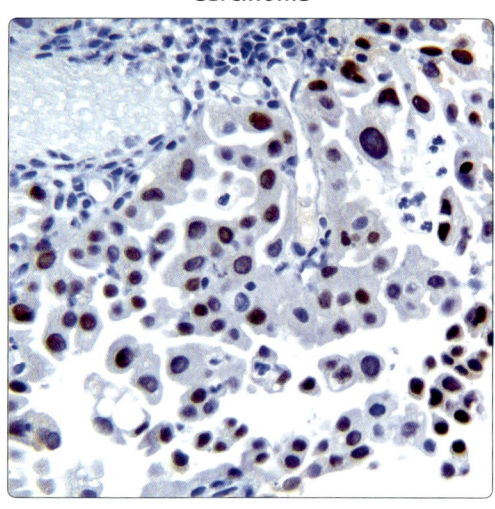

(Left) Metastatic papillary serous carcinoma of the ovary may simulate micropapillary urothelial carcinoma. Clinical presentation is helpful as ovarian carcinomas typically have large adnexal masses and peritoneal spread. **(Right)** Nuclear pax-8 expression is common in ovarian surface epithelial tumors, such as this metastatic ovarian papillary serous carcinoma. This nuclear transcription factor is not entirely specific and may occasionally be expressed in urothelial neoplasms, particularly in the upper urinary tract.

Endometrioid Adenocarcinoma of Uterus

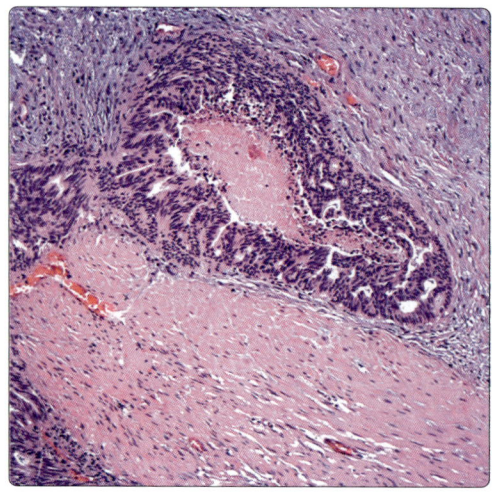

Endometrioid Adenocarcinoma of Uterus With Mucinous Features

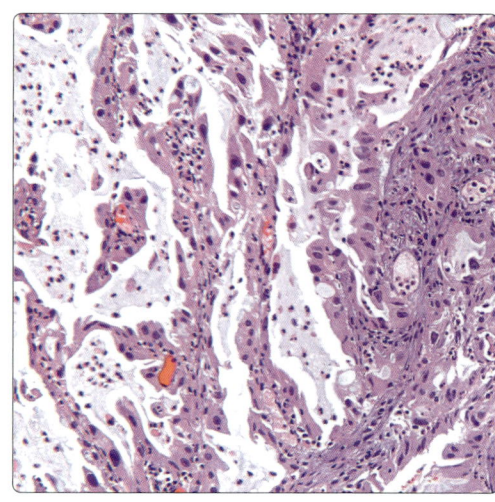

(Left) Uterine endometrioid adenocarcinoma may involve the muscularis propria by direct extension. This may be morphologically indistinguishable from primary bladder adenocarcinoma. Pattern of growth, lamina propria or muscularis propria predominant growth without surface involvement is helpful. **(Right)** Other histologic patterns of endometrioid adenocarcinoma, such as mucinous differentiation, may also mimic primary adenocarcinoma of the urinary bladder.

Metastatic and Secondary Carcinomas

Melanoma
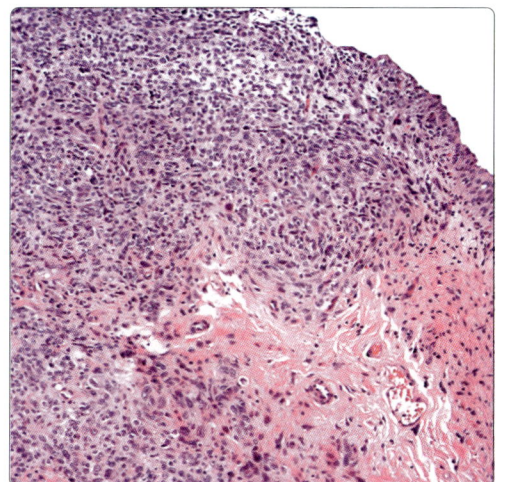

Melanoma
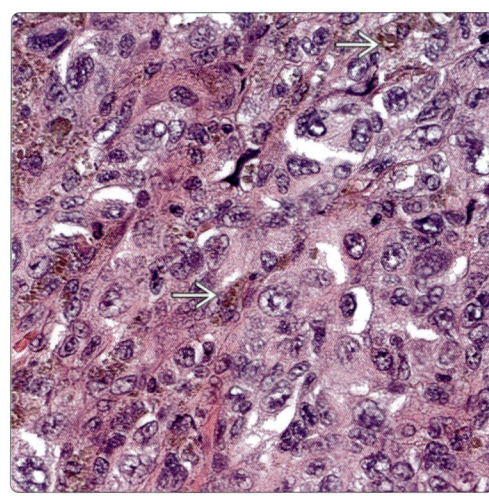

(Left) Melanoma may have epithelioid or spindled features and can mimic a variety of primary bladder neoplasms. Consideration of melanoma is important when choosing a panel of immunostains for screening poorly differentiated neoplasms. (Right) Metastatic melanoma in the bladder may resemble any undifferentiated malignancy, such as poorly differentiated urothelial carcinoma. Obvious melanin pigment ⇨ may not be present. S100 protein is the most sensitive screening marker for melanoma.

Metastatic Breast Adenocarcinoma
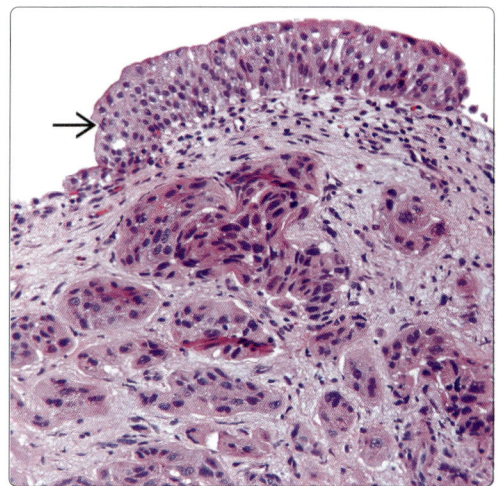

Metastatic Breast Adenocarcinoma
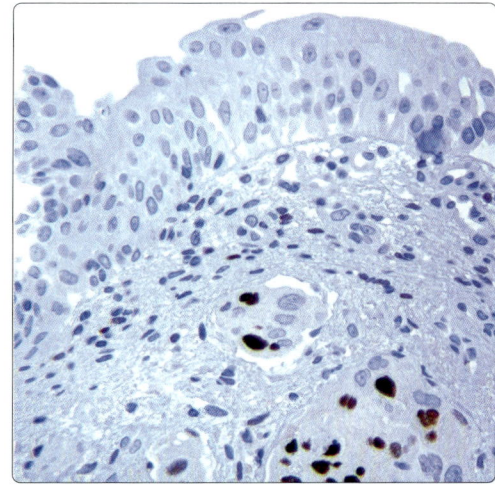

(Left) Metastatic ductal adenocarcinoma from the breast may closely resemble invasive urothelial carcinoma. Preservation of the overlying urothelium ⇨ or predominant intravascular growth should suggest the possibility of metastasis. (Right) Nuclear immunoreactivity for ER is often maintained by metastatic breast cancer, as in this metastatic ductal carcinoma of breast origin in the superficial lamina propria of the bladder.

Metastatic Breast Adenocarcinoma
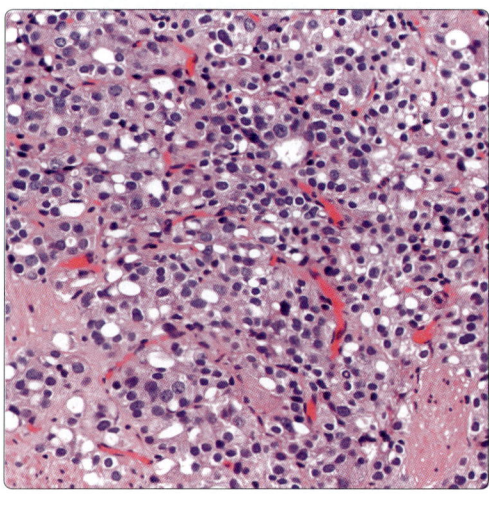

GATA3: Metastatic Breast Adenocarcinoma
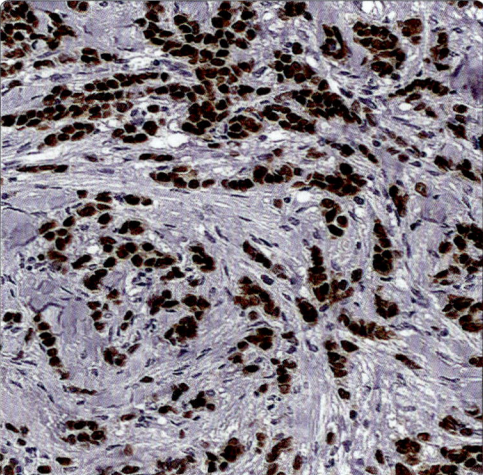

(Left) Metastatic lobular carcinoma of the breast may have significant morphologic overlap with some morphologic variants of invasive urothelial carcinoma (such as plasmacytoid variant). ER, mammaglobin, and GCDFP-15 are helpful stains. (Right) Adenocarcinomas of breast origin, particularly low grade ductal and lobular carcinomas, commonly show diffuse immunoreactivity with GATA3. This represents a potential diagnostic pitfall. Inclusion of ER, PR, and uroplakin-2 will be helpful.

Diverticula

KEY FACTS

TERMINOLOGY
- Bladder diverticula are outpouchings of urothelial lining through congenital or acquired weakness in muscular bladder wall (detrusor muscle)
- Usually consist of thin-walled sac with narrow neck or ostium communicating with bladder lumen

CLASSIFICATION
- Acquired diverticula are devoid of muscularis propria (may be considered pseudodiverticula)
- Congenital diverticula are less common, observed more frequently in boys

ETIOLOGY/PATHOGENESIS
- In adults, most diverticula are acquired, resulting from congenital weakness of bladder wall
- Congenital diverticula result from congenital disarrangement of muscle fibers at ureterovesical junction

CLINICAL ISSUES
- Most diverticula are asymptomatic
- In adults, most common presentation is hematuria, urinary retention, or urinary tract infection
- In pediatric diverticula, urinary tract infection is most common presentation
- Cystoscopic assessment of diverticula is essential
- Biopsy of diverticula, important to assess presence of neoplastic or nonneoplastic conditions
- Surgical treatment approaches include transurethral resection (TUR), diverticulectomy, partial cystectomy, or radical cystectomy

MICROSCOPIC
- Most diverticula show chronic inflammatory infiltrates but also acute and granulomatous inflammation
- Other findings include: Cystitis cystica et glandularis, intestinal metaplasia, squamous metaplasia, and nephrogenic adenoma (metaplasia)

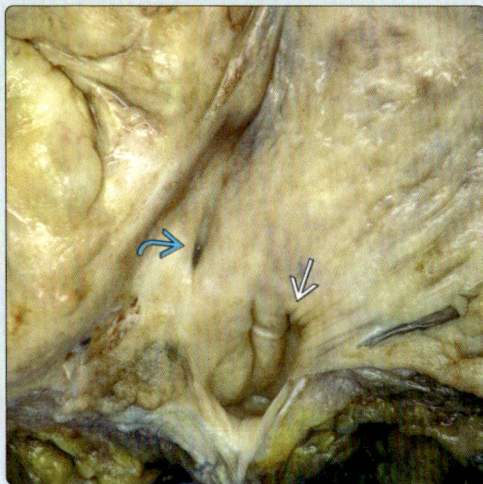

Bladder Diverticulum

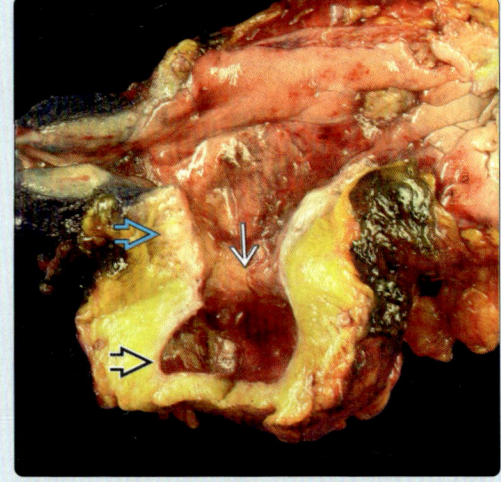

Bladder Diverticulum: Opened

(Left) This is an open cystectomy specimen with a diverticulum ➡ located on the lateral wall. The diverticular opening is close to the ureteral orifice ➡. (Right) This is a cystectomy specimen with a diverticulum ➡ on the left lateral wall adjacent to the left ureter. Note the difference in wall thickness between the diverticulum ➡ (devoid of muscularis propria) and the adjacent bladder ➡ (intact muscularis propria). Basically, the mucosa is separated from perivesical fat only by the lamina propria.

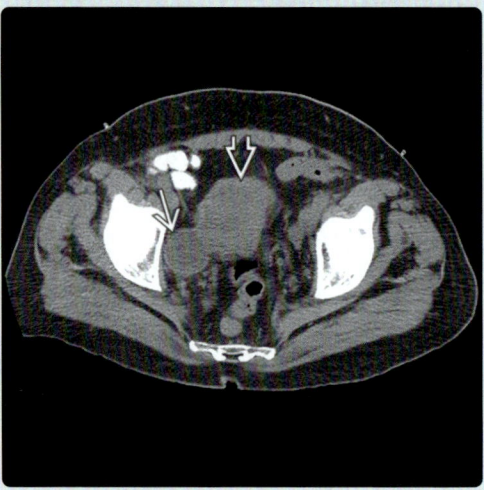

Bladder Diverticulum: CT Scan

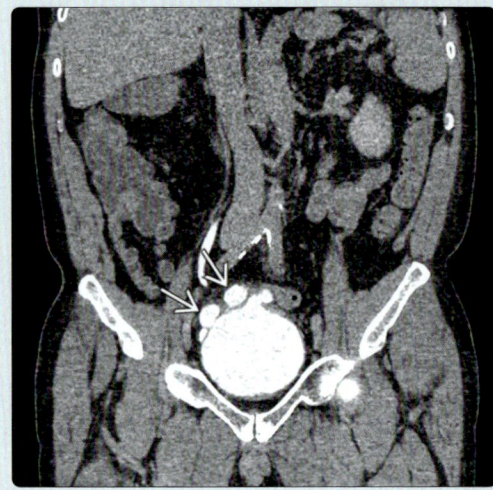

Bladder Diverticula: Multiple

(Left) Cross-sectional radiologic image shows the pelvis with a large and solitary vesical diverticulum ➡ connected to the right lateral wall of the bladder ➡. Note how close the diverticular wall is to the bony pelvic side wall. (Right) Coronal MR with contrast media shows multiple bladder diverticula located at the dome and right lateral wall ➡. Note the narrow areas connecting the diverticulum to the lumen of the bladder.

Diverticula

TERMINOLOGY

Synonyms
- Bladder diverticula, vesical diverticula

Definitions
- Bladder diverticula are outpouchings of urothelial lining through muscularis layer of bladder wall, through congenital or acquired weakness in muscular bladder wall (detrusor muscle)
  o Usually consist of thin-walled sac with narrow neck or ostium communicating with bladder lumen
  o Acquired diverticula are devoid of muscularis propria (may be considered pseudodiverticula)
  o Congenital diverticula are less common, observed more frequently in boys
    – Considered true diverticula due to presence of all layers of bladder in diverticular wall (including muscularis propria)
    – Hutch diverticulum is congenital bladder diverticulum seen at vesicoureteral junction

ETIOLOGY/PATHOGENESIS

Developmental Anomaly
- In adults, most diverticula are acquired, resulting from congenital weakness of bladder wall at level of ureterovesical junction (UVJ)
  o UVJ represents embryological junction of ureteric bud with urogenital sinus
  o Increased intravesical pressure can cause herniation of mucosa and submucosa through bladder wall to form pseudodiverticulum (devoid of muscularis propria)
  o Any condition that results in increased intravesical pressure may lead to development of diverticula
    – Most commonly secondary to bladder outlet obstruction due to prostatic enlargement, bladder neck stricture, or neurogenic bladder
    – Bladder outlet obstruction causes compensatory muscle hypertrophy and eventual mucosal herniation in areas of weakness
- Congenital diverticula result from congenital disarrangement of muscle fibers at ureterovesical junction

CLINICAL ISSUES

Presentation
- Most diverticula are asymptomatic
- Most common presentation is hematuria, urinary retention, or urinary tract infection
- In pediatric diverticula, urinary tract infection is most common presentation
  o Pediatric diverticula may be associated with other features of congenial syndromes

Treatment
- Surgical approaches
  o Cystoscopic assessment of diverticulum is essential, primarily to rule out neoplasms
    – May be difficult due to narrow diverticular ostium
  o Biopsy to investigate presence of neoplasms
  o Transurethral resection (TUR) for suspected neoplasms and for complete removal of intradiverticular tumors
    – For noninvasive, low-grade tumor without presence of carcinoma in situ
    – Biopsy and TUR of bladder diverticula carry risk of perforation, due to lack of proper muscle layer
  o Diverticulectomy or partial cystectomy
    – For bulky tumors, incomplete removal of tumor by TUR, or for risk of perforation
  o Radical cystectomy
    – For locally advanced tumors, high-grade tumors in diverticulum and synchronous intravesical multifocal tumors or extensive carcinoma in situ, or multifocal disease associated with poor bladder function

Prognosis
- Bladder diverticula are associated with urinary stasis
  o May increase risk of urinary tract infection, bladder calculi, and neoplasms

IMAGING

Radiographic Findings
- Bladder diverticula can be detected by ultrasound, CT (± contrast), and MR
- Ultrasound may also assess how well diverticulum empties after voiding

MACROSCOPIC

General Features
- Vesical diverticula can be single or multiple
- Diverticular size can range from subcentimeter up to 18 cm
- Most common locations: Adjacent to ureteral orifices, bladder dome, and region of internal urethral orifice

MICROSCOPIC

Histologic Features
- Lining urothelium may be denuded, ulcerated, reactive, or unremarkable
- Wall of diverticulum consists of urothelium and underlying connective tissue (similar to bladder lamina propria, including muscularis mucosae, and perivesical fat)
  o Absent muscularis propria; muscle fascicles of muscularis mucosae may be identified and can be hypertrophic
- Most diverticula show chronic inflammatory infiltrates
  o Chronic inflammation may be prominent and extensive
  o Acute inflammation may be seen
  o Granulomatous inflammation, occasionally with giant cells; likely related to prior treatment with BCG
- Other nonneoplastic conditions include
  o Cystitis cystica et glandularis ± intestinal metaplasia
  o Squamous metaplasia ± keratinization
  o Nephrogenic adenoma (metaplasia)

SELECTED REFERENCES

1. Walker NF et al: Diagnosis and management of intradiverticular bladder tumours. Nat Rev Urol. 11(7):383-90, 2014
2. Idrees MT et al: The spectrum of histopathologic findings in vesical diverticulum: implications for pathogenesis and staging. Hum Pathol. 44(7):1223-32, 2013
3. Kong MX et al: Histopathologic and clinical features of vesical diverticula. Urology. 82(1):142-7, 2013
4. Tamas EF et al: Histopathologic features and clinical outcomes in 71 cases of bladder diverticula. Arch Pathol Lab Med. 133(5):791-6, 2009

Diverticula

(Left) Low-power view shows vesical diverticulum devoid of muscular layer in wall. Note the close proximity of perivesical fat to the surface urothelium ⇒ where it is only separated by lamina propria. Portions of muscularis propria are present at mouth of diverticulum ⇒. **(Right)** Section shows diverticular wall with thick and intersecting bundles of smooth muscle ⇒ consistent with hypertrophic muscularis mucosae. There is no muscularis propria and only perivesical fat can be seen deep in section ⇒.

Bladder Diverticulum: Panoramic View
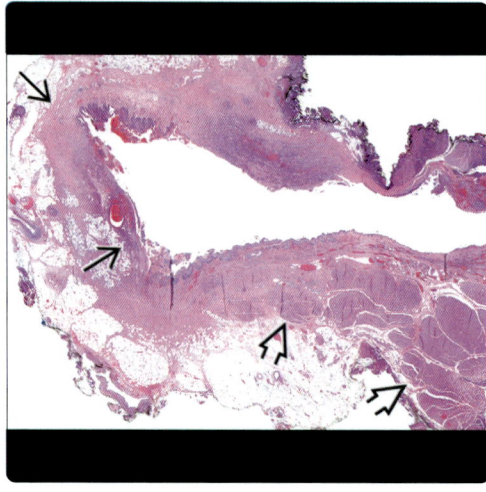

Bladder Diverticulum: Hypertrophic Muscularis Mucosae
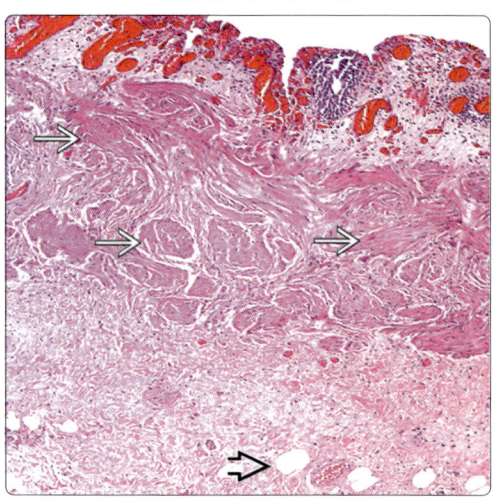

(Left) In this section of diverticular wall, a fragment of hypertrophic muscularis mucosae is identified ⇒. Discontinuous bundles of muscles are commonly seen in diverticular wall, and, oftentimes, they may be hypertrophic but should not be mistaken for muscularis propria. **(Right)** In this section taken from a bladder diverticulum near the opening, there are a few thick and organized bundles of smooth muscle ⇒ that represent residual muscularis propria from the bladder wall adjacent to the diverticulum.

Bladder Diverticulum: Muscularis Propria
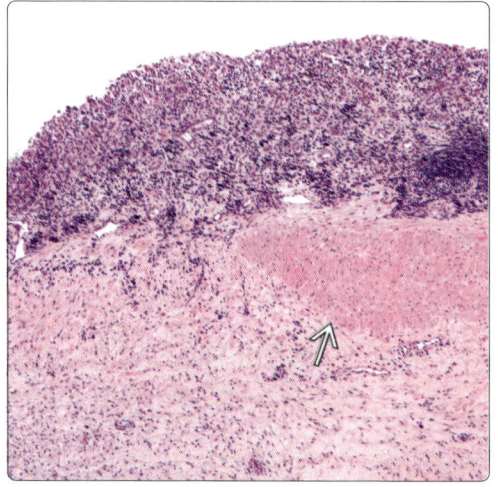

Bladder Diverticulum: Near Ostium
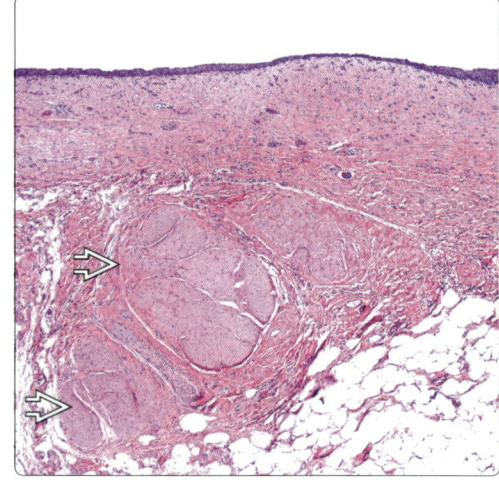

(Left) This is a section of diverticular mucosa that is extensively denuded and inflamed. Note the presence of a mixture of plasma cells and lymphocytes as well as the prominent vascular proliferation. **(Right)** In this section taken from the base of a diverticulum, there is extensive ulceration and denudation of the mucosa and prominent fibrosis and hyalinization of the subepithelial connective tissue ⇒ that blends into the perivesical fat ⇒.

Bladder Diverticulum: Inflamed and Denuded
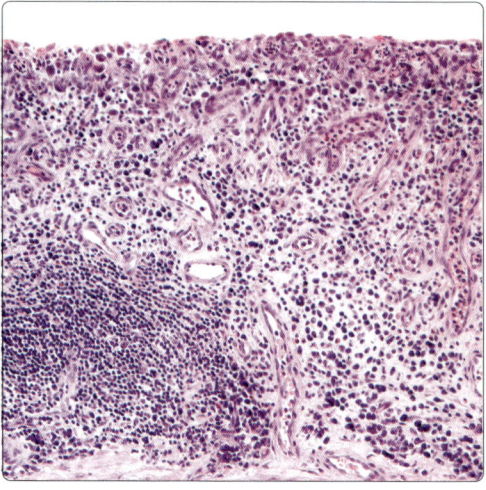

Bladder Diverticulum: Fibrotic Wall
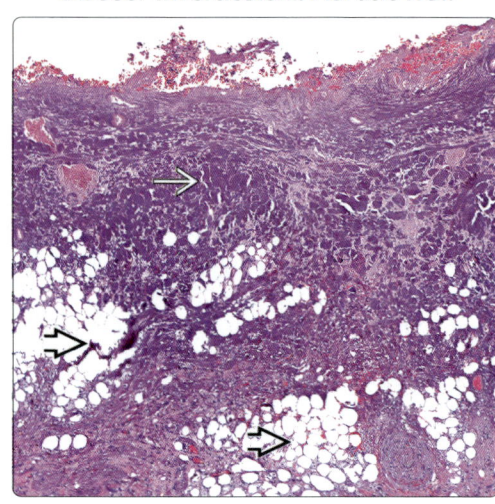

Diverticula

Bladder Diverticulum: Inflammation and Fibrosis

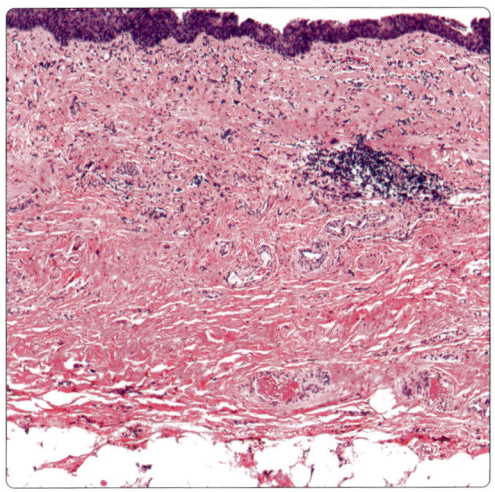

Bladder Diverticulum: Extensive Inflammation

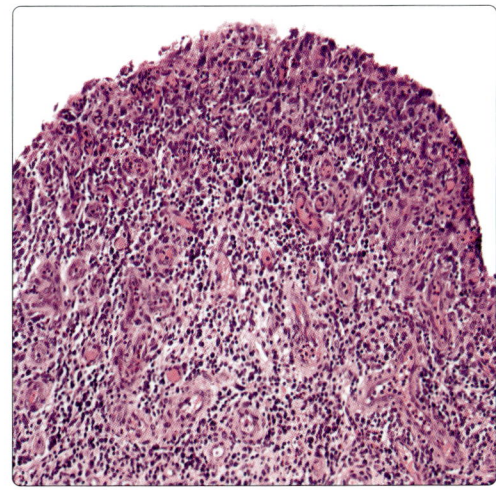

(Left) In this section from a bladder diverticulum, the surface urothelium is unremarkable and the lamina propria contains clusters and sprinkling of lymphocytes. Note the absence of any noticeable muscular tissue in this section. (Right) In this superficial section of bladder diverticulum, there is intense inflammation, primarily chronic, with many lymphocytes and plasma cells. Note the prominent vascular proliferation and granulation tissue formation.

Bladder Diverticulum: Cystitis Cystica

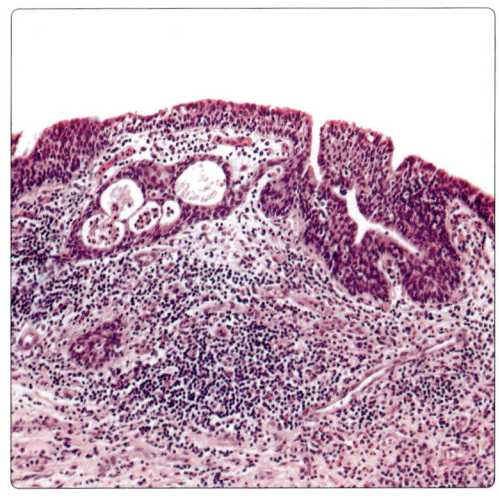

Bladder Diverticulum: Intestinal Metaplasia

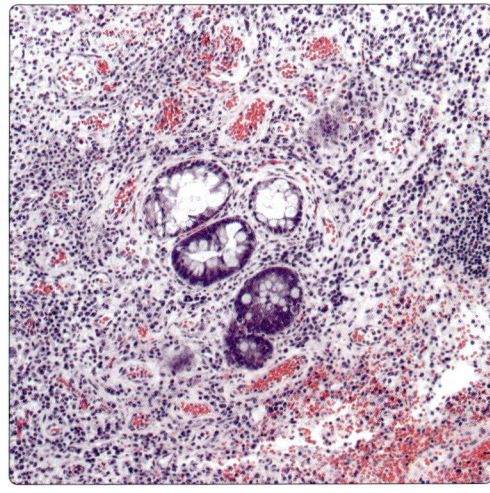

(Left) This section shows proliferative cystitis characterized by the marked inflammation in the lamina propria and the dilation of some of the Brunn nests. These are classical features of cystitis cystica that may develop in diverticula of the bladder. (Right) In this diverticular biopsy, in addition to the intense chronic inflammation and extravasation of red blood cells, there is a cluster of glands with enteric features and goblet cells, consistent with intestinal metaplasia.

Bladder Diverticulum: Squamous Metaplasia

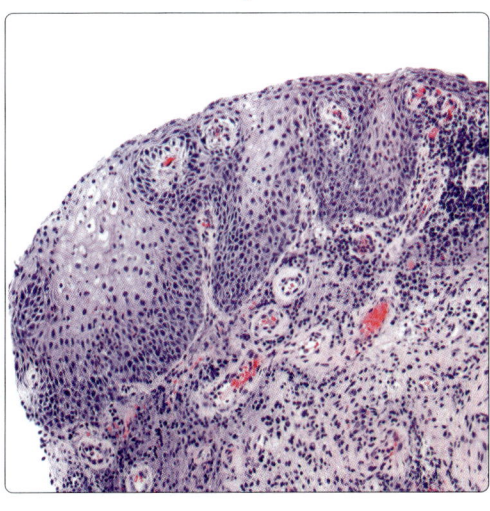

Bladder Diverticulum: Nephrogenic Adenoma (Metaplasia)

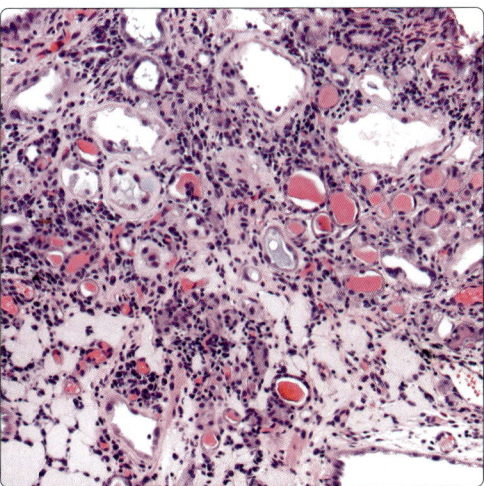

(Left) Other forms of metaplasia have been reported in vesical diverticula, including squamous metaplasia, as seen in this image. Keratinization, although not seen in this case, has been reported in some cases of bladder diverticula. (Right) As a reactive/metaplastic lesion, nephrogenic adenoma (metaplasia) has been reported in bladder diverticula, as in this case. The morphologic features are identical to those seen in the bladder and are almost always associated with inflammation.

Diverticular-Associated Neoplasia

KEY FACTS

TERMINOLOGY
- Tumors arising in diverticula of bladder

CLINICAL ISSUES
- Intradiverticular bladder tumors are rare, accounting for ~ 1% of all bladder tumors
  - True prevalence not known, as most are asymptomatic
- Most patients present in 7th decade (range 27-92 years)
- 11-12x more common in men than in women
- 5-year survival for all patients is 72%, and for those with pT3 disease it is 45%
- Urine cytology, ultrasonography, and cystoscopy should be used in initial assessment of suspected intradiverticular bladder tumors
- Bladder conservation treatments include transurethral resection, diverticulectomy, or partial cystectomy ± intravesical adjuvant therapy for low-grade, low-volume, noninvasive disease
- Radical cystectomy, ± systemic neoadjuvant or adjuvant therapy, is required for patients with large, invasive tumors or tumors that are associated with poor bladder function (chronic retention)

IMAGING
- Cross-sectional imaging (CT scan, MR, etc.) may complement these techniques, provide vital information, and may also be important in staging

STAGING
- There is no muscularis propria in diverticular wall; therefore, stage pT2 cannot be assigned to invasive tumors arising in bladder diverticula
- Invasive tumors go from invading lamina propria (pT1) to invading perivesical fat (pT3)
- Hypertrophy of muscularis mucosae is common and should not be mistaken for muscularis propria (definitionally absent in this setting)

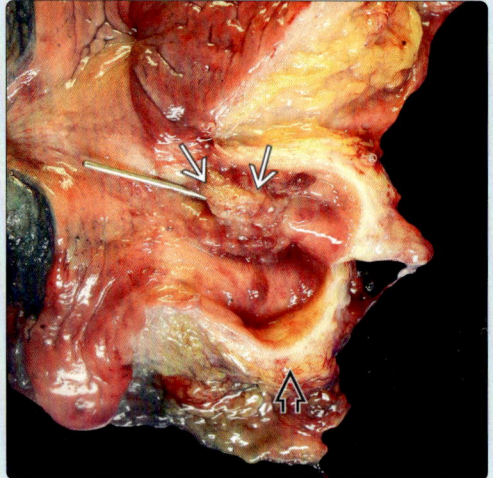

Intradiverticular Tumor, Gross Image

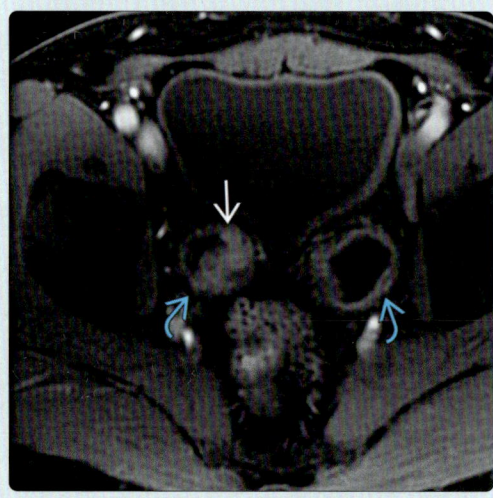

Intradiverticular Tumor, CT Scan

(Left) This is a cystectomy specimen removed for invasive intradiverticular urothelial carcinoma. The diverticulum is opened to reveal the tumor ➡ and its location adjacent to the opening of the left ureter (probe). Note the absence of muscularis propria in the diverticular wall ➡. (Right) In this CT radiograph, there are 2 diverticula on either side of the bladder ➡. The 1 on the patient's right side ➡ contains a filling defect with heterogeneous density and irregular borders, later confirmed as invasive urothelial carcinoma.

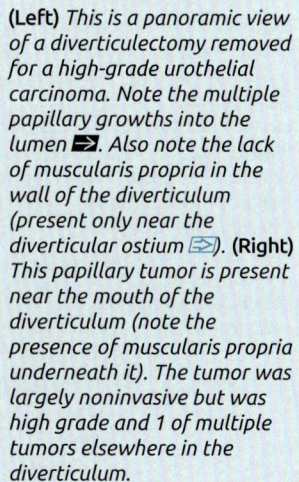

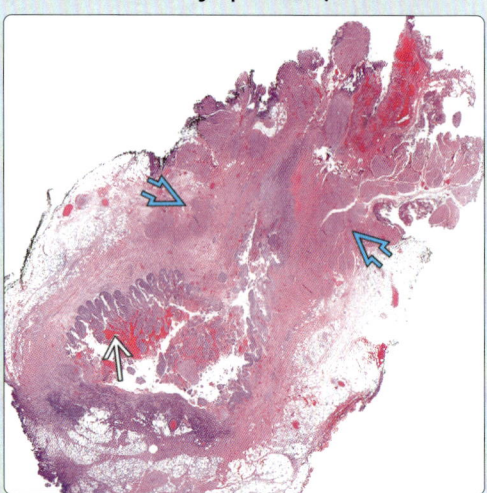

Diverticulectomy Specimen, With Tumor

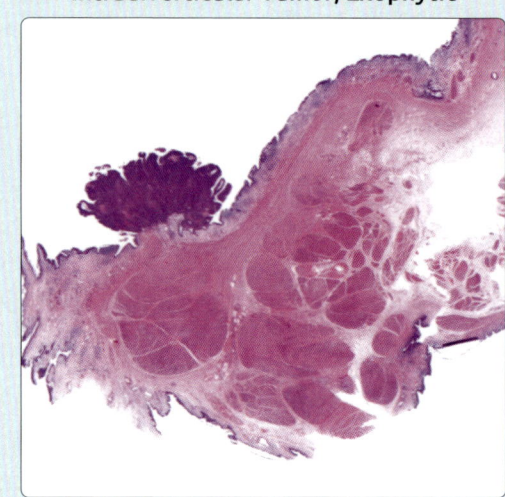

Intradiverticular Tumor, Exophytic

(Left) This is a panoramic view of a diverticulectomy removed for a high-grade urothelial carcinoma. Note the multiple papillary growths into the lumen ➡. Also note the lack of muscularis propria in the wall of the diverticulum (present only near the diverticular ostium ➡). (Right) This papillary tumor is present near the mouth of the diverticulum (note the presence of muscularis propria underneath it). The tumor was largely noninvasive but was high grade and 1 of multiple tumors elsewhere in the diverticulum.

Diverticular-Associated Neoplasia

TERMINOLOGY

Definitions
- Tumors arising in diverticula of bladder

CLINICAL ISSUES

Epidemiology
- Tumors arising within bladder diverticulum are uncommon
  - True prevalence of bladder diverticula and neoplasia not known, as most are asymptomatic
  - Reported incidence ranging from 0.8-10.0%
  - Carcinomas arising in vesical diverticula constitute ~ 1.5% of all bladder carcinoma
  - Most patients present in 7th decade
    - Reported age range from 27–92 years
  - Vesical intradiverticular tumors are 11–12x more common in men than in women
    - In one study, M:F ratio was 26:1

Presentation
- Most common presentation: Hematuria, urinary retention, urinary tract infection
  - Other reported presentations include: Urinary incontinence, dysuria, and frequency

Treatment
- Cystoscopic evaluation of diverticulum is essential, primarily to rule out neoplastic process
  - Cystoscopy may be difficult to perform due to narrow diverticular mouth
- Biopsy to investigate presence of, or to rule out, neoplasms
- Transurethral resection (TUR) for complete removal of intradiverticular tumors
  - For noninvasive low-grade tumor without presence of carcinoma in situ
  - Biopsy and TUR of bladder diverticula carry risk of perforation, due to lack of proper muscle layer
- Diverticulectomy or partial cystectomy
  - For bulky tumors, incomplete removal of tumor by TUR, or for risk of perforation
  - Radical cystectomy
    - For locally advanced tumors, high-grade tumors in diverticulum, synchronous intravesical multifocal tumors, extensive carcinoma in situ, or multifocal disease associated with poor bladder function

Prognosis
- Overall, survival for patient with vesical intradiverticular cancers is similar to that of bladder cancer when compared stage for stage
- 5-year survival for all patients is 72%, and for those with pT3 disease it is 45%

Diagnostic Procedures
- Urine cytology, cystoscopy, and ultrasonography may be used in initial assessment of suspected intradiverticular neoplasms
- CT scan ± contrast and MR may be important complementary tests
  - Can also be important in staging
  - CT imaging features may also provide prognostic information and association with clinical outcomes

MACROSCOPIC
- Bladder diverticula can be single or multiple
- Diverticular size can range from subcentimeter up to 18 cm
- Most common locations: (1) lateral walls adjacent to ureteral orifices, (2) bladder dome, and (3) region of internal urethral orifice

MICROSCOPIC

Histologic Features
- Histologic patterns of intradiverticular tumors recapitulates those of bladder
- Coexisting carcinoma in bladder may be seen in up to 20% of cases in which diverticula were involved by urothelial carcinoma
  - In 1 series, rate of concurrent or subsequent urothelial carcinoma in nondiverticular bladder was 53%
- Most common tumor type is urothelial carcinoma
  - May be either pure or associated with variant histology
  - Other tumor types include: Squamous cell carcinoma, adenocarcinoma (including clear cell adenocarcinoma), small cell carcinoma, sarcomatoid carcinoma
  - Some studies reported increased incidence of nonurothelial carcinomas in this setting
- Within urothelial carcinoma group, most tumors are high grade (both papillary and flat carcinoma in situ) and invasive
  - Low-grade papillary carcinoma is present in ~ 20% of cases
  - Most invasive tumors are limited to subepithelial soft tissue (lamina propria, pT1)
  - Invasion into perivesical soft tissue is present in ~ 1/5 of cases (pT3)
- 1 important aspect of staging intradiverticular cancer is absence of proper muscle layer (no muscularis propria)
  - As result, stage pT2 cannot be assigned to such tumors
  - After pT1, these tumors invade perivesical soft tissue and are assigned pT3 stage
  - Muscularis mucosae may become hypertrophic, superficially resembling muscularis propria
    - This distinction is very important due to prognostic implications related to stage determination and risk stratification

SELECTED REFERENCES

1. Di Paolo PL et al: Intradiverticular bladder cancer: CT imaging features and their association with clinical outcomes. Clin Imaging. 39(1):94-8, 2015
2. Walker NF et al: Diagnosis and management of intradiverticular bladder tumours. Nat Rev Urol. 11(7):383-90, 2014
3. Idrees MT et al: The spectrum of histopathologic findings in vesical diverticulum: implications for pathogenesis and staging. Hum Pathol. 44(7):1223-32, 2013
4. Kong MX et al: Histopathological and clinical features of vesical diverticula. Urology. 82(1):142-7, 2013
5. Tamas EF et al: Histopathologic features and clinical outcomes in 71 cases of bladder diverticula. Arch Pathol Lab Med. 133(5):791-6, 2009
6. Golijanin D et al: Carcinoma in a bladder diverticulum: presentation and treatment outcome. J Urol. 170(5):1761-4, 2003

Diverticular-Associated Neoplasia

Intradiverticular Tumor, Noninvasive, Papillary

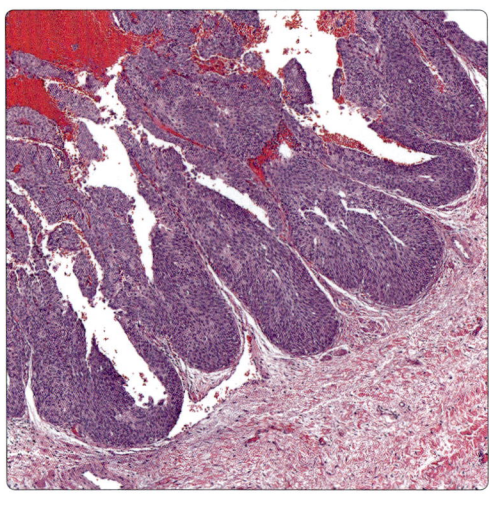

Intradiverticular Tumor, Endophytic

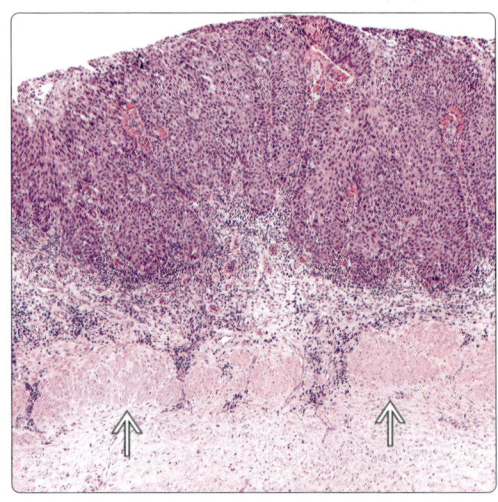

(Left) This section contains a papillary tumor taken from a diverticulectomy specimen. The underlying soft tissue is fibrotic and devoid of a muscular layer. (Right) This is an intradiverticular high-grade urothelial carcinoma that is suspicious for lamina propria invasion. Note the prominent muscle bundles of the muscularis mucosae ➡. Perivesical fat is separated by a fibrotic connective tissue layer from these muscle bundles. Muscularis propria is not present.

Intradiverticular High-Grade Urothelial Carcinoma

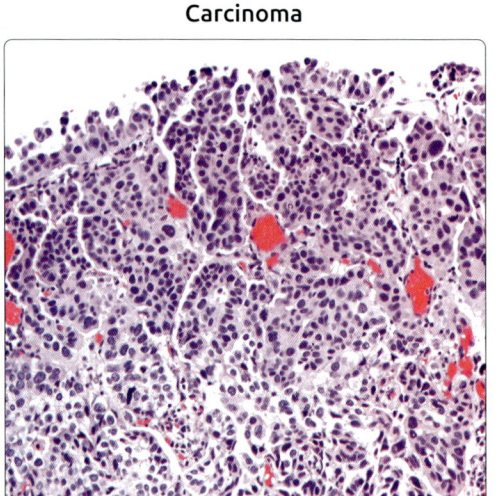

Intradiverticular Urothelial Carcinoma In Situ

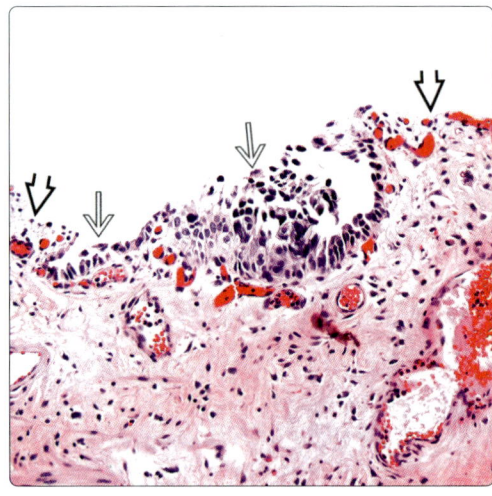

(Left) This is a high-grade urothelial carcinoma, not otherwise specified, detected on biopsy from a mass-containing bladder diverticulum. There is evidence of invasive disease, but the depth of invasion cannot be determined from this superficial biopsy. (Right) In this section taken from a diverticular biopsy with positive urine cytology, parts of the surface urothelium are covered by highly atypical cells ➡ consistent with flat urothelial carcinoma (in situ). Other areas of the mucosa are partially denuded ➡.

Intradiverticular Urothelial Carcinoma, Invasive

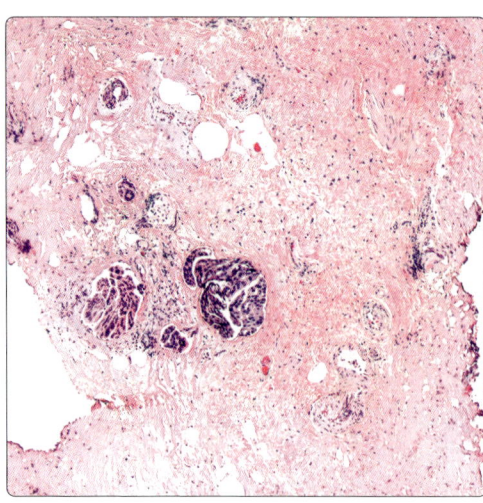

Intradiverticular Tumor, Thermal Artifact

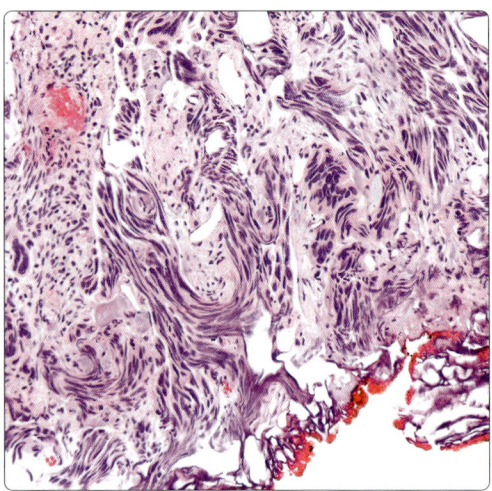

(Left) In this biopsy section from a diverticular mass, there are invasive tumor clusters in the middle of fibroconnective tissue that also seems to be surrounded by some retraction. Sometimes it is difficult to determine whether this represents lymphovascular invasion or simply invasion of connective tissue. (Right) This is a cystoscopic biopsy taken from a diverticular mass. While a tumor is seen in this material, the presence of a marked thermal artifact precludes any definitive diagnosis in regard to tumor type and stage.

Diverticular-Associated Neoplasia

Intradiverticular Urothelial Carcinoma, Invasive Into Perivesical Fat

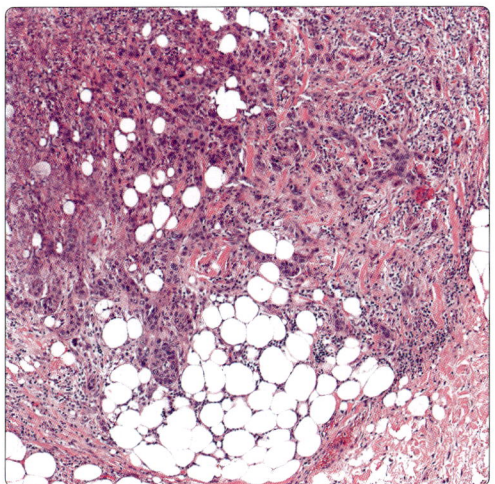

Intradiverticular Urothelial Carcinoma, Superficial Tumor

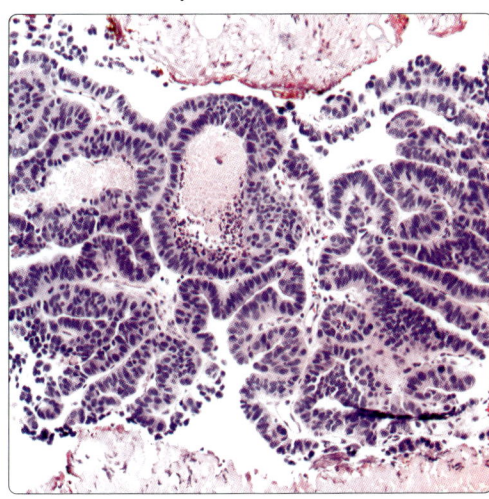

(Left) This is an intradiverticular urothelial carcinoma that is locally advanced, extending into the perivesical adipose tissue (pT3). The absence of muscularis propria is significant, as these tumors go from pT1 to pT3 directly. **(Right)** This biopsy shows fragments of frank high-grade urothelial carcinoma that is detached from underlying soft tissue. This makes it impossible to assess for invasion though the treatment decision may not always depend on the presence or absence of invasion.

Intradiverticular Urothelial Carcinoma, Lymphovascular Invasion

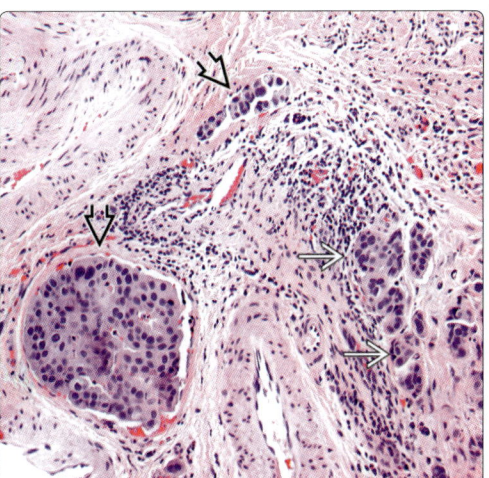

Lymph Node Metastasis, Intradiverticular Urothelial Carcinoma

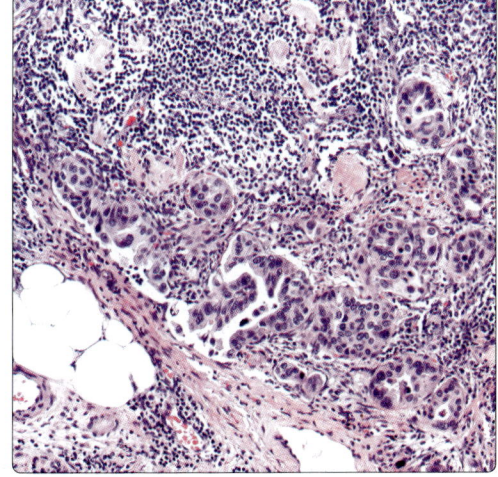

(Left) In this diverticular biopsy for a mass, there is invasive urothelial carcinoma ➡. In addition, there are variable tumor clusters in retraction spaces ➡ that are highly suspicious for lymphovascular invasion. **(Right)** This lymph node contains metastatic urothelial carcinoma. It was taken as part of lymph node dissection along with diverticulectomy from the same patient. Lymph node metastasis is associated with worse prognosis for patients with intradiverticular cancer.

Intradiverticular Urothelial Carcinoma, With Glandular Differentiation

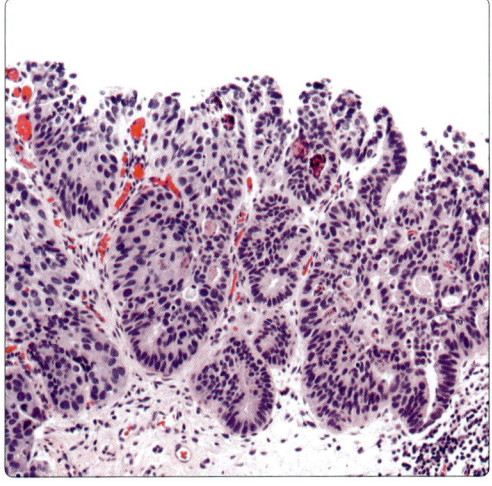

Intradiverticular Squamous Cell Carcinoma

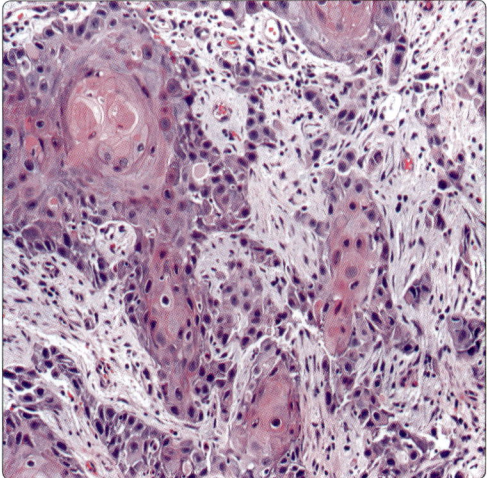

(Left) The spectrum of morphologies seen in intradiverticular tumors may recapitulate that of bladder tumors. In this case, this is an intradiverticular urothelial carcinoma with glandular differentiation. **(Right)** Any tumor type that occurs in the bladder can develop in a vesical diverticulum. In this example, a keratinizing squamous cell carcinoma developed in a bladder diverticulum. The tumor is invasive, and radical surgical resection is warranted in this situation.

Inflammatory Lesions of Urethra

KEY FACTS

CLASSIFICATION

- **Urethritis**
  - Inflammatory response seen histologically involving urethra, or clinically based on symptomatology, cultures, and smears
  - Reiter syndrome is presentation of reactive arthritis, postinfectious syndrome that may involve many sites
  - Reiter syndrome is classic triad of urethritis, conjunctivitis, and arthritis
- **Urethral caruncle**
  - Prolapsing polypoid lesion at distal urethral meatus, predominantly in women
  - Urethral prolapse represents circumferential mucosal prolapse
- **Papillary/polypoid urethritis**
  - Nonneoplastic reactive lesion analogous to papillary/polypoid cystitis
  - 1 or multiple papillary to polypoid-appearing luminal evaginations of edematous, usually myxoinflammatory lamina propria
  - Related to chronic localized trauma
- **Pseudosarcomatous myofibroblastic proliferation**
  - Marked myofibroblastic stromal reaction with myxoinflammatory background and rich vascularity
  - Raises morphologic differential with inflammatory sarcoma and sarcomatoid carcinoma
- **Malakoplakia**
  - Rare, idiosyncratic inflammatory lesion composed of mixed inflammation with prominent histiocytes (von Hansemann cells)
  - Scattered cells with Michaelis-Gutmann bodies, laminated calcospherites

Lymphofollicular Urethritis
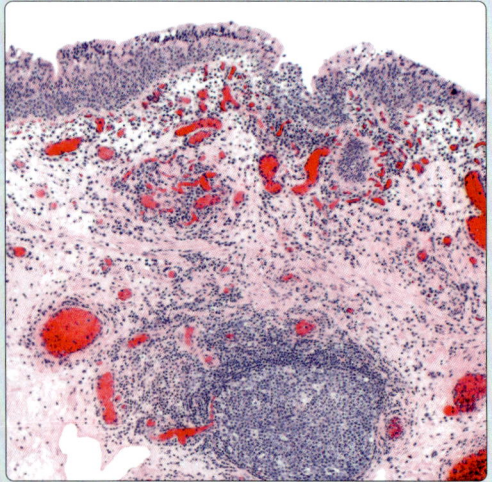

Proliferative Urethritis
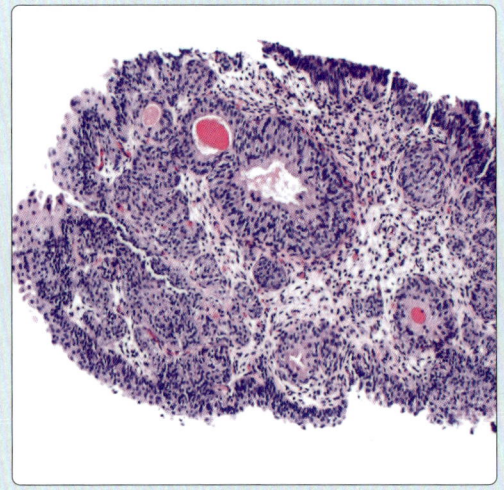

(Left) *Biopsies of the urethra may present the same spectrum of proliferative changes as the urinary bladder, here with brisk active chronic lymphofollicular urethritis, involving the prostatic urethra.* (Right) *Similarly, biopsy fragments of the proximal urethra may show the same spectrum of proliferative changes as other sites, here von Brunn nests and urethritis cystica et glandularis.*

Papillary/Polypoid Urethritis
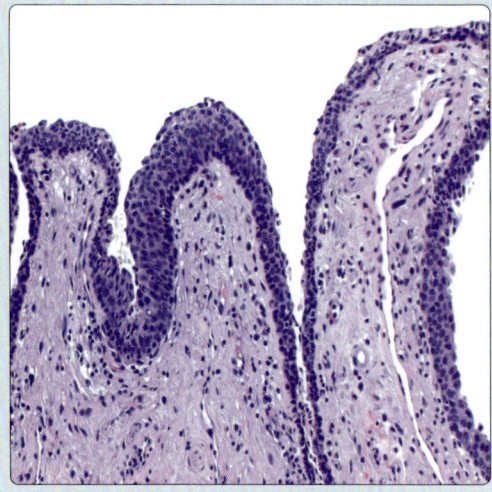

Papillary/Polypoid Urethritis
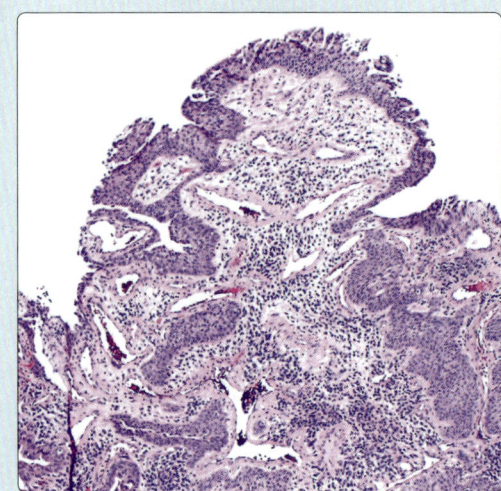

(Left) *Chronic local insults to the urethra may result in papillary/polypoid urethritis (PPU), in this case showing broad papillae with chronically inflamed edematous and myxoid stroma with overlying reactive urothelium.* (Right) *Lesions of papillary/polypoid urethritis often appear worrisome endoscopically to urologists and may be resected for suspicion of recurrent carcinoma. Despite the architectural complexity and redundance of the stroma, the urothelial atypia is in the range of reactive changes.*

Inflammatory Lesions of Urethra

TERMINOLOGY

Abbreviations
- Pseudosarcomatous myofibroblastic proliferation (PMP)
- Papillary/polypoid urethritis (PPU)

Synonyms
- PMP, inflammatory myofibroblastic tumor, pseudosarcomatous fibromyxoid tumor, postoperative spindle cell nodule

Urethritis
- Inflammatory response seen histologically involving urethra or clinically based on symptomatology, cultures, and smears
- Reiter syndrome is presentation of reactive arthritis, postinfectious syndrome that may involve many sites
  - Reiter syndrome is classic triad of urethritis, conjunctivitis, and arthritis

Urethral Caruncle
- Prolapsing polypoid lesion at distal urethral meatus, predominantly in women
- Urethral prolapse represents circumferential mucosal prolapse

Papillary/Polypoid Urethritis
- Nonneoplastic reactive lesion analogous to papillary/polypoid cystitis
- 1 or multiple papillary to polypoid-appearing luminal evaginations of edematous, usually myxoinflammatory lamina propria
- Related to chronic localized trauma

Pseudosarcomatous Myofibroblastic Proliferation
- Marked myofibroblastic stromal reaction with myxoinflammatory background and rich vascularity
- Raises morphologic differential with inflammatory sarcoma and sarcomatoid carcinoma

Malakoplakia
- Rare, idiosyncratic inflammatory lesion composed of mixed inflammation with prominent histiocytes (von Hansemann cells)
- Scattered cells with Michaelis-Gutmann bodies, laminated calcospherites

ETIOLOGY/PATHOGENESIS

Urethritis
- May be related to number of infectious agents, including sexually transmitted agents *Neisseria gonorrhoeae*, *Chlamydia trachomatis*, *Trichomonas vaginalis*
- Additionally *Gardnerella vaginalis*, *Ureaplasma urealyticum*, *Mycoplasma hominis*, *Candida* sp.
- Reiter syndrome may also be preceded by infection with *Chlamydia trachomatis*, *Yersinia*, *Salmonella*, *Shigella*, *Campylobacter*, *Escherichia coli*, *Clostridium difficile*, and *Chlamydia pneumoniae*, whether at GI or GU sites

Urethral Caruncle
- Thought to be caused by mucosal prolapse, which may be age or estrogen deficiency-related in females
- Prolapsed mucosa becomes chronically inflamed, eroded, infected due to local trauma
- Subsets of cases with history of irradiation, recent data implicating IgG4 in a subset of lesions

Malakoplakia
- Contemporary understanding is that infection may trigger the inflammatory reaction
- Histiocytic phagosomal digestion defects result in accumulation of degenerated bacterial fragments, which calcify

Pseudosarcomatous Myofibroblastic Proliferation
- ~ 1/2 of cases have prior history of instrumentation and may represent postoperative spindle cell nodule-type changes
- Subset of cases demonstrate activating gene rearrangements of ALK locus, or recently detected rearrangements of ROS1 in ALK(-) cases

CLINICAL ISSUES

Presentation
- **Urethritis**
  - Men are usually asymptomatic, diagnosed by purulent discharge or urethral smear
  - Women are usually symptomatic, with dysuria, urgency, frequency, or purulent discharge/smear
  - Reiter syndrome exhibits
    - Days to weeks between urethral infection and reactive arthritis and conjunctivitis
    - Usually mono or oligoarticular arthritis of lower extremities
- **Urethral caruncle**
  - Essentially lesion of females
  - Prolapsing lesion at urethral meatus, which may involve partial urethra (caruncle) or circumferential urethra (urethral prolapse)
  - Women may be asymptomatic or show dysuria, frequency, or obstructive symptoms
  - May simulate carcinoma clinically
- **PPU**
  - Has not been associated with indwelling catheter, unlike cystitis
  - Often found near the verumontanum in prostatic urethra
    - May be incidental papillary-appearing finding on endoscopic follow-up for urothelial carcinoma
- **PMP**
  - May or may not be preceded by identifiable inciting event, such as instrumentation
  - Pain, obstructive symptoms
- **Malakoplakia**
  - Characteristically among female, middle-aged patients (F:M ratio: 4:1)
  - Debility, immunosuppression, multiple medical comorbidities
  - Appear as plaque-like mucosal lesions
  - May result in significant morbidity with strictures or obstructive symptoms

Treatment
- **Urethritis** treated symptomatically and with etiologically specific antibiosis

Inflammatory Lesions of Urethra

- **Urethral caruncle** treated warm sitz baths, topical estrogen creams, topical antiinflammatory drugs
  - Biopsy and surgical excision if failed conservative treatment
- **PPU** and **PMP** are usually resected at diagnosis
- **Malakoplakia** is treated through management of inciting infection, usually including antibiotics
  - Resection of obstructive lesions

Prognosis

- **Urethral caruncle** may recur in subset of cases
- **PPU** generally does not recur unless inciting factor continues
- **PMP** typically stable or regressive after resection, minority recur, while rare cases progress to inflammatory sarcoma
- **Malakoplakia** may cause significant morbidity in immunocompromised

MICROSCOPIC

Histologic Features

- **Urethritis**
  - Variable active/acute inflammatory infiltrate to chronic inflammatory patterns, including lymphofollicular, xanthogranulomatous, mixed, and plasma cell-rich
  - Depends on underlying injury or infectious agent
- **Urethral caruncle**
  - Older studies stress 3 predominant patterns, granulation predominant, papillomatous with lobulated epithelial growth, and angiomatous with vascular ectasias
  - Frequently mixed urothelial and squamous epithelium with reactive hyperplasia
  - Variably fibrotic, edematous, myxoid, inflamed stroma
  - Folds and invaginations of urothelium into the stroma in more than 2/3 of cases
  - Epithelial nests with appearance of urethritis cystica et glandularis
- **PPU**
  - 2 archetypes: Broad polypoid examples with features of bullous cystitis and examples with finer folded/papillary appearance
  - Polypoid examples with broad bulbous projections of lamina propria
  - Papillary examples of thinner projections with edematous fibrovascular cores simulate low-grade urothelial neoplasms (though no or rare branching)
  - Edematous, chronically inflamed stroma demonstrated by both
- **PMP**
  - Lesions composed of plump, fusiform, or stellate reactive-appearing myofibroblasts
  - Fasciitis-like tissue culture appearance in short fascicles, may appear infiltrative
  - Myofibroblasts with abundant eosinophilic to amphophilic cytoplasm and nuclei with nucleoli
  - Prominent intralesional microvasculature
  - Stroma with variably prominent active chronic inflammation, often containing plasma cells
- **Malakoplakia**
  - Plaque-like lesion, usually in superficial lamina propria with overlying reactive epithelial hyperplasia
  - Admixture of large, eosinophilic to amphophilic histiocytic population with intracytoplasmic and intercellular calculospherules
  - Histiocytes are designated Von Hansemann cells, which are interspersed among active chronic inflammation
  - E. coli and other gram-negative bacteria identified within histiocytic populations by electron microscopy
  - Calculospherules are composed of laminated calcium phosphate crystals, positive on iron/calcium stains

DIFFERENTIAL DIAGNOSIS

Urethral Carcinoma

- Urothelial carcinoma, squamous cell carcinoma, or adenocarcinoma, may appear similar endoscopically to these inflammatory lesions
- Papillary urothelial carcinoma demonstrates fine fibrovascular cores, often ramifying, and distinct cytologic atypia
- Squamous cell carcinoma demonstrates squamous atypia, dyskeratosis
- Adenocarcinoma demonstrates cytologic atypia, ductal differentiation, and stratified or columnar epithelium

Sarcomatoid Carcinoma

- May pose morphologic differential diagnosis with PMP
- Sarcomatoid carcinoma best recognized by carcinoma from which it arises, or adjacent dysplasia
- Greater cytologic atypia, greater nuclear hyperchromasia
- Foci of admixed epithelioid component
- Lack vascular network of PMP, lack myxoedematous stroma of PMP, lacks ALK positivity, p63, HMWCK(+)

SELECTED REFERENCES

1. Kesan KV et al: Posterior urethral polyp with type I posterior urethral valves: a rare association in a neonate. Urology. 83(6):1401-3, 2014
2. Lovly CM et al: Inflammatory myofibroblastic tumors harbor multiple potentially actionable kinase fusions. Cancer Discov. 4(8):889-95, 2014
3. Regmi SK et al: An unusual cause of urinary retention in a young female: a case report. Urol Int. 93(1):122-4, 2014
4. Rasouly HM et al: Lower urinary tract development and disease. Wiley Interdiscip Rev Syst Biol Med. 5(3):307-42, 2013
5. Williamson SR et al: Urethral caruncle: a lesion related to IgG4-associated sclerosing disease? J Clin Pathol. 66(7):559-62, 2013
6. Conces MR et al: Urethral caruncle: clinicopathologic features of 41 cases. Hum Pathol. 43(9):1400-4, 2012
7. Kumar A et al: Genito-urinary polyps: summary of the 10-year experiences of a single institute. Int Urol Nephrol. 40(4):901-7, 2008
8. Lane Z et al: Polypoid/papillary cystitis: a series of 41 cases misdiagnosed as papillary urothelial neoplasia. Am J Surg Pathol. 32(5):758-64, 2008
9. Harik LR et al: Pseudosarcomatous myofibroblastic proliferations of the bladder: a clinicopathologic study of 42 cases. Am J Surg Pathol. 30(7):787-94, 2006
10. Hirsch MS et al: ALK expression in pseudosarcomatous myofibroblastic proliferations of the genitourinary tract. Histopathology. Apr;48(5):569-78, 2006
11. Montgomery EA et al: Inflammatory myofibroblastic tumors of the urinary tract: a clinicopathologic study of 46 cases, including a malignant example inflammatory fibrosarcoma and a subset associated with high-grade urothelial carcinoma. Am J Surg Pathol. 30(12):1502-12, 2006
12. Love KD et al: Urethral stricture associated with malacoplakia: a case report and review of the literature. Urology. 57(1):169, 2001

Inflammatory Lesions of Urethra

Urethral Caruncle

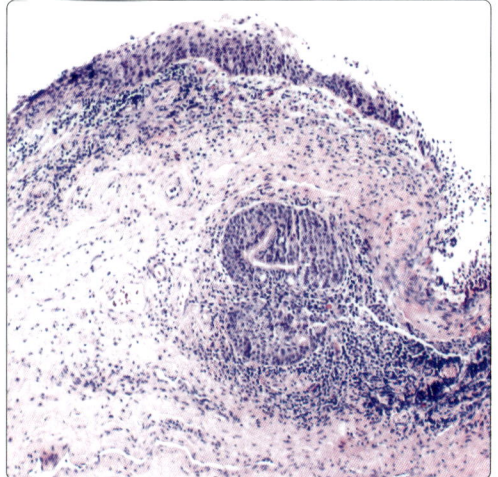

Urethral Caruncle

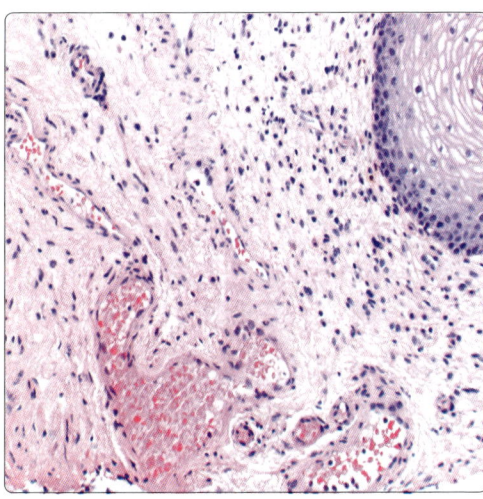

(Left) Urethral caruncle demonstrates reactive epithelial changes with ulceration and hyperplasia. Invagination of the epithelium with proliferative cystitis-like appearance has been described, as have other metaplastic changes. *(Right)* Another urethral caruncle shows squamous epithelium of the distal urethra overlying fibrotic stroma with angiomatous morphology with prominent vessels, some with thrombosis, and scattered hyperchromatic stromal cells.

Pseudosarcomatous Myofibroblastic Proliferation

Pseudosarcomatous Myofibroblastic Proliferation

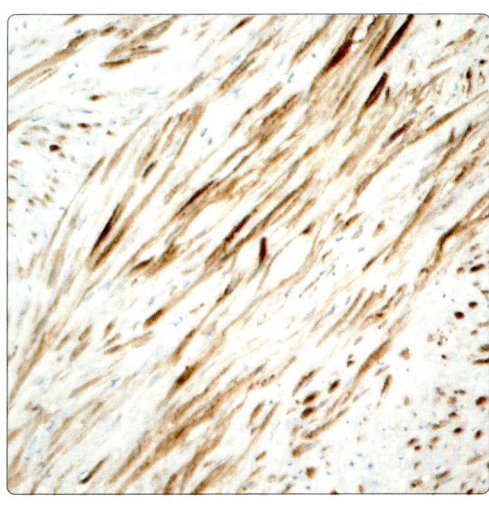

(Left) A pseudosarcomatous myofibroblastic proliferation (PMP) of the urethra presented with obstructive changes post instrumentation. The lesional cells show fusiform myofibroblastic morphology with abundant cytoplasm, myxoid stroma, and scattered plasma cells. *(Right)* A subset of PMPs are positive for ALK by immunohistochemistry, which is correlated with rearrangements of this gene. Recent scholarship also identifies a subset with rearrangements of ROS1.

Malakoplakia

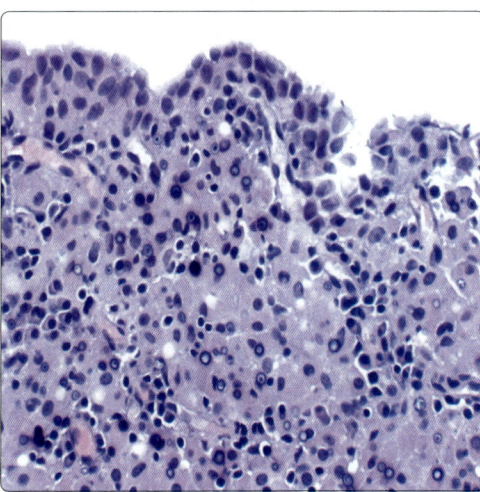

Malakoplakia

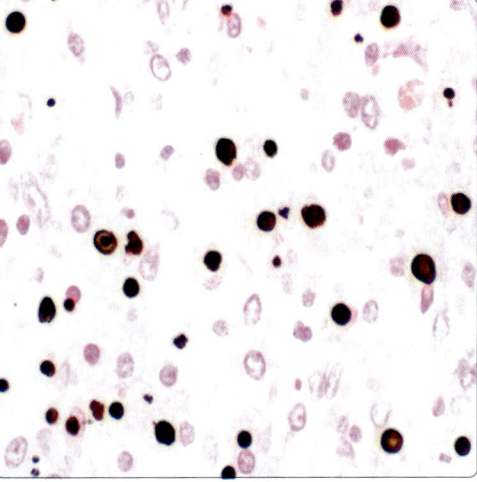

(Left) Malakoplakia of the urethra demonstrates a histiocytic infiltrate composed of plump von Hansemann cells with intracytoplasmic lamellated calculospherules underlying reactive urothelium. *(Right)* On histochemical stain for calcium, the Michaelis-Gutmann bodies of malakoplakia stand out as dark brown, targetoid spherules in tissue sections. Seldom are special stains necessary as these are readily identified on H&E.

Carcinoma of Urethra

KEY FACTS

CLINICAL ISSUES

- Primary urethral carcinomas (UCs) are rare compared to secondary involvement of urethra by bladder UC
  - ~ 10-20% of bladder UC patients with urethral involvement
- Primary UC age range and mean onset similar to bladder UC
- Wide range; mean: 7th decade
- Squamous cell carcinoma (SCC), UC, and adenocarcinoma occur with anatomic and sex-specific distribution
- In women
  - Prevalence by histology: 3/4 SCC, remaining 1/4 are UC or adenocarcinoma
  - Carcinomas arising in proximal 1/3 of urethra are generally UC
  - Carcinomas arising in distal 2/3 are generally SCC
- In men
  - Carcinomas arising in proximal/prostatic urethra are usually UC
  - Carcinomas arising in bulbomembranous and penile urethra are usually SCC

MICROSCOPIC

- Urothelial neoplasia
  - Full spectrum of papillary neoplasms as occur elsewhere, including exophytic and endophytic papilloma, PUNLMP, low- and high-grade UC
  - Full spectrum of flat neoplasia as occur elsewhere, including urothelial hyperplasia, dysplasia, and carcinoma in situ
- SCC
  - Conventional, verrucous, basaloid, and sarcomatoid variants
- Adenocarcinoma
  - Variable morphologies, arising either from the surface, from accessory glands (Littre or Skene), or in association with diverticulum
  - Clear cell adenocarcinoma (CCA)

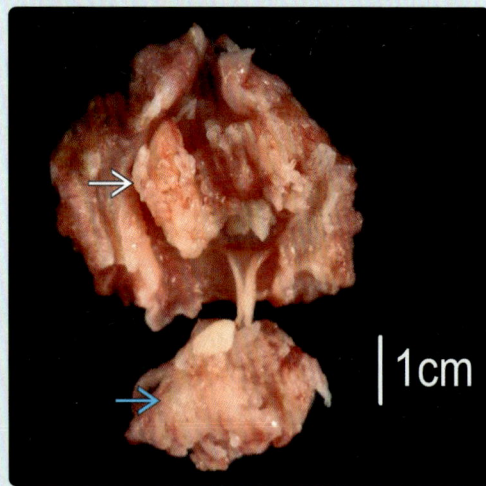

Squamous Cell Carcinoma: Urethrectomy

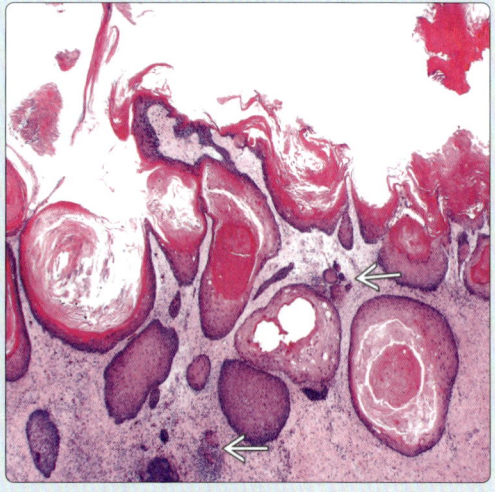

Urethral Squamous Cell Carcinoma

(Left) An opened urethrectomy specimen of a female with squamous cell carcinoma (SCC) demonstrates a friable exophytic mass protruding from the mucosa of the proximal urethra ➔. More distal involvement is also apparent ➔. Careful prosection and surgical correlation is essential for staging and margins. *(Right)* The previous case showed an invasive, moderately to well-differentiated, keratinizing SCC. Irregular angulated nests of SCC with dyskeratosis infiltrate the lamina propria ➔.

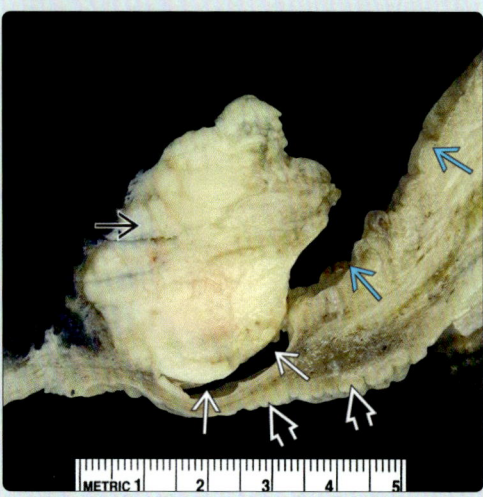

Clear Cell Adenocarcinoma: Diverticulum

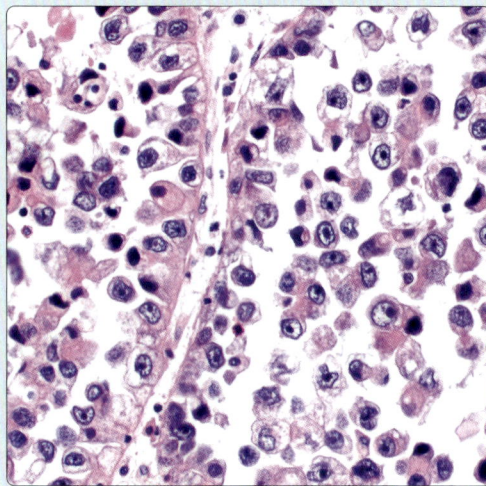

Clear Cell Adenocarcinoma

(Left) Section in the sagittal plane of a bulbous, nodular clear cell adenocarcinoma ➔ arising in and filling the lumen of a urethral diverticulum ➔, with adjacent proximal urethra ➔ and extending close to vaginal mucosa ➔, is shown. Careful fixation and prosection were necessary to show these anatomic relationships. *(Right)* Clear cell adenocarcinoma shows a friable carcinoma with high-grade cytology, clear to palely eosinophilic cytoplasm, hobnailed cells, and a papillary to tubulocystic architecture.

Carcinoma of Urethra

TERMINOLOGY

Synonyms
- Clear cell adenocarcinoma (CCA): Mesonephric adenocarcinoma

CLINICAL ISSUES

Presentation
- Primary urethral carcinomas are rare compared to secondary involvement of urethra by bladder urothelial carcinoma (UC)
  - Secondary involvement most prevalent in patients with multifocal papillary UC or carcinoma in situ (CIS)
    - ~ 10-20% of male and female patients
- Primary urethral carcinoma age range and mean onset similar to bladder UC (7th decade)
- Squamous cell carcinoma (SCC) and UC occur with anatomic and sex-specific distribution
- Adenocarcinomas of varying morphology occur in both sexes; distinctive CCA variant occurs more commonly in women
- Some SCCs may be related to human papillomavirus oncogenesis, limited data
- **In women**
  - Primary urethral carcinoma is rare, more prevalent than men
  - Presenting symptoms related to frequency, dysuria, hematuria, obstruction, new onset fistula
  - Prevalence by histology: 3/4 SCC, remaining 1/4 are UC or adenocarcinoma
  - Carcinomas arising in proximal 1/3 of urethra are generally UC
  - Carcinomas arising in distal 2/3 are generally SCC
    - Include well-differentiated, keratinizing SCC and verrucous carcinoma
    - Exclusion of vulvar SCC secondarily involving distal urethra is requisite
- **In men**
  - Primary urethral carcinoma is rare
  - Dysuria, hematuria, alteration in urine stream, history of infection, stricture, fistulas
  - Carcinomas arising in proximal/prostatic urethra are usually UC
    - Proximal urethral carcinomas often present higher stage, prostatic stromal involvement
    - Staged by AJCC as UC of prostate, different than urethral carcinoma in females
  - Carcinomas arising in bulbomembranous and penile urethra are usually SCC
    - Diagnosis at earlier stage than proximal urethral carcinoma
    - Exclusion of penile lesion is requisite
- **Adenocarcinoma, in either men or women**
  - More common in women than men
  - Generally represents on 3 processes
    - Adenocarcinoma arising from surface in setting of longstanding inflammatory insult, diverticulum, or stricture with metaplasia
    - Rare adenocarcinomas arising from periurethral glands of Littre or Cowper glands (men) or Skene glands (women)
    - Unusual cases of CCA arising almost always in women and of uncertain histogenesis
  - Symptomatology related to hematuria, obstruction, essentially independent of which type
  - Determination of anatomic site of origin requires careful clinicopathologic correlation, as large masses may have obliterated their site of origin (e.g., periurethral glands)
  - Adenocarcinomas of other primary sites (gynecologic, enteric, prostatic) involving urethra must be excluded in work-up
  - Adenocarcinoma is most common histologic type of urethral carcinoma arising in setting of diverticulum

Treatment
- **In women**
  - Proximal urethral carcinomas treated by total urethrectomy
    - Pelvic and inguinal lymphadenectomy as metastatic pattern may be variable
  - Distal urethral carcinoma may by treated by distal urethrectomy only
    - Inguinal lymphadenectomy, as generally distal lesions metastasize to inguinal lymph nodes
- **In men**
  - Proximal urethral carcinomas treated by cystoprostatectomy, same as UC of prostatic urethra
    - Carcinoma may extend extensively into prostate by pagetoid involvement of prostatic ducts or by direct invasion
    - Securing negative margins may be difficult in locally advanced lesions
  - Distal urethral carcinomas treated by partial penectomy ± inguinal lymph node dissection

Prognosis
- **In men**
  - Proximal urethral carcinoma has worse prognosis
  - Distal urethral carcinoma has superior prognosis at any stage
  - Multivariate analysis finds younger age, nodal status, and lower histologic grade associated with better prognosis
  - Lymph nodes positive in 6%, metastases at presentation in 5%
  - SEER data report cancer-specific survival: 68% at 5 years, 60% at 10 years
- **In women**
  - Stage of primary tumor, nodal stage, and anatomic site independent prognostic factors
    - Proximal worse than distal, just as in males
  - Tumors < 2 cm and in distal urethra: 60% survival at 5 years
  - Tumors > 4 cm in proximal urethra: 13% survival at 5 years

Carcinoma of Urethra

MACROSCOPIC

General Features
- Resection specimens are frequently large and complex, requiring careful correlation with surgical team to ensure appropriate margin sampling
- Detailed prosection may provide best indication of site of origin of carcinomas
  - Sections showing relationship to urinary bladder may reveal bladder primary
  - May demonstrate site of diverticulum or stricture
  - Sampling adjacent to lesion may show metaplastic, dysplastic, or in situ precursor lesion
  - Relationship to any attached gynecologic and gastrointestinal organs key for adenocarcinoma, for exclusion of secondary involvement and for staging purposes

MICROSCOPIC

Histologic Features
- Papillary urothelial neoplasms, often more proximal in urethra, demonstrate full spectrum of lesions at any site in urinary tract
  - Urothelial papilloma with nonhyperplastic, nonatypical urothelium arrayed on fibrovascular cores
  - Papillary urothelium neoplasm of low malignant potential characterized by hyperplastic, essentially nonatypical urothelium arrayed on fibrovascular cores
  - Low-grade papillary UC with distinct, low-grade cytologic atypia and some maintenance of polarization and maturation
  - High-grade papillary UC with loss of polarization, disordered maturation, and often pleomorphism
  - Though rare in this setting, full spectrum of histologic variants of UC (e.g., plasmacytoid, micropapillary) are possible
  - UC with squamous differentiation raises differential with primary SCC
- Flat urothelial neoplasms include, as in other sites
  - Urothelial hyperplasia (increased in thickness &/or cell density) without cytologic atypia
  - Urothelial dysplasia (low grade but distinct cytologic atypia) in flat lesion with preserved polarization
  - UC in situ (high-grade cytologic atypia) with loss of order and polarity
- SCC
  - Typical SCC graded on 3-tiered system, well differentiated, moderately differentiated, and poorly differentiated
  - Variants include verrucous carcinoma, basaloid SCC, and sarcomatoid SCC
- Adenocarcinoma
  - CCA: Distinctive cytology of flat, cuboidal to hobnailed cells with clear to palely eosinophilic cytoplasm
    - Multiple patterns, often admixed, include tubulocystic, papillary, and diffuse (solid)
    - Tubulocystic is most common, with tubules of varying sizes with basophilic to eosinophilic luminal secretions
    - Papillary examples show fibrovascular cores with very frequent, extensive hyalinization
    - Atypia is high grade, mitotic activity is brisk
  - Non-CCAs include mucinous, including colloid, signet ring cell, and conventional not otherwise specified
    - Atypical columnar epithelium with varying degrees of mucin production and variable degree of enteric type morphology
      - Urethritis cystica et glandularis or dysplasia arising in this process may be seen adjacent to the tumor
  - Rare adenocarcinomas of accessory glands (Littre or Skene glands) may show similar features to adenocarcinomas arising from surface or show tubular or micropapillary growth with variable cuboidal to columnar cytology

DIFFERENTIAL DIAGNOSIS

Urothelial Carcinoma of Urinary Bladder With Extension Into Urethra
- By far, more frequent than primary urethral carcinoma
- Exclude rigorously clinically (exam and history) and histologically

Squamous Cell Carcinoma of Penis or Vulva With Extension Into Distal Urethra
- Exclude by exam and by history

Adenocarcinoma From Adjacent Anatomic Site
- Exclude by exam, history, imaging, and careful prosection of specimens
- In enteric-type adenocarcinoma, nucleocytoplasmic β-catenin expression (as opposed to membranocytoplasmic expression) supports GI primary

Nephrogenic Adenoma: Differential With Clear Cell Adenocarcinoma
- Does not have high-grade cytologic atypia
- Less mitosis and lower Ki-67 proliferative index
- Less cellular, less solid, more haphazard tubules
- At present, no reliable immunostains to distinguish from clear cell, both may be racemase and pax-8(+)

SELECTED REFERENCES
1. Gakis G et al: EAU guidelines on primary urethral carcinoma. Eur Urol. 64(5):823-30, 2013
2. Champ CE et al: Prognostic factors and outcomes after definitive treatment of female urethral cancer: a population-based analysis. Urology. 80(2):374-81, 2012
3. Rabbani F: Prognostic factors in male urethral cancer. Cancer. 117(11):2426-34, 2011
4. McKenney JK et al: Protocol for the examination of specimens from patients with carcinoma of the urethra. Arch Pathol Lab Med. 134(3):345-50, 2010
5. Nixon RG et al: Carcinoma in situ and tumor multifocality predict the risk of prostatic urethral involvement at radical cystectomy in men with transitional cell carcinoma of the bladder. J Urol. 167(2 Pt 1):502-5, 2002
6. Dalbagni G et al: Female urethral carcinoma: an analysis of treatment outcome and a plea for a standardized management strategy. Br J Urol. 82(6):835-41, 1998

Carcinoma of Urethra

CIS of Urethra

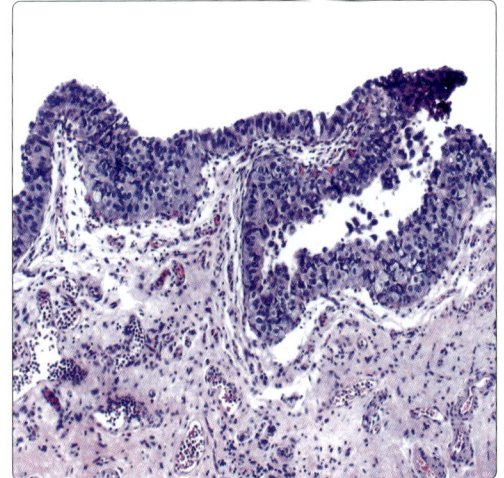

Bladder CIS Involving Urethra

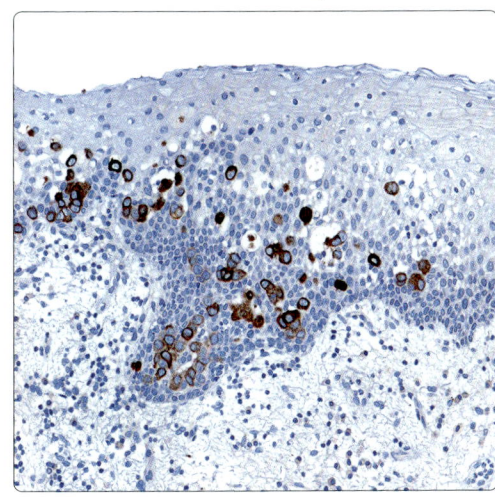

(Left) Here, an unusual case of primary urethral CIS is seen overgrowing reactive urothelium with the appearance of papillary/polypoid urethritis. Secondary involvement from a bladder primary, which is much more frequent, was excluded by history and cystoscopy. (Right) Here, uroplakin-2 immunostain highlights CIS from a bladder cancer patient, secondarily involving the squamous mucosa of the penile urethra in a Pagetoid intraepithelial manner.

Urothelial Neoplasms: Urethra

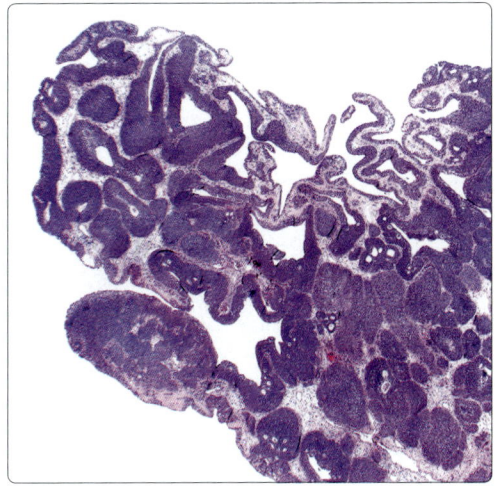

Urothelial Neoplasms: Urethra

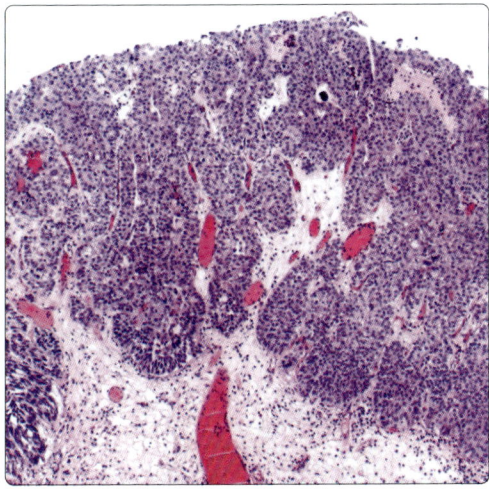

(Left) This urethral papillary urothelial neoplasm of low malignant potential shows prominent inverted architecture. A full spectrum of urothelial neoplasia ranging from benign papillomas to malignant, high-grade UCs occur in the urethra, most frequently the proximal portion in both sexes. (Right) Here, a high-grade papillary urothelial carcinoma arising in the urethra also demonstrates areas of noninvasive, inverted architecture. Review of deeper sections and all tissue is indicated to exclude invasion.

Adenocarcinoma of Urethra

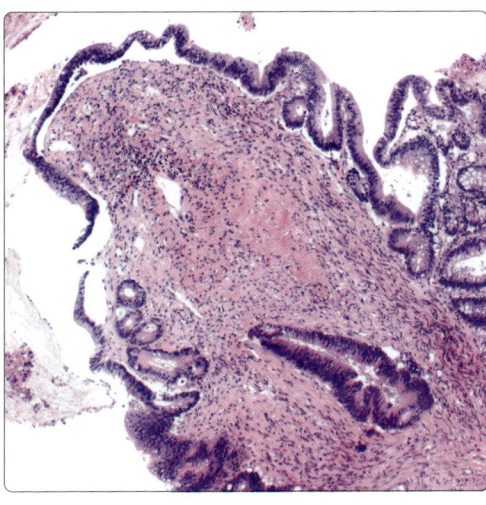

Adenocarcinoma of Urethra

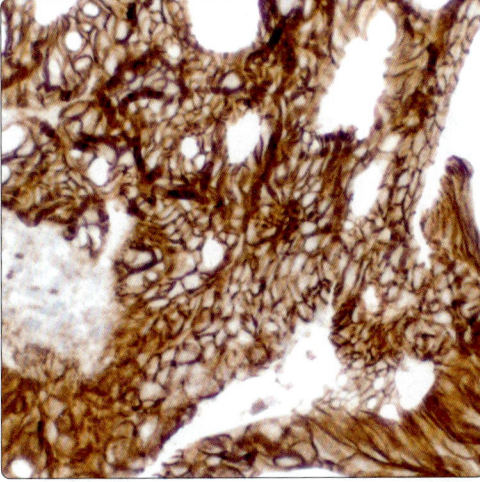

(Left) Here, an adenocarcinoma with prominent enteric differentiation is seen involving the prostatic urethra in a male patient. Exclusion of a GI primary is required to make this diagnosis. (Right) Here, a β-catenin immunostain done in the same case demonstrates prominent membranocytoplasmic staining that is excluded from the nucleus, which in addition to absence of a GI primary is supportive of a noncolorectal primary (which would be expected to have nuclear accumulation).

Other Tumors and Tumor-Like Lesions of Urethra

KEY FACTS

CLASSIFICATION

- **Urethral valves**: Congenital abnormality of redundant mucosal folds that may cause obstruction, hematuria, or recurrent infections
  - Rarely presents specimen for surgical pathology
- **Urethral diverticula**: Pathologic herniation or outpouching of urethral mucosa
  - Associated with recurrent infections, stricture, lithiasis
  - May be lined by urothelium with variable metaplasia
  - Significantly associated with cancer, urothelial, squamous, or adenocarcinoma (frequently clear cell adenocarcinoma)
- **Fibroepithelial polyp**: Rare congenital lesion most commonly of prostatic urethra, near verumontanum
- **Nephrogenic adenoma**: Common, benign proliferative lesion in reactive settings
  - Often associated with prior infection, instrumentation
  - May simulate carcinoma clinically and histologically
- **Amyloidosis**: Plaque-like stromal deposition of amorphous, homogeneous pink, Congophilic material identical to deposition at other sites
- **Prostatic-type polyp/ectopic prostate tissue**: Exophytic lesions protruding into prostatic urethra composed of prostatic acinar and ductal epithelium, often admixed with urothelium
  - If beyond prostatic urethra into penile urethra, considered ectopic prostate tissue
- **Polypoid prostatic adenocarcinoma involving urethra**
  - Rarely, ductal or even acinar adenocarcinoma of prostate may protrude into urethral lumen and be sampled with concern for primary urethral lesion
- **Condyloma acuminatum**: HPV-related papillomatous squamous neoplasm
  - Frequent lesion of distal urethra and genital skin
  - Extension into urethra in as many as 20% of cases

Fibroepithelial Polyp

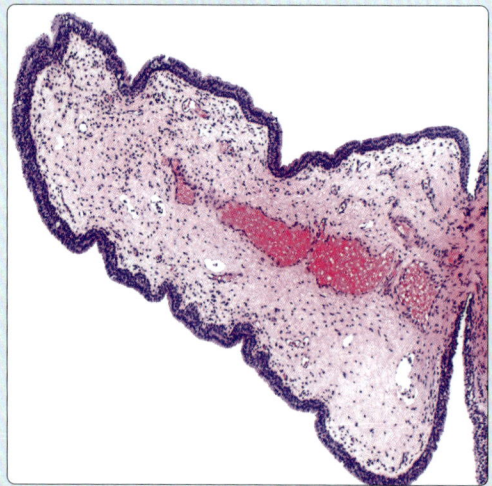

(Left) *A rare anterior urethral polyp in a young male demonstrates stratified columnar epithelium overlying edematous myxoinflammatory stroma with prominent vascular ectasia.* (Right) *Like condylomata of other sites, urethral condyloma acuminatum is a papillary squamous lesion with fibrovascular cores lined by squamous epithelium with koilocytic atypia. Such cases are strongly associated with synchronous or antecedent condylomata of the external genital skin.*

Condyloma Acuminatum

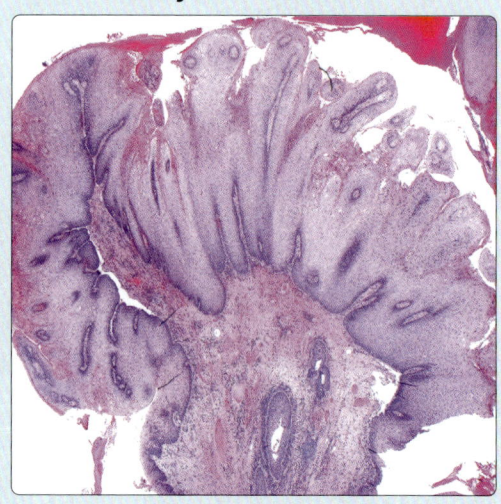

Urethral Diverticulum: Male

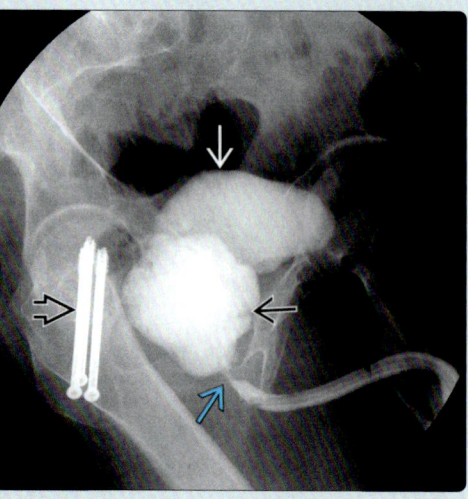

(Left) *Rare urethral diverticulum of the membranous urethra in a male patient shows a 7-cm diverticulum just proximal to a bulbar urethral stricture, which clinically was suspected as a cause. The bladder is partially distended but compressed by this large lesion. The orthopedic hardware visible to the side is incidental.* (Right) *Urethral diverticulum excised from a female patient for recurrent infections shows marked chronic inflammation and granulation tissue replacing denuded urothelium.*

Urethral Diverticulum: Histology

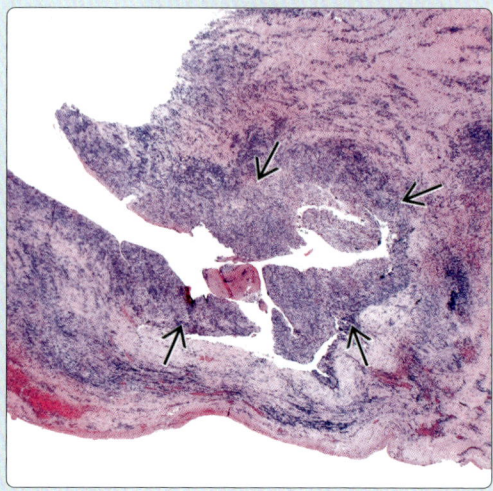

Other Tumors and Tumor-Like Lesions of Urethra

TERMINOLOGY

Synonyms
- Fibroepithelial polyp: Congenital urethral polyp
- Nephrogenic adenoma: Nephrogenic metaplasia

Definitions
- **Urethral valves**: Congenital abnormality of redundant mucosal folds that may cause obstruction, hematuria, or recurrent infections
- **Urethral diverticula**: Pathologic herniation or outpouching of urethral mucosa
  - Associated with recurrent infections, stricture, lithiasis
  - May be lined by urothelium with variable metaplasia
  - Significantly associated with cancer, urothelial, squamous, or adenocarcinoma (frequently clear cell adenocarcinoma)
- **Fibroepithelial polyp**: Rare congenital lesion most commonly of prostatic urethra
- **Nephrogenic adenoma**: Common, benign proliferative lesion in reactive settings
  - Often associated with prior infection, instrumentation
  - May simulate carcinoma clinically and histologically
- **Amyloidosis**: Plaque-like stromal deposition of amorphous, homogeneous pink, Congophilic material identical to deposition at other sites
- **Prostatic-type polyp/ectopic prostate tissue**: Exophytic lesions protruding into prostatic urethra composed of prostatic acinar and ductal epithelium
  - If beyond prostatic urethra into penile urethra (or bladder), considered ectopic prostate tissue
- **Polypoid prostatic adenocarcinoma involving urethra**
  - Rarely, ductal or even acinar adenocarcinoma of prostate may protrude into urethral lumen and be sampled with concern for primary urethral lesion
- **Condyloma acuminatum**: HPV-related neoplasm
  - Frequent lesion of distal urethra and genital skin
  - Extension into urethra in as many as 20% of cases

ETIOLOGY/PATHOGENESIS

Urethral Valves and Fibroepithelial Polyps
- Congenital/developmental anomalies

Urethral Diverticula
- Thought to be either congenital or acquired, adult cases sequelae of infection, calculi, obstruction

Nephrogenic Adenoma
- Studies suggest autotransplantation of renal tubular cells into areas of local injury with subsequent proliferation

Amyloidosis
- Localized buildup of abnormally folded protein fragments

Prostatic-Type Polyp
- Urethral examples probably represent polypoid hyperplasia overgrowing urothelium
- Proximal (bladder) or distal (penile urethra) may represent developmental anomalies, metaplasia, or implantation

Condyloma Acuminatum
- Caused by human papillomavirus subtypes 6, 11, 16, and 18

CLINICAL ISSUES

Presentation
- **Urethral valves**: Posterior urethral valves are most common etiology of urinary obstruction in newborn male
  - Often asymptomatic
  - Risk of obstruction, hydronephrosis and hydroureter, recurrent infection, cystic renal dysplasia (prenatal) and ongoing kidney injury
- **Urethral diverticulum**: Most commonly affects females
  - Asymptomatic to painful, irritative symptoms
  - May be tumefacient, palpable through vagina
  - May present due to recurrent infection, stone formation, obstruction, or development of associated carcinoma
- **Fibroepithelial polyp**: Nearly exclusively of males, usually children
  - Polypoid lesion adjacent to the verumontanum: Posterior urethral polyp
  - Polypoid lesion of the penile urethra: Anterior urethral polyp; rare
  - Obstructive symptoms, hematuria, infection
  - Female examples probably represent prolapsing epithelium
- **Nephrogenic adenoma**: Often incidental finding on endoscopy for surveillance or other reason
- **Amyloidosis**: Hematuria, irritative voiding symptoms, obstruction
- **Prostatic-type polyp**: Often incidental finding on endoscopy for other reason
- **Condyloma acuminatum**: Hematuria, irritative voiding symptoms
  - Often associated with prior/synchronous external lesions

Prognosis
- **Urethral valves**: Benign lesion, but clinically troublesome; 15-20% progress to end-stage kidney disease
- **Urethral diverticulum**: Individual prognoses related to causes of diverticulum and whether involved by carcinoma
- **Fibroepithelial polyp**: Do not recur after surgical excision
- **Nephrogenic adenoma**: Benign, rarely recurs
- **Amyloidosis**: Excised for control of local lesion, prognosis related to systemic disease
- **Condyloma acuminatum**: Present challenging local control with frequent recurrence after transurethral resection, laser, or cryotherapy
  - Low but real risk of development of dysplasia and progression to invasive squamous cell carcinoma

MICROSCOPIC

Histologic Features
- **Urethral valves**: Reactive urothelium overlies folded stroma with chronic inflammation
- **Urethral diverticulum**
  - Variable histology based on size and location
  - Varied, reactive and metaplastic epithelial changes
  - Squamous and glandular metaplasia are common
  - Stromal fibrosis and variable chronic inflammatory infiltrate
  - Carcinoma arises in 2-15% of symptomatic diverticula

Other Tumors and Tumor-Like Lesions of Urethra

- Most frequently squamous cell carcinoma or adenocarcinoma
- Clear cell carcinoma may present papillary, tubular, microcystic, or solid morphology
- Unlike gynecologic clear cell carcinoma, it is unrelated to DES exposure
- **Fibroepithelial polyp**
  - Club-like projections into lumen associated with proliferative urethritis or squamous metaplasia
  - Broad core of fibrovascular stroma may show atypical stromal cells, calcification, or vascular ectasia
- **Nephrogenic adenoma**
  - Notoriously variable morphology, with papillary, tubular, solid, flat, and fibromyxoid variants
  - Papillary examples show complex ramifying architecture with cuboidal to hobnailed epithelium with variable eosinophilic to basophilic to foamy cytoplasm
  - Nuclei with reactive-appearing micronucleoli
  - Tubular variant with infiltrative-appearing tubules with luminal contents, eosinophilic to basophilic
    - Compact examples can resemble signet ring cells
  - Fibromyxoid variant consisting of compressed spindled cells present in fibromyxoid stroma with rare tubules or cords of cells
  - Positive for pax-8 and pax-2, less helpfully CK7
  - Often positive for AMACR and S100A1
  - Rarely PSA and GATA3 positivity raise differential with prostatic lesions and urothelial neoplasia, respectively
- **Amyloidosis**
  - Amorphous, homogeneous, eosinophilic, afibrillar material deposited into lamina propria
  - May extend to involve superficial muscle fibers
  - Less frequently can show perivascular orientation similar to other sites
  - Congo red positive
  - Apple green birefringence on polarized microscopy
- **Condyloma acuminatum**
  - Broad, fusing papillae consisting of mildly atypical squamous cells with multifocal clearing cytoplasm
  - Nuclear atypia, in form of raisinoid or koilocytic atypia present but less prominent than cervical lesions
  - In situ hybridization for high- and low-risk HPV

DIFFERENTIAL DIAGNOSIS

Other Cystic Lesions of Urethra: Differential vs. Urethral Diverticula

- Urethral duplication
  - Rare developmental anomaly may be associated with bladder duplication
  - Complete or incomplete, asymptomatic or symptomatic with infections
- Prostatic utricle cyst
  - Midline, arising from utricle, connected to the urethra but not prostatic ducts
  - Often incidental findings, asymptomatic
  - Lined by epithelium positive for PSA and resembling prostatic ducts and acini
- Cowper gland duct cyst: Children and young males
  - Irritative or obstructive voiding symptoms
  - Cystic dilatation of the duct, with fibrosis, denudation of epithelium
  - Diagnosis secured on urethrography, rarely produce surgical specimen
- Skene duct cyst: Females
  - Dysuria or asymptomatic
  - Squamous lining
  - Cystourethrography and MR distinguish based on anatomy

Other Exophytic Lesions of Urethra: Differential vs. Polypoid Lesions

- Verumontanum mucinous gland hyperplasia
  - Polypoid overgrowth of mucinous acini
  - Prominent corpora amylacea with concentric lamellations seen
- Cowper gland hyperplasia
  - Increased number of histologically normal Cowper glands
  - PAS-positive mucins, negative of PSA and PAP

SELECTED REFERENCES

1. Humphrey PA: Prostatic-type epithelial polyp of the urethra. J Urol. 193(6):2095-6, 2015
2. Gordetsky J et al: Pseudopapillary features in prostatic adenocarcinoma mimicking urothelial carcinoma: a diagnostic pitfall. Am J Surg Pathol. 38(7):941-5, 2014
3. McDaniel AS et al: Immunohistochemical staining characteristics of nephrogenic adenoma using the PIN-4 cocktail (p63, AMACR, and CK903) and GATA-3. Am J Surg Pathol. 38(12):1664-71, 2014
4. McKenney J and Oliva E: Chapter 7. Pathology of the Male and Female Urethra. In: Urological Pathology. Amin MB et al. Ed. Philadelphia: Wolters Kluwer, 2014
5. López JI et al: Nephrogenic adenoma of the urinary tract: clinical, histological, and immunohistochemical characteristics. Virchows Arch. 463(6):819-25, 2013
6. Kumar A et al: Genito-urinary polyps: summary of the 10-year experiences of a single institute. Int Urol Nephrol. 40(4):901-7, 2008
7. Thomas AA et al: Urethral diverticula in 90 female patients: a study with emphasis on neoplastic alterations. J Urol. 180(6):2463-7, 2008
8. Hansel DE et al: Fibromyxoid nephrogenic adenoma: a newly recognized variant mimicking mucinous adenocarcinoma. Am J Surg Pathol. 31(8):1231-7, 2007
9. Samaratunga H et al: Prostatic ductal adenocarcinoma presenting as a urethral polyp: a clinicopathological study of eight cases of a lesion with the potential to be misdiagnosed as a benign prostatic urethral polyp. Pathology. 39(5):476-81, 2007
10. Tsuzuki T et al: Fibroepithelial polyp of the lower urinary tract in adults. Am J Surg Pathol. 29(4):460-6, 2005

Other Tumors and Tumor-Like Lesions of Urethra

Polypoid Ductal Prostatic Adenocarcinoma

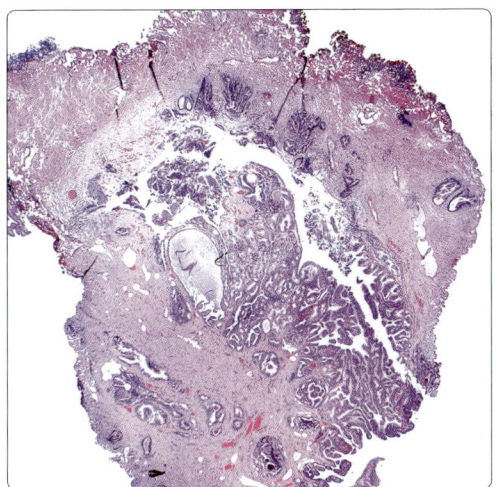

Polypoid Ductal Prostatic Adenocarcinoma

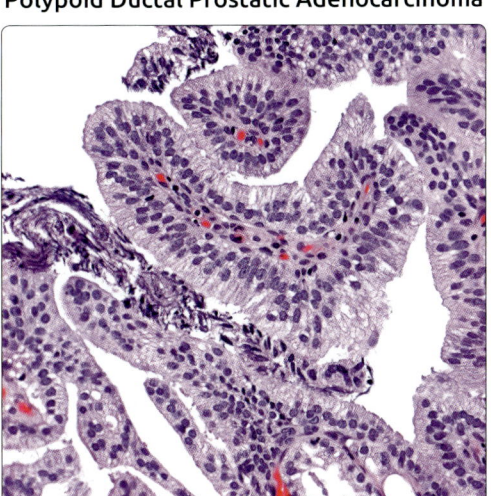

(Left) Ductal adenocarcinoma of the prostate was encountered in the urethra on transurethral resection for obstruction. At low power, a prostatic-type polyp might also be considered. *(Right)* At high power, the distinctive cytologic atypia of ductal carcinoma is apparent with nucleomegaly and macronucleoli. As is the case with all prostatic lesions, nuclear atypia is key. PIN cocktail demonstrates predominant lack of a basal cell layer, while ERG is positive, PTEN negative, in more than half of ductal cases.

Prostatic-Type Polyp

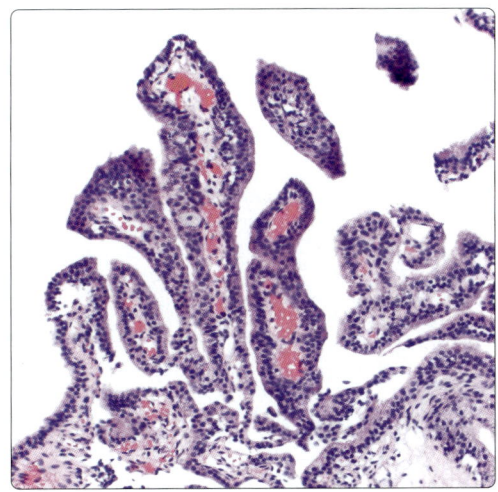

Nephrogenic Adenoma: Papillary/Tubular

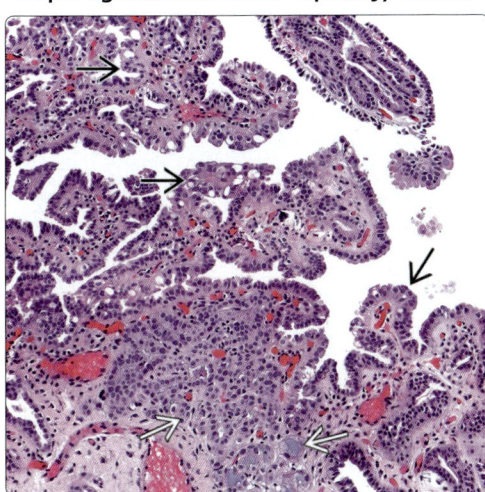

(Left) Prostatic-type polyp excised from the urethra as an incidental finding during surveillance for urothelial carcinoma demonstrates fine papillae and tubules lined by non-atypical prostatic acinar and ductal-type epithelium. PSA is positive in these lesions. *(Right)* This urethral biopsy taken on cystoscopy for recurrent urinary tract infections shows papillary ⇨ as well as tubular ⇨ morphology of nephrogenic adenoma.

Nephrogenic Adenoma: Fibromyxoid

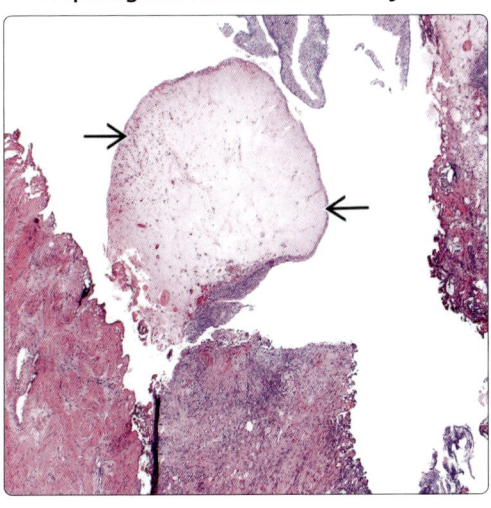

Nephrogenic Adenoma: Fibromyxoid

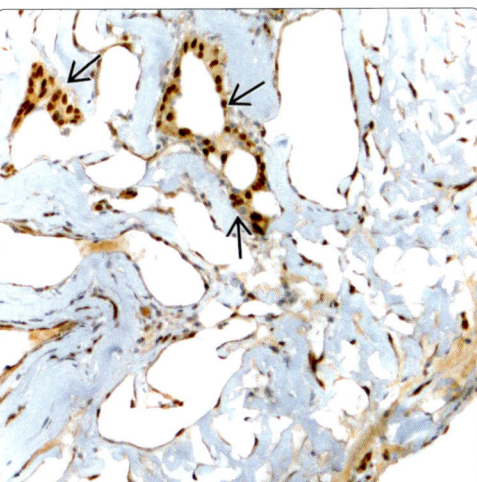

(Left) A recently appreciated variant of nephrogenic adenoma is the fibromyxoid variant. Here, it presents as a tumefacient polypoid mass ⇨ in the urethra, thought clinically to represent polypoid urethritis. *(Right)* Cases with fibromyxoid morphology demonstrate pax-8 nuclear positivity among the lesional cells, which show a distinctive compressed, spindled morphology, coursing through myxohyaline matrix. Helpfully, most examples with this morphology show at least focal tubular morphology ⇨.

Urothelial Carcinoma of Ureter

KEY FACTS

TERMINOLOGY
- Urothelial carcinoma of ureter: Malignant neoplasm of urothelial (transitional cell) origin involving ureter

ETIOLOGY/PATHOGENESIS
- Tobacco smoking is important risk factor
- Blackfoot disease, endemic to region in southwest Taiwan, form of vasculitis caused by chronic exposure to arsenic pollution of water
  - More common in women than in men
  - More common in ureter than renal pelvis
- History of previous lower urinary tract carcinoma is predisposing factor
- Increased risk of ureteral carcinoma in patients of Lynch syndrome

CLINICAL ISSUES
- Incidence: < 1% of all urothelial tumors
- Age at presentation usually 6th or 7th decades
- Usually younger in patients with Lynch syndrome
- More common in men than in women
- Patients present with hematuria, flank pain, or hydronephrosis

IMAGING
- Filling defect or obstructive mass associated with hydronephrosis or urolithiasis

MACROSCOPIC
- Mostly predominantly papillary or polypoid or infiltrative mass with thickening of pelvic wall
- Multiple tumors may be seen throughout ureter

MICROSCOPIC
- Histopathological features of urothelial carcinoma of ureter are similar to those in urinary bladder and renal pelvis, including variant histologies
- High-grade tumors are more common
- Assessment of invasion may be difficult

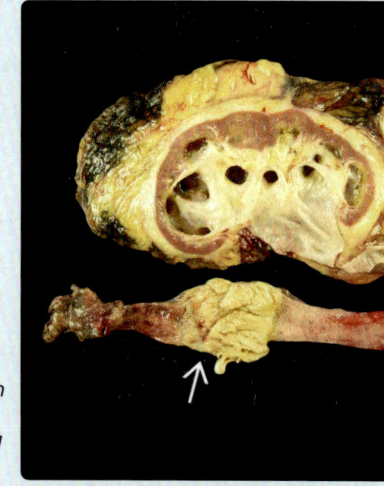

Urothelial Carcinoma of Ureter

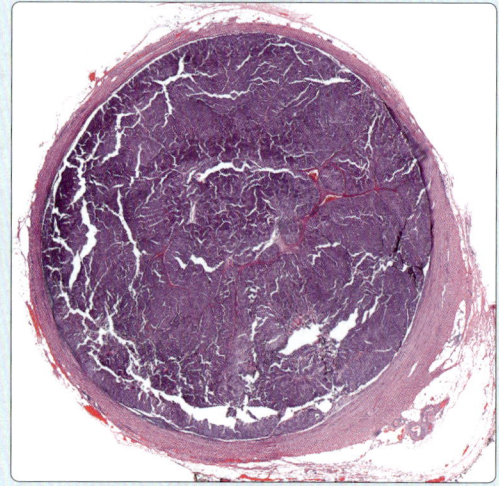

Urothelial Carcinoma of Ureter: Cross Section

(Left) This gross photograph shows a bulky exophytic papillary tumor in the distal 1/3 of the ureter ➡. The ureteral mucosa proximal to the tumor is hyperemic. Note the dilated renal pelvis and proximal ureter with thinning of the renal cortex. (Right) This is a cross section from a ureterectomy specimen containing a bulky tumor filling and expanding the ureteral lumen. This tumor is papillary, but due to limited space to grow such tumors can take on a more inverted appearance. Note the thinning of the ureteral wall.

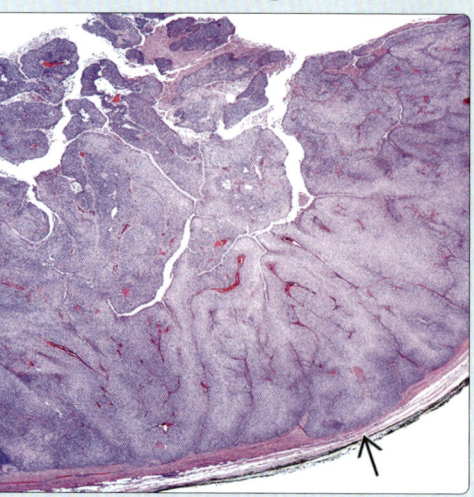

Urothelial Carcinoma of Ureter: Pushing Tumor Edge

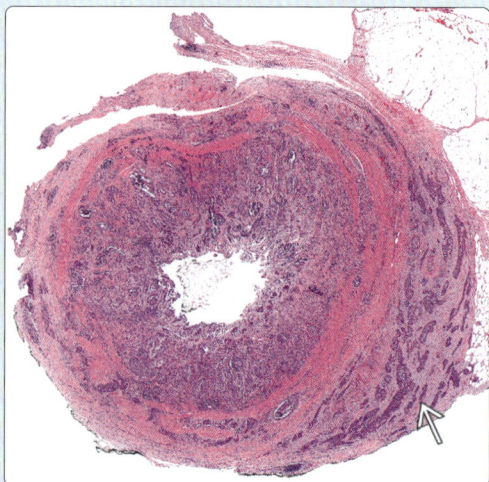

Invasive Urothelial Carcinoma of Ureter

(Left) This is another bulky exophytic papillary tumor expanding the ureteral lumen. The ureteral wall is markedly thinned by the tumor compression and the tumor is coming into near contact with the periureteral soft tissue ➡. Despite this, assessing invasion may be very difficult in such tumors. (Right) This is a cross section of a ureter with extensive involvement by a high-grade urothelial carcinoma. The tumor is invasive through the different layers of the ureteral wall into periureteral soft tissue ➡.

Urothelial Carcinoma of Ureter

TERMINOLOGY

Definitions
- Urothelial carcinoma of ureter
  - Malignant neoplasm of urothelial (transitional cell) origin involving ureter

ETIOLOGY/PATHOGENESIS

Environmental Exposure
- Tobacco smoking is important risk factor
  - Lifetime risk increases with increased consumption and intensity of smoking
- Blackfoot disease (BFD), endemic to region in southwest Taiwan, has been associated with increased risk of developing upper tract tumors, particularly in ureter
  - More common in women than men (2:1)
  - Tumors develop more in ureters (2x more common in ureter than in renal pelvis)
  - BFD is form of vasculitis caused by chronic exposure to arsenic pollution of water in artesian wells

Other Risk Factors
- History of previous lower urinary tract carcinoma is predisposing factor
  - Most patients have prior, concurrent, or subsequent carcinoma of bladder
- Increased risk of ureteral carcinoma in patients of Lynch syndrome
- Other possible risk factors include: Urolithiasis and chronic urinary tract infections

Molecular Features
- Generally similar to that of urothelial carcinomas of bladder
- Frequent mutations in fibroblastic growth factor receptor 3 (*FGFR3*) gene
  - Common primarily in tumors with papillary morphology
  - Relative incidences of *FGFR3* mutations suggest that noninvasive papillary tumors do progress, although infrequently
  - Tumors with *FGFR3* mutations may have lower risk for progression than those without
  - Other common mutations detected in chromatin-modifying genes (*KDM6A*, *KMT2D*, *KMT2C*, *CREBBP*, *ARID1A*)
  - *TP53* mutations are less frequent, and *RB1* mutations are rare
- Microsatellite instability and loss of mismatch repair proteins MSH2, MLH1, or MSH6 present in upper urinary tract tumors
  - Rare in sporadic cases but more common in patients with Lynch syndrome
    - Incidence in upper tract tumors (renal pelvis and ureter) is more common than in bladder tumors
  - Upper urinary tract tumors are 3rd most common tumors with microsatellite instability
    - Colonic and endometrial carcinoma are 2 most common tumors reported within hereditary nonpolyposis colorectal cancer (HNPCC)/Lynch syndrome patients

CLINICAL ISSUES

Epidemiology
- Incidence: < 1% of all urothelial tumors
- In upper tract, ureteral carcinoma is significantly outnumbered by that of renal pelvis
  - ~ 9:1 = pelvic:ureteral tumors
  - Reports suggesting ureteral tumors to be originating from tumors of renal pelvis as "drop metastases" with flow of urine
    - Supporting fact includes significantly higher incidence of renal pelvic tumors compared to ureteral tumors
    - Cannot explain ureteric tumors developing without prior renal pelvic tumors
- Age at presentation usually 6th or 7th decades
  - Usually younger in patient with Lynch syndrome
- More common in men than in women

Presentation
- Hematuria
- Hydronephrosis
- Flank pain

Treatment
- Segmental ureterectomy with ureteral reimplantation
  - Usually for distal uretal tumors, generally of lower grade and stage
- Nephroureterectomy with bladder cuff
  - Primarily for proximal ureteral tumors (close to renal pelvis)
  - Or when associated with severe hydronephrosis and afunctional kidney

Prognosis
- Most ureteral tumors have been studied grouped with renal pelvic tumors (combined upper urinary tract tumors)
  - Exact prognostic information and risk stratification difficult to ascertain from reported literature
- Generally, pathologic stage is single most important prognostic factor for urothelial carcinomas of upper urinary tract
- On univariate analysis, significant prognostic indicators include
  - Tumor size
  - Tumor grade
  - Pathologic stage
    - pTa: Papillary noninvasive carcinoma
    - pTis: Flat noninvasive urothelial carcinoma (in situ)
    - pT1: Tumor invades subepithelial connective tissue
    - pT2: Tumor invades muscularis
    - pT3: Tumor invades beyond muscularis into periureteric fat
    - pT4: Tumor invades adjacent organs
  - Lymphovascular invasion
- On multivariate analysis, stage is only significant prognostic factor for survival

IMAGING

Radiographic Findings
- Ureteral tumors usually present as filling defect, or
  - Obstructive mass associated with hydronephrosis

Urothelial Carcinoma of Ureter

- Renal/ureteral stones

MACROSCOPIC

General Features

- Most of these tumors are predominantly papillary or polypoid, but some tumors grow as infiltrative masses with thickening of ureteral wall
  - Tumors with predominant papillary or polypoid appearance
    - Usually expand and fill ureteral lumen
    - Tend to be noninvasive or are associated with limited invasion
    - Require ample sampling after proper fixation, which is important for accurate staging
  - Infiltrative tumors may extensively involve ureter wall and periureteric tissue or adjacent organs
  - Multiple tumors may be seen throughout resected ureteral segment

MICROSCOPIC

Histologic Features

- Histopathological features of ureteral urothelial carcinoma are similar to those in urinary bladder and renal pelvis
  - Papillary urothelial neoplasms of low malignant potential (PUNLMP) extremely uncommon in ureter
  - Low-grade carcinoma relatively less common, compared to that in bladder
- High-grade tumors are more common, and invasion should be thoroughly investigated, because it may not always be readily identifiable
- Assessing invasion should include stalks of papillary structure as well as deeper and advancing parts of tumor
- Due to limited space available to grow, papillary tumors may quickly fill and expand ureteral lumen
  - As a result, tumor edge will come into close proximity with muscularis layer
    - Muscle layer may become attenuated, bringing tumor into contact with fibrous and adipose tissue of periureteric space
    - Assessment of invasion may be very difficult in these situations, especially if tumor edge is smooth and pushing (tumor may appear inverted)
- Histopathologic diversity with morphologic variants/aberrant differentiations similar to that in bladder, although perhaps less frequent
- Variant morphologies seen, among others, include
  - Micropapillary variant
  - Lymphoepithelioma-like carcinoma
  - Squamous differentiation and squamous cell carcinoma
  - Sarcomatoid differentiation
  - Signet ring cell or plasmacytoid features
  - Small cell/neuroendocrine carcinomatous features

Margins

- Important to carefully examine for presence of carcinoma
- Positive margins may not necessarily increase risk of recurrence or progression
  - Skip lesions are known to occur in ureter

Lymph Nodes

- Most generated data are from reports of combined ureteral and renal pelvic tumors as upper tract tumors
  - Overall lymph node involvement reported to be ~ 10%
  - Reported incidence is not based on cases where lymph nodes were removed at time of nephroureterectomy
  - Rates of lymph node metastasis are close to 25% among cases where lymph node dissection was performed

ANCILLARY TESTS

Frozen Sections

- Frozen sections may be requested primarily to assess status of margins
- Positive margins may prompt surgeon to submit additional margin(s) if surgically possible
- Positive margin may not necessarily increase risk of recurrence or progression
- Negative (benign) margin does not necessarily mean that there is no tumor in other parts of ureter that have not been resected

Immunohistochemistry

- Uroplakin-2, CK7, and GATA3 diffusely positive
- HMWCK and p63 often strongly and diffusely positive
- CK20 at least focally positive in most cases
- pax-8 may be positive

DIFFERENTIAL DIAGNOSIS

Urothelial Carcinoma of Renal Pelvis

- Main distinguishing feature is location in pelvicalyceal system
  - May become issue if it located in distal pelvis close to ureteropelvic junction
  - Not particularly significant clinically

Urothelial Carcinoma of Bladder

- May become diagnostic challenge in tumors located in distal ureter
  - May present diagnostic challenges particularly when assigning stage to tumors involving muscle (muscularis layer of intramural ureter vs. muscularis propria or even muscularis mucosa of bladder surrounding intramural ureter)

SELECTED REFERENCES

1. Sfakianos JP et al: Genomic characterization of upper tract urothelial carcinoma. Eur Urol. 68(6): 970-7, 2015
2. Cosentino M et al: Upper urinary tract urothelial cell carcinoma: location as a predictive factor for concomitant bladder carcinoma. World J Urol. 31(1):141-5, 2013
3. Cha EK et al: Predicting clinical outcomes after radical nephroureterectomy for upper tract urothelial carcinoma. Eur Urol. 61(4):818-25, 2012
4. Colin P et al: Environmental factors involved in carcinogenesis of urothelial cell carcinomas of the upper urinary tract. BJU Int. 104(10):1436-40, 2009
5. Margulis V et al: Outcomes of radical nephroureterectomy: a series from the Upper Tract Urothelial Carcinoma Collaboration. Cancer. 115(6):1224-33, 2009

Urothelial Carcinoma of Ureter

Invasive Urothelial Carcinoma of Ureter: Infiltrating Growth

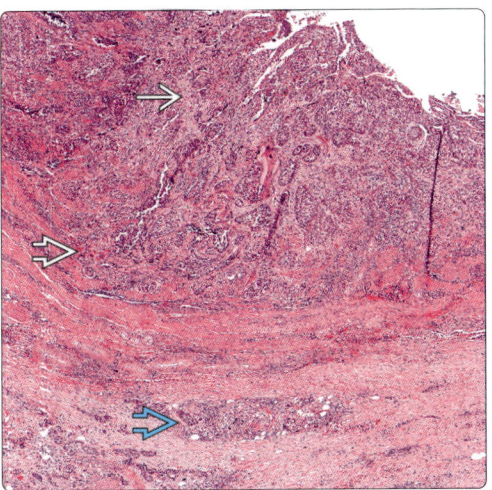

Urothelial Carcinoma of Ureter: In Situ and Invasive

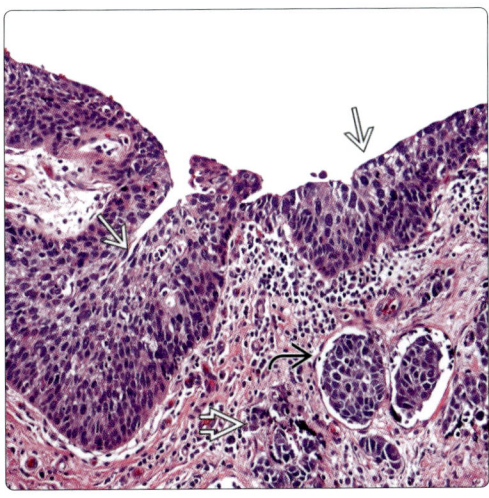

(Left) This urothelial carcinoma of the ureter shows a transmural infiltrating pattern with tumor foci expanding the lamina propria ⇥, invading the muscular layer ⇥, and reaching the periureteral soft tissue ⇥. *(Right)* In this section of a ureter, there is both urothelial carcinoma in situ (flat) ⇥ as well as invasive urothelial carcinoma into the lamina propria ⇥. There are tumor foci consistent with tumor spread into lymphovascular space ⇥.

Papillary Urothelial Carcinoma of Ureter: Invasion Within Papillary Fronds

Urothelial Carcinoma of Ureter: Inverted With Pushing Borders

(Left) This is a papillary urothelial carcinoma of ureter. The advancing edge of tumor is rounded and pushing, but superficial lamina propria invasion is present in the stalks of papillary structures ⇥. *(Right)* This is a urothelial carcinoma of ureter with a prominent inverted pattern. It is in close contact with bundles of the muscular layer, consistent with invasion ⇥. This pattern of invasion is not common and can be difficult to corroborate.

Urothelial Carcinoma of Ureter: Poor Fixation

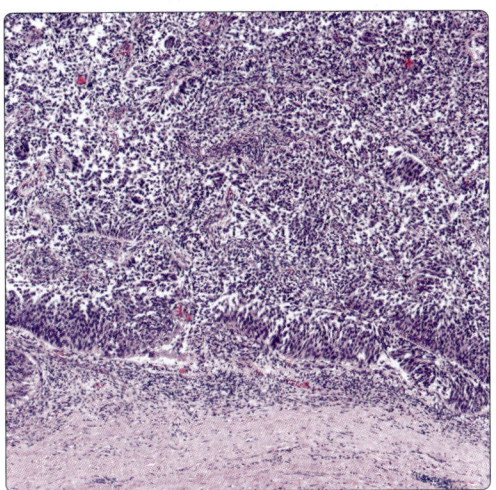

Urothelial Carcinoma of Ureter: Lynch Syndrome (MSH2 Immunostain)

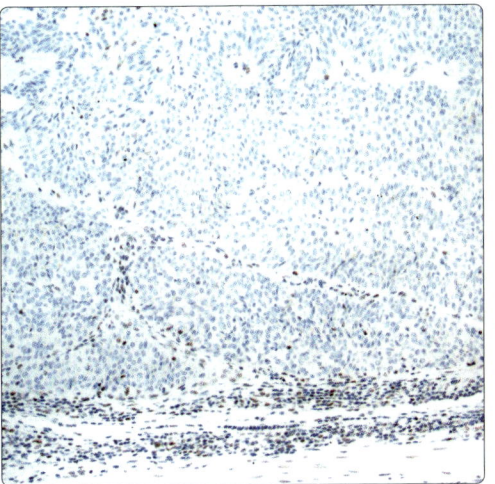

(Left) In this ureteral tumor, the section is not well prepared as the tissue was not well preserved or fixed. It is important to open these specimens and start the fixation process as soon as possible to ensure proper sample preparation and histopathologic assessment. *(Right)* This is a papillary urothelial carcinoma from a patient with known Lynch syndrome (MSH2 germline mutation). By MSH2 immunostain, the tumor completely lacks expression whereas the infiltrating lymphocytes are positive.

Other Tumors and Tumor-Like Lesions of Ureter

KEY FACTS

TERMINOLOGY
- Neoplasms other than usual urothelial carcinoma involving upper urinary tract

CLASSIFICATION
- Benign or malignant epithelial neoplasms of nonurothelial histology
- Benign mesenchymal or fibroepithelial neoplasms
- Malignant mesenchymal neoplasms
- Metastatic or secondary neoplasms

CLINICAL ISSUES
- Most carcinomas with nonurothelial cell features in ureter exist in association with usual urothelial carcinomas
- Pure nonurothelial carcinomas of ureter are very rare

MICROSCOPIC
- Squamous cell carcinoma usually accompanied by extensive squamous metaplasia of urothelium and squamous cell carcinoma in situ
- Adenocarcinoma shows various phenotypes, including glandular NOS, enteric, clear cell, signet ring, mucinous
- Inverted papilloma with endophytic interconnected trabeculae and cords of urothelium, extensively invaginating from surface into lamina propria
- Nephrogenic metaplasia/adenoma shows multiple architectural patterns, including papillary, tubular/glandular, cystic, sheet-like, and hyalinized
  - Typically, thick basement membrane/hyalinized sheath surrounding epithelium
- Benign nonepithelial tumors include fibroepithelial polyp, inflammatory myofibroblastic tumor, hemangioma, angiomyolipoma, leiomyoma, neurofibroma

TOP DIFFERENTIAL DIAGNOSES
- Urothelial carcinoma with divergent differentiation
- Urothelial carcinoma with inverted growth pattern
- Metastatic tumors
- Soft tissue tumors secondarily involving ureter

Fibroepithelial Polyp of Ureter: Gross
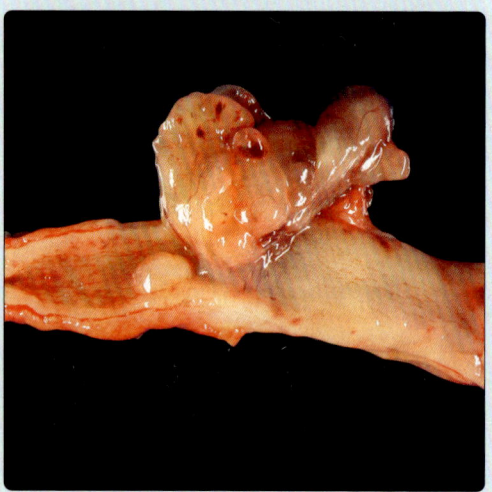

Fibroepithelial Polyp of Ureter: Microscopic
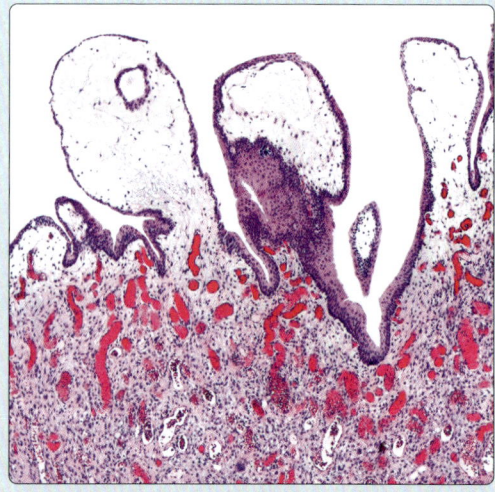

(Left) This is a fibroepithelial polyp removed by segmental ureterectomy in a 35-year-old woman. The lesion is lobulated and congested, and the outer surface is shiny. Despite the clinical suspicion for a malignant process, histopathologic evaluation was consistent with a benign lesion. (Right) Fibroepithelial polyps consist of proliferation and expansion of subepithelial stroma, often accompanied by prominent vascularity and inflammatory infiltrate. The stroma is loose, and occasional atypical pleomorphic stromal cells can be seen.

Inflammatory Myofibroblastic Tumor of Ureter
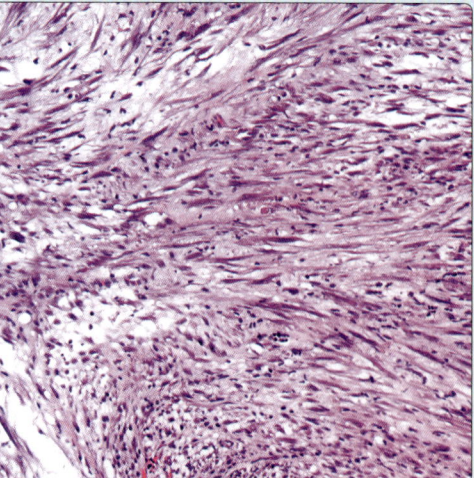

Nephrogenic Metaplasia/Adenoma of Ureter
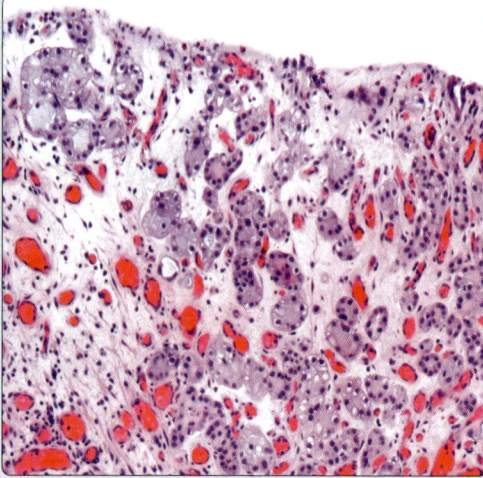

(Left) Inflammatory myofibroblastic tumor of the ureter is rare and morphologically similar to that occurring at other sites, including the bladder. Note the alternating loose and hypercellular areas and scattered inflammatory cell infiltrate. (Right) Nephrogenic metaplasia/adenoma often shows a mixture of architectural patterns. In this example, is it predominantly tubular. Loose stroma, inflammation, and vascular proliferation and congestion are characteristic features, as seen here.

Other Tumors and Tumor-Like Lesions of Ureter

TERMINOLOGY

Definitions
- Neoplasms other than usual urothelial carcinoma involving ureter

ETIOLOGY/PATHOGENESIS

Nephrolithiasis and Repeated Infections
- Squamous cell carcinoma and adenocarcinoma often occur in background of urolithiasis and metaplastic changes following chronic irritation

Bladder Cancer
- Most cases of ureteral urothelial (transitional cell) carcinoma are associated with prior, concurrent, or subsequent bladder or renal pelvis carcinoma
  - However, for nontransitional cell carcinomas of upper tract, such association is not commonly observed

CLINICAL ISSUES

Epidemiology
- Incidence
  - Most of what is reported in literature groups tumors of ureter with those of renal pelvis
    - It is therefore difficult to derive conclusion about true incidence and clinical outcome
  - Most carcinomas with nonurothelial cell features (variants) in ureter coexist with usual urothelial carcinoma
  - Pure nonurothelial carcinomas of ureter are very rare
  - Squamous cell carcinoma is 2nd most common carcinoma of upper tract
    - Most of what is reported in literature likely includes cases of urothelial carcinomas with squamous differentiation
    - Recent studies report combined incidence of < 1% for squamous cell carcinoma and adenocarcinoma of upper tract
    - All other types of carcinoma in literature exist as case reports or small case series
  - Benign epithelial, mesenchymal, and other tumors are also very rare
    - Fibroepithelial polyps, although more common in adults, are most common benign polypoid ureteral tumors in children
- Age
  - Carcinomas: 41-87 years (mean: 66)
  - Fibroepithelial polyps: 7-73 years (mean: 40)
  - Inverted papillomas: 19-89 years (mean: 64)
  - Primitive neuroectodermal tumors: Mostly young adults/adolescents; 10-60 years (mean: 27)
  - Other tumors: Variable, mostly older adults

Presentation
- Most common presentations are flank pain &/or hematuria
  - Obstruction with resultant hydronephrosis
  - Episodic colicky pain, mimicking or complicated by urolithiasis

Treatment
- Surgical approaches
  - Usually nephroureterectomy performed for carcinomas of proximal ureter
  - Malignant tumors of more distal ureter may be amenable to ureterectomy
  - Small or polypoid benign tumors, particularly fibroepithelial polyps, may be resected endoscopically

Prognosis
- Most pure nontransitional cell (variants), as well as urothelial carcinomas with divergent/aberrant differentiation, are high-grade and high-stage tumors
- Most patients with advanced tumor (pT3 or pT4) die of disease, and 5-year survivals are extremely uncommon
- Some benign tumors may cause obstruction and resultant hydronephrosis with related complications

MACROSCOPIC

General Features
- Carcinomas
  - Usually large tumors, filling and expanding ureteral lumen, ± periureteral soft tissue invasion
- Fibroepithelial polyps, hemangiomas, squamous papillomas, and nephrogenic adenomas
  - Mostly polypoid lesions in ureter
  - Size usually small (mean: 2 cm; mostly 0.5-4.0 cm in maximum diameter); larger tumors are rare
- Inverted papilloma
  - Smooth surface, broad based, sessile, rarely pedunculated
- Malignant mesenchymal tumors
  - Often arising in periureteral or perirenal soft tissue, and secondarily involving ureter

MICROSCOPIC

Histologic Features
- Benign epithelial tumors/lesions
  - Inverted papilloma
    - Endophytic interconnected trabeculae and cords of urothelium, extensively invaginating from surface into lamina propria
    - Covered by flat-surfaced urothelium
    - Periphery is smooth and pushing; typically shows palisading of basal nuclei
    - Small glandular or microcystic structures may be seen
  - Nephrogenic metaplasia/adenoma
    - Shows wide spectrum of architectural patterns, often mixed patterns (papillary, tubular/glandular, cystic, single cells, and sheet-like)
    - Lining epithelial cells are cuboidal and single layered, occasionally hobnailed; prominent nucleoli may be present
    - Cytoplasm varies from eosinophilic to clear
    - Some areas with single cells, may show minute lumina, closely mimicking blood vessels or signet ring cells
    - Frequently, thick basement membrane/hyalinized sheath surrounds epithelium
    - Often associated with inflammatory infiltrate
  - Villous adenoma
    - Similar to villous adenoma of colorectal region

Other Tumors and Tumor-Like Lesions of Ureter

- Biopsy-based diagnosis of villous adenoma should not be made, as adenocarcinoma in vicinity may be missed
  - Other exquisitely rare benign epithelial lesions include squamous and urothelial papilloma, endometriosis
- Malignant epithelial tumors
  - Squamous cell carcinoma
    - More common in renal pelvis than ureter; often associated with nephrolithiasis
    - Usually accompanied by extensive squamous metaplasia of urothelium and squamous cell carcinoma in situ
    - Often high stage, frequently with renal parenchymal invasion
  - Adenocarcinoma
    - Variable morphologic appearance, similar to that in bladder (glandular NOS, enteric, clear cell, signet ring, mucinous, etc.)
    - Often accompanied by glandular and intestinal metaplasia of surrounding urothelium or occasionally by villous adenoma
    - Usually high-stage tumors, often with invasion of periureteral soft tissue
  - Other rare types of carcinoma include
    - Small cell and large cell neuroendocrine, lymphoepithelioma-like, sarcomatoid, hepatoid, and rhabdoid
- Benign nonepithelial tumors/lesions
  - Fibroepithelial polyp
    - Usually solitary but sometimes multifocal
    - Proliferation and expansion of subepithelial stromal cells with prominent vascularity, inflammatory infiltrate, and edema
    - Stromal cells usually loosely arranged, but there may be hypercellular, compact areas
    - Atypical and giant forms of stromal cells may be present
    - Mitotic activity uncommon
    - Covering urothelium is benign; usually flat but may show papillary or polypoid fronds and may be ulcerated, hyperplastic, and reactive
  - Hemangioma
    - Usually solitary and polypoid but may be multifocal
    - Often cavernous type but may be capillary or venous type
    - Covered by benign, often ulcerated, urothelium
  - Other reported benign mesenchymal lesions include
    - Inflammatory myofibroblastic tumor, angiomyolipoma, leiomyoma, neurofibroma, hibernoma, and lipoma
- Malignant nonepithelial tumors
  - Leiomyosarcoma most common
  - Rhabdomyosarcoma, including botryoides type, angiosarcoma, fibrosarcoma, Ewing sarcoma, malignant peripheral nerve sheath tumor are other unusual types
  - Sarcomatoid carcinoma always needs to be excluded in all malignant spindle cell neoplasms of ureter

ANCILLARY TESTS

Immunohistochemistry

- Usually not helpful for most of these tumors

DIFFERENTIAL DIAGNOSIS

Metastatic Tumors

- Metastatic tumors to ureter are very uncommon
  - Morphologic feature of primary ureteral squamous cell carcinoma or adenocarcinoma are similar to those that are metastatic to this location
  - Metastatic tumors are often multifocal and bilateral
    - Not associated with in situ component
    - Usually show prominent vascular invasion
  - Clinical history and radiologic findings are often critical
  - Both primary and metastatic small cell carcinomas share morphologic and immunohistochemical features
    - In particular, TTF-1 positivity may be seen in both
    - Presence of at least focal urothelial component (even in situ) strongly favors primary origin

Urothelial Carcinoma With Inverted Growth

- Important distinction from inverted papilloma
- Presence of following features favors urothelial carcinoma with inverted growth pattern
  - Cytologic atypia, solid, nested or nontrabecular growth
  - Presence of adjacent in situ or papillary (noninvasive) carcinoma may be very helpful, if identified

DIAGNOSTIC CHECKLIST

Pathologic Interpretation Pearls

- Adequate sampling is important to identify components that may be crucial to correct diagnosis
- For all unusual ureteral carcinomas, clinical history is necessary to exclude metastasis
- Immunohistochemistry may be helpful in specific situations but generally is of limited value in work-up of most of these lesions

SELECTED REFERENCES

1. Luo JD et al: Upper urinary tract inverted papillomas: Report of 10 cases. Oncol Lett. 4(1):71-74, 2012
2. Childs MA et al: Fibroepithelial polyps of the ureter: a single-institutional experience. J Endourol. 23(9):1415-9, 2009
3. Volkmer BG et al: Upper urinary tract recurrence after radical cystectomy for bladder cancer--who is at risk? J Urol. 182(6):2632-7, 2009
4. Holmäng S et al: Squamous cell carcinoma of the renal pelvis and ureter: incidence, symptoms, treatment and outcome. J Urol. 178(1):51-6, 2007
5. Frickmann H et al: [Villous adenoma of the renal pelvis and ureter.] Urologe A. 45(11):1435-7, 2006
6. Ford TF et al: Adenomatous metaplasia (nephrogenic adenoma) of urothelium. An analysis of 70 cases. Br J Urol. 57(4):427-33, 1985

Other Tumors and Tumor-Like Lesions of Ureter

Squamous Cell Carcinoma of Ureter

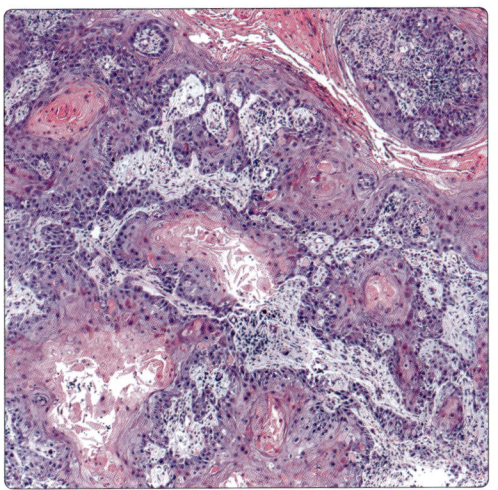

Small Cell/Neuroendocrine Carcinoma of Ureter

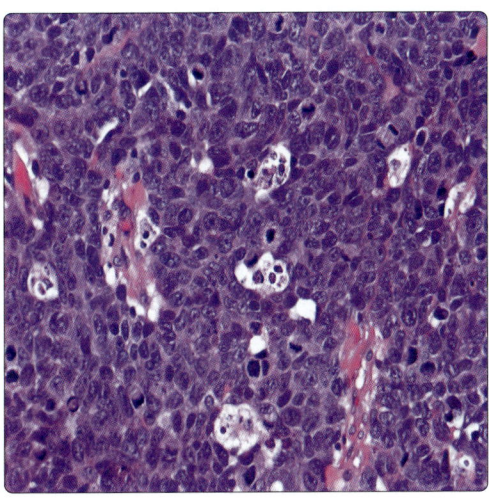

(Left) This section is taken from a bulky ureteral tumor with obstruction and hydronephrosis. The tumor consists of infiltrating malignant cells of squamous cell carcinoma, with evidence of keratinization. (Right) Pure small cell carcinomas of the ureter are quite rare. At both the morphological and immunophenotypic levels, they are similar to small cell carcinomas of the lung and other sites. Immunostains may not help in determining site of origin, but the presence of a urothelial component is diagnostic for primary tumor.

Clear Cell Carcinoma of Ureter

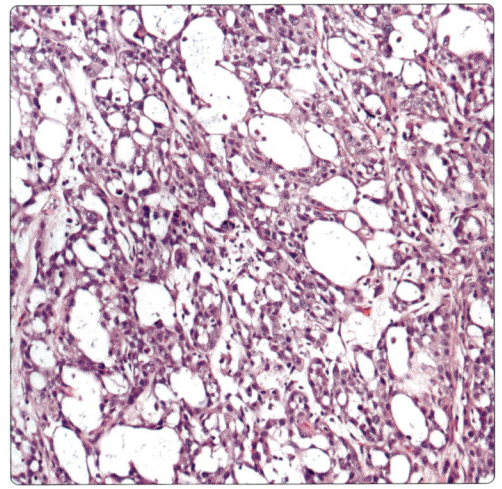

Secondary Involvement of Ureter by Bladder Cancer

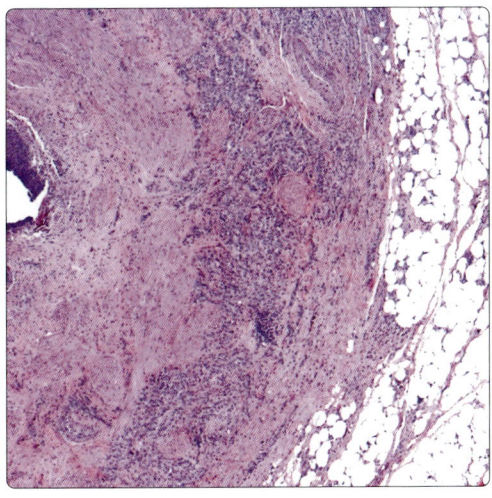

(Left) Virtually the entire spectrum of bladder tumors can arise in the ureter, as in this example of clear cell carcinoma that developed in a 38-year-old woman. This rare form of adenocarcinoma is identical to its counterpart in the bladder and gynecologic tract. (Right) In some cases, tumors primary in the bladder can extend to and invade the ureter. In this example, a primary bladder plasmacytoid carcinoma showed extensive involvement of the ureteral wall, primarily along the periureteral tissue and muscular layer.

Sarcomatoid Carcinoma of Ureter

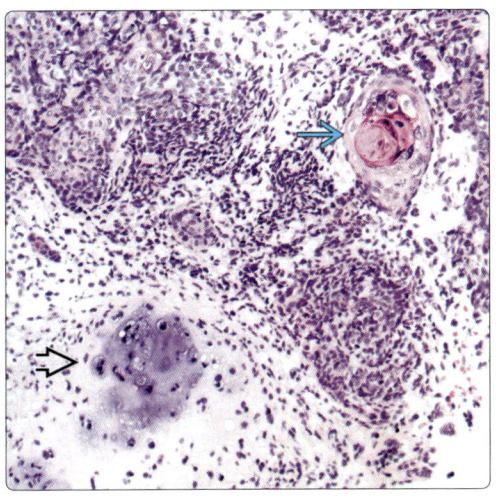

Endometriosis of Ureter

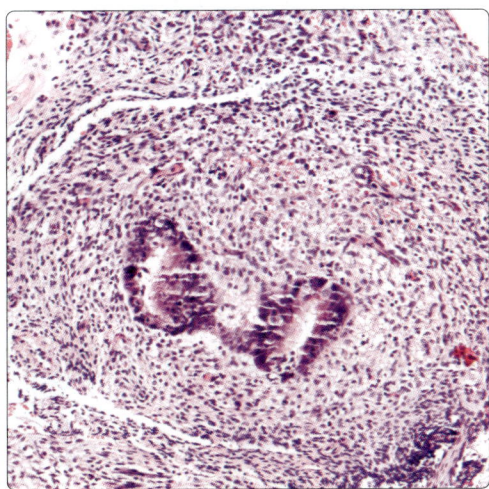

(Left) This section is taken from a bulky distal ureteral tumor from an elderly patient. The tumor was heterogeneous and contained areas of anaplastic spindle and round cells throughout but also areas of squamous ⇨ as well as heterologous differentiation in the form of chondrosarcoma ⇨. (Right) Rare benign lesions in the ureter may be symptomatic, as is the case in this patient who suffered from cyclical pelvic pain. Ureteral biopsy identified components of endometriosis (glands and stroma) that was causing ureteral stricture.

Urothelial Carcinoma of Renal Pelvis

KEY FACTS

TERMINOLOGY
- Malignant neoplasm of urothelial (transitional cell) origin involving renal pelvicalyceal system
- Urothelial carcinoma of renal pelvis

ETIOLOGY/PATHOGENESIS
- Tobacco smoking is important risk factor
- Long-term use of analgesics, especially phenacetin, also implicated as independent risk factor
- Increased risk in patients with Lynch syndrome

CLINICAL ISSUES
- 4-5% of all urothelial tumors
- Pathologic stage is single most important prognostic factor for urothelial carcinomas of upper urinary tract

MACROSCOPIC
- Predominantly papillary or polypoid, but also infiltrative mass with thickening of pelvic wall

MICROSCOPIC
- Papillary urothelial neoplasms of low malignant potential extremely uncommon in upper tract
- Low-grade carcinoma relatively less common, compared to that in bladder
- Overall lymph node involvement reported to be ~ 10%

TOP DIFFERENTIAL DIAGNOSES
- Collecting duct carcinoma
- Renal cell carcinoma, unclassified type
- Metastatic carcinoma

DIAGNOSTIC CHECKLIST
- Collecting duct and urothelial carcinomas; both may show extensive desmoplasia in renal parenchyma
- Morphologic and immunophenotypic features may not be absolutely reliable in distinguishing these 2 entities

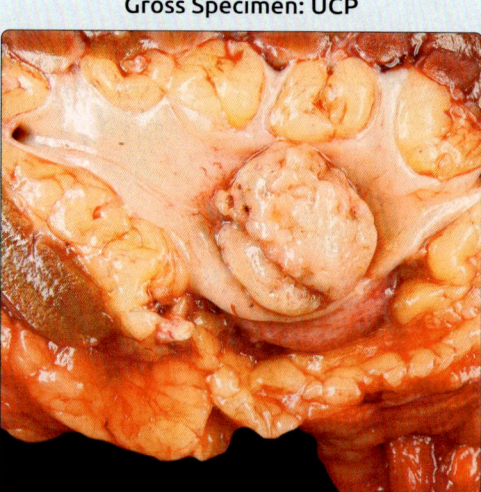

Gross Specimen: UCP

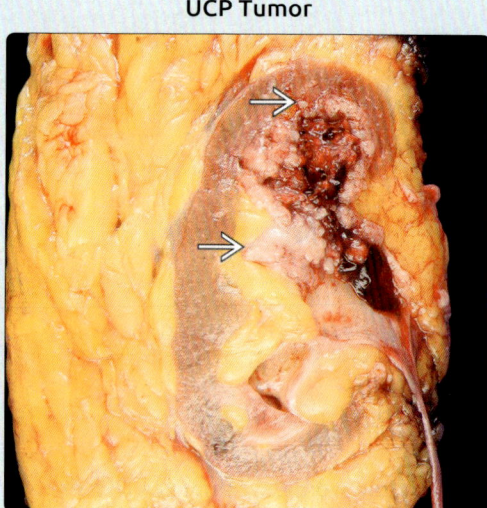

UCP Tumor

(Left) Gross specimen of urothelial carcinoma of the renal pelvis (UCP) shows polypoid lesions with a solid, smooth surface. This size of tumor might block urine flow from an entire segment of pelvicalyceal system & cause segmental renal injury. (Right) The tumor nearly completely occupies upper pelvicalyceal system, much of which is exophytic, but there are areas suggestive of involvement of renal parenchyma or renal sinus ➡. Microscopic determination of invasion is very important to accurately determine tumor stage.

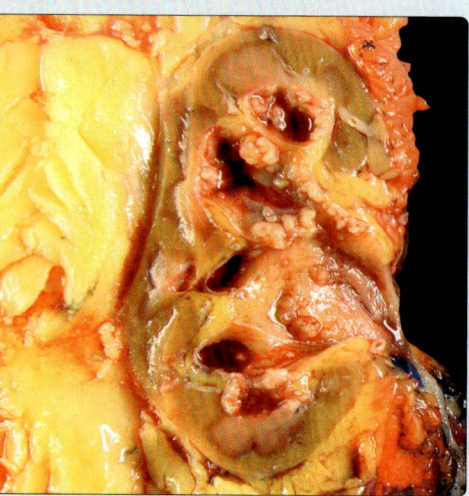

UCP: Multifocal Tumor

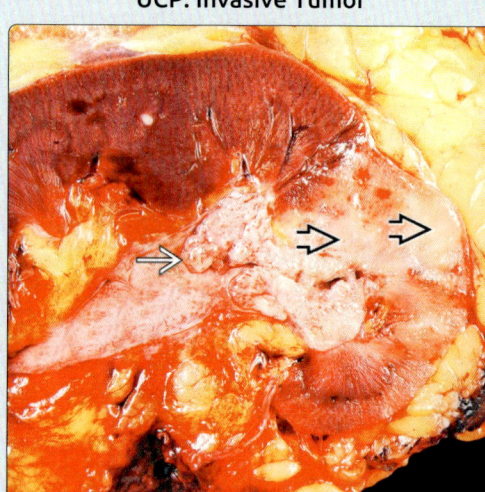

UCP: Invasive Tumor

(Left) This tumor is multifocal and involves multiple areas throughout the pelvicalyceal system and proximal ureter. Although most of the tumor foci are exophytic and polypoid, it is important to extensively sample them in order to identify potential foci of invasion. (Right) This tumor is predominantly invasive, with extensive involvement of the full thickness of the renal parenchyma ➡. A noninvasive component is also identified protruding into the lumen of the renal pelvis ➡.

Urothelial Carcinoma of Renal Pelvis

TERMINOLOGY

Abbreviations
- Urothelial carcinoma of renal pelvis (UCP)

Definitions
- Malignant neoplasm of urothelial (transitional cell) origin involving renal pelvicalyceal system

ETIOLOGY/PATHOGENESIS

Risk Factors
- Tobacco smoking is important risk factor
  - Lifetime risk increases with increased consumption and intensity of smoking
- Long-term use of analgesics, especially phenacetin, implicated as independent risk factor
  - With decrease in usage of phenacetin, it is less significant risk factor
- Other risk factors include Balkan nephropathy and occupational exposures
  - Petrochemicals, plastic materials, coal, asphalt, tar, and thorium-containing contrast media
- History of previous lower urinary tract carcinoma is predisposing factor
  - > 2/3 have prior, concurrent, or subsequent bladder carcinoma
- Increase risk in patients of Lynch syndrome

Molecular Features
- Generally similar to that of urothelial carcinomas of bladder
- Frequent mutations in fibroblastic growth factor receptor 3 (*FGFR3*) gene and *HRAS* gene
  - Primarily in tumors with papillary morphology
  - Relative incidences of *FGFR3* mutations suggest that noninvasive papillary tumors do progress, although infrequently
    - Tumors with *FGFR3* mutations have lower risk for recurrence than those without
- Common mutations in chromatin-modifying genes (*KDM6A*, *KMT2D*, *KMT2C*, *CREBBP*, *ARID1A*)
- *TP53* mutations are less frequent and *RB1* mutations are rare
- Microsatellite instability and loss of mismatch repair proteins MSH2, MLH1, or MSH6 present in upper urinary tract tumors
  - Rare in sporadic cases, but more common in patients with Lynch syndrome
    - Incidence in upper tract is many times more common than in bladder tumors
  - Upper urinary tract tumors form 3rd most common tumor with microsatellite instability
    - Colon and endometrium are 2 most common sites within hereditary nonpolyposis colorectal cancer-related tumors

CLINICAL ISSUES

Epidemiology
- Incidence
  - 4-5% of all urothelial tumors
  - Most common type of tumor in pelvicalyceal location (90%)
- Age
  - Mean: 67-70 years (range: 34-93 years)
- Sex
  - More common in males; M:F = 1.7-2:1

Presentation
- Flank pain
- Hematuria

Treatment
- Nephroureterectomy, including removal of bladder cuff, ± neoadjuvant chemotherapy

Prognosis
- Pathologic stage is single most important prognostic factor for urothelial carcinomas of upper urinary tract
- On univariate analysis, significant prognostic indicators include
  - Size
  - Tumor grade
  - Pathologic stage
    - pTa: Papillary noninvasive carcinoma
    - pT1: Tumor invades subepithelial connective tissue
    - pT2: Tumor invades muscularis
    - pT3: Tumor invades (for renal pelvis): Beyond muscularis in peripelvic fat/renal parenchyma; (for ureter): Beyond muscularis in periureteric fat
    - pT4: Tumor invades adjacent organs or through kidney to perinephric fat
  - Lymphovascular invasion
- However, on multivariate analysis, stage is only significant prognostic factor for survival
  - Based on multiple studies, 5-year survival > 99% for pTa, 91% for pT1, 72% for pT2, 40% for pT3, and 16% for patients with metastasis

IMAGING

Radiographic Findings
- Filling defect, obstructive mass associated with hydronephrosis, renal stones

MACROSCOPIC

General Features
- Either predominantly papillary or polypoid, or infiltrative mass with thickening of pelvic wall
  - Tumors that primarily appear as papillary or polypoid
    - May expand and fill pelvicalyceal system
    - Tend to be noninvasive or are associated with limited invasion
    - Systematic sampling after fixation and maintaining relationship to underlying structures important for accurate staging
  - Infiltrative tumors may extensively involve renal parenchyma, mimicking primary renal parenchymal tumor
    - Occasionally may arise from minor calyx and grossly appear cortical in location

Urothelial Carcinoma of Renal Pelvis

- Equivocal radiographic localization may warrant intraoperative assessment of urothelial vs. renal parenchymal origin
  - Surgical approaches quite different in these 2 situations
  - Radical nephroureterectomy for urothelial vs. partial, total, or radical nephrectomy for renal cortical tumors

MICROSCOPIC

Histologic Features

- Histopathological features of upper tract urothelial tumors similar to those in urinary bladder
  - However, papillary urothelial neoplasms of low malignant potential extremely uncommon in upper tract
  - Low-grade carcinoma relatively less common, compared to that in bladder
- High-grade tumors are most common, and invasion should be diligently looked for if not obvious
- Histopathologic diversity with morphologic variants/aberrant differentiations similar to that in bladder
- Variant morphologies seen, among others, include
  - Micropapillary variant
  - Lymphoepithelioma-like carcinoma
  - Squamous differentiation and squamous cell carcinoma
  - Sarcomatoid differentiation
  - Signet ring cell or plasmacytoid features
  - Small cell/neuroendocrine carcinomatous features
- Renal parenchymal invasion requires destructive invasive beyond renal tubules
  - Tumors often extend inside kidney within tubules
    - May, at times, form grossly identified expansile nodules
    - For staging purposes of renal parenchymal invasion, tumor cells have to invade out of well-defined tubular structures

Lymph Nodes

- Overall lymph node involvement reported to be ~ 10%
  - Reported incidence is not based on cases where lymph nodes were removed at time of nephroureterectomy
  - Rates of lymph node metastasis close to 25% among cases where lymph nodes were removed at surgery

Predominant Cell/Compartment Type

- Epithelial, urothelial

ANCILLARY TESTS

Immunohistochemistry

- CK7 and GATA3 diffusely positive
- HMWCK and p63 often strongly and diffusely positive
- CK20 at least focally positive in ~ 1/2 to 2/3 of cases
- pax-8 may be positive and may not be helpful in distinguishing upper tract urothelial carcinoma from renal cell carcinoma (RCC); usually not diffuse
- S100p positive

DIFFERENTIAL DIAGNOSIS

Collecting Duct Carcinoma (CDC)/Unclassified RCC

- Highly infiltrative neoplasm extensively involving renal parenchyma may mimic high-grade RCC, undifferentiated, or CDC
  - Features in favor of urothelial carcinoma include carcinoma in situ or papillary tumor involving pelvicalyceal system
    - Predominantly nested or solid architecture with variable squamous or glandular differentiation also favors urothelial carcinoma
  - CDC is primarily high-grade carcinoma, usually with glandular architecture
  - Immunohistochemical staining may not be useful in distinction
    - CDC often positive for CK7, HMWCK(34βE12), and occasionally CK20
    - Role of CK20 in distinction not known at present
    - Unclassified RCC may show variable immunophenotype, as likely not uniform single entity

Metastatic Carcinoma

- Features favoring metastatic carcinoma over urothelial carcinoma include
  - Known history of nonurothelial carcinoma
  - Histology not conforming to any known subtypes of RCC or typical urothelial carcinoma
  - Extensive interstitial growth
  - Multifocality both grossly and microscopically
  - Extensive vascular-lymphatic invasion
  - Immunophenotype, matching tumor in primary site and is different from that in urothelial carcinomas

DIAGNOSTIC CHECKLIST

Pathologic Interpretation Pearls

- Collecting duct and urothelial carcinomas; both may show extensive desmoplasia in renal parenchyma
- Morphologic and immunophenotypic features may not be absolutely reliable in distinguishing these 2 entities
- Adequate sampling of urothelial mucosa to identify urothelial carcinoma in situ is crucial to definitively diagnose urothelial carcinoma

SELECTED REFERENCES

1. Sfakianos JP et al: Genomic characterization of upper tract urothelial carcinoma. Eur Urol. 68(6):970-7, 2015
2. Amin MB: Histological variants of urothelial carcinoma: diagnostic, therapeutic and prognostic implications. Mod Pathol. 22 Suppl 2:S96-S118, 2009
3. Colin P et al: Environmental factors involved in carcinogenesis of urothelial cell carcinomas of the upper urinary tract. BJU Int. 104(10):1436-40, 2009
4. Ferriero M et al: Re: Lymphovascular invasion predicts poor outcome of urothelial carcinoma of the renal pelvis after nephroureterectomy. BJU Int. 103(8):1143, 2009
5. Margulis V et al: Outcomes of radical nephroureterectomy: a series from the upper tract urothelial carcinoma collaboration. Cancer. 115(6):1224-33, 2009
6. Gupta R et al: Neoplasms of the upper urinary tract: a review with focus on urothelial carcinoma of the pelvicalyceal system and aspects related to its diagnosis and reporting. Adv Anat Pathol. 15(3):127-39, 2008
7. Olgac S et al: Urothelial carcinoma of the renal pelvis: a clinicopathologic study of 130 cases. Am J Surg Pathol. 28(12):1545-52, 2004

Urothelial Carcinoma of Renal Pelvis

UCP
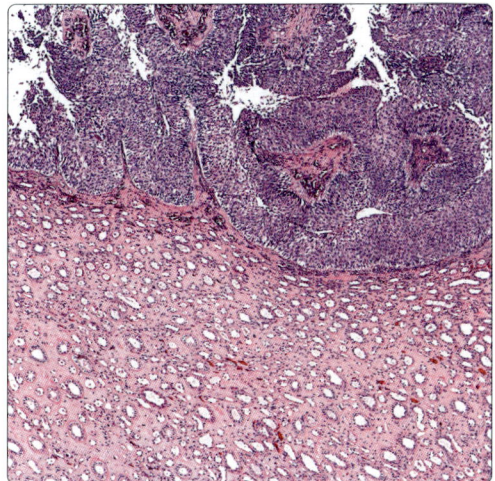

Papillary UCP
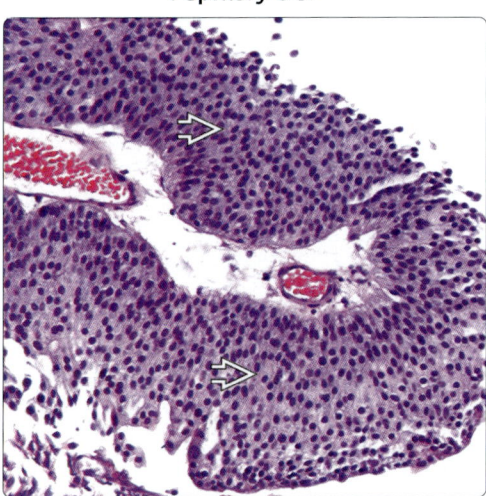

(Left) An exophytic tumor involving the renal pelvis is shown. Note the papillary architecture and the close proximity to the distal renal tubules. There is virtually no lamina propria separating the urothelium and the renal parenchyma, which may have important implications on tumor staging in the presence of invasion. **(Right)** Similar to those in the bladder, papillary tumors may show morphology of a low-grade urothelial carcinoma (UC) ➡. However, high-grade carcinomas are more frequent in the upper urinary tract.

Papillary UCP
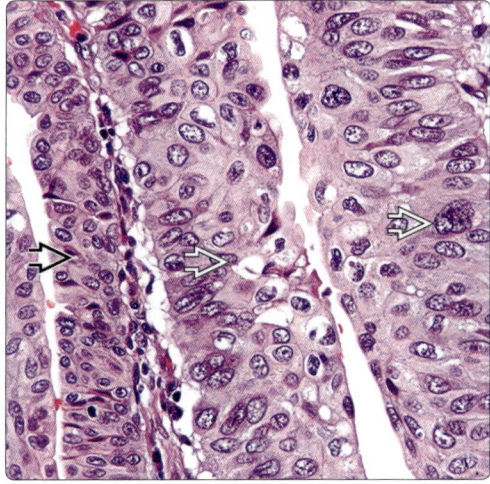

Invasive UCP
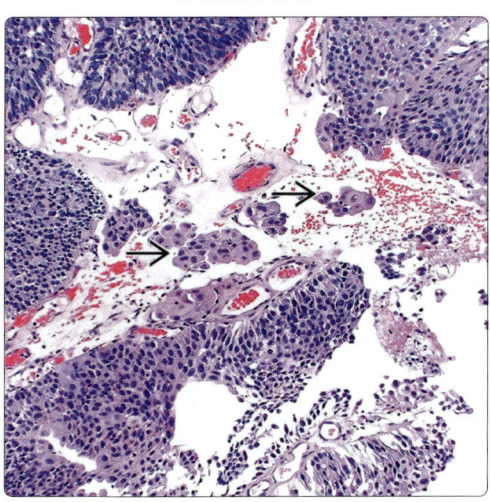

(Left) This tumor has both low- ➡ and high-grade ➡ features. Similar to bladder tumors, carcinomas with a combination of tumor grades are graded according to the highest grade in the lesion. This phenomenon is more common in the upper tract than in the bladder. **(Right)** Invasion of the lamina propria in upper tract UC ➡ is much less common than that in the bladder. Criteria for invasion are similar to those in the bladder; in this tumor, irregular tumor nests in clear space are in retraction and paradoxical differentiation.

Invasive UCP With Tumor Nests
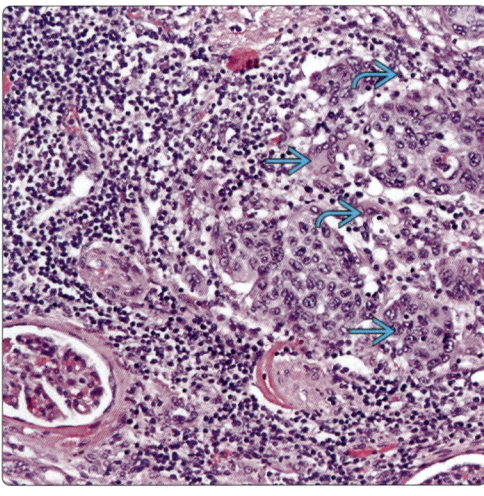

Parenchymal Invasive UCP
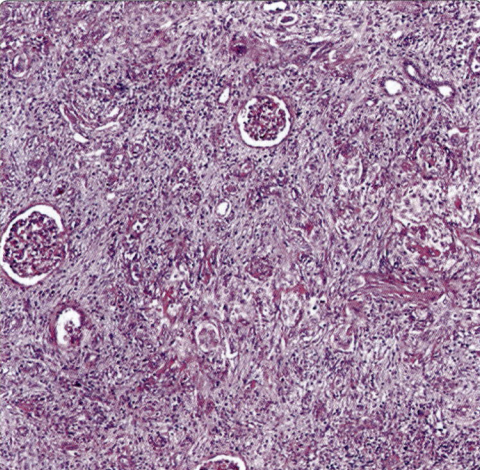

(Left) Invasion of renal parenchyma characterized by irregular tumor nests ➡ along with inflammatory stromal response ➡ are shown. The presence of tumor adjacent to a glomerulus is further evidence of invasion into the renal parenchyma, a major upstage for this tumor. **(Right)** UC with extensive parenchymal invasion and desmoplasia may mimic collecting duct carcinoma. Solid nests and squamoid features favor UC, but definitive diagnosis requires the presence of in situ carcinoma in the pelvis.

Urothelial Carcinoma of Renal Pelvis

UCP Tumor With Autolytic Changes

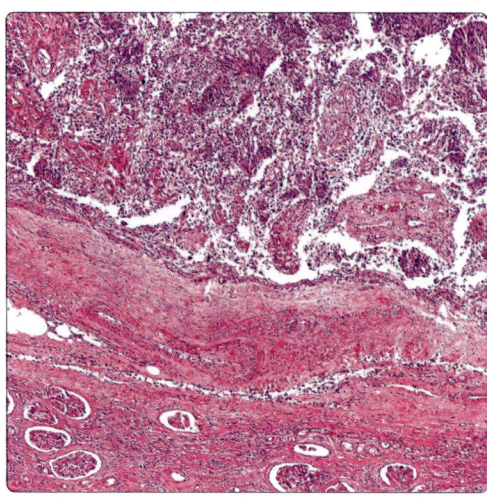

UCP: Papillary Tumors

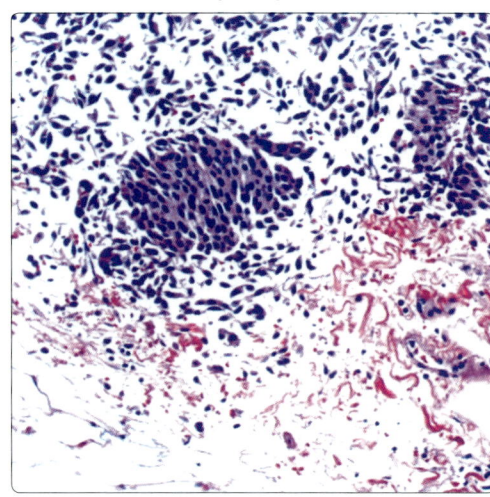

(Left) This tumor exhibits marked autolytic changes primarily due to insufficient fixation. This can greatly affect tumor grading and staging. Opening the renal pelvis and exposing the tumors to fixatives as soon as possible is key to ensuring proper fixation and histopathologic evaluation. (Right) Papillary tumors are friable and prone to fragmentation and displacement, precluding accurate staging in some cases. The prevalence of autolytic changes necessitates adequate fixation prior to prosecting in these tumors.

UCP Tumor Invading Renal Parenchyma

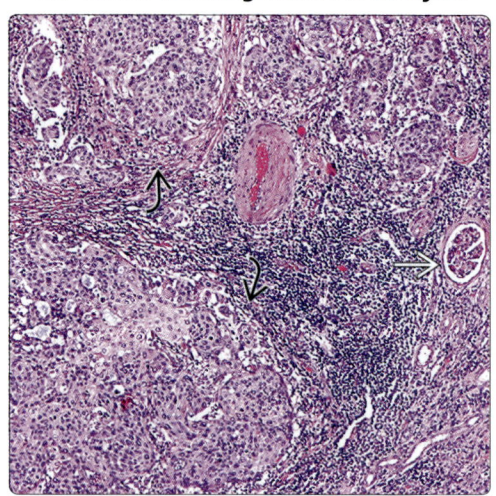

UCP Tumor Invading Renal Sinus Fat

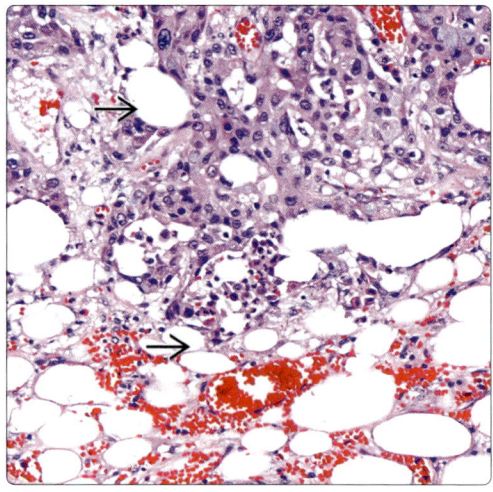

(Left) In this section, the tumor invaded both the renal parenchyma (note the glomerulus ➡) and the renal sinus ➡. Note the presence of a brisk inflammatory infiltrate, which could represent host response to the infiltrating tumor. (Right) This tumor invades renal sinus fat ➡. Such tumors, & those invading renal parenchyma, are both regarded as pT3 tumors and seem to have similar clinical outcomes. Tumor invasion of the perinephric fat (after complete invasion through the renal parenchyma) is staged as pT4.

UCP With Renal Sinus Invasion

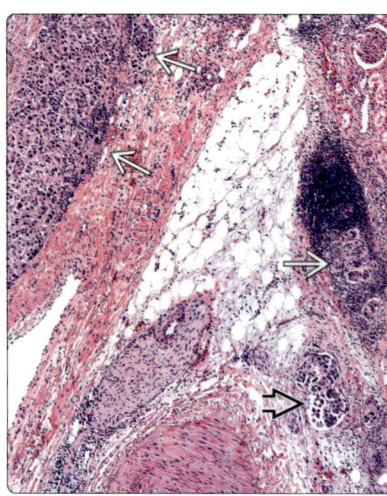

UCP: Inverted Growth Pattern

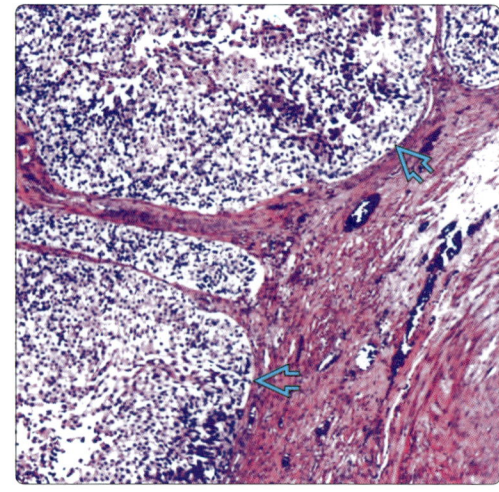

(Left) Extensive involvement of the renal sinus ➡ by invasive urothelial carcinoma is seen here. Although in some areas lymphovascular invasion is suspected ➡, this could also be a retraction artifact, which is commonly associated with invasive UC. (Right) An inverted growth pattern of papillary UC may cause difficulty in staging. The uniform, broad tumor edge ➡ and lack of stromal reaction argue against invasion. Additional sampling and careful search for small irregular foci of invasion is imperative in such cases.

Urothelial Carcinoma of Renal Pelvis

Noninvasive Urothelial Carcinoma

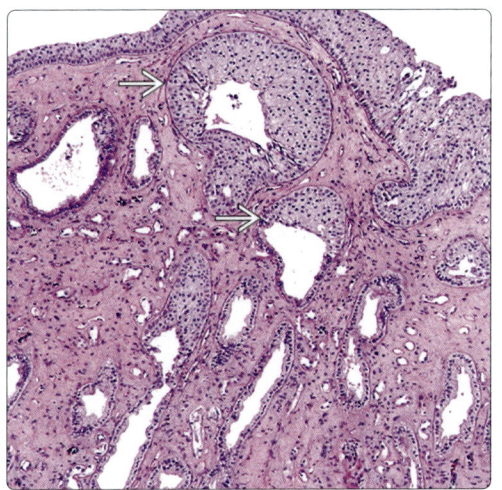

UCP Tumor Staging

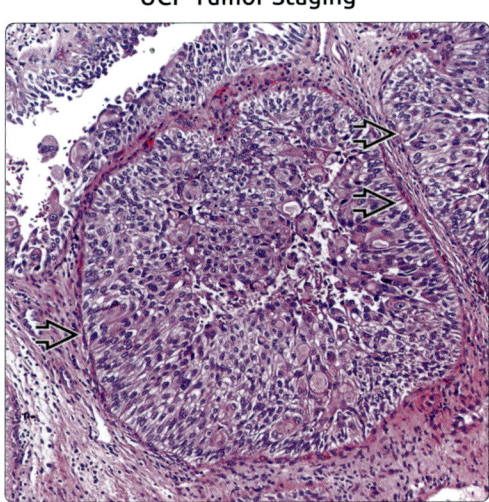

(Left) In this section, only a noninvasive urothelial carcinoma is identified, which involves the renal pelvic lining and also extends to the distal renal tubules and collecting system ➡. The smooth and rounded borders indicate the absence of invasion into the renal parenchyma in this case. (Right) An important staging issue among papillary UC is the invasion of renal parenchyma. The tumor commonly involves, and may expand, distal renal tubules (not invasion) ➡. Generous tumor sampling is needed to definitively assess invasion.

UCP Tumor

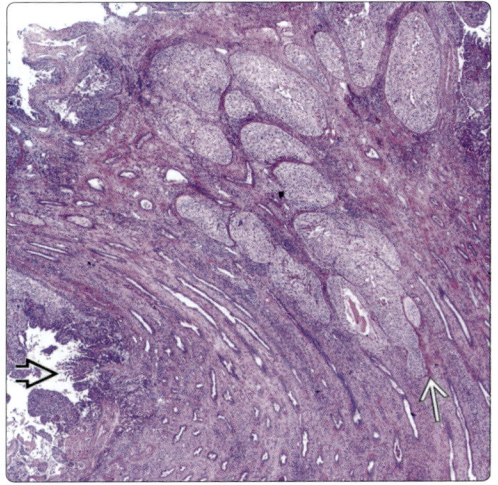

UCP: pT3 Stage

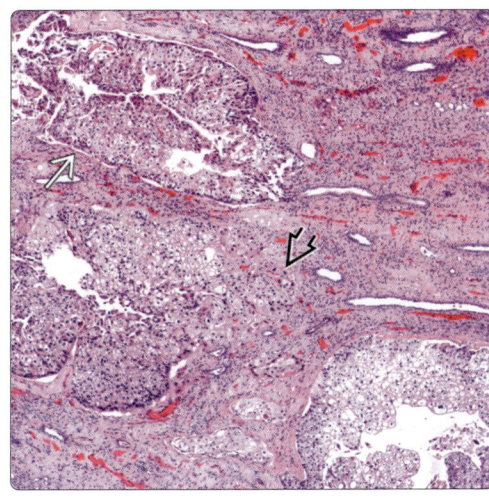

(Left) This tumor exhibits extensive involvement of the distal renal tubules rather deep into the renal parenchyma ➡, which still does not constitute invasion. Note the presence of the exophytic papillary component ➡. (Right) In this section, in addition to the noninvasive tumor involving the distal renal tubules ➡, there is unequivocal invasion of the renal parenchyma in the form of irregular tumor clusters ➡ to warrant a pT3 stage.

Endoscopic Biopsy of Renal Pelvis

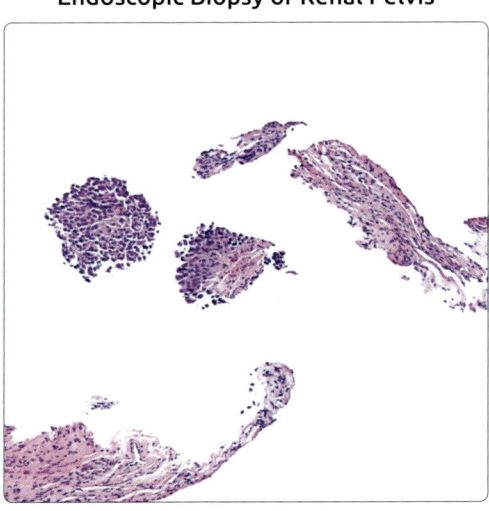

Endoscopic Biopsy of Renal Pelvis

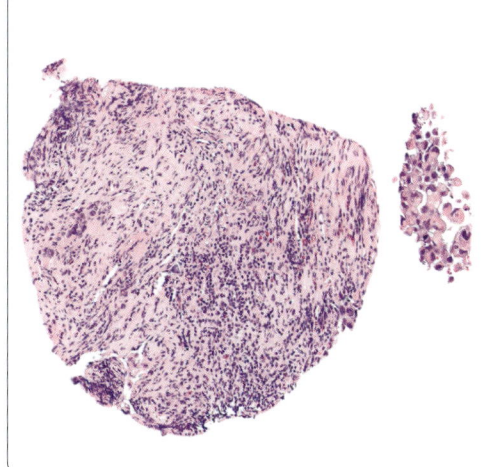

(Left) Endoscopic biopsies from renal pelvic tumors often yield limited material and the pathologist's role is primarily to document a urothelial tumor. Grade and invasion status may not always be evaluable. (Right) Renal pelvic biopsy shows a detached cluster of malignant cells. Determining invasion or a papillary tumor is often difficult in limited material but usually does not influence further management, i.e., nephroureterectomy, as long as a malignant (high-grade) diagnosis is rendered on this material.

Urothelial Carcinoma of Renal Pelvis

(Left) Assessing invasion may be challenging in some cases, despite adequate sampling, as demonstrated in this case. The presence of stromal reaction is suggestive of invasion but the smooth borders and basement membrane material around tumor nests argues against invasion. **(Right)** Lymph node metastasis is not very common in the upper tract (reported to be ~ 10%). This rate, however, is higher (up to 25%) in studies when lymph node dissection was performed. The morphology of the metastasis may resemble low-grade carcinoma in some cases.

UCP: Stromal Reaction

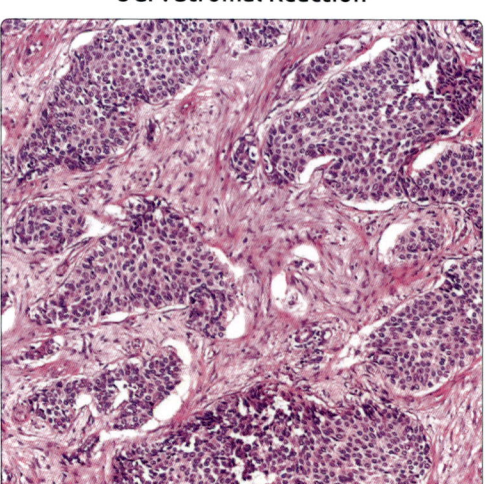

Lymph Node Metastasis: UCP

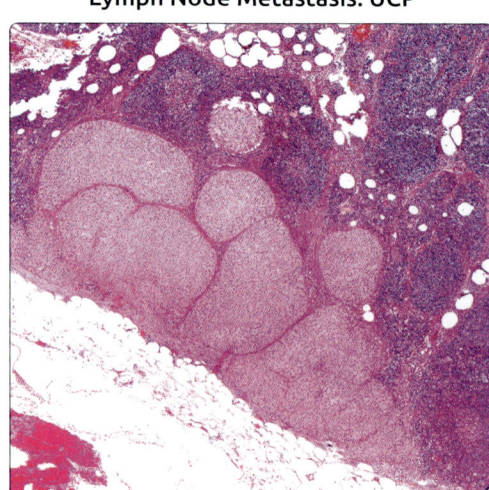

(Left) This is a UC in a patient who has confirmed Lynch syndrome with confirmed germline mutation in MSH2. The tumor is associated with fibrosis, hyalinization, and inflammation, but the patient received neoadjuvant chemotherapy prior to nephroureterectomy. **(Right)** There is absence of expression of MSH2 by tumor cells (some of the infiltrating and surrounding lymphocytes are positive). This tumor was also negative for MSH6 but retained expression of MLH1 and PMS2.

UCP in Lynch Syndrome

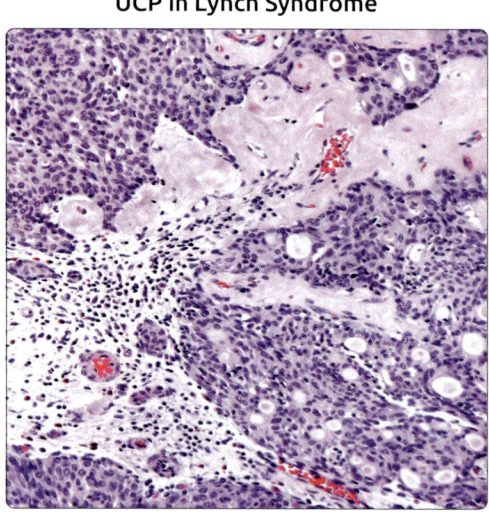

UCP in Lynch syndrome

(Left) In this section, there is a high-grade malignant neoplasm infiltrating the renal parenchyma. The tumor consists of areas of spindle ➡ and epithelial cells ➡, which is consistent with a sarcomatoid UC. **(Right)** This is another section of the tumor shown in the previous image. There is UC in situ of the renal pelvis and distal tubules of the collecting system. Identifying this component confirms the urothelial origin of the sarcomatoid carcinoma.

Sarcomatoid UCP

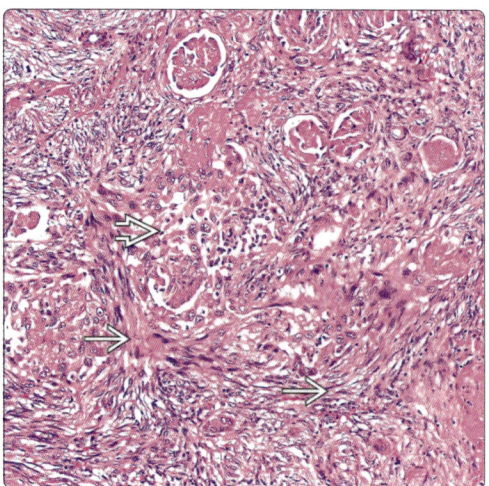

Urothelial Carcinoma In Situ of Renal Pelvis

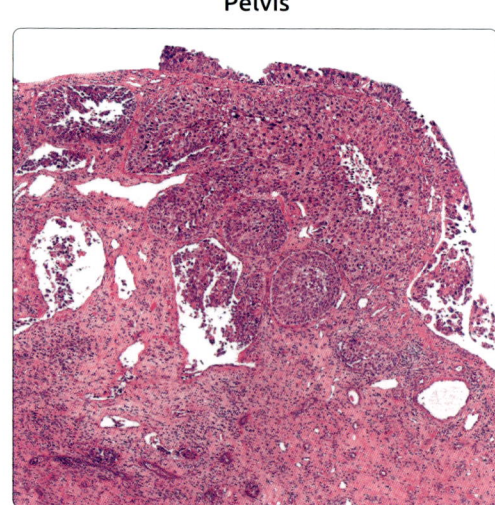

Urothelial Carcinoma of Renal Pelvis

UCP: Micropapillary Variant

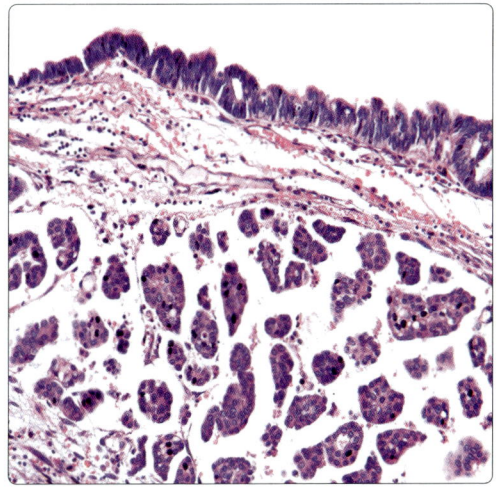

Undifferentiated UC With Giant Cells of Renal Pelvis

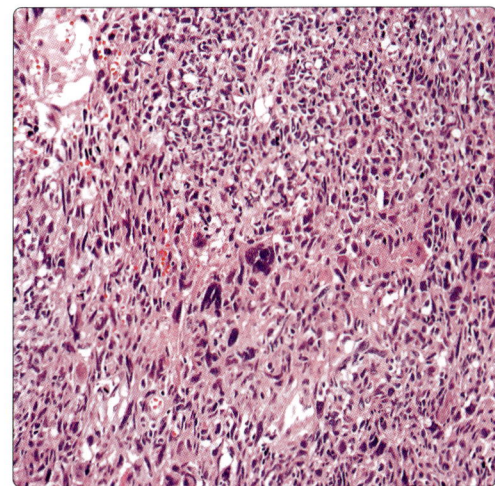

(Left) This tumor exhibits classical features of micropapillary carcinoma (multiple small clusters of tumor in large lacunar spaces and absence of fibrovascular cores). There is evidence of UC in situ in the surface urothelium. (Right) This is an undifferentiated carcinoma with extensive pleomorphic cells, spindle cells, and occasional giant cells. These tumors are rare but in the same morphologic spectrum of tumors that are seen in the bladder that may be encountered in the renal pelvis.

UC With Trophoblastic Differentiation, Involving Renal Pelvis

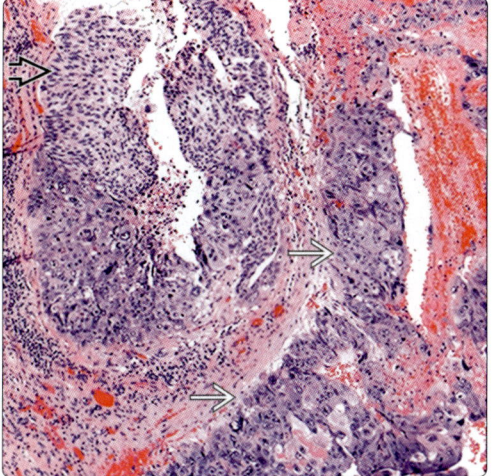

Collecting Duct Carcinoma

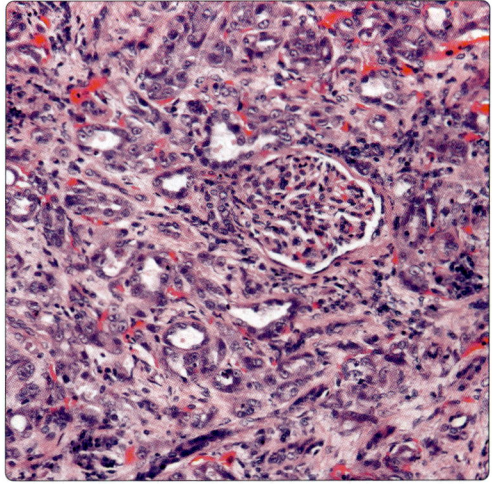

(Left) Consistent with the wide spectrum of variant histology in UC, this tumor has areas of syncytiotrophoblastic differentiation ⇒ (note association with hemorrhage). Foci of classical UC may be also appreciated in this tumor ⇒. (Right) Collecting duct carcinoma (CDC) may sometimes mimic UCP by having a destructive and infiltrating pattern of invasion into the renal parenchyma. The presence of tubular morphology, as seen in this example, may favor the diagnosis of CDC.

Renal Cell Carcinoma: Unclassified Type

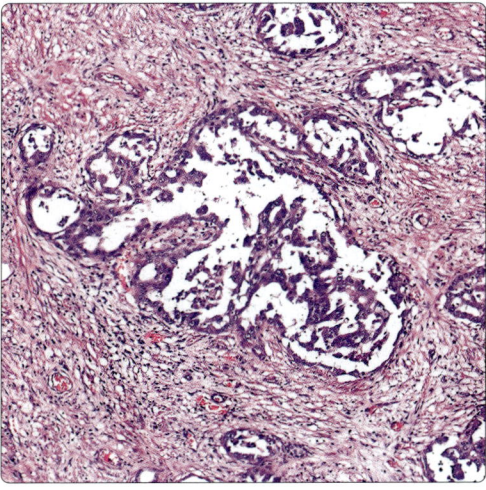

Metastatic Squamous Cell Carcinoma of Kidney

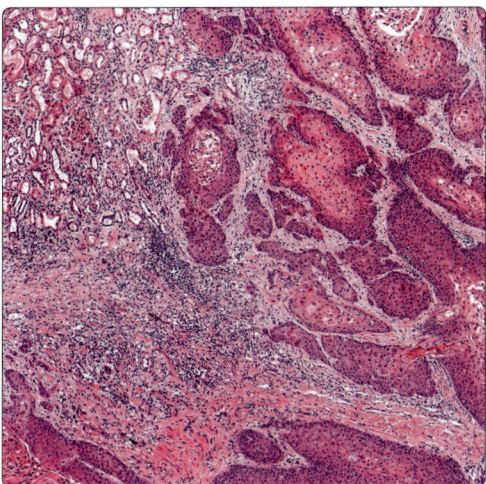

(Left) This tumor exhibits complex cystic and papillary infiltrating morphology. This glandular histology, along with the lack of identifiable UC in situ and lack of immunoprofile typical for UC, may help in establishing the nonurothelial nature of the tumor. (Right) This is a metastatic squamous cell carcinoma of the kidney. Awareness of the presence of a primary tumor elsewhere is crucial to render the correct diagnosis, especially since squamous differentiation is common in UC.

Other Tumors and Tumor-Like Lesions of Renal Pelvis

KEY FACTS

TERMINOLOGY
- Neoplasms other than usual urothelial carcinoma involving upper urinary tract

CLINICAL ISSUES
- Most carcinomas with nontransitional (nonurothelial or variants) cell features in renal pelvis exist in association with usual urothelial (transitional cell) carcinomas
- Pure nonurothelial carcinomas of pelvis are very rare

MICROSCOPIC
- Squamous cell carcinoma usually accompanied by extensive squamous metaplasia of urothelium and squamous cell carcinoma in situ
- Adenocarcinoma shows various phenotypes, including glandular NOS, enteric, signet ring, mucinous
- Inverted papilloma with endophytic interconnected trabeculae and cords of urothelium, extensively invaginating from surface into lamina propria
- Nephrogenic metaplasia/adenoma shows multiple architectural patterns, including papillary, tubular/glandular, cystic, sheet-like, and hyalinized
    - Typically, thick basement membrane/hyalinized sheath surrounding epithelium
- Benign nonepithelial tumors include fibroepithelial polyp, inflammatory myofibroblastic tumor, hemangioma, angiomyolipoma, leiomyoma, neurofibroma

TOP DIFFERENTIAL DIAGNOSES
- Metastatic tumors
- Urothelial carcinoma with inverted growth pattern
- Renal tumors extending to renal pelvis

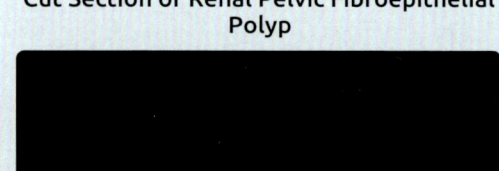

Fibroepithelial Polyp of Renal Pelvis

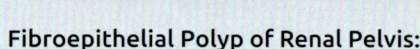

Cut Section of Renal Pelvic Fibroepithelial Polyp

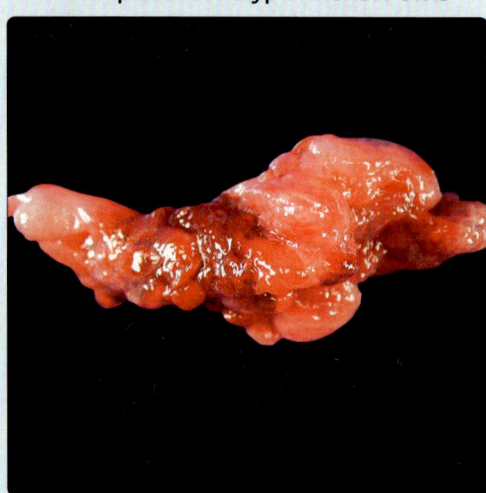

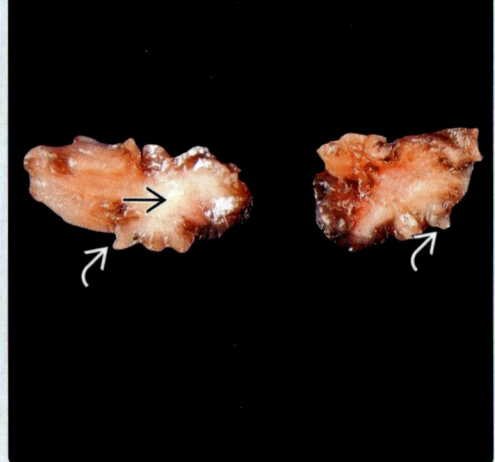

(Left) This fibroepithelial polyp presented as mass in the renal pelvis in a 35-yr-old woman. The lesion is lobulated and congested and the outer surface is shiny. Despite the clinical suspicion for a malignant process, histopathologic evaluation was consistent with a benign lesion. (Right) This polypoid mass in the renal pelvis has sclerotic white ⇨ cores. The outer surface is lobulated and nodular and may show papillary excrescences ➡.

Fibroepithelial Polyp of Renal Pelvis: Papillary Projections

Fibroepithelial Polyp of Renal Pelvis: Stromal Cell Atypia

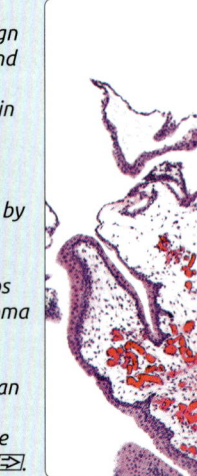

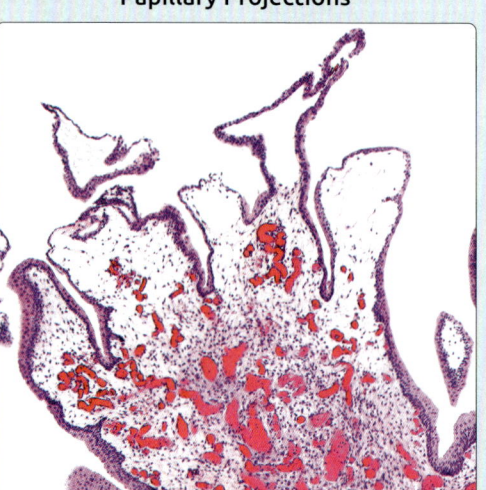

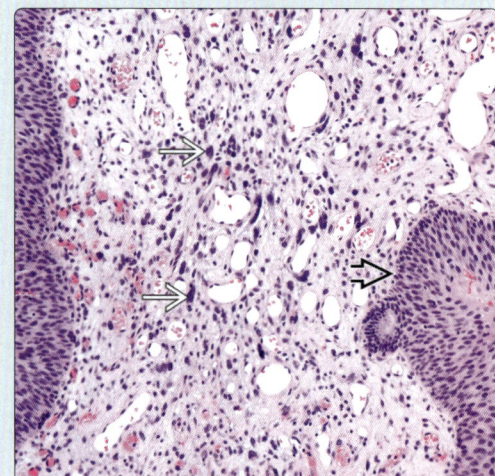

(Left) Fibroepithelial polyps are relatively common benign lesions of the renal pelvis and ureter in the pediatric population, but most occur in adults. They predominantly consist of proliferation and expansion of subepithelial stroma, often accompanied by prominent vascularity and inflammatory infiltrate. (Right) Fibroepithelial polyps generally contain loose stroma with rich vascularity. Occasionally, atypical pleomorphic stromal cells can be seen ➡, but this is not a sign of malignancy. Note the normal looking urothelium ⇨.

Other Tumors and Tumor-Like Lesions of Renal Pelvis

TERMINOLOGY

Definitions
- Neoplasms other than usual urothelial carcinoma involving renal pelvis

ETIOLOGY/PATHOGENESIS

Nephrolithiasis and Repeated Infections
- Squamous cell carcinoma and adenocarcinoma often occur in background of nephrolithiasis and metaplasia

Bladder Cancer
- Most cases of renal pelvic urothelial (transitional cell) carcinoma are associated with prior, concurrent, or subsequent bladder carcinoma
- However, for nontransitional cell carcinomas of upper tract, such association is not observed

CLINICAL ISSUES

Epidemiology
- Incidence
  - Most carcinomas with nontransitional cell features (variants) in pelvis coexist with usual urothelial (transitional cell) carcinomas of pelvis
  - Pure nonurothelial carcinomas of renal pelvis are very rare
    - Squamous cell carcinoma is 2nd most common carcinoma of renal pelvis
    - Incidence of 10% of renal pelvic cases is reported in older study; likely includes urothelial carcinomas with squamous differentiation
    - More recent studies report a combined incidence of < 1% for squamous cell carcinomas and adenocarcinomas of renal pelvis
    - All other types of carcinoma in literature exist as case reports or small case series
  - Benign epithelial, mesenchymal, and other tumors are also very rare
    - Fibroepithelial polyps, although more common in adults, are most common benign polypoid pelvic tumors in children
- Age
  - Carcinomas: Range 41-87 yr (mean: 66 yr)
  - Fibroepithelial polyps: Range 7-73 yr (mean: 40 yr)
  - Inverted papillomas: Range 19-89 yr (mean: 64 yr)
  - Primitive neuroectodermal tumors: Mostly young adults/adolescents; range 10-60 yr (mean: 27 yr)
  - Other tumors: Variable, mostly older adults

Presentation
- Flank pain &/or hematuria common presentations
- Ureteral or pelviureteric junction obstruction with resultant hydronephrosis also not uncommon
- Episodic colicky pain, especially in tumors of ureter

Treatment
- Surgical approaches
  - Usually nephroureterectomy performed for carcinomas of pelvis or proximal ureter
  - Malignant tumors of more distal ureters may be amenable to ureterectomy
  - Polypoid smaller benign tumors, particularly fibroepithelial polyps, may be resected endoscopically

Prognosis
- Most pure nontransitional cell (variants), as well as urothelial carcinomas with divergent/aberrant differentiation, are high-grade and high-stage tumors
- Most patients with pT3 or pT4 tumors die of disease; 5-year survival is extremely uncommon
- Some benign tumors may cause obstruction and resultant hydronephrosis, with related complications

MACROSCOPIC

General Features
- Carcinomas
  - Usually large tumors, filling pelvicalyceal system, ± renal parenchymal and renal sinus soft tissue invasion
- Fibroepithelial polyps, hemangiomas, squamous papillomas, and nephrogenic adenomas
  - Mostly polypoid lesions in pelvis or ureter
  - Size usually small (mean: 2 cm; mostly 0.5-4 cm in maximum diameter); rare tumors are much larger
- Inverted papillomas
  - Smooth surface, broad based, sessile, rarely pedunculated
- Malignant mesenchymal tumors
  - Often arising in perirenal and renal hilar soft tissues, and secondarily involving pelvicalyceal system and renal parenchyma

MICROSCOPIC

Histologic Features
- Benign epithelial tumors/lesions
  - Inverted papilloma
    - Endophytic interconnected trabeculae and cords of urothelium, extensively invaginating from surface into lamina propria
    - Covered by flat-surfaced urothelium
    - Periphery is smooth and pushing; typically shows palisading of basal nuclei
    - Small glandular or microcystic structures may be seen
  - Nephrogenic metaplasia/adenoma
    - Shows wide spectrum of architectural patterns, often mixed patterns (papillary, tubular/glandular, cystic, single cells, and sheet-like)
    - Lining epithelial cells are cuboidal and single layered, or occasionally hobnailed
    - Cytoplasm varies from eosinophilic to clear; prominent nucleoli may be present
    - In single cell areas, cells may show minute lumina, and closely mimic blood vessels or signet ring cells
    - Frequently, thick basement membrane/hyalinized sheath surrounds epithelium
    - Often associated with inflammatory infiltrate
  - Villous adenoma
    - Similar to villous adenomas of colorectum
    - Biopsy-based diagnosis of villous adenoma should not be made, as adenocarcinoma in vicinity may be missed
  - Other exquisitely rare benign epithelial lesions include squamous and urothelial papillomas

Other Tumors and Tumor-Like Lesions of Renal Pelvis

- Malignant epithelial tumors
  - Squamous cell carcinoma
    - More common in renal pelvis than ureter; often associated with nephrolithiasis
    - Usually accompanied by extensive squamous metaplasia of urothelium and squamous cell carcinoma in situ
    - Often high stage, frequently with renal parenchymal invasion
  - Adenocarcinoma
    - Variety of morphologic phenotypes seen, similar to that in bladder (glandular NOS, enteric, signet ring, mucinous, etc.)
    - Often accompanied by glandular and intestinal metaplasia of surrounding urothelium, or occasionally by villous adenoma
    - Usually high-stage tumors, often with renal parenchymal invasion
  - Other rare types of carcinoma include
    - Small cell and large cell neuroendocrine, lymphoepithelioma-like, sarcomatoid, hepatoid, and rhabdoid
- Benign nonepithelial tumors/lesions
  - Fibroepithelial polyp
    - Usually solitary but sometimes multifocal
    - Consist of proliferation and expansion of subepithelial stromal cells with prominent vascularity, inflammatory infiltrate, and edema
    - Stromal cells usually loosely arranged but may have hypercellular, compact areas
    - Atypical and giant forms of stromal cells may be present
    - Mitotic activity uncommon, and proliferation index as judged by immunostaining is very low
    - Covering urothelium is benign; usually flat but may show papillary or polypoid fronds and may be ulcerated, hyperplastic, and reactive
  - Hemangioma
    - Usually solitary and polypoid but may be multifocal
    - Often cavernous type but may be capillary or venous-type
    - Covered by benign, often ulcerated urothelium
  - Other reported benign mesenchymal lesions include
    - Inflammatory myofibroblastic tumor, angiomyolipoma, leiomyoma, neurofibroma, hibernoma, and lipoma
- Malignant nonepithelial tumors
  - Leiomyosarcoma most common
  - Rhabdomyosarcoma, including botryoides type, angiosarcoma, fibrosarcoma, Ewing tumor, malignant peripheral nerve sheath tumor are other unusual types
  - Sarcomatoid carcinoma always needs to be excluded in all malignant spindle cell neoplasms of ureter and pelvis

DIFFERENTIAL DIAGNOSIS

Metastatic Tumors

- Based on histologic features alone, distinction of primary squamous cell or adenocarcinoma from metastases is very difficult, though metastases are rare
- Immunohistochemical stains are usually not helpful
- Metastatic tumors are often multifocal and bilateral, lack in situ component, have interstitial growth, and usually show prominent vascular invasion
- Clinical history and radiologic findings are often critical
- Both primary and metastatic small cell carcinomas share morphologic and immunohistochemical features
  - In particular, TTF-1 positivity may be seen in both
  - Presence of at least focal urothelial component strongly favors primary origin

Urothelial Carcinoma With Inverted Growth

- Distinction from inverted papilloma is critical
- Presence of following features favors urothelial carcinoma with inverted growth pattern
  - Significant cytologic atypia, solid, nested or nontrabecular growth
  - Adjacent in situ or papillary (noninvasive) carcinoma may be very helpful, if identified

DIAGNOSTIC CHECKLIST

Pathologic Interpretation Pearls

- For all unusual renal pelvic carcinomas, clinical history is a must to exclude metastasis
- Immunohistochemistry often not useful in this distinction
- Adequate sampling is important to identify components that may be crucial to correct diagnosis

SELECTED REFERENCES

1. Guo CC et al: Micropapillary variant of urothelial carcinoma in the upper urinary tract: a clinicopathologic study of 11 cases. Arch Pathol Lab Med. 133(1):62-6, 2009
2. La Rosa S et al: Primary small cell neuroendocrine carcinoma of the kidney: morphological, immunohistochemical, ultrastructural, and cytogenetic study of a case and review of the literature. Endocr Pathol. 20(1):24-34, 2009
3. Volkmer BG et al: Upper urinary tract recurrence after radical cystectomy for bladder cancer--who is at risk? J Urol. 182(6):2632-7, 2009
4. Gupta R et al: Neoplasms of the upper urinary tract: a review with focus on urothelial carcinoma of the pelvicalyceal system and aspects related to its diagnosis and reporting. Adv Anat Pathol. 15(3):127-39, 2008
5. Holmäng S et al: Squamous cell carcinoma of the renal pelvis and ureter: incidence, symptoms, treatment and outcome. J Urol. 178(1):51-6, 2007
6. Tamas EF et al: Lymphoepithelioma-like carcinoma of the urinary tract: a clinicopathological study of 30 pure and mixed cases. Mod Pathol. 20(8):828-34, 2007
7. Frickmann H et al: [Villous adenoma of the renal pelvis and ureter.] Urologe A. 45(11):1435-7, 2006
8. Perez-Montiel D et al: High-grade urothelial carcinoma of the renal pelvis: clinicopathologic study of 108 cases with emphasis on unusual morphologic variants. Mod Pathol. 19(4):494-503, 2006
9. Darras J et al: Synchronous inverted papilloma of bladder and renal pelvis. Urology. 65(4):798, 2005
10. Kapusta LR et al: Inflammatory myofibroblastic tumors of the kidney: a clinicopathologic and immunohistochemical study of 12 cases. Am J Surg Pathol. 27(5):658-66, 2003
11. Raghavendran M et al: Stones associated renal pelvic malignancies. Indian J Cancer. 40(3):108-12, 2003
12. Nowak MA et al: Benign fibroepithelial polyps of the renal pelvis. Arch Pathol Lab Med. 123(9):850-2, 1999
13. Ford TF et al: Adenomatous metaplasia (nephrogenic adenoma) of urothelium. An analysis of 70 cases. Br J Urol. 57(4):427-33, 1985

Other Tumors and Tumor-Like Lesions of Renal Pelvis

Nephrogenic Adenoma/Metaplasia

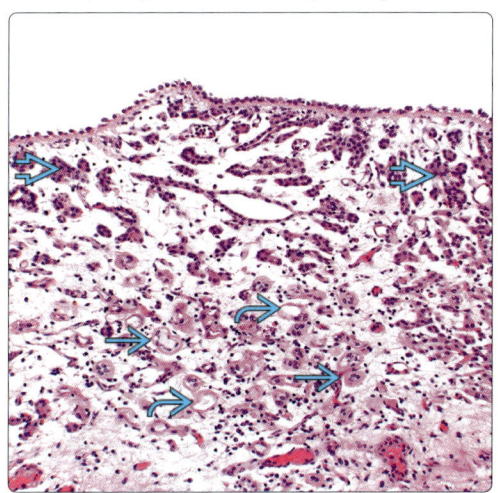

Nephrogenic Adenoma/Metaplasia: Papillary Morphology

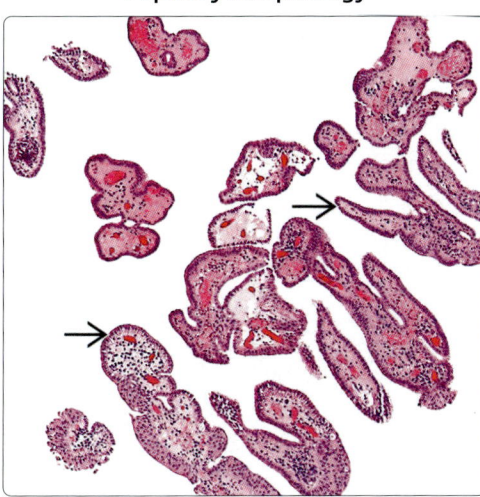

(Left) Nephrogenic metaplasia often shows a mixture of architectural patterns, including tubular ➡ and nested ➡, as seen here. A prominent basement membrane ➡ surrounding the epithelial nests is a characteristic feature. (Right) Compared to the bladder, nephrogenic metaplasia is relatively rare in the renal pelvis. Many lesions appear polypoid or papillary, raising the suspicion of a papillary neoplasm. Typically, the lining cells in nephrogenic metaplasia are cuboidal and single layered ➡.

Inverted Papilloma

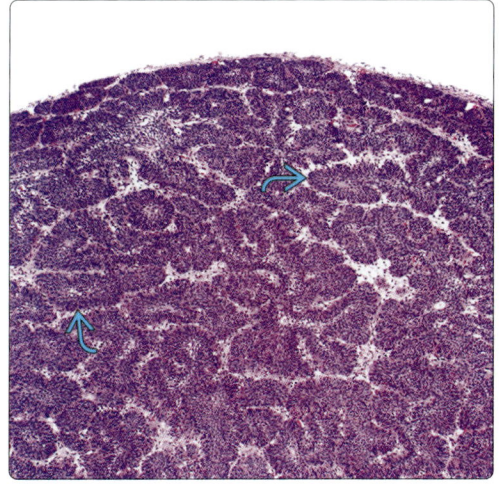

von Brunn Nest Hyperplasia

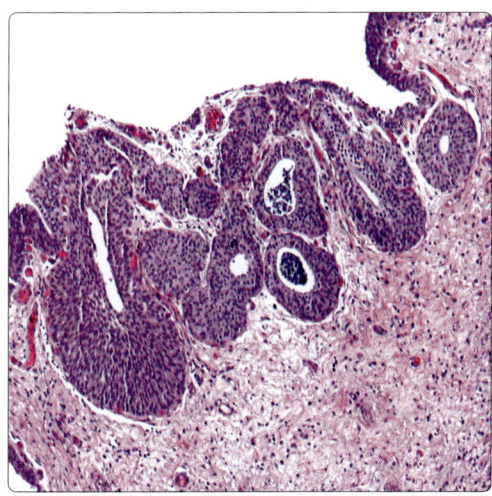

(Left) Inverted papilloma is very rare in the upper urinary tract. It shows interconnecting cords/trabeculae invaginated into the lamina propria, with a flat surface urothelium. The periphery of cords typically show nuclear palisading ➡. (Right) The equivalent to proliferative cystitis may occur in the renal pelvis and the term "proliferative pyelitis" may apply. Clusters of von Brunn nests with cystic changes are typical finding. When florid, this finding may be confused with malignancy such as nested variant of urothelial carcinoma.

Villous Adenoma: Renal Pelvis

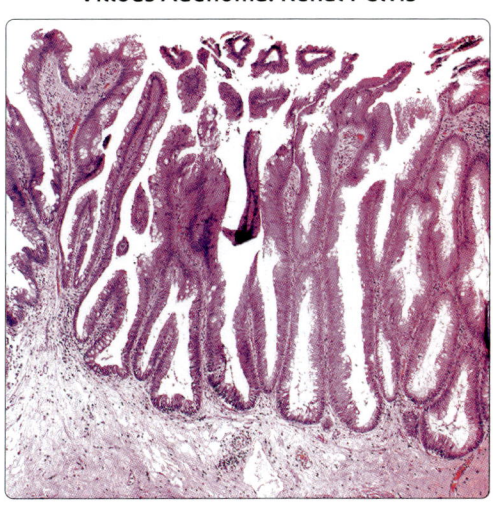

Clear Cell Renal Cell Carcinoma Involving Renal Pelvis

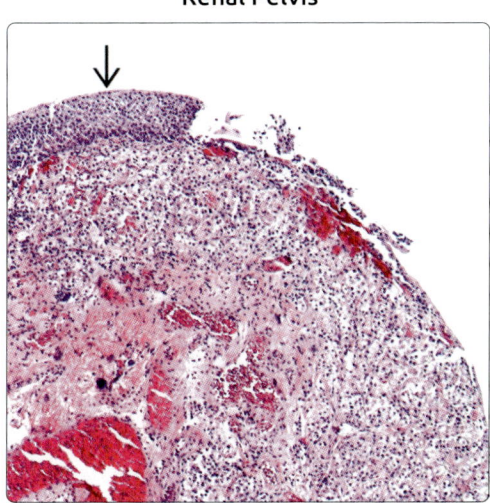

(Left) Villous adenoma is morphologically identical to its more common colorectal counterpart. This neoplasm is characterized by prominent thin papillae, lined by dysplastic mucin-producing columnar epithelium. (Right) This is a renal cell carcinoma, clear cell type with involvement of the renal pelvis. This tumor presented as a more centrally located mass that obliterated the medullary portion of the kidney, involved the renal sinus, and protruded into the renal pelvis. Surface urothelium is noted ➡ and is nonneoplastic.

Other Tumors and Tumor-Like Lesions of Renal Pelvis

Small Cell/Neuroendocrine Carcinoma

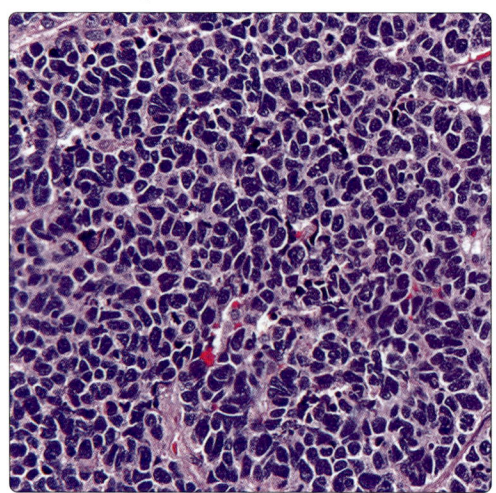

Small Cell/Neuroendocrine Carcinoma and Urothelial Carcinoma In Situ

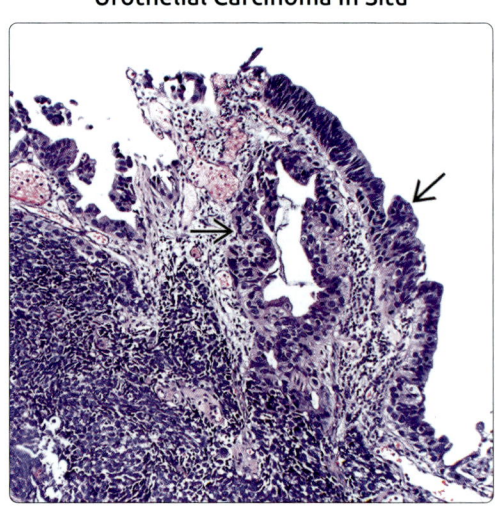

(Left) Pure small cell carcinomas, although quite rare, may be seen in the renal pelvis. At both the morphological and immunophenotypic levels, they are similar to small cell carcinomas of the lung and other sites. Thus, immunostains, including TTF-1, do not discriminate between primary and metastatic tumors. (Right) In most cases, small cell carcinoma, including that of renal pelvis, is associated with a urothelial component. This may be invasive or noninvasive ⇥ as in this example.

Schwannoma

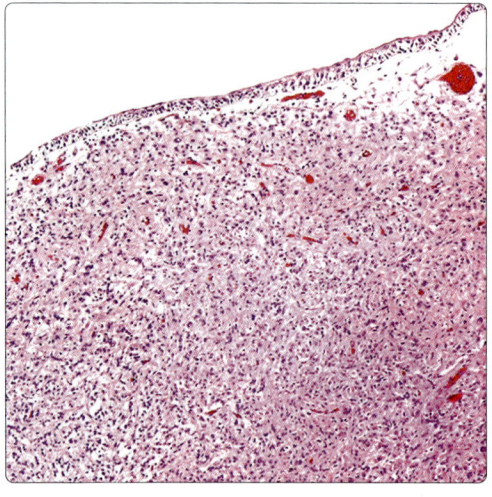

Schwannoma: S100 Immunostain

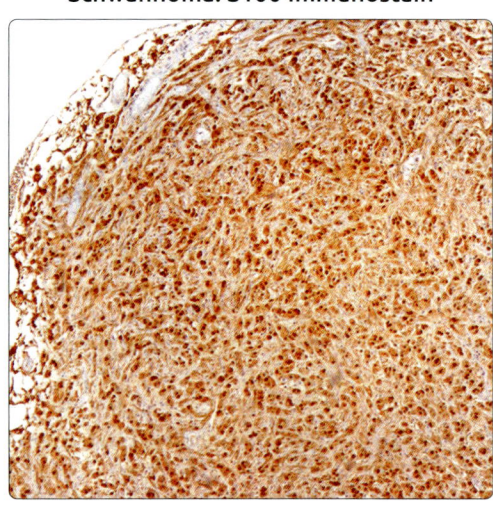

(Left) Benign mesenchymal tumors involving, or arising from, the pelvis are very uncommon. These include schwannoma (as shown here), hemangioma, lipoma, myxoma, and leiomyoma, among others. For any spindle cell neoplasm of the pelvis, the possibility of a sarcomatoid urothelial carcinoma must be excluded. (Right) This image shows diffuse cytoplasmic and nuclear labeling with S100 antibody in the tumor cells, supporting the diagnosis of a schwannoma.

Inflammatory Myofibroblastic Tumor: Renal Pelvis

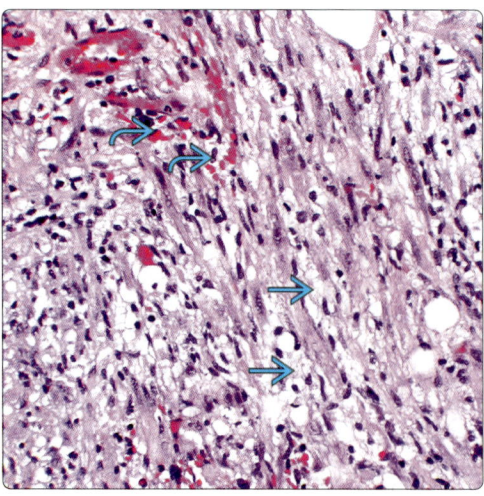

Inflammatory Myofibroblastic Tumor: ALK Immunostain

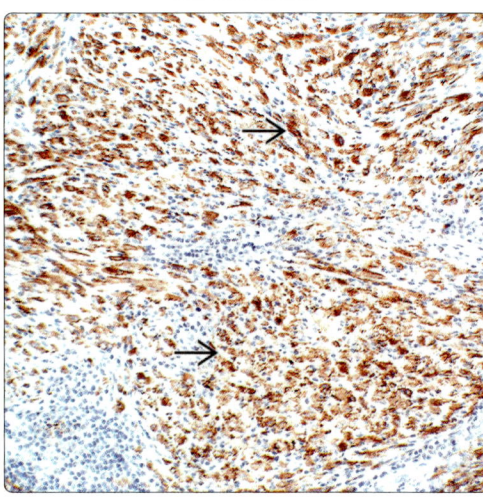

(Left) Inflammatory myofibroblastic tumor of the renal pelvis is rare and morphologically similar to that occurring at other sites, including the bladder. Notice alternating loose ⇥ and hypercellular areas, with extravasated red blood cells ⇥, and scattered inflammatory cell infiltrate. (Right) Most of the inflammatory myofibroblastic tumors of the renal pelvis are reported in the pediatric age group. Rare reported cases at this site also show immunoreactivity ⇥ for ALK.

Other Tumors and Tumor-Like Lesions of Renal Pelvis

Lymphoepithelioma-Like Carcinoma: Renal Pelvis

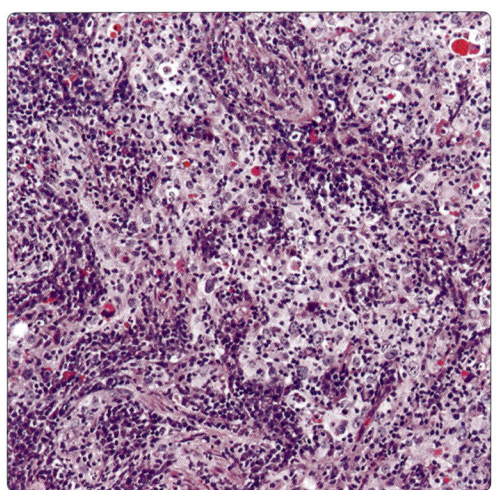

Adenocarcinoma: Renal Pelvis

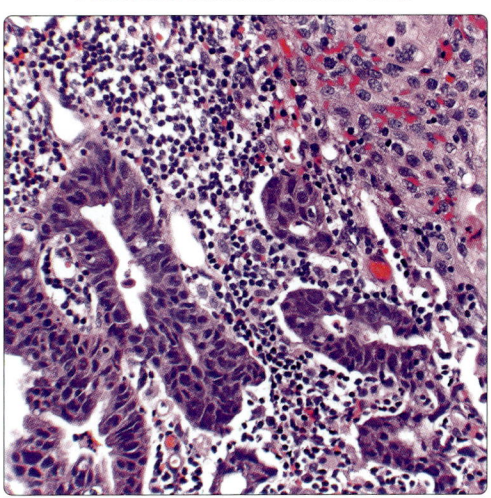

(Left) Lymphoepithelioma-like carcinomas are extremely rare in the renal pelvis. Like their bladder counterparts, they are not associated with Epstein-Barr virus (EBV), although the morphologic features are similar to EBV-associated nasopharyngeal tumors. (Right) The entire spectrum of divergent differentiation of urothelial carcinoma seen in the bladder may be seen in the upper tract. Adenocarcinoma may be pure but often appears in association with a urothelial component.

Squamous Cell Carcinoma: Renal Pelvis

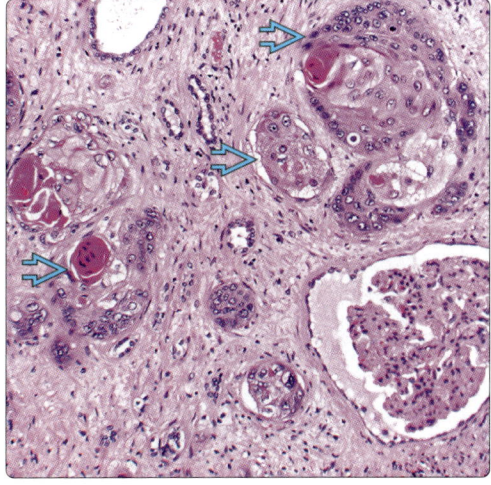

Urothelial Carcinoma: Renal Pelvis

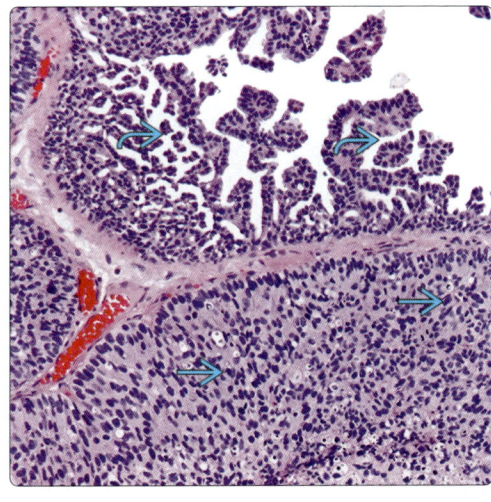

(Left) Squamous cell carcinoma, seen here invading the renal parenchyma ⇒, is the 2nd most common carcinoma in the pelvis. Most cases occur as aberrant differentiation in urothelial carcinoma, but pure forms may be seen. (Right) As in the bladder, a variety of morphologic features of urothelial carcinoma may be seen in the upper urinary tract. This image shows a noninvasive micropapillary component ⇒ in otherwise typical urothelial carcinoma ⇒.

Sarcomatoid Carcinoma of Renal Pelvis: Panoramic View

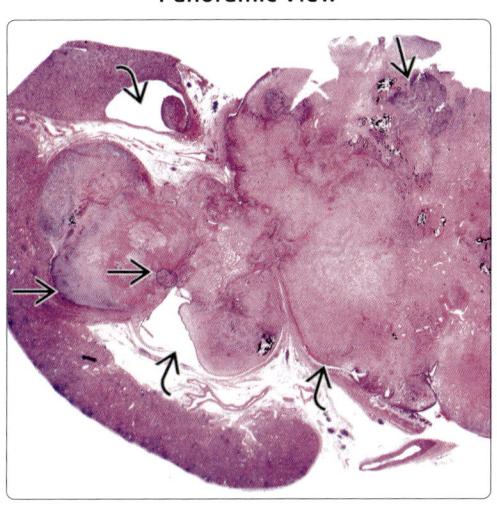

Sarcomatoid Carcinoma With Heterologous Elements (Chondrosarcoma)

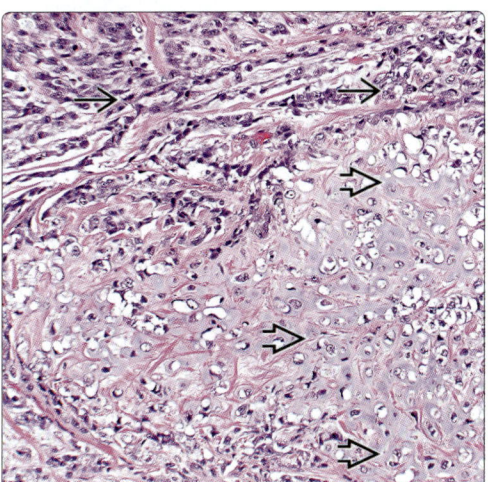

(Left) This whole-mount shows a large exophytic tumor mass, completely filling a markedly dilated ⇒ pelvicalyceal system. The blue and gray areas ⇒ are suggestive of chondromatous differentiation. Sarcomatoid carcinoma and sarcomas may present with large bulky and polypoidal intraluminal masses. (Right) This renal pelvic tumor shows chondrosarcomatous ⇒ differentiation. In all sarcomatous tumors of the pelvis, the possibility of sarcomatoid carcinoma ⇒ must always be excluded.

Urachal Remnants

KEY FACTS

TERMINOLOGY

- Urachus
  - Fibrous cord, known also as median umbilical ligament
  - Apex of bladder to umbilicus, between peritoneum and deep abdominal fascia
- Urachal remnant may be used to describe incidental histologic finding
  - Tubular remnants, either obliterated lumen or with variable, usually urothelial, lining
  - Dense connective tissue surrounded by bundles of muscularis, then adventitia
- Urachal remnant may also be used to describe clinically evident anomaly
  - Completely patent urachus: Urine may flow from bladder and be expressed via umbilicus
  - Umbilicourachal sinus: Blind-ended sinus tract open at umbilicus
  - Vesicourachal sinus: Blind-ended sinus tract opening into apex of bladder
  - Urachal cyst: Patent urachus with closure of both umbilical and vesical ends

ETIOLOGY/PATHOGENESIS

- Defective obliteration of lumen of allantois in later development

CLINICAL ISSUES

- True incidence is unknown, male predominance
- High prevalence of histologic remnants, low prevalence of clinically significant anomalies
- Prominent association with other genitourinary developmental anomalies and syndromes
  - Trigger work-up for associated anomalies
- Consideration of excision, particularly if symptomatic

TOP DIFFERENTIAL DIAGNOSES

- Mucinous cystic urachal tumors
  - Mostly unilocular or multilocular cystic lesion, clinically tumefacient

Clinical Anomalies: Cyst and Patency

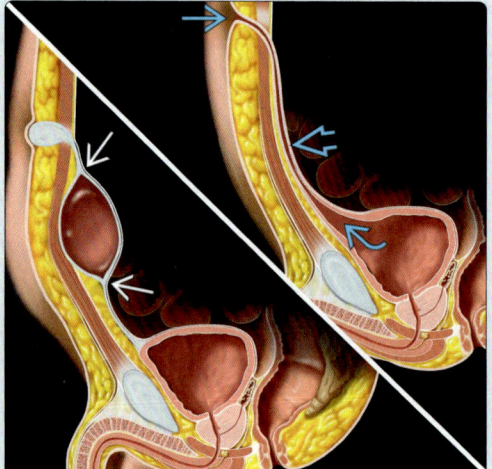

Clinical Anomalies: Sinuses

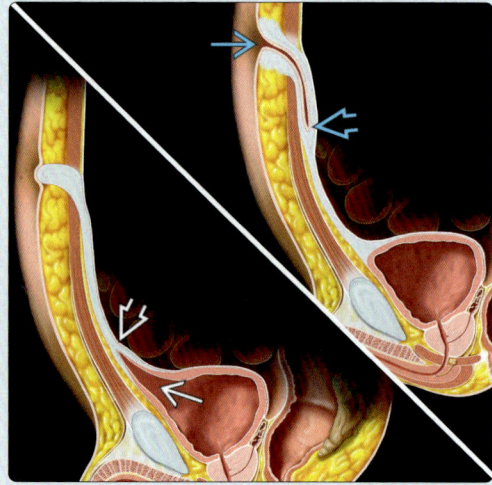

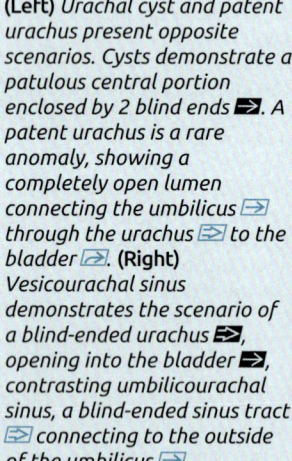

(Left) Urachal cyst and patent urachus present opposite scenarios. Cysts demonstrate a patulous central portion enclosed by 2 blind ends ➡. A patent urachus is a rare anomaly, showing a completely open lumen connecting the umbilicus ➡ through the urachus ➡ to the bladder ➡. (Right) Vesicourachal sinus demonstrates the scenario of a blind-ended urachus ➡, opening into the bladder ➡, contrasting umbilicourachal sinus, a blind-ended sinus tract ➡ connecting to the outside of the umbilicus ➡.

Histology: Incidental Urachal Remnant

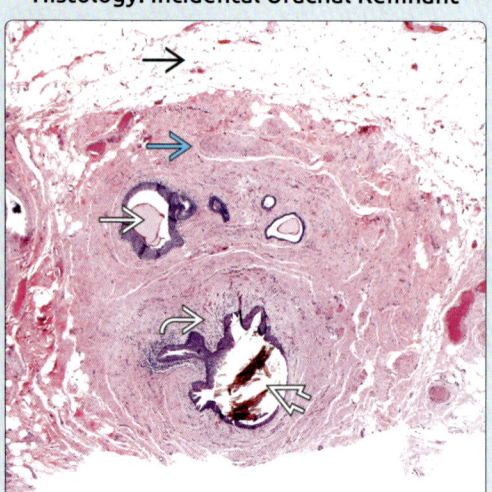

Histology: Symptomatic Urachal Cyst

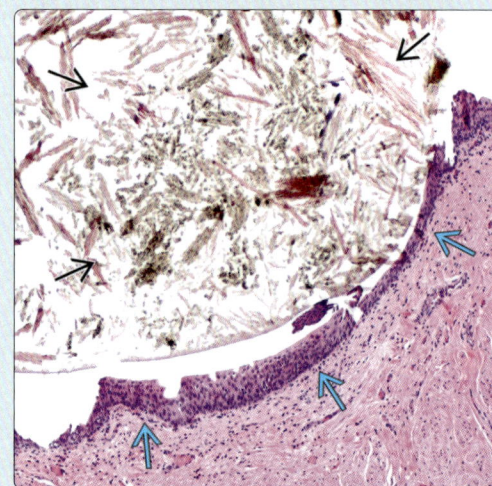

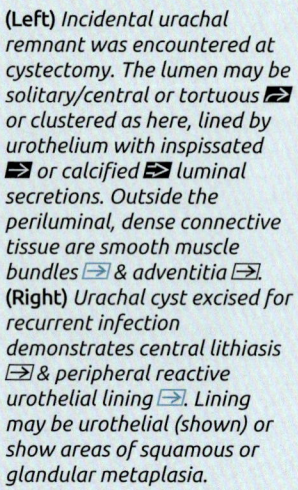

(Left) Incidental urachal remnant was encountered at cystectomy. The lumen may be solitary/central or tortuous ➡ or clustered as here, lined by urothelium with inspissated ➡ or calcified ➡ luminal secretions. Outside the periluminal, dense connective tissue are smooth muscle bundles ➡ & adventitia ➡. (Right) Urachal cyst excised for recurrent infection demonstrates central lithiasis ➡ & peripheral reactive urothelial lining ➡. Lining may be urothelial (shown) or show areas of squamous or glandular metaplasia.

Urachal Remnants

TERMINOLOGY

Definitions

- **Urachus**
  - Fibrous cord, known also as median umbilical ligament, which runs from apex of bladder to umbilicus, coursing in space of Retzius between transversalis fascia and peritoneum
  - Product of regression of allantois and most rostral aspect of bladder apex
  - In many adults, this structure represents only fibrous cord, though in subset, it is identifiable tubular remnant
  - Segments include supravesical (between bladder and umbilicus), intramural (within muscular wall of bladder), and mucosal (at opening to lumen of bladder, if present)
- **Urachal remnant may be used to describe incidental histologic finding**
  - Urachal remnants consist of central tubular lumen, which may be obliterated or lined by variable, usually transitional, epithelium (urothelium), surrounded by dense connective tissue, then by large/compact muscle bundles, then by soft tissue adventitia
  - Tubular remnants have been classified into type I (simple, straight tube), type II (tube with saccular dilatations), type III (complex/convoluted tube with dilatations)
- **Urachal remnant may also be used to describe clinically evident anomaly**
  - Completely patent urachus: Urine may flow from bladder and be expressed via umbilicus
  - Umbilicourachal sinus: Blind-ended sinus tract open at umbilicus
  - Vesicourachal sinus: Blind-ended sinus tract opening into apex of bladder
  - Urachal cyst: Patent urachus with closure of both umbilical and vesical ends

ETIOLOGY/PATHOGENESIS

Developmental Anomaly

- Defective obliteration of lumen of allantois in later development

CLINICAL ISSUES

Epidemiology

- True incidence is unknown; prevalence depends on whether considering histologic incidental remnants or clinically detectable anomalies
  - For instance, autopsy series suggest at least 30% of adult bladders contain identifiable remnant structure (urachal remnant)
- In contrast, clinically identifiable remnants or anomalies are rare in general population
  - 1 retrospective cohort studying all urachal anomalies identified **radiologically** reported their prevalence as 1% of pediatric population
    - Vast majority are asymptomatic; 89% urachal remnants, 9% urachal cysts, and 1.5% patent urachus, with mean age of 6.2 years, male predominance
- In series based on diagnosis rather than imaging findings, higher prevalence of symptomatic lesions
- High association with other genitourinary tract developmental anomalies; should trigger work-up

Presentation

- Patients with completely patent urachus have unobstructed tract between bladder and umbilicus
  - Most are male; umbilical expression of urine, urinary tract infections, association with prune belly syndrome
- Umbilicourachal sinus presents with inflammatory umbilical polyp reactive to inflammation and infection of accumulated debris
- Vesicourachal sinus presents as bladder diverticulum
  - Infection, ureteral obstruction, accumulation of cellular debris, lithiasis
- Urachal cyst presents as mass
  - Older children and adults with palpable mass, often infected, with infraumbilical abdominal pain, erythema, swelling

Treatment

- Traditionally, surgical excision of entire structure, extending from mucosal segment, through mural segment, to supravesical segment, to ostensibly prevent adenocarcinoma
- Contemporary studies of urachal remnants, particularly asymptomatic urachal anomalies, question excision
  - Urachal adenocarcinoma is vanishingly rare and unclear if it is preceded by urachal remnants
  - Emerging evidence that many asymptomatic/incidental urachal remnants involute over time in follow-up studies

MICROSCOPIC

Histologic Features

- Recent review identifies epithelium in majority of excised remnants, whether symptomatic or asymptomatic
  - Majority were urothelial lined, but squamous and enteric-type glandular epithelia are identified, may be admixed

DIFFERENTIAL DIAGNOSIS

Mucinous Cystic Urachal Tumors

- Mostly unilocular or multilocular cystic lesion, clinically tumefacient
  - Not tubular remnant with foci of glandular metaplasia
- Diffuse mucinous epithelium with variable atypia
- Fibrotic wall, extravasated mucin, dystrophic calcification

SELECTED REFERENCES

1. Gleason JM et al: A comprehensive review of pediatric urachal anomalies and predictive analysis for adult urachal adenocarcinoma. J Urol. 193(2):632-6, 2015
2. Naiditch JA et al: Current diagnosis and management of urachal remnants. J Pediatr Surg. 48(10):2148-52, 2013
3. Copp HL et al: Clinical presentation and urachal remnant pathology: implications for treatment. J Urol. 182(4 Suppl):1921-4, 2009
4. Bostwick et al: Nonneoplastic disorders of the urinary bladder. In Urologic Surgical Pathology. 3rd ed. Elsevier, 2014

Tumors of Urachus

KEY FACTS

CLASSIFICATION

- **Urachal carcinoma**
- Primary, invasive carcinoma of **any morphologic type**, fulfilling criteria
  - Tumor primarily located in dome of or anterior wall of bladder
  - Epicenter of carcinoma is in muscularis propria of bladder, with sharp demarcation between tumor and underlying bladder mucosa
  - Lack of extensive cystitis cystica et glandularis in bladder
  - Absence of carcinoma of similar histology at another primary site
- Most examples are adenocarcinoma, but infrequent urothelial and squamous carcinomas occur as well
- **Mucinous cystic tumors (MCT) of urachus**
- Recently proposed classification for lower grade, cystic glandular tumors by analogy to mucinous cystic ovarian epithelial tumors
- Tumors having prominent cystic component, elaboration of luminal mucin, and fibrotic stroma
- Mucinous cystadenoma
- MCT of low malignant potential (LMP)
- MCT of LMP with intraepithelial carcinoma
- Mucinous cystadenocarcinoma with microinvasion
- Mucinous cystadenocarcinoma with frank invasion

CLINICAL ISSUES

- Both urachal carcinoma and MCTs very rare
- Hematuria, mass lesion, or mucusuria symptoms
- Both tumor types treated by partial or radical cystectomy ± umbilectomy and excision of urachal tract
- Prognosis is variable
  - Invasive urachal carcinoma quite aggressive
  - MCTs quite indolent

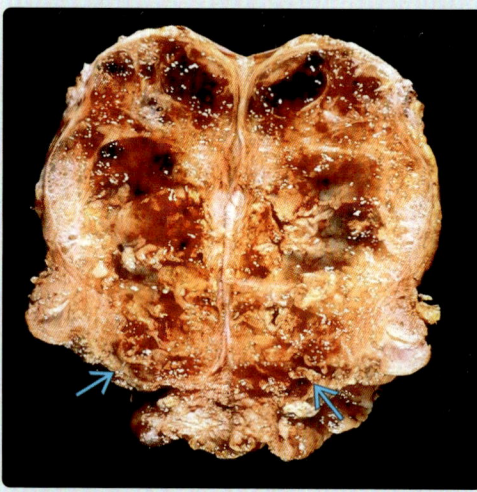

Urachal Adenocarcinoma

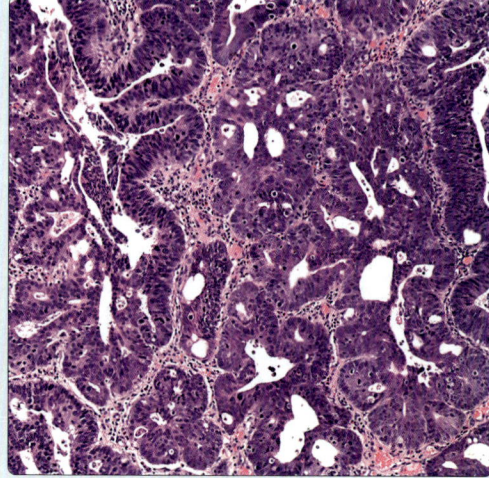

Enteric-Type Urachal Adenocarcinoma

(Left) Gross micrograph of a partial cystectomy-orchectomyorchectomy specimen, "butterfly" bisected, shows a diffusely invasive mucinous tumor invading in the space of Retzius and the bladder wall and eroding into the dome of the bladder ➡. *(Right)* Invasive, enteric-type adenocarcinoma demonstrates high-grade cytology and tubular and cribriform growth based in the wall of the dome of the bladder.

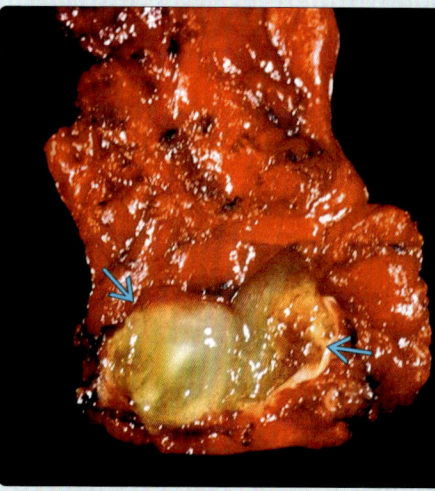

Mucinous Cystic Tumor of Urachus

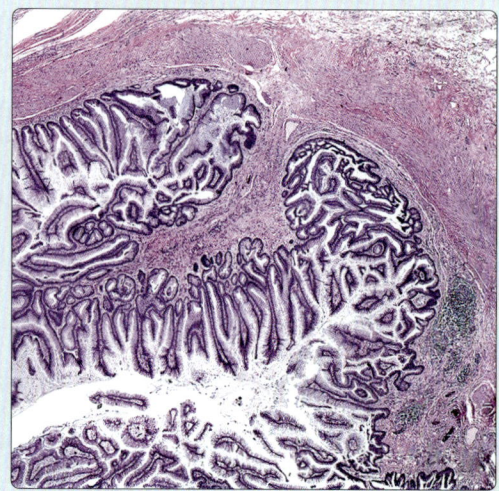

Urachal Mucinous Cystic Tumor of Low Malignant Potential

(Left) A rare gross micrograph of a urachal mucinous cystic tumor (MCT) of low malignant potential (LMP), also bisected ➡, shows a prominent, unilocular cyst with mucinous luminal contents within a orchectomyorchectomy specimen. *(Right)* Micrograph of the same case demonstrates a glandular neoplastic lining with intestinal-type mucinous cytology, villous architecture, and low-grade dysplasia lining the entire cyst wall. The perilesional stroma is chronically inflamed and fibrotic, as is characteristic.

Tumors of Urachus

TERMINOLOGY

Abbreviations
- Mucinous cystic tumor (MCT)
- Low malignant potential (LMP)

CLASSIFICATION

Urachal Carcinoma
- Primary, invasive carcinoma of **any morphologic type** originating from urachus and fulfilling following clinicopathologic criteria
  - Tumor primarily located in dome of or anterior wall of bladder
  - Epicenter of mass is in wall (muscularis propria) of bladder, with sharp demarcation between urachal tumor and underlying bladder mucosa
  - Lack of extensive cystitis cystica et glandularis in bladder
  - Absence of tumor of similar histology at another primary site
- Most examples are adenocarcinoma (enteric, colloid, mixed, or not otherwise specified)
- Urothelial and squamous carcinomas also arise as primary to urachus

Mucinous Cystic Tumors of Urachus
- Prior examples diagnosed under variety of terms and criteria
- Recently proposed classification based on analogy to MCTs of ovary
  - Overall, group of lower grade of glandular tumors, most without invasion or with limited invasion
  - Tumors having prominent cystic component, elaboration of luminal mucin, and fibrotic stroma
- Categories proposed include
  - **Mucinous cystadenoma**
    - Cyst lined by mucinous columnar epithelium, lacking atypia or epithelial complexity
  - **MCT of LMP**
    - Cyst showing areas of epithelial proliferation, with papillation and low-grade cytologic atypia
  - **MCT of LMP with intraepithelial carcinoma**
    - Cyst showing significant epithelial atypia, often with complexity, stroma-poor papillae, and cribriform growth
  - **Mucinous cystadenocarcinoma with microinvasion**
    - Mucinous cystic adenocarcinoma with stromal invasion < 2 mm and comprising < 5% of tumor
  - **Mucinous cystadenocarcinoma with frank invasion**
    - Mucinous cystic adenocarcinoma with more extensive invasion than microinvasion as defined above

ETIOLOGY/PATHOGENESIS

Developmental Anomaly
- Urachal remnants
  - May undergo glandular metaplasia and eventual malignant transformation
  - Contemporary studies emphasize vanishing rarity of malignant transformation of incidental urachal remnants

CLINICAL ISSUES

Epidemiology
- Incidence
  - Rare, both urachal carcinoma and MCTs
- Age
  - 5th and 6th decades for both urachal carcinoma and MCTs
- Sex
  - Urachal adenocarcinoma more common in men (M:F = > 2:1)
  - MCTs of urachus with slight female preponderance but limited data

Site
- Dome and anterior wall of urinary bladder
  - Anatomic location of urachus

Presentation
- Urachal adenocarcinoma
  - Hematuria (> 60%)
  - Suprapubic mass
  - Mucusuria seen among ~ 25% of cases
  - Irritative bladder symptoms, such as voiding difficulties
- Urachal MCTs
  - Incidental (32%), mass lesion (32%)
  - Hematuria (24%)
  - Mucusuria (12%), pain (12%)

Treatment
- For urachal carcinoma, partial or radical cystectomy, usually with excision of urachal tract and umbilectomy, is treatment of choice
  - Cohort data suggest higher local recurrence when only partial cystectomy performed
  - Adjuvant therapy depends on stage, may include chemo- or radiotherapy
- For urachal MCTs, no comparative studies of treatments
  - Most prevalent treatments in largest series include partial cystectomy (50%), partial cystectomy with orchectomyorchectomy (23%), orchectomyorchectomy/umbilectomy only (9%), transurethral resection (5%)

Prognosis
- Invasive urachal carcinoma is aggressive tumor with poor prognosis
  - Usually diagnosed at advanced stage
  - 5-year survival rate reported from 25-61%
- MCTs are comparatively very indolent, but limited data
  - In limited cases with reported outcomes no recurrence or metastasis

IMAGING

CT Findings
- Urachal carcinoma demonstrates thickened bladder dome
  - Tumor may extend along urachus to umbilicus
- Urachal MCTs may present, often incidentally, as cystic masses or cystic urachal remnants

Tumors of Urachus

MACROSCOPIC

General Features
- Urachal adenocarcinoma
  - Underlying bladder mucosa is intact in early stages
    - Becomes ulcerated as tumor grows endophytically
  - Mass localized to dome of bladder, infiltrative in muscle
- MCTs are unilocular or multilocular cysts, often with indurated, fibrotic walls

MICROSCOPIC

Histologic Features
- Urachal carcinoma
  - Adenocarcinoma or urothelial, squamous, and other rarer carcinomas
    - Enteric, mucinous, signet ring, mixed, or not otherwise specified histology of adenocarcinoma
- MCT
  - Unilocular or multilocular cyst with fibrotic stroma in walls, often extravasated mucin, dystrophic calcification, or even metaplastic ossification
  - Epithelium ranges from entirely bland, nonatypical columnar intestinal type glandular epithelium in mucinous cystadenoma, to distinct low-grade atypia/dysplasia in L tumors, to cytologically malignant in MCT with intraepithelial carcinoma and cystadenocarcinoma

ANCILLARY TESTS

Immunohistochemistry
- Both urachal carcinomas and MCTs share much immunophenotypic overlap with colorectal adenocarcinomas
  - CK7 and CK20 are both variably positive in urachal carcinomas
    - CK7 expression is more frequent in urachal than colorectal carcinomas
  - CDX2 expression highly prevalent among all these tumors
- Only β-catenin may provide help distinguishing urachal carcinoma from gastrointestinal (GI) primaries (but not bladder)
  - Strong nuclear (and, usually, cytoplasmic) positivity supports GI primary
  - Membranocytoplasmic positivity sparing nucleus supports urachal (or bladder) primary

DIFFERENTIAL DIAGNOSIS

Primary Adenocarcinoma of Urinary Bladder
- Many have associated adenocarcinoma in situ in surrounding urothelial mucosa
- Usually based on posterior wall or trigone; history of chronic irritation
- Requires close clinical and imaging correlation

Invasive Urothelial Carcinoma With Glandular Differentiation
- Usually located in trigone or posterior wall
- Prior or concurrent typical urothelial carcinoma helpful
  - Adjacent urothelial carcinoma in situ
  - Papillary urothelial neoplasia in bladder

Colonic Adenocarcinoma (or Other Secondary Adenocarcinoma)
- Clinicopathologic correlation is critical
  - Not typically based in dome, bowel may be adherent
- Recommend colonoscopy to detect primary in difficult cases
- Other primary carcinomas may also directly invade bladder
  - Gynecologic tract or even prostatic adenocarcinoma
    - Endometrial, ovarian, or cervical carcinomas most common

Villous Adenoma of Urachus
- Localized, papillary proliferation of columnar intestinal-type epithelium arising in urachus
- Distinguished conceptually from MCTs by its distinctly localized nature rather than as diffuse mucinous epithelial process lining unilocular or multilocular cystic neoplasm
- Varying degree of epithelial dysplasia, many reported with dysplasia in range seen in villous adenomas of GI tract
- Historically, some cases of MCT of LMP of urachus may have been labeled villous adenomas

REPORTING

Staging
- No AJCC TNM staging system accepted for use for urachal carcinomas
  - While other systems have been proposed, Sheldon Staging System (Sheldon et al, 1984) remains best known and most used for urachal carcinoma
    - pT1: No invasion beyond urachal mucosa
    - pT2: Invasion confined to urachus
    - pT3: Local extension to
      - Bladder
      - Abdominal wall
      - Viscera other than bladder
    - pT4: Metastasis
      - Regional lymph nodes
      - Distant sites

SELECTED REFERENCES

1. Busto Martín L et al: Urachal adenocarcinoma of the bladder, our experience in 20 years. Arch Esp Urol. 68(2):178-182, 2015
2. Amin MB et al: Glandular neoplasms of the urachus: a report of 55 cases emphasizing mucinous cystic tumors with proposed classification. Am J Surg Pathol. 38(8):1033-45, 2014
3. Gopalan A et al: Urachal carcinoma: a clinicopathologic analysis of 24 cases with outcome correlation. Am J Surg Pathol. 33(5):659-68, 2009
4. Herr HW et al: Urachal carcinoma: contemporary surgical outcomes. J Urol. 178(1):74-8; discussion 78, 2007
5. Molina JR et al: Predictors of survival from urachal cancer: a Mayo Clinic study of 49 cases. Cancer. 110(11):2434-40, 2007
6. Cheng L et al: Villous adenoma of the urinary tract: a report of 23 cases, including 8 with coexistent adenocarcinoma. Am J Surg Pathol. 23(7):764-71, 1999

Tumors of Urachus

Urachal Carcinoma: Gross
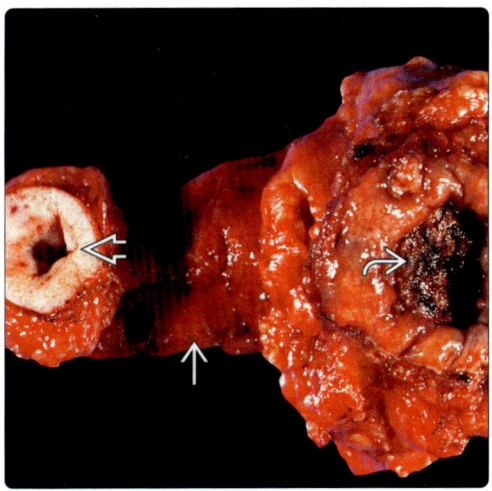

Urachal Adenocarcinoma: Enteric Type
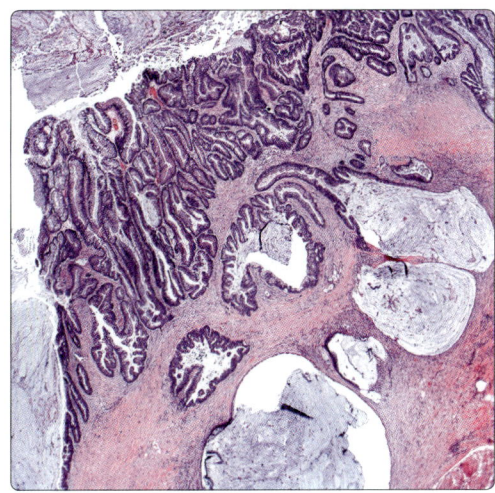

(Left) This gross specimen from a partial cystectomy umbilicourachectomy shows an ulcerative tumor eroding into the bladder ⊋, the excised urachal tract ➔, and the attached umbilicus ⇨. (Right) An adenocarcinoma, with hyperchromatic, predominantly enteric morphology and pools of extravasated mucin, is seen invading in the wall of the bladder. It is imperative to rule out a metastatic carcinoma.

Urachal Adenocarcinoma, Not Otherwise Specified
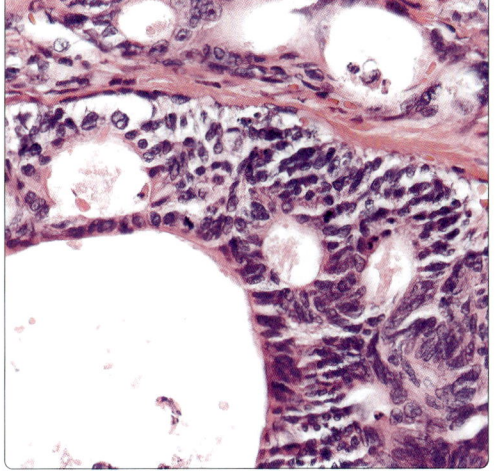

Urachal Adenocarcinoma: Mucinous Type
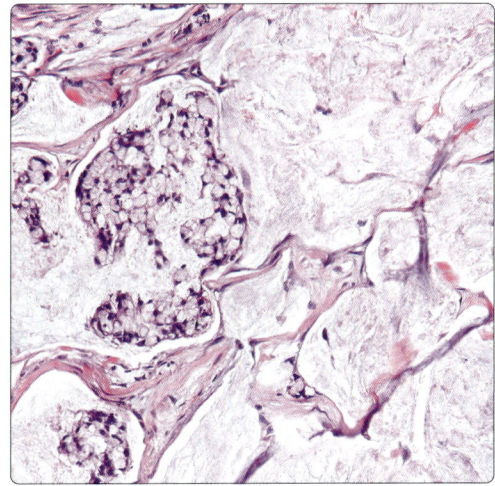

(Left) Within the not otherwise specified variants of urachal adenocarcinoma are examples showing cribriform architecture that may mimic endometrioid-type endometrial adenocarcinoma. Clinical correlation is essential to rule out uterine or colorectal origin. (Right) Mucinous adenocarcinoma may arise within urachal remnants at the dome of the bladder. Correlation with clinical/imaging evaluation is critical to establish a urachal origin.

Urachal Adenocarcinoma: Enteric Type
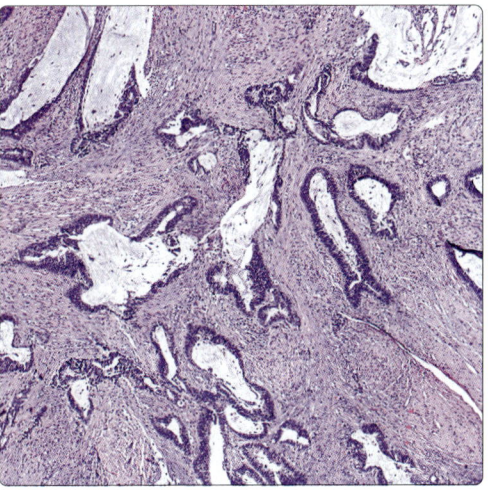

Urachal Adenocarcinoma, Not Otherwise Specified
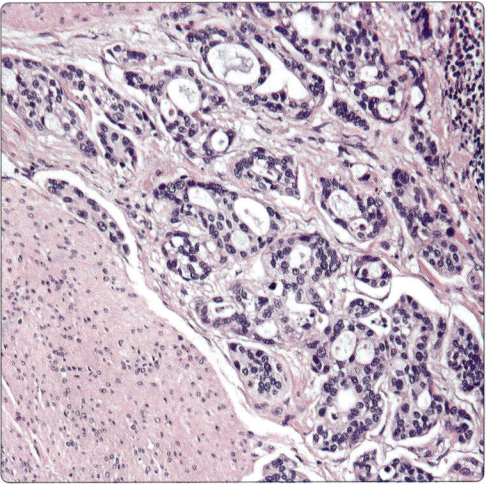

(Left) Some urachal adenocarcinomas have an enteric phenotype that is morphologically indistinguishable from primary vesical adenocarcinoma and secondary involvement from a colorectal adenocarcinoma. In males, prostatic ductal adenocarcinoma may bear consideration. (Right) H&E shows the morphologic spectrum of primary urachal carcinomas as would be designated adenocarcinoma, not otherwise specified. Such cases could morphologically mimic metastases from a variety of anatomic locations.

Tumors of Urachus

Urachal Carcinoma: Urothelial Type
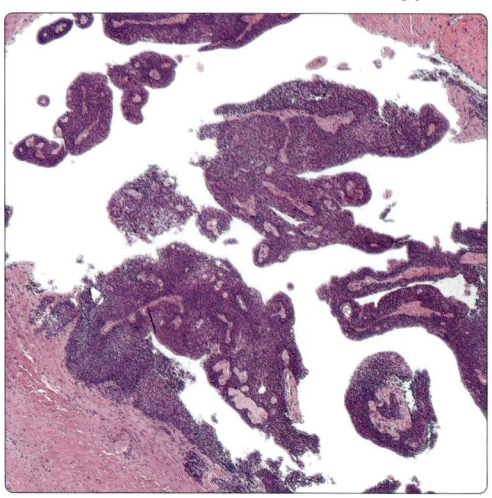

Urachal Carcinoma: Urothelial Type
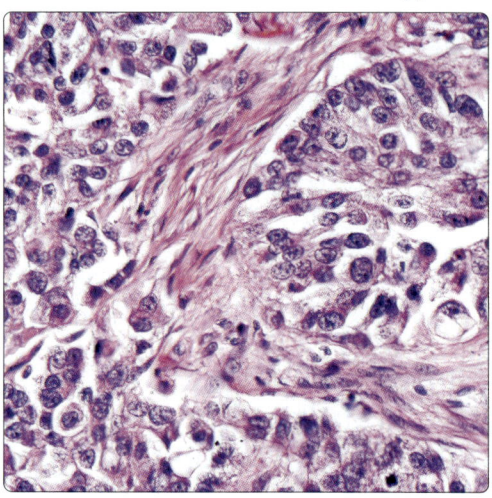

(Left) Primary urachal carcinomas may also have purely urothelial differentiation. This example of a carcinoma arising in the urachus is a noninvasive, high-grade papillary urothelial carcinoma. The distinction from a urinary bladder primary is based entirely on the anatomic location of the tumor. (Right) This primary urachal carcinoma with pure urothelial differentiation has high-grade cytology and lacks gland formation or intracytoplasmic mucin.

Mucinous Cystic Tumor: CDX2 IHC
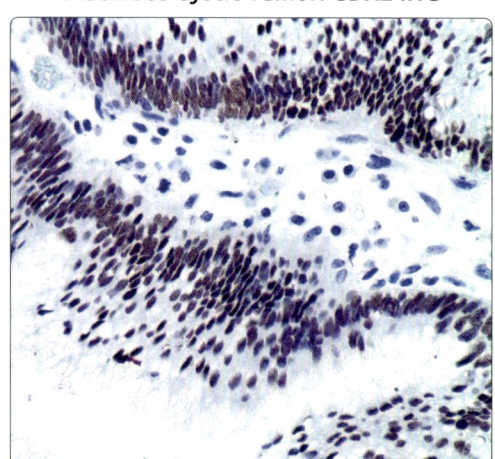

Urachal Carcinoma: CK7 IHC
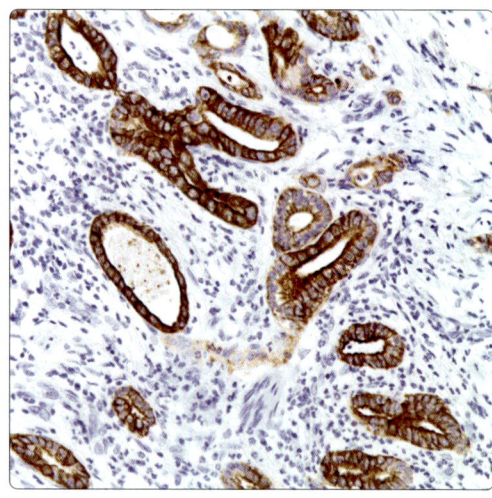

(Left) In both MCTs (pictured) and urachal carcinomas, CDX2 positivity is very prevalent, providing no discrimination between these lesions and colorectal carcinomas. (Right) This urachal adenocarcinoma demonstrates tubular morphology and diffuse expression of CK7. CK7 in urachal carcinoma and in MCTs is usually more than in colorectal adenocarcinomas but is not a reliable discriminant.

Urachal Carcinoma: CK20 IHC
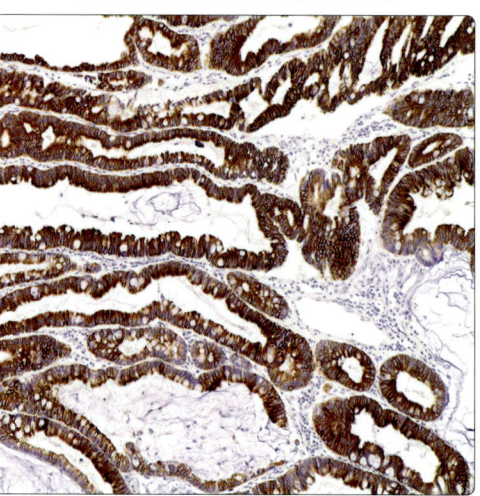

Colorectal Carcinoma: β-Catenin IHC
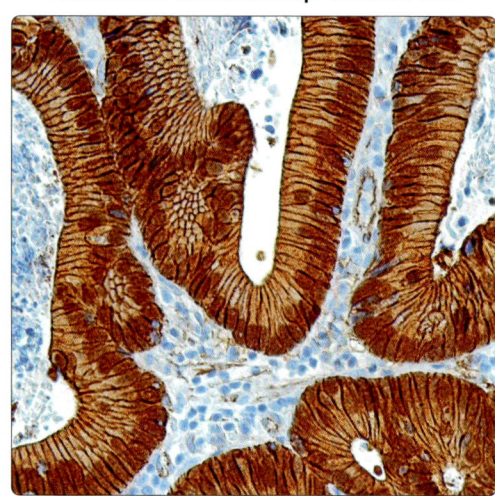

(Left) A urachal adenocarcinoma with enteric morphology shows diffuse CK20 expression. This feature is unfortunately highly prevalent in urachal adenocarcinomas, urachal MCTs, and colorectal carcinomas. (Right) This colorectal adenocarcinoma invading the bladder shows strong nuclear positivity for β-catenin. Nuclear reactivity to β-catenin is specific for colonic primary carcinomas and is not reported in urachal carcinomas or MCTs. It is the only known useful IHC in this differential.

Tumors of Urachus

Mucinous Cystadenoma

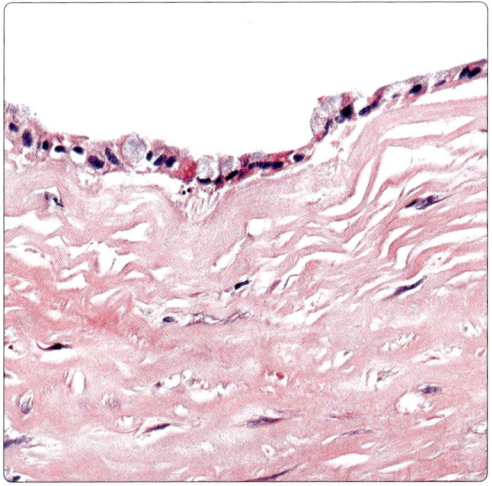

Mucinous Cystic Tumor of Low Malignant Potential

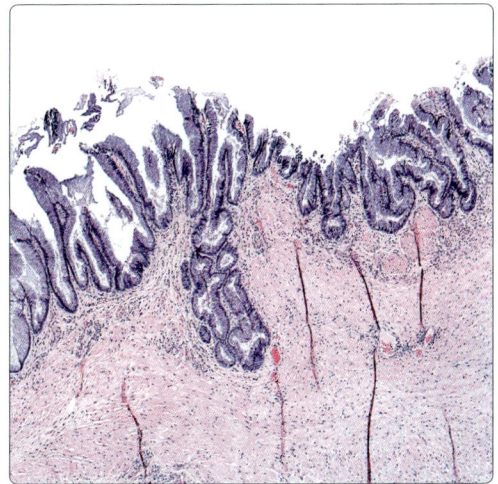

(Left) A high-power micrograph of the attenuated, nonatypical, nonproliferative lining of a urachal mucinous cystadenoma, with underlying fibrotic stroma, similar to those seen in the ovary, is shown. Distinct atypia or papillary growth would trigger a MCT of low malignant potential designation. *(Right)* Glandular epithelial proliferation in the form of stroma-poor papillae and any degree of significant epithelial cytologic atypia/dysplasia merits classification as a MCT of LMP.

Mucinous Cystic Tumor of Low Malignant Potential

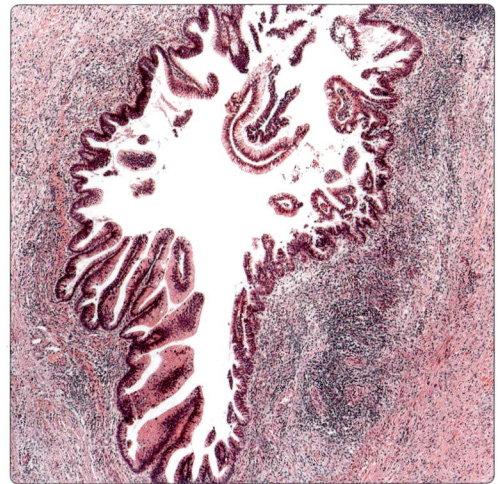

Mucinous Cystic Tumor of Low Malignant Potential With Intraepithelial Carcinoma

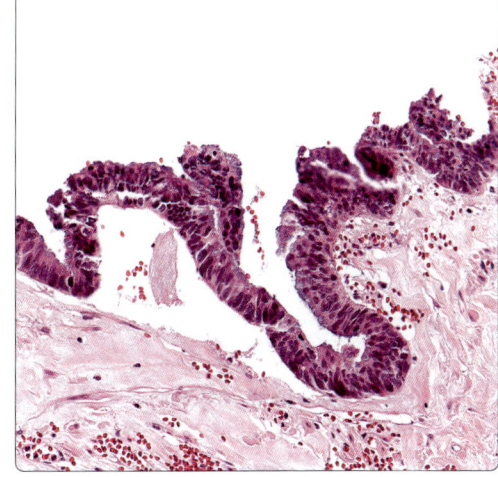

(Left) Another MCT of LMP diffusely lines a smaller cystic tumor, with papillary architecture, and demonstrates dysplasia in the range of that seen in villous adenomas of the gastrointestinal tract. *(Right)* Here, marked cytologic atypia is seen in the lining of a MCT. Such cases, with high-grade dysplasia or noninvasive cribriform growth, are designated MCT of LMP with intraepithelial carcinoma. Generous sampling is important to rule out invasion.

Mucinous Cystic Tumor of Low Malignant Potential With Intraepithelial Carcinoma

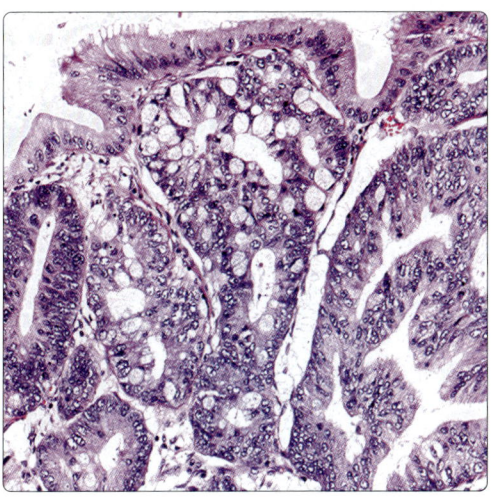

Cystadenocarcinoma With Microinvasion

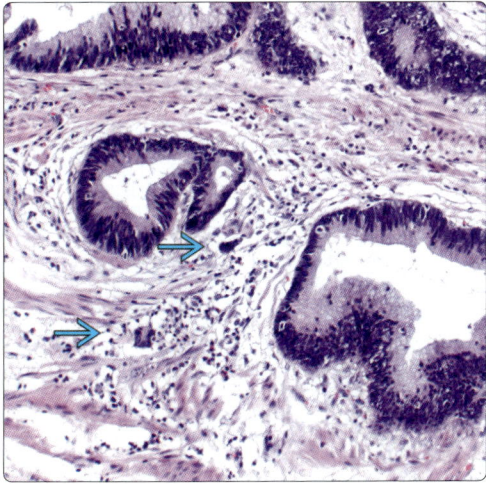

(Left) Another noninvasive MCT of LMP with intraepithelial carcinoma shows cribriform growth and high-grade cytologic atypia within the epithelial lining. *(Right)* Here, a focus at the periphery of a large cyst (lumen above, out of field) demonstrates a focus of several small glands surrounded by desmoplastic stromal reaction and tiny invasive nests ➔, invasive < 2 mm and < 5% of the tumor. Generous sampling is recommended as greater invasion is designated as frank invasion.

Immunohistochemistry, Urinary Tract

Markers Used in Flat Urothelial Lesions

Antibody/Protein Detected	Normal Urothelium	Reactive Atypia	CIS
CK20 (cytoplasmic)	Limited to umbrella cells	Limited to umbrella cells	Aberrant expression through all cell layers; may be full thickness
CD44(s)	Limited to basal cells	Increased reactivity in all cell layers	Absent in atypical cells
p53 (nuclear, brown)	Absent or weak, scattered basal positivity	Absent or weak, scattered basal positivity	Strong and intense positivity in atypical cells (or conspicuous, complete negativity)

Several commercial and laboratory developed tests combining these markers into a cocktail are employed, generally using p53 and CD44(s) detection with brown chromogen and CK20 with red chromogen. CIS = carcinoma in situ.

Adapted from Amin MB et al: Best practices recommendations in the application of immunohistochemistry in the bladder lesions: report from the International Society of Urologic Pathology consensus conference. Am J Surg Pathol. 38(8):e20-34, 2014; Epstein JI et al: Best practices recommendations in the application of immunohistochemistry in the prostate: report from the International Society of Urologic Pathology consensus conference. Am J Surg Pathol. 38(8):e6-e19, 2014.

More Common Spindle Cell Lesions of Bladder

Entity	Typical Immunophenotype
PMP	AE1/AE3(+), SMA(+), Desmin (+/-), ALK1(+/-), p63/HMWCK/CK5/6(-)
LMS	SMA/Desmin (+), p63/HMWCK/CK5/6(-/+), AE1/AE3(+/-), ALK(-)
Sarcomatoid UC	AE1/AE3(+), p63/HMWCK/CK5/6(+/-), SMA(-/+), ALK(-)
RMS	Desmin (+), Keratin (-), p63/HMWCK/CK5/6(-), SMA(+), ALK(-/+)

PMP = pseudosarcomatous myofibroblastic proliferation; LMS = leiomyosarcoma; UC = urothelial carcinoma; RMS = rhabdomyosarcoma.

Adapted from Amin MB et al: Best practices recommendations in the application of immunohistochemistry in the bladder lesions: report from the International Society of Urologic Pathology consensus conference. Am J Surg Pathol. 38(8):e20-34, 2014; Epstein JI et al: Best practices recommendations in the application of immunohistochemistry in the prostate: report from the International Society of Urologic Pathology consensus conference. Am J Surg Pathol. 38(8):e6-e19, 2014.

Marker Positivity in Types of Spindle Cell Proliferations

Antibody/Protein Detected	PMP	Sarcomatoid UC	LMS (Nonbladder Series in Parentheses)	RMS (Nonbladder Series in Parentheses)
ALK1	20-89%	0%	0-10%	20%
Muscle-Associated Markers				
SMA	63-100%	15-80%	43-100%	97%
Desmin	27-80%	0-40%	0-60% (35-75%)	97-100%
h-caldesmon	0-67%	ND	100% (18-57%)	0%
Calponin	89%	ND	100% (57-90%)	0%
MyoD1	0	0	ND (0%)	100%
Myogenin/*MYF4*	0	0	0	76-100%
Epithelial Markers				
PAN-CK (AE1/AE3)	36-89%	67-100%	0-58%	ND (6%, focal)
EMA/MUC1	0-50%	50-100%	0-12%	ND (6%, focal)
p63	0%	50-58%	23%	ND (5%, focal/weak)
HMWCK (34βE12)	0%	0-27%	0%	ND
CK5/6	0%	27-65%	0%	ND
OSCAR	70%	68%	54%	ND

PMP = pseudosarcomatous myofibroblastic proliferation (including inflammatory myofibroblastic tumor, inflammatory pseudotumor, pseudosarcomatous fibromyxoid tumor, and pseudosarcomatous spindle cell proliferation); ND = no data; LMS = leiomyosarcoma; UC = urothelial carcinoma; RMS = rhabdomyosarcoma.

Adapted from Amin MB et al, Am J Surg Pathol. 38(8):e20-34, 2014; Epstein JI et al, Am J Surg Pathol. 38(8):e6-e19, 2014.

Immunohistochemistry, Urinary Tract

Urothelial Markers in UC vs. PCa Differential

Antibody/Protein Detected	Advantages	Disadvantages
Thrombomodulin	Widely used	Lack of sensitivity: Only positive in ~ 63% of high-grade UC; some lack of specificity as focal positive in 5% of PCa
Uroplakin-3	Negative in PCa, exquisitely specific	Lack of sensitivity: Only positive in ~ 60% of high-grade UC
GATA3	High degree of specificity, sensitivity in > 80% of UC	Expression in non-urothelial entities (breast, paraganglioma, weak in lower genital tract squamous lesions)

Markers Used for Urothelial Lesions: Review of State of the Art

Antibody/Protein Detected	Positivity in Urothelial Lesions	Considerations in Differential Diagnosis
HMWCK (34βE12)	65-97%	6-10% of prostate cancers, nearly all squamous cell carcinomas
Uroplakin-2	60-80%, membranous and cytoplasmic	Brenner tumors of the ovary likely also positive
Uroplakin-3	20-60%, membranous	0% of prostate cancers, 100% of Brenner tumors
Thrombomodulin	49-91%	Weak expression in up to 5% of prostate carcinomas (differential where it is most useful); expressed in subset of squamous cell carcinoma, mesothelioma, and adenocarcinomas of bladder, lung, pancreatic, ovary and breast, limiting use in metastatic setting
p63	81-92%	Useful in differential with prostate cancer but is expressed in nearly all squamous cell carcinomas and basal cell carcinomas of all sites
S100p (placental S100)	88-93%	May be useful in differential with lower genital tract squamous lesions, which only show 9% expression
GATA3	67-90%	67-91% of ductal carcinomas of breast, up to 100% of lobular carcinomas of breast, most benign and neoplastic trophoblastic lesions, skin adnexal tumors, and subset of yolk sac, mesothelial, and pancreaticobiliary tumors
CK7	87-100%	Sensitive but nonspecific: Highly prevalent expression in multitude of other carcinomas
CK20	25-67%	Neither sensitive nor specific: As few as 44% of invasive or metastatic UCs express CK20, while multitude of other carcinomas do as well
CK7 and CK20 coexpression	50-62%	Coexpression in other tumors, particularly pancreaticobiliary carcinomas

Enteric-Type Adenocarcinoma Involving Bladder: Useful Markers

Antibody/Protein Detected	Primary Bladder Adenocarcinoma	GI Primary Invading the Bladder
Cytokeratins 7 and 20, and Combinations		
CK7 and CK20 coexpression	24%	8%
CK7 only	41%	0%
CK20 only	29%	82%
Neither CK7 nor CK20	6%	10%
Other Markers[1]		
β-catenin (strong nuclear positivity)	0%	81%
CDX2	47-100%	99-100%
Villin	65-100%	82-98%
Thrombomodulin	59%	0%

[1]β-catenin may be only useful one.

Immunohistochemistry, Urinary Tract

Flat Urothelial Lesions
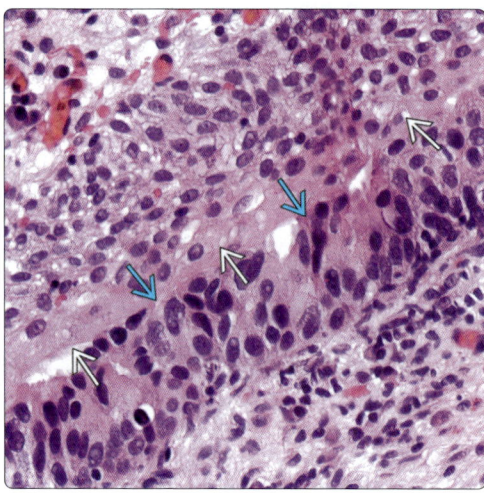

Triple Cocktail for Flat Urothelial Lesions
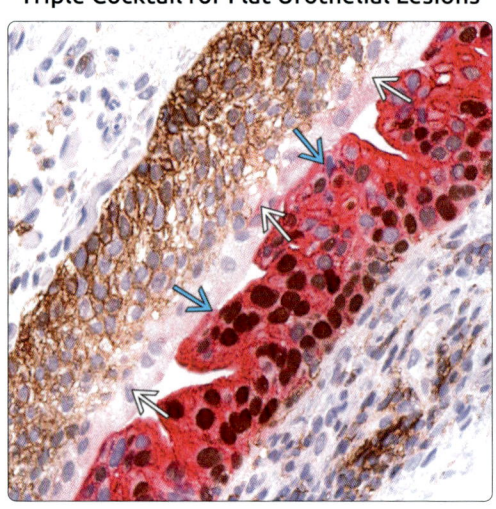

(Left) Here, two urothelial lesions are closely apposed along the center diagonal. A urothelium with reactive atypia is at upper left ⇨, while urothelial carcinoma in situ is seen lower right ⇨. (Right) Same field stained for triple urothelial cocktail, including the stem cell associated CD44s (brown chromogen), shows full-thickness expression in the reactive urothelium ⇨, while CK20 (red chromogen) shows full-thickness expression and p53 nuclear accumulation (brown) in the atypical cells of carcinoma in situ ⇨.

Triple Cocktail for Flat Urothelial Lesions
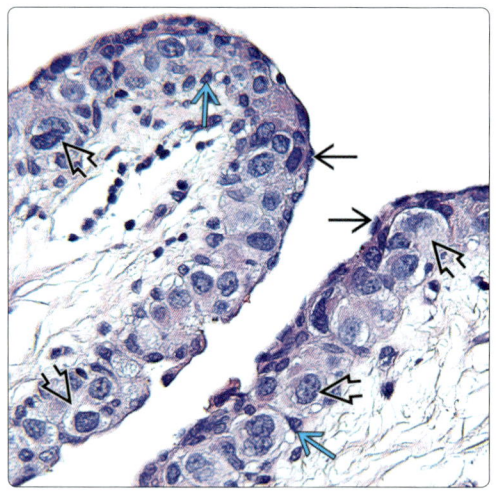

Triple Cocktail for Flat Urothelial Lesions
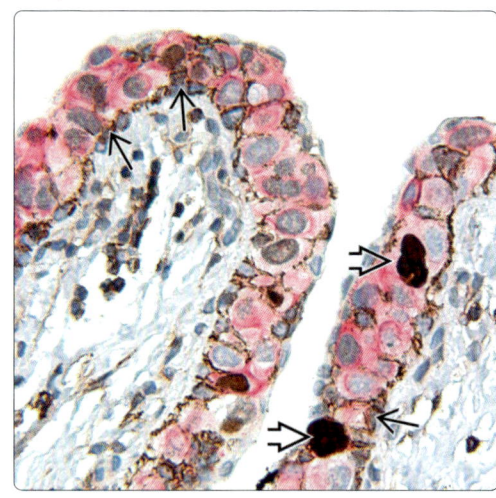

(Left) This example of urothelial carcinoma in situ has a pagetoid pattern with individual cytologically malignant intraepithelial CIS cells ⇨ infiltrating amongst intact umbrella cells ⇨ and basal cells ⇨. (Right) Here, pagetoid CIS shows diffuse staining for CK20 (red). Retained basal cells are CD44s positive (brown ⇨). Scattered CIS cells show strong nuclear reactivity for p53 ⇨, albeit among a subset; p53 is overall less sensitive and specific than CK20 and only diffuse, strong positive staining in atypical cells is most helpful.

CK20 in CIS
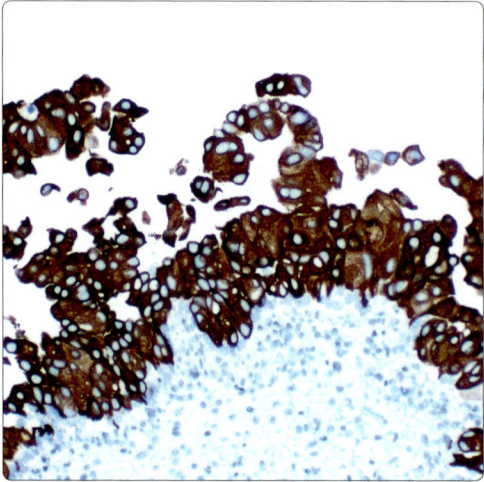

AMACR in CIS
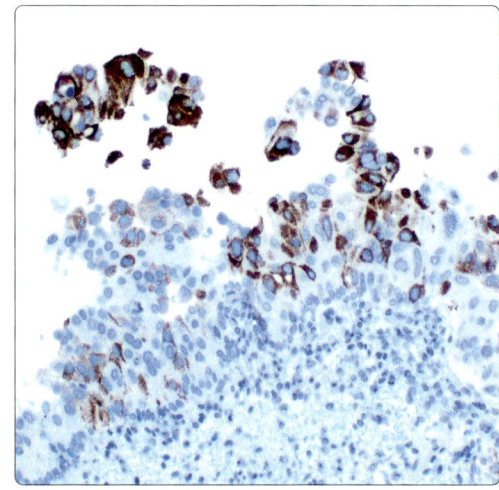

(Left) CK20 remains perhaps the best ancillary marker of CIS, in this case nonpleomorphic CIS with fragmentation. Diffuse, strong, full-thickness expression is characteristic. (Right) An emerging marker of CIS, validated in the setting of surveillance post treatment, is AMACR (racemase, p504S). In this same lesion as left, racemase positivity at all levels of the urothelium is taken as further support for classification as CIS.

Immunohistochemistry, Urinary Tract

Spindle Cell Lesions: PMP

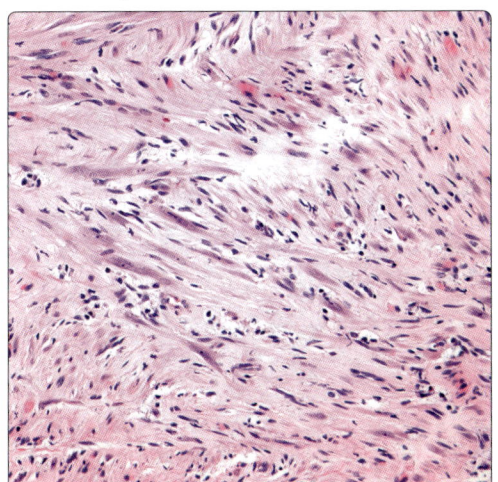

Spindle Cell Lesions: PMP

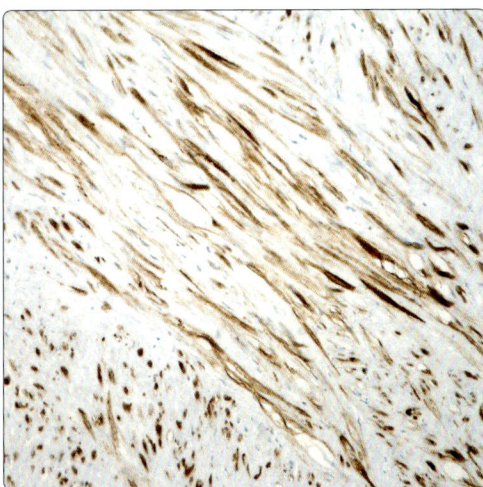

(Left) Here a pseudosarcomatous myofibroblastic proliferation demonstrates spindle cells with myofibroblastic morphology coursing through myxocollagenous stroma with chronic inflammation. Such a lesion engenders consideration of a PMP vs. sarcomatoid UC vs. smooth muscle neoplasm. *(Right)* ALK expression (pictured) is positive in a subset of PMPs, particularly among the young (newer ALK antibodies are more sensitive). Diffuse SMA and scattered pancytokeratin positivity is characteristic.

Spindle Cell Lesions: Sarcomatoid UC

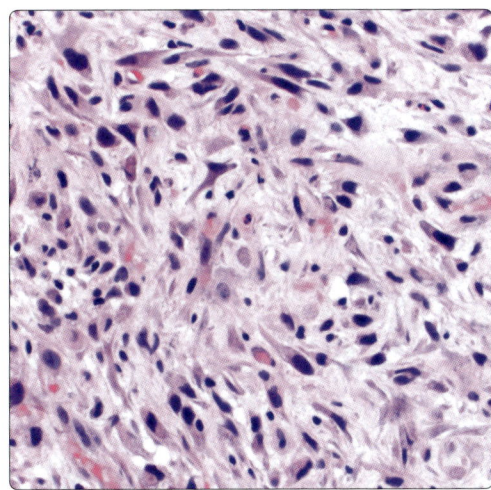

Spindle Cell Lesions: Sarcomatoid UC

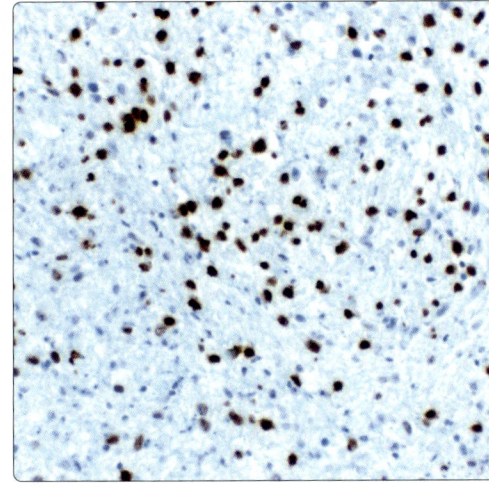

(Left) Sarcomatoid UC characterized by proliferation of overtly atypical stellate to spindled cells is shown. The differential includes pseudosarcomatous stromal reaction and primary bladder sarcoma. *(Right)* IHC work-up for this lesion includes broad spectrum and high molecular weight keratins as well as p63 (pictured). The nuclear positivity for p63 is most helpful given its nearly absent expression in mesenchymal lesions.

Spindle Cell Lesions: Rhabdomyosarcoma

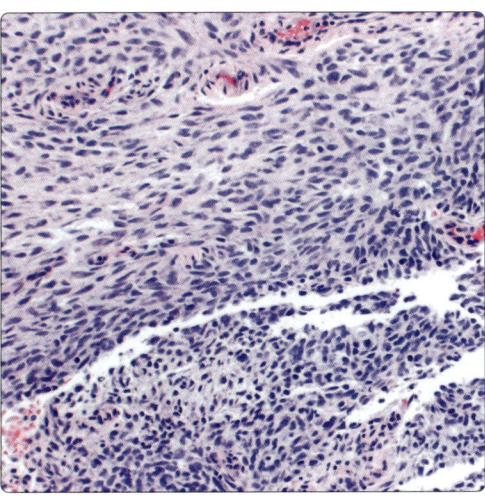

Spindle Cell Lesions: Rhabdomyosarcoma

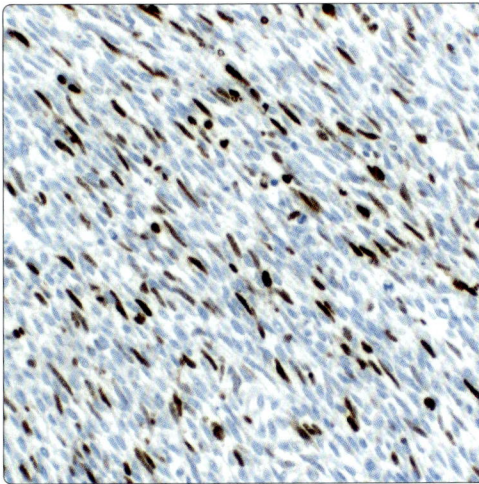

(Left) A spindle cell sarcoma with fibrosarcomatous morphology from the bladder dome and urachus of a pediatric patient is shown. The differential is broad but includes rhabdomyosarcoma. *(Right)* Nuclear staining for myogenin (MYF4) IHC is sensitive and specific for all types of rhabdomyosarcoma, in this case embryonal type. MyoD1 showed a similar pattern, while a smaller subset of cells also showed induction of desmin expression.

Immunohistochemistry, Urinary Tract

(Left) Absent observation of an in situ or conventional UC component, signet ring and plasmacytoid lesions present an archetype of IHC work-up for site of origin, as they may be primaries of bladder, stomach, or breast, among other sites. (Right) GATA3 nuclear positivity is helpful in favoring urothelial histogenesis if a breast primary is relatively excluded (e.g., male patient, negative imaging). It also relatively excludes a gastric primary.

Urothelial-Associated Markers

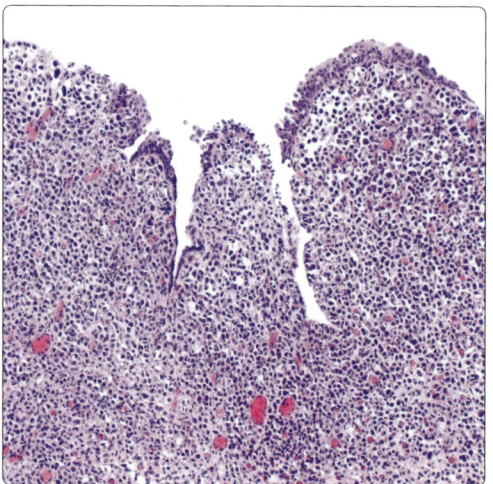

Urothelial-Associated Markers

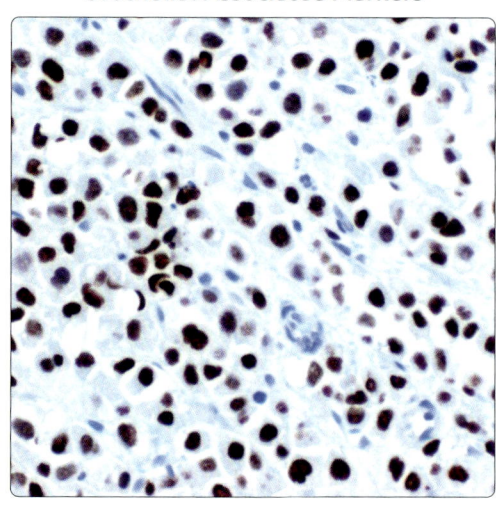

(Left) S100p, or placental S100, is an emerging marker used in urothelial histogenesis, positive in urothelial and pancreaticobiliary primaries. Nucleocytoplasmic positivity has been established to strongly favor UC over prostatic adenocarcinoma in that differential, while other differentials require further study. (Right) Nuclear p63 staining remains a bulwark of the IHC work-up of poorly differentiated UC vs. prostate and other lesions, with the caveat that its expression is expected in all squamous lesions.

Urothelial-Associated Markers

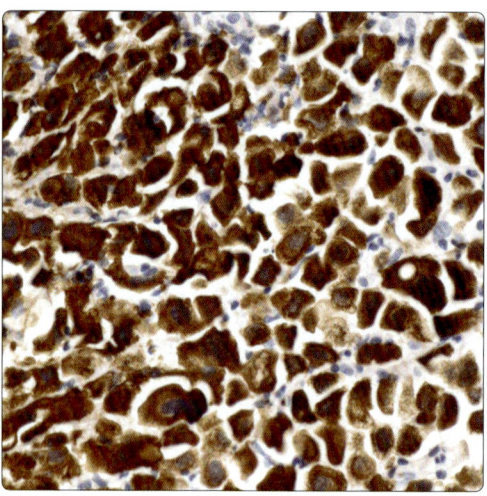

Urothelial-Associated Markers

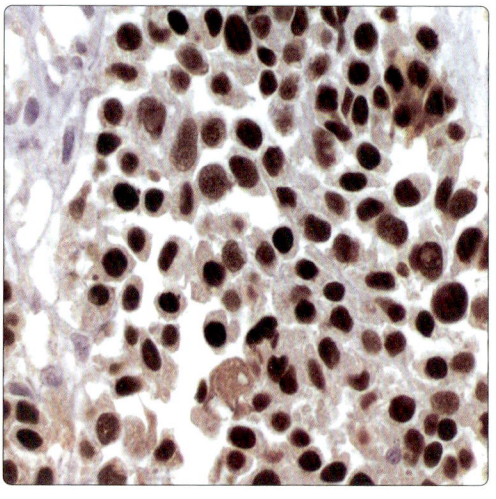

(Left) Uroplakin-3 is exquisitely specific for urothelial neoplasms when scored for plaque-like membranous positivity ⮕. Essentially only Brenner tumors (themselves of transitional differentiation) have shown expression beyond UC. Sensitivity, however, has proven disappointing. (Right) Uroplakin-2 antibodies have been recently introduced and show greater sensitivity with retained specificity for UC. Diffuse membranocytoplasmic positivity is counted as positive, as seen here.

Uroplakins: Highly Specific

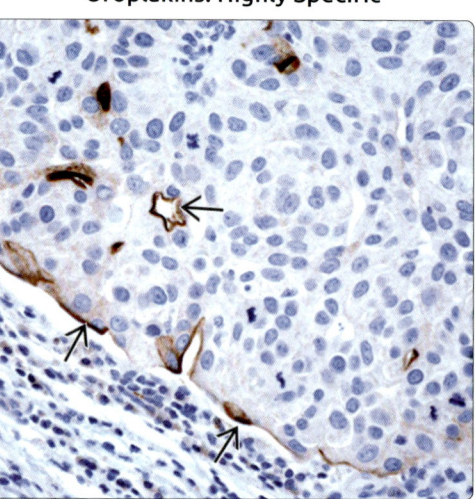

Uroplakins: Highly Specific

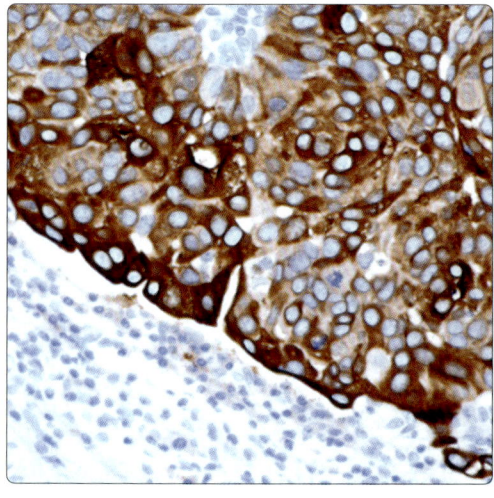

Immunohistochemistry, Urinary Tract

Paraganglioma: Pitfall With GATA3

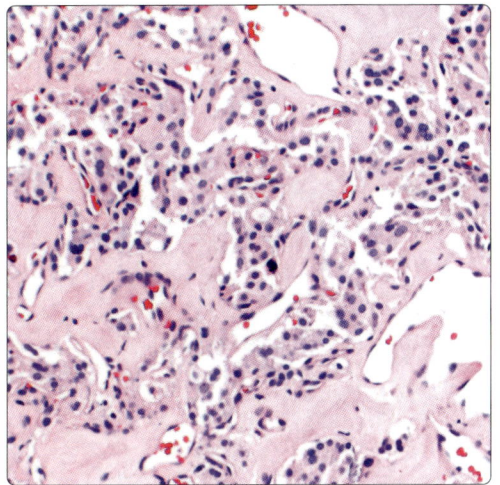

Paraganglioma: Pitfall With GATA3

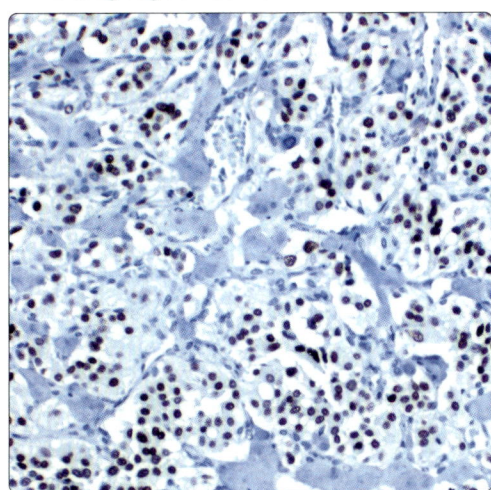

(Left) *Paragangliomas arise infrequently in the wall of the bladder and show nested and trabecular morphology that simulates UC. Helpfully, keratins and p63 should be negative, while chromogranin and synaptophysin positive, with S100 positive sustentacular cells.* **(Right)** *A majority of paragangliomas of the bladder and other sites show GATA3 nuclear positivity. Absent an appropriate context and other markers, GATA3 should not be taken to establish unequivocal diagnosis of UC.*

Enteric-Type Adenocarcinoma

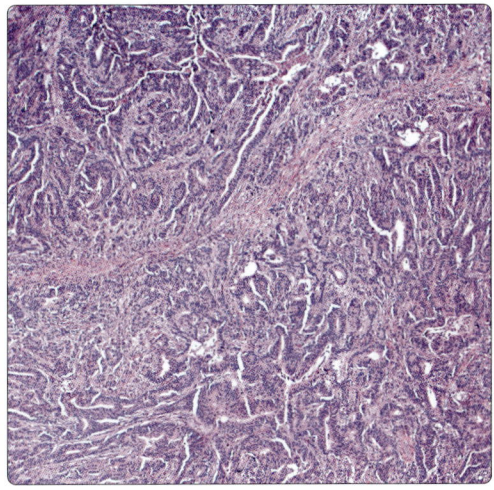

Enteric-Type Adenocarcinoma

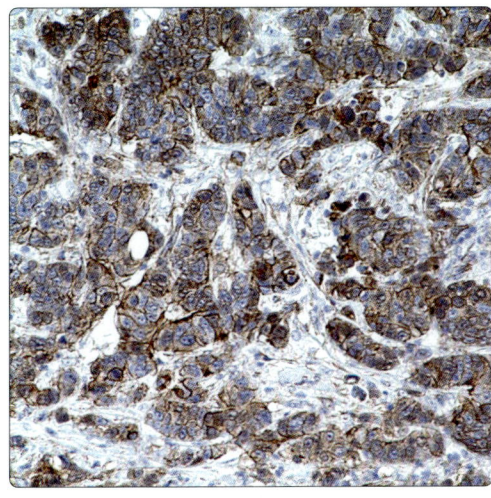

(Left) *A moderately differentiated enteric-type adenocarcinoma is seen in the bladder dome. While "dirty necrosis" is not prominent, the differential remains between a bladder or urachal primary (rare tumors) or secondary involvement by a GI primary.* **(Right)** *β-catenin is the only marker reported to be helpful in the differential between a bladder or urachal primary adenocarcinoma and a colorectal primary. In a bladder/urachal primary, membranous accentuation with relative nuclear sparing (pictured) is expected.*

Enteric-Type Adenocarcinoma

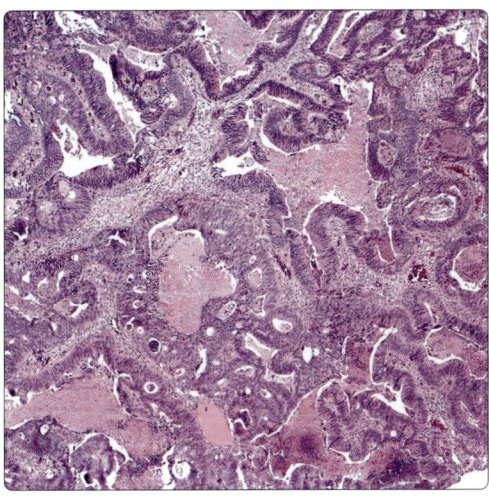

Enteric-Type Adenocarcinoma

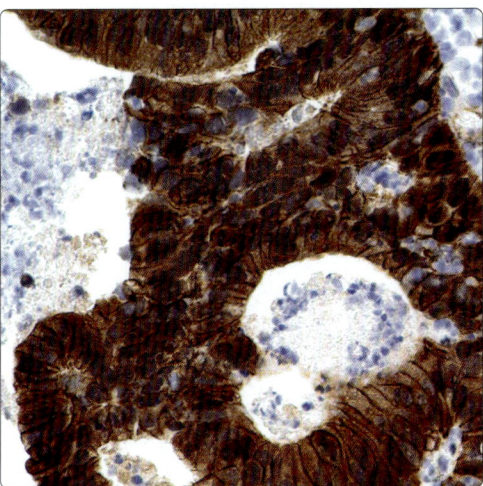

(Left) *In this adenocarcinoma invading the bladder, prominent dirty necrosis and columnar features favor a GI primary; a bladder or urachal primary should be excluded given staging and prognostic differences.* **(Right)** *β-catenin shows diffuse membranous, cytoplasmic and, most importantly, nuclear accumulation favoring enteric primary. β-catenin is positive in the majority of colorectal primaries, reflective of prevalent oncogenic activation of WNT signaling.*

SECTION 3
Prostate Gland and Seminal Vesicle

Introduction and Overview

Classification of Prostate Tumors and Tumor-Like Lesions	536
General Concepts, Prostate	538
Microanatomy and Zonal Variations	544

Nonneoplastic Lesions

Prostatitis	554
Prostate Hyperplasia	558
Adenosis	566
Atrophy and Its Variants	570
Hyperplasia of Mesonephric Remnants	576
Verumontanum Mucosal Gland Hyperplasia	580
Nephrogenic Adenoma (Metaplasia) of Prostatic Urethra	582

Putative Premalignant Lesions and Lesions Falling Short of Malignant Diagnosis

Prostatic Intraepithelial Neoplasia	590

Prostate Neoplasms

General Concepts, Prostate Carcinoma	600
Acinar Adenocarcinoma	608
Acinar Adenocarcinoma Variants	626
Atypical Small Acinar Proliferations	638
Intraductal Carcinoma	644
Ductal Adenocarcinoma	650
Urothelial Carcinoma Involving Prostate Gland	658
Prostate Carcinoma With Neuroendocrine Differentiation	664
Basal Cell Carcinoma	672
Sarcomatoid Carcinoma of Prostate	678
Carcinomas With Squamous Differentiation	684
Stromal Tumors	690
Mesenchymal Tumors of Prostate	698
Melanocytic Lesions of Prostate	706
Hematopoietic Neoplasms of Prostate	710
Secondary Tumors of Prostate	714

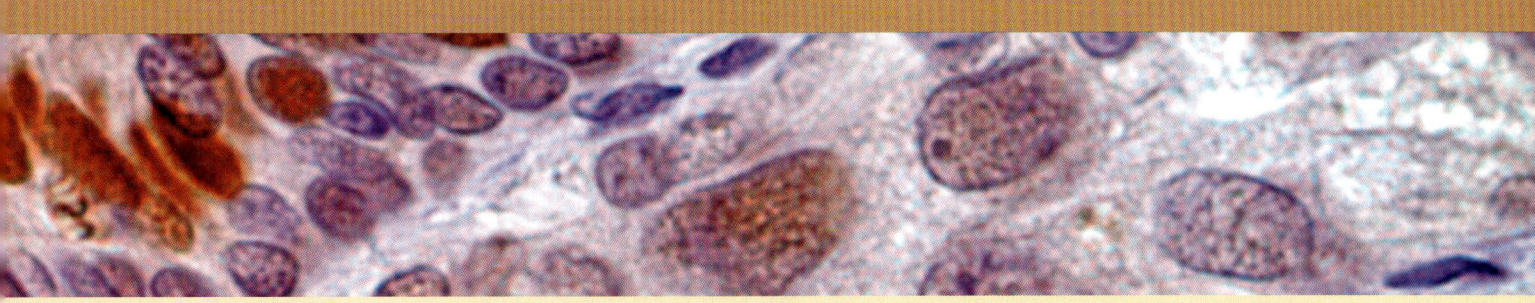

Tumors of Seminal Vesicle

Cystadenoma and Epithelial Stromal Tumor 718
Seminal Vesicle Adenocarcinoma 722

Immunohistochemical Profiles for Tumors and Tumor-Like Lesions Involving Prostate Gland

Immunohistochemistry, Prostate 724

Classification of Prostate Tumors and Tumor-Like Lesions

NONNEOPLASTIC LESIONS

Inflammation (Prostatitis)
- Granulomatous prostatitis
  - Nonspecific granulomatous prostatitis
  - Postprocedural granuloma
  - Inflammatory granulomatous prostatitis
  - Systemic granulomatous prostatitis
- Prostatitis syndromes (NIH classification)
  - Class I, acute bacterial prostatitis
  - Class II, chronic bacterial prostatitis
  - Class III, chronic prostatitis/chronic pelvic pain syndrome
    - Type A, inflammatory
    - Type B, noninflammatory
  - Class IV, asymptomatic inflammatory prostatitis

Atrophy
- Simple atrophy
- Simple atrophy with cyst formation
- Post atrophic hyperplasia
- Partial atrophy
- Sclerotic atrophy

Hyperplasia
- Benign nodular hyperplasia
  - Usual pattern
    - Epithelial predominant hyperplasia
    - Stromal predominant hyperplasia
    - Mixed epithelial and stromal hyperplasia
  - Special pattern
    - Epithelial
      - Small glandular hyperplasia
      - Cribriform hyperplasia
      - Basal cell hyperplasia
      - Adenoid cystic-like hyperplasia
    - Stromal
      - Fibrous hyperplasia
      - Fibromuscular hyperplasia
      - Leiomyomatous hyperplasia
    - Mixed epithelial and stroma
      - Fibroadenoma-like hyperplasia
      - Phyllodes-type hyperplasia
- Veromontanum mucosal gland hyperplasia
- Mesonephric remnant hyperplasia
- Transitional cell hyperplasia

Metaplasia
- Transitional metaplasia
- Squamous metaplasia
- Mucinous metaplasia

Pigments (Other Than Melanocytic)
- Lipofuscin
- Hemosiderin
- Ochronosis (homogentisic acid)

Other Tumor-Like Lesions
- Retention cysts
- Sclerosing adenosis
- Amyloid
- Endometriosis
- Postneedle biopsy changes
- Radiation atypia
- Paraganglia

NEOPLASMS

Benign Epithelial Tumors
- Cystadenoma
- Nephrogenic adenoma of prostatic urethra

Putative Premalignant Lesions
- Atypical adenomatous hyperplasia (adenosis)
- Prostatic intraepithelial neoplasia (PIN)
  - Low-grade PIN
  - High-grade PIN
    - Tufted PIN
    - Micropapillary PIN
    - Cribriform PIN
    - Flat PIN
    - Uncommon types
      - Signet ring PIN
      - Mucinous PIN
      - Foamy PIN
      - Inverted or hobnail PIN
      - Small cell neuroendocrine PIN

Acinar Adenocarcinoma
- Usual (conventional) adenocarcinoma
  - Atypical small acinar proliferation
  - Intraductal carcinoma
  - With therapy-related changes
    - Radiation therapy effects
    - Hormonal therapy effects
- Ductal adenocarcinoma
- Mucinous (colloid) carcinoma
- Signet ring cell carcinoma
- Pseudohyperplastic carcinoma
- Atrophic carcinoma
- Foamy gland (xanthomatous) carcinoma
- Stratified/double cell layer/PIN-like carcinoma
- Lymphoepithelioma-like carcinoma
- Oncocytic carcinoma
- Pleomorphic giant cell adenocarcinoma
- Sarcomatoid carcinoma (carcinosarcoma)
- Microcystic carcinoma
- Cystadenocarcinoma
- Carcinoid-like carcinoma
- Adenocarcinoma with aberrant p63 expression

Other Carcinomas
- Urothelial carcinoma of prostate (including prostatic urethra)
  - Usual (conventional) urothelial carcinoma
  - Urothelial carcinoma variants
- Neuroendocrine tumors of prostate
  - Usual carcinoma with neuroendocrine differentiation
  - Carcinoma with Paneth cell-like neuroendocrine differentiation
  - Carcinoid tumor
  - Small cell carcinoma
  - Large cell neuroendocrine carcinoma

Classification of Prostate Tumors and Tumor-Like Lesions

- - Mixed neuroendocrine carcinoma/acinar adenocarcinoma
  - Carcinoma with overlapping features of small cell carcinoma and acinar carcinoma (provisional category)
- Basal cell carcinoma (adenoid cystic carcinoma)
- Carcinomas with squamous differentiation
  - Squamous cell carcinoma
  - Adenosquamous carcinoma
- Undifferentiated carcinoma

Tumors of Specialized Prostatic Stroma

- Stromal proliferation of uncertain malignant potential
  - Degenerative atypia
  - Hypercellular stroma
  - Myxoid
  - Phyllodes type
- Prostatic stromal sarcoma
  - Stromal sarcoma
  - Malignant phyllodes tumor

Benign Mesenchymal Tumors

- Leiomyoma
- Inflammatory myofibroblastic tumor (IMT, pseudosarcomatous myofibroblastic proliferation)
- Solitary fibrous tumor (SFT), benign
- Paraganglioma (extraadrenal pheochromocytoma), benign
- Rhabdomyoma
- Tumors with neural differentiation
  - Neurofibroma
  - Schwannoma
  - Ganglioneuroma
- Hemangioma (including posterior urethral hemangioma)
- Osteogenic and chondrogenic tumors
- Malakoplakia

Malignant Mesenchymal Tumors

- Leiomyosarcoma
- Malignant IMT
- Malignant SFT
- Malignant paraganglioma (extraadrenal pheochromocytoma)
- Rhabdomyosarcoma
- Vascular tumors
  - Epithelioid hemangioendothelioma
  - Angiosarcoma
- Malignant peripheral nerve sheath tumor
- Malignant fibrous histiocytoma
- Sarcoma, not otherwise specified

Tumors of Uncertain Origin

- Synovial sarcoma
- Primitive neuroectodermal tumor/Ewing sarcoma
- Angiomyolipoma/perivascular epithelioid cell tumor

Secondary Tumors of Prostate

- Metastatic solid tumors
  - Lung cancer
  - Cutaneous cancer
  - Other primary visceral cancers
- Direct spread from adjacent organs
  - Urinary bladder cancer
  - Colorectal cancer
  - Gastrointestinal stromal tumors

Hematopoietic Tumors

- Lymphoma (primary or secondary)
  - Non-Hodgkin lymphoma
    - B-cell lymphomas
      - Small cell lymphoma/chronic lymphocytic leukemia
      - Diffuse large B-cell lymphoma
      - Marginal zone lymphoma
      - Follicular lymphoma
      - Mucosa-associated lymphoid tissue lymphoma
      - Intravascular large B-cell lymphoma
      - Burkitt lymphoma
    - T-cell lymphomas
  - Hodgkin disease
- Leukemia
  - Myeloid (including granulocytic sarcoma)
  - Lymphoblastic
- Multiple myeloma (including plasmacytoma)

Melanocytic Tumors

- Blue nevus
- Melanosis
- Melanoma

Germ Cell Tumors

- Pure germ cell tumor (GCT)
  - Pure seminoma
  - Pure yolk sac tumor
- Mixed GCT

Tumors of Seminal Vesicles

- Cystadenoma
- Mixed epithelial-stromal tumor
- Seminal vesicle adenocarcinoma

General Concepts, Prostate

ANATOMIC FEATURES

Prostate Gland

- Exocrine compound tubuloalveolar gland
- Located in true pelvis
  - Surrounded by urinary bladder superiorly, transverse urogenital diaphragm inferiorly, inferior aspect of symphysis pubis anteriorly, and rectum posteriorly
- Inverted conical shape: Base is broad superior region, and apex is tapered inferior region
  - **Base** contiguous with bladder neck superiorly and seminal vesicle attachment posteriorly
    - Distinguished histologically by presence of smooth muscle bundles
  - **Apex** blends with striated muscle of transverse urogenital diaphragm
    - Distinguished histologically by presence of skeletal muscle often seen blending with prostatic glands and Cowper gland
- Normal prostate in men (21-30 yr old), weighs ~ 20 g (range: 14-26 g)
- In adults, usually measures 4 x 3 x 2 cm
  - Widest at transverse dimension of base
  - Prostates resected for cancer are usually larger because of commonality of benign prostatic hyperplasia in older adults
- McNeal anatomic model divides prostate into **glandular** and **nonglandular** components
  - Glandular component
    - **Peripheral zone (PZ), central zone (CZ), transition zone (TZ), periurethral gland region**
  - Nonglandular component
    - Anterior fibromuscular stroma, preprostatic sphincter, striated sphincter
- Receives arterial supply from inferior vesical and middle rectal arteries, branches of internal iliac artery
- Prostatic venous plexus lies partly within prostatic fascial sheath and drains into internal iliac vein

Handling of Radical Prostatectomy Specimen

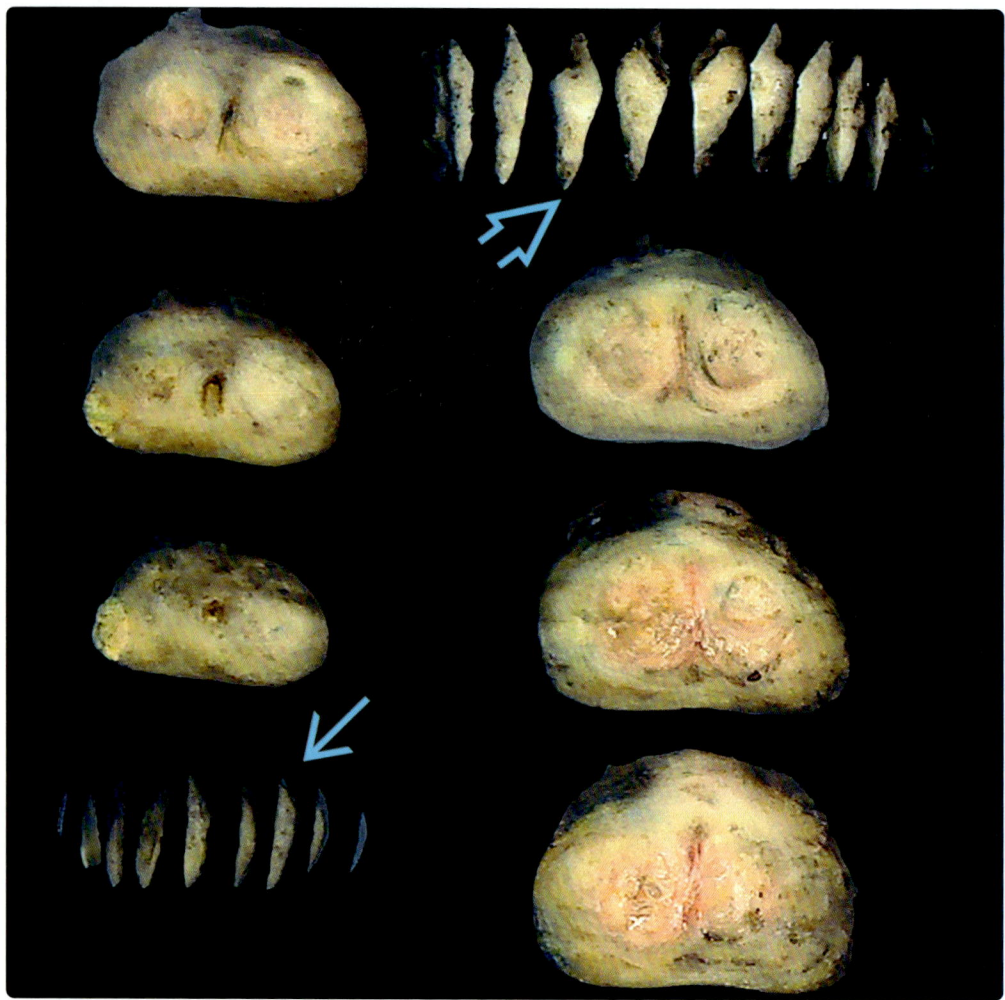

Apex ⇥ and base ⇥ margins are transected and submitted as a series of parasagittal (perpendicular) sections. Shaving of the apex (en face margin) is not recommended due to risk of false-positivity. The remaining prostate is coronally sectioned at 3- to 5-mm intervals and submitted sequentially. Submission of prostate ranges from systematic partial sampling (at least 50%) to entire gland processing. Most institutions in USA submit the middle sections in quadrants. Whole-mount sections provide ease in determining location of extraprostatic extension and positive margin but are technically demanding and require special filing and storage. (Courtesy E. Drinka, MD.)

General Concepts, Prostate

- Primary lymphatics drain into regional lymph nodes in true pelvis
  - Hypogastric, obturator, internal and external iliac, and sacral lymph nodes

Prostatic Urethra

- ~ 3 cm in length and begins at internal urethral orifice at apex to bladder trigone
- Courses through prostate, makes anteriorly concave 35° bend, ends as urethra penetrates fascia of urogenital diaphragm and enters perineum
- Continues distally as membranous urethra
- Posterior wall of prostatic urethra has several unique features related to prostatic secretory function
  - Contains longitudinal ridge (urethral crest) lined by 2 adjacent grooves (prostatic sinuses)
  - Prostatic ductules enter urethra predominantly in sinuses with fewer entering along lateral aspects of crest
  - Urethral crest also has midline protuberance (verumontanum or colliculus seminalis)

Verumontanum (Colliculus Seminalis)

- Protrusion of prostatic tissue from posterior wall of urethra at angulation, tapers distally as crista urethralis
- Contains epithelium-lined blind sac (utricle) between openings of paired ejaculatory ducts
- Prostate carcinoma may protrude from ejaculatory duct as urethral polyp along verumontanum, particularly with ductal adenocarcinoma
- Important landmark in congenital posterior urethral valve anomaly

Ejaculatory Ducts

- Passes through central zone entering at cephalad aspect
- Both ducts open into prostatic urethra at verumontanum, lateral to prostatic utricle

Seminal Vesicles

- Attached to superior-posterior aspect of prostate and bladder base
- Paired, highly coiled epithelial-lined tubes with irregular outpouchings
- Contains smooth muscle wall
- Small intraprostatic portion is seen
- Excretory duct connects anteriorly with ampullary portion of vas deferens forming ejaculatory duct
- In adults, average 6 x 2 cm and contains up to 5 mL milky fluid, which forms bulk of ejaculatory volume

Periprostatic Structures

- Resected prostate may include adjoining tissues, such as adipose tissue, neurovascular bundle, paraganglia, Denonvilliers fascia, and lateral prostatic fascia
  - Potency-sparing prostatectomy preserves neurovascular bundle, site of cavernous nerves important for erection

SPECIMEN TYPES AND HANDLING

Needle Core Biopsy

- Indication is for histologic diagnosis of prostate cancer and evaluation of mass lesion or hypoechoic region
- Performed for elevated serum PSA level &/or abnormal digital rectal examination (DRE)
- Increasing use for active surveillance of men with low-volume, low-grade prostate cancer
- Performed more commonly via transrectal ultrasound (TRUS)-guided using 18-gauge needle as outpatient procedure
- May also be performed perineally or transurethrally
- Different prostate biopsy sampling schemes
  - **Sextant biopsy** (6 cores)
    - Use remains widespread despite becoming less preferred technique
    - Samples bilateral base, midgland, and apex
  - **Extended biopsy** (10-12 cores)
    - Preferred initial diagnostic procedure
    - Demonstrated increased cancer detection rate without increase in morbidity
    - False-negativity rate of 5% (vs. ~ 25% for sextant biopsy)
    - Optimal extended biopsy includes standard sextant area plus cores that target mid and lateral PZ
    - TZ biopsy is not usually recommended at initial biopsy due to low detection rate
  - **Saturation biopsy** (≥ 20 cores)
    - Considered in men with persistently elevated PSA and several prior negative biopsies
    - Not commonly performed
  - **MR-ultrasound (US) fusion biopsy**
    - Gaining popularity; MR higher sensitivity
    - Multiparametric MR detects suspicious areas and targeted by biopsy under US
    - Shown to be 3x more likely to identify cancer vs. systematic biopsy (21% vs. 7%)
    - Allows follow-up biopsy of specific cancer sites in men undergoing active surveillance
- **Handling of biopsy specimen**
  - If possible, avoid accessioning prostate biopsy specimens in sequence
  - Count and document number of cores per container
    - Ideally core(s) submitted in 1 container per site (> 3 is detrimental for evaluation)
  - Formalin fixative is preferred
    - Bouin solution is not preferred, as it may enhance nucleoli in benign glands
  - Hematoxylin or other indelible dye makes tissue cores more visible when cutting paraffin blocks
  - Ideally, submit only 1-2 tissue cores per block to maximize tissue representation
    - More cores per block often leads to undesired tissue loss
  - Prospectively cut intervening unstained slides to ensure presence of atypical focus for adjunctive immunostains
    - Levels 1, 3, and 5 for H&E staining
    - Save unstained levels 2, 4, and 6 for potential immunohistochemistry (IHC) or H&E stains
    - Attempting immunostains on subsequent deeper levels more frequently results in loss of atypical focus
  - Multiple sections (ideally 3) should be present on each H&E slide to enhance sampling
  - Most tissue in block from superficial to deep should be included in sections

General Concepts, Prostate

Fine-Needle Aspiration Biopsy
- Rarely performed in USA
  - Advocates claim aspiration cytology is cheaper, faster, easier to use, and has less morbidity
  - Major drawback is lack of cancer architecture that precludes histologic grading and distinction from high-grade prostatic intraepithelial neoplasia (HGPIN)
    - Inability to provide important information for planning therapy and prognostication

Transurethral Resection of Prostate (TURP) or Subtotal Prostatectomy
- TURP is surgical treatment option for benign prostatic hyperplasia (BPH)
- Open simple prostatectomy may be performed for bulky BPH
- Incidental prostate cancer encountered in ~ 10%
- TURP specimen consists of elongated rubbery fragments called prostate chips
  - Includes TZ and areas around proximal prostatic urethra
  - Cancer if present is more often secondary cancer extending from PZ or less commonly is primary TZ cancer
- **Handling of TURP specimen**
  - Specimens ≤ 12 g: Submit entirely
  - For > 12 g: Submit initial 12 g (6-8 cassettes) and 1 cassette for every additional 5 g
  - Sensitivity for cancer detection may be increased by selectively submitting chips that are firm, yellow, or grossly suspicious for cancer
  - If incidental prostate cancer comprises < 5% of tissues examined, entire remaining tissue should be submitted

Radical Prostatectomy (RP)
- Most common treatment for localized prostate cancer (cT1-T2), when life expectancy is > 10 yr
- Robotic-assisted, laparoscopic, retropubic, or perineal
  - Robotic-assisted prostatectomy is now considered most dominant technique
  - Major complications include incontinence (damage at sphincter) and impotence (damage at neurovascular bundle)
  - Robotic-assisted surgery may have less blood loss and small improvement in erectile dysfunction
- **Handling of RP specimen**
  - Weigh and measure specimen in 3 dimensions
  - Unless being sampled for research, fix in 10%-buffered formalin for 18-24 hr
    - May use microwave-assisted technique to facilitate fixing
  - Ink entire outer surface using 2 colors to identify right and left sides
  - Apex, base, and seminal vesicles should be handled in standardized fashion
  - Apical margin
    - Apex amputated (should not be thinly shaved) and subsequently sectioned perpendicular to inked surface
    - Perpendicular apex sections may be taken in series of parallel (parasagittal) sections (preferred) or radial manner (similar to cervical cone)
    - Shaved (en face) margin not recommended, as it may lead to false-positive margin
    - Urethra often retracts, and urothelium may not be present in apical margin sections
  - Base margin
    - Submit either as perpendicular or shaved (en face) section(s)
    - Perpendicular sections recommended because they avoid possibility of false-positive margin
  - Middle portion serially sectioned coronally at 3- to 5-mm intervals and sections submitted in quadrants
    - Sections submitted from remainder of gland range from systematic partial sampling to entire prostate submission
  - Partial sampling should be systematic to allow for assessment of volume, multifocality, and orientation
    - Random sampling precludes tumor measurements, evaluation of dominant mass features, focality determination, and location of margin and EPE positivity
  - Grossly evident tumor should be sampled with adjacent extraprostatic tissue and margins
  - Seminal vesicle
    - Sections of prostatic tissue at base, including adjacent attached seminal vesicle, are needed to demonstrate direct tumor extension
    - Not necessary to submit entire seminal vesicle tissue
    - Margins of vas deferens optional since cancer spread through this route is highly unusual
  - Few institutions in US process whole-mount prostate sections
    - Advocates report ease in assessing tumor volume and assigning more precise primary Gleason score in multifocal tumors
    - Location of extraprostatic extension and positive margins easier to determine
    - Drawbacks: Expensive, technically cumbersome, and requires special filing and storage

Frozen Section (FS)
- Currently, there is no standard for intraoperative FS in patients undergoing RP
  - Performed mostly to assess
    - Margins of resection
      - Mainly for apical margin, bladder neck margin, and posterolateral aspect of prostate for monitoring neurovascular bundle
    - Status of regional lymph nodes
  - Also depends on surgeon's preference and preoperative or intraoperative findings
- Good correlation between FS and permanent section interpretations
  - High positive predictive value
- FS artifacts may compromise interpretation particularly of Gleason 3 pattern carcinoma
- Overall, has low sensitivity (42%) in identifying positive margins due to sampling bias
- Utility of FS in improving functional outcomes and biochemical control has not been shown

General Concepts, Prostate

IMMUNOHISTOCHEMISTRY

General Principles
- Use of IHC in prostate cancer is primarily for following scenarios
  - Confirming diagnosis of carcinoma in biopsy materials containing atypical glands, treated carcinoma, or unusual morphology
  - Diagnosis of prostatic origin of tumor, whether in prostate or at distant metastatic site
- Principles of IHC used in prostate carcinoma diagnosis
  - Confirm absence of basal cell layer
    - Carcinoma should not contain basal cells
  - Demonstrate overexpression of proteins (AMACR and ERG) upregulated in prostate cancer
  - Diagnosis of carcinoma should always be made in conjunction with H&E morphology

Basal Cell Markers
- Include HMCK (34βE12), CK5/CK6, CK14, p63, and antibody cocktails
  - HMCK (34βE12) labels intermediate filaments in basal cell cytoplasm
    - Does not stain prostatic secretory cells
  - p63 labels basal cell nuclei
    - Comparable to HMCK (34βE12), although some studies suggested p63 has higher sensitivity
  - Basal cell marker cocktails [HMCK (34βE12) or CK5/CK6 & p63] provide more intense basal cell staining, combination of nuclear and cytoplasmic
- Interpretation
  - Complete lack of immunoreactivity in suspicious atypical glandular focus is supportive of carcinoma diagnosis
    - All morphologically atypical glands must be identified by H&E, and corresponding glands on IHC slide should be completely negative
    - Consistency of staining reaction should preferably be demonstrated on subsequent section included on same slide (if available)
- Potential pitfalls
  - Main drawback is staining pattern supportive of carcinoma diagnosis is based on negative staining
    - Absence of basal cell staining is not entirely diagnostic of cancer, as some benign glands may show patchy, discontinuous, or absent staining
    - Weak or nonreactive in 5-23% of benign glands
    - May be absent (up to 24%) in small foci of partial atrophy, postatrophic hyperplasia, and up to 50% of atypical adenomatous hyperplasia (adenosis)
  - Rare aberrant nuclear p63 staining may occur in malignant secretory cells of acinar adenocarcinoma
  - Several preanalytic and analytic factors may interfere with immunoreactivity
    - Should be run with appropriate positive and negative controls

α-methylacyl-CoA-racemase (AMACR, P504S)
- Overexpressed in prostate cancer with marked differential staining between malignant (positive) and benign (negative or weak expression) glands
  - Identified in gene expression array studies
- Highly sensitive, reportedly positivity in ~ 75-95% of carcinomas
- Potential pitfalls
  - Similar immunoreactivity pattern seen in HGPIN (reported 56-100%)
  - Negative or weakly expressed in some prostatic carcinomas: 5-25% typical, 30% atrophic, 32-38% foamy gland, 23-30% pseudohyperplastic, and up to 29% hormone-treated carcinomas
  - Expressed in benign lesions: 35-58% nephrogenic adenoma, up to 29% luminal staining in partial atrophy and postatrophic hyperplasia, 2-36% benign glands, 18% atypical adenomatous hyperplasia
  - Not specific for prostatic origin in metastatic setting
    - Expressed by variety of other malignancies

Dual Chromogen Antibody Cocktails
- More commonly used
- Combine 1 or 2 basal cell markers with AMACR
- Maximize tissue preservation, which may be critical in small foci of carcinoma
  - May be performed on single unstained or destained section if required
- Utilizes 2 chromogens, usually red for AMACR and brown for basal cell marker
  - AMACR(+) complements negative basal cell markers in carcinoma

Epithelial Marker
- CK-PAN (AE1/AE3)
  - Aids distinction of poorly differentiated prostate carcinoma cells from nonepithelial process (e.g., inflammatory cells, lymphoma)
  - In posttreatment setting, highlights individual atrophic prostate cancer cells

Prostate Lineage-Specific Markers
- PSA and PAP
- New markers include prostate-specific membrane antigen, proPSA, P501S (prostein) and NKX3.1
- Positive in benign and malignant prostatic epithelium
  - Aid in exclusion of nonprostatic lesions that mimic carcinoma
    - Seminal vesicle/ejaculatory duct, mesonephric glands, nephrogenic adenoma, Cowper gland, and paraganglionic tissue
  - Differential diagnosis of unusual variants of prostate carcinoma (e.g., ductal, mucinous, signet ring) vs. secondary tumors involving prostate
- Intensity of expression usually inversely proportional to Gleason grade
  - Gleason pattern 5 tumors may exhibit weak or negative staining (up to 13%)
- In metastatic setting, strong expression of PSA and PAP is strongly suggestive of prostate primary
  - PSA and PAP are not entirely specific for prostate carcinoma

SELECTED REFERENCES
1. Egevad L et al: International society of urological pathology consensus conference on handling and staging of radical prostatectomy specimens. Adv Anat Pathol. 18(4):301-5, 2011

General Concepts, Prostate

Prostate in True Pelvis

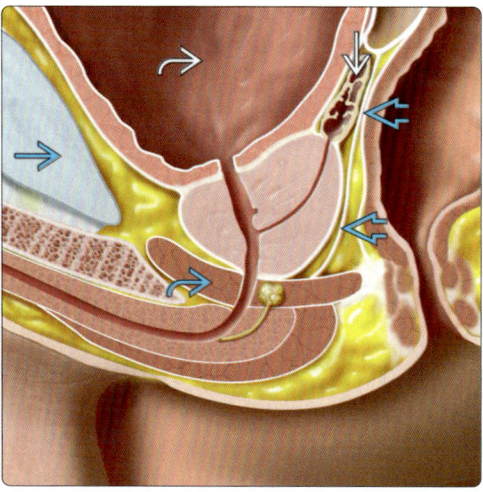

Robotic-Assisted Laparoscopic Radical Prostatectomy

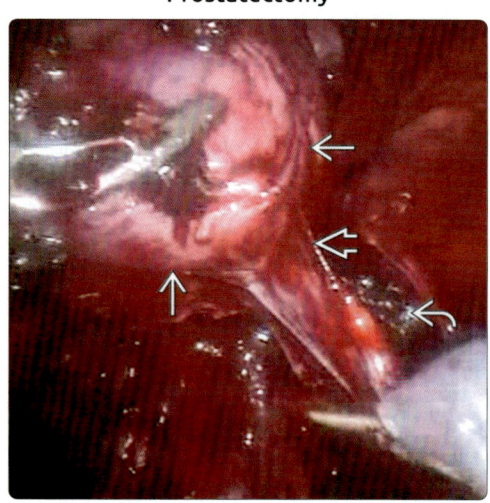

(Left) Prostate is situated in true pelvis surrounded by urinary bladder superiorly ➡, urogenital diaphragm inferiorly ➡, inferior aspect of symphysis pubis anteriorly ➡, and rectum posteriorly, with intervening Denonvilliers fascia ➡, which hinders prostate cancer spread to rectum. Seminal vesicles ➡ are attached posterosuperiorly. **(Right)** Robotic prostatectomy shows lateral-posterior prostate ➡ being dissected from neurovascular bundle ➡ along lateral prostatic fascia ➡. (Courtesy M. Woods, MD.)

External Gross Appearance of Prostate

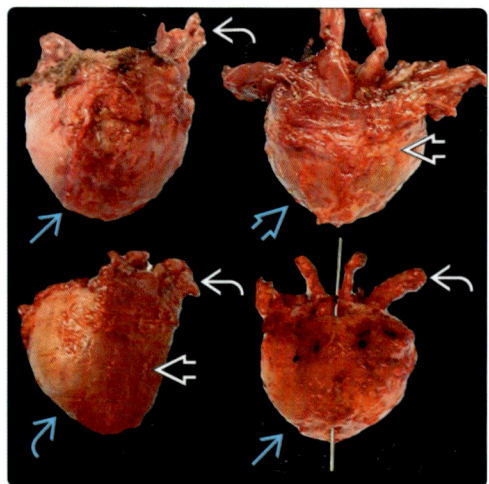

Prostate Microanatomy

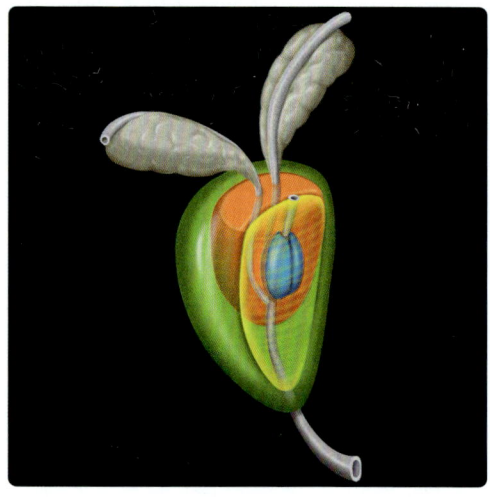

(Left) Anterior ➡, posterior ➡, and posterolateral ➡ views show an inverted conical gland with broad base and tapered apex. Seminal vesicles ➡, vas deferens, & relatively flatter posterior surface ➡ are orientation landmarks. **(Right)** McNeal anatomic model of prostate depicts the internal structural relationship of peripheral (green), central (orange), and transition (blue) zones, and the anterior fibromuscular stroma (yellow). The prostatic urethra and ejaculatory duct can be used as landmarks to identify these different zones histologically.

Prostate Base, Seminal Vesicles and Vas Deferens

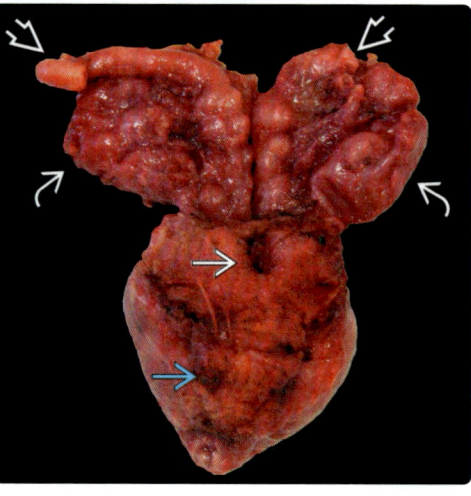

Handling of Prostate Specimen

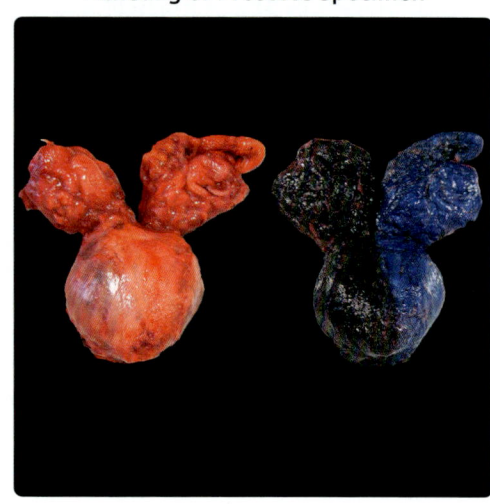

(Left) Anterior-superior view shows the urethra ➡ at the base. Paired bilateral seminal vesicles ➡ are attached to the posterior aspect of the base, lateral to the tubular vas deferens ➡. Note the muscular condensation anteriorly ➡. (Courtesy S. Fidai, MD.) **(Right)** The entire outer prostate surface must be inked for assessment of margins. Right and left sides are designated by different colors. Knowledge of prostate microanatomy and landmarks allows histologic orientation of submitted sections. (Courtesy S. Fidai, MD.)

General Concepts, Prostate

Prostate at Verumontanum

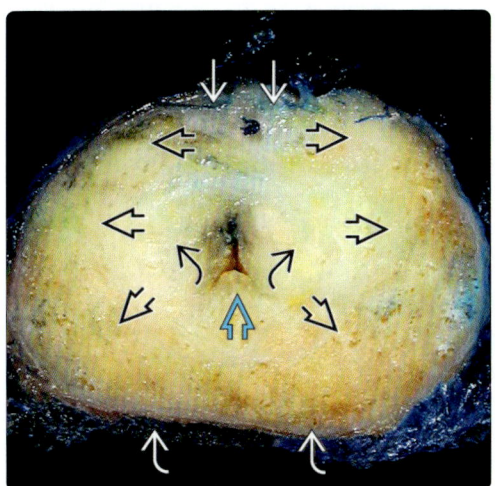

Gross Appearance of Prostate Zones

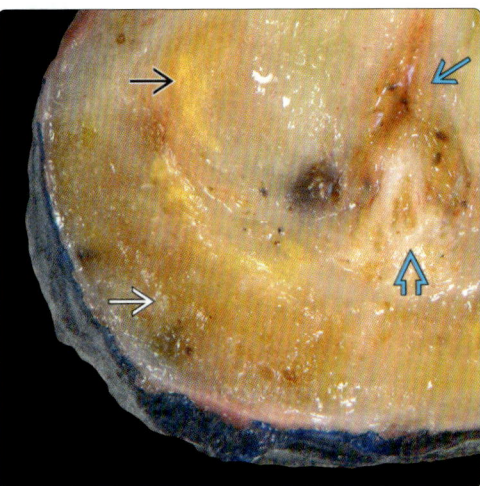

(Left) This coronal section of prostate at verumontanum ➡ shows the peripheral zone ➡ extending from posterior (PZ) ➡, surrounding part of the transition zone (TZ) ➡, and abutting ("anterior horn") the anterior fibromuscular stroma ➡. The central urethra is enveloped by the TZ. (Right) PZ ➡ exhibits a spongy consistency. TZ ➡ has nodularity due to BPH, which compresses the urethra ➡. Prostatic urethral promontory/verumontanum ➡ are landmarks pointing anteriorly. (Courtesy S. Fidai, MD.)

Sextant Biopsy Sampling

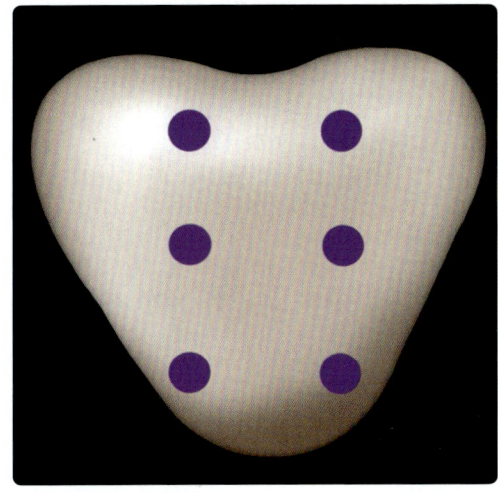

Extended Biopsy Sampling

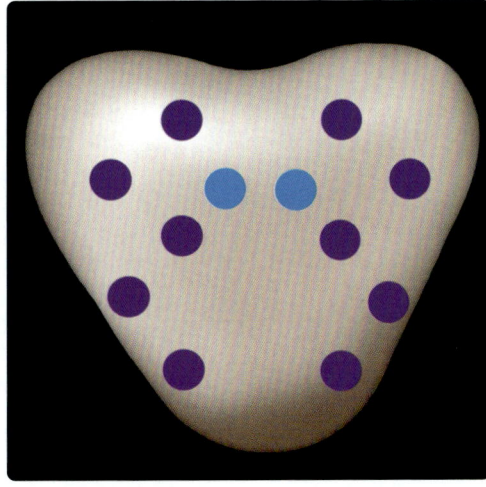

(Left) This anterior view of the prostate shows targets for the classic sextant biopsy scheme, which samples bilateral base, midgland, and apex. (Right) The extended biopsy scheme includes standard sextant biopsies with more laterally directed biopsies and is preferred due to a lower false-negative rate. Biopsy of the TZ (blue) is not recommended at initial biopsy; the saturation biopsy scheme is reserved for persistent indication and negative prior biopsies. This systematic biopsy scheme is now the preferred approach.

Handling of Prostate Biopsy

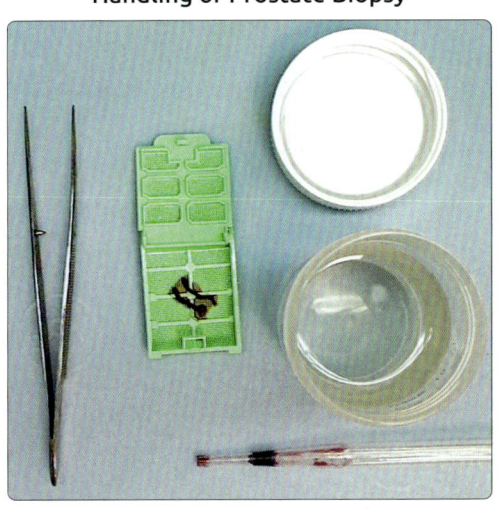

Handling of Prostate Biopsy

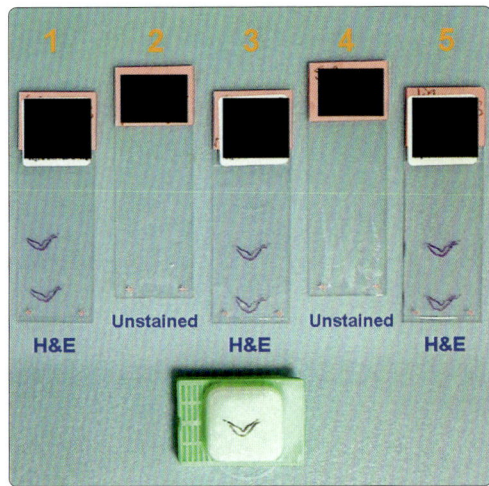

(Left) The prostate cores are ideally submitted with only 1-2 cores per cassette. Too many cores per block may cause tissue loss since cores may be cut at different levels. Inked cores are more visible and aid in the optimal cutting of the tissue within the paraffin blocks. (Right) Prospective intervening unstained slides are recommended for possible immunohistochemical studies or additional H&E stains. This approach ensures representation of the focus of interest that may be lost in subsequent deeper levels.

Microanatomy and Zonal Variations

DUCTAL ACINAR UNIT

Ducts and Acini
- Primarily lined by prostatic secretory cells, except at proximal ducts close to prostatic urethra (PU) where epithelium is urothelial
- Main cell types: Secretory, basal, and endocrine-paracrine cells
- Cross section of ducts and acini cannot be reliably distinguished histologically, except when longitudinal dimension of duct is appreciated
- All ducts originate from PU and end near capsule, except main transition zone (TZ) duct, which ends at extraprostatic tumor extension (AFS)
- Very rarely, acini may lie within perineural space

Secretory or Acinar Cells
- Typically cuboidal to columnar with clear to pale cytoplasm and basally located round regular nuclei
- May appear multilayered depending on plane of section
- PSA, PSAP, PSMA, NKX3.1, prostein (+)
- HMCK(34βE12), p63, CK5/6, CK14 (-)

Basal Cells
- Believed to be stem cell compartment of acini that divides and matures into secretory cells
- Lack muscle filaments, thus not identical to myoepithelial cells in breast ducts and lobules
- Located between secretory cells and acinar basement membrane and should be internal to gland outline
- Cuboidal, flattened, attenuated, or triangular cells with long axis parallel to basement membrane
- Contains little or no discernible cytoplasm, dark round-to-oval nuclei, and occasional small nucleoli
- May not be obvious on H&E or may appear discontinuous or absent, unless highlighted by immunohistochemistry
- PSA, PSAP, PSMA, NKX3.1, prostein (-)
- p63, HMCK(34βE12), CK5/6, CK14 (+)

Endocrine-Paracrine Cells
- Typically isolated or irregularly distributed in acini
- May not be readily identifiable on H&E, demonstrable only by immunohistochemistry or special stains
- Contain hormones, such as serotonin, neuron-specific enolase, somatostatin, calcitonin, and bombesin
- Include argentaffin and Paneth-like cells
  - Argentaffin cells contain finer eosinophilic granules situated between secretory cells, rest on basal cells, and usually do not reach lumen
  - Paneth-like cell contains larger intensely eosinophilic granules and extends to luminal aspect of acini
- Exact function not known

Nonglandular &/or Metaplastic Cells
- **Urothelial cells**
  - Lining epithelium of proximal prostatic urethra (PPU), proximal part of distal prostatic urethra (DPU), and proximal portion of prostatic ducts
  - Unlike in bladder, urothelium of PU and ducts have scant cytoplasm, and maturation into surface umbrella cells is variable
  - May be seen in deep ducts and acini presumably as metaplastic process
  - Seen in up to 34% of prostate biopsies
  - May undergo exuberant hyperplasia that may mimic urothelial carcinoma
- **Mucinous metaplasia**
  - May occur in benign prostate glands
  - Reported in nodular hyperplastic epithelium, transitional cell metaplasia, basal cell hyperplasia, sclerotic atrophy, and postatrophic hyperplasia
  - Postulated to arise from metaplasia of basal cells
  - Mucinous cells contain foamy cytoplasm and basally oriented bland nuclei
  - Contain both neutral and acid mucin [PASD, mucicarmine, Alcian blue (+)]
  - Nonreactive to PSA/PSAP
- **Squamous metaplasia**
  - Prostate glands may undergo squamous metaplasia in response to infarction and estrogen
  - Postulated to arise directly from proliferative basal cells

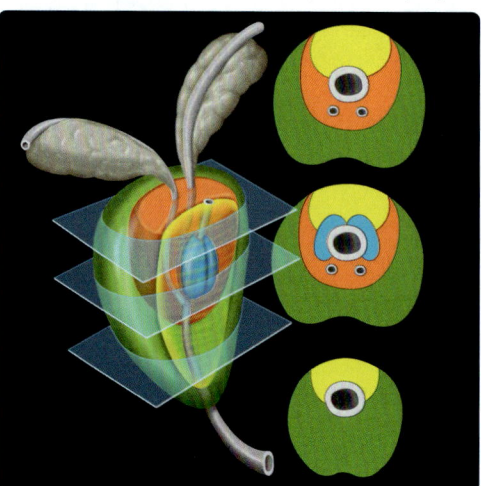

McNeal Model of Prostate Zones (PZ)

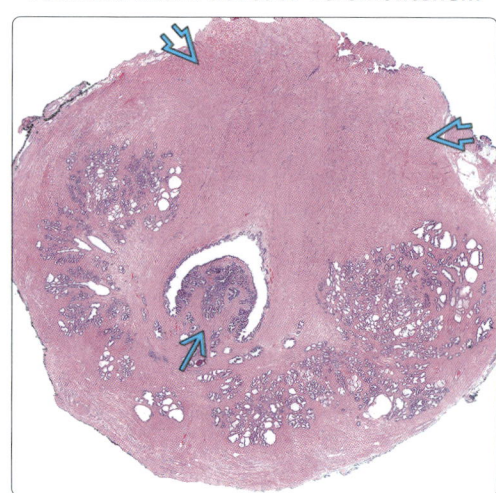

Prostate Below Level of Verumontanum

(Left) McNeal model uses PU as a key anatomic landmark and divides prostate glandular component into PZ (green), CZ (orange), TZ (blue), and PUGR (white). The AFS (yellow) comprises midanterior portion. (Right) Coronal section below the verumontanum shows the PZ forming the posterior and lateral aspects of the gland. The promontory ➡ points anteriorly toward the AFS, a nonglandular area consisting of fibromuscular tissue ➡ intermingled with skeletal muscle. The promontory and AFS are useful landmarks for histologic orientation.

Microanatomy and Zonal Variations

- Reduces or loses ability to express prostate-associated antigens [PSA/PSAP (-)]
- Differential diagnosis for rare squamous cell carcinoma of prostate, which in contrast has marked atypia and infiltrative growth

PROSTATE ANATOMIC ZONES

Peripheral Zone

- Comprises about 70% of glandular compartment
- Accounts for all glandular tissues surrounding DPU
- Forms prostate bulk posteriorly and laterally and tapers anteriorly at both sides (anterior horn)
- Surrounds central zone (CZ) and peripheral zone (PZ) posteriorly, laterally, and inferiorly
- Ducts exit in double row at posterolateral aspect of DPU extending from verumontanum to apex
- Ducts extend laterally within PZ, major branches curve anteriorly, and minor branches curve posteriorly
- Most common origin for prostate carcinoma (70-75%)
- Most susceptible to inflammation and most common to undergo atrophy

Central Zone

- Comprises about 25% of glandular compartment
- Inverted conical shape with its base comprising entire base of prostate
- Ducts arise around ejaculatory duct (ED) opening at verumontanum, follow course of ED, and fan out posteriorly to base
- Relatively resistant to prostate carcinoma and inflammation

Transition Zone

- Comprises about 5% of glandular compartment
- 2 separate small paraurethral lobes at mid prostate
- Ducts of both TZ lobes arise posterolaterally from PPU at lower border of preprostatic sphincter just above urethral angulation
- Main ducts extend laterally around preprostatic sphincter and curve sharply anteriorly
- Most common site for BPH and atypical adenomatous hyperplasia (AAH)/adenosis
- Zone resected in TURP for BPH

Periurethral Gland Region

- Series of tiny ducts and abortive acini embedded within longitudinal smooth muscle of preprostatic sphincter organized around PPU
- Possible origin of uncommon pure primary urothelial carcinoma of prostate

ZONAL VARIATIONS IN HISTOLOGY

Prostatic Ducts and Acini

- PZ and TZ acini are identical
  - Small, usually 0.15-0.3 mm, with slight luminal undulations
  - TZ acini are less numerous than in PZ
  - Secretory cells of PZ and TZ are evenly spaced, uniform columnar cells, with pale cytoplasm and small, more basally situated nuclei
- CZ acini are larger, up to 0.6 mm, and more complex
  - Luminal borders are uneven, with individual secretory cells protruding into lumen
  - Contain cribriform formations, "Roman bridging," and papillary infolding
  - May be confused with prostatic intraepithelial neoplasia or BPH glands
  - Secretory cells of CZ have more crowded columnar cells, more granular or darker cytoplasm, and relatively larger nuclei at varying levels within cells
- Urothelial cells variably line PUGR glands

Prostatic Stroma

- PZ stroma is loose with random muscle bundles
- TZ stroma is relatively more compact than PZ with interlacing, smooth muscle bundles that blend with preprostatic sphincter and AFS
- CZ stroma is more compact but with a lower stroma:acini ratio than PZ and TZ
- Contrast of stromal quality is more abrupt between PZ and CZ than with TZ

LUMINAL AND CELLULAR DEPOSITS

Corpora Amylacea

- Common in lumen of benign prostate glands and verumontanum glands
- Present in benign acini of 25% of men ages 20-40 years and frequency increases with age
- Reported in 32% of atypical AAH, 75% of postatrophic hyperplasia cases, and 20% of needle biopsies with infarcts
- Very rare in prostate carcinoma
- Round pink-purple concretions often with concentric lamination
- Thought to be related to cellular desquamation and degeneration

Intraluminal Crystalloids

- Seen in 5% of benign glands and up to 41% of prostate carcinoma; usually associated with carcinoma if present
- Bright, eosinophilic, refractile, with sharp borders and variety of shapes
- When seen in benign glands, not significant risk factor for subsequent diagnosis of prostate cancer

Intraluminal Secretions

- Occasionally present in gland lumina consisting of light eosinophilic amorphous material on H&E
- Contains neutral mucin [PAS/PASD(+)]

Pigments

- Lipofuscin
  - Ubiquitously present in seminal vesicle (SV) and ED epithelium
  - May also be seen within benign prostatic secretory cells and rarely in basal and stromal cells especially in CZ
    - Awareness is important and should not be sole criterion to identify SV and ED epithelium
    - Golden-yellow pigment usually subnuclear or at basal aspect of secretory cells
    - Usually finely granular and sparse although may have coarse clumping where it is abundant
    - Varies from inconspicuous to diffuse and may be found in all prostate zones

Microanatomy and Zonal Variations

- Exhibits yellow autofluorescence
- Pigment within basal cells more likely artifactual overlap of pigment from secretory cells
- Rare pigment in stroma is scant and appears as isolated clusters
  ○ May be found in epithelium of BPH, prostatic intraepithelial hyperplasia, and adenocarcinoma
  ○ SV and ED lipofuscin pigment is more uniformly yellow, coarsely granular to globular, more refractile, and found in luminal aspect of cytoplasm
- Melanin
  ○ Seen rarely in prostatic stromal cells (blue nevus)
  ○ Finely granular brown or black pigment
  ○ Stromal cells show melanosomes at different stages of differentiation by electron microscopy
  ○ Pigmented stromal cells are S100(+)
  ○ Pigment may be seen in adjacent glandular epithelia, which are S100(-) and due to pigment transfer
  ○ Pigment may also be dispersed extracellularly among cells and collagen fibers

NONGLANDULAR PROSTATE

Anterior Fibromuscular Stroma

- Comprises anterior 1/3 of prostate, at anteromedial aspect extending from bladder neck to apex
- Laterally, covers most anterior aspect of PZ
- Deep aspect always in contact with PU, proximally with preprostatic sphincter and TZ, and distally with striated sphincter
- Composed of large compact smooth muscle bundles similar to bladder neck although more haphazard and some separated by fibrous tissue
- Occasionally may contain benign acini; complicates assessment for extraprostatic tumor extension (EPE)
- Fat cells may be present anterior to AFS; involvement by cancer definitive for EPE

Preprostatic Sphincter

- Circular smooth muscle fibers surrounding PU, which prevents retrograde ejaculation
- Located preprostatic or proximal to openings of ducts from main glandular areas
- More compact at urethra posteriorly, but fibers dispersed more laterally to mingle with TZ ducts and acini
- Not complete anteriorly, where it blends with AFS

Striated Sphincter

- Semicircular cap over anterior and anterolateral surface of gland
- Surrounds distal urethra anteriorly but incomplete posterolaterally where fibers continue to anterior margin of PZ
- Thin, consisting of small, compact, striated muscle fibers

Prostatic "Capsule"

- Prostate does not have true capsule but outer condensation of fibromuscular tissue that is inseparable component of prostatic stroma
- For convenience, this fibromuscular band is referred to in literature as prostate capsule
- Covers most of posterior and lateral surfaces of prostate
- Blends anteriorly with AFS
- Not well defined or absent at anterolateral aspect of apex and at bladder neck, where prostatic stroma blends with bladder musculature
  ○ Complicates interpretation of EPE at these sites
- Outer surface of this fibromuscular band gives rise to few fibromuscular bands that blend into periprostatic connective tissue

NONPROSTATIC STRUCTURES

Prostatic Urethra

- PPU lined by urothelium with variable umbrella cells and merges imperceptibly with DPU
- Distal aspect of DPU lined by pseudostratified or stratified columnar cells

Verumontanum (Colliculus Seminalis)

- Elevation from posterior wall at PU angulation
- Contains a mid, blind, epithelial-lined sac known as utricle and opening of ED at both sides
- Contains closely apposed small to medium-sized glands, which often contain corpora amylacea or orange-brown luminal secretions
- Gland has 2 layers consisting of glandular cells and readily discernible basal cells
- Glandular cells are cuboidal to low columnar containing clear to eosinophilic cytoplasm and round regular nuclei
- May undergo florid glandular hyperplasia, which may be confused with prostate carcinoma

Ejaculatory Duct

- Paired ducts cross CZ and exit in PU at both sides of prostatic utricle in verumontanum
- Similar to SV, shows complex luminal papillation
- Identical lining epithelium to SV, including presence of lipofuscin pigment and random pleomorphism

Cowper Glands (Bulbourethral Glands)

- Paired tubuloalveolar gland situated in striated muscles of urogenital diaphragm lateral to membranous urethra
- Because of its proximity, may be inadvertently sampled by transurethral resection or rarely by needle biopsy of apex
- May mimic low-grade prostate carcinoma
- Lobular arrangement of numerous mucinous acini with excretory ducts that end in posterior aspect of bulbous urethra
- Acinar structures contain single layer of bland cuboidal to columnar cells with abundant mucin and basally located small nuclei
- Acinar structures contain myoepithelial cells that are not easily discernible on H&E
- PSA/PSAP (-)
- SMA strongly stains myoepithelial cells around acini

PERIPROSTATIC STRUCTURES

Adipose Tissue

- Involvement by prostate cancer constitutes EPE
- Present in periprostatic region in about 1/2 of radical prostatectomy specimens

Microanatomy and Zonal Variations

- Distribution around radical prostatectomy specimen varies: Most frequent in lateral region (57-59%), lowest at posterior surface (36%)
- Nerve-sparing radical prostatectomy contains lesser periprostatic adipose tissue
- Fat within prostate is exceedingly rare

Neurovascular Bundle

- Has short distance anterior to plane of rectal surface
- Consists of nerves and blood vessels in varying amounts of fibroadipose tissue and contains several autonomic ganglia
- Bundle formation not always present and may be seen spreading to lateral surface, although larger nerves and vessels tend to be at posterolateral region
- Ganglion cells may be present within prostate in region of neurovascular bundle

Paraganglia

- Present in a ~ 8% of radical prostatectomy specimens
- Primarily situated in loose connective and adipose tissue immediately external to prostate
- Mostly located in lateral to slightly posterior extraprostatic tissues, closer to base than apex, and often in association with neurovascular bundle
- Rare in anterior aspect of prostate
- Range from ~ 100.0 µm to 1.7 mm (median: 0.9 mm)
- Lobular or zellballen pattern of cells with prominent stromal vascular component
- Cells typically have abundant clear to slightly granular, basophilic to amphophilic cytoplasm with centrally placed small round to oval nuclei
- Rarely, may have more solid configuration, show single cell infiltrative pattern, or contain larger cells
- May mimic prostate carcinoma with hypernephroid features
- Synaptophysin, chromogranin, neuron-specific enolase (+)

Denonvilliers Fascia

- Single avascular fascial sheath sometimes referred to as "prostoperitoneal membrane" situated behind prostate, covering posterior surface and SV
- Fused layers of collagenous fibers and occasional muscle
- Often fused with midposterior portion of prostate capsule, separated laterally by investing adipose tissue
- Usually dissected with prostate in radical and nerve-sparing radical prostatectomy, being plane of dissection in latter

Lateral Prostatic Fascia

- Collagenous fascia at variable distance from lateral aspect of prostate
- Either completely separate or fused with prostate capsule with very little adipose tissue in between
- Usually at lateral border of prostate near base; this area overlies boundary of CZ and PZ
- Usually dissected with prostate in radical prostatectomy and spared with preservation of neurovascular bundle

Urinary Bladder Neck

- Bladder neck smooth musculature blends imperceptibly with fibromuscular stroma of superior prostate
  - CZ of prostate adjacent to bladder neck has more muscular stroma than PZ or TZ
- Boundary is ill defined
  - Cancer involvement of bladder neck tissue with no benign prostatic glands is considered EPE (microscopic bladder neck involvement)

SEMINAL VESICLE

SV Glands

- Adult SV mucosa contains papillary projections and invaginating ducts surrounded by glands in vaguely lobular configuration
- Surrounding glands are small to medium and elongated or slit-like
- Papillae are lined by single layer of cuboidal to columnar secretory cells and underlying basal cells
- Secretory cells
  - Not uniform
  - Randomly contain pseudomalignant pleomorphic cells with nucleomegaly, hyperchromasia, and multinucleation
  - Lipofuscin granules frequent in cytoplasm
  - Nuclei may contain occasional pseudoinclusions
- Secretory cells are PSA/PSAP (-), pax-2(+), and basal cells are basal cell marker (+)
- Localized amyloid deposits seen in subepithelial region and around vessels in 4-12% of SV, usually incidental or identified at autopsy

SV Wall

- Thick inner circular layer and thin outer longitudinal fibromuscular layer
- Thinner at prostate base
- Contain round eosinophilic hyaline bodies thought to be degenerating smooth muscle cells

SELECTED REFERENCES

1. Fine SW et al: Anatomy of the prostate revisited: implications for prostate biopsy and zonal origins of prostate cancer. Histopathology. 60(1):142-52, 2012
2. Fine SW et al: Anatomy of the anterior prostate and extraprostatic space: a contemporary surgical pathology analysis. Adv Anat Pathol. 14(6):401-7, 2007
3. Christian JD et al: Corpora amylacea in adenocarcinoma of the prostate: incidence and histology within needle core biopsies. Mod Pathol. 18(1):36-9, 2005
4. Hong H et al: Anatomic distribution of periprostatic adipose tissue: a mapping study of 100 radical prostatectomy specimens. Cancer. 97(7):1639-43, 2003
5. Anton RC et al: The significance of intraluminal prostatic crystalloids in benign needle biopsies. Am J Surg Pathol. 22(4):446-9, 1998
6. Saboorian MH et al: Distinguishing Cowper's glands from neoplastic and pseudoneoplastic lesions of prostate: immunohistochemical and ultrastructural studies. Am J Surg Pathol. 21(9):1069-74, 1997
7. Amin MB et al: Pigment in prostatic epithelium and adenocarcinoma: a potential source of diagnostic confusion with seminal vesicular epithelium. Mod Pathol. 9(7):791-5, 1996
8. Villers A et al: Anatomy of the prostate: review of the different models. Eur Urol. 20(4):261-8, 1991
9. Ayala AG et al: The prostatic capsule: does it exist? Its importance in the staging and treatment of prostatic carcinoma. Am J Surg Pathol. 13(1):21-7, 1989
10. McNeal JE: Normal histology of the prostate. Am J Surg Pathol. 12(8):619-33, 1988

Microanatomy and Zonal Variations

Significance of Normal Histoanatomic Structures in Prostate Pathology

Structures	Remarks
Peripheral zone	Most common origin for prostate carcinoma (70-75%)
	Most susceptible to inflammation and most common to undergo atrophy
	Uncommon site for BPH
Transition zone	Most frequent site for BPH and its myriad morphologic patterns
	Common site for atypical adenomatous hyperplasia
	Less commonly, site of origin of prostate carcinoma (15-20%), which tends to be lower grade
Central zone	Relatively resistant to prostate carcinoma and inflammation
	Mimic glands of BPH and prostatic intraepithelial neoplasia
Periurethral gland region	Possible origin of uncommon pure primary urothelial carcinoma of prostate
Corpora amylacea	Common in benign prostate glands and rarely seen in carcinoma
Intraluminal crystalloids	Common in prostate carcinoma but may also be seen in benign glands
	Presence in benign glands not risk factor for subsequent diagnosis of prostate carcinoma
Lipofuscin pigment	Not exclusive for SV and ED epithelium and may also be seen uncommonly in benign and malignant prostate glands
Striated muscles in AFS and apical region	Benign glands may be seen admixed with striated muscles and thus not necessarily invasive or malignant feature
	Adenocarcinoma involving striated muscles at these sites does not constitute EPE
Prostate capsule	Although not true capsule, serves as histoanatomic boundary for organ-confined prostate cancer
	Absent in base and not clearly defined in apex, complicating interpretation of EPE at these sites
Nerve	Perineural glands not exclusively associated with carcinoma, unless glands are completely circles or are present within nerve
	One of pathways for EPE by carcinoma
Prostatic urethra	May give rise to urothelial carcinoma (common), squamous carcinoma, adenocarcinoma of prostate, and primary of urethra
	Florid nephrogenic adenoma from this site may extend to prostate and mimic prostate carcinoma
	Urothelial carcinoma of PU invading prostate may occur in patients with bladder urothelial carcinoma and should not be staged as pT4 bladder cancer
Verumontanum	May undergo florid glandular hyperplasia, which may be confused with prostate carcinoma
Seminal vesicle	Rare site for primary malignancy
	Secondary involvement by prostate carcinoma relatively more common and denotes higher tumor stage (pT3b)
	Pseudomalignant features of epithelium may be confused with malignancy in limited sample
Ejaculatory duct	Involvement by cancer in needle biopsy should not be confused as SV involvement, which denotes higher tumor stage
	Pseudomalignant features of epithelium may be confused with malignancy in limited sample
	Distinction from SV is based on absence of distinct smooth muscle wall
Cowper gland	Resembles minor salivary gland tissue, may mimic low-grade prostate carcinoma
Periprostatic adipose tissue	Involvement by prostate carcinoma constitutes EPE, including in needle biopsy specimens
	May be absent over large areas of prostatic surface in prostatectomy specimen, making evaluation of EPE difficult
Bladder neck	Bladder wall smooth muscle bundles blend imperceptibly with prostate fibromuscular stroma at superior prostate
	Cancer involvement of bladder neck tissue without prostate glands considered EPE (microscopic bladder neck involvement)
Paraganglia	May mimic prostate carcinoma with hypernephroid features
	Involvement by carcinoma not always equivalent to EPE since it may be present rarely within prostate

AFS = anterior fibromuscular stroma; SV = seminal vesicle; ED = ejaculatory duct; EPE = extraprostatic tumor extension; PU = prostatic urethra.

Microanatomy and Zonal Variations

McNeal Model of Prostate Zones

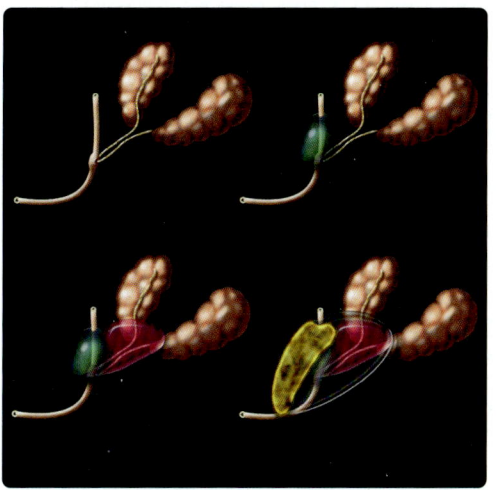

Prostate at Level of Verumontanum

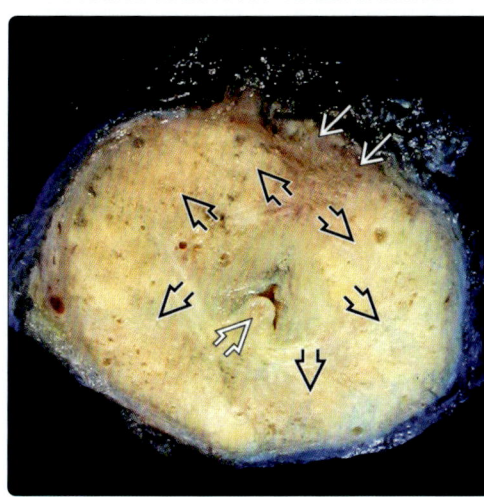

(Left) PU is divided into PPU and DPU by a mid angulation. TZ (blue) and CZ (magenta) encase PPU and ED, respectively. PZ (transparent) surrounds CZ and DPU posteriorly. AFS (yellow) is situated anteriorly and extends to both urethral openings. (Right) Coronal section of prostate at level of verumontanum ⇨ shows PZ ⇨ located posteriorly and extending anteriorly abutting the AFS ⇨. The verumontanum is at urethral angulation midway between base and apex, and where both EDs exit into PU.

Anterior Fibromuscular Stroma (AFS)

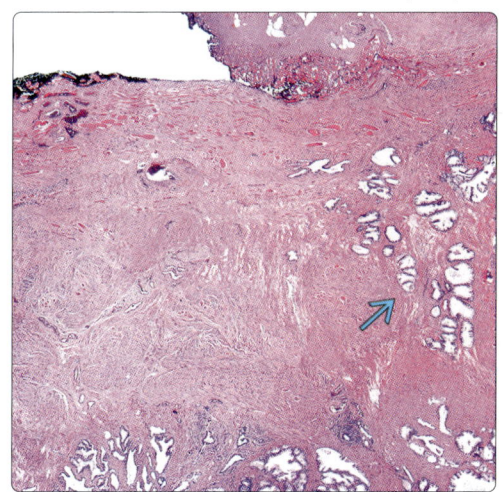

Benign Glands Within Skeletal Muscles

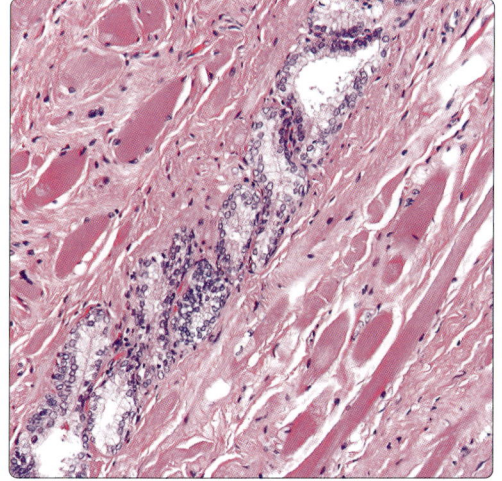

(Left) Low power view of AFS shows condensation of fibromuscular tissue and skeletal muscles devoid of glands. Lateral to the AFS is the anterior PZ ⇨. AFS is continuous cephalad with the preprostatic sphincter and caudal with the striated sphincter. (Right) This H&E section shows benign glands present in between striated muscle. This may be seen in AFS and apical regions and must not be interpreted as an invasive feature. The presence of glands in striated muscle complicates interpretation of EPE by cancer at these sites.

Verumontanum

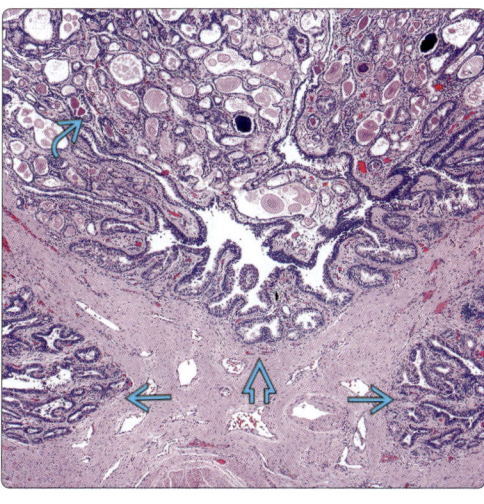

Verumontanum Mucosal Glands

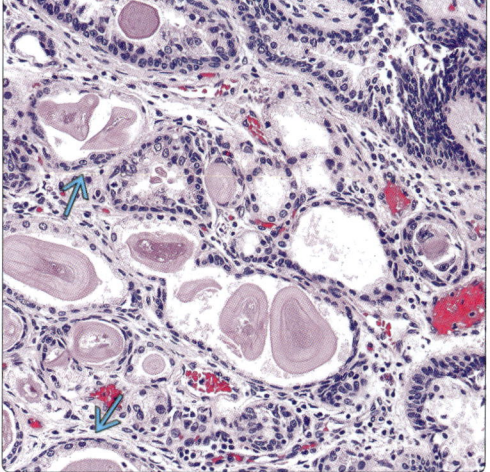

(Left) Low-power view of the verumontanum shows the paired EDs ⇨ situated lateral to the invagination of the prostatic utricle ⇨. Note the hyperplasia of verumontanum mucosal glands, which frequently contain corpora amylacea in their lumina ⇨. The verumontanum forms an elevation at the PU angulation to the DPU. (Right) Verumontanum mucosal glands show 2 layers of cells, including distinct basal cells ⇨ and intraluminal corpora amylacea. Hyperplasia of these glands may mimic prostate carcinoma.

Microanatomy and Zonal Variations

Benign Prostatic Acini

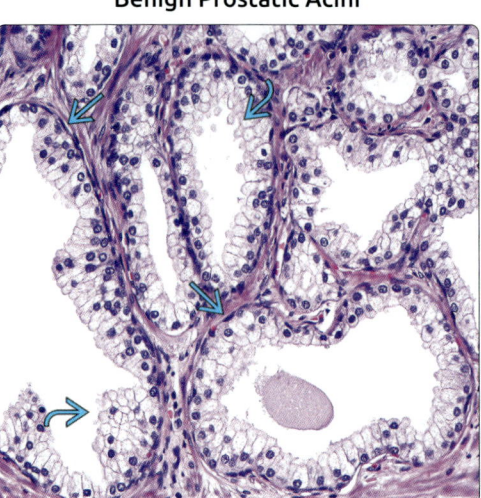

Benign Prostatic Duct

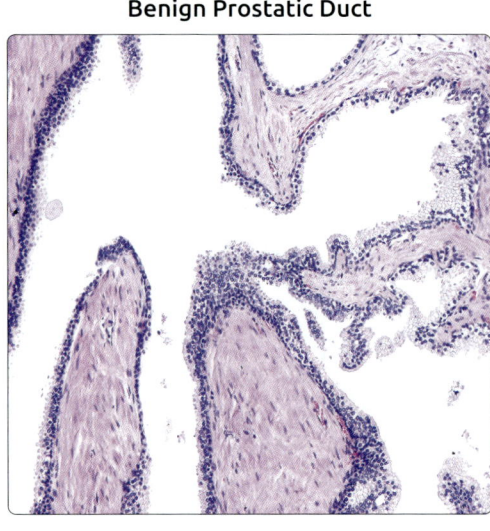

(Left) Typical benign acini show columnar cells with pale cytoplasm and round, regular, basally oriented nuclei, with indistinct nucleoli. Basal cells ⇨ are situated internal to the glandular basement membrane outline and with scant cytoplasm. The glands are variable in size, and the luminal outline is usually not sharp or rigid ⇨. (Right) The lining of the duct is similar to the acini lined by secretory and basal cells. On cross section, ducts and acini are not reliably distinguished unless the longitudinal dimension of the duct is appreciated.

Corpora Amylacea

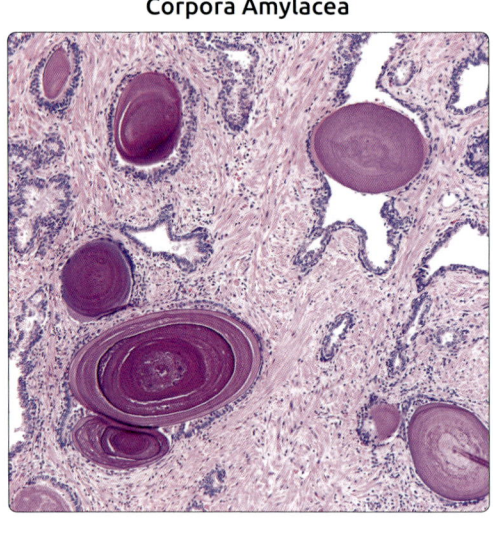

Luminal Secretions

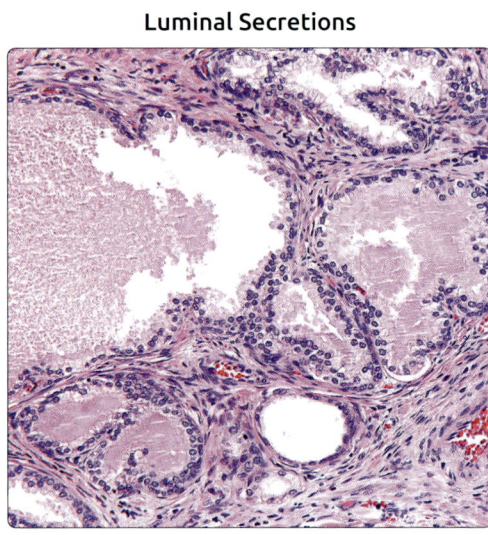

(Left) Benign glands contain corpora amylacea with its distinctive magenta color and circular lamellation. Corpora amylacea are frequent in benign prostate and verumontanum glands and may only rarely be seen in prostate carcinoma. These concretions are thought to be related to cellular degeneration. (Right) Benign glands show intraluminal pink amorphous secretions. Prostatic secretions are a minor component of ejaculatory volume and contain enzymes, which enhance sperm viability.

Crystalloids

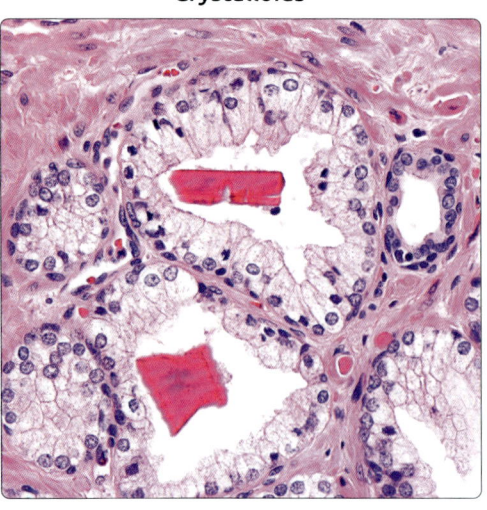

Cytoplasmic Pigments

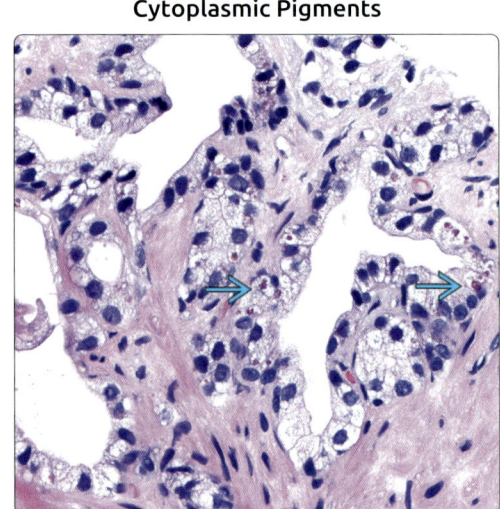

(Left) Benign glands show bright refractile eosinophilic crystals with sharp borders. Intraluminal crystalloids are common in prostate carcinoma and may be seen uncommonly in benign glands. Presence in benign glands is not a risk factor for carcinoma. (Right) Benign glands show intracytoplasmic golden-yellow pigment ⇨. The presence of pigment granules should not be used as sole criterion to distinguish seminal vesicle (SV) and ED from prostatic epithelium. SV/ED granules are coarser and more abundant.

Microanatomy and Zonal Variations

Peripheral Zone
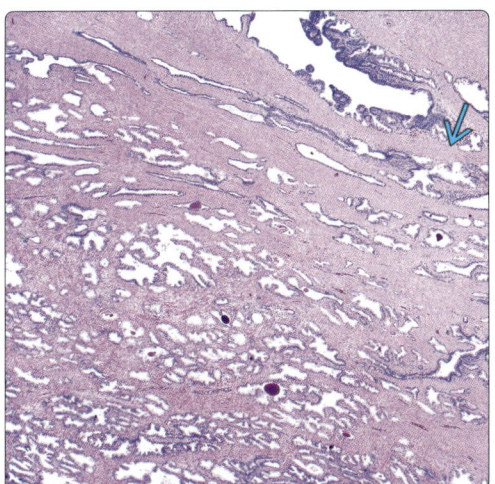

Peripheral Zone
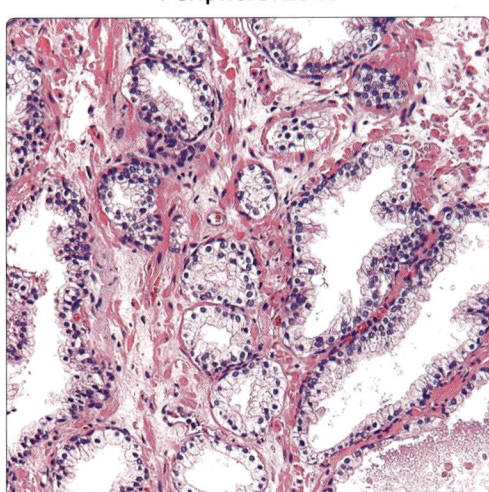

(Left) Ducts ➡ of the PZ arise from the verumontanum, the major branches curve anteriorly, and minor branches curve posteriorly. The longitudinal axis of the glands is usually oriented circumferentially toward the anterior. Most carcinomas of the prostate arise from the PZ. (Right) Normal PZ shows glands that have a smaller caliber compared to CZ glands. The stroma is loose and less compact. Note the luminal undulations, 2 cell layers, small nuclei, and absence of prominent nucleoli in these benign glands.

Central Zone
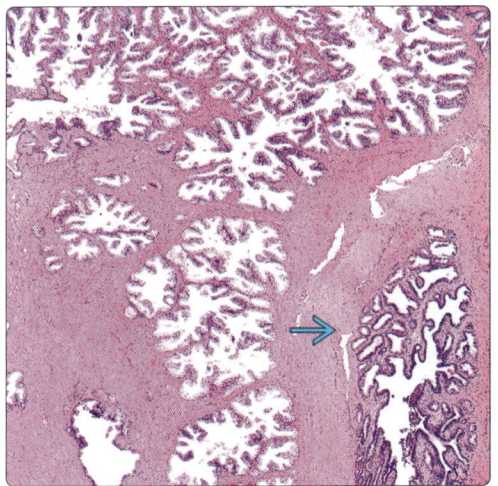

Central Zone
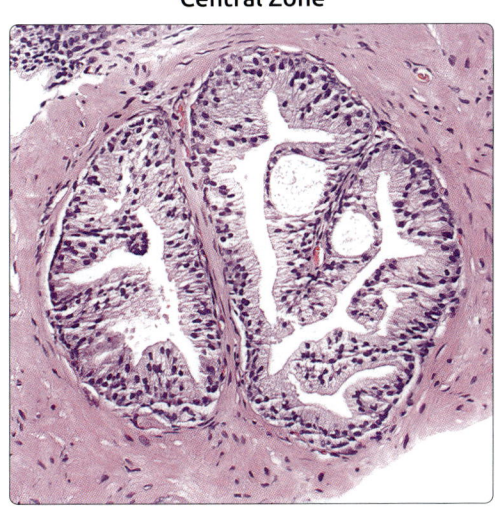

(Left) Low-power view shows CZ glands around the ED ➡. The CZ glands are larger and more complex than glands in the PZ. The stroma of CZ is distinctively more muscular and is contiguous with the bladder base. CZ is the least common site for carcinoma. (Right) The glands of central zone are innately larger. There are multilayering, intraluminal ridges, epithelial arches, & papillary infoldings. These features overlap with benign prostatic hyperplasia & high-grade PIN; awareness is important particularly in needle biopsy.

Ducts of Prostate Zones
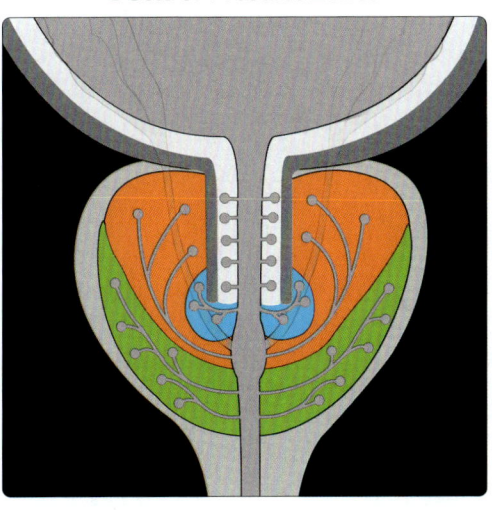

Periurethral Glands
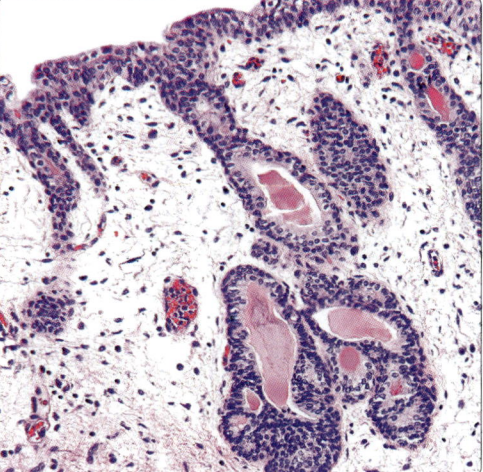

(Left) Ducts of PZ (green) exit in DPU and extend laterally within PZ. Ducts of CZ (orange) arise at verumontanum and fan out posteriorly. Ducts of TZ (blue) arise at lower PPU. PUGR is seen as series of ducts and acini in PPU. (Right) PU shows surface urothelium and underlying glands forming the PUGR (McNeal's model). These abortive ducts and acini are often lined by urothelium and may give rise to primary urothelial carcinoma of the prostate. The more distal portions are occasionally lined by prostatic acinar cells.

Microanatomy and Zonal Variations

Periurethral Prostatic Duct

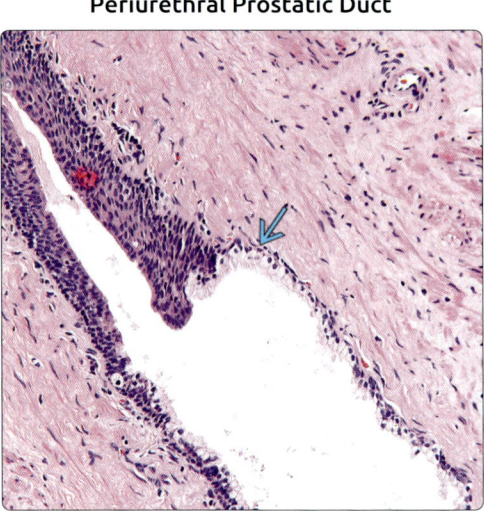

Urothelial Cells in Acini

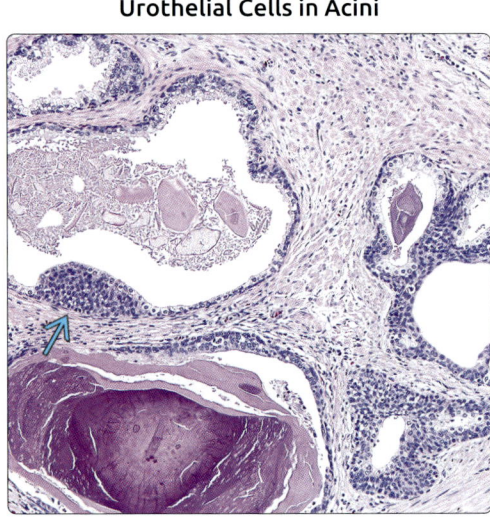

(Left) The periurethral prostatic duct shows urothelium lining its proximal aspect and secretory cells more distally ⇨. Urothelial carcinoma that arises primarily within the prostate is believed to originate from these cells. The presence of urothelium in the peripheral prostate indicates metaplasia. Note the transition of the lining to prostatic acinar and secretory cells. (Right) Peripheral prostatic glands show urothelial metaplasia ⇨ of the basal cells. The rest of the gland retained its secretory and basal cell lining.

Benign Glands Adjacent to Nerve

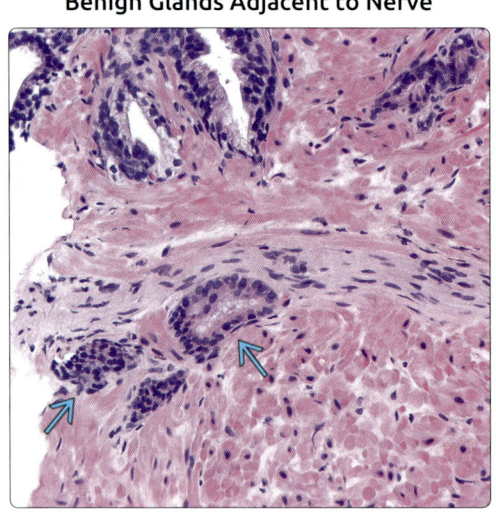

Prostatic Capsule

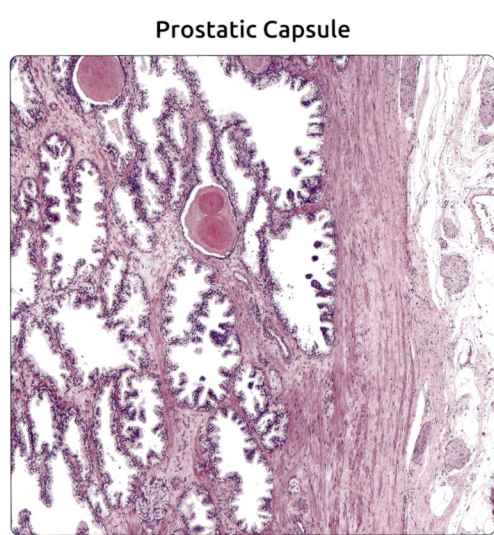

(Left) Perineural glands show intimate associate with benign glands ⇨ to nerve; this feature should not be used as an absolute criterion for malignancy. Circumferential or intraneural invasion is more diagnostic for cancer. (Right) The prostate capsule is not a true capsule but a condensation of fibromuscular tissue that is an inseparable component of the prostatic stroma. Periprostatic adipose tissues and nerves are present outside the capsule. Involvement of adipose tissue by prostatic carcinoma constitutes EPE.

Cowper Gland

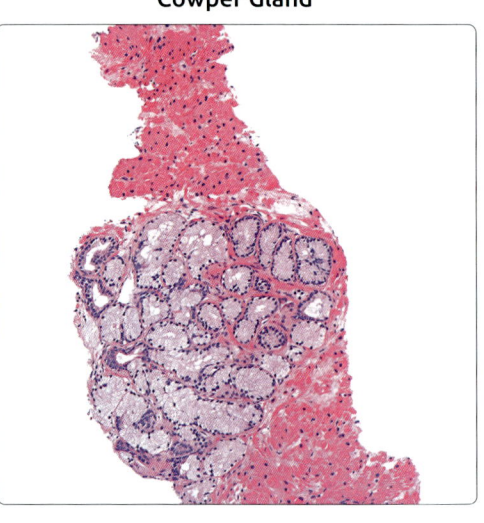

Cowper Gland

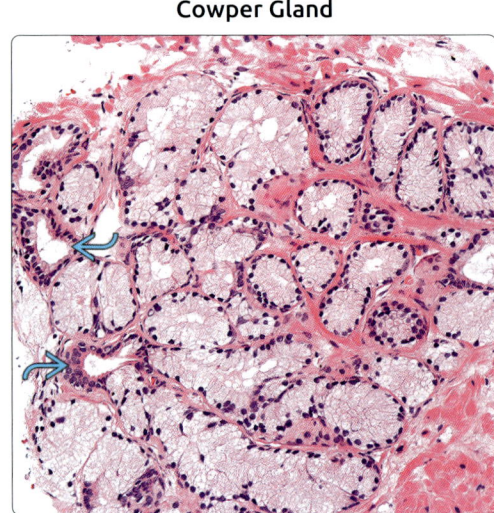

(Left) Cowper glands may occasionally be included in a needle biopsy from the apex. These are tubuloalveolar glands situated within striated muscle. The abundant clear cytoplasm and the crowded lobular architecture of these glands overlap with adenocarcinoma of prostate. (Right) Clues to the recognition of Cowper glands include the presence of excretory duct-like structures ⇨ as well as glands with abundant, voluminous, and mucinous cytoplasm. Skeletal muscle is often present around the glands.

Microanatomy and Zonal Variations

Paraganglion
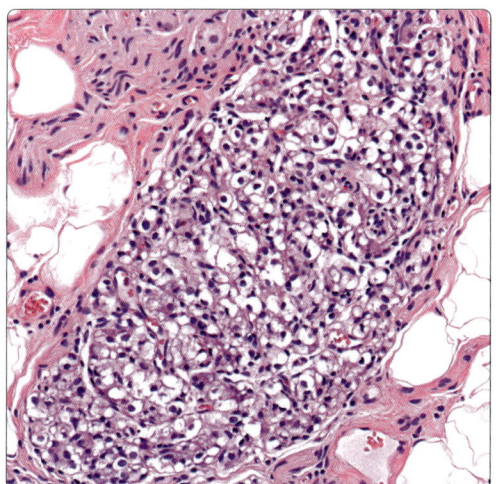

Paraganglion
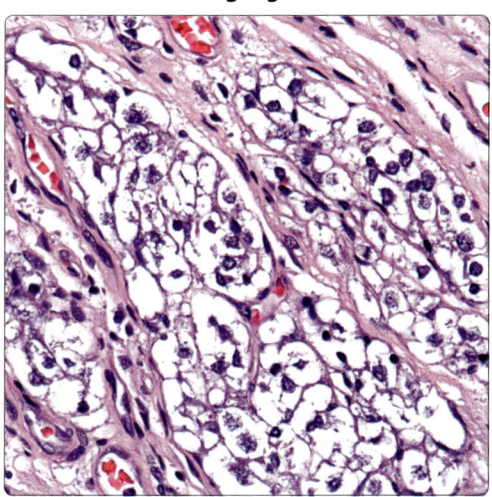

(Left) Paraganglion shows lobular configuration of cells with clear to slightly granular cytoplasm and round regular nuclei. Location in periprostatic fat, as in this case, and identification of sinusoidal vasculature are useful for accurate recognition. (Right) Paraganglia have cells with amphophilic, granular to clear cytoplasm and are associated with a delicate, characteristic vascular pattern. Paraganglia may mimic hypernephroid prostate carcinoma and, if misdiagnosed, may lead to upstaging as EPE.

Seminal Vesicle Lumina
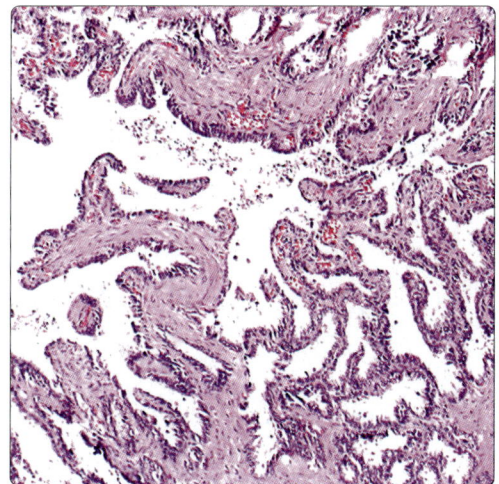

Seminal Vesicle Wall
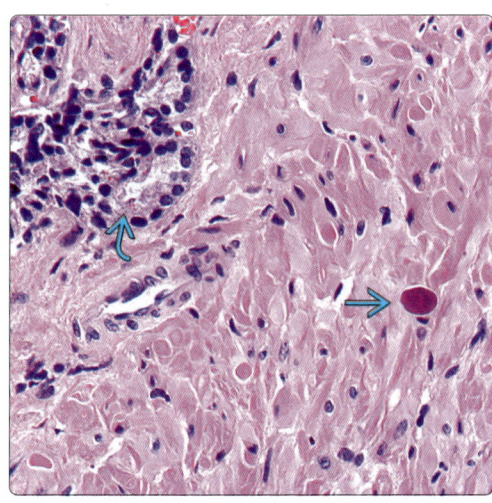

(Left) Seminal vesicles show a central lumen with invaginations and branching of elongated, cleft- and slit-like primary and secondary ducts that extend into a thick muscular coat of 2 cell layers. When the peripheral glands are tangentially sectioned, they may mimic adenocarcinoma of prostate. (Right) A hyaline body ➡ within the SV wall represents degenerating smooth muscle cell. Involvement of the muscular wall of the SV by carcinoma is required to diagnose SV invasion. Note the pigment in SV epithelium ➡.

Seminal Vesicle Epithelium
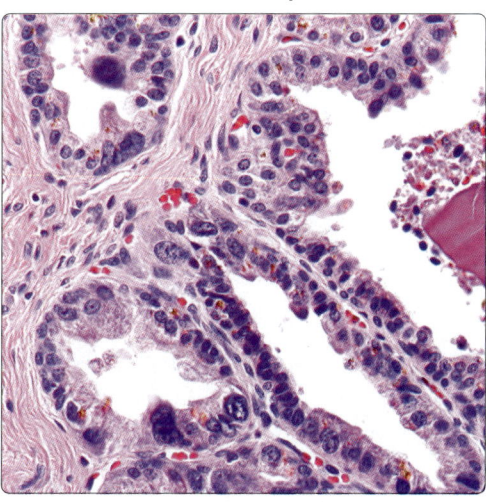

Seminal Vesicle Amyloid
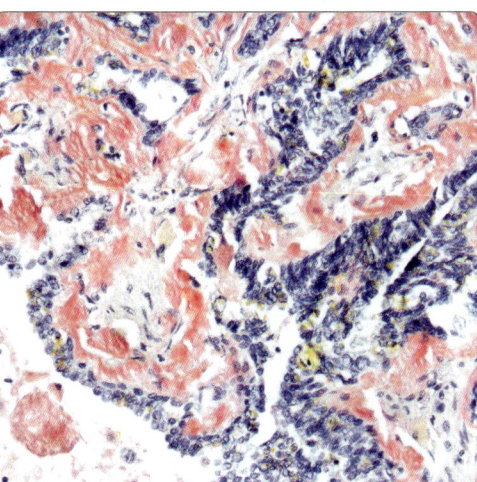

(Left) SV epithelium shows prominent cytoplasmic, coarse, golden-yellow granules. The epithelium is not uniform and contains random, markedly pleomorphic cells containing enlarged hyperchromatic nuclei. Intranuclear inclusions are another hallmark of SV epithelium. (Right) Congo red stain of SV lumina shows abundant subepithelial amyloid deposits (red), which may be seen in up to 12% of SV, mostly as an incidental finding. These are localized deposits and not a component of systemic amyloidosis.

Prostatitis

KEY FACTS

TERMINOLOGY
- Prostatitis syndromes, classified by National Institutes of Health (NIH) system
  - Group of inflammatory and noninflammatory conditions of prostate characterized by genitourinary or pelvic pain
  - NIH classification: I: Acute bacterial prostatitis; II: Chronic bacterial prostatitis; III: Chronic prostatitis/chronic pelvic pain syndrome; IV: Asymptomatic inflammatory prostatitis
- Granulomatous prostatitis (GP)
  - Includes nonspecific GP (NSGP), postprocedural granuloma (PPG), infectious GP (IGP), and systemic GP

CLINICAL ISSUES
- Prostatitis syndromes account for about 1/4 of male clinic visits with genitourinary complaints
  - Clinical and microbiologic work-up, without biopsy
- GP seen in 0.8% of benign prostate specimens
  - NSGP most common, comprising 50-78% of GP

MICROSCOPIC
- NSGP
  - Expansile, nodular infiltrates usually involving entire lobules
  - Epithelioid histiocytes, lymphocytes, plasma cells, neutrophils, variable often prominent eosinophil infiltrates
- Infectious GP (IGP)
  - Granulomatous inflammation with clinical, serologic, microbiologic, or histologic pathogen
- PPG
  - Necrobiotic granulomas or central fibrinoid necrosis surrounded by palisaded histiocytes; previous procedure
- Prostatitis syndromes as defined by NIH are clinical, not histologic, diagnoses
  - Acute or chronic inflammation in prostate biopsies should **not** be labeled as prostatitis

Acute Inflammation
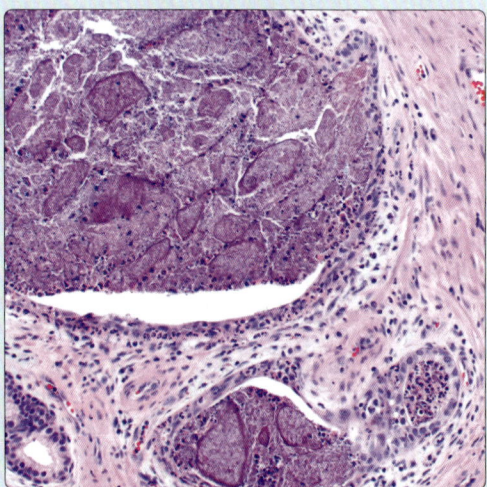

Chronic Inflammation
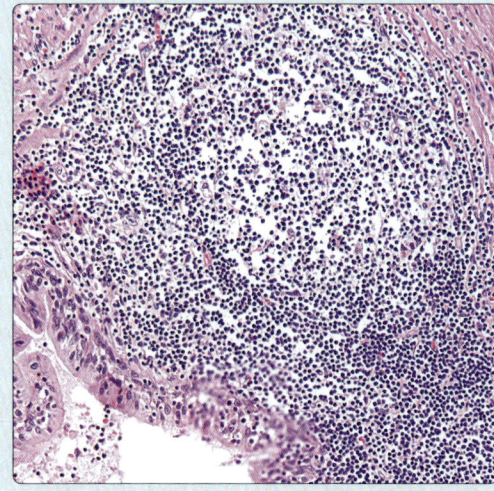

(Left) Several acini distended by acute inflammation are shown; the atrophic epithelial lining shows reactive cytoplasmic amphophilia and nuclear micronucleoli. Such foci should not be diagnosed as acute prostatitis if observed incidentally in biopsies for other reasons. (Right) Periglandular chronic inflammation of the prostate shows reactive germinal center formation. Again, chronic inflammation in prostate is observed frequently incidentally and should not be routinely labeled as chronic prostatitis.

Inflammation Simulating Carcinoma
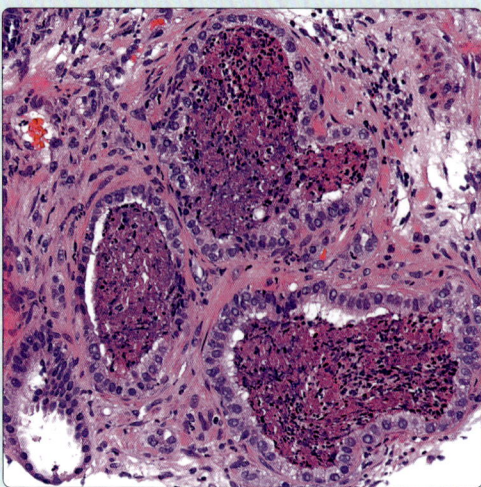

Inflammation and Carcinoma
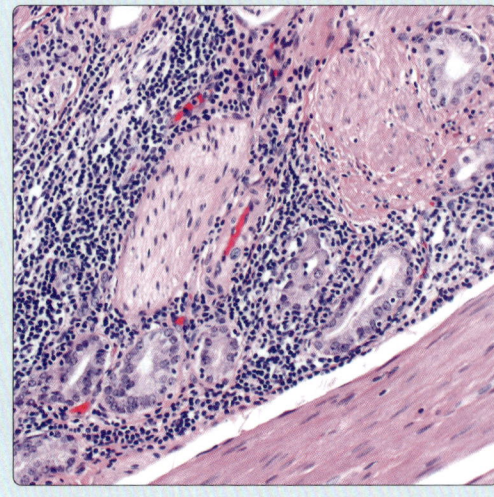

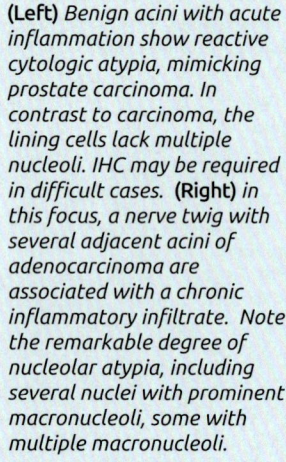

(Left) Benign acini with acute inflammation show reactive cytologic atypia, mimicking prostate carcinoma. In contrast to carcinoma, the lining cells lack multiple nucleoli. IHC may be required in difficult cases. (Right) In this focus, a nerve twig with several adjacent acini of adenocarcinoma are associated with a chronic inflammatory infiltrate. Note the remarkable degree of nucleolar atypia, including several nuclei with prominent macronucleoli, some with multiple macronucleoli.

Prostatitis

TERMINOLOGY

NIH Classification of Prostatitis Syndromes

- USA National Institutes of Health (NIH) convened International Prostatitis Collaborative Network to standardize definitions/terminology
- Class I: Acute bacterial prostatitis: Symptomatic and evidence of bacterial infection
- Class II: Chronic bacterial prostatitis: Chronic/recurrent symptoms and evidence of infection
- Class III: Chronic prostatitis/chronic pelvic pain syndrome
  - Type A: Inflammatory: Chronic/recurrent symptoms with inflammation but not bacterial infection
  - Type B: Noninflammatory: Chronic/recurrent symptoms without inflammation or bacterial infection
- Class IV: Asymptomatic inflammatory prostatitis: Absence of symptoms, inflammation found incidentally
  - Often biopsy for another purpose
- Evidence of infection detected from expressed prostatic secretions, postprostate massage urine, or seminal fluid
- Granulomatous prostatitis (GP): Histopathologic diagnosis not in NIH Classification of Prostatitis Syndromes
  - Inflammation of prostate containing granulomata
  - Nonspecific, infectious, and systemic causes

ETIOLOGY/PATHOGENESIS

Infectious Prostatitides

- Acute and chronic bacterial prostatitis (NIH I & II)
  - Gram-negative rods, including *E. coli* in vast majority
  - Also *E. faecalis, K. pneumoniae, P. mirabilis, P. aeruginosa*, occasionally gram-positive *S. aureus* and *Streptococcus* sp.
- Rare cases of fungi and mycobacteria, especially in exposed/immune-suppressed populations, may be granulomatous

Nonspecific Granulomatous Prostatitis

- Inflammatory reaction to altered prostatic acini &/or secretions from duct blockade, bacterial products, or refluxed urine is suggested
- Possibly autoimmune based
  - HLA-DR15-linked T-cell response against proteins in prostatic secretion, principally PSA

Postprocedural Granulomatous Prostatitis

- Inflammatory response to traumatic injury

CLINICAL ISSUES

Epidemiology

- Incidence
  - GP
    - 0.8% of benign prostate specimens, 0.36% of prostate needle biopsies
    - Nonspecific GP (NSGP) most common (50-78% of GP)
    - Posttransurethral resection GP (21-24% of GP)
    - Infectious GP (3.5-8.0% of GP)
    - Systemic GP exceedingly rare, Sarcoid and Wegener
  - Bacillus Calmette-Guérin (BCG)-related GP
    - Seen in at least 1.3% of patients with BCG treatment
    - Intravesical instillation performed 3-55 months (average ~ 1 yr) before diagnosis of GP
  - Chronic prostatitis/chronic pelvic pain syndrome; NIH Classification IV
    - Accounts for about 1/4 of male clinic visits for genitourinary complaints
- Age
  - GP
    - 18-86 yr old; mean and median: 62 yr
    - 2/3 of patients between 50 and 70 yr old

Presentation

- GP
  - Irritative voiding symptoms of urgency, frequency, and dysuria
  - Fever and chills common, infrequently asymptomatic (11%)
  - Systemic symptoms of allergy in allergic GP
  - Upper and lower respiratory involvement in Wegener granulomatosis
  - May have firm, fixed nodules on digital rectal exam
    - Clinical suspicion of carcinoma in 60% of cases
  - Concomitant prostate carcinoma in 10-14% of cases
- Prostatitis syndromes
  - Acute and chronic bacterial prostatitis (I & II) diagnosed based on symptomatology and cultures
    - Generally not biopsied for diagnosis
  - Chronic bacterial prostatitis (II) experiences recurrent, documented bacterial urinary tract infection
  - Chronic prostatitis/chronic pelvic pain syndrome (III) clinically identical to chronic bacterial prostatitis but negative cultures
    - Characterized by genitourinary or pelvic pain
  - Asymptomatic inflammatory prostatitis (IV) diagnosed in patients without genitourinary tract complaints
    - e.g., incidental inflammation encountered in prostate needle biopsy for prostate carcinoma work-up
- Much of inflammation encountered in routine biopsies for cancer falls under asymptomatic inflammatory prostatitis (IV)
  - Histologic classification of prostatitis based on pattern of inflammation seen in tissues
  - Determination if it fits into clinical class requires clinicopathologic correlation

Laboratory Tests

- Prostate inflammation common cause for serum PSA elevation
- Microbiology cultures, e.g., postprostatic massage secretions
- GP
  - Elevated serum PSA level in 84% of NSGP), 45% of infectious GP
  - Majority of patients have pyuria &/or hematuria, leukocytosis, or eosinophilia

Treatment

- GP
  - Majority (NSGP) require no treatment
  - Rarely prostatectomy to relieve obstructive symptoms in refractory cases
  - Distinction of NSGP from infectious GP and systemic GP important because of different management
    - Antibiotics for infectious GP

– Chemotherapy and steroids for systemic GP

MICROSCOPIC

Syndromal Prostatitides, National of Health Classes I-IV

- Diagnosis of specific classes of prostatitis syndrome requires clinical, microbiological, and laboratory correlation
  - Acute or chronic inflammation encountered in prostate biopsies should **not** be labeled as acute prostatitis or chronic prostatitis
  - Only descriptive diagnosis should be made for prostate parenchymal inflammation in absence of symptoms related to prostatitis syndrome
    - Such findings define asymptomatic inflammatory prostatitis (IV)
- Acute inflammation of prostate due to acute bacterial prostatitis overlaps with that due to noninfectious causes
  - Thus requirement of clinical and microbiologic correlation
- Histologic changes of chronic inflammation of prostate similar in
  - Chronic bacterial prostatitis (II)
  - Chronic prostatitis/chronic pelvic pain syndrome inflammatory type (IIIA)
  - Asymptomatic inflammatory prostatitis (IV)

Granulomatous Prostatitis

- NSGP
  - Expansile nodular infiltrates usually involving entire lobules; discrete granulomas rare
  - Epithelioid histiocytes, lymphocytes, plasma cells, neutrophils, and variable eosinophil infiltrates
  - Well-formed noncaseating granulomas and multinucleated giant cells may rarely be seen
  - Periglandular/periductal pattern of inflammation
  - Dilated and ruptured ducts/acini may be identified
- Postprocedural GP
  - Resembles rheumatoid nodules
  - Necrobiotic granulomas or central fibrinoid necrosis surrounded by palisaded histiocytes
  - Noncaseating granulomas and multinucleated giant cells frequent in surrounding tissues
  - Multinucleated giant cells may appear to engulf damaged prostatic epithelium
  - Granulomas vary in shape; may be wedge-shaped or long and tortuous
- Infectious GP (IGP)
  - Granulomas may be caseating or noncaseating
  - Specific infectious agent identified by combination of history, serologies, cultures, and special stains
  - BCG-related GP
    - Multiple caseating and noncaseating granulomas
    - May be accompanied by extensive necrosis and parenchymal destruction
    - Caseating necrosis more frequent in larger granulomas
    - Acid-fast bacilli demonstrable in up to 38% of cases, seen in areas of caseation
- Allergic GP
  - Necrobiotic granulomas surrounded by palisaded histiocytes containing eosinophil infiltrates
  - Presence of increased eosinophils not specific for allergic GP
- Xanthogranulomatous prostatitis
  - Predominant or pure collections of lipid-laden histiocytes in prostate
  - Histiocytes have abundant xanthomatous cytoplasm and small nuclei with inconspicuous nucleoli
  - Other type of inflammatory cells may be minimal

DIFFERENTIAL DIAGNOSIS

Prostate Carcinoma

- Prostate carcinoma glands may be mimicked by benign acini with reactive inflammatory atypia
  - Typically lacks background inflammation
  - Contains nucleomegaly, prominent and multiple nucleoli
  - Lacks basal cell layer
- High-grade (Gleason pattern 5 single-cell pattern) prostate carcinoma or small cell carcinoma may be mimicked by crushed inflammatory lymphocytic infiltrate
  - CK-PAN(AE1/AE3)(+), synaptophysin (+, if small cell carcinoma)
  - CD45(LCA)(-), CD3(-), CD30(-)
- High-grade (Gleason pattern 5, solid) or foamy gland prostate carcinoma may be mimicked by sheets of epithelioid histiocytes or xanthoma cells
  - CK-PAN(AE1/AE3)(+), CD68(-)

Malakoplakia

- Michaelis-Gutman bodies and von Hassman cells
- Calcium and iron stains may be necessary

DIAGNOSTIC CHECKLIST

Pathologic Interpretation Pearls

- Acute or chronic inflammation in prostate biopsies should not be labeled as prostatitis because prostatitis syndrome requires clinical diagnostic criteria
  - May represent asymptomatic inflammatory prostatitis
- Clinical history important in diagnosis of GP and distinction of NSGP, infectious GP, and systemic GP

SELECTED REFERENCES

1. Warrick J et al: Nonspecific granulomatous prostatitis. J Urol. 187(6):2209-10, 2012
2. Uzoh CC et al: Granulomatous prostatitis. BJU Int. 99(3):510-2, 2007
3. Krieger JN et al: NIH consensus definition and classification of prostatitis. JAMA. 282(3):236-7, 1999
4. Oppenheimer JR et al: Granulomatous prostatitis on needle biopsy. Arch Pathol Lab Med. 121(7):724-9, 1997
5. Bryan RL et al: Granulomatous prostatitis: a clinicopathological study. Histopathology. 19(5):453-7, 1991
6. Oates RD et al: Granulomatous prostatitis following bacillus Calmette-Guerin immunotherapy of bladder cancer. J Urol. 140(4):751-4, 1988
7. Stillwell TJ et al: The clinical spectrum of granulomatous prostatitis: a report of 200 cases. J Urol. 138(2):320-3, 1987

Prostatitis

Histiocytes Simulating Carcinoma
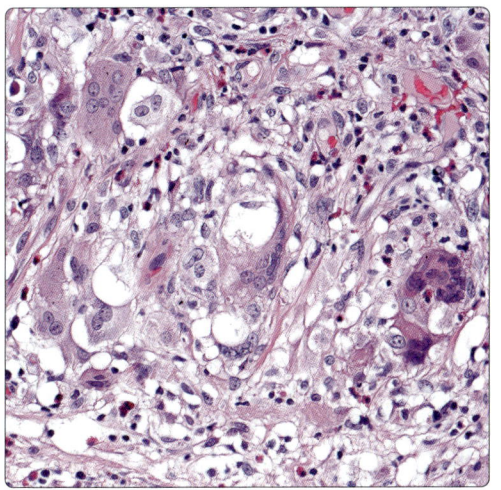

BCG-Related Granulomatous Prostatitis
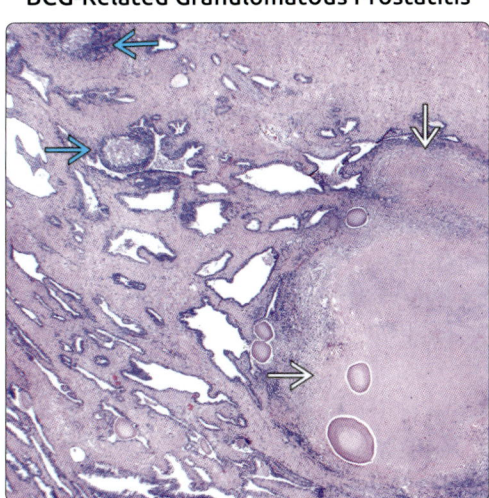

(Left) In this example of postprocedural granulomatous prostatitis (GP), multinucleated giant cells and epithelioid histiocytes show nuclear enlargement and nucleoli that could simulate a high-grade carcinoma. These histiocytes will be positive for CD68 and CD163 but negative for keratins and prostate lineage markers like PSA. (Right) Prior intravesical therapy with BCG for urothelial carcinoma results frequently in GP characterized by numerous caseating ➡ and noncaseating ➡ granulomas.

Inflammation With Schistosomiasis
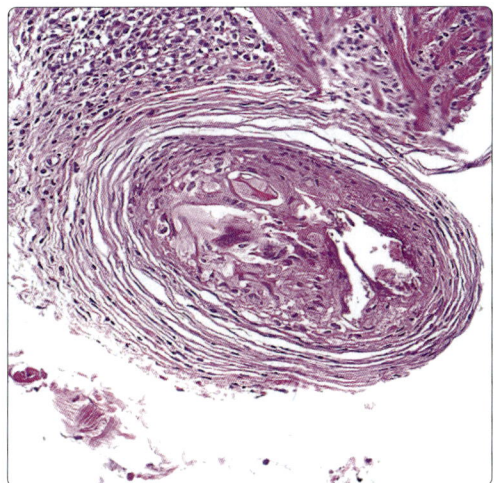

Granulomas and Blastomyces
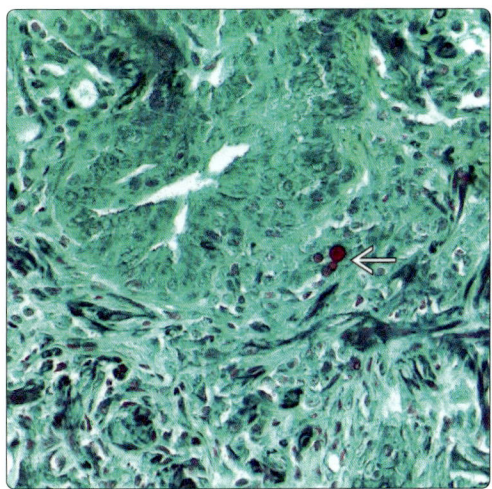

(Left) Prostate needle biopsy shows Schistosoma ova with associated inflammation. Schistosoma infestation of bladder and association with squamous cell carcinoma is well documented; prostate involvement is exceedingly rare. (Right) GMS stain in infectious granulomatous prostatitis (IGP) shows budding yeast forms of Blastomyces dermatitidis ➡. IGP may be caused by fungal, bacterial, parasitic, and viral infections. Mycobacterium tuberculosis (miliary form) is most common etiologic agent for IGP.

Coccidioidomycosis of Prostate
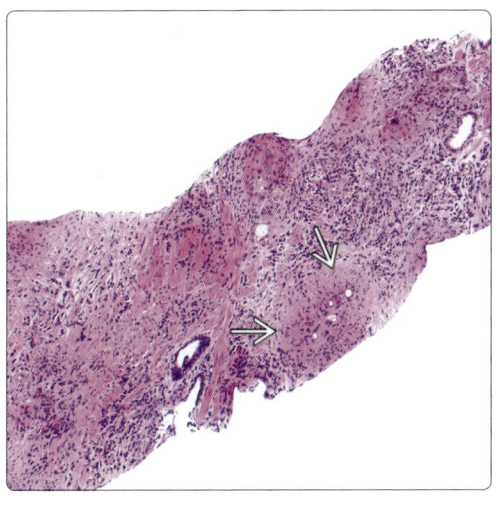

Coccidioides, PAS Stain
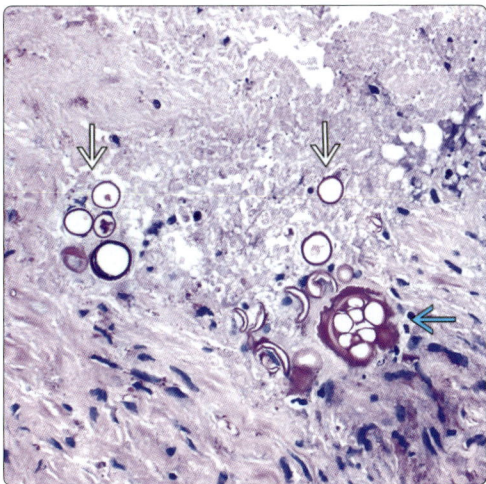

(Left) This biopsy demonstrates IGP due to disseminated infection from Coccidioides immitis. In this example, a tight noncaseating epithelioid granuloma is seen in the background of a prostate biopsy showing atrophy and active chronic inflammation. The granuloma contains several spherules of Coccidioides ➡. (Right) In this caseating granuloma, spherules of Coccidioides ➡, including an enlarged spherule with endospore formation ➡, are highlighted by PAS stain.

Prostate Hyperplasia

KEY FACTS

TERMINOLOGY
- Nodular prostate enlargement due to cellular proliferation of prostatic glands and stroma associated with lower urinary tract symptoms (LUTS)

CLINICAL ISSUES
- A leading cause of morbidity in elderly men
- Seen in 50% of men in their 50s, up to 80-90% of men in their 70s and 80s
- Most common noncancerous cause of serum PSA elevation
- Medical therapy is most frequently used approach
- Surgery is more effective in terms of controlling LUTS
- Without associated LUTS, features of glandular and stromal proliferation in needle biopsies should **not** be labeled as benign prostatic hyperplasia (BPH)

MACROSCOPIC
- Hallmark of BPH is nodular prostatic enlargement
- Hyperplastic nodules are mainly centered on proximal prostatic urethra involving transition zone and submucosal compartment

MICROSCOPIC
- Epithelial predominant hyperplasia shows nodules composed of tightly clustered expanded ductal acinar elements
- Stromal predominant hyperplasia composed of bland spindle cells with little cytoplasm and plump nuclei seen surrounding small blood vessels
- Morphologic variants: Small glandular, cribriform, basal cell, leiomyomatous nodule, and phyllodes-type hyperplasia
- Differential diagnosis for epithelial hyperplasia: Pseudohyperplastic variant of acinar carcinoma, atypical adenomatous hyperplasia
- Differential diagnosis for stromal hyperplasia: Specialized stromal tumors of prostate, smooth muscle tumors, solitary fibrous tumors

Prostate Hyperplasia
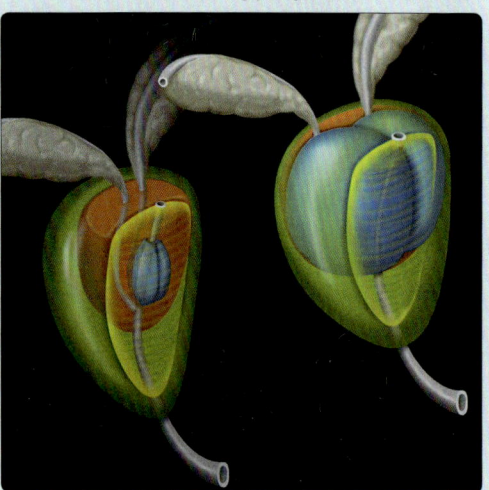

Prostate Hyperplasia
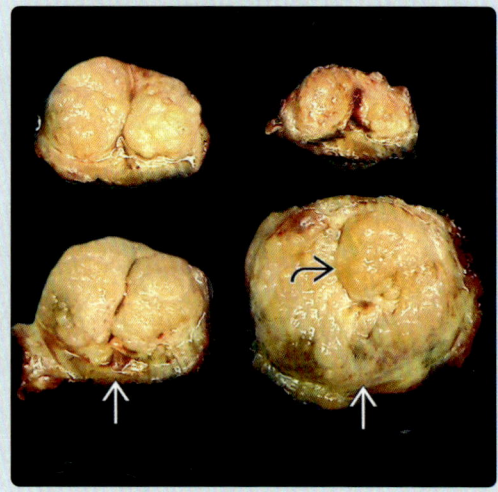

(Left) Graphic compares normal prostate (left) and BPH (right), which shows enlargement of prostatic transition zone (blue). BPH mainly involves transition zone and submucosal compartment around proximal prostatic urethra. (Right) Cross section of BPH shows marked nodular enlargement of transition zone compressing the prostatic urethra ⇨ that results in bladder-obstructive symptoms. Peripheral zone ⇨ is compressed and attenuated by the hyperplastic transition zone, causing secondary diffuse atrophy.

Hyperplastic Nodule
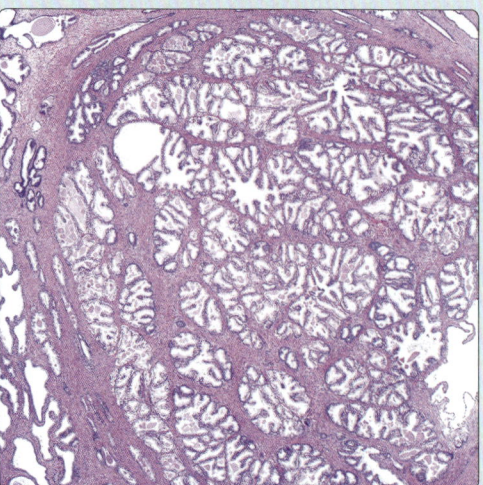

Hyperplastic Glands
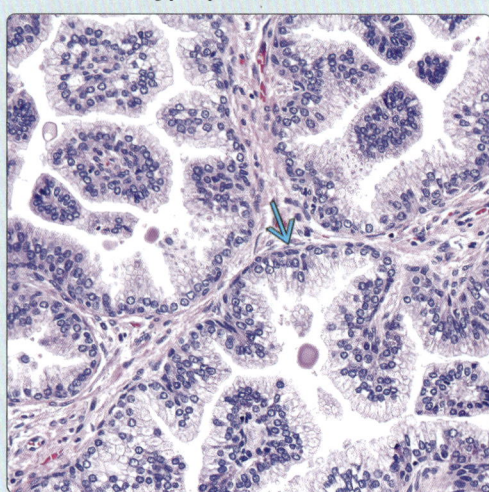

(Left) Low-power view shows a well-circumscribed, proliferative nodule composed of medium to large glands with complex architecture. There is compression of glands immediately surrounding the hyperplastic nodule. (Right) Hyperplastic glands exhibit luminal undulations and papillary infoldings and are lined by columnar cells with clear to pale cytoplasm. The nuclei are regular with open chromatin and often show stratification. The basal cell layer is easily discernible ⇨. The stroma between glands shows bland spindle cells.

Prostate Hyperplasia

TERMINOLOGY

Abbreviations
- Benign prostatic hyperplasia (BPH)

Synonyms
- Benign prostatic hypertrophy

Definitions
- Nodular prostate enlargement due to cellular proliferation of prostatic glands and stroma associated with lower urinary tract symptoms (LUTS)

ETIOLOGY/PATHOGENESIS

Origin
- Prostatic glandular hyperplasia
  - Acinar cells and basal cells
- Prostatic stromal hyperplasia
  - Undifferentiated mesenchyme, fibroblasts, and smooth muscle cells

Etiology
- Pathophysiology remains poorly understood
- Hormonal alteration plays central role
  - Cellular accumulation of testosterone, particularly active metabolite dihydrotestosterone (DHT)
  - Castrated patients with BPH experience significant decrease in prostate size
- Known risk factors include aging and family history
- No association with tobacco use, weight, sexual libido, diabetes mellitus, hypertension, or cirrhosis

CLINICAL ISSUES

Epidemiology
- A leading cause of morbidity in elderly men
- Increasing incidence with age, particularly in men > 50 years of age
  - Seen in 50% of men in their 50s and up to 80-90% of men in their 70s and 80s
    - In contrast, seen in only 8% of men in their 40s and rarely in younger men

Site
- Mainly in tissues surrounding proximal prostatic urethra
  - Transition zone, submucosal compartment, specialized mesenchyme of preprostatic sphincter
- Peripheral zone uncommonly involved, reported in 2-15% of prostatectomies

Presentation
- LUTS
  - Obstructive symptoms, such as hesitancy, straining, weak flow, prolonged voiding, retention, and overflow incontinence
  - Irritative symptoms, such as frequency, urgency, nocturia, painful urination, and dribbling
- Digital rectal palpation of enlarged, nodular, often symmetric and rubbery prostate
- No correlation between histology and symptoms
  - Only 50% with histologic disease have clinical prostatic enlargement; 50% of these have symptoms
- Without associated LUTS, features of glandular and stromal proliferation in needle biopsies should not be labeled as BPH

Laboratory Tests
- Most common noncancerous cause of serum PSA elevation

Treatment
- Medical therapy is most frequently used approach
  - α-adrenergic blockers or 5-α-reductase inhibitors
  - 25-30% patients do not respond
- Surgery is more effective in terms of controlling LUTS
  - Transurethral resection of prostate (TURP) is standard surgical procedure
  - Open (simple) prostatectomy for very bulky prostate

Prognosis
- Benign course

IMAGING

General Features
- CT, US, and MR can visualize BPH
- Evidence of urinary retention, dilated bladder, hydroureter, or hydronephrosis in advanced cases

MACROSCOPIC

General Features
- Nodular prostatic enlargement is hallmark of BPH
- Hyperplastic nodules identifiable in prostatic chips or more readily in prostatectomy specimens
  - Vary from millimeters to large bulging masses; sometimes prostate can be massively enlarged
  - Typically firm and white-tan but can be spongy due to cystically dilated glands
- Hyperplastic nodules are mainly centered on proximal prostatic urethra involving submucosal compartment and transition zone
- Hyperplastic transition zone compresses peripheral zone, which can be markedly attenuated or atrophic
- Uncommon peripheral zone hyperplasia more often presents as solitary hyperplastic nodule

Sections to Be Submitted
- TURP specimen
  - For ≤ 12 g, submit entirely (usually 6-8 cassettes)
  - For > 12 g, submit initial 12 g plus 1 cassette for every additional 5 g

MICROSCOPIC

Histologic Features
- Epithelial predominant hyperplasia
  - Proliferative nodules composed of tightly clustered expanded ductal acinar elements
  - Glands are medium to large or sometimes cystically enlarged
  - Enlarged glands usually show architectural complexity and papillary infoldings
  - Distinct acinar and basal cell layers present
  - Acinar cells are usually columnar or cuboidal to flat when cystic

Prostate Hyperplasia

- o Cytoplasm is abundant and pale
- o Nuclei are regular with open chromatin
- **Stromal predominant hyperplasia**
  - o Early stromal nodule seen around urethral submucosal connective tissue
  - o Bland spindle cells with little cytoplasm and plump nuclei containing open chromatin
  - o Contains abundant small capillaries and spindle cells typically condensed around these vessels
  - o Occasionally can be very cellular with dense collagen around small capillaries
  - o Increasing smooth muscle component with increasing nodule size
- **Mixed epithelial and stromal hyperplasia**
  - o Both glandular and stromal proliferations substantially present
- **Special morphologic variants**
  - o Can be seen within overall spectrum of BPH
- **Small glandular hyperplasia**
  - o Composed of proliferation of relatively small glands in fibromuscular stroma
  - o Acinar cells are more cuboidal, and basal cells are more prominent than in usual hyperplasia
- **Cribriform hyperplasia**
  - o Unique form of nodular hyperplasia wherein glandular component is composed of medium to large glands with cribriform architecture
  - o May have clear cytoplasm (clear cell cribriform hyperplasia)
- **Basal cell hyperplasia**
  - o Usually seen, but not exclusively, in cases of BPH
  - o Can also be seen associated with glandular atrophy, typically involving peripheral zone, in setting of androgen ablation therapy
  - o Proliferation can be incomplete (preserving acinar cells) or complete (imparting solid nests)
  - o May have cribriform architecture (adenoid cystic-like hyperplasia)
  - o May undergo squamous metaplasia
  - o May show nuclear atypia (atypical basal cell hyperplasia)
  - o Basal cell markers [p63 or HMCK(34βE12)] helpful in diagnosis of challenging cases
- **Leiomyomatous nodule**
  - o Stromal predominant hyperplasia with prominent smooth muscle component
  - o Unlike leiomyoma, usually small (< 1 cm), blends into surrounding stroma, contains fibroblastic component, and is sometimes multinodular
- **Fibroadenoma-like hyperplasia**
  - o Glandular and stromal proliferations are architecturally arranged to mimic fibroadenoma of breast
- **Phyllodes-type hyperplasia**
  - o Stromal predominant proliferation with cleft-like spaces and intramural stromal projections covered peripherally by glandular epithelium
  - o In contrast to phyllodes-like tumor of prostate, is focal, lacks significant atypia, and seen in background of BPH

ANCILLARY TESTS

Immunohistochemistry
- Reactivity similar to normal benign glands
- Not routinely needed for diagnosis

DIFFERENTIAL DIAGNOSIS

Pseudohyperplastic Variant of Acinar Adenocarcinoma
- Large, dilated glands ± papillary fronds
- Single cells with basally aligned nuclei and prominent nucleoli
- Lumina often contain amorphous eosinophilic secretions and variable crystalloids
- Often associated with conventional adenocarcinoma at periphery

Atypical Adenomatous Hyperplasia
- Differential diagnosis for small glandular hyperplasia in limited sample, such as needle biopsy
- No associated stromal proliferation
- Less uniform glands with presence of parent duct

Specialized Stromal Tumors of Prostate
- **Stromal tumors of uncertain malignant potential**
  - o Diagnosis may be made when sampling is limited
  - o Hypercellular stroma that often shows degenerate-type nuclear atypia
  - o May be admixed with benign glands, with myxoid change, or with phyllodes-type pattern
  - o Lacks typical intermixed small blood vessels; may lack multinodularity of BPH
- **Stromal sarcoma**
  - o Shows greater degree of cellularity, significant atypia, increased mitosis, and presence of necrosis

Smooth Muscle Tumors
- Differential diagnosis for hyperplastic leiomyomatous nodule
- Leiomyoma is more cellular, lacks stromal vessels, and occurs without background BPH
- Leiomyosarcoma contains significant cytologic atypia that is often high grade with increased mitotic activity and shows coagulative necrosis

Solitary Fibrous Tumor of Prostate
- Uniform bland spindle cells with haphazard patternless pattern, dense ropey collagen, more variable cellularity, and staghorn vessels
- Borderline and malignant cases with increasing cellularity, mitotic activity, presence of necrosis, and infiltrative growth
- Positive for CD34, Bcl-2, and CD99

SELECTED REFERENCES

1. Bechis SK et al: Personalized medicine for the management of benign prostatic hyperplasia. J Urol. 192(1):16-23, 2014
2. Viglione MP et al: Should the diagnosis of benign prostatic hyperplasia be made on prostate needle biopsy?. Hum Pathol. 33(8):796-800, 2002

Prostate Hyperplasia

Prostate Hyperplasia on CT

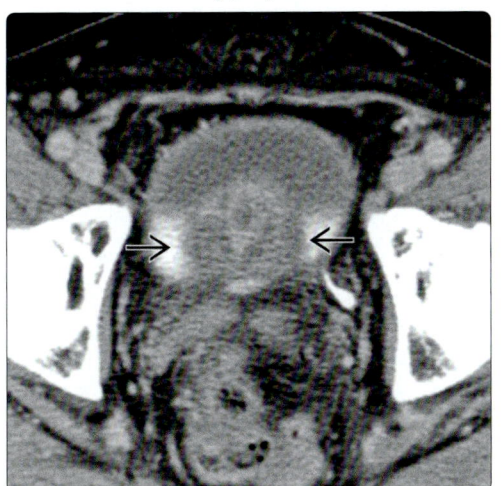

Prostate Hyperplasia

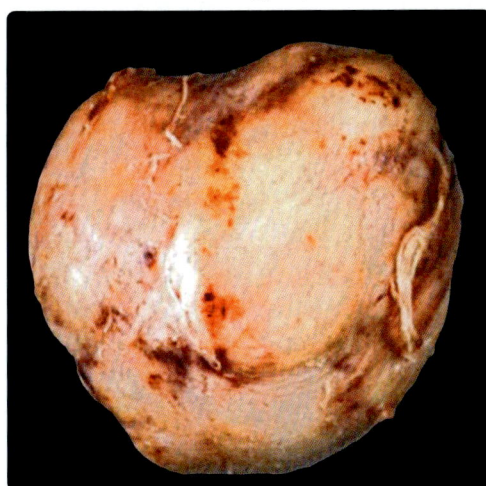

(Left) Axial CECT shows BPH. Note medial lobe hypertrophy of prostate pressing on the base of the bladder ➡. Advanced BPH may show evidence of urinary retention and dilated bladder. Pathologic diagnosis of BPH, particularly in limited samples, requires clinical correlation and must be reserved in absence of lower urinary tract symptoms (LUTS). *(Right)* BPH shows an asymmetrically enlarged prostate due to bulging hyperplastic nodules as seen from external surface. The prostate may be massively enlarged in BPH.

Hyperplastic Nodules

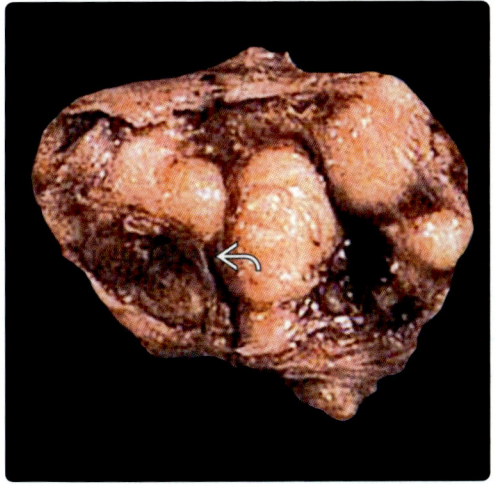

Epithelial Predominant Hyperplasia

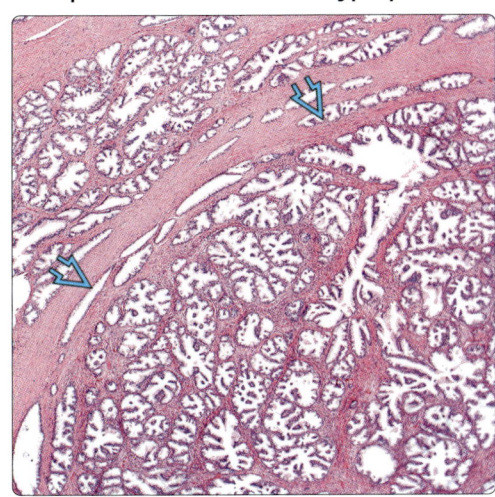

(Left) Cross section of prostate with BPH shows multiple bulging hyperplastic nodules in transition zone compressing prostatic urethra ➡. BPH commonly presents with multiple macro- and microscopic hyperplastic nodules that vary in size. Uncommon peripheral zone hyperplasia more often presents with solitary nodule. *(Right)* Epithelial predominant hyperplastic nodule ➡ shows well-circumscribed expansile cluster of medium to large complex glands. Note the stroma within the nodule is more cellular.

Hyperplastic Glands

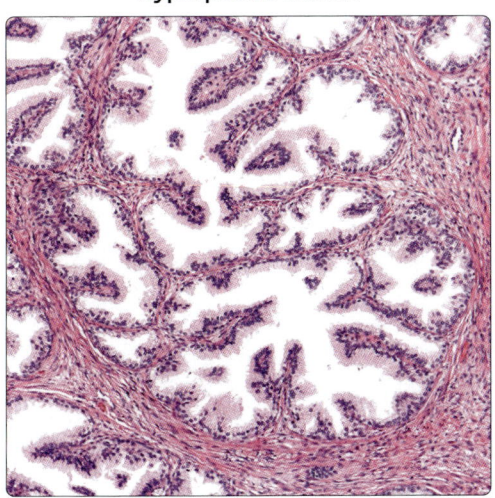

Hyperplastic Glands

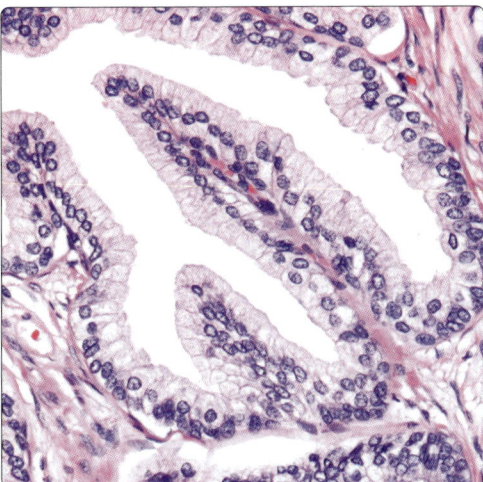

(Left) Hyperplastic glands typically show papillary infoldings imparting inverted image of luminal branchings. Stromal cells follow the contour of hyperplastic glands. *(Right)* BPH gland shows columnar cells with abundant pale to clear cytoplasm and round nuclei with open chromatin. Nucleoli are not prominent. Architecture mimics normal central zone glands and high-grade prostatic intraepithelial neoplasia (HGPIN) glands. Central zone glands are less crowded, and HGPIN contains greater nuclear atypia.

Prostate Hyperplasia

Stromal Hyperplasia

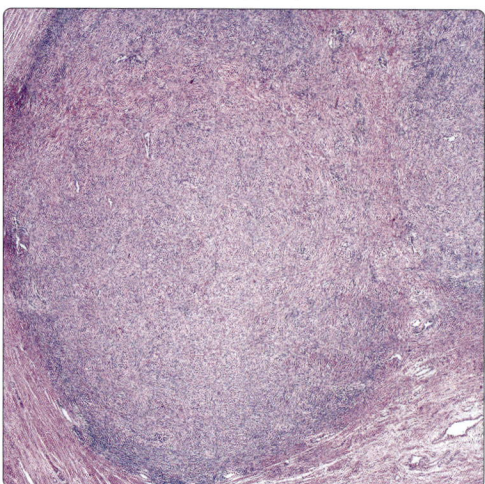

Stromal Hyperplasia

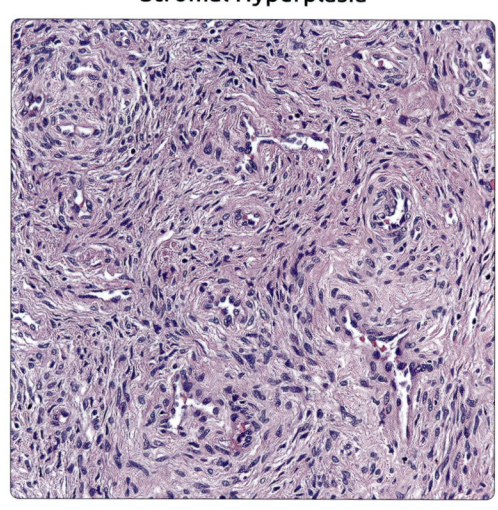

(Left) Circumscribed stromal predominant hyperplastic nodule shows sheets of spindle cells containing abundant capillaries dispersed throughout the stroma. (Right) High-power magnification of stromal-predominant hyperplasia shows bland spindle cells often condensed around small blood vessels following their contour. These small blood vessels are not typically seen in STUMP, a main differential diagnosis. In contrast to BPH, STUMP is often solitary and involves both peripheral and transition zones.

Early Stromal Hyperplasia

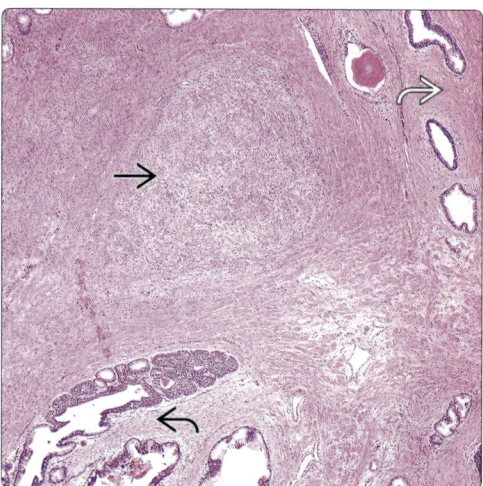

Stromal Hyperplasia

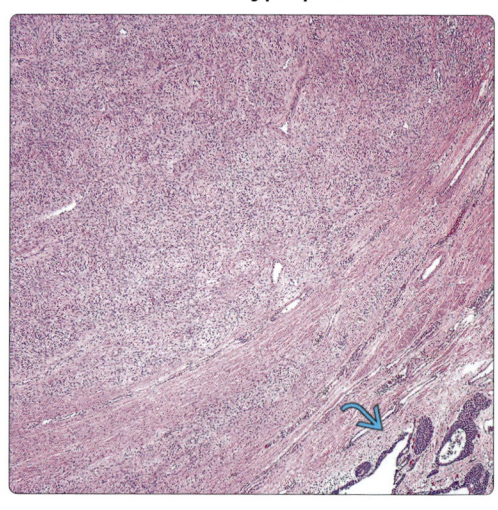

(Left) An early stromal nodule ➡ is seen in submucosal compartment of proximal urethra ➡ adjoining the transition zone ➡, a.k.a. estrogen-sensitive zone. (Right) A large stromal nodule is shown adjacent to and compressing the prostatic urethra ➡. BPH nodules are believed to begin as pure stromal nodules and later acquire epithelial component with growth. Proximity of proximal prostatic urethra results in obstruction and LUTS with nodule enlargement.

Leiomyomatous Stromal Hyperplasia

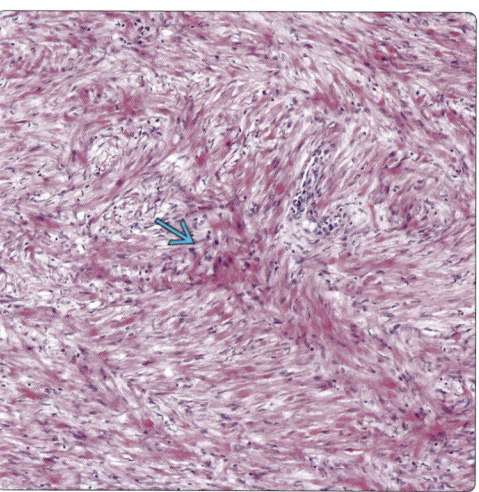

Stromal and Glandular Hyperplasia

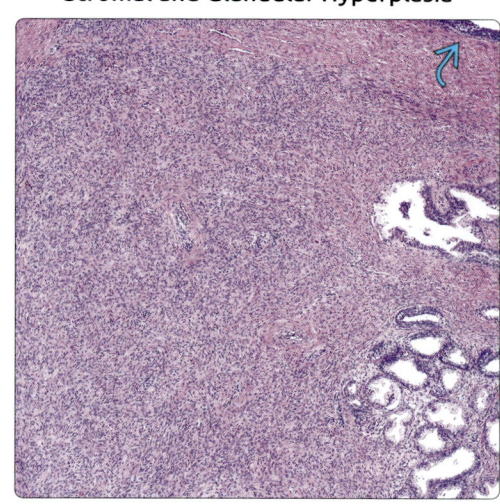

(Left) Stromal-predominant hyperplastic nodule shows myoid component ➡ admixed with stromal elements. Myoid component usually becomes much more prominent with increasing size of the hyperplastic nodule. Occasionally, myoid component may become abundant, imparting myomatous appearance. (Right) Hyperplastic nodule with substantial proliferation of stromal and glandular elements is seen adjacent to prostatic urethra ➡. Note the small blood vessels within the hyperplastic stroma.

Prostate Hyperplasia

Hyperplastic Nodule in TURP

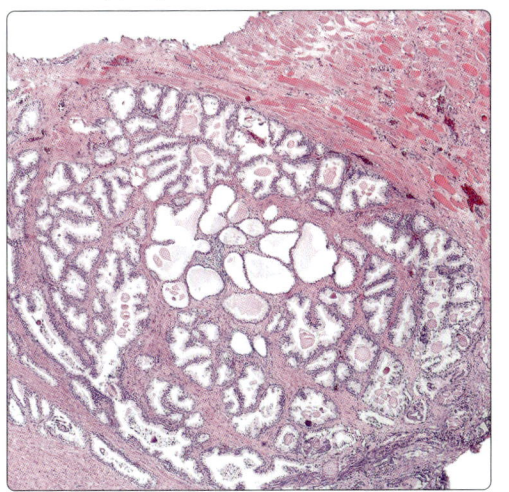

Hyperplastic Nodule in TURP

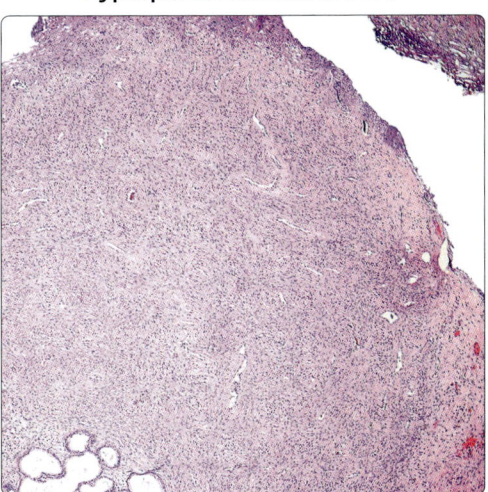

(Left) TURP chip shows an epithelial-predominant hyperplastic nodule adjacent to skeletal muscles situated anterior to the transition zone. **(Right)** TURP chip shows a stromal-predominant hyperplastic nodule. In limited samples, pathologic diagnosis of BPH requires clinical evidence of LUTS. Unlike in needle biopsy containing epithelial &/or stromal proliferation, pathologic diagnosis of BPH is readily rendered in TURP specimens since TURP is performed as therapeutic procedure for clinically diagnosed BPH.

Secondary Atrophy of Peripheral Zone

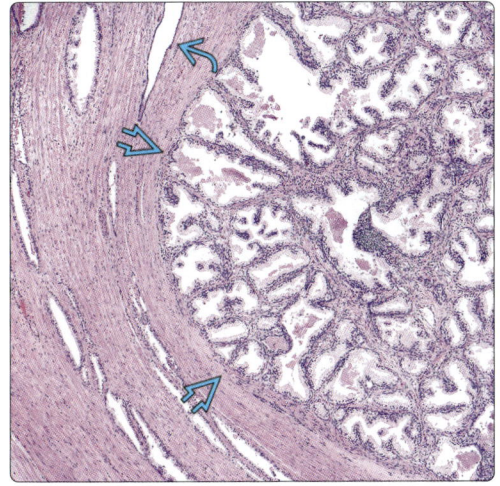

Hyperplastic Nodule Extending to Bladder

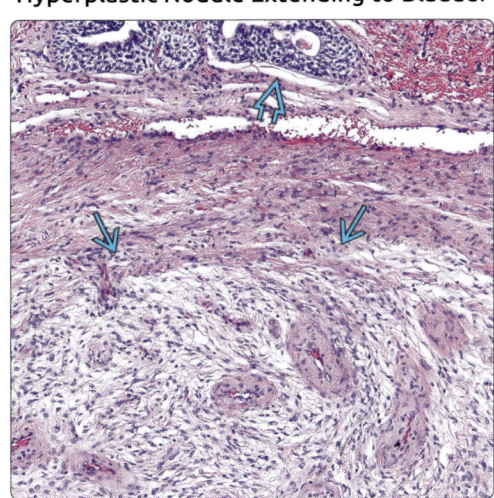

(Left) BPH nodule arising from transition zone ⇨ shows compression with secondary atrophy of the surrounding peripheral zone ⇨. The hyperplastic glands are much larger, showing luminal undulations and papillary infoldings, and the hyperplastic stroma is denser compared with peripheral zone. **(Right)** This hyperplastic nodule ⇨ is seen close to the urothelial surface of the bladder neck ⇨. BPH may sometimes extend into the bladder outlet and protrudes into the bladder lumina (median lobe).

Small Glandular Hyperplasia

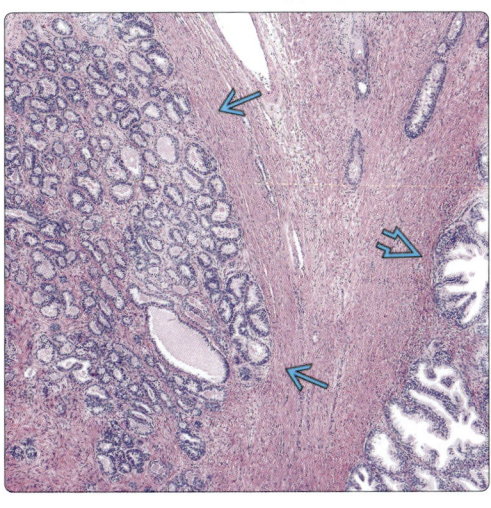

Small Glandular Hyperplasia

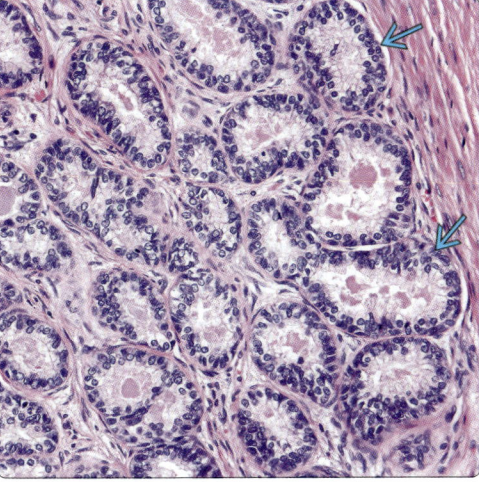

(Left) Small-gland hyperplasia ⇨ shows a well-defined proliferation of relatively small-sized crowded glands adjacent to usual epithelial-predominant hyperplasia ⇨. Small glandular hyperplasia exhibits crowding and may mimic AAH. AAH has no associated stromal proliferation, often contains parent duct, and occurs with or without background BPH. **(Right)** Small-gland hyperplasia shows relatively more cuboidal secretory cells and prominent basal cells ⇨. Note the hyperplastic stroma between the glands.

Prostate Hyperplasia

Cribriform Hyperplasia

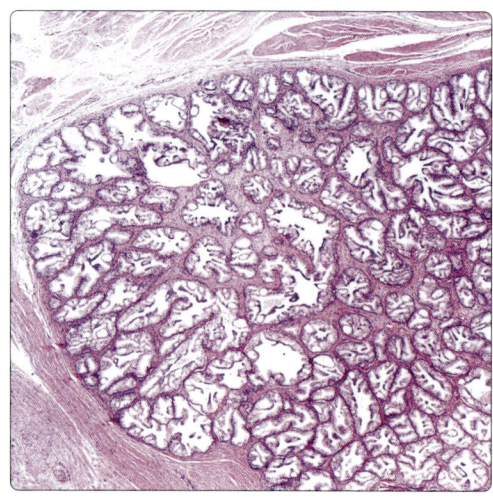

Cribriform Hyperplasia

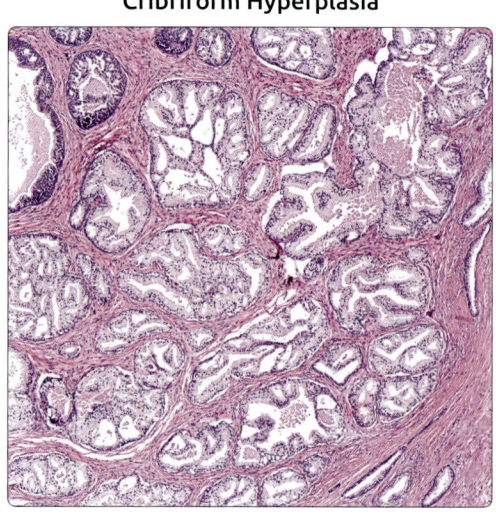

(Left) Cribriform hyperplasia shows a dense nodular cluster of complex glands showing cribriform architecture and papillary infoldings. *(Right)* Cribriform hyperplasia composed of large glands shows distinctive cribriform or "Roman bridging" architecture. The glandular complexity may mimic cribriform acinar adenocarcinoma, ductal carcinoma, and HGPIN. In contrast, cribriform hyperplasia lacks cytologic atypia or other features associated with malignant glands.

Cribriform Hyperplasia

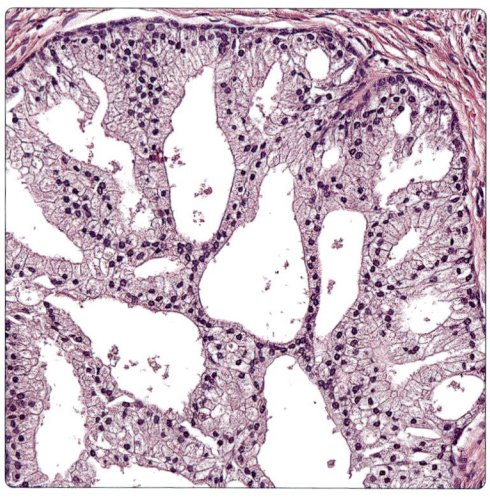

Basal Cell Hyperplasia

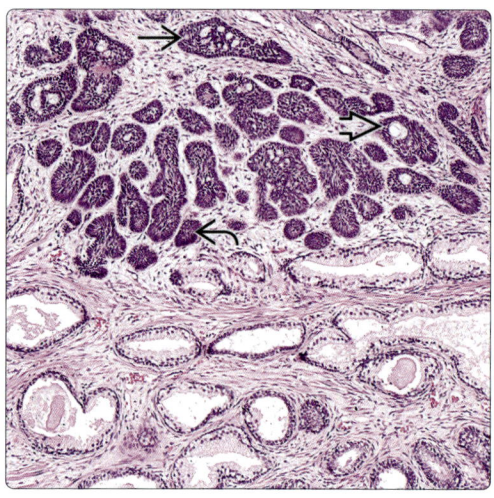

(Left) Cribriform hyperplasia gland shows bland acinar cells with abundant pale to clear cytoplasm and round, regular nuclei lacking atypia. Presence of pale cytoplasm is often distinctive (clear cell cribriform hyperplasia). Note the prominent basal cell layer. *(Right)* Basal cell hyperplasia may be seen uncommonly within spectrum of BPH. Basal cell proliferation is either complete ⇒, imparting solid nests, or incomplete ⇒, retaining lumen. Rarely, cribriform pattern ⇒ may be seen (adenoid cystic-like hyperplasia).

Basal Cell Hyperplasia

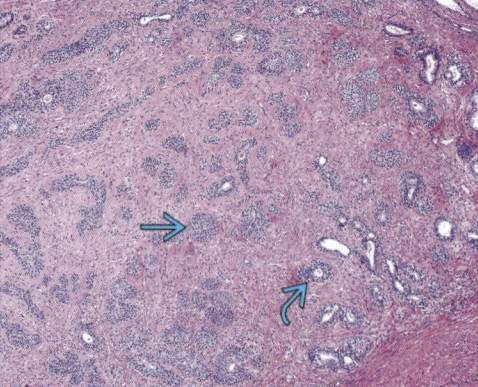

Basal Cell Hyperplasia

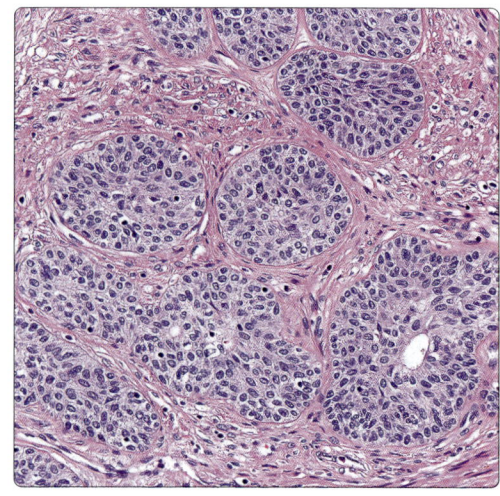

(Left) Low-power view of basal cell hyperplasia shows nodular proliferation consisting of admixture of complete ⇒ and incomplete ⇒ basal cell nests. *(Right)* Basal cell hyperplasia shows proliferation of basaloid cells with high nuclear:cytoplasmic ratio. Basal cell hyperplasia when exuberant may mimic basal cell carcinoma (BCC). In contrast to BCC, basal cell hyperplasia exhibits lobular growth and lacks invasive features. Basal cell hyperplasia and BCC have similar immunostaining pattern.

Prostate Hyperplasia

Basal Cell Hyperplasia With Squamous Metaplasia

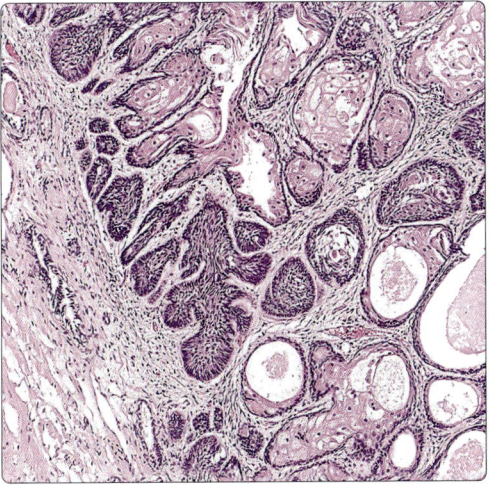

Basal Cell Hyperplasia With Squamous Metaplasia

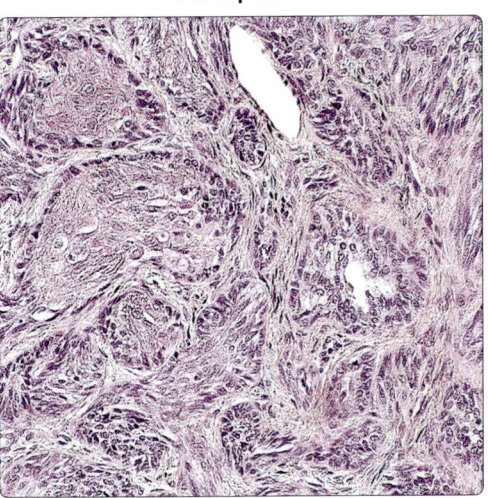

(Left) Basal cell hyperplasia with squamous metaplasia shows some nests containing squamous cells with abundant glassy cytoplasm surrounded peripherally by basal cells. Some cellular nests contain central lumen, and some contain pure basal cell hyperplasia. (Right) Basal cell hyperplasia with squamous metaplasia shows transition of centrally placed squamous cells and peripherally situated basal cells. Squamous cells lack cytologic atypia or mitosis. Squamous cell metaplasia arises from the proliferative basal cells.

Fibroadenoma-Like Hyperplasia

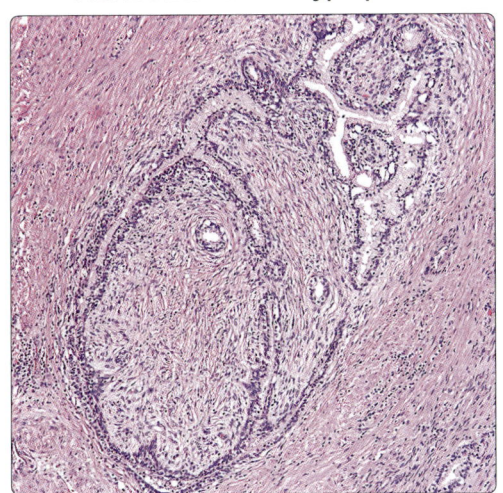

Phyllodes-Type Hyperplasia

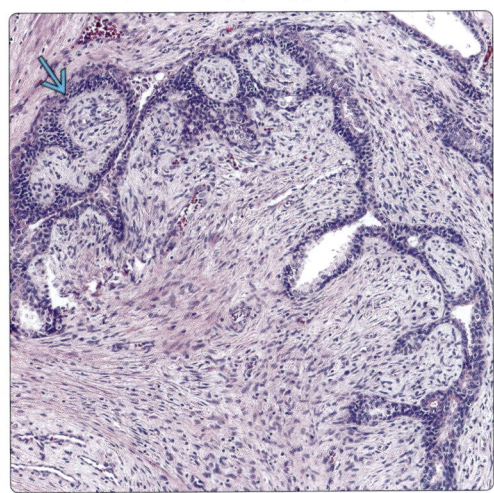

(Left) Fibroadenoma-like hyperplasia shows stromal proliferation surrounding compressed hyperplastic acini, which morphologically mimics mammary fibroadenoma. The spindle and epithelial cells have bland cytology. This process is typically focal and seen in background of BPH. (Right) Phyllodes-type hyperplasia shows stromal proliferation with cleft-like spaces and intramural stromal projections surrounded by glandular epithelium ➡. This is often focal and lacks atypia in contrast to phyllodes-like tumor of the prostate.

Leiomyomatous Hyperplasia

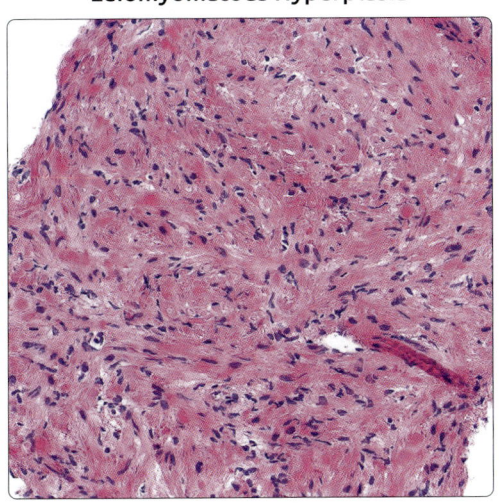

HMCK in Basal Cell Hyperplasia

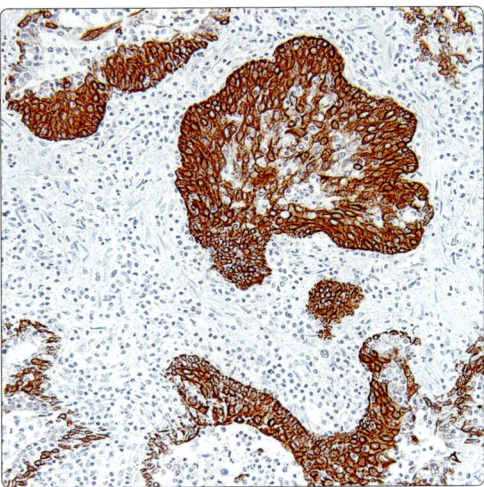

(Left) Leiomyomatous hyperplasia in prostate biopsy shows prominent myoid elements admixed with stromal cells. Distinction from benign smooth muscle tumor may be difficult. Leiomyomatous hyperplasia is less cellular, may contain abundant small stromal vessels, and may have background typical stromal &/or epithelial hyperplasia. (Right) Basal cell hyperplasia shows basal cells diffusely positive for HMCK(34βE12). Central acinar cells are negative. Basal cells are negative for PSA and PAP.

Adenosis

KEY FACTS

TERMINOLOGY
- Atypical adenomatous hyperplasia (AAH)
- Small- to medium-sized acinar proliferation usually forming well-circumscribed nodule in prostate transition zone
- Does not fulfill cytologic criteria of carcinoma and possesses basal cell layer

CLINICAL ISSUES
- Evidence (weak) suggests that AAH may represent preneoplastic entity, particularly for low-grade, transition zone adenocarcinoma
- Comes to attention in routine practice as prostate cancer mimic in needle biopsy or TURP

MICROSCOPIC
- Well-circumscribed proliferation of small- to medium-sized glands in transition zone
- Usually mixed with typical hyperplastic nodules

- Variable size and shape of glands; similar cytology of surrounding hyperplastic glands
- More dilated parent gland may be centrally located
- Some peripheral AAH glands minimally infiltrate surrounding stroma but tend to merge with adjacent benign glands
- Acinar cells with clear cytoplasm, round uniform nuclei with inconspicuous nucleoli
- Fragmented basal cell layer, often requires immunostains for detection

ANCILLARY TESTS
- Basal cell markers frequently show discontinuous basal cell layer
- AMACR is focally positive in 7% and may be diffusely positive in up to 10% of cases
- ERG immunostain is typically negative
- In sclerotic variant (sclerosing adenosis), basal cells may stain with myoepithelial markers (S100, calponin)

Histochemistry

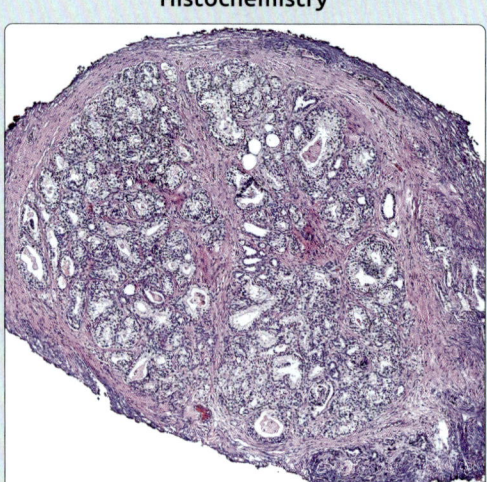

Immunohistochemistry

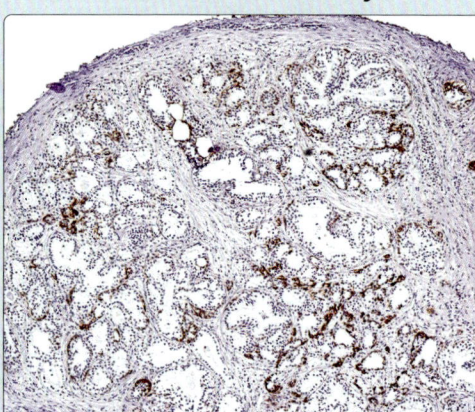

(Left) Atypical adenomatous hyperplasia (AAH) in TURP chip shows a well-circumscribed nodule of small acinar proliferation containing glands of variable size and shape. Most AAH are encountered in TURP specimens since the majority of these lesions arise in the transition zone. A low-grade prostate adenocarcinoma is the main differential diagnosis on low-power magnification. (Right) AAH typically shows patchy positivity with HMCK(34βE12), which is typical for this lesion.

Centrally Dilated Gland

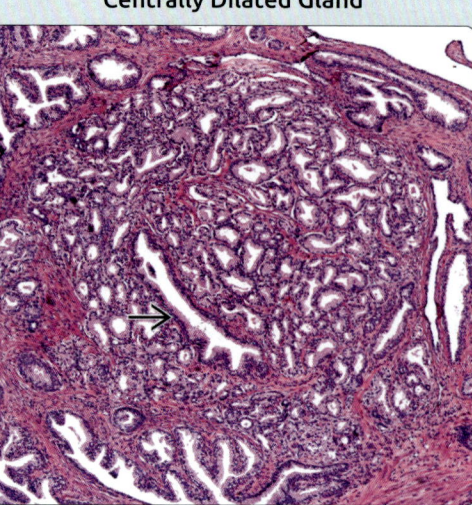

Panoramic View

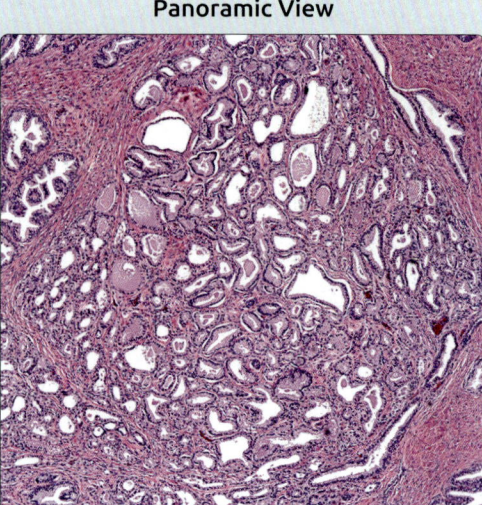

(Left) Adenosis (AAH) shows relatively well-circumscribed proliferation of variably sized acini. Note the presence of a larger parent duct ➡ in the central aspect of the lesion. The background is that of a BPH. (Right) Variable size of acini is a key low-power feature of AAH. The overall circumscribed architecture raises concern for low-grade carcinoma. Some experts propose that some of the original Gleason pattern 1 or 2 tumors may have represented AAH.

Adenosis

TERMINOLOGY

Synonyms
- Atypical adenomatous hyperplasia (AAH)
  - 1994 consensus statement by expert GU pathologists recommended use of term AAH
  - Both AAH and adenosis are used interchangeably

Definitions
- Small- to medium-sized acinar proliferation usually forming well-circumscribed nodule in transition zone of prostate
  - Basal cells are present, and cytologic criteria of carcinoma are lacking

CLINICAL ISSUES

Epidemiology
- Incidence
  - Present in 1.5-19.6% of transurethral resections of prostate (TURP) specimens
  - Seen in up to 33% of radical prostatectomies
  - Uncommon in needle core biopsies (< 2%) since transition zone is not often sampled

Presentation
- Asymptomatic, incidental histologic finding

Treatment
- No treatment is currently warranted

Prognosis
- Weak evidence suggests AAH may represent preneoplastic entity, particularly for low-grade, transition zone adenocarcinoma
- Evidence is circumstantial, mostly based on morphologic findings and little molecular or clinical supporting data

MICROSCOPIC

Histologic Features
- On low power, AHH is relatively well circumscribed, consists of small- to medium-sized glands in transition zone, usually mixed with typical hyperplastic nodules
- Some peripheral AAH glands minimally infiltrate surrounding stroma, merge with adjacent benign glands
- More dilated parent gland may be centrally located
- Variable size and shape of glands, with similar cytology of surrounding hyperplastic glands
- Acinar cells with clear cytoplasm, round uniform nuclei, and inconspicuous nucleoli
- Fragmented basal cell layer, often requires immunostains for detection; some glands may completely lack basal cell layer
- Occasionally crystalloids, amorphous eosinophilic secretions, corpora amylacea, or mucin may be found intraluminally

Predominant Pattern/Injury Type
- Hyperplasia

Predominant Cell/Compartment Type
- Epithelial, glandular

ANCILLARY TESTS

Immunohistochemistry
- Basal cell markers: p63, HMCK(34βE12), and CK5/6
- AMACR focally positive (can rarely be diffusely positive)
- ERG immunostain is typically negative

DIFFERENTIAL DIAGNOSIS

Benign Prostatic Hyperplasia
- Benign prostatic hyperplasia nodules are better circumscribed with no peripheral infiltration by glands
- Glands are larger with papillary infoldings and consistent double cell layer

Sclerosing Adenosis
- Associated with dense fibrotic cellular stroma
- Thickened basement membrane or hyalinized stroma around glands may be present
- Poorly formed budding glands and individual cells
- Basal cell layer usually easy to recognize, may stain with myoepithelial markers (S100, calponin)

Mesonephric Remnants
- Presence of colloid material within lumina
- Less nodular, more haphazardly arranged

Low-Grade Acinar Adenocarcinoma
- May demonstrate infiltrative growth
- Characteristic cytologic features of carcinoma (macronuclei, multiple nucleoli, amphophilic cytoplasm)
- Absent basal cell layer (confirmed by immunostains in difficult or ambiguous cases)

DIAGNOSTIC CHECKLIST

Pathologic Interpretation Pearls
- Well-circumscribed proliferation of glands in transition zone frequently seen in TURP specimens, which on close inspection lack cytologic features for cancer
- Immunohistochemistry shows discontinuous basal cell marker staining and uncommonly may show focal or diffuse AMACR staining

REPORTING

Key Elements to Report
- Absence or presence of coexistent adenocarcinoma
- Not required to include AAH in final diagnosis report

SELECTED REFERENCES

1. Humphrey PA: Atypical adenomatous hyperplasia (adenosis) of the prostate. J Urol. 188(6):2371-2, 2012
2. Srigley JR: Benign mimickers of prostatic adenocarcinoma. Mod Pathol. 17(3):328-48, 2004
3. Yang XJ et al: Expression of alpha-Methylacyl-CoA racemase (P504S) in atypical adenomatous hyperplasia of the prostate. Am J Surg Pathol. 26(7):921-5, 2002
4. Epstein JI: Adenosis (atypical adenomatous hyperplasia): histopathology and relationship to carcinoma. Pathol Res Pract. 191(9):888-98, 1995
5. Bostwick DG et al: Consensus statement on terminology: recommendation to use atypical adenomatous hyperplasia in place of adenosis of the prostate. Am J Surg Pathol. 18(10):1069-70, 1994
6. Bostwick DG et al: Atypical adenomatous hyperplasia of the prostate: morphologic criteria for its distinction from well-differentiated carcinoma. Hum Pathol. 24(8):819-32, 1993

Adenosis

(Left) The peripheral small acini show a crowded pattern and bland cytology (nucleomegaly and prominent nucleoli are absent). Distinction may be difficult if the entire lesion (boundaries) is not visualized. **(Right)** Intraluminal proteinaceous material and crystalloids may occasionally be seen in AAH. The presence of both these features in atypical glands compounds the diagnostic difficulty (vs. cancer). Use of pertinent immunostains is often necessary in challenging cases.

Histochemistry
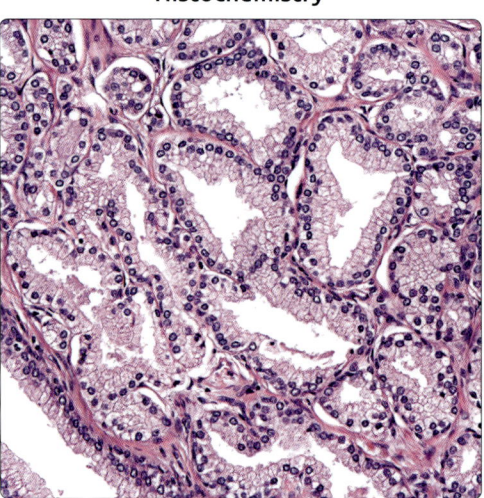

Luminal Contents
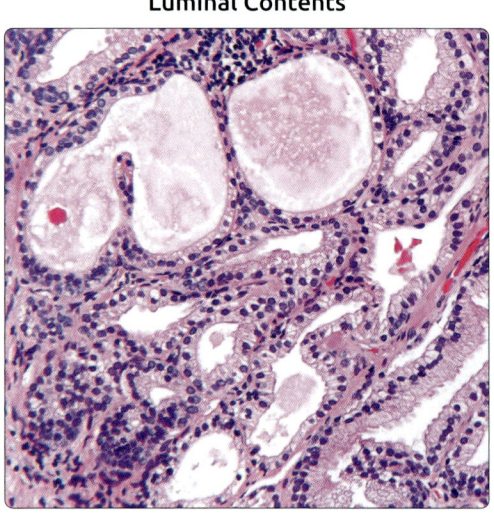

(Left) Some AAH glands may show rigid configuration ➡ and uniformity of caliber closely mimicking cancer. However, other glands in the same focus vary considerably in size and shape. This feature along with overall nodularity would suggest AAH. **(Right)** Crystalloids are not infrequently present in AAH. However, the glandular cells lack the cellular atypia and prominent nucleoli of adenocarcinoma. Basal cells ➡ are discernible on H&E stain in this particular example.

Histochemistry
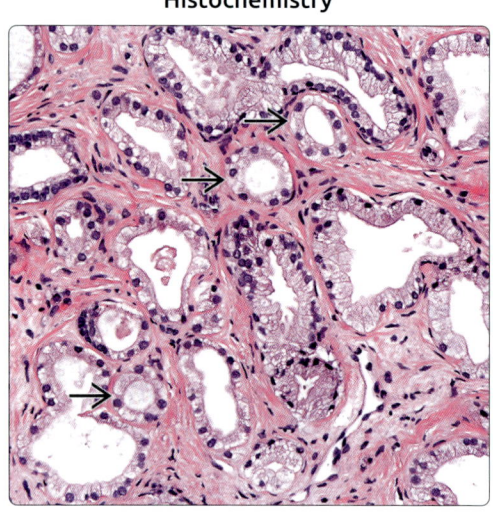

Intraluminal Crystalloids
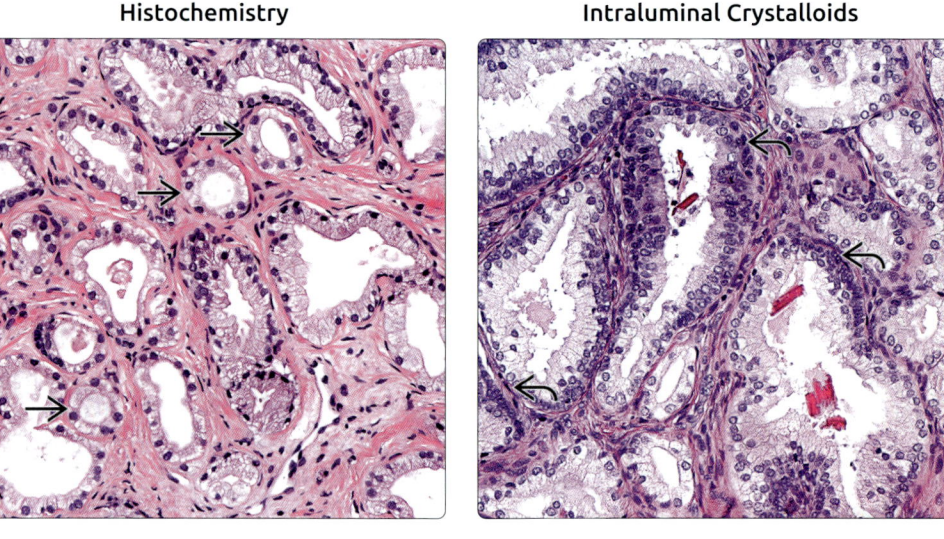

(Left) The peripheral aspect of AAH shows small atypical glands, which may mimic microacinar adenocarcinoma. Lack of cytologic features of malignancy is helpful in the diagnosis, but immunostains are often needed to differentiate the 2 entities. **(Right)** Staining for basal-associated markers HMCK (34βE12) and p63 as well as AMACR shows discontinuous basal cell layer ➡ and overexpression of AMACR. Immunostaining must be evaluated in aggregate and not for individual acini.

Glandular Atypia
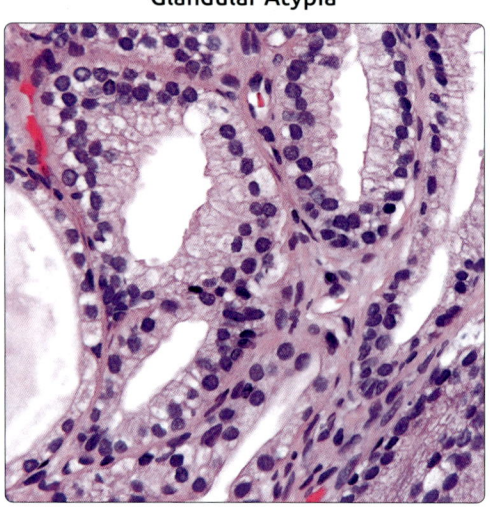

Immunostain Cocktail
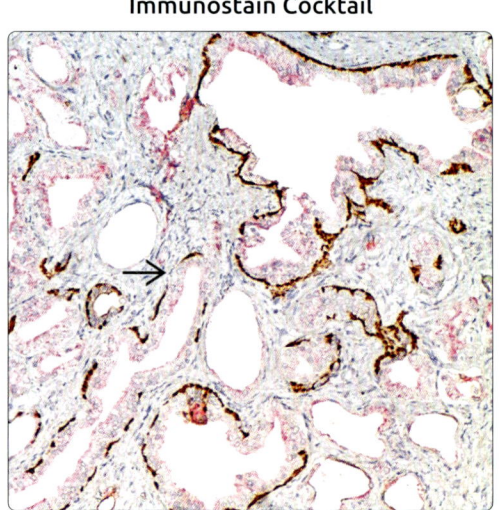

Adenosis

Circumscribed Border
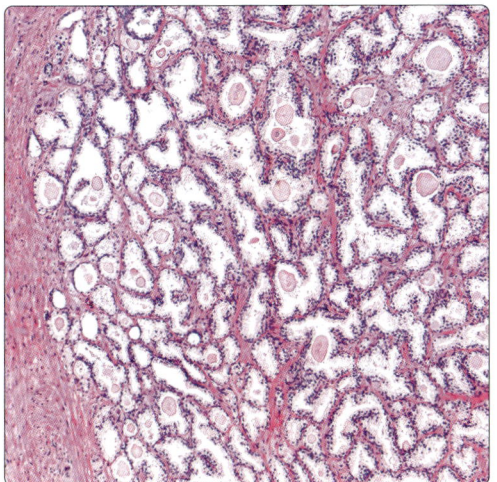

Sclerosing Adenosis
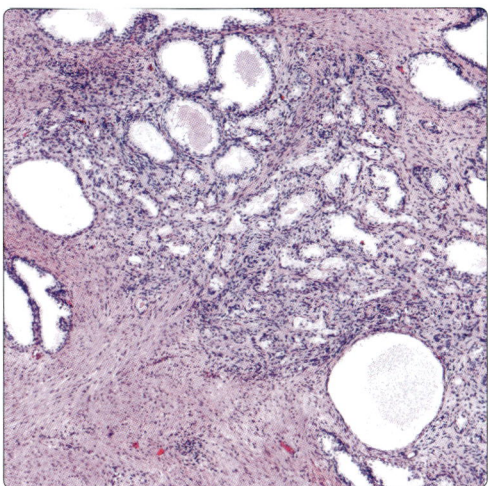

(Left) Low-power view of AAH shows a relatively well-circumscribed border without infiltration or other atypical features. The glands are back to back with very little intervening stroma. *(Right)* This lesion consists of irregular glands that are haphazardly arranged and surrounded by hypercellular stroma of spindle cells. The lesion appears to be infiltrating at the edges. Both sclerosing adenosis and AAH are benign, and most are in the spectrum of BPH.

Clear Cells
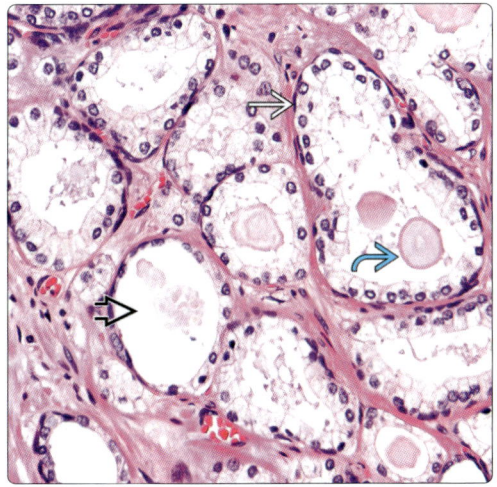

Immunostain Cocktail
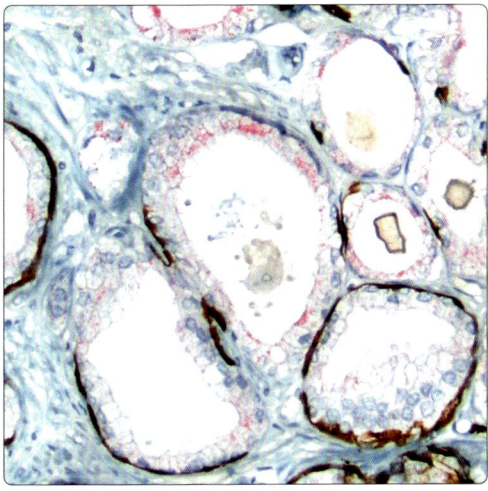

(Left) The glands in this high-power view are back to back and consist of bland-looking cells with clear cytoplasm. Basal cells can be appreciated ➡. Note the presence of intraluminal secretions ➡ and corpora amylacea ➡. *(Right)* This field shows back-to-back glands of AAH with discontinuous basal cells and overexpression of AMACR. This immunoprofile is common in many AAH lesions and essentially rules out the malignant diagnosis.

Sclerosing Adenosis: Immunostain Cocktail
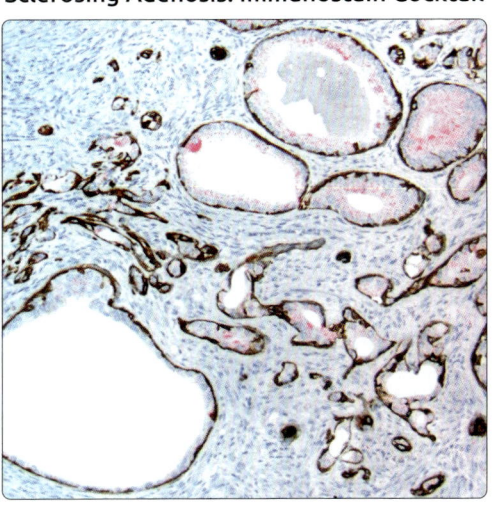

Sclerosing Adenosis: S100
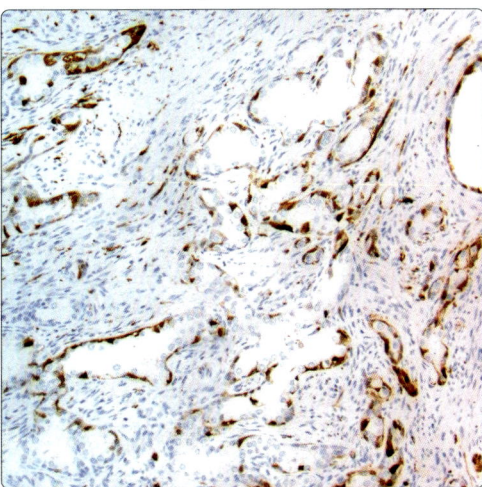

(Left) In this PIN4 cocktail of a sclerosing adenosis lesion, the glands are irregular and haphazardly arranged. The basal cell layer is maintained in most of these glands. AMACR is overexpressed in most glands. Note the hypercellular stroma surrounding the glands. *(Right)* S100 immunostain in sclerosing adenosis highlights the basal cells, which also acquired a myoepithelial phenotype. The same cells were also positive for calponin (another myoepithelial marker).

Atrophy and Its Variants

KEY FACTS

TERMINOLOGY
- Cellular shrinkage with loss of cytoplasmic volume of prostatic ductal acinar unit and surrounding stroma

CLINICAL ISSUES
- Frequency increases with age; more common after 6th decade of life
- Remarkable in routine practice as morphologic mimicker of adenocarcinoma in prostate biopsy

MICROSCOPIC
- Most commonly involves peripheral zone
- All patterns of atrophy are characterized by acinar cells with scant cytoplasm producing higher nuclear:cytoplasmic ratio
- Glands contain crowded and hyperchromatic nuclei, imparting more basophilic appearance
- Atrophy may be diffuse or widespread; linked to aging, androgen deprivation, and radiotherapy
- Main morphologic types of focal atrophy include simple atrophy (SA), SA with cyst formation, postatrophic hyperplasia (PAH), and partial atrophy (PA)
- SA consists of atrophic acini that are spaced relatively similarly to normal glands
- SA with cyst formation shows cystic dilatation of atrophic acini
- PAH consists of proliferative atrophic acini arranged in lobules, often surrounding central larger dilated duct
- Unlike other forms of atrophy, PA contains relatively modest amount of pale or clear cytoplasm and has less crowded nuclei
- Most are positive for basal cell markers; PA and PAH may have patchy or absent staining
- Main differential diagnosis is prostate adenocarcinoma with atrophic features
- PA is common reason for consultations of atypical glands concerning for cancer in biopsies

Simple Atrophy
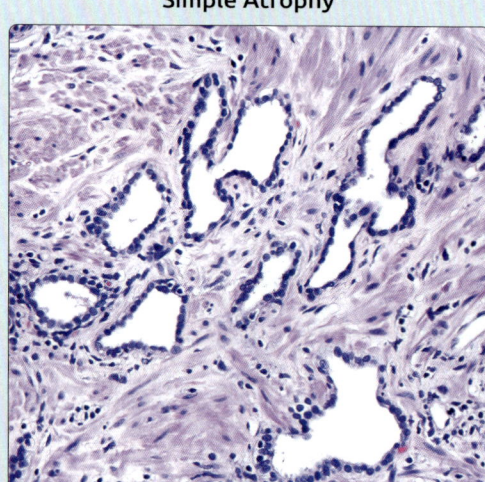

Partial Atrophy
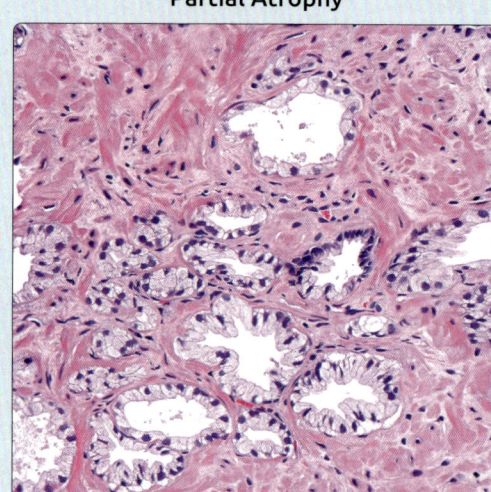

(Left) Simple atrophy (SA) consists of attenuated atrophic acini spaced relatively similarly to normal benign glands. The lumen of acini is usually irregular or angulated. Atrophic glands are characterized by cells with scant cytoplasm that impart basophilic appearance on low magnification. **(Right)** Partial atrophy (PA) is characterized by small glands with irregular lumina and cells with modest pale to clear cytoplasm. PA is 1 of the most common benign reasons for consultation needle biopsies with concern for small cancer focus.

Simple Atrophy With Cyst Formation
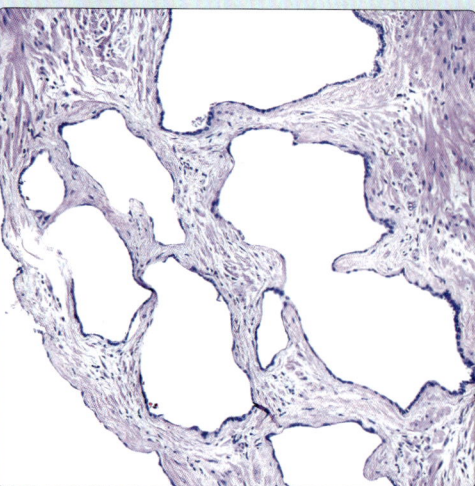

Diffuse Atrophy
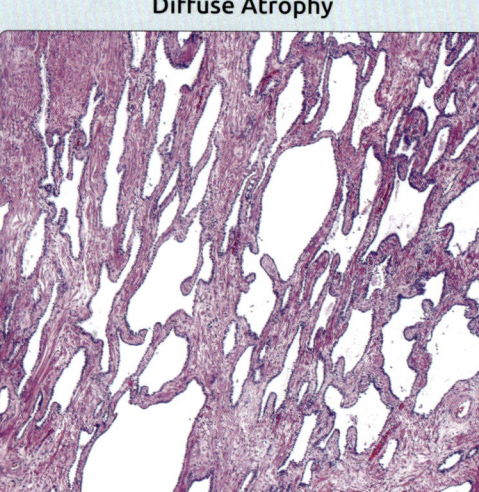

(Left) These atrophic glands are enlarged and cystically dilated, lined mainly by flattened atrophic cells. SA with cyst formation is usually not a diagnostic challenge because it bears no close resemblance to cancer in needle biopsies. **(Right)** Low-power view shows diffuse atrophy of peripheral zone ducts and glands. These ducts and acini maintain their longitudinal axis of orientation in the peripheral zone. Diffuse atrophy of the acini may be caused by hormonal or radiation therapy and is also linked to aging.

Atrophy and Its Variants

TERMINOLOGY

Definitions
- Cellular shrinkage with loss of cytoplasmic volume of prostatic ductal acinar unit and surrounding stroma

ETIOLOGY/PATHOGENESIS

Causes
- Diffuse atrophy linked to aging, androgen deprivation, and radiotherapy
- Secondary compression by benign prostate hyperplasia (BPH) nodule, e.g., peripheral zone atrophy in BPH of transition zone
- End result of severe chronic inflammation (postinflammatory atrophy)
- Chronic local ischemia has also been suggested

CLINICAL ISSUES

Epidemiology
- Very common; seen in 85% of prostates in autopsies of men > 40 years of age
- Frequency increases with age; more common after 6th decade of life

Presentation
- Asymptomatic; incidental histologic finding
- Remarkable in routine practice as morphologic mimicker of adenocarcinoma in prostate biopsy

Prognosis
- Benign course

MICROSCOPIC

Histologic Features
- Characterized by acinar cells with scant cytoplasm imparting higher nuclear:cytoplasmic ratio
- Maintains overall lobular configuration with angular or slit-like glands, occasionally with parent duct
- Glands contain crowded and hyperchromatic nuclei, imparting more basophilic appearance
- Since secretory cells have minimal to no cytoplasm, they resemble basal cells and impart single-cell type appearance
- Surrounding stroma with variable amount of fibrosis
- Chronic inflammation may be seen in association with atrophic acini

Diffuse Atrophy
- Widespread, shows uniform involvement of all glands
- Basal cells are relatively prominent

Focal Atrophy
- Localized or patchy atrophy of glands

Morphologic Types of Focal Atrophy
- Simple atrophy (SA)
  - Atrophic acini are spaced relatively similarly to normal glands
  - Glands are about normal in caliber but may be larger and are often irregular in shape
- SA with cyst formation
  - SA associated with cystic dilatation of atrophic acini
  - Dilated glands closely apposed with little amount of intervening stroma and show rounded configuration
- Postatrophic hyperplasia (PAH)
  - Atrophic acini arranged in lobules often surrounding central larger dilated duct
  - Acini can be oval, slit-like, or stellate-shaped
  - Nuclei typically bland but occasionally may be enlarged with distinct nucleoli
  - Admixed with variable amount of hyperplastic acini containing clear or pale cytoplasm
- Partial atrophy (PA)
  - PA is most common reason for consultations of atypical glands concerning for cancer in biopsies
  - Has relatively modest amount of pale to clear cytoplasm and less crowded nuclei
  - Acini are small- to medium-sized and round or undulating in contour
  - Nucleoli are occasionally moderately enlarged
- Sclerotic atrophy
  - Atrophy containing dense fibrotic stroma
  - Atrophic glands are more angulated or irregular

ANCILLARY TESTS

Immunohistochemistry
- Positive for basal cell markers [p63 or HMWK (34βE12)]
  - Rare glands within PAH focus may be completely negative (23%)
  - PA shows patchy staining in 73-87% and has completely absent staining in 6%
- Underexpresses or negative for AMACR
  - 10% of PA shows stronger staining than benign glands
  - 24% of PA shows combination of AMACR positivity and basal cell marker negativity

DIFFERENTIAL DIAGNOSIS

Acinar Adenocarcinoma
- Malignant acini are relatively smaller, more rigid, or less irregular in contour
- Shows nucleomegaly and presence of prominent &/or multiple nucleoli; most helpful particularly if appreciated in several cells
- Completely negative for basal cell markers and strong circumferential staining with AMACR

Prostate Adenocarcinoma With Atrophic Features
- Carcinoma that is architecturally similar in appearance to atrophic benign glands
- Retains cytologic and other features of adenocarcinoma and is occasionally admixed with more typical carcinoma histology

SELECTED REFERENCES

1. Billis A et al: Focal prostatic atrophy: morphologic classification and immunohistochemistry. Anal Quant Cytopathol Histpathol. 36(2):71-81, 2014
2. De Marzo AM et al: A working group classification of focal prostate atrophy lesions. Am J Surg Pathol. 30(10):1281-91, 2006
3. Amin MB et al: Postatrophic hyperplasia of the prostate gland: a detailed analysis of its morphology in needle biopsy specimens. Am J Surg Pathol. 23(8):925-31, 1999

Atrophy and Its Variants

Simple Atrophy

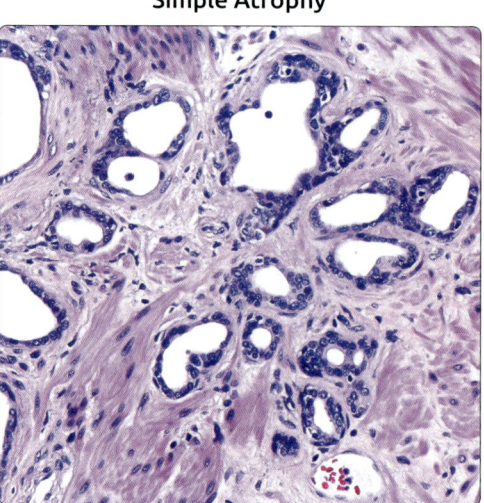

Simple Atrophy

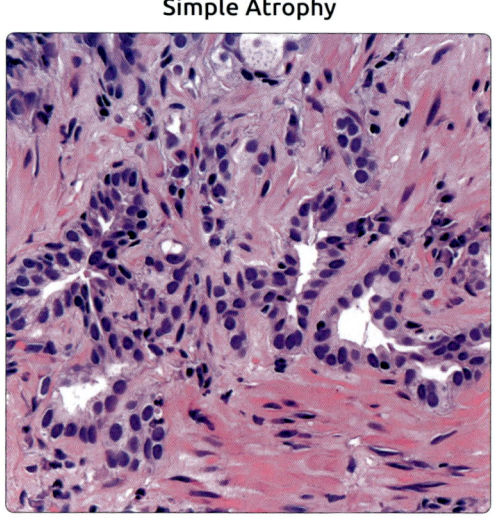

(Left) SA shows normally spaced atrophic acini lined by cuboidal to flattened cells. Like in most forms of atrophy, the nuclei are bland and appear crowded from the loss of cytoplasmic volume. Nuclear atypia (seen in adenocarcinoma), such as nucleomegaly, prominent nucleoli, multiple nucleoli, and mitosis, are not seen in atrophic glands. **(Right)** SA shows nuclear crowding from loss of cytoplasmic volume. Unlike adenocarcinoma, these atrophic glands are more irregular and angulated and do not exhibit nuclear atypia.

p63 in Atrophy

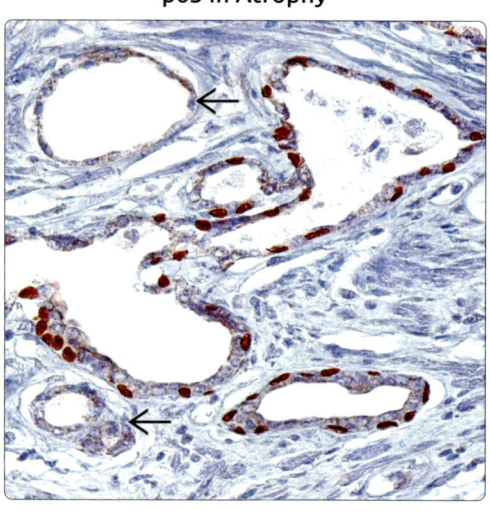

HMWK in Atrophy

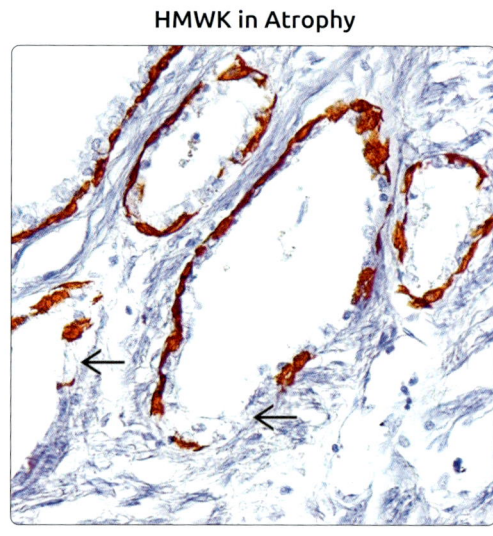

(Left) Basal cells within the atrophic benign acini exhibit nuclear p63 positivity. Note few benign glands within the atrophic focus are completely negative for p63 ➡. Focal p63 positivity is sufficient to rule out cancer diagnosis. **(Right)** HMWK immunostain highlights the basal cells within these atrophic benign glands. Note the patchy discontinuous (+) staining in portions of the glands ➡. In contrast, adenocarcinoma (not shown) demonstrates complete lack of basal cell staining in all the atypical acini within a suspicious focus.

Simple Atrophy With Cyst Formation

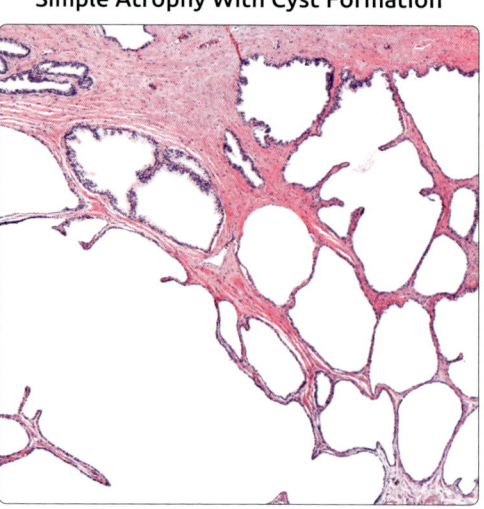

Simple Atrophy With Cyst Formation

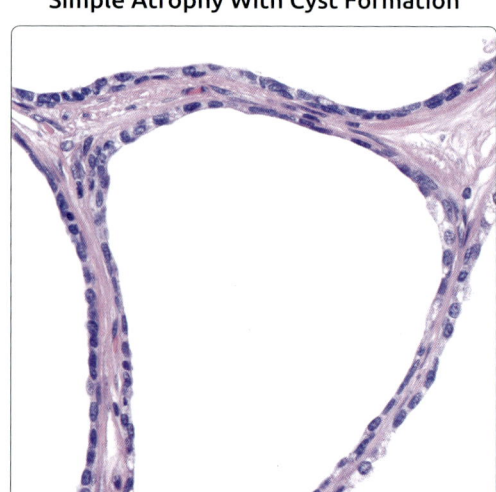

(Left) SA with cyst formation shows cluster of cystically dilated glands, which exhibit nodular configuration. There is relatively less stroma in between the clusters of atrophic acini. In comparison, some relatively normal-sized glands with nonatrophic cells are seen on the left upper side of the image. **(Right)** High-power view of SA with cyst formation shows the dilated acini lined by flattened to cuboidal cells. Like in most forms of atrophy, the nuclei are relatively crowded with overlapping and do not show atypicality.

Atrophy and Its Variants

Partial Atrophy

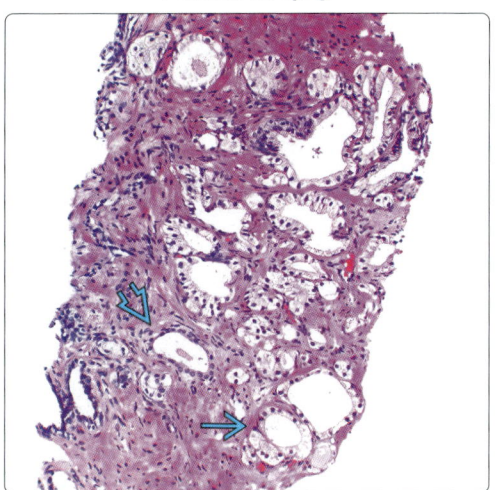

Partial Atrophy

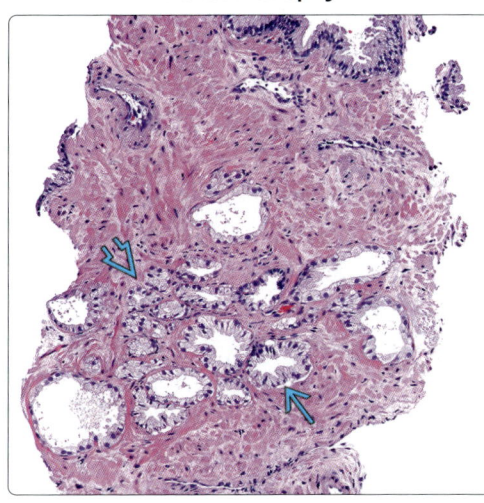

(Left) PA, in contrast to other forms of atrophy, shows a relatively ample amount of pale to clear cytoplasm and less crowded nuclei. Most of the glands have irregular lumina, but some may exhibit rigidity ⇨, raising the concern for carcinoma. Completely atrophic acini with more flattened cells are often seen at periphery of PA ⇨. (Right) Focus of PA in biopsy shows the characteristic undulated glands with irregular (star-like) lumina and cells with modest pale cytoplasm ⇨. Some of the acini are small ⇨, raising concern for carcinoma.

Partial Atrophy

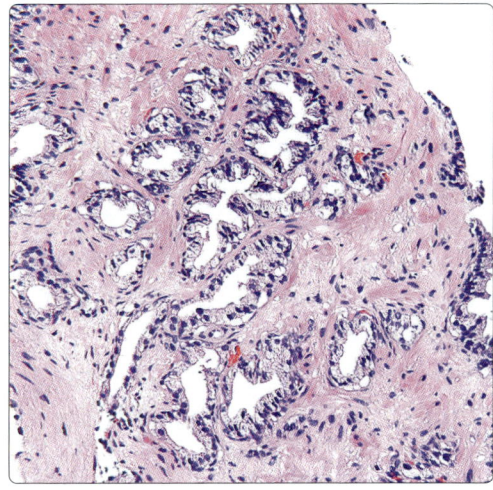

p63 in Partial Atrophy

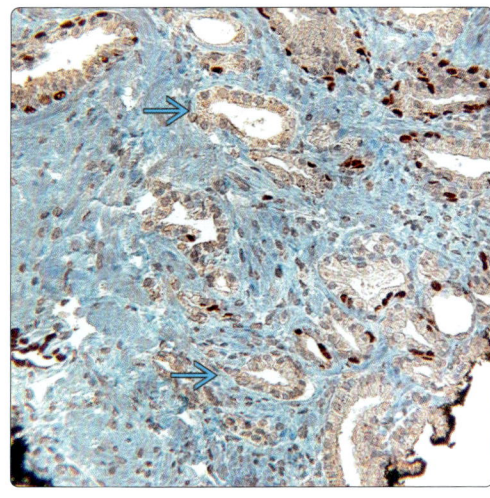

(Left) PA consists of small- to medium-sized glands with pale to clear cytoplasm. In contrast to adenocarcinoma, these glands are more irregular and lack nuclear features of malignancy. However, nucleoli may occasionally be moderately enlarged in PA, compounding distinction from carcinoma. Use of IHC stains is helpful in challenging cases. (Right) This cluster of partially atrophic glands shows the usual patchy nuclear reactivity for p63 in some glands. Note that some glands have no p63 staining ⇨, compounding its distinction from cancer.

Postatrophic Hyperplasia

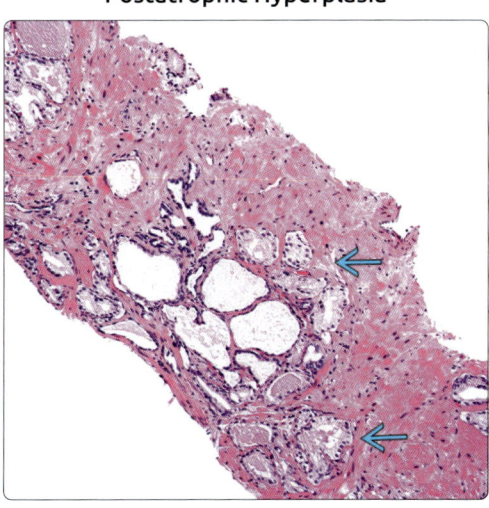

Postatrophic Hyperplasia

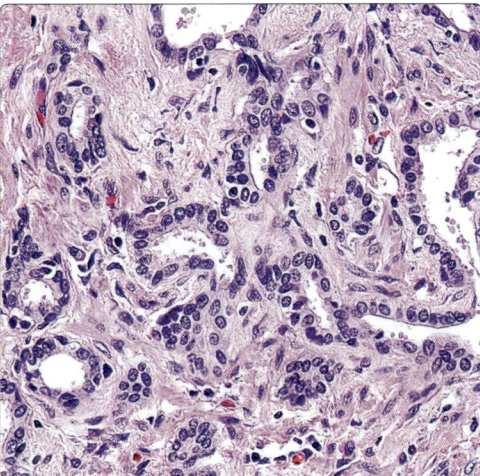

(Left) Postatrophic hyperplasia (PAH) encountered in needle biopsy is shown, an important differential diagnosis for atypical small acinar proliferation in needle biopsy. The diagnosis is less challenging if the entire architecture is seen, as in this case. Note the more atypical glands at the periphery of PAH ⇨ (Right) At the periphery of PAH, glands are small and may resemble carcinoma. In contrast to adenocarcinoma, these atrophic acini are more irregular and lack nuclear atypia, such as nucleomegaly and prominent nucleoli.

Atrophy and Its Variants

Postatrophic Hyperplasia

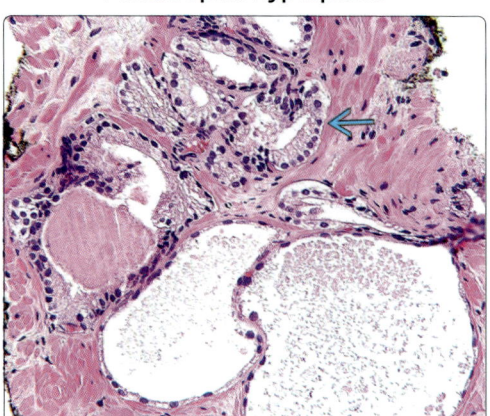

Postatrophic Hyperplasia

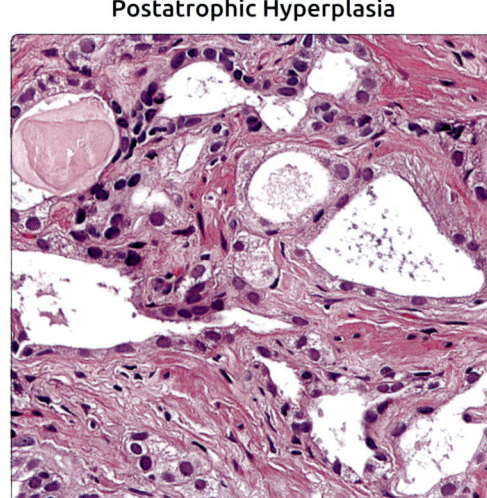

(Left) PAH in needle biopsy is seen. Sometimes admixed with the atrophic acini are hyperplastic acini with relatively abundant pale to clear cytoplasm and less crowded nuclei ➡. Note some glands have completely atrophic flattened cells, and the nuclei lack atypicality. (Right) The nuclei of PAH typically have inconspicuous nucleoli; however, they may occasionally be prominent. In challenging cases, use of IHC stains, particularly basal cell markers, may be helpful in establishing definitive diagnosis of PAH.

Postatrophic Hyperplasia

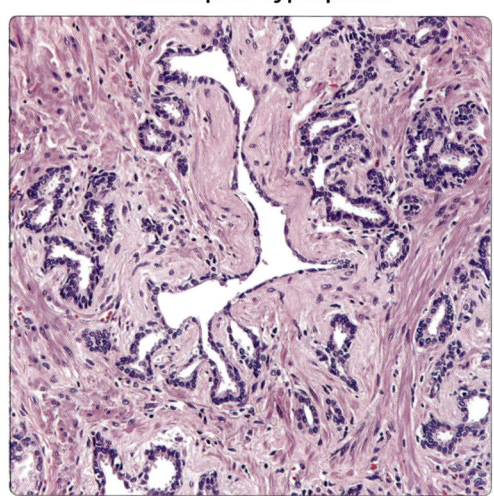

Postatrophic Hyperplasia

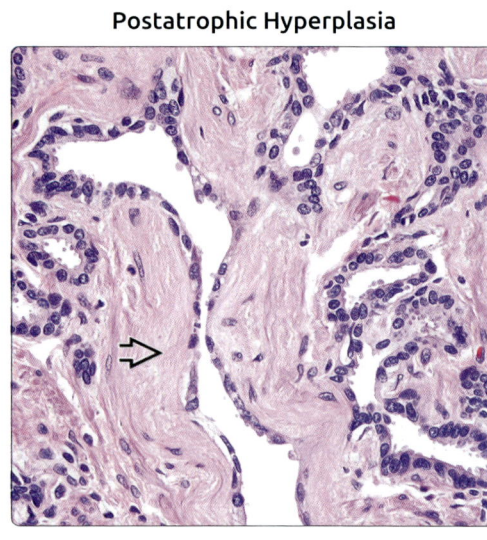

(Left) PAH shows a lobular configuration of atrophic acini surrounding a larger central atrophic duct. These smaller glands, particularly if the lesion is not appreciated in its entirety, may mimic prostate adenocarcinoma. (Right) High-power magnification PAH in the same patient shows the duct and acini are lined by cuboidal to flattened cells with nuclear crowding. Note the presence of sclerotic stroma within the atrophic lobule ➡. In contrast to carcinoma, these glands are more irregular and lack nuclear atypia.

PIN4 in Postatrophic Hyperplasia

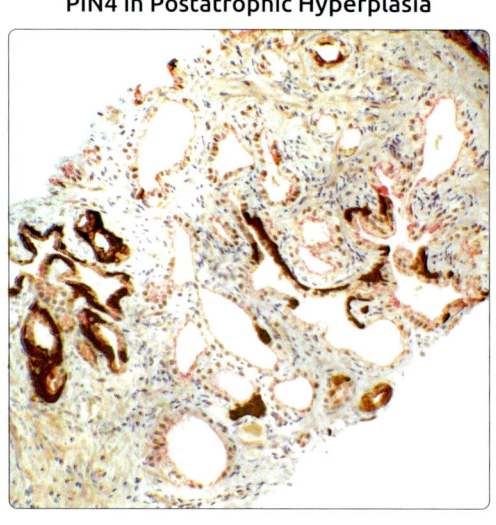

Sclerotic Atrophy

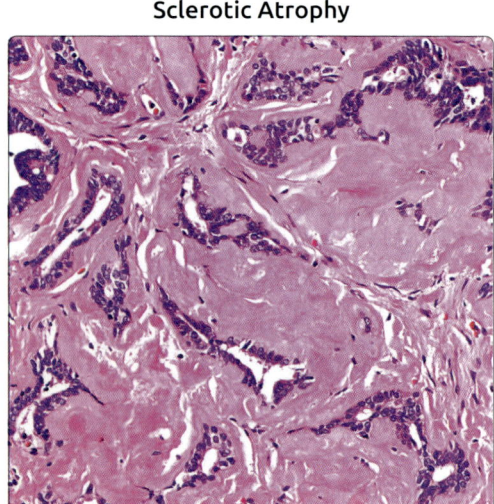

(Left) PAH shows patchy to absent basal cell markers (brown) and weak AMACR (red) staining in benign glands. Unlike PAH or PA, prostate carcinoma (not shown) shows uniformly absent basal cell markers staining in all glands within the suspicious focus and has more intense and circumferential staining for AMACR. (Right) Sclerotic atrophy shows dense fibrotic stroma surrounding angulated atrophic glands. The atrophic glands show typical features of atrophy, including irregular contour, basophilia, nuclear crowding, and bland nuclei.

Atrophy and Its Variants

Proliferative Inflammatory Atrophy

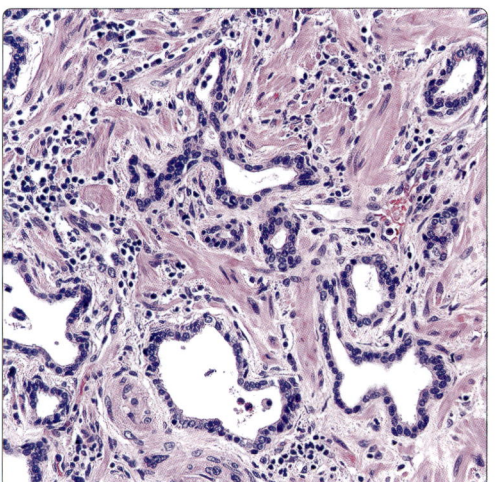

Diffuse Atrophy

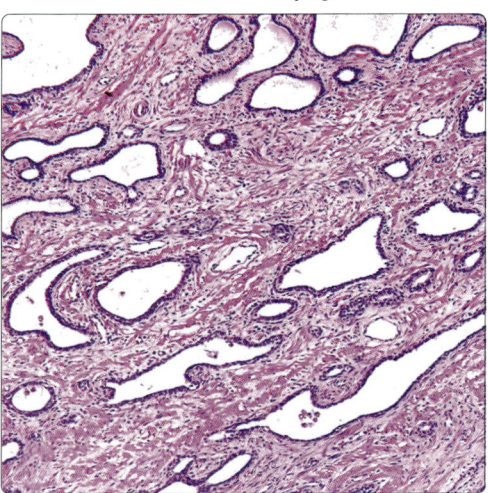

(Left) Atrophic acini associated with chronic inflammation show glands with usual features of atrophy such as angulation, scant cytoplasm, basophilia, and no nuclear atypia. Ki-67 (not shown) shows increased nuclear staining in proliferative inflammatory atrophy, suggested by some authors to be a risk for prostate cancer. (Right) Diffuse atrophy shows widespread cell shrinkage of all glands. This type of atrophy is linked to aging, androgen deprivation, and radiotherapy or can be secondary to compression by a BPH nodule.

Diffuse Atrophy

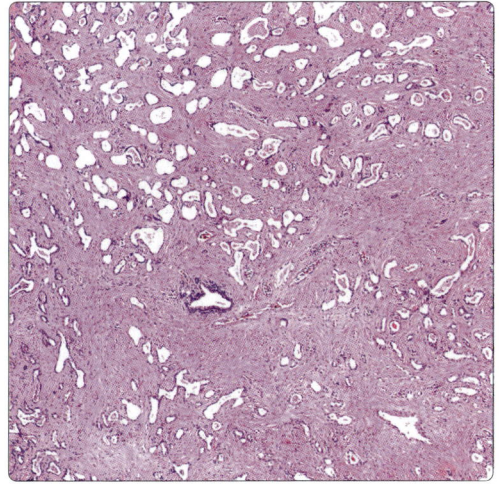

Diffuse Atrophy

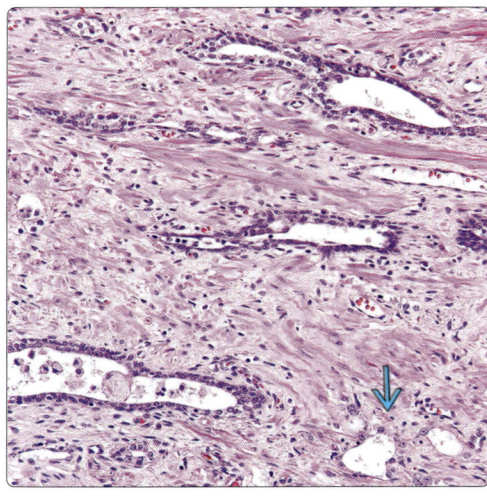

(Left) Diffuse glandular atrophy secondary to therapy for adenocarcinoma shows attenuated glands with variably irregular or angulated lumen. (Right) Diffuse glandular atrophy secondary to androgen ablation therapy for adenocarcinoma is shown. Few residual treated adenocarcinoma glands are present ⇨, which are markedly shrunken as a result of hormonal deprivation. Diffuse atrophy should alert for possible prior hormone ablation and careful search for treated cancer, which may not be readily discernible.

Diffuse Atrophy of Central Zone

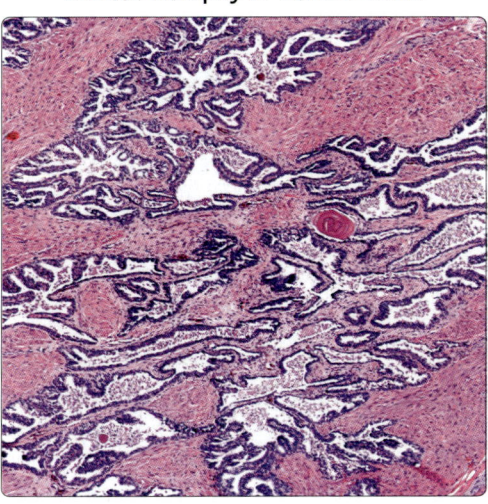

Diffuse Atrophy of Central Zone

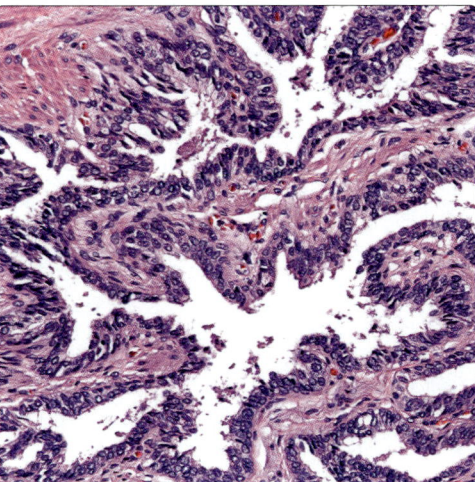

(Left) Diffuse atrophy involving the prostate central zone shows involvement of all central zone glands. These atrophic glands maintain their overall architectural complexity typical for glands from this zone, including luminal papillary infoldings. Note the densely muscular stroma between glands, which is typical for central zone. (Right) High-power view of the same central zone atrophy to the left shows large glands with loss of cytoplasmic volume and nuclear crowding. The nuclei do not show atypicality.

Hyperplasia of Mesonephric Remnants

KEY FACTS

TERMINOLOGY
- Tubular or acinar proliferation of putative mesonephric duct remnants containing characteristic intraluminal colloid-like material

ETIOLOGY/PATHOGENESIS
- During embryogenesis, mesonephric or wolffian duct gives rise to rete testis, epididymis, vas deferens, and seminal vesicles
- Mesonephric remnants may undergo proliferation

CLINICAL ISSUES
- Very rare, seen in 0.6% of TURP specimens
- Mean age: 67 years; range: 50-85 years
- Incidental histologic finding
- Typically in anterior gland or periphery at base, but can extend into bladder neck and periprostatic soft tissues

MICROSCOPIC
- Lobular or infiltrative growth of tubules that often contain dense eosinophilic colloid-like material
- Lined by single layer of bland cuboidal cells with scant cytoplasm imparting "atrophic" appearance
- Nuclei are regular, round, and typically with inconspicuous nucleolus
- Hyperplasia may be florid; tubules may appear to infiltrate between bladder neck muscle bundles and into periprostatic connective tissues
- Tubules may be seen intimately associated with nerves or ganglions

ANCILLARY TESTS
- Colloid-like material is PAS(+) and PASD(+)
- pax-8(+), PSA/PAP(-)
- Most are HMWCK(34βE12)(+)

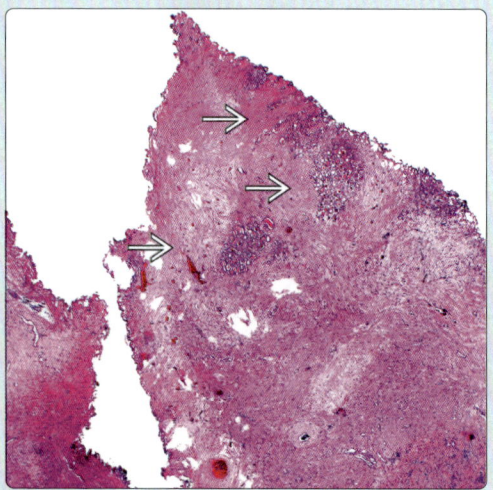

Mesonephric Hyperplasia: TURP Case

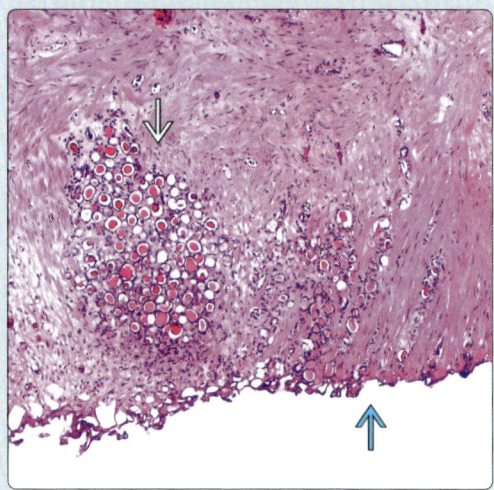

Mesonephric Hyperplasia: TURP Case

(Left) A focus of hyperplasia of mesonephric remnants, appearing crowded and perhaps infiltrative, is seen in fragments of a transurethral resection of prostate performed for BPH ➡. (Right) At the cauterized edge, this lesion shows a crowded, lobular proliferation of tiny acini with atrophic-appearance and colloid-like luminal material ➡. Involving < 1% of TURPs, these foci may simulate carcinoma by appearing to proliferate between muscle slips ➡.

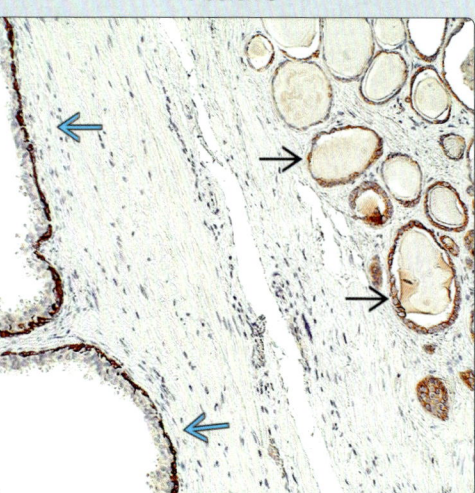

Mesonephric Hyperplasia: HMWCK Positive

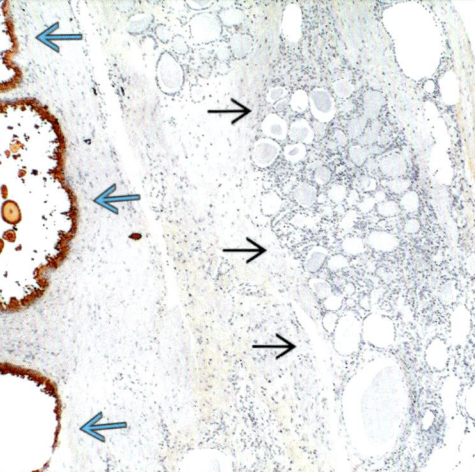

Mesonephric Hyperplasia: PSA Negative

(Left) Mesonephric remnant tubules ➡ show HMWCK (34βE12) positivity in the tubular cells, in contrast to the basal cell-only positivity in adjacent prostate glands ➡. Carcinoma, of course, would lack the HMWCK(+) basal cells. (Right) An adjacent section, stained for PSA, shows the PSA(-) mesonephric hyperplasia ➡ juxtaposed to the PSA(+) benign glands ➡. HMWCK and PSA, along with pax-8, are quite helpful in this differential.

Hyperplasia of Mesonephric Remnants

TERMINOLOGY

Definitions
- Benign, tubuloacinar proliferation of putative mesonephric duct remnants with characteristic intraluminal colloid-like material
- Histologically similar to mesonephric remnants that are well recognized in female genital tract

ETIOLOGY/PATHOGENESIS

Origin
- During embryogenesis, mesonephric or wolffian duct gives rise to rete testis, epididymis, vas deferens, and seminal vesicles
- Mesonephric duct remnants may undergo proliferation or hyperplasia, the cause of which is not known

CLINICAL ISSUES

Epidemiology
- Incidence
  - Very rare, 0.6% of transurethral resection (TUR) specimens
- Age
  - Mean: 67 years; range: 50-85 years

Site
- TURs show lobular mesonephric hyperplasia around and between bladder neck smooth muscle bundles
- Prostatectomy-based studies suggest that mesonephric hyperplasia is mostly found in
  - Anterior fibromuscular stroma of prostate and adjacent anterolateral periprostatic tissue
    - Which may merge with bladder neck smooth muscle toward base, correlating TUR findings
  - Toward base posteriorly and posterolaterally, either within gland periphery or in periprostatic and periseminal vesicle soft tissues

Presentation
- Usually as rare, incidental histologic finding, in TUR for obstruction due to BPH

MACROSCOPIC

Size
- Measures 0.1-0.7 cm in TURP specimens, usually not grossly apparent

MICROSCOPIC

Histologic Features
- Composed of tubules or acini arranged in somewhat lobular clusters, with distinctive, dense, colloid-like luminal material
- Tubules are lined by single layer of bland cuboidal, flattened, or low columnar cells
- Cytoplasm is typically scant and pale pink, imparting atrophic appearance
- Nuclei are round, regular, and typically with inconspicuous nucleoli, although occasionally they may be prominent
- Tubules may have infiltrative-appearing growth pattern or may show intraluminal papillary fronds
- Hyperplasia may be florid; tubules may appear to infiltrate between bladder neck muscle bundles and into periprostatic connective tissues
- Tubules may be seen intimately associated with nerves and ganglia
- May contain infiltrative-appearing cords of microacini that lack colloid-like material and, along with prominent nucleoli, may mimic prostate cancer
- Infrequently may appear as nodules of ill-formed small glands intermixed with spindle cells, mimicking sclerosing adenosis or higher grade prostate cancer

ANCILLARY TESTS

Immunohistochemistry
- Diffuse nuclear positivity for pax-8, PSA/PAP(-)
- Most, but not all are HMCK(34βE12)(+)

DIFFERENTIAL DIAGNOSIS

Verumontanum Mucosal Gland Hyperplasia
- Microacinar proliferation along verumontanum and adjacent urethra at openings of utricle and ejaculatory ducts
- Tubules are lined by single layer of cuboidal to columnar cells with underlying basal cell layer and abundant intraluminal corpora amylacea or concretions

Nephrogenic Adenoma
- Also pax-8(+) lesion, but associated with reactive/reparative/inflammatory milieu
- Mainly periurethral in location, only secondarily extending into prostate
- Cystic tubules may contain colloid-like material in subset
- Shows thickened peritubular hyaline sheath and characteristic hobnail cell lining
- May have exophytic papillary growth overlying tubular parenchyma
- May be PSA/PAP(+), may be AMACR(+)

Benign Small Acinar Proliferations
- Benign prostatic lesions in differential of atypical small acinar proliferations, including small glandular BPH, adenosis, atrophy, and sclerosing adenosis
- PSA/PAP(+), pax-8(-), p63/HMWCK(+) basal cell layer, lack luminal colloid-like material

Acinar Adenocarcinoma
- Malignant glands are more atypical (nucleomegaly, nucleoli) and infiltrative, lacking lobular pattern of mesonephric hyperplasia
- PSA/PAP(+), pax-8(-), ERG (+, 30-50%), lack p63/HMWCK(+) basal cell layer

SELECTED REFERENCES
1. Chen YB et al: Mesonephric remnant hyperplasia involving prostate and periprostatic tissue: findings at radical prostatectomy. Am J Surg Pathol. 35(7):1054-61, 2011
2. Yacoub M et al: Mesonephric remnant hyperplasia: an unusual benign mimicker of prostate cancer. Ann Diagn Pathol. 13(6):402-4, 2009
3. Bostwick DG et al: Mesonephric remnants of the prostate: incidence and histologic spectrum. Mod Pathol. 16(7):630-5, 2003
4. Gikas PW et al: Florid hyperplasia of mesonephric remnants involving prostate and periprostatic tissue. Possible confusion with adenocarcinoma. Am J Surg Pathol. 17(5):454-60, 1993

Hyperplasia of Mesonephric Remnants

Mesonephric Hyperplasia: Biopsy Sample

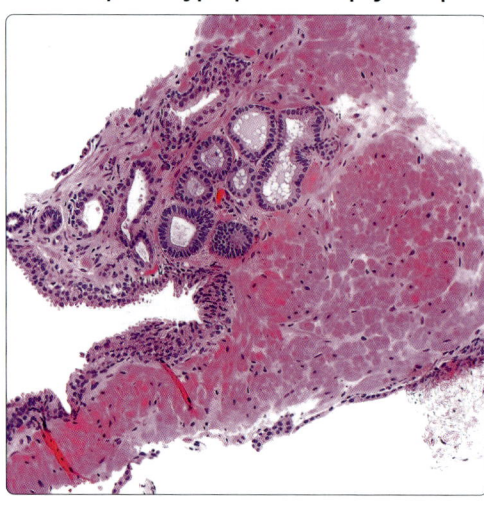

Diffuse pax-8 Positivity

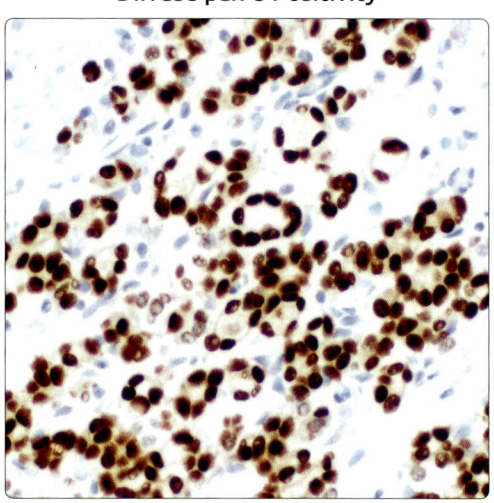

(Left) Prostate needle biopsy shows mesonephric remnant tubules. The tight clustering and rigid appearance of these tubules simulate prostate cancer on low-power magnification. Lack of cytologic atypia and the presence of luminal secretions in these glands are key in making the diagnosis. (Right) Pax-8 IHC is very helpful, as PCa is uniformly negative, while mesonephric hyperplasia is uniformly, diffusely nuclear positive. pax-8 may be more reliable than HMWCK, as some mesonephric hyperplasias may be HMWCK(-).

Lobular Architecture

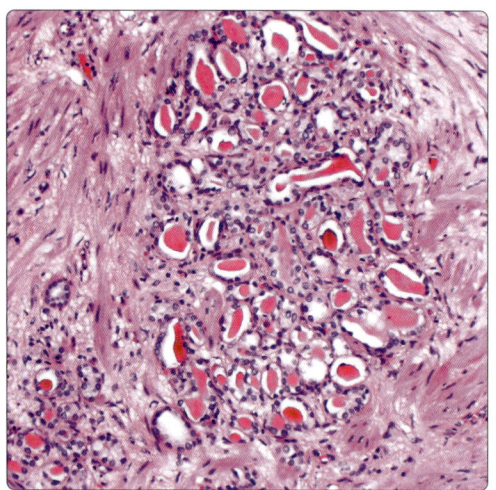

Variably Sized, Dilated Acini

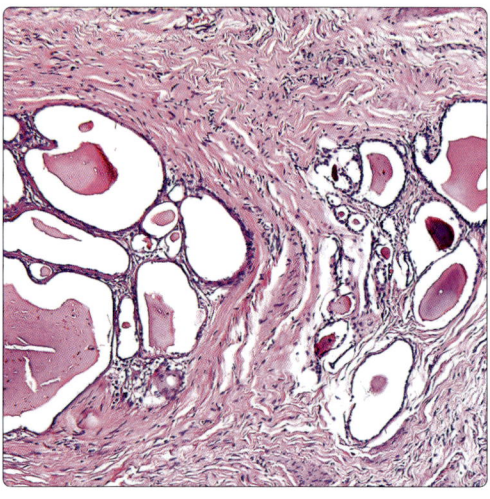

(Left) An example of mesonephric hyperplasia demonstrates a dense proliferation of small tubules with colloid-like luminal material and bland attenuated lining epithelium. (Right) Mesonephric hyperplasia is seen arranged in lobular configuration, though some tubules show luminal dilation reminiscent of cystic atrophy.

Mesonephric Hyperplasia: Crowding

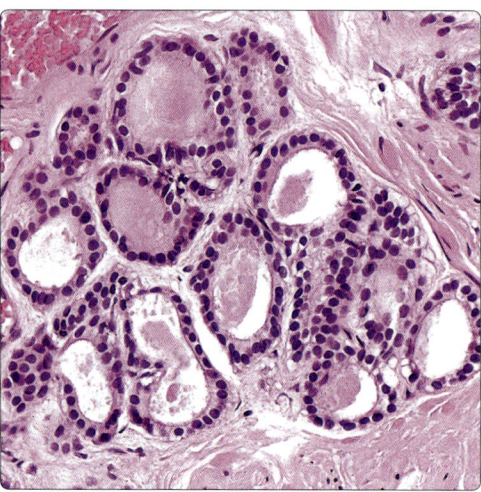

Mesonephric Hyperplasia: No Atypia

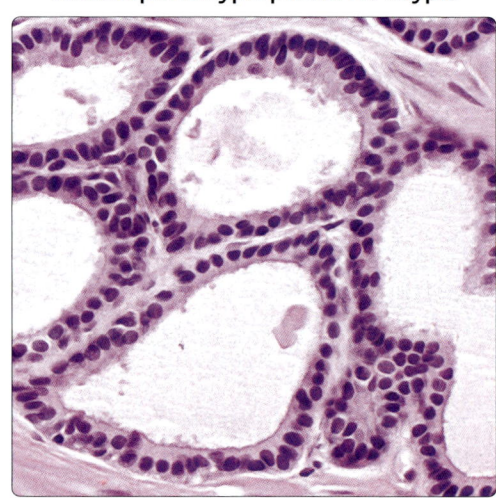

(Left) A cluster of mesonephric remnant tubules mimics PCa. These glands are tightly clustered, small, regular, and show monolayer of cells, which are all worrisome features for PCa. However, the lack of nuclear atypia and presence of intraluminal eosinophilic material in some of the tubules is helpful in making the diagnosis. (Right) Close inspection of the same mesonephric remnant tubules does not reveal the nuclear atypia of malignancy.

Hyperplasia of Mesonephric Remnants

Frequent Anterior Gland Involvement

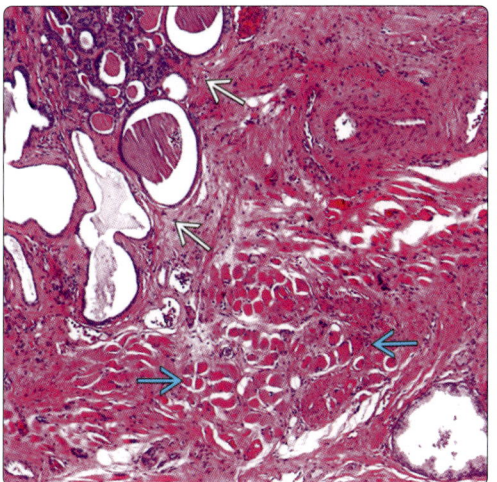

Basolateral/Peripheral Gland Involvement

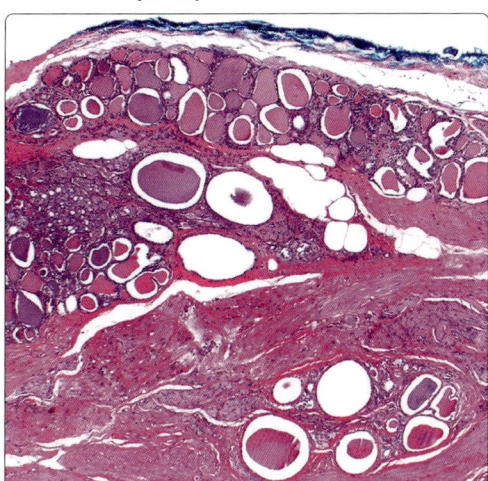

(Left) Prostatectomy-based series suggests mesonephric hyperplasia ➡ quite often involves the anterior fibromuscular stroma Note the skeletal muscle ➡ of the gland. *(Right)* Mesonephric hyperplasia also often involves the basolateral prostate, with periprostatic soft tissue involvement that shows clusters of variably sized tubules arranged in lobular configuration. Despite this worrisome architectural pattern and presence outside of the prostate, the lesion is benign.

Luminal Papillation

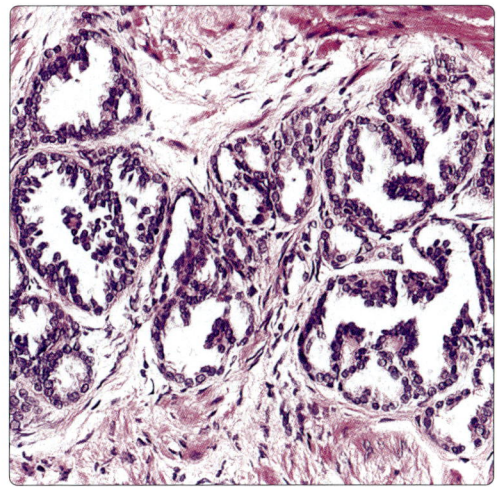

Hyperplasia Involving Ganglion

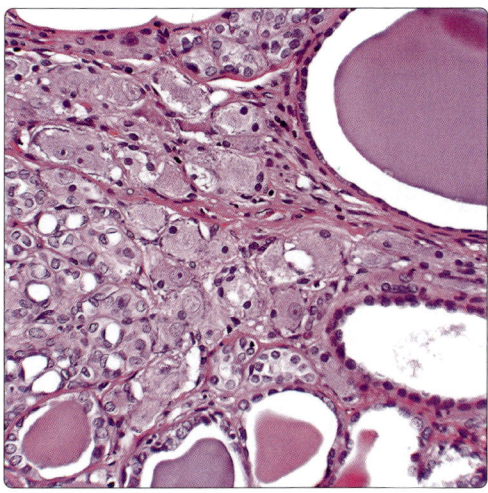

(Left) Mesonephric tubules occasionally may contain intratubular papillary fronds, which may be seen admixed with more typical-appearing mesonephric remnant tubules. *(Right)* Mesonephric remnant tubules show intimate association with a ganglion. Awareness of this occasional finding in mesonephric hyperplasia is important to avoid misdiagnosis of carcinoma with perineural or ganglionic invasion.

Differential: Nephrogenic Adenoma

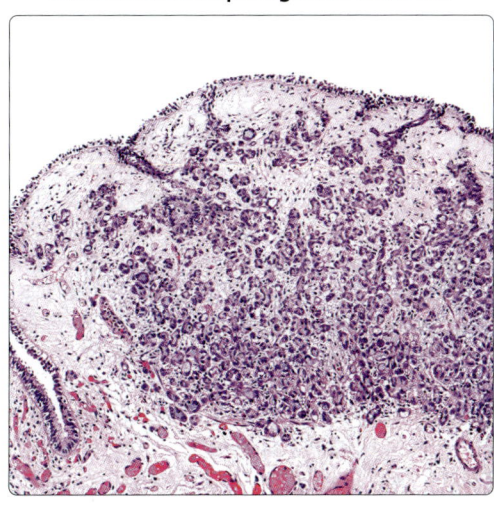

Differential: Nephrogenic Adenoma

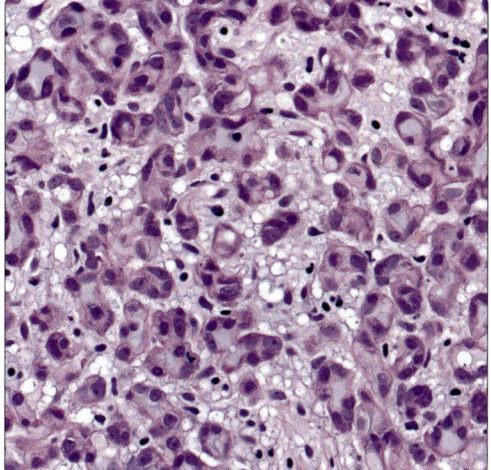

(Left) Nephrogenic adenoma is also a benign pax-8(+) lesion that may involve the prostate. However, even in cases appearing infiltrative, a periurethral orientation of the lesion is identified. *(Right)* Also, rather than arising in the setting of a noninflamed, nonreactive developmental rest, nephrogenic adenoma instead often has myxoinflammatory stroma and granulation tissue-like stromal vascular pattern such as seen in the reparative setting of prior instrumentation.

Verumontanum Mucosal Gland Hyperplasia

KEY FACTS

TERMINOLOGY
- Benign proliferation of glands indigenously situated along verumontanum of posterior prostatic urethra

CLINICAL ISSUES
- Encountered as incidental histologic finding more commonly in prostatectomies
- Significant as morphologic mimic of adenocarcinoma in prostate biopsy specimens

MICROSCOPIC
- Seen along ejaculatory or prostatic ducts (67%), utricle (19%), or adjacent urethral mucosa (14%)
- Composed of relatively well-circumscribed proliferations of closely packed glands
- Frequently contain corpora amylacea or orange-red concretions
- Glandular cells usually are cuboidal to low columnar, and basal cell layer is readily discernible
- Adjacent urethral urothelium or ejaculatory duct epithelium helpful in identification

ANCILLARY TESTS
- Glandular cells are PSA(+)
- Basal cells are HMCK(34βE12)(+)

TOP DIFFERENTIAL DIAGNOSES
- Nephrogenic adenoma
  - PSA/PAP(-), pax-2/pax-8(+)
- Mesonephric hyperplasia
  - PSA/PAP(-)
- Low-grade acinar adenocarcinoma
  - Lacks basal cell layer

DIAGNOSTIC CHECKLIST
- Diagnosis of benign nature is usually straightforward, based on nuclear features and presence of basal cell layer

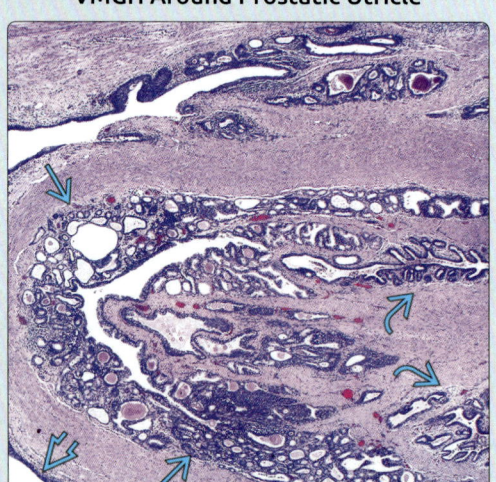

VMGH Around Prostatic Utricle

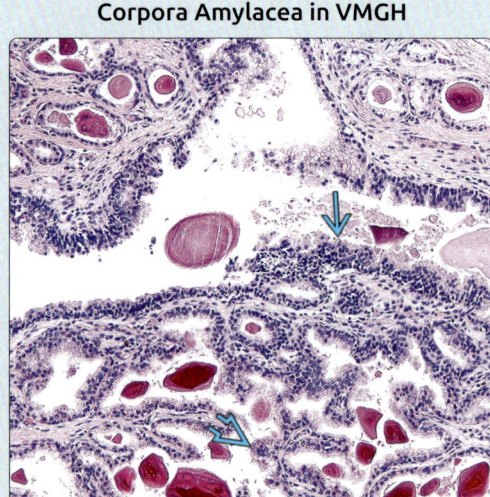

Corpora Amylacea in VMGH

(Left) Low magnification of verumontanum mucosal gland hyperplasia (VMGH) shows tightly clustered glands around the prostatic utricle ➡. Prostatic urethral surface ➡ and both ejaculatory ducts are visible ➡. The glandular proliferation is relatively circumscribed following the outline of the utricle. (Right) H&E shows abundant corpora amylacea in the lumina of small to medium-sized, closely packed glands ➡. Closer inspection of the glands may also reveal cytoplasmic lipofuscin pigments ➡.

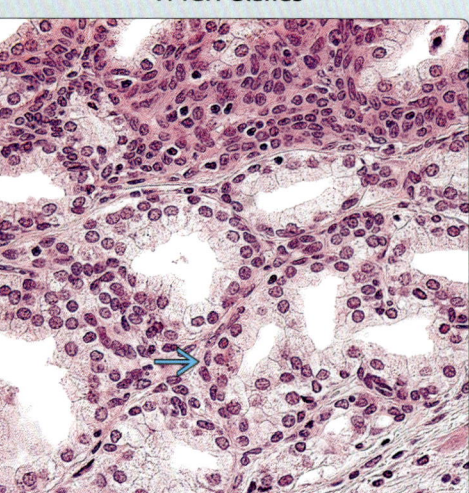

VMGH Glands

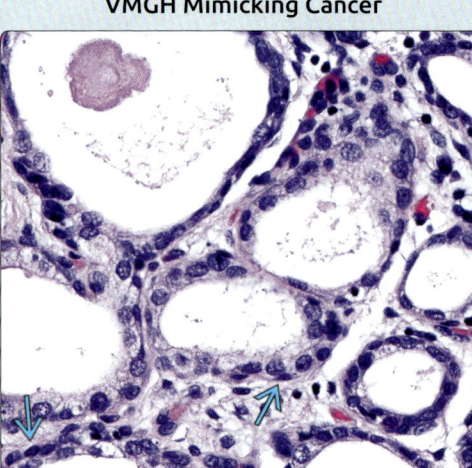

VMGH Mimicking Cancer

(Left) VMGH glands are often small and back to back; basal cells are readily discernible in some of these glands ➡. (Right) VMGH may show tightly packed, small, rigid glands that may mimic low-grade prostatic adenocarcinoma. However, the basal cells are readily discernible in some of the glands in this focus excluding cancer ➡. Also, the glandular cells do not exhibit nucleomegaly and lack prominent nucleoli. Note the presence of corpora amylacea.

Verumontanum Mucosal Gland Hyperplasia

TERMINOLOGY

Abbreviations
- Verumontanum mucosal gland hyperplasia (VMGH)

Definitions
- Benign proliferation of glands indigenously situated along verumontanum of prostatic urethra; usually > 5 glands in a focus is considered hyperplastic
- Verumontanum or seminal colliculus is located at posterior prostatic urethral wall where utricle and bilateral ejaculatory ducts merge with prostatic urethra

ETIOLOGY/PATHOGENESIS

Origin
- Morphologic evidence suggests origin from urethral mucosal glands, which occupy most distal portion of prostatic ducts, ejaculatory ducts, and utricle
- Another possibility is origin from utricle since this structure developmentally acquires morphological and functional features of prostate
  - However, presence of VMGH exclusively along prostatic urethra argues against this theory

CLINICAL ISSUES

Epidemiology
- Incidence
  - Reported in 14-32% of prostatectomy specimens
- Age
  - Older patients (range: 47-87 years)

Presentation
- Clinically asymptomatic, encountered as incidental histologic lesions more commonly in prostatectomy and less often in needle biopsy specimens
  - Unlikely to be seen in transurethral resection of prostate specimens, since verumontanum is spared in this procedure
- Significance in routine practice: Morphologic mimic of prostatic adenocarcinoma in biopsy

Treatment
- None

Prognosis
- Benign course, histologic variation

MICROSCOPIC

Histologic Features
- Situated along openings of ejaculatory or prostatic ducts (67%), utricle (19%), or adjacent urethral mucosa (14%)
- Seen subjacent to urothelium, demonstrating expansile circumscription
- Composed of relatively well-circumscribed proliferation of small to medium-sized, closely packed glands
- Glands are often back to back with minimal interglandular stroma
- Glandular cells are cuboidal to low columnar and rarely may be flattened
  - Cytoplasm is clear to eosinophilic
  - Nuclei are round and regular with indistinct nucleoli and absent mitoses
  - Cytoplasmic lipofuscin pigment is often present
- Basal cell layer is readily identifiable in routine H&E stained sections
- Characteristically, lamellated eosinophilic concretions typical of corpora amylacea are seen
- Uncommonly, intraluminal orange-red fragmented concretions may be seen
- True crystalloids or luminal mucin are typically not present
- Adjacent urethral urothelium or ejaculatory duct epithelium helpful in identification

Predominant Pattern/Injury Type
- Hyperplasia

Predominant Cell/Compartment Type
- Epithelial, glandular

Immunohistochemistry
- Glandular cells are PSA(+)
- Basal cells are HMCK(34βE12)(+)

DIFFERENTIAL DIAGNOSIS

Nephrogenic Adenoma
- Located in suburethral prostatic stroma
- Tubules lined by cuboidal, flattened, or hobnailed cells
- May have thickened or prominent peritubular basement membranes
- May contain intraluminal eosinophilic secretions
- May have exophytic papillary component overlying tubular proliferation
- PSA/PAP(-), pax-2/pax-8(+)

Mesonephric Hyperplasia
- May be situated along urethral aspect of prostate
- Tubules arranged in somewhat lobular and infiltrative-appearing growth pattern
- Characteristically contain dense eosinophilic colloid-like material
- PSA/PAP(-)

Low-Grade Acinar Adenocarcinoma and Its Mimics
- Cytologic features of malignancy, including prominent nucleoli
- Demonstrates infiltrative or expansile growth pattern
- Lacks basal cell layer
  - Basal cell markers useful in challenging cases
- May contain intraluminal crystalloids and mucin
- Corpora amylacea are very rare

DIAGNOSTIC CHECKLIST

Pathologic Interpretation Pearls
- Diagnosis of benign nature is usually straightforward, based on nuclear features and presence of basal cell layer

SELECTED REFERENCES
1. Srigley JR: Benign mimickers of prostatic adenocarcinoma. Mod Pathol. 17(3):328-48, 2004

Nephrogenic Adenoma (Metaplasia) of Prostatic Urethra

KEY FACTS

TERMINOLOGY

- Nephrogenic adenoma (NA)
  - Tubulopapillary proliferations along urothelial mucosa that resemble immature renal tubules

ETIOLOGY/PATHOGENESIS

- Renal tubular cell seeding hypothesis
- Nephrogenic metaplasia hypothesis

CLINICAL ISSUES

- Most are incidental findings and may cause diagnostic problems in prostatic specimens

MICROSCOPIC

- Most common as small round to oval tubules
- Thickened peritubular basement membrane
- May contain intraluminal basophilic or eosinophilic secretions
- Other architectural patterns include cystic, papillary-polypoid, solid growth, and rare fibromyxoid or flat subtype
- Monolayer of cuboidal, flattened, or hobnailed cells
- Scanty to modest eosinophilic to clear cytoplasm
- Nuclei with minimal atypia, inconspicuous nucleoli, and absent to rare mitosis; rarely, nuclear atypia may be due to features of reactive changes with prominent nucleoli
- Tubules may be very small, simulating signet ring cells
- Admixture of these different patterns is common
- Polypoid-papillary growth when present is always seen with underlying tubular proliferation
- Extension of tubules into subjacent prostatic fibromuscular stroma is common

ANCILLARY TESTS

- pax-2/pax-8(+), AMACR(+), PSA/PAP(-) in majority of cases

TOP DIFFERENTIAL DIAGNOSES

- Prostatic acinar adenocarcinoma
- Urethral papillary neoplasms
- Clear cell adenocarcinoma

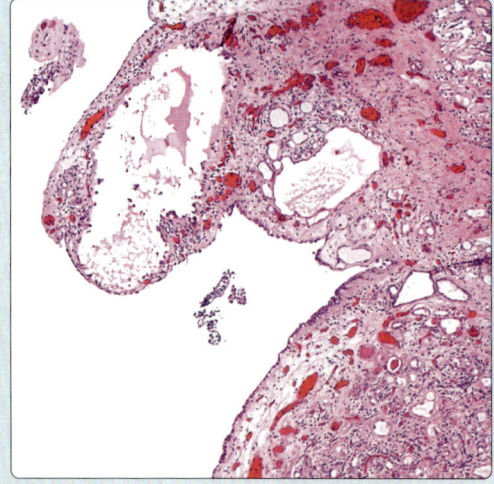

Nephrogenic Adenoma (NA) at Prostatic Urethra

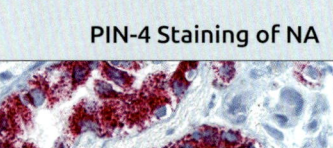

Biphasic Polypoid and Tubular NA

(Left) Low-power magnification of nephrogenic adenoma (NA) of the prostatic urethra shows polypoid growth with subjacent tubular and cystic proliferations in the lamina propria. (Right) H&E shows typical biphasic growth of NA exhibiting surface polypoid architecture and underlying tubular proliferations. Cells lining the tubules are similar to those at the surface including with hobnail appearance. Note the thick basement membrane material underneath the tubular and surface cells ➡.

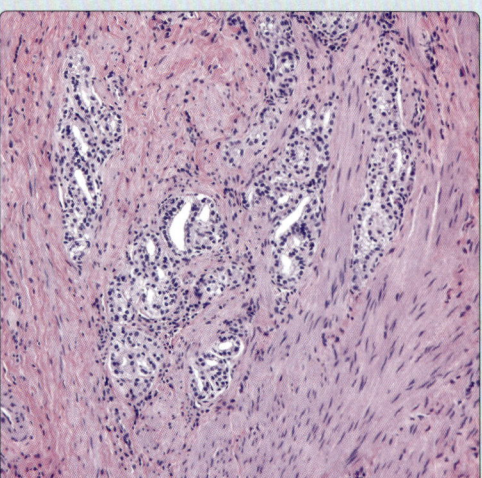

NA Tubules in Prostatic Stroma Mimicking Prostate Cancer

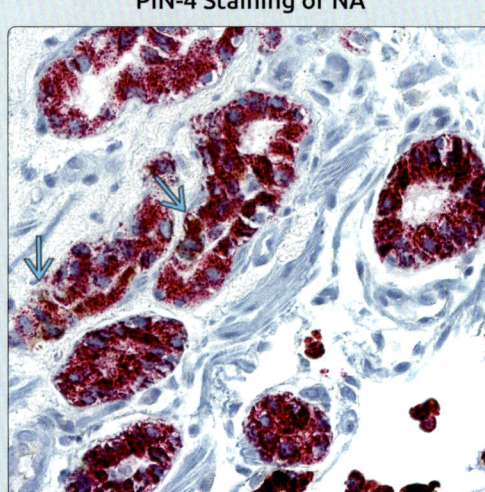

PIN-4 Staining of NA

(Left) Clusters of small tubules of NA with an infiltrative growth are shown in the fibromuscular stroma, mimicking prostatic adenocarcinoma. (Right) PIN-4 shows diffuse cytoplasmic staining for AMACR (red) in NA tubules. This intense staining compounds the morphologic overlap of NA and prostatic adenocarcinoma. Note that some of the same cells show scattered HMCK staining (brown) overcome by the intense red chromogen of AMACR ➡. Focal HMCK is commonly expressed in NA, unlike in prostate cancer.

Nephrogenic Adenoma (Metaplasia) of Prostatic Urethra

TERMINOLOGY

Abbreviations
- Nephrogenic adenoma (NA)

Synonyms
- Nephrogenic metaplasia
- Adenomatoid metaplasia

Definitions
- Benign epithelial lesion of urethra characterized by tubular, glandular, &/or papillary growth patterns
  - Tubuloglandular growth is morphologic and immunohistochemical mimic of prostatic adenocarcinoma

ETIOLOGY/PATHOGENESIS

Renal Tubular Cell Seeding Hypothesis
- In renal transplant patients, NA cells have been shown to have same sex chromosome status with allografted kidneys and not with surrounding bladder tissue in opposite gender recipients
- May represent seeding implantation and growth of renal tubular cells in injured urothelial mucosa

Nephrogenic Metaplasia Hypothesis
- Metaplastic alteration of urothelium in response to insult or injury

CLINICAL ISSUES

Epidemiology
- Age
  - Mean: 66 years; range: 4-81 years
  - ~ 10% seen in children
- Sex
  - M:F = 2:1

Site
- Vast majority of NA encountered in urinary bladder (~ 80%)
- Prostatic urethra is involved in ~ 15% of cases and may extend into subjacent prostate stroma
- ~ 5% occurs in ureter or renal pelvis

Presentation
- Most are incidental findings
  - Mainly seen in transurethral resection of prostate (TURP) specimens for benign prostatic hyperplasia
  - May cause diagnostic challenge when encountered in prostatic specimens

Natural History
- Majority of cases with preceding genitourinary surgery, instrumentation, urinary tract infection, or calculi
- A subset is seen in patients with renal transplant or Bacillus Calmette-Guérin therapy
- Rarely seen in association with urothelial neoplasms

Treatment
- None required

Prognosis
- Benign but with high "recurrence" rate (37%) if inciting etiology persists

MACROSCOPIC

General Features
- Only about 1/3 may assume macroscopic proportions, which may be seen at cystourethroscopy as exophytic papillary or polypoid lesions

Size
- Generally < 1 cm; average: 0.3 cm

MICROSCOPIC

Histologic Features
- Architectural patterns
  - Commonly as small round to oval tubules in laminar fashion
    - Some tubules characteristically have thickened or prominent peritubular basement membrane
    - May contain intraluminal basophilic or eosinophilic secretions, the latter imparting resemblance of tubules to thyroid follicles
    - Tubules lined by flattened cells may resemble small vessels
    - Tubules may be very small, simulating signet ring cells
    - Extension of tubules into subjacent prostatic fibromuscular stroma common
  - Cystically dilated tubules
  - Papillary-polypoid pattern
    - Single layer of lining epithelium
    - Usually with minimal branching
    - With stromal edema
    - Does not show fusion of papillae
  - Uncommon solid or diffuse growth
  - Rare fibromyxoid appearance with spindled cells
  - Rare surface flat pattern merging with adjacent urothelium or with Pagetoid growth
  - Admixture of these different patterns is common; polypoid-papillary, when present, is always seen with underlying tubular proliferation
- Cytological features
  - Usually monolayer of bland cuboidal, flattened, or hobnailed cells
    - Surface flat pattern may have multiple cell layers
  - Scanty to modest amount of eosinophilic to clear cytoplasm
  - Small nuclei with minimal atypia (in range of reactive) and inconspicuous to rarely prominent nucleoli
  - Absent to rare mitotic figures
- Additional findings
  - Stromal edema
  - Inflammatory cell infiltrates
  - Dilated vessels
  - Occasional microcalcifications

Predominant Pattern/Injury Type
- Metaplastic

Nephrogenic Adenoma (Metaplasia) of Prostatic Urethra

Predominant Cell/Compartment Type

- Epithelial, tubular

ANCILLARY TESTS

Immunohistochemistry

- Key panel: pax-8(+), PSA/PAP(-) in majority of cases; rare focal positivity is pitfall
  - Other (+) markers
    - S100-A1, pax-2, CK7, EMA/MUC1, HMCK(34βE12) (variable and focal), pancytokeratin
    - MIB1 (low index)
    - AMACR (pitfall)
    - GATA3; (+) in 40% of NA (pitfall)
  - Other (-) markers: p63
  - PIN-4 cocktail
    - AMACR(+) in 56%; HMWK(+) in 97%; p63(-) in > 98% and is never diffuse (+)
      - AMACR and HMWK staining present on same cells; lacks basal cell pattern of staining

Genetic Testing

- Monosomy 9 (24% of cells), trisomy 7 (8% of cells)

DIFFERENTIAL DIAGNOSIS

Prostatic Acinar Adenocarcinoma

- In contrast to NA, which is commonly at edge of specimen, prostate cancer may diffusely involve specimen
- Monotonous small acinar pattern (tubular, cystic, surface papillary, or flat components are absent)
- Hobnail cells, eosinophilic secretions, stromal edema, and inflammation are rare to absent
- PSA/PAP/NKX-3.1/ PSMA(+), pax-2/pax-8(-), and S100-1A(-)

Urethral Papillary Neoplasms

- Papillae lined by multilayered urothelium; presence and extent of atypia determines grade
  - Denudation may occur in high-grade neoplasms resulting in few cell layers like in NA
- May have complex papillae including multiple branching and fusion
- Lacks concomitant tubular growth
- GATA3(+); maker is also expressed in 40% of NA (a pitfall)
- p63(+), uroplakin II (+), and pax-2/pax-8(-)

Clear Cell Adenocarcinoma

- Exhibits high-grade cytology including nuclear pleomorphism and with increased mitotic activity
- More cellular and shows greater complexity in its tubulopapillary architecture
- May have solid growth of clear cells
- Frequently forms clinically conspicuous mass
- Immunophenotype may overlap significantly with NA
- High proliferation index (Ki-67)

Urethral Flat Urothelial Lesions With Atypia

- Mimicked by rare flat NA with multiple cell layers growing contiguously with adjacent urothelium
- Lacks concomitant tubular growth
- p63(+) and pax-2/pax-8(-)

DIAGNOSTIC CHECKLIST

Pathologic Interpretation Pearls

- Proliferation of small round tubules and cysts lined by bland monolayered cuboidal or hobnail epithelial cells, often with concomitant surface papillary or polypoid growth
- In TURP and needle biopsies, usually seen near or at terminal end (representing urethral surface)
- AMACR and HMWK staining present on same cells; lacks basal cell pattern of staining
- Eosinophilic secretions, thickened basement membranes, and appreciation of multiple patterns are helpful

SELECTED REFERENCES

1. McDaniel AS et al: Immunohistochemical staining characteristics of nephrogenic adenoma using the PIN-4 cocktail (p63, AMACR, and CK903) and GATA-3. Am J Surg Pathol. 38(12):1664-71, 2014
2. López JI et al: Nephrogenic adenoma of the urinary tract: clinical, histological, and immunohistochemical characteristics. Virchows Arch. 463(6):819-25, 2013
3. Piña-Oviedo S et al: Flat pattern of nephrogenic adenoma: previously unrecognized pattern unveiled using PAX2 and PAX8 immunohistochemistry. Mod Pathol. 26(6):792-8, 2013
4. Quinones W et al: Immunohistochemical markers for the differential diagnosis of nephrogenic adenomas. Ann Diagn Pathol. 17(1):41-4, 2013
5. Kunju LP: Nephrogenic adenoma: report of a case and review of morphologic mimics. Arch Pathol Lab Med. 134(10):1455-9, 2010
6. Cossu-Rocca P et al: S-100A1 is a reliable marker in distinguishing nephrogenic adenoma from prostatic adenocarcinoma. Am J Surg Pathol. Epub ahead of print, 2009
7. Fromont G et al: Revisiting the immunophenotype of nephrogenic adenoma. Am J Surg Pathol. 33(11):1654-8, 2009
8. Tong GX et al: Expression of PAX8 in nephrogenic adenoma and clear cell adenocarcinoma of the lower urinary tract: evidence of related histogenesis?. Am J Surg Pathol. 32(9):1380-7, 2008
9. Hansel DE et al: Fibromyxoid nephrogenic adenoma: a newly recognized variant mimicking mucinous adenocarcinoma. Am J Surg Pathol. 31(8):1231-7, 2007
10. Rahemtullah A et al: Nephrogenic adenoma: an update on an innocuous but troublesome entity. Adv Anat Pathol. 13(5):247-55, 2006
11. Xiao GQ et al: Nephrogenic adenoma: immunohistochemical evaluation for its etiology and differentiation from prostatic adenocarcinoma. Arch Pathol Lab Med. 130(6):805-10, 2006
12. Skinnider BF et al: Expression of alpha-methylacyl-CoA racemase (P504S) in nephrogenic adenoma: a significant immunohistochemical pitfall compounding the differential diagnosis with prostatic adenocarcinoma. Am J Surg Pathol. 28(6):701-5, 2004
13. Mazal PR et al: Derivation of nephrogenic adenomas from renal tubular cells in kidney-transplant recipients. N Engl J Med. 347(9):653-9, 2002
14. Gilcrease MZ et al: Clear cell adenocarcinoma and nephrogenic adenoma of the urethra and urinary bladder: a histopathologic and immunohistochemical comparison. Hum Pathol. 29(12):1451-6, 1998
15. Oliva E et al: Nephrogenic adenoma of the urinary tract: a review of the microscopic appearance of 80 cases with emphasis on unusual features. Mod Pathol. 8(7):722-30, 1995
16. Malpica A et al: Nephrogenic adenoma of the prostatic urethra involving the prostate gland: a clinicopathologic and immunohistochemical study of eight cases. Hum Pathol. 25(4):390-5, 1994
17. Young RH: Nephrogenic adenomas of the urethra involving the prostate gland: a report of two cases of a lesion that may be confused with prostatic adenocarcinoma. Mod Pathol. 5(6):617-20, 1992
18. Martin SA et al: Adenomatoid metaplasia of prostatic urethra. Am J Clin Pathol. 75(2):185-9, 1981

Nephrogenic Adenoma (Metaplasia) of Prostatic Urethra

NA Tubules and Surface Cells

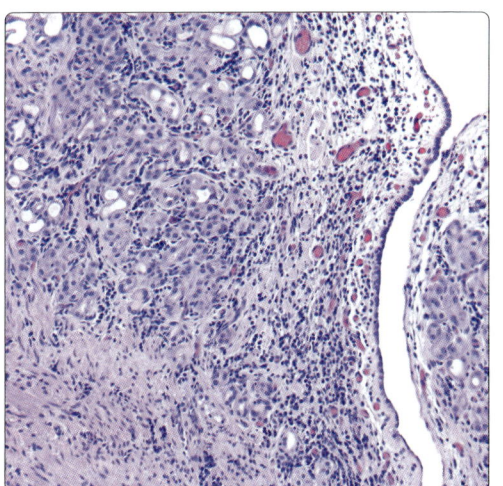

Hobnail Cells in NA

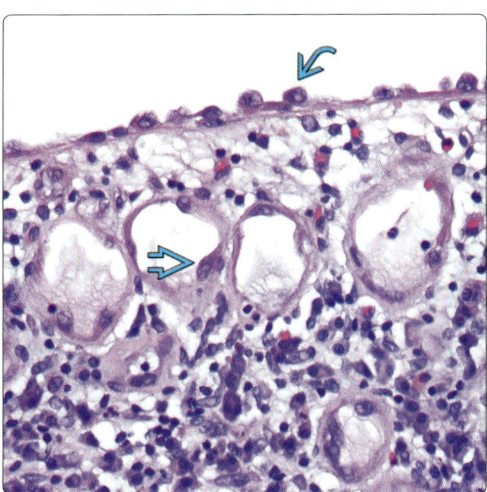

(Left) H&E shows a florid tubular proliferation underneath the surface, which is lined by a monolayer of NA cells. Note the presence of concomitant inflammation. (Right) H&E shows NA tubules lined by flattened cells with hobnail nuclei protruding in the lumen ➡. Similar cells are seen in the surface lining ➡. Note the presence of chronic inflammation in the background. Identification of the relationship of a small glandular proliferation in the prostate to the urethra is an important clue to diagnose NA.

NA Tubules

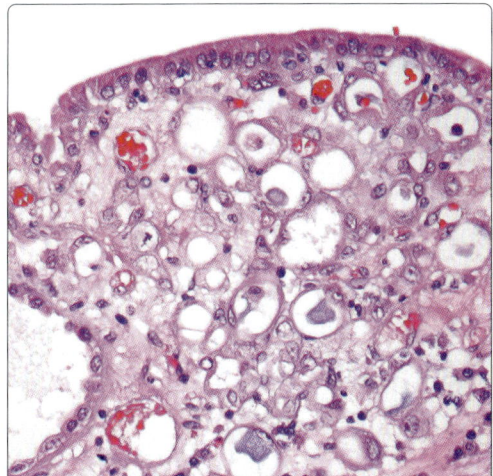

NA Tubules

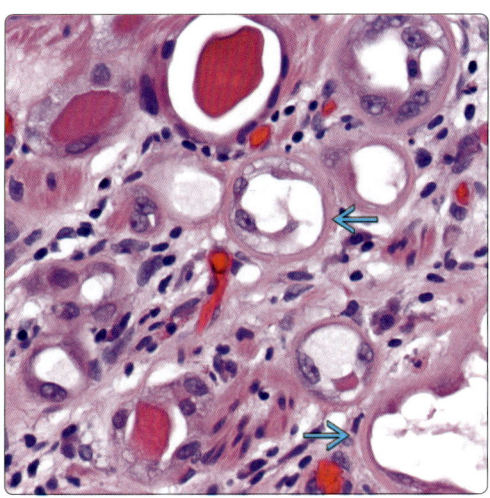

(Left) H&E of NA shows a tight cluster of hollow tubules mimicking a florid vascular proliferation. Occasional true capillaries (containing RBCs) are seen in this cluster, which may add to the false impression. (Right) High-power magnification of NA shows variably sized round hollow tubules with characteristic thickened basement membrane ➡. Some of the tubules contain intraluminal eosinophilic secretions that impart resemblance to thyroid follicles.

NA Tubules

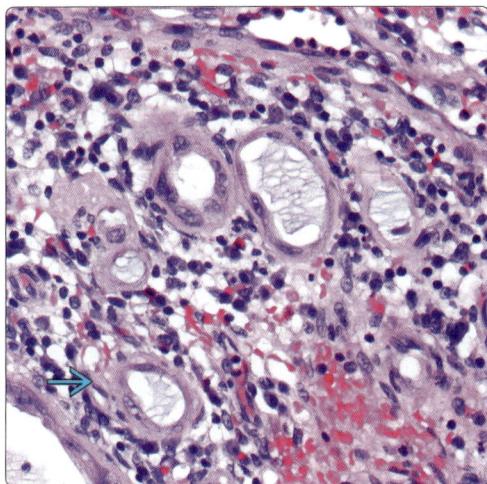

NA Tubules

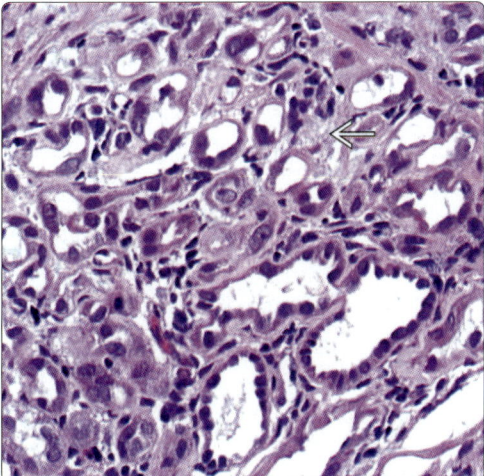

(Left) H&E shows NA tubules with intraluminal basophilic secretions. Note the characteristic thickened basement membrane ➡ around the tubules, which may be highlighted with PAS stain. (Right) H&E shows NA tubules lined by hobnail cells, some tubules are smaller in caliber and contain scant intraluminal basophilic secretions. Some of the tubules resemble capillary vessels. Note the basophilic hue of extracellular mucinous material in the stroma ➡ along with the background inflammation.

Nephrogenic Adenoma (Metaplasia) of Prostatic Urethra

(Left) H&E shows that there is marked variation in the size and shape of the tubules, a feature that is rare in prostatic carcinoma. The cytoplasm is eosinophilic and the nuclei have a hobnail appearance. There is accompanying inflammation. (Right) H&E of NA shows numerous tubules lined by clear cells. Presence of clear cells raises concern for clear cell adenocarcinoma (CCA) or prostatic carcinoma. In contrast to NA, CCA is less common in males and shows obvious cytologic atypia and features of malignancy.

NA Tubules
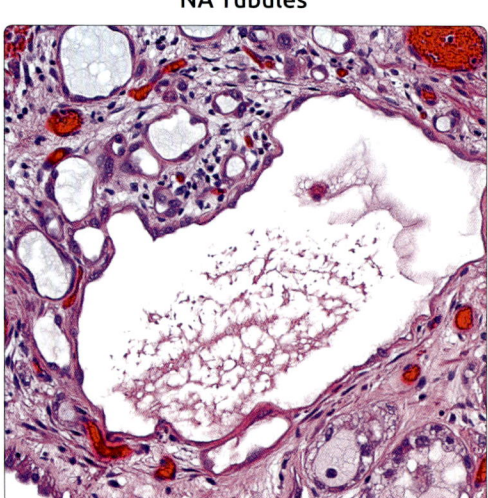

NA Tubules
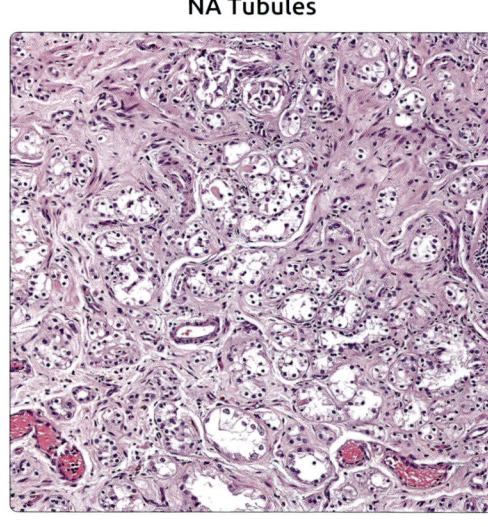

(Left) Occasionally, NA tubules can be very tiny, showing small lumina with a single nucleus and may contain basophilic mucin, mimicking signet ring cells ➡. This H&E shows the presence of extracellular basophilic mucin in the stroma. (Right) Solid or diffuse pattern of NA is shown. This pattern usually occurs as a minor component and is often admixed with other architectural patterns. Observation of a range of architectural patterns in the same lesion should raise the possibility of NA.

NA Tubules and Signet Ring Cells
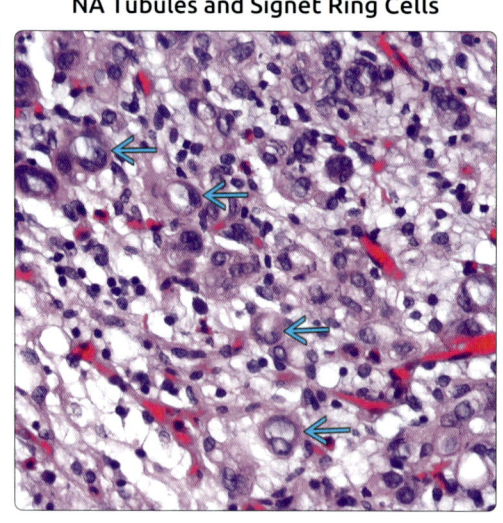

NA Tubules and Solid Growth
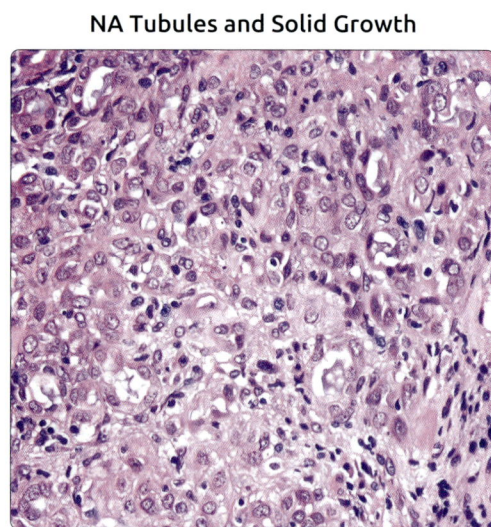

(Left) H&E shows fibromyxoid stromal background and occasional elongated and spindled cells of NA ➡. Note the presence of typical NA tubule with hobnail nuclei ➡. (Right) H&E shows a flat NA at the urethral surface consisting of multiple layers of cells with crowded and overlapping nuclei. No tubules are present in the lamina propria. This rare pattern of NA can be contiguous with the urothelium and may mimic a flat urothelial lesion. Note the characteristic thick basement membrane underneath the NA cells ➡.

Fibromyxoid NA
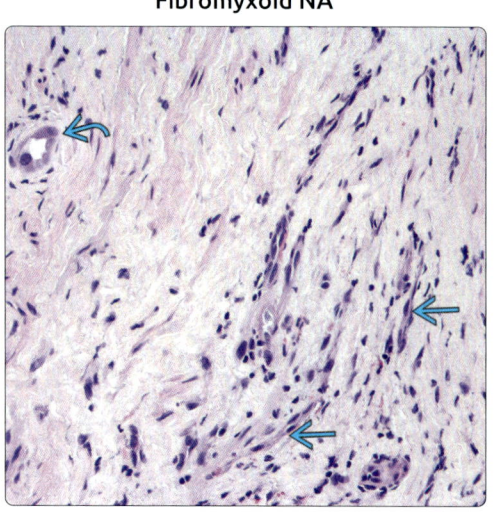

Flat NA
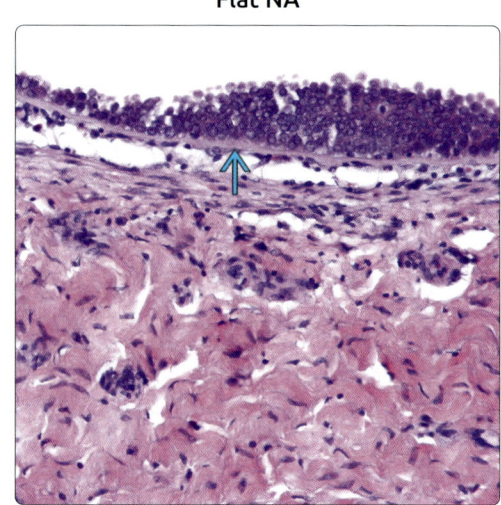

Nephrogenic Adenoma (Metaplasia) of Prostatic Urethra

NA Tubules Mimicking Prostate Cancer

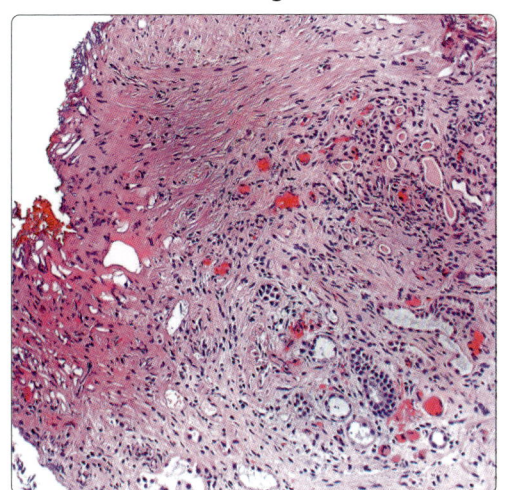

NA Tubules Mimicking Prostate Cancer With Atrophic Pattern

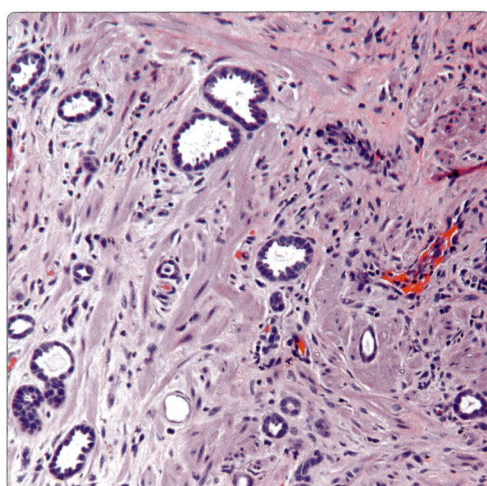

(Left) NA tubules are shown in a TURP chip. Extension of urethral NA into the prostatic fibromuscular stroma is common and may enter into the differential diagnosis of atypical glandular proliferations of the prostate. *(Right)* Several rigid NA tubules in the prostate stroma are shown. In contrast to prostate adenocarcinoma, these NA tubular cells show frequent hobnail nuclei and do not exhibit nucleomegaly and prominent nucleoli. The differential diagnosis is the atrophic pattern of prostatic cancer.

NA Tubules With Occasional Nucleoli

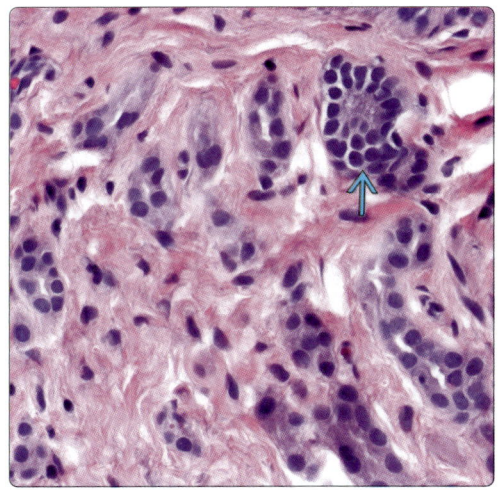

NA Tubules With Infiltrative Appearance

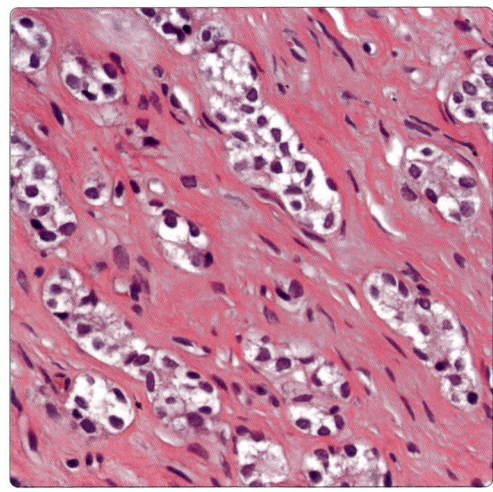

(Left) High-power view shows small NA tubules lined by cuboidal cells with eosinophilic cytoplasm. Note some of the nuclei contain a discrete nucleolus ➡. This pattern of NA resembles Gleason pattern 3 prostate carcinoma and distinction, compounded by the overlap in immunohistochemical staining, can be difficult in a needle biopsy. *(Right)* Cluster of NA tubules and cords with clear to eosinophilic cytoplasm show pseudoinfiltrative growth pattern in the prostate stroma, mimicking microacinar prostate adenocarcinoma.

NA Tubules Mimicking High-Grade Prostate Cancer

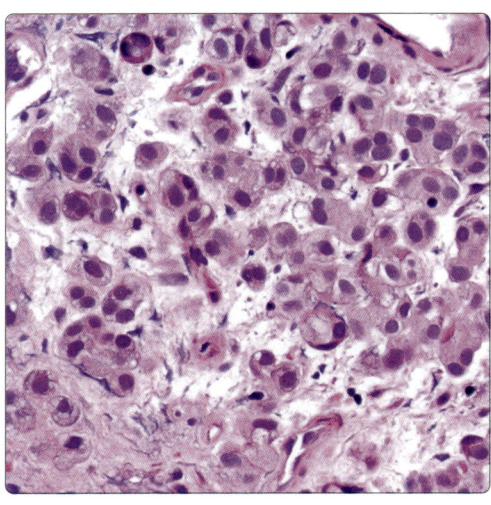

NA Tubules Mimicking Prostate Cancer

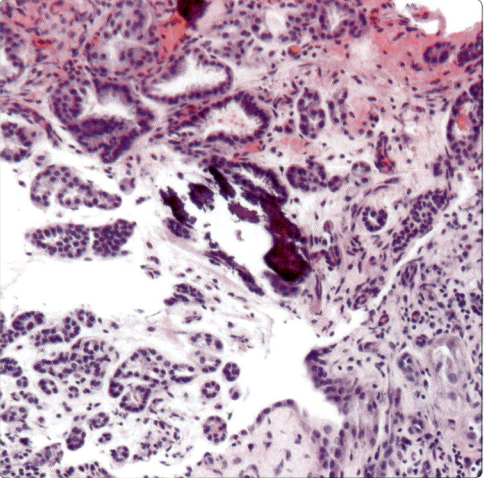

(Left) NA shows clusters of small, poorly formed tubules and occasional separate single cells, mimicking Gleason pattern 4 and 5 prostate adenocarcinoma, respectively. In challenging cases, appropriate immunohistochemical stains [PSA/PAP(-) and pax-8(+)] may be helpful. *(Right)* Rarely, microcalcifications may be seen in NA. The background stroma is edematous. The variation in the size & shape of the tubules plus stromal edema helps distinguish NA from the atrophic pattern of prostatic adenocarcinoma.

Nephrogenic Adenoma (Metaplasia) of Prostatic Urethra

NA Papillae

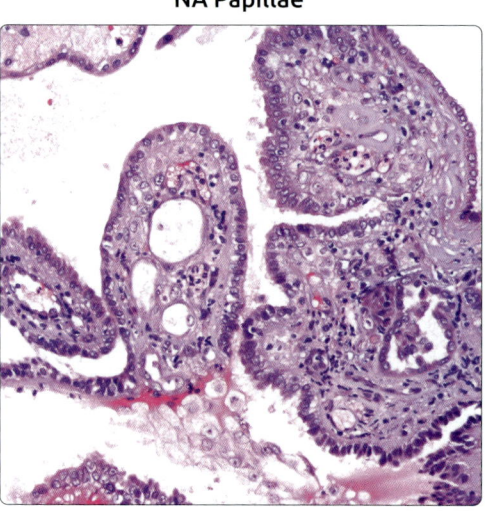

NA Papillae

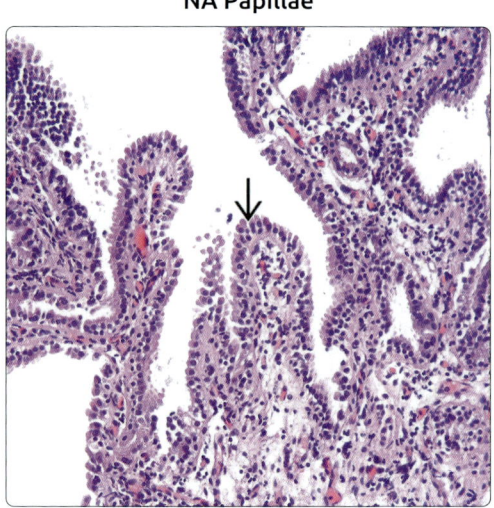

(Left) H&E shows simple NA papillae with few tubules lined by flattened cells in the fibrovascular cores. Presence of single cell layer and tubules distinguish this NA from papillary urothelial neoplasm. (Right) Exophytic papillary projections of NA show papillae that are nonbranching or have minimal branching. Papillae, when present, are frequently accompanied by subepithelial tubular proliferations. These papillae are lined by a monolayer of cells ➡ similar to those in tubules.

NA Papillae

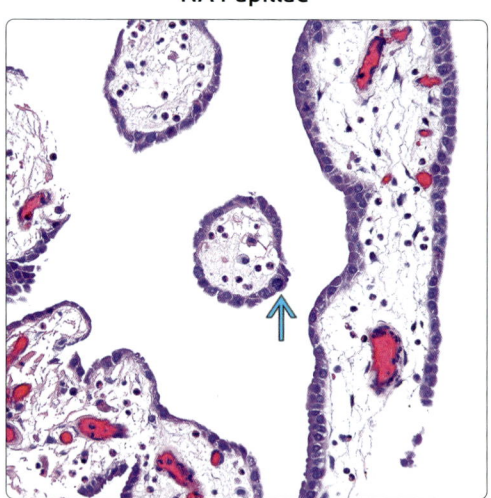

NA Papillae

(Left) Simple NA papillae are evident without branching, and are lined by single layer of cuboidal to flattened cells. Note the presence of mitosis ➡, which is rare in NA. Overall, the cells do not exhibit cytologic atypia. The papillary core shows stromal edema and scattered acute inflammatory cells. (Right) Uncommonly, the papillary growth may be florid & show more complex branching. These papillae may mimic a papillary urothelial neoplasm (PUN). Distinction is tenable, as PUN is typically multilayered.

NA and Papillary Urothelial Carcinoma

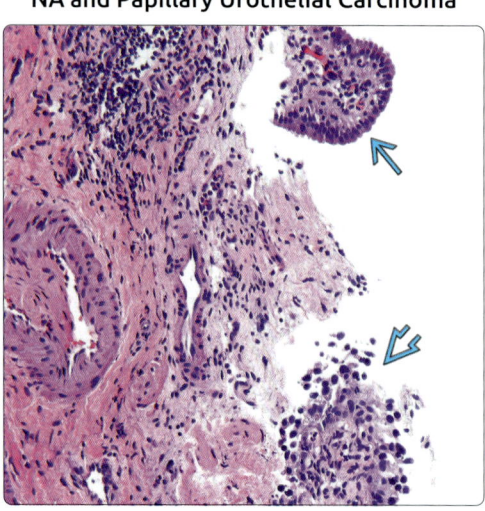

Concomitant Papillary Urothelial Neoplasm and NA

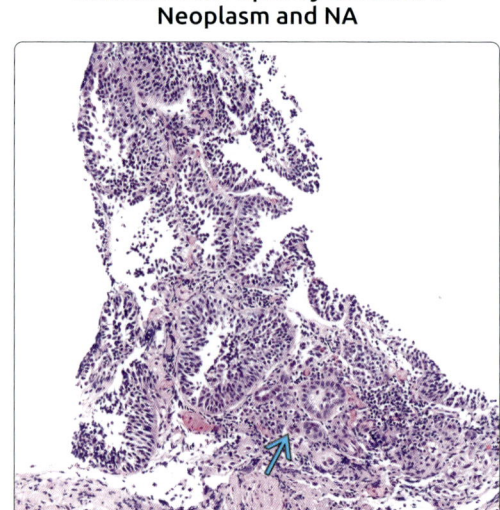

(Left) NA papilla ➡ is adjacent to a focus of urothelial carcinoma in situ (CIS) ➡. NA papilla is monolayered and shows only minimal cytologic atypia. In contrast, the focus of CIS shows multiple layers of hyperchromatic pleomorphic cells. (Right) Low-power view shows papillary urothelial neoplasm of low malignant potential (PUNLMP) and underlying tubules of NA ➡. The NA tubules may simulate a glandular change in a urothelial neoplasm. Note the presence of luminal basophilic secretions in the glands.

Nephrogenic Adenoma (Metaplasia) of Prostatic Urethra

p63 in NA

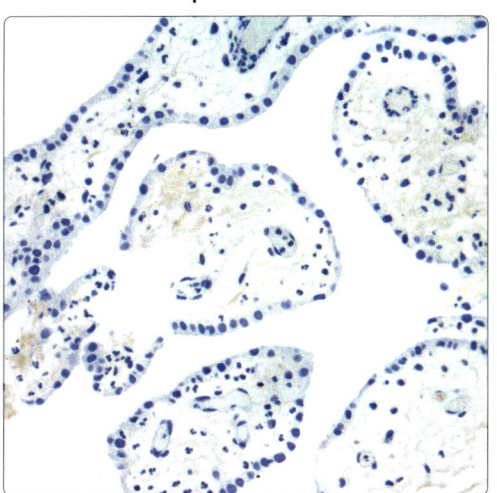

AMACR in NA

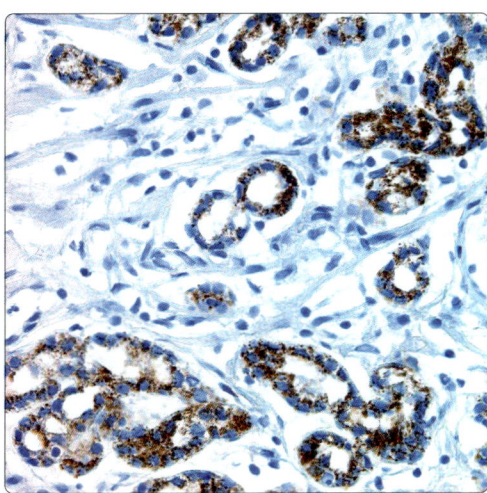

(Left) p63 shows lack of staining in NA. p63 is expressed in papillary urothelial neoplasm (PUN) and can be helpful in their distinction from NA. Distinction of papillary NA from PUN may often be made by morphology alone. The other commonly used urothelial marker GATA3 is expressed by some NA and is less helpful compared to p63. **(Right)** Granular cytoplasmic AMACR positivity in NA tubules is shown. Awareness of this pitfall is important in the differential diagnosis of prostate adenocarcinoma.

PIN-4 in NA

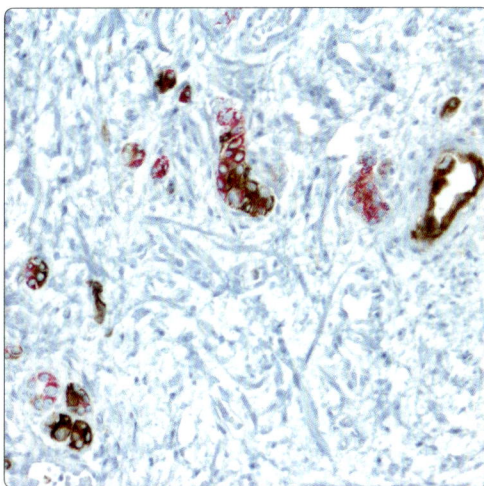

pax-8 in NA

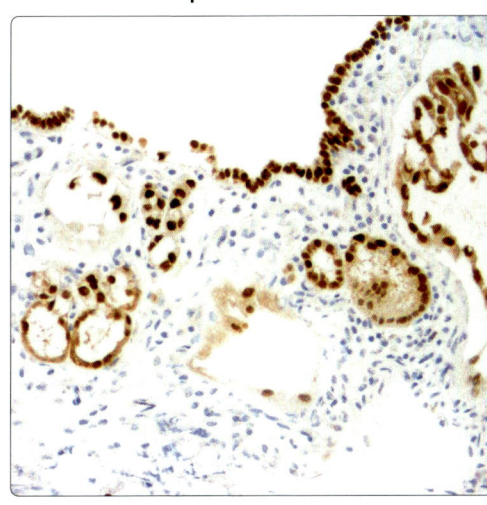

(Left) PIN-4 staining in NA shows admixture of AMACR (red) and HMCK (brown) positivity in the same glands. HMCK is commonly positive in NA unlike in prostate adenocarcinoma. NA does not show basal HMCK staining exhibited by benign prostatic glands. Occasionally, HMCK positivity in NA is masked by the intense red AMACR staining. **(Right)** pax-8 shows diffuse nuclear positivity in NA. This marker is useful in distinguishing NA from prostatic adenocarcinoma. Note the similar positivity in the surface monolayer of cells.

S100-A1 in NA

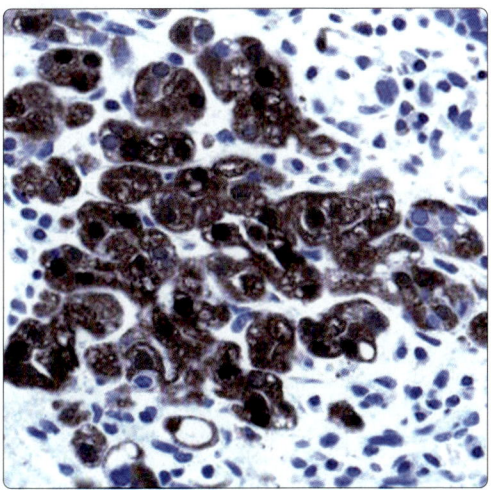

PSA in NA

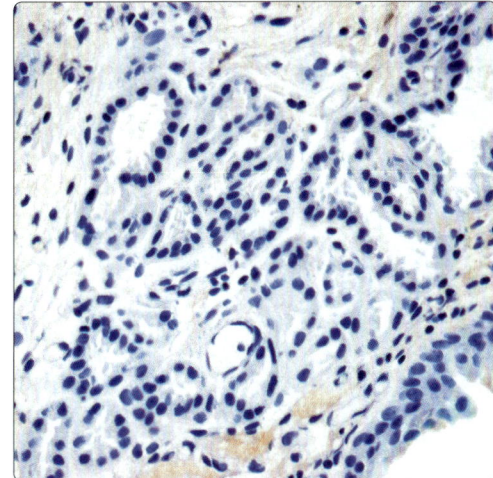

(Left) S100-A1, a marker associated with renal tubular differentiation, is positive (nuclear and cytoplasmic) in NA. It is not expressed in prostate adenocarcinoma and is helpful in the differential diagnosis. **(Right)** NA shows negative reaction to PSA, which complements positivity to pax-8 and S100-A1 in NA [PSA(-) and pax-8/S100-A1(+)] vs. prostate adenocarcinoma [PSA(+) and pax-8/S100-A1(-)]. Rare and focal positivity for PSA and PAP has been reported in NA such that a panel of markers should be employed in their distinction.

Prostatic Intraepithelial Neoplasia

KEY FACTS

TERMINOLOGY

- High-grade prostatic intraepithelial neoplasia (HGPIN)
  - Noninvasive neoplastic transformation of lining epithelium of existing prostatic ducts and acini characterized by severe nuclear atypia

ETIOLOGY/PATHOGENESIS

- Generally similar to that of prostatic adenocarcinoma
  - *TMPRSS-ERG* fusion (and ERG expression by IHC) may be seen in minority of HGPIN

CLINICAL ISSUES

- HGPIN is present as isolated diagnosis in 4-16% of needle core biopsies and < 5% in transurethral resection specimens
- Present in over 80% of prostate glands harboring adenocarcinoma vs. 43% of age-matched controls
- Incidence ↑ with age, reaching up to 67% in 8th decade
- Median risk of cancer following diagnosis of HGPIN is ~ 21% in more recent series

MICROSCOPIC

- Preexistent ducts and acini are lined by crowded epithelial cells with abnormal cytologic features
  - Enlarged monomorphic nuclei, prominent nucleoli, hyperchromasia, nuclear overlap, amphophilic cytoplasm
- Preserved or discontinuous basal cell layer may be readily identified on H&E or rarely only with basal cell-specific immunostains
- 4 major architectural patterns: Tufted, micropapillary, cribriform, and flat
- Other uncommon types: Signet ring, mucinous, foamy, inverted or hobnail, small cell (neuroendocrine)

TOP DIFFERENTIAL DIAGNOSES

- Central zone glands
- Intraductal carcinoma
- PIN-like adenocarcinoma
- Urothelial carcinoma involving prostatic ducts

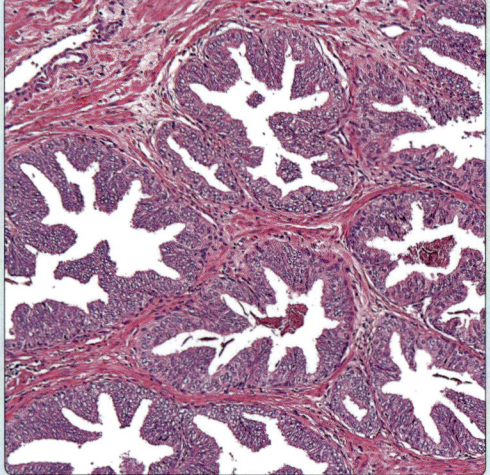

High-Grade PIN

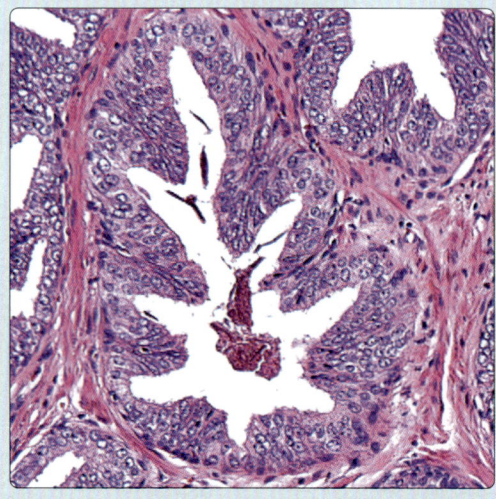

PIN: Tufted Pattern

(Left) *High-grade prostatic intraepithelial neoplasia (HGPIN) shows large- and medium-sized glandular structures, which appear expanded and crowded but retain their rounded contours. Basal cell layer in HGPIN is often discernible on H&E-stained sections.* **(Right)** *A tufted pattern of HGPIN shows stratification of acinar cells causing luminal undulations or folds. These glands retain their rounded contour, and basal cell layer is discernible. The lesions are hyperchromatic due to nuclear stratification.*

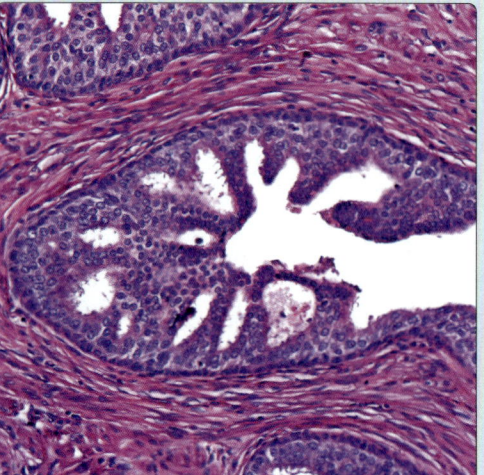

PIN: Cribriform Pattern

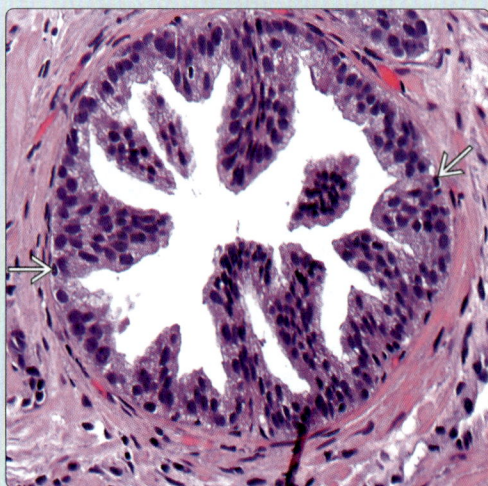

PIN: Micropapillary Pattern

(Left) *A cribriform pattern of HGPIN shows luminal cellular proliferation characterized by the presence of multiple irregular or rounded lumina. The glands retain their rounded contours, and the basal cell layer is discernible.* **(Right)** *In this pattern, the epithelial proliferation takes the form of slender and long papillary projections without fibrovascular cores. Basal cells are readily identifiable in some areas ➡.*

Prostatic Intraepithelial Neoplasia

TERMINOLOGY

Abbreviations
- Prostatic intraepithelial neoplasia (PIN)

Definitions
- PIN: Noninvasive neoplastic transformation of lining epithelium of preexisting prostatic ducts and acini
  - Historically categorized into low-grade or high-grade PIN (HGPIN), but currently only high-grade lesions are reported
- HGPIN: Characterized by severe nuclear atypia (as in carcinoma) and varied architectural patterns

ETIOLOGY/PATHOGENESIS

Genetics
- Provides evidence of association between HGPIN and prostate carcinoma (PCa)
- *TMPRSS-ERG* fusion
  - Seen in 19% of HGPIN intermingling with cancer foci vs. 48.5% for clinically localized PCa
  - Much less common in HGPIN cases not associated with invasive carcinoma
- Aneuploid DNA seen in 32-58% of cases
- Nuclear morphometric studies show characteristics intermediate between cancer and benign glands
- Deletions of chromosome 8p most common allelic loss, detected in both HGPIN and adenocarcinoma
- Increased expression of *CDKN2A* (p16), *TP53* (p53), *AMACR*, *BCL2*, and *MYC* genes
- Intact expression of *PTEN*
- Hypermethylation of glutathionine S-transferase

CLINICAL ISSUES

Epidemiology
- Incidence
  - HGPIN is present as isolated diagnosis in up to 16% of needle core biopsies (usually 5-6%) and 1-5% in transurethral resection specimens
  - Present in 80-100% of prostate glands harboring adenocarcinoma vs. 43% of age-matched controls
- Age
  - May be seen as early as 3rd decade; incidence increases with age, reaching up to 67% by 8th decade
- Ethnicity
  - Lesion is usually more diffuse and presents earlier in African Americans compared to Caucasians

Presentation
- Asymptomatic, commonly encountered as incidental histologic finding
- May have abnormal serum PSA level

Treatment
- Surgical approaches
  - No aggressive treatment (i.e., surgery, radiation) is warranted with diagnosis of HGPIN, unless concomitant adenocarcinoma is documented
- Risk of cancer
  - In contemporary data, with extended sampling biopsy, median risk of cancer following diagnosis of HGPIN is ~ 21%
    - This is not significantly different from risk following benign diagnosis (~ 19%)
      - Thus, recommendations on follow-up of diagnosis of HGPIN are currently controversial
  - Patients with multifocal (i.e., > 3 cores), bilateral HGPIN and that associated with atypical foci have higher risk of harboring concomitant PCa and should be more aggressively followed

IMAGING

Ultrasonographic Findings
- May be associated with hypoechoic lesion in peripheral zone

MACROSCOPIC

General Features
- Not associated with recognizable gross findings

Sections to Be Submitted
- If only HGPIN (without invasive foci) detected in transurethral resection
  - Submit entire specimen for histologic evaluation or obtain deeper levels of block with HGPIN
  - Biopsy of peripheral zone may be option, particularly in younger males
- If only HGPIN (without invasive foci) detected in prostate needle biopsy specimen
  - May consider deeper levels if extensive or associated with atypical small acinar proliferation (ASAP)

MICROSCOPIC

Histologic Features
- Preexisting ducts and acini, usually of medium to large size, lined by crowded epithelial cells with abnormal cytologic features
  - Hyperchromasia
  - Nuclear overlap
  - Enlarged relatively monomorphic nuclei
  - Prominent nucleoli (easily observed at 20x magnification)
  - Amphophilic cytoplasm
- Preserved or discontinuous basal cell layer may be readily identified on routine slides or only with basal cell-specific immunostains
- 4 major architectural patterns of HGPIN
  - **Tufted**: Stratification of acinar cells imparting luminal undulations or folds
  - **Micropapillary**: Nuclear stratification forming slender filiform projections and cellular budding
  - **Cribriform**: Complex proliferation resulting in multiple irregular or round punched-out lumina
    - May show "cellular maturation," as peripheral cells show greater nuclear atypia (i.e., nucleomegaly, prominent nucleoli) than cells at luminal aspect
  - **Flat**: Lacks cellular stratification (1 or 2 cell layers)
- Other uncommon types
  - Signet ring

Prostatic Intraepithelial Neoplasia

- o Mucinous
- o Foamy
- o Inverted or hobnail
- o Small cell
- Multiple patterns frequently seen concurrently
- Variety of other architectural and cytologic features may be observed in HGPIN
  - o Luminal cytoplasmic blebs, epithelial arches, cellular trabecular epithelial bars, "Roman bridges," partial gland involvement, and basal cell layer disruption with glandular budding
    - Uncommonly, large cystic gland pattern, involvement in nodular hyperplasia and mucinous metaplasia
- Variety of luminal features may be observed in HGPIN
  - o Proteinaceous secretions, corpora amylacea, and exfoliated cells of PIN
  - o Uncommonly, microcalcifications and crystalloids; comedonecrosis is extremely rare

Predominant Pattern/Injury Type
- Neoplastic

Predominant Cell/Compartment Type
- Epithelial, glandular

Grade
- Low-grade PIN
  - o Tufted or micropapillary pattern
  - o Nuclear crowding, stratification, and irregular spacing
  - o Mild nuclear enlargement, with inconspicuous to rare prominent nucleoli
  - o Diagnostic reproducibility is very low and has questionable relationship to PCa
  - o Should not be diagnosed in needle core biopsies, as management and significance are uncertain
- HGPIN
  - o Cellular proliferation within medium to large glands
  - o Increased basophilia or amphophilia readily detected at low power
  - o Hyperchromasia, nucleomegaly, nuclear membrane irregularity, macronucleoli
  - o Greater reproducibility among pathologists and more established relationship to concomitant or subsequent adenocarcinoma

ANCILLARY TESTS

Immunohistochemistry
- Basal cell markers [p63, HMCK(34βE12)] highlight intact or frequently discontinuous basal cell layer around involved ducts
- Due to discontinuous basal cell layer, these cells may not be apparent in particular plane of section, compounding differential diagnosis with PCa
- AMACR variably stains acinar cells (56-100%)
- PSA/PSAP(+) in acinar cells
- ERG may be positive in minority of cases

DIFFERENTIAL DIAGNOSIS

Prostate Central Zone Glands
- Show architectural complexity, including cribriforming and "Roman bridges," but lack nuclear changes of HGPIN

Seminal Vesicle/Ejaculatory Duct Epithelium
- No prominent nucleoli
- More pleomorphism than HGPIN
- Nuclear pseudoinclusions
- Degenerative nuclear atypia
- Intracellular coarse lipofuscin pigment

Prostate Glands With Reactive Atypia (Inflammation, Infarction, or Radiation)
- Diagnosis of HGPIN should require more stringent criteria or should be questioned in areas of infarction, inflammation, or in previously radiated glands
- Architectural features of HGPIN tend to be absent in mimics

Transitional Cell Metaplasia
- Multilayered cells or solid nests that lack typical patterns of HGPIN
- Uniform, elongated cells with nuclear grooves; secretory cell layer may be focally present

Benign Prostate Hyperplasia Nodule With Prominent Papillary Fronds
- Located in transition zone, background BPH
- Architectural complexity but lack atypical cytology of HGPIN

Cribriform Hyperplasia
- Located in transition zone
- Frequently clear cytoplasm with no amphophilia
- Lack of nuclear changes of HGPIN

Atypical Basal Cell Hyperplasia
- Atypical nuclei are in basal and not secretory cells; usually architectural patterns of HGPIN absent
- Frequently lumina are obliterated

Low-Grade Acinar Adenocarcinoma
- Small glands adjacent to HGPIN may pose particularly difficult differential diagnosis
- May not be possible to determine whether small glands represent adjacent invasive adenocarcinoma or tangentially sectioned outpouching of HGPIN glands
- Immunostains are useful only if basal cells are demonstrated in small glands, indicating outpouching
- Even in absence of basal cell markers, small glands could still represent HGPIN, as basal cell layer may frequently be discontinuous or markedly attenuated
- Such cases may be diagnosed as HGPIN with atypical focus suspicious, but not diagnostic, for carcinoma

High-Grade Acinar Adenocarcinoma With Cribriform Pattern (Gleason Pattern 4 or 5)
- Greater architectural complexity, including consistent cribriforming, back-to-back glands, and solid nests
- Confluence of cribriform structures
- Absent basal cell layer with IHC

PIN-Like Adenocarcinoma
- Some adenocarcinomas may have stratified epithelium and may form medium-sized glands
- Numerous atypical glands with absence of basal cell layer; may be associated with typical acinar pattern

Prostatic Intraepithelial Neoplasia

Ductal Adenocarcinoma

- Commonly involves prostatic urethra and periurethral region; involvement may be diffuse
- Shows expansile large glandular pattern
- Papillae contain true fibrovascular stalks; maturation not present
- Nuclei frequently pseudostratified with elongated appearance; mitoses may be frequent
- Invasive features present, such as crowded back-to-back glands, stromal fibrosis, perineural invasion, extraprostatic extension
- Majority lacks basal cell layer confirmed by use of basal cell markers [p63 and HMCK(34βE12)]

Basal Cell/Adenoid Cystic Carcinoma

- Basaloid-appearing cells with smaller nuclei with adenoid cystic pattern; infiltrative architecture
- Basement membrane material may be present
- p63 &/or HMCK(34βE12)(+)
- Typically PSA/PSAP(-)

Urothelial (Transitional Cell) Carcinoma Involving Prostatic Ducts and Acini

- Significant cellular pleomorphism and mitotic activity within large glandular structures
- Cytoplasm is densely eosinophilic and may show squamoid features
- Pagetoid growth by neoplastic cells with elevation and preservation of normal secretory cells
- PSA or PSAP (-); p63, HMCK(34βE12) (+)
- Clinical history of bladder urothelial neoplasm is often present

Intraductal Carcinoma of Prostate

- Controversial nomenclature when it is exclusive finding in needle core biopsy
- Suggested to represent either intraductal or intraacinar spread of invasive prostate carcinoma or intraluminal carcinomatous progression of HGPIN
- *TMPRSS-ERG* fusion more common in intraductal carcinoma than HGPIN
- *PTEN* loss more common in intraductal carcinoma (*PTEN* loss not identified in HGPIN)
- Similar loss of heterozygosity seen with Gleason pattern 4 and 5 adenocarcinoma
- Multivariate analysis confirms independent adverse prognostic value of intraductal carcinoma over Gleason grade, stage, tumor volume, and treatment failure
- Proposed criteria for diagnosing atypical intraductal lesions exceeding HGPIN but lacking features of invasive carcinoma include
  - Major criteria
    - Large glands (> 2x normal), presence of basal cells (confirmed by immunohistochemistry), cytologically malignant cells (enlarged nuclei, prominent nucleoli) with frequent mitosis, cells spanning gland lumen, comedonecrosis
  - Minor criteria
    - Irregular (angled) gland branching, round smooth gland contour, frequently 2 populations of cells
    - Solid or extensive cribriform architecture
- Basal cell layer is present, similar to HGPIN; often continuous
- Without invasive foci, may be impossible to differentiate vs. HGPIN in limited biopsy material or when lesion is not extensive
- Limited number of cases with follow-up show that virtually all cases have invasive carcinoma in rebiopsy or prostatectomy
- Closely associated with large volume and high-grade invasive adenocarcinoma (Gleason pattern 4 or 5)

DIAGNOSTIC CHECKLIST

Pathologic Interpretation Pearls

- Screen for HGPIN on low-power magnification and confirm cytologic features on high-power view
- If cytologic threshold for diagnosis is doubtful or borderline, probably not HGPIN
- If features exceed HGPIN, consider intraductal carcinoma

REPORTING

Key Elements to Report

- Look for suspicious small glands for invasive cancer adjacent to foci of HGPIN
- Presence or absence of concomitant adenocarcinoma
- Number of biopsy cores involved by HGPIN
- Number of foci of HGPIN (e.g., isolated, focal, multifocal, extensive)
- Associated atypical small acinar proliferation suspicious for cancer

SELECTED REFERENCES

1. Lotan TL et al: Cytoplasmic PTEN protein loss distinguishes intraductal carcinoma of the prostate from high-grade prostatic intraepithelial neoplasia. Mod Pathol. 26(4):587-603, 2013
2. Singh PB et al: Risk of prostate cancer after detection of isolated high-grade prostatic intraepithelial neoplasia (HGPIN) on extended core needle biopsy: a UK hospital experience. BMC Urol. 9:3, 2009
3. Delatour NL et al: Positive predictive value of high-grade prostatic intraepithelial neoplasia in initial core needle biopsies of prostate adenocarcinoma--a study with complete sampling of hemi-prostates with corresponding negative biopsy findings. Urology. 72(3):623-7, 2008
4. Cohen RJ et al: A proposal on the identification, histologic reporting, and implications of intraductal prostatic carcinoma. Arch Pathol Lab Med. 131(7):1103-9, 2007
5. Perner S et al: TMPRSS2-ERG fusion prostate cancer: an early molecular event associated with invasion. Am J Surg Pathol. 31(6):882-8, 2007
6. Egevad L et al: Current practice of diagnosis and reporting of prostatic intraepithelial neoplasia and glandular atypia among genitourinary pathologists. Mod Pathol. 19(2):180-5, 2006
7. Epstein JI et al: Prostate needle biopsies containing prostatic intraepithelial neoplasia or atypical foci suspicious for carcinoma: implications for patient care. J Urol. 175(3 Pt 1):820-34, 2006
8. Netto GJ et al: Widespread high-grade prostatic intraepithelial neoplasia on prostatic needle biopsy: a significant likelihood of subsequently diagnosed adenocarcinoma. Am J Surg Pathol. 30(9):1184-8, 2006
9. Bishara T et al: High-grade prostatic intraepithelial neoplasia on needle biopsy: risk of cancer on repeat biopsy related to number of involved cores and morphologic pattern. Am J Surg Pathol. 28(5):629-33, 2004
10. McNeal JE et al: Spread of adenocarcinoma within prostatic ducts and acini. Morphologic and clinical correlations. Am J Surg Pathol. 20(7):802-14, 1996
11. Sakr WA et al: The frequency of carcinoma and intraepithelial neoplasia of the prostate in young male patients. J Urol. 150(2 Pt 1):379-85, 1993

Prostatic Intraepithelial Neoplasia

(Left) In this pattern of HGPIN, there are 1 or 2 layers of neoplastic cells without papillation or cribriform morphology. Note the features of the neoplastic cells (large nuclei and prominent nucleoli). Basal cells were identified by immunostains. **(Right)** This is the same case of flat HGPIN in which the basal cells were highlighted by a high molecular weight cytokeratin. This immunostain is very helpful in identifying basal cells in difficult or ambiguous cases.

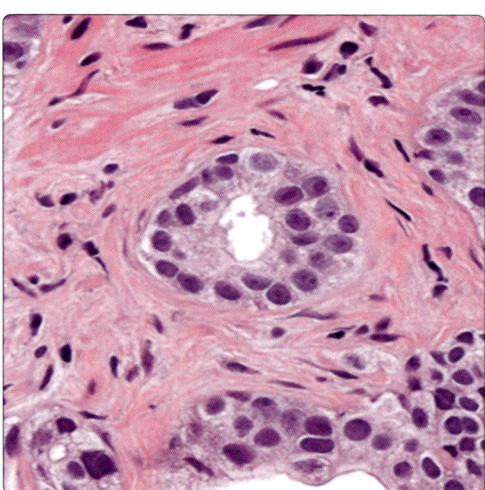

PIN: Flat Pattern

PIN: Immunostain (Basal Cell Marker)

(Left) HGPIN shows nuclear enlargement, nuclear overlap, hyperchromasia, prominent nucleoli, and amphophilic cytoplasm. Prominent nucleoli in HGPIN may easily be observed at 20x magnification. Discontinuous basal cell layer ➡ is identifiable. **(Right)** Cribriform pattern of HGPIN shows "cellular maturation," wherein the peripheral cells ➡ show greater nuclear atypia (i.e., nucleomegaly, prominent nucleoli) than cells at the luminal aspect ➡.

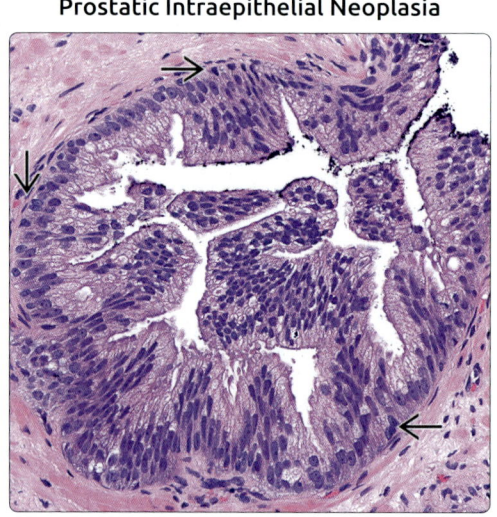
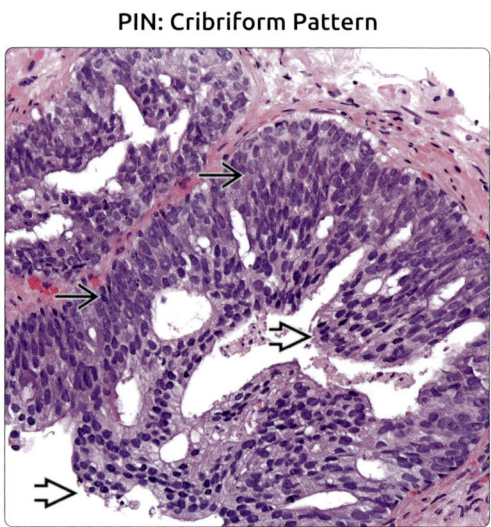

Prostatic Intraepithelial Neoplasia

PIN: Cribriform Pattern

(Left) A micropapillary pattern of HGPIN shows stratification of acinar cells forming slender filiform projections. Detached cellular budding may be seen distally. There are no fibrovascular cores (pseudopapillae). **(Right)** In this HGPIN, there is a population of small cells in the center of the lumen, reminiscent of small cell neuroendocrine carcinoma. This unusual pattern does not always express neuroendocrine markers.

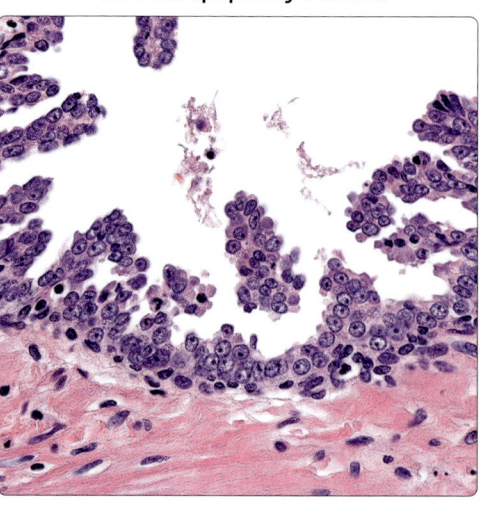
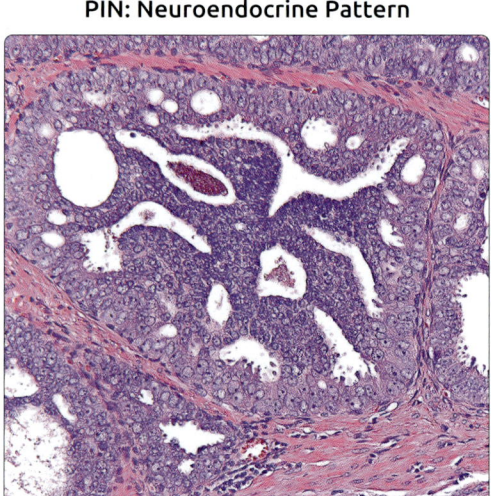

PIN: Micropapillary Pattern

PIN: Neuroendocrine Pattern

Prostatic Intraepithelial Neoplasia

PIN: Inverted Pattern
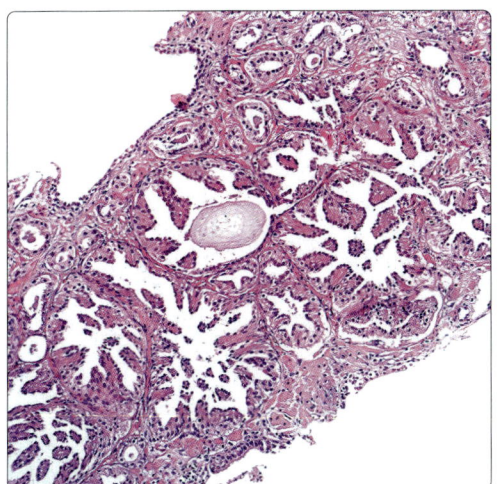

PIN: Inverted Pattern
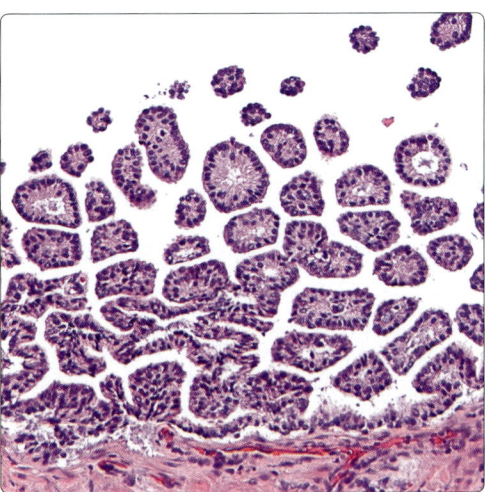

(Left) An inverted gland flat pattern of HGPIN is admixed with small glands of prostate carcinoma in a needle biopsy, as seen here. (Right) In this pattern of inverted HGPIN, detached tufts of neoplastic cells are present and characterized by nuclei with reversed polarity (they line the luminal aspect of the gland). This is also referred to as a hobnail pattern of HGPIN.

PIN: Hobnail Inverted Pattern
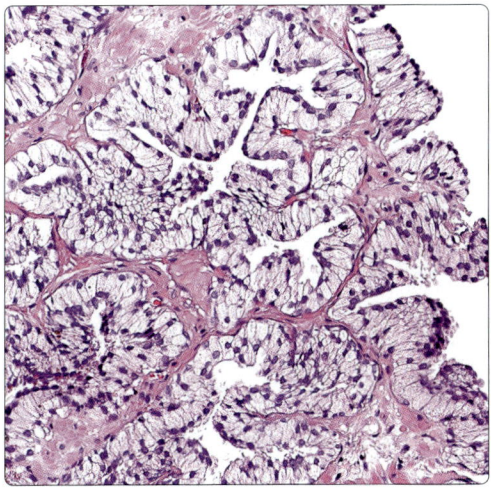

PIN: Flat Pattern
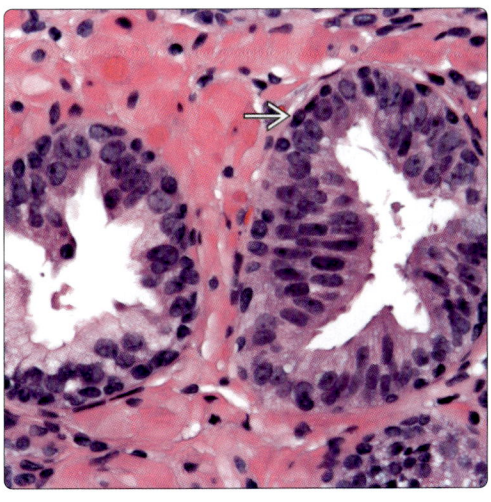

(Left) In this HGPIN with hobnail or inverted pattern, the nuclei are characteristically aligned along the luminal aspect of the gland. The glands with HGPIN additionally contain abundant foamy cytoplasm. (Right) The glands in this section are small with minimal stratification, but the nuclear and cytoplasmic features requisite for HGPIN are present (nucleomegaly, prominent nucleoli, amphophilic cytoplasm). Basal cells are also identifiable ➡.

PIN: Invasive Carcinoma, Adjacent Atypical Glands
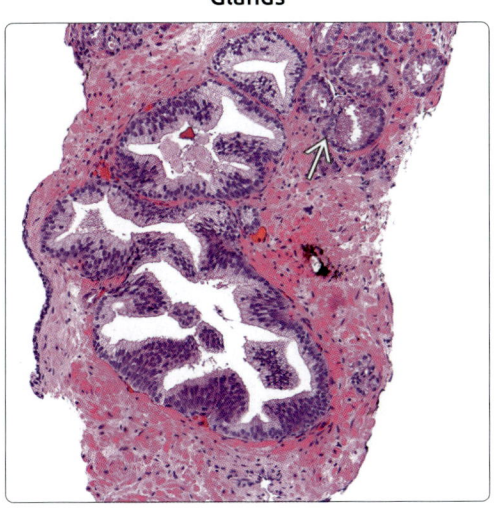

PIN and Adjacent Atypical Glands
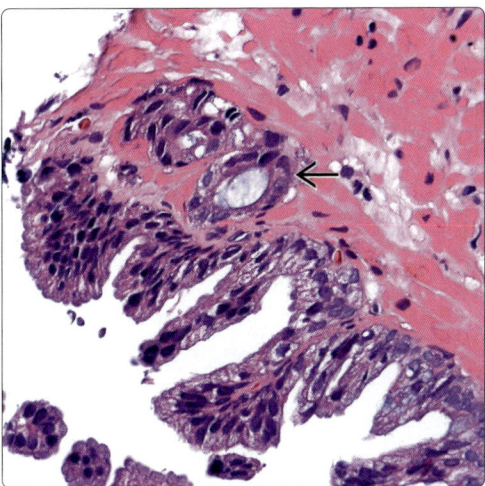

(Left) HGPIN is frequently associated with invasive carcinoma ➡ characterized by tight clusters of small glands adjacent to HGPIN glands. Careful examination is important to rule out outpouching from the adjacent HGPIN. (Right) Occasionally, small glands ➡ adjacent to HGPIN may be too close and too few to ascertain whether they represent a focus of adenocarcinoma, adjacent acini involved by HGPIN, or tangentially sectioned outpouchings of convoluted HGPIN.

Prostatic Intraepithelial Neoplasia

PIN and Adjacent Atypical Glands

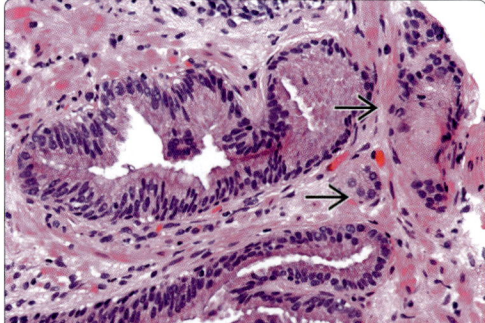

(Left) In this biopsy, the small glands ➡ raise the possibility of invasive cancer or outpouching of glands involved by adjacent HGPIN. (Right) A triple PIN cocktail stain shows absence of a basal cell layer around the smaller glands, suspicious for a diagnosis of invasive cancer ➡ adjacent to HGPIN. Other features that should be factored in to rule out outpouching include overall gland configuration and the spatial relationship with HGPIN. Deeper levels may also be helpful.

Triple PIN Cocktail Stain

PIN: Needle Biopsy

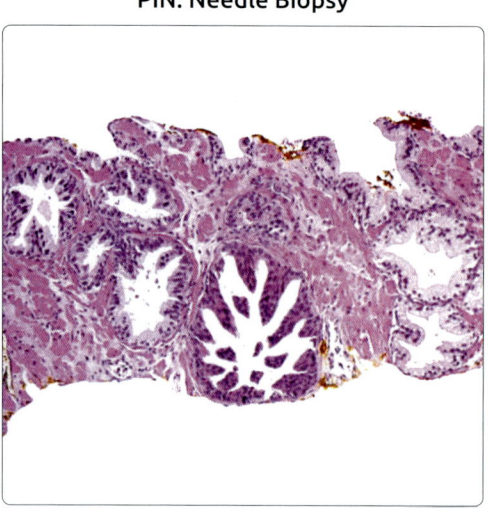

(Left) In a needle biopsy with HGPIN, the glands should be screened at low power. HGPIN glands stand out from the surrounding benign glands due to their architecture, size, and cellular quality. (Right) HGPIN may extend to involve smaller glands with lobular architecture. The resulting small glandular pattern should not be confused with acinar adenocarcinoma, as basal cells are preserved. This pattern of HGPIN may also be designated as flat pattern of HGPIN.

PIN Involving Small Acini

PIN: Partial Gland Involvement

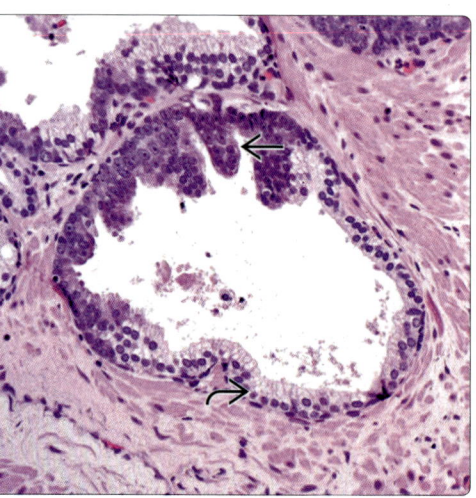

(Left) In partial involvement of a glandular structure by HGPIN, the gland is focally lined by cells displaying hyperchromasia, nuclear enlargement, and prominent nucleoli ➡ compared to the cytologic features of the benign aspect of the gland ➡. (Right) This needle biopsy with HGPIN shows the nuclear enlargement and prominent nucleoli are evident, as well as the darker and more abundant cytoplasm. Despite the inconspicuous basal cells, the round contour and cellular maturation within the lumen indicate HGPIN.

PIN: Partial Gland Involvement

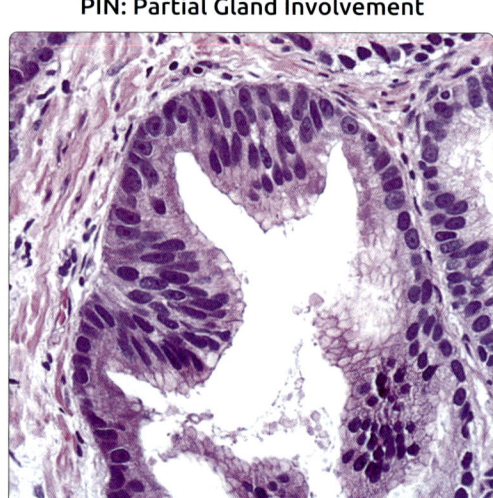

Prostatic Intraepithelial Neoplasia

PIN: Complex Glands

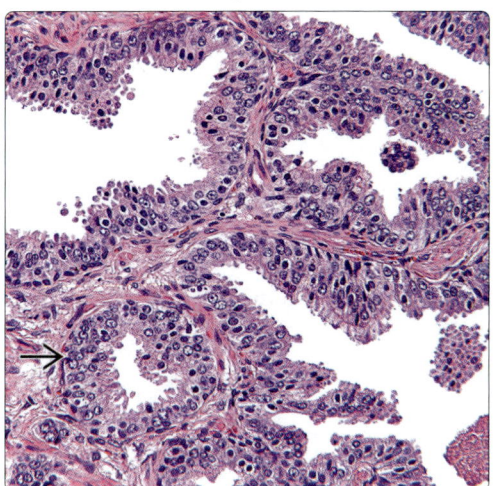

PIN With Smaller Atypical Glands

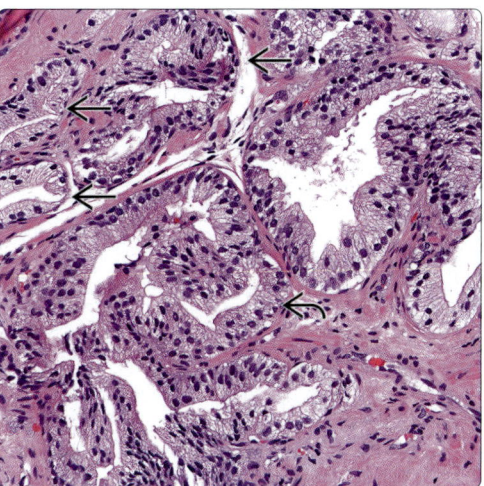

(Left) Tangential sectioning of convoluted HGPIN glands may result in smaller glands adjacent to HGPIN ⇒. (Right) HGPIN ⇒ is shown with smaller atypical glands ⇒. Without immunohistochemical support, it may be difficult to distinguish invasive carcinoma from outpouching of glands involved by HGPIN; such a distinction is not always possible. To be designated as invasive, the small glands should be spatially away from HGPIN glands.

Needle Biopsy: Atypical and Complex Glandular Proliferation

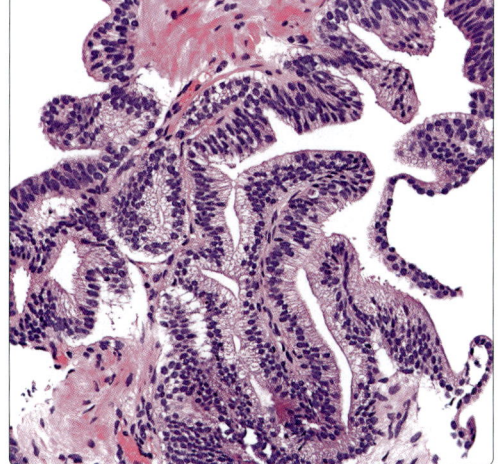

Immunostain Cocktail: Atypical and Complex Glandular Proliferation

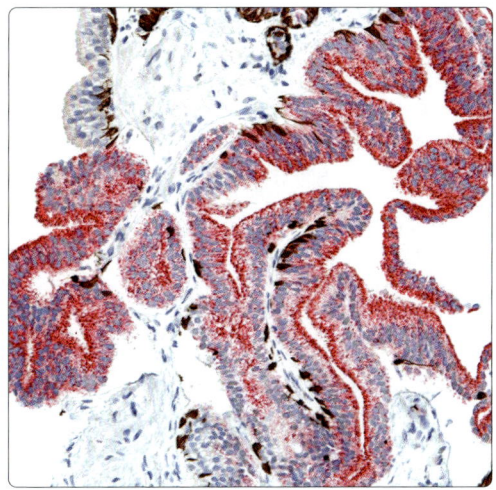

(Left) Needle biopsy shows an isolated focus of atypical large glands with branching and papillary projections. It is difficult to differentiate whether this represents HGPIN or ductal adenocarcinoma. (Right) Triple PIN cocktail stain shows strong AMACR expression (red) with scattered basal cells (brown). This pattern may be seen in HGPIN and intraductal adenocarcinoma. Therefore, a diagnosis of atypical large glandular proliferation is rendered with a comment.

Ductal Adenocarcinoma

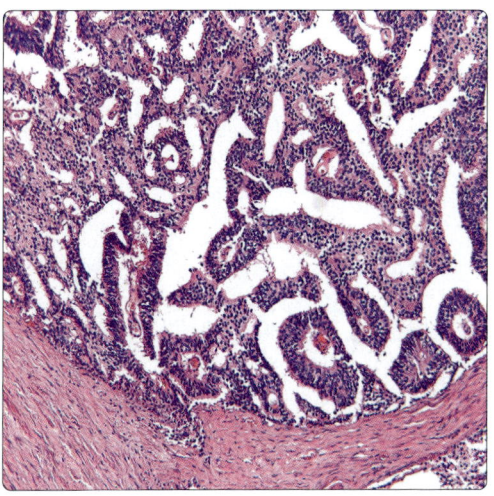

Intraductal Carcinoma

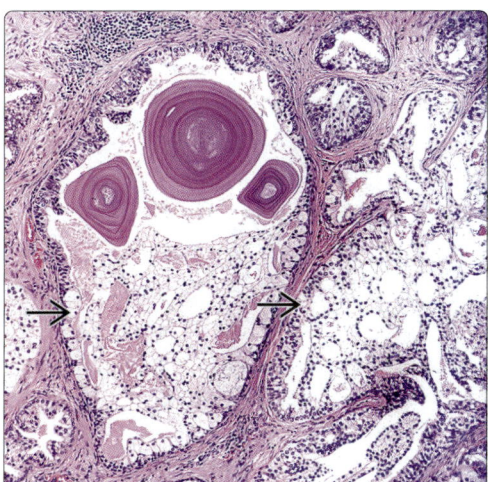

(Left) In this tumor, the ducts are greatly expanded and the architecture is complex with evident papillary and cribriform patterns. Nuclear stratification is easily recognizable as well. (Right) This is an example of intraductal spread ⇒ by foamy gland carcinoma. This growth pattern is usually associated with high-grade and high-volume disease at prostatectomy.

Prostatic Intraepithelial Neoplasia

Intraductal Carcinoma

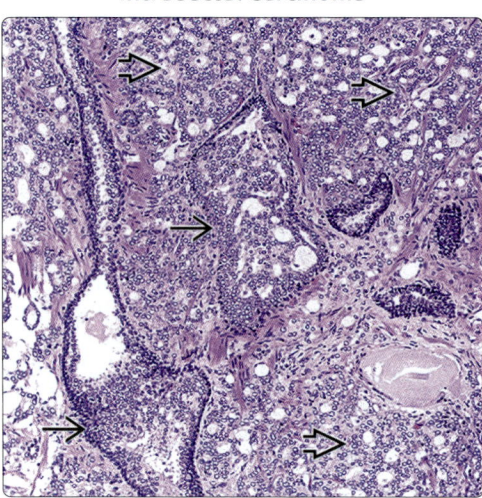

Intraductal Carcinoma: Immunostain (Basal Cell Marker)

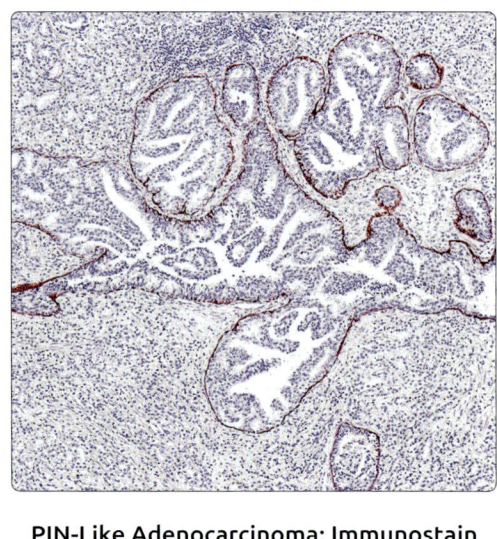

(Left) The terminology of intraductal carcinoma is controversial when seen in a needle biopsy. In this prostatectomy, within an area of invasive carcinoma ⇒, there is an intraglandular proliferation spanning the entire lumen of the ducts ⇒ with easily discernible basal cells indicating intraductal growth or extension of carcinoma. (Right) HMCK(34βE12) highlights the outline of the ducts and confirms the intraluminal proliferation of the high-grade carcinoma cells.

PIN-Like Adenocarcinoma

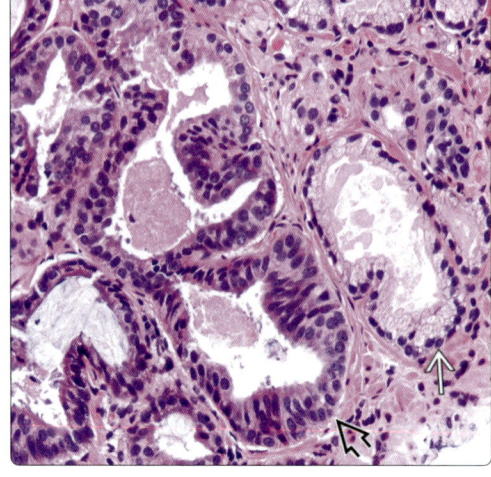

PIN-Like Adenocarcinoma: Immunostain Cocktail

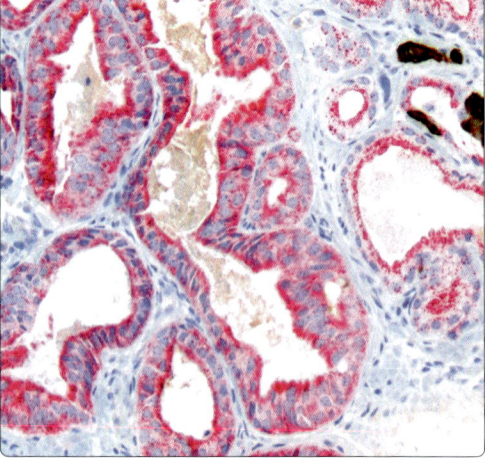

(Left) This tumor consists of 2 components of invasive glands: Conventional acinar carcinoma ⇒ and a stratified multilayered component that strongly mimics HGPIN ⇒. Basal cells are not visible on the H&E preparation. (Right) The presence of invasive carcinoma is confirmed by the lack of basal cells in all the glands; the simple single-layer-lined as well as multilayered stratified glands. AMACR is equally overexpressed in both types of glands.

Ejaculatory Duct/Seminal Vesicle Tissue

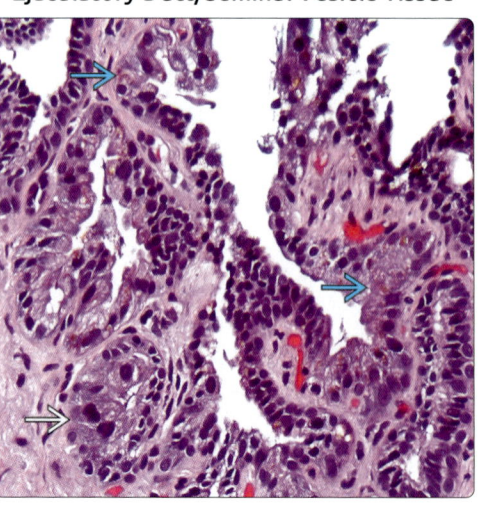

Urothelial Carcinoma Involving Prostatic Ducts and Acini

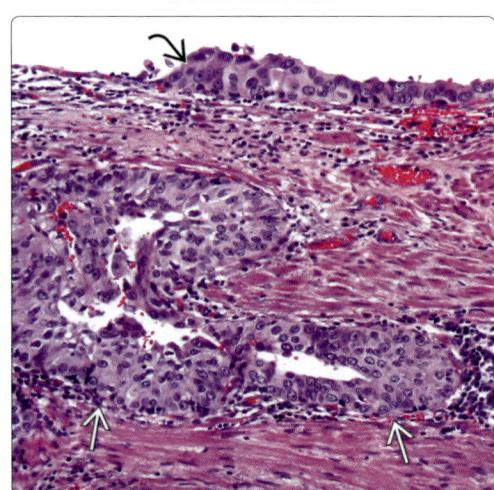

(Left) The enlarged nuclei and occasional stratification may cause confusion with HGPIN. The presence of atypical and pleomorphic nuclei ⇒ and yellow/brown pigments ⇒ are clues to the correct identification of this tissue. (Right) In this example, the prostatic ducts are enlarged by intraluminal proliferation with oval to round cells with occasional distinct nucleoli ⇒. The history of urothelial carcinoma and the presence of urothelial carcinoma in situ in the urethra ⇒ help resolve the diagnosis.

Prostatic Intraepithelial Neoplasia

Clear Cell Cribriform Hyperplasia

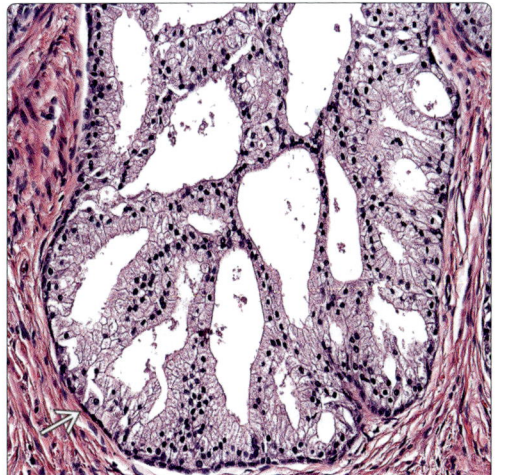

Nodular (Glandular) Hyperplasia

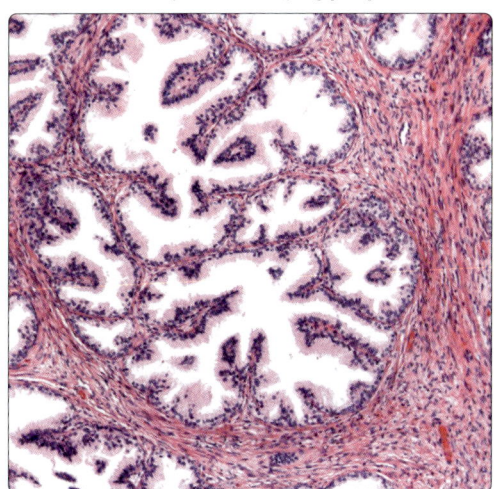

(Left) Clear cell cribriform hyperplasia consists of cribriform glands with clear cytoplasm. There is typically no nuclear atypia. Basal cells are prominent ➡ in the majority of cases, at least in parts of the glands, as seen in this example. (Right) Glandular hyperplasia may superficially resemble HGPIN by having intraluminal projections and occasional complex architecture. Typically, the hyperplastic glands lack any significant hyperchromasia and nuclear atypia and also retain basal cells.

Central Zone Glands

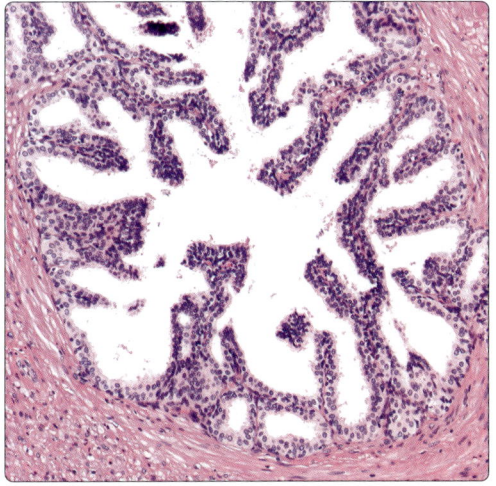

Transitional Cell Metaplasia

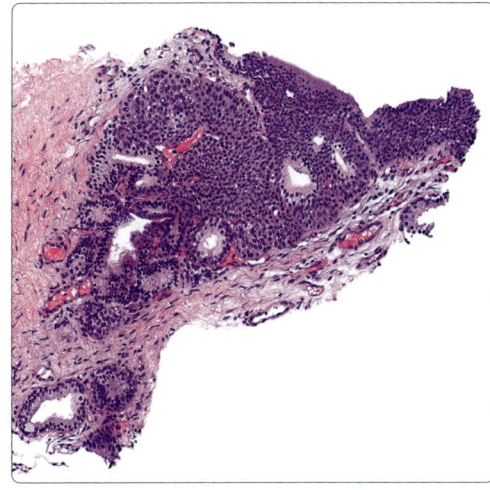

(Left) Central zone glands, typically present at the base of the prostate, may display long papillary architecture (with bridging between adjacent papillae), nuclear pseudostratification, and eosinophilic cytoplasm. Unlike HGPIN, nuclear atypia and prominent nuclei are not identified. (Right) This normal finding in many prostate biopsies and resection specimens is characterized by multilayered cells or solid nests of small uniform oval cells with nuclear grooves that lack typical patterns of HGPIN.

Basal Cell Hyperplasia

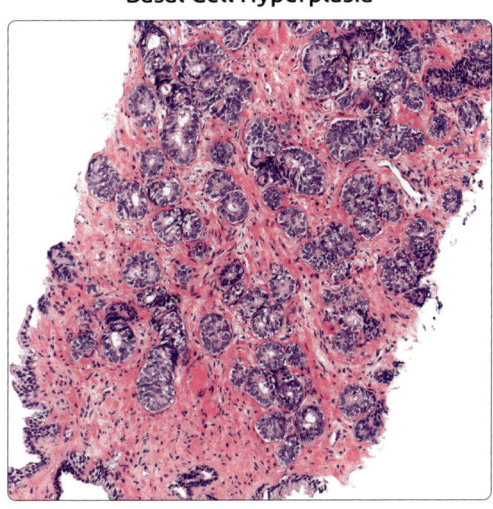

Basal Cell Hyperplasia: Immunostain Cocktail

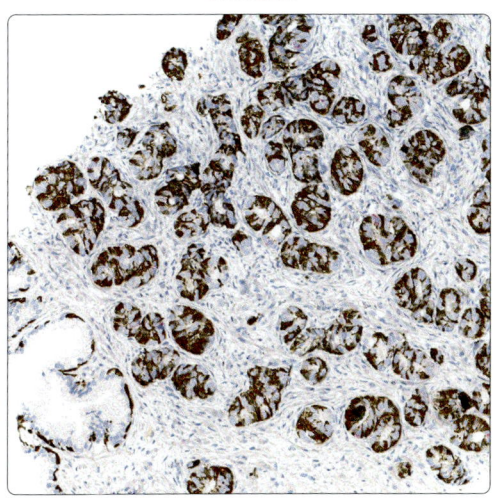

(Left) In this biopsy with tight clusters of atypical cells, the nuclei are distinctly darker than what is seen in HGPIN. The acini are not markedly enlarged, and the luminal space is obliterated in many glands. (Right) The main cellular proliferation in this lesion was proven to be of the basal cell component of the glands, as supported by both HMCK and p63. AMACR was essentially negative in these glands. This is consistent with basal cell hyperplasia.

General Concepts, Prostate Carcinoma

TERMINOLOGY

Synonyms
- Prostate carcinoma (PCa), prostatic adenocarcinoma, adenocarcinoma of prostate

Definitions
- Term prostate cancer/carcinoma has been used loosely to describe varying histologic subtypes
  - Acinar adenocarcinoma and is morphologic variants, ductal adenocarcinoma, adenosquamous and squamous cell carcinoma, basal cell carcinoma/adenoid cystic carcinoma
  - Prostatic adenocarcinoma with neuroendocrine differentiation (including large and small cell carcinoma) and sarcomatoid carcinoma
- However, in > 95% of cases it is used to designate conventional/usual adenocarcinoma, acinar type

EPIDEMIOLOGY

Age Range
- Common in elderly men; low incidence in < 50 years
- PCa incidence increases dramatically with age; > 75% occur in patients ≥ 65 years
- Mortality from prostate cancer also increases with age
  - 2nd and 3rd cause of cancer death in ages 60-79 years and ages 80 yr or older, respectively
  - Not 1 of top 5 causes of cancer mortality for ages 40-59 years

Incidence
- 4th most common cancer in the world, even across both sexes, with 1.1 million men diagnosed in 2012
- Incidence varies > 25 fold across different parts of the world, greatest in developed nations
  - Ethnic/racial differences, environmental factors, and detection rates contribute to this degree of variation
- Highest rates seen in Australasia, then North America, then Europe, particularly Northern and Western Europe
  - Attributed to widespread use of PSA testing, though Southern Africa, Caribbean, and South America also show high rates
  - Low rates in Asia and North Africa
- In USA, prostate cancer is most commonly diagnosed cancer and 2nd most lethal
  - In 2014, > 230,000 estimated new cases, and nearly 30,000 deaths

Ethnicity Relationship
- In USA, African Americans have highest incidence and mortality rates, up to 70% higher than Caucasians
  - Higher prevalence of PCa in anterior prostate gland that are difficult to sample via biopsy in African Americans
- Increased upgrading and upstaging at prostatectomy questions active surveillance for African Americans
- Lower rates in Asian Americans than Caucasians

Diet
- Strong positive association with diets rich in animal products, red meat, due to heterocyclic amines
- Fruits and vegetables may have protective effect
- Weak association with obesity
  - Healthy weight and diet low in total fat associated with lower risk for PCa

ETIOLOGY/PATHOGENESIS

General Concepts
- Migration studies demonstrate that immigrants from low incidence areas acquire intermediate-risk levels after migrating to high-risk areas
  - Suggests role for environmental and genetic factors
- Proposed higher risk with environmental exposures
- Vitamin D deficiency implicated and may explain geographic differences due to light exposure
- Prior controversy regarding potential pathogenic role for xenotropic murine leukemia virus-related virus (XMRV)
  - Now understood to be contaminant/artifact only

(Left) Infiltrating PCa, usual acinar variant, characterized by crowded malignant acini showing predominantly well-formed glands (Gleason pattern 3 ➡) with scattered cribriform glands (Gleason pattern 4 ➡). (Right) Same focus as at left, stained by ERG and SPINK1 dual immunohistochemistry. 40-50% of PCas show fusion of the genes TMPRSS2 and ERG ➡, while < 10% shows outlier overexpression of SPINK1 ➡.

Prostatic Adenocarcinoma
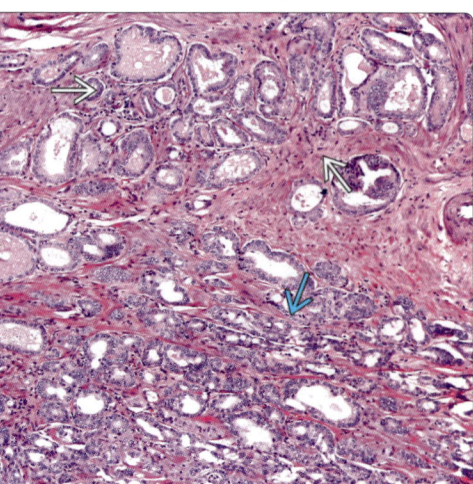

Molecular Subtypes
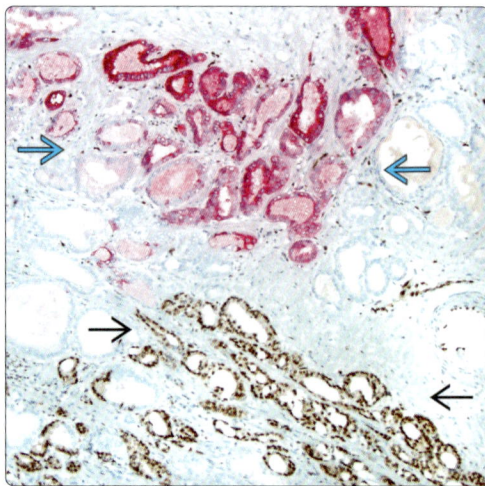

General Concepts, Prostate Carcinoma

Familial Prostate Cancer

- Well-documented familial association, with 5-10x increased risk in men with multiple affected 1st-degree relatives
- Recent scholarship identifies role for germ line mutations of genes *HOXB13*, *BRCA1*, *BRCA2*, and mismatch repair (MMR) proteins
  o *HOXB13* (G84E) germ line variant associated with significantly increased risk of PCa
  o Odds ratios depend on ethnic background and degree of familial history, ~ 4fold in recent metaanalysis across all groups tested

Molecular Pathogenesis

- Typical, peripheral zone PCa thought to arise from high-grade prostatic intraepithelial neoplasia (HGPIN)
  o Not all cases arise from HGPIN, especially low-grade PCa in central zone and transition zone
- 1/2 of PCa harbor oncogenic rearrangements of ETS family protooncogenic transcription factors
  o Most commonly fuse androgen-responsive gene *TMPRSS2* and *ERG*, driving proliferation, invasion
  o Other androgen responsive genes and ETS family members (*ETV1*, *ETV4*, *ETV5*) in < 10% of cases
  o May provide highly prostate specific molecular target for diagnostic testing
- 1/2 of PCa are ETS rearrangement negative
  o *SPINK1* serine protease outlier expression defines subgroup, ~ 10-20% of ETS negative
  o *SPOP* and *CHD1* mutated and deleted cases, ~ 10-30% of ETS negative cases
- Proportions of these molecular groups vary between ethnicities
  o Lower proportion of *TMPRSS2-ERG* rearranged cases among individuals of African, Asian ancestry

CLINICAL IMPLICATIONS

Clinical Presentation

- Majority of PCa in USA are diagnosed in asymptomatic patients due to PSA screening
- Main indications for prostate biopsy
  o Increased serum PSA level
  o Abnormal digital rectal examination (DRE), palpable nodules, induration asymmetry
    – Majority of prostate cancer (70-75%) in posterior zone, which is accessible by DRE
    – Low sensitivity, low positive predictive value, still used for clinical staging
- When symptomatic, prostate cancer presents with signs or symptoms of advanced disease
  o Obstructive bladder symptoms in transition zone cancers
  o Pelvic pain due to local extension
  o Bone pain and tenderness, spinal cord compression, or adenopathy due to metastatic disease
- Paraneoplastic syndrome more common in certain carcinoma subtypes (i.e., small cell carcinoma)
- ~ 10% of transurethral resection of prostate (TURP) specimens for lower urinary tract obstruction contain incidental prostate cancer

Laboratory Tests

- Prostate specific antigen (PSA): Synthesized by benign or malignant prostatic glands and ducts
  o Traditional cut off is 4 ng/mL, over which prostate biopsies are recommended
  o PSA serum level above 4 ng/mL has sensitivity of ~ 20% and specificity of 60-70% for PCa
  o PSA density: Serum PSA/prostate gland volume; > 0.15 prompts biopsy
  o Age-specific ranges, with higher PSA allowed for older groups (e.g., 2.5 ng/mL for men 40-49 years vs. 6.5 ng/mL for men 70-79 years)
  o PSA velocity: Change in PSA value over time - Increase of > 0.75 ng/mL per year would prompt prostate biopsy
    – Useful in monitoring patients after treatment for prostate cancer
- Emergence of PCA3 and combination PCA3/TMPRSS2-ERG molecular testing
  o PCA3 is noncoding RNA that is highly expressed in prostate cancer with significant specificity but lower sensitivity than PSA
    – May be detected by amplification from urine collected after vigorous DRE
    – Test calculates ratio of PCA3 RNA:PSA RNA to generate PCA3 score
    – Approved by USA FDA for risk assessment in men with prior negative biopsy
    – May also have value in risk assessment of men undergoing initial biopsy
  o TMPRSS2-ERG fusion gene transcript expression is 99.99% specific to prostate cancer
    – Similarly, may be tested from urine, with ratio of TMPRSS2-ERG RNA:PSA RNA
  o TMPRSS2-ERG and PCA combination testing
    – Conceptual appeal of adding TMPRSS2-ERG specificity to PCA3 sensitivity
    – Validated retrospectively and prospectively in multicenter setting to add independent predictive value beyond predictions of PCA3 and European Randomised Study of Screening for Prostate Cancer (ERSPC) risk calculator
    – Associations with cancer volume, Gleason score, upgrading and upstaging at prostatectomy
    – Studies demonstrate test may offer potential to avoid many biopsies in patients with elevated PSA

Screening Guidelines

- In 2012 the United States Preventative Services Task Force (USPSTF) updated its recommendations to categorically recommend against screening for prostate cancer by PSA
  o Argued that screening results in detection and treatment of many cancers that would not progress
  o Assessment that risks of over treatment outweigh benefits of detection
  o Triggered much controversy among urologists, patients, public health experts
- American Urological Association (AUA) Updated Recommendations, 2013
  o AUA recommends against PSA screening men younger than 40 yr

General Concepts, Prostate Carcinoma

- AUA recommends shared decision-making for screening in the key age range of 55-69 years
- AUA recommends screening interval of 2 years, if screening and individualization of subsequent screening intervals based on baseline PSA level

Imaging Findings

- Traditional radiographic studies: Ancillary tool only
  - More useful for staging and detection of metastases
    - Bone scan performed for localized disease with PSA > 20 ng/mL, Gleason score (GS) ≥ 8, or symptomatic T3 or T4 disease
    - Osteoblastic bone metastasis most common for acinar carcinoma
    - Pelvic CT or MR performed for T3 or T4 disease or in localized cancer with high nomogram probability for lymph node involvement
- Ultrasonography
  - Until recently, prostate gland has remained only human organ biopsied, essentially blindly
  - Transrectal ultrasound (TRUS) may guide anatomic sampling but ability to localize lesions is limited
    - Has use in measuring prostate gland volume and to estimate prostate cancer size
    - Most prostate cancers are hypoechoic (40%) but may be hyper- (30%) or isoechoic (30%)
  - Some techniques under study to improve sensitivity: Contrast-enhanced transrectal US (CETRUS) using gas filled microbubbles
- Multiparametric (MP) MR: Rapidly advancing toward routine use in clinical care
  - MP MR uses anatomical and functional sequences of T1-weighted, T2-weighted, diffusion-weighted, dynamic contrast-enhanced MR
    - Some approaches use magnetic resonance spectroscopy as well
  - Best established use is to screen for clinically significant carcinomas that may be missed by TRUS and standard sampling templates
    - MP MR shows superior detection of clinically significant carcinomas with lower detection of clinically insignificant carcinomas and less biopsy cores sampled
    - Studies demonstrate MP MR predicts clinically significant carcinoma with higher accuracy than clinical nomograms
    - When biopsies are undertaken, they may be done either "in bore" (within and during MR) or outside the magnet, either transrectal or transperineal
      - May be targeted using cognitive fusion where operator targets area identified by prior MP MR without live guidance
      - May be performed "in bore" within MR under sedation, or use emerging MR/ultrasound "fusion" guided direct targeting using prior MR images
  - Also, established use in staging carcinoma preprostatectomy, identifying extraprostatic extension (extracapsular extension)
    - Less sensitive for microscopic extraprostatic extension, but overall exceeds Partin tables for predicting extraprostatic disease

RISK ASSESSMENT AND TREATMENT OPTIONS

Contemporary Emphasis on Avoidance of Overtreatment

- Significant data suggest that thousands of patients have been overtreated and suffer from side effects
  - NCCN Guidelines 2015.1: Risk assessment for whether PCa diagnosed is clinically significant disease
    - Very low risk: Clinical stage T1c, and biopsy Gleason ≤ 6, and PSA < 10ng/mL, and < 3 cores involved, and ≤ 50% of any core, and PSA density < 0.15
    - Low risk: Clinical stage T1 to T2a, and Gleason ≤ 6, and serum PSA < 10ng/mL
    - Intermediate risk: Clinical stage T2b-T2c, or Gleason = 7, or PSA 10-20ng/mL
    - High risk: Clinical stage T3a, or Gleason 8-10, or PSA > 20ng
    - Very high risk: Clinical stage T3b or T4, or predominant Gleason pattern 5, or > 4 cores with Gleason 8-10
  - Treatment recommendations from many organizations, but emphasis on active surveillance for very low risk and low risk strata
- Active surveillance: Postponement of definitive treatment until evidence of disease progression
  - Subset of very low- and low-risk cancers are unlikely to progress and harms of treatment may be avoided
  - Optimal inclusion criteria, surveillance protocols, and criteria for failure have not been defined and vary by institution
  - Several protocols involve
    - Serum PSA checked every 3-6 months
    - DRE and rebiopsy at 6- to 12-month intervals
    - Failure of active surveillance defined by either pathologic criteria (Gleason score > 6, increased number cores involved, percentage involvement per core) or clinical criteria (PSA doubling time < 3 years)
    - Some protocols decrease frequency of biopsy and PSA check over time
  - Some data suggest that active surveillance protocols as currently exist are suboptimal for African American men
  - Potential use of MP MR to complement biopsy protocols in surveillance

Treatment Options

- Primary androgen deprivation therapy
  - Recommended for metastatic disease or with radiation for locally advanced carcinoma
  - Not recommended for localized disease due to increased all cause mortality
- Focal therapy/ablative techniques
  - Controversy, limited data for cryotherapy
  - High-intensity focused ultrasound (HIFU) not available in USA
- Brachytherapy
  - High-dose brachytherapy performed inpatient with temporary insertion of radiation source
  - Low-dose brachytherapy permanent implantation of radiation source
- Radical prostatectomy ± pelvic lymph node dissection
- Primary androgen deprivation therapy?

General Concepts, Prostate Carcinoma

Predictive Tables and Nomograms

- Clinical tools for integrating several clinicopathologic variables to predict prostate cancer progression
  o Partin tables: Preoperative parameters (tPSA, GS, and clinical stage) predictive of stage at prostatectomy
- Several pre- or postprostatectomy models are proposed
  o Documentation of key prognostic variables from biopsy or RP specimens crucial
    – e.g., GS (primary, secondary, and sum), cancer volume, EPE, margins, seminal vesicle invasion, lymph node involvement

Grade Groups: Emerging Prognostic System

- Acknowledgment of need for more intuitive grading system for patient understanding
- Reassignment of total Gleason scores to grade groups 1-5 to more intuitively reflect prognosis
- Gleason score 6 (or less), the lowest risk/lowest grade assigned at biopsy designated grade group 1
- Gleason 3+4=7 and 4+3=7 form grade groups 2 and 3, reflective of their true prognostic differences
- Gleason score 8 designated grade group 4, separating it from Gleason 9-10 (grade group 5)
- Recommendation that Gleason score still be included in reporting in near term

KEY FEATURES IN EXAMINATION OF PROSTATE CANCER SPECIMENS

Key Elements to Report

- **Gleason grade and Gleason score: Enduring prognostic marker**
  o Based on histoarchitectural patterns of disease, which reflect degree of differentiation of adenocarcinoma
  o Gleason score (GS) is sum of 2 most prevalent patterns, though approach differs between biopsy and resections
  o 2014 International Society of Urological Pathology Consensus recommends reporting both Gleason score and corresponding grade group
  o Grade groups, whether evaluated at needle biopsy or at prostatectomy correlate with biochemical recurrence-free survival
  o Each successive increasing grade group is associated with increasing hazard ratios as compared to grade group 1
    – Grade groups 2-5 show hazard ratios of 2.2, 7.3, 12.3, and 23.9, respectively, in validation set of 20,845 prostatectomies
- **Tumor quantity**
  o Tumor volume in core needle biopsy
    – Studies show correlation with RP stage, tumor volume, GS, margin status, neurovascular bundle involvement, and posttreatment progression
    – Small amount of tumor in biopsy is not always indicative of small tumor volume in RP
    – Recommended to report as number of positive cores and estimated proportion (percentage) &/or linear extent of tumor in millimeters
    – Recommended to report positive core with greatest tumor percentage
  o Tumor volume in TURP
    – Should always be reported, as tumor volume is determinant of substaging T1 in TURP
    – Should report number of involved chips and ratio or percentage of involved to total chips
  o Tumor volume in RP and subtotal prostatectomy
    – Studies show correlation with disease progression; although inconsistently as independent factor
    – Percentage of tumor involvement may be estimated by visual inspection
    – Size of dominant tumor nodule may be provided as linear measurement
- **Extraprostatic extension (EPE)**
  o Preferred term over capsular penetration or extracapsular extension since prostate does not have true capsule
  o Reported in ~ 36% of prostatectomy specimens
  o Definitions
    – Tumor involvement of fat; intraprostatic fat exceedingly rare
    – In cases with no direct contact to fat, tumor seen in loose connective tissues in plane of fat
    – Peri-/intraneural invasion within or in plane of fat
  o Amount of fat varies with paucity of fat in apex, anterior part of prostate, or base
    – EPE in these 3 regions suggested as tumor outside glandular confines of prostate
    – Rarely, fat may be seen around apex
  o Comment on extent and if positive margin at site of EPE; location is optional
  o EPE descriptors and definitions: Recommended reporting but variable criteria used
    – Focal EPE: Tumor extension < 1 HPV and not in > 2 sections
      □ Also 5 glands or less used as criterion
    – Nonfocal or established EPE: More extensive tumor spread
    – Size estimate is optional; greatest linear dimension ± number of blocks involved
  o Comment of EPE may be made in needle biopsy or TURP showing fat involvement by tumor
  o Involvement of striated muscles (anterior or apex) &/or ganglion cells alone does not constitute EPE
- **Margin status**
  o Positive if tumor cells touch ink; report extent of positive margin in mm
  o Positive margin reported in 16-41% of RP
  o Should report location of positive margin
    – Most common in posterolateral aspect of prostate
  o 2 types of positive margins
    – Iatrogenic or capsular incision (pT2+ or pT2x): Tumor transected within prostate
    – Noniatrogenic: Tumor transected at EPE
  o Higher progression-free probability with negative (81-83%) than positive (58-64%) RP margin
  o Reporting size, focality (unifocal or multifocal), and presence of benign glands at margin is optional
- **Perineural invasion (PNI)**
  o Defined as presence of prostate cancer juxtaposed intimately along, around, or within nerve
  o Most studies have shown prognostic significance in univariate analysis only
  o Some studies suggest strong correlation of PNI in biopsy with EPE on RP

General Concepts, Prostate Carcinoma

Prognostic Grade Groups and Risk of Biochemical Recurrence

Prognostic Grade Groups	Corresponding Gleason Score	Hazard Ratio	BCRFS
Grade group 1	Gleason score ≤ 6	1.0	96%
Grade group 2	Gleason score 3+4=7	2.2	88%
Grade group 3	Gleason score 4+3=7	7.3	63%
Grade group 4	Gleason score = 8	12.3	48%
Grade group 5	Gleason score = 9-10	23.9	26%

Biochemical recurrence-free survival = BCRFS.

Adapted from ISUP Companion Meeting, 2015 USCAP Meeting, Epstein JI et al: Eur Urol 2015, Epstein et al: Am J Surg Pathol, in press.

- o PNI present in fat is considered as EPE
- o PNI ubiquitously present in RP
- o PNI in needle biopsy has been correlated with recurrence after radiation therapy
- **Lymphovascular invasion (LVI)**
  - o Several studies have shown LVI as independent predictor of disease progression
  - o Reporting of LVI in RP is required
- **Seminal vesicle (SV) invasion**
  - o Defined as PCa involving muscular wall of SV
  - o 3 mechanisms of SV involvement by PCa
    - Direct spread along ejaculatory duct tissue into SV
    - Direct extra- or intraprostatic spread into SV
    - Noncontiguous metastasis to SV, often by lymphovascular invasion
  - o Portion of SV may be intraprostatic; only extraprostatic SV involvement should be considered
  - o Should note SV involvement if seen in needle biopsy
    - Caution not to overinterpret ejaculatory duct involvement as SV invasion
- **High-grade prostatic intraepithelial neoplasia (HGPIN) and atypical small acinar proliferation (ASAP)**
  - o HGPIN or ASAP are predictive of subsequent cancer in 21-31% and 40-50% of patients, respectively; prognostic significance being questioned
  - o Extent of HGPIN on biopsy is more predictive of subsequent cancer, particularly if multifocal and/or bilateral
  - o Reporting of HGPIN optional in biopsy, and RP is optional when PCa is present

STAGING

General Principles

- American Joint Committee on Cancer (AJCC) tumor node metastasis (TNM) universally accepted staging for prostate cancer
  - o Stage T1 is clinical stage
  - o Formal pathologic staging at prostatectomy, starting with pT2
  - o AJCC anatomic stage/prognostic groups incorporate PSA level and GS in addition to TNM stage

T1: Clinically Inapparent Tumor

- Neither palpable, nor visible by imaging
- T1a: Incidental carcinoma in transurethral resection, involves < 5% of tissue
- T1b: Incidental carcinoma, involves > 5% of tissue
- T1c: Carcinoma detected in needle core biopsy

pT2: Organ-Confined Disease

- pT2a: Unilateral carcinoma involves < 50% of 1 lobe
- pT2b: Unilateral carcinoma involves > 50% of 1 lobe
- pT2c: Carcinoma involves both lobes of prostate

pT3: Extraprostatic Extension of Disease

- pT3a: Extraprostatic extension, unilateral or bilateral, including bladder neck
- pT3b: Seminal vesicle invasion

pT4: Invasion of Adjacent Organs Beyond Seminal Vesicle

- Rectum, levator ani group musculature, pelvic side wall
- Diagnosis often requires clinicopathologic correlation as these tissues are not generally present in prostatectomy

SELECTED REFERENCES

1. Bouchelouche K et al: Advances in imaging modalities in prostate cancer. Curr Opin Oncol. 27(3):224-31, 2015
2. Epstein JI et al: A Contemporary Prostate Cancer Grading System: A Validated Alternative to the Gleason Score. Eur Urol. 69(3):428-35, 2015
3. Siegel RL et al: Cancer statistics, 2015. CA Cancer J Clin. 65(1):5-29, 2015
4. Amin MB et al: The critical role of the pathologist in determining eligibility for active surveillance as a management option in patients with prostate cancer: consensus statement with recommendations supported by the College of American Pathologists, International Society of Urological Pathology, Association of Directors of Anatomic and Surgical Pathology, the New Zealand Society of Pathologists, and the Prostate Cancer Foundation. Arch Pathol Lab Med. 138(10):1387-405, 2014
5. Carroll PR et al: Prostate cancer early detection, version 1.2014. Featured updates to the NCCN Guidelines. J Natl Compr Canc Netw. 12(9):1211-9; quiz 1219, 2014
6. Loeb S: Guideline of guidelines: prostate cancer screening. BJU Int. 114(3):323-5, 2014
7. Tomlins SA: Urine PCA3 and TMPRSS2:ERG using cancer-specific markers to detect cancer. Eur Urol. 65(3):543-5, 2014
8. Samaratunga H et al: International Society of Urological Pathology (ISUP) Consensus Conference on Handling and Staging of Radical Prostatectomy Specimens. Working group 1: specimen handling. Mod Pathol. 24(1):6-15, 2011
9. Tomlins SA et al: ETS gene fusions in prostate cancer: from discovery to daily clinical practice. Eur Urol. 56(2):275-86, 2009
10. Lilja H et al: Prostate-specific antigen and prostate cancer: prediction, detection and monitoring. Nat Rev Cancer. 8(4):268-78, 2008

General Concepts, Prostate Carcinoma

Imaging by Ultrasound

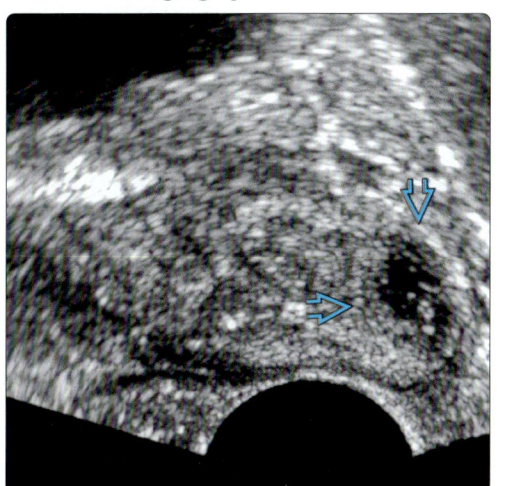

Peripheral Zone PCa: Gross Appearance

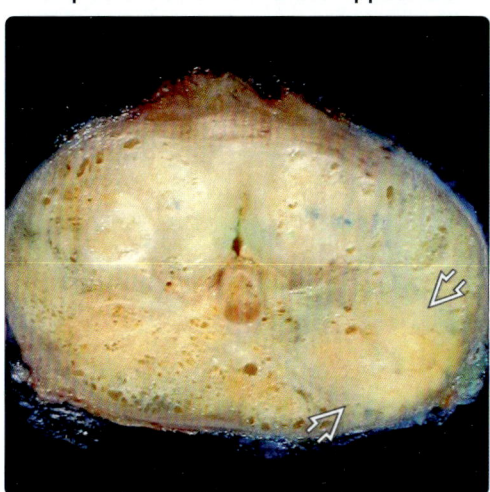

(Left) Longitudinal TRUS shows a small, hypoechoic lesion ⇨ in the peripheral zone, confirmed as PCa by biopsy. A nodule of benign hyperplasia or infarction may also mimic PCa. **(Right)** PCa shows a relatively dense, homogeneous solid area ➡ at the posterolateral aspect of the peripheral zone. PCa most commonly occurs at this site. Most PCas are multifocal.

Clinical Stage T1: Incidental PCa

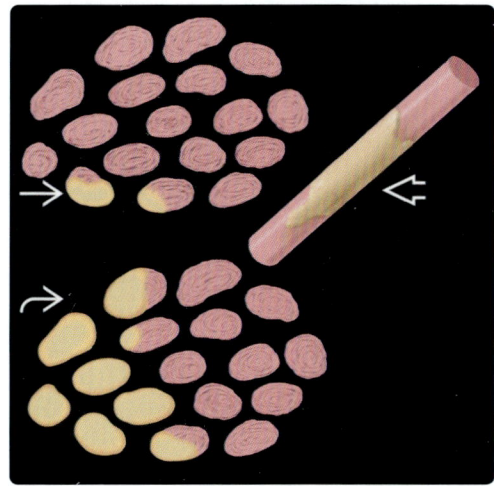

Pathologic Staging: pT2a

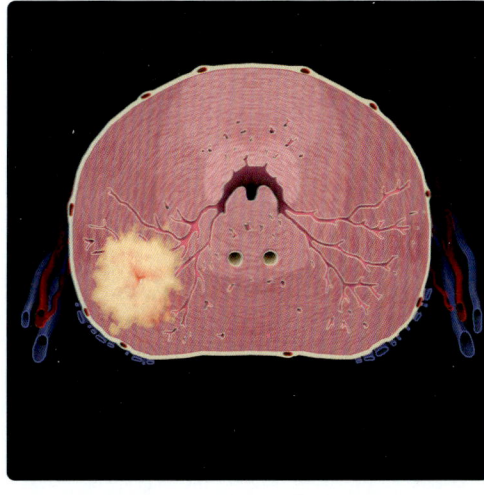

(Left) Clinical staging of incidental (T1) PCa, including T1a [5% tumor in tissue resected (TURP) ➡] and T1b [> 5% tumor in tissue resected (TURP) ➡]. If incidental PCa is identified in tissue submitted and is < 5%, all tissue should be submitted for histologic evaluation. Stage T1c is for carcinoma identified on needle biopsy ➡. **(Right)** Pathologic staging for PCa, performed at prostatectomy, starts with pT2a, where carcinoma involves no more than 1/2 of only 1 lobe of the prostate.

Pathologic Staging: pT2b

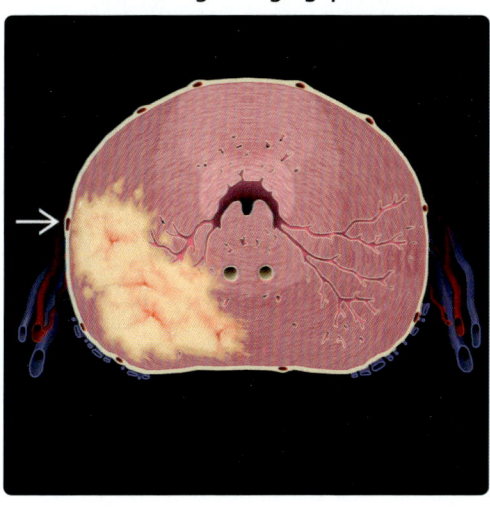

Pathologic Staging: pT2c

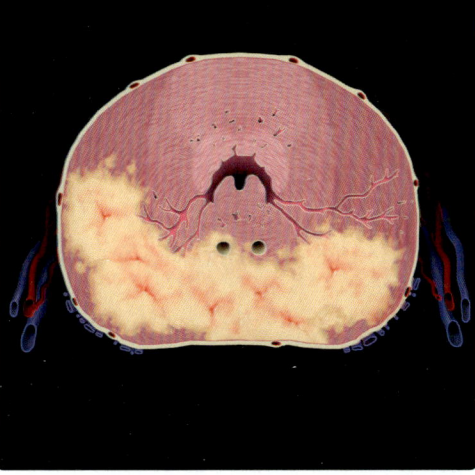

(Left) In stage pT2b, PCa, while still confined to 1 lobe, involves more than 1/2 ➡ of 1 lobe of prostate. This pattern of tumor involvement is uncommon, since PCa is usually located at the posterior aspect and larger tumors tend to involve bilateral posterior sides (pT2c), even without anterior involvement. **(Right)** Stage pT2c is for organ-confined PCa involving both lobes of prostate. pT2 subdivisions may act as surrogate for estimating PCa volume, which correlates with disease relapse.

General Concepts, Prostate Carcinoma

Pathologic Staging: Extraprostatic pT3a

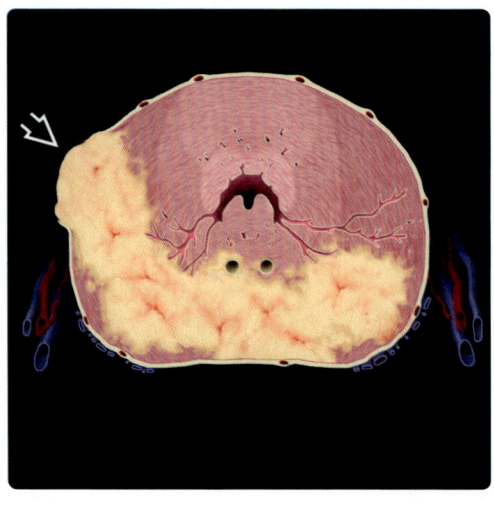

Histologic Features of pT3a

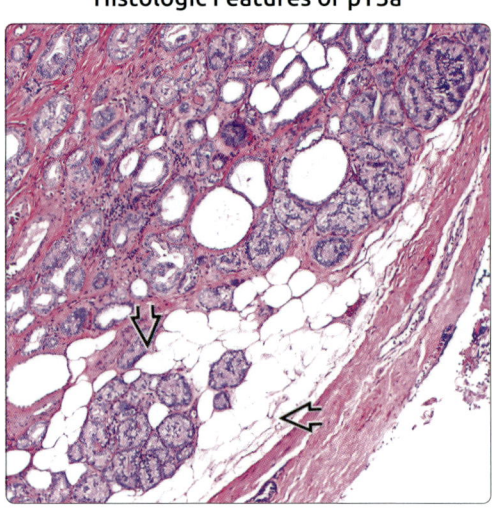

(Left) Stage pT3 signals extraprostatic disease. Stage pT3a denotes PCa extending outside of the prostate to involve periprostatic soft tissue ➡ or microscopic invasion of the bladder neck. Detection of EPE is most reliably made by histologic examination. DRE and radiographic studies are not sensitive in detecting EPE. Up to 36% of RP have EPE. (Right) Stage pT3a carcinoma showing PCa infiltrating into the plane of periprostatic adipose tissue ➡.

Pathologic Staging: pT3b SV Involvement

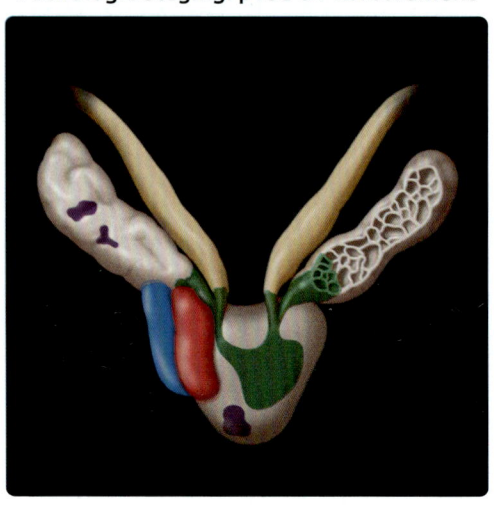

Histologic Features of pT3b

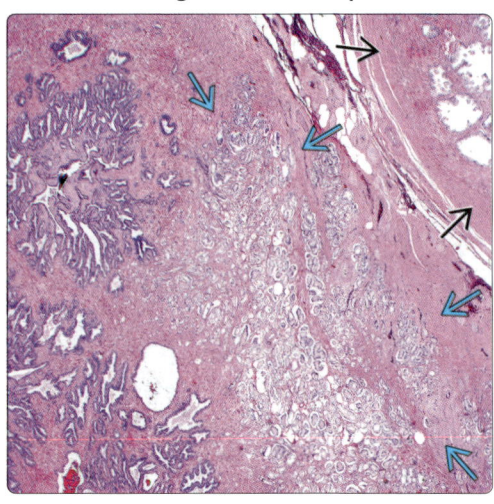

(Left) Mechanisms of seminal vesicle (SV) involvement by PCa includes spread via (1) ejaculatory duct tissue into SV (green), (2) direct extra- (blue) or intraprostatic (red) spread into SV, or (3) noncontiguous metastasis to SV (purple). (Right) True seminal vesicle involvement is demonstrated histologically by carcinoma invading the muscular coat of the extraprostatic SV ➡, here seen adjacent to the base of the prostate gland ➡.

Metastatic PCa

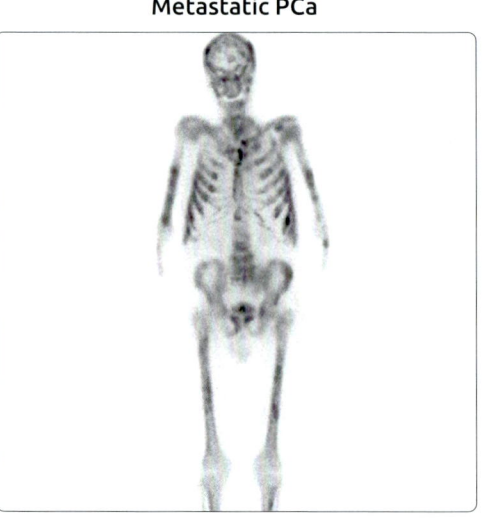

Metastatic PCa: Histology

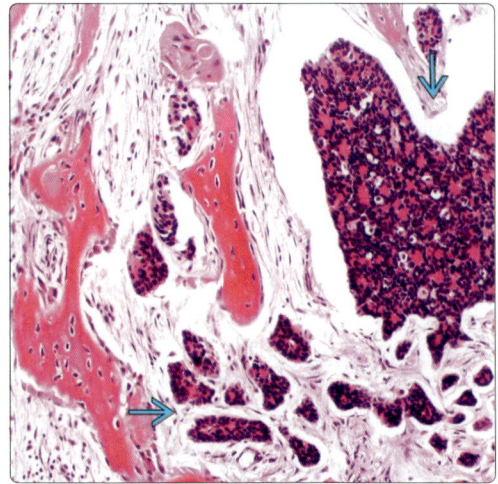

(Left) Anterior bone scan shows multiple osseous metastases by PCa (stage M1 disease), including to the calvaria, bilateral humeri, multiple ribs, sternum, lumbar spine, pelvis, and both femurs. Bone metastasis by PCa is usually osteoblastic. (Right) Metastatic PCa to bone shows cribriform morphology ➡ interspersed with reactive marrow fibrosis juxtaposed between trabeculae of woven bone. Immunohistochemical markers, such as PSA, p501S, NKX3.1, and ERG, can help establish prostatic origin in poorly differentiated cases.

General Concepts, Prostate Carcinoma

Skeletal Muscle in Anterior Gland
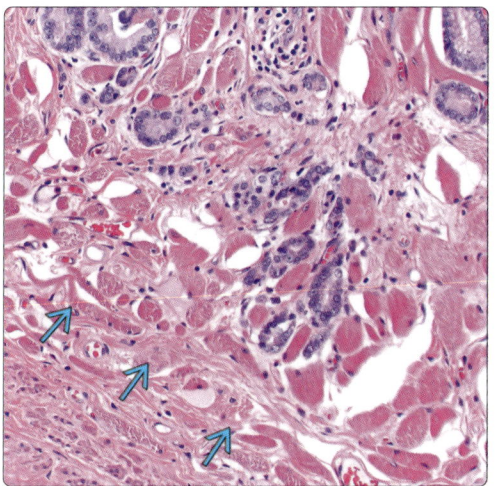

True EPE in Anterior Gland
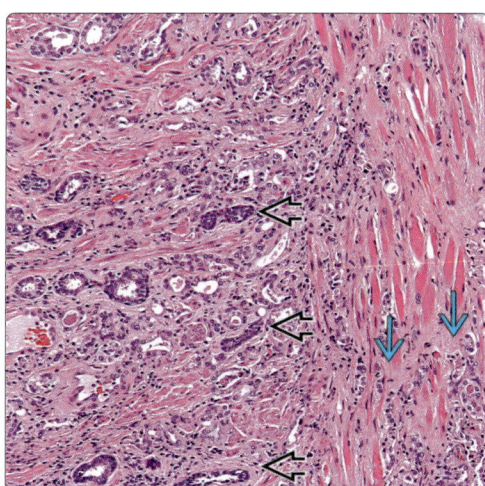

(Left) In the anterior gland, bands of skeletal (striated) muscle ⇨ may be invaded by PCa well within the confines of the prostate. This focus was seen within the contours of the gland and does not constitute extraprostatic extension (EPE). (Right) In contrast, in stage pT3a, PCa invades striated muscle ⇨, beyond the outermost limits of the anterior gland (entrapped normal ducts ⇨). Because fat is often absent in the anterior, diagnosis of EPE requires careful correlation of the depth of invasion to the contours of the gland.

Microscopic Bladder Neck Invasion pT3a
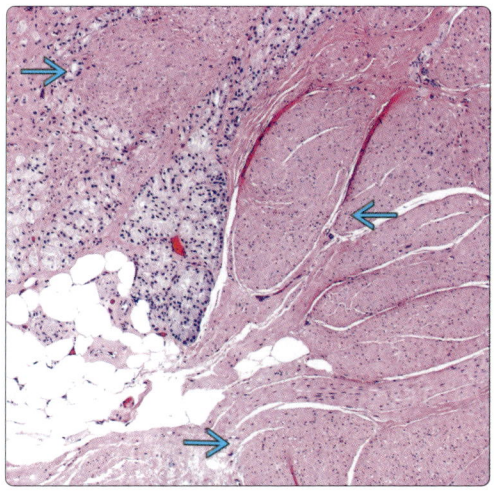

Focal Extraprostatic Extension pT3a
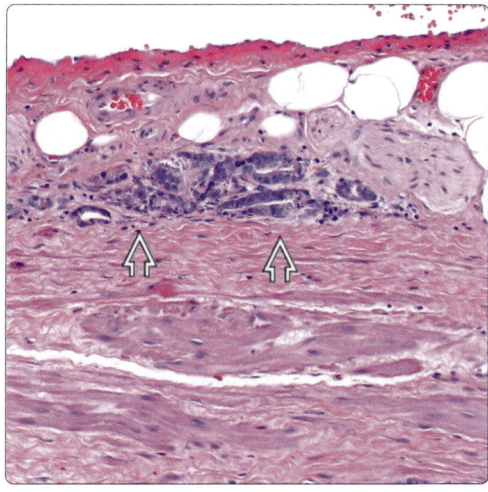

(Left) Microscopic involvement of bladder neck shows PCa involving large caliber slips of smooth muscle bundles ⇨ with interspersed fat. Invasion of these muscles, lacking the confluent morphology of prostatic stroma, signal microscopic bladder neck invasion, which is also pathologic stage (pT3a). (Right) Focal extraprostatic extension demonstrates a small group of invading acini of PCa ⇨ outside of the contours of the prostate, at the level of the plane of extraprostatic adipose tissue, pathologic stage pT3a.

Ejaculatory Duct Invasion Remains pT2
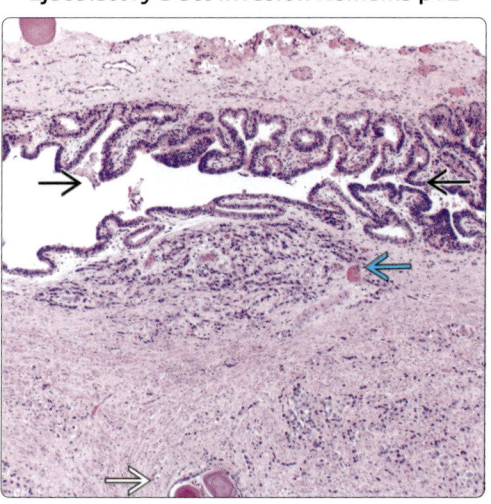

Seminal Vesicle Invasion pT3b
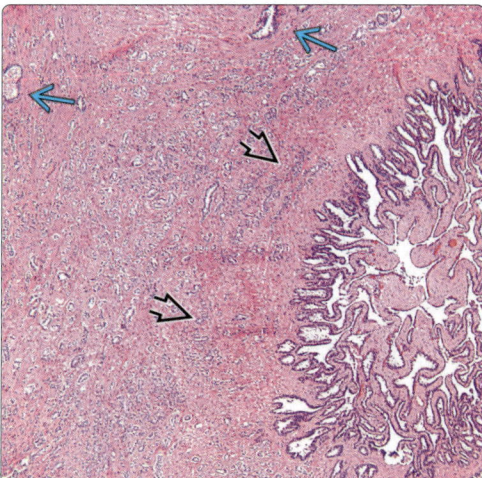

(Left) If PCa ⇨ invades adjacent to the ejaculatory duct (ED) ⇨, it remains staged as organ confined (pT2). While the epithelium of the ED is similar to the seminal vesicle (SV), it does not show the thick muscular coat of the SV. Adjacent prostatic glands are apparent nearby ⇨. (Right) True seminal vesicle invasion shows invasion of the SV muscular wall ⇨ and is stage pT3b. This may occur by direct extension of PCa from the prostate (nearest benign glands ⇨). Recognition of invasion of the muscular wall of the SV organ is paramount.

Acinar Adenocarcinoma

KEY FACTS

TERMINOLOGY
- Malignant neoplasm of prostatic secretory cells

ETIOLOGY/PATHOGENESIS
- ~ 50% PCa harbor *TMPRSS2* and *ETS1* gene fusion
- Loss of *PTEN* suggested as late event in PCa carcinogenesis
- *SPOP* mutation seen in up to 13% of PCa and is mutually exclusive of *TMPRSS2* and *ETS1* rearrangement

MACROSCOPIC
- 75-80% of PCas arise in PZ; ~ 15-25% arise in TZ

MICROSCOPIC
- Diagnosis based on constellation of architectural, nuclear, cytoplasmic, and intraluminal features
- Crowded uniform glands that infiltrate between preexisting benign glands
  - Small caliber, crowded clusters, rigid or sharp lumina, tinctorial staining of cytoplasm distinct from adjacent benign glands
- Malignant glands lack basal cells by immunohistochemistry
- Nuclear enlargement and hyperchromasia with prominently enlarged &/or multiple and peripherally located nucleoli
- Pathognomonic features for malignant glands
  - Glomerulations or collagenous micronodules
  - Circumferential perineural/intraneural invasion or growth within fat
- Less differentiated tumors have poorly formed, fused, cribriform or glomeruloid glands
- Poorly differentiated tumors may grow as infiltrative single cells or solid sheets
- Treated PCa glands usually poorly formed but retain infiltrative appearance
- 2014 ISUP grading condenses GS 2-10 into 5 prognostic grade groups (1-5) and is recommended to use in conjunction with Gleason grading system

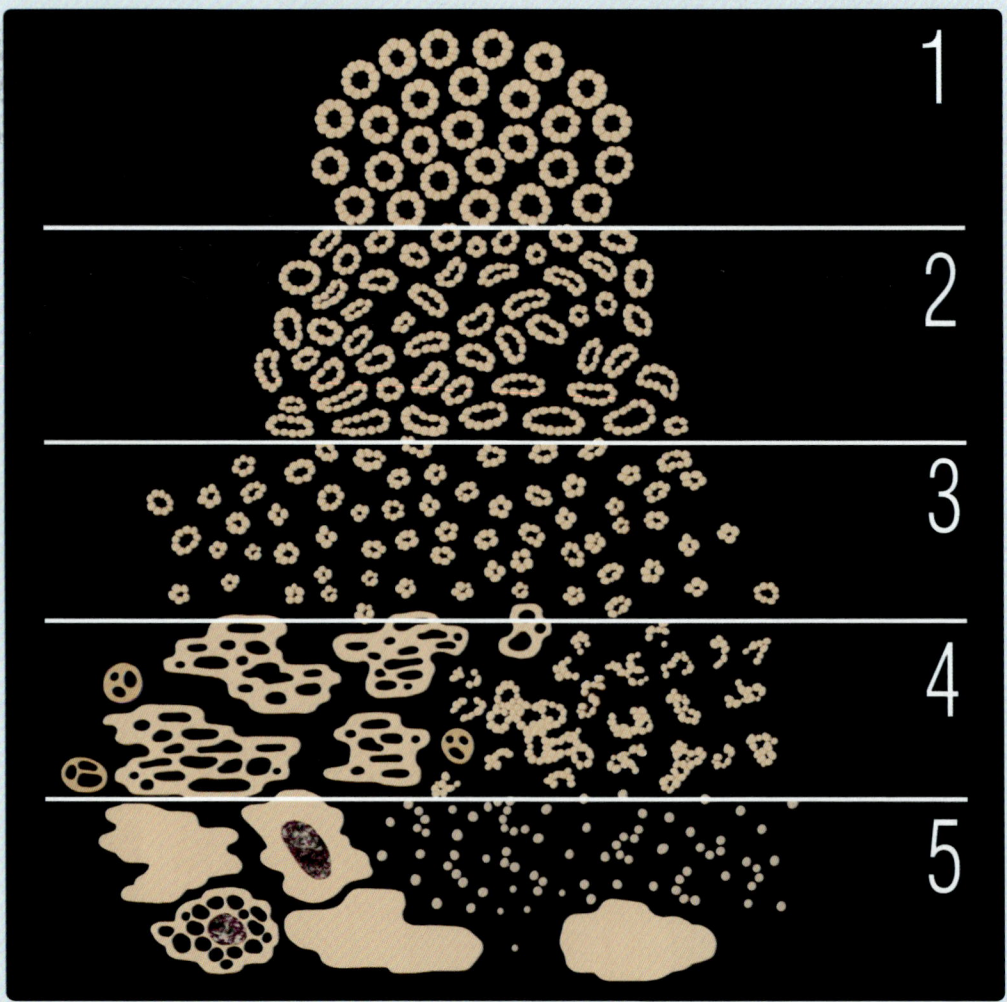

Contemporary Gleason Grading System

Schematic diagram shows modified Gleason grading system for PCa. The Gleason score is a powerful prognostic variable in predicting PCa behavior. This grading system is based purely on glandular architectural patterns, divided into 5 histologic categories or grades with decreasing differentiation. First developed in 1966 by Dr. Donald F. Gleason, it underwent refinements in 1974 and 1977 and had its latest modification by ISUP in 2005 and 2014. This grading scheme is universally accepted and recognized by WHO and by AJCC as the grading system of choice for PCa. This modified Gleason grading is the foundation for the new 2014 ISUP grading system.

Acinar Adenocarcinoma

TERMINOLOGY

Abbreviations
- Prostate adenocarcinoma (PCa)

Synonyms
- Prostatic adenocarcinoma

Definitions
- Malignant neoplasm of prostatic secretory cells

ETIOLOGY/PATHOGENESIS

Cell of Origin
- Recent in vitro studies in animal models suggests that PCa more likely arises from basal cells that develop secretory cell phenotype

Molecular Genetics
- TMPRSS2 and ETS gene fusion
  - Most common recurrent arrangement identified
  - ~ 50% PCa harbor these recurrent gene fusions; individual estimates vary between 15-78%
  - TMPRSS2 encodes for serine protease secreted by prostatic cells in response to androgen exposure
  - ETS family of transcription factors include *ERG*, *ETV1*, *ETV4*, and *ETV5*
  - *TMPRSS2:ERG* gene fusion most common (~ 90%)
    - ERG brought under control of androgen-regulated promoter causing protein overexpression
  - Intra- and interchromosomal genetic rearrangements lead to creation of fusion transcript
    - In ~ 2/3 of cases, fusion results from deletion (intervening 3 Mb between *TMPRSS2* and *ERG*)
    - Fusion may also occur by more complex rearrangement, such as translocation
    - > 20 *TMPRSS2:ERG* variants now described
  - Morphological features of PCa associated with *TMPRSS2:ERG* gene fusion
    - Blue-tinged mucin, cribriform pattern, intraductal spread, macronucleoli, and signet ring cells
      - 93% of tumors with ≥ 3 features have translocation vs. 24% for those without these features
  - Clinical significance of this gene fusion not yet fully understood
    - Conflicting reports in literature
- PTEN
  - Mutated in ~ 20-40% of PCa, often 10q23 deletion
  - Mutation more often identified in advanced prostate cancer, suggesting late genetic event in carcinogenesis
  - Present in normal prostate epithelium and is reduced in cancer
  - Significant cooccurrence with *TMPRSS2:ERG*
- SPOP
  - Mutation detected in 6-13% of PCca
  - Interestingly, occurrence mutually exclusive of *TMPRSS2:ERG*, suggesting that those harbor *SPOP* mutation may represent different class of PCa
- Hereditary prostate cancer
  - Compelling evidence suggests familial predisposition to prostate cancer in some cases
  - High-risk alleles identified with either autosomal dominant or x-linked mode of inheritance
  - 3 candidates genes identified: *HPC2/ELAC2* on 17p, *RNASEL* on 1q25, and *MSR1* on 8p22-23
- Other genes and molecular alterations
  - Most common chromosomal alterations in prostate cancer are losses at 1p, 6q, 8p, 10q, 13q, 16q, and 18q and gains at 1q, 2p, 7, 8q, 18q, and Xq
  - Genes implicated in PCa include *GSTP1*, *NKX3-1*, *AMACR*, *HPN* (hepsin), *KLF6*, *EZH2*, *PSMD9* (p27), *CDH1* (E-cadherin)
  - Mutations in androgen receptor gene may promote cancer growth at lower circulating androgen levels
  - Hedgehog pathway has been shown to play role in growth and metastasis of PCa

MACROSCOPIC

General Features
- Unlike most other visceral organ tumors, PCa often has no reliably distinguishable gross mass lesion
  - Grossly evident tumors are usually pT3, ≥ Gleason score (GS) 8, or ≥ 1 cm size tumors
    - Indurated yellow to yellow-tan homogeneous areas
    - More dense or firmer than surrounding benign spongy parenchyma
  - Typically lack necrosis or hemorrhage
  - Tumor border blends imperceptibly with benign parenchyma
  - Lesions < 5 mm generally inapparent
  - Tumors often larger when examined by microscopy than when measured grossly
  - False-positivity rate in gross identification up to 19%
- Tumors usually in posterior or posterolateral aspect [peripheral zone (PZ)] of gland
- Anterior tumors more difficult to recognize as they are usually admixed with nodular hyperplasia

Site
- 75-80% of PCas arise in PZ, and 15-25% arise in transition zone (TZ)
- Central zone is usually only secondarily involved
- Multifocal tumors present in > 50% of PCas

MICROSCOPIC

Histologic Features
- Diagnosis based on constellation of architectural, nuclear, cytoplasmic, and intraluminal features
  - Some individual features may also be seen in benign glands
- Architectural features
  - Better differentiated tumors consist of compact or loose collections of well-formed glands
    - Small crowded uniform glands infiltrate between preexisting benign glands
  - Malignant glands usually differ in appearance from surrounding benign glands
    - Smaller caliber glands
    - Crowded or compact gland clusters
    - Rigid or sharp glandular lumina
    - May have periglandular clefts

Acinar Adenocarcinoma

- o Malignant glands should lack basal cells
- o Less differentiated tumors consist of poorly formed, fused, or large cribriform glands
- o Poorly differentiated tumors may grow as infiltrative single cells or solid sheets
- **Nuclear features**
  - o Nuclear enlargement and hyperchromasia
  - o Prominently enlarged nucleoli
  - o Multiple and peripherally located nucleoli
  - o Parachromatin clearing
  - o Mitoses are rare; highly suggestive of malignancy if present
  - o Apoptotic bodies (rare)
  - o Nuclei commonly uniform, nonpleomorphic
- **Cytoplasmic features**
  - o Typically cuboidal to columnar cells with modest cytoplasm
  - o Amphophilic, clear or pale granular cytoplasm
  - o Taller cells with clear to pale pink cytoplasm and basally located nuclei more common in TZ
- **Intraluminal features**
  - o Blue mucin
    - Usually prominent collection of wispy, blue-tinged intracellular mucin
  - o Eosinophilic amorphous secretions
    - Granular eosinophilic luminal material
  - o Crystalloids
    - Geometric bright eosinophilic rhomboid to prismatic structures with sharp edges, usually associated with eosinophilic amorphous secretions
    - Present in up to 41% of PCas
    - Seen in atypical adenomatous hyperplasia and uncommonly in benign glands
  - o Corpora amylacea are extremely rare in PCa, should strongly suggest benign glands
  - o Intraluminal necrosis may be present in high-grade tumors, highly indicative of malignancy
- **Pathognomonic features for malignant glands**
  - o Glomerulations
    - Cribriform cellular luminal proliferations in otherwise well-formed glands attached to 1 pole
  - o Collagenous micronodules (mucinous fibroplasia)
    - Hyalinized eosinophilic material usually associated with abundant intraluminal blue mucin
    - Often imparts anastomosing epithelial pattern
  - o Circumferential perineural or intraneural invasion
    - Gland should completely surround nerve or be seen within nerve
    - Benign glands may focally touch or indent nerve; very rarely may be intraneural
  - o Growth within adipose tissue
    - Intraprostatic fat is exceedingly rare
    - Indicates extraprostatic extension

Gleason Grading System

- Widely accepted grading system for PCa
- Assessment of glandular architectures (patterns) at low/intermediate magnification: Classified into 5 basic grades
  - o Each grade/pattern may arise de novo without progression from lower grade
- In resection specimens, GS is sum of primary and secondary Gleason patterns
  - o Primary pattern is most prevalent pattern and secondary is 2nd most common pattern
- International Society of Urological Pathology (ISUP) proposed several modifications and guidelines in 2005 and 2014
  - o In needle biopsies, include tertiary pattern in GS if it is higher than secondary pattern
    - Similar rule applies for transurethral resection and enucleation (simple prostatectomy) specimens
    - In high-grade cancers, ignore lower grade pattern if < 5% (e.g., 4 + 4, if pattern 3 is < 5%)
    - For cancers with > 1 pattern, include higher grade even if it is < 5% (e.g., 3 + 4, even if pattern 4 is < 5%)
  - o Assign individual GS to all cores as an aggregate if submitted in 1 container; assign GS to each core separately designated (e.g., ink or separately submitted) by urologist
  - o In radical prostatectomy, provide GS (primary and secondary pattern); separately mention tertiary pattern
    - Tertiary pattern upgraded as secondary pattern if > 5%
  - o Assign separate GS to dominant tumor(s) for multifocal tumors in radical prostatectomy
  - o Individualized Gleason grading approach for some PCa morphologic variants and subtypes
- **Gleason pattern 1**
  - o Circumscribed nodule of tightly packed, uniform, round to oval, well-formed glands, with no or minimal infiltration of adjacent parenchyma
  - o Using these strict criteria, controversial and disregarded in current practice
    - Those described preimmunohistochemistry were likely atypical adenomatous hyperplasia
  - o Condensed with Gleason pattern 3 in 2014 ISUP grading system under grade group 1
- **Gleason pattern 2**
  - o Nodular with minimal peripheral infiltration, less uniform and more loosely arranged glands
  - o Very rare and typically found in TZ; perhaps tumor conforming to nodular stroma
  - o GS < 6 should rarely, if ever, be diagnosed in needle biopsy specimens
    - Architecture cannot be assessed in its entirety
    - Poor reproducibility among experts
    - Poor correlation with grade in subsequent prostatectomy (i.e., undergrading)
    - May misguide clinicians and patients with assumption of indolent tumor
  - o Condensed with Gleason pattern 3 in 2014 ISUP grading system under grade group 1
- **Gleason pattern 3**
  - o Most common pattern
  - o Predominantly well-formed, individual glands that infiltrate between benign ducts and acini
  - o Includes smaller but well-formed glands (microacini)
  - o Glands typically smaller but may also be enlarged and elongated
  - o Glands may have branching
- **Gleason pattern 4**

Acinar Adenocarcinoma

- Most commonly fused, poorly formed glands
  - Tangentially sectioned pattern 3 glands may mimic fused pattern 4 glands
  - Common cause of overgrading
- 2nd most common pattern is cribriform structures with either regular or irregular outlines
  - By 2014 ISUP consensus, any cribriform gland is now considered Gleason pattern 4
- Uncommon hypernephromatoid pattern, consists of solid sheets of cells with optically clear cytoplasm
- Glomeruloid pattern now included under pattern 4 based on 2014 ISUP consensus
- For diagnosis, needs to be seen at 10x magnification
  - Occasional seemingly poorly formed or fused glands in between well-formed glands are insufficient

- **Gleason pattern 5**
  - Lacks glandular differentiation: Manifests as solid sheets, cords, or single infiltrative tumor cells
  - Also includes solid, cribriform, or papillary structures with central comedo-type necrosis
  - 2014 ISUP consensus added small solid cylinders and solid, medium to large nests with rosette-like spaces

Prognostic Grade Groups

- One aim of 2014 ISUP consensus conference was to adopt new grading system for PCa
- New grading system was based on following observations
  - New grade groupings have better stratification of prostate cancer patients than current Gleason grading
  - Grading simplified to 1-5 with improved gradation than GS 2-10
  - Lowest grade is 1 and not 6, as in GS (middle of scale), and may not lead to possible overtreatment
  - New grading system is based on ISUP modified Gleason grading system, which bears little resemblance to original Gleason system
- Grade should be used in conjunction with Gleason system [e.g., GS 3 + 3 = 6 (grade group 1)]

Therapy-Related Changes

- **Radiation therapy**
  - Treated PCa glands usually poorly formed glands that retain their infiltrative appearance
    - Foamy vacuolated cytoplasm and pleomorphic nuclei; changes vary from mild to marked
    - Marked radiation effect may artifactually produce architecture resembling GS 9 or 10 cancers
    - Luminal features of malignancy may be retained
  - Cytologic atypia and pleomorphism more pronounced in benign than malignant glands
  - Residual treated PCa with minimal or no radiation effect has higher chance of recurrence
  - CK-PAN(AE1/AE3) useful to highlight treated PCa
- **Hormonal therapy**
  - Treated PCa may be shrunken glands or single cells
  - Glands show xanthomatous cytoplasm, pyknotic and fragmented nuclei, and mucin extravasation
  - Empty spaces representing remnants of shrunken glands may be present
  - Marked atrophy, basal cell hyperplasia, or squamous metaplasia in adjacent benign glands
  - CK-PAN(AE1/AE3) useful to highlight treated PCa

DIFFERENTIAL DIAGNOSIS

General Features

- Given broad morphologic spectrum, differential diagnosis for PCa ranges from innocuous benign normal structures to secondary high-grade cancers
- PCa most often mimicked by benign prostatic glandular lesions; difficulty enhanced in limited samples (e.g., biopsy)
  - Use of ancillary immunohistochemistry helpful in some scenarios
  - Pattern-based approach facilitates work-up and judicious selection of adjuvant stains

Atypical Small Acinar Proliferation

- Focal atypical glands that are suspicious but quantitatively &/or qualitatively insufficient for diagnosis or exclusion of PCa
- Most common differential diagnostic scenario for PCa
- Differential diagnosis includes focal PCa and benign glandular lesions
- Immunohistochemistry may be helpful
  - PCa lacks basal cell staining and often overexpresses AMACR
    - In some cases, definitive diagnosis of PCa is not possible even with carcinoma staining pattern

SELECTED REFERENCES

1. Epstein JI et al: The 2014 International Society of Urological Pathology (ISUP) Consensus Conference on Gleason Grading of Prostatic Carcinoma: Definition of Grading Patterns and Proposal for a New Grading System. Am J Surg Pathol. 40(2):244-52, 2015
2. Epstein JI et al: A Contemporary Prostate Cancer Grading System: A Validated Alternative to the Gleason Score. Eur Urol. 69(3):428-35, 2015
3. Samaratunga H et al: The prognostic significance of the 2014 International Society of Urological Pathology (ISUP) grading system for prostate cancer. Pathology. 47(6):515-9, 2015
4. Epstein JI et al: Best practices recommendations in the application of immunohistochemistry in the prostate: report from the International Society of Urologic Pathology consensus conference. Am J Surg Pathol. 38(8):e6-e19, 2014
5. Pierorazio PM et al: Prognostic Gleason grade grouping: data based on the modified Gleason scoring system. BJU Int. 111(5):753-60, 2013
6. Gottipati S et al: Usual and unusual histologic patterns of high Gleason score 8 to 10 adenocarcinoma of the prostate in needle biopsy tissue. Am J Surg Pathol. 36(6):900-7, 2012
7. Ross HM et al: Do adenocarcinomas of the prostate with Gleason score (GS) ≤6 have the potential to metastasize to lymph nodes? Am J Surg Pathol. 36(9):1346-52, 2012
8. Epstein JI: An update of the Gleason grading system. J Urol. 183(2):433-40, 2010
9. Van der Kwast TH et al: Variability in diagnostic opinion among pathologists for single small atypical foci in prostate biopsies. Am J Surg Pathol. Epub ahead of print, 2010
10. Gopalan A et al: TMPRSS2-ERG gene fusion is not associated with outcome in patients treated by prostatectomy. Cancer Res. 69(4):1400-6, 2009
11. Latour M et al: Grading of invasive cribriform carcinoma on prostate needle biopsy: an interobserver study among experts in genitourinary pathology. Am J Surg Pathol. 32(10):1532-9, 2008
12. Epstein JI et al: The 2005 International Society of Urological Pathology (ISUP) Consensus Conference on Gleason Grading of Prostatic Carcinoma. Am J Surg Pathol. 29(9):1228-42, 2005
13. Tomlins SA et al: Recurrent fusion of TMPRSS2 and ETS transcription factor genes in prostate cancer. Science. 310(5748):644-8, 2005
14. Varma M et al: Morphologic criteria for the diagnosis of prostatic adenocarcinoma in needle biopsy specimens. A study of 250 consecutive cases in a routine surgical pathology practice. Arch Pathol Lab Med. 126(5):554-61, 2002
15. Baisden BL et al: Perineural invasion, mucinous fibroplasia, and glomerulations: diagnostic features of limited cancer on prostate needle biopsy. Am J Surg Pathol. 23(8):918-24, 1999

Acinar Adenocarcinoma

ISUP Grading System for Prostatic Adenocarcinoma

ISUP Grade	Definition	Gleason Score
1	Only individual discrete well-formed glands	3 + 3 = 6
2	Predominantly well-formed glands with lesser component of poorly formed/fused/cribriform glands* (record percent of lesser component)	3 + 4 = 7
3	Predominantly poorly formed/fused/cribriform glands with lesser component of well-formed glands*+ (record percent of greater component)	4 + 3 = 7
4	Only poorly formed/fused/cribriform glands+ OR predominantly well-formed glands and lesser component lacking glands OR predominantly lacking glands and lesser component of well-formed glands+	8
5	Lack gland formation (or with necrosis) ± poorly formed/fused/cribriform glands+	9 - 10

*A < 5% component of no gland formation is denoted as a minor high-grade pattern (i.e. tertiary pattern). Grades 2 and 3, with > 5% no gland formation, are reassigned grades 4 and 5, respectively.
+ For cases with > 95% poorly formed/fused/cribriform glands or lack of glands on a core or at RP, the component of < 5% well-formed glands is not factored into the grade.

Derived from Epstein JI et al. Am J Surg Pathol, 2015.

Differential Diagnosis for Prostate Carcinoma

Histologic Pattern	Prostate Carcinoma	Main Differential Diagnoses
Small glandular proliferation	Glandular Gleason pattern 3	Crowded benign glands, not otherwise specified
	Atrophic pattern	Simple atrophy, partial atrophy, postatrophic hyperplasia
	Posttreatment cancer	Atypical adenomatous hyperplasia (adenosis), sclerosing adenosis, basal cell hyperplasia
		Outpouching of high-grade PIN
		Seminal vesicle epithelium, ejaculatory duct, Cowper glands
		Nephrogenic adenoma, mesonephric remnants, verumontanum mucosal gland hyperplasia
		Radiation atypia
Atypical large glandular proliferation	Cribriform Gleason patterns 3, 4, and 5	High-grade PIN
	Ductal adenocarcinoma	Urothelial carcinoma involving prostatic ducts and acini
	Pseudohyperplastic pattern	Colorectal carcinoma involving prostate
		Cribriform hyperplasia, squamous metaplasia, urothelial metaplasia
Infiltrative single cell pattern	Single cell Gleason 5 pattern	Dense inflammation, granulomatous prostatitis
	Posttreatment carcinoma	Lymphoma, small cell carcinoma
Clear cell pattern	Hypernephroid Gleason pattern 4	Prostatic xanthoma
	Glandular Gleason pattern 3	
Oncocytic pattern	Gleason pattern 4	Paraganglion/paraganglioma
		Carcinoid tumor
Poorly to undifferentiated carcinoma	Solid Gleason pattern 5	Urothelial carcinoma
Spindle cell pattern	Sarcomatoid carcinoma	Pseudosarcomatous myofibroblastic proliferation
		Stromal sarcoma, leiomyosarcoma
Small cell pattern	Small cell carcinoma	Lymphoma, rhabdomyosarcoma

PIN = prostatic intraepithelial neoplasia.

Modified from Paner et al: Arch Pathol Lab Med;132:1388-96, 2008.

Acinar Adenocarcinoma

Gross Appearance of Prostate Cancer

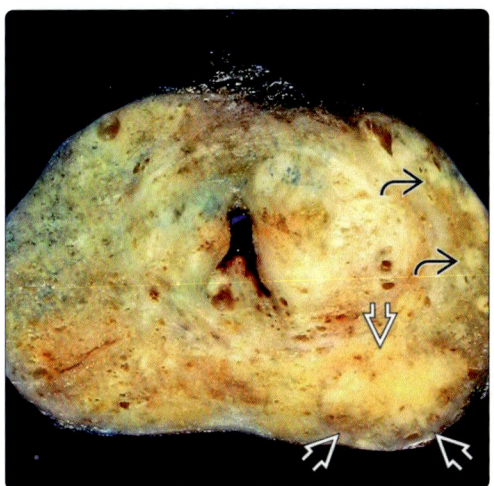

Gross Appearance of Prostate Cancer

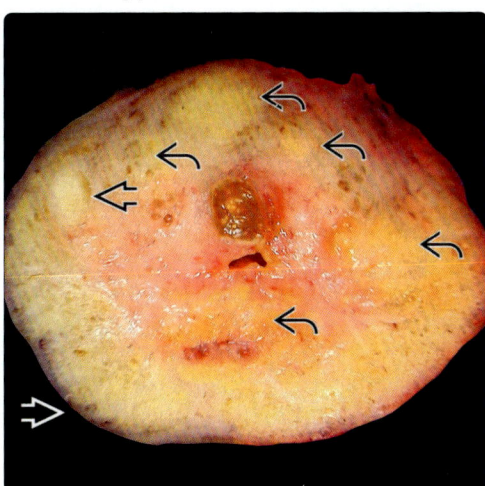

(Left) This coronal section of the prostate shows multifocal PCa predominantly involving the left lobe with a dominant nodule ➡ at the posterolateral aspect and additional smaller tumor foci ➡ at the lateral aspect of the peripheral zone (PZ). *(Right)* Coronal section of prostate shows a focus of PCa ➡ involving the anterior aspect of PZ. Several hyperplastic nodules ➡ are seen in the adjacent transition zone (TZ). Note the absence of grossly visible tumor in posterior and posterolateral aspect of the PZ ➡.

Prostate Cancer at Peripheral Zone

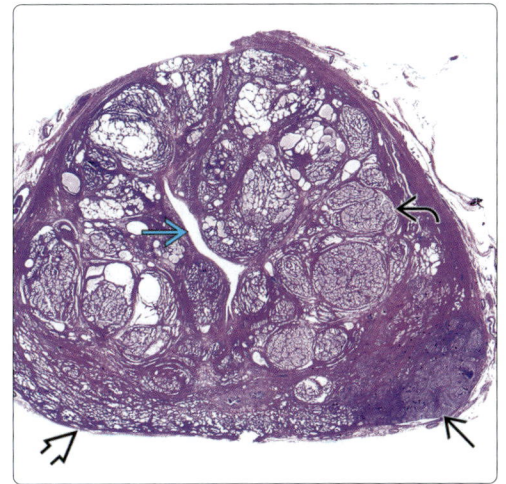

Prostate Cancer at Peripheral Zone

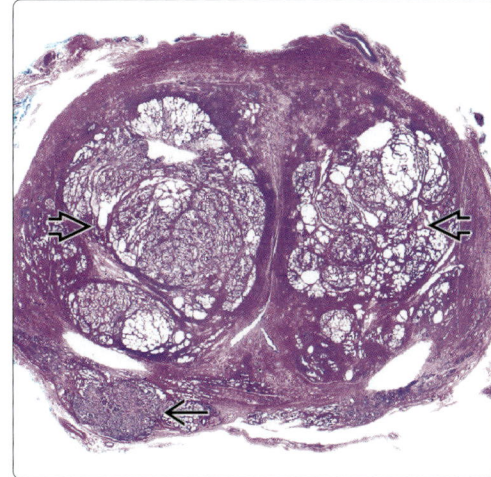

(Left) Coronal section of the prostate shows the urethra ➡ pushed to the left due to prominent benign fibromuscular and glandular hyperplasia ➡. The PZ shows evidence of prominent atrophy ➡ and a carcinoma ➡ involving the posterolateral aspect. *(Right)* Whole mount coronal section of the prostate shows evidence of prominent fibromuscular hyperplasia ➡ in the TZ compressing the urethra and a focus of adenocarcinoma ➡ in the PZ.

Prostate Cancer at Peripheral Zone

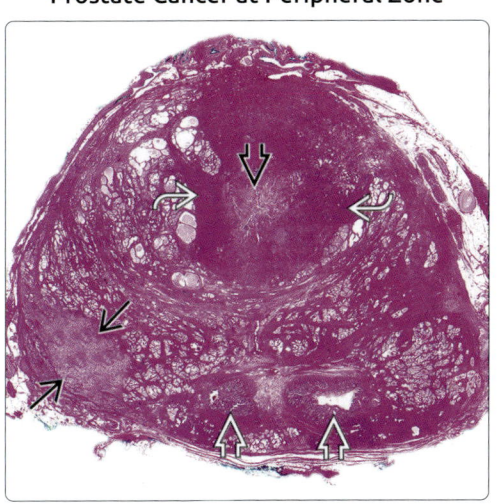

Prostate Cancer at Peripheral Zone

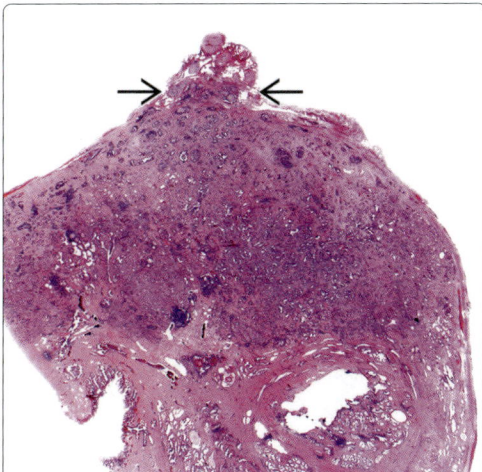

(Left) A nodule of adenocarcinoma ➡ is present in the right posterolateral aspect of the PZ. There is also prominent stromal hyperplasia ➡ in the TZ, which compresses the urethra ➡. The intraprostatic portion of the seminal vesicles ➡ is also seen. *(Right)* This macrosection shows extensive adenocarcinoma replacing much of the PZ. Extraprostatic extension ➡ is present in the neurovascular bundle. Note the uncommon desmoplastic response to PCa seen in this case.

Acinar Adenocarcinoma

(Left) *In contrast to most carcinomas, stromal reaction is rare in PCa; infiltration is therefore difficult to define. Most commonly, it is identified as infiltration of small glands between larger, normal, benign glands ⇒. Well-formed glands of PCa on low-power view may closely resemble benign glands.* (Right) *This poorly differentiated PCa is characterized by crowded, poorly formed glands infiltrating between normal large-caliber glands ⇒. Glandular crowding is another key feature in the recognition of adenocarcinoma.*

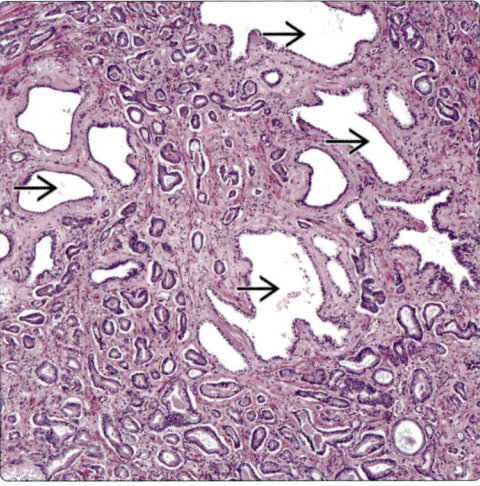
Prostate Cancer Architecture

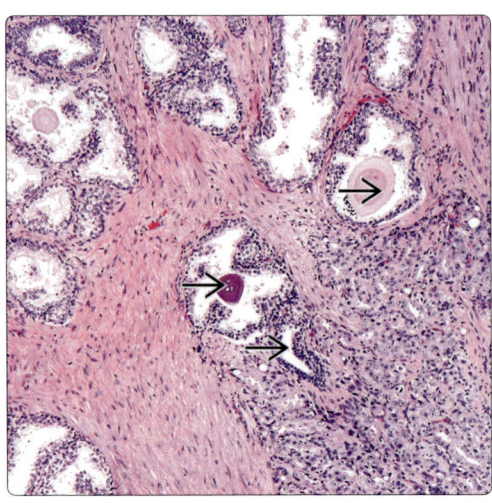
Prostate Cancer Architecture

(Left) *This low-power magnification of focal PCa shows a collection of tightly clustered, small, crowded glands ⇒. Despite the absence of infiltrative growth, these features warrant closer examination to evaluate for adenocarcinoma.* (Right) *This PCa is characterized by crowded medium-caliber glands with extensive retraction spaces surrounding the individual carcinoma glands. This periglandular clearing is not specific but is relatively rare in benign glands.*

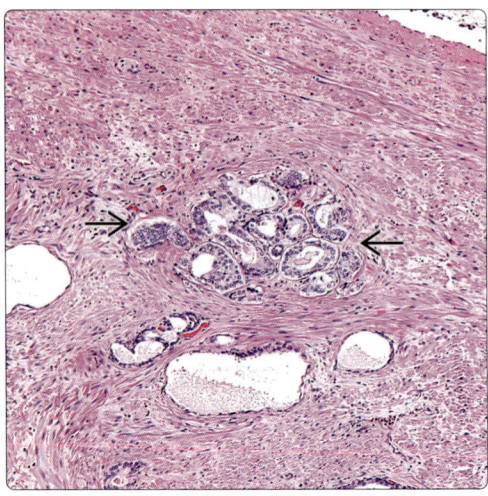
Prostate Cancer Architecture

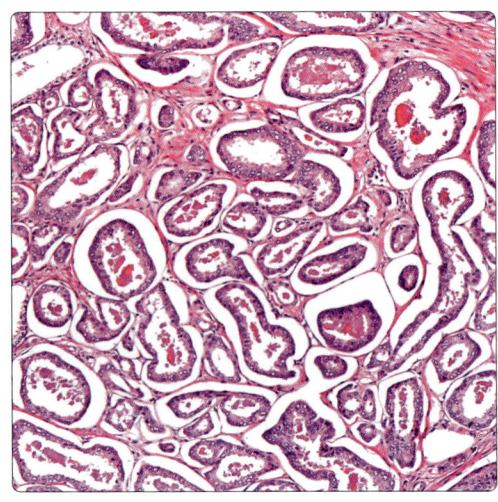
Prostate Cancer Architecture

(Left) *PCa in biopsy may show linear alignment of glands ⇒ that course perpendicular to the long axis of the core. This architectural growth pattern is highly suggestive of adenocarcinoma.* (Right) *PCa glands are tightly clustered and oriented in a linear arrangement. Cytologic features of PCa are not readily apparent. The focus lacked basal cells by immunohistochemistry with p63 and also had strong luminal racemase/AMACR immunoreactivity, features supporting the diagnosis of PCa.*

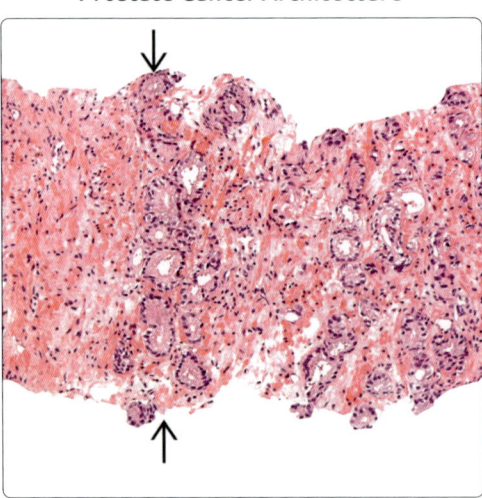
Prostate Cancer Architecture

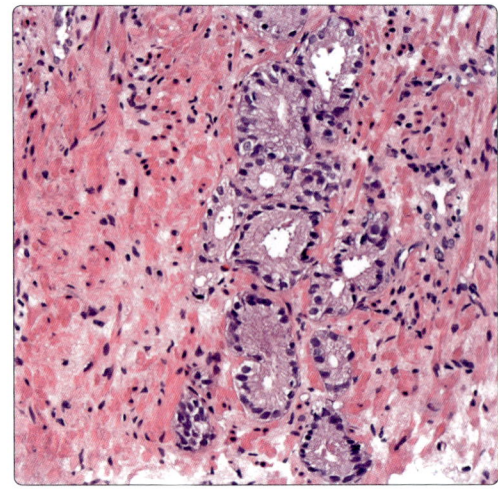
Prostate Cancer Architecture

Acinar Adenocarcinoma

Prostate Cancer Cytologic Features

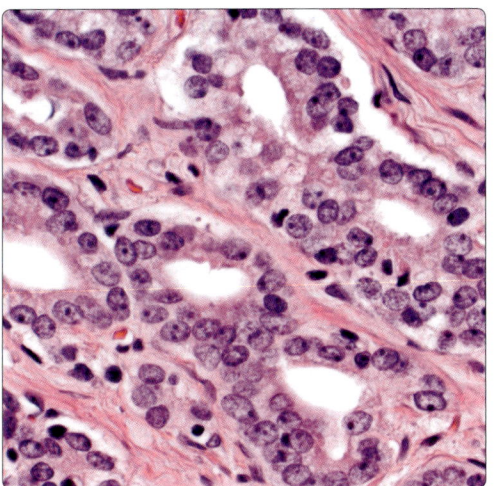

Prostate Cancer Cytologic Features

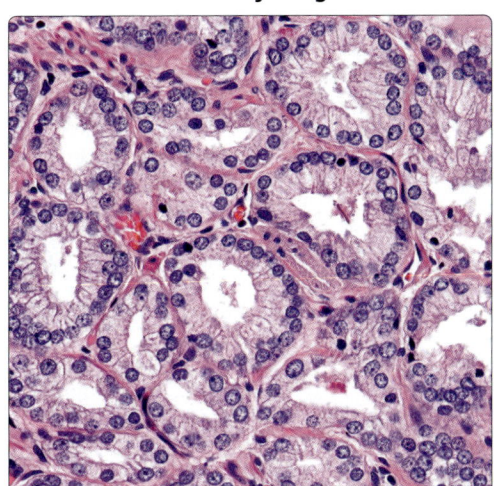

(Left) Prominent nucleoli, as seen here, are characteristic of PCa, but they are not always required for the diagnosis. In addition, nuclei larger than the adjacent nuclei of benign glands and those with double nucleoli and with parachromatin clearing or mitosis are helpful features. **(Right)** PCa shows pale granular cytoplasm and monotonous-appearing round nuclei. PCa nuclei are typically homogeneous. Nuclear pleomorphism should suggest the possibility of a nonprostatic lesion.

Prostate Cancer Cytologic Features

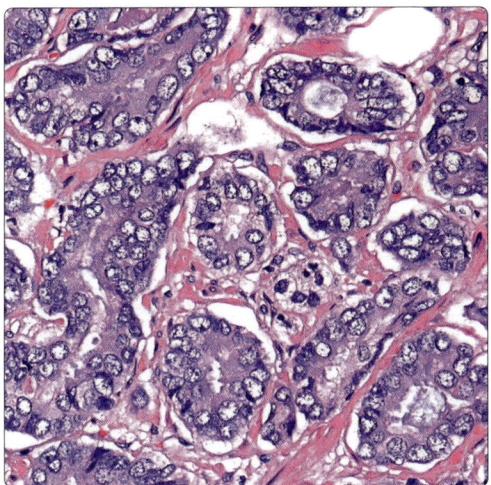

Prostate Cancer Cytologic Features

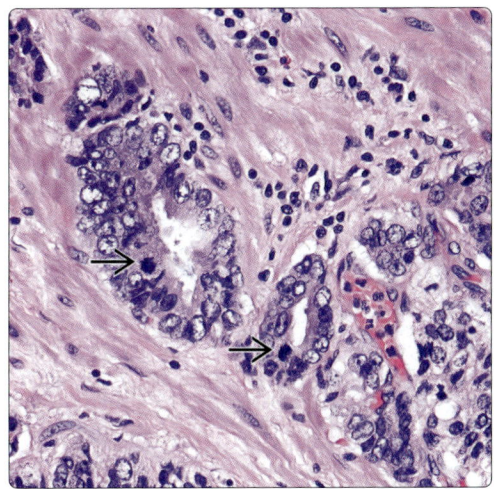

(Left) PCa glands commonly show parachromatin clearing in the malignant nuclei. These nuclei also show a mild degree of nuclear variability and crowding not typically seen in most PCa. PCa nuclei are usually very round and monotonous. Note the absence of any stromal reaction. **(Right)** PCa shows readily identifiable mitotic figures ➡ within the malignant glands. Mitotic figures are very rare in PCa; however, their presence is highly suggestive of adenocarcinoma.

Prostate Cancer Cytologic Features

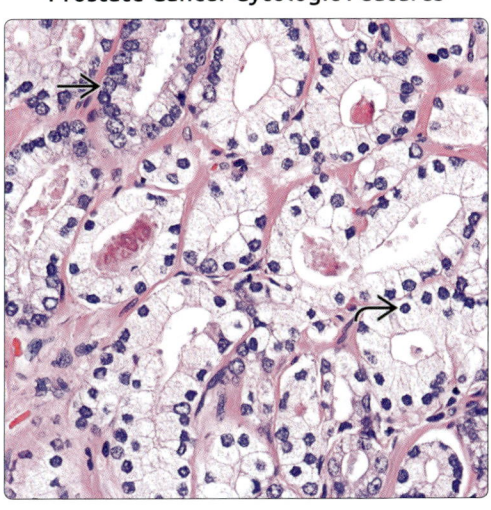

Prostate Cancer Cytologic Features

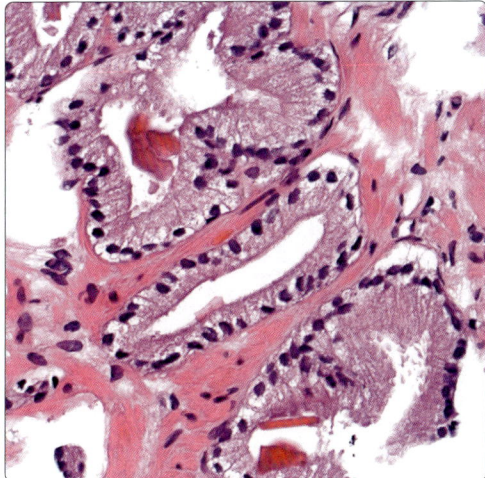

(Left) PCa shows columnar cells with pale cytoplasm and basally situated nuclei. Some nuclei are large with prominent nucleoli ➡, while others are more condensed ➡. The size of the nuclei and prominence of nucleoli may vary considerably within the same tumor. **(Right)** Some PCa have relatively bland nuclear features, as seen in this case. The presence of obvious nucleoli is not required for a diagnosis of adenocarcinoma if other sufficient features are present. Gland rigidity and crystalloids in this case are helpful in the diagnosis.

Acinar Adenocarcinoma

Prostate Cancer Luminal Features

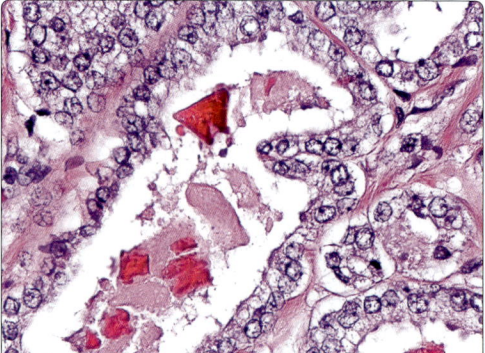

(Left) PCa shows abundant intraluminal crystalloids. Luminal crystalloids are relatively more common in PCa than in benign glands; however, abundant crystalloids may be seen in atypical adenomatous hyperplasia (adenosis) and some other small glandular proliferations. **(Right)** Intraluminal blue mucin ➡ is another feature that, while not entirely specific, is highly suggestive of adenocarcinoma. Glands with luminal mucin should be carefully evaluated for other features of carcinoma.

Prostate Cancer Luminal Features

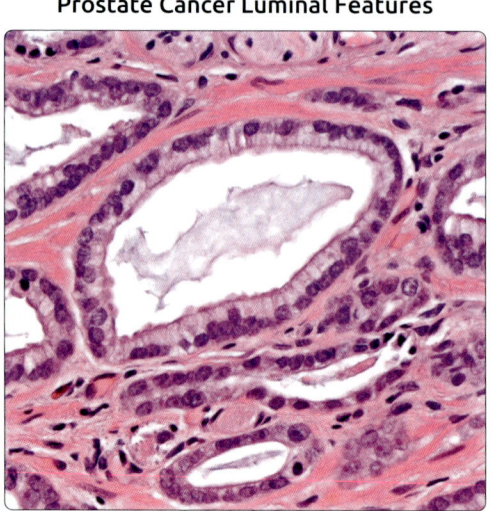

(Left) PCa with intraluminal pale mucin has a sharp luminal contour, which is distinct from the undulating or tufted luminal surface typical of benign glands. This PCa also shows basal orientation of the nuclei; in normal glands, nuclei have more variation in their relation to the lumen. **(Right)** This PCa has both corpora amylacea ➡ and crystalloids ➡ within the lumina. Despite their presence here, corpora amylacea are very rare in PCa glands and should prompt careful exclusion of a benign process.

Prostate Cancer Luminal Features **Lymphovascular Invasion**

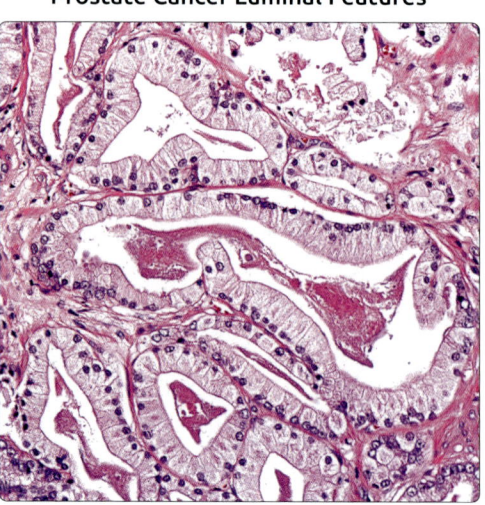 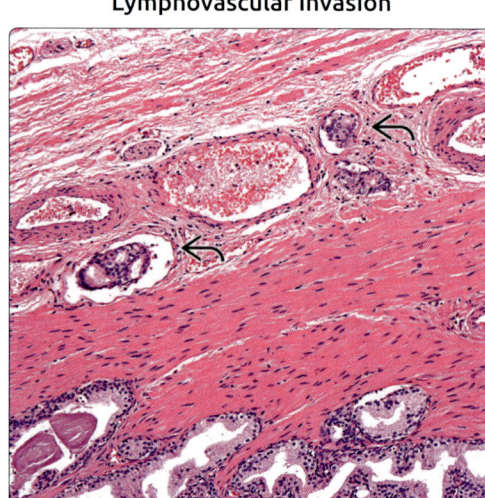

(Left) Intraluminal eosinophilic secretions, while not entirely specific, are commonly seen in PCa. This PCa also shows basally oriented nuclei and prominent luminal cytoplasm, other histologic features that are suggestive of malignancy. **(Right)** This PCa shows multiple foci of lymphovascular invasion ➡. Retraction artifact may closely mimic lymphovascular invasion, but definite involvement of vascular spaces is diagnostic of malignancy. This finding is rare in needle biopsy.

Acinar Adenocarcinoma

Prostate Cancer Pathognomonic Features

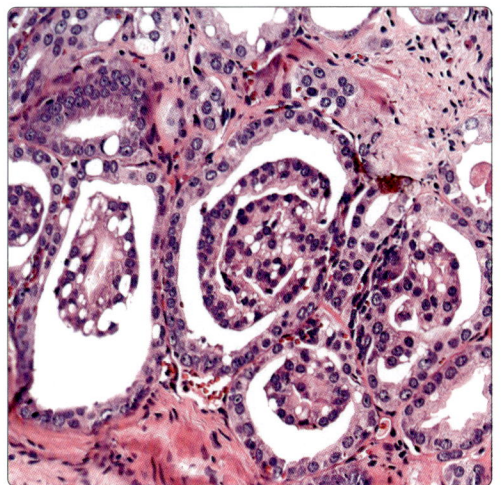

Prostate Cancer Pathognomonic Features

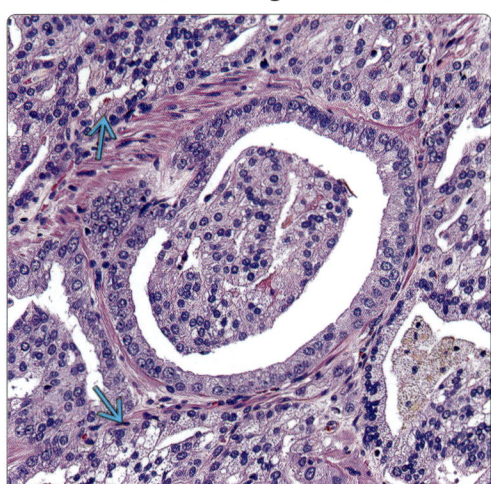

(Left) The presence of glomerulations, defined as a cribriform cellular luminal proliferation attached to 1 pole of the lumen, is diagnostic of adenocarcinoma. **(Right)** High-power view of a PCa gland with a glomerulation shows the cribriform cellular luminal proliferation attached at 1 pole. Based on the 2014 ISUP consensus, glomerulation should be regarded as Gleason pattern 4. Glomerulation is usually associated with other higher grade patterns, such as the fused gland patterns ➡ seen in this case.

Prostate Cancer Pathognomonic Features

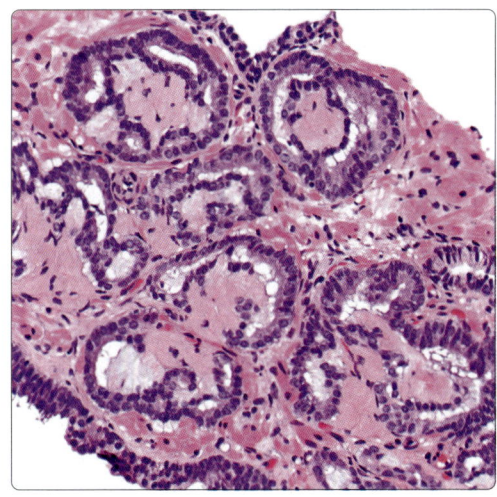

Prostate Cancer Pathognomonic Features

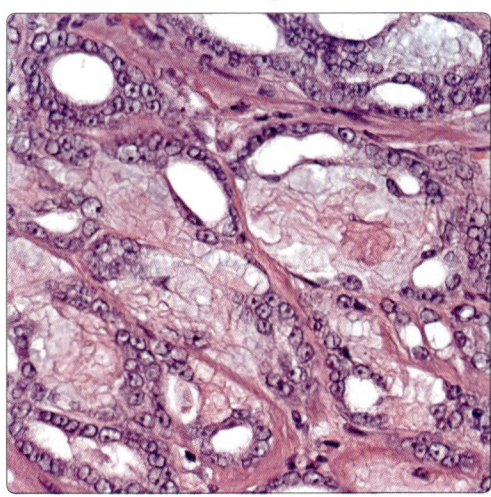

(Left) Collagenous micronodules (mucinous fibroplasia) are a pathognomonic feature of PCa. They are typically associated with mucin and are characterized by dense nodules of fibrous tissue and fibroblasts associated with the epithelium. **(Right)** In early collagenous micronodules, the fibrous tissue is scant and more mucin is seen. Although the epithelium often assumes a complex architecture, mucinous fibroplasia is typically assigned a 3 + 3 = 6 Gleason score (GS).

Prostate Cancer Pathognomonic Features

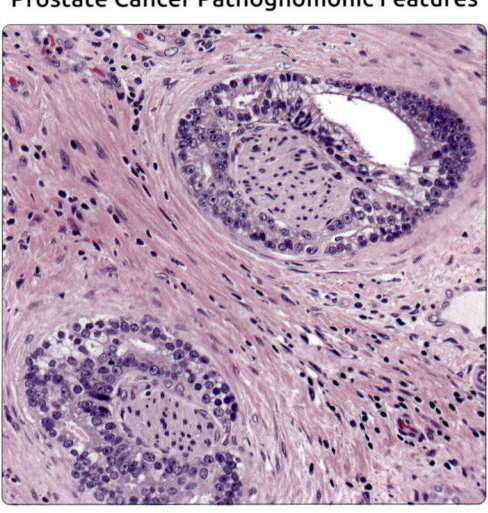

Prostate Cancer Pathognomonic Features

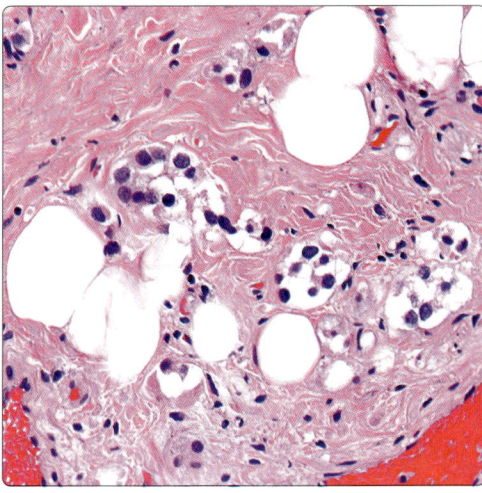

(Left) Circumferential (or intraneural) involvement is required if perineural invasion is used as a diagnostic adjunct. Some benign lesions, such as postatrophic hyperplasia, may contain glands with focal, noncircumferential indentation of a nerve. When present, perineural invasion is supportive of a diagnosis of PCa. **(Right)** This PCa shows invasion into adipose tissue, which is considered by most as a diagnostic feature of adenocarcinoma since intraprostatic fat is exceedingly rare.

Acinar Adenocarcinoma

Gleason Patterns 2-3

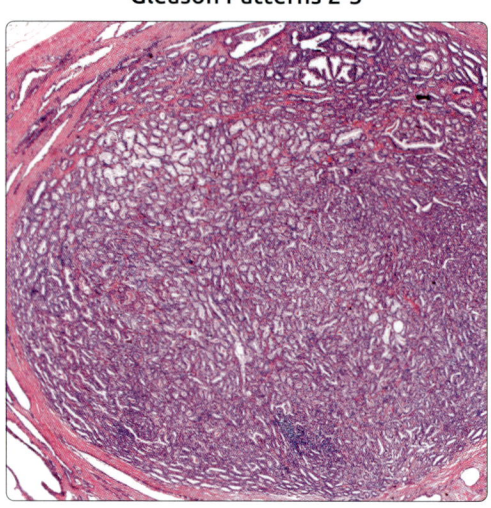

Gleason Patterns 2-3

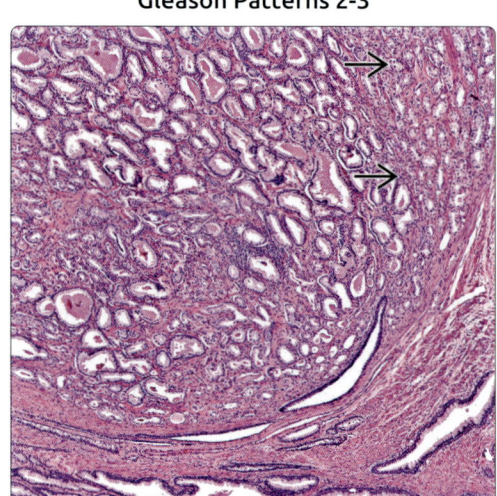

(Left) This GS 2 + 2 = 4 PCa is characterized by a circumscribed nodule of mainly medium-sized glands with minimal peripheral infiltration. This pattern is rare and seen almost exclusively in TZ. Low-grade patterns (GS 2-4) are now condensed with GS 6 under prognostic grade group 1. (Right) This GS 2 + 3 = 5 PCa shows a relatively circumscribed large nodule composed of mostly medium-sized glands (Gleason pattern 2) with focal peripheral infiltration by smaller glands (Gleason pattern 3) ➡.

Gleason Patterns 2-3

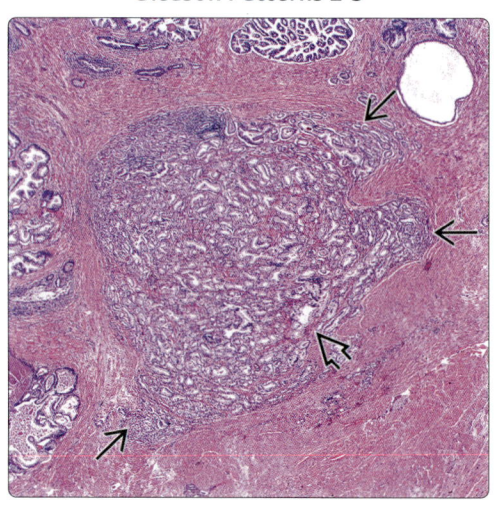

Gleason Pattern 3

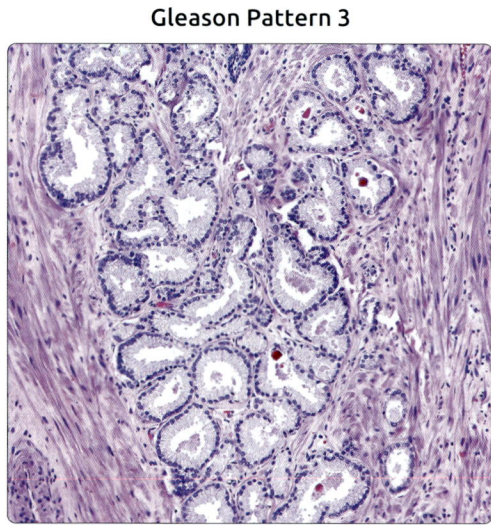

(Left) This GS 3 + 2 = 5 PCa contains more prominent foci of peripheral infiltration by smaller glands (Gleason pattern 3) ➡. PCa cluster shows overall nodular configuration with relatively larger sized glands (Gleason pattern 2) ➡. Low-grade patterns (GS 2-4) are now condensed with GS 6 under prognostic grade group 1. (Right) Gleason pattern 3 PCa shows discrete, well-formed glands. These glands are crowded and have infiltrative pattern. Gleason grade 3 is the most common pattern in the Gleason grading scheme.

Gleason Pattern 3

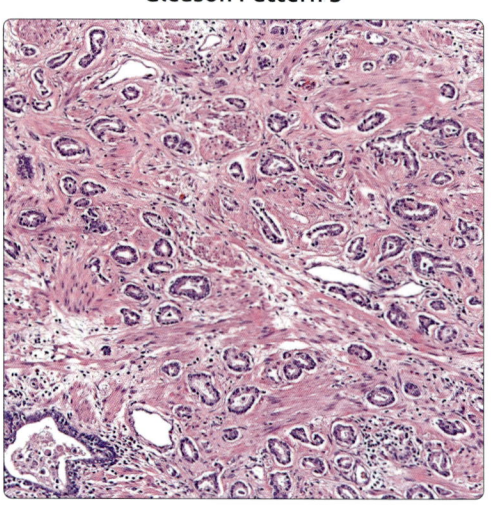

Gleason Pattern 3

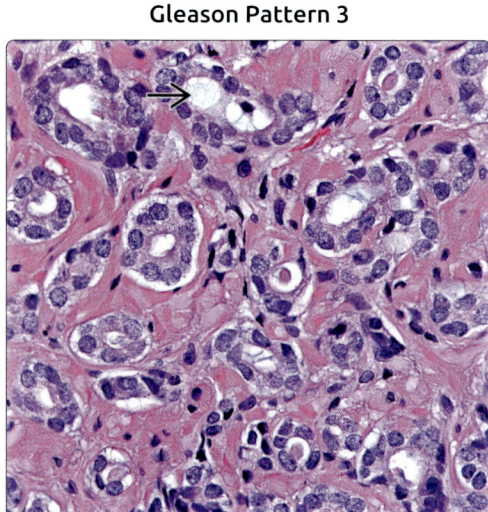

(Left) This Gleason pattern 3 PCa shows well-formed glands with marked variation in gland size and shape, as well as diffuse infiltrative growth without formation of a discrete nodule. Note the large benign gland with 2 cell layers. (Right) High-power view of Gleason pattern 3 PCa shows clusters of small to minute glands (microacinar pattern). These glands have a continuous cell lining around central lumina. Some of these glands display luminal rigidity and contain blue-tinged mucin ➡, typical of PCa.

Acinar Adenocarcinoma

Gleason Pattern 4

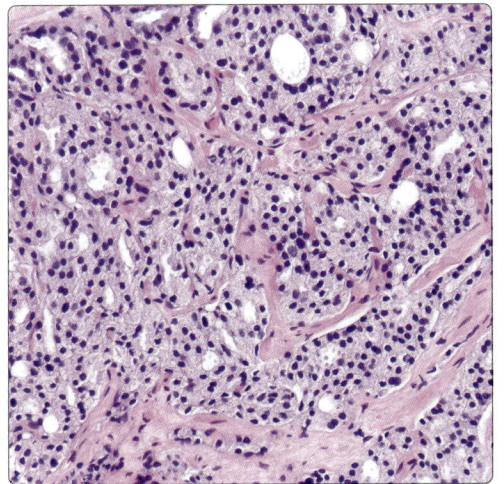

Gleason Pattern 4

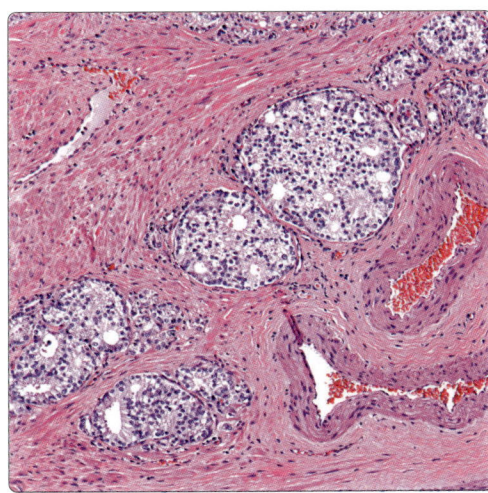

(Left) PCa with extensive confluent anastomosing growth (or fusion) indicates Gleason pattern 4. Fused glands are complex, such that an imaginary line cannot be easily drawn around the individual glands. **(Right)** This GS 4 + 4 = 8 PCa shows large tumor nodules with a well-developed internal cribriform structure. Based on 2014 ISUP consensus, any cribriform pattern should be designated as Gleason pattern 4, and cribriform intraductal carcinoma and high-grade prostatic intraepithelial neoplasia should be excluded.

Gleason Pattern 4

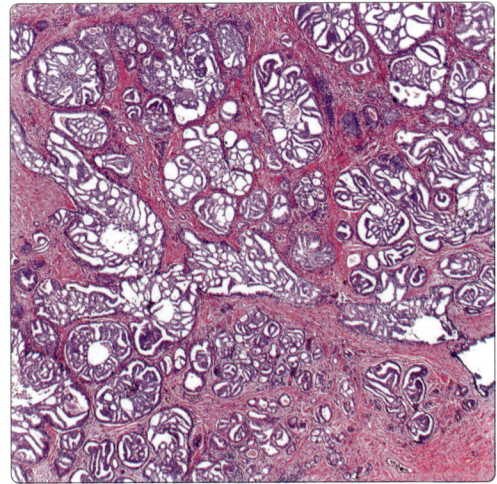

Gleason Pattern 4

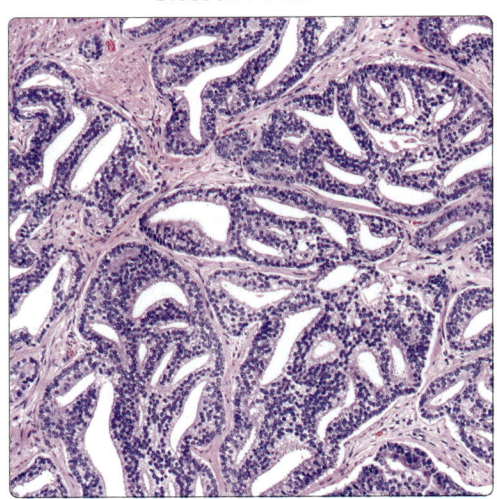

(Left) Most cribriform growth represents Gleason pattern 4, and this may include intraductal growth, especially in high-volume cancer. Central necrosis in any of the glands would indicate pattern 5. **(Right)** This Gleason pattern 4 cribriform pattern shows large glands with irregular outline containing multiple lumina separated by cellular bridges. The presence of tumor cell necrosis or solid growth in a cribriform gland (not seen here) would warrant designation as Gleason pattern 5.

Gleason Pattern 4

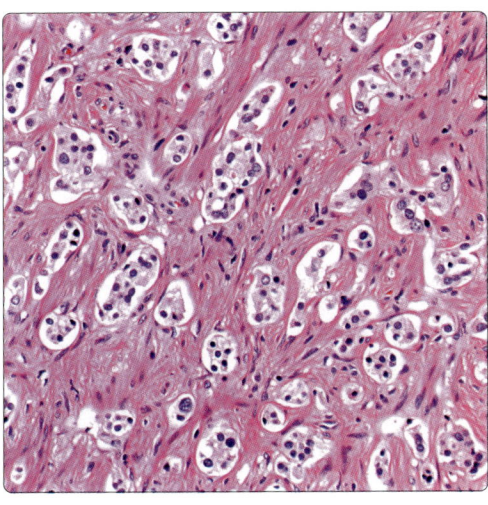

Gleason Pattern 3 Tunneling

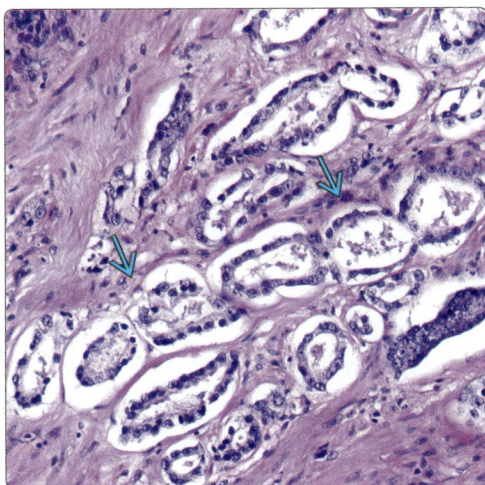

(Left) Irregular clusters of PCa shows no well-formed glands (Gleason 4 pattern). It is important to rule out tangential sectioning (follow on deeper cuts) and the architecture of accompanying PCa glands. **(Right)** This GS 3 + 3 = 6 PCa has tangentially sectioned, elongated, undulating glands (tunneling) ➡ identified by the linear direction of the lumina. The series of luminal compartments represent part of a single continuous lumina (hence not pattern 4), which is not evident in one H&E plane.

Acinar Adenocarcinoma

(Left) Solid, diffuse or sheet-like growth without luminal formation is considered Gleason pattern 5. Note the prominent nucleoli. **(Right)** This Gleason pattern 5 PCa with comedonecrosis shows a large, partly cribriform gland with a central collection of necrotic tumor ghost cells ⮕. The comedonecrosis of Gleason pattern 5 may also be surrounded by solid or papillary growth of cells. Comedonecrosis should be distinguished from amorphous secretions with pyknotic nuclei, which may be seen in Gleason pattern 3 glands.

Gleason Pattern 5
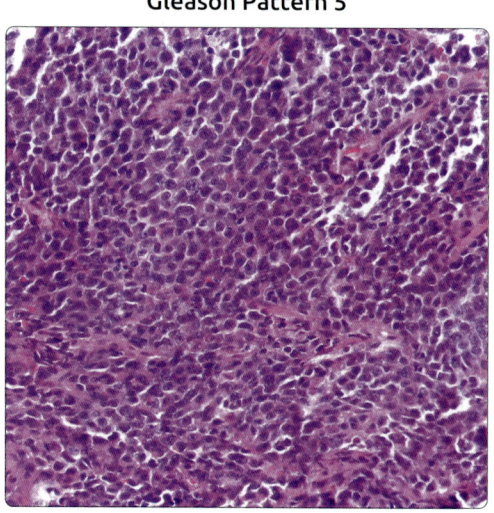

Gleason Pattern 5
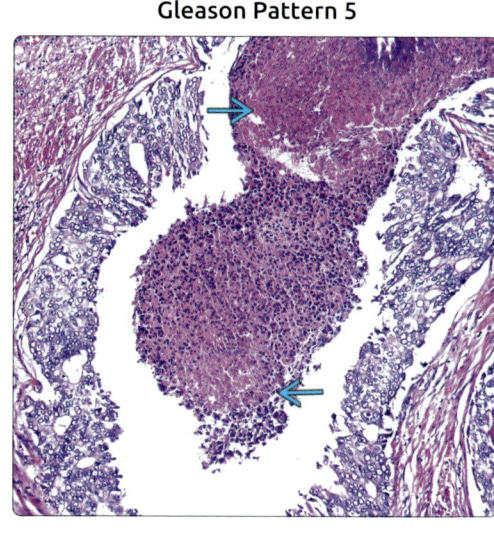

(Left) Gleason pattern 5 PCa solid architecture shows diffuse, sheet-like growth without lumina. This pattern may be difficult to distinguish from urothelial carcinoma involving the prostate. Use of GATA3, p63, &/or HMCK(34βE12) immunostains complemented by PSA &/or PAP are helpful in making this distinction. **(Right)** Gleason pattern 5 PCa with central comedonecrosis shows a large, irregular, cribriform gland with central area of necrotic tumor cells ⮕. Stringent criteria should be used in identifying tumor cell necrosis.

Gleason Pattern 5
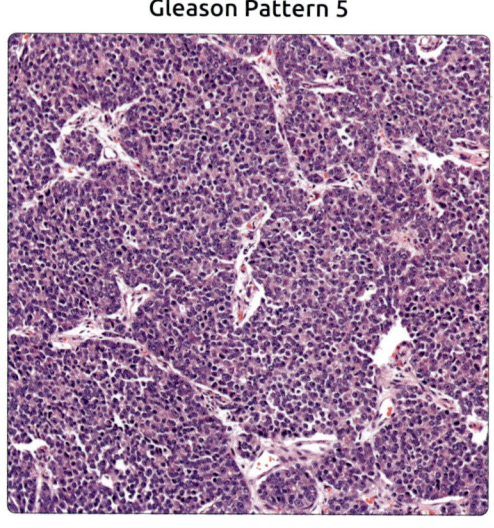

Gleason Pattern 5
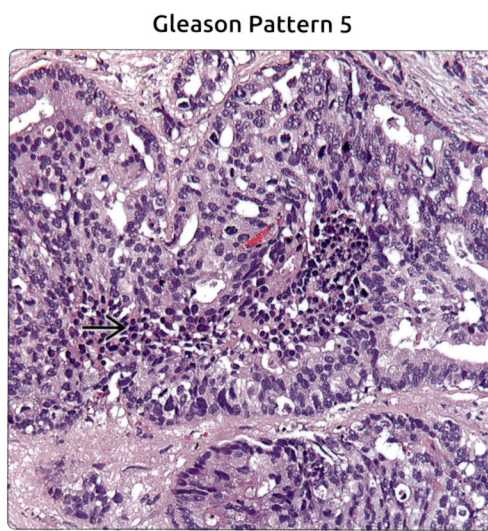

(Left) This needle core biopsy shows infiltration of poorly differentiated PCa as linear or trabecular chains and individual single cells and is designated as Gleason pattern 5. **(Right)** This PCa shows prominent cytoplasmic vacuoles, which should not be considered signet ring differentiation (Gleason pattern 5). The ISUP consensus recommends discounting the vacuoles while assigning a grade. In this case, the underlying architecture of the vacuolated cells is that of Gleason pattern 4, poorly formed glands.

Gleason Pattern 5
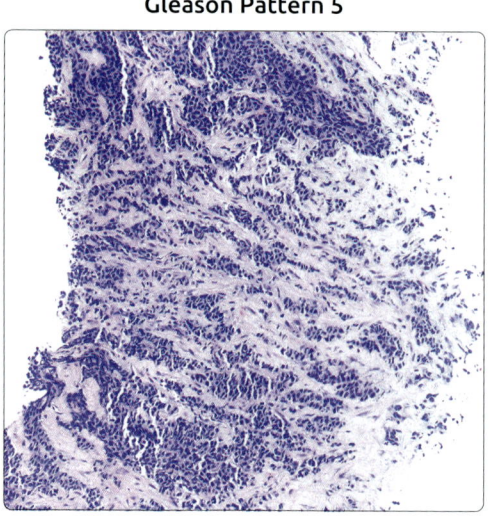

Prostate Cancer With Vacuolations
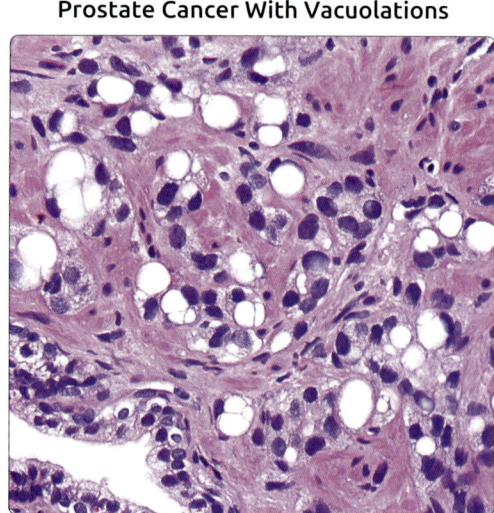

Acinar Adenocarcinoma

Gland Architecture in Perineural Invasion

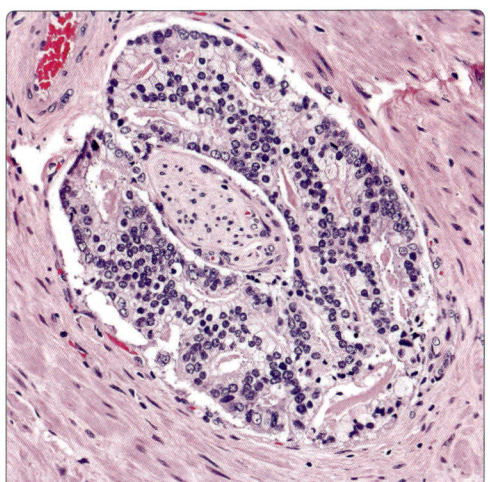

PIN4 Immunostaining in Prostate Cancer

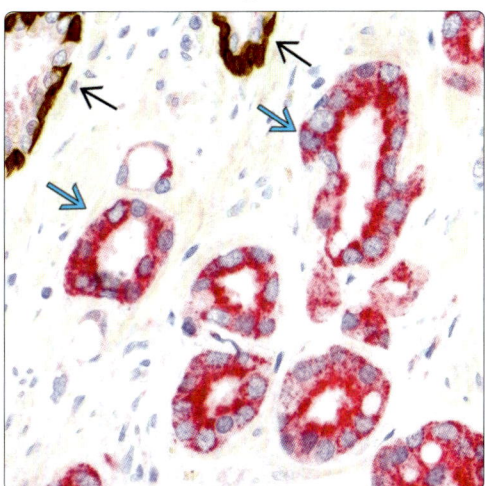

(Left) This PCa is seen surrounding a nerve and exhibits architecture reminiscent of cribriform gland. Perineural invasion may form complex architecture and should not be assigned a grade. (Right) PIN4 shows ➡ PCa with strong diffuse cytoplasmic expression of AMACR (red) and complete absence of basal cell layer (brown). Note adjacent benign glands ➡ with preserved basal cells exhibiting weak AMACR staining. IHC can be helpful to distinguish small focus of cancer vs. benign glands in needle biopsy.

Prostate Cancer With Radiotherapy Effects

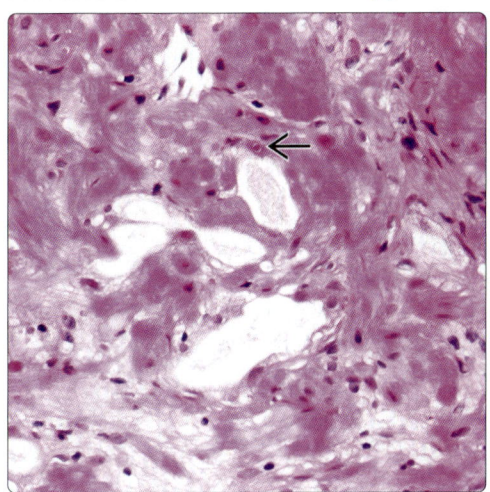

Prostate Cancer With Radiotherapy Effects

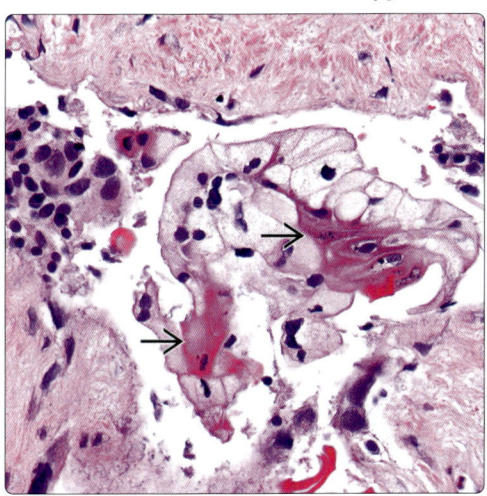

(Left) PCa with radiation effects shows poorly formed, atrophic glands with foamy or vacuolated cytoplasm and nucleolomegaly ➡. Gleason grading is not recommended for PCa with treatment effect. Marked radiation effect may artifactually produce an architecture resembling GS 9 or 10 PCa. Awareness of prior therapy is important. (Right) PCa with radiation effects shows voluminous foamy cells with focal squamous differentiation ➡. Radiation may induce squamous differentiation in both primary and metastatic foci of PCa.

Prostate Cancer With Radiotherapy Effects

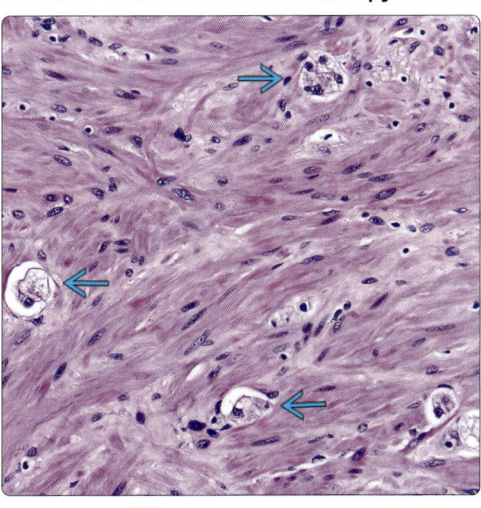

PIN4 in Radiated Prostate Cancer

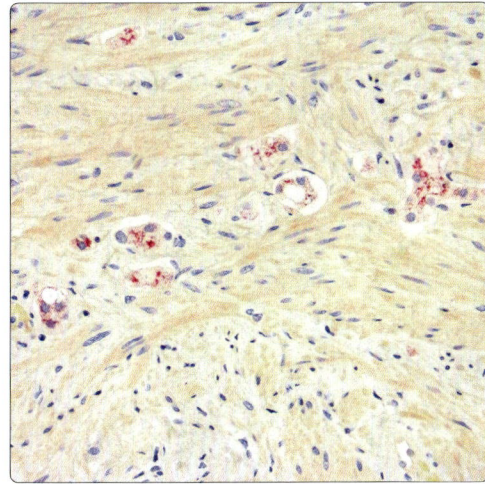

(Left) Residual PCa after radiotherapy shows scattered foamy and vacuolated tumor cells ➡ consistent with marked treatment effects. This distortion of PCa does not correlate with poor outcome and should not be graded. Treated cancer may not be readily visible or may resemble inflammatory cells on H&E and may necessitate use of epithelial markers. (Right) This treated PCa shows AMACR (red) expression and no basal cell markers staining. AMACR expression of PCa may be diminished with therapy-related changes.

Acinar Adenocarcinoma

Prostate Cancer With Radiotherapy Effects

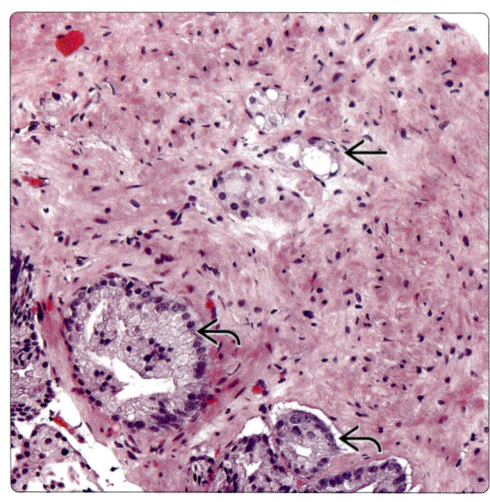

Prostate Cancer With Hormonal Therapy Effects

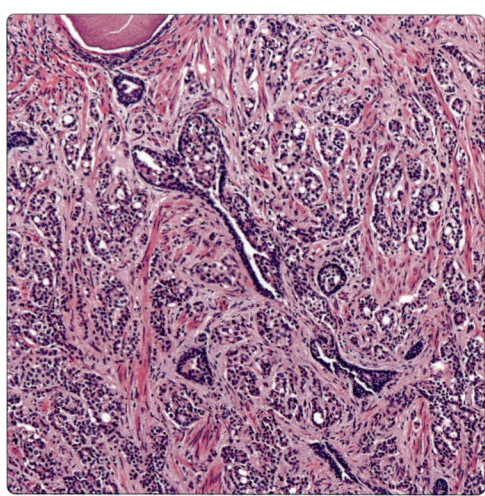

(Left) PCa with radiation effect may show atrophic changes and vacuolated cytoplasm ⮕. Adjacent PCa glands ⮕ show minimal radiation effect in this case. The effects of radiation in PCa are variable. Minimal or no radiation effect following radiotherapy portends a poorer prognosis. The carcinoma without treatment effect should be graded as usual. (Right) PCa with hormonal therapy effects shows shrunken PCa glands. Some PCa cells may resemble inflammatory cells and histiocytes.

Prostate Cancer With Hormonal Therapy Effects

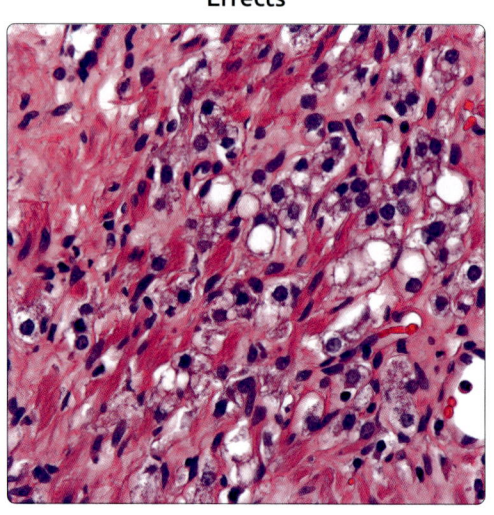

Prostate Cancer With Hormonal Therapy Effects

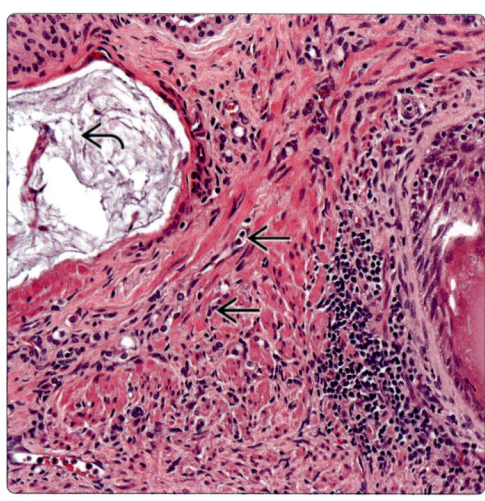

(Left) PCa with hormonal therapy effects shows shrunken cells with vacuolated and xanthomatous cytoplasm. Some cells display pyknotic nuclei. AMACR staining is variable and proportional to the degree of therapy effect. (Right) PCa with hormonal therapy effects shows shrunken PCa cells ⮕, not readily identifiable on low power, that may mimic inflammatory cells. Use of CK-PAN(AE1/AE3) helps to facilitate detection of residual PCa. Cystic spaces ⮕ may also be seen following therapy.

Prostate Cancer With Hormonal Therapy Effects

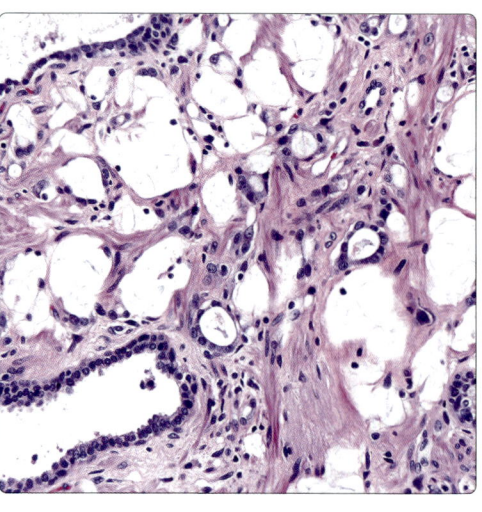

Prostate Cancer With Hormonal Therapy Effects

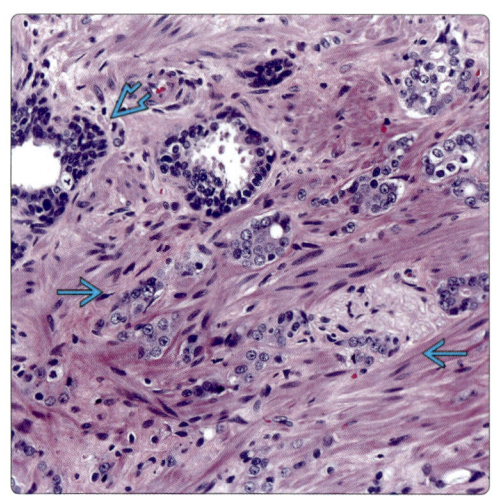

(Left) PCa after hormonal therapy shows widespread cystic change with extravasation of mucin and shrinkage of tumor cells. It is important not to misinterpret this change as mucinous carcinoma. (Right) PCa after hormone therapy shows infiltrating tumor cells with modest to scant cytoplasm ⮕. Adjacent benign gland ⮕ shows prominent and hyperplastic basal cells and atrophic acinar cells. This pattern suggests prior hormonal therapy and clinical history should be investigated to avoid overgrading of PCa.

Acinar Adenocarcinoma

Differential Diagnosis

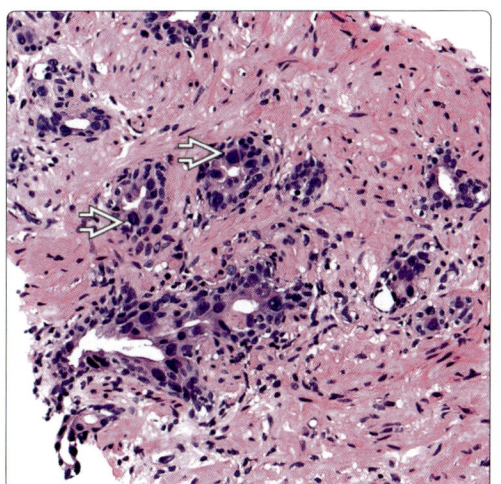

Differential Diagnosis

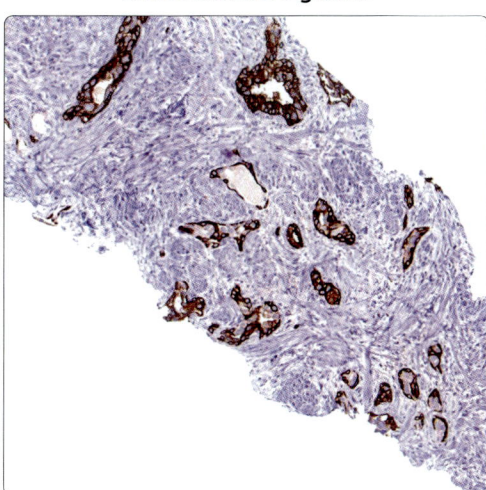

(Left) These benign prostatic glands with radiation therapy effect show marked nuclear pleomorphism ➡. The pleomorphism is due to variable effect on benign basal cells and secretory cells. Nuclear pleomorphism is extremely uncommon in PCa. (Right) Following local radiation therapy, benign glands invariably show strong and diffuse cytoplasmic immunoreactivity for HMCK, unlike PCa, which is negative. This makes the distinction from malignancy relatively straightforward with immunostaining.

Differential Diagnosis

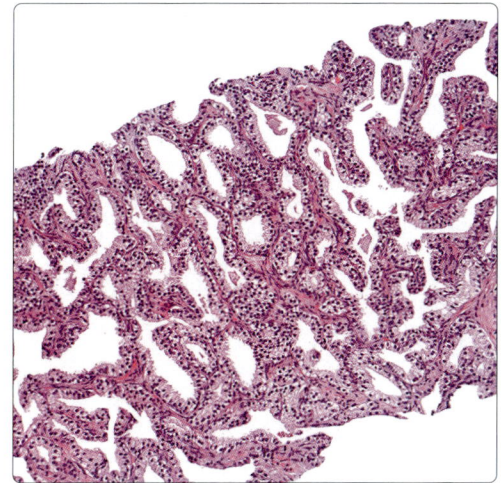

Differential Diagnosis

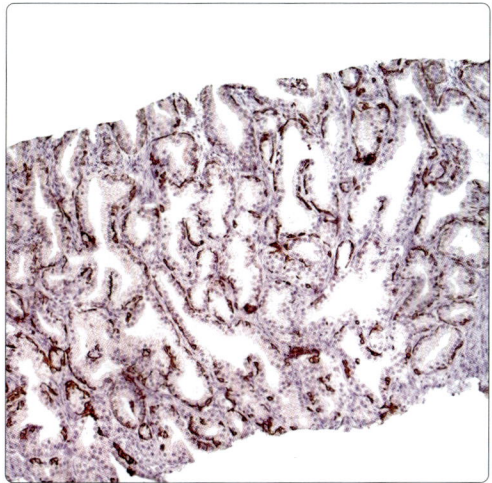

(Left) Atypical adenomatous hyperplasia (adenosis) is characterized by crowded glands, but varying caliber glands with normal cytology and luminal infolding and tufting are common. This lesion occurs mostly within the TZ, so it is relatively uncommon on needle biopsy. (Right) The HMCK(34βE12) staining in this atypical adenomatous hyperplasia (adenosis) demonstrates basal cells. In atypical adenomatous hyperplasia, the basal layer may be patchy or even absent in some acini.

Differential Diagnosis

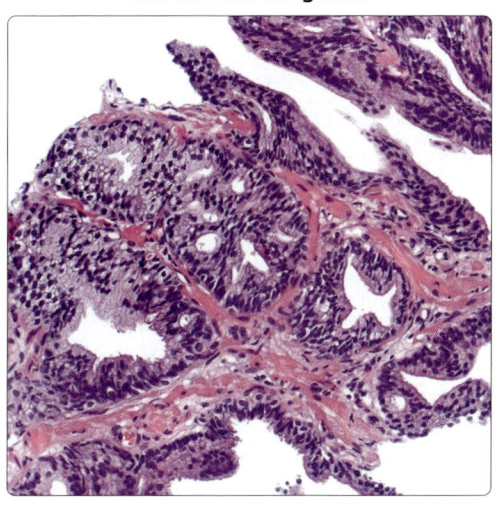

Differential Diagnosis

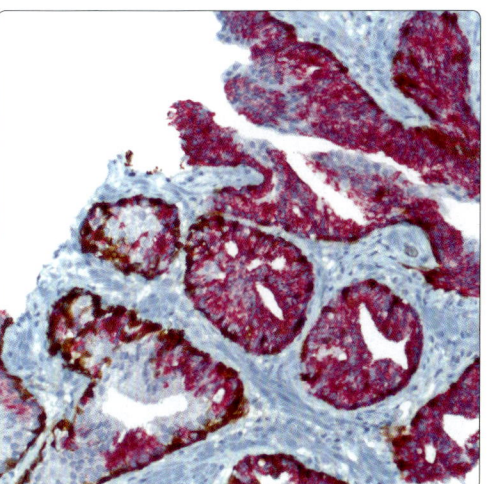

(Left) Cribriform high-grade prostatic intraepithelial neoplasia, as seen in this example, may closely mimic invasive adenocarcinoma with a cribriform pattern (Gleason pattern 4). Central zone glands and clear cell cribriform hyperplasia are also mimics. (Right) In this AMACR/p63/HMCK immunostain cocktail, there is strong luminal AMACR reactivity, but the basal layer remains intact, features expected in high-grade prostatic intraepithelial neoplasia.

Acinar Adenocarcinoma

(Left) Partial atrophy, atrophy, and postatrophic hyperplasia are the most common mimics of PCa encountered in daily practice and can be problematic in needle biopsy. The loss of luminal cytoplasm with preserved lateral cytoplasm is characteristic. **(Right)** This HMCK(34βE12) immunostain highlights a patchy discontinuous basal cell layer, a pattern typical for partial atrophy. Some glands in partial atrophy may completely lack basal cells ⇒, but the overall staining in the entire focus should be interpreted.

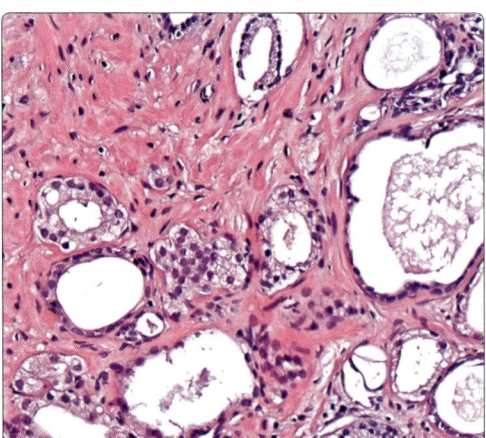
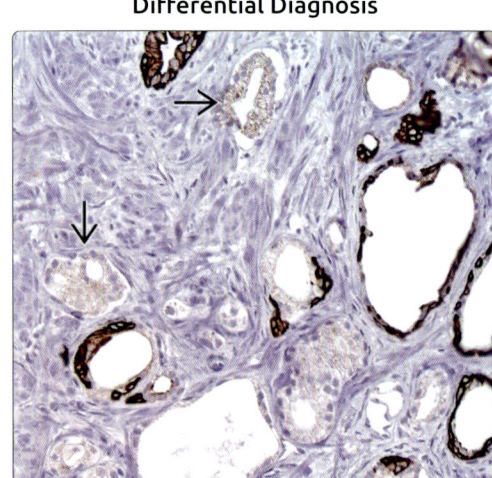

(Left) Verumontanum gland hyperplasia is typically adjacent to the prostatic urethra epithelium and is characterized by a back-to-back collection of varying sized benign prostate glands. Intraluminal secretions and corpora amylacea are common. **(Right)** On high-power examination, this example of verumontanum gland hyperplasia shows varying caliber glands, luminal undulation, and a preserved basal cell layer that may be confirmed by immunohistochemistry. Note the corpora amylacea.

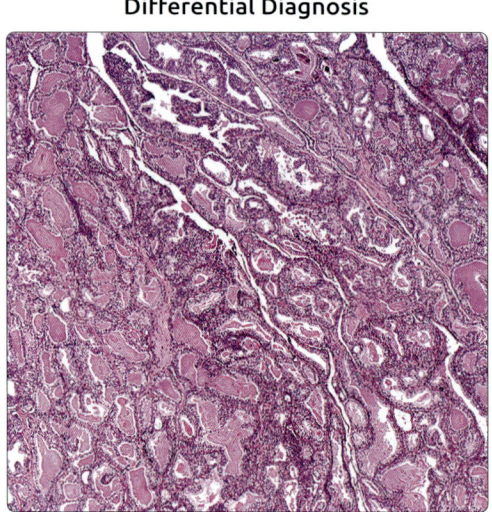
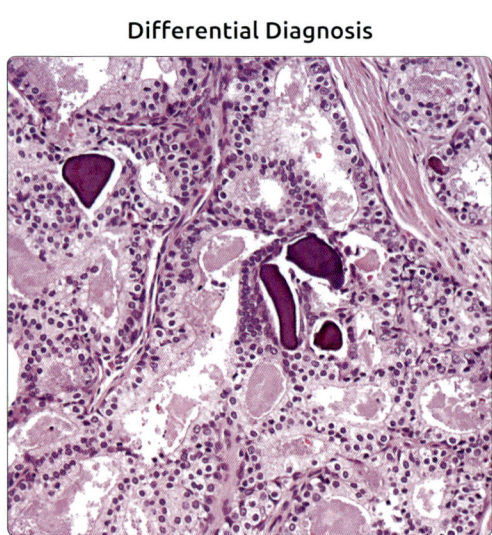

(Left) Seminal vesicle (SV) epithelium commonly has scattered pleomorphic cells, intranuclear inclusions, and intracytoplasmic coarse yellow pigment, which all aid in the distinction from PCa. It is extraordinarily rare for PCa to show marked nuclear pleomorphism. **(Right)** This pax-2 immunostaining shows strong nuclear reactivity in SV epithelium but not in the neoplastic cell population of PCa. This staining pattern is useful, as PSA, PAP, and AMACR may show nonspecific reaction in SV.

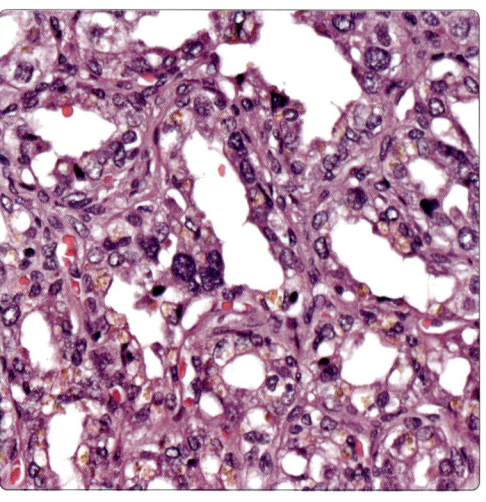
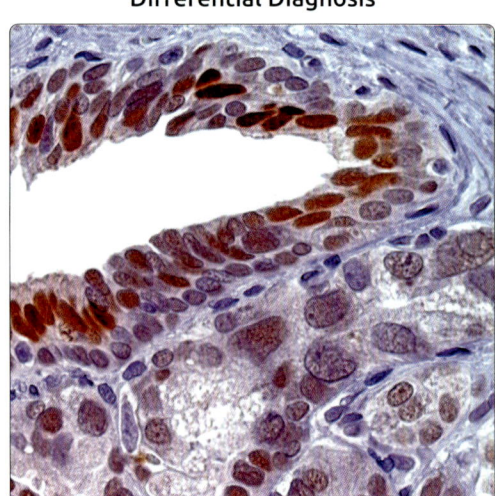

Acinar Adenocarcinoma

Differential Diagnosis

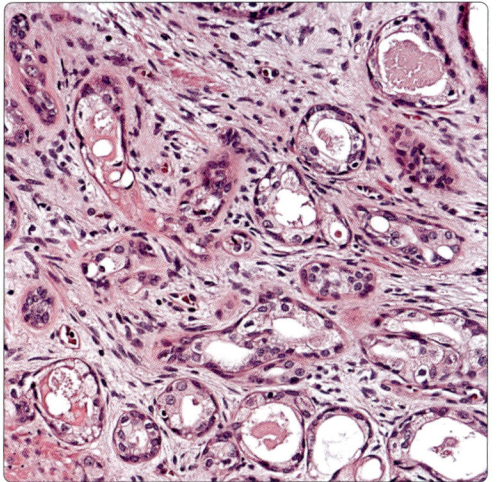

Differential Diagnosis

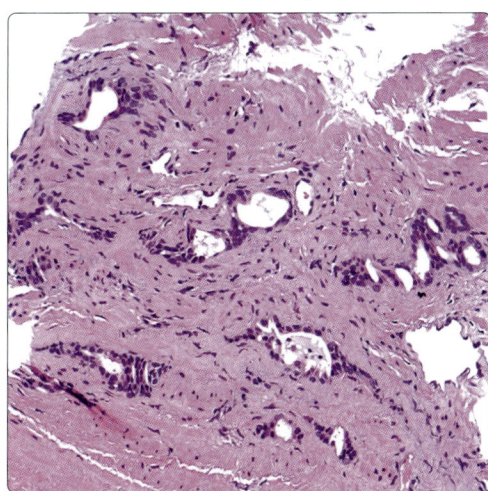

(Left) *Sclerosing adenosis is rare and is seen most commonly in the TZ. It is characterized by crowded benign glands with an associated cytologically benign spindle cell component. The spindle cells commonly have a myoepithelial phenotype not typically found in prostatic basal cells.* (Right) *Sclerotic atrophy may closely mimic the invasive growth of PCa. Nevertheless, the irregular angulated glands with scant cytoplasm, lack of nuclear atypia, and the dense fibrotic stroma are distinctive.*

Differential Diagnosis

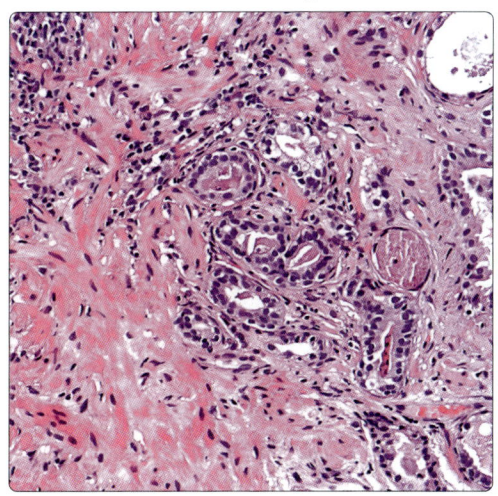

Differential Diagnosis

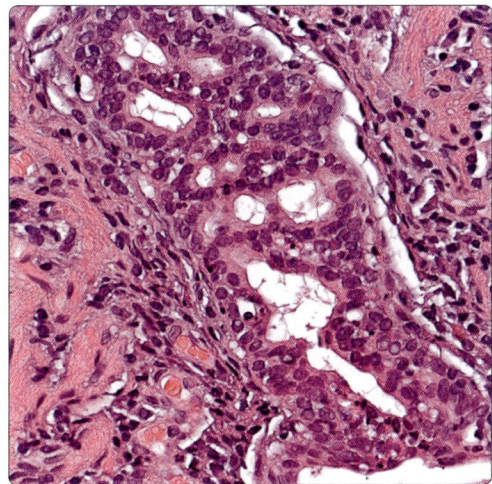

(Left) *When associated with inflammatory infiltrates, benign glands may appear crowded and hyperchromatic. In addition, luminal secretions may be present. A diagnosis of malignancy should be rendered with great caution in the setting of inflammatory infiltrates.* (Right) *Benign glands may also show a pseudoneoplastic cribriform pattern when associated with significant inflammation. Reactive atypia with nucleoli in the epithelium further compounds the diagnostic dilemma.*

Differential Diagnosis

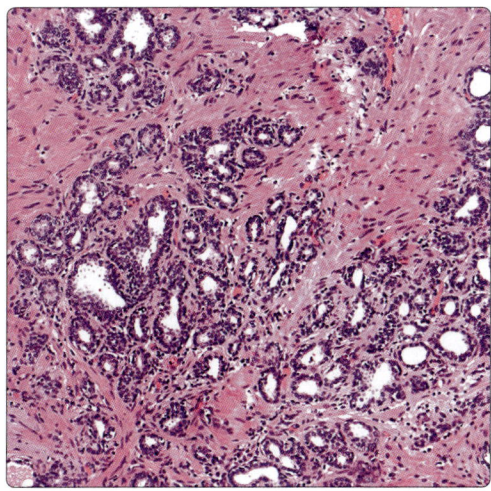

Differential Diagnosis

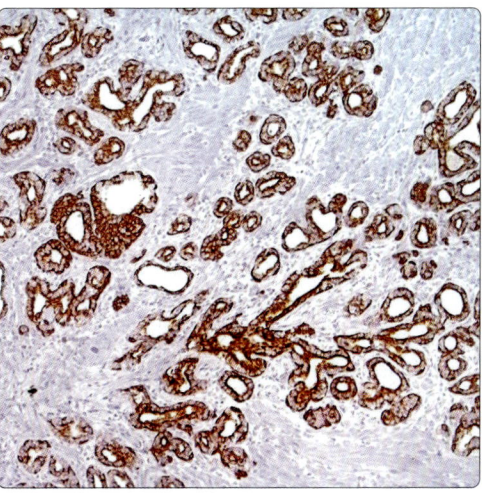

(Left) *Postatrophic hyperplasia is characterized by an aggregate of small, crowded benign glands with atrophic features. The glands are usually situated in a lobular arrangement and may have an associated central larger caliber duct. Lobular architecture and variation in size and shape of the glands are useful diagnostic features.* (Right) *With HMCK(34BE12) immunostaining, postatrophic hyperplasia typically shows strong and diffuse basal cell positivity, as illustrated, in contrast to PCa, which shows absent staining in basal layer.*

Acinar Adenocarcinoma Variants

KEY FACTS

TERMINOLOGY
- Carcinomas of prostatic acinar type with morphologies divergent from usual adenocarcinoma

CLINICAL ISSUES
- Age group and presentation similar to conventional acinar adenocarcinoma
- May mimic benign processes or nonprostatic carcinomas including in metastatic sites
- Some variants associated with higher grade and stage, leading to poorer prognosis

MICROSCOPIC
- **Mucinous carcinoma**: ≥ 25% of tumor cells floating in copious extracellular mucin
- **Signet ring cell carcinoma**: Tumor cells contain optically clear vacuoles displacing nuclei and are usually widely infiltrative
- **Pseudohyperplastic carcinoma**: Tumor architecturally and to certain extent, cytologically resembles hyperplasia
- **Atrophic carcinoma**: Glands lined by tumor cells with scant cytoplasm, resembling atrophy on low-power magnification
- **Foamy gland carcinoma**: Tumor cells with abundant foamy cytoplasm
- **PIN-like carcinoma**: Malignant glands exhibit stratification (≥ 2 layers) of tumor cells
- **Lymphoepithelioma-like carcinoma**: Characterized by syncytial growth amid dense lymphocytic background
- **Oncocytic carcinoma**: Tumor cells with abundant granular eosinophilic cytoplasm, ultrastructurally contains abundant mitochondria
- **Pleomorphic giant cell adenocarcinoma**: Characterized by large anaplastic bizarre tumor cells
- **Adenocarcinoma with aberrant p63 expression**: Tumor cells with diffuse nuclear expression of p63
- **Other unusual variants**: Cystadenocarcinoma, microcystic carcinoma, carcinoid-like carcinoma

Mucinous Carcinoma
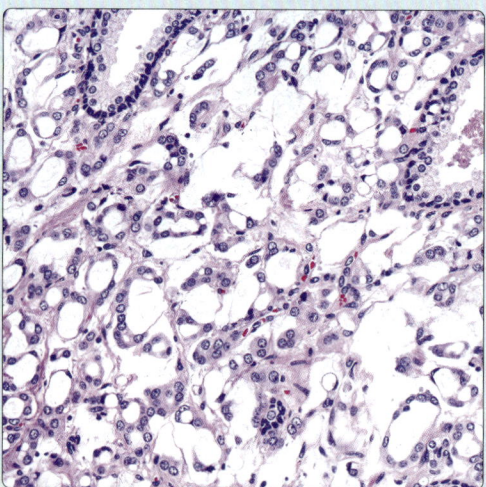

Pseudohyperplastic Carcinoma
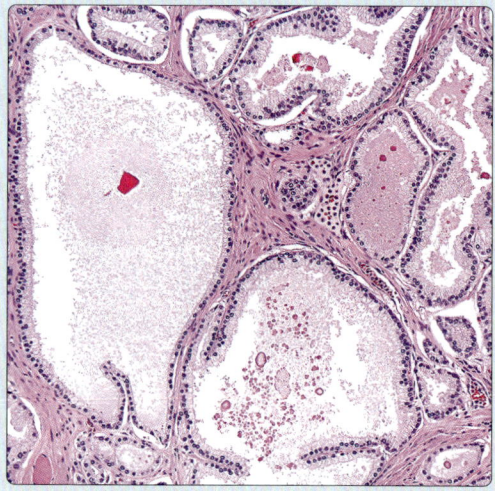

(Left) Mucinous carcinoma exhibits tumor cells floating in abundant extracellular mucin. The tumor should have at least 25% of this feature to make the diagnosis. Intraluminal mucin is not accounted, and metastasis from other primary should be ruled out. *(Right)* Pseudohyperplastic carcinoma shows medium to large glands with luminal infoldings reminiscent of benign hyperplasia. This tumor typically has basally oriented nuclei and luminal eosinophilic amorphous materials and may have crystalloids.

Atrophic Carcinoma
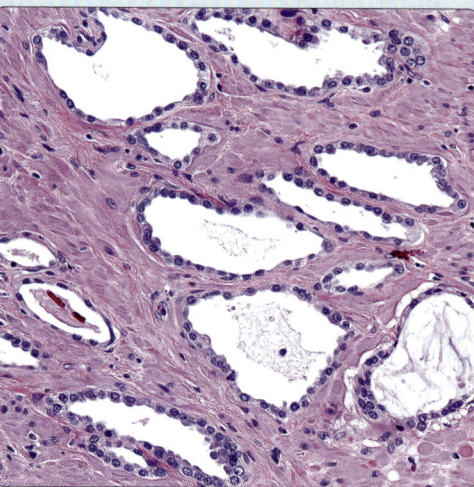

Foamy Gland Carcinoma
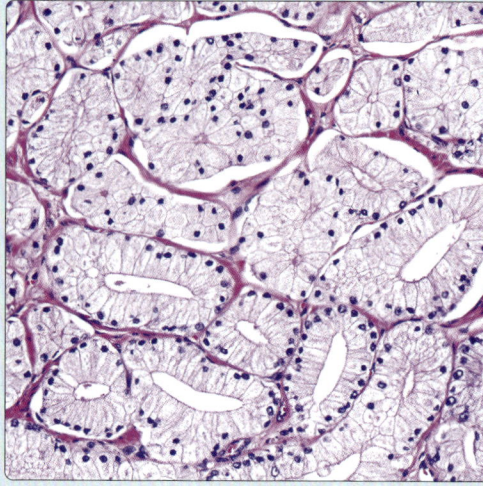

(Left) This PCa consists of irregular and angulated glands and cells having scant cytoplasm, reminiscent of benign glandular atrophy. However, unlike atrophy, nuclei are enlarged and have prominent nucleoli. The lumen also contains amorphous materials, mucin, and crystalloids, supportive of carcinoma. *(Right)* This PCa consists of tumor cells with abundant foamy or xanthomatous cytoplasm. Unlike other PCa variants, foamy gland carcinomaS typically have nuclei that are small or pyknotic-appearing.

Acinar Adenocarcinoma Variants

TERMINOLOGY

Definitions
- Carcinomas of prostatic acinar type with morphologies divergent from usual adenocarcinoma
  - Ductal adenocarcinoma and sarcomatoid carcinoma covered in separate chapters

CLINICAL ISSUES

Presentation
- Age group and presentation similar to conventional acinar adenocarcinoma
- Knowledge of variants is important
  - May mimic benign processes or lesions in prostate
  - May mimic nonprostatic carcinomas in prostate or metastatic sites
  - Aberrant immunohistochemical staining (e.g., p63-positive adenocarcinoma)
  - Modified grading approach for some variants
  - Some are associated with higher grade and stage, leading to poorer prognosis

DIAGNOSTIC CHECKLIST

Mucinous (Colloid) Carcinoma
- Comprises 0.38-0.43% of PCas
- Criteria
  - ≥ 25% tumor cells floating in extracellular mucin
  - Intraluminal mucinous material in dilated or nondilated glands not included
  - Extraprostatic origin must be excluded
- Diagnosis should be made only in resection specimen, as needle biopsy specimen may not show exact proportion of mucinous component
  - In needle biopsy, may be diagnosed as carcinoma with mucinous features
- Grossly, may have mucoid or gelatinous appearance particularly if mucin is abundant
- Tumor cells exhibit cribriform, anastomosing nests, tubules or cords floating in mucin
- Amount of mucin varies from 25-90% (mean: 52%)
- Mucin is positive for PAS, mucicarmine, and Alcian blue pH 2.5; special staining often not necessary
- ERG positive in 47%, about similar to conventional adenocarcinoma
- With strict diagnostic criteria, suggested to have similar features and behavior with conventional PCa
- ISUP recommend to grade according to underlying architecture
  - Most are Gleason grade 4; ~ 78% are Gleason score 7 or higher
- Positive for PSA and PAP; immunohistochemistry is helpful for diagnosis in metastatic setting
- Differential diagnosis
  - Mucinous carcinoma of bladder, urachus, urethra, and large bowel
    - Negative for PSA and PAP
  - Mucinous metaplasia of benign glands
    - Mucin intracellular and focal, cells with bland nuclei and basal cell layer discernible
  - Cowper gland
    - Lobular arrangement of glands with intracellular mucin encountered in apex often intermingled with skeletal muscles

Signet Ring Cell Carcinoma
- Rare, estimated incidence of 30 per 100,000 prostate cancers
- ≥ 25% of resected tumor shows signet ring cell (arbitrary definition); no uniform cut-off in literature
- Tumor cells contain optically clear vacuoles displacing nuclei and are widely infiltrative
- Usually associated with typical high-grade (Gleason grade 4 and 5) PCa
  - Signet ring cells may comprise up to 80% of tumor
- May be mucin-producing carcinoma (mucinous carcinoma with signet ring cells)
  - Not clear if nonmucinous (mucicarmine negative) signet ring PCa is distinct clinically
- Gleason score ranges from 6-10, most commonly 8 (33%)
- May be associated with high-grade prostatic intraepithelial neoplasia (PIN) with optically clear vacuoles
- Clinical presentation similar to conventional adenocarcinoma but with tendency to present at higher stage
  - One study showed 34% stage IV disease at presentation
  - Prognosis reported poor with mean survival of only 29 months
- Differential diagnosis
  - Signet ring cell carcinomas of bladder or stomach
    - Not admixed with acinar adenocarcinoma and negative for PSA and PAP
  - Signet ring cell change in prostatitis and lymphoma
    - Positive for CD45 and negative for PSA and PAP

Pseudohyperplastic Carcinoma
- Carcinoma that architecturally and to certain extent, cytologically, resembles benign hyperplasia
  - Diagnosis problematic in needle biopsy and TURP
    - Incidental finding in TURP performed for BPH
    - 1 study showed 1.3% of pseudohyperplastic carcinoma misdiagnosed as hyperplasia
- ~ 1/2 involves transition zone
- Histology
  - Large-sized or dilated glands, with branching and papillary infolding
  - Tall columnar cells with abundant pale to slight granular luminal cytoplasm
  - Basally located nuclei along basement membrane
  - Commonly with luminal eosinophilic amorphous secretions and may have crystalloids
  - Diagnostic malignant nuclear features retained, in contrast to benign hyperplastic glands
  - Corpora amylacea may be seen in lumen of ~ 20% of cases, further compounding similarity with hyperplasia
- Commonly coexists and shows continuity with acinar adenocarcinoma
  - Amount of pseudohyperplastic carcinoma ranges from 2-80% (mean: 22%)
- AMACR overexpressed in 70-83%, and basal markers are negative; helpful in distinguishing from hyperplasia
- ISUP recommends grade of 3 + 3 = 6

Acinar Adenocarcinoma Variants

Atrophic Carcinoma
- Carcinoma with glands lined by cells with scant cytoplasm, resembling atrophy on low-power magnification
- Reported in 2% of carcinomas in prostate needle biopsy and 3-16% of carcinomas in radical prostatectomy
- Infiltrative growth
- Cytology of malignancy
  - Nucleomegaly and prominent nucleoli
- Luminal features of malignancy
  - Eosinophilic proteinaceous materials, blue mucin and crystalloids
- AMACR is positive in ~ 70%
- Usually admixed with nonatrophic prostate cancer
- Differential diagnosis
  - Benign atrophic glands
    - Caution: ~ 30% of atrophic cancers are negative for AMACR
    - Typically have dense hyperchromatic nuclei and lobular growth
    - Have basal cells that can be highlighted by basal cell markers in contrast to atrophic carcinoma
  - Diffuse atrophy of adenocarcinoma and benign glands may also be seen in posttreatment setting, particularly with antiandrogen therapy

Foamy Gland (Xanthomatous) Carcinoma
- PCa with abundant foamy cytoplasm
- Relatively common among variants
  - Seen in ~ 20% of carcinomas in prostate biopsy, mostly admixed with acinar adenocarcinoma
    - Foamy gland ranges from 5-100%
  - Admixed in acinar adenocarcinoma in 14-23% in RP
    - Foamy gland ranges from 1-90%
- Malignant nuclear features not always present, as nuclei may be small and pyknotic
- Presence of infiltrative pattern; may require immunostains
- May form discrete well-formed glands, fused or ill-formed glands, cribriform structures and nests, or confluent cells
- Erg positive in 42% of cases
- ISUP recommends discounting foamy cytoplasm and assigning grade based on architecture
  - Most are Gleason score 3 + 3 = 6 (80%)
- Unclear if uncommon foamy high-grade PIN is associated with foamy gland carcinoma
- Differential diagnosis
  - Xanthoma
    - Occurs purely as single or cluster or cells and does not form glands
    - ~ 10% or less may show nonspecific staining to PSA, PAP, or AMACR
    - Negative for epithelial markers
  - Other benign mimickers such as Cowper gland, mucinous metaplasia, clear cell cribriform hyperplasia

Carcinoma With Stratified Epithelium (PIN-Like)
- Glands exhibit stratification (≥ 2 layers) of malignant cells
- May resemble high-grade PIN
- Reported incidence of 1.3% in needle biopsy containing carcinoma
- Glands may be flat, tufted, micropapillary, or admixture of these architectures
- Tumor cells are mostly tall columnar cells with amphophilic cytoplasm and round to elongated nuclei
  - Predominance of stratified tall columnar cells give resemblance to ductal adenocarcinoma
    - Considered by some as pattern of ductal adenocarcinoma (high-grade PIN-like ductal adenocarcinoma)
- Typically lacks solid growth, necrosis, true papillae, and marked pleomorphism
- Often seen admixed with acinar adenocarcinoma, mostly Gleason 3 + 3 = 6
- Suggested to be graded as Gleason grade 3, score 6
- Differential diagnosis
  - Flat, tufted, or micropapillary PIN
    - Contains basal cells that can be highlighted by basal cell markers
  - Ductal adenocarcinoma
    - Includes those with true papillae or cribriform patterns

Lymphoepithelioma-Like Carcinoma
- Exceedingly rare
- As in other organ systems particularly head and neck, characterized by syncytial growth amid dense lymphocytic background
- Tumor cells are high grade with vesicular nuclei, prominent nucleoli, and abundant mitoses
- Carcinoma cells in background of dense, mostly lymphoplasmacytic cells and some eosinophils and neutrophils
- Hematopoietic cells are polyclonal or nonneoplastic
- No Epstein-Barr virus association reported
- Admixed acinar adenocarcinoma often present
  - Lymphoepithelioma-like carcinoma component comprises 10-90% of tumor
- Suggested to have aggressive outcome

Oncocytic Carcinoma
- Exceptionally rare
- Prostate carcinoma with abundant granular eosinophilic cytoplasm
- Like other oncocytic tumors, ultrastructurally contains abundant mitochondria
- Reported cases exhibit infiltrating glands, nests, or cords with round, small to medium nuclei
- Clinical significance still unclear

Pleomorphic Giant Cell Adenocarcinoma
- Characterized by presence of large anaplastic bizarre cells
- May occur admixed with high-grade adenocarcinoma (mostly Gleason score 9) and other histologies such as ductal, squamous, or small cell carcinoma
- Staining of PSA and PAP inconsistent
- Suggested to have aggressive morphology

Adenocarcinoma With Aberrant p63 Expression
- Carcinoma with diffuse (usually 100%) nuclear expression of p63
- Usually forms atrophic or ill-formed glands with multilayered, spindled, or basaloid nuclei
- Often mixed with conventional adenocarcinoma (~ 85% of cases)

Acinar Adenocarcinoma Variants

Main Mimics of Variants of Prostate Adenocarcinoma

Variant Carcinoma	Main Mimic
Mucinous	Mucinous carcinoma of bladder, urachus, urethra, and large bowel
Signet ring cell	Bladder or gastric signet ring cell carcinoma
Pseudohyperplastic	Benign glandular hyperplasia
Atrophic	Benign glandular atrophy
Foamy gland	Xanthoma
Ductal	High-grade PIN and intraductal carcinoma
Lymphoepithelioma-like	Chronic inflammation and lymphoma

PIN = prostatic intraepithelial neoplasia.

Gleason Grading of Prostate Carcinoma Variants

Variant Carcinoma	Gleason Grade
Mucinous	Based on underlying growth pattern; mostly grade 4
Signet ring cell	Mostly grade 4 or 5
Pseudohyperplastic	Grade 3
Atrophic	Grade 3
Foamy gland	Mostly grade 3 (~ 80%)
Ductal	Grade 4; 5 if with necrosis
PIN-like	Grade 3
Carcinoma with aberrant p63 expression	Optional; suggested to have favorable findings at RP

- If graded, most are Gleason score 6 (~ 2/3)
- Basal cells are absent, confirmed by HMWK negativity
- Positive for PSA, confirming acinar cell type
- Most are AMACR positive
- Suggested to be molecularly distinct from acinar adenocarcinoma
    o Shows mixed luminal and basal immunophenotype
    o ERG gene rearrangement not demonstrated so far
    o Cases do not show PTEN loss
    o Frequent expression of GSTP1
- Has favorable features in radical prostatectomy; some have suggested not to assign Gleason grade
- Differential diagnosis
    o Basal cell hyperplasia
        – Prominence and increased layers of basal cells in glands usually in transition zone
        – Cells have high nuclear:cytoplasmic ratio and lack nuclear atypicality
        – Positive for p63 but are also HMWK(+) and PSA and PAP (-)
    o Basal cell carcinoma
        – Either have nests or cords of basaloid cells with peripheral palisading or adenoid cystic-like architecture with basement membrane-like material
        – Positive for p63, but are also HMWK(+) and PSA and PAP(-)

Other Unusual Variants
- Cystadenocarcinoma
- Microcystic carcinoma
- Carcinoid-like carcinoma

SELECTED REFERENCES

1. Arista-Nasr J et al: Pseudohyperplastic prostate carcinoma: histologic patterns and differential diagnosis. Ann Diagn Pathol. 19(4):253-60, 2015
2. Tan HL et al: Prostate adenocarcinomas aberrantly expressing p63 are molecularly distinct from usual-type prostatic adenocarcinomas. Mod Pathol. 28(3):446-56, 2015
3. Koca SB et al: Foamy gland carcinoma in core needle biopsies of the prostate: clinicopathologic and immunohistochemical study of 56 cases. Ann Diagn Pathol. 18(5):271-4, 2014
4. Giannico GA et al: Aberrant expression of p63 in adenocarcinoma of the prostate: a radical prostatectomy study. Am J Surg Pathol. 37(9):1401-6, 2013
5. Johnson H et al: ERG expression in mucinous prostatic adenocarcinoma and prostatic adenocarcinoma with mucinous features: comparison with conventional prostatic adenocarcinoma. Hum Pathol. 44(10):2241-6, 2013
6. Warrick JI et al: Foamy gland carcinoma of the prostate in needle biopsy: incidence, Gleason grade, and comparative α-methylacyl-CoA racemase vs. ERG expression. Am J Surg Pathol. 37(11):1709-14, 2013
7. Wu A et al: Prostate cancer with aberrant diffuse p63 expression: report of a case and review of the literature and morphologic mimics. Arch Pathol Lab Med. 137(9):1179-84, 2013
8. Fine SW: Variants and unusual patterns of prostate cancer: clinicopathologic and differential diagnostic considerations. Adv Anat Pathol. 19(4):204-16, 2012
9. Hudson J et al: Foamy gland adenocarcinoma of the prostate: incidence, Gleason grade, and early clinical outcome. Hum Pathol. 43(7):974-9, 2012
10. Humphrey PA: Histological variants of prostatic carcinoma and their significance. Histopathology. 60(1):59-74, 2012
11. Fiandrino G et al: Prostatic adenocarcinoma with oncocytic features. J Clin Pathol. 64(2):177-8, 2011
12. Warner JN et al: Primary signet ring cell carcinoma of the prostate. Mayo Clin Proc. 85(12):1130-6, 2010
13. Yaskiv O et al: Microcystic adenocarcinoma of the prostate: a variant of pseudohyperplastic and atrophic patterns. Am J Surg Pathol. 34(4):556-61, 2010
14. Han B et al: Characterization of ETS gene aberrations in select histologic variants of prostate carcinoma. Mod Pathol. 22(9):1176-85, 2009
15. Lopez-Beltran A et al: Lymphoepithelioma-like carcinoma of the prostate. Hum Pathol. 40(7):982-7, 2009

Acinar Adenocarcinoma Variants

Mucinous Carcinoma

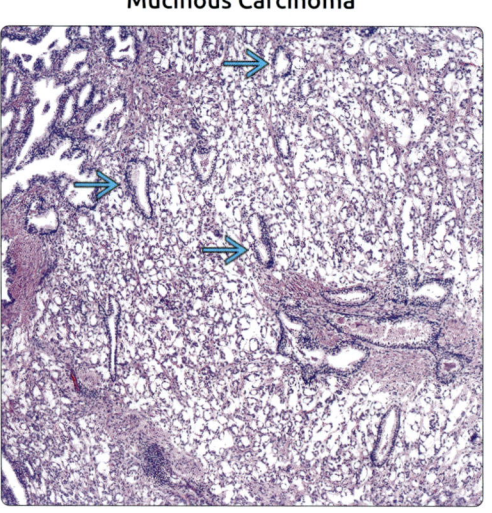

Mucinous Carcinoma

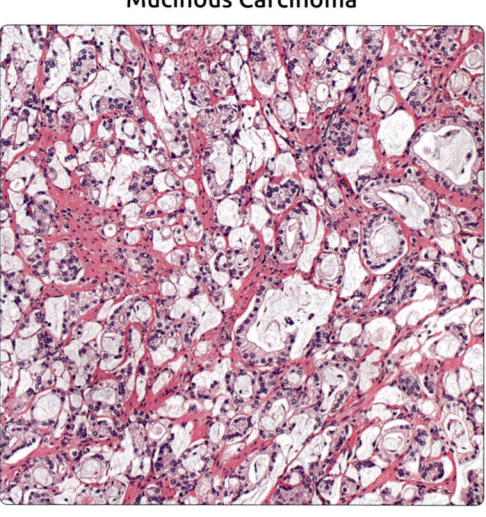

(Left) Low magnification shows abundant extracellular mucin with floating tumor cells infiltrating between benign glands ➡. In this resection, almost all of the tumor is mucinous, and diagnosis of mucinous carcinoma is rendered; 25% cut-off is required. (Right) Low-power view shows tumor cells admixed with abundant mucin. Because of this unusual feature, possibility of metastasis to prostate should always be excluded. The tumor cells retain their expression of PSA and PAP, which is helpful in the metastatic setting.

Mucinous Carcinoma

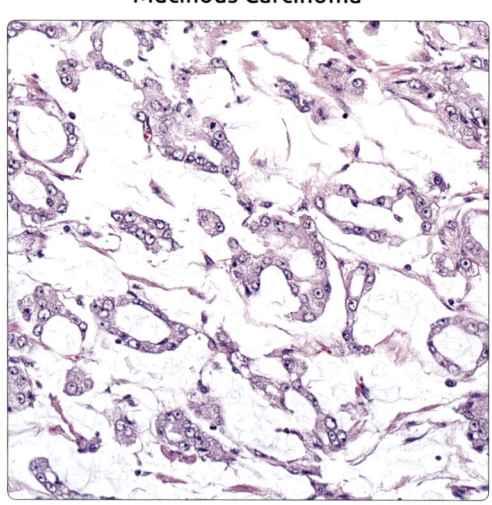

Mucinous Carcinoma

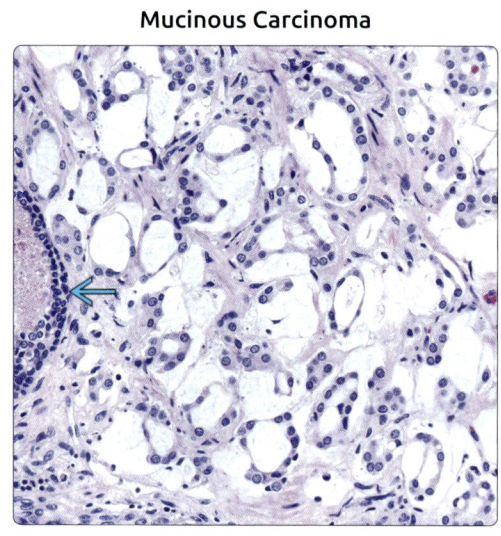

(Left) Mucinous carcinoma is characterized by the presence of malignant epithelium floating in abundant extracellular mucin. This is distinct from the intraluminal mucin seen in more typical forms of PCa. (Right) This mucinous PCa exhibits well-formed glands admixed with mucin. ISUP consensus suggests grading this tumor based on the underlying tumor architecture. In this case, the tumor is predominantly Gleason pattern 3. Note the benign gland with bland nuclei for comparison ➡.

Mucinous Carcinoma

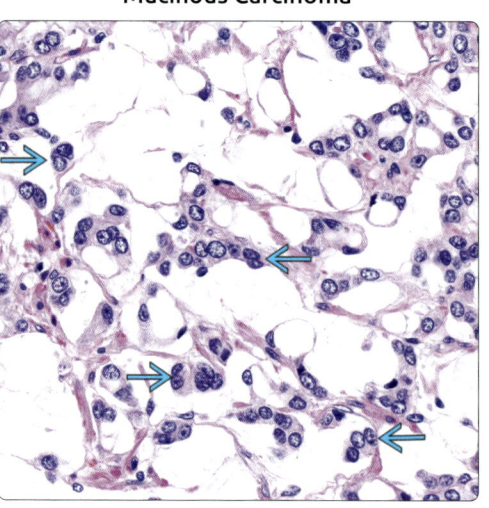

Mucinous Carcinoma

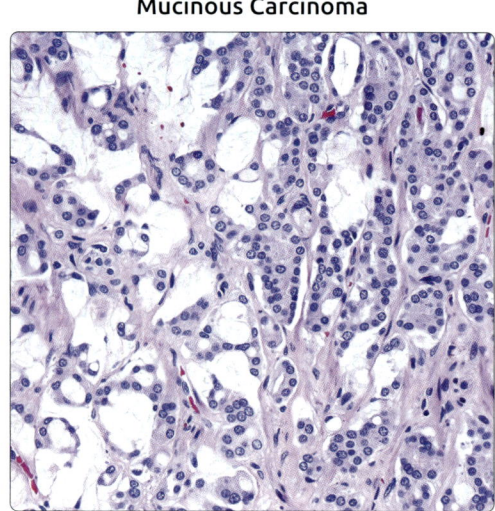

(Left) This mucinous carcinoma exhibits some tight clusters of tumor cells without forming a lumen (Gleason pattern 4) ➡. Most mucinous carcinoma are Gleason grade 3 or 4. (Right) This case shows mucinous PCa (left) admixed with nonmucinous conventional adenocarcinoma (right). The nuclei of mucinous carcinoma cells exhibit nucleomegaly and prominent nucleoli similar to the nuclei of conventional adenocarcinoma. In cases of mixed morphology, entire tumor is graded with the mucin pools discounted.

Acinar Adenocarcinoma Variants

Signet Ring Cell Carcinoma

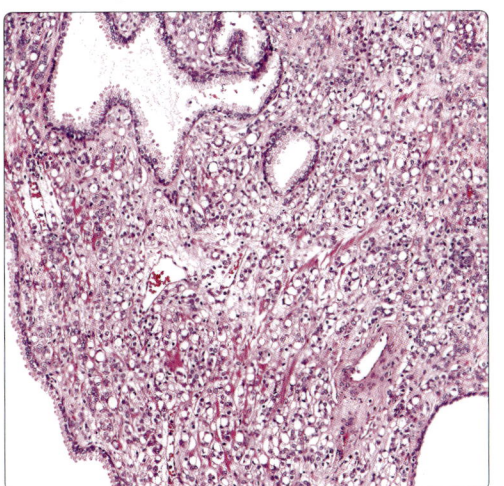

Signet Ring Cell Carcinoma

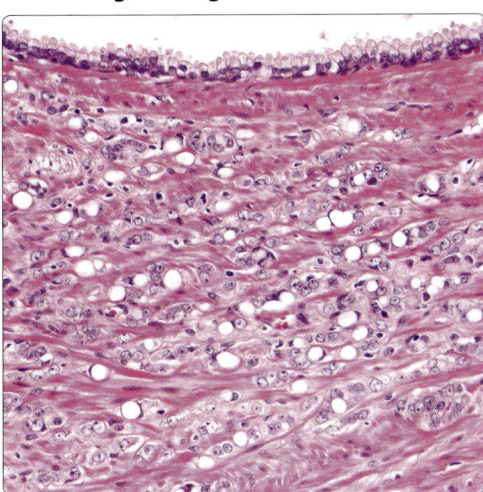

(Left) This RP shows diffuse infiltration of signet ring cell carcinoma, including between benign glands. This PCa variant usually exhibits diffuse infiltration and is associated with high-grade PCa. *(Right)* The signet ring cell carcinoma cells have optically clear cytoplasmic vacuoles that displace and indent the nuclei to the side. The tumor cells exhibit the usual malignant nuclear features, such as enlargement and prominent nucleoli. In this case, the tumor cells show linear arrangement, consistent with Gleason pattern 5.

Signet Ring Cell Carcinoma

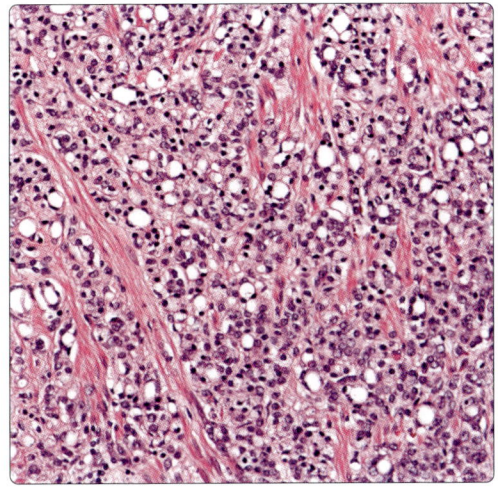

Signet Ring Cell Carcinoma

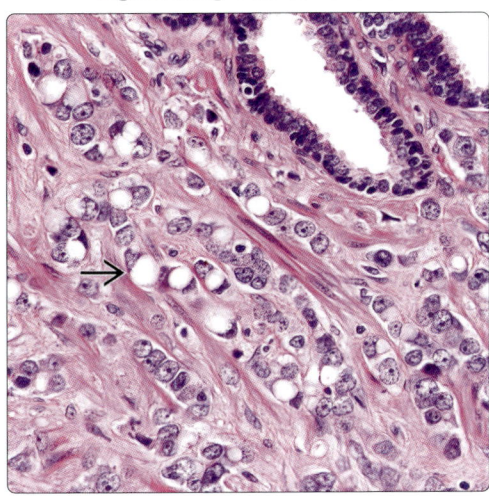

(Left) This signet ring cell PCa is composed of sheets of dyscohesive round cells with scattered vacuoles displacing the nuclei peripherally. Signet ring cell features may be seen in lymphocytes, rarely in stromal nodular BPH and sarcomas involving the prostate. *(Right)* Signet ring cell variant of PCa shows diffuse infiltrates of individual cells that include some with optically clear vacuoles displacing the nuclei peripherally ⇒. This carcinoma is usually high grade (Gleason patterns 4 and 5).

Signet Ring Cell Carcinoma

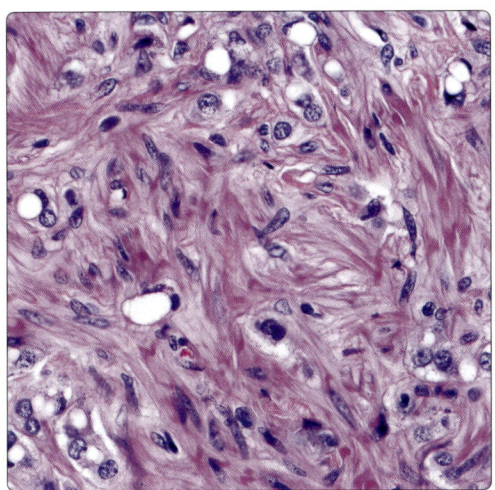

Signet Ring Cell Carcinoma

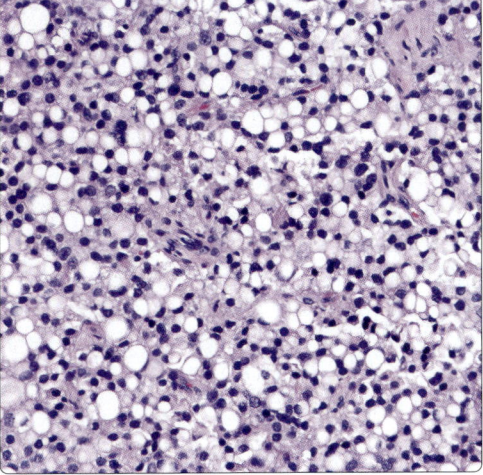

(Left) This PCa shows cells with optically clear cytoplasmic vacuoles. The signet ring cells are dispersed individually (Gleason pattern 5). Cytoplasmic vacuoles may also occur in prostatic lymphoma and chronic inflammatory cells (prostatitis) that may mimic this PCa. *(Right)* This signet ring cell carcinoma shows diffuse solid growth (Gleason pattern 5). Secondary signet ring cell carcinoma, such as from the bladder, urachus, and stomach, should be excluded. PSA &/or PAP staining confirms prostate primary.

Acinar Adenocarcinoma Variants

Pseudohyperplastic Carcinoma

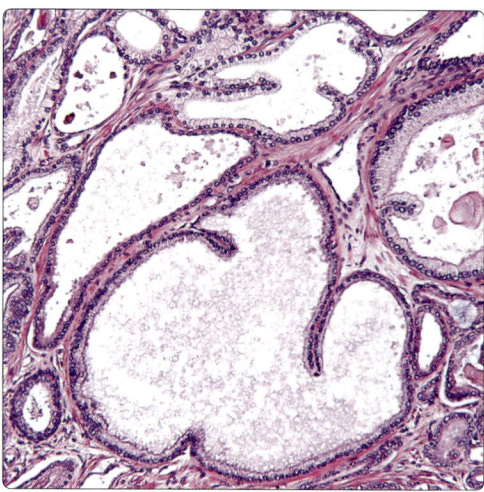

Pseudohyperplastic Carcinoma

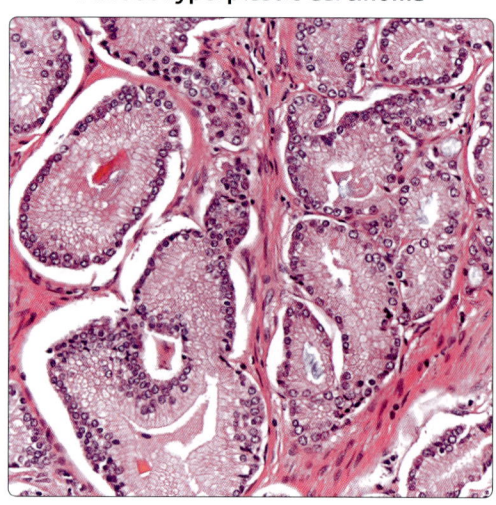

(Left) The pseudohyperplastic variant of PCa shows medium to large dilated glands with papillary infoldings and luminal eosinophilic secretions. These glands are deceptively benign on low-power view and may be mistaken for hyperplastic benign glands. *(Right)* The abundant cytoplasm and larger-caliber glands admixed with smaller glands may impart a deceptively benign appearance. In this case, the intraluminal mucin, amorphous material, and crystalloids should raise additional suspicion for PCa.

Pseudohyperplastic Carcinoma

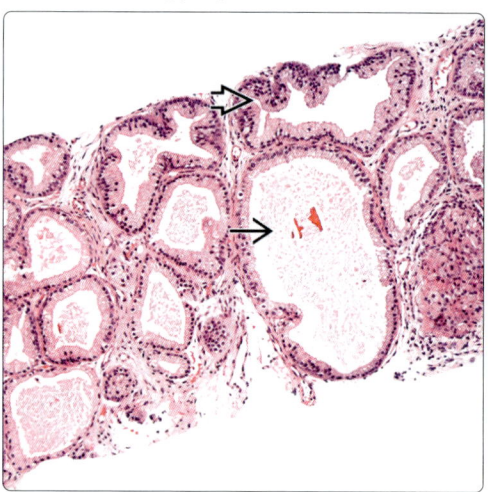

Pseudohyperplastic Carcinoma

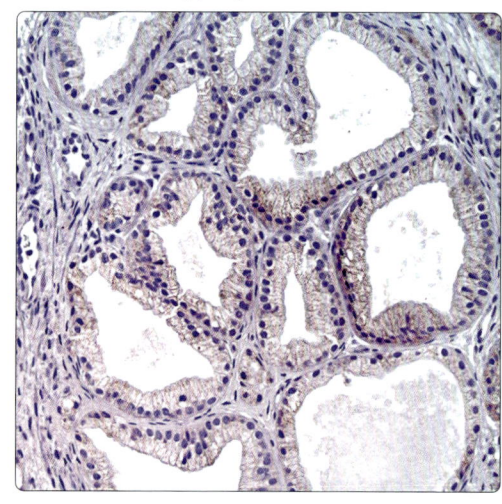

(Left) Prostate biopsy shows a morphologically subtle, pseudohyperplastic PCa characterized by evenly dispersed large-caliber glands with papillary infoldings ⇒ and intraluminal eosinophilic secretions with rare crystalloids ⇒. *(Right)* HMWCK(34βE12) documents complete absence of basal cells in pseudohyperplastic PCa. Internal positive controls were present in basal cells of benign glands. AMACR staining (not shown here) may be negative in many cases with this pattern.

Pseudohyperplastic Carcinoma

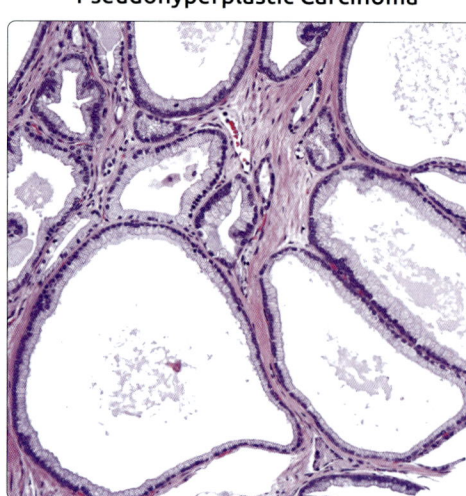

Pseudohyperplastic Carcinoma

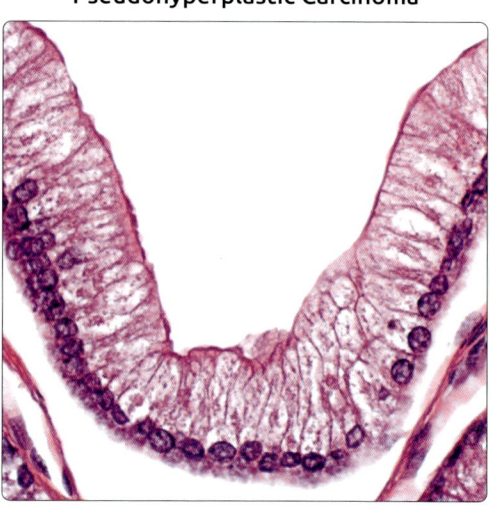

(Left) This pseudohyperplastic PCa also has large-caliber glands, but the abundant luminal cytoplasm and basally oriented nuclei suggest the diagnosis of malignancy at low power. Adjunctive immunohistochemistry (AMACR/p63/HMWCK) is often used to confirm histologically subtle patterns of adenocarcinoma. *(Right)* Pseudohyperplastic PCa often has abundant luminal cytoplasm, and nuclei may show alignment at the basal layer, as seen in this example. Nuclei features of carcinoma are retained in this tumor.

Acinar Adenocarcinoma Variants

Pseudohyperplastic Carcinoma

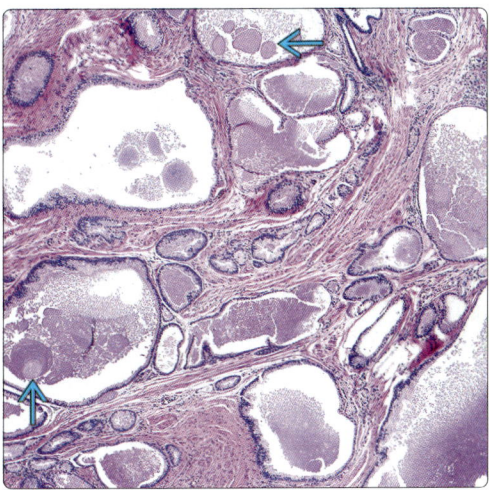

Pseudohyperplastic Carcinoma

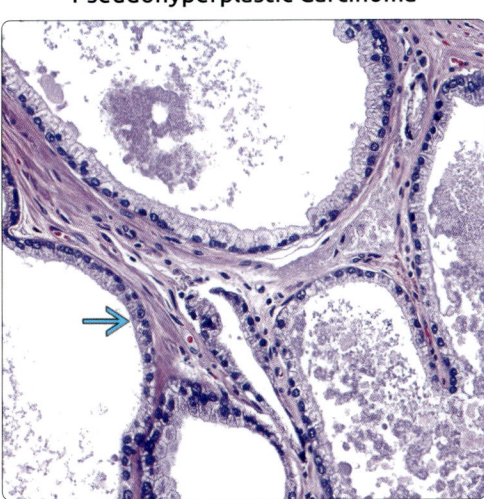

(Left) Low-power view shows pseudohyperplastic carcinoma with large dilated glands, luminal amorphous materials and corpora amylacea ➡. Despite these large-size glands, this tumor is designated as Gleason 3 + 3 = 6. (Right) Basally oriented nuclei are a salient feature of pseudohyperplastic carcinoma. Despite the architectural resemblance to hyperplasia, the nuclei retain their malignant features including prominent nucleoli ➡. The amorphous material is a helpful clue at screening to prompt further examination.

Pseudohyperplastic Carcinoma

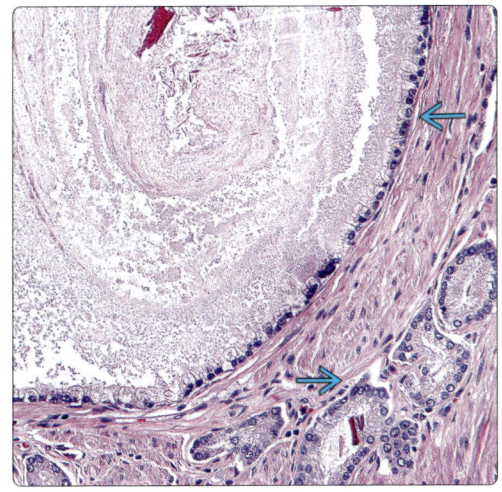

Atrophic Carcinoma

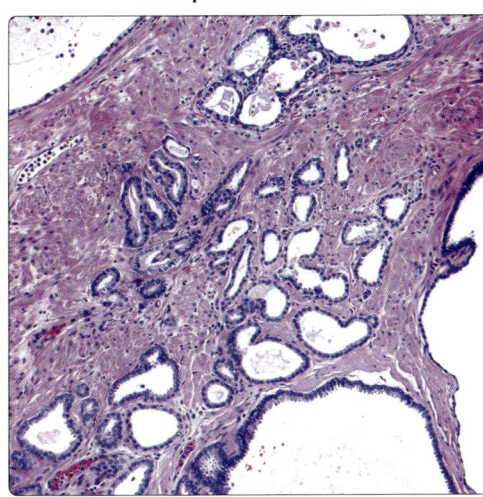

(Left) Pseudohyperplastic carcinoma commonly coexists with conventional adenocarcinoma ➡. Both tumor types show similar nuclear features and have luminal crystalloids. (Right) Lower-power view shows a focus of atrophic carcinoma. The glands are variable, irregular, and angulated, and the tumor cells have scant cytoplasm. The somewhat lobular configuration of this focus further compounds its mimicry to benign atrophy. Higher-power view examination will reveal the malignant nuclear features.

Atrophic Carcinoma

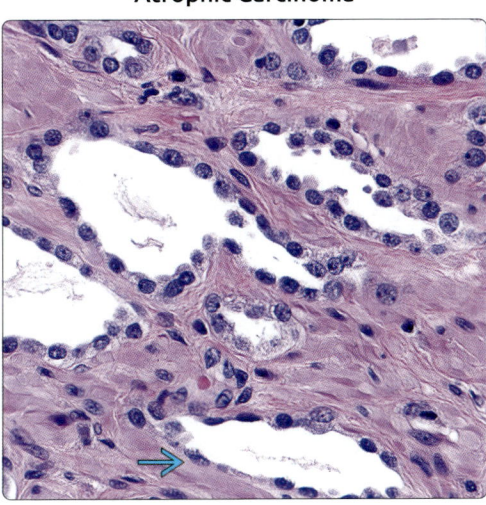

Atrophic Carcinoma

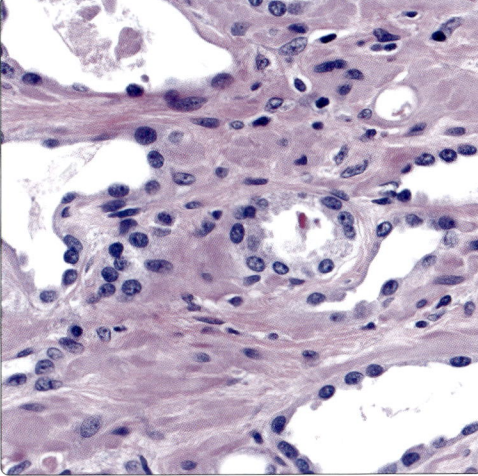

(Left) High-power view shows atrophic carcinoma with angulated glands and tumor cells with scant cytoplasm, and some are flattened ➡. In contrast to benign atrophy, these glands have enlarged nuclei and prominent nucleoli. (Right) Luminal features of cancer, as in this case, can be helpful in identifying atrophic carcinoma focus on screening magnification. These atrophic glands exhibit luminal crystalloids and amorphous eosinophilic materials. Immunohistochemistry may be needed to confirm the diagnosis of carcinoma.

Acinar Adenocarcinoma Variants

(Left) The atrophic variant of PCa shows infiltration of malignant glands with scant cytoplasm, resembling atrophy. There is often heterogeneity with some markedly atrophic forms ➡. **(Right)** The atrophic variant of PCa shows acini lined by cells with attenuated cytoplasm. Helpful features indicative of malignancy include malignant nuclear features (e.g., nucleomegaly, prominent nucleoli), nonlobular or infiltrative growth, luminal features of malignancy, and admixed usual PCa morphology.

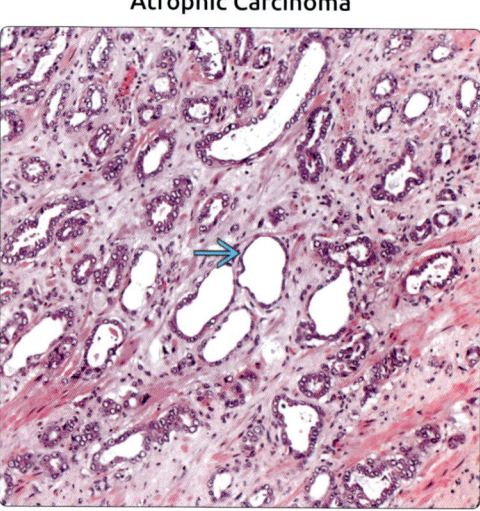
Atrophic Carcinoma

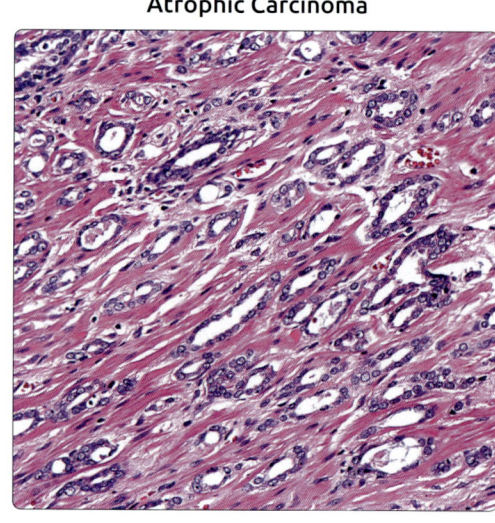
Atrophic Carcinoma

(Left) This PCa with an atrophic morphology allows comparison of the smaller irregular infiltrating carcinoma glands ➡ with the larger benign atrophic glands ➡. A nonlobular architecture is key to recognize this subtle carcinoma variant. **(Right)** At high-power magnification, the nucleomegaly and occasional nucleoli may be appreciated in the cuboidal to flattened cells of this atrophic PCa ➡. In contrast, the adjacent benign glands ➡ have smaller nuclei without distinct nucleoli and an intact basal cell layer.

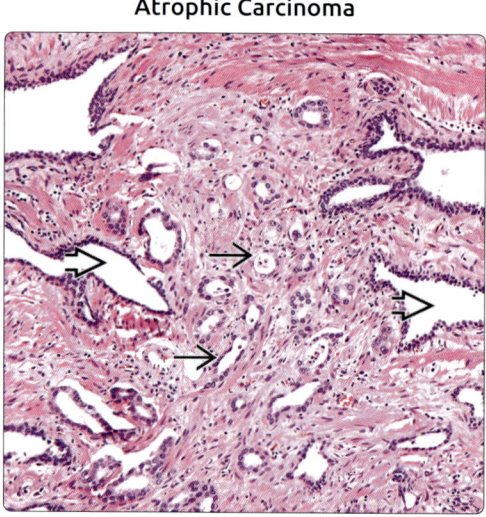
Atrophic Carcinoma

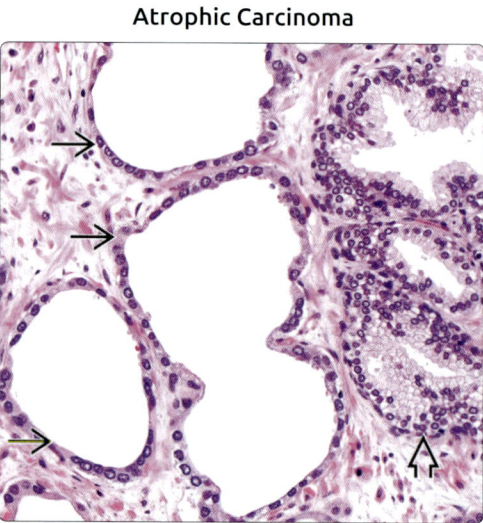
Atrophic Carcinoma

(Left) This example of PCa shows an admixture of both typical ➡ and markedly atrophic ➡ carcinoma glands. The nonlobular growth and admixture with more typical areas of PCa are helpful in this case. **(Right)** As expected, the AMACR/p63/HMWCK cocktail immunostain shows an absence of basal cells, even in the markedly atrophic-appearing large glands ➡ (with strong internal control in benign glands ➡). The carcinoma glands also show strong luminal AMACR immunoreactivity.

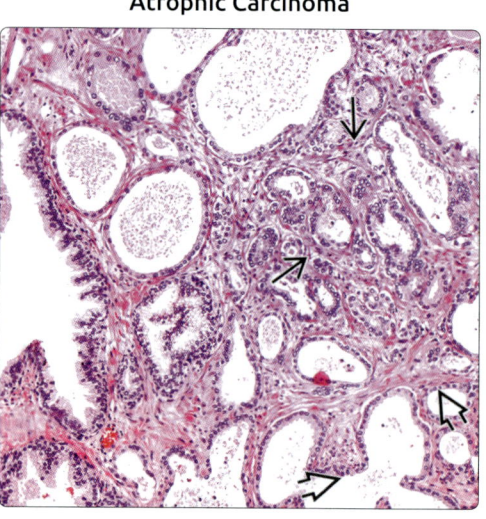
Atrophic Carcinoma

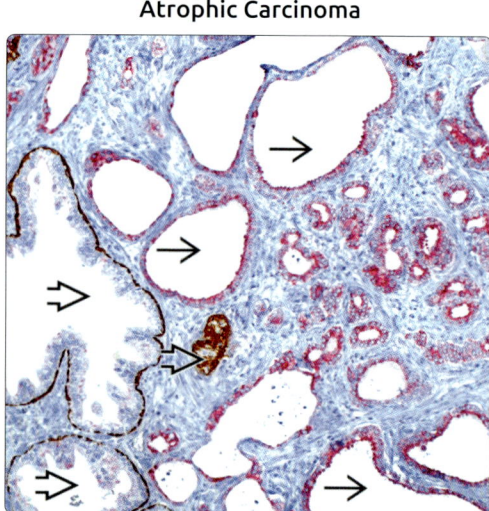
Atrophic Carcinoma

Acinar Adenocarcinoma Variants

Foamy Gland Carcinoma

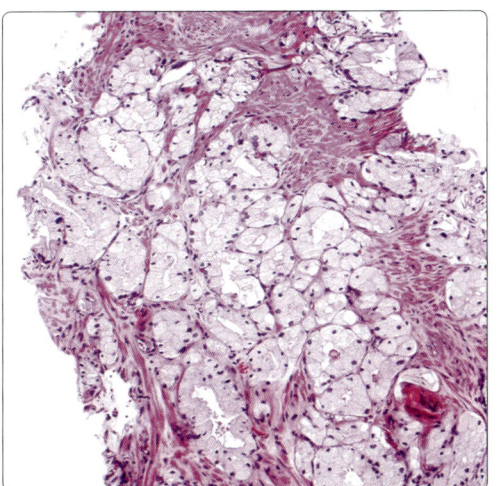

Foamy Gland Carcinoma

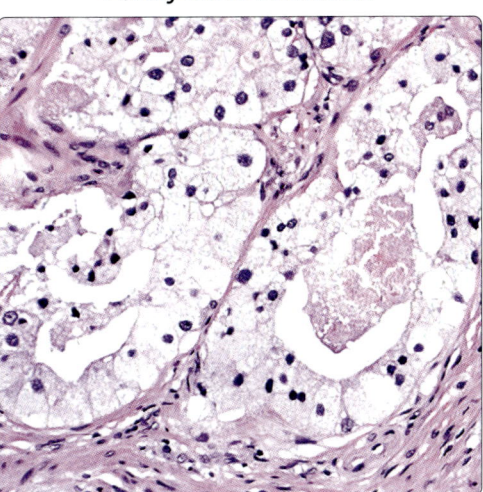

(Left) Invasive foamy carcinoma of the prostate is characterized by abundant xanthomatous cytoplasm. *(Right)* The foamy gland variant of PCa shows cells with abundant xanthomatous cytoplasm, small to pyknotic nuclei, and eosinophilic luminal secretions. The typical malignant nuclear features of PCa may not be present, making recognition as PCa difficult. Infiltrative growth, negativity for basal cell markers, and familiarity with the unique features are helpful in diagnosis.

Foamy Gland Carcinoma

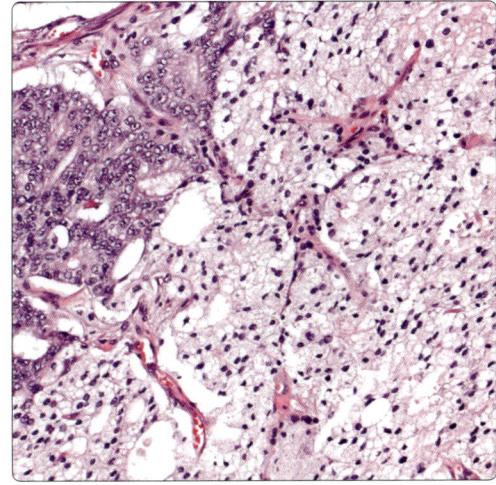

Foamy Gland Carcinoma

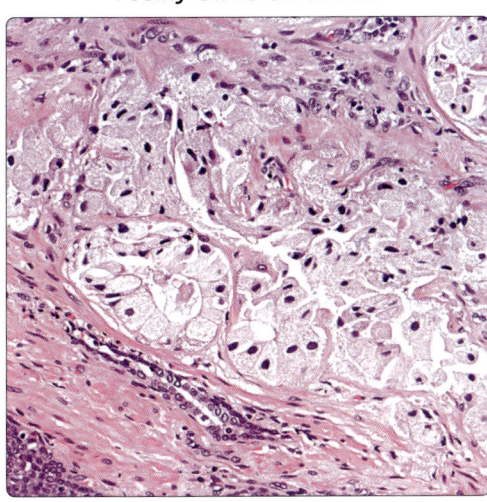

(Left) This photomicrograph contrasts the small, relatively pyknotic nuclei of the foamy gland carcinoma with the large nucleoli in the more conventional acinar PCa. *(Right)* Some studies suggest that foamy gland carcinoma, as seen in this photomicrograph, potentially has a worse prognosis than conventional acinar PCa, although the prognostic significance is debatable. AMACR staining is less frequently positive (32-38%) in foamy gland carcinoma.

Foamy Gland Carcinoma

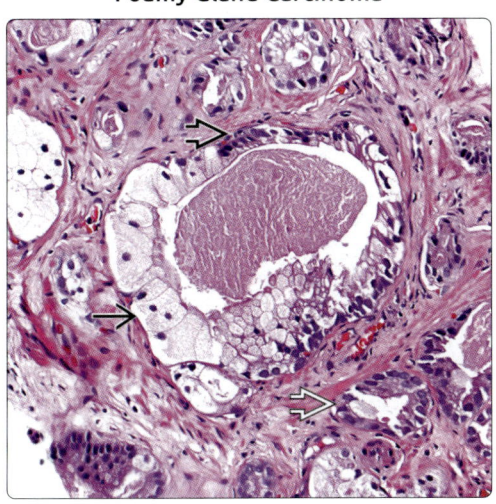

Foamy Gland Carcinoma

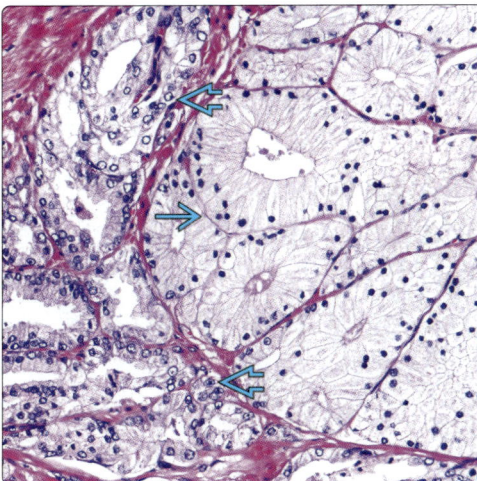

(Left) The central gland in this PCa shows a mixture of foamy features ➡ and conventional morphology ➡ within the same gland. Adjacent typical PCa is present ➡. This combination is not infrequent and contributes to difficulty in defining this variant and its prognostic significance. *(Right)* Foamy PCa cells with small pyknotic ➡ nuclei set in a xanthomatous cytoplasm are highlighted and contrasted with adjacent focus of conventional PCa showing more typical nuclear features including enlargement and prominent nucleoli ➡.

Acinar Adenocarcinoma Variants

(Left) This is an unusual example of the morphologically subtle PIN-like invasive PCa. On low-power evaluation, the architecture suggests normal glands but with some degree of hyperchromasia in the lining cells. **(Right)** The epithelium is pseudostratified columnar, which has led some authors to regard this as a pattern of ductal carcinoma. These PIN-like invasive PCas do not seem to be as aggressive as conventional ductal PCa. Immunostaining is necessary to confirm the diagnosis.

Carcinoma With Stratified Epithelium

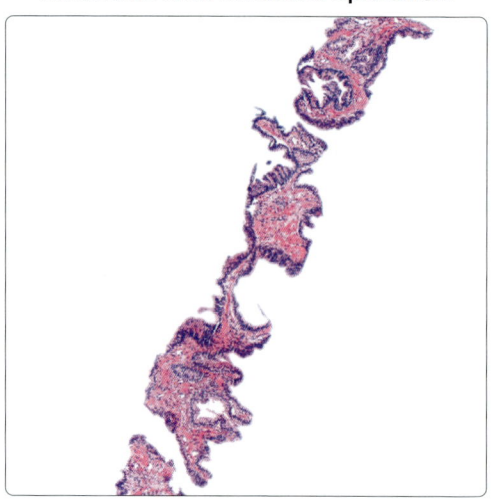

Carcinoma With Stratified Epithelium

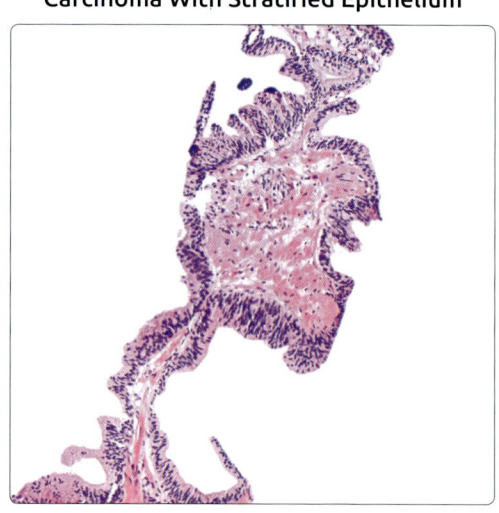

(Left) At high-power magnification, the hyperchromasia and pseudostratified columnar lining of PIN-like invasive PCa ⇒ are distinct from the adjacent benign glands with the usual round nuclei ⇒. Immunohistochemistry confirmed an absence of basal cells. **(Right)** Rare examples of invasive PCa have a multilayered or stratified epithelial layer, as seen here, that closely mimics HGPIN with apparent basal cells. This case mimics the flat pattern of high-grade PIN.

Carcinoma With Stratified Epithelium

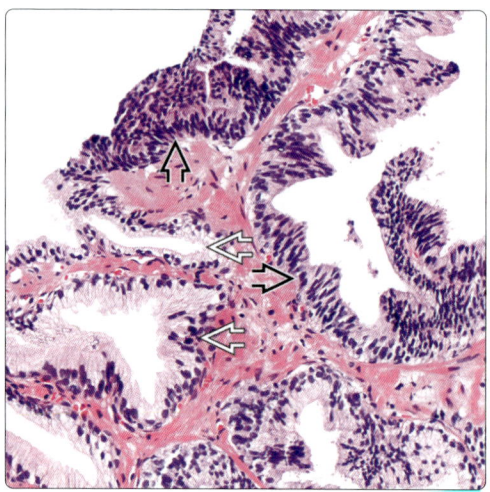

Carcinoma With Stratified Epithelium

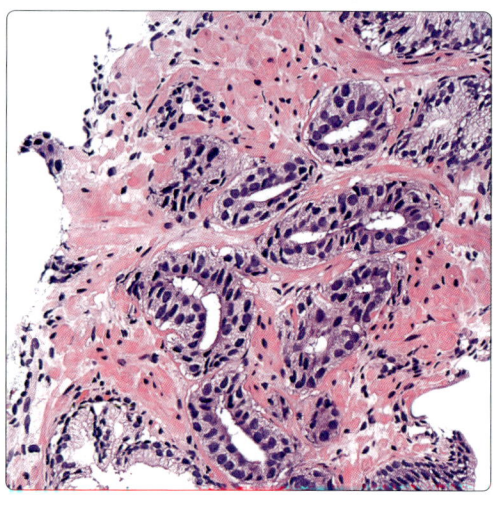

(Left) Unusual PCa pattern with acini shows several layers of secretory cells ⇒ with malignant nuclear features similar to that of usual PCa. The architecture and cytology may mimic flat or tufted HGPIN glands, requiring adjunctive confirmatory immunostaining. **(Right)** This p63/HMWCK(34βE12) cocktail confirms an absence of basal cells in this PCa ⇒ with an unusual stratified appearance. There is a strong internal control staining in the basal cells of adjacent benign glands ⇒.

Carcinoma With Stratified Epithelium

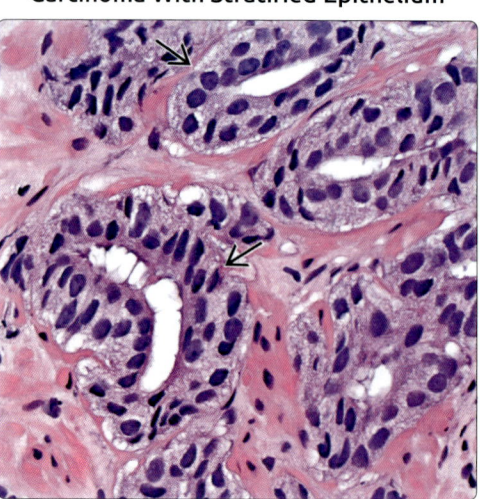

Carcinoma With Stratified Epithelium

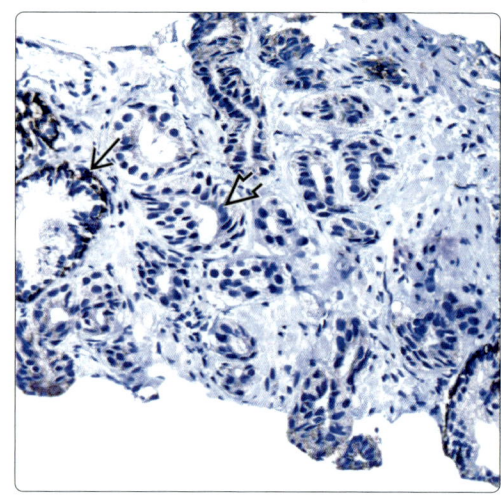

Acinar Adenocarcinoma Variants

Adenocarcinoma With Aberrant p63
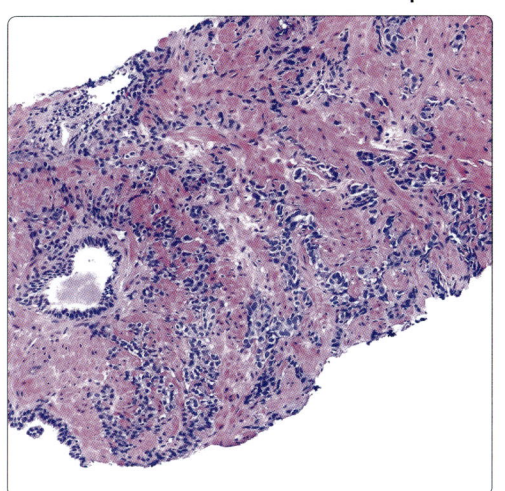

Adenocarcinoma With Aberrant p63
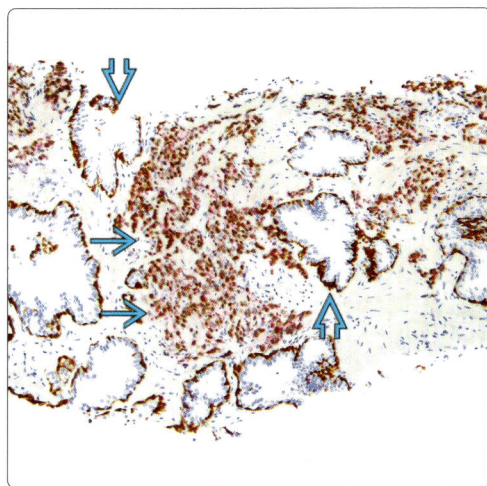

(Left) Prostate biopsy shows infiltrative growth by carcinoma with a poorly formed gland pattern. These tumor cells were shown to be positive for PSA, confirming secretory-type cells. (Right) The same case stained with p63/HMWK/AMACR cocktail immunostain shows diffuse nuclear p63 positivity in the tumor cells ➡. Red staining (AMACR) can also be seen in the cytoplasm of the same tumor cells. In contrast, surrounding benign glands ➡ exhibit basal layer positivity for HMWK and p63 with no AMACR expression.

Adenocarcinoma With Aberrant p63
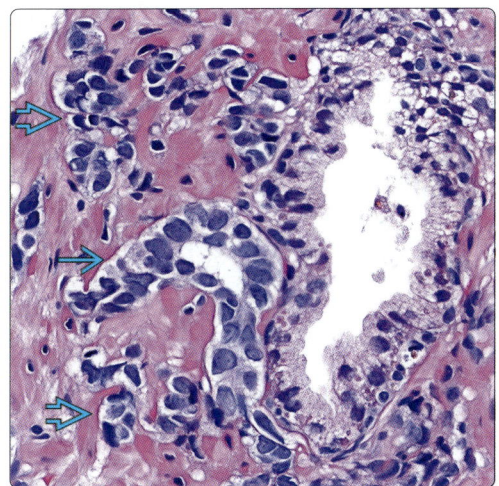

Adenocarcinoma With Aberrant p63
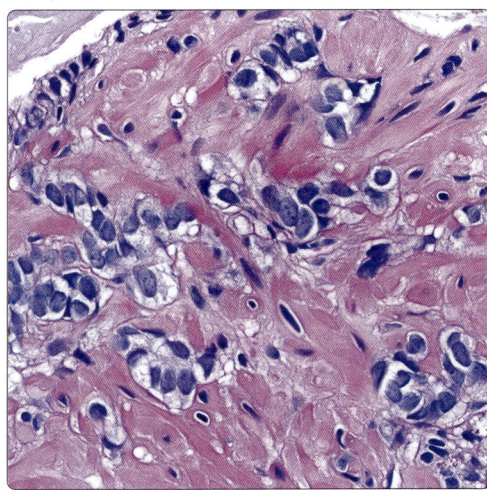

(Left) This PCa with aberrant nuclear p63 shows an admixture of well-formed ➡ and ill-formed glands ➡. Tumor cells have enlarged nuclei showing some basaloid features (e.g., modest to scant cytoplasm with perinuclear clearing). However, most of this PCa variant exhibits morphology similar to usual PCa, and the only manner of distinction is by nuclear positivity for p63. (Right) This PCa with aberrant p63 consists of poorly formed glands. The tumor cells have enlarged, overlapping nuclei and dispersed chromatin.

Adenocarcinoma With Aberrant p63
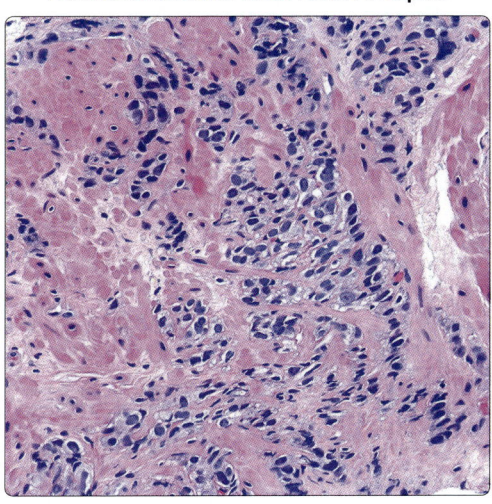

Adenocarcinoma With Aberrant p63
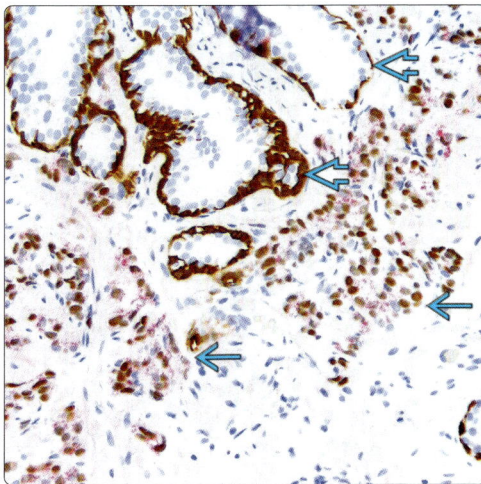

(Left) This PCa with aberrant p63 shows infiltrative tumor cells arranged in loose clusters and single file, equivalent to Gleason 4 + 5 = 9. However, it is suggested by some experts that Gleason grade should not be assigned to this variant because of its favorable findings in RP despite the high-grade pattern. (Right) Cocktail of p63/HMWK/AMACR shows diffuse nuclear p63 (brown) and AMACR (red) expression in the tumor cells ➡. In contrast, the benign glands ➡ show p63/HMWK (brown) positivity in basal cells only.

Atypical Small Acinar Proliferations

KEY FACTS

TERMINOLOGY
- Focus of atypical glands in needle biopsy
  - Quantitatively &/or qualitatively insufficient for definitive diagnosis of or exclusion of prostatic carcinoma
- Not diagnostic entity
  - Includes undersampled cancer and various benign mimics in which cancer cannot be reliably excluded
  - Represents descriptive diagnosis to aid in subsequent clinical management

CLINICAL ISSUES
- Reported in 5% of prostate needle biopsies (0.7-9%)
- Atypical small acinar proliferations (ASAP) diagnosis should prompt rebiopsy
  - Including area designated ASAP
- Carries higher risk of finding PCa in rebiopsy
  - Mean: 40%; range: 17-70%

MICROSCOPIC
- Atypical small glands that either are too few in number or do not show minimum morphologic features for definite diagnosis as PCa
- IHC with AMACR and basal cell markers may be helpful
  - Being cognizant of overlap with benign lesions in small foci
  - ERG IHC may be of value in select cases

TOP DIFFERENTIAL DIAGNOSES
- Benign
  - Partial atrophy
  - Atypical adenomatous hyperplasia (adenosis)
  - Crowded benign glands
- Malignant
  - Prostatic acinar adenocarcinoma

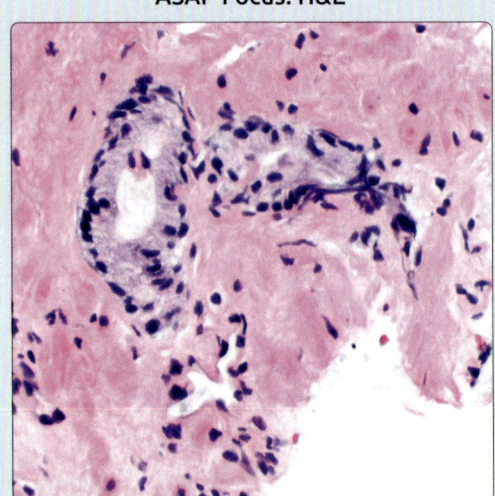

ASAP Focus: H&E

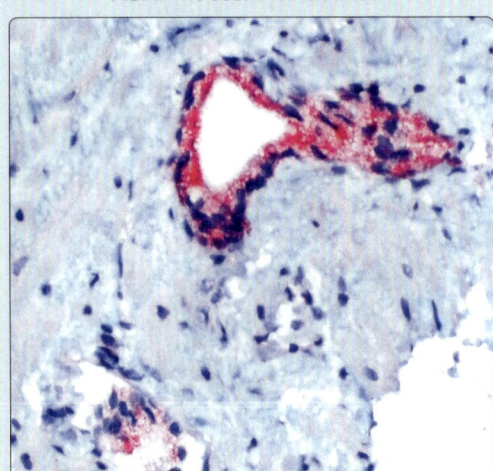

ASAP Focus: PIN Cocktail

(Left) A focus of 2 small glands appears crowded and irregularly sized, with areas of rigid luminal borders surrounding a hint of mucin. Though the nuclei palisade basally around the lumen, the crush artifact precludes assessment of nucleolar atypia. A PIN cocktail work-up is indicated. (Right) A PIN cocktail [AMACR (red, positive here) with p63/HMWCK (brown, negative here)] confirms lack of basal cells. These acini are worrisome for carcinoma but not diagnostic (ASAP), and near-term rebiopsy is recommended.

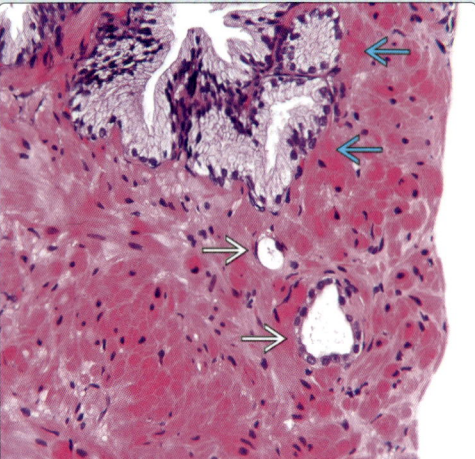

ASAP With Atrophic Morphology: H&E

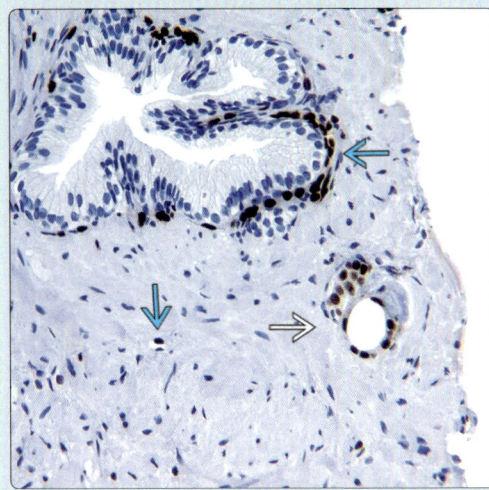

ASAP With Atrophic Morphology: ERG IHC

(Left) Here, 2 acini with atrophic morphology ➡ but apparent, prominent macronuclei appear adjacent to unequivocally benign glands ➡ (that conspicuously lack atrophy). On morphologic grounds, this focus is worrisome for carcinoma with atrophic features. (Right) ERG IHC shows strongly nuclear positivity in suspicious atrophic acini ➡; capillary endothelial cells subjacent to benign glands and elsewhere in section ➡ provide internal positive control. Highly specific to cancer, ERG can be helpful in challenging cases.

Atypical Small Acinar Proliferations

TERMINOLOGY

Abbreviations
- Atypical small acinar proliferation (ASAP)

Synonyms
- Suspicious for cancer
- Focal glandular atypia
- Atypical glands

Definitions
- Focus of atypical glands in needle biopsy quantitatively &/or qualitatively insufficient for definitive diagnosis or exclusion of prostate carcinoma (PCa)
- ASAP is **not entity**
  o Represents descriptive diagnosis to guide subsequent clinical management
    – Includes undersampled PCa and various benign mimics of PCa
- ASAP introduced in 1993 and is well-accepted descriptive diagnosis in contemporary practice
  o Term ASAP not entirely accurate as some atypical foci may not be acinar, small, or proliferative
    – Some atypical glandular lesions suspicious for carcinoma are comprised of large caliber glands (e.g., pseudohyperplastic carcinoma)

CLINICAL ISSUES

Epidemiology
- Incidence
  o Reported in 5% of prostate needle biopsies (individual series vary from 0.7-9%)
    – Threshold for establishing PCa diagnosis has interobserver variability
    – Variation, even amongst experts, dependent on experience and training

Presentation
- Biopsy performed for standard PCa biopsy indications
- Multiparametric MR image guided prostate biopsy, increasingly prevalent

Treatment
- Patient with ASAP diagnosis should be rebiopsied in near term, with extended sampling, including site where ASAP found previously

Prognosis
- ASAP carries higher risk of finding PCa in rebiopsy (40-50%)
  o Lower, ~ 25% if original biopsy was MR guided
- Subsequent PCa may also be identified in contralateral side (up to 27%)
- When adjacent to high-grade prostatic intraepithelial neoplasia (HGPIN) (HGPIN and ASAP), much higher risk of carcinoma than HGPIN alone
- Most PCa detected on subsequent rebiopsy are Gleason score 6 (up to 80%)
  o May be ≥ Gleason score 8 in some cases (up to 10%)

MACROSCOPIC

Importance of Grossing, Histology Protocols, and Diagnostic Approach
- Multiple levels (ideally 3) should be on each H&E slide to enhance representation of atypical focus
- Deeper levels, particularly if atypical focus is present in last level, may produce more diagnostic features
- Ancillary IHC helpful in resolving some ASAP cases as PCa or benign glands
  o Prospectively obtaining intervening unstained slides is important and beneficial
- When atypical glands are present in conjunction with separate cores showing definitive cancer, there may be need for further evaluation if diagnosis of PCa would upstage tumor (e.g., bilateral involvement)
- Confirming number of foci of cancer is also important for active surveillance
- Internal &/or external expert consultation may help resolve issue of diagnostic uncertainty
  o For some cases, ASAP remains best diagnosis

MICROSCOPIC

Histologic Features
- Typically group of small crowded glands that do not meet threshold for definitive carcinoma diagnosis
  o Either too few glands or insufficient degree of atypia
- Quantitative factors associated with ASAP diagnosis
  o Inadequate number of glands
    – No absolute cut-off in number of glands is formal criteria for diagnosis of PCa
    – In absence of pathognomonic features, minimum requirement for PCa varies between expert genitourinary pathologists
    – Most authors do not recommend diagnosis of PCa on single atypical gland; others favor presence of at least 3 glands
    – Threshold largely dependent on extent of other associated qualitative features: Infiltrative growth, cytologic atypia, intraluminal mucin, nucleoli, crystalloids
  o Small size of atypical glandular focus: Linear extend < 0.8 mm
- Qualitative factors associated with ASAP diagnosis
  o Features may suggest PCa but are insufficient to reach diagnostic threshold for PCa
    – Architecture may not show definite infiltration
    – May lack significant nuclear atypia (i.e., absence of nucleomegaly &/or nucleolomegaly)
    – Glandular lumina may have smooth, sharp contour (no luminal irregularity or infolding) or basal palisading of nuclei without other features
    – Diagnostic threshold for PCa may be more stringent when certain histologic findings are present: Atrophic features, pseudohyperplastic appearance, or foamy cytoplasm
  o ASAP frequently does not have any pathognomonic features of PCa
    – Glomerulations
    – Collagenous micronodules (mucinous fibroplasia)

Atypical Small Acinar Proliferations

- Circumferential perineural or intraneural invasion
- Invasion of adipose tissue or seminal vesicle
○ Confounding features
- Presence at edge of biopsy
- Poor cytologic detail, such as crush artifact
- Obscuring inflammation
- Loss of atypical focus on subsequent (and intervening) levels precluding adjunctive IHC
- When adjacent to HGPIN, makes distinction from noninvasive outpouchings of HGPIN difficult

ANCILLARY TESTS

Immunohistochemistry

- 2 general approaches (philosophies) to interpreting adjunctive IHC in diagnosis of focal PCa
  ○ Use to establish definitive diagnosis as PCa
    - To confirm very strong impression of carcinoma
    - To confirm carcinoma of morphologically subtle subtype
  ○ Use to exclude benign process, which would preclude ASAP designation
    - Typically in cases with less diagnostic certainty
    - When partial atrophy and other mimics are considered
    - In this setting, presence of basal cells would determine diagnosis as benign (positive) or ASAP (negative)
  ○ Decision not to render definitive PCa diagnosis is made on H&E evaluation
    - If qualitative threshold is not met on H&E review, IHC supportive for PCa may not be sufficient to confidently make diagnosis of PCa
    - In cases with absence of basal cells, biopsy is diagnosed as ASAP
- Circumferential, strong, luminally accentuated AMACR overexpression typical of carcinoma
  ○ Definitive diagnosis of PCa does not require AMACR expression
    - AMACR may be completely negative or show weak noncircumferential staining
  ○ False-negative AMACR immunoreactivity, including 5-25% typical PCa (usually < 10%)
    - Morphologic variants more commonly negative include 30% atrophic PCa, 32-38% foamy gland PCa, 23-30% pseudohyperplastic PCa, and 29% of hormone ablation treated PCa
  ○ False-positive AMACR immunoreactivity (usually weaker noncircumferential staining)
    - 2-36% benign glands, 10% atypical adenomatous hyperplasia (adenosis), up to 40% partial atrophy and post atrophic hyperplasia, 35-58% nephrogenic adenoma, 56-100% of HGPIN (usually 50-60%), pure intraductal carcinoma (common)
- Absence of basal cell markers [p63, HMCK(34βE12), or CK5/6] required in carcinoma
  ○ Presence of focal or patchy basal cells argues against diagnosis of invasive carcinoma
  ○ False-negative PCa staining pattern (absence of basal cells by IHC)
    - ~ 5-20% benign glands, ~ 20-25% partial atrophy, up to 50% of atypical adenomatous hyperplasia (adenosis)

- Nuclear Expression of ETS-related gene, *ERG* helpful in some cases
  ○ ~ 50% of PCa harbor gene fusions of *TMPRSS2* and *ERG*
  ○ International Society of Urological Pathology best practices recommendations for IHC consider ERG optional in work-up of limited carcinoma at biopsy
  ○ Accumulating data confirm that PCa mimics postatrophic hyperplasia, partial atrophy, and adenosis are uniformly negative
  ○ Consideration that 5-15% of HGPIN may show ERG positivity, strongly associated with concomitant carcinoma
  ○ Principle advantage is exquisite specificity to HGPIN and PCa over nonneoplastic lesions; disadvantage is lower sensitivity
    - Prevalence of ERG positivity lower in smaller foci/ASAP, ~ 15-30%
  ○ Quadruple stain cocktail proposed using ERG, AMACR, p63, and HMWCK (optional; not recommended)

DIFFERENTIAL DIAGNOSIS

Prostatic Carcinoma

- ASAP, in most instances, represents PCa in which fully diagnostic features are not sampled
- Minimal volume PCa: Quantitatively insufficient glands
- PCa variants
  ○ Foamy gland variant may have small pyknotic nuclei
  ○ Atrophic variant may have significant histologic overlap with partial atrophy
- Presence of well-described pathognomonic features of carcinoma in small foci are often diagnostic of cancer regardless of extent
  ○ Collagenous micronodules (mucinous fibroplasia), circumferential perineural invasion, glomerulations, or invasion of adipose tissue
- Clear presence of Gleason pattern 4 or higher warrants definitive diagnosis of carcinoma

Normal Structures

- Benign crowded glands
  ○ Lack nuclear features of PCa, AMACR only patchy, basal cells by IHC
- Seminal vesicles/ejaculatory duct epithelium
  ○ Prominent nuclear pleomorphism, scattered hyperchromatic cells, "monster cells"
  ○ Coarse lipofuscin pigmentation, intranuclear inclusions
  ○ Nuclear pax-2 expression, less intense in ejaculatory duct than SV
- Cowper's glands, especially apical biopsies
  ○ Lobular architecture, admixture of mucinous acini and ducts, pax-8
  ○ PSAP(-), may be focal PSA
- Verumontanum mucosal gland hyperplasia
  ○ Noninfiltrative closely packed glands of variable caliber
  ○ Usually closely oriented to urothelium, abundant corpora amylacea, and luminal concretions
  ○ HMCK(34βE12) typically highlights numerous basal cells
- Paraganglia
  ○ Found in 8% of radical prostatectomies
  ○ Usually located in periprostatic soft tissue of posterolateral region; associated with nerves

Atypical Small Acinar Proliferations

- Prominent vasculature delineates nests of cells
  - Express synaptophysin, chromogranin, often GATA3 by IHC; cytokeratin (-)

Proliferative Lesions
- Outpouching of HGPIN
  - Nuclear features of carcinoma, basal cells seen or confirmed on IHC
- Atypical adenomatous hyperplasia (adenosis)
  - More common in transition zone
  - Crowded glands with lobular configuration, small glands admixed with larger, convoluted, more benign glands
  - Adenosis glands show similar histology to adjacent unequivocally benign glands
  - May contain abundant crystalloids (up to 39% of cases), corpora amylacea, intraluminal mucin rare and focal
  - Contains patchy basal cell layer by IHC
    - May be present in as few as 10% of total glands
    - Individual glands may have only 1 or 2 basal cells
- Mesonephric remnant hyperplasia: Identical to GYN tract lesions
  - More atrophic glands with dense intraluminal colloid secretions
  - PSA and PSAP (-), basal cells by IHC
- Sclerosing adenosis: Rare in needle biopsies
  - Occurs in transition zone
  - Glands characteristically associated with intimately admixed spindle cell population
  - Hyaline membranes around glands
  - Contain basal cells by IHC
- Basal cell hyperplasia
  - Prominent nucleoli common
  - Strongly reactive for p63, CK5/6, &/or HMWCK (34βE12)

Atrophy Variants
- Simple atrophy
  - Glands retain lobular architecture
  - Cells with scant cytoplasm imparting basophilic appearance on low-power view
  - Contains basal cell layer confirmed by IHC
- Post atrophic hyperplasia
  - More crowded acinar units than simple atrophy
  - Large "feeder" duct may be identified
  - Numerous basal cells are typically obvious by IHC
- Partial atrophy
  - Most common and closest morphologic mimic of PCa
  - Slightly more disorganized architecturally than other atrophy variants
  - Comprised of secretory cells with scant pale clear to eosinophilic luminal cytoplasm
    - Often have abundant cytoplasm lateral to nucleus
  - Typically have undulating luminal surface
  - Usually bland nuclear features, but small nucleoli seen in up to 20%
  - Immunohistochemistry interpretation may be difficult
    - Presence of any basal cells is diagnostic of benign lesion
    - Basal cells are typically patchy, but in some small foci they may not be identifiable
    - In 24% of cases, small foci of partial atrophy may show both AMACR reactivity and absence of basal cells

Inflammatory/Reactive Lesions
- Nephrogenic adenoma
  - Variably sized tubules with thick basement membrane; hobnail cells and inflammation
  - May have mixed papillary &/or solid growth
  - Helpfully pax-2/pax-8 (+)
    - AMACR (frequent +) and PSA/PSAP (infrequent +) are pitfalls
  - More common in TURP chips

DIAGNOSTIC CHECKLIST
Pathologic Interpretation Pearls
- In small focus not fulfilling diagnostic criteria for PCa, there should be consideration for benign mimics
  - Benign lesions should be excluded by IHC if at all possible
    - Avoids overuse of ASAP diagnosis and unnecessary rebiopsy
- ASAP should not be used for lesions with only patchy basal cells
  - Leads to unnecessary rebiopsy
  - Should be diagnosed as benign in appropriate morphologic context

REPORTING
Recommendations
- Some authors recommend qualifying ASAP, such as suspicious or highly suspicious for cancer
  - No known difference in risk of PCa on follow-up biopsy between ASAP qualifiers
  - May aid in understanding of ASAP diagnosis
  - Some clinicians may be unaware of conveyed risk in ASAP diagnosis and need for rebiopsy
    - Some authors advocate detailed comment relaying risk of subsequent cancer on rebiopsy

SELECTED REFERENCES
1. Dorin RP et al: Prostate atypia: Does repeat biopsy detect clinically significant prostate cancer? Prostate. 75(7):673-8, 2015
2. Raskolnikov D et al: The role of image guided biopsy targeting in patients with atypical small acinar proliferation. J Urol. 193(2):473-8, 2015
3. Andrews C et al: Utility of ERG versus AMACR expression in diagnosis of minimal adenocarcinoma of the prostate in needle biopsy tissue. Am J Surg Pathol. 38(7):1007-12, 2014
4. Epstein JI et al: Best practices recommendations in the application of immunohistochemistry in the prostate: report from the International Society of Urologic Pathology consensus conference. Am J Surg Pathol. 38(8):e6-e19, 2014
5. Green WM et al: Immunohistochemical evaluation of TMPRSS2-ERG gene fusion in adenosis of the prostate. Hum Pathol. 44(9):1895-901, 2013
6. Tomlins SA et al: Antibody-based detection of ERG rearrangements in prostate core biopsies, including diagnostically challenging cases: ERG staining in prostate core biopsies. Arch Pathol Lab Med. 136(8):935-46, 2012
7. Tolonen TT et al: Routine dual-color immunostaining with a 3-antibody cocktail improves the detection of small cancers in prostate needle biopsies. Hum Pathol. 42(11):1635-42, 2011
8. Van der Kwast TH et al: Variability in diagnostic opinion among pathologists for single small atypical foci in prostate biopsies. Am J Surg Pathol. Epub ahead of print, 2010
9. Wang W et al: Partial atrophy on prostate needle biopsy cores: a morphologic and immunohistochemical study. Am J Surg Pathol. 32(6):851-7, 2008
10. Epstein JI et al: Prostate needle biopsies containing prostatic intraepithelial neoplasia or atypical foci suspicious for carcinoma: implications for patient care. J Urol. 175(3 Pt 1):820-34, 2006

Atypical Small Acinar Proliferations

(Left) Recognition of ASAP at low power may be challenging, demonstrated by this focus admixed with inflammation ➡. (Right) At higher power, a collection of small acini are seen infiltrating between benign glands ➡; though the number of atypical acini would be sufficient to diagnose carcinoma, the quality of the atypia is not unequivocal and diagnostically unreliable in the background of inflammation.

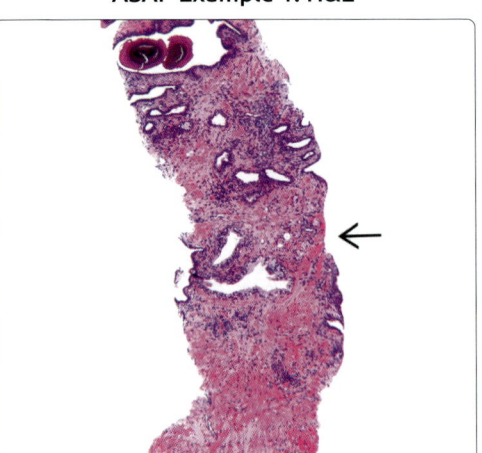

ASAP Example 1: H&E

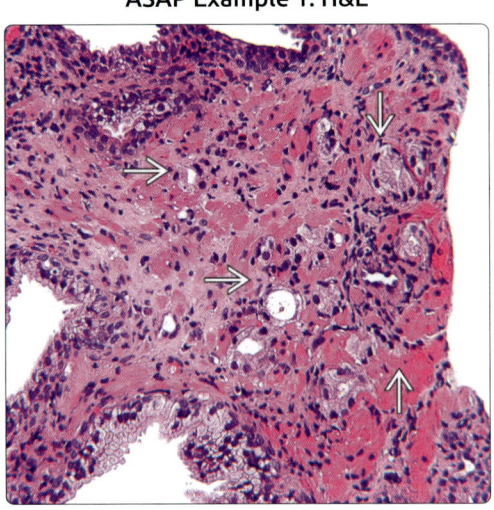

ASAP Example 1: H&E

(Left) The ASAP focus shows complete lack of basal cells and luminally accentuated overexpression of AMACR ➡, while adjacent benign acini ➡ provide helpful internal negative and positive controls, respectively. The diagnosis was upgraded to adenocarcinoma. (Right) Here a focus of 3-4 acini with an infiltrative appearance, amorphous pink luminal secretions, and variably enlarged nuclei with nucleoli ➡ are seen adjacent to acini appearing to harbor basal cells ➡.

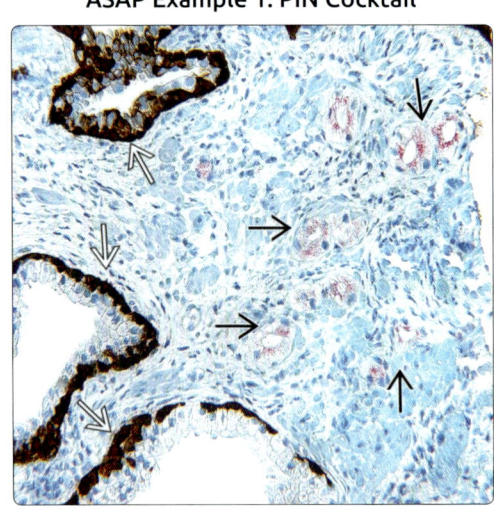

ASAP Example 1: PIN Cocktail

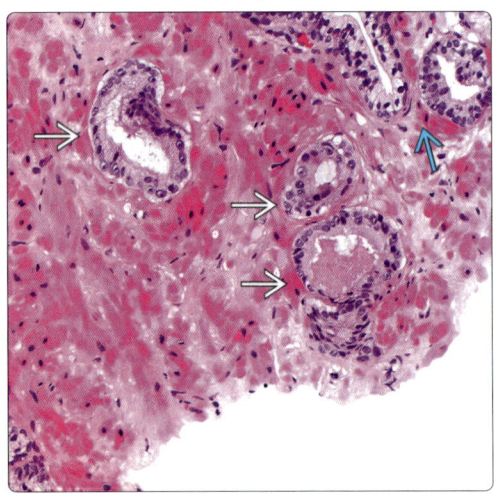

ASAP Example 2: H&E

(Left) ASAP in the same case shows positive nuclear ERG ➡ supportive of carcinoma. The upper acini with a multilayered appearance ➡ are ERG(+) HGPIN, an infrequent (10%) finding mostly associated with adjacent carcinoma. (Right) However, ASAP designation was retained due to scattered basal cells in one atypical acinus ➡, while the others lack basal cells and show AMACR induction ➡. The HGPIN acini ➡ are confirmed to harbor basal cells.

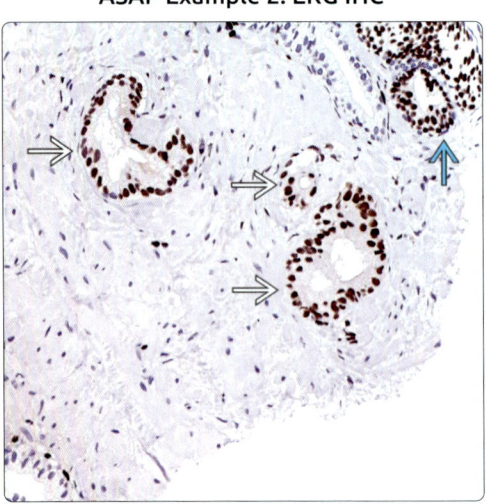

ASAP Example 2: ERG IHC

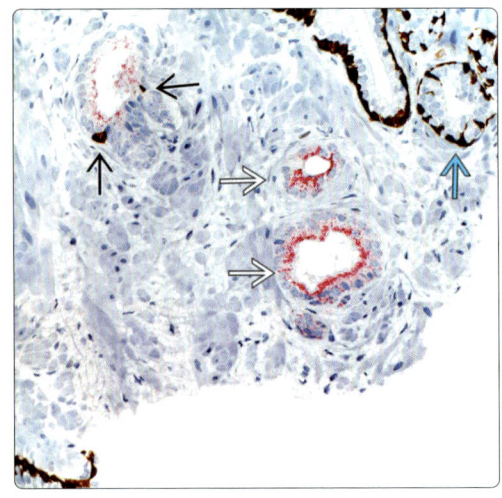

ASAP Example 2: PIN Cocktail

Atypical Small Acinar Proliferations

HGPIN With Adjacent ASAP: PINATYP

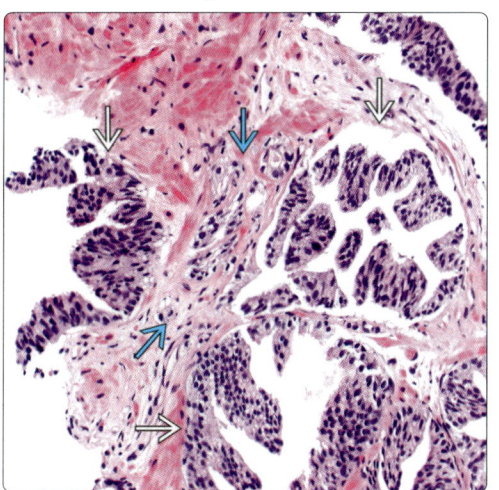

PINTATYP: PIN Cocktail

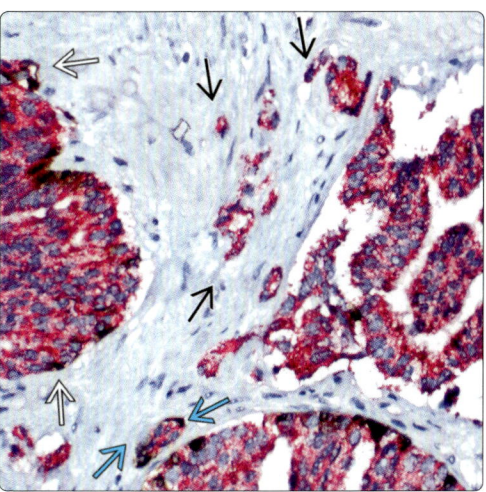

(Left) HGPIN ➡ with adjacent ASAP ➡, also known as "PINATYP" on needle biopsy, is associated with a 40-60% risk of subsequent cancer diagnosis and bears recommendation of near-term rebiopsy. (Right) The same focus as at left, shows atypical small acini with AMACR positivity and lacking basal cells ➡ adjacent to AMACR(+) and basal cell (+) HGPIN ➡. Outpouchings of HGPIN cannot be excluded, underscored by 1 small acinus with basal cells ➡.

Atypical Focus Proven To Be Adenosis

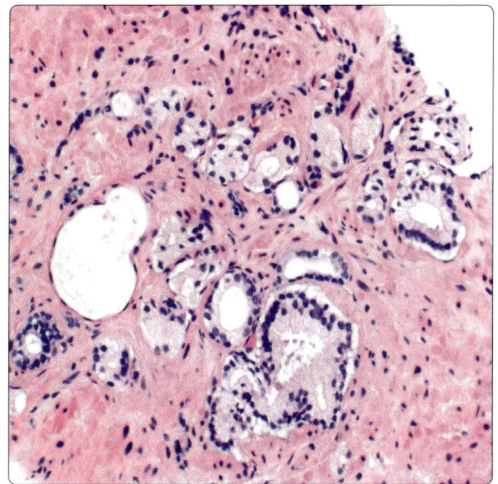

Adenosis: PIN Cocktail

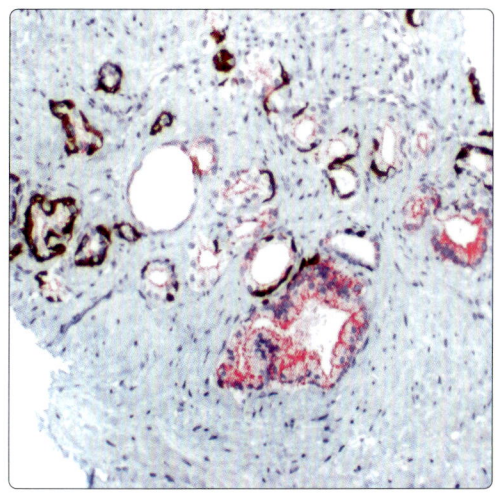

(Left) Here, an atypical focus of crowded, variably sized glands with foamy cytoplasm, mild nuclear enlargement, basally oriented nuclei, and variably rigid luminal boarders is seen at biopsy. (Right) The same focus demonstrates scattered p63/HMWCK (+) basal cells throughout the focus, confirming adenosis. Approximately 10% of adenosis may overexpress AMACR, as seen here, a pitfall in use of this stain alone.

Atypical Focus Proven Benign

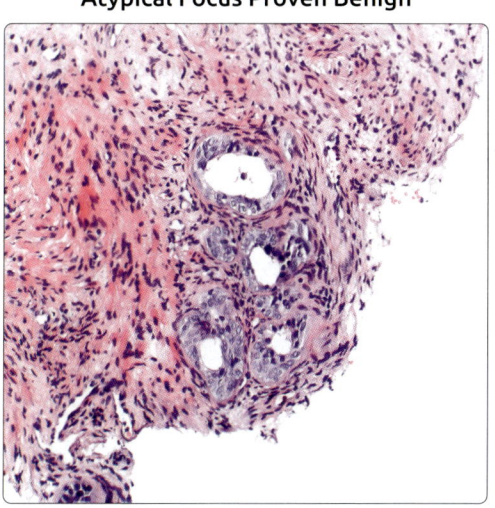

Atypical Focus Proven Benign: PIN Cocktail

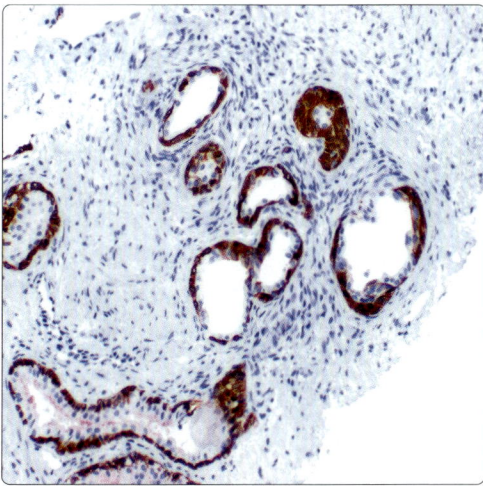

(Left) An atypical focus of 4 or 5 glands with a crowded appearance, rigid luminal borders, cytoplasmic hyperchromasia and amphophilia, and scattered nucleoli raises consideration of a focus of PCa. (Right) PIN cocktail performed on a deeper section of this focus confirms presence of p63/HMWCK (+) basal cells with hyperplastic appearance and lack of AMACR positivity in the relevant acini. The cellular stroma raises consideration of sclerosing adenosis. Carcinoma is excluded.

Intraductal Carcinoma

KEY FACTS

TERMINOLOGY
- Intraductal carcinoma of prostate (IDC-P) is proliferation of malignant epithelial cells, most commonly in form of cribriform or solid growth patterns, which fill and markedly enlarge large acini and prostatic ducts with preservation of basal cells

ETIOLOGY/PATHOGENESIS
- In vast majority of cases, IDC-P is associated with invasive acinar prostatic adenocarcinoma
- Rarely, pure IDC-P may be present as only evidence of cancer in prostate (i.e., no associated invasive carcinoma)
- *TMPRSS-ERG* fusion and loss of *PTEN* cytoplasmic expression in subset of cases

CLINICAL ISSUES
- IDC-P is rare in needle biopsy specimens (up to 0.3% when without associated invasive carcinoma and 2.8% when associated with invasive carcinoma)
- IDC-P more common in radical prostatectomies
- 20-40% of prostatectomy specimens
- Associated with high-grade, high-volume, and high-stage acinar prostatic adenocarcinoma
- Pure IDC-P (without associated invasive carcinoma) very rare in prostatectomy specimens

MICROSCOPIC
- Major criteria for diagnosis of IDC-P include
  - (1) Solid or dense cribriform architecture (tumor cells filling 50–70% of involved glands)
  - (2) Marked nuclear atypia and pleomorphism with nucleomegaly (6x normal nuclei)
  - (3) Nonfocal comedonecrosis
- Basal cells are typically prominent at periphery of involved glands but may be partially or sporadically present
- Other features include involvement of many glands (> 6), irregular glands branching at right angles, and with frequent mitoses

Intraductal Carcinoma of Prostate

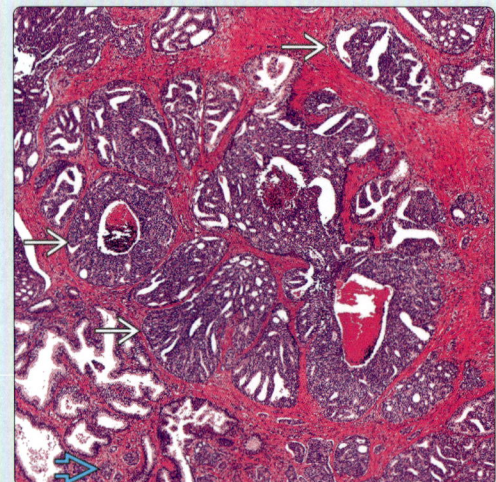

(Left) *A low-power view showing extensive involvement of many prostatic ducts and acini ⇨ by prostate cancer. Cribriform and complex architecture is evident. Note the presence of usual acinar adjacent invasive carcinoma ⇨. (Right) In this needle biopsy, the intraductal growth is primarily solid in many of the involved ducts. The duct in the center is expanded and enlarged and additionally exhibits unusual branching at a right angle.*

Intraductal Carcinoma of Prostate: Solid Growth

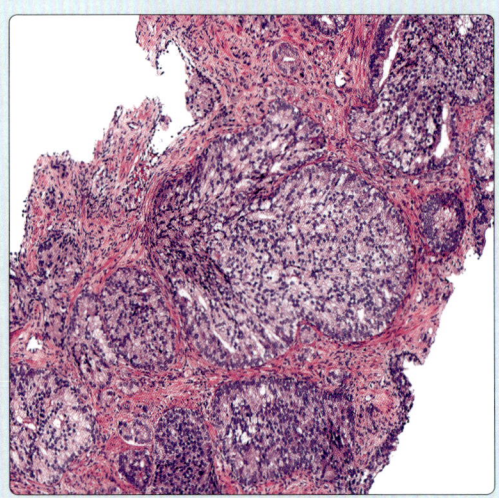

Intraductal Carcinoma of Prostate: Comedonecrosis

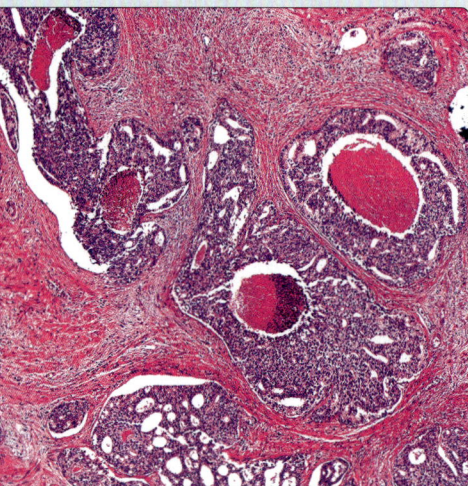

(Left) *In this section, tumors fill and expand many ducts, typical of intraductal carcinoma of prostate (IDC-P). Many of the ducts exhibit central comedo-type necrosis, which is also a typical feature of IDC-P. The presence of basal cells was confirmed by IHC in this case. (Right) This is a needle biopsy with IDC-P with cribriform and micropapillary architecture. There are multiple tumors cells with marked nuclear atypia and hyperchromasia ⇨. The presence of basal cells was confirmed by IHC in this case.*

Intraductal Carcinoma of Prostate: Nuclear Atypia

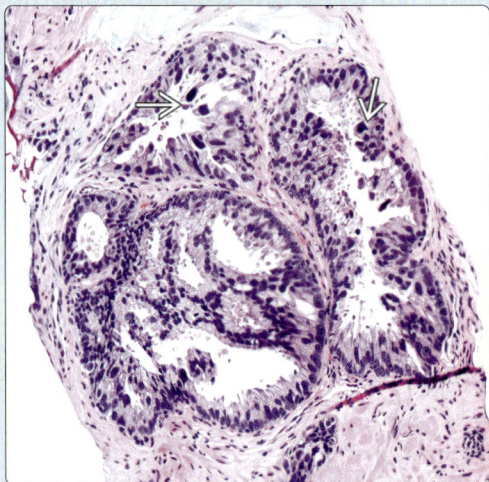

Intraductal Carcinoma

TERMINOLOGY

Abbreviations
- Intraductal carcinoma of prostate (IDC-P)

Definitions
- IDC-P is proliferation of malignant epithelial cells, most commonly in form of cribriform or solid growth patterns, which fill and markedly enlarge large acini and prostatic ducts with preservation of basal cells

ETIOLOGY/PATHOGENESIS

Pathogenesis
- In vast majority of cases, IDC-P is associated with invasive acinar prostatic adenocarcinoma
- Rarely, pure IDC-P may be present as only evidence of cancer in prostate
- Possible scenarios for development
  o IDC-P represents intraductal spread of adjacent invasive high-grade prostate cancer
  o IDC-P represents precursor of invasive high-grade prostate cancer
  o Or combination of above 2 scenarios
- Origin and pathogenesis of IDC-P still controversial and requires further studies
- Potential continuum between high-grade prostatic intraepithelial neoplasia (HGPIN) and IDC-P has been proposed but needs further validation

Genetics
- There is evidence of similar frequencies of loss of heterozygosity in IDC-P and in Gleason pattern 4/5 carcinomas
- By comparative genomic hybridization, IDC-P has more chromosomal imbalances than HGPIN
  o Loss of heterozygosity of *TP53*, *RB1*, and *PTEN* more common than in HGPIN
- Common *TMPRSS-ERG* fusion in IDC-P
  o Cytoplasmic *PTEN* loss in subset of IDC-P
    – May help in distinguishing IDC-P from HGPIN

CLINICAL ISSUES

Epidemiology
- Incidence
  o IDC-P is rare in needle biopsy specimens
    – 0.1% to 0.3% of biopsy cases when in isolation (without associated invasive adenocarcinoma)
    – 2.8% of biopsy cases when associated with invasive adenocarcinoma
  o IDC-P more common in radical prostatectomy
    – 20-40% of prostatectomy specimens
      □ Generally located in peripheral zone admixed with high-grade, high-volume, and high-stage acinar prostatic adenocarcinoma
      □ Pure IDC-P (without associated invasive carcinoma) in prostatectomies is very rare
- Age
  o Wide age distribution, similar to prostatic adenocarcinoma (range 46 to 93)
- Ethnicity
  o No strong ethnic association has yet been reported

Presentation
- Asymptomatic, discovered during regular work-up for prostate cancer
- Elevated serum prostate-specific antigen may be present

Treatment
- Surgical approaches
  o Radical prostatectomy is treatment of choice after identification in needle biopsy
  o Rebiopsy may be attempted when IDC-P is diagnosed without associated invasive carcinoma
- Drugs
  o Androgen deprivation therapy may be attempted
    – Generally poor response to hormonal therapies
- Limited information about radiation therapy for this tumor

Prognosis
- Generally, IDC-P is associated with high-risk features and considered to follow aggressive course
  o After needle biopsy diagnosis of IDC-P, radical prostatectomy usually shows adverse features
    – Higher Gleason scores (median score 8)
    – More advanced stage; high rate of extraprostatic extension and seminal vesicle involvement
    – That is true even in absence of associated invasive carcinoma component in needle biopsy
      □ Recent reports of adverse pathological findings on prostatectomy when even Gleason score 6 invasive carcinoma was associated with IDC-P on biopsy

MACROSCOPIC

General Features
- Not associated with specific gross findings
  o May form distinct nodule(s)
  o Primarily located in peripheral zone

MICROSCOPIC

Histologic Features
- IDC-P consists of florid and expansile proliferation of prostatic adenocarcinoma cells within native prostatic ducts with at least partially intact basal cell layer
  o Glands involving IDC-P are usually large with irregular and branching contour
  o Architecture of IDC-P may be solid, dense cribriform, loose cribriform, micropapillary, or flat (rare)
    – Comedonecrosis very common
  o Tumor cells can be cuboidal or columnar; typically with large nuclei and marked nuclear pleomorphism
    – Nuclei may be up to 6 times larger than adjacent nonneoplastic nuclei
  o Basal cells typically prominent at periphery of involved glands but may be partially or sporadically present
- Major criteria for diagnosis of IDC-P include (presence of any criterion is diagnostic for IDC-P)
  o (1) Solid or dense cribriform architecture (tumor cells filling 50–70% of involved glands)
  o (2) Marked nuclear atypia and pleomorphism with nucleomegaly (6x normal nuclei)
  o (3) Nonfocal comedonecrosis

Intraductal Carcinoma

- Other morphologic features of IDC-P include (often present and helpful but not diagnostic)
  - (1) Involvement of many glands (typically > 6 glands in prostatectomy specimen)
  - (2) Irregular glands, branching at right angles
  - (3) Frequent mitoses
  - (4) 2 cell populations (tall pleomorphic and mitotically active cells at periphery and cuboidal monomorphic less mitotically active cells more centrally located)

Predominant Pattern/Injury Type
- Neoplastic

Predominant Cell/Compartment Type
- Epithelial, glandular

Grade
- IDC-P is high grade by definition

ANCILLARY TESTS

Immunohistochemistry
- Basal cell markers [p63, HMCK(34βE12)] highlight intact basal cell layer around involved ducts (generally prominent but may be only focal or discontinuous)
- AMACR generally overexpressed by intraductal tumor cells
- PSA/PSP/PSMA (+) in intraductal tumor cells
- Nuclear ERG expression in subset of cases
- Loss of cytoplasmic PTEN expression in some cases

DIFFERENTIAL DIAGNOSIS

High-Grade Prostatic Intraepithelial Neoplasia
- May be difficult to distinguish from IDC-P
  - Both entities may have cribriform or papillary/micropapillary architecture
  - Both entities retain basal cell layer
- Architectural and cytologic atypia are less severe in HGPIN than in IDC-P
  - HGPIN glands typically smooth with rounded contours
  - HGPIN glands typically similar in size or slightly larger than adjacent, benign glands
  - HGPIN cells lack marked nuclear atypia or pleomorphism
  - Rare mitoses in HGPIN
  - Rare (or absent) comedonecrosis in HGPIN
- *TMPRSS-ERG* fusion more common in IDC-P than in HGPIN
- Cytoplasmic PTEN loss in subset of IDC-P but not in HGPIN

High-Grade Acinar Adenocarcinoma With Cribriform Pattern (Gleason Pattern 4 or 5)
- Absent basal cell layer with IHC
- Greater architectural complexity, more infiltration
- Comedonecrosis much less common than in IDC-P

Ductal Adenocarcinoma
- Commonly involves prostatic urethra and periurethral region; involvement may be diffuse
- Shows expansile large glandular and true papillary patterns
- Nuclei frequently pseudostratified with elongated appearance; mitoses may be frequent
- Majority lacks basal cell layer confirmed by use of basal cell markers [p63 and HMCK(34βE12)]
- Has invasive and intraductal component

Urothelial (Transitional Cell) Carcinoma Involving Prostatic Ducts and Acini
- Significant cellular pleomorphism and mitotic activity within large glandular structures
- Densely eosinophilic cytoplasm, may be squamoid
- Pagetoid growth by neoplastic cells with elevation and preservation of normal secretory cells
- PSA(-)/PSP(-)/ERG(-); p63/HMCK(34βE12) (+)
  - Caveat: Some IDC-P cases may stain with HMCK(34βE12) and/or CK7 (typically focally)

DIAGNOSTIC CHECKLIST

Pathologic Interpretation Pearls
- IDC-P should be suspected whenever there are large irregular ducts with florid/cribriform luminal proliferation of highly atypical cells
- Presence of comedonecrosis should prompt investigation for IDC-P, confirmation by IHC for basal cell markers
- Reporting presence of IDC-P is important due to more aggressive nature of disease
- IDC-P without invasive cancer is not graded

REPORTING

Key Elements to Report
- Presence of IDC-P explicitly mentioned in report in addition to invasive carcinoma
- Presence or absence of concomitant invasive adenocarcinoma and Gleason grading of invasive cancer

SELECTED REFERENCES

1. Haffner MC et al: Molecular evidence that invasive adenocarcinoma can mimic prostatic intraepithelial neoplasia (PIN) and intraductal carcinoma through retrograde glandular colonization. J Pathol. 238(1):31-41, 2015
2. Humphrey PA: Intraductal carcinoma of the prostate. J Urol. 194(5):1434-5, 2015
3. Khani F et al: Prostate biopsy specimens with Gleason 3+3=6 and intraductal carcinoma: radical prostatectomy findings and clinical outcomes. Am J Surg Pathol. 39(10):1383-9, 2015
4. Magers M et al: Intraductal carcinoma of the prostate: morphologic features, differential diagnoses, significance, and reporting practices. Arch Pathol Lab Med. 139(10):1234-41, 2015
5. Morais CL et al: Utility of PTEN and ERG immunostaining for distinguishing high-grade PIN from intraductal carcinoma of the prostate on needle biopsy. Am J Surg Pathol. 39(2):169-78, 2015
6. Tsuzuki T: Intraductal carcinoma of the prostate: a comprehensive and updated review. Int J Urol. 22(2):140-5, 2015
7. Iczkowski KA et al: Intraductal carcinoma of the prostate: interobserver reproducibility survey of 39 urologic pathologists. Ann Diagn Pathol. 18(6):333-42, 2014
8. Watts K et al: Incidence and clinicopathological characteristics of intraductal carcinoma detected in prostate biopsies: a prospective cohort study. Histopathology. 63(4):574-9, 2013
9. Robinson B et al: Intraductal carcinoma of the prostate. Arch Pathol Lab Med. 136(4):418-25, 2012
10. Robinson BD et al: Intraductal carcinoma of the prostate without invasive carcinoma on needle biopsy: emphasis on radical prostatectomy findings. J Urol. 184(4):1328-33, 2010
11. Cohen RJ et al: A proposal on the identification, histologic reporting, and implications of intraductal prostatic carcinoma. Arch Pathol Lab Med. 131(7):1103-9, 2007
12. Guo CC et al: Intraductal carcinoma of the prostate on needle biopsy: Histologic features and clinical significance. Mod Pathol. 19(12):1528-35, 2006
13. Dawkins HJ et al: Distinction between intraductal carcinoma of the prostate (IDC-P), high-grade dysplasia (PIN), and invasive prostatic adenocarcinoma, using molecular markers of cancer progression. Prostate. 44(4):265-70, 2000

Intraductal Carcinoma

Intraductal Carcinoma of Prostate: Partial Duct Involvement

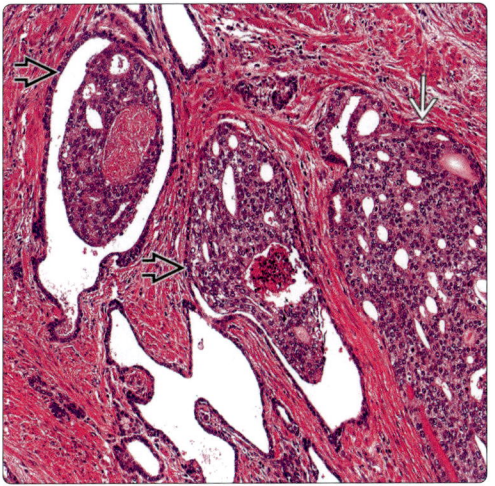

Intraductal Carcinoma of Prostate: Adjacent Invasive Carcinoma

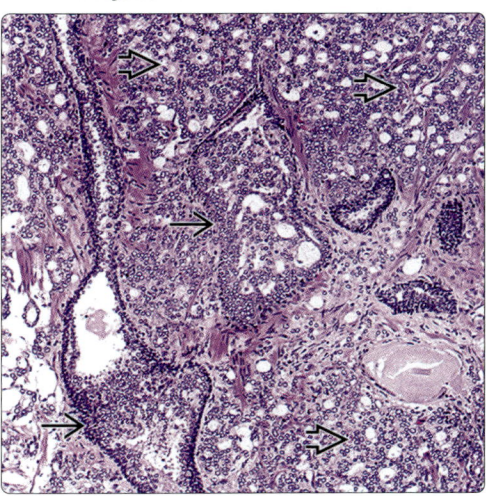

(Left) In this photomicrograph, in addition to the duct that is filled by carcinoma ➡, there are multiple ducts that are partially involved by tumor spread into the duct lumen ➡, leaving parts of the ducts uninvolved. (Right) There is invasive high-grade carcinoma ➡ adjacent to and surrounding areas of intraductal proliferation, spanning the entire lumen of the ducts ➡ with easily discernible basal cells, indicating intraductal growth or extension of carcinoma.

Intraductal Carcinoma of Prostate: Ductal and Acinar Involvement

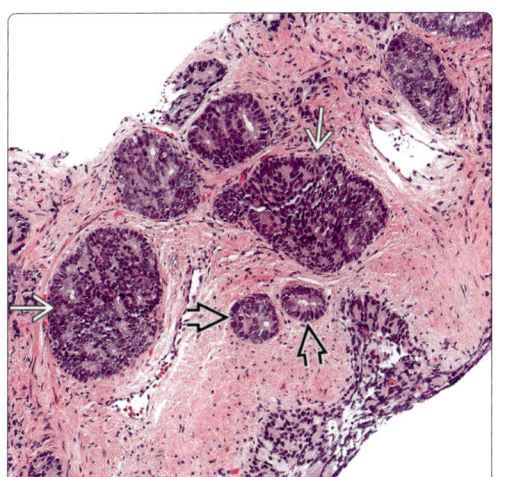

IDC-P: Ductal and Acinar Involvement (Immunostains)

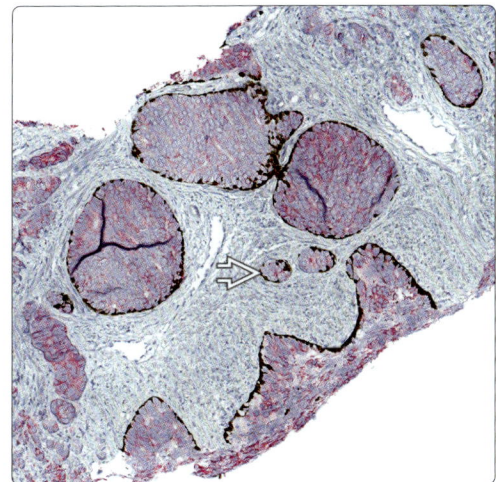

(Left) In this needle biopsy, the presence of expanded ducts with cribriform and solid tumor growth is evident ➡. There are adjacent smaller ducts with similar malignant features that are suggestive of invasive acinar adenocarcinoma ➡. (Right) Immunostain cocktail highlights the basal cells. In addition to the enlarged and expanded ducts, adjacent smaller acini ➡ retained a discontinuous basal cell layer, supporting the presence of both ductal and acinar involvement by IDC-P.

Intraductal Carcinoma of Prostate: Heterogeneous Tumor Cellularity

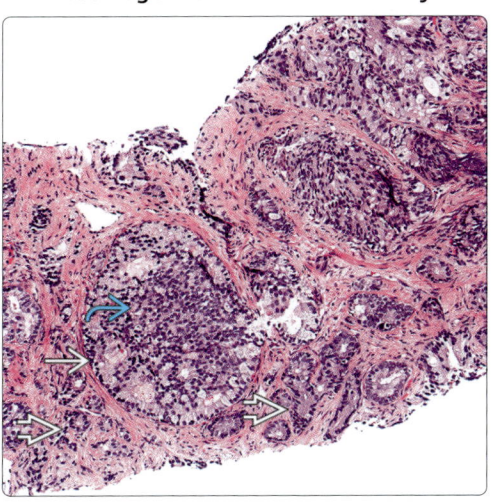

IDC-P: Ductal and Acinar Involvement (Immunostains)

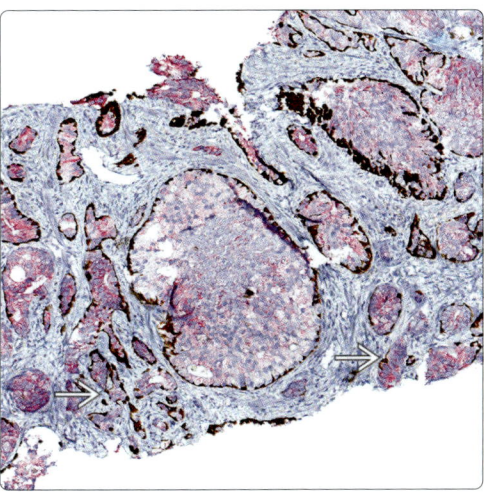

(Left) This IDC-P exhibits enlarged and expanded duct with columnar cells and more cytoplasm at the periphery ➡ and rounded cells with scant cytoplasm in the center ➡. Note the presence of smaller infiltrating glands indicative of invasive carcinoma ➡. (Right) By immunostain cocktail PIN4, the presence of basal cell layer is confirmed. Also, most of the small infiltrating glands adjacent to the expanded central gland retain a basal cell layer ➡, consistent with acinar involvement by IDC-P.

Intraductal Carcinoma

IDC-P and Invasive Prostatic Adenocarcinoma (Immunostain)

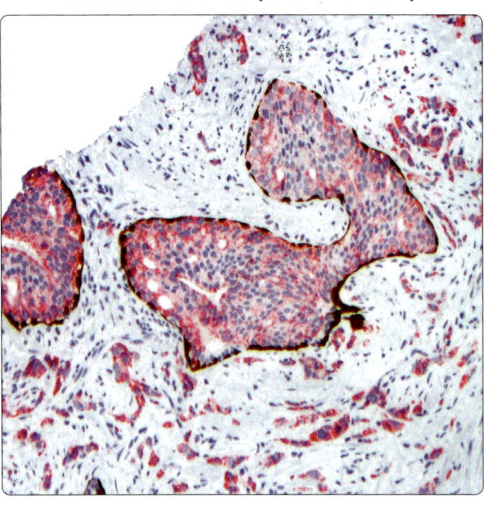

(Left) This section shows expanded and distorted ducts of IDC-P with angulation and branching, surrounded by numerous infiltrating glands of typical acinar adenocarcinoma. Basal cell markers highlight the intraductal component and confirm the presence of invasive tumor.

Intraductal Carcinoma of Prostate: Pleomorphism and Mitoses

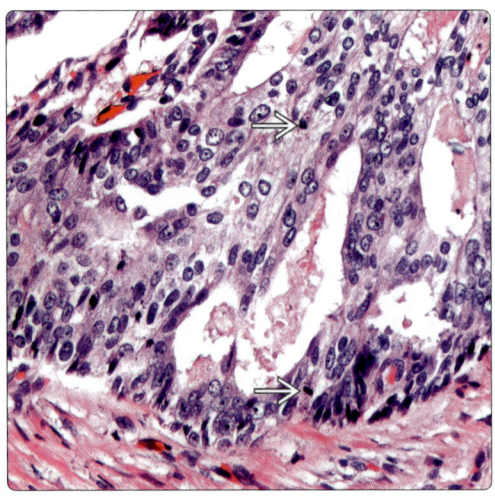

(Right) This section from an IDC-P is characterized by nuclear atypia and pleomorphism. It also features multiple mitotic figures throughout multiple layers of the tumor ➡, which is characteristic of IDC-P.

Intraductal Carcinoma of Prostate: Prominent Basal Cells

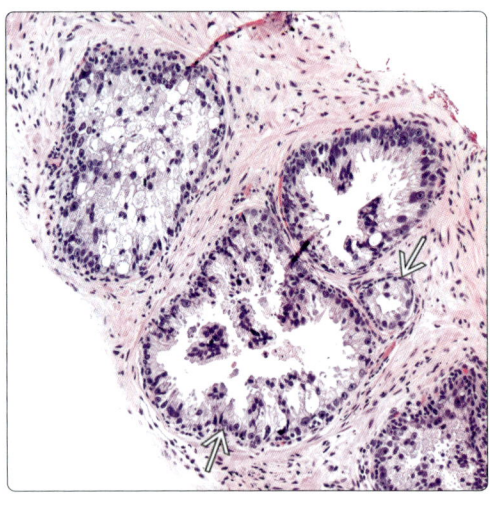

(Left) There is a prominent basal cell layer ➡ at the periphery of glands that contain highly atypical malignant cells with pleomorphism and prominent nucleoli. Additionally, the enlarged ducts exhibit solid, cribriform, and papillary growth patterns, typical for IDC-P.

Intraductal Carcinoma of Prostate: Prominent Basal Cells (Immunostain)

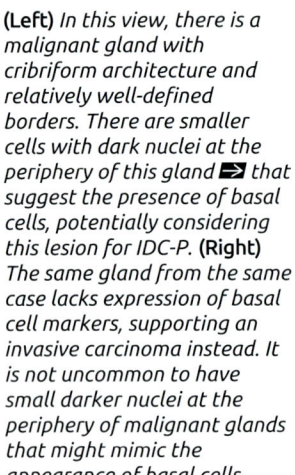

(Right) The presence of basal cells in this section was further confirmed by immunostain cocktail PIN4; AMACR is overexpressed throughout the tumor. Distinction from high-grade prostatic intraepithelial neoplasia can be hard.

Invasive Adenocarcinoma With Cribriform Architecture

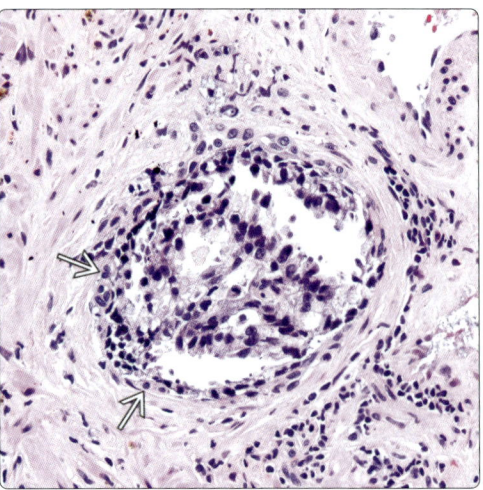

(Left) In this view, there is a malignant gland with cribriform architecture and relatively well-defined borders. There are smaller cells with dark nuclei at the periphery of this gland ➡ that suggest the presence of basal cells, potentially considering this lesion for IDC-P.

Invasive Prostatic Adenocarcinoma (Immunostain)

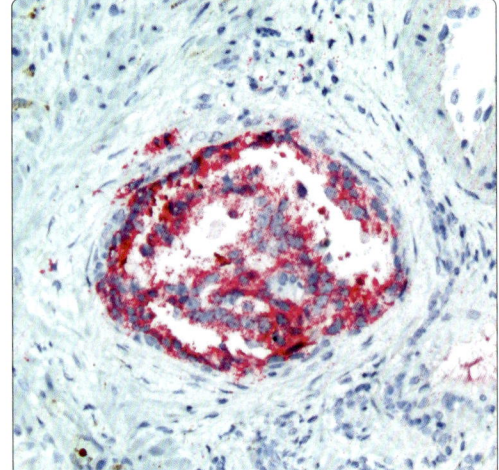

(Right) The same gland from the same case lacks expression of basal cell markers, supporting an invasive carcinoma instead. It is not uncommon to have small darker nuclei at the periphery of malignant glands that might mimic the appearance of basal cells.

Intraductal Carcinoma

Intraductal Carcinoma of Prostate: Adjacent HGPIN

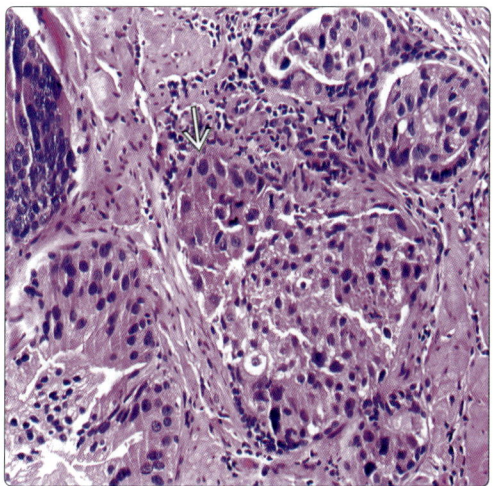

Intraductal Carcinoma of Prostate: Loss of PTEN Expression

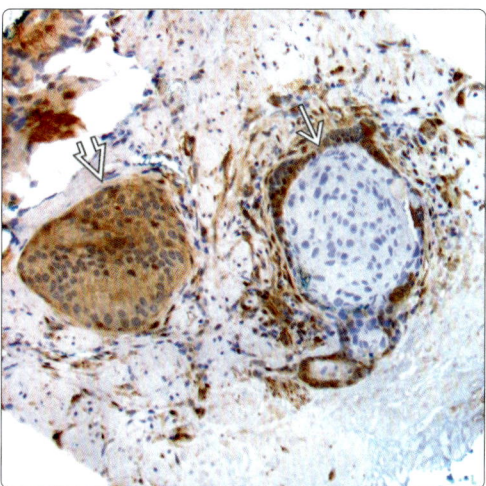

(Left) In this field, there is a focus of IDC-P ➡ with the typical features of nuclear atypia and pleomorphism with solid growth and possible necrosis. There is partial gland involvement as well (top right). (Right) The focus of IDC-P ➡ identified in the same case exhibits complete loss of cytoplasmic expression of PTEN. Note PTEN expression retained in the adjacent gland that does not contain IDC-P ➡ as well as the basal cells surrounding the IDC-P.

High-Grade Prostatic Intraepithelial Neoplasia

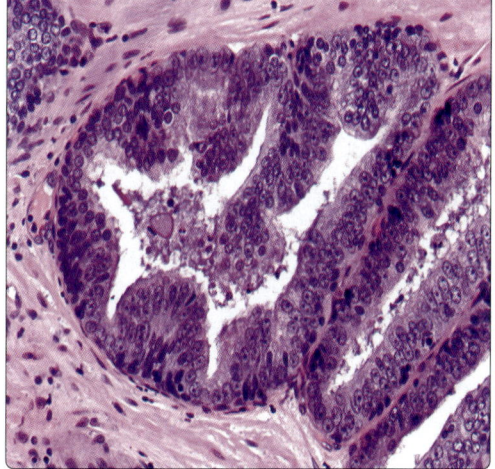

Ductal Adenocarcinoma of Prostate

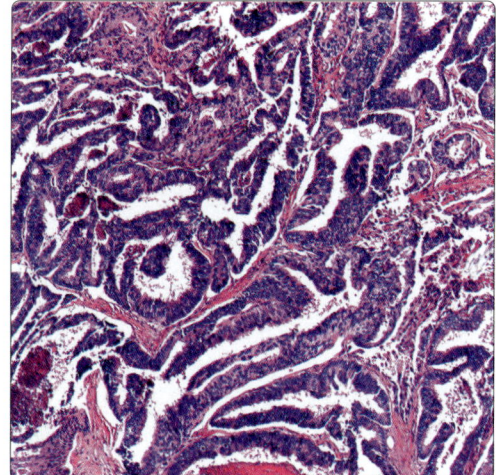

(Left) One of the main differential diagnoses with IDC-P is HGPIN, depicted here. Unlike IDC-P, the gland here is not expanded and has a smooth contour, and the nuclei are more uniform and rounded with prominent nucleoli, with no cribriform architecture or comedonecrosis. (Right) In this other differential diagnosis with IDC-P, prostatic ductal adenocarcinoma, the tumor exhibits prominent papillary morphology. There is marked branching and obvious nuclear stratification, and the nuclei are typically more oval.

Invasive Prostatic Adenocarcinoma With Cribriform Features

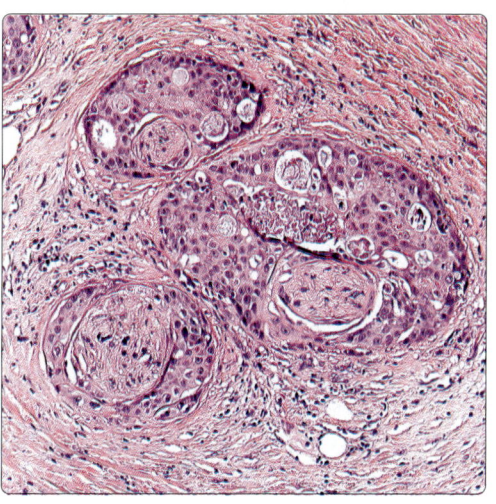

Urothelial Carcinoma Involving Prostatic Ducts

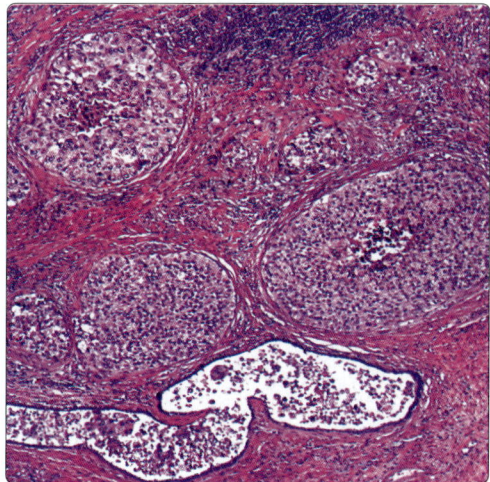

(Left) In some instances, an acinar adenocarcinoma may take the shape of expanded glands with cribriform morphology, but the obvious perineural invasion negates the presence of IDC-P, particularly when it is located outside the confines of the prostate, as in this case. (Right) Another differential diagnosis with IDC-P is urothelial carcinoma that extended into prostatic ducts, as depicted in the photomicrograph. Here, tumor cells have more eosinophilic cytoplasm and may be more pleomorphic.

Ductal Adenocarcinoma

KEY FACTS

TERMINOLOGY

- Adenocarcinoma of prostatic epithelial cell origin with large glandular and papillary architecture lined by tall columnar cells, often with pseudostratified growth
- Must comprise predominant (> 80%) or pure histology in radical prostatectomy or transurethral resection of prostate (TURP)
  - Diagnosis not tenable in needle biopsy (adenocarcinoma of prostate with ductal features)

CLINICAL ISSUES

- Pure ductal adenocarcinoma accounts for 0.2-1.3% of all prostate cancers
- Mixed ductal and acinar adenocarcinoma reported in 1.7%-5% of prostate cancers
- Majority of patients have elevated serum PSA level; 2.4x likely to have PSA < 4 ng/mL than acinar adenocarcinoma
- Most studies suggest more aggressive clinical behavior than acinar adenocarcinoma

MACROSCOPIC

- Centrally located tumors can have exophytic friable fronds protruding in urethral lumen
- Peripheral tumors are more often posteriorly situated as firm, gray-white parenchymal mass

MICROSCOPIC

- Main architectural patterns: Papillary, cribriform, individual glands (PIN-like), solid
- Tall columnar cells in single or pseudostratified growth pattern; frequent mitosis
- Cytoplasm usually amphophilic and nucleus oblongated with usually prominent nucleolus
- Can grow intraluminally into preexisting ducts retaining native basal cell layer
- Majority has no detectable basal cells by p63 or HMCK (34βE12)
- Recommends grading as Gleason grade 4 except if necrosis is present (grade 5)

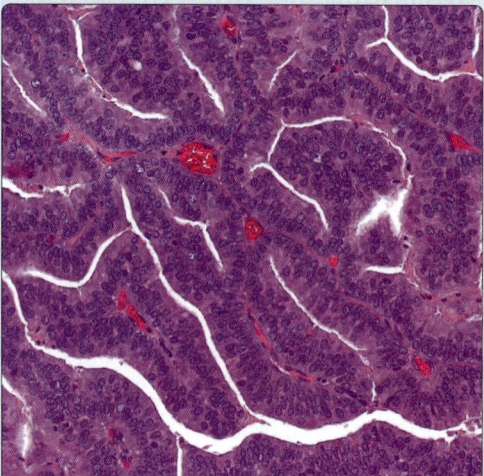

Ductal Adenocarcinoma, Papillary Pattern

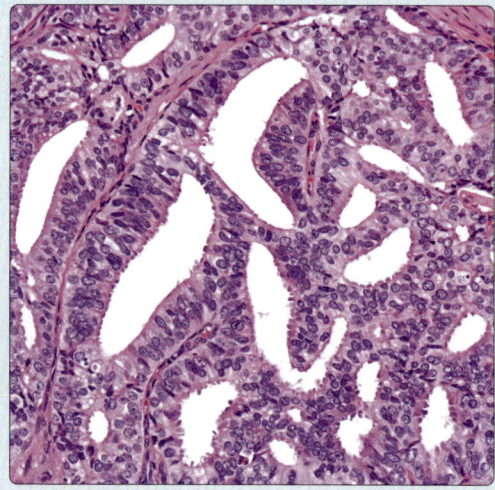

Ductal Adenocarcinoma, Cribriform Pattern

(Left) This ductal adenocarcinoma exhibits papillary architectures lined by tall columnar cells exhibiting pseudostratification. This is the most distinctive pattern of ductal adenocarcinoma. The papillae show a central, delicate fibrovascular core. The tumor cells typically have elongated nuclei and prominent nucleoli. (Right) Ductal adenocarcinoma, cribriform pattern, shows multiple luminal spaces and bridges lined by tall columnar cells. Ductal adenocarcinoma without necrosis are graded as Gleason pattern 4.

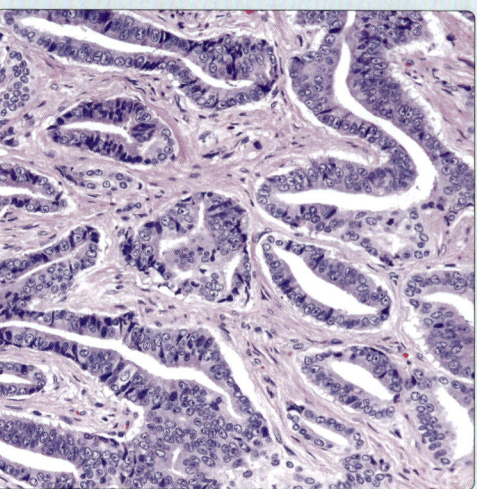

Ductal Adenocarcinoma, Individual Glands

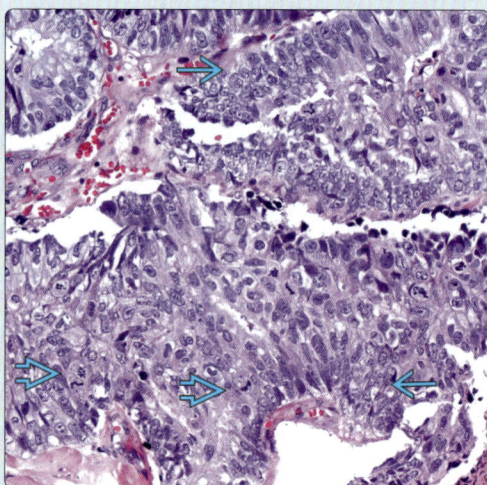

Ductal Adenocarcinoma, Solid Pattern

(Left) This ductal adenocarcinoma consists of glands lined by tall columnar cells with pseudostratification. This rare pattern of ductal adenocarcinoma may resemble high-grade PIN and may necessitate IHC for distinction. (Right) Solid pattern of ductal adenocarcinoma is rare. In this case, the tall pseudostratified columnar cells are most recognizable at the periphery of the solid nests ➡. Note the high-grade nuclei and brisk mitotic activity ➡.

Ductal Adenocarcinoma

TERMINOLOGY

Synonyms
- Prostatic duct adenocarcinoma
- Endometrioid carcinoma of prostate (outdated term)

Definitions
- Adenocarcinoma of prostatic epithelial cell origin with large glandular and papillary architecture lined by tall columnar cells, often with pseudostratified growth
- Features comprising predominant (> 80%) or pure histology of carcinoma in transurethral resection of prostate (TURP) or radical prostatectomy
- Occurs either as pure ductal adenocarcinoma or, more commonly, in combination with acinar adenocarcinoma in microscopy

ETIOLOGY/PATHOGENESIS

Origin
- Prostatic glandular epithelial cell origin
- Previously postulated to arise from müllerian-derived prostatic utricle due to its morphologic resemblance to adenocarcinoma of endometrium

CLINICAL ISSUES

Epidemiology
- Incidence
  - Pure ductal adenocarcinoma accounts for 0.2-1.3% of all prostate cancers
  - Mixed ductal and acinar adenocarcinoma reported in 1.7%-5% of prostate cancers
  - Contemporary studies report 0.5% to 12.7% ductal component in prostate cancers
- Age
  - Mean: 63-72 years; range: 41-89 years; similar to acinar adenocarcinoma

Site
- May be central &/or peripheral in location
- Central tumors occur in periurethral area and involve transition zone and TURP specimens
- Peripheral tumors involve prostate peripheral zone and can extend to transition zone

Presentation
- Central/periurethral tumors: Obstructive symptoms, hematuria
- Peripherally located tumors: Abnormal digital rectal examination, elevated serum PSA levels
- Bone metastasis are osteoblastic

Laboratory Tests
- Majority of patients have elevated serum PSA level, but 2.4x likely to have PSA < 4 ng/mL than acinar adenocarcinoma

Treatment
- Reported response to treatment options for prostate acinar adenocarcinoma, including hormonal manipulation

Prognosis
- Data suggests that tumors are more aggressive than acinar adenocarcinoma; SEER data suggests similar behavior to Gleason 4 + 4 acinar adenocarcinoma
  - Overall 5-year survival rate of 15-24% in older series
- Presence in biopsies indicate more advanced cancer at prostatectomy and shortened progression time than Gleason 7 or less acinar adenocarcinoma
- Extraprostatic extension and seminal vesicle involvement seen in 63% and 10% of prostatectomy specimens, respectively
- Metastasis in 12-50% of cases, mostly to lymph nodes, bones and lungs

MACROSCOPIC

General Features
- Centrally located tumors
  - Can have exophytic friable fronds protruding in urethral lumen around prostatic utricle or verumontanum
  - Cystoscopic visualization possible
- Peripherally located tumors
  - More often posteriorly situated
  - Firm, gray-white parenchymal mass, similar to acinar adenocarcinoma

MICROSCOPIC

Histologic Features
- Main architectural patterns
  - Papillary, cribriform, individual glands (PIN-like), solid
- Papillary and cribriform patterns seen in 65% and 59% of peripherally situated ductal adenocarcinoma, respectively
- > 1 architectural pattern is typical; combination of papillary and cribriform patterns seen in 36% of tumors
- Papillary tumors are often centrally located
- Peripheral tumors are often papillary and cribriform
- Neoplastic cells
  - Tall columnar cells
  - Single or pseudostratified cell layer
  - Cytoplasm usually amphophilic but can be pale or clear
  - Nucleus typically elongated
  - Usually prominent nucleolus
  - Occasional to frequent mitoses present
  - Greater degree of chromatin irregularities compared to usual acinar prostate adenocarcinoma
- Can grow intraluminally into preexisting ducts retaining native basal cell layer
  - Invasive component must be present to be diagnosed as ductal adenocarcinoma
  - Negativity for basal cell marker immunohistochemistry is a must in invasive component
- Glands can be very large, expansile, and crowded back to back
- Background stromal fibrosis often present
- Perineural invasion may be seen
- Almost 1/2 admixed with acinar adenocarcinoma
- Concomitant acinar adenocarcinoma usually microacinar Gleason pattern 3, seen in 48% of tumors

Ductal Adenocarcinoma

- Rare patterns include cystic, foamy gland, mucinous with goblet cells, micropapillary and associated with Paneth cell-like neuroendocrine

Predominant Pattern/Injury Type
- Neoplastic

Predominant Cell/Compartment Type
- Epithelial, glandular

Genetics
- *TMPRSS2-ERG* gene fusion
  - Less frequent in pure ductal adenocarcinoma (11%) and mixed ductal acinar adenocarcinoma (5%) than pure acinar adenocarcinoma (45%)
  - When present, mostly through deletion
- 1 study of ductal and acinar adenocarcinomas show striking similarities with only 25 gene transcripts deferentially expressed
  - Prolactin receptor expressed 5-27 fold in ductal adenocarcinoma
- *SPINK1*, which is suggested to be unfavorable clinical parameter, is overexpressed in 22% of ETS fusion-negative ductal adenocarcinoma

ANCILLARY TESTS

Immunohistochemistry
- Positive for PSA and PAP
- Positive for AMACR in 77% of cases
- Majority lacks basal cell layer
  - Negative for p63 or HMCK (34βE12)
  - 31% have detectable basal cells by p63 or HMCK (34βE12), staining in patchy discontinuous or continuous distribution (intraductal growth)

DIFFERENTIAL DIAGNOSIS

High-Grade Prostatic Intraepithelial Neoplasia
- Micropapillary, cribriform, and flat high-grade prostatic intraepithelial neoplasia (HGPIN) can mimic ductal adenocarcinomas due to overlap in architecture
- Distinction can be very difficult in limited samples
- Typically lacks predominance of tall columnar cells
- Lacks expansile large glandular growth pattern
- No invasive features such as crowded back-to-back glands, stromal fibrosis, or perineural invasion
- Micropapillary HGPIN cellular fronds lack true fibrovascular core
- Occasionally, cells at center of cribriform HGPIN glands tend to have lower grade nuclei (maturation)
- Consistently contains basal cell layer highlighted by basal cell markers, such as p63 or HMCK(34βE12)

Cribriform Hyperplasia
- Unusual form of benign prostatic hyperplasia composed of crowded cribriform glands
- Nodular pattern of growth
- Composed of cells with uniformly bland cytology, often with clear cytoplasm and absent nucleoli
- Contains basal cell layer

Cribriform Gleason Pattern 4 and 5 Acinar Adenocarcinoma
- Overlap and continuum of ductal adenocarcinoma and cribriform acinar carcinoma
- Similar to ductal adenocarcinoma, shows invasive features, including large expansile growth and glandular crowding
- Morphologic definition limited to invasive large cribriform glands lacking true papillary component and tall columnar cells

Prostatic Urethral Polyp
- Reactive papillary lesions growing along urethra lined by cuboidal to columnar prostatic acinar cells
- More commonly seen in younger patients
- Bland cytology

DIAGNOSTIC CHECKLIST

Pathologic Interpretation Pearls
- Presence of large prostatic glandular proliferations lined by pseudostratified tall columnar cells generally lacking basal cells and showing invasive features
- High-grade tumor morphology compared to acinar adenocarcinoma

GRADING

Criteria
- Ductal adenocarcinoma must be graded as Gleason score 4 + 4 = 8
- If solid nests or necrosis are present, upgraded to 5
- In mixed ductal and acinar adenocarcinoma, ductal component to be assigned with
- Retain diagnostic term when grading, i.e., ductal adenocarcinoma (Gleason score 4 + 4 = 8), prognostic grade group 4

SELECTED REFERENCES

1. Meeks JJ et al: Incidence and outcomes of ductal carcinoma of the prostate in the USA: analysis of data from the Surveillance, Epidemiology, and End Results program. BJU Int. 109(6):831-4, 2012
2. Amin A et al: Pathologic stage of prostatic ductal adenocarcinoma at radical prostatectomy: effect of percentage of the ductal component and associated grade of acinar adenocarcinoma. Am J Surg Pathol. 35(4):615-9, 2011
3. Lee TK et al: Rare histological patterns of prostatic ductal adenocarcinoma. Pathology. 42(4):319-24, 2010
4. Morgan TM et al: Ductal adenocarcinoma of the prostate: increased mortality risk and decreased serum prostate specific antigen. J Urol. 184(6):2303-7, 2010
5. Samaratunga H et al: Any proportion of ductal adenocarcinoma in radical prostatectomy specimens predicts extraprostatic extension. Hum Pathol. 41(2):281-5, 2010
6. Lotan TL et al: TMPRSS2-ERG gene fusions are infrequent in prostatic ductal adenocarcinomas. Mod Pathol. 22(3):359-65, 2009
7. Herawi M et al: Immunohistochemical antibody cocktail staining (p63/HMWCK/AMACR) of ductal adenocarcinoma and Gleason pattern 4 cribriform and noncribriform acinar adenocarcinomas of the prostate. Am J Surg Pathol. 31(6):889-94, 2007
8. Bock BJ et al: Does prostatic ductal adenocarcinoma exist? Am J Surg Pathol. 23(7):781-5, 1999
9. Brinker DA et al: Ductal adenocarcinoma of the prostate diagnosed on needle biopsy: correlation with clinical and radical prostatectomy findings and progression. Am J Surg Pathol. 23(12):1471-9, 1999

Ductal Adenocarcinoma

Ductal Adenocarcinoma
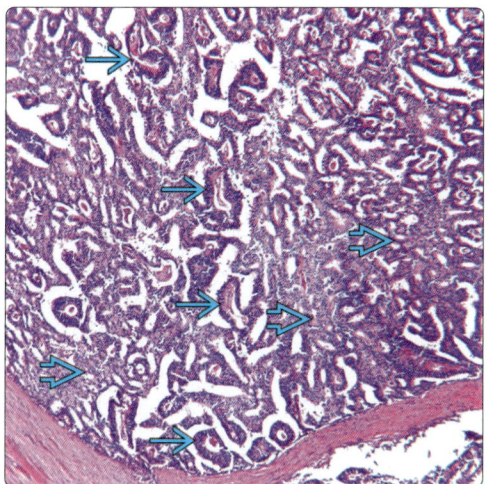

Ductal Adenocarcinoma, Papillary Pattern
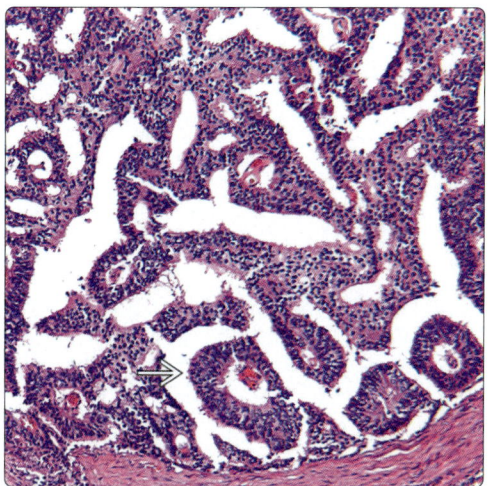

(Left) Ductal adenocarcinoma shows numerous papillae containing a fibrovascular core ➡ (true papillae). Part of this tumor consists of cribriform architecture ➡. Admixture of papillary and cribriform patterns is common in ductal adenocarcinoma. **(Right)** Ductal adenocarcinoma, papillary pattern, shows distinctive papillary architecture with a fibrovascular core lined by pseudostratified tall columnar cells ➡. The nuclei appears crowded and dark on low-power magnification.

Ductal Adenocarcinoma, Papillary Pattern
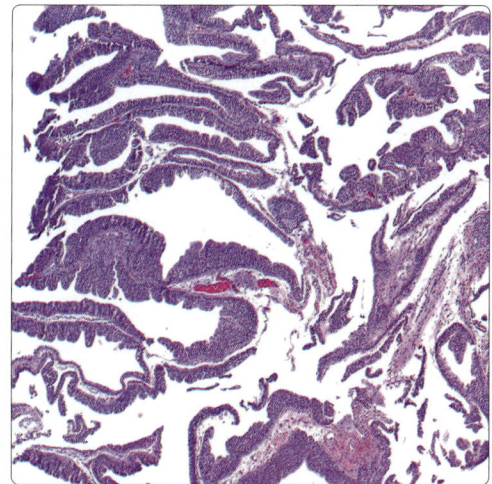

Ductal Adenocarcinoma, Papillary Pattern
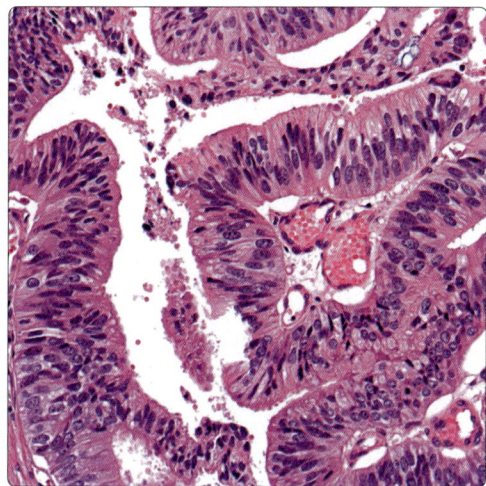

(Left) Ductal adenocarcinoma, papillary pattern, encountered in a TURP specimen shows multiple papillary fragments lined by tall columnar cells. Papillary architecture is relatively more common in tumors that arise in the central region of the prostate. **(Right)** Ductal adenocarcinoma, papillary pattern, shows a cell lining composed of tall columnar cells with pale cytoplasm and elongated nuclei, exhibiting pseudostratification. Presence of a tall columnar cell lining is a distinguishing feature of ductal adenocarcinoma.

Ductal Adenocarcinoma, Papillary Pattern
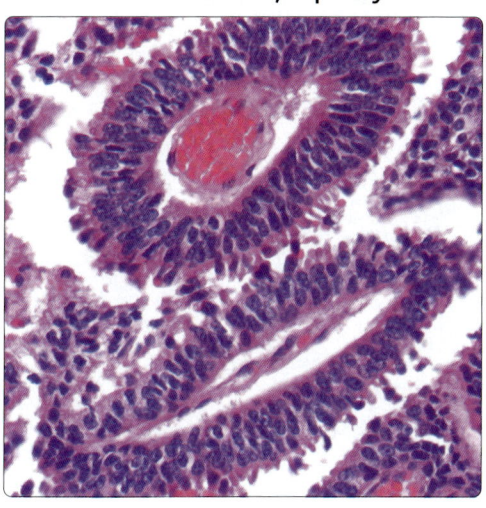

Ductal Adenocarcinoma, Papillary Pattern
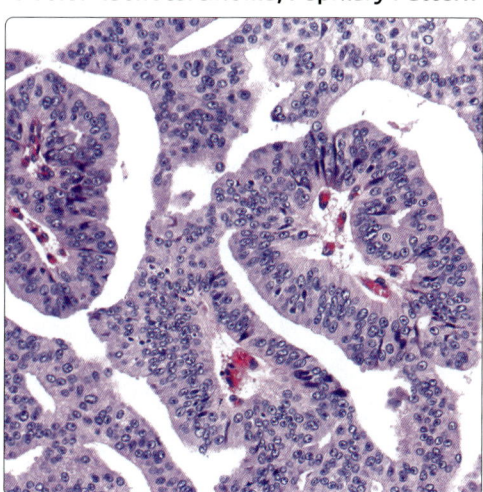

(Left) High-power magnification of ductal adenocarcinoma, papillary pattern, shows nuclei with dense irregular chromatin and occasional prominent nucleoli. Ductal adenocarcinoma nuclei are typically of higher grade compared to conventional prostate adenocarcinoma. **(Right)** This ductal adenocarcinoma shows layers of nuclei that are overlapping, enlarged, ovoid, and with prominent nucleoli. Higher grade nuclei is typical for ductal adenocarcinoma and is common for all the different ductal patterns.

Ductal Adenocarcinoma

(Left) Ductal adenocarcinoma, cribriform pattern, shows large glands with cribriform architecture imparting multiple lumina lined by pseudostratified tall columnar cells. **(Right)** Low-power magnification of ductal adenocarcinoma, cribriform pattern, in a prostatectomy specimen shows large glands containing multiple lumina separated by cell bridges. Note the presence of comedonecrosis ➡, which indicates Gleason grade 5 carcinoma. Central necrosis must show necrotic tumor cells (ghost cells).

Ductal Adenocarcinoma, Cribriform Pattern

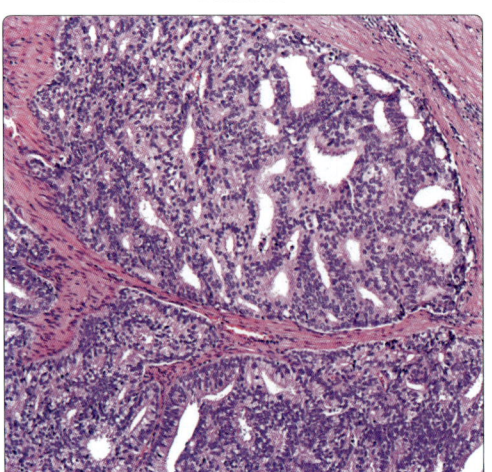

Ductal Adenocarcinoma, Comedonecrosis

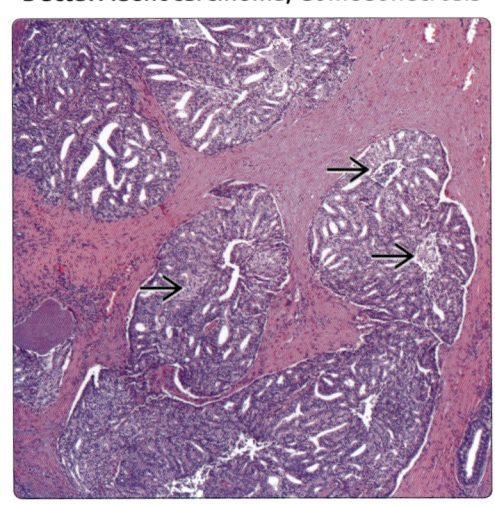

(Left) Ductal adenocarcinoma, cribriform pattern, shows pseudostratified hyperchromatic nuclei. In contrast, cribriform HGPIN lacks large expansile growth, back-to-back glands, and contains basal cell layer that can be confirmed immunohistochemically. **(Right)** Ductal adenocarcinoma, cribriform pattern, shows peripheral lumina lined by tall columnar cells with pale eosinophilic cytoplasm. In contrast, cribriform acinar adenocarcinoma are lined by nontall columnar cells.

Ductal Adenocarcinoma, Pseudostratification

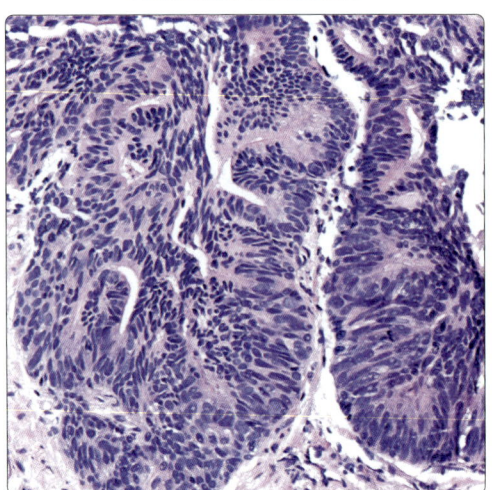

Irregular Cribriform Gland

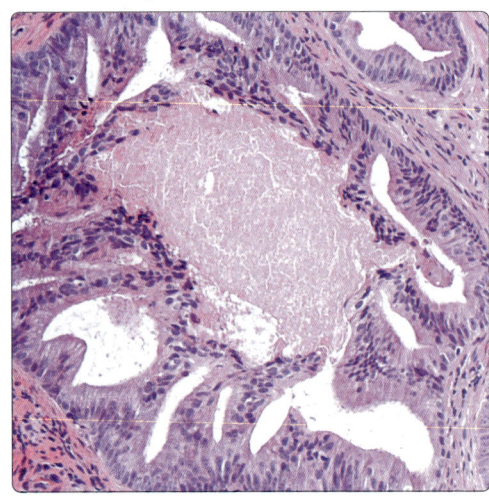

(Left) Ductal adenocarcinoma, cribriform pattern, shows large glands with multiple lumina containing tall columnar cells, some exhibiting atypical nuclear rounding. **(Right)** High-power view of ductal adenocarcinoma, cribriform pattern, shows tall columnar cells with pale cytoplasm and high-grade, oval to elongated nuclei. In contrast, cribriform acinar adenocarcinoma is composed of nontall columnar cells with rounder nuclei of a relatively lower grade. Mitotic activity is less frequent.

Ductal Adenocarcinoma, Pseudostratification

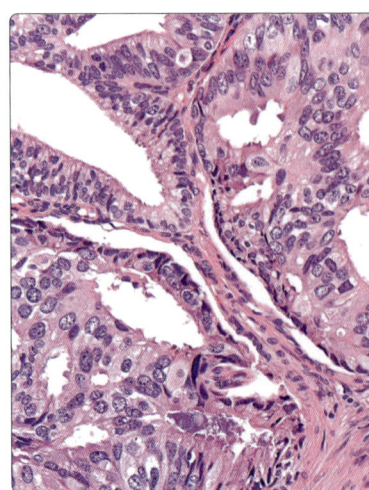

Ductal Adenocarcinoma, Tall Columnar Cells

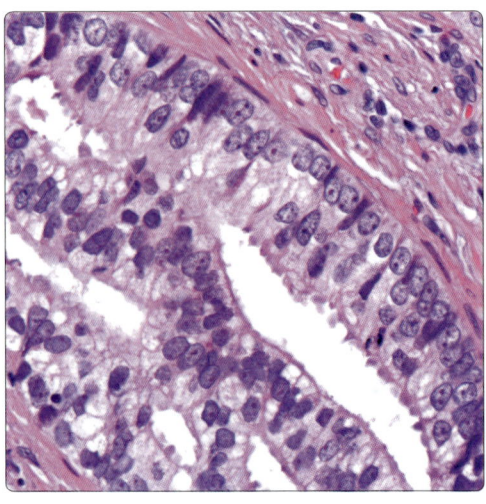

Ductal Adenocarcinoma

Ductal Adenocarcinoma, Individual Glands

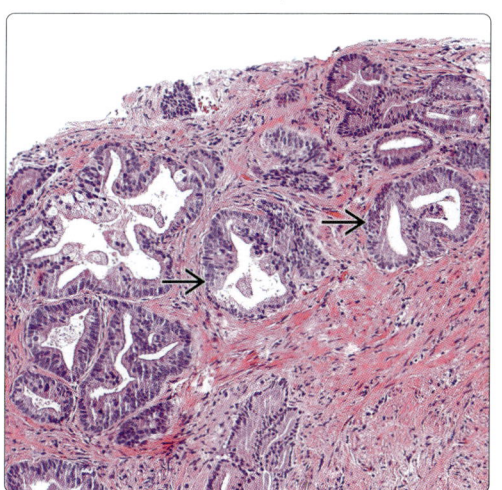

Ductal Adenocarcinoma, Solid Pattern

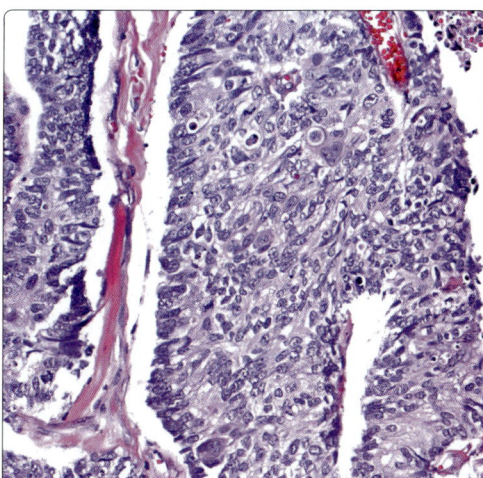

(Left) Ductal adenocarcinoma, individual glands pattern ⇒, shows well-formed glands lined predominantly by a single layer of tall columnar cells. The tall columnar cell lining distinguishes these glands from microacinar adenocarcinoma glands and absence of basal cell layer from flat HGPIN, aided by immunohistochemistry. **(Right)** Ductal adenocarcinoma, solid growth pattern, shows solid nests of columnar cells with crowded elongated nuclei, some with palisaded growth. Solid growth indicates Gleason pattern 5.

Ductal Adenocarcinoma With Necrosis

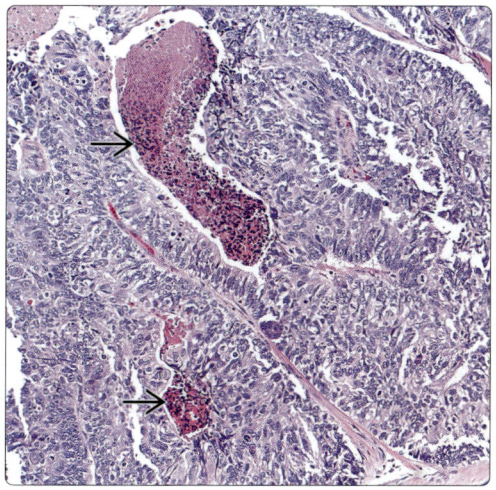

Ductal Adenocarcinoma With Necrosis

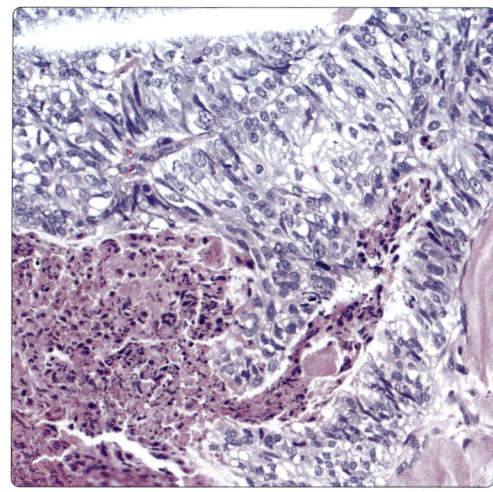

(Left) Ductal adenocarcinoma shows large cribriform and solid glands containing tall columnar cells and contains comedonecrosis ⇒. **(Right)** High-power view of ductal adenocarcinoma with comedonecrosis is characterized by luminal collection of necrotic ghost cells and nuclear debris. Presence of comedonecrosis warrants designation of Gleason pattern 5 for these glands. Without necrosis, this ductal adenocarcinoma should be designated as Gleason pattern 4.

Ductal Adenocarcinoma in Transurethral Resection

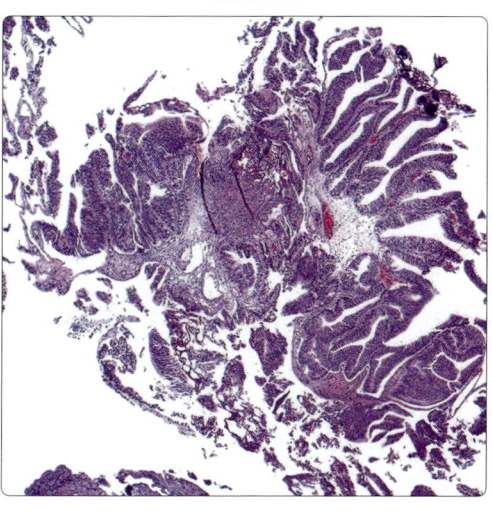

Ductal Adenocarcinoma in Needle Biopsy

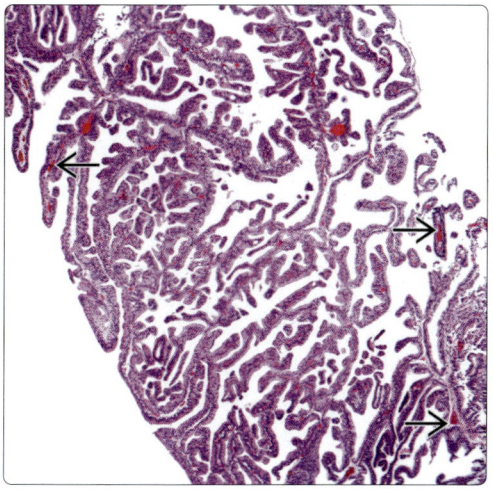

(Left) TUR of urethral mass shows ductal adenocarcinoma with mainly papillary pattern. The tumor may protrude along the verumontanum and can be visualized cystoscopically as a urethral polyp. **(Right)** Adenocarcinoma with ductal features, papillary pattern, in a needle biopsy shows multiple papillae with fibrovascular cores ⇒. In contrast to micropapillary high-grade PIN, these glands are large with expansile growth and papillae contains fibrovascular core. Ductal adenocarcinoma diagnosis is not tenable in needle biopsy.

Ductal Adenocarcinoma

Mixed Ductal and Acinar Adenocarcinoma

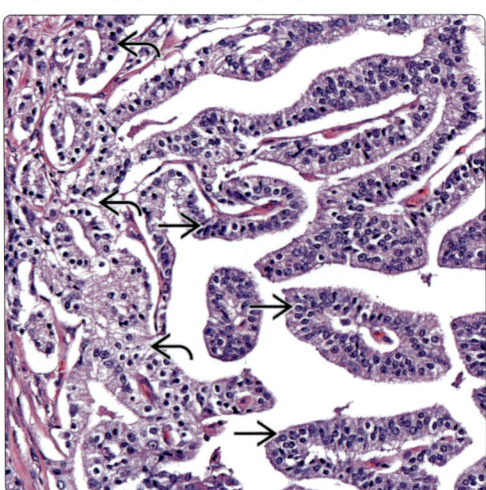

Mixed Ductal and Acinar Adenocarcinoma

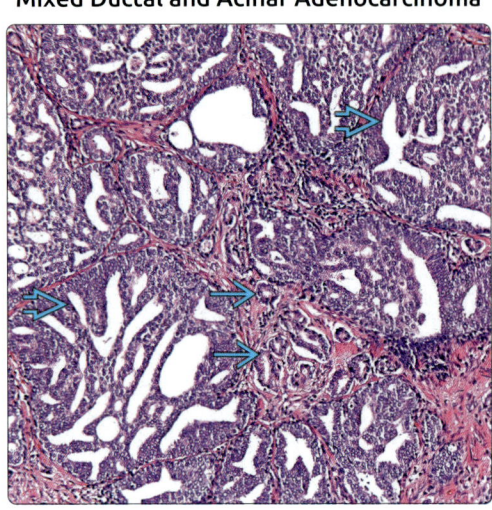

(Left) Mixed acinar (left side) and ductal (right side) adenocarcinoma shows that acinar adenocarcinoma cells are relatively more cuboidal ⇨, while ductal adenocarcinoma cells are taller and contain larger and more hyperchromatic nuclei ⇨. (Right) Mixed ductal and acinar adenocarcinoma shows acinar adenocarcinoma component consisting of individual Gleason 3 pattern glands ⇨ interspersed between larger cribriform glands of ductal adenocarcinoma ⇨.

Mixed Ductal and Acinar Adenocarcinoma

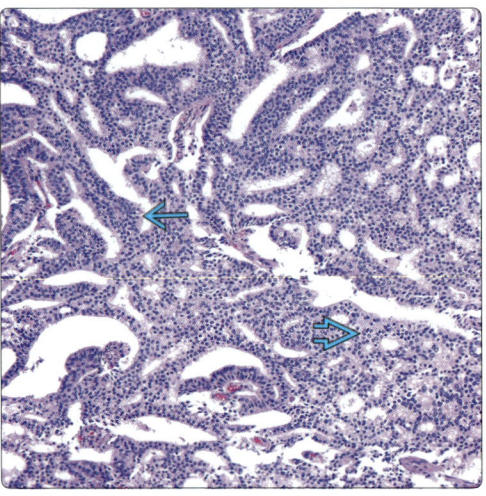

Mixed Ductal and Acinar Adenocarcinoma

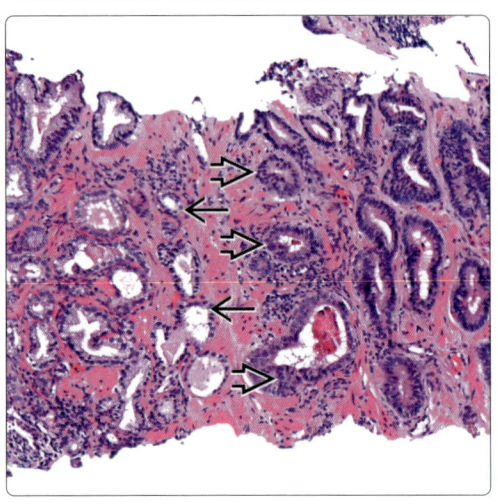

(Left) Low-power view shows the transition between ductal adenocarcinoma ⇨ and acinar adenocarcinoma ⇨. Approximately 1/2 of ductal adenocarcinomas are mixed with acinar adenocarcinoma. In prostatectomy specimens, > 80% ductal features are required for diagnosis of ductal adenocarcinoma. (Right) Adenocarcinoma with mixed acinar ⇨ and ductal ⇨ features in a needle biopsy shows individual glands of acinar adenocarcinoma and ductal adenocarcinoma lined by cuboidal and tall columnar cells, respectively.

Perineural Invasion by Ductal Adenocarcinoma

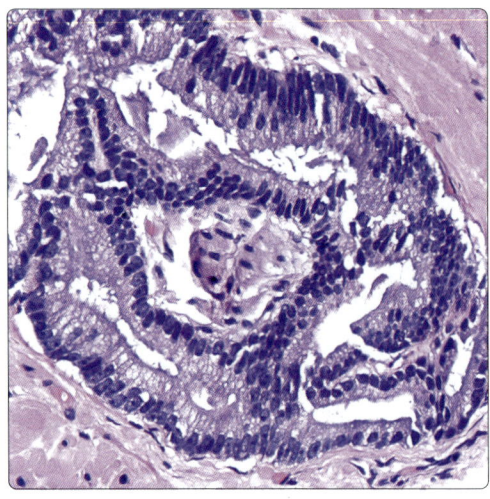

Extraprostatic Extension by Ductal Adenocarcinoma

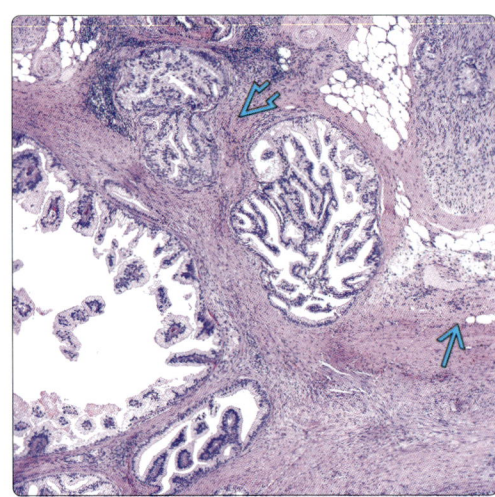

(Left) Ductal adenocarcinoma shows a cribriform gland of tall columnar cells with complete perineural invasion. (Right) Low-power view shows established (nonfocal) EPE by ductal adenocarcinoma. The tumor nests exhibiting papillary architecture are seen infiltrating beyond the plane of fat cells ⇨ and are seen within the loose connective tissue of the neurovascular bundle ⇨. Presence of ductal morphology in biopsy has higher risk for EPE on radical prostatectomy compared to acinar adenocarcinoma.

Ductal Adenocarcinoma

Ductal Adenocarcinoma With Treatment Effects

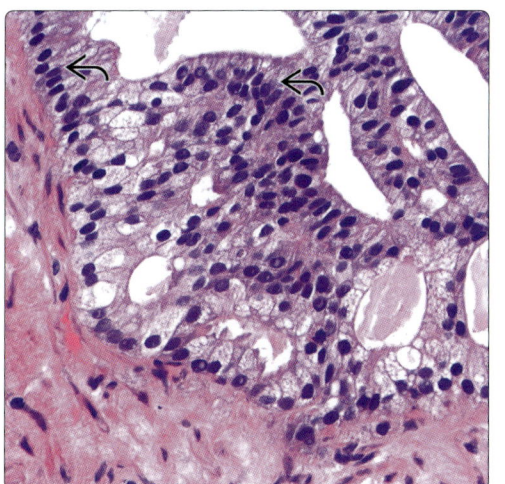

PIN4 in Ductal Adenocarcinoma

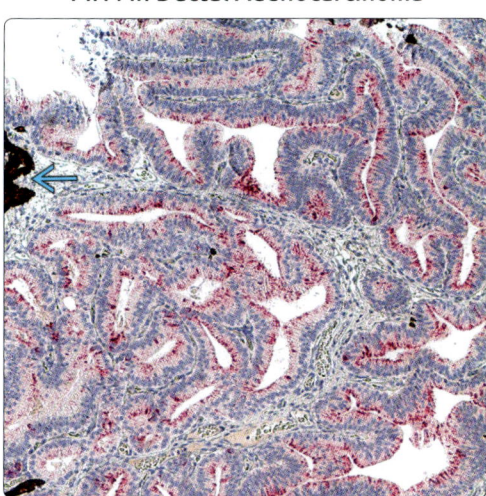

(Left) Ductal adenocarcinoma, cribriform pattern with radiation treatment effects, shows a foamy appearance of cytoplasm. The tall columnar and palisaded appearance can still be appreciated ➡. Data suggests that ductal adenocarcinoma has a more aggressive clinical behavior than acinar adenocarcinoma. (Right) PIN4 shows diffuse cytoplasmic expression of AMACR (red) and complete absence of basal cell marker staining (brown) in this ductal adenocarcinoma. Note the adjacent benign glands with basal cell staining (brown) ➡.

PIN4 in Ductal Adenocarcinoma

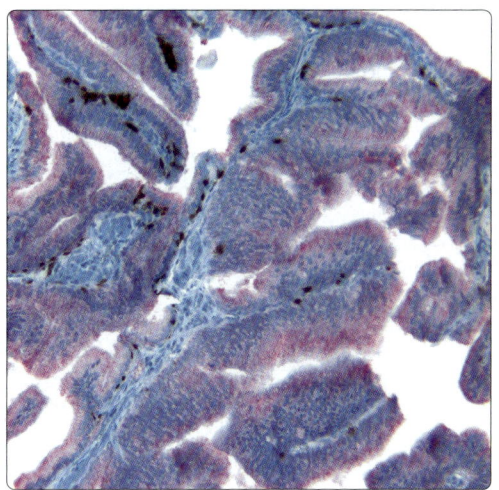

PSA in Ductal Adenocarcinoma

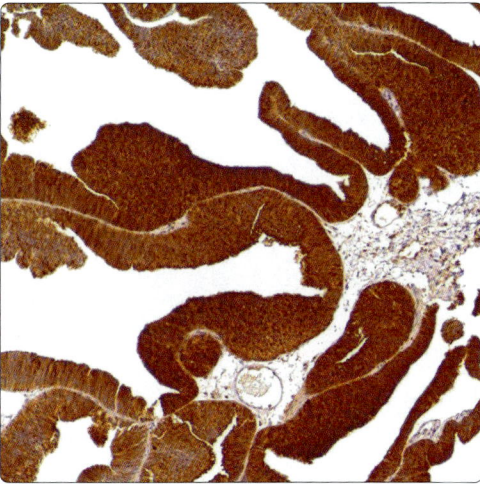

(Left) PIN4 shows diffuse cytoplasmic expression of AMACR (red) and some basal cell marker (brown) staining in this ductal adenocarcinoma. Focal basal cell staining may occur in ductal adenocarcinoma. (Right) Ductal adenocarcinoma, papillary pattern, shows diffuse PSA positivity. PSA is helpful in distinguishing ductal adenocarcinoma from other tumors with similar architecture, such as the rare seminal vesicle papillary adenocarcinoma, which is PSA(-) or in metastatic setting.

Ductal Adenocarcinoma in Biopsy

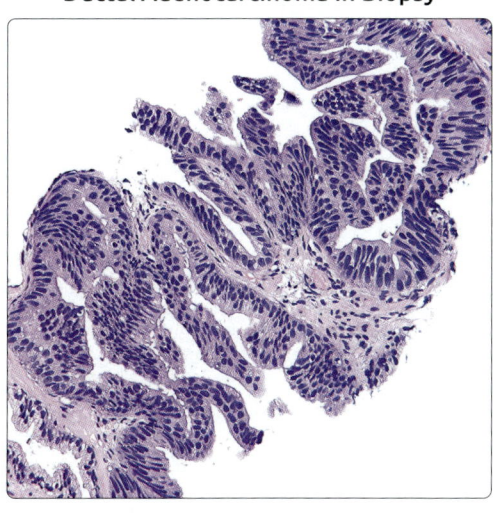

PIN 4 in Ductal Adenocarcinoma

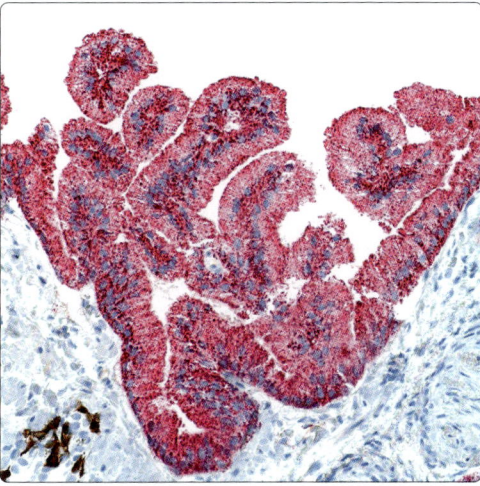

(Left) Adenocarcinoma of prostate with ductal features in a needle biopsy shows several large glands with high-grade nuclei. Distinction from high-grade PIN can be difficult and may necessitate use of IHC to confirm absence of basal cells. (Right) This focus of ductal adenocarcinoma in needle biopsy shows diffuse and strong cytoplasmic staining with AMACR (red) and with complete absence of basal cell markers (brown) staining. High-grade PIN will also show positivity for AMACR but with no basal cell marker reactivity.

Urothelial Carcinoma Involving Prostate Gland

KEY FACTS

CLASSIFICATION
- **Urothelial carcinoma (UC) of urinary bladder secondarily involving prostate** refers to urothelial carcinoma arising primarily in bladder but extending to involve prostatic urethra or prostatic glandular parenchyma by either direct invasion, intraepithelial pagetoid spread, or by combination of these processes
- **Primary UC of prostate** refers to either UC arising primarily in prostatic urethra or arising in more distal, suburethral ducts and glands of prostate itself

CLINICAL ISSUES
- **UC of urinary bladder secondarily involving prostate** is relatively more common, ranging from 12-58% at cystoprostatectomy
- **Primary UC of prostate** is uncommon, comprising 1-4% of prostate cancers in adults
- Similar in age distribution to bladder UC
- Bladder UC involving prostate presents due to bladder symptoms
- Most primary prostatic UCs present with obstructive symptoms
- Among primary UCs of prostate
  - Much superior prognosis for in situ lesions of urethra and periurethral ducts
  - Much inferior prognosis for lesions invasive of prostatic stroma
  - Prostatic stromal invasion associated with higher incidence of nodal metastasis
- Among UCs of bladder secondarily involving prostate
  - Survival rate substantially poorer for UC invading prostate transmurally or extravesically (pT4)
  - Survival rate substantially better for UC invading prostate stroma secondarily from intraurethral spread

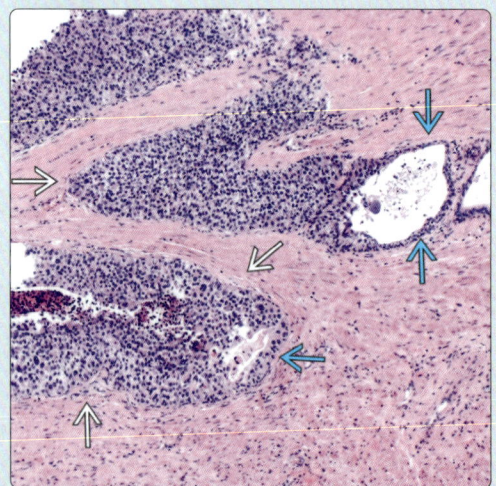

Urethral CIS Involving Prostatic Ducts

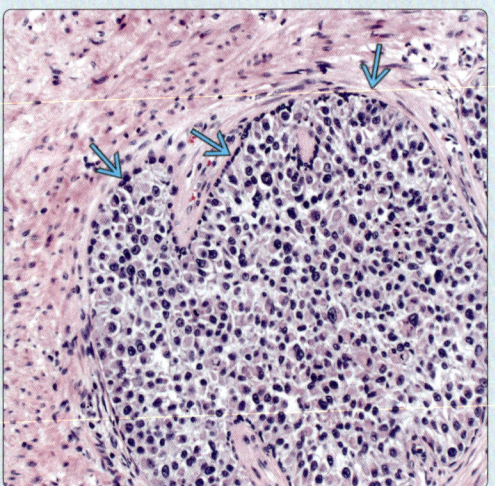

Urethral CIS Involving Prostatic Ducts

(Left) In this case, a bladder urothelial carcinoma (UC) has extended to involve the prostate in a pagetoid manner, with CIS involving prostatic ducts and acini. Rounded, dilated ducts ➡ do not show diagnostic features of invasion, and the preservation of lobular ductal architecture is confirmed by identification of as yet uninvolved areas ➡. (Right) Also helpful in confirming involvement of prostatic ducts by CIS is identification of a preserved, though often discontinuous, layer of basal cells ➡.

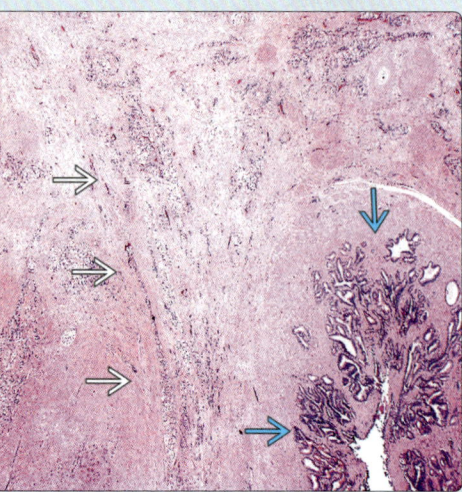

Primary UC of Prostate

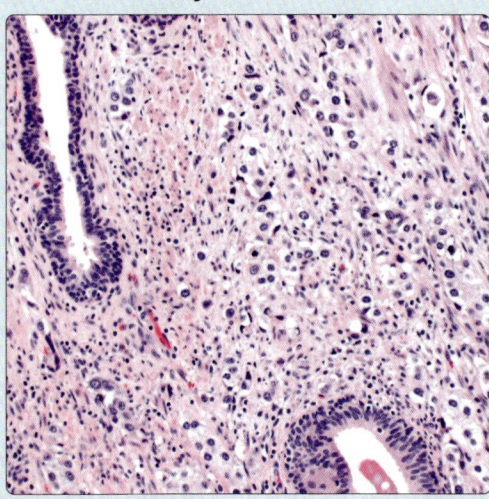

Primary UC of Prostate

(Left) In this case of primary UC of the prostate, which arose deep in suburethral prostatic ducts, diffusely invasive cords of carcinoma ➡ with desmoplastic stromal reaction are seen adjacent to ejaculatory duct ➡. (Right) Higher power view of the same case shows single cells, small nests, and cords of UC invading between prostatic acini. High-grade prostatic carcinoma must be excluded in cases with this morphology, but use of IHC with or without supportive observation of an in situ urothelial component is helpful.

Urothelial Carcinoma Involving Prostate Gland

TERMINOLOGY

Abbreviations
- Urothelial carcinoma (UC)
- Carcinoma in situ (CIS)

Definitions
- **UC of urinary bladder secondarily involving prostate** refers to UC arising primarily in bladder but extending to involve prostatic urethra or prostatic glandular parenchyma by either direct invasion, intraepithelial pagetoid spread, or by combination of these processes
- **Primary UC of prostate** refers to either UC arising primarily in prostatic urethra or arising in more distal, suburethral ducts and glands of prostate itself

CLASSIFICATION

UC Seen Histologically Invading Prostate Gland
- May represent any of 3 scenarios
  - Urinary bladder UC involves prostate gland secondarily by direct invasion &/or intraepithelial spread
  - Primary prostatic urethral UC, ± invasion of prostatic stroma
  - Primary prostatic UC arising in more distal, suburethral prostatic ducts

Staged as UC of Urinary Bladder Secondarily Involving Bladder
- UC arising primarily in urinary bladder and secondarily involving prostate
  - Staged as a primary UC of urinary bladder
  - Recent scholarship describes 3 routes to involvement of prostate by primary bladder UC
    - UC may spread from bladder to prostatic urethra in pagetoid manner and then invade subepithelial prostatic stroma (excluded from pT4a)
    - UC may invade from bladder into prostate directly through wall of bladder (stage pT4a)
    - UC may invade through bladder into perivesical fat and then into prostate gland (stage pT4a)

Staged as Primary UC of Prostate
- UC arising in prostatic urethra
  - Staged as UC of prostate, substaged based on presence/absence and degree of invasion
- UC arising in more distal suburethral prostatic ducts and acini
  - Staged as UC of prostate, substaged based on presence/absence and degree of invasion
- Both have been lumped together as primary prostate UC historically and in large clinical series
  - Most data on UC of prostate combine these 2 patterns for study
  - Staging system for UC of prostate is described in urethra section in AJCC 7th Edition

CLINICAL ISSUES

Epidemiology
- Incidence
  - Primary prostate UC is uncommon, comprising < 5% of prostate cancers in adults
  - Majority have concomitant bladder urothelial CIS
  - Minority have no prior or concurrent invasive or in situ bladder UC
  - Secondary involvement of prostate by bladder UC is relatively more common, ranging from 12-58% of cystoprostatectomies
    - UC invading prostate from prostatic urethra and ducts comprises 76-87%
    - UC invading through bladder wall or perivesical fat into prostate comprises 13-24%
- Age
  - Similar in age distribution to UC of urinary bladder
  - Mean: 66 years; range: 52-87 years

Presentation
- UC secondarily involving prostate is most commonly detected in cystoprostatectomies for bladder UC
  - Presentation for these cases was based on symptomatology at primary bladder site
- In contrast, primary prostatic UCs present with obstructive urinary symptoms, such as hesitancy, slowed stream, frequency, and dysuria
  - May have rapid progression of obstruction, usually < 6 months
- Other symptoms include hematuria, prostatism, weight loss, and rectal pain
- Prostate may be large on rectal examination, and may be mistaken clinically as benign prostatic hyperplasia, prostatitis, or prostate cancer
- Symptomatic cases more often encountered in transurethral resection of prostate (TURP) specimens performed for obstructive symptoms

Laboratory Tests
- Serum PSA level typically not elevated except in cases where prostate biopsy done for elevated PSA
- May have elevated serum alkaline phosphatase level, due to bone metastasis

Treatment
- Depends on extent, location, and stage of disease
  - **For bladder UC secondarily involving prostate**, treatment is driven by bladder primary stage
    - If prostate is invaded transmurally or from extravesical disease, higher stage may trigger adjuvant chemotherapy
  - **For primary prostatic urethral UC** in TURP specimens
    - Prostatic urethral UC with minimal or superficial prostatic acinar involvement without stromal involvement may be treated with bacillus Calmette-Guérin (BCG)
    - Cystoscopy should be performed to determine presence of bladder neoplasia
    - 1 study reported 87% complete response rate for BCG, but only 17% of these had prostatic acinar involvement and none had stromal invasion
  - **For primary prostatic UC of suburethral prostatic ducts** and invasion of prostatic stroma and peripheral zone
    - Radical cystoprostatectomy is treatment of choice
    - Chemotherapy and radiotherapy may have role

Urothelial Carcinoma Involving Prostate Gland

Prognosis
- Depends on extent, location, and stage of disease

Prevalence of Involvement in Reported Series
- **For bladder primary UC secondarily involving prostate gland (~ 30% of cases at prostatectomy)**
  - 40-50% show noninvasive involvement of prostate, consisting of
    - CIS of prostatic urethra: ~ 20%
    - CIS of suburethral prostatic ducts: ~ 50%
    - CIS of both urethral and prostatic ducts: ~ 33%
  - 50-60% show invasive involvement of prostate, consisting of
    - Invasion of lamina propria of urethra in ~ 30%
    - Invasion of prostatic stroma in ~ 30%
    - Extraprostatic extension in ~ 15%
    - Transmural/extravesical route of prostate invasion ~ 25%
- **For primary prostatic UC**
  - Noninvasive CIS of prostatic urethra: ~ 10%
  - Noninvasive CIS of suburethral prostatic ducts and acini: ~ 30%
  - UC invading prostatic stroma: ~ 40%
  - UC with extraprostatic extension: ~ 5%
  - Lymph node metastasis: ~ 15%

Prognosis by Pattern of Involvement
- **For bladder UC secondarily involving prostate**
  - Bladder UC ± prostatic involvement
    - Bladder UC patients without prostatic involvement 5-year survival rate: 64%
    - Bladder UC patients with either prostatic CIS and urethral lamina propria invasion 5-year survival rate: 44%
    - Bladder UC patients with prostatic stromal/periprostatic/seminal vesical invasion 5-year survival rate: 32%
  - Prostate involvement decreases survival of bladder UC, which varies predominantly according to primary stage of bladder cancer
  - Age, degree of prostate invasion, and lymph node involvement are independent prognostic variables
  - Primary bladder UC involving prostate through subepithelial stromal invasion from urethra and ducts has much better prognosis than transmural/extravesical routes
    - Validates AJCC 7th Edition exclusion of subepithelial invasion from pT4a
- **For primary UC of prostatic urethra or suburethral prostatic ducts**
  - 5-year disease-specific survival
    - Prostatic urethral CIS and CIS involving prostatic ducts and acini without stromal invasion (100%)
    - Prostatic stromal invasion: 45%
    - Extraprostatic extension: 0%
    - Lymph node extension: 30%
    - Prostate primary UC overall: 52%
  - Concurrent prostatic adenocarcinoma seen in 8%
  - Subsequent UC of upper urinary tract seen in 6%
  - Metastases most commonly occur in bone, lung, and liver

IMAGING
Radiographic Findings
- Abnormal excretory urograms in > 1/2 of patients
- Hydronephrosis and enlarged prostatic impression in more advanced disease

Bone Scan
- Bone metastasis is lytic in > 70%

MACROSCOPIC
General Features
- Indistinguishable from prostate adenocarcinoma
- Prostate may be enlarged, firm, and fixed with more advanced spread

Cystoscopy
- Majority of prostatic urethral UC are flat lesions (86%) and 14% have papillary component

MICROSCOPIC
Histologic Features
- Diagnostic criteria identical to those of UC of any other site in GU tract
  - **Noninvasive papillary UC involving prostatic urethra**
    - Low-grade or high-grade histology
    - Low-grade papillary UC defined by urothelium demonstrating distinct atypia, crowding, nuclear rounding, nuclear grooves, and nucleoli, arrayed along fine fibrovascular cores with maintenance of polarization, analogous in degree to flat urothelial dysplasia
    - High-grade papillary UC defined by urothelium demonstrating marked atypia, crowding, nuclear rounding, anisonucleosis, macronucleoli, chromatin irregularity, loss of polarization, dyscohesion and cellular or nuclear pleomorphism, analogous in degree to urothelial CIS
  - **Prostatic urethral CIS**
    - CIS may spread from prostatic urethra, involve ducts and acini, or grow along ejaculatory ducts to seminal vesicle
    - May exhibit different CIS patterns identical to bladder, including large cell pleomorphic, large cell nonpleomorphic, small cell, clinging, pagetoid, and undermining types
    - High-grade dysplastic urothelium confined to urethral basement membrane
    - Invasion of stroma may arise along this pagetoid intraepithelial spread
  - **Prostatic urethral CIS with invasion of lamina propria**
    - Destructive invasion by nests or single cells through urethral basement membrane often accompanied by desmoplasia or inflammation
  - **UC involving prostatic duct and acini/CIS without stromal invasion**
    - High-grade dysplastic urothelium confined within expanded prostatic ducts or acini
    - Ducts/acini often completely filled by neoplastic cells
    - Ducts/acini have rounded contours and are rimmed by basal cells

Urothelial Carcinoma Involving Prostate Gland

- Surrounding basal cells may be highlighted by more intense, and contiguous HMWCK/34bE12 staining; lesional cells also frequently positive with these markers
- May contain central area of necrosis
- Uncommonly, may exhibit pagetoid spread of UC within ducts or acini
○ Prostatic stromal invasion
- Destructive invasion by nests or single cells through ductal/acinar basement membranes often accompanied by desmoplasia or inflammation
- Less commonly may have lymphovascular invasion
- Invasion may be in absence of duct/acinar involvement
- Invasive UC typically forms small nests with marked nuclear pleomorphism and increased mitosis
- Invasive UC may have squamous differentiation
- Typically with associated desmoplastic stromal response or inflammation
- Perineural invasion is not typical finding

ANCILLARY TESTS

Immunohistochemistry

- HMWCK, p63, CK5/6: Lesional cells (±), native basal cells (+)
- CK7(+/-) and CK20(+/-): ~ 50-70% double (+)
- Positive in UC but not basal cells: GATA3, uroplakin-2, uroplakin-3, S100, thrombomodulin
- PSA/PAP(-), p501S(-), NKX3.1(-), PSMA, ERG(-)
- AMACR(+); not helpful vs. prostate adenocarcinoma

DIFFERENTIAL DIAGNOSIS

Poorly Differentiated Adenocarcinoma of Prostate, ± Intraductal Growth

- Intraductal growth of acinar carcinoma ± comedonecrosis
- Usually associated with invasive Gleason pattern 4 and 5 carcinoma
- Focally may contain glandular formations
- Stromal desmoplasia and inflammatory response to tumor is less common
- Less mitotically active, squamous differentiation is unusual, and perineural invasion is frequent
- Mostly PSA/PAP(+), p501S/NKX3.1(+) even in high grade
- ERG(+) and PTEN(-) in most intraductal carcinoma of prostate

High-Grade Prostatic Intraepithelial Neoplasia

- Mimics UC involving prostatic ducts and acini
- Atypical cells are prostatic acinar in nature [(+) prostatic markers]
- Although atypical, including prominent nucleoli, pleomorphism and mitoses are not common

GRADING

Criteria

- WHO 2004/International Society of Urological Pathologists classification for flat and papillary lesions
  ○ Applicable for prostatic urethral UCa
  ○ Full spectrum from papilloma, PUNLMP, low-grade and high-grade carcinoma applies to lesions primary to prostatic urethra or suburethral prostatic ducts

STAGING

Criteria

- American Joint Committee on Cancer/International Union Against Cancer 2009
  ○ UC of prostate has separate TNM staging system from prostate or bladder cancer
    - Either UC of urethra involving prostate or primary UC of prostatic ducts
  ○ Bladder UC transmurally invading through vesical wall and extending into prostate is staged under bladder cancer TNM staging (pT4 bladder UC)
- UC involving prostate stroma may occur as result of extension from UC primary to bladder
  ○ Subepithelial stromal invasion; not staged as bladder primary pT4
  ○ Direct transmural or extravesical invasion of prostate; staged as bladder primary pT4
- UC involving prostate stroma may occur as result of extension from involvement of prostatic ducts and acini
  ○ Staged as pT2, whether urethral primary or suburethral prostatic ductal primary

SELECTED REFERENCES

1. Epstein JI et al: Best practices recommendations in the application of immunohistochemistry in the prostate: report from the International Society of Urologic Pathology consensus conference. Am J Surg Pathol. 38(8):e6-e19, 2014
2. Patel AR et al: Validation of new AJCC exclusion criteria for subepithelial prostatic stromal invasion from pT4a bladder urothelial carcinoma. J Urol. 189(1):53-8, 2013
3. Chuang AY et al: Immunohistochemical differentiation of high-grade prostate carcinoma from urothelial carcinoma. Am J Surg Pathol. 31(8):1246-55, 2007
4. Shen SS et al: Prostatic involvement by transitional cell carcinoma in patients with bladder cancer and its prognostic significance. Hum Pathol. 37(6):726-34, 2006
5. Njinou Ngninkeu B et al: Transitional cell carcinoma involving the prostate: a clinicopathological retrospective study of 76 cases. J Urol. 169(1):149-52, 2003
6. Oliai BR et al: A clinicopathologic analysis of urothelial carcinomas diagnosed on prostate needle biopsy. Am J Surg Pathol. 25(6):794-801, 2001
7. Cheville JC et al: Transitional cell carcinoma of the prostate: clinicopathologic study of 50 cases. Cancer. 82(4):703-7, 1998
8. Esrig D et al: Transitional cell carcinoma involving the prostate with a proposed staging classification for stromal invasion. J Urol. 156(3):1071-6, 1996
9. Mahadevia PS et al: Prostatic involvement in bladder cancer. Prostate mapping in 20 cystoprostatectomy specimens. Cancer. 58(9):2096-102, 1986
10. Sawczuk I et al: Primary transitional cell carcinoma of prostatic periurethral ducts. Urology. 25(4):339-43, 1985

Urothelial Carcinoma Involving Prostate Gland

(Left) UC involving prostatic ducts expands and fills preexisting acini ➡, as seen here. Stromal invasion may arise anywhere along these ducts, and on occasion obtaining additional levels may be indicated for accurate staging. **(Right)** Here, a preexisting prostatic duct is expanded by intraductal growth UC with a central area of necrosis, which may simulate Gleason pattern 5 prostatic adenocarcinoma with comedonecrosis. In UC involving prostatic ducts, periductal inflammation is often prominent.

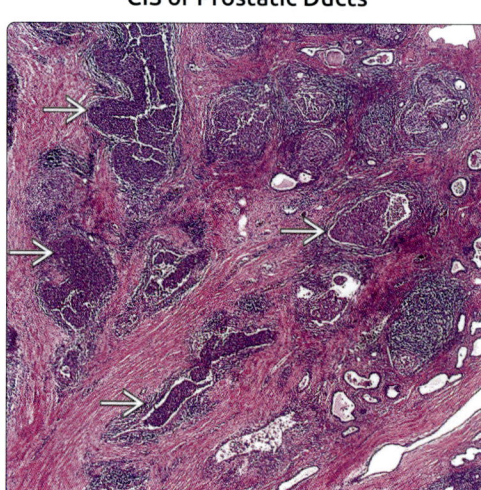
CIS of Prostatic Ducts

CIS of Prostatic Ducts

(Left) UC involving prostatic ducts and acini with stromal invasion is shown. At low power, there is ↑ complexity than mere expansion of preexisting ducts & acini; this pattern should raise concern for invasion. **(Right)** UC involving prostatic ducts may be associated with stromal invasion. Small irregular nests with desmoplasia and associated inflammatory response are shown. Solid invading small nests ➡ are unusual for prostatic adenocarcinoma. Retraction ➡, as seen in early invasion in bladder cancer, is present.

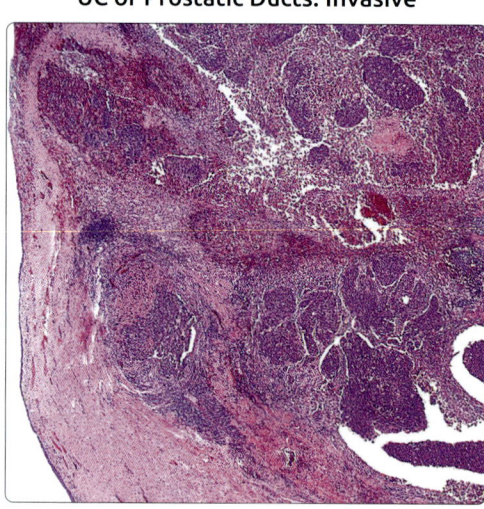
UC of Prostatic Ducts: Invasive

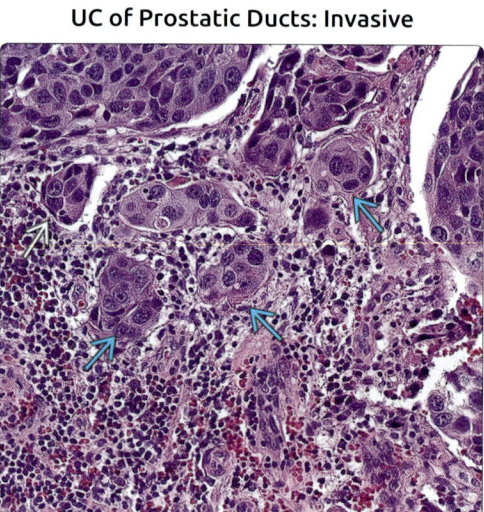
UC of Prostatic Ducts: Invasive

(Left) An unusual case of low-grade papillary UC ➡, arising in and expanding periurethral glands, is seen adjacent to suburethral prostatic glands ➡. The full spectrum of urothelial neoplasia may arise in the prostate, though papillary lesions are distinctly unusual here. **(Right)** A higher power view of low-grade papillary UC shows areas of inverted and exophytic luminal papillary growth ➡ juxtaposed to compressed, adjacent prostatic acini ➡.

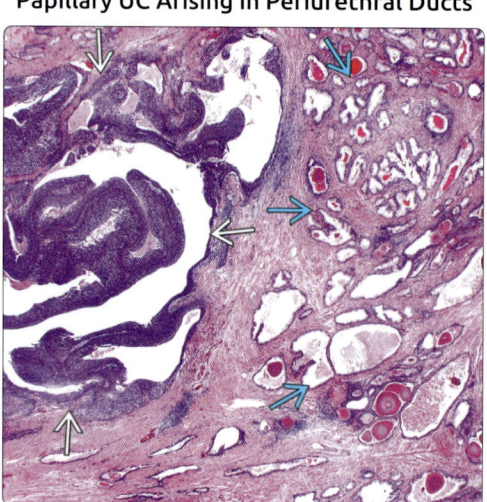
Papillary UC Arising in Periurethral Ducts

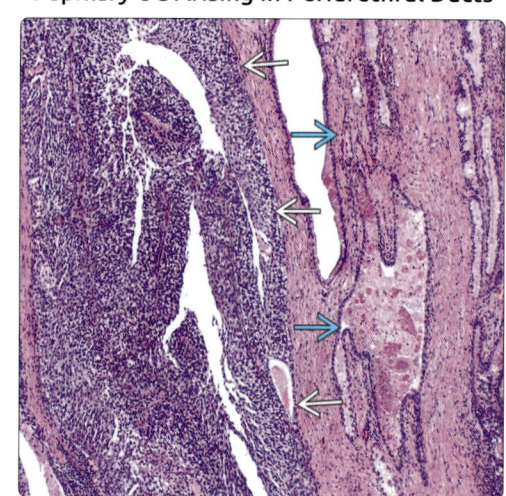
Papillary UC Arising in Periurethral Ducts

Urothelial Carcinoma Involving Prostate Gland

Prostatic UC With Extraprostatic Extension

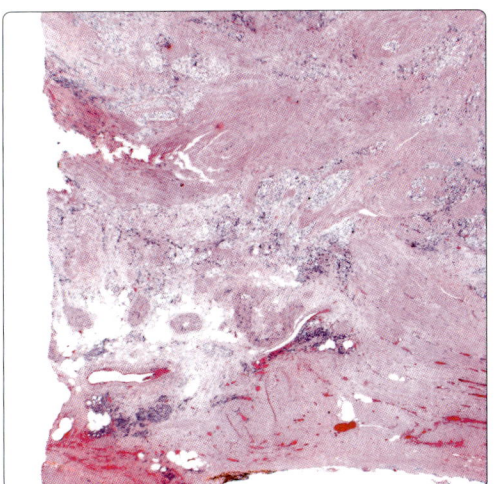

Prostatic UC With Extraprostatic Extension

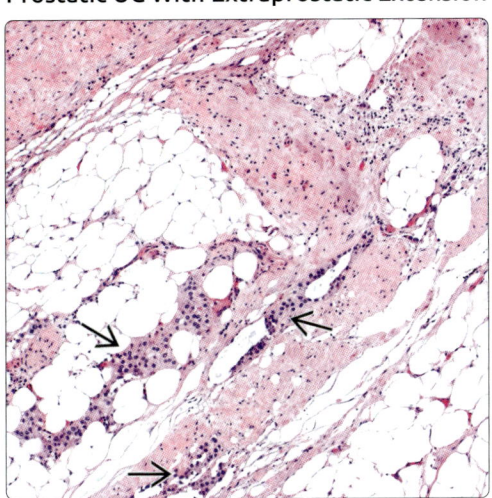

(Left) An aggressive subset (~ 5%) of primary prostatic UCs demonstrates extraprostatic invasion, which portends a generally poor prognosis. *(Right)* Invasive cords and nests of UC are seen in the plane of periprostatic fat ➡. It is important to determine if the invasive carcinoma is secondary to a bladder primary or secondary to a UC arising in the prostate. Depending on the situation, the appropriate staging system should be used.

Pagetoid CIS Involving Ejaculatory Duct

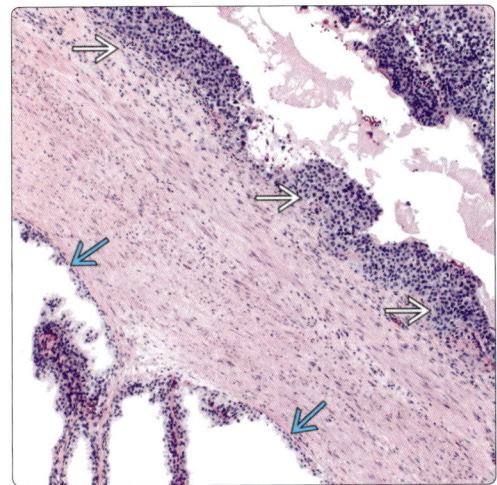

Pagetoid CIS Involving Ejaculatory Duct

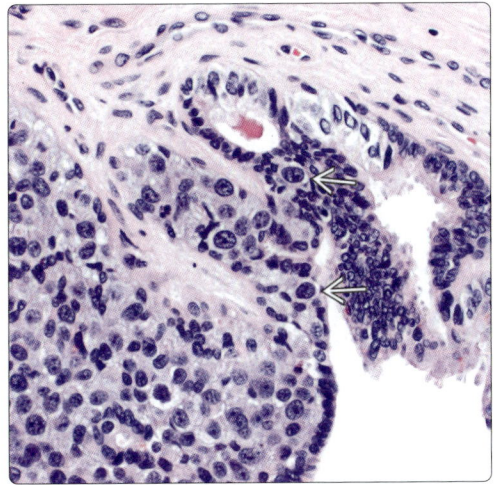

(Left) Prostatic urethral UC demonstrates extensive pagetoid involvement, extending all the way into the ejaculatory duct ➡, seen adjacent to central zone glands ➡. *(Right)* At the leading edge of CIS involving the ejaculatory duct, pagetoid atypical single cells of UC are seen growing into the ejaculatory duct epithelium ➡. Seminal vesicle epithelium may also be involved by pagetoid CIS.

Prostate UC vs. High-Grade PCa

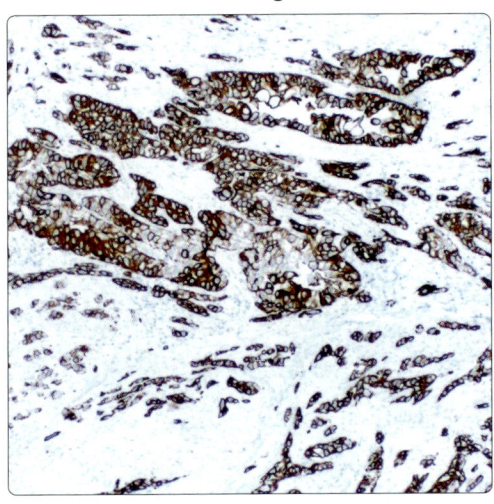

Prostate UC vs. High-Grade PCa

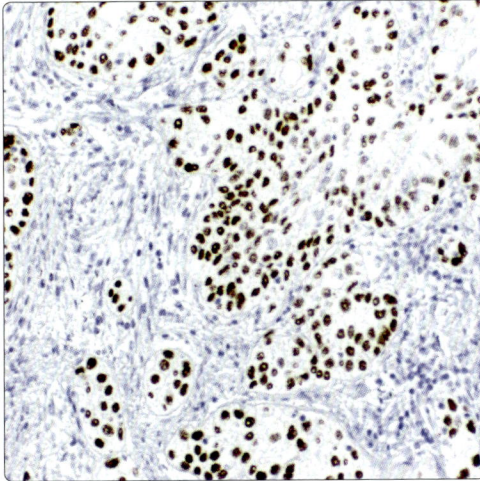

(Left) High molecular weight cytokeratin is a helpful marker for UC in poorly differentiated cases of UC where PCa might be in the morphologic differential. *(Right)* The immunostain p63 is very helpful in the differential between UC and PCa, as are newer urothelial markers GATA3, uroplakin-2, and S100. Useful prostate markers are PSA, PAP, PSMA, p501s or NKX3.1; not all markers are necessary.

Prostate Carcinoma With Neuroendocrine Differentiation

KEY FACTS

CLASSIFICATION

- **Usual prostate carcinoma (PCa) with neuroendocrine differentiation (NED)**
  - Morphologically conventional PCa with varying proportions of cells IHC positive for markers of NED
- **PCa with Paneth cell-like NED**
  - PCa with varying proportions of bright red granulated cells reminiscent of Paneth cells
  - New paucigranular variant, pale to amphophilic cytoplasm
- **Carcinoid tumor**
  - Rare, morphologically similar to those of other organs, must exclude metastasis from other sites
  - Syndromal associations with multiple endocrine neoplasia
- **Small cell carcinoma (SCC)**
  - Defined by cytologic features of high nuclear:cytoplasmic ratio, molding, crush artifact, lack of nucleoli, brisk mitosis, necrosis
- **Large cell neuroendocrine carcinoma (LCNEC)**
  - Defined by sheet-like or nested organoid growth, peripheral palisading, necrosis
  - Nucleoli present, coarser chromatin, larger cells, abundant cytoplasm
- **Mixed neuroendocrine carcinoma/acinar adenocarcinoma**
  - Admixture of recognizable conventional PCa, usual high grade, with either SCC or LCNEC
- **PCa with overlapping features of SCC and acinar PCa**
  - New provisional category referring to examples showing hybrid/overlapping morphology between high-grade PCa and SCC rather than admixture

CLINICAL ISSUES

- Rare forms of PCa, may be increasing in prevalence
- Variable NED in otherwise usual PCa of uncertain significance, often with high-grade disease
- SCC & LCNEC, mixed or pure, are aggressive tumors

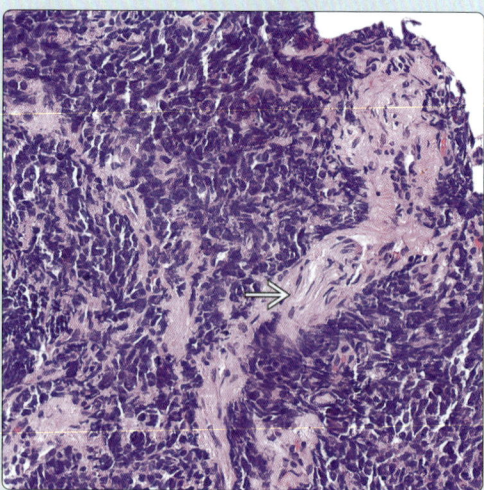

Small Cell Carcinoma

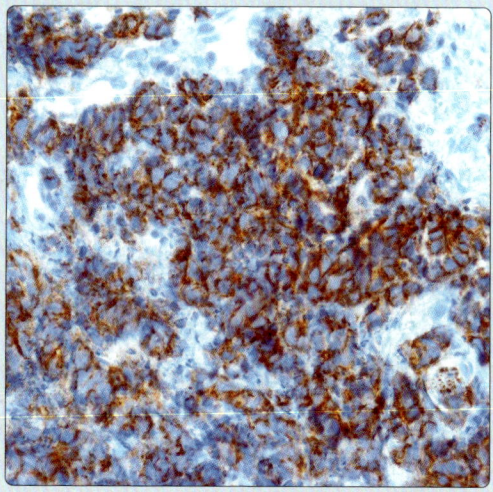

Small Cell Carcinoma

(Left) Small cell carcinoma (SCC) shows sheets of small cells with extensive crush artifact. This finding is a low-power feature helpful in the prospective recognition of SCC of the prostate, just as at other sites. Note the presence of perineural invasion ➡. *(Right)* This SCC shows strong and diffuse expression of chromogranin. Studies have shown that synaptophysin and CD56 stains are more sensitive than chromogranin.

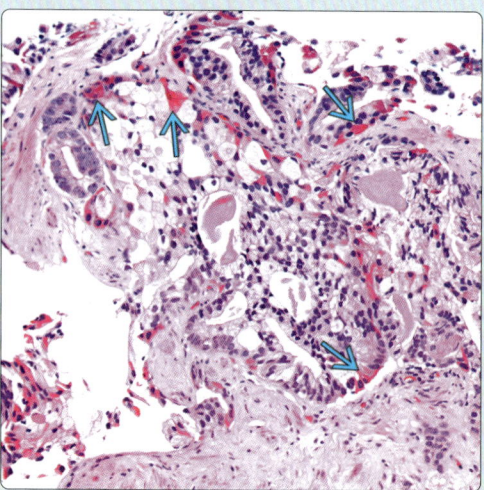

PCa With Paneth Cell-Like NED

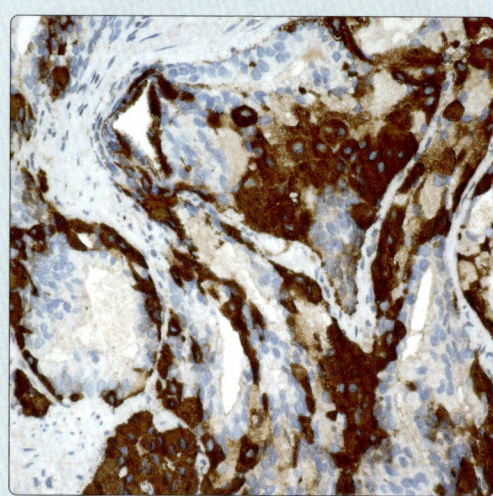

PCa With Paneth Cell-Like NED

(Left) This biopsy sample shows a prostate carcinoma (PCa) with Paneth cell-like neuroendocrine differentiation (NED), evinced by bright red polygonal granular cells, often accentuated at the periphery of the acinus ➡. Most data suggest these cases are relatively indolent; Gleason grading may not be relevant to the Paneth cell-like component. *(Right)* The same patient shows chromogranin immunostain, which highlights the granular Paneth cell-like cells.

Prostate Carcinoma With Neuroendocrine Differentiation

TERMINOLOGY

Abbreviations
- Neuroendocrine (NE) differentiation (NED)
- Prostatic adenocarcinoma (PCa)

Synonyms
- Small cell carcinoma (SCC): Small cell NE carcinoma, poorly differentiated NE carcinoma, small cell anaplastic carcinoma, oat cell carcinoma

CLASSIFICATION

Usual PCa With NED
- Conventional PCa, whether acinar or ductal in origin, of any grade, where NED is demonstrated by IHC using markers of NED

PCa With Paneth Cell-Like NED
- Conventional PCa, where brightly eosinophilic cytoplasmic granules apparent on routine H&E stain are identifiable in variable number of cells
- Variation of this morphology includes examples where some or all of these cells are paucigranulated, demonstrating instead bland cords to spindled collections of cells with amphophilic or pale cytoplasm
- Both granulated and ungranulated examples demonstrate diffuse NED by IHC

Carcinoid Tumor
- Well-differentiated NE tumor, arising as primary of prostate, but which shows morphologic features of carcinoid tumor such as rise at other sites, like lung and GI tract
- These are vanishingly rare tumors that require rigorous criteria, including
  - Exclusion of secondary involvement from another pimary site
  - IHC evidence of NED and lack of PSA expression
  - Absence of closely associated usual PCa

Small Cell Carcinoma
- High-grade NE carcinoma
- Defined by characteristic cytology, particularly nuclear features
  - Lack of prominent nucleoli
  - Nuclear molding and fragility, crush artifact
  - High nuclear:cytoplasmic ratio
  - High mitotic activity, apoptotic debris, and karyorrhexis
  - Geographic necrosis

Large Cell Neuroendocrine Carcinoma
- High-grade NE carcinoma showing morphologic evidence of NED
  - Large, often organoid nests with palisading cells
  - Geographic necrosis
  - Nuclear features not typical of small cell, with nucleoli, vesicular chromatin, more abundant cytoplasm
- NED must be supported by diffuse expression of at least 1 IHC marker of NED

Mixed Neuroendocrine Carcinoma/Acinar Adenocarcinoma
- Biphasic carcinoma demonstrating readily identifiable different morphologic populations of usual PCa and NE carcinoma
- NE carcinoma may be either SCC or large cell neuroendocrine carcinoma (LCNEC)
  - Most cases encountered are mixed SCC and acinar PCa
  - Reported examples of mixed LCNEC and acinar PCa
- Most examples show abrupt, very distinct populations of NE carcinoma and usual PCa, usually high grade

PCa With Overlapping Features of SCC and Acinar PCa: Provisional Category
- Provisional term for cases of PCa, usually high grade, that show significant areas of overlapping morphology with PCa
- Significant areas of hybrid morphology, in contradistinction to admixture of 2 components
- Cytologic features that are intermediate between usual PCa and SCC raise concern for SCC
- Generally diffuse expression of IHC markers of NED

ETIOLOGY/PATHOGENESIS

Origin
- Differing theories regarding origin of NED
  - Transdifferentiation of PCa into cells with NED driven by therapy
  - Older theories of de novo transformation from prostatic NE cells and NE cells facilitating transdifferentiation

CLINICAL ISSUES

Epidemiology
- Incidence
  - Focal to variable NED is reported in 10-100% of adenocarcinomas, depending on IHC marker
  - PCa with NED, outside of usual PCa with NED, is unusual
  - SCC and mixed SCC/acinar PCa accounts for ~ 1% of all prostate cancers
  - Limited data regarding prevalence of other variants
    - Carcinoid exorbitantly rare, with only < 10 cases reported
      - Subset associated with multiple endocrine neoplasia type 2B
    - LCNEC rare, particularly pure LCNEC
  - Little data on PCa with overlapping features of SCC
  - PCa with NED, especially pure and mixed SCC, LCNEC, and PCa with overlapping features with SCC may be increasing
    - Increased longevity, higher-potency androgen-deprivation therapy, or increased awareness/biopsy protocols hypothesized as causes
- Age
  - Most PCa with NED occurs predominantly in elderly patients
  - SCC and mixed SCC/acinar PCa
    - Mean: 69 years; range: 30-92 years
  - Carcinoid tumors in younger populations, syndromal association

Prostate Carcinoma With Neuroendocrine Differentiation

Presentation

- **Pure SCC and mixed SCC/acinar PCa**
  - Rapid-onset urinary tract obstructions, such as dysuria, nocturia, or urgency, are main presenting symptoms
  - Previous diagnosis of adenocarcinoma in 42-67% cases, some with history of prior hormonal therapy
    - Interval from adenocarcinoma to diagnosis of SCC ranges from 1 to 300 months; mean: 59 months
  - Lack of clinically evident hormone production in most cases
  - Paraneoplastic syndromes: ACTH or antidiuretic hormone production, Eaton-Lambert syndrome, and others
  - Most patients present with extraprostatic extension, large primary tumor masses, advanced-stage disease, and distant metastases
- **Pure LCNEC and mixed LCNEC/acinar PCa**
  - Most patients with initial diagnosis of acinar adenocarcinoma and prior androgen-deprivation therapy
    - Interval from adenocarcinoma to diagnosis of LCNEC ranges from 2 to 12 years; mean: 4.7 years
  - Advanced stage at time of diagnosis
  - Clinical and therapeutic significance of distinguishing LCNEC from SCC in prostate is not established

Laboratory Tests

- Serum PSA level variable, may be normal
- May show significant drop in serum PSA, as NE component predominates over acinar adenocarcinoma component
- Serum chromogranin-A and progastrin-releasing peptide levels
  - May be diagnostically and prognostically useful in prostate cancers with focal NE differentiation
  - May be useful particularly in androgen-independent cancers

Treatment

- Therapeutic significance of usual PCa with NED is unclear
- SCC and mixed SCC/acinar SCC treated aggressively
  - Clinically localized prostate SCC treated with multimodal therapy, including surgery, androgen-deprivation therapy, chemotherapy, and radiotherapy
  - Metastatic SCC of prostate treated with platinum-based chemotherapy with similar regiments to lung SCC
- Optimum therapies for carcinoid tumors, LCNEC not established
  - LCNEC has been treated similarly to SCC

Prognosis

- Prognostic significance of focal NE differentiation in acinar adenocarcinoma is controversial
  - Some studies show negative effect on prognosis, whereas some studies show no relationship
  - Paneth cell-like NED in adenocarcinoma does not portend poor prognosis
- Prognosis of SCC is poor with mean survival of < 1 year after development of SCC component
  - No difference in prognosis between pure SCC and SCC admixed with adenocarcinoma
  - Response to available treatment modalities is poor
  - Common metastatic sites include bone, liver, lung, and lymph nodes
- Prognosis of carcinoid tumor is uncertain because of few cases reported
  - Some tumors with clinically aggressive behavior may represent prostate adenocarcinoma (carcinoid-like adenocarcinoma)
  - True carcinoid is suggested to have indolent behavior although cases reported are limited
- Prognosis of LCNEC is similar to SCC
  - Most common metastatic site is bone; other sites of metastasis include lung, liver, lymph nodes

MOLECULAR

Emerging Molecular Pathology

- Recent scholarship identifies N-MYC and Aurora-A kinase amplifications as key mediators of PCa with NED
  - May be present in cases susceptible to progression as PCa with NED
- Similar to other PCa, at least 1/2 of PCa with NED harbors oncogenic rearrangements of E26-transformation-specifc family of transcription factors

MICROSCOPIC

Histologic Features

- **Usual PCa with NED**
  - Characterized by varying proportion of cells positive by IHC for markers of NED
  - May be focal (most common) or diffuse, latter more often in higher-grade PCa
- **SCC**
  - Histologically similar to SCC of lung
  - Predominantly diffuse sheet-like growth; may form clusters, trabeculae, cords, and single-cell patterns
  - Small blue cell tumor
    - Scant cytoplasm, high nuclear:cytoplasm ratio
    - "Salt and pepper" chromatin without prominent nucleoli
    - Brisk mitotic activity
    - Nuclear molding, crush and smear artifacts
    - Single-cell necrosis or geographic necrosis
    - Frequent apoptosis
  - 2 cell types, classic "oat cell" and intermediate types, may be admixed
    - "Oat cell" carcinoma consists of small cells (up to 2x size of lymphocytes), pyknotic round to oval nuclei, and indistinct nucleoli
    - Intermediate cell histology with overall less uniformity, containing slightly larger nuclei, visible nucleoli, relatively more cytoplasm, and polygonal or fusiform cells
  - Rosette-like structures formed in ~ 30%, giant tumor cells seen in ~ 20%
  - Perineural invasion and lymphovascular invasion may be seen
- **Mixed SCC and acinar PCa**
  - About 50% of SCCs have distinct, recognizable acinar adenocarcinoma component
  - Most admixed adenocarcinomas are high grade: 85% are Gleason score 8 or higher
- **Carcinoid tumor**
  - Histologically similar to carcinoid tumor at other sites

Prostate Carcinoma With Neuroendocrine Differentiation

- Nests, trabecular pattern, cords, or mixed architectural patterns
- Uniform round or polygonal cells with round, regular nuclei containing "salt and pepper" chromatin; nucleoli are indistinct
- Rare to low mitotic activity and absent necrosis
- LCNEC
  - Histologically similar to LCNEC of lung
  - Organoid nests and sheets of cells with suggestion of peripheral palisading
  - Tumor cells contain large, hyperchromatic nuclei with coarse to vesicular chromatin and visible nucleoli
  - Geographic necrosis often prominent, mitosis brisk

ANCILLARY TESTS

Immunohistochemistry

- Spectrum of positivity of IHC markers of NED predominantly studied in SCC, limited data for LCNEC
- No systematic data for PCa with overlapping features, etc.
- Up to 90% of SCC and LCNEC are positive for IHC markers of NED
- Reported NE marker immunoreactivity in SCC
  - Synaptophysin 84-89% (+)
  - Chromogranin 61-75% (+)
  - CD56 83-92% (+)
  - NSE 85% (+)
  - CD44 has been proposed as sensitive, specific marker of SCC but has failed validation studies
- < 20% express prostate-specific markers (PSA, PAP, NKX3.1) or are positive for ERG
- ~ 50% of SCC are TTF-1(+)
- Basal cell markers (p63 and HMWK) typically (-), 1/2 of SCC are AMACR(+)
- AR typically (-)
- SCC may show typical paranuclear dot-like immunoreactivity with PAN-CK (AE1/AE3)

In Situ Hybridization

- In metastatic SCC of unknown primary setting, positive ERG break-apart FISH establishes prostatic primary

DIFFERENTIAL DIAGNOSIS

SCC Secondarily Involving Prostate

- Primary and secondary NE tumors of prostate are histologically and immunohistochemically indistinguishable
- Use of lung marker TTF-1 is not helpful, as about 1/2 of prostate or bladder primary SCCs are positive
- Distinction from SCC of urinary bladder is based on clinical/anatomic grounds, correlation with history of PCa, hormone therapy, PSA level
- ERG IHC, if positive, confirms prostatic origin; ERG FISH more sensitive

Poorly Differentiated Acinar Adenocarcinoma (Gleason Pattern 5)

- High-grade adenocarcinoma with solid sheet and single-cell infiltration
- Does not have typical architectural and cytologic features of SCC
- Strong prostatic markers, PSA, p501S, AR, NKX3.1, favor high-grade PCa
- May lack expression of other NE markers (chromogranin, CD56)
- PAN-CK (AE1/AE3) shows diffuse positivity, in contrast to SCC, which may show dot-like positivity
- Very difficult distinction from cases of PCa with overlapping features of SCC and usual PCa

Poorly Differentiated Urothelial Carcinoma

- Crush artifact in urothelial carcinoma may cause it to mimic SCC on low magnification
- Does not have typical cytologic features of SCC
- Typically diffusely p63(+), HMWK (34βE12) (+), CK7(+), and CK20(+)
- Negative for NE markers

Basal Cell Carcinoma

- Similar to SCC, tumor cells have scant cytoplasm, high nuclear:cytoplasmic ratio, and form nests, cords, or trabeculae
- Negative for NE markers
- Typically diffusely (+) for basal cell markers [p63 and HMWK (34βE12)]

REPORTING

Gleason Grading

- Not applicable for SCC or LCNEC
- May be provided for admixed usual PCa component if mixed neuroendocrine carcinoma/usual PCa
- Likely not applicable for areas of Paneth cell-like NED

Staging

- AJCC Staging System applies for SCC of prostate

SELECTED REFERENCES

1. Tsai H et al: Cyclin D1 loss distinguishes prostatic small cell carcinoma from most prostatic adenocarcinomas. Clin Cancer Res. 21(24):5619-29, 2015
2. Wang CC et al: Overlap of CD44 expression between prostatic small cell carcinoma and acinar adenocarcinoma. Hum Pathol. 46(4):554-7, 2015
3. Beltran H et al: Aggressive variants of castration-resistant prostate cancer. Clin Cancer Res. 20(11):2846-50, 2014
4. Epstein JI et al: Proposed morphologic classification of prostate cancer with neuroendocrine differentiation. Am J Surg Pathol. 38(6):756-67, 2014
5. Lugnani F et al: The role of neuroendocrine cells in prostate cancer: a comprehensive review of current literature and subsequent rationale to broaden and integrate current treatment modalities. Curr Med Chem. 21(9):1082-92, 2014
6. So JS et al: Variant of prostatic adenocarcinoma with Paneth cell-like neuroendocrine differentiation readily misdiagnosed as Gleason pattern 5. Hum Pathol. 45(12):2388-93, 2014
7. Wang W et al: Small cell carcinoma of the prostate. A morphologic and immunohistochemical study of 95 cases. Am J Surg Pathol. 32(1):65-71, 2008
8. Evans AJ et al: Large cell neuroendocrine carcinoma of prostate: a clinicopathologic summary of 7 cases of a rare manifestation of advanced prostate cancer. Am J Surg Pathol. 30(6):684-93, 2006
9. Tamas EF et al: Prognostic significance of paneth cell-like neuroendocrine differentiation in adenocarcinoma of the prostate. Am J Surg Pathol. 30(8):980-5, 2006
10. Yao JL et al: Small cell carcinoma of the prostate: an immunohistochemical study. Am J Surg Pathol. 30(6):705-12, 2006
11. Yashi M et al: Small cell/neuroendocrine carcinoma may be a more common phenotype in advanced prostate cancer. Urol Int. 69(2):166-8, 2002

Prostate Carcinoma With Neuroendocrine Differentiation

Usual PCa With NED

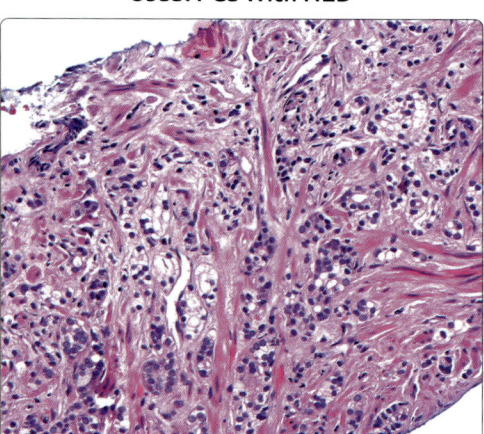

Usual PCa With NED

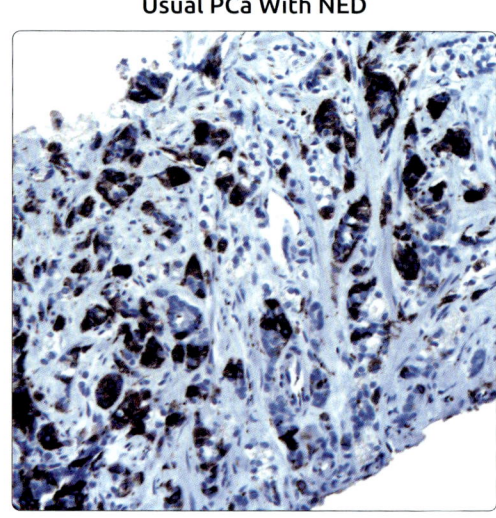

(Left) Conventional PCa may demonstrate IHC evidence of NED in many cases. A body of data suggests that this feature is more prevalent among higher grade tumors, like this one. (Right) Synaptophysin IHC performed on the same patient shows multifocal positivity although, in the setting of convincing conventional morphology, this finding is of questionable significance. Routine staining for neuroendocrine markers is not recommended in such cases.

Usual PCa With NED

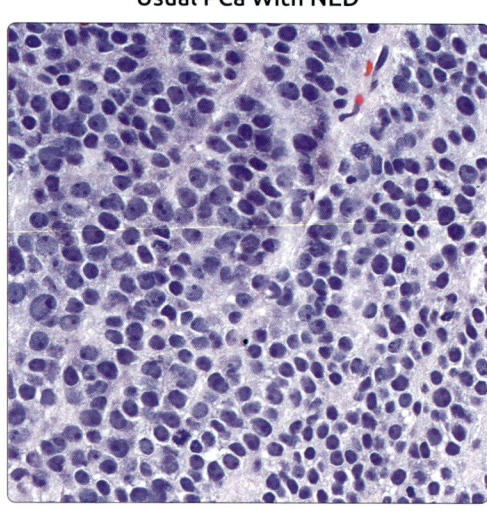

Usual PCa With NED

(Left) Another high-grade PCa shows convincing cytologic features of PCa, including prominent nucleoli, without cytologic features of SCC. (Right) Chromogranin IHC demonstrates scattered positivity, which absent an appropriate morphologic context should not be construed as establishing a diagnosis of SCC. PSA and AR immunostains are positive in contrast to SCC.

PCa With Paneth Cell-Like NED

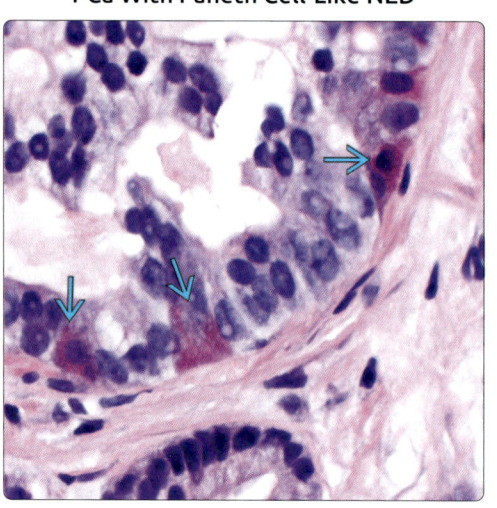

Paucigranular Paneth Cell-Like NED

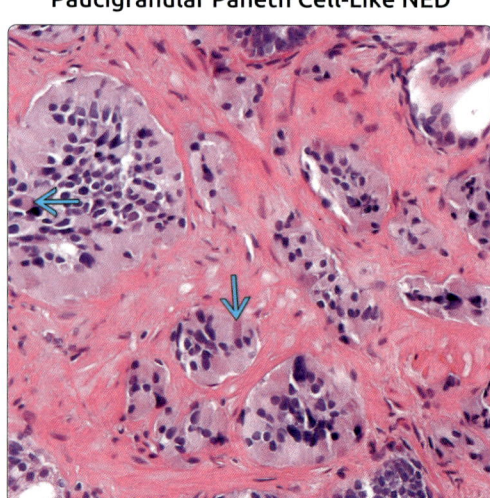

(Left) Several bright pink, granulated peripheral cells ➡ reminiscent of the Paneth cells of the GI tract are apparent. This incidental pattern of differentiation is seen in a small subset of carcinomas, and emerging data implicate Aurora-A kinase amplifications. (Right) Some cases show only focal ➡ or absent granules, simulating high-grade (Gleason 5) PCa. Synaptophysin remains diffusely positive, allowing identification of these much less aggressive cases. (Courtesy Dr. Jonathan Epstein.)

Prostate Carcinoma With Neuroendocrine Differentiation

Small Cell Carcinoma, Classic

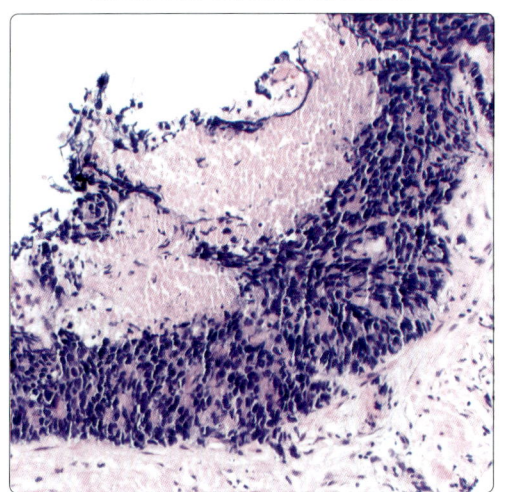

Small Cell Carcinoma, Classic

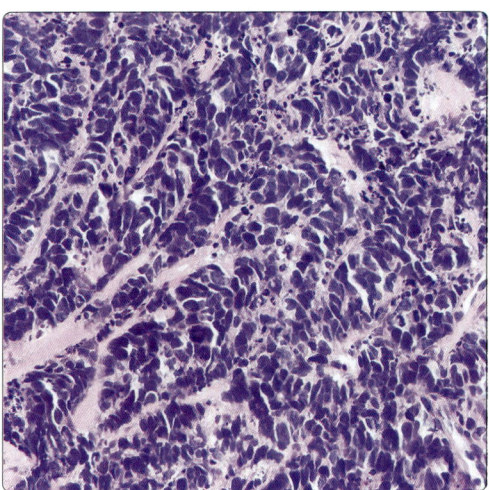

(Left) Classic SCC of the prostate at biopsy demonstrates "oat cell" morphology of small cells, up to twice the size of lymphocytes, without nucleoli, with scant cytoplasm, brisk mitosis, geographic necrosis, and crush artifact. (Right) At higher power, the nuclear "molding" of SCC is apparent, demonstrating the cellular fragility of this variant. Also, the typical high mitotic index and karyorrhectic debris are well represented here.

Small Cell Carcinoma, Intermediate

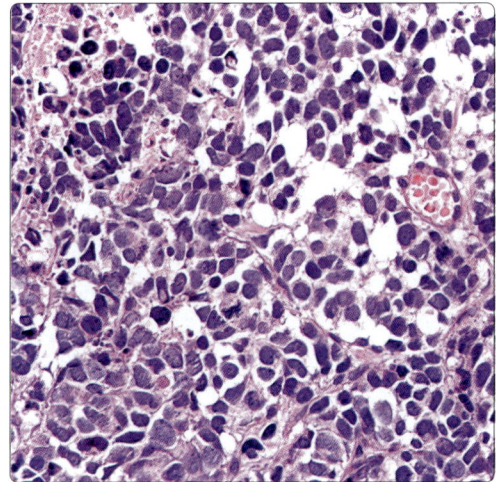

Mixed SCC/Acinar Adenocarcinoma

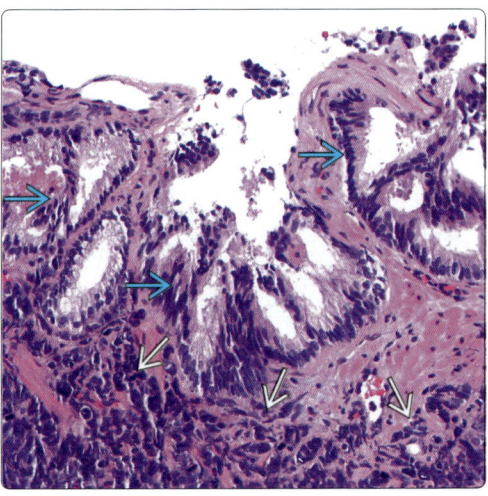

(Left) Many examples of SCC of the prostate show a so-called intermediate morphology with slightly larger cells, more cytoplasm, and indistinct nucleoli. Mitosis and necrosis remain prominent. This variation is significant only in as much as it must be recognized as SCC. (Right) A needle biopsy shows SCC ➡ admixed with tubular and cribriform patterns of acinar adenocarcinoma ➡. Approximately half of SCCs demonstrate synchronous or prior diagnosis of a conventional acinar PCa.

SCC, Rosette-Like Structures

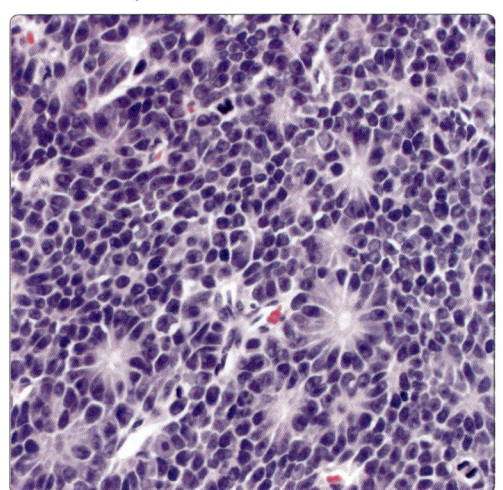

SCC, Extraprostatic Extension

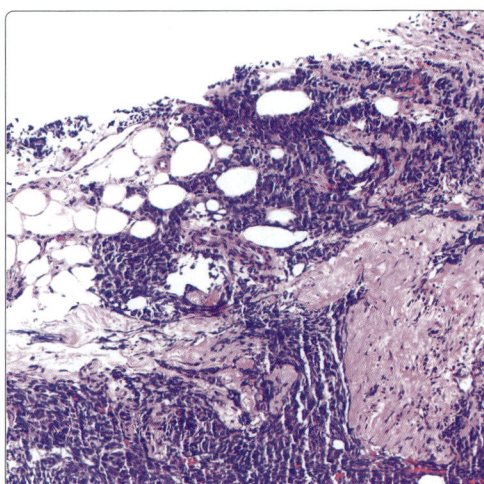

(Left) As many as 30% of SCCs may demonstrate formation of rosettes, which may cause diagnostic consideration of either cribriform acinar carcinoma or an extraskeletal Ewing sarcoma. This case, showing prominent nucleoli, showed ERG rearrangement by FISH. (Right) SCC shows extraprostatic extension by tumor cells (pT3a disease) characterized by infiltration of periprostatic adipose tissue. The majority of SCCs present with advanced tumor stage, and the prognosis is poor with an aggressive disease course.

Prostate Carcinoma With Neuroendocrine Differentiation

(Left) SCC shows diffuse and strong expression of synaptophysin. The majority of SCCs are positive for multiple NE markers, such as synaptophysin, chromogranin, CD56, and less specific NSE. Strong positivity for PSA or other prostatic markers is unusual in these tumors. **(Right)** Needle biopsy with SCC shows completely negative staining with PSA ➡. SCCs are typically negative for prostate-specific markers, such as PSA, PAP, and PSMA. Note benign prostatic glands in adjacent core are strongly PSA(+).

Markers of NED, Synaptophysin
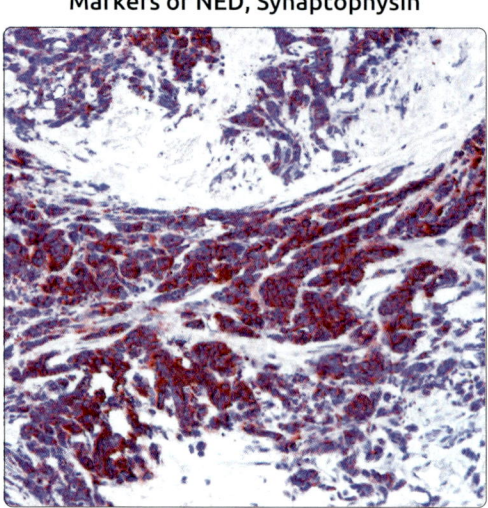

Prostatic Markers Lost in NED, PSA
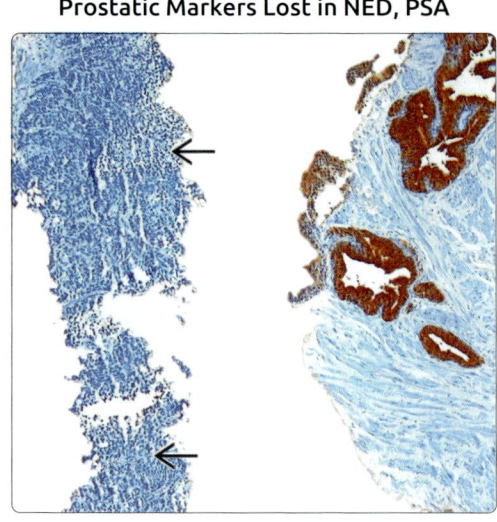

(Left) CK-PAN (AE1/AE3) expression in SCC may show dot-like cytoplasmic positivity, which is associated with prostatic and other NE neoplasms. TTF-1 may be positive. **(Right)** PIN cocktail (AMACR, p63, and HMWK) in prostate needle biopsy with SCC ➡ shows SCC tumor cells with modest AMACR staining (red) patchy with basal cell markers (brown). Note adjacent benign glands showing basal cell marker positivity ➡ and AMACR negativity.

Dot-Like Cytokeratin Positivity
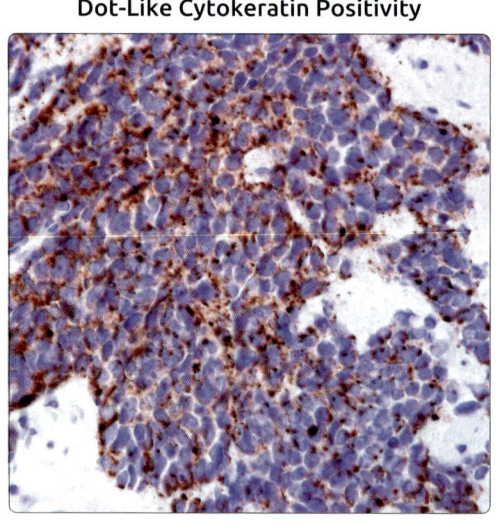

PIN Cocktail, Pattern of SCC
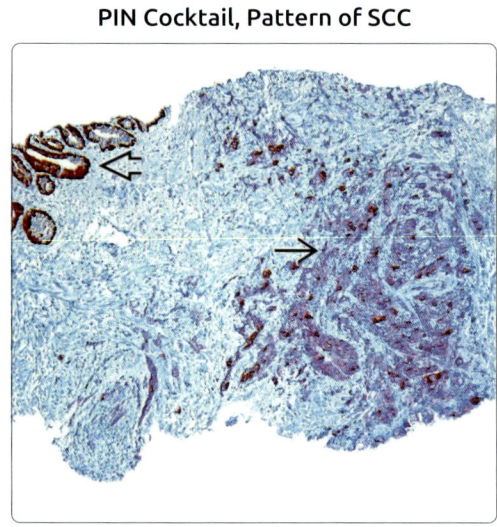

(Left) PCa with overlapping features of SCC and acinar PCa, proposed in the 2013 PCF Consensus, is characterized by a tumor with areas of hybrid patterns; here islands of recognizable prostatic differentiation ➡ are seen blending into areas of SCC-like cytology with crush artifact and lack of macronucleoli ➡. **(Right)** Synaptophysin IHC performed on the same patient shows that this marker was diffusely positive, supportive of the morphologic interpretation as overlapping with SCC.

Overlapping Features, SCC & Acinar PCa
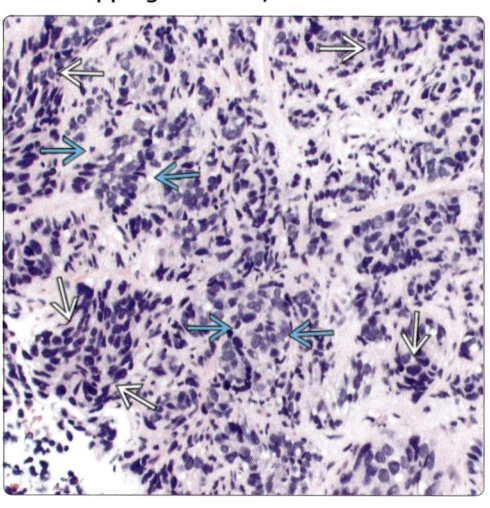

Overlapping Features, SCC & Acinar PCa
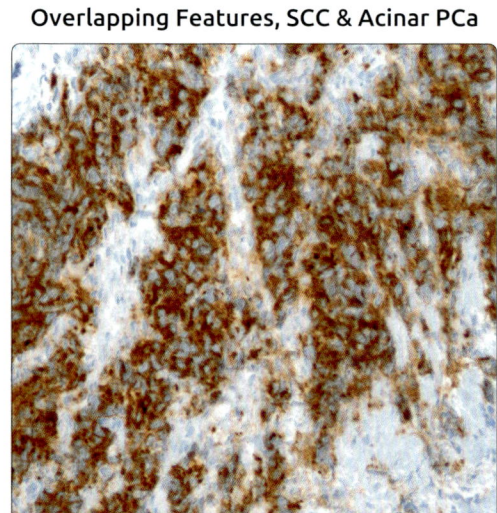

Prostate Carcinoma With Neuroendocrine Differentiation

Overlapping Features, SCC & Acinar PCa

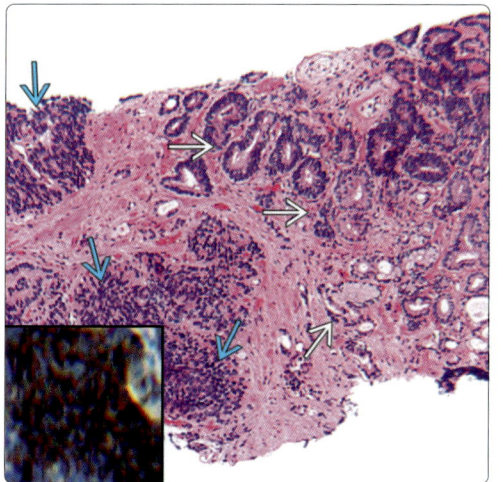

Overlapping Features, SCC & Acinar PCa

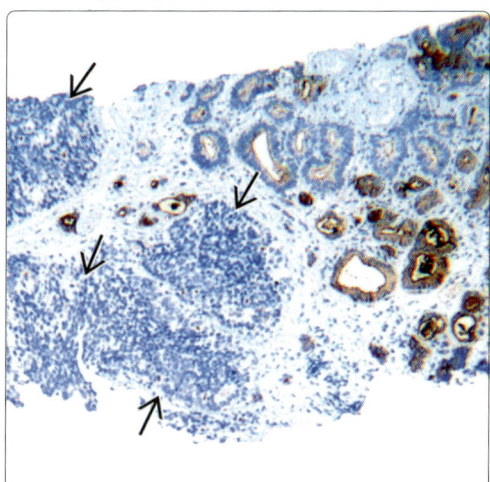

(Left) Another example shows PCa with overlapping features between SCC and acinar PCa; here areas of Gleason pattern 3 and 4 PCa ⇒ are juxtaposed to areas with morphology overlapping between high-grade acinar PCa (glandular differentiation) and SCC ⇒, with brisk IHC evidence of NED (chromogranin, inset). (Right) Areas of overlapping morphology between SCC and high-grade acinar PCa ⇒ are most often associated with predominant loss of markers of prostatic differentiation, in this case PSA.

Large Cell Neuroendocrine Carcinoma

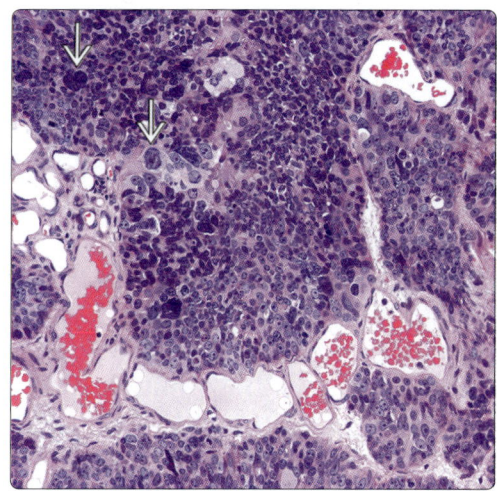

Large Cell Neuroendocrine Carcinoma

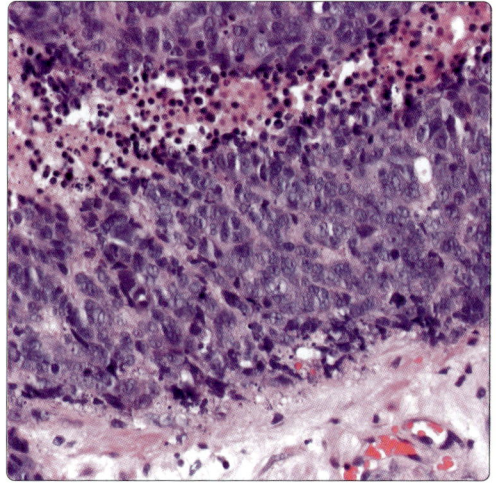

(Left) Here, a rare case of large cell neuroendocrine carcinoma (LCNEC) demonstrates organoid growth and prominent nucleoli. Similar to a subset of SCCs, scattered so-called giant cells are apparent ⇒. (Right) LCNEC demonstrates prominent necrosis, similar to that seen in SCC. Often this imparts the appearance of peripheral palisading of the cells at the periphery of sheet-like growth. This diagnosis should be made with caution, as Gleason 5+5 adenocarcinoma is in the differential.

LCNEC, Synaptophysin IHC

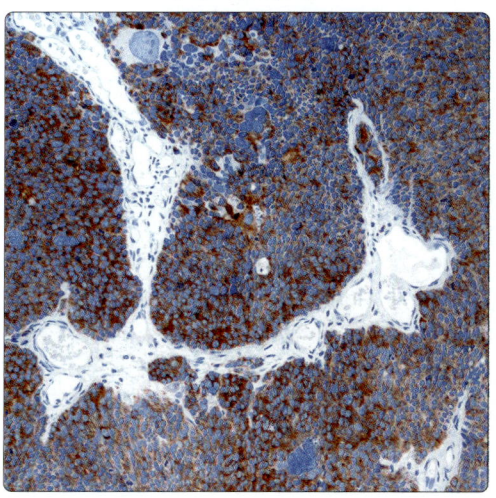

LCNEC, ERG IHC

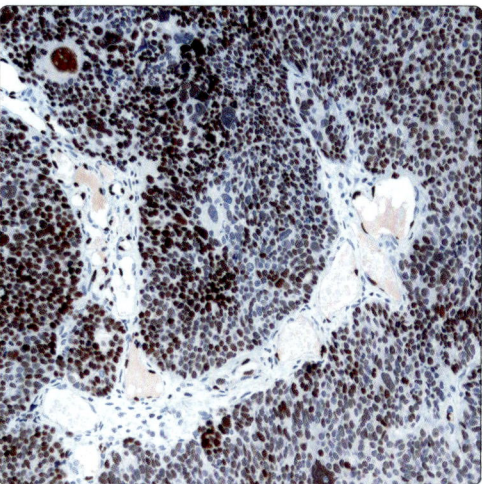

(Left) LCNEC demonstrates diffuse expression of synaptophysin, supportive of its NED. IHC evidence of NED is a requirement for this diagnosis, given the overlap with high-grade conventional acinar PCa. (Right) In this example of LCNEC, ERG expression was diffusely positive, supportive of prostatic histogenesis rather than urothelial histogenesis, given the potential for overlap with the LCNEC variant of urothelial carcinoma.

Basal Cell Carcinoma

KEY FACTS

TERMINOLOGY
- Malignant neoplasm composed primarily of basaloid cells arising putatively from prostatic basal cells

CLINICAL ISSUES
- Wide age range (28-89 years) but majority occur in older men
- Most commonly presents with obstructive urinary symptoms
- Normal serum PSA level
- Local recurrence, metastasis, and death from disease reported in ~ 30-50% of cases

MACROSCOPIC
- White and fleshy tumor with ill-defined infiltrative edges, may have microcystic features
- Tumor primarily centered in transition zone, with variable peripheral zone and periprostatic involvement

MICROSCOPIC
- Basaloid tumor cells have scant cytoplasm, high nuclear:cytoplasmic ratio, and irregular or angulated nuclei with open chromatin
- Infiltration of adjacent parenchyma (diffuse, nonlobular growth) is hallmark feature for diagnosis of malignancy
- 2 main histologic patterns
  - BCC consisting of variably sized solid nests, cords, or trabeculae with peripheral palisading of cells
  - Adenoid cystic carcinoma (ACC) consisting of infiltrative nests with prominent cribriform architecture

ANCILLARY TESTS
- Basal cell markers (+) and usually PSA/PSAP(-)

TOP DIFFERENTIAL DIAGNOSES
- Adenoid cystic pattern of basal cell hyperplasia
- Small cell carcinoma
- Poorly differentiated urothelial carcinoma

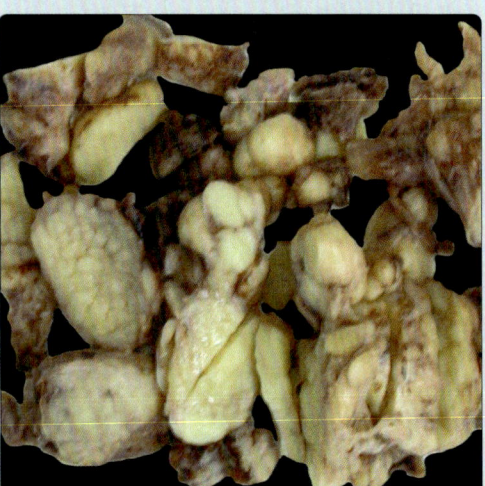

Basal Cell Carcinoma: Gross

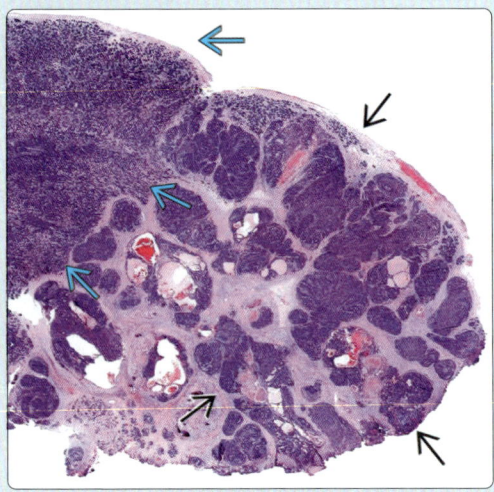

Basal Cell Carcinoma: Low Power

(Left) A gross photograph of a prostate enucleation specimen of basal cell carcinoma (BCC) demonstrates multiple nodular fragments with an indurated, rubbery gross texture. **(Right)** A low-power micrograph of BCC demonstrates a biphasic pattern, including a multinodular/septate growth pattern of sheets of cells ➡ corresponding to the BCC pattern and a 2nd smaller nested pattern ➡ corresponding to the ACC pattern.

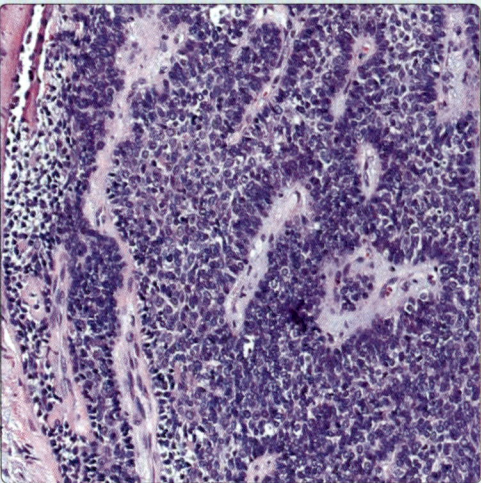

Basal Cell Carcinoma Pattern

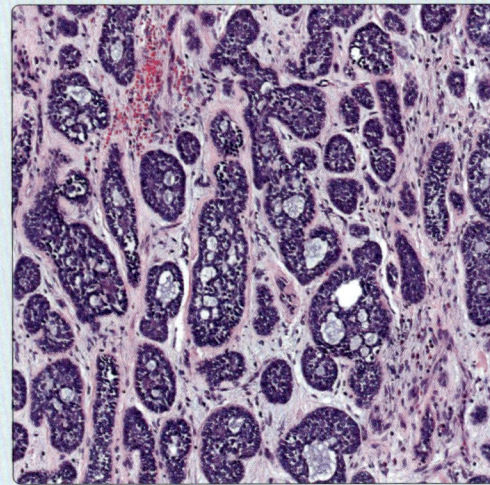

Adenoid Cystic Pattern

(Left) The BCC pattern consists of variably sized solid nests, cords, or trabeculae of small cells with high nuclear:cytoplasmic ratio, vesicular cytoplasm, and hyperchromatic, angulated nuclei. Peripheral palisading of basaloid cells is characteristic. **(Right)** The adenoid cystic pattern is characterized by nests of cells with similar cytologic features to the BCC pattern, but with prominent cribriform architecture and eosinophilic, hyaline, basement membrane-like, or mucinous material present in lumina.

Basal Cell Carcinoma

TERMINOLOGY

Abbreviations
- Basal cell carcinoma (BCC)

Synonyms
- Adenoid cystic carcinoma (ACC), adenoid basal cell tumor, adenoid cystic-like tumor of prostate

Definitions
- Malignant neoplasm composed primarily of basaloid cells arising putatively from prostatic basal cells

ETIOLOGY/PATHOGENESIS

Origin
- Considered to arise from basal cells along prostatic ducts and acini
- Recent series of 9 cases studied does not identify any rearrangements of *ERG* proto-oncogene, unlike other prostate cancers
- No data regarding t(6;9) MYB-NFIB translocations seen in ACC of salivary, skin adnexa, or lung

CLINICAL ISSUES

Epidemiology
- Incidence
  - Uncommon: ~ 75 cases reported in literature
- Age
  - Wide age range (28-89 years) but majority occur in older men

Presentation
- Most commonly presents with obstructive urinary symptoms
  - Thus most cases diagnosed on transurethral resection of prostate (TURP) specimens
- Perianal pain
- Few examples incidentally encountered in needle biopsy during work-up for elevated serum PSA level for other causes

Laboratory Tests
- Serum PSA levels may be normal, elevated if coincident conventional prostate carcinoma

Treatment
- Most reported cases treated with TURP, with subset undergoing radical prostatectomy
- Advanced stage treated with adjuvant radiotherapy or chemotherapy

Prognosis
- Limited data available on clinical behavior
- Local recurrence, metastasis, and death from disease reported in ~ 30-50% of cases
- Metastases commonly to lung and liver
- Bone metastasis rare compared to acinar adenocarcinoma
- Presence of large solid nests with central necrosis, high Ki-67 staining, and less immunoreactivity to basal cell markers suggested to be associated with aggressive behavior

MACROSCOPIC

General Features
- Grossly apparent tumor that is white and fleshy with ill-defined infiltrative edges
- May have microcystic features

Site of Involvement
- Tumor widely involving prostate, including peripheral zone; many invade bladder neck or periprostatic adipose tissue

MICROSCOPIC

Histologic Features
- Basaloid tumor cells have scant cytoplasm, high nuclear:cytoplasmic ratio, and irregular or angulated nuclei with open chromatin
- Basaloid cells may exhibit nuclear and cytoplasmic microvacuolation
- Infiltration of adjacent parenchyma (diffuse nonlobular growth) is hallmark feature of BCC
- BCC pattern
  - Variably sized solid nests, cords, or trabeculae with peripheral palisading of basaloid cells
  - May be associated with extensive central necrosis
- ACC pattern
  - Tumor grows in nests with prominent cribriform architecture
  - Eosinophilic, hyaline, basement membrane-like material may be present
  - Basophilic mucinous secretions may be present in lumina
- Additionally, tubuloglandular pattern with collagenous rim and basal cell hyperplasia-like patterns may occur
- **Combination of these different architectural patterns is often (> 80%) encountered**
- Usually associated with desmoplastic stromal response, which may be fibromyxoid or myxoid
- Rarely acinar, sebaceous, or squamous cell differentiation may be present
- Perineural invasion, angiolymphatic invasion, or necrosis may be present
- Extraprostatic extension is present in majority of cases, involving bladder neck, adipose tissue, or seminal vesicle
- Tumor involvement of thick bladder neck muscles detected in most TURP specimens
- Subset may have synchronous or metachronous prostate cancer, such as acinar adenocarcinoma, sarcomatoid carcinoma, or small cell carcinoma

ANCILLARY TESTS

Immunohistochemistry
- Usually PSA/PSAP(-), or at most focally (+), subset AR(+), all ERG(-)
- Basal cell markers (+), including p63 or HMWCK (34βE12)
  - May stain multiple layers of cells, only peripheral aspect of tumor clusters, or in only few scattered tumor cells
- Typically CK20(-) /CK7(+)
  - CK7 exhibits luminal (+) staining in ACC pattern, inverse to HMWCK (34βE12), which stains peripheral aspect
  - CK7(-) in pure solid basal cell nests
- Only minority (27%) of tumors are AMACR(+)

Basal Cell Carcinoma

- Variable proportions of cells stain for p53 in 2/3 of cases
- Synaptophysin (-/+), chromogranin (-)
- Bcl-2 staining is strongly and diffusely (+)
- High proliferative rate with Ki-67 nuclear staining, > 20% (+)

DIFFERENTIAL DIAGNOSIS

Adenoid Cystic Pattern of Basal Cell Hyperplasia

- Occurs in background of benign prostatic hyperplasia (BPH) and basal cell hyperplasia (BCH)
- When florid may mimic BCC
- Cribriform architecture may be present; glands typically smaller
- Many previously reported BCC may correspond to exuberant examples of adenoid cystic pattern of basal cell hyperplasia (AC-BCH)
- Exhibits nodular, well-circumscribed or lobulocentric growth, predominantly in transition zone
- In contrast to orderly arranged clusters of BCH, BCC shows haphazard, widespread, or single gland infiltration
- Distinction from BCC based mainly on absence of invasive features
  - Absent desmoplasia, perineural invasion, or necrosis; stroma is cellular, as in BPH
  - Lack of infiltration between normal prostatic glands or extraprostatic extension
- Luminal aspect of AC-BCH is bounded by acinar cells
- Bcl-2 stains more diffusely and strongly in BCC than BCH
- Ki-67 usually labels > 20% of cells in BCC, compared to < 5% in BCH

Acinar Adenocarcinoma of the Prostate With Aberrant p63 Expression

- Rare examples of acinar prostatic adenocarcinoma demonstrate diffuse, aberrant nuclear expression of p63
- These cancers may be encountered on PIN cocktail work-up of small foci or carcinomas with variant morphology
- Such carcinomas may also demonstrate basaloid or atrophic morphology
- Some cases with multilayered or spindled cytomorphology
- Infiltrative architecture with small gland pattern
- These cases are HMWCK(-) as may be demonstrated on single stain for this antibody

Small Cell Carcinoma

- Sheets of small cells with high nuclear:cytoplasmic ratio exhibiting nests, cords, or trabecular growth
- Nuclear molding, salt and pepper chromatin, abundant single cell necrosis, and crush artifact
- Neuroendocrine markers (+) and basal cell markers (-)

Poorly Differentiated Acinar Adenocarcinoma (Gleason Pattern 5)

- High-grade adenocarcinoma composed of cribriform and solid nodules may mimic ACC
- Often with markedly elevated serum PSA level
- Basal cell markers (-), PSA/PSAP(+)

Cribriform Pattern Acinar Adenocarcinoma (Gleason Pattern 3 and 4)

- May mimic ACC on low magnification
- Acinar cells have more cytoplasm and exhibit nucleomegaly with prominent nucleoli
- May contain luminal crystalloids
- Basal cell markers (-), PSA/PSAP(+)

Poorly Differentiated Urothelial Carcinoma

- Like BCC/ACC, are p63 &/or HMWCK (34βE12) (+)
- Invasive nests with cells containing abundant cytoplasm and higher degree of pleomorphism
- Carcinoma in situ may be present along prostatic urethra, prostatic ducts, or bladder mucosa

Anal Cloacogenic Carcinoma and Adenoid Cystic Carcinoma of Cowper Glands

- Histological and immunohistochemical overlap with BCC; cloacogenic carcinoma indistinguishable from BCC and ACC of Cowper glands similar to ACC of prostate
- Distinction based on epicenter of tumor, with prostate being only secondarily involved

DIAGNOSTIC CHECKLIST

Pathologic Interpretation Pearls

- Infiltrative solid or cribriform nests of basaloid cells showing invasive features

GRADING

Criteria

- Gleason grading is not applicable for BCC and ACC of prostate

STAGING

American Joint Committee on Cancer (AJCC) 7th Edition Cancer Staging Manual

- Though not specifically endorsed in AJCC prostate TNM system, it is widely used in reported literature

SELECTED REFERENCES

1. Simper NB et al: Basal cell carcinoma of the prostate is an aggressive tumor with frequent loss of PTEN expression and overexpression of EGFR. Hum Pathol. 46(6):805-12, 2015
2. Chang K et al: Basal cell carcinoma of the prostate: clinicopathologic analysis of three cases and a review of the literature. World J Surg Oncol. 11(1):193, 2013
3. Wu A et al: Prostate cancer with aberrant diffuse p63 expression: report of a case and review of the literature and morphologic mimics. Arch Pathol Lab Med. 137(9):1179-84, 2013
4. Halat SK et al: Adenoid cystic/basal cell carcinoma of the prostate. J Urol. 179(4):1576, 2008
5. Ali TZ et al: Basal cell carcinoma of the prostate: a clinicopathologic study of 29 cases. Am J Surg Pathol. 31(5):697-705, 2007
6. McKenney JK et al: Basal cell proliferations of the prostate other than usual basal cell hyperplasia: a clinicopathologic study of 23 cases, including four carcinomas, with a proposed classification. Am J Surg Pathol. 28(10):1289-98, 2004
7. Iczkowski KA et al: Adenoid cystic/basal cell carcinoma of the prostate: clinicopathologic findings in 19 cases. Am J Surg Pathol. 27(12):1523-9, 2003
8. Mastropasqua MG et al: Basaloid cell carcinoma of the prostate. Virchows Arch. 443(6):787-91, 2003
9. Devaraj LT et al: Atypical basal cell hyperplasia of the prostate. Immunophenotypic profile and proposed classification of basal cell proliferations. Am J Surg Pathol. 17(7):645-59, 1993

Basal Cell Carcinoma

Adenoid Cystic Pattern

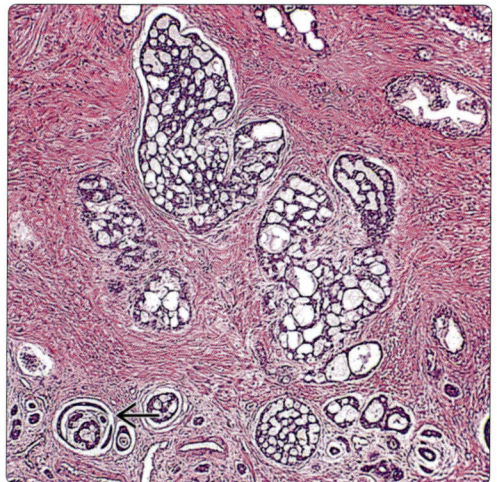

Adenoid Cystic Pattern

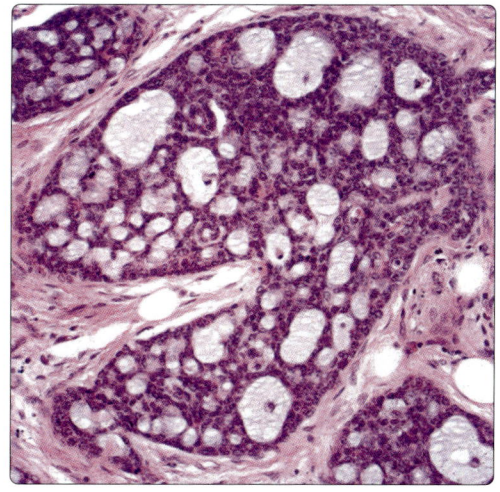

(Left) ACC pattern is characterized by infiltrative nests of basaloid tumor cells with prominent cribriform architecture, resembling ACC of the salivary gland. Note the perineural invasion ➡. The growth pattern is haphazard, and the cribriform nests are large and irregular. *(Right)* Cribriform architecture of ACC with several lumina is separated by cellular bridges formed by thin strands of basaloid cells. The lumina contain basophilic mucinous material. The basaloid cells in ACC are similar to those seen in BCC pattern.

Adenoid Cystic Pattern

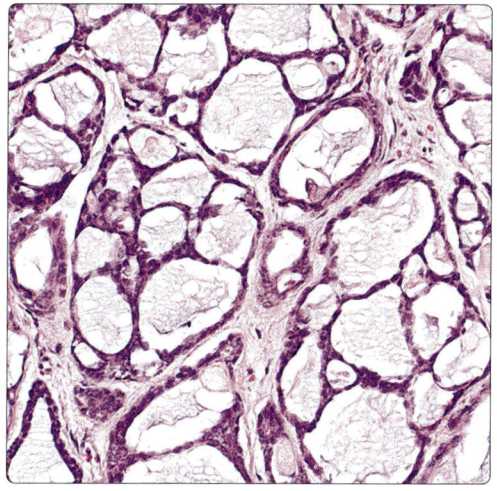

Mixed Adenoid Cystic Carcinoma and Basal Cell Carcinoma Patterns

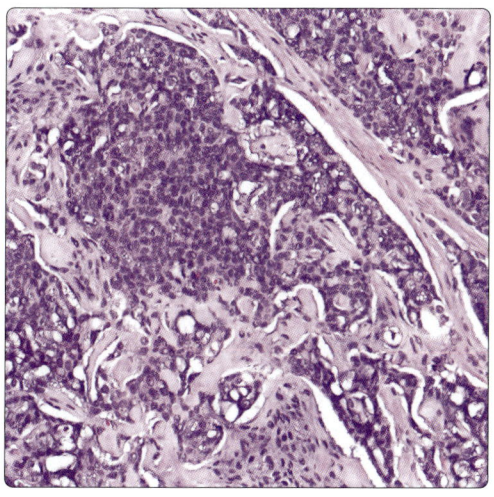

(Left) The ACC pattern is characterized by large, invasive nests with cribriform architecture containing multiple lumina resembling ACC at other sites. BCC and ACC patterns may coexist in the same tumor. *(Right)* A combination of BCC and ACC patterns is shown. Most cases, in fact, demonstrate both patterns (> 80% of cases). In contrast to basal cell hyperplasia (BCH), the nests are irregular and anastomosing and the stroma is desmoplastic.

Basal Cell Carcinoma Pattern

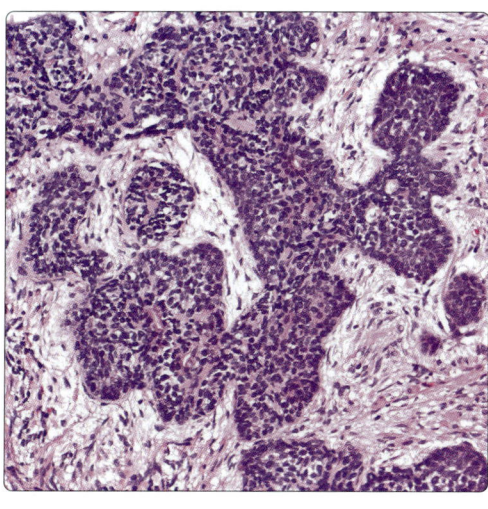

Basal Cell Carcinoma Pattern: Cytology

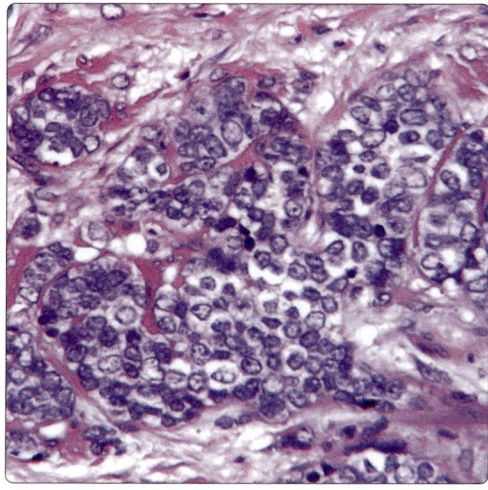

(Left) The BCC pattern is shown consisting of basaloid cells arranged in infiltrative large and small solid nests with peripheral palisading. The basaloid tumor cells have scant cytoplasm and are crowded, imparting a basophilic appearance. Note the stromal desmoplasia, which is helpful in excluding BCH. *(Right)* At higher power, BCC shows crowded basaloid cells with high a nuclear to cytoplasmic ratio, irregular nuclei, open chromatin, and nuclear overlapping. Mitotic activity is variable but often increased versus BCH.

Basal Cell Carcinoma

(Left) The tumor shows infiltrative, small, irregular nests of basaloid cells with desmoplastic stromal response. This particular BCC must be carefully distinguished from potential mimics, such as poorly differentiated adenocarcinoma and small cell carcinoma. **(Right)** HMWCK (34βE12) is typically positive in BCC but may be more variable, peripheral, or only scattered positive in some cases. HMWCK positivity is useful in exclusion of acinar PCa, which is negative.

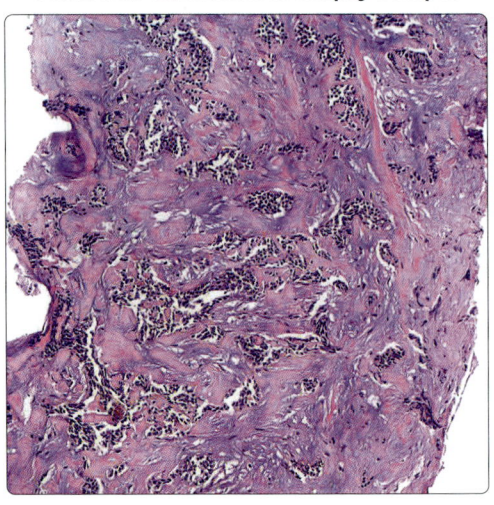
Basal Cell Carcinoma in Biopsy Sample

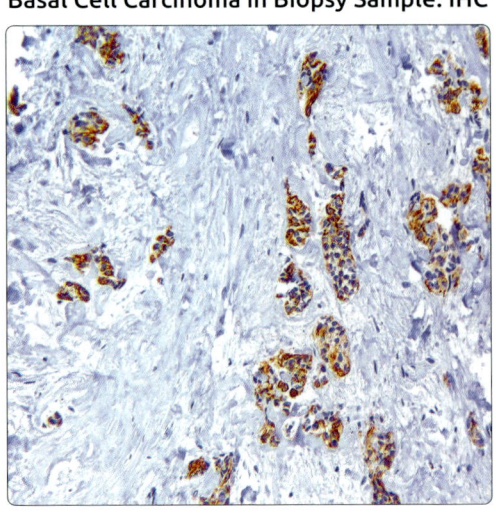
Basal Cell Carcinoma in Biopsy Sample: IHC

(Left) Rare cases of conventional acinar adenocarcinoma showing p63 positivity may demonstrate an atrophic or basaloid appearance, simulating BCC. **(Right)** p63/HMWCK dual immunostain performed on the acinar adenocarcinoma at left within image, demonstrating diffuse nuclear p63 positivity, is shown. Fortunately, these cases lack the HMWCK positivity characteristic of BCC. These atrophic prostatic adenoca are PSA (+).

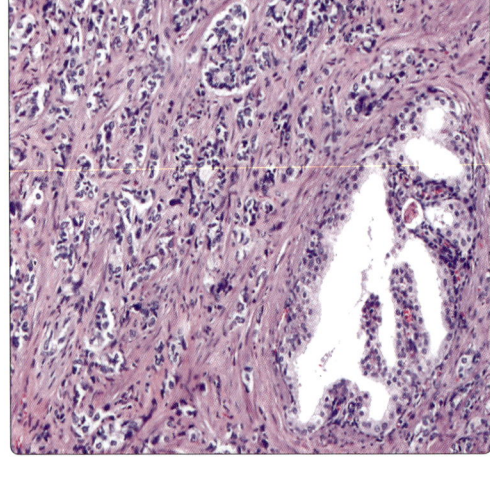
p63(+) Acinar Adenocarcinoma

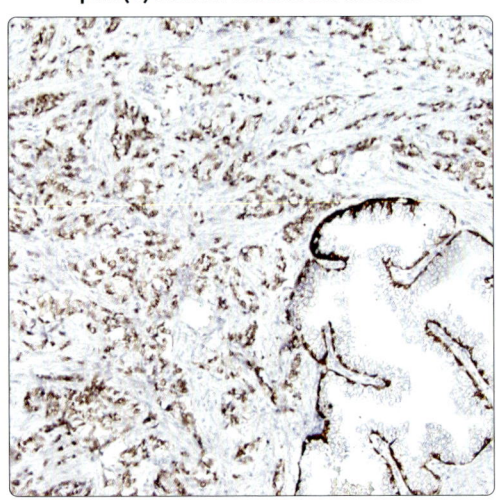
p63(+) Acinar Adenocarcinoma

(Left) BCC shows little to no expression of PSA, which is only apparent in an entrapped prostatic duct ➡ in this example. This property is useful in the differential diagnostic consideration with high-grade acinar adenocarcinoma. **(Right)** This BCC demonstrates diffuse, weak blush positivity for the NE marker synaptophysin. Such expression should not be interpreted as supportive of diagnosis of small cell carcinoma.

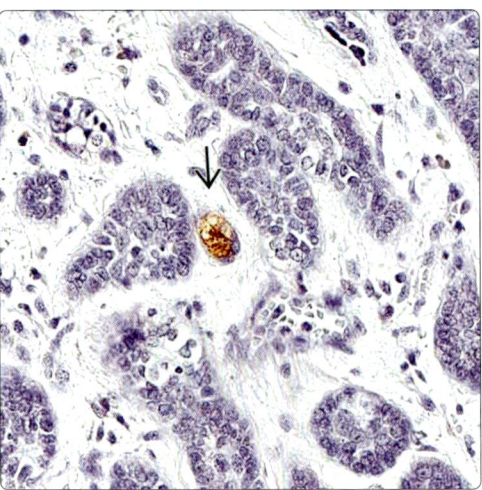
Basal Cell Carcinoma IHC: PSA

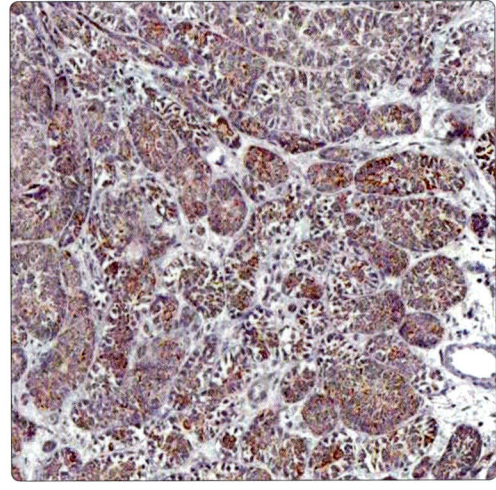
Basal Cell Carcinoma IHC: Synaptophysin

Basal Cell Carcinoma

Differential Diagnosis: Basal Cell Hyperplasia vs. Basal Cell Carcinoma

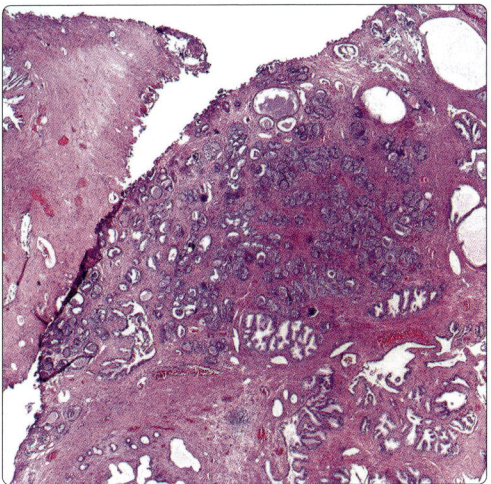

Differential Diagnosis: Basal Cell Carcinoma vs. Basal Cell Hyperplasia

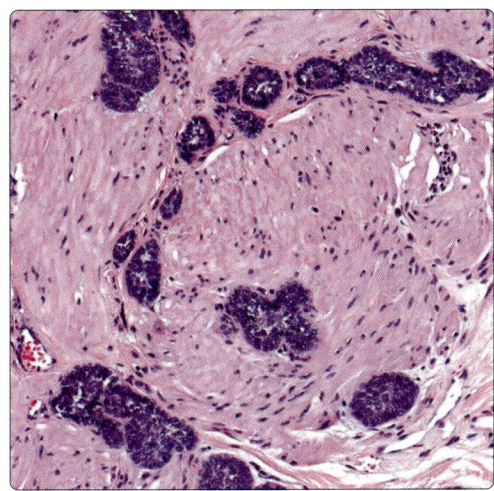

(Left) Florid basal cell hyperplasia (BCH), though demonstrating hyperchromasia and cellularity that may appear alarming, generally retains a lobular configuration at low power, confined to preexisting ducts and acini. *(Right)* Here, a BCC is shown invading around smooth muscle bundles of the bladder neck. Though BCH may be florid, it is lobular, noninfiltrative, and confined to the prostate, while most BCCs show infiltrative growth in prostatic parenchyma and extraprostatic disease.

Differential Diagnosis: Basal Cell Hyperplasia vs. Basal Cell Carcinoma

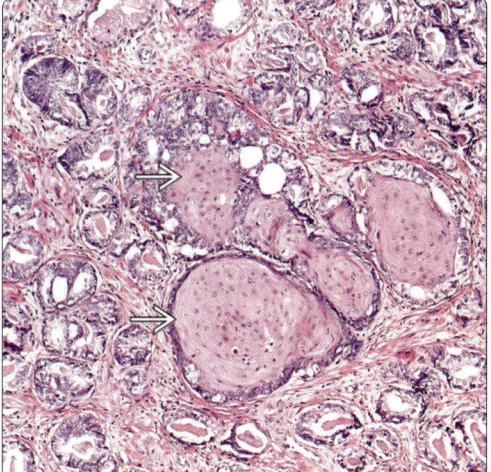

Differential Diagnosis: Basal Cell Carcinoma vs. Basal Cell Hyperplasia

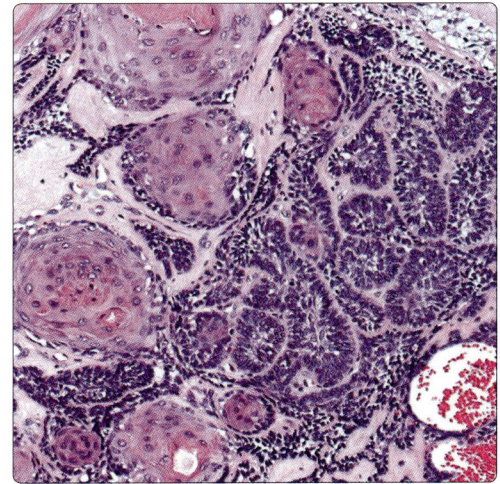

(Left) BCH, shown here, may appear cribriform and show foci of squamous metaplasia ➡. Though florid, a lobular configuration of background BPH must be observed on low power. *(Right)* BCC with squamous differentiation may appear similar to BCH, but the degree of anastomosis between invading trabeculae of hyperchromatic cells with peripheral palisading is marked in this example. To diagnose as Ca, infiltration of prostatic parenchyma in a nonlobular pattern is required.

Basal Cell Carcinoma vs. Basal Cell Hyperplasia: BCL2 IHC

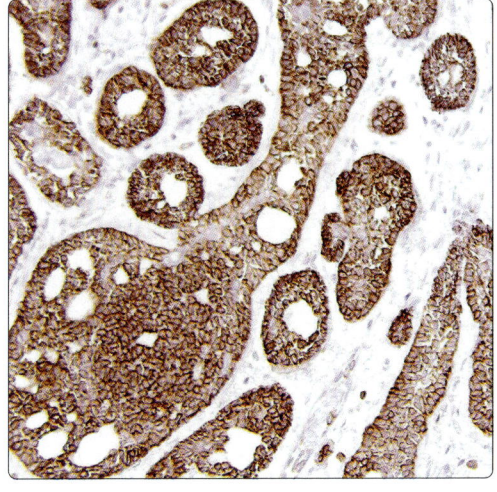

Basal Cell Carcinoma vs. Basal Cell Hyperplasia: Ki-67 IHC

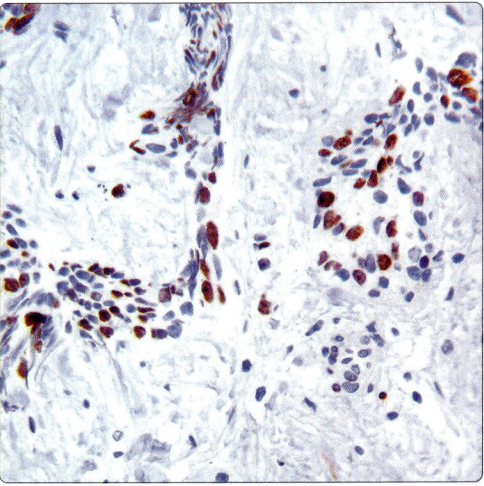

(Left) BCC shows prevalent, extensive expression of BCL2, which may also be helpful in supporting a diagnosis of BCC vs. florid BCH. *(Right)* BCC is shown with increased Ki-67 nuclear positivity. BCC usually exhibits higher Ki-67 (> 20%) than BCH (typically < 5%). Infiltrative (nonlobular) architecture, cytologic atypia, mitotic activity, stromal desmoplasia, or EPE when present are features indicative of carcinoma over BCH.

Sarcomatoid Carcinoma of Prostate

KEY FACTS

TERMINOLOGY
- Malignant biphasic or monophasic neoplasm of prostate demonstrating evidence of epithelial and mesenchymal differentiation and admixture with identifiable adenocarcinomatous component in most all cases
- Rationale for considering sarcomatoid carcinoma (SC) and carcinosarcoma (CS) as single entity is due to similar clinicopathologic features, prognosis, and molecular lesions

CLINICAL ISSUES
- Rare; only about 100 cases described in literature

MICROSCOPIC
- Overall histology falls into 3 categories
  - Carcinoma admixed with sarcomatoid spindle cell component (most common)
  - Carcinoma admixed with sarcomatous component containing heterologous elements
  - Monophasic spindle cell tumor with immunohistochemical &/or electron microscopic evidence of epithelial differentiation
- Acinar adenocarcinoma pattern most commonly admixed
- Sarcomatoid component frequently composed of hypercellular high-grade spindle cells (undifferentiated spindle cell sarcoma)
- Heterologous elements, most commonly osteosarcomatous, present in 20-30% of cases
- Carcinoma typically (+) for PSA/PSAP/prostein/NKX3.1, at least focally
- Spindle cells at least focally (+) for at least 1 epithelial marker

TOP DIFFERENTIAL DIAGNOSES
- Primary sarcomas of prostate
- Pseudosarcomatous myofibroblastic proliferation of prostate

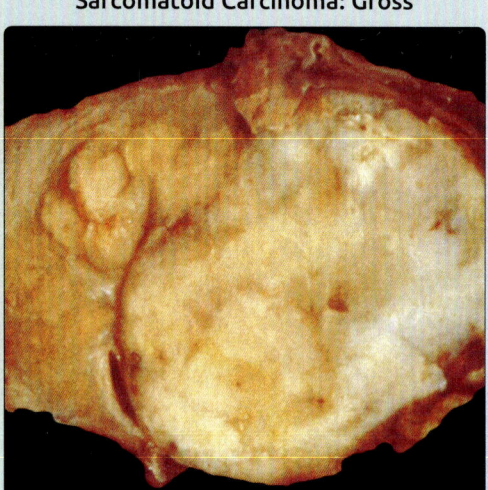

Sarcomatoid Carcinoma: Gross

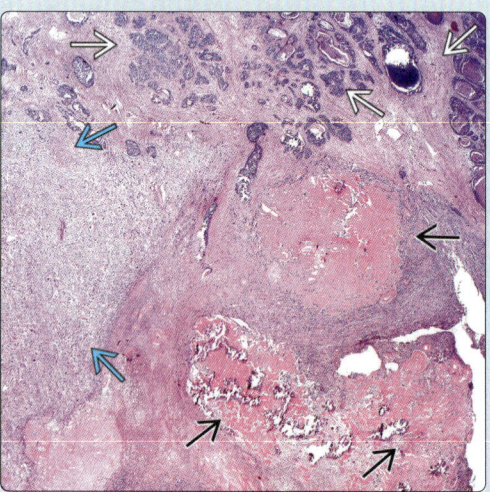

Sarcomatoid Carcinoma

(Left) Gross photograph of sarcomatoid carcinoma (SC) shows extensive involvement of peripheral and transition zones of prostate. The tumor is tan-white and yellow, fleshy (sarcoma-like) with ill-defined edges. (Right) In this low-power view, marked heterogeneity is seen, including a high-grade conventional adenocarcinoma ➡, a cellular, undifferentiated sarcomatous morphology ➡, and nodules of an osteosarcomatous component ➡.

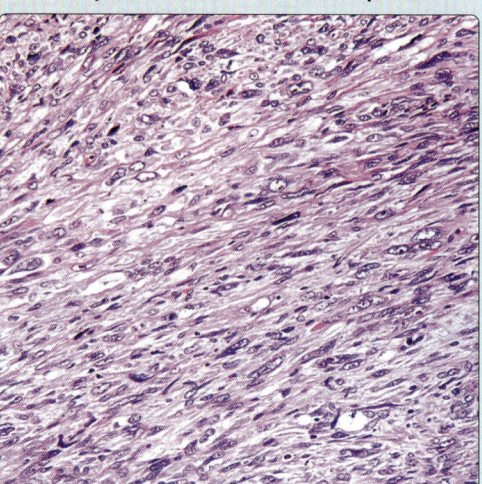

Monophasic Sarcomatoid Component

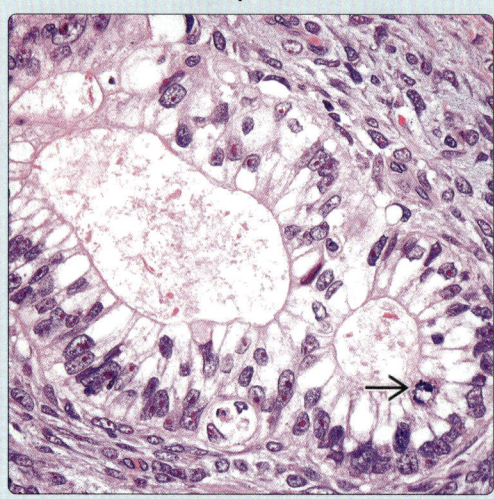

Admixed Acinar Adenocarcinoma Component

(Left) SC with monophasic malignant spindle cell morphology is shown. Other areas of this neoplasm showed typical high-grade adenocarcinoma of the prostate with acinar histology. (Right) Adjacent to the sarcomatoid component at left, an adenocarcinomatous component of SC shows prominent nucleoli, mitoses ➡, and absence of basal cell layer.

Sarcomatoid Carcinoma of Prostate

TERMINOLOGY

Abbreviations
- Sarcomatoid carcinoma (SC)
- Carcinosarcoma (CS)

Definitions
- Malignant sarcomatoid biphasic or monophasic neoplasm of prostate, demonstrating evidence of epithelial and mesenchymal differentiation by light microscopy and immunohistochemistry
  - CS has been employed previously for tumors with heterologous sarcomatous elements
  - Rationale for considering SC and CS as single entity is due to similar clinical features, prognosis, and molecular findings

ETIOLOGY/PATHOGENESIS

Origin
- Sarcomatoid dedifferentiation in prostatic carcinoma
  - High proportion (~ 2/3) of SCs have prior diagnosis of prostate adenocarcinoma
    - Essentially all have admixed adenocarcinoma at time of CS diagnosis
  - Focal immunohistochemical expression of PSA &/or PAP may be demonstrated in spindle cells
  - Loss-of-heterozygosity studies show that carcinomatous and sarcomatoid components are clonally related
  - Recent data demonstrate identical ERG rearrangements in acinar and sarcomatoid components
  - Model systems implicate role for loss of PTEN and p53 tumor suppressor function in SC

Risk Factors
- Vast majority with history of radiotherapy or hormonal therapy

CLINICAL ISSUES

Epidemiology
- Incidence
  - Rare
  - Only ~ 100 cases described in literature
- Age
  - Mean: 70 years; range: 43-91 years

Presentation
- Majority present with obstructive urinary symptoms or metastatic disease
- Uncommonly, tumors are detected in patients with elevated serum PSA level or palpable nodule on digital rectal examination (DRE)

Laboratory Tests
- PSA serum level may be normal or elevated

Natural History
- Prior diagnosis of conventional prostate adenocarcinoma seen in 48-66%
  - Interval to diagnosis of SC ranging from 6 months to 16 years (mean: 6.8 years)
- ~ 1/3 of cases arise de novo with no prior history of prostate adenocarcinoma and radiation &/or hormonal therapy

Treatment
- Current therapies remain ineffective, including multimodal treatment

Prognosis
- Poor outcomes, with 20% risk of death within 1 year of diagnosis
- Aggressive clinical course with local recurrences and metastasis (~ 40%)
- 1 study reports 5-year cancer-specific survival of 41% and 7-year survival of 14%
- Systemic metastases in majority of patients are to lungs and bone
  - Other reported sites include brain, lymph node, liver, peritoneum, and skin

MACROSCOPIC

General Features
- Most tumors are encountered in transurethral resection of prostate (TURP) specimens for obstructive urinary symptoms
- Large gray-white to yellow-tan with prominent necrosis, hemorrhage, and infiltrative growth
- Tumors extend extraparenchymally into periprostatic soft tissues or adjacent organs, such as seminal vesicles and urinary bladder

MICROSCOPIC

Histologic Features
- Carcinomatous and sarcomatoid components are intimately admixed
- Overall histology falls into 3 categories
  - Carcinoma admixed with sarcomatoid spindle cell component (most common)
  - Carcinoma admixed with sarcomatous component containing heterologous elements
  - Monophasic spindle cell tumor with ancillary evidence of epithelial differentiation (IHC, EM)
- Proportion of components vary, and sarcomatoid elements may range from 5-99% of tumor
  - Florid sarcomatoid overgrowth may be mistaken as pure sarcoma of prostate
- **Carcinomatous component**
  - Variable and may be admixture of the following patterns
  - **Acinar adenocarcinoma**
    - Most frequent epithelial pattern, often high grade
  - **Uncommon prostate adenocarcinoma patterns**
    - Foamy gland, ductal, adenosquamous, and signet ring cell carcinoma
  - **Uncommon nonglandular prostate carcinoma pattern**
    - Small cell, basaloid, squamous, and transitional (urothelial) carcinoma
  - **Discrete polygonal cell**
    - Seen intimately admixed with spindle cells, highlighted by epithelial markers
  - **Monophasic spindle cell morphology**

Sarcomatoid Carcinoma of Prostate

- Rare, evidence of epithelioid differentiation demonstrated only by immunohistochemistry or electron microscopy
  o Nuclei are often enlarged and can be markedly pleomorphic
- **Sarcomatoid/sarcomatous component**
  o Spindle cell morphology (most frequent)
    - Typically composed of hypercellular fusiform cells lacking specific lineage differentiation (undifferentiated spindle cell sarcoma)
    - Architecture may show storiform, fascicular growth, or patternless appearance
    - Majority are high-grade cells with large hyperchromatic nuclei
    - Mitotic activity is usually brisk
    - May contain bizarre nuclei and tumor giant cells resembling undifferentiated pleomorphic sarcoma
    - Rarely, spindle cells are less cellular with background myxoid stroma
  o May contain heterologous elements (20-30%) that resemble
    - Osteosarcoma (most frequent), leiomyosarcoma, chondrosarcoma, rhabdomyosarcoma, angiosarcoma
    - Combination of these heterologous elements is common
    - Heterologous elements typically merge with spindle cells
- Necrosis is frequent
- Histology of metastatic tumors is usually carcinomatous, although less commonly both components may be present

Predominant Pattern/Injury Type

- Neoplastic

Predominant Cell/Compartment Type

- Epithelial
- Mesenchymal

ANCILLARY TESTS

Immunohistochemistry

- Carcinomatous component
  o Typically PSA/PAP/prostein/NKX3.1, PSMA (+), at least weakly
  o Epithelial markers (PAN-CK, CAM5.2, EMA) (+)
  o Vimentin (-)
- Sarcomatoid spindle cell component
  o PSA/PAP usually negative; may be focally positive
  o Positive for PAN-CK, HMWCK, CK5/6, p63, at least focally
  o Vimentin (+), desmin and SMA variably (+); ALK-1(-)
- Heterologous sarcomatous elements
  o PSA/PAP(-), epithelial markers (-)
  o Vimentin (+)
  o SMA(+) in leiomyosarcoma
  o Desmin, myogenin (+) in rhabdomyosarcoma
  o S100(+) in chondrosarcoma

DIFFERENTIAL DIAGNOSIS

Primary Sarcomas of Prostate

- Overgrowth of any heterologous sarcomatous component of SC may simulate their pure sarcoma counterpart
- Most common prostate sarcomas are leiomyosarcoma and stromal sarcoma
  o Stromal sarcomas with phyllodes growth: Epithelial component is benign
  o Stromal sarcomas are positive for CD34 and PR; cytokeratin is typically negative
  o Leiomyosarcoma may occasionally show focal positivity for cytokeratin, although diffuse positivity is rare
- Other rare prostate sarcomas include rhabdomyosarcoma, undifferentiated pleomorphic sarcoma, solitary fibrous tumor, angiosarcoma, osteosarcoma, malignant peripheral nerve sheath tumor, and synovial sarcoma
  o These entities lack carcinomatous component and have clinicopathological features distinct from SC
- These tumors will not harbor rearrangements of ERG detectable by FISH

Pseudosarcomatous Myofibroblastic Proliferations of Prostate

- Includes inflammatory myofibroblastic tumors and postoperative spindle cell nodule
- Bland spindle cell proliferation with nodular fascitis/tissue culture appearance
- Lack significant cytologic atypia (no nuclear hyperchromasia or pleomorphism)
- Typical granulation tissue-type vascularity with scattered inflammatory cells
- Morphologic features, including necrosis, infiltrative growth, cellularity, and mitotic activity, overlap with sarcomatoid carcinoma
- Tumor cells may demonstrate strong and diffuse positivity for cytokeratin, further compounding the diagnostic difficulty
- Subset with ALK rearrangements positive by FISH or IHC; negative for p63, HMWCK, and CK5/6

Gastrointestinal Stromal Tumor

- Tumors of gastrointestinal origin or pelvic soft tissue may secondarily involve prostate, mimicking prostatic primary
- CD117, DOG-1, and CD34 are positive

DIAGNOSTIC CHECKLIST

Pathologic Interpretation Pearls

- Differential diagnosis of malignant spindle cell neoplasm of prostate should always include sarcomatoid carcinoma

SELECTED REFERENCES

1. Rodrigues DN et al: Sarcomatoid carcinoma of the prostate: ERG fluorescence in-situ hybridization confirms epithelial origin. Histopathology. 66(6):898-901, 2015
2. Martin P et al: Prostate epithelial Pten/TP53 loss leads to transformation of multipotential progenitors and epithelial to mesenchymal transition. Am J Pathol. 179(1):422-35, 2011
3. Huan Y et al: Sarcomatoid carcinoma after radiation treatment of prostatic adenocarcinoma. Ann Diagn Pathol. 12(2):142-5, 2008
4. Hansel DE et al: Spindle cell lesions of the adult prostate. Mod Pathol. 20(1):148-58, 2007
5. Hansel DE et al: Sarcomatoid carcinoma of the prostate: a study of 42 cases. Am J Surg Pathol. 30(10):1316-21, 2006
6. Ray ME et al: Clonality of sarcomatous and carcinomatous elements in sarcomatoid carcinoma of the prostate. Urology. 67(2):423, 2006
7. Perez N et al: Carcinosarcoma of the prostate: two cases with distinctive morphologic and immunohistochemical findings. Virchows Arch. 446(5):511-6, 2005

Sarcomatoid Carcinoma of Prostate

Sarcomatoid Carcinoma

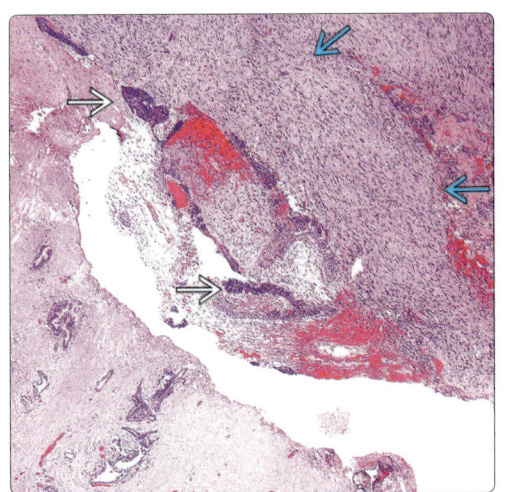

Sarcomatoid Carcinoma

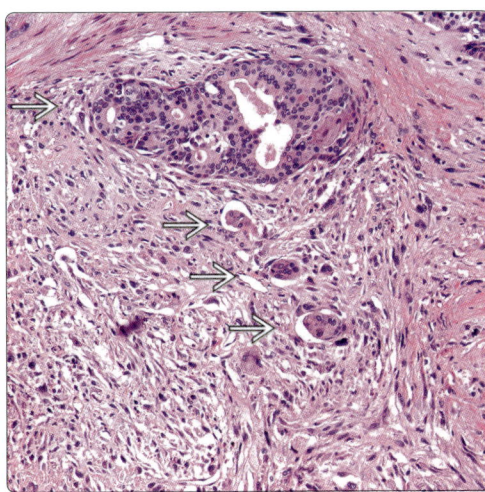

(Left) SC in prostatic chip of TURP specimen shows intimate admixture of malignant epithelial ➡ and stromal ➡ cell populations. The spindle cell component is hypercellular and markedly atypical, establishing the diagnosis of SC. *(Right)* The biphasic nature of SC is apparent as malignant glands of high-grade acinar PCa ➡ are closely juxtaposed to a malignant sarcomatoid spindle cell component.

Sarcomatoid Carcinoma

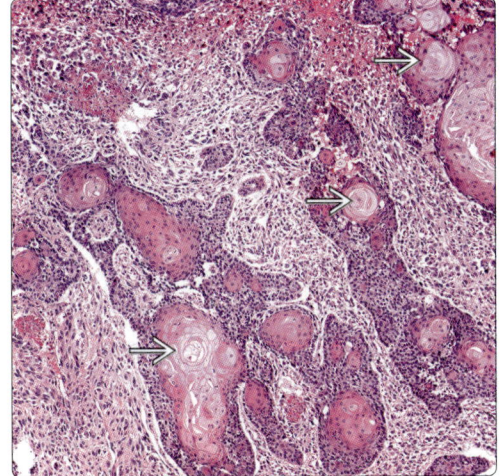

Sarcomatoid Carcinoma

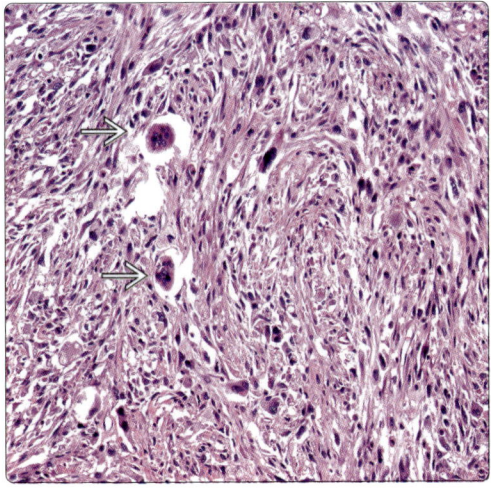

(Left) In this case, adenosquamous differentiation is prominent in the malignant epithelial component, with patches of keratinization including keratin pearls ➡. The intimate admixture of the malignant spindle cell and malignant epithelial component is helpful to establish this diagnosis. *(Right)* Another case shows a high-grade sarcomatous morphology reminiscent of that of undifferentiated pleomorphic sarcoma. Osteoclast-type giant cells are admixed ➡.

Heterologous Elements

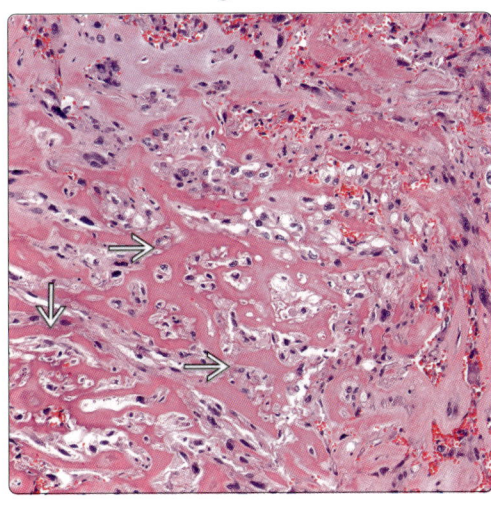

Heterologous Elements

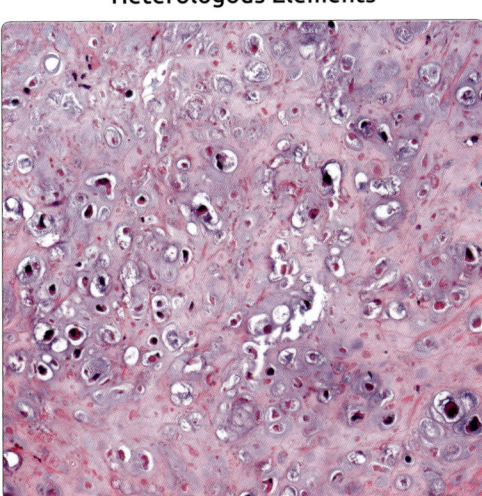

(Left) Heterologous osteosarcoma is seen in this focus of sarcomatoid carcinoma. Osteosarcoma is apparent as lacy trabeculae of malignant bone ➡ being laid by malignant spindle cells with marked nuclear hyperchromasia. *(Right)* In this focus, overt heterologous chondrosarcomatous differentiation is seen in the sarcomatoid component. Up to 30% of SCs show heterologous elements.

Sarcomatoid Carcinoma of Prostate

(Left) In this SC, a malignant cribriform acinar adenocarcinoma ➡ is seen intimately admixed with a malignant stromal component ➡. (Right) In the same focus of SC, strong expression of pancytokeratin OSCAR is seen in the epithelial component ➡, with attenuated keratin expression in scattered cells ➡ of the malignant sarcomatoid component.

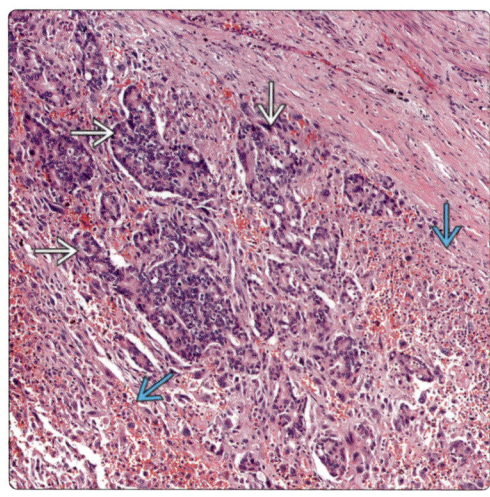
Sarcomatoid Carcinoma: H&E

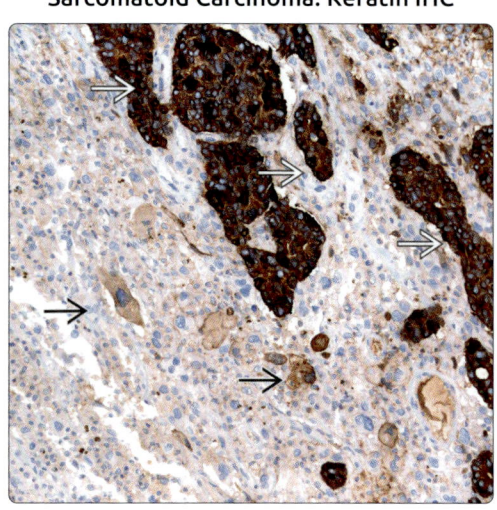
Sarcomatoid Carcinoma: Keratin IHC

(Left) In the same focus of SC, p501S/prostein expression (perinuclear/Golgi pattern) is maintained in the malignant adenocarcinoma component ➡, with only scattered cells in the admixed spindle cell component. (Right) In SC, expression of prostate lineage marker NKX3.1 (nuclear) ➡ is maintained in the epithelial component but lost in all but scattered cells of the sarcomatoid component.

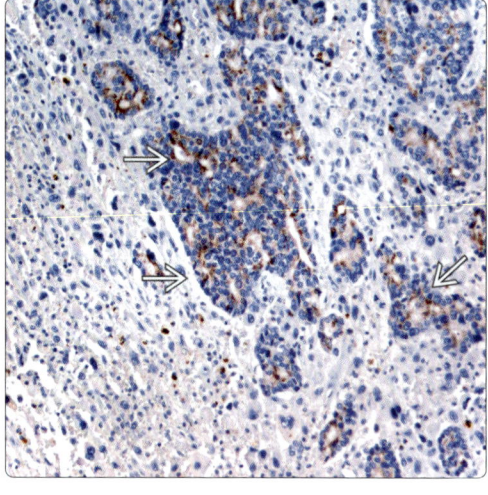
Sarcomatoid Carcinoma: Prostein IHC

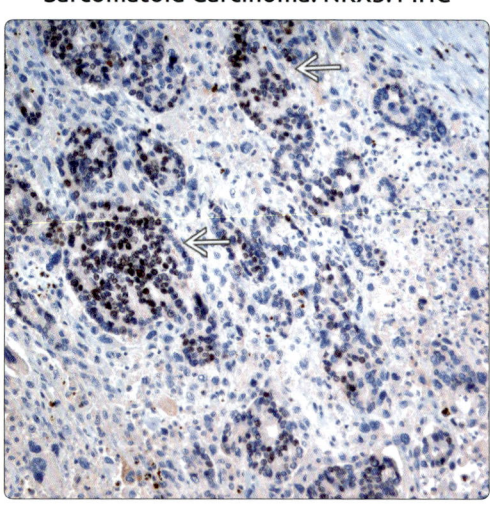
Sarcomatoid Carcinoma: NKX3.1 IHC

(Left) In this SC, PSMA (prostate-specific membrane antigen) is expressed only on the luminal aspect ➡ of the acinar component. (Right) In treated carcinomas, including this SC, ERG expression is often weaker; it is maintained with patchy nuclear expression in the acinar component ➡, with widely scattered sarcomatoid nuclei positive ➡, supporting the shared origin of both. Endothelium is a useful internal positive control ➡.

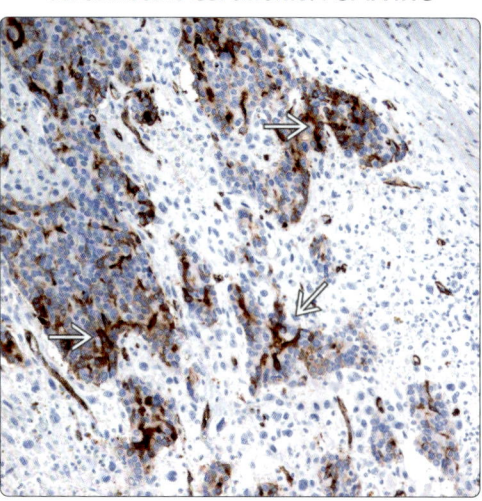
Sarcomatoid Carcinoma: PSMA IHC

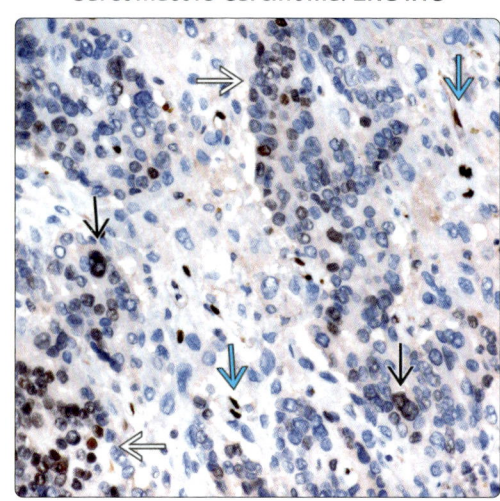
Sarcomatoid Carcinoma: ERG IHC

Sarcomatoid Carcinoma of Prostate

Sarcomatoid Carcinoma: Biopsy

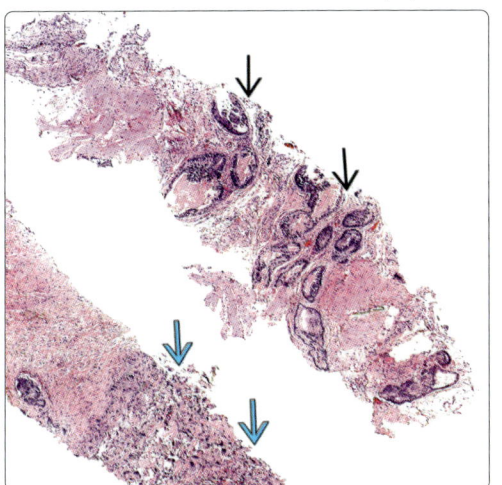

Sarcomatoid Carcinoma vs. Desmoplasia

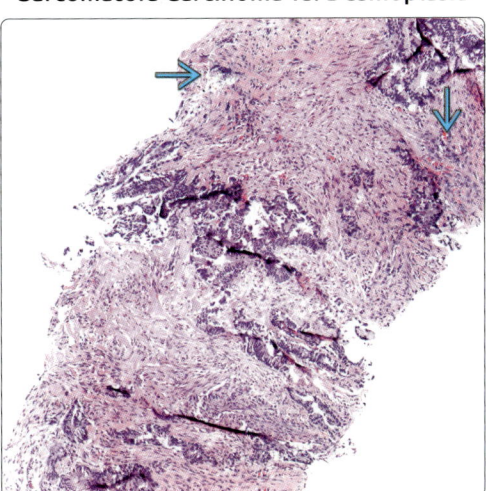

(Left) In this SC sampled by transrectal biopsy, a high-grade carcinoma is evident in 1 core fragment ➡, while a second malignant sarcomatoid component is evident in the other fragment ➡. *(Right)* PCa does not generally elicit marked desmoplastic stromal response. The degree of stromal cellularity adjacent to cribriform acini of high-grade carcinoma is worrisome, while scattered atypical spindle cells ➡ help establish the diagnosis of sarcomatoid carcinoma. Overt sarcomatoid transformation was apparent in other foci, as below.

Sarcomatoid Carcinoma: Biopsy

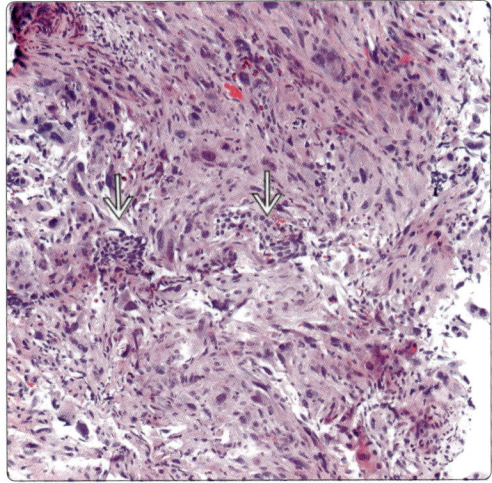

Sarcomatoid Carcinoma: Biopsy

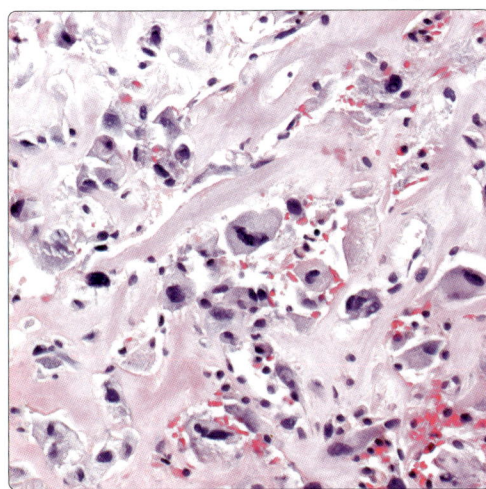

(Left) Sarcomatoid dedifferentiation is apparent as a malignant, sarcomatoid spindle cell proliferation, overrunning entrapped nests of high-grade carcinoma ➡. *(Right)* High-power micrograph shows that marked atypia, pleomorphism, and mitosis are all apparent. CK, high molecular weight cytokeratin, p63, and CK5/6 are frequently positive in malignant stromal cell component.

SC Biopsy: Pancytokeratin IHC

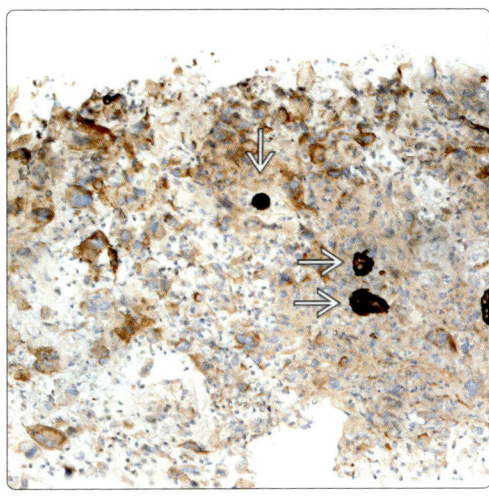

SC Biopsy: PSA IHC

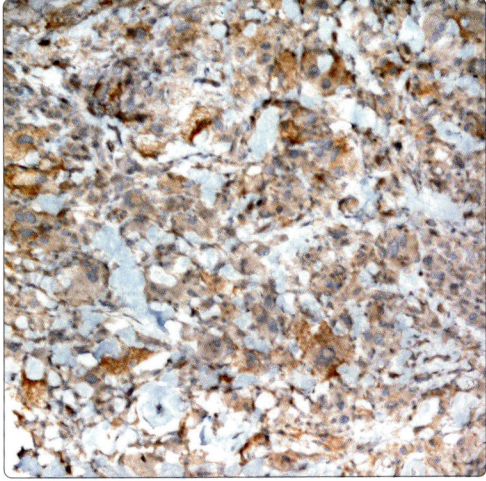

(Left) Pancytokeratin CAM5.2 highlights the entrapped epithelial component with strong diffuse positivity ➡ but is more attenuated in expression among the malignant sarcomatoid background, reflecting the epithelial mesenchymal transition of these cells. *(Right)* In this biopsy case, without prior treatment, weak PSA expression was maintained in the sarcomatoid component. Morphology with malignant biphasic histology is most diagnostic.

Carcinomas With Squamous Differentiation

KEY FACTS

TERMINOLOGY
- Primary carcinomas of prostate with squamous cell features and include pure SCC and adenocarcinoma admixed with SCC (ASC)
- Requires exclusion of secondary SCC involving prostate from other anatomic sites

ETIOLOGY/PATHOGENESIS
- Both SSC and ASC may arise de novo or preceded by prostate adenocarcinoma ± radiation or hormonal treatment

CLINICAL ISSUES
- Incidence: < 0.6% of all prostate cancers
- Serum PSA or acid phosphatase level typically normal, even with advanced disease
- More aggressive than prostate adenocarcinoma
- Generally poor response to surgical, hormonal, chemotherapeutic, or radiation therapies
- Bone metastasis is osteolytic, in contrast to osteoblastic metastasis in acinar adenocarcinoma

MICROSCOPIC
- Pure SCC similar to SCC of other anatomic sites
- Well to poorly differentiated with variable cytologic atypia
- Glandular component of ASC similar to acinar adenocarcinoma and tends to be higher grade
- Squamous and glandular components intermingled

ANCILLARY TESTS
- SCC: Negative for PSA and PAP and positive for HMCK (34βE12)
- Glandular component of ASC: Positive for PSA and PAP and negative for HMCK (34βE12)

TOP DIFFERENTIAL DIAGNOSES
- Secondary SCC involving prostate, secondary urothelial carcinoma with squamous differentiation, and squamous metaplasia of benign prostatic glands

Squamous Cell Carcinoma
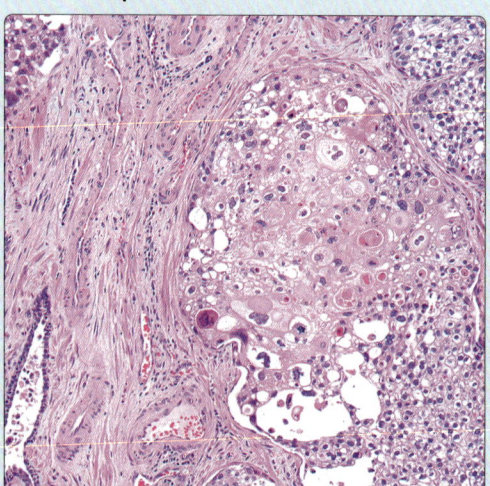

Squamous Cell Carcinoma
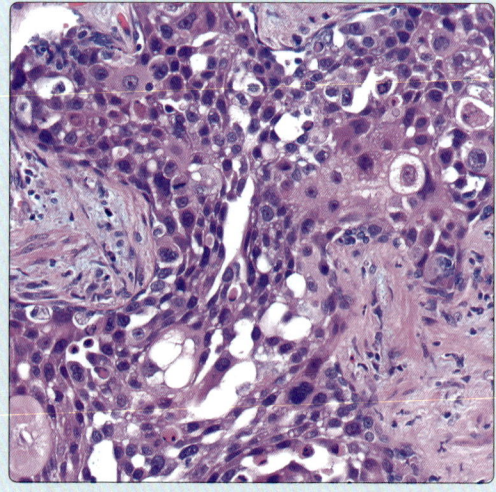

(Left) Infiltrating nests of SCC of the prostate are distinguished by cells with abundant glassy cytoplasm and keratin production. SCC of the prostate resembles SCC of other anatomic sites. Diagnosis as prostatic primary requires exclusion of secondary SCC from extraprostatic sites. (Right) Higher magnification of SCC shows polygonal cells with abundant glassy cytoplasm, distinct boundary, and intercellular bridges. The nuclei are pleomorphic, with prominent nucleoli and mitosis.

Adenosquamous Carcinoma
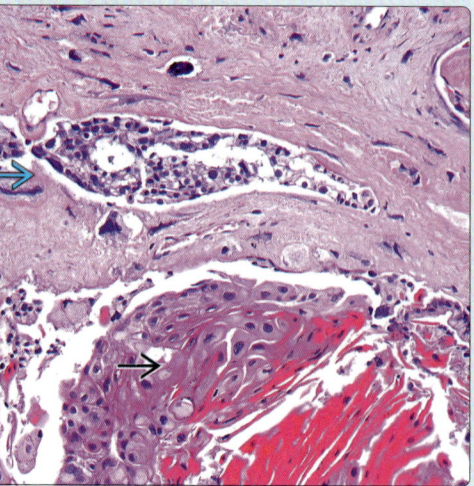

Adenosquamous Carcinoma
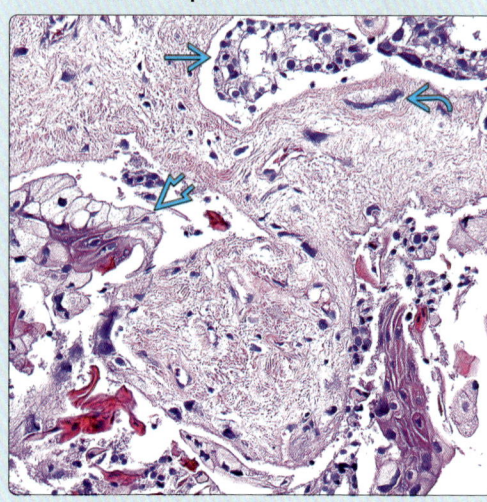

(Left) Adenocarcinoma of prostate treated with radiotherapy shows juxtaposition of acinar adenocarcinoma ➡ and atypical squamous cells with keratinization ➡. Both glandular and squamous components exhibit nuclear atypia. (Right) This ASC in postradiation setting shows the glandular component with foamy cytoplasm due to treatment effects ➡. Intimately associated are high-grade cells with keratin production ➡. Note atypia in stromal cells consistent with radiation effects ➡.

Carcinomas With Squamous Differentiation

TERMINOLOGY

Abbreviations
- Squamous cell carcinoma (SCC)
- Adenosquamous carcinoma (ASC)

Synonyms
- SCC: Epidermoid carcinoma
- ASC: Mixed adenocarcinoma and SCC, adenocarcinoma with squamous differentiation, adenoacanthoma (outdated term)

Definitions
- Primary prostate carcinoma with squamous cell features, including pure SCC and adenocarcinoma admixed with SCC (ASC)
  - Definition requires exclusion of secondary SCC involving prostate from other anatomic sites
  - Prostatic urothelial carcinoma with squamous differentiation and sarcoma admixed with SCC not included

ETIOLOGY/PATHOGENESIS

Risk Factors
- Prior history of prostate adenocarcinoma
  - May uncommonly give rise to SCC or ASC 3-10 years after adenocarcinoma diagnosis
- Radiation or hormonal therapy
  - May influence squamous differentiation in primary as well as metastatic adenocarcinoma
  - Greater proportion of ASC (~ 2/3) than SCC reported post therapy
- Genitourinary schistosomiasis has been proposed
- May also arise de novo without radiation or hormonal therapy or prior prostate adenocarcinoma history

Origin
- Precise cell of origin remains controversial
- Considered to be derived from prostatic glandular cells that show ability to differentiate toward squamous cells
  - Both acinar and basal glandular cells proposed as cell of origin
- Other proposed theories of cell derivation
  - Urothelium of prostatic urethra or periurethral ducts
  - Malignant transformation in squamous metaplasia of benign glands
  - Pluripotential stem cells capable of multidirectional differentiation
  - For ASC: Collision-type tumor with de novo origin for SCC and adenocarcinoma

CLINICAL ISSUES

Epidemiology
- Incidence
  - Very rare; < 0.6% of all prostate cancers
    - ~ 60 cases of pure SCC reported
    - ASC rarer; < 50 cases reported including 25 cases from SEER database
- Age
  - Mean: 68 years; range: 49-86 years

Presentation
- Presenting symptoms resemble advanced prostate adenocarcinoma
- Obstructive urinary symptoms
  - Majority encountered in TURP specimens
- Hematuria
- Bone pain from metastasis
- Most cases with palpable disease on rectal examination at time of presentation

Laboratory Tests
- Serum PSA or acid phosphatase level may be normal, even with advanced disease
  - PSA elevation occurs more often in ASC
- Serum SCC antigen marker elevated; may be useful in monitoring disease

Natural History
- Both SCC and ASC may arise de novo or be preceded by prostate adenocarcinoma ± radiation or hormonal treatment
- Relatively greater proportion of ASC (than SCC) encountered in patients with prior adenocarcinoma
- No established relationship with squamous metaplasia of benign prostatic glands

Treatment
- Generally poor response to surgical, hormonal, chemotherapeutic, or radiation therapy
- Multimodal therapy appears to be most promising

Prognosis
- More aggressive than prostate adenocarcinoma
  - Median postdiagnosis survival time for SCC is ~ 14 months
  - Median cancer-specific survival for ASC is 16 months
- Metastasis occurs in ~ 1/3 of cases, most commonly to bones and lung
- Bone metastasis is osteolytic, in contrast to osteoblastic metastasis in acinar adenocarcinoma

MACROSCOPIC

General Features
- Tends to be more localized in transition zone or central region of prostate
- Firm grayish white tumor
- Tumor may be bulky and extend into adjacent organs, such as seminal vesicles and rectum

MICROSCOPIC

Histologic Features
- Pure squamous cell carcinoma
  - Similar to SCC of other anatomic sites
  - By definition does not contain glandular elements
  - Infiltrating nests and sheets of polygonal cells with intercellular bridges
  - Abundant eosinophilic glassy cytoplasm or keratin pearls in better differentiated tumors
- Adenosquamous carcinoma
  - Squamous component similar to pure SCC

Carcinomas With Squamous Differentiation

- Glandular component demonstrates range seen in morphology of acinar adenocarcinoma
- Squamous and glandular components intermingled with no distinct transition
- Amount of adenocarcinoma varies from 5-95% of tumor (average 40%)
- Adenocarcinoma tends to be higher grade (Gleason score 7 or higher)
- Perineural invasion may be seen
- May have extraprostatic extension

Grade
- SCC
  - Well to poorly differentiated with variable cytologic atypia (Broder grade)
- Glandular component of ASC
  - Tends to be higher grade (Gleason score 7 or higher)

ANCILLARY TESTS

Immunohistochemistry
- SCC
  - Negative for PSA and PAP
  - Positive for HMCK (34βE12)
- Glandular component of ASC
  - Positive for PSA and PAP
  - Negative for HMCK (34βE12)
  - Newer markers: PSMA, NKX3.1, prostein (+)

Flow Cytometry
- DNA analysis
  - Similarity in DNA peaks observed in both squamous and glandular components of ASC

Electron Microscopy
- SCC demonstrates microvilli lining intercellular spaces and variable desmosomes

DIFFERENTIAL DIAGNOSIS

Secondary Squamous Cell Carcinoma Involving Prostate
- Direct extension from urinary bladder or anal SCC
- Histologic distinction is difficult, if not impossible, especially in limited tissue samples
- Distinction may require clinicopathologic correlation
- SCC metastatic to prostate from distant anatomic sites exceedingly rare, encountered mainly in autopsies

Secondary Urothelial Carcinoma With Squamous Differentiation
- Urinary bladder or prostatic urethral urothelial carcinoma with squamous differentiation may invade into prostate
- Differentiation may be difficult in limited tissue samples
- Admixed invasive urothelial carcinoma ± glandular (nonprostatic type) differentiation
- Presence of urothelial carcinoma in situ or papillary neoplasm in bladder mucosal surface
- Acinar component absent (vs. ASC)
- Distinction may require clinicopathologic correlation

Squamous Metaplasia of Benign Prostatic Glands ± Inflammation
- Occurs as response to infarction and hormonal or radiation therapy
- Similar to SCC, does not express PSA and PAP
- Lacks cytologic atypia and invasive features of SCC
- Clinical history or recognition of adjacent infarcted prostatic tissue helpful in diagnosis

DIAGNOSTIC CHECKLIST

Pathologic Interpretation Pearls
- Neoplastic squamous growth displaying cytologic atypia and invasive features
- Diagnosis requires clinicopathologic exclusion of secondary carcinomas with squamous differentiation from other sites (mainly urinary bladder)

GRADING

Types
- Gleason grading
  - Applied to glandular component of ASC
  - Not applicable for SCC component
- Broder grading system for SCC of other anatomic sites
  - Applied to prostate SCC
  - Based on degree of squamous differentiation (i.e., keratinization of tumor cells) and nuclear atypicality
  - Well to differentiated tumors (grades I to IV)

REPORTING

Key Elements to Report
- Biopsy, microscopic evaluation
  - Histologic type (SCC or ASC)
  - Grade (Gleason grade &/or Broder grade)
  - Local invasion: Prostatic fat; seminal vesicles
  - Additional findings, if present
- Prostatectomy, microscopic evaluation
  - Histologic type (SCC or ASC)
  - Grade (Gleason grade &/or Broder grade)
  - Location
  - Extent of local invasion: Prostatic fat; seminal vesicle
  - Margins (location and extent of margins involved with tumor)
  - Regional lymph node status
  - Additional findings, if present

SELECTED REFERENCES

1. Fine SW: Variants and unusual patterns of prostate cancer: clinicopathologic and differential diagnostic considerations. Adv Anat Pathol. 19(4):204-16, 2012
2. Humphrey PA: Histological variants of prostatic carcinoma and their significance. Histopathology. 60(1):59-74, 2012
3. Arva NC et al: Diagnostic dilemmas of squamous differentiation in prostate carcinoma case report and review of the literature. Diagn Pathol. 6:46, 2011
4. Malik RD et al: Squamous cell carcinoma of the prostate. Rev Urol. 13(1):56-60, 2011
5. Wang J et al: Clinical features and outcomes of 25 patients with primary adenosquamous cell carcinoma of the prostate. Rare Tumors. 2(3):e47, 2010
6. Guo CC et al: Prostate cancer invading the rectum: a clinicopathological study of 18 cases. Pathology. 41(6):539-43, 2009
7. Parwani AV et al: Prostate carcinoma with squamous differentiation: an analysis of 33 cases. Am J Surg Pathol. 28(5):651-7, 2004

Carcinomas With Squamous Differentiation

Squamous Cell Carcinoma

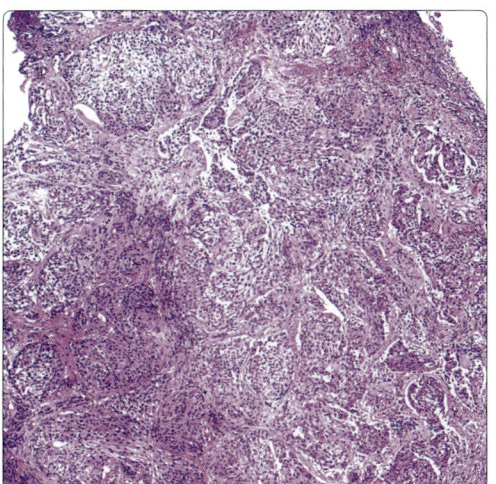

Squamous Cell Carcinoma

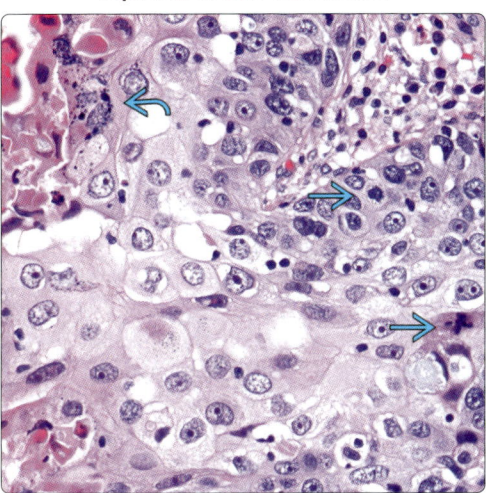

(Left) Pure SCC in TURP consists of infiltrating nests of malignant squamous cells amidst a desmoplastic stroma. Before diagnosis of pure SCC is rendered, extensive sampling is required to rule out acinar component. (Right) Pure SCC of the prostate shows cells containing abundant glassy eosinophilic cytoplasm with well-defined borders. Mitosis is frequent ⇨. Note the keratohyaline granules ⇨ next to keratinized cells. Squamous differentiation may occur in urothelial carcinoma and should be distinguished from pure SCC.

Squamous Cell Carcinoma

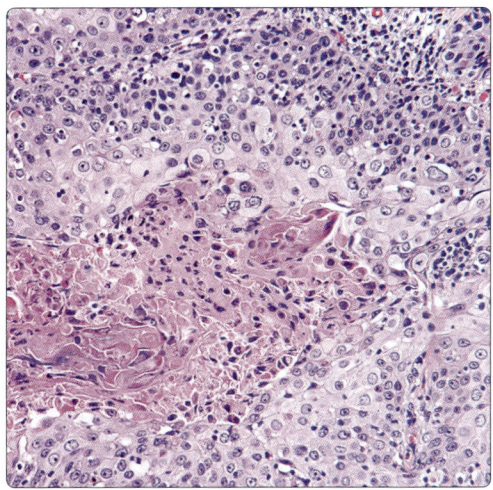

Squamous Cell Carcinoma

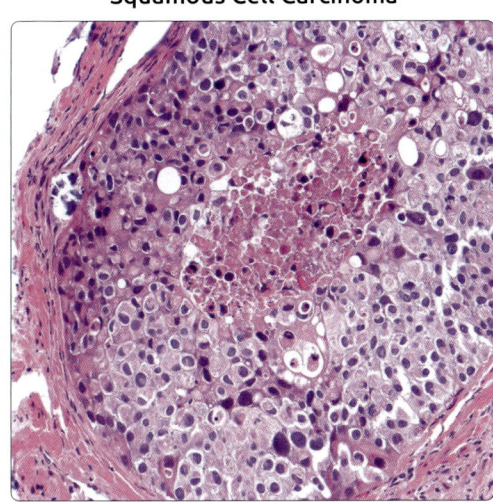

(Left) Invasive pure SCC of the prostate shows evidence of squamous differentiation including abundant keratinization. SCC in prostate is graded similar to usual SCC, and abundant keratin indicates a better differentiated tumor. (Right) This SCC in a prostate biopsy shows pure squamous histology. In needle biopsy, distinction from secondary SCC or urothelial carcinoma with squamous differentiation is often not possible. Clinicopathological correlation is required to establish the primary site of this tumor.

Adenosquamous Carcinoma

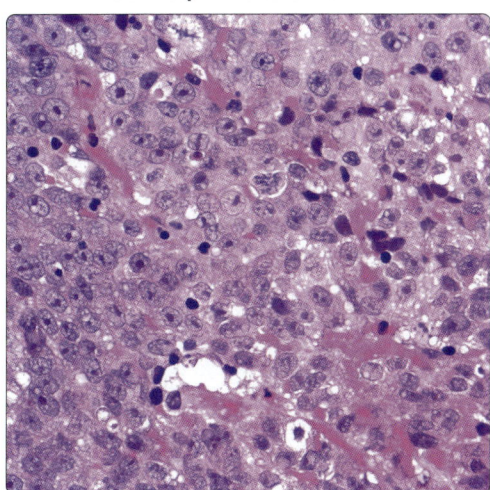

Adenosquamous Carcinoma

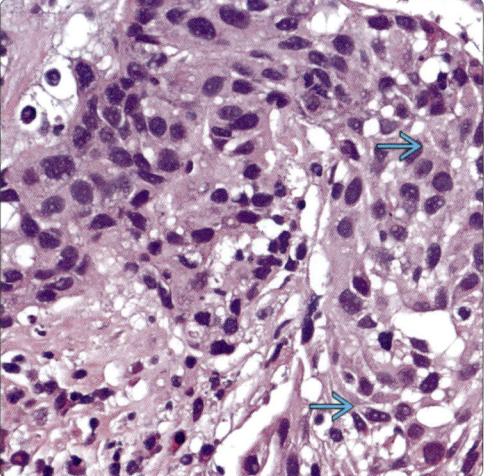

(Left) ASC of the prostate with a poorly differentiated adenocarcinoma component shows high-grade cells with nucleomegaly lacking glandular lumina (Gleason pattern 5). This component was positive for PSA. (Right) ASC of the prostate in the same patient shows malignant squamous cells with intercellular bridges ⇨. In ASC, the glandular component is typically of higher grade (Gleason score 7 or higher). About 2/3 of ASC has a prior history of adenocarcinoma treated with radiation or hormonal therapy.

Carcinomas With Squamous Differentiation

(Left) ASC of prostate in a needle biopsy shows nests of abrupt squamous differentiation, including keratin pearl ⇒ formation, present within cribriform Gleason score 9 prostate adenocarcinoma. **(Right)** ASC of the prostate shows squamous differentiation ⇒ within high-grade adenocarcinoma of prostate ⇒. There is a separate focus of conventional acinar carcinoma, which helps in the distinction from primary SCC, secondary SCC, or urothelial carcinoma with squamous differentiation.

Adenosquamous Carcinoma
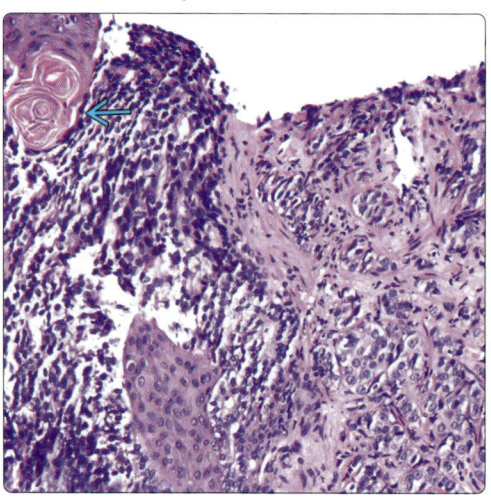

Adenosquamous Carcinoma
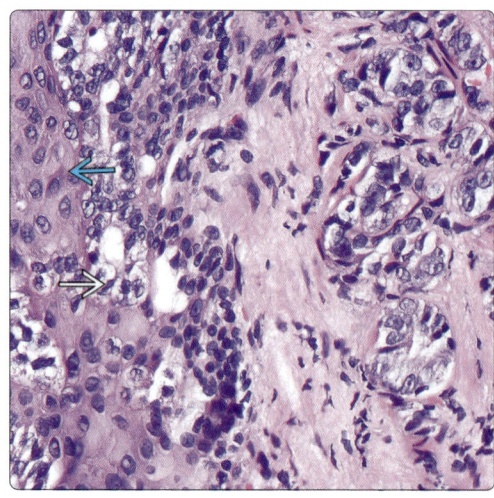

(Left) Urothelial carcinoma in situ along the prostatic urethra shows focal squamous differentiation. Presence of this feature is a helpful clue in distinguishing invasive urethral urothelial carcinoma with squamous differentiation from pure SCC of prostate. **(Right)** The invasive component from the same patient maintains squamous differentiation, including the presence of occasional intracytoplasmic keratin ⇒.

Urothelial Carcinoma With Squamous Differentiation From Urethra
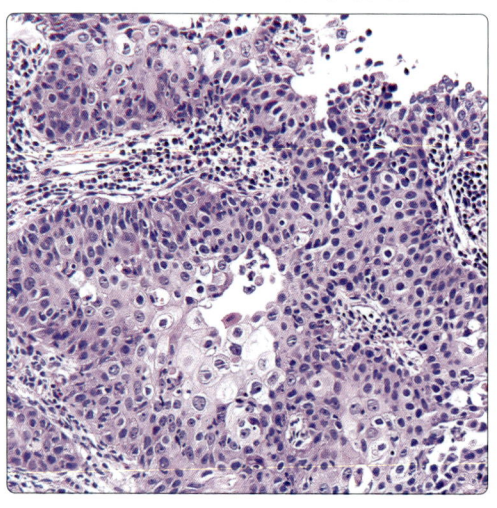

Urothelial Carcinoma With Squamous Differentiation From Urethra
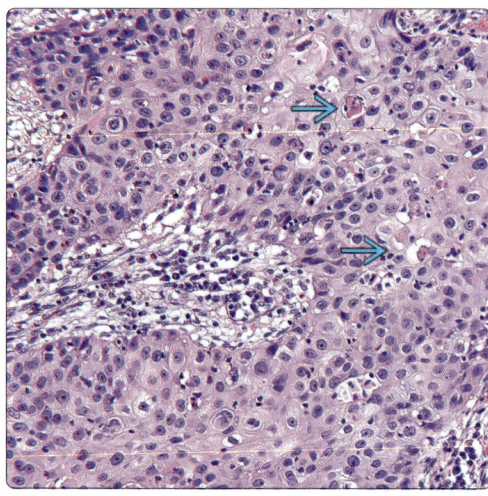

(Left) Bladder urothelial carcinoma with squamous differentiation invades the prostatic stroma. The invasive squamous component is adjacent to prostatic glands ⇒. Urinary bladder carcinoma directly invading the prostatic stroma denotes high-stage bladder cancer (pT4). **(Right)** Concomitant urothelial carcinoma with squamous differentiation and prostatic acinar adenocarcinoma is shown. The malignant glands are distinct from the squamous component in contrast to ASC, where there is intimate admixture.

Urothelial Carcinoma With Squamous Differentiation From Bladder
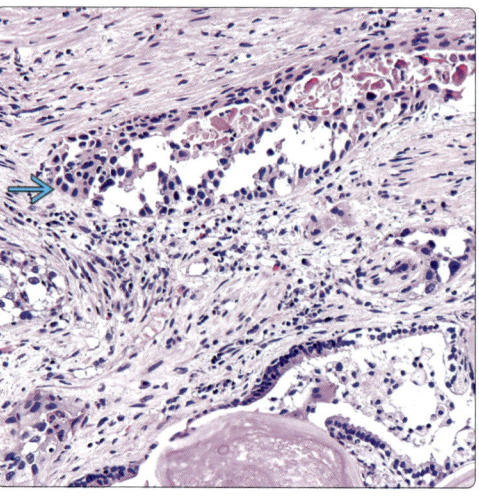

Urothelial Carcinoma With Squamous Differentiation From Bladder
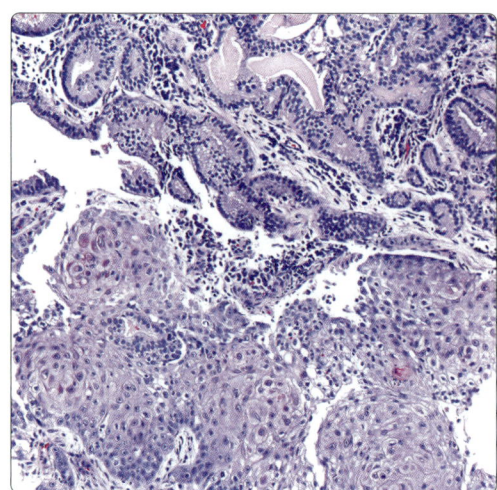

Carcinomas With Squamous Differentiation

Squamous Metaplasia
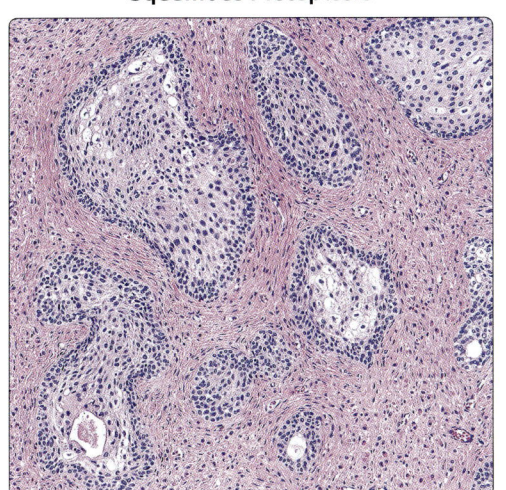

Squamous Metaplasia
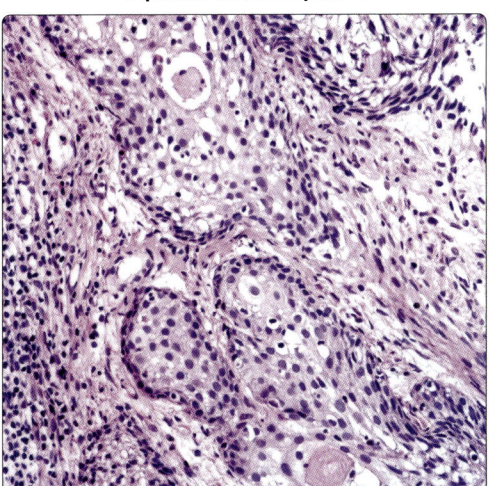

(Left) Florid squamous metaplasia of benign prostatic glands. The squamous epithelium lacks atypia and shows a distinct basal cell layer. Squamous metaplasia does not express PSA and PAP. **(Right)** Squamous metaplasia of benign prostatic glands may be seen adjacent to an area of infarction and in patients with prior TURP, hormonal, or radiation therapy. Areas of better squamous differentiation may be seen in squamous nests. Associated inflammation and resultant atypia may compound the diagnostic difficulty.

Squamous Metaplasia
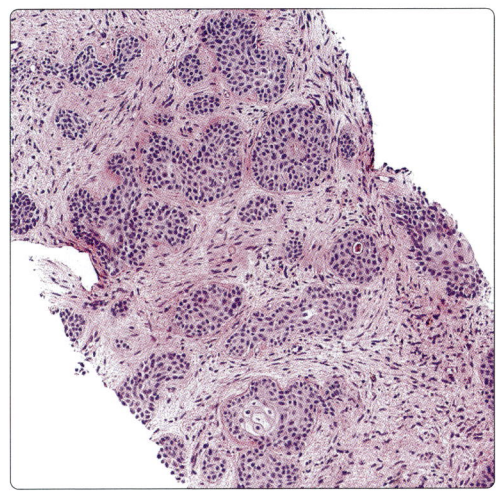

Squamous Metaplasia and Adenocarcinoma of Prostate
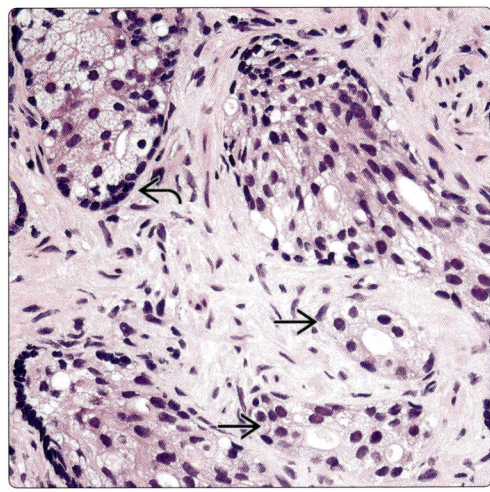

(Left) Needle core biopsy from a patient with prior radiation treatment for adenocarcinoma shows florid squamous metaplasia in benign prostatic epithelium. There is a maintenance of overall architecture and regular spacing between metaplastic glands arguing against an invasive process. **(Right)** Prostatic adenocarcinoma ⇒ adjacent to benign glands with squamous metaplasia is shown. Benign glands show a distinct basal cell layer ⇒. Histology does not represent ASC of the prostate.

PSA in Adenosquamous Carcinoma
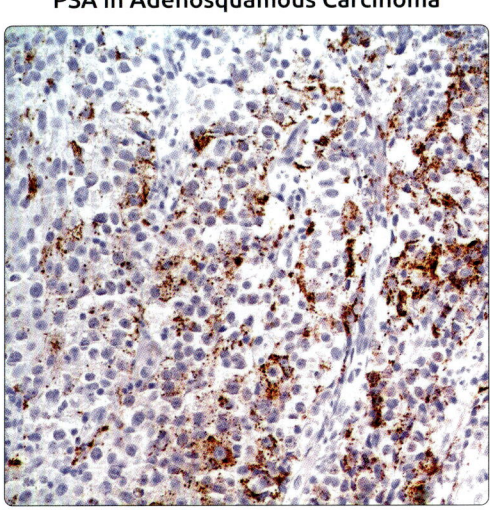

p63 in Squamous Cell Carcinoma
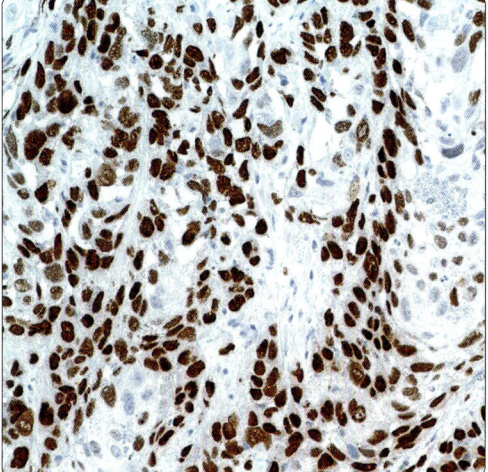

(Left) Poorly differentiated prostatic adenocarcinoma component of ASC shows patchy positivity with PSA immunostaining. PAP and PSMA may be alternatively used. Differentiated squamous component is negative for these markers and positive for keratin 34βE12. **(Right)** Pure SCC of the prostate exhibits diffuse nuclear reactivity with p63. Both primary and secondary SCC involving the prostate are positive for p63. p63 immunoreactivity is not expected in poorly differentiated prostatic adenocarcinoma.

Stromal Tumors

KEY FACTS

TERMINOLOGY
- Tumors putatively derived from specialized stroma of prostate and include pure mesenchymal and mixed epithelial stromal (phyllodes) tumors
- Classified into **STUMP** and **PSS**

ETIOLOGY/PATHOGENESIS
- PR frequently expressed supporting derivation from hormonally responsive mesenchyme of prostate
- Loss in chr 13, 14, and 10 common in STUMP and PSS

CLINICAL ISSUES
- Mean: 58 years old; range: 25-86 years
- More than 1/2 of patients with PSS are younger than 50 years old
- Majority presents with lower urinary tract symptoms
- STUMP generally has good prognosis since mostly confined to prostate, but it may recur and uncommonly can adhere to adjacent organ
- PSS has high recurrence rate, locally aggressive, and can metastasize

MICROSCOPIC
- STUMP lacks significant cellular atypia, mitotic activity, necrosis, or extraprostatic growth
- 4 histologic patterns of STUMP, including **degenerative atypia**, **hypercellular stroma**, **myxoid**, and **phyllodes type**
- PSS is characterized by stromal overgrowth, greater cellularity, pleomorphism, presence of increased mitosis, and necrosis
- Biphasic phyllodes tumor with sarcomatous stroma included in this group
- Stromal cells CD34(+) and PR(+)
- Epithelial component (phyllodes tumor) PSA/PAP(+)
- Main differentials include sarcomatoid carcinoma, BPH, smooth muscle tumors, GIST, solitary fibrous tumor, and seminal vesicle epithelial stromal tumor

Prostatic STUMP
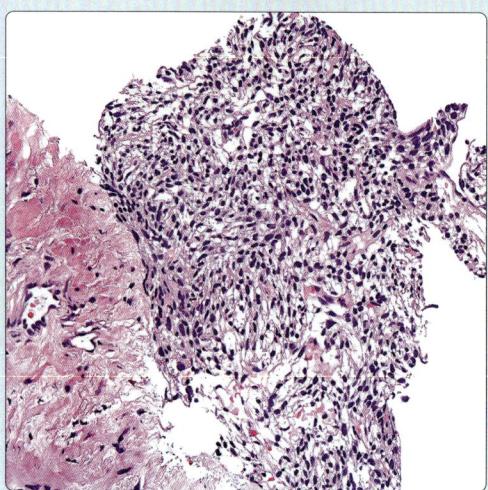

Prostatic STUMP
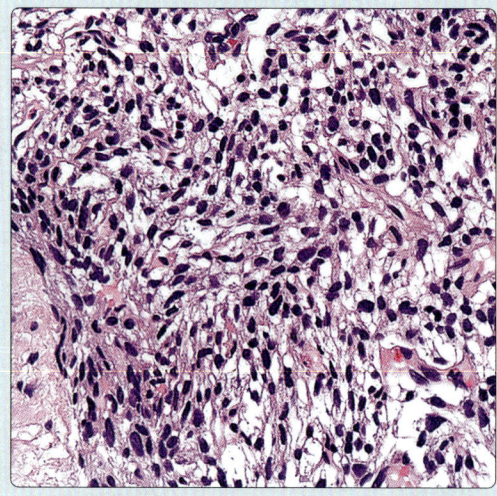

(Left) Low-power magnification of STUMP in needle biopsy specimen shows cellular stroma without associated glands. There is no pleomorphism, and proliferation appears circumscribed in sampled tissue. **(Right)** Higher power magnification of STUMP shows mild nuclear atypia of stromal cells. Other features of malignancy, including nuclear anaplasia, necrosis and increased mitotic activity, are lacking. Definitive categorization of stromal tumors may not be always possible in needle biopsy.

Prostatic Stromal Sarcoma
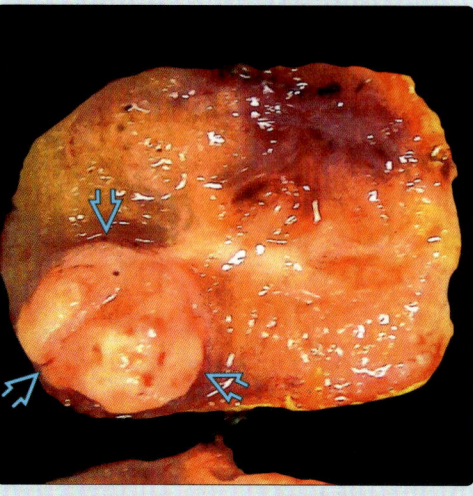

Prostatic Stromal Sarcoma
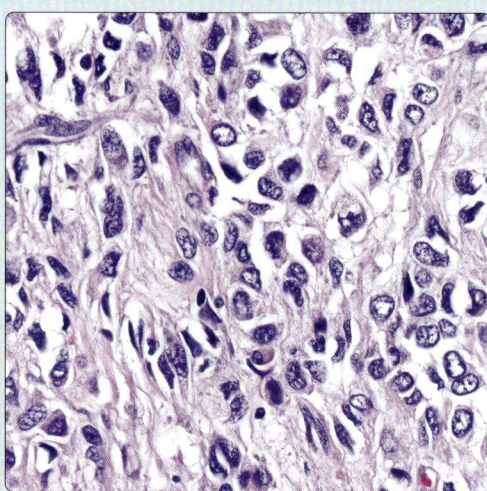

(Left) Cut section of prostate shows a PSS involving the peripheral zone. Tumor is circumscribed, pale tan, and more solid in consistency than surrounding benign prostatic parenchyma. Stromal tumors, in contrast to BPH nodules, are usually solitary and more commonly arise from the peripheral zone. **(Right)** High-grade PSS shows nondescript stromal overgrowth of spindle and epithelioid cells with cell crowding and marked nuclear pleomorphism. The histologic pattern is different from other sarcomas of distinct histogenesis.

Stromal Tumors

TERMINOLOGY

Abbreviations
- Prostatic stromal tumors of uncertain malignant potential (STUMP)
- Prostatic stromal sarcoma (PSS)

Synonyms
- Atypical stromal hyperplasia
- Prostatic stromal hyperplasia with atypia (PSHA)
- Prostatic stromal proliferation of uncertain malignant potential
- Phyllodes type of hyperplasia
- Phyllodes tumor of prostate
- Phyllodes type of atypical hyperplasia
- Cystic epithelial stromal tumor
- Cystadenoleiomyofibroma
- Cystosarcoma phyllodes
- Sarcoma of specialized prostatic stroma

Definitions
- Tumors putatively derived from specialized stroma of prostate and include pure mesenchymal and mixed epithelial stromal (phyllodes) tumors
- Classified into **STUMP** and **PSS**
  - Biphasic phyllodes tumors of prostate are categorized into STUMP and PSS based on degree of stromal atypia
- STUMP encompasses cellular spindle cell lesions of specialized prostatic stroma ± epithelial component
  - Lack significant cellular atypia, mitotic activity, necrosis, or extraprostatic growth
- PSS, low grade or high grade, is malignant cellular spindle cell lesion of specialized prostatic stroma with potential for local invasion or metastasis

ETIOLOGY/PATHOGENESIS

Origin
- PR is frequently expressed in STUMP and PSS, supporting derivation from hormonally responsive mesenchyme of prostate
- Epithelial component of phyllodes pattern of STUMP and PSS expresses PSA and PAP, confirming its prostatic acinar origin

Clonality
- Clonal but dissimilar loss of heterozygosity patterns observed in epithelial and stromal components of phyllodes tumor
- Both epithelial and stromal components of phyllodes tumor are neoplastic but suggested to have different clonal origins

Chromosomal Abnormality
- Loss in chromosomes 13, 14, and 10 common in STUMP and PSS

CLINICAL ISSUES

Epidemiology
- Incidence
  - Rare: ~ 100 STUMP and < 50 PSS reported
  - Clinicopathologic characterization of these lesions mainly based on 3 major series published to date; largest series included 50 cases
- Age
  - Mean: 58 years; range: 25-86 years
  - More than 1/2 of patients with PSS are younger than 50 years
  - 1/5 of patients with STUMP are younger than 50 years

Presentation
- Majority present with lower urinary tract symptoms
- Abnormal digital rectal examination (DRE), hematuria, hematospermia, acute urinary retention, secondary renal dysfunction may be present
- May be asymptomatic; lesion detected upon work-up for elevated serum PSA level

Natural History
- PSS suggested to rarely arise from STUMP but may arise de novo without prior STUMP

Treatment
- STUMP
  - Appropriate treatment approach currently unknown
  - Transurethral resection of prostate to relieve lower urinary tract symptoms
  - Additional sampling to rule out presence of higher grade lesion
  - Proposed recommendation for definitive resection to be based on patient age, treatment preference, and size or extent of lesion
  - Active surveillance proposed for elderly patients with limited lesion on biopsy and with no discernible mass on DRE or imaging studies
- PSS
  - Radical prostatectomy, cystoprostatectomy, or pelvic exenteration for locally aggressive tumors
  - Multimodal therapy, including chemotherapy for advanced and metastatic tumors may be of value
    - Complete remission reported in PSS metastatic to lung using anthracycline and alkylating agent-based regimen followed by metastasectomy

Prognosis
- STUMP
  - Generally has good prognosis since tumors are confined to prostate; they may recur
  - Has more rapid growth compared to nodules of benign prostatic hyperplasia (BPH)
  - Rarely may progress to PSS
    - STUMP is uncommonly seen in association with PSS, including in previous biopsies or resection of subsequent PSS
    - Progression to PSS in subset of STUMP with interglandular growth, particularly under those described as PSHA, is controversial
- PSS
  - High recurrence rate: 65% of cases reported to recur in 1 series, with 2 years average time to 1st recurrence
  - Locally aggressive and may directly invade seminal vesicle, urinary bladder, colon, pelvis, and perineum
  - May metastasize, more frequently in high-grade PSS

Stromal Tumors

- Reported metastatic sites include lung (most common), bone, abdominal wall, and retroperitoneum

MACROSCOPIC

General Features
- STUMP
  - Solid or partially cystic mass, latter corresponding to phyllodes pattern of STUMP
  - Solid tumors are firm, white, tan, or yellow
  - Partially cystic tumors are multilobated, with variably sized cysts that may contain bloody, mucinous, or clear fluid
  - Most tumors arise from peripheral zone and transition zone, or may involve both zones
- PSS
  - Solid or partially cystic mass, latter corresponding to phyllodes pattern of PSS
  - Solid tumors are gray, tan-yellow circumscribed or infiltrative mass
  - Solid-cystic mass of phyllodes pattern of PSS has relatively more evident solid component and may contain necrosis

Size
- STUMP: Range: 0.7-15 cm
- PSS: Range: 2-18 cm

MICROSCOPIC

Histologic Features
- STUMP
  - 4 histologic patterns
    - Pure mesenchymal: Degenerative atypia, hypercellular stroma, and myxoid patterns; may exhibit interglandular pattern of growth
    - Phyllodes type: Biphasic with both stromal and epithelial proliferation
    - Admixture of different patterns may be seen
    - Mitotic activity is absent to rare in all patterns
    - Necrosis is absent
    - Proliferation may be seen between benign normal glands
  - Degenerative atypia
    - Normal to mildly hypercellular stroma with scattered atypical degenerative-appearing cells surrounding benign prostatic glands
    - Atypical stromal cells contain enlarged, single, or multiple pleomorphic nuclei with degenerate-type smudgy chromation
    - Most common pattern of STUMP (50%)
  - Hypercellular stroma
    - Moderately hypercellular, cytologically bland, fusiform stromal cells surrounding benign prostatic glands
    - Resembles florid mixed epithelial and stromal hyperplasia of BPH
    - In contrast to BPH, greater degree of cellularity and stromal cells have more eosinophilic cytoplasm
  - Myxoid
    - Extensive stromal overgrowth of stromal cells often embedded in myxoid stroma and often lacking benign glands
    - May resemble stromal-predominant BPH but lacks multinodularity
  - Phyllodes-type growth
    - Leaf-like growth with compressed, slit-like pattern of benign glandular epithelium containing hypocellular to hypercellular stroma
    - Resembles benign phyllodes tumor of breast
    - Epithelial cells are low cuboidal to columnar and show distinct layer of basal cells
    - Spindle cells tend to be more cellular or condensed around cystic or glandular epithelium
  - Admixture of different STUMP patterns may occur
  - Common concomitant epithelial abnormalities are glandular crowding (50%), prominent basal cell layer (46%), and papillary infoldings
- PSS
  - Stromal overgrowth with overt infiltration, increased cellularity, pleomorphism, increased mitoses, necrosis, and extraprostatic extension
    - Diagnosis of sarcoma based on presence of many or all of these features
  - Biphasic phyllodes tumor with sarcomatous stroma is included in this group
  - Sarcomatous growth: Spindled cells ± epithelioid component
  - Spindled component: Herringbone, short fascicles, or patternless
  - Grading PSS as high grade or low grade, as proposed in AFIP fascicle, is preferred by authors
    - High-grade tumors based on increased cellularity, frequent mitoses, cytologic atypia, necrosis, and stromal overgrowth
    - Low-grade tumors are less atypical; prominent cellularity, appreciable mitoses, nuclear atypia, necrosis, and extraprostatic spread indicate malignant nature
  - 3-tier grading system for phyllodes tumors has been proposed
  - Low grade
    - Low to moderate stromal cellularity
    - Absent or rare cytological atypia
    - Mitosis < 2/10 HPF; absent necrosis
    - Low or mildly hypercellular stroma lined by complete epithelium with frequent leaf-like pattern
  - Intermediate grade
    - Moderate to high stromal cellularity
    - Intermediate number of atypical cells with moderate to marked atypia
    - Mitosis 2-5/10 HPF; absent necrosis
  - High grade
    - Moderate to high cellularity, marked anaplasia
    - Mitosis > 5/10 HPF; necrosis may be present
    - High, markedly hypercellular stroma with scattered lining epithelium, infrequent leaf-like pattern
  - Recurrent tumor of PSS may show higher grade features than initial tumor

Stromal Tumors

Immunohistochemistry
- Stromal cells
  - Vimentin (+), CD34(+), PR(+)
  - Desmin, SMA, and actin-HHF-35 shows variable (±) reactivity
  - S100(-), CD117(-), ER mostly positive
- Epithelial component (phyllodes tumor)
  - PAN-CK(AE1/AE3)(+), PSA/PAP(+)

DIFFERENTIAL DIAGNOSIS

Sarcomatoid Carcinoma
- May be associated with malignant glandular component
- May be associated with history of prostatic adenocarcinoma with radiation/hormone treatment
- Cytokeratin, HMCK(34βE12), CK5/6, and p63 may be positive in spindle cell component
- PSA/PAP(+) in malignant glandular component

Benign Prostate Hyperplasia
- STUMP with hypercellular stromal pattern mimics mixed epithelial stromal BPH
- STUMP with myxoid pattern mimics stromal predominant BPH
- Uncommon in younger patients
- Typical multinodular growth, unlike STUMP, which is often solitary
- Most commonly arises from transition zone, unlike STUMP, which may involve both transition and peripheral zones
- In contrast to STUMP, stromal predominant BPH shows abundant stromal capillaries and may show condensation of stromal cells around vessels
- In contrast to STUMP with hypercellular stroma, glands of mixed epithelial stromal BPH are hyperplastic, and stromal cells are less eosinophilic

Smooth Muscle Tumors
- Includes leiomyoma and leiomyosarcoma of prostate
- Leiomyosarcoma is most common sarcoma involving adult prostate
- Leiomyosarcoma vary from those resembling smooth muscle cells with moderate atypia and increased mitotic activity to pleomorphic tumors
- Leiomyosarcoma may exhibit epithelioid features
- Leiomyoma may contain atypical symplastic nuclei, but nevertheless remain with benign clinical behavior
- May be PR(+), similar to stromal tumors, thus, not helpful in differential diagnosis
- May exhibit distinct fascicular growth characteristic of smooth muscle cells
- CD34 is usually negative, and desmin is strongly positive in smooth muscle tumors

Gastrointestinal Stromal Tumor
- Gastrointestinal stromal tumor from colorectal region may invade into prostate and may even present as intraprostatic mass
- CD34(+) similar to stromal tumors
- Diffusely and strongly positive for CD117 and DOG1

Solitary Fibrous Tumor
- Ropey collagen and thick-walled, irregular or hemangiopericytomatous blood vessels
- May arise primarily from prostate or from pelvis with secondary involvement of prostate
- ~ 1/2 of cases are malignant
- CD34 and bcl-2(+)

Seminal Vesicle Epithelial Stromal Tumor
- Histologically similar to phyllodes tumor of prostate
- Tumor is grossly and histologically intimately associated with seminal vesicle and often separated from prostate/prostatectomy specimen
- Unlike prostatic phyllodes tumor, epithelial component is PSA and PAP (-)

DIAGNOSTIC CHECKLIST

Pathologic Interpretation Pearls
- Spindle cell proliferations of specialized prostatic stroma that span spectrum from monophasic to biphasic (phyllodes-type) tumors
- Classified based on stromal cellularity, stromal overgrowth, cellular atypia, mitoses, necrosis, infiltrative growth, and extraprostatic extension
- Categorized based on histologic features
  - STUMP
    - Includes lesions of PSHA
  - PSS, low grade
  - PSS, high grade
- Positive for CD34 and PR; SMA and desmin variable
- Definitive categorization as PSS may not be possible in needle biopsies or transurethral resection specimens
  - In such cases, diagnostic terminology, such as "at least stromal tumor of unknown malignant potential," may be used
  - Definitive characterization be recommended only on basis of examination of additional tissue or from prostatectomy specimen, if performed

SELECTED REFERENCES

1. Murer LM et al: Stromal tumor of uncertain malignant potential of the prostate. Arch Pathol Lab Med. 138(11):1542-5, 2014
2. Pan CC et al: Common chromosomal aberrations detected by array comparative genomic hybridization in specialized stromal tumors of the prostate. Mod Pathol. 26(11):1536-43, 2013
3. Tavora F et al: Mesenchymal tumours of the bladder and prostate: an update. Pathology. 45(2):104-15, 2013
4. Paner GP et al: Non-epithelial neoplasms of the prostate. Histopathology. 60(1):166-86, 2012
5. Egevad L et al: Atypical stromal hyperplasia of the prostate. Scand J Urol Nephrol. 42(5):484-7, 2008
6. Hossain D et al: Prostatic stromal hyperplasia with atypia: follow-up study of 18 cases. Arch Pathol Lab Med. 132(11):1729-33, 2008
7. Herawi M et al: Specialized stromal tumors of the prostate: a clinicopathologic study of 50 cases. Am J Surg Pathol. 30(6):694-704, 2006
8. Bostwick DG et al: Phyllodes tumor of the prostate: long-term followup study of 23 cases. J Urol. 172(3):894-9, 2004
9. McCarthy RP et al: Molecular genetic evidence for different clonal origins of epithelial and stromal components of phyllodes tumor of the prostate. Am J Pathol. 165(4):1395-400, 2004
10. Lam KC et al: Chemotherapy induced complete remission in malignant phyllodes tumor of the prostate metastasizing to the lung. J Urol. 168(3):1104-5, 2002
11. Gaudin PB et al: Sarcomas and related proliferative lesions of specialized prostatic stroma: a clinicopathologic study of 22 cases. Am J Surg Pathol. 22(2):148-62, 1998

Stromal Tumors

Prostatic STUMP

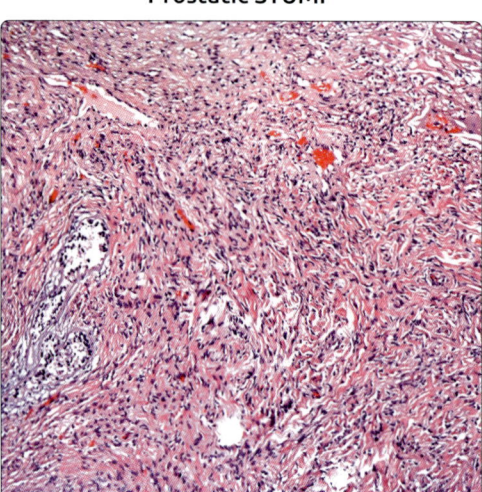

Prostatic STUMP: Cellular Stroma

(Left) Low-power magnification shows STUMP with hypercellular stroma surrounding benign prostatic glands. This pattern of STUMP may resemble florid mixed epithelial and stromal hyperplasia of BPH. *(Right)* High-power view of STUMP shows moderately hypercellular stroma composed of bland fusiform cells. Note the absence of appreciable mitosis. In contrast to BPH, the growth is usually solitary, with a greater degree of cellularity. The cells have more eosinophilic cytoplasm.

Prostatic STUMP: Needle Biopsy

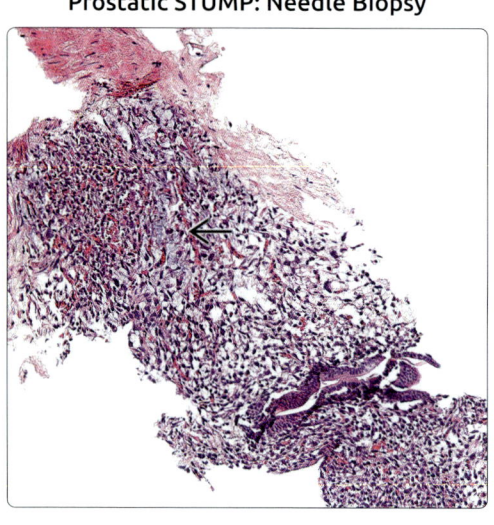

Prostatic STUMP: Bland Cellular Stroma

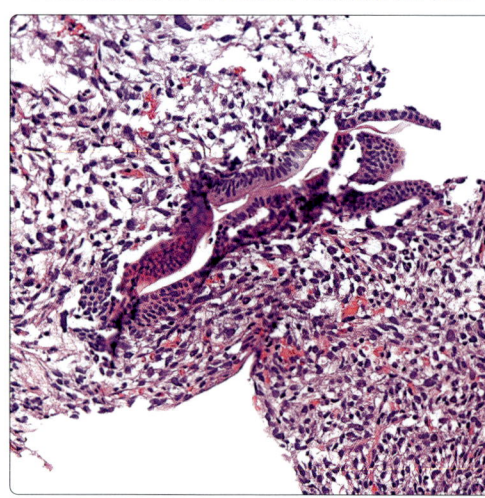

(Left) STUMP in a needle biopsy specimen shows cellular spindle cell stroma focally with a myxoid background ➡. There is no evidence of necrosis. The spindle cells have nondescript patternless growth. *(Right)* Higher power of STUMP shows cellular stromal cells surrounding a benign gland. The spindle cells are focally dense, have uniform nuclear contours, lack chromatin abnormalities, and do not show increase in mitotic activity. STUMP may rarely progress to PSS or may show PSS in an excision specimen.

Prostatic STUMP: Absent Anaplasia and Necrosis

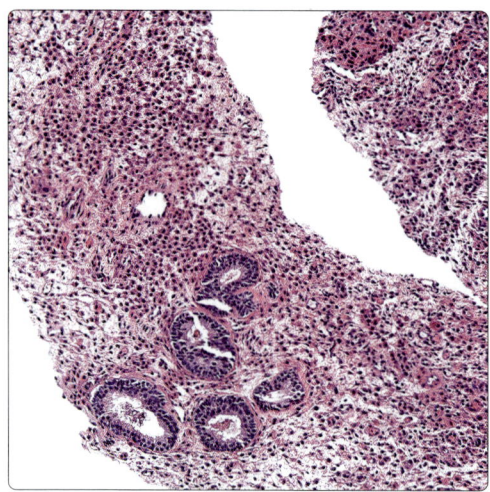

Prostatic STUMP: Cytology

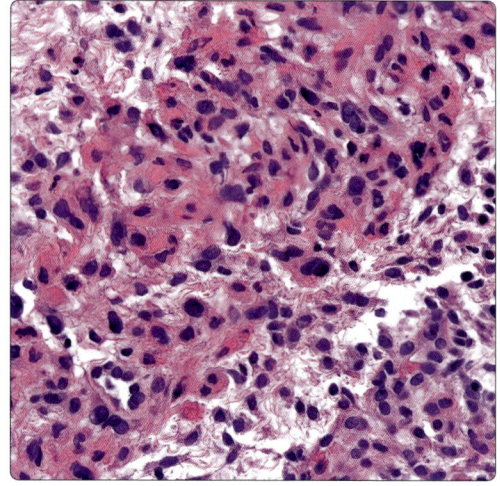

(Left) Low-power magnification of STUMP in a needle biopsy specimen shows cellular stroma with atypical cells in between benign glands. There is marked stromal overgrowth. Necrosis and marked pleomorphism are lacking. *(Right)* Higher power magnification shows atypia within stromal cells and no mitotic activity. Stromal cells are more cellular and plumper with more eosinophilic cytoplasm than in BPH. Diagnosis of malignancy (PSS) is based on the accumulative assessment of multiple adverse pathologic features.

Stromal Tumors

Prostatic Stromal Sarcoma: Low Grade

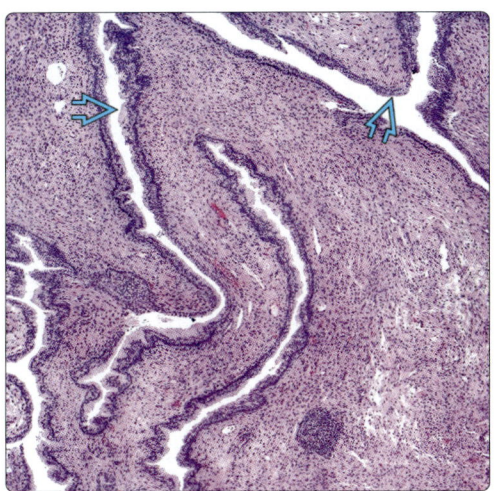

Prostatic Stromal Sarcoma: Low Grade

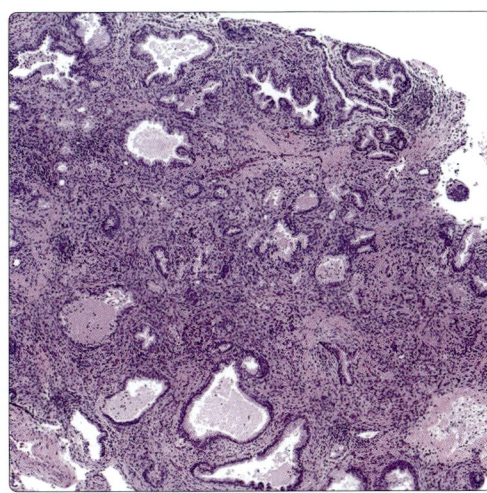

(Left) Low-grade PSS phyllodes pattern exhibits leaf-like growth of epithelial glandular cells ➡ with an investing spindle cell stroma with increased cellularity. Some large cystic glands amid the stromal proliferation are compressed or slit-like in appearance. This epithelial component shows 2 cell types and is immunohistochemically positive for PSA and PAP. (Right) Low-grade PSS shows hypercellular stroma in between benign prostatic glands. Greater cellularity is appreciated surrounding the glands.

Prostatic Stromal Sarcoma: Low Grade With Spindle Cells

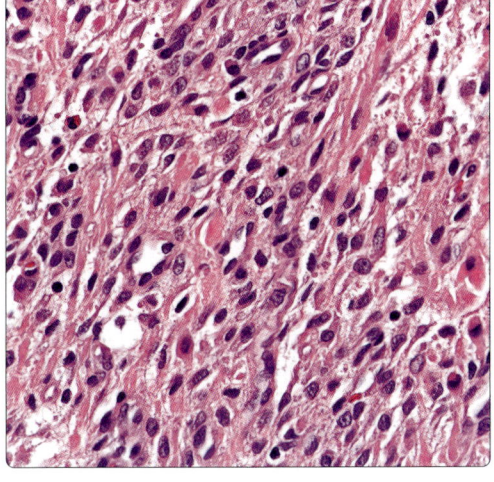

Prostatic Stromal Sarcoma: Low Grade With Epithelioid Cells

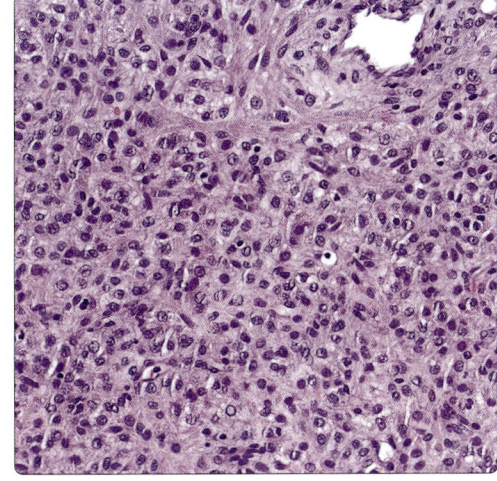

(Left) High-power magnification of low-grade PSS shows fusiform spindle cells. No distinct growth pattern, such as fascicular, storiform, or herringbone, is seen in this tumor. Cytoplasm of spindle cells is compact and not fibrillar. (Right) Low-grade PSS consists of hypercellular sheets of epithelioid cells. There is moderate nuclear atypia. Admixture of epithelioid and spindle cells is not uncommon. Differential diagnosis includes sarcomatoid carcinoma, solitary fibrous tumor, and GIST.

Prostatic Stromal Sarcoma: Necrosis

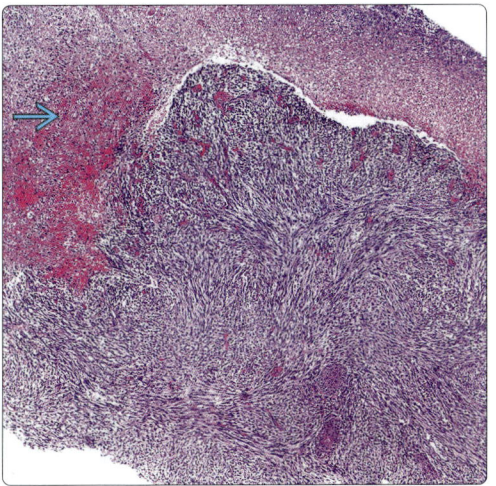

Prostatic Stromal Sarcoma: Cellular Atypia

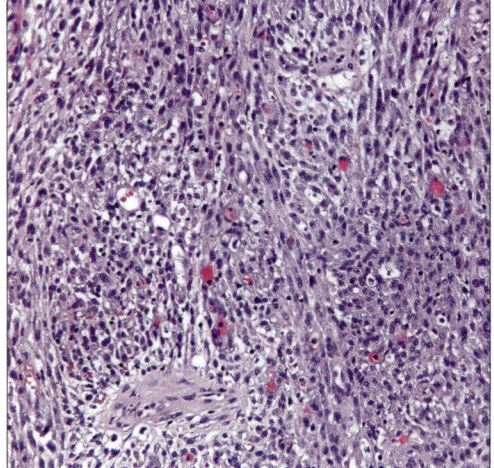

(Left) PSS in TURP associated with broad necrosis ➡ is shown. The tumor is markedly hypercellular, consisting of atypical spindle cells. Presence of hypercellularity, pleomorphism, increased mitosis, & tumor-related necrosis are used for sarcoma designation. (Right) High-grade PSS shows spindle cells with a focal fascicular growth pattern. PSS may demonstrate variable architecture not distinctive of other sarcomas involving prostate, including leiomyosarcoma, malignant solitary fibrous tumor, and GIST.

Stromal Tumors

Prostatic Stromal Sarcoma: High Grade With Spindle Cells

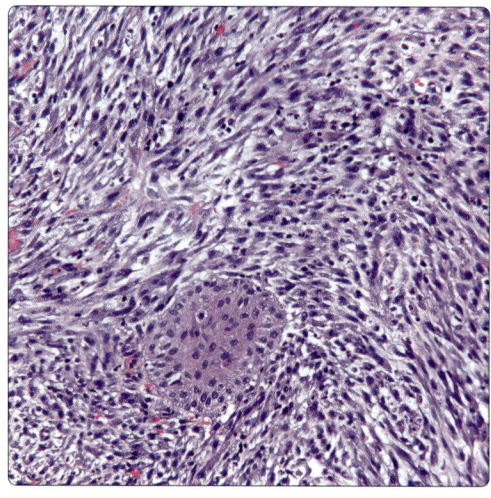

Prostatic Stromal Sarcoma: High Grade With Spindle Cells

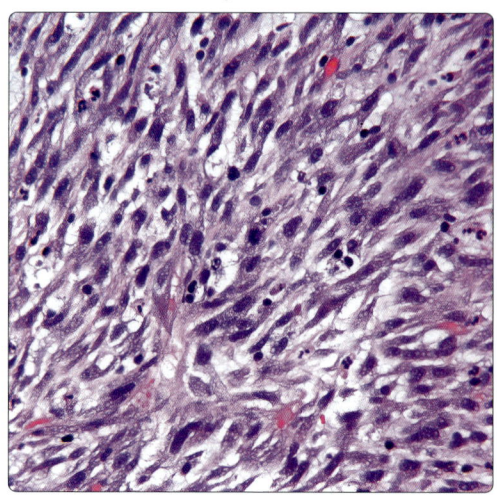

(Left) PSS, high grade, is shown with spindle cells overgrowth and an entrapped benign prostatic epithelium. Pattern of spindle cell varies and may exhibit short, fascicular, herring bone or patternless growth. Other spindle cell lesions of the prostate may mimic stromal tumors and distinction can often be made by morphology and judicious immunostaining. (Right) High-grade PSS shows nondescript growth of spindle cells with marked hypercellularity, mitosis, nuclear hyperchromasia, and pleomorphism.

Prostatic Stromal Sarcoma: High Grade With Epithelioid Cells, Demarcation

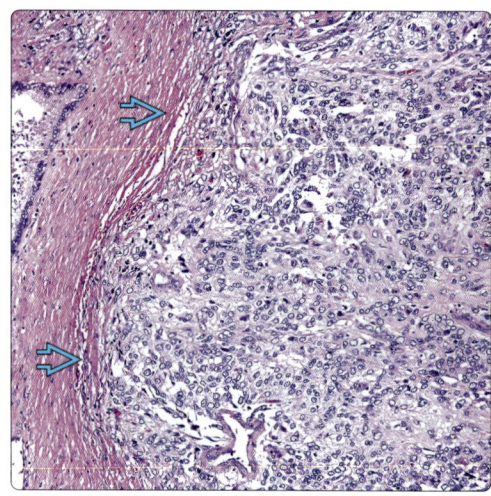

Prostatic Stromal Sarcoma: High Grade With Epithelioid Cells, Cytologic Atypia

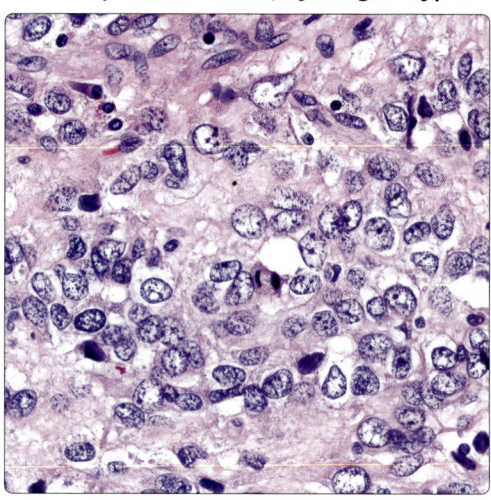

(Left) Low-power view of high-grade PSS shows a well-demarcated tumor ⇨ that exhibits increased in cellularity. Stromal tumors are typically well-circumscribed and solitary. (Right) High-grade PSS consisting of plump epithelioid cells that show nuclear enlargement, crowding, and overlapping, with irregular nuclear outlines and mitoses is shown. The cytoplasm is light eosinophilic and relatively abundant. Approach to such malignant proliferations requires a judicious immunohistochemical panel.

Prostatic Stromal Sarcoma: High Grade With Myxoid Stroma

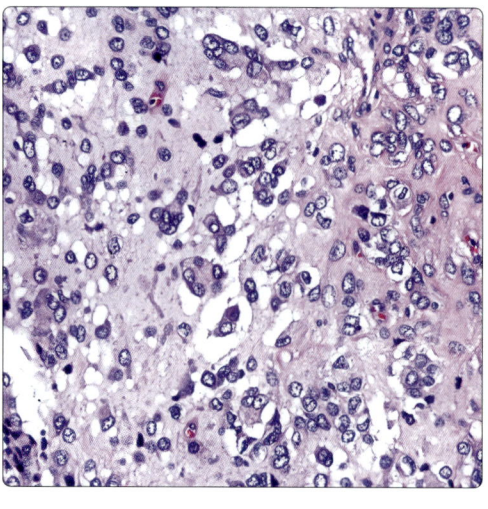

Prostatic Stromal Sarcoma: High Grade With Rhabdoid Cells

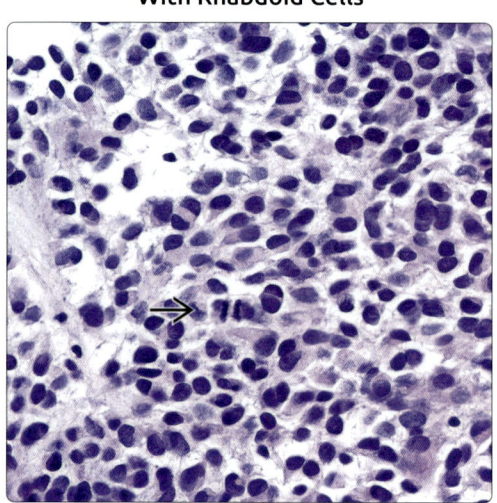

(Left) This high-grade PSS shows pleomorphic tumor cells amidst stromal mucin. This myxoid stromal change may also be seen in STUMP, including in rare examples that transformed to PSS. Note the presence of multinucleated tumor cells. (Right) High-power view of PSS, high grade, shows marked atypia and mitotic activity ⇨ in cells exhibiting rhabdoid morphology. This cellular phenotype is very rare and suggests an aggressive behavior. Rhabdoid PSS does not exhibit loss of INI1 expression.

Stromal Tumors

PR in Prostatic Stromal Tumor
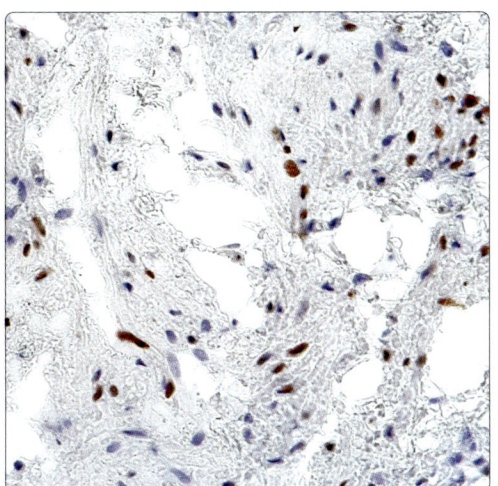

SMA in Prostatic Stromal Tumor
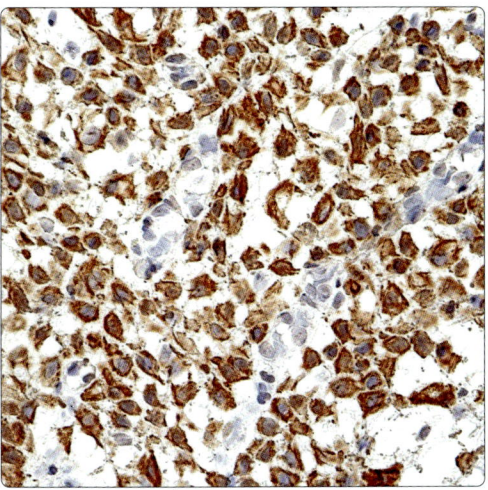

(Left) STUMP exhibits nuclear PR positivity, supporting derivation from the hormonally responsive specialized mesenchyme of the prostate. PR may also be expressed by smooth muscle tumors; hence, CD34 is more discriminatory. (Right) Low-grade PSS with epithelioid features shows diffuse SMA staining. Stromal tumors show variable immunoreactivity to SMA. Thus, this stain is not helpful in distinguishing stromal tumors from smooth muscle tumors. This diffuse positivity is unusual for sarcomatoid carcinomas.

Leiomyomatous Stromal Benign Prostatic Hyperplasia
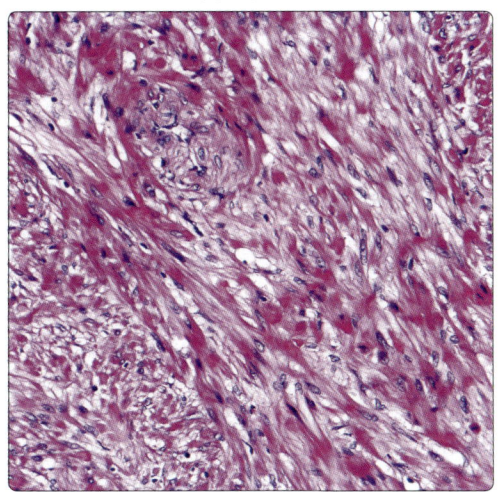

Gastrointestinal Stromal Tumor
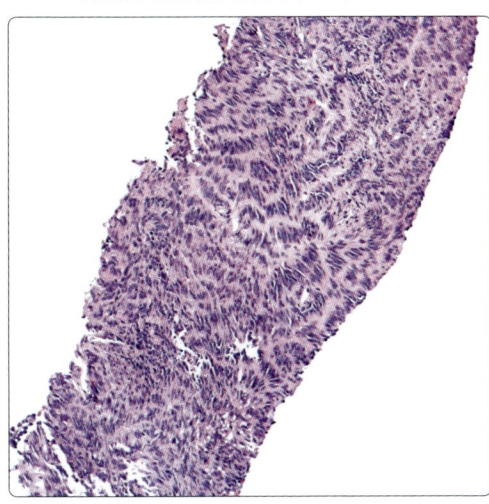

(Left) This leiomyomatous stromal hyperplasia may resemble STUMP. BPH nodules, unlike STUMP, are typically multinodular, more commonly arise from the transition zone, and are uncommon in younger patients. (Right) This GIST diagnosed on prostate biopsy arises from the rectum and has invaded into the prostate, presenting as intraprostatic tumor. GIST and prostatic stromal tumor are both CD34(+). GIST is distinguished from prostatic stromal tumors by CD117 and DOG1 positivity.

Leiomyoma
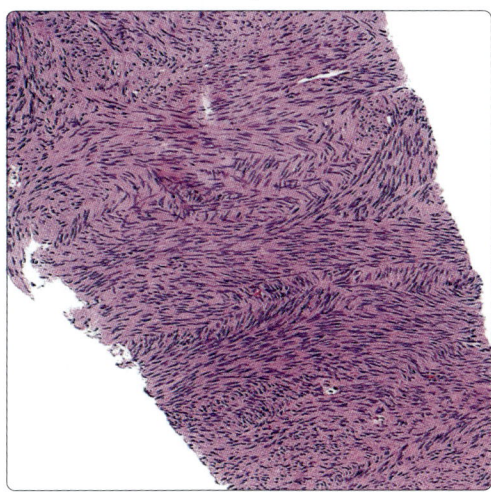

Leiomyosarcoma
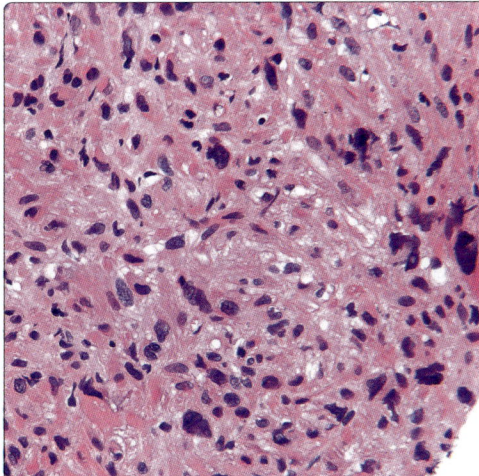

(Left) Cellular leiomyoma of the prostate in a needle biopsy shows fascicular growth of bland-appearing spindle cells reminiscent of smooth muscle bundles. Additional assessment of the tumor revealed lack of mitotic activity and necrosis. (Right) High-grade leiomyosarcoma in prostate biopsy shows marked nuclear anaplasia in spindle cells. It shares smooth muscle actin, desmin, and PR positivity with PSS but is negative for CD34. Leiomyosarcoma is the most common sarcoma in the adult prostate.

Mesenchymal Tumors of Prostate

KEY FACTS

TERMINOLOGY
- Prostatic neoplasms arising from innate prostatic &/or periprostatic mesenchymal elements
- Includes tumors arising from fibromuscular stroma, smooth muscle, blood vessels, paraganglia, and nerves
  - Includes smooth muscle tumors, IMT, SFT, paraganglioma, RMS, vascular tumors, neural tumors, MFH, osteogenic or chondrogenic tumors
- Origin of some mesenchymal tumors uncertain such as SS, PNET, and PEComa

CLINICAL ISSUES
- Rare, represents < 1% of all prostatic tumors
- Most common adult prostate sarcomas are LMS and RMS
- Adult prostate sarcomas in general have poor prognosis
  - ~ 25% have metastasis at presentation
  - 1 study showed median cancer-specific survival (CSS) of 2.9 years and for cases with metastasis CSS of 1.5 years
- Malignant mesenchymal tumors treated surgically &/or by multimodality therapy
- Benign mesenchymal tumors treated conservatively

MICROSCOPIC
- Similar histology to counterpart mesenchymal tumors from extraprostatic sites
- Most prostatic mesenchymal tumors exhibit spindle cell morphology; some with epithelioid cells or biphasic histology
  - Overlap in morphology common, particularly with spindle cell lesions
    - Differential diagnosis includes stromal BPH, prostatic stromal tumors, GIST, and sarcomatoid carcinoma
  - Use of IHC panel and identification of some genetic alterations helpful in diagnosis
    - *NAB2-STAT6* fusion in SFT, *EWSR1* transcript in PNET, *SS18-SSX* fusion in SS and *PAX3-FOXO1* or *PAX7-FOXO1* fusion in alveolar RMS

Leiomyosarcoma
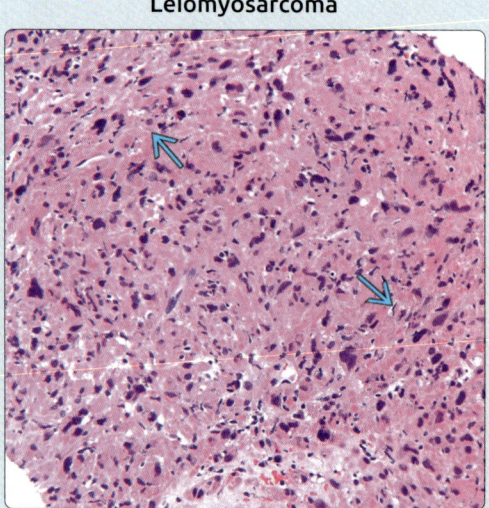

Rhabdomyosarcoma
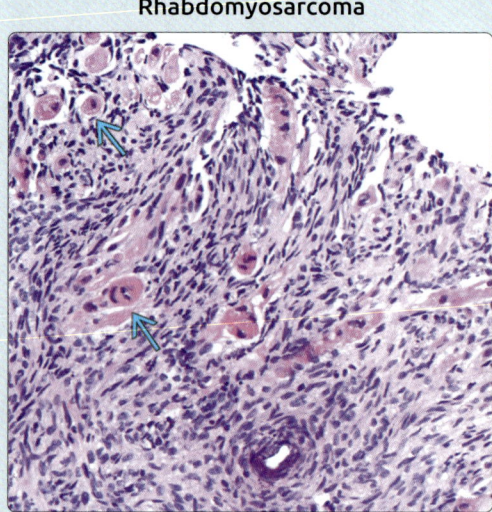

(Left) Prostate needle biopsy shows LMS exhibiting vague fascicles ➡ of neoplastic spindle cells with markedly pleomorphic nuclei. Diagnosis of LMS can be confirmed by expression of smooth muscle markers. LMS is most predominant sarcoma in adult prostate. *(Right)* Prostate needle biopsy shows RMS with densely packed spindle & small round cells admixed with rhabdomyoblasts ➡. Diagnosis can be confirmed by desmin &/or myogenin positivity. RMS in adult prostate is more aggressive than pediatric RMS.

Angiosarcoma (AS)
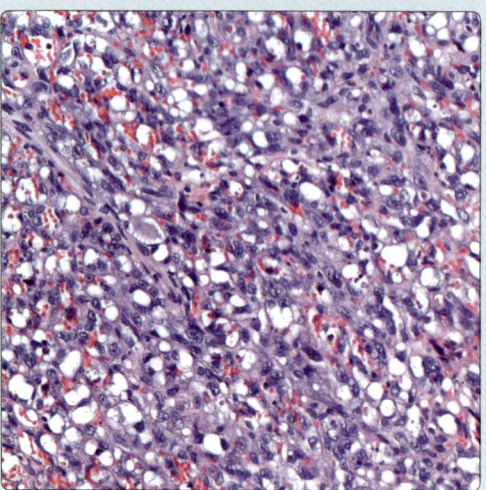

Solitary Fibrous Tumor
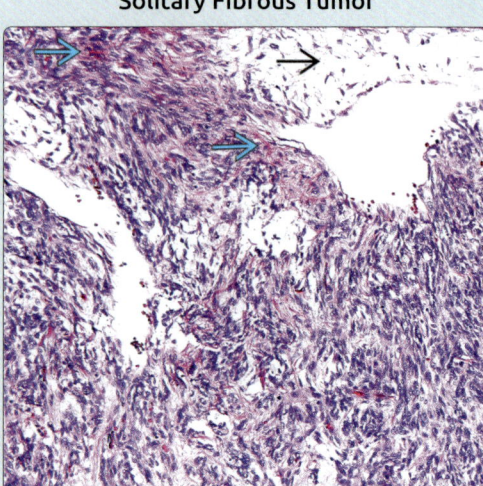

(Left) AS shows vasoformation with malignant endothelial cells showing nuclear pleomorphism. Association of prior radiotherapy for prostatic adenocarcinoma to AS is still controversial. *(Right)* Low power view of SFT shows alternating sparsely cellular ➡ and hypercellular areas of spindle cells intimately associated with thick, "ropey" collagen bundles ➡ and with "patternless" pattern. Note the large staghorn vessels; also a characteristic feature of SFT. Mitosis, nuclear pleomorphism, and necrosis are absent in this benign SFT.

Mesenchymal Tumors of Prostate

TERMINOLOGY

Synonyms
- Inflammatory myofibroblastic tumor (IMT): Pseudosarcomatous myofibroblastic proliferation, pseudosarcomatous fibromyxoid tumor, postoperative spindle cell nodule (PSCN), inflammatory pseudotumor
- Paraganglioma: Extraadrenal pheochromocytoma

Definitions
- Prostatic neoplasms arising from innate prostatic &/or periprostatic mesenchymal elements
  - Includes tumors arising from fibromuscular stroma, smooth muscle, blood vessels, paraganglia, and nerves
    - Tumors of specialized prostatic stroma not included in this chapter
  - Except for prostatic stromal tumors, all have similar histology to extraprostatic mesenchymal tumors
  - Origin of some mesenchymal tumors uncertain
    - Synovial sarcoma (SS), primitive neuroectodermal tumor (PNET), perivascular epithelioid cell tumor (PEComa)

CLINICAL ISSUES

Epidemiology
- Incidence
  - Rare, represents < 1% of all prostatic tumors
  - Most predominant prostate sarcoma in adults is leiomyosarcoma (LMS) followed by rhabdomyosarcoma (RMS)

Presentation
- Large or bulky tumors present with compressive or lower urinary tract symptoms, hematuria, &/or urinary retention
- Most adult prostate sarcomas present with locally aggressive disease, and ~ 25% have metastasis at presentation

Treatment
- Malignant tumors treated surgically &/or by multimodality therapy
- Benign tumors treated conservatively

Prognosis
- Vary depending on tumor type (histology), grade, and extent (stage)
- Adult prostate sarcomas in general have poor prognosis
  - 1 study showed median cancer-specific survival (CSS) of 2.9 years
    - CSS of 7.7 years for clinically localized disease
    - CSS of 1.5 years for metastatic disease

DIAGNOSTIC CHECKLIST

Smooth Muscle Tumors
- **Leiomyoma (LM)**
  - Suggested to arise from smooth muscle elements of periglandular tissues, prostate capsule, or müllerian duct remnants
  - < 100 cases of prostatic LM reported
  - Most occur in 6th decade of life
  - Most present with obstructive urinary symptoms, abnormal DRE, and less often hematuria
    - May be clinically mistaken as BPH and encountered in TURP to relieve symptoms of prostatism
  - Typically solitary mostly 2-7 cm in size, but can be bulky (> 10 cm)
  - Gross and microscopic features similar to extraprostatic LM
    - Well delineated, circumscribed, and white to yellow-tan with smooth external surface
    - Fascicles of interlacing smooth muscle cells that may whorl around blood vessels
    - With cigar-shaped nuclei or degenerative nuclear atypia and absent to rare mitosis
    - No prostatic glands seen in between tumor cells
    - May exhibit distinct nuclear atypia (LM with atypia) consisting of atypical and bizarre giant cells
      - Nuclei can be multiple, vacuolated, with smudgy chromatin, inconspicuous nucleolus, and lack mitosis
      - Important not to misdiagnose as LMS
    - May rarely assume epithelioid morphology (leiomyoblastoma)
    - Positive for smooth muscle markers and AR(+)
  - Main differential diagnosis includes leiomyomatous BPH, hypercellular STUMP, GIST, solitary fibrous tumor (SFT), and sarcomatoid carcinoma
    - LMs previously described as BPH are perhaps leiomyomatous BPH
      - Occurs in background of BPH, less cellular, and lacks typical vessels of LM
    - LM in background BPH has to be disproportionately large (> 10 cm) and grossly distinct from BPH including peripheral zone location
  - Benign behavior
  - Treated with TUR or prostatectomy for larger tumors
- **Leiomyosarcoma**
  - Comprises < 0.1% of prostatic malignancies
    - Most predominant sarcoma in adult prostate
  - Most occur in 4th-7th decades of life but may occur in young adults and children
  - Most present with obstructive urinary symptoms as well as perineal pain, constipation, local mass effect, hematuria, and weight loss
  - Usually large, reported range of 3.3-21 cm (mean: 9 cm)
  - Gross and microscopic features similar to extraprostatic LMS
    - May have tumor necrosis and cystic degeneration
    - Vague fascicles of spindle cells with range of nuclear atypia, mitotic activity, and necrosis
      - Can be low or high grade
      - High-grade tumors have increased cellularity, vague fasciculation, pleomorphism, and brisk mitotic activity
    - May have epithelioid morphology (epithelioid LMS)
    - Positive for smooth muscle markers
  - Main differential diagnosis includes LM, sarcomatoid carcinoma, stromal sarcoma, GIST, and SFT
    - Distinction can be made with aid of IHC
    - ~ 25% of LMS may express keratin; can be mistaken as sarcomatoid carcinoma

Mesenchymal Tumors of Prostate

- Sarcomatoid carcinoma may show adenocarcinoma component that can be highlighted by PSA and PAP
- Aggressive behavior
  - 1 series of 14 patients had 4 with metastasis and 10 died within 3 years after diagnosis

Inflammatory Myofibroblastic Tumor (Pseudosarcomatous Myofibroblastic Proliferation)

- Well recognized in bladder; those in prostate occur either as secondary extension or as primary tumor and are extremely rare
  - ~ 12 cases of prostatic IMT reported
- Most occurs in 4th-7th decades of life
- Most present with obstructive urinary symptoms, hematuria, abnormal DRE
- Some discovered incidentally in prostates with carcinoma
- Similar in bladder, subset may have prior surgery (postoperative spindle cell nodule) or trauma
- Histology similar to bladder IMTs
  - Relatively uniform bland spindle cells of variable cellularity in loose myxoid stroma (cell culture appearance)
  - Prominent inflammatory cell infiltrates and often contains granulation tissue-type vascularity
  - Cells have elongated cytoplasmic processes with regular nuclei with fine chromatin and occasionally prominent nucleoli
  - Commonly positive for SMA, broad spectrum and low molecular weight keratins; usually negative for high molecular weight keratins such as keratin 34βE12, CK5, and CK6
  - ALK1(+), reported range varies from 20-75%; FISH for ALK gene alteration positive in up to 72% of cases
- Main differential diagnosis includes sarcomatoid carcinoma and sarcoma
  - Distinction can be made with aid of IHC
  - Sarcomatoid carcinoma may show adenocarcinoma component that can be highlighted by PSA and PAP
- Most reported cases were treated with TUR and had no progression or metastasis
  - 1 case with usual IMT histology developed metastasis to groin lymph nodes and lungs

Solitary Fibrous Tumor

- ~ 30 cases of prostatic SFT reported; largest series had 13 cases
  - SFT and hemangiopericytoma now considered part of same spectrum
- Most tumors arise in prostate; small subset are from extraprostatic tissues or secondary extension to prostate
- Patients' age: 21-75 yr (mean: 58 yr)
- Most present with obstructive urinary symptoms and abnormal DRE
- Gross and microscopic features similar to extraprostatic SFT
  - Size range from 2.4-15.0 cm
  - Well circumscribed, firm, or rubbery, with white-to-tan solid-cut surface
  - Spindle cells with scant cytoplasm haphazardly arranged (patternless pattern) or admixed with thick collagen (ropey or keloid-like)
  - Cellularity varies with hypo- and hypercellular areas
  - Vessels are abundant from small to hemangiopericytomatous (staghorn vessels)
  - Other growth patterns include storiform, herringbone, hemangiopericytic, and neural-like
  - Most are positive for CD34, CD99, and Bcl-2
  - FISH may detect characteristic NAB2-STAT6 gene fusion
  - May have malignant features
    - Criteria extrapolated from SFT of pleural sites; so far inconsistent in prostatic SFT
    - Combination of size (> 10 cm), mitosis (> 4/10 HPF), pleomorphism, infiltrative borders, and necrosis
- Main differential diagnosis includes stromal-predominant BPH, stromal tumor, smooth muscle tumors, sarcomatoid carcinoma, SS, and GIST
  - Stromal-predominant BPH occurs in background of BPH, has spindle cells following vessel contour, and lacks thick collagen and hemangiopericytomatous vessels
  - Both stromal tumor and SFT express CD34; stromal tumor lacks thick collagen, hemangiopericytomatous vessels, and variable architectural patterns
- To date, all prostatic SFTs, including those considered histologically malignant, have favorable outcome

Paraganglioma

- ~ 15 cases of prostatic and periprostatic paraganglioma reported
- Believed to arise from extraadrenal chromaffin cells present in ganglia
  - Mainly situated in immediate extraprostatic tissue particularly lateral neurovascular bundle
- May also arise within prostatic urethra as obstructive urethral polyp
- Most patients are young with mean age of 28 yr (range 8-63 yr)
- When functional, may present with catecholamine-related symptoms such as hypertension, tachycardia, headache, and palpitations
- Nonfunctional paraganglioma presents with localized GU symptoms such as urinary obstruction and hematuria
- Diagnosis facilitated by measurement of catecholamine levels in blood or urine
- Consists of polygonal cells with abundant granular cytoplasm and minimal pleomorphism arranged in distinctive nested (zellballen) pattern
- Positive for neuroendocrine markers such as synaptophysin, chromogranin, and CD56; S100 highlights sustentacular cells
- Most reported cases with favorable outcome
  - 2 reported cases developed metastasis
  - Histologic criteria for malignancy inconsistent
  - Presence of metastasis only reliable criterion for malignancy

Adult Rhabdomyosarcoma

- Most common tumor of lower GU tract in pediatric patients
- Rare in adults, with ~ 75 cases reported in literature
  - 2nd most predominant sarcoma in adult prostate after LMS
- Patients' age: 18-89 yr
- Histology similar to extraprostatic RMS
  - Most are embryonal subtype (58%)

Mesenchymal Tumors of Prostate

- May also present initially as polypoid urethral mass mimicking fibroepithelial polyp
- Positive for desmin, myogenin, and MYOD1
- Alveolar RMS can be confirmed by detection of t(2;13) and t(1;13) or *PAX3-FOXO1* and *PAX7-FOXO1* gene fusions
- Clinically very aggressive in contrast to pediatric RMS
  - Has poorer CSS when compared to prostatic LMS
  - Has rapid growth and typically forms large pelvic mass and disseminates to lungs, bone, liver, and serosa
  - Poor response to multimodality therapy, in contrast to pediatric RMS

Vascular Tumors

- **Hemangioma**
  - Mostly identified arising along posterior urethra (posterior urethral hemangioma)
    - Presents with hematuria and hematospermia
    - Patients' age: 29-80 yr (mean: 57 yr)
    - Most are cavernous hemangioma
    - Benign course; treated with fulguration or resection
  - Much rarer are intraprostatic hemangiomas
    - Only 3 cases reported in patients 52-84 yr
    - May present with lower urinary tract symptoms or incidentally discovered in radical prostatectomy
    - Multiple hemorrhagic nodules with spongy bloody areas
- **Epithelioid hemangioendothelioma**
  - Reported in 69-year-old patient with 3.5-cm mass attached to prostate/seminal vesicles
  - Histology similar to extraprostatic EHE including epithelioid cells with intracytoplasmic vacuoles containing red blood cells and positivity for endothelial markers
- **Angiosarcoma**
  - < 15 cases reported in literature
  - Patients' age: 31-79 yr (mean: 62 yr)
  - Causal relationship of prior radiotherapy for prostatic adenocarcinoma controversial
  - Most present with lower urinary tract symptoms as well as pain and hematuria
  - May form large masses extending into bladder or extraprostatic tissues
  - Histology similar to extraprostatic AS
    - Proliferative vascular channels lined by atypical cells
    - Diagnosis confirmed by expression of endothelial markers such as CD34, CD31, and ERG
  - Aggressive clinical course
    - May develop widespread metastasis
    - Distant metastasis to lungs and liver may bleed causing hemothorax and hemoperitoneum, respectively
    - May cause significant hematuria requiring multiple blood transfusions

Tumors With Neural Differentiation

- Probably arises from adjacent pelvic autonomic plexus
- Most often in patients with neurofibromatosis 1 (NF1)
  - 11 neurofibromas, 1 ganglioneuroma, and 1 malignant peripheral nerve sheath tumor (MPNST) reported in NF1 patients
  - Mostly young patients (1 month to 35 yr)
  - Most have neurofibromas in other organs including skin
  - Prostate involvement presents with mass lesion or obstructive urinary symptoms
  - Concomitant bladder and prostate involvement by neurofibroma common; 1/5 have only prostatic involvement
- Prostatic schwannoma and MPNST described in non-NF1 patients
  - Older patients explains lack of association to NF1
- Histology similar to extraprostatic neural tumors
- Diagnosis confirmed by S100 positivity

Malignant Fibrous Histiocytoma

- < 10 cases of prostatic malignant fibrous histiocytoma (MFH) reported
- Patients' aged: 25-80 yr (mean: 58 yr)
- Tumors are large, presenting with obstructive urinary symptoms and abnormal DRE
- Histologically similar to extraprostatic MFH
- Clinically aggressive course
  - 3 of 5 patients with follow-up died of disease

Osteogenic and Chondrogenic Tumors

- Malignant osteoid or chondroid neoplasm usually heterologous component of sarcomatoid carcinoma
- Sporadic bone or cartilage prostatic tumors reported
  - 2 aggressive and lethal pleomorphic undifferentiated tumors with osteoid formation devoid of epithelial differentiation were reported; may represent primary prostatic osteosarcoma
  - Uneventful prostate chondroma within BPH has been reported

Synovial Sarcoma

- < 12 cases of prostatic SS reported
- Patients' aged: 28-63 yr
- Most present with obstructive urinary symptoms
- Suggested to arise from prostatic parenchyma and prostatic fascia
- Large tumors (5-12 cm) with frequent necrosis and extension to pelvic organs or soft tissues
- Histology similar to extraprostatic SS
  - Most with pure spindle cell (monophasic) morphology
  - Some with biphasic epithelioid cell and spindle cell morphology
  - Positive for CD99
  - Diagnosis can be confirmed by detection of t(X;18) or *SS18-SSX* fusion transcript
- Of 10 patients with follow-up, 5 died of disease mostly from recurrence &/or metastasis

Primitive Neuroectodermal Tumor/Ewing Sarcoma

- ~ 10 cases of prostatic PNET reported
- Patients were young ranging from 20-37 yr
- Main symptoms include pain during micturition, pelvic discomfort, and dysuria
- Tumor usually large (6.7-10.0 cm) and extraprostatic extension common with involvement of bladder &/or seminal vesicles
- Histology similar to extraprostatic PNET
  - Small, round blue cells

Mesenchymal Tumors of Prostate

Differential Diagnosis for Spindle Cell Lesion of the Prostate

Lesions/Neoplasms	Histology
Stromal-predominant BPH	Multinodular growth of bland cells with abundant capillaries exhibiting stromal cell condensation around vessels
STUMP	Degenerate atypia, hypercellular, myxoid, phyllodes-type patterns
PSS	Solid growth of spindle or epithelioid cells or biphasic phyllodes-type growth with hypercellular stroma showing range of nuclear atypia, mitotic activity, and necrosis; infiltrative
LM	Well-defined fascicles and whorls of interlacing smooth muscle cells with cigar-shaped nuclei or degenerative nuclear atypia and absent to rare mitosis; circumscribed
LMS	Vague to well-defined fascicles and whorls of interlacing smooth muscle cells with range of nuclear atypia, mitotic activity, and necrosis; infiltrative
RMS	Mostly embryonal type, consisting of spectrum of primitive or undifferentiated cells to larger round or spindled rhabdomyoblasts
IMT	Reactive-appearing uniform myofibroblastic cells in loose myxoid stroma with fine chromatin, occasional prominent nucleoli, and variable mitotic activity
SFT	Haphazardly arranged (patternless) bland spindle cells with scant cytoplasm admixed with thick (ropey or keloid-like) collagen and small to hemangiopericytomatous (staghorn) vessels
GIST	Fascicle of spindle cells with occasional perinuclear vacuoles
SC	High-grade spindle cells ± heterologous elements that may be admixed with distinct epithelioid (adenocarcinoma) component

STUMP = stromal tumor of unknown malignant potential; PSS = prostatic stromal sarcoma; LM = leiomyoma; LMS = leiomyosarcoma; RMS = solitary fibrous tumor; IMT = inflammatory myofibroblastic tumor; SFT = solitary fibrous tumor; GIST = gastrointestinal stromal tumor; SC = sarcomatoid carcinoma.

Modified from Paner GP, et al. Histopathology. 60:166-186. 2012.

Immunohistochemical Staining of Spindle Cell Tumors of the Prostate

Neoplasm	CD34	SMA	Desmin	ALK1	CD117	PR	Pankeratin	PSA/PAP	Myogenin
STUMP	+	-/+	-/+	-	-	+	-	-	-
PSS	+	-/+	-/+	-	-	+	-	-	-
SMT	-	+	+	-	-	+/-	-/+	-	-
IMT	-	+	+	+/-	+/-	-	+/-	-	-
SFT	+	-	-	-	-	+/-	-	-	-
GIST	+	+/-	+/-	-	+	-	-	-	-
SC	-	-/+	-/+	-	-	-	+*/-	+*/-	-
RMS	-	+	+	-	-	-	-	-	+

SMT = smooth muscle tumor; *positivity more intense in better differentiated carcinoma cells.

Derived from Paner GP, et al. Histopathology; 60:166-186, 2012.

- Positive for CD99 and FLI-1
- Diagnosis can be confirmed by detection of t(11;22) or EWSR1 (EWS/FLI1) transcript

Angiomyolipoma/Perivascular Epithelioid Cell Tumor

- 3 cases of prostatic PEComas reported
- Patients' aged: 36-54 yr
- Presentations include obstructive urinary symptoms and hematospermia
- Tumor causes prostatic enlargement (up to 8.5 cm)
- Contains epithelioid cells with clear to eosinophilic granular cytoplasm, ± admixed spindle cells, arranged in vascularized solid nests or sheets
- Positive for HMB-45
- 2 of 3 cases had metastasis, and 1 died of disease

SELECTED REFERENCES

1. Ball MW et al: Multimodal therapy in the treatment of prostate sarcoma: The Johns Hopkins Experience. Clin Genitourin Cancer. 13(5):435-40, 2015
2. Musser JE et al: Adult prostate sarcoma: the Memorial Sloan Kettering experience. Urology. 84(3):624-8, 2014
3. Sohn M et al: Histologic variability and diverse oncologic outcomes of prostate sarcomas. Korean J Urol. 55(12):797-801, 2014
4. Tavora F et al: Mesenchymal tumours of the bladder and prostate: an update. Pathology. 45(2):104-15, 2013
5. Wang X et al: Twenty-five cases of adult prostate sarcoma treated at a high-volume institution from 1989 to 2009. Urology. 82(1):160-5, 2013
6. Paner GP et al: Non-epithelial neoplasms of the prostate. Histopathology. 60(1):166-86, 2012
7. Dotan ZA et al: Adult genitourinary sarcoma: the 25-year Memorial Sloan-Kettering experience. J Urol. 176(5):2033-8; discussion 2038-9, 2006

Mesenchymal Tumors of Prostate

Leiomyosarcoma
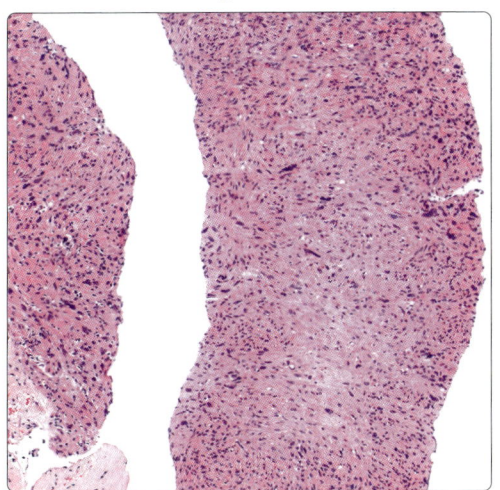

Leiomyosarcoma
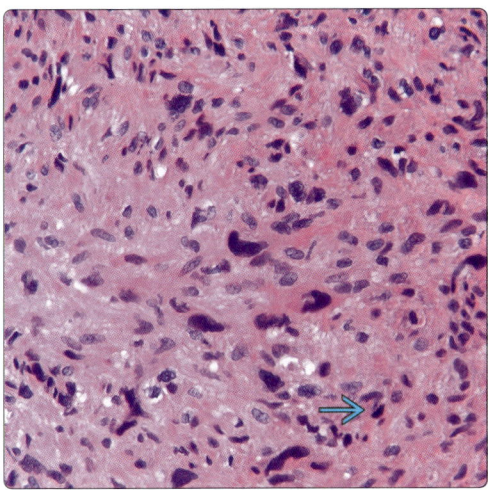

(Left) LMS in needle biopsy cores shows spindle cells with bright eosinophilic cytoplasm. This tumor is cellular, and diffuse pleomorphism is obvious even in low-power magnification. Both cores are completely involved by LMS. Prostatic LMS are usually large bulky tumors. *(Right)* High-power view of LMS shows enlarged, irregular, and hyperchromatic nuclei. Note presence of mitosis ➡. Other features associated with malignancy include increased mitosis and presence of coagulative necrosis, features that are not present in LM.

Epithelioid Leiomyosarcoma
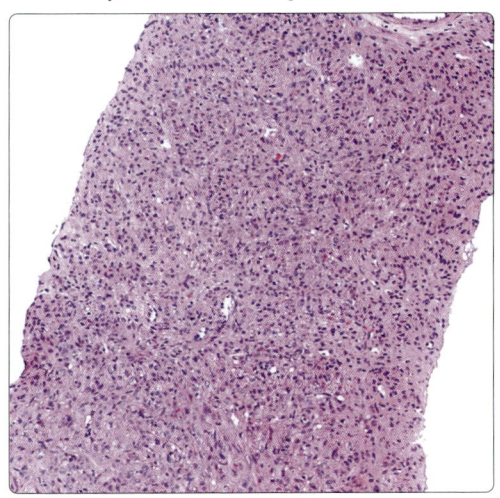

Epithelioid Leiomyosarcoma: Smooth Muscle Actin
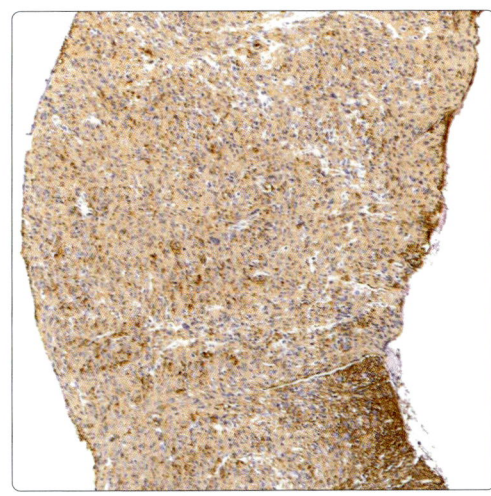

(Left) Prostate needle biopsy shows LMS that is highly cellular with predominance of epithelioid cells containing eosinophilic cytoplasm and exhibiting nuclear atypia. *(Right)* Diagnosis of epithelioid LMS in this prostate biopsy is confirmed by diffuse expression of smooth muscle markers including SMA and desmin. GIST, including epithelioid type, from colorectal area may mimic LMS. GIST may also express smooth muscle markers. Unlike LMS, GIST shows strong diffuse expression of CD117 and DOG1.

Leiomyoma
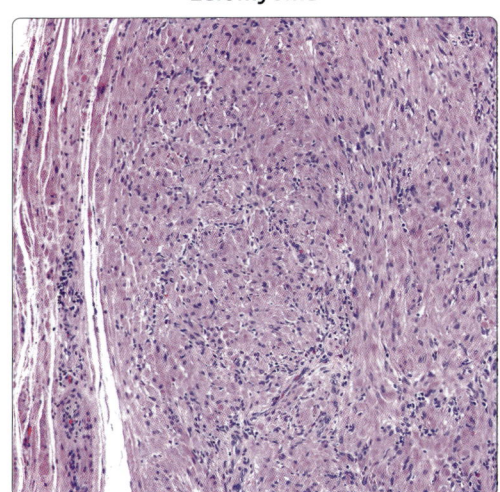

Inflammatory Myofibroblastic Tumor (IMT)
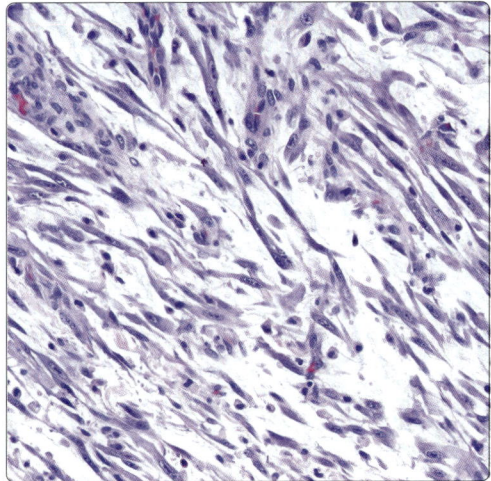

(Left) Well-circumscribed LM containing fascicles of bland neoplastic smooth muscle cells devoid of nuclear atypia, mitosis, or necrosis. *(Right)* This IMT shows characteristic spindle cells with elongated cytoplasmic processes in a myxomatous stroma. Most prostatic IMTs are secondary involvement from bladder IMT and may morphologically overlap with sarcomatoid carcinoma and spindle cell sarcomas. Diagnosis of IMT can be confirmed by ALK1 positivity; however, reported expression of this protein varies from 20-75%.

Mesenchymal Tumors of Prostate

Solitary Fibrous Tumor

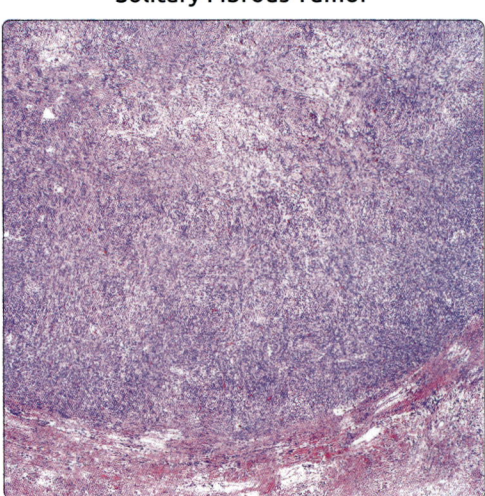

Solitary Fibrous Tumor

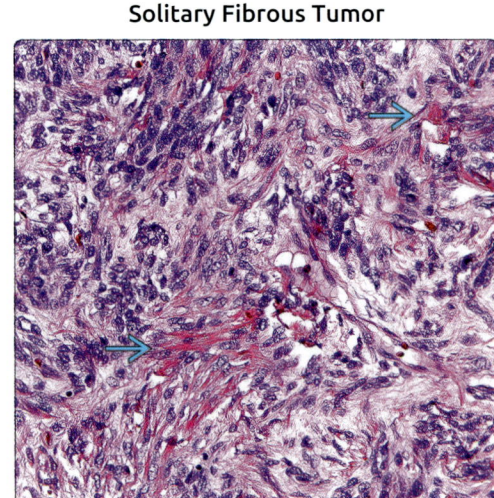

(Left) Low-power view of SFT in radical prostatectomy shows well-circumscribed tumor involving the prostate. Although most SFTs arise within the prostate, a subset may arise from adjacent extraprostatic tissues and extends into prostate. (Right) High-power view of SFT shows haphazardly arranged spindle cells with oval nuclei and modest cytoplasm. Bundles of collagen are seen intimately associated with the tumor cells ➡. This SFT lacks nuclear pleomorphism and mitosis. Most SFTs are positive for CD34, CD99, or Bcl-2.

Paraganglioma

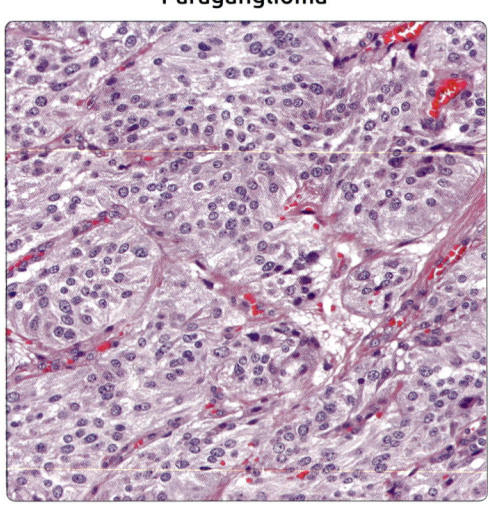

Rhabdomyosarcoma

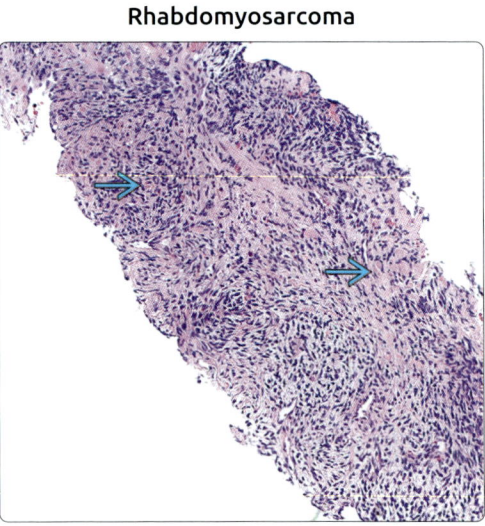

(Left) Paraganglioma shows characteristic solid nested architecture (zellballen) surrounded by a network of delicate vessels. Tumor cells have granular cytoplasm, and nuclei show mild atypia. Paraganglioma can be functional and may cause symptoms related to elevated levels of catecholamines such as hypertension, tachycardia, and dizziness. (Right) Prostate needle biopsy shows RMS consisting mainly of poorly differentiated small cells with hyperchromatic nuclei. Occasional rhabdomyoblasts ➡ are discernible.

Rhabdomyosarcoma

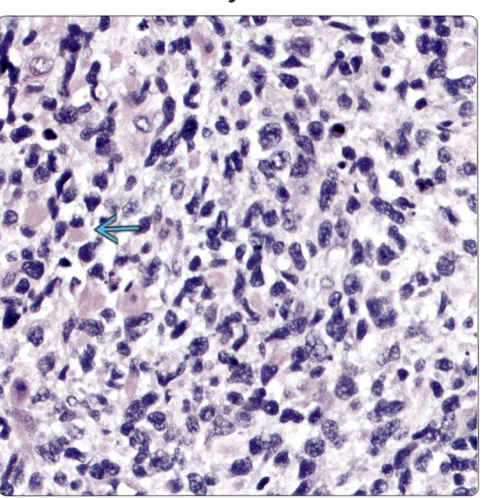

Rhabdomyosarcoma

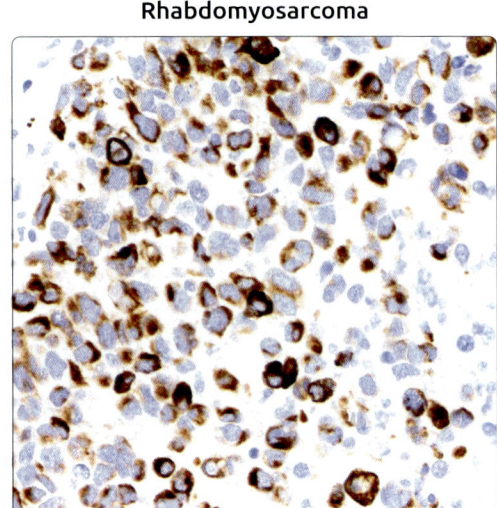

(Left) RMS shows predominance of primitive-appearing cells with hyperchromatic nuclei. Rhabdomyoblasts ➡ have more abundant eosinophilic cytoplasm, and nuclei are often eccentrically situated. (Right) RMS shows cytoplasmic positivity for desmin. These cells are positive for nuclear myogenin and MYOD1. RMS in an adult prostate should also raise sarcomatoid carcinoma (SC) with heterologous elements in the differential diagnosis. Unlike RMS, SC shows a carcinoma component that may express PSA or PAP.

Mesenchymal Tumors of Prostate

Angiosarcoma

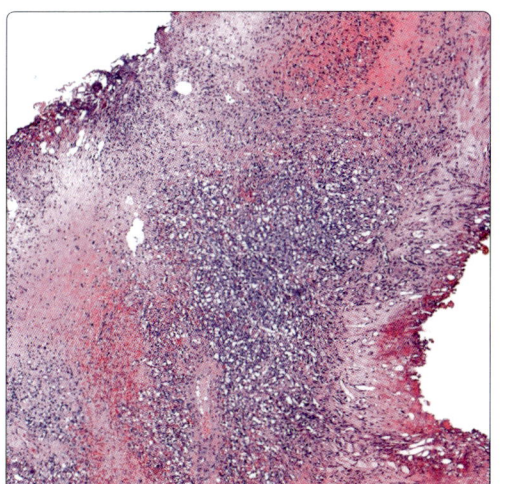

Angiosarcoma

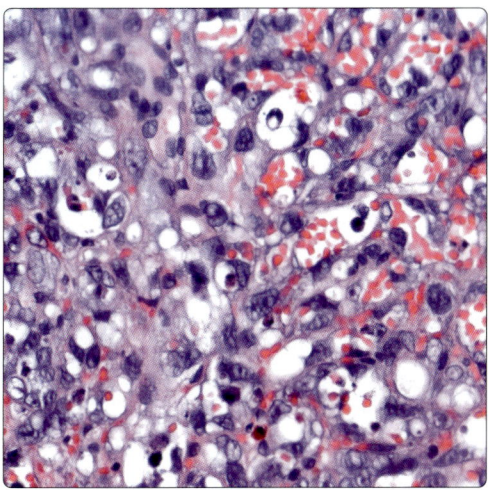

(Left) TURP chip shows involvement by AS exhibiting areas of hemorrhage and necrosis. The cellular tumor exhibits multiple luminal formations. (Right) High-power view of AS shows malignant endothelial cells with prominent nuclear atypia. The tumor cells form luminal spaces, some intracytoplasmic, that contain erythrocytes. AS may also exhibit solid growth, making the diagnosis more challenging. Diagnosis of AS may be confirmed by its expression of endothelial markers such as CD34 or CD31.

Synovial Sarcoma (SS)

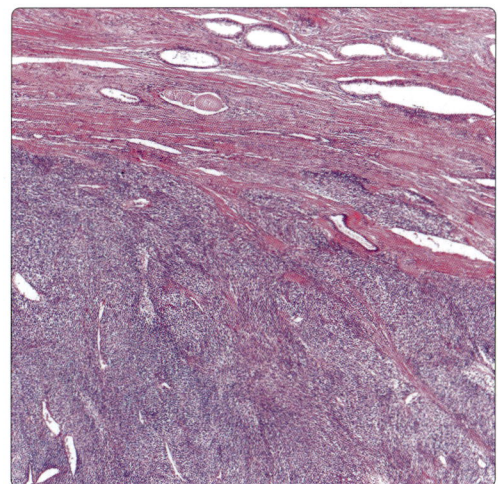

Synovial Sarcoma

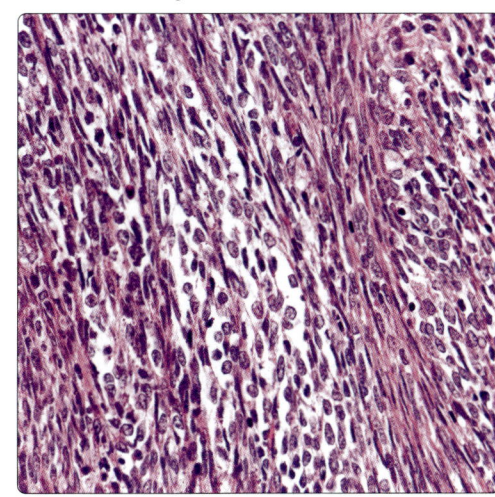

(Left) Low-power view shows SS involving the prostate. The tumor in this case is well delineated and is highly cellular. SS is extremely rare in prostate. (Courtesy C. Pan, MD.) (Right) SS shows intertwining spindle cells with overlapping ovoid-to-elongated vesicular nuclei showing moderate atypia. This particular prostatic SS is positive for CD99 and Bcl2 and confirmed to have the SYT-SSX fusion transcript. SS can be purely spindled or may have admixed epithelial differentiation (biphasic SS). (Courtesy C. Pan, MD.)

PNET

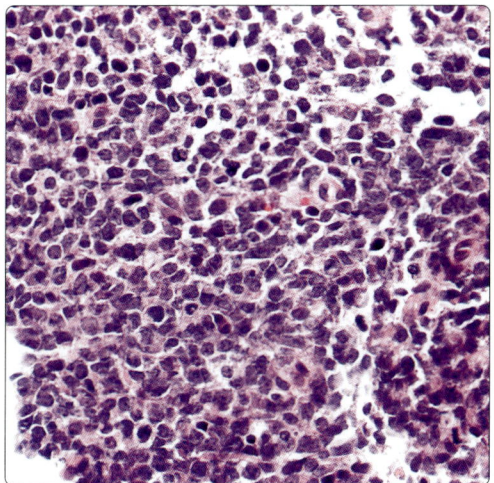

PNET

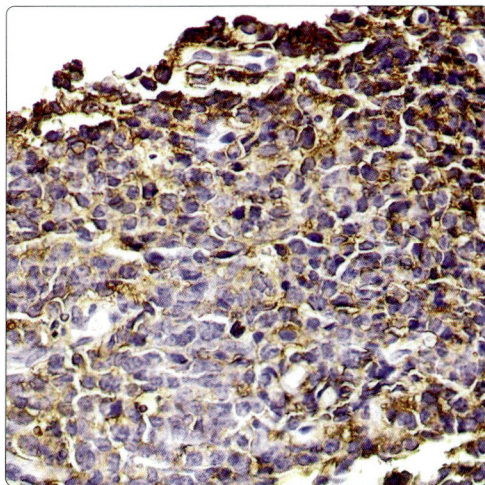

(Left) PNET shows solid sheet of closely packed tumor cells. The cells are relatively monotonous, have scant cytoplasm, round nuclei, fine dispersed chromatin, and inconspicuous nucleoli. (Courtesy T. Shibuya.) (Right) Prostatic PNET with diffuse positivity for CD99. Other markers that may be positive are caveolin-1, Bcl-2, NSE, and CD57. Translocation involving ES breakpoint region 1 at chromosome 22q12 was demonstrated in this case, confirming the diagnosis of SS. (Courtesy T. Shibuya.)

Melanocytic Lesions of Prostate

KEY FACTS

TERMINOLOGY
- **Blue nevus**: Benign lesion wherein melanocytes are present only in prostatic stroma
- **Melanosis**: Benign lesion with recognizable melanin in prostatic epithelium ± stromal involvement
- **Melanoma**: Malignant melanocytic neoplasm that may primarily or secondarily involve prostate

ETIOLOGY/PATHOGENESIS
- Origin of melanocytes within prostate is controversial
- Melanoblasts entrapped ectopically in prostate during migration from neural crest cells to superficial sites
- Primary melanoma of prostate may arise from melanocytes along prostatic urethral epithelium

CLINICAL ISSUES
- Rare: ~ 32 blue nevus, ~ 20 melanosis, and < 10 primary melanoma of prostate reported
- Blue nevus and melanosis are incidental findings
- Melanoma may present with obstructive urinary symptoms, hematuria, and abnormal DRE due to large mass

MACROSCOPIC
- Blue nevus and melanosis appear as black streaks or nodules in prostate, which are often unifocal

MICROSCOPIC
- Blue nevus characterized by stromal melanocytes containing abundant fine granular brown to black pigment
- Melanosis shows melanin pigments in glandular epithelium, often together with stromal melanocytes
- Melanoma contains pleomorphic cells with prominent nucleoli and abundant mitosis

ANCILLARY TESTS
- Melanocytes: S100(+), HMB-45(-), CD68(-)
- Melanoma: S100(+), HMB-45(+)
- Fontana-Masson highlights melanin pigments
- EM: Melanosomes at different stages of differentiation

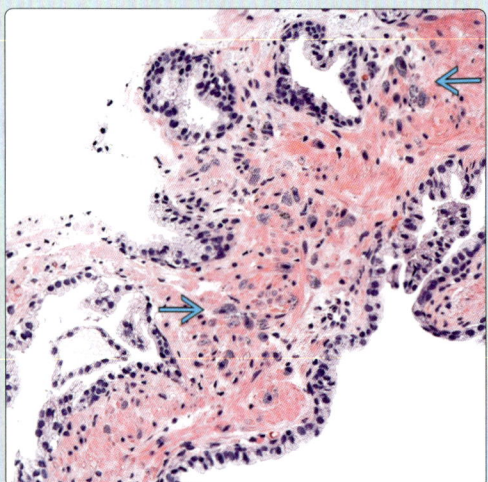

Stromal Melanosis in Biopsy

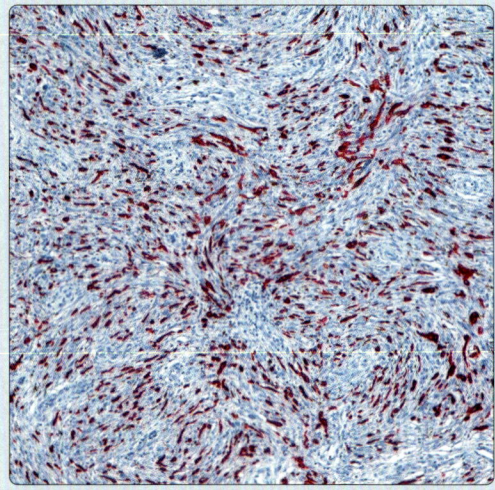

S100 in Blue Nevus

(Left) Needle biopsy of prostate shows melanocytes ➡ in stroma containing fine granular brown black pigments in the cytoplasm. Melanin in blue nevus are present only in the stroma and not in prostatic glandular cells, unlike in melanosis. (Right) The stromal melanocytes in this blue nevus are highlighted by strong S100 immunostaining. The melanocytic cells are spindled with elongated processes and are arranged haphazardly. These cells do not express HMB-45 and CD68. (Courtesy M.R. Raspollini, MD, PhD.)

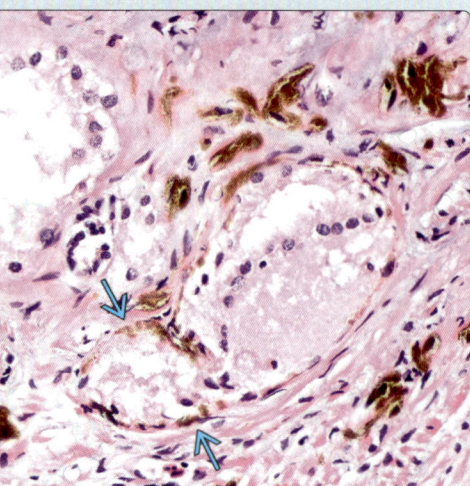

Melanosis

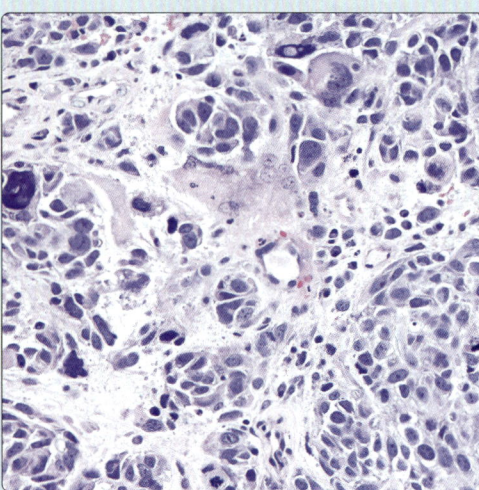

Melanoma

(Left) This melanosis shows pigmented melanocytes in the stroma between glands. Brown pigment is also present in the cytoplasm of benign acinar cells ➡. The pigment in epithelial cells is suggested to result from secondary uptake of melanin from the stromal melanocytes. (Courtesy H. Gucer, MD.) (Right) This melanoma exhibits marked pleomorphism with bizarre and multinucleated tumor cells. Melanoma may arise along the urethra and extend into prostate. Melanocytic lineage can be confirmed by its HMB-45 positivity.

Melanocytic Lesions of Prostate

TERMINOLOGY

Synonyms
- Blue nevus and melanosis: Pigmented melanocytosis, prostatic nevohyperplasia

Definitions
- **Blue nevus**: Benign lesion wherein melanocytes are present only in prostatic stroma
- **Melanosis**: Benign lesion with recognizable melanin in prostatic epithelium ± stromal involvement
  o Blue nevus and melanosis may be part of 1 disease spectrum; terminologies interchanged by few authors
- **Melanoma**: Malignant melanocytic neoplasm that may primarily or secondarily involve prostate

ETIOLOGY/PATHOGENESIS

Origin of Melanocytes in Prostate
- Controversial
  o Melanoblasts entrapped ectopically in prostate during migration from neural crest cells to superficial sites
  o Epithelial melanin in melanosis suggested to result from secondary uptake from adjacent pigmented stromal cells
- Primary melanoma of prostate may arise from melanocytes along prostatic urethral epithelium

CLINICAL ISSUES

Epidemiology
- Incidence
  o Rare: ~ 32 blue nevus, ~ 20 melanosis, and < 10 primary melanoma of prostate reported
- Age
  o Blue nevus and melanoma: Range 20-85 years; most > 50
  o Primary melanoma reported in men 37-85 years old; encountered also in patients young for prostate cancer

Presentation
- Blue nevus and melanosis are incidental findings, commonly in patients treated for benign prostatic hyperplasia (BPH) or uncommonly in patients diagnosed with prostate carcinoma
  o Both should not cause serum PSA elevation; higher levels likely due to BPH or other causes
- Melanoma may present with obstructive urinary symptoms, hematuria, and abnormal DRE due to large mass
  o In absence of melanoma in situ lesion, prior or concomitant cutaneous or noncutaneous melanoma should be ruled out for diagnosis as prostate primary

Treatment
- Blue nevus and melanosis require no therapy
- Advanced melanoma has poor response to surgery and systemic therapy

Prognosis
- Blue nevus and melanosis are benign lesions with no increased risk for malignancy
- Few reported cases of primary prostatic melanoma had very poor prognosis
  o 1 case did not recur or metastasize after 7 years follow-up attributed to resection of tumor at early stage

MACROSCOPIC

General Features
- Blue nevus and melanosis appear as black streaks or nodules in prostate, which are often unifocal
  o Blue nevus range from 0.1-2.0 cm in size
- Melanoma may diffusely involve prostate gland and extend to adjacent structures

MICROSCOPIC

Histologic Features
- **Blue nevus**
  o Similar to its cutaneous counterpart, stromal melanocytes contain abundant fine granular brown to black pigment lacking birefringent features
  o Pigmented stromal cells are often fusiform with dendritic cytoplasmic processes but may also be round to polygonal
  o Bland nuclei often covered by the dense melanin
  o Stromal melanosis is more appropriate term of accumulation in stromal macrophages
- **Melanosis**
  o In addition to stromal melanocytes, melanin pigments present in the glandular epithelium
  o Uncommonly pigments may be present in concomitant adenocarcinoma glands
  o Only 1 instance of melanosis with pigment present only in epithelium
- **Melanoma**
  o Frankly malignant or pleomorphic cells with prominent nucleoli and abundant mitosis
  o Melanoma in situ may be seen along urethra

ANCILLARY TESTS

Histochemistry
- Fontana-Masson highlights melanin pigment and can be bleached with potassium permanganate

Immunohistochemistry
- Melanocytes: S100(+), HMB-45(-), CD68(-)
- Melanoma: S100(+), HMB-45(+)

Electron Microscopy
- Melanosomes at different stages of differentiation

DIFFERENTIAL DIAGNOSIS

Blue Nevus and Melanosis
- Lipofuscin: Ziehl-Neelsen, Sudan black B, or PAS stain (+)
- Hemosiderin: Prussian blue stain (+)
- Ochronosis: Homogentisic acid deposition

Melanoma
- Sarcoma and poorly differentiated carcinoma: HMB-45(-)

SELECTED REFERENCES
1. Tosev G et al: Primary melanoma of the prostate: case report and review of the literature. BMC Urol. 15:68, 2015
2. Gucer H et al: Prostatic melanosis. Urol Ann. 6(4):384-6, 2014
3. Dailey VL et al: Blue nevus of the prostate. Arch Pathol Lab Med. 135(6):799-802, 2011

Melanocytic Lesions of Prostate

Blue Nevus in Resection

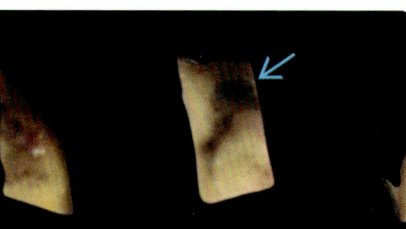

Blue Nevus in Resection

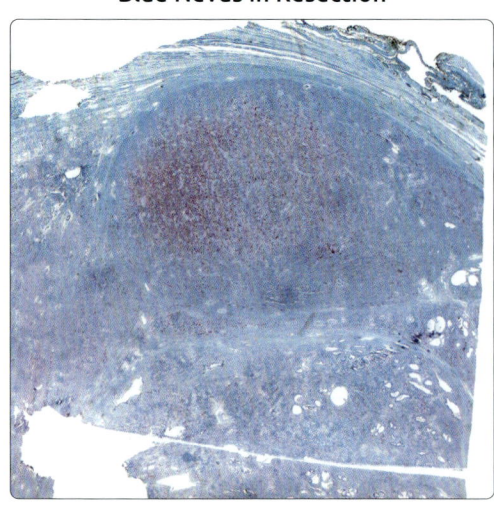

(Left) Prostate resection shows a grossly visible darkly pigmented nodule of blue nevus ➡. This lesion is usually unifocal and may also manifest as streaks or nodules of dark discoloration. The nodule may be up to 2 cm in size. (Courtesy M.R. Raspollini, MD, PhD.) (Right) The blue nevus nodule at the left is highlighted by diffuse S100 immunopositivity (red color). Blue nevus of the prostate are typically asymptomatic and have no potential for malignant transformation. (Courtesy M.R. Raspollini, MD, PhD.)

Blue Nevus in Resection

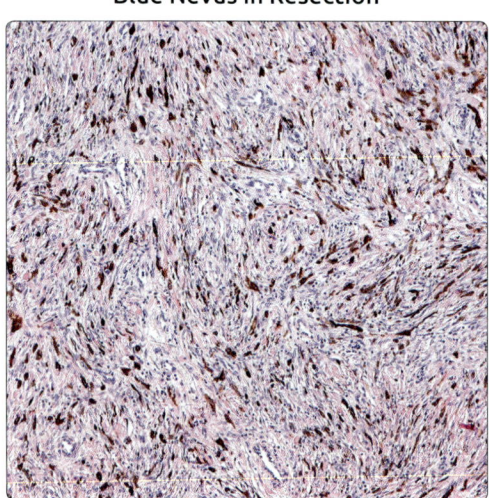

Stromal Melanosis in Biopsy

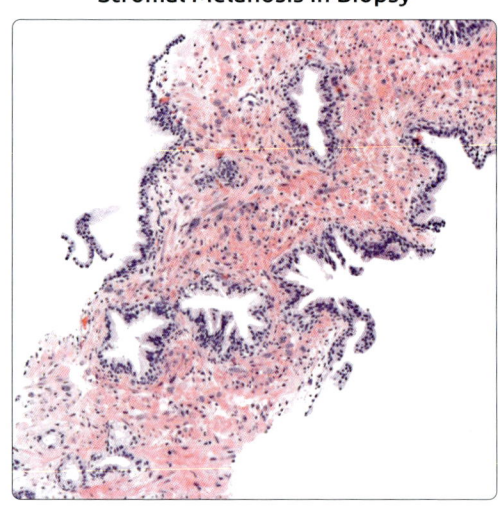

(Left) This prostate resection shows abundant darkly pigmented melanocytes haphazardly dispersed in the stroma. The cells have dendritic appearance and are densely loaded with brown-black pigment obscuring the cellular details. (Courtesy M.R. Raspollini, MD, PhD.) (Right) This needle core biopsy shows occasional melanocytes in the prostatic stroma. The density of melanocytic cells may vary. These benign melanocytes are suggested to be entrapped in the prostate during its migration from the neural crest to superficial sites.

Stromal Melanosis in Biopsy

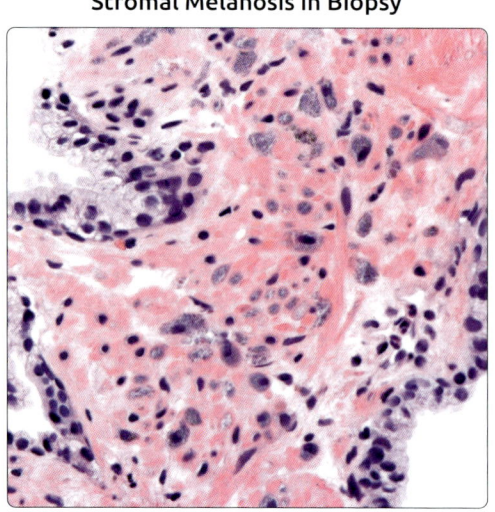

Fontana-Masson in Stromal Melanosis

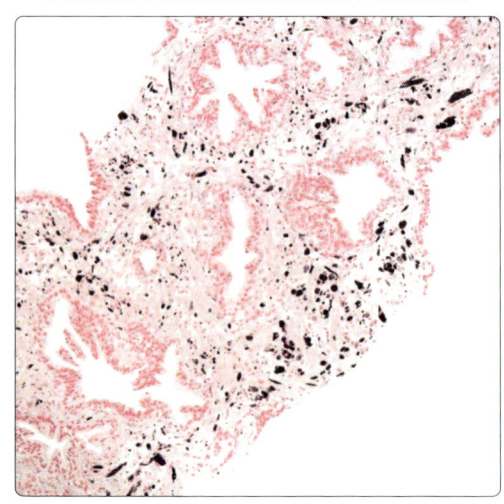

(Left) The scattered melanocytes blend with the fibromuscular stromal cells. These cells have bland nuclei and no atypia or increase in mitotic activity. These pigmented cells can be subtle and may be overlooked on routine histologic sections. (Right) The melanin pigment in the stroma are highlighted in black by a Fontana-Masson stain. This dark discoloration may be bleached with potassium permanganate. Hemosiderin does not stain with Fontana-Masson and may be highlighted by Prussian blue reaction.

Melanocytic Lesions of Prostate

Melanosis
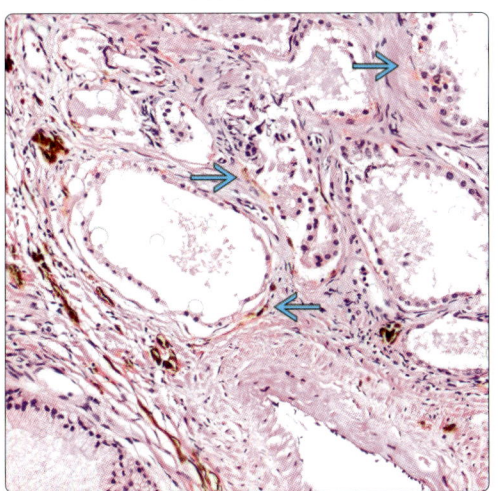

Melanosis
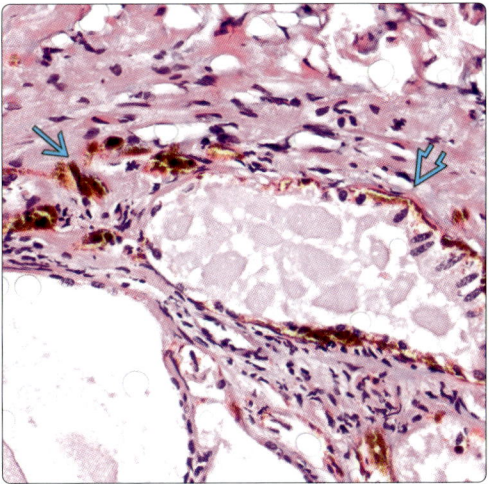

(Left) This melanosis shows pigment in both stroma and benign glandular cells ➡. Most melanosis involve both stroma and epithelium. Pure epithelial involvement is exceedingly rare. Likewise, the presence of melanin pigment in malignant or carcinomatous glands is also rare. (Courtesy H. Gucer, MD.) (Right) Stromal melanocytes ➡ are densely loaded with fine granular brown melanin pigments that obscure the nuclei. In benign glands, the pigments are less dense and do not cover the nuclei ➡. (Courtesy H. Gucer, MD.)

Melanoma of Urethra
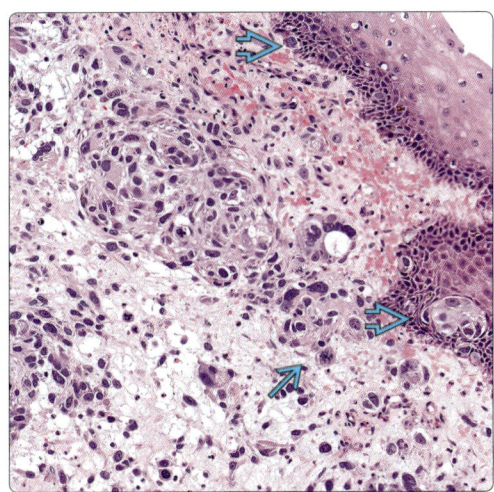

HMB-45 in Melanoma
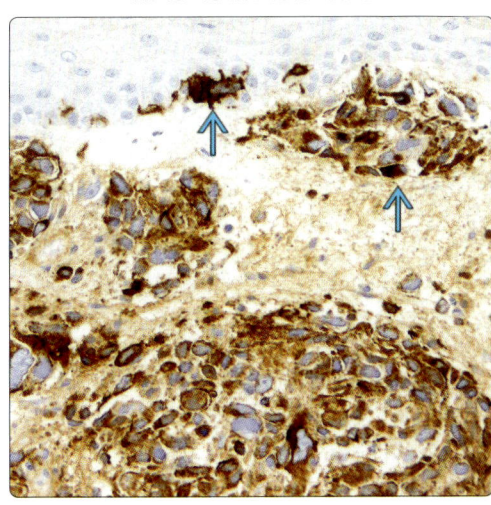

(Left) This melanoma in stark contrast to blue nevus and melanosis is more cellular and exhibits marked nuclear pleomorphism and abundant mitosis ➡. Note the presence of melanoma in situ within the surface epithelium ➡. (Right) Melanoma with strong and diffuse positivity with HMB-45, including in the in situ component ➡. Melanoma involving the prostate is highly aggressive and may be primary or more rarely, a secondary metastasis from another site. Presence of an in situ lesion confirms a primary melanoma at this site.

Lipofuscin in Seminal Vesicle
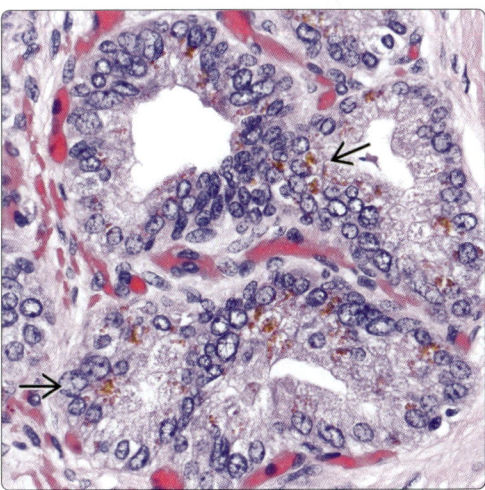

Lipofuscin in Benign Prostatic Glands
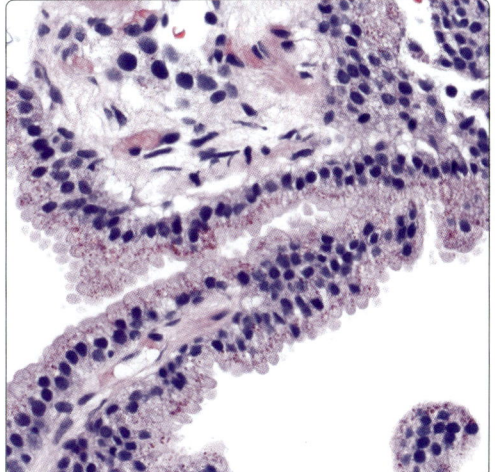

(Left) Seminal vesicle and ejaculatory duct epithelium are characterized by its unusual nuclear atypicality and presence of densely granular golden yellow lipofuscin pigment ➡. These features are helpful in distinguishing this epithelium in needle core biopsy. (Right) Benign acinar cells uncommonly contain cytoplasmic pigments. These deposits are less dense than in seminal vesicle epithelium. Unlike in melanosis, this pigment is golden yellow and no melanin laden cells are present in adjacent stroma.

Hematopoietic Neoplasms of Prostate

KEY FACTS

TERMINOLOGY
- Hematopoietic neoplasms primarily or secondarily involving prostate
- Criteria for diagnosis of primary lymphoma of prostate
  - Lymphoma involves prostatic tissue with absence or minimal involvement of periprostatic tissue
  - Symptoms of disease attributable to enlargement of prostate
  - Lack of involvement of hematopoietic system (peripheral blood, lymph nodes, liver, and spleen) within 1 month of diagnosis

CLINICAL ISSUES
- Lymphoma encountered in 0.3-0.8% of prostate specimens
- Secondary involvement more common than primary prostate lymphoma
- Symptomatic lymphoma cases presents mainly with obstructive symptoms and occasionally hematuria
- Incidental lymphoma may be identified in biopsy and TUR specimens and in lymph nodes dissected during radical prostatectomies

MICROSCOPIC
- Majority of incidental and secondary prostatic lymphomas are low grade B-cell lymphomas and DLBCL
- B-cell lymphomas reported in prostate include SLL/CLL, DLCBL, MZL, follicular lymphoma, mantle cell lymphoma, MALT lymphoma, intravascular large B-cell lymphoma, and Burkitt lymphoma
- Other hematologic neoplasms reported are lymphoblastic lymphoma/leukemia, myeloid leukemia (granulocytic sarcoma), multiple myeloma, Hodgkin disease, and T-cell lymphoma

ANCILLARY TESTS
- Lymphomas: Positive for CD45, CD20, CD79-a, or CD3
- Myeloid leukemia: Myeloperoxidase (+)
- Plasma cell dyscrasia: CD138(+)

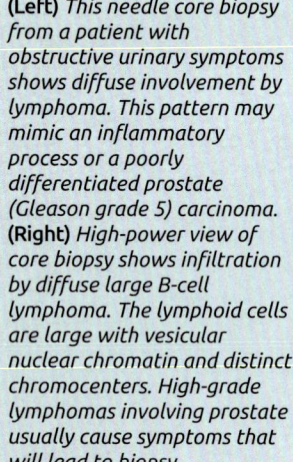
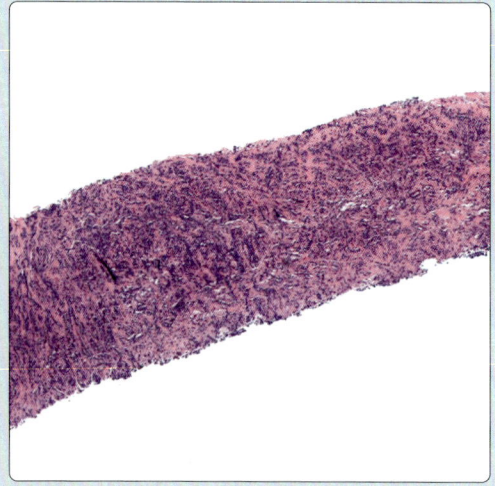
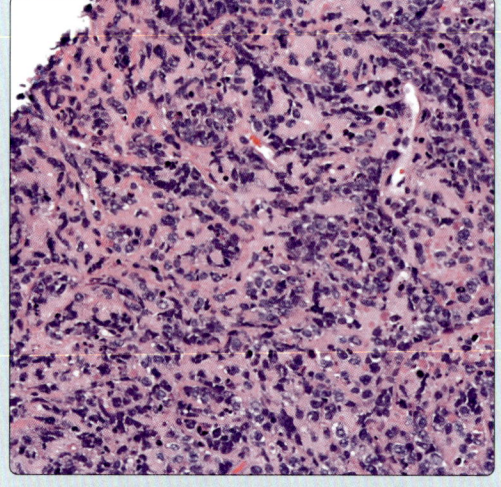

Lymphoma in Prostate Biopsy | **Lymphoma in Prostate Biopsy**

(Left) This needle core biopsy from a patient with obstructive urinary symptoms shows diffuse involvement by lymphoma. This pattern may mimic an inflammatory process or a poorly differentiated prostate (Gleason grade 5) carcinoma. (Right) High-power view of core biopsy shows infiltration by diffuse large B-cell lymphoma. The lymphoid cells are large with vesicular nuclear chromatin and distinct chromocenters. High-grade lymphomas involving prostate usually cause symptoms that will lead to biopsy.

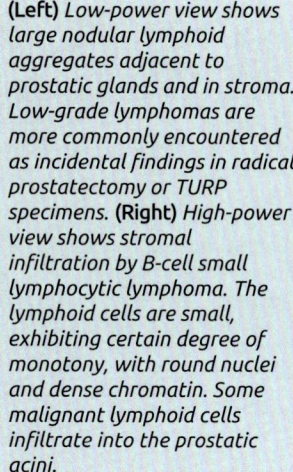
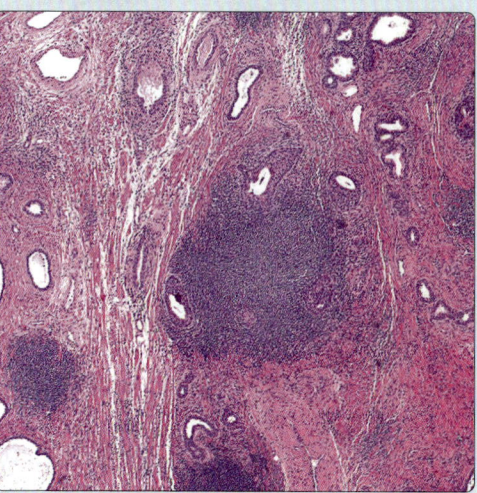
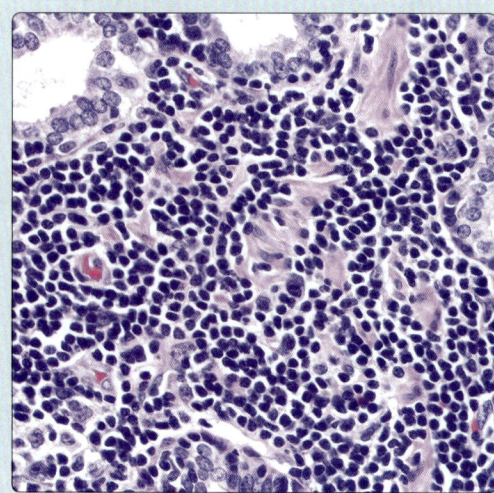

Lymphoma in Prostate Resection | **Lymphoma in Prostate Resection**

(Left) Low-power view shows large nodular lymphoid aggregates adjacent to prostatic glands and in stroma. Low-grade lymphomas are more commonly encountered as incidental findings in radical prostatectomy or TURP specimens. (Right) High-power view shows stromal infiltration by B-cell small lymphocytic lymphoma. The lymphoid cells are small, exhibiting certain degree of monotony, with round nuclei and dense chromatin. Some malignant lymphoid cells infiltrate into the prostatic acini.

Hematopoietic Neoplasms of Prostate

TERMINOLOGY

Definitions

- Hematopoietic neoplasms primarily or secondarily (with hematopoietic system disease) involving prostate
- Proposed criteria for diagnosis of **primary lymphoma** of prostate
  - Lymphoma involves prostatic tissue with absence or minimal involvement of periprostatic tissue
  - Symptoms of disease attributable to enlargement of prostate
  - Lack of involvement of hematopoietic system (peripheral blood, lymph nodes, liver, and spleen) within 1 month of diagnosis

CLINICAL ISSUES

Epidemiology

- Incidence
  - Rare; most are B-cell lymphomas
    - Lymphoma encountered in 0.3-0.8% of prostate specimens
  - Secondary involvement more common than primary prostate lymphoma
  - Other types of hematopoietic neoplasm (e.g., T cell, lymphoblastic, myeloid, or plasma cell) much rarer
- Age
  - Primary lymphoma: Mean: 66 years (range: 32-89 years)
  - Secondary lymphoma: Mean: 60 years (range: 5-86 years)

Presentation

- Symptomatic lymphoma cases mainly obstructive symptoms and occasionally hematuria
- Incidental lymphoma may be identified in biopsy and transurethral resection (TUR) specimens and in lymph nodes dissected during radical prostatectomies
- Occasionally, lymphoma is identified concomitantly in specimens of prostate with adenocarcinoma
- Cystoscopically, lymphoma may show urethral luminal narrowing and bladder trabeculation indistinguishable from those seen secondary to nodular hyperplasia

Treatment

- Systemic (nonsurgical) therapy based on hematopoietic tumor type, grade, and spread

Prognosis

- Prognosis depends on hematopoietic neoplasm lineage, subtype, and grade
  - 1 series of 43 patients showed lymphoma-specific survival in 1 and 5 years at 64% and 33%, respectively
  - Longer survival expected for indolent lymphomas, such as asymptomatic small lymphocytic lymphoma/chronic lymphocytic leukemia (SLL/CLL)

MICROSCOPIC

Histologic Features

- **B-cell lymphoma**
  - Majority of incidental and secondary prostatic lymphomas are low-grade B-cell lymphomas
    - Series of 8 incidental lymphomas included 7 low-grade B-cell lymphomas [5 SLL/CLL and 2 marginal zone lymphomas (MZL)] and 1 diffuse large B-cell lymphoma (DLBCL)
      - In cases of MZL, lymphoma cells may infiltrate prostatic acini and form characteristic lymphoepithelial lesions
    - Same series had 7 secondary prostate lymphomas that included 6 low-grade B-cell lymphomas (3 B-cell SLLs/CLLs, 1 follicular lymphoma, 2 mantle cell lymphomas) and 1 DLBCL
  - Other series however showed DLBCL as more common
    - Series showed most prostatic lymphomas were DLBCLs (55% of primary and 37% of secondary) and SLLs/CLLs (18% of primary and 27% of secondary)
    - Another series with 8 prostatic lymphomas showed 4 DLBCL, 3 SLLs/CLLs, and 1 follicular lymphoma
  - Other types of B-cell prostatic lymphoma reported include extranodal MALT lymphoma, intravascular large B-cell lymphoma, and Burkitt lymphoma
- **Lymphoblastic lymphoma/leukemia** may involve prostate in pediatric and young adult patients, either as 1st manifestation or as site of relapse
- **Myeloid leukemia** may rarely involve prostate as
  - Secondary site of leukemic infiltration
  - Initial site of relapse
  - Much rarely, as initial presentation of mass lesion (granulocytic sarcoma)
- **Multiple myeloma** initially diagnosed on prostate biopsy has been reported
- **Hodgkin disease** and **T-cell lymphoma** exceedingly rare

ANCILLARY TESTS

Immunohistochemistry

- Lymphoma
  - Positive for CD45, CD20, CD79-a, or CD3
  - Negative for CK-PAN (AE1/AE3)
- Myeloid leukemia: Myeloperoxidase (+)
- Plasma cell dyscrasia: CD138(+)

DIFFERENTIAL DIAGNOSIS

Chronic Prostatitis

- Shows polymorphous population of cells (mature T and B cells, large activated B cells, plasma cells, and histiocytes)
- Has nodular infiltrates with pushing borders, and is often periglandular in location

Poorly Differentiated Carcinomas

- Positive for CK-PAN (AE1/AE3)
- Negative for CD45, CD20, CD79-a, or CD3

SELECTED REFERENCES

1. Schniederjan SD et al: Lymphoid neoplasms of the urinary tract and male genital organs: a clinicopathological study of 40 cases. Mod Pathol. 22(8):1057-65, 2009
2. Chu PG et al: Incidental and concurrent malignant lymphomas discovered at the time of prostatectomy and prostate biopsy: a study of 29 cases. Am J Surg Pathol. 29(5):693-9, 2005
3. Bostwick DG et al: Malignant lymphoma involving the prostate: report of 62 cases. Cancer. 83(4):732-8, 1998

Hematopoietic Neoplasms of Prostate

Diffuse Large B-Cell Lymphoma in Biopsy

Diffuse Large B-Cell Lymphoma in Biopsy

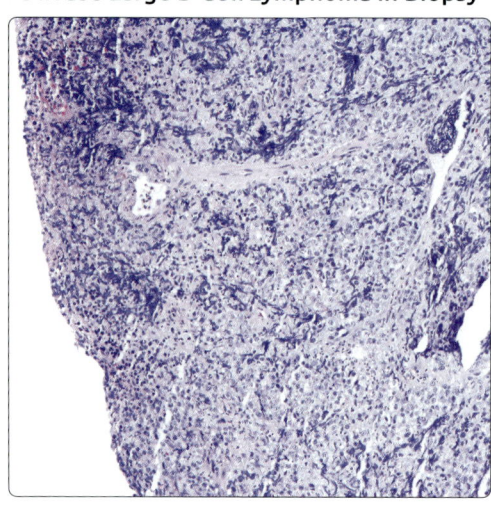
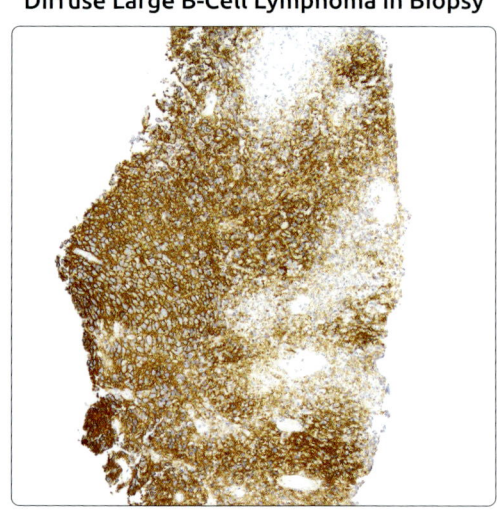

(Left) This core biopsy is diffusely infiltrated by large lymphoid cells with foci of tumor cell necrosis and smearing artifacts. Lymphoma is highly suspected with this morphology; however, definitive exclusion of poorly differentiated carcinoma can only be made with the aid of immunohistochemistry. **(Right)** CD20 shows diffuse or sheet-like staining supporting the diagnosis of diffuse large B-cell lymphoma. This lymphoma is the most common high-grade lymphoma diagnosed in the prostate.

Diffuse Large B-Cell Lymphoma in Biopsy

Diffuse Large B-Cell Lymphoma in Biopsy

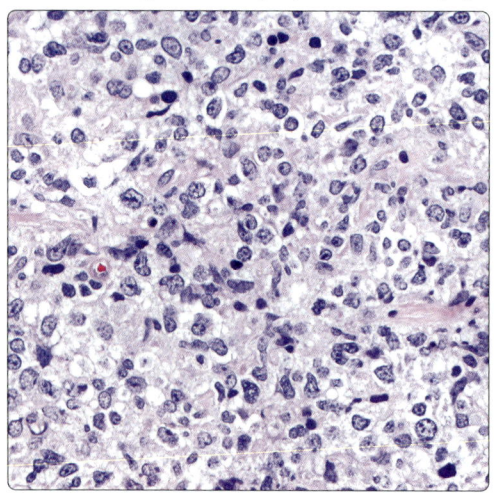
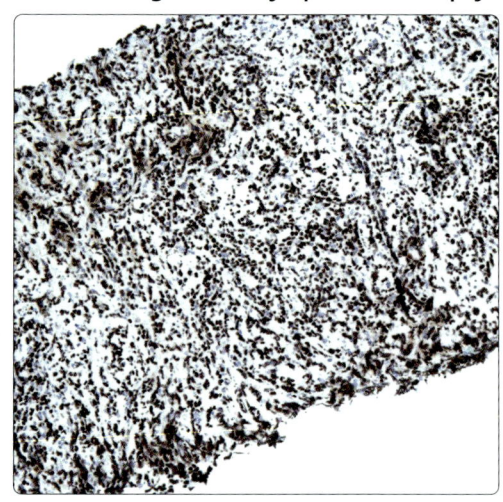

(Left) High-power view shows large nuclei with vesicular chromatin and contain 1 or multiple chromocenters (centroblastic type). This morphology contrasts the smaller nuclei with more clumped chromatin that characterize the low-grade lymphomas. **(Right)** This diffuse large B-cell lymphoma shows high nuclear ki-67 staining, which correlates with its aggressiveness. In this case, ~ 80% of the nuclei exhibits staining. Burkitt lymphoma, which is very rare in prostate, typically shows nearly 100% ki-67 nuclear staining.

Small Lymphocytic Lymphoma in Biopsy

Small Lymphocytic Lymphoma in Biopsy

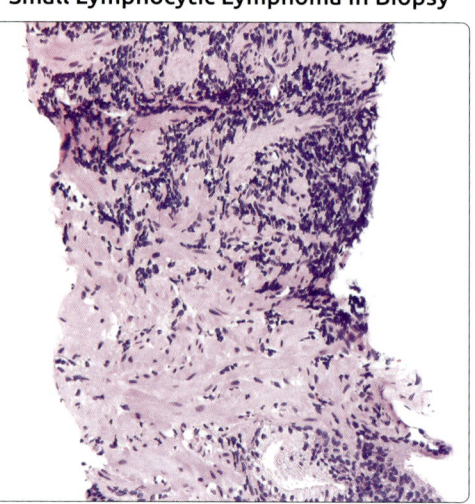
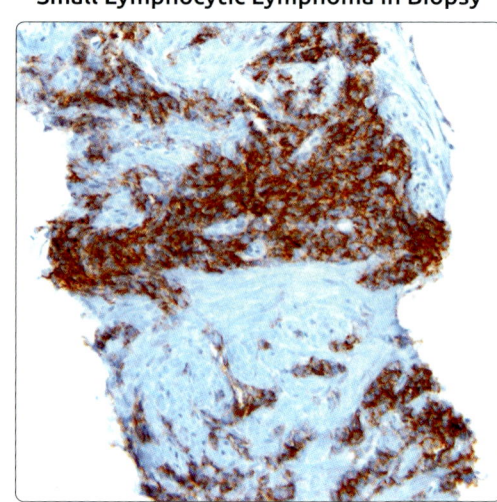

(Left) Needle biopsy shows prostate with involvement by B-cell small lymphocytic lymphoma. This low-grade lymphoma is often encountered incidentally. The small lymphoid cells when present as patchy infiltrates can easily be dismissed as benign chronic inflammation. Immunohistochemistry for CD20 and CD3 may give hint to its clonality. **(Right)** Despite the patchy nature of this infiltrates, CD20 is able to demonstrate clonality by showing diffuse positivity in (almost all) the lymphoid cells.

Hematopoietic Neoplasms of Prostate

Small Lymphocytic Lymphoma Involving Prostate

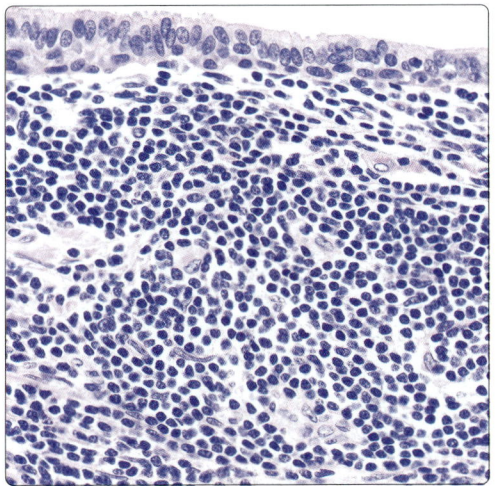

Mantle Cell Lymphoma Involving Prostate

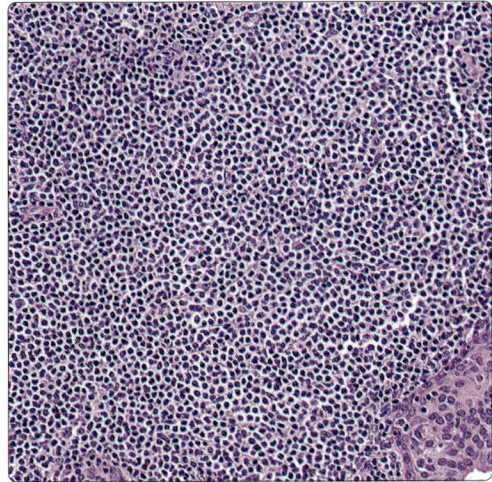

(Left) B-cell small lymphocytic lymphoma is characterized by small lymphoid cells with round nuclei and clumped chromatin. This lymphoma is the most common low-grade lymphoma in prostate. *(Right)* Mantle cell lymphoma consists of small monomorphous lymphoid cells with nuclei slightly more irregular than in small lymphocytic lymphoma. Both lymphoma types coexpress CD20 and CD5. Mantle cell lymphoma is usually negative for CD23 and expresses cyclin D1, in contrast to small lymphocytic lymphoma.

Small Lymphocytic Lymphoma in Pelvic Lymph Node

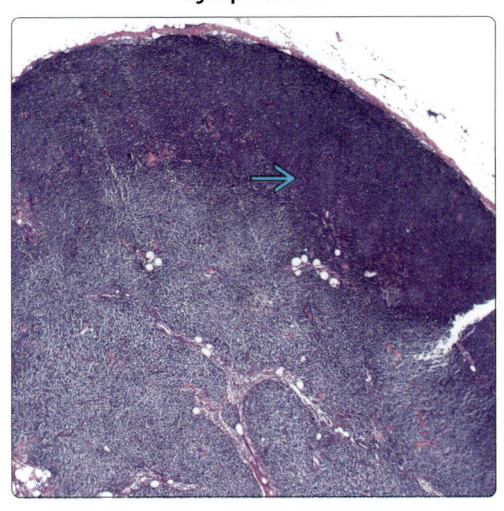

Benign Lymphoid Aggregate

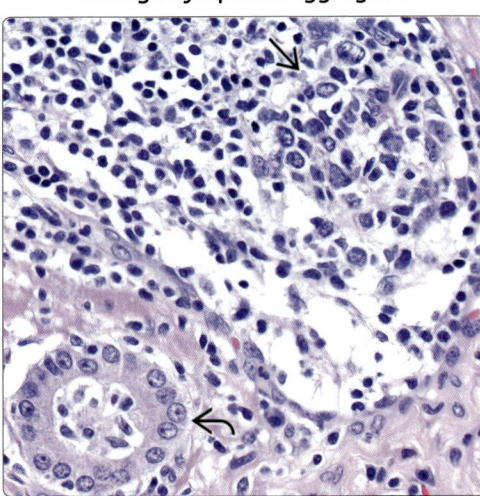

(Left) Diagnosis of low-grade lymphomas in radical prostatectomies are more often apparent in concomitant pelvic lymph nodes. In this case, the lymph node architecture is effaced ➡ by infiltrates forming distinctive proliferative centers, a feature of B-cell small lymphocytic lymphoma. *(Right)* This benign lymphoid aggregate consists of polymorphous cells, including plasma cells and mature lymphocytes and with a germinal center ➡. Note the adjacent carcinoma gland with nucleomegaly and prominent nucleoli ➡.

Nonspecific Granulomatous Prostatitis

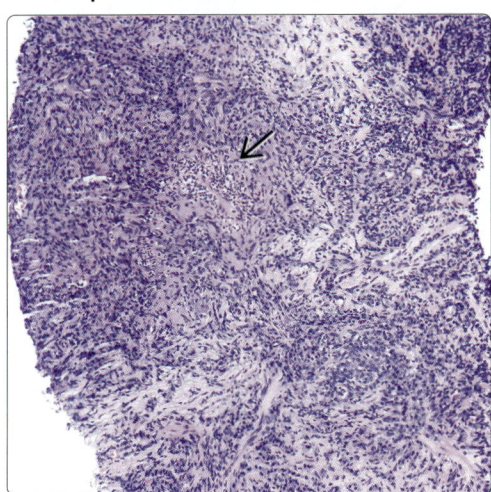

Poorly Differentiated Prostate Carcinoma

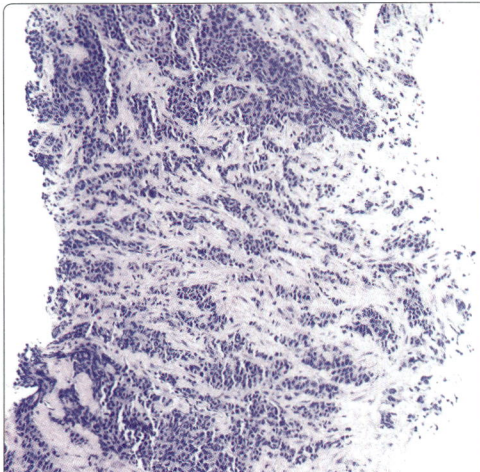

(Left) This prostate biopsy shows dense hematopoietic cell infiltrates. Unlike lymphoma, the cells are polymorphous consisting of lymphocytes, plasma cells, histiocytes, and with few clusters of acute inflammatory cells ➡. *(Right)* This biopsy from a patient with markedly elevated PSA shows Gleason grade 5 prostate carcinoma consisting of poorly differentiated cells in small sheet-like growth and cords. This pattern may resemble lymphoma and can be distinguished by its positivity to epithelial markers.

Secondary Tumors of Prostate

KEY FACTS

TERMINOLOGY
- Neoplasms involving prostate through direct spread from adjacent organs or metastasis from distant sites

CLINICAL ISSUES
- Seen in 5.6% of male autopsies with malignancies and 0.2% of prostate resections and biopsies
- Mostly encountered as incidental autopsy findings
- Involvement of prostate by metastasis indicates late or widely disseminated stage of disease
- Rarely, gastrointestinal stromal tumors (GIST) may invade into prostate and present as intraprostatic mass

IMAGING
- Radiologic work-up helpful in investigating unknown primary origin

MICROSCOPIC
- Distant solid metastasis mostly originates from lungs (49%), skin (24%), and pancreaticobiliary (9%)
- Direct tumor spread predominantly from urinary bladder (85%) and rectum (15%)
- Differential diagnosis of poorly differentiated prostate vs. bladder urothelial and rectal cancers may be very difficult in limited sample (i.e., biopsy)
- Distinction important due to differing therapies (i.e., hormonal for prostate cancer, chemotherapy for bladder cancer, and radiotherapy for rectal cancer)

ANCILLARY TESTS
- Use of immunohistochemistry can be crucial in differential diagnosis of primary vs. secondary tumors of prostate
  - Poorly differentiated prostate carcinoma: PSA(+/-) and PAP(+/-) and (-) for p63, HMCK, CDX-2, and β-catenin
  - Poorly differentiated urothelial carcinoma: p63, GATA3 and HMCK(34βE12) (+)
  - Poorly differentiated rectal adenocarcinoma: CDX-2 and β-catenin nuclear (+)
  - GIST: (+) for CD117 (diffuse), DOG1, and CD34

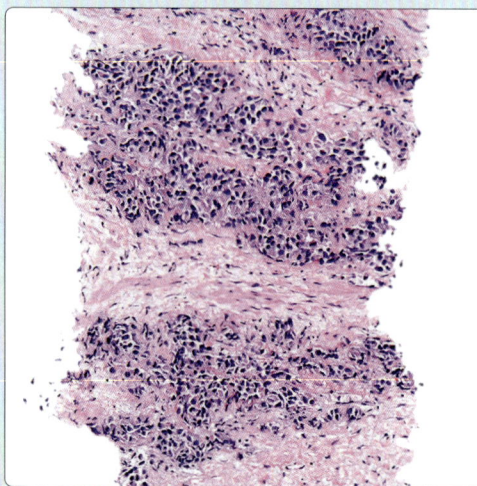

Bladder Urothelial Carcinoma Invading Prostate

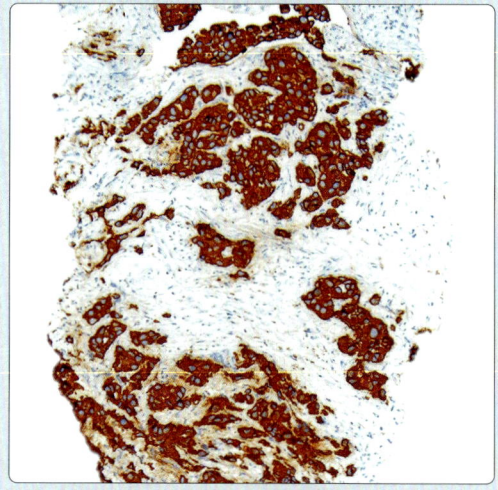

CK7 in Bladder Urothelial Carcinoma Invading Prostate

(Left) Needle biopsy shows high-grade urothelial carcinoma from the urinary bladder invading the prostate. Bladder carcinoma is the most common malignancy to invade the prostate via direct extension. (Right) Bladder urothelial carcinoma involving the prostate in a needle biopsy shows diffuse positivity to CK7. Urothelial carcinomas are typically CK7(+) and CK20(+/-); however, these stains alone are not confirmatory in distinguishing from prostate carcinoma. GATA3 or p63 (+) supports urothelial carcinoma.

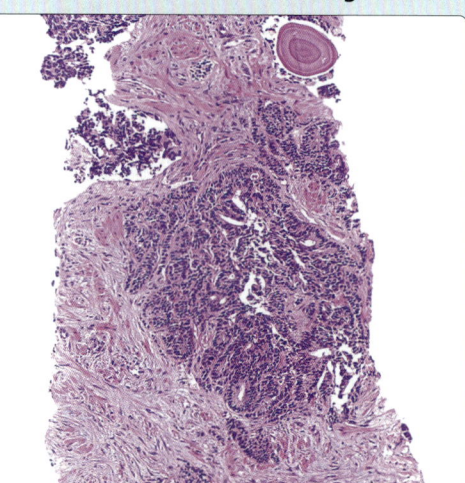

Rectal Adenocarcinoma Invading Prostate

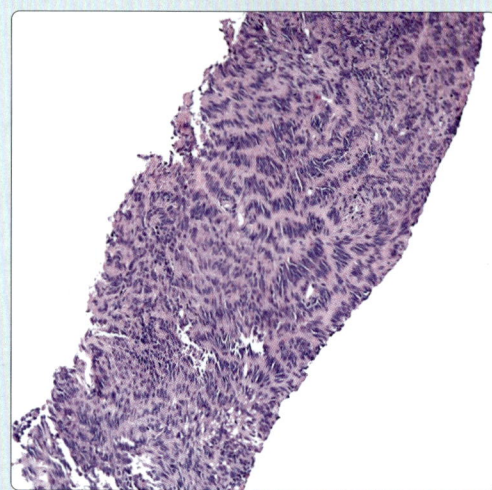

GIST Involving Prostate

(Left) Prostate needle biopsy shows infiltrating moderately differentiated adenocarcinoma of colorectal primary invading the prostate. Prostate involvement by rectal adenocarcinoma denotes high-stage rectal cancer (pT4). (Right) Needle biopsy shows GIST with spindled cell morphology. Most GIST in prostate are extension of tumor arising from rectal area, although very rare instances of prostatic GIST with no rectal or perirectal involvement are reported, and considered by some as primary prostatic GIST.

Secondary Tumors of Prostate

TERMINOLOGY

Definitions
- Neoplasms involving prostate through direct spread from adjacent organs or metastasis from distant sites
  - Hematopoietic neoplasms not included in this chapter

ETIOLOGY/PATHOGENESIS

Pattern of Spread
- Most distant metastases reach prostate through arterial (rather than venous) dissemination
- Direct prostate invasion of cancers arising from urinary bladder or colorectal region

Origin
- Most common origin of distant solid tumor metastasis
  - Lungs (49%), laryngotracheal (2%)
  - Skin, including melanoma (24%)
  - Pancreaticobiliary (9%), gastrointestinal tract (7%)
  - Isolated cases from kidney, penis, thyroid, breast, and eye
- Direct tumor spread
  - Urinary bladder (85%)
  - Rectum (15%)
    - Rectal carcinoma
    - Rarely, gastrointestinal stromal tumors (GIST) may invade into prostate and present as intraprostatic mass (although rare primary prostatic cases do occur)

CLINICAL ISSUES

Epidemiology
- Incidence
  - Very rare, encountered in only 0.2% of male autopsies
  - Seen in 5.6% of male autopsies with malignancies
    - 44% via direct spread and 56% via distant metastasis
  - Seen in 0.2% of prostate resections and biopsies
    - 93% via direct spread and 7% via distant metastasis
- Age
  - Median: 66 years; range: 39-83 years

Presentation
- Distant metastases to prostate are mostly incidental autopsy findings of disseminated tumors
- Clinical presentation of distant metastasis to prostate prompting urologic work-up is very rare
  - Few reported examples presented with obstructive uropathy and inflammatory symptoms
- Metastasis to prostate as initial histologic diagnosis of malignancy seen in only 2% of cases
- In surgical pathology specimens, direct spread is more frequently encountered than distant metastasis
- Bladder and rectal tumors also present with urinary and lower GI tract symptoms, respectively

Treatment
- Systemic therapy or supportive care; may require surgical management as palliation for obstructive symptoms
- GIST may have good response to resection and imatib mesylate

Prognosis
- Generally poor; involvement of prostate by metastasis indicates late or widely disseminated stage of tumor
- Distant metastasis to prostate is almost invariably associated with carcinomatosis to other organs
  - Mainly involves liver (90%), lungs (79%), kidneys (77%), adrenal glands (61%)

IMAGING

General Features
- Radiologic work-up helpful in investigating unknown primary origin

MICROSCOPIC

Histologic Features
- Similar to primary tumors from organ of origin

ANCILLARY TESTS

Immunohistochemistry
- May be crucial in differential diagnosis of primary vs. secondary tumors of prostate
- Poorly differentiated carcinomas
  - Poorly differentiated prostate carcinoma
    - PSA(+/-) and PAP(+/-)
    - Negative for p63, HMCK, CDX-2, and β-catenin
    - CK7(+/-) and CK20(+/-)
    - Other (+) markers: P501S, PSMA, NKX3.1, pPSMA
  - Poorly differentiated urothelial carcinoma
    - Positive for p63 and HMCK(34βE12)
    - Negative for PSA or PAP, CDX-2, and β-catenin
    - CK7(+/-) and CK20(+/-)
    - Other (+) markers: GATA3, thrombomodulin, CK5/6, uroplakin-2
    - AMACR also positive and is not helpful
  - Poorly differentiated rectal adenocarcinoma
    - Positive for CDX-2 and β-catenin (nuclear)
    - CK7(-) and CK20(+)
    - Negative for PSA or PAP, p63, and HMCK
- Spindle cell tumors involving prostate
  - GIST
    - Positive for CD117 (diffuse), DOG1, and CD34
    - S100 negative; often negative for actin-sm and desmin
  - Primary prostatic mesenchymal tumors
    - Prostatic stromal tumors are CD34 and PR (+)
    - Smooth muscle tumors are actin-sm and desmin (+)
    - SFT positive for CD34

SELECTED REFERENCES

1. Huh JS et al: Diagnosis of a gastrointestinal stromal tumor presenting as a prostatic mass: a case report. World J Mens Health. 32(3):184-8, 2014
2. Morichetti D et al: Secondary neoplasms of the urinary system and male genital organs. BJU Int. 104(6):770-6, 2009
3. Herawi M et al: Gastrointestinal stromal tumors (GISTs) on prostate needle biopsy: A clinicopathologic study of 8 cases. Am J Surg Pathol. 30(11):1389-95, 2006
4. Bates AW et al: Secondary solid neoplasms of the prostate: a clinico-pathological series of 51 cases. Virchows Arch. 440(4):392-6, 2002
5. Zein TA et al: Secondary tumors of the prostate. J Urol. 133(4):615-6, 1985

Secondary Tumors of Prostate

Bladder Poorly Differentiated Urothelial Carcinoma Invading Prostate

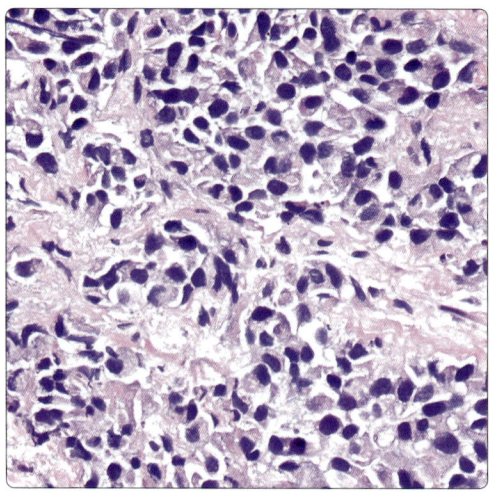

Bladder Urothelial Carcinoma Invading Prostate Stroma

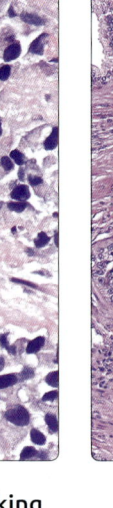

(Left) Needle biopsy of prostate with bladder urothelial carcinoma shows infiltrating poorly differentiated carcinoma cells. Differentiation between bladder urothelial carcinoma and high-grade prostate carcinoma can be very difficult. Distinction is important due to different treatment modalities, particularly in tumors with high stage. (Right) Prostate resection with infiltrating urothelial carcinoma from the bladder is shown. Urothelial carcinoma may also arise from prostatic urethra and ducts.

Bladder Urothelial Carcinoma Mimicking Prostate Carcinoma

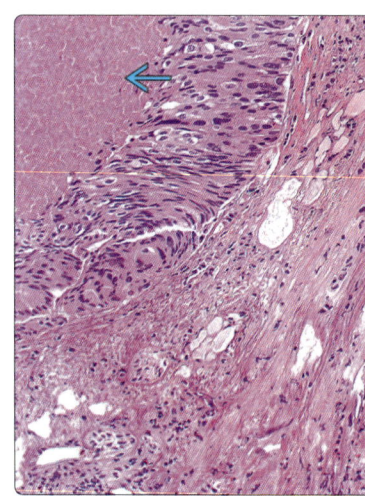

p63 in Bladder Urothelial Carcinoma Invading Prostate

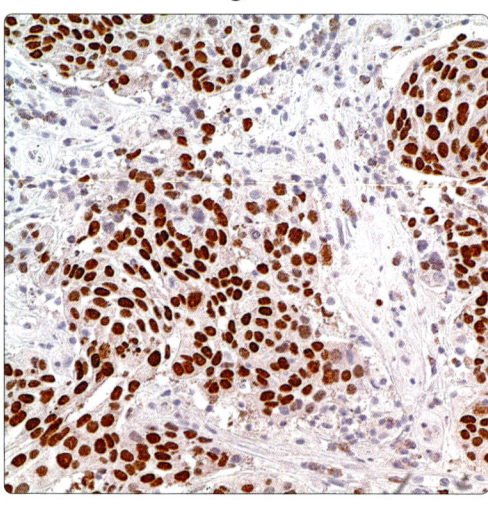

(Left) Invasive urothelial carcinoma is seen in a TURP specimen. The tumor is high grade with tumor cell necrosis ➔ simulating a comedo-type prostate carcinoma. Direct extension of the prostatic stroma by bladder cancer denotes high-stage cancer (pT4). (Right) p63 immunohistochemical stain shows diffuse nuclear positivity in urothelial carcinoma. p63 and GATA3 are useful in distinguishing urothelial carcinoma vs. prostate carcinoma, which is typically negative.

Bladder Urothelial Carcinoma and Prostate Carcinoma

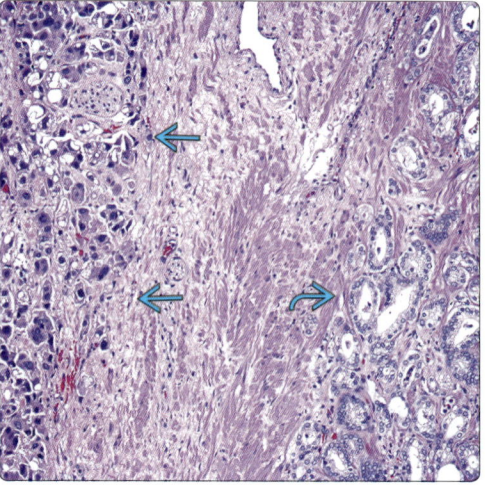

PIN4 in Bladder Urothelial Carcinoma Invading Prostate

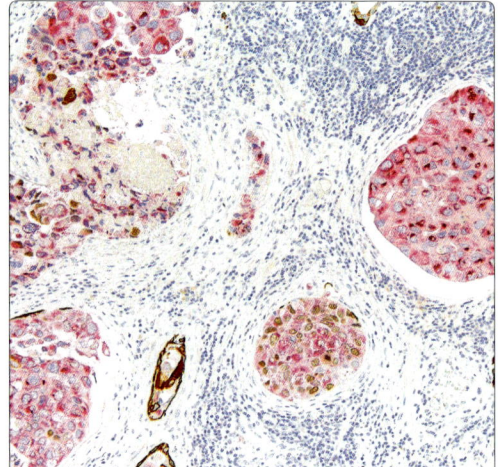

(Left) Poorly differentiated urothelial carcinoma ➔ from bladder invades into prostate. There is concomitant prostatic adenocarcinoma adjacent to urothelial carcinoma ➔. In this case of 2 tumors, immunohistochemistry is important to confirm the urothelial lineage of the poorly differentiated tumor. (Right) PIN4 immunostain shows AMACR (red) expression in urothelial carcinoma similar to prostatic adenocarcinoma. However, nuclear reactivity to p63 (brown) is evident, supporting urothelial carcinoma.

Secondary Tumors of Prostate

Bladder Adenocarcinoma Invading Prostate

Rectal Adenocarcinoma Invading Prostate

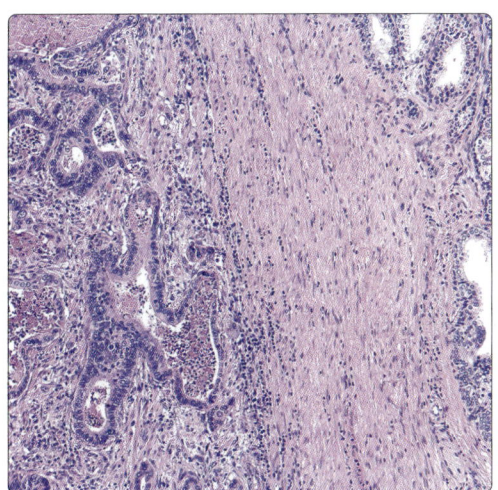
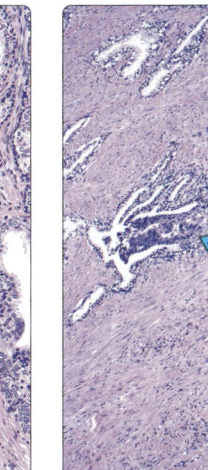

(Left) This bladder adenocarcinoma exhibits intestinal morphology, indistinguishable from colorectal adenocarcinoma. Immunohistochemistry is not always helpful and clinical correlation (e.g., rectosigmoidoscopy, cystoscopy) is imperative in this situation. (Right) This adenocarcinoma from the rectum shows glands with tall columnar cells, pallisading nuclei and "dirty" necrosis ⇨, characteristic of intestinal type adenocarcinoma. Note the tumor extension into prostatic gland ⇨.

CDX-2 in Rectal Adenocarcinoma Invading Prostate

β-catenin in Rectal Adenocarcinoma Invading Prostate

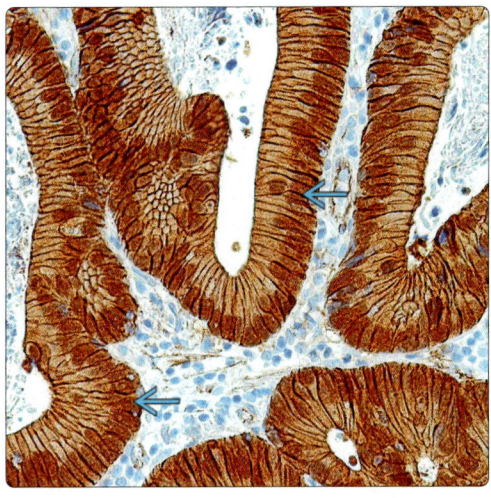

(Left) CDX-2 ⇨ immunohistochemical stain shows strong nuclear immunoreactivity in colonic adenocarcinoma. CDX-2 is helpful in distinguishing colonic carcinoma from prostate carcinoma, which is typically negative. PSA, PAP, and PSMA are also useful. (Right) β-catenin stain shows nuclear positivity ⇨ in colonic adenocarcinoma. In contrast to prostate carcinoma and primary bladder adenocarcinoma that may invade the prostate, colonic adenocarcinoma is commonly nuclear positive.

GIST Involving Prostate

CD117 in GIST Involving Prostate

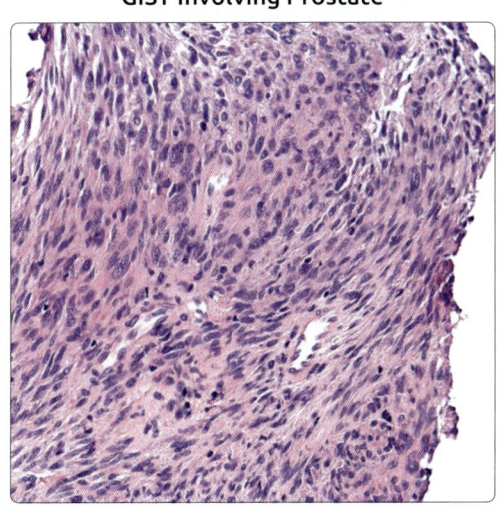
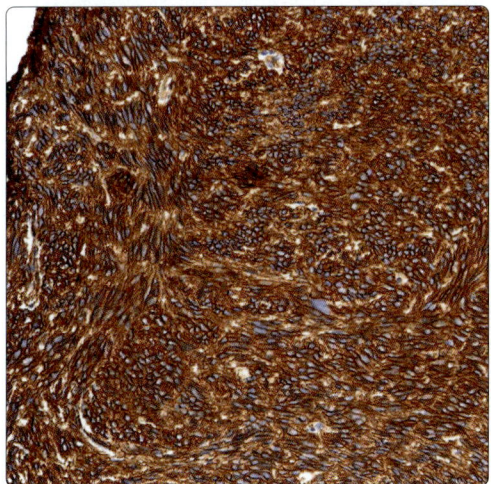

(Left) GIST secondarily involving the prostate shows spindle cells mimicking primary prostatic sarcomas. GIST is strongly positive for CD117, in contrast to the common primary mesenchymal tumors of the prostate that are negative. (Right) The majority of GIST will show strong and diffuse reactivity to CD117. This immunostain is negative in stromal tumors, smooth muscle tumors, solitary fibrous tumors, and other rare mesenchymal tumors that may arise from the prostate.

Cystadenoma and Epithelial Stromal Tumor

KEY FACTS

TERMINOLOGY
- Synonyms
  - Cystadenoma: Multilocular cyst
  - Epithelial stromal tumors: Mesonephric hamartoma, fibroepithelial tumor, cystomyoma, mesenchymoma

CLINICAL ISSUES
- Rare; < 30 reported cases within this spectrum
- Obstructive symptoms most common presentation, solid and cystic pelvic mass on imaging
- Cystadenoma and low-grade epithelial stromal tumors have benign course but may recur
- 2 reports of high-grade epithelial stromal tumors with mets

MICROSCOPIC
- Cystadenoma pattern
  - Consists of multiple variably sized cystic and glandular formations lined by single to few layers of bland cuboidal to low columnar epithelial cells
  - Variable amount of stroma that resembles usual seminal vesicle fibromuscular stroma
- Epithelial stromal tumor pattern
  - Consist of neoplastic proliferation of both glandular and stromal elements
  - May have broad, leaf-like growth consisting of epithelium with investing spindle cell stroma (phyllodes-like growth)
  - Histologic spectrum of benign to malignant tumors defined by degree of atypicality of stromal component
  - Includes low-grade fibroadenoma/adenomyoma and high-grade epithelial stromal tumors
  - High-grade tumors contain frank sarcomatous areas, including marked stromal overgrowth, pleomorphism, frequent mitosis, and necrosis

ANCILLARY TESTS
- Epithelial component PSA/PAP(-), consistent with seminal vesicle origin

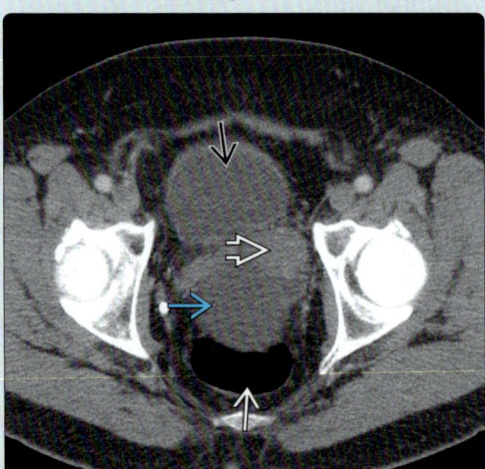

CT Scan: Cystadenoma

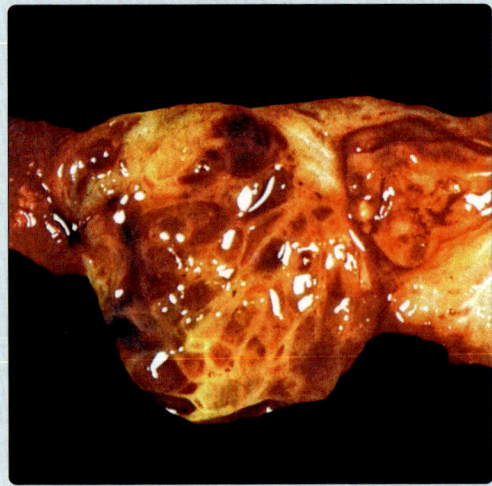

Gross: Mixed Epithelial-Stromal Tumor

(Left) CT shows a cystadenoma [low-grade mixed epithelial-stromal tumor (MEST)] of the seminal vesicle (SV), presenting as a pelvic mass with solid ➡ and cystic ➡ components seen between the bladder ➡ and rectum ➡. This large example arose from the left SV and recurred post vesiculectomy. (Courtesy A.S. McDaniel, MD, PhD.) (Right) Gross photograph of SV epithelial stromal tumor shows multicystic cut surface. (Courtesy E.C. Jones, MD.)

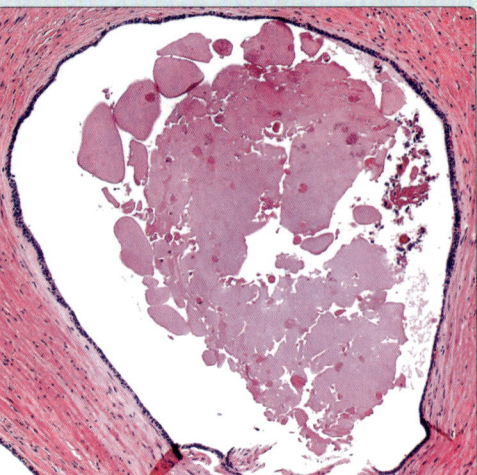

Cystadenoma: Cystic Mixed Epithelial-Stromal Tumor

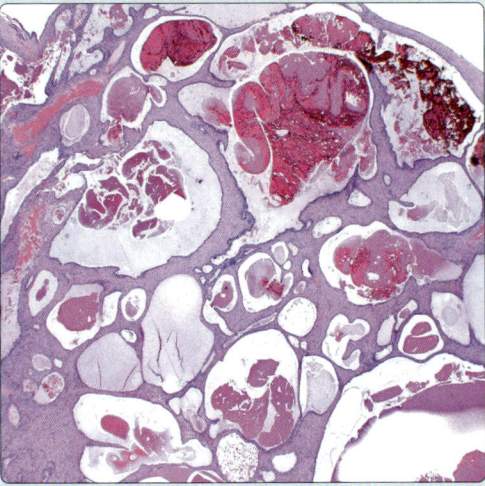

Mixed Epithelial-Stromal Tumor

(Left) Seminal vesicle cystadenoma (cystic MEST) consists of cysts lined by single to few layers of epithelial cells and underlying fibromuscular stroma. The cyst lumen contains amorphous eosinophilic material. (Right) In low-grade MEST, a biphasic neoplasm of both glands and stroma is appreciated, though many cases show a spectrum of solid and cystic components. Mixed mucinous and eosinophilic amorphous cystic material is prominent.

Cystadenoma and Epithelial Stromal Tumor

TERMINOLOGY

Synonyms
- Cystadenoma: Multilocular cyst
- Epithelial stromal tumors
  - Mesonephric hamartoma, fibroepithelial tumor, cystomyoma, mesenchymoma, phyllodes tumor, cystosarcoma phyllodes, müllerian adenosarcoma-like tumor

Definitions
- **Cystadenoma**
  - Benign cystic epithelial neoplasm of seminal vesicle
  - Tumor lacking significant stromal proliferation or containing only usual seminal vesicle-type stroma
- **Epithelial stromal tumor**
  - Seminal vesicle neoplasm with proliferation of both glandular and stromal elements
  - Considerable overlap in literature with use of terminology regarding cystadenoma and low-grade epithelial stromal tumor
- **Mixed epithelial-stromal tumor (MEST) of seminal vesicle: Proposed unifying terminology**
  - Encompass both "cystadenoma," "epithelial stromal tumor," and prior reported variants
  - Low-grade, intermediate-grade, and high-grade designations based on
    - Presence or absence of stromal atypia
    - Presence or absence of mitoses
    - Nuclear atypia and pleomorphism
    - Necrosis

ETIOLOGY/PATHOGENESIS

Developmental Anomaly
- No association with ureter or renal developmental anomalies, in contrast to that noted in nonneoplastic congenital seminal vesicle cysts

CLINICAL ISSUES

Epidemiology
- Incidence
  - Very rare; < 30 reported seminal vesicle cystadenoma and epithelial stromal tumors
- Age
  - Mean: 51 years; range: 33-70 years

Presentation
- Obstructive symptoms most common: Retention, decreased stream, hesitancy, frequency, dysuria
- Other symptoms include lower abdominal pain, painful ejaculation, constipation, fever
- Few cases are asymptomatic &/or detected as pelvic or rectal mass on physical examination

Laboratory Tests
- Normal serum PSA level
- Normal serum CA125 level (in contrast to seminal vesicle adenocarcinoma, which may have elevated level)

Treatment
- Tumor resection with vesiculectomy, prostatectomy, or cystoprostatectomy
- Systemic chemotherapy for malignant epithelial and stromal tumor, particularly if metastatic

Prognosis
- Cystadenoma has benign course but may recur
- No metastasis reported in epithelial stromal tumors lacking high-grade features but may recur
- Rare reports of high-grade epithelial stromal tumors with metastasis to lung and even death

IMAGING

General Features
- CT and MR show multilocular cystic or solid-cystic pelvic mass centered in region of seminal vesicle between rectum and urinary bladder or prostate
- Large mass often compresses or displaces urinary bladder and prostate
- Imaging may be key to determine origin (seminal vesicle vs. prostate), particularly in biopsy specimens

MACROSCOPIC

General Features
- Lobulated mass with glistening, smooth, tan surface and multilocular or solid-cystic cut surface
  - Cysts may contain gelatinous to serous fluid
  - Malignant tumors are relatively more solid, reflecting marked sarcomatous overgrowth
- Mass located at seminal vesicle bed; may be seen contiguous with identifiable seminal vesicle remnants
- May be completely separable from prostate or bladder in radical excision specimens
- Most gross reports document unilateral mass

Size
- Range: 3-16 cm in largest dimension; mean: 8.9 cm

MICROSCOPIC

Histologic Features
- **Cystadenoma: Cystic neoplasm of glandular elements**
  - Multiple variably sized cystic and glandular formations
  - Lined by single to few layers of bland cuboidal to low columnar epithelial cells
  - Nuclei are round, regular, with inconspicuous nucleoli
  - Cysts and glands may contain homogeneous or amorphous eosinophilic material
  - Variable amount of stroma that resembles usual seminal vesicle fibromuscular stroma
- **Epithelial stromal tumors: Neoplasm of both glandular and stromal elements**
  - May have broad, leaf-like growth consisting of epithelium with investing spindle cell stroma (phyllodes-like growth)
    - This architectural pattern may not be seen in all cases; therefore, term epithelial stromal tumor is preferred over phyllodes tumor
  - Epithelial component

Cystadenoma and Epithelial Stromal Tumor

- Cysts and glands vary in size and shape, sometimes branching, distorted, or slit-like
- Lining epithelium consists of single to few layers of cuboidal or low columnar cells, generally lacking marked atypia
- Occasionally, 2 cell layers may be seen, consisting of inner layer of cuboidal or low columnar cells and basal layer of cuboidal or flattened cells
- Focal cellular stratification may be present
- Lipofuscin pigment may rarely be appreciated
o **Stromal component**
- Stroma composed of spindled cells with varying degree of cellularity
- Tendency of spindle cells to be more cellular or condensed around cysts and glandular formations
- Rare case with myomatous (adenomyoma) or myxomatous stroma with spindle cells
- Less cellular areas may show pale basophilic stroma
o Cysts and glands may contain homogeneous or amorphous eosinophilic materials, mucinous material, or, rarely, eosinophilic crystalline debris
o Blending of cystic tumor with seminal vesicle fibromuscular wall and lining epithelium, which contains lipofuscin pigment, may be present
o Degree of atypia of stromal component is key distinction between benign and malignant examples
o Biphasic tumor containing benign myomatous stroma (adenomyoma) has been reported
- **MEST: Proposed classification and criteria**
o Includes both lesions previously designated "cystadenoma" and "epithelial stromal tumor" as above
o **Low-grade MEST**
- Epithelial and stromal proliferation without stromal atypia or mitotic activity
- No more than mild nuclear pleomorphism; no necrosis
o **Intermediate-grade MEST**
- Epithelial and stromal proliferation with increased stromal cellularity and low mitotic activity
- Nuclear atypia and pleomorphism are present; no necrosis
o **High-grade MEST**
- Increased stromal cellularity and significant mitotic activity
- Marked nuclear atypia and pleomorphism
o Of cases reported to date, ~ 80% are of low-grade category

ANCILLARY TESTS

Immunohistochemistry
- Epithelial component
  o Pancytokeratin (AE1/AE3) (+), CK7 often (+)
  o High molecular weight cytokeratin (34βE12) may show patchy basal cells (+)
  o PSA/PSAP(-), CA125(-)
- Stromal component
  o Vimentin (+)
  o CD34(+)

DIFFERENTIAL DIAGNOSIS

Congenital or Developmental Seminal Vesicle Cysts
- Most are congenital and associated with ipsilateral ectopic ureter and renal dysplasia or agenesis
- Acquired cysts may be due to genitourinary infection, prostate surgery, or ejaculatory duct lithiasis
- Cyst is usually unilocular but may be multilocular
- Easily evacuated by needle puncture
- Histologically resembles dilated seminal vesicle with attenuated epithelial lining
- Cyst contents may include spermatozoa debris, blood, or inflammatory cells

Phyllodes Tumor of Prostate
- Histologically similar to phyllodes-type epithelial stromal tumor of seminal vesicle
- Tumor is grossly and histologically intimately associated with prostatic parenchyma
- Glandular epithelial component PSA/PAP(+)

Prostatic Stromal Tumor of Uncertain Malignant Potential and Prostatic Stromal Sarcoma
- Tumor centered in prostate
- Lacking neoplastic epithelial component

DIAGNOSTIC CHECKLIST

Pathologic Interpretation Pearls
- Imaging, intraoperative, gross findings, and microscopy (including absent PSA staining) key to distinguish seminal vesicle from prostatic lesions of similar histology
- Seminal vesicle cystadenoma
  o Benign multilocular cyst lined by single to few layers of bland, cuboidal, or columnar cells lacking significant stromal proliferation
- Seminal vesicle epithelial and stromal tumor
  o Neoplasm consisting of mixed epithelial and stromal proliferation, sometimes exhibiting phyllodes-like growth, with varying stromal atypia ranging from benign to frank sarcomatous features

SELECTED REFERENCES

1. Reikie BA et al: Mixed epithelial-stromal tumor (MEST) of seminal vesicle: a proposal for unified nomenclature. Adv Anat Pathol. 22(2):113-20, 2015
2. Monica B et al: Low grade epithelial stromal tumour of the seminal vesicle. World J Surg Oncol. 6:101, 2008
3. Son HJ et al: Phyllodes tumor of the seminal vesicle: case report and literature review. Pathol Int. 54(12):924-9, 2004
4. Abe H et al: Cystosarcoma phyllodes of the seminal vesicle. Int J Urol. 9(10):599-601, 2002
5. Laurila P et al: Mullerian adenosarcomalike tumor of the seminal vesicle. A case report with immunohistochemical and ultrastructural observations. Arch Pathol Lab Med. 116(10):1072-6, 1992
6. Mazur MT et al: Cystic epithelial-stromal tumor of the seminal vesicle. Am J Surg Pathol. 11(3):210-7, 1987
7. Damjanov I et al: Cystadenoma of seminal vesicles. J Urol. 111(6):808-9, 1974

Cystadenoma and Epithelial Stromal Tumor

Cystadenoma: Epithelium

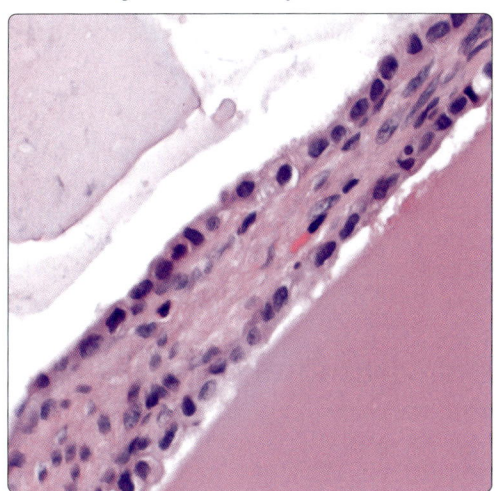

Low-Grade MEST: Stroma

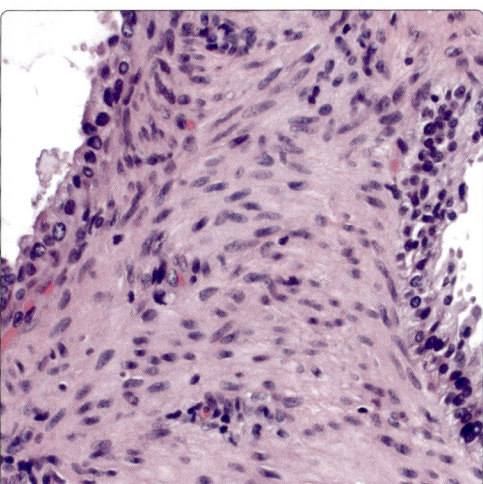

(Left) The epithelium is characteristically bland and single layered, with cuboidal to columnar cytomorphology. HMWCK(+) basal cells may be apparent by immunostain. (Right) The stromal features are key to grading these tumors. This low-grade MEST shows proliferation of a moderately cellular myoid stroma analogous to the normal stroma of the seminal vesicle. Atypia, mitoses, and pleomorphism are absent.

MEST: Adjacent to Seminal Vesicle

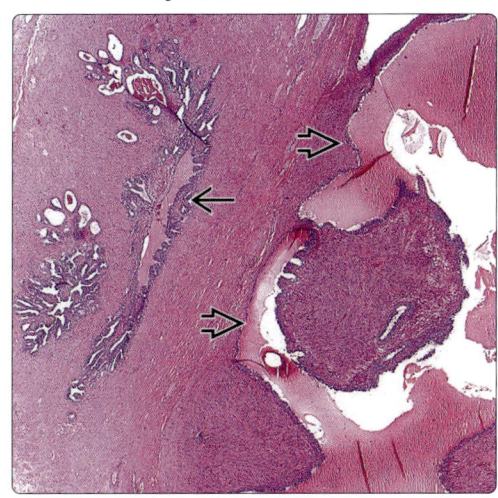

Phyllodes-Like Growth Pattern

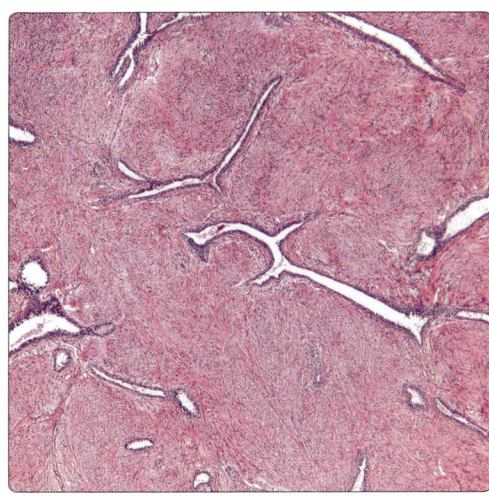

(Left) MEST ⇒ contiguous with the seminal vesicle fibromuscular wall is shown. Normal seminal vesicle glandular epithelium is present ⇒ adjacent to a dilated neoplastic cyst with polypoid growth and stromal cellularity. (Right) Some epithelial, stromal tumors show branching, slit-like glands surrounded by a spindle cell stromal proliferation, or phyllodes-like growth. The spindle cell stroma may vary in cellularity. The degree of stromal atypia defines the histologic (and biologic) spectrum of this tumor.

Cellular Stroma: MEST

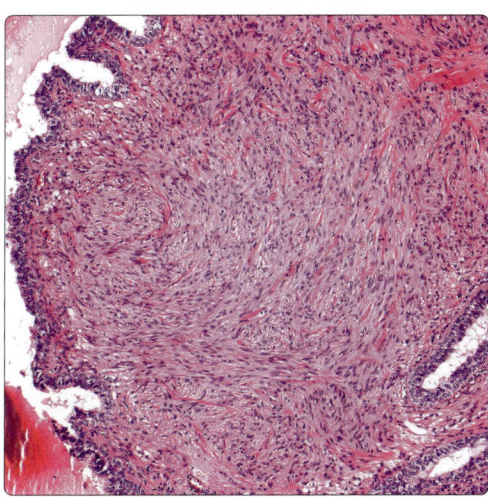

Low-Grade MEST

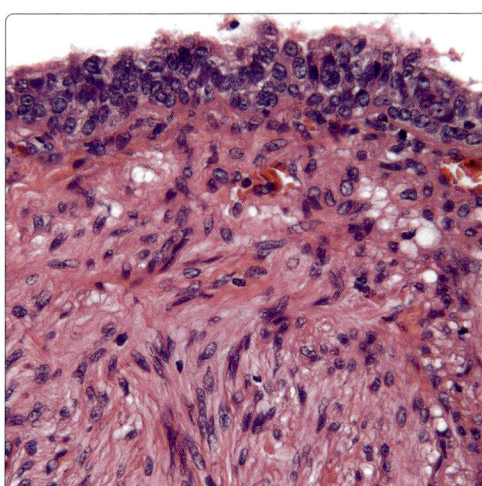

(Left) SV MEST shows phyllodes-like growth pattern consisting of epithelium with investing cellular spindle cell stroma. (Right) Low-grade MEST shows a few layers of bland polygonal cell epithelial lining and subjacent spindle cell stroma, lacking both cellular atypia and mitoses. Lipofuscin pigment and atypia innately seen in SV epithelium may be seen.

Seminal Vesicle Adenocarcinoma

KEY FACTS

TERMINOLOGY
- Malignant neoplasm of seminal vesicle glandular epithelial cell origin

CLINICAL ISSUES
- Rare; ~ 60 acceptable published cases
- Mean age: 63 years; range: 19-90 years
- Nonspecific symptoms at advanced stage, such as bladder outlet obstruction, hematuria, hematospermia, and pelvic or perineal pain
- Serum CA125 elevated; PSA and PAP normal
- Extremely poor; ~ 95% of patients die in < 3 years
- Majority of patients with metastasis at time of diagnosis

MACROSCOPIC
- Usually large and invades adjacent bladder or rectum
- Solid or cystic mass
- Bilateral involvement in 8% of cases

MICROSCOPIC
- Papillary pattern lined by columnar cells most recognized feature
- May be glandular or poorly differentiated tumor with solid, nested, or cord-like growths
- May have clear cells or hobnail morphology similar to clear cell adenocarcinoma in female genital tract
- Mucin production present, sometimes copious
- Carcinoma in situ may be seen, which is helpful in poorly differentiated cases
- Typically pax-2(+), CA125(+), PSA/PAP(-), CK7(+)/CK20(-), CDX2(-)

TOP DIFFERENTIAL DIAGNOSES
- Seminal vesicle cystadenoma
- Prostate adenocarcinoma
- Urinary bladder adenocarcinoma
- Colorectal adenocarcinoma

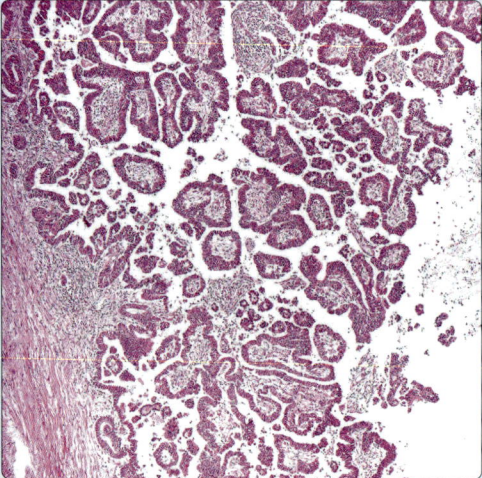

Seminal Vesicle Adenocarcinoma: Papillary Growth

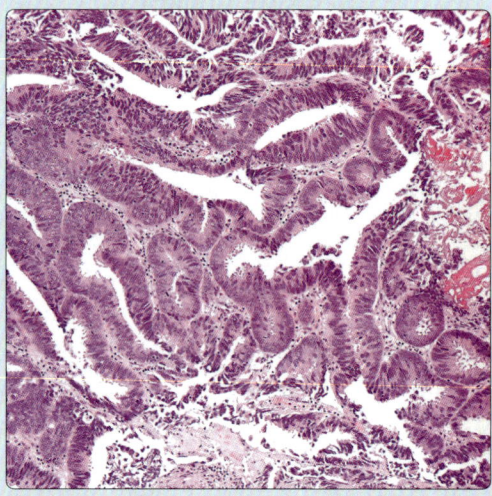

Seminal Vesicle Adenocarcinoma: Glandular Growth

(Left) Seminal vesicle adenocarcinoma is shown with papillary architecture, which is the most recognized feature of this tumor. The papillae contains fibrovascular stalk lined by high-grade, tall columnar cells. (Courtesy L. Egevad, MD, PhD.) (Right) This seminal vesicle adenocarcinoma exhibits glandular growth composed of high-grade columnar cells with nuclear palisading and may resemble prostatic ductal adenocarcinoma and bladder or colonic adenocarcinomas. (Courtesy L. Egevad, MD, PhD.)

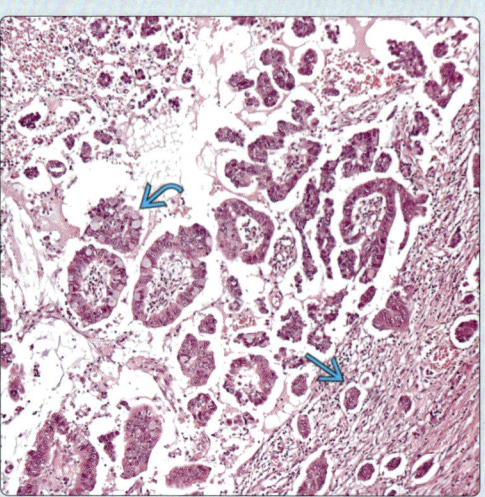

Invasive Seminal Vesicle Adenocarcinoma

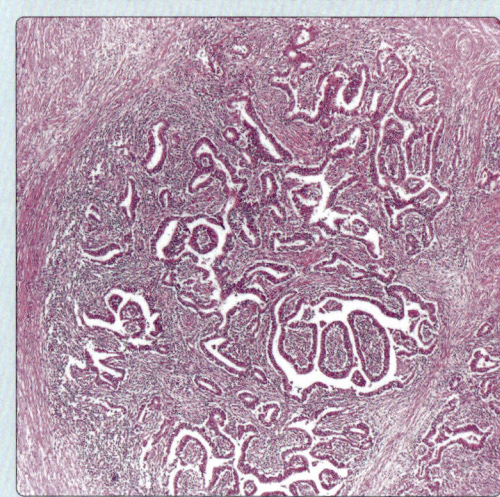

Invasive Seminal Vesicle Adenocarcinoma

(Left) This seminal vesicle adenocarcinoma shows variably sized papillae lined by high-grade columnar cells associated with infiltrative nests in the stroma ➡. Note the presence of occasional goblet cells in the papillae ➡. (Courtesy L. Egevad, MD, PhD.) (Right) Seminal vesicle adenocarcinoma shows tubulopapillary formations with associated stromal fibrosis. This pattern may resemble prostatic ductal adenocarcinoma, which can be distinguished by PSA(+) and PAP(+) and CA125(-). (Courtesy L. Egevad, MD, PhD.)

Seminal Vesicle Adenocarcinoma

TERMINOLOGY

Synonyms
- Papillary adenocarcinoma of seminal vesicle

Definitions
- Malignant neoplasm of seminal vesicle glandular epithelial cell origin

CLINICAL ISSUES

Epidemiology
- Incidence
  - Rare; ~ 60 acceptable published cases
- Age
  - Mean: 63 years; range: 19-90 years
  - 1/5 of patients younger than 40 years

Presentation
- May be asymptomatic at early stage
- Nonspecific symptoms at advanced stage, such as bladder outlet obstruction, hematuria, hematospermia, and pelvic or perineal pain
- Mostly palpable as nontender mass above or contiguous with prostate on digital rectal examination

Laboratory Tests
- Serum CA125 elevated
  - Can be useful in monitoring disease
- Serum PSA and PAP levels normal
- Serum CEA can be elevated

Natural History
- Manifests with advanced symptomatic disease

Treatment
- Mainstay is surgical resection with negative margin; offers best survival
- Adjuvant radiotherapy or androgen deprivation able to prolong survival in some patients

Prognosis
- Extremely poor; ~ 95% of patients die in < 3 years
- Although ~ 1/2 of cases in recent reports are free of recurrence after 1-4 years
- Majority of patients with metastasis at time of diagnosis

IMAGING

General Features
- Computed tomography scan and transrectal ultrasound helpful in diagnosis
- Solid or partly cystic mass centered at seminal vesicle area between rectum and bladder or prostate

MACROSCOPIC

General Features
- Usually large and invades adjacent bladder or rectum
- Irregular, firm, gray-white to brown tumor nodules
- May be partly cystic
- Bilateral involvement in 8% of cases

MICROSCOPIC

Histologic Features
- Variable histologic pattern
- Papillary architecture lined by columnar cells is most recognized feature
- May be glandular or poorly differentiated tumor with solid, nested, or cord-like growth
- May have clear cells or hobnail morphology
  - Similar to clear cell adenocarcinoma of female genital tract
- Mucin production present, sometimes may be copious
- Desmoplasia seen around infiltrating glands
- Carcinoma in situ may be seen
  - Helpful in poorly differentiated cases

ANCILLARY TESTS

Immunohistochemistry
- pax-2(+), CA125(+)
- PSA(-) and PAP(-); CDX2(-)
- Typically CK7(+)/CK20(-)
- CEA variably (+)

DIFFERENTIAL DIAGNOSIS

Seminal Vesicle Cystadenoma
- Very rare benign tumor
- Cystically dilated glandular spaces with pale intraluminal secretions lined by few layers of cuboidal or columnar cells surrounded by spindle cell stroma
- Lacks cytologic atypia and invasive features

Prostate Adenocarcinoma
- Secondary involvement of seminal vesicle considerably more common than primary adenocarcinoma
- Ductal adenocarcinoma with papillary architecture mimics seminal vesicle adenocarcinoma
- Unusual to have cystic growth
- Stromal desmoplastic response not typical
- PSA/PAP(+), CA125(-)

Urinary Bladder Adenocarcinoma
- Correlation of clinical, radiologic, and gross findings critical
- CA125(-); most are CK7(+)/CK20(+)

Colorectal Adenocarcinoma
- Correlation of clinical, radiologic, and gross findings critical
- Typically invasive intestinal-type glands with abundant necrosis (dirty necrosis)
- CA125(-), CDX2(+); most are CK7(-)/CK20(+)

SELECTED REFERENCES

1. Campobasso D et al: Primary bilateral seminal vesicle carcinoma: description of a case and literature review. Int J Surg Pathol. 20(6):633-5, 2012
2. Stenzel P et al: Primary seminal vesicle carcinoma. Int J Surg Pathol. 19(3):401-4, 2011
3. Egevad L et al: Primary seminal vesicle carcinoma detected at transurethral resection of prostate. Urology. 69(4):778, 2007
4. Thiel R et al: Primary adenocarcinoma of the seminal vesicles. J Urol. 168(5):1891-6, 2002
5. Ormsby AH et al: Primary seminal vesicle carcinoma: an immunohistochemical analysis of four cases. Mod Pathol. 13(1):46-51, 2000

Immunohistochemistry, Prostate

Markers for Diagnosis of Limited PCa on Needle Biopsy

Antibody/Protein Detected	Advantages	Disadvantages
p63	Nuclear marker, less nonspecific staining	Discontinuous basal cell layers (and therefore p63) may appear absent in benign mimics of PCa; a rare subset of PCa aberrantly expresses p63
HMWCK	No diffuse aberrant HMWCK positive PCa	Increased nonspecific staining compared to p63; discontinuous basal cell layers (and therefore HMWCK) may appear negative in benign mimics of PCa
HMWCK/p63 Cocktail	Conserves tissue, both proteins tested may help detect basal cells in the setting of atrophy.	May not recognize PCa with aberrant p63 expression; evolving concerns regarding multiplex stain reimbursement
AMACR (racemase)	Sensitive, positive in > 80% of PCa	Often positive in mimics, including adenosis
AMACR/p63 Cocktail	Conserves tissue, see both in same section	If both antibodies use same chromogen, it can be hard to see p63 positive basal cells; evolving concerns regarding multiplex stain reimbursement
Triple p63/AMACR/HMWCK Cocktail	AMACR and dual basal cell stain in same section	Dual-color stain may require more extensive work-up and validation; p63 positive aberrant cancer may be missed; evolving concerns regarding multiplex stain reimbursement
ERG	Exquisite specificity to PCa, and rarely, its immediate precursor HGPIN	Sensitivity limited to ~ 40% of PCa; subset of HGPIN may be positive but is frequently associated with concomitant or subsequent PCa

PCa = prostatic adenocarcinoma; HMWCK = high molecular weight cytokeratin 34βE12/CK903; AMACR = alpha-methylacyl-CoA racemase; ERG = ETS-related gene; HGPIN = high-grade prostatic intraepithelial neoplasia.

Adapted from Epstein JI et al: Best practices recommendations in the application of immunohistochemistry in the prostate: report from the International Society of Urologic Pathology consensus conference. Am J Surg Pathol. 38(8):e6-e19, 2014.

Markers Used in Differential of PCa vs. UC

Antibody/Protein Detected	Advantages	Disadvantages
PSA	Widely available; 85-90% of PCas, including Gleason score 10 PCas are positive; negative in urothelial carcinoma	Negative in subset of high-grade PCas; variation between monoclonal and polyclonal antibody preparations and technical performance; weak, nonspecific cytoplasmic positivity is frequently interpreted incorrectly as positive; loss of expression in androgen deprivation-treated carcinomas
PSAP	85-90% of PCas, including Gleason score 10 PCas are positive; negative in urothelial carcinoma	Negative in subset of high-grade PCas; variation between monoclonal and polyclonal antibody preparations and technical performance; weak, nonspecific cytoplasmic positivity is frequently interpreted incorrectly as positive; loss of expression in androgen deprivation-treated carcinomas
p501S (prostein)	Expression retained in many PCas that lose PSA; punctate cytoplasmic staining provides further specificity	Less widely available; punctate cytoplasmic staining pattern may be more difficult to interpret for some observers
NKX3.1	Expression retained in many PCas that lose PSA; nuclear stain reduces false-positivity	Less widely available
AR	High sensitivity for PCa	Expression by subset of UCs
AMACR	High sensitivity for PCa	Expression by many UCs
PSMA	High sensitivity for PCa	Expression by 14% of UCs
CK7 and CK20, stained separately	Negative CK7, positive CK20 phenotype favors PCa; both are widely available	Some PCas may coexpress both, like UC
p63	Less false-positive in PCa than HMWCK; diffuse positivity in high-grade cancer rules out PCa	Infrequent subset of UCs are negative; rare PCas may show aberrant p63 expression

Immunohistochemistry, Prostate

Markers Used in Differential of PCa vs. UC (Continued)

Antibody/Protein Detected	Advantages	Disadvantages
HMWCK	Diffuse, strong positivity rules out PCa	Infrequent subset of UCs are negative; occasional false-positive staining is seen in PCas

PCa = prostatic adenocarcinoma; UC = urothelial carcinoma; HMWCK = high molecular weight cytokeratin 34βE12/CK903; AMACR = alpha-methylacyl-CoA racemase; PSA = prostate specific antigen; PSAP = prostate specific acid phosphatase; AR = androgen receptor; PSMA = prostate specific membrane antigen.

Adapted from Epstein JI et al: Best practices recommendations in the application of immunohistochemistry in the prostate: report from the International Society of Urologic Pathology consensus conference. Am J Surg Pathol. 38(8):e6-e19, 2014.

Markers in Differential PCa vs. Bladder Adenocarcinoma

Antibody/Protein Detected	Advantages	Disadvantages
PSA	High sensitivity, high specificity with monoclonal	7-13% of high-grade PCas are negative, while 13% of bladder adenocarcinomas are positive with polyclonal
PSAP	High sensitivity, high specificity	5% of Gleason score 8-10 carcinomas are negative, 33% of bladder adenocarcinomas are positive with polyclonal
p501S (prostein)	High sensitivity, high specificity	Data limited; none pitfalls reported
NKX3.1	High sensitivity, high specificity in general	Not well studied in this differential
Villin	High specificity for bladder adenocarcinoma	Approximately 35% of bladder adenocarcinomas are negative
Thrombomodulin	95% negative in PCa	Only 60% sensitive in bladder adenocarcinomas
CDX2	94% negative in PCa	Sensitivity 47% for bladder adenocarcinoma
Monoclonal CEA	> 95% negative in PCa	Sensitivity 52% for bladder adenocarcinoma

PCa = prostatic adenocarcinoma; PSA = prostate specific antigen; PSAP = prostate specific acid phosphatase; CEA = carcinoembryonic antigen.

Adapted from Epstein JI et al: Best practices recommendations in the application of immunohistochemistry in the prostate: report from the International Society of Urologic Pathology consensus conference. Am J Surg Pathol. 38(8):e6-e19, 2014.

Markers Used in Metastatic Setting to Prove PCa

Antibody/Protein Detected	Advantages	Disadvantages
PSA	97% sensitive in metastases, high specificity	In Gleason 9-10, only rare cells may be positive; expression is decreased with hormonal therapy; salivary gland tumors, bladder adenocarcinomas, and melanoma may be positive
PSAP	99% sensitive in metastases	Less specific than PSA and may also be positive in neuroendocrine tumors; similar to PSA it may be decreased in hormone therapy
p501S (prostein)	99% sensitive in metastases; expression does not decrease with hormone therapy	Limited studies relative to other markers
NKX3.1	94% sensitive in metastases	Lobular breast cancer may be positive

PCa = prostatic adenocarcinoma; PSA = prostate specific antigen; PSAP = prostate specific acid phosphatase.

Adapted from Epstein JI et al: Best practices recommendations in the application of immunohistochemistry in the prostate: report from the International Society of Urologic Pathology consensus conference. Am J Surg Pathol. 38(8); Amin et al: Am J Surg Pathol. Aug;38(8):1017-22, 2014.

Markers for PCa vs. Prostatic Small Cell Carcinoma

Antibody/Protein Detected	Advantages	Disadvantages
CD56	Sensitive, 83-92% of small cell carcinomas; specific as high-grade PCa is negative	Limited studies generalizing these findings
TTF-1	Specific for small cell, high-grade PCa positive in only 1%	Limited sensitivity in 52% of small cell carcinomas

Immunohistochemistry, Prostate

Markers for PCa vs. Prostatic Small Cell Carcinoma (Continued)

Antibody/Protein Detected	Advantages	Disadvantages
Ki-67	~ 83% proliferative index in small cell carcinoma	~ 10% proliferative index in high-grade PCa
NE stains: Synaptophysin and chromogranin	Sensitive: Synaptophysin positive in 85% and chromogranin positive in 75% of small cell carcinomas	Approximately 10% of conventional high-grade PCa with strong positive staining
Prostate markers: PSA, p501S, NKX3.1	95%-100% positive in conventional high-grade PCa	~ 25% of small cell carcinomas positive, usually only focally
AR	Sensitive: 90% of high-grade PCa	Lack of specificity, ~ 17% of small cell carcinomas positive

PCa = prostatic adenocarcinoma; TTF1 = thyroid transcription factor 1; NE = neuroendocrine; PSA = prostate specific antigen; AR = androgen receptor.

Adapted from Epstein JI et al: Best practices recommendations in the application of immunohistochemistry in the prostate: report from the International Society of Urologic Pathology consensus conference. Am J Surg Pathol. 38(8); Amin et al: Am J Surg Pathol. Aug;38(8):1017-22, 2014.

Markers, Prostatic Sarcoma vs. Sarcomatoid Carcinoma

Antibody/Protein Detected	Advantages	Disadvantages
Desmin	Positive in leiomyosarcoma, may be diffuse	Some staining in sarcomatoid carcinoma, while stromal sarcomas are generally negative
Vimentin	Sensitive for sarcomas	Nonspecific
SMA	Positive in stromal sarcomas and leiomyosarcomas	Focal positivity in some sarcomatoid carcinomas
CD34	Positive in most stromal sarcomas, negative in sarcomatoid carcinomas	Only 8% of leiomyosarcomas are positive
Pancytokeratin	Generally negative in sarcomas	Positive in up to 27% of prostatic leiomyosarcomas and 71% of sarcomatoid carcinomas, yet may be only focal; limited data characterize prevalence of positivity in stromal sarcomas
HMWCK	Sometimes more sensitive than pancytokeratin (no prostate data)	Negative in bladder leiomyosarcomas (no prostate data)
p63	One of the most sensitive markers for sarcomatoid carcinomas, no positivity in leiomyosarcoma in 1 large study	No data for stromal sarcomas; 1 study showed 23% of bladder leiomyosarcomas may be positive
Prostate markers: PSA, p501S, NKX3.1	Negative in sarcomas; positive in epithelial component if present	Usually not very helpful as carcinoma component should generally be apparent by H&E and strongly favors sarcomatoid carcinoma if present

SMA = smooth muscle actin; HMWCK = high molecular weight cytokeratin 34βE12/CK903; PSA = prostate-specific antigen.

Adapted from Epstein JI et al: Best practices recommendations in the application of immunohistochemistry in the prostate: report from the International Society of Urologic Pathology consensus conference. Am J Surg Pathol. 38(8); Amin et al: Am J Surg Pathol. Aug;38(8):1017-22, 2014.

Immunohistochemistry, Prostate

Markers: Minimal PCa Work-Up

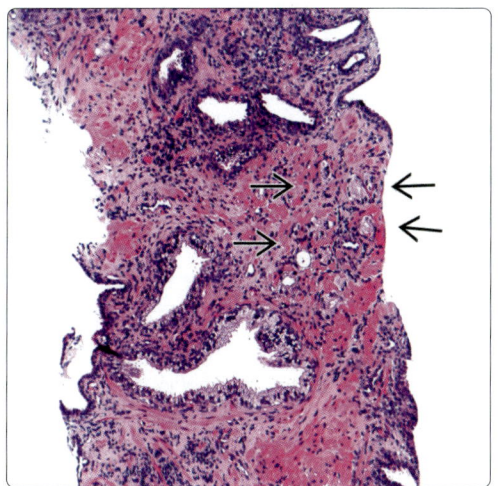

Markers: Minimal PCa Work-Up

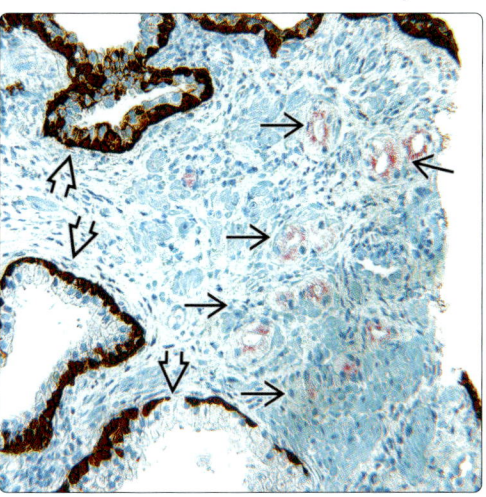

(Left) An atypical focus consisting of 5-8 small acini with an atrophic appearance ⇒ are seen against an obscuring inflammatory background. (Right) A contemporary PIN cocktail employs AMACR (red chromogen) as a positive marker overexpressed with some specificity in PCa ⇒, while basal cell markers p63 (nuclear, brown) and HMWCK (cytoplasmic, brown) identify benign glands ⇒. Even a scattered or discontinuous basal cell would contraindicate unequivocal diagnosis of PCa.

Markers: PCa Work-Up

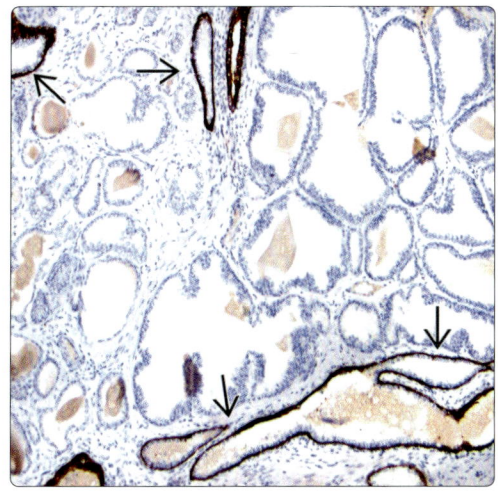

Markers: PCa Work-Up

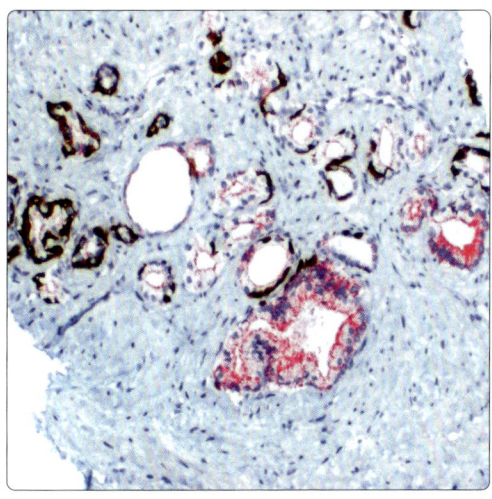

(Left) Some labs employ just a cocktail of basal cell markers p63 and HMWCK, as seen here, identifying scattered benign glands ⇒ amongst a carcinoma with pseudohyperplastic features. (Right) A focus of atypical adenomatous hyperplasia is identified, supported by a present but discontinuous layer of basal cells (p63/HMWCK brown). Aberrant AMACR expression (red) is seen in a subset of adenosis and presents a pitfall without the triple stain.

Markers: PCa Work-Up

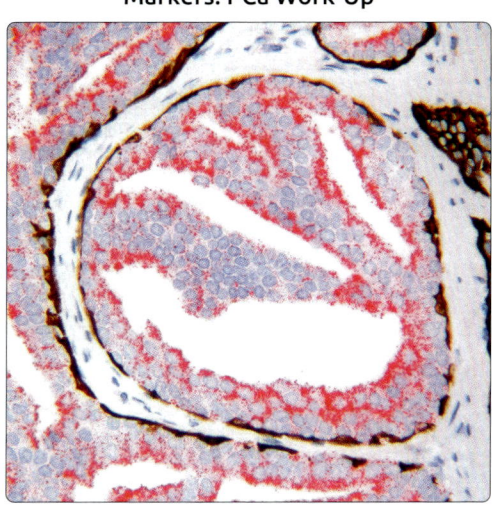

Markers: Limited PCa Work-Up

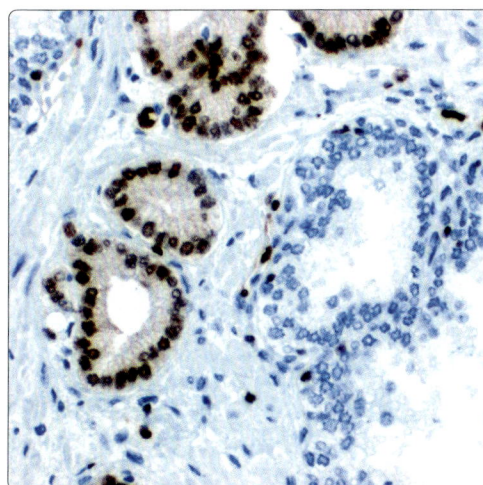

(Left) PIN cocktail in HGPIN shows AMACR overexpression in acinar cells (red) and positivity for basal cell markers (brown). (Right) An emerging marker supporting diagnosis for prostate cancer is ERG, which is exquisitely specific to cancer as opposed to benign mimics. Expression of this marker is reflective of oncogenic fusions involving the ERG locus, usually fused to the androgen-responsive gene, TMPRSS2. The marker is limited by its sensitivity.

Immunohistochemistry, Prostate

Markers: PIN Cocktail and ERG

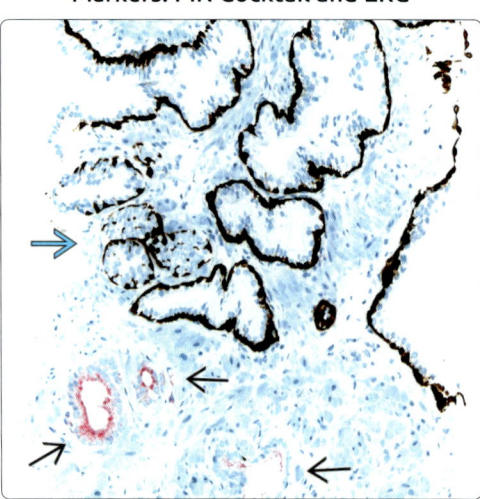

Markers: PIN Cocktail and ERG

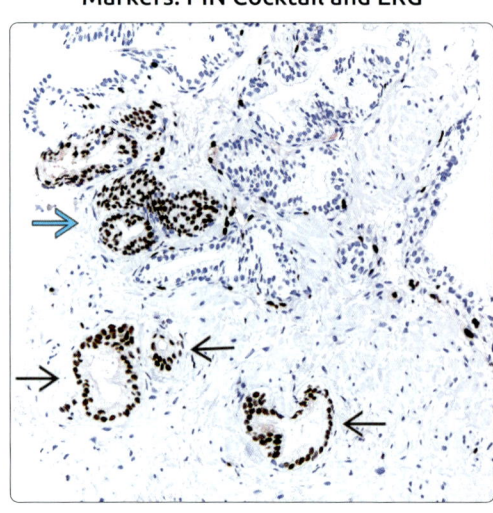

(Left) A focus of 2 or 3 acini of PCa lacking basal cells and overexpressing AMACR ⇒ are highlighted by PIN4 cocktail. Note the basal cell markers at the indicated focus ⇒. *(Right)* Same focus as at left but with ERG immunostain, clearly highlighting the invading acini of adenocarcinoma ⇒. Note this rare example of ERG-positive HGPIN in the focus with the basal cells demonstrated at left ⇒. This presents a pitfall without PIN cocktail but is nearly always seen adjacent to unequivocal PCa.

Markers: Prostatic Histogenesis

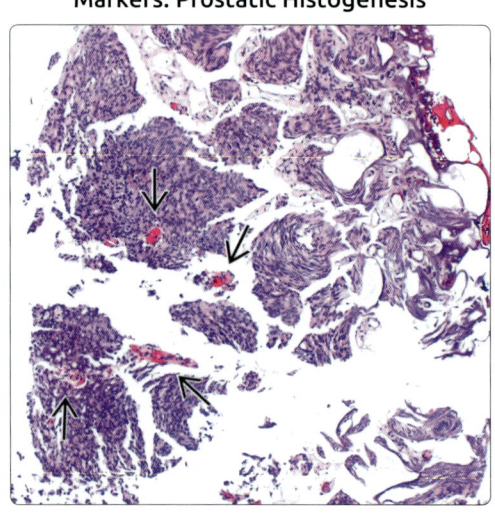

Markers: Prostatic Histogenesis

(Left) Heavily cauterized biopsy of a papillary lesion seen in the bladder of a patient with longstanding androgen oblation-treated PCa. The cautery and appearance of fibrovascular cores ⇒ raises consideration of UC. *(Right)* PSA is negative in this case, as is often true in high-grade carcinomas treated with contemporary androgen ablation regimens.

Markers: Prostatic Histogenesis

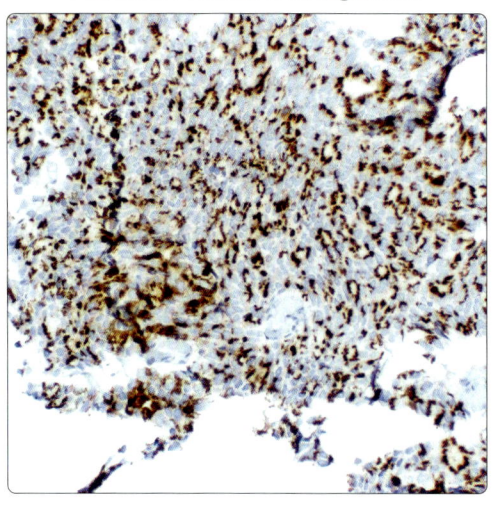

Markers: Prostatic Histogenesis

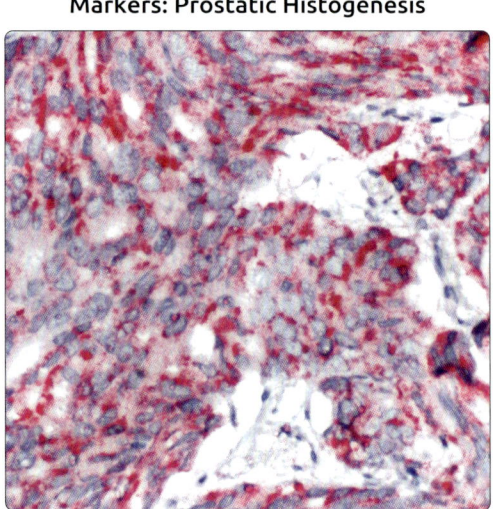

(Left) The same case where p501S expression is retained in a punctate, cytoplasmic pattern, confirming high-stage prostate cancer invading into lumen of the bladder. This marker is retained better than PSA and PSAP despite treatment. *(Right)* The same stained by PIN cocktail is shown here. AMACR expression (red chromogen) supports PCa diagnosis but may be expressed by UCs. More useful, however, is the lack of p63 and HMWCK (brown) expression, which would have supported UC over PCa.

Immunohistochemistry, Prostate

Markers: Small Cell Carcinoma

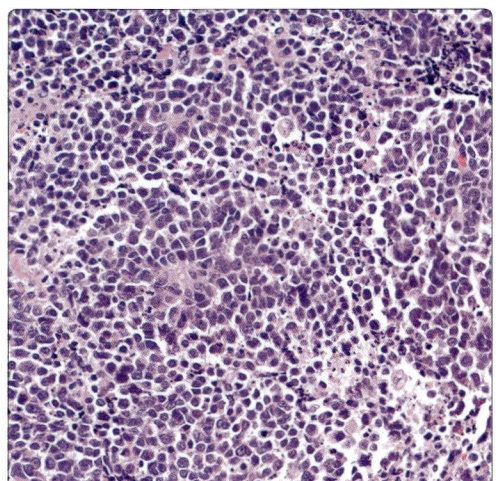

Markers: Small Cell Carcinoma

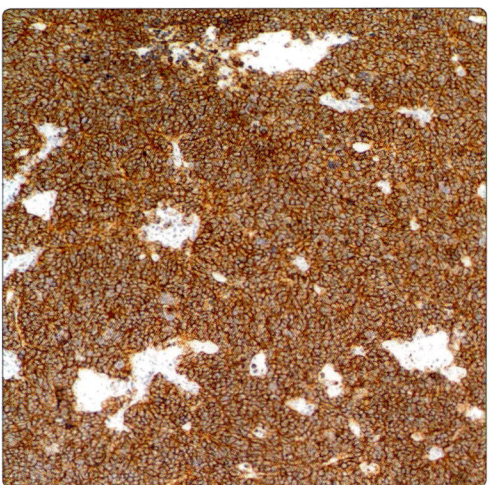

(Left) Small cell carcinoma of prostate shows undifferentiated small cells with abundant mitosis, apoptosis, and nuclear molding. (Right) Synaptophysin is a sensitive marker for small cell carcinoma of the prostate, though it may also be strongly expressed in high-grade, non-small cell PCa and PCa with overlapping features with small cell PCa, emphasizing the need for a panel of markers and interpretation in the morphologic context.

Markers: Prostatic Histogenesis

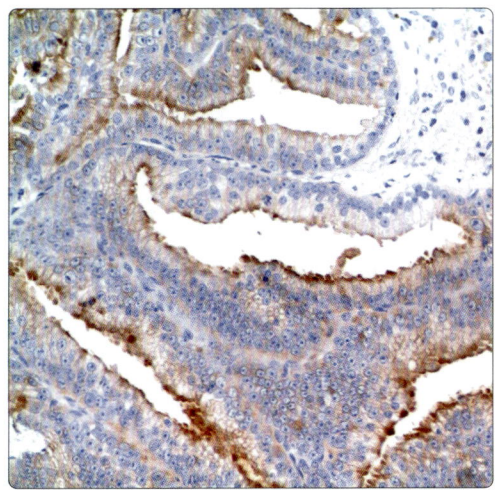

Markers: Prostatic Histogenesis

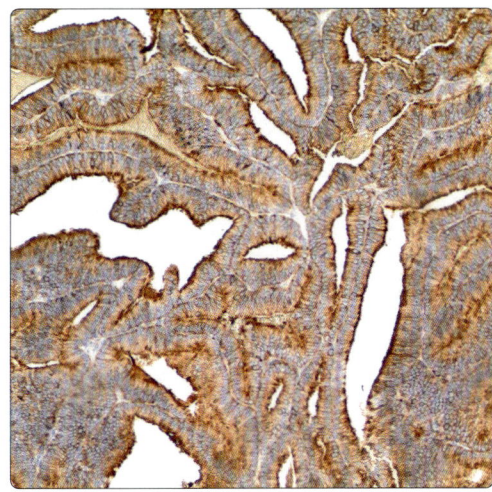

(Left) PSA remains a widely available, useful, and specific marker of prostate cancer, in this case supporting a high-grade PCa with ductal features over a bladder adenocarcinoma, only a subset of which would be expected to show positivity. (Right) PSAP remains also a useful and relatively specific marker of prostatic origin; however, polyclonal preparations lack specificity in the differential with bladder adenocarcinoma, of which 1/3 may show positivity.

Markers: Sarcoma vs. Sarcomatoid PCa

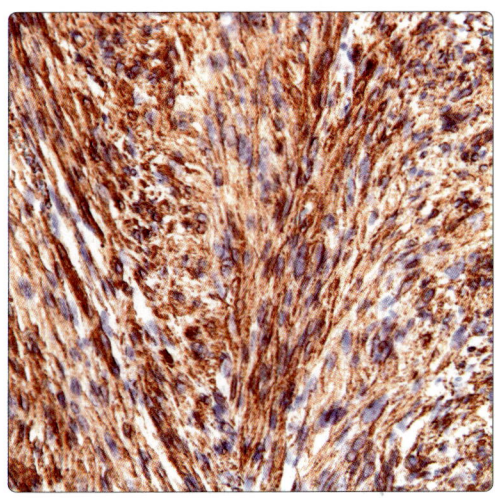

Markers: Sarcoma vs. Sarcomatoid PCa

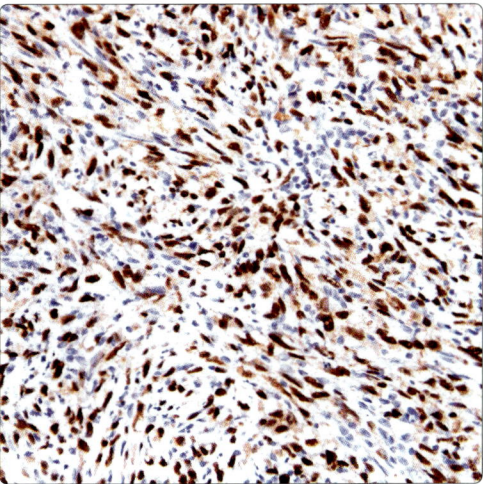

(Left) SMA shows diffuse positivity in leiomyosarcoma of prostate. SMA is more focal or negative in prostatic stromal sarcoma and sarcomatoid carcinoma. Positivity for p63 and pancytokeratin (AE1/AE3) helps distinguish sarcomatoid carcinoma. (Right) p63 shows nuclear positivity in sarcomatoid carcinoma of prostate. Though conventional PCa is nearly always p63 negative, expression of p63 is helpful in identifying sarcomatoid PCa, usually seen in the more epithelioid population of cells.

SECTION 4
Testis and Paratesticular Structures

Introduction and Overview
Classification of Testis and Paratestis Tumors and Tumor-Like Lesions — **732**

Nonneoplastic Lesions
Cryptorchidism — **734**
Sertoli Cell-Only Syndrome — **738**
Nontuberculous Infections — **742**
Nonspecific Granulomatous Orchitis — **744**
Tuberculous Epididymo-Orchitis — **746**

Germ Cell Tumors
General Concepts, Germ Cell Tumors — **748**

Germ Cell Tumors Related to Germ Cell Neoplasia In Situ
Germ Cell Neoplasia In Situ — **756**
Seminoma — **762**
Embryonal Carcinoma — **770**
Yolk Sac Tumor — **776**
Choriocarcinoma and Variants — **784**
Teratoma, Adult Type — **790**
Mixed Germ Cell Tumors — **794**
Somatic-Type Malignancy in Germ Cell Tumor — **798**
Burnt-Out (Regressed) Germ Cell Tumor — **800**

Germ Cell Tumors Unrelated to Germ Cell Neoplasia In Situ
Spermatocytic Tumor — **802**
Teratoma, Prepubertal Type — **806**
Yolk Sac Tumor, Prepubertal Type — **810**
Carcinoid Tumor — **814**

Sex Cord-/Gonadal Stromal Tumors
General Concepts, Sex Cord-/Gonadal Stromal Tumors — **818**
Leydig Cell Tumors — **824**
Sertoli Cell Tumors — **828**
Large Cell Calcifying Sertoli Cell Tumor — **834**

Granulosa Cell Tumor	838
Juvenile Granulosa Cell Tumor	842
Testicular Tumor of Adrenogenital Syndrome	846
Sex Cord-Stromal Tumor, Mixed/Unclassified	850
Gonadoblastoma	854

Hematopoietic Tumors

Lymphoma/Leukemia/Plasmacytoma	858

Tumors of Paratesticular Structures

Adenomatoid Tumor	864
Malignant Mesothelioma	868
Adenocarcinoma of Rete Testis/Epididymis	872
Papillary Serous Carcinoma, Müllerian Subtype	874
Liposarcoma	878
Melanotic Neuroectodermal Tumor	882
Embryonal Rhabdomyosarcoma	886
Other Sarcomas	890

Metastatic Tumors, Testis and Paratesticular Structures

Metastatic Tumors, Testis and Paratesticular Structures	894

Immunohistochemical Profiles for Tumors Involving Testis and Paratesticular Structures

Immunohistochemistry, Testis	898

Classification of Testis and Paratestis Tumors and Tumor-Like Lesions

NONNEOPLASTIC LESIONS

Tumor-Like Lesions
- Sertoli cell-only syndrome
- Cryptorchidism
- Torsion/infarct
- Hematoma/hematocoele
- Pyogenic epididymo-orchitis
- Nonspecific granulomatous orchitis
- Juvenile xanthogranuloma
- Tuberculous epididymo-orchitis
- Necrotizing vasculitis
- Malakoplakia
- Other infections
  - Syphilis, leprosy, etc.
- Sarcoidosis
- Sperm granuloma
- Leydig cell hyperplasia
- Sertoli cell nodule
  - Pick adenoma
- Testicular appendages and Walthard nests
- Inflammatory pseudotumor
- Hyperplasia of rete testis
- Adrenal cortical rests
- Mesothelial hyperplasia
- Cysts
  - Parenchymal
  - Rete testis
  - Epididymal
- Cystic dysplasia
- Ectopic spleen

NEOPLASMS

Germ Cell Tumors
- Precursor lesions
  - Germ cell neoplasia in situ
- Germ cell neoplasia in situ with microinvasion
- Seminoma
  - With syncytiotrophoblastic cells
- Nonseminomatous germ cell tumor
  - Embryonal carcinoma
  - Yolk sac tumor, postpubertal type
  - Choriocarcinoma and variants
    - Monophasic
    - Placental site trophoblastic tumor
    - Epithelioid trophoblastic tumor
    - Cystic trophoblastic tumor
  - Teratoma, adult type
    - Somatic-type malignancy in germ cell tumor
  - Mixed germ cell tumor
    - Specialized mixed germ cell tumors
      - Polyembryoma
      - Diffuse embryoma
  - Burnt-out (regressed) germ cell tumor
- Spermatocytic tumor
  - Sarcomatoid variant
- Teratoma, prepubertal type
  - Dermoid cyst
  - Epidermoid cyst
  - Carcinoid tumor
    - Monodermal teratoma
- Yolk sac tumor, prepubertal type

Sex Cord-/Gonadal Stromal Tumors
- Fibroma/thecoma
- Leydig cell tumors
- Sertoli cell tumors
  - Sertoli cell tumor, not otherwise specified (NOS)
  - Sclerosing Sertoli cell tumor
  - Large cell calcifying Sertoli cell tumor
  - Intratubular large cell calcifying Sertoli cell tumor
- Sertoli-Leydig cell tumor
- Granulosa cell tumor
  - Adult
  - Juvenile
- Sex cord-stromal tumor, mixed/unclassified
- Myoid gonadal stromal tumor
- Gonadoblastoma
- Tumors of adrenogenital syndrome

Hematopoietic Tumors
- Myeloid sarcoma
- Diffuse large B-cell lymphoma
- Follicular lymphoma
- Primary MALT lymphoma
- Extranodal NK-/T-cell lymphoma
- Burkitt lymphoma
- Plasmacytoma
- Rosai-Dorfman disease

Tumors of Rete Testis
- Calcifying nodule
- Cystic dilatation (transformation)
- Inflammatory pseudotumor
- Adenomatous hyperplasia
- Cystadenoma
- Adenocarcinoma

Tumors of Paratesticular Structures
- Adenomatoid tumor
- Malignant mesothelioma
- Squamous cell carcinoma
- Paratesticular multicystic mass of wolffian origin

Ovarian-Type Tumors
- Brenner tumor
- Mucinous cystadenocarcinoma
- Papillary serous carcinoma, müllerian subtype

Epididymal Tumors
- Idiopathic granulomatous epididymitis
- Spermatocele
- Adenomatoid tumor
- Papillary cystadenoma
- Cribriform hyperplasia
- Rhabdomyoma
- Melanotic neuroectodermal tumor
  - Retinal anlage tumor
- Adenocarcinoma
- Mesothelioma

Classification of Testis and Paratestis Tumors and Tumor-Like Lesions

Spermatic Cord
- Vasitis nodosa
- Proliferative funiculitis
- Papillary cystadenoma
- Hemangioma
- Lipoma
- Vascular myxolipoma
- Aggressive angiomyxoma
- Angiomyofibroblastoma
- Solitary fibrous tumor
- Paraganglioma
- Liposarcoma
- Malignant fibrous histiocytoma

Other Tumors
- Hemangioendothelioma
- Angiosarcoma
- Kaposi sarcoma
- Fibrosarcoma
- Chondrosarcoma
- Osteosarcoma
- Ossified intratesticular mucinous tumor
- Melanotic neuroectodermal tumor
  - Retinal anlage tumor
- Leiomyosarcoma
- Embryonal rhabdomyosarcoma
- Desmoplastic small round cell tumor

Metastatic Tumors of Testis and Paratestis
- Prostate adenocarcinoma
- Lung adenocarcinoma
- Kidney renal cell carcinoma
- Colon adenocarcinoma
- Bladder urothelial carcinoma
- Malignant melanoma
- Neuroblastoma
- Others
  - Pancreas
  - Stomach
  - Esophagus
  - Small intestine

Cryptorchidism

KEY FACTS

TERMINOLOGY
- 1 or both testes present outside scrotum with failure to descend into scrotum (empty scrotum)

CLINICAL ISSUES
- Most common birth defect of male genitalia
- 1% of infants have incompletely descended testes 12 months after birth
- Cryptorchidism increases risk of testicular cancer 4-10x
- Most common problem caused by cryptorchidism is infertility
- 90% can be palpable in inguinal canal (10% in abdomen or nonexistent, truly hidden, or anorchia)
- Most will descend into scrotum without any intervention during 1st year of life
- Medical or surgical correction are both effective

MACROSCOPIC
- Abnormal location and usually smaller sized testis than normal or contralateral testis

MICROSCOPIC
- Variable degrees of decreased diameter of seminiferous tubules
- Tubules with hypospermatogenesis to complete lack of spermatogenesis (resembling Sertoli cell-only syndrome)
- Presence of ring-shaped tubules or megatubules
- Interstitial (Leydig cells) cells usually spared and may show hyperplasia or Pick adenoma (Sertoli cell nodule)
- Thickening and hyalinization of tubular basement membranes and interstitial edema
- Presence of eosinophilic bodies or microliths
- Germ cell neoplasia in situ (GCNIS) may be present

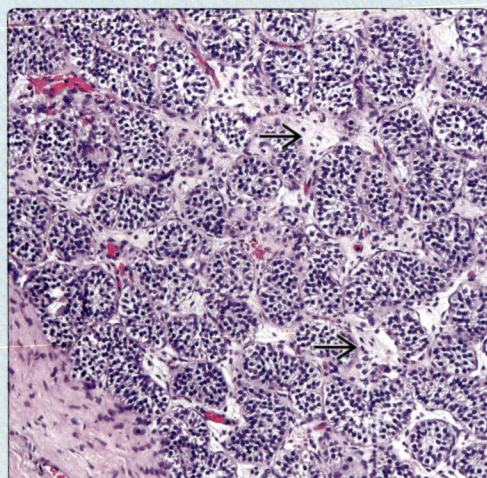
Cryptorchid Testis: Low Power

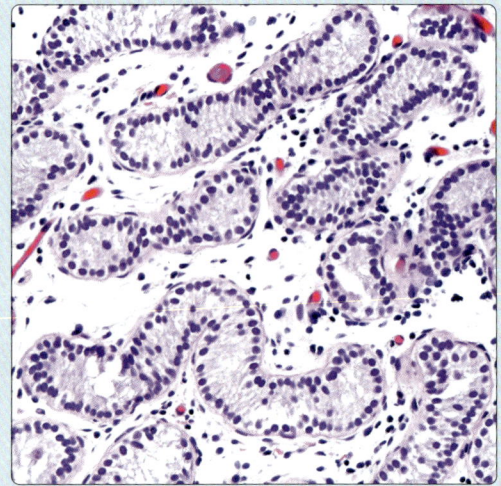
Cryptorchid Testis: Sertoli Cells Only

(Left) Low-power photomicrograph shows cryptorchid testis with crowded seminiferous tubules with no spermatogenesis and decreased tubular size, filled with immature germ cells. The interstitium is edematous ➡. (Right) This photomicrograph from a cryptorchid testis shows seminiferous tubules with no spermatogenesis and marked interstitial edema. The tubules are lined by Sertoli cells only.

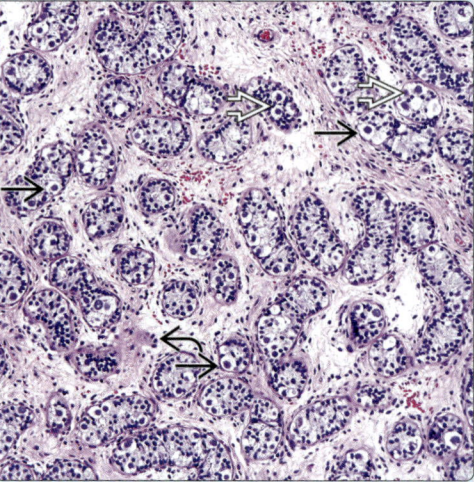
Cryptorchid Testis: Immature Spermatogenesis

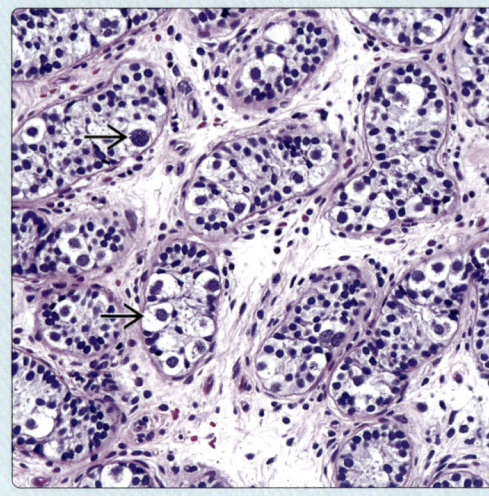
Cryptorchid Testis: Large Spermatogonia

(Left) Cryptorchid testis shows seminiferous tubules with immature spermatogenesis with an isolated spermatogonium ➡ or clusters ➡. There is interstitial fibrosis and scattered primitive Leydig cells ➡. (Right) Cryptorchid testis shows large spermatogonia ➡ with clear cytoplasm resembling those of germ cell neoplasia in situ (GCNIS). Podoplanin (D2-40) and OCT3/4 immunostains are helpful to make the distinction. GCNIS is positive for these stains, but normal germ cells are negative.

Cryptorchidism

TERMINOLOGY

Synonyms
- Undescended testis

Definitions
- 1 or both testes present outside scrotum with failure to descend into scrotum (empty scrotum)

ETIOLOGY/PATHOGENESIS

Developmental Anomaly
- Idiopathic
- Anomalies in anatomic development
- Defect in fetal androgens or excess maternal estrogen
- Associated with congenital malformation syndromes, such as Prader-Willi, Noonan, and cloacal exstrophy

Acquired Cryptorchidism
- Postoperative trapped testis (iatrogenic) or spontaneous ascent

CLINICAL ISSUES

Epidemiology
- Incidence
  - Most common birth defect of male genitalia
  - 3% of full-term newborns have undescended testis/testes
  - 1% of infants have incompletely descended testes 12 months after birth
  - More common in premature infants (30% of boys born before 30 weeks gestational age)
  - True cryptorchidism accounts for 25% of cases of empty scrotum

Presentation
- No particular symptoms; empty scrotal sac usually detected by parents
- ~ 2/3 unilateral and 1/3 bilateral
- 90% may be palpable in inguinal canal (10% in abdomen or nonexistent, truly hidden, or anorchia)
- Testis may be found anywhere along path of descent from retroperitoneum to inguinal ring
- Rarely located outside of path of descent (ectopic), such as outside of inguinal canal, perineum, opposite scrotum, femoral canal, or under skin

Natural History
- Predisposition to testicular germ cell neoplasia
  - Cryptorchidism increases risk of testicular cancer by 4-10x
  - Orchiopexy facilitates self-examination and may decrease risk of germ cell tumor
- Infertility
  - Most common problem caused by cryptorchidism; 75-85% of cryptorchid males have sperm count below normal
  - Tubular fertility index (number of germ cells per cross-sectioned tubule) is most important factor
- Increased risk of torsion

Treatment
- Hormone injection (β-HCG or testosterone) may be administered to try bringing testicle into scrotum
- If medical treatment is unsuccessful, early orchiopexy (~ 1 year old) should be performed to prevent irreversible damage to testicle

Prognosis
- Most will descend into scrotum without any intervention during 1st year of life
- Medical or surgical correction are both effective
- ~ 5% of patients with undescended testicles do not have testicles at surgery (vanished or absent testis)

IMAGING

Ultrasonographic Findings
- Snowstorm pattern by ultrasonography if severe microlithiasis

MACROSCOPIC

General Features
- Testicle in abnormal location; size is usually smaller than normal testis and comparatively smaller than contralateral testis

MICROSCOPIC

Histologic Features
- Variable degree of decreased diameter of seminiferous tubules
- Tubules with hypospermatogenesis to complete lack of spermatogenesis (resembling Sertoli cell-only syndrome)
- Presence of ring-shaped tubules or megatubules
- Abnormal giant spermatogonia with dark nuclei
- Interstitial (Leydig cells) cells usually spared and may show hyperplasia or Pick adenoma (Sertoli cell nodule)
- Thickening and hyalinization of tubular basement membranes and interstitial edema
- Presence of eosinophilic bodies or microliths
- May have dysgenetic features with nondescriptive undifferentiated sex cord-stromal tissue and nests resembling that of immature seminiferous tubules
- Contralateral descended testis may show regressive changes
- Germ cell neoplasia in situ (GCNIS) may be present

DIAGNOSTIC CHECKLIST

Pathologic Interpretation Pearls
- Abnormal testis location and variable development or maturation of testicular parenchyma
- In biopsies and orchiectomy specimens, it is important to look for GCNIS
  - Sampling and immunohistochemistry may be necessary

SELECTED REFERENCES

1. Kolon TF et al: Evaluation and treatment of cryptorchidism: AUA guideline. J Urol. 192(2):337-45, 2014
2. Cendron M et al: Anatomical, morphological and volumetric analysis: a review of 759 cases of testicular maldescent. J Urol. 149(3):570-3, 1993

Cryptorchidism

Cryptorchid Testis: Microlith

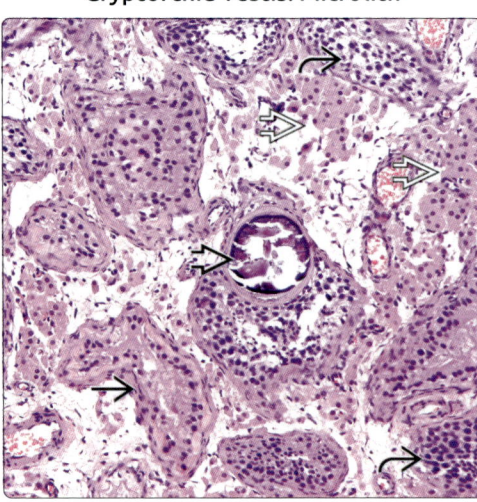

Cryptorchid Testis: Microlith

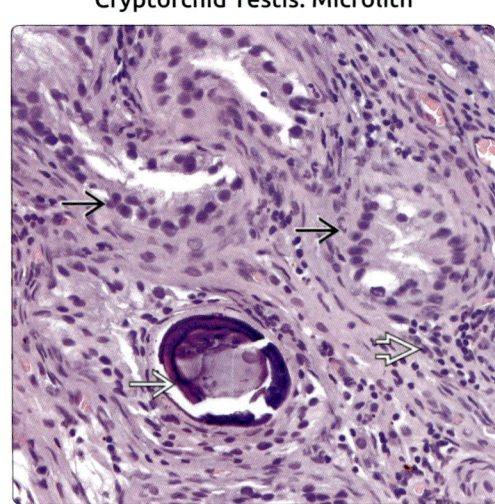

(Left) Cryptorchid testis shows seminiferous tubules with uneven maturation. Some tubules lack spermatogenesis ⇨ and others have incomplete spermatogenesis ⇨. Intratubular microlith ⇨ and Leydig cell hyperplasia ⇨ are seen. (Right) Cryptorchid testis is shown composed of seminiferous tubules with Sertoli cell only pattern ⇨ and an intratubular microlith ⇨. There is peritubular fibrosis and chronic inflammatory cell infiltration in the interstitium ⇨.

Cryptorchid Testis: Interstitial Edema

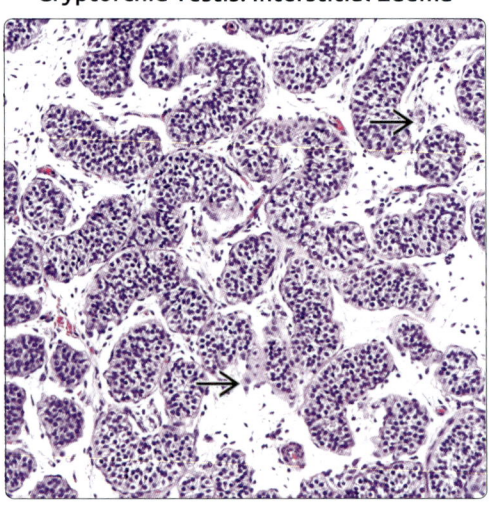

Cryptorchid Testis: Sertoli Cells

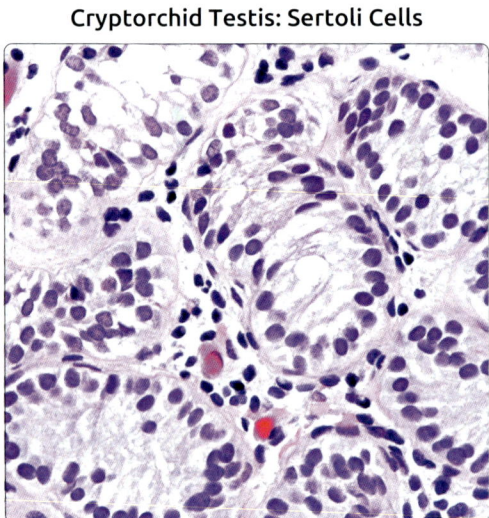

(Left) This low-power photomicrograph shows cryptorchid prepubertal testis with seminiferous tubules filled with primitive germ cells. The tubules are small, and there is marked interstitial edema. A few scattered Leydig cells are observed ⇨. (Right) Cryptorchid testis shows seminiferous tubules filled with Sertoli cells and no spermatogenesis. The interstitium shows scattered chronic inflammatory cells. Adequate sampling is necessary in postpubertal specimens for GCNIS.

Cryptorchid Testis: Megatubules

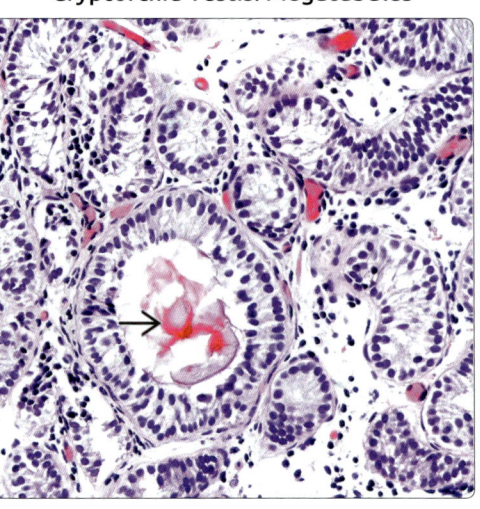

Cryptorchid Testis: Atrophy

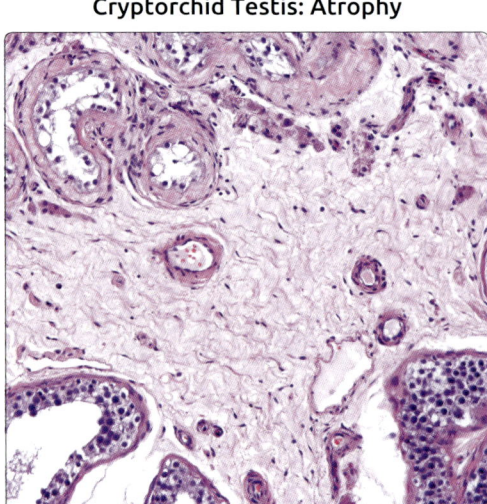

(Left) This is an example of cryptorchid testis with marked germinal hypoplasia and a megatubule with eosinophilic bodies ⇨. The interstitium shows edema and a few lymphocytes. (Right) This photomicrograph shows testicular parenchyma with marked hypoplasia in a patient with cryptorchid testis. There is marked testicular atrophy with hyalinized and edematous stroma. Some seminiferous tubules are entirely devoid of spermatogenesis and others are hypoplastic with immature spermatogenesis.

Cryptorchidism

Cryptorchid Testis: Dysgenetic Features
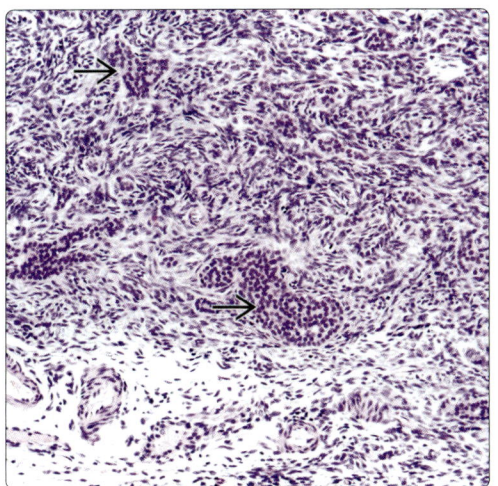

Cryptorchid Testis: Dysgenetic Features
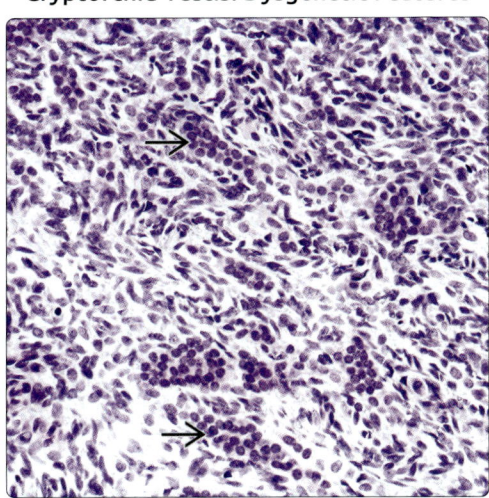

(Left) This low-power photomicrograph shows cryptorchid testis with marked dysgenetic features with nondescriptive, undifferentiated sex cord, stromal tissue and nests resembling that of immature seminiferous tubules ➡. (Right) Higher power view of cryptorchid testis shows undifferentiated sex cord, stromal tissue and nests resembling immature seminiferous tubules ➡. The absence of a mass lesion on gross examination argues against a sex cord, stromal neoplasm.

Cryptorchid Testis: Dysgenetic Features
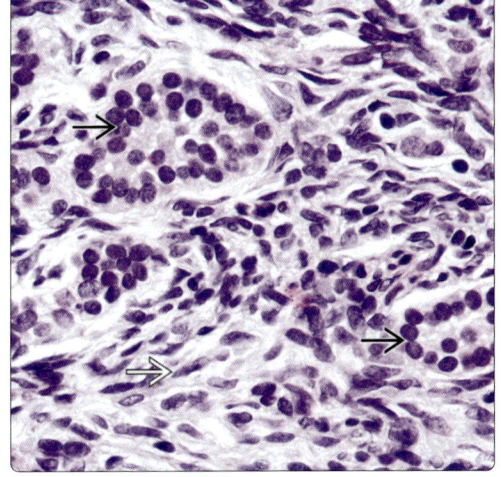

Cryptorchid Testis: Paratesticular
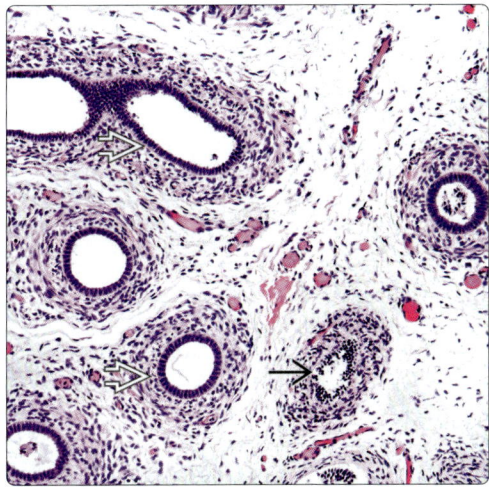

(Left) High-power view shows undifferentiated sex cord spindle cells with elongated nuclei ➡ and pale cytoplasm. Poorly formed tubules filled with round to ovoid cells resembling Sertoli cells in seminiferous tubules ➡ are also present. (Right) This photomicrograph from a cryptorchid testis shows immature paratesticular tissue, including efferent ductules ➡ and epididymis ➡ surrounded by immature spindle cells with eosinophilic cytoplasm.

Sertoli Cell Nodule (Pick Adenoma)
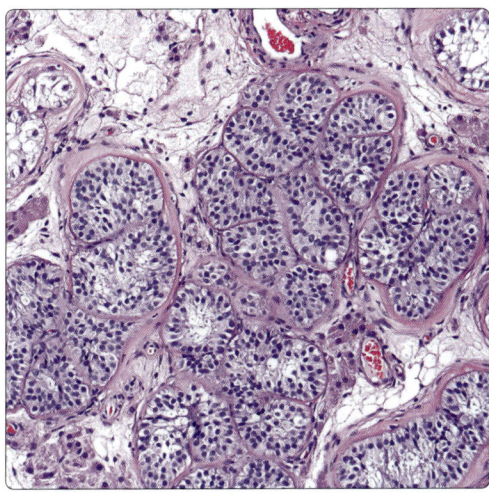

Cryptorchid Testis: Leydig Cell Hyperplasia
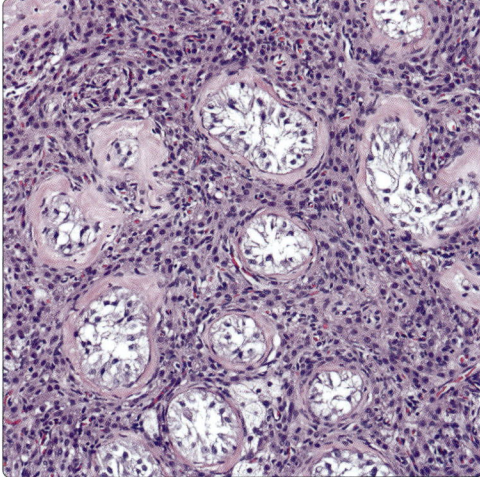

(Left) This photomicrograph shows a Sertoli cell nodule (Pick adenoma) in a patient with cryptorchid testis. The nodule is small and well demarcated from the surrounding seminiferous tubules. Formation of a nodule (adenoma) is the main difference from Sertoli cell-only pattern testis. (Right) This photomicrograph shows marked interstitial Leydig cell hyperplasia in a patient with cryptorchid testis. The seminiferous tubules are atrophic with hyalinization of basement membranes and contain Sertoli cells only.

Sertoli Cell-Only Syndrome

KEY FACTS

TERMINOLOGY
- Germ cell aplasia
- All azoospermias in which seminiferous epithelium consists of only Sertoli cells

CLINICAL ISSUES
- Infertility, azoospermia, &/or hypogonadism
- Usually present between ages 20-40 years for evaluation of infertility
- 5-10% of infertile men are due to Sertoli cell-only syndrome
- Well-developed secondary male sexual characteristics
- Normal virilization with no gynecomastia
- Gonadotropins may be increased or decreased depending on type of syndrome

MACROSCOPIC
- Testes are usually normal, smaller, or atrophic

MICROSCOPIC
- Seminiferous tubules contain only Sertoli cells and 5 histologic variants have been described
  - Immature Sertoli cells
  - Dysgenetic Sertoli cells
  - Adult Sertoli cells
  - Involuting Sertoli cells
  - Dedifferentiated Sertoli cells

TOP DIFFERENTIAL DIAGNOSES
- Germ cell neoplasia in situ (GCNIS)
  - Atypical germ cells positive for podoplanin (D2-40), PLAP, OCT3/4 (do not use SALL4 or CD117)
- Maturation arrest or hypospermatogenesis
  - Presence of spermatogonia or maturating spermatocytes
- Tubular hyalinization
  - Variable degree of hyalinized tubules
  - Isolated tubules containing germ cells or Sertoli cells

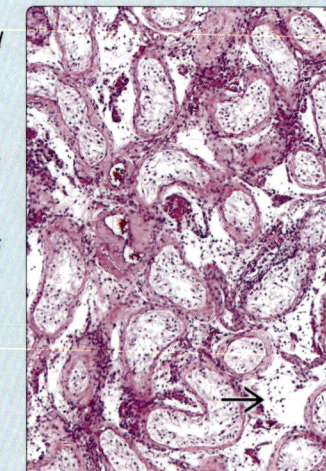

Sertoli Cell-Only Syndrome: Low Power

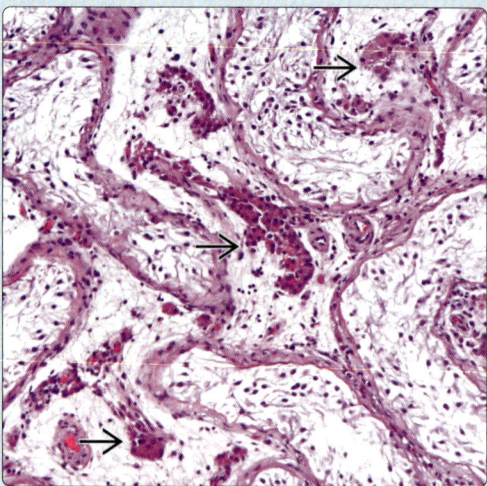

Sertoli Cell-Only Syndrome: Intermediate Power

(Left) Sertoli cell-only syndrome shows smaller sized seminiferous tubules containing Sertoli cells and lack of spermatogenesis. The tubular tunica propria is hyalinized and thickened, and the interstitium is edematous ➡. (Right) Sertoli cell-only syndrome shows seminiferous tubules with thickened tunica propria layer and containing Sertoli cells only with abundant pale eosinophilic cytoplasm. No germ cells are seen. Clusters of Leydig cells ➡ are present.

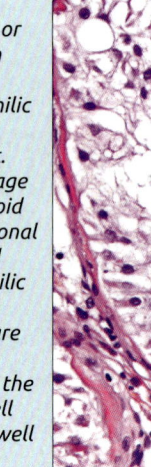

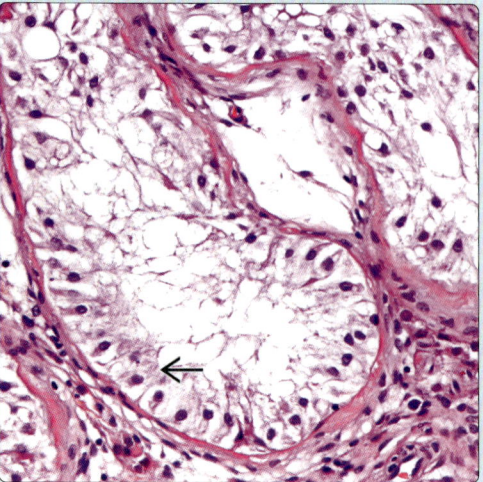

Sertoli Cell-Only Syndrome: High Power

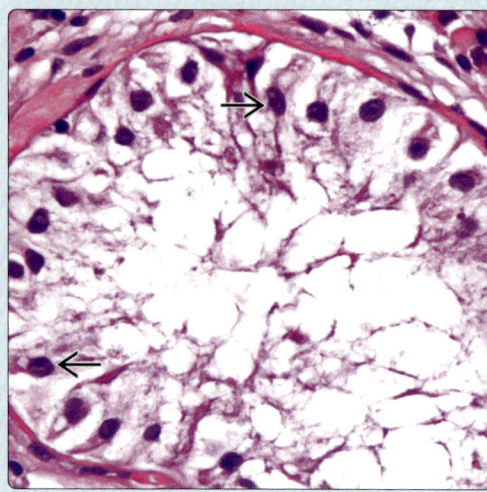

Sertoli Cell-Only Syndrome: High Power

(Left) Sertoli cell-only syndrome shows columnar or pyramidal Sertoli cells with oval to round nuclei and abundant clear to eosinophilic cytoplasm ➡. No spermatogenesis is present. (Right) This high-power image shows Sertoli cells with ovoid or elongated nuclei, occasional prominent nucleoli ➡, and abundant pale to eosinophilic cytoplasm. No germ cell component is present. In rare cases the nuclei may have prominent nucleoli, raising the possibility of GCNIS. The cell borders, however, are not well defined in most cases.

Sertoli Cell-Only Syndrome

TERMINOLOGY

Synonyms
- Germ cell aplasia
- Del Castillo syndrome (old term, now replaced by specific subtypes)

Definitions
- All azoospermias in which seminiferous tubules lack germ cells and contain Sertoli cells only

ETIOLOGY/PATHOGENESIS

Developmental Anomaly
- Sertoli cell-only syndrome with immature Sertoli cells caused by deficiency of both FSH and LH
- Sertoli cell-only syndrome with dysgenetic Sertoli cells has Sertoli cells that proceed to pubertal maturation but variably deviate from normal maturation
  - Associated with cryptorchidism, Y chromosome abnormalities, Klinefelter syndrome (47XXY), and idiopathic infertility
- Sertoli cell-only syndrome with mature Sertoli cells is thought to be due to failure of migration of germ cells

Environmental Exposure
- Sertoli cell-only syndrome with involuting Sertoli cells may be secondary to irradiation, cytotoxic therapy, hormonal therapy for prostate cancer, chemical/toxin exposure, and viral infection
- Sertoli cell-only syndrome with dedifferentiated Sertoli cells is associated with androgen deprivation therapy, estrogen treatment for transsexuality, and platinum chemotherapy agents

CLINICAL ISSUES

Epidemiology
- Age
  - Range: 20-40 years

Presentation
- Infertility, azoospermia, &/or hypogonadism
- 5-10% of infertility in men is due to Sertoli cell-only syndrome
- Well-developed secondary male sexual characteristics with no gynecomastia

Laboratory Tests
- Gonadotropins may be increased or decreased depending on type of syndrome
- Most common types (dysgenetic, adult, and involuting) have elevated FSH, normal or elevated LH, and normal or decreased testosterone
- Immature type has decreased FSH and LH beginning in childhood

Treatment
- No known effective treatment options
- Immature Sertoli cell type may be treated with hormone therapy to recover some degree of spermatogenesis
- Secondary Sertoli cell-only syndrome may be reversible after elimination of specific etiology

Prognosis
- Extensive fine-needle aspiration may recover some spermatozoa in some types

MACROSCOPIC

General Features
- Testes are normal, small, or atrophic

MICROSCOPIC

Histologic Features
- Seminiferous tubules contain only Sertoli cells and 5 histologic variants have been described
  - Immature Sertoli cells
    - Immature prepubertal appearance with pseudostratification
    - Increased cellularity with small tubules often lacking lumina
  - Dysgenetic Sertoli cells
    - Morphology varies within and between tubules
    - Nuclei have mature and immature features
    - Hyalinized tubules are frequent
  - Adult Sertoli cells
    - Mature Sertoli cells with increased numbers
    - Small diameter tubules
  - Involuting Sertoli cells
    - Lobulated nuclei with irregular outlines
    - Seminiferous tubules have variable thickening of basement membrane
    - Leydig cells variably involuted
  - Dedifferentiated Sertoli cells
    - Immature Sertoli cells in otherwise mature tubules
    - Tubule wall thickened with increased elastic fibers and collagen
    - Markedly decreased tubular diameter

DIFFERENTIAL DIAGNOSIS

Germ Cell Neoplasia In Situ
- Normal spermatogenesis may be present
- Concurrent invasive malignant germ cell tumor
- Atypical germ cells positive for podoplanin (D2-40), PLAP, OCT3/4 (do not use SALL4 or CD117)

Maturation Arrest or Hypospermatogenesis
- Presence of spermatogonia or maturating spermatocytes

Tubular Hyalinization
- Variable degree of hyalinized tubules
- Isolated tubules containing germ cells or Sertoli cells
- Caused by dysgenetic, ischemic, postinflammatory, obstructive etiologies

SELECTED REFERENCES

1. Lardone MC et al: Histological and hormonal testicular function in oligo/azoospermic infertile men. Andrologia. 45(6):379-85, 2013
2. Venkatachala S et al: Testicular biopsies–histomorphologic patterns in male infertility. Indian J Pathol Microbiol. 50(4):726-9, 2007
3. Nistal M et al: Sertoli cell types in the Sertoli-cell-only syndrome: relationships between Sertoli cell morphology and aetiology. Histopathology. 16(2):173-80, 1990

Sertoli Cell-Only Syndrome

Atrophic Tubules

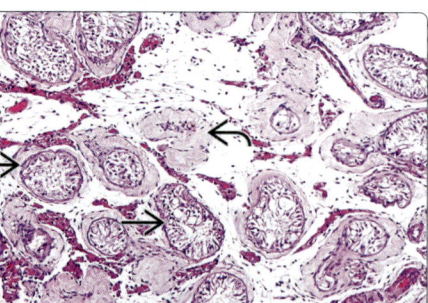

Leydig Cell Hyperplasia

(Left) This low-power view of Sertoli cell-only syndrome shows atrophic seminiferous tubules; some are filled with only Sertoli cells ⇨ and others are entirely sclerotic ⇨. (Right) This photomicrograph shows seminiferous tubules filled with Sertoli cell-only pattern and surrounded by extensive Leydig cell hyperplasia.

Thickened Basement Membranes

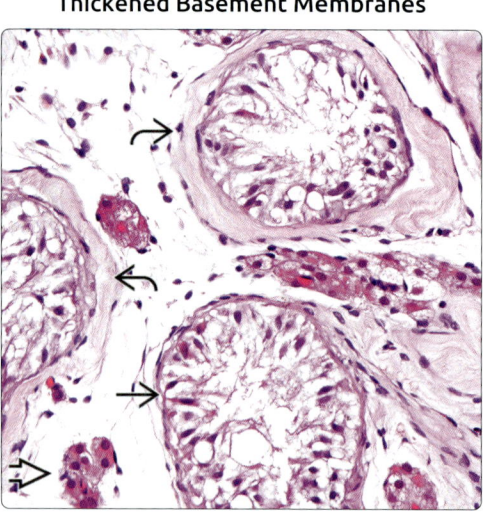

Wind-Swept Appearance

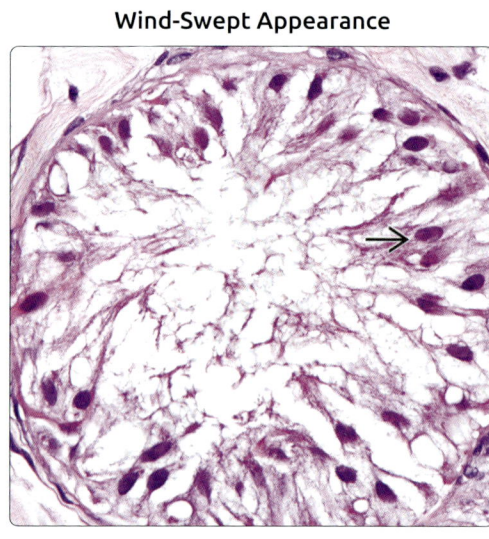

(Left) This photomicrograph shows seminiferous tubules filled entirely with Sertoli cells. 2 tubules ⇨ have markedly thickened tunica propria. 1 tubule has normal thickness of tunica propria ⇨. Clusters of Leydig cells ⇨ are present within the interstitium. (Right) Seminiferous tubule is filled entirely with Sertoli cells, which have ovoid or elongated nuclei, prominent nucleoli ⇨, and abundant pale to eosinophilic cytoplasm. This appearance has been referred to as a wind-swept appearance.

Klinefelter Syndrome

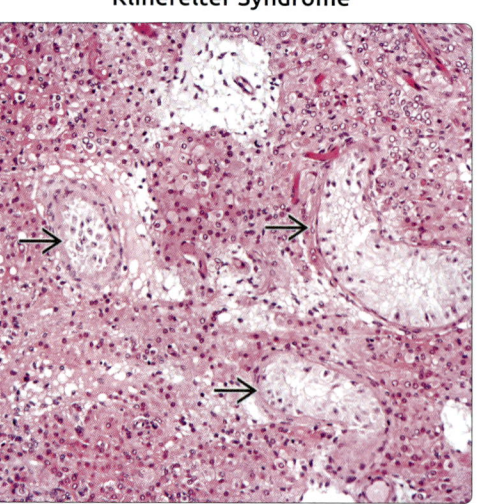

Klinefelter Syndrome

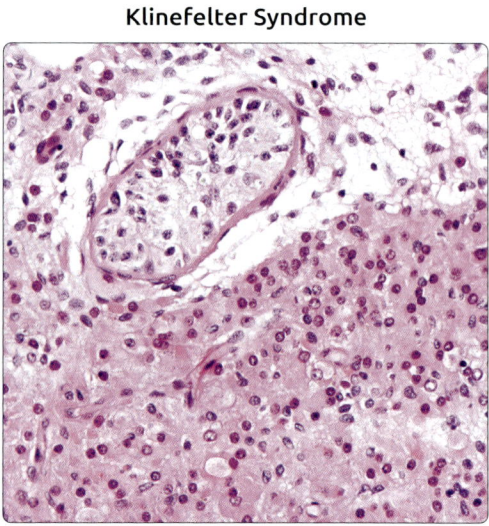

(Left) This image is from a testicular biopsy of a patient with Klinefelter syndrome. There is marked interstitial Leydig cell hyperplasia and few seminiferous tubules with Sertoli cells only ⇨. No germ cells are seen in these tubules. (Right) High-power photomicrograph of testicular biopsy of a patient with Klinefelter syndrome shows interstitial Leydig cell hyperplasia and one seminiferous tubule filled with only Sertoli cells. No spermatogenesis is present.

Sertoli Cell-Only Syndrome

Tubular Atrophy

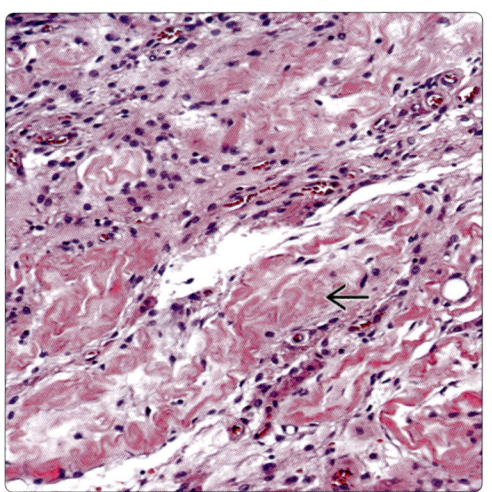

Tubular Hyalinization

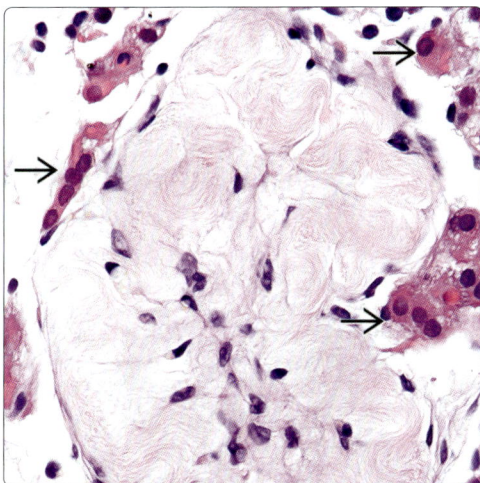

(Left) An example of a hyalinized seminiferous tubule is shown. The tubules are completely sclerotic with intratubular and peritubular hyalinization ⇨. No germ cells or Sertoli cells are present. **(Right)** This photomicrograph shows an entirely sclerotic seminiferous tubule surrounded by clusters of Leydig cells ⇨. When the entire or most of the tubule shows sclerosis, the terms end-stage testis or tubular sclerosis are applied. No Sertoli cells are seen.

Normal Seminiferous Tubule

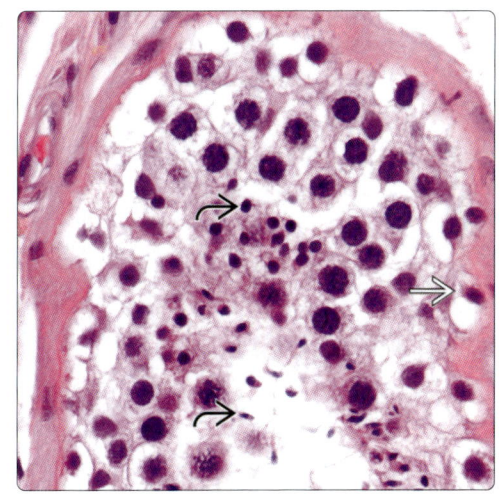

Germ Cell Neoplasia In Situ

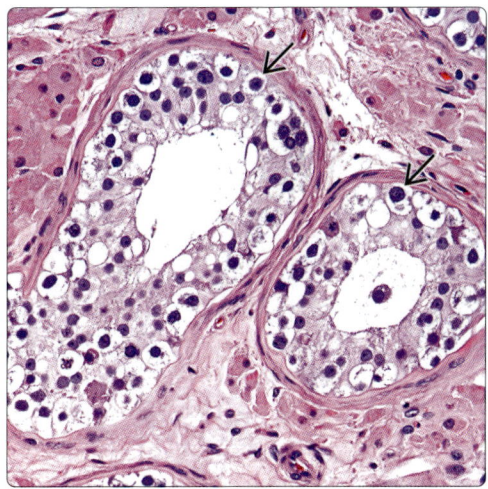

(Left) Normal seminiferous tubule with appropriate spermatogenesis with mature forms ⇨ is shown. Normally the Sertoli cells ⇨ account for 8-10% of the cellularity within a tubule (germ cell/Sertoli cell ratio of 13:1), and there is an average of 10-12 Sertoli cells per tubule. **(Right)** GCNIS is characterized by large, atypical cells with clear cytoplasm situated at the periphery of the tubules ⇨. GCNIS is commonly seen in association with germ cell tumors. These atypical germ cells are positive for D2-40, OCT3/4, and PLAP.

Maturation Arrest

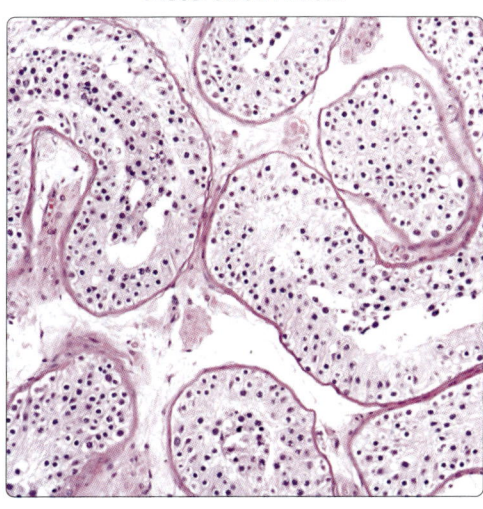

Maturation Arrest

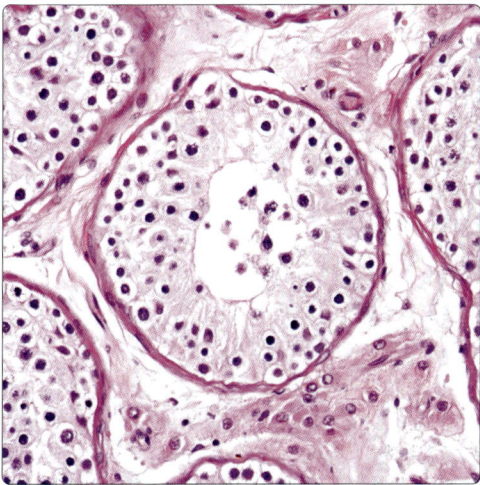

(Left) Low-power view of maturation arrest shows multiple tubules filled with spermatogonia and spermatocytes, but no spermatids or spermatozoa in most of tubules. Sertoli cells are admixed. **(Right)** Maturation arrest shows spermatogonia and spermatocytes, but no mature forms, such as spermatids or spermatozoa, are present. This condition should be differentiated from Sertoli cell-only syndrome.

Nontuberculous Infections

KEY FACTS

TERMINOLOGY
- Inflammatory process of testis or epididymis due to microorganisms (bacteria, fungus, virus, etc.)

ETIOLOGY/PATHOGENESIS
- Bacteria, virus, fungus or parasites

CLINICAL ISSUES
- Painful mass or swelling
- Fever and other systemic signs of infection
- Mumps orchitis occurs in 15-30% of adult cases but is rare before puberty
- Surgery is not indicated unless infarction occurs

MACROSCOPIC
- General enlargement of testicle
- Mass lesion with pus, hemorrhagic cut surface

MICROSCOPIC
- Variable mixed acute, chronic, or granulomatous inflammation
- Abscess formation and seminiferous tubule necrosis
- Acute bacterial orchitis causes abscesses with acute inflammation
- Syphilitic orchitis is usually granulomatous and has abundant plasma cells
- Mump orchitis characterized by interstitial edema, vascular congestion, inflammatory infiltrate consisting mainly of lymphocytes and plasma cells
- Fungal infection characterized by mixed inflammation ± necrosis

TOP DIFFERENTIAL DIAGNOSES
- Testicular trauma or torsion
- Sarcoidosis
- Seminoma or other germ cell neoplasm

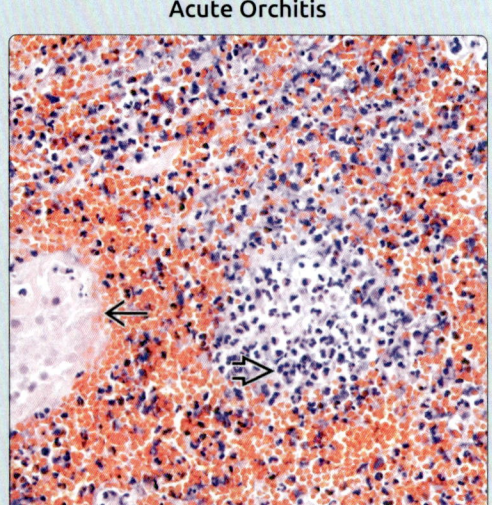
Acute Orchitis

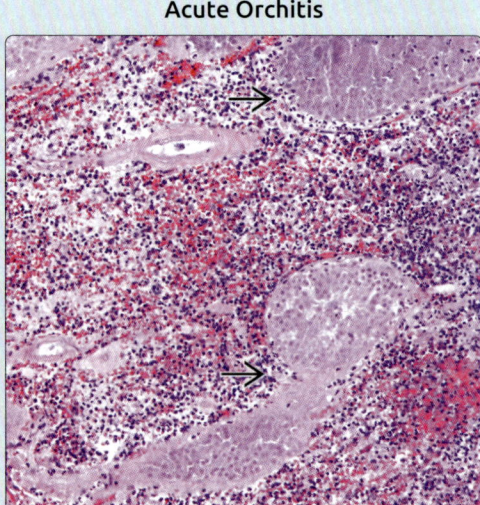
Acute Orchitis

(Left) This image shows acute bacterial orchitis with neutrophils and necrosis of seminiferous tubule ⇨. Microabscess ⇨ with numerous neutrophils and associated hemorrhage is seen in the interstitium. (Right) Interstitial acute inflammation and necrosis of seminiferous tubules ⇨ is shown. Predominantly neutrophilic infiltration is seen with extensive hemorrhage. The tubules are totally necrotic with preservation of their architecture (ghost tubules).

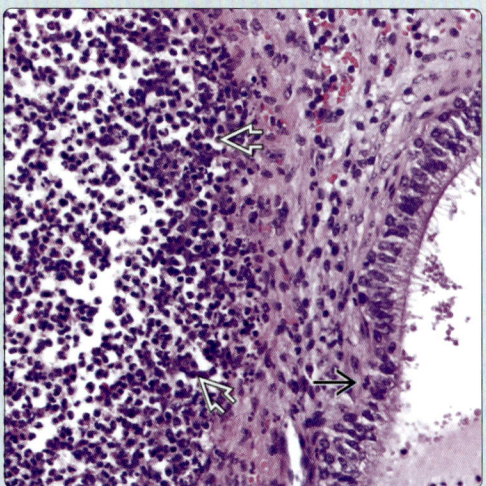
Acute Epididymitis

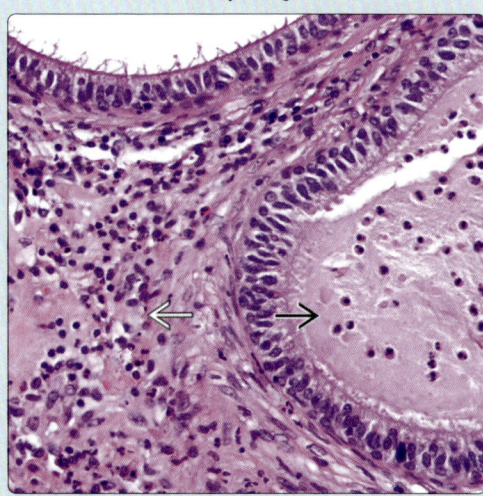
Acute Epididymitis

(Left) Acute epididymitis with abscess formation ⇨ is seen, adjacent to epididymal epithelium ⇨. There is a localized acute suppurative inflammation extending to the epididymal epithelium and stroma. (Right) Hematoxylin & eosin shows acute epididymitis with neutrophilic infiltration within the lumen of epididymal lumen ⇨ and stroma ⇨.

Nontuberculous Infections

TERMINOLOGY

Synonyms
- Orchitis, epididymitis, epididymoorchitis

Definitions
- Inflammatory process of testis or epididymis due to microorganisms (bacteria, fungus, virus, etc.)

ETIOLOGY/PATHOGENESIS

Infectious Agents
- Bacteria
  - In younger men (< 35 years), sexually transmitted bacterial pathogens are most common cause
    - *Chlamydia trachomatis* antigen is detected in 30% of cases of epididymitis and 11-35% of cases of epididymoorchitis
    - *Neisseria gonorrhoeae* is also common
  - In older men (> 35 years), urinary tract pathogens, such as *Escherichia coli*, are most common bacterial cause of epididymitis and secondary orchitis
  - Chronic orchitis with microabscesses may be due to many types of bacteria
  - Tertiary syphilis
  - *Brucella* associated with ingestion of raw milk and contact with animals
  - *Mycobacterium leprae*
  - Tuberculosis: *Mycobacterium tuberculosis*
- Virus
  - Mumps: Epididymoorchitis occurs in 15-30% of adult cases of mumps but is rare before puberty
  - Coxsackie B
  - Uncommonly: Influenza, echovirus, Epstein-Barr virus, adenovirus, and others
- Fungus
  - Fungal orchitis is rare but may be caused by Candida, Aspergillus, *Coccidioides*, *Histoplasma*, and *Cryptococcus*
- Parasites
  - Injury is secondary to vascular lesions
  - Main organisms are *Schistosoma*, filarial worms, *Leishmania*, *Toxoplasma*, *Echinococcus*, *Trichomonas*, *Entamoeba*

CLINICAL ISSUES

Presentation
- General
  - Painful mass or swelling
  - Fever and other systemic signs of infection
- Mumps orchitis occurs in 15-30% of adult cases but is rare before puberty
  - Bilateral in 15-30% of cases
  - Onset 4-8 days after parotiditis

Treatment
- Surgical approaches
  - Not indicated unless infarction occurs
- Drugs
  - Antiviral, antibiotics, antifungal, or agents against parasites

Prognosis
- With medical treatment, response is relatively good
- Pyogenic orchitis can cause testicular infarction
- May cause oligospermia, or azoospermia if bilateral

MACROSCOPIC

General Features
- General enlargement of testicle
- Mass lesion with pus, hemorrhagic cut surface

MICROSCOPIC

Histologic Features
- Variable mixed acute, chronic, or granulomatous inflammation
- Abscess formation and seminiferous tubule necrosis
- Acute bacterial orchitis causes abscesses with acute inflammation
  - Lepromatous leprosy causes granulomatous orchitis and usually has macrophages filled with acid-fast bacilli
  - Brucellosis has dense lymphohistiocytic inflammation with noncaseating granulomas
  - Chlamydia inflammation may involve urethra, epididymis, and testicular parenchyma
- Syphilitic orchitis is usually granulomatous and has abundant plasma cells
  - Interstitial inflammation with sclerotic tubules and endarteritis obliterans leading to fibrosis
  - Gummatous orchitis has well-delineated zones of necrosis with lymphocytes, plasma cells, and giant cells
- Mump orchitis characterized by interstitial edema, vascular congestion, inflammatory infiltrate consisting mainly of lymphocytes and plasma cells
- Fungal infection characterized by mixed inflammation ± necrosis

DIFFERENTIAL DIAGNOSIS

Testicular Trauma or Torsion
- History and lack of fever

Sarcoidosis
- Noncaseating granulomatous inflammation
- Special stains negative for microorganisms

Seminoma or Other Germ Cell Neoplasm
- Seminoma may have intense sarcoid-like granulomatous reaction
- Presence of tumor cells

SELECTED REFERENCES

1. Walker NA et al: Managing epididymo-orchitis in general practice. Practitioner. 257(1760):21-5, 2-3, 2013
2. Trojian TH et al: Epididymitis and orchitis: an overview. Am Fam Physician. 79(7):583-7, 2009
3. Cunningham KA et al: Male genital tract chlamydial infection: implications for pathology and infertility. Biol Reprod. 79(2):180-9, 2008
4. Hviid A et al: Mumps. Lancet. 371(9616):932-44, 2008
5. Garthwaite MA et al: The implementation of European Association of Urology guidelines in the management of acute epididymo-orchitis. Ann R Coll Surg Engl. 89(8):799-803, 2007

Nonspecific Granulomatous Orchitis

KEY FACTS

TERMINOLOGY
- Mixed chronic and granulomatous orchitis with no specific etiology

ETIOLOGY/PATHOGENESIS
- Trauma, infection, extravasated sperm, and autoimmune disease have been postulated as possible pathogenetic mechanisms

CLINICAL ISSUES
- Rare; more common in African Americans
- Range: 29-79 years old (average: 55 years old)
- Usually unilateral testicular enlargement
- May be accompanied by tenderness, fever, or heaviness
- Symptomatic control or surgical resection

MACROSCOPIC
- Unilateral, solid nodular enlargement of testis or thickened tunica layer
- Testis may be totally or partially involved

MICROSCOPIC
- Early stage: Mainly intratubular infiltration of histiocytes with destruction of predominantly germ cells, but also Sertoli cells (lesser extent)
- Late stage: Tubular destruction and atrophy with extensive fibrosis
- Intratubular aggregation of epithelioid histiocytes, plasma cells, and lymphocytes
- No well-formed granulomas or necrosis

TOP DIFFERENTIAL DIAGNOSES
- Infectious orchitis due to specific infections
- Sarcoidosis
- Seminoma
- Malignant lymphoma
- Sperm granuloma
- Malakoplakia

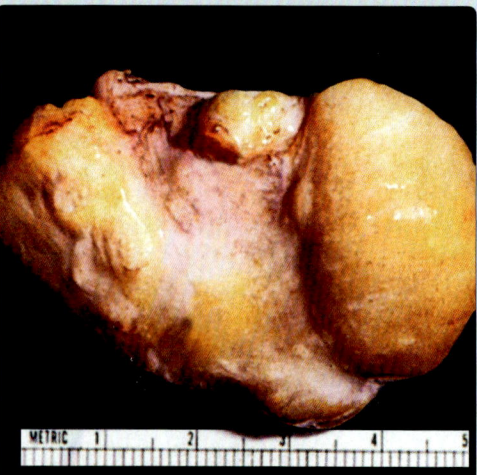

Gross Pathology

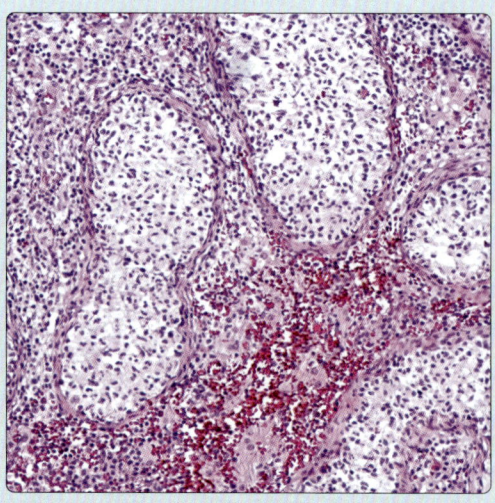

Characteristic Low Power

(Left) Nonspecific granulomatous orchitis is shown. Bivalved testis with ill-defined nodules variably involve the testis and paratestis. Due to the pseudotumorous firm consistency, malignancy is mimicked. (Right) Typical features of early stage are characterized by intratubular histiocytic infiltration with a few lymphocytes, mimicking granulomas. Special stains for microorganisms are typically negative.

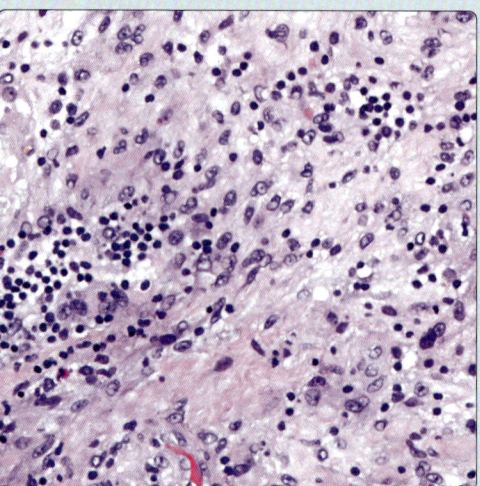

Late-Stage Disease

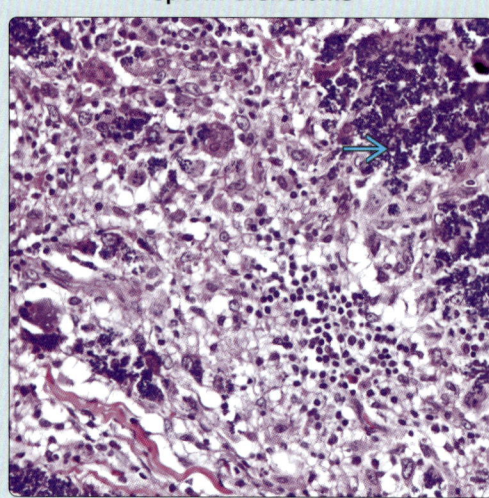

Sperm Granuloma

(Left) Late-stage nonspecific granulomatous orchitis with complete destruction of seminiferous tubules shows dense fibrosis and mixed inflammation with histiocytes and lymphocytes. (Right) This is an example of longstanding sperm granulomas with collections of histiocytes, lymphocytes, and sperm ➡.

Nonspecific Granulomatous Orchitis

TERMINOLOGY

Definitions
- Mixed chronic and granulomatous orchitis with no specific etiology; may be autoimmune or posttraumatic reaction

ETIOLOGY/PATHOGENESIS

Unknown Causes
- Trauma, infection, extravasated sperm, and autoimmune disease have been postulated as possible pathogenetic mechanisms
  - May be associated with urinary tract infection, history of prostatectomy, and inguinal hernia repair
  - Autoimmune reaction to sperm antibodies
  - Vascular compromise with ischemia or infarction
  - Share some features with IgG4-related disease

CLINICAL ISSUES

Epidemiology
- Incidence
  - Rare; more common in African Americans
- Age
  - Range: 29-79 years old (average: 55 years old)

Presentation
- Usually unilateral testicular enlargement (more common in right side) but can be bilateral
- May be accompanied by tenderness, fever, or heaviness
- Ipsilateral or contralateral hydrocele
- May be associated with gram-negative urinary tract infection

Treatment
- Symptomatic control or surgical resection
- In cases with bilateral involvement with 1 testis already removed, steroid treatment may be an option

MACROSCOPIC

General Features
- Unilateral, solid nodular enlargement of testis or thickened tunica layer
- Testis may be totally or partially involved
- Poorly defined nodules with variable, yellowish or tan-white, hard cut surface
- Epididymis and tunics may be involved concurrently

MICROSCOPIC

Histologic Features
- Early stage: Mainly intratubular infiltration of histiocytes with destruction of predominantly germ cells, but also Sertoli cells (lesser extent)
- Late stage: Tubular destruction and atrophy with extensive fibrosis
- Variable degree of intratubular aggregation of epithelioid histiocytes, plasma cells, and lymphocytes
- No well-formed granulomas or necrosis
- Giant cells and dystrophic calcification may be present
- May be associated with sperm granuloma

ANCILLARY TESTS

Histochemistry
- Gram stain: Negative
- Ziehl-Neelsen stain: Negative
- GMS (Gomori methenamine silver): Negative

DIFFERENTIAL DIAGNOSIS

Infectious Orchitis Due to Specific Infections
- Syphilis may cause granulomatous orchitis, interstitial orchitis, or gummatous orchitis
  - Abundant plasma cells and endarteritis obliterans; Warthin-Starry stain may demonstrate spirochetal organisms
- Lepromatous leprosy
  - Early stage shows perivascular lymphocytic inflammation and interstitial macrophages filled with acid-fast bacilli
  - Late stage shows tubular atrophy, clustering of Leydig cells, endarteritis obliterans, fibrosis
- Brucellosis
  - Dense lymphohistiocytic inflammation with noncaseating granulomas in interstitium
- Tuberculosis
  - Necrotizing granulomatous inflammation with Langhans giant cells due to acid-fast bacilli

Sarcoidosis
- Confluent well-formed granulomas; systemic involvement and diagnosis of exclusion

Seminoma
- Clinical history; abnormal serum tumor markers; presence of tumor cells

Malignant Lymphoma
- Predominantly interstitial infiltrative pattern of uniform lymphoma cells

Sperm Granuloma
- Presence of sperm; positive AFB stain in sperm may be misinterpreted as mycobacteria

Malakoplakia
- Presence of Michaelis-Gutmann bodies (may be highlighted by von Kossa or iron stains)

SELECTED REFERENCES

1. Karram S et al: Idiopathic granulomatous orchitis: morphology and evaluation of its relationship to IgG4 related disease. Hum Pathol. 45(4):844-50, 2014
2. Dhand S et al: Idiopathic granulomatous orchitis. J Urol. 186(4):1477-8, 2011
3. Roy S et al: Idiopathic granulomatous orchitis. Pathol Res Pract. 207(5):275-8, 2011
4. Varma R et al: Acute syphilitic interstitial orchitis mimicking testicular malignancy in an HIV-1 infected man diagnosed by Treponema pallidum polymerase chain reaction. Int J STD AIDS. 20(1):65-6, 2009
5. Wegner HE et al: Granulomatous orchitis--an analysis of clinical presentation, pathological anatomic features and possible etiologic factors. Eur Urol. 26(1):56-60, 1994
6. Perimenis P et al: Idiopathic granulomatous orchitis. Eur Urol. 19(2):118-20, 1991
7. Sporer A et al: Granulomatous orchitis. Urology. 19(3):319-21, 1982
8. Kahn RI et al: Granulomatous disease of the testis. J Urol. 123(6):868-71, 1980

Tuberculous Epididymo-Orchitis

KEY FACTS

TERMINOLOGY
- Infection of testis and epididymis due to *Mycobacterium tuberculosis*

ETIOLOGY/PATHOGENESIS
- *Mycobacterium tuberculosis*
- Most tuberculous epididymo-orchitis are associated with other genitourinary tract involvement

CLINICAL ISSUES
- Affects any age but mainly adults (> 72% are older than 35 years)
- Mild testicular enlargement and scrotal pain

MACROSCOPIC
- Epididymis is almost always primary site of involvement with secondary spread to testis
- Irregular mass with foci of caseating necrosis

MICROSCOPIC
- Multiple granulomas with central caseating necrosis
- Aggregates of epithelioid cells with peripheral rim of lymphocytes
- Destruction of epididymis, seminiferous tubules, and interstitium by necrotizing (caseating necrosis) or nonnecrotizing granulomatous inflammation
- Langhans giant cells may be present
- Late stage with fibroblastic response with scar formation

ANCILLARY TESTS
- Acid-fast bacteria stain positive

TOP DIFFERENTIAL DIAGNOSES
- Nonspecific granulomatous orchitis
- Seminoma with extensive granulomatous inflammation
- Malakoplakia
- Sperm granuloma
- Other infectious granulomatous epididymo-orchitis

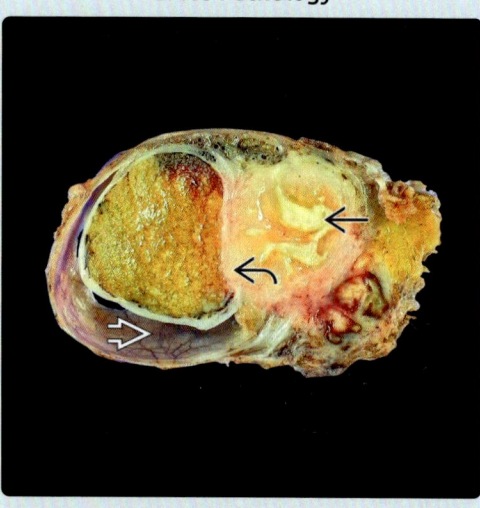

Gross Pathology

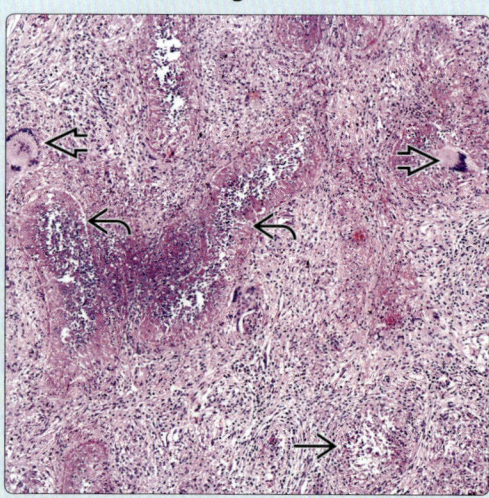

Necrotizing Granulomas

(Left) *Gross photo shows tuberculous epididymo-orchitis with predominant involvement of the epididymis with focal extension into the testis ⮕. Large areas of geographic necrosis ⮕ are present. There is a secondary hydrocele ⮕.* (Right) *This image shows testicular tuberculosis with nonnecrotizing granulomas ⮕, multinucleated Langhans giant cells ⮕, and necrotizing granulomas destroying the seminiferous tubules ⮕. In contrast, the inflammatory infiltrate in nonspecific granulomatous orchitis is intratubular.*

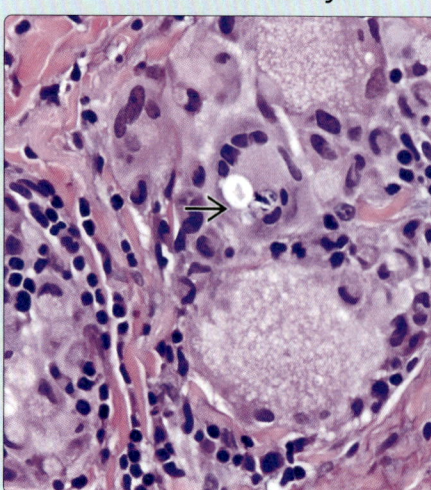

Schaumann Body

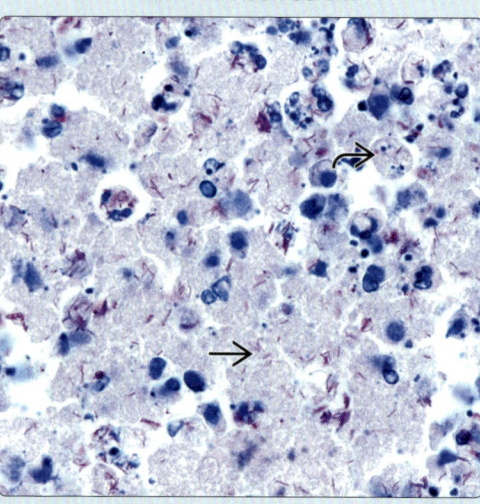

Ziehl-Neelsen Strain

(Left) *High-power photomicrograph shows a basophilic, shell-like structure (Schaumann body) ⮕ in the cytoplasm of multinucleated giant cells of a granuloma. This finding is not specific for tuberculosis and may occur in most other types of granulomatous disease.* (Right) *Ziehl-Neelsen technique shows acid-fast bacilli within the necrotic debris ⮕ and in histiocytes ⮕. Correlation with microbiology cultures is essential for speciating the type of tuberculous infection.*

Tuberculous Epididymo-Orchitis

TERMINOLOGY

Definitions
- Infection of testis and epididymis due to *Mycobacterium tuberculosis*

ETIOLOGY/PATHOGENESIS

Infectious Agents
- *M. tuberculosis*
- Most cases of tuberculous epididymo-orchitis are associated with other sites genitourinary tract involvement
- In adults, almost all are result of tuberculous prostatitis
- In children, > 1/2 of patients have advanced pulmonary tuberculosis and miliary spread

CLINICAL ISSUES

Epidemiology
- Incidence
  - High in developing countries, immigrants, and immunocompromised patients
  - May be late manifestation of intravesical Bacillus Calmette-Guérin (BCG) therapy
- Age
  - Affects any age but mainly adults (> 72% are older than 35 yr)

Presentation
- Mild testicular enlargement and scrotal pain
- Associated with other constitutional symptoms of tuberculous infection
- Commonly associated with tuberculosis of lung and other genitourinary tracts
- Bilateral involvement (30%), formation of abscess or sinus tract (50%), or secondary hydrocele (30%)

Treatment
- Surgical resection and systemic antituberculous therapy

Prognosis
- Excellent with modern antituberculous treatment

IMAGING

General Features
- Nonspecific heterogeneous or homogeneous mass of epididymis or testis on ultrasonography

MACROSCOPIC

General Features
- Epididymis is almost always primary site of involvement with secondary spread to testis
- Irregular mass with foci of caseating necrosis
- When testis is involved, swollen and nodular
- Late stages: Extensive cystic change due to necrosis

MICROSCOPIC

Histologic Features
- Destruction of epididymis/seminiferous tubules with caseating or noncaseating granulomatous inflammation
- Multiple confluent granulomas with central caseating necrosis
- Aggregates of epithelioid cells with peripheral rim of lymphocytes
- Langhans giant cells (fusion of epithelioid cells with nuclei arranged in horseshoe-shaped pattern, often pointing toward necrosis)
- Schaumann (basophilic, shell-like, lamellated calcified conchoidal bodies) and asteroid bodies may be present
- Late stage with fibroblastic response with scar formation

ANCILLARY TESTS

Histochemistry
- Ziehl-Neelsen (acid-fast bacillus): Positive

DIFFERENTIAL DIAGNOSIS

Nonspecific Granulomatous Orchitis
- Lack of necrosis or well-formed granuloma
- Predominantly intratubular location of granulomas
- Special stains negative for microorganisms; caution requires false-positive due to sperm staining with AFB

Seminoma With Extensive Granulomatous Inflammation
- Presence of large tumor cells
- Large cells positive for PLAP, CD117, podoplanin (D2-40), SAL4, and OCT3/OCT4
- Serum tumor markers (LDH and HCG) may be elevated (but not for AFP)

Malakoplakia
- Diffuse infiltrate of macrophages with granular eosinophilic cytoplasm; well-formed granulomas absent
- Presence of typical Michaelis-Gutmann bodies and von Hansemann cells

Sperm Granuloma
- History of vasectomy is common
- Granulomatous inflammation with sperms

Other Infectious Granulomatous Epididymo-Orchitis
- Caused by fungi and parasites
- Organisms may be visualized with GMS or PAS stains

SELECTED REFERENCES

1. Shenoy VP et al: Isolated tuberculous epididymo-orchitis: an unusual presentation of tuberculosis. J Infect Dev Ctries. 6(1):92-4, 2012
2. Harving SS et al: Granulomatous epididymo-orchitis, a rare complication of intravesical bacillus Calmette-Guérin therapy for urothelial cancer. Scand J Urol Nephrol. 43(4):331-3, 2009
3. Jacob JT et al: Male genital tuberculosis. Lancet Infect Dis. 8(5):335-42, 2008
4. Wise GJ et al: An update on lower urinary tract tuberculosis. Curr Urol Rep. 9(4):305-13, 2008
5. Ramdial PK et al: Tuberculids as sentinel lesions of tuberculous epididymo-orchitis. J Cutan Pathol. 34(11):830-6, 2007
6. Muttarak M et al: Tuberculous epididymitis and epididymo-orchitis: sonographic appearances. AJR Am J Roentgenol. 176(6):1459-66, 2001
7. Chung JJ et al: Sonographic findings in tuberculous epididymitis and epididymo-orchitis. J Clin Ultrasound. 25(7):390-4, 1997

General Concepts, Germ Cell Tumors

TERMINOLOGY

Synonyms
- Germ cell tumor (GCT), seminoma, nonseminomatous germ cell tumor (NSGCT), mixed germ cell tumor (MGCT)

Definitions
- Diverse group of tumors arising from totipotential germ cells with embryonic or extraembryonic differentiation

EPIDEMIOLOGY

Age Range
- Most GCTs occur between 20-50 yr of age with peak incidence at 30 yr
- Seminoma occurs at age ranging 35-45 yr
- NSGCTs occur at age ranging 25-35 yr (10 years younger than seminoma)

Ethnicity Relationship
- Incidence is higher in Western and Northern Europe, Australia/New Zealand, and North America (5.4-7.9 per 100,000)
- Incidence is lower in Africa, Caribbean, and Asia (2 per 100,000)

Incidence
- Estimated 8,430 new cases and 380 deaths from testicular cancer in USA in 2015
- ~ 49,000 new cases and 9,000 deaths each yr worldwide (2002 data)
- Worldwide incidence has more than doubled in last 40 yr

Natural History
- Germ cell neoplasia in situ (GCNIS) is precursor to most GCTs except for spermatocytic tumor and infantile germ cell tumors
- NSGCTs are more likely than seminomas to present with metastasis
- Choriocarcinoma often presents with early hematogenous spread to lung, liver, and bone
  - May present with choriocarcinoma syndrome (hemorrhagic cannonball metastasis)
- Metastasis of GCTs occurs in stepwise pattern of lymphatic spread through testicular mediastinum to retroperitoneal lymph nodes

ETIOLOGY/PATHOGENESIS

Histogenesis
- Exact causes of GCT are not completely understood
- No known genetic abnormalities are found in most patients with GCT
- Estimated 25% of GCTs may have genetic susceptibility

Cytogenetic Changes
- GCTs arising in prepubertal gonads (teratoma and yolk sac tumor) are usually diploid
- GCTs in postpubertal men typically have 1 or more copies of chromosome 12p [most commonly i(12p)] and other forms of 12p abnormalities and aneuploidy
- ~ 80% of GCTs have at least 1 isochromosome 12 [i(12p)]
- Other genetic changes in postpubertal men include loss of chromosome 11, 13, 18, and Y, and gains of 7, 8, and X
- Spermatocytic tumor may be either diploid or aneuploid and may show loss of chromosome 9

Risk Factors
- Prior history of GCT
- Positive family history of GCT
- Cryptorchidism
- Testicular dysgenesis
- Klinefelter syndrome
- Infertility

CLINICAL IMPLICATIONS

Clinical Presentation
- Often unilateral painless testicular swelling or mass (bilaterality is rare: < 2%)
- Gynecomastia or exophthalmos may be presenting symptom [related to human chorionic gonadotropin (hCG) production]

Testis and Paratestis

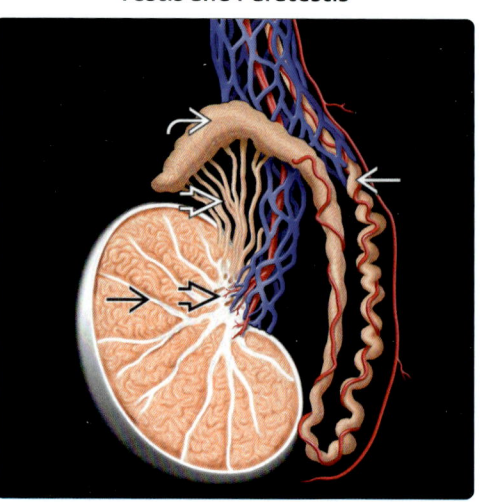

Seminiferous Tubule

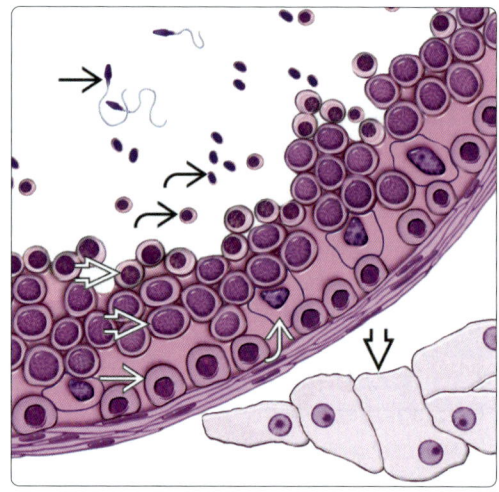

(Left) Schematic diagram of testis and paratestis is shown. The testicular parenchyma is separated by fibrous septa ➡. The tubules converge and exit to the rete testis ➡, efferent ducts ➡, epididymis ➡, and vas deferens ➡. *(Right)* Schematic diagram shows seminiferous tubule with spermatogenesis (spermatogonia ➡, spermatocytes ➡, spermatids ➡, spermatozoa ➡). Sertoli cells ➡ and Leydig cells ➡ are also shown.

General Concepts, Germ Cell Tumors

- ~ 10% may present with symptoms related to metastasis at initial presentation
- Elevation of serum tumor markers, including lactate dehydrogenase (LDH), α-fetoprotein (AFP), hCG

Laboratory Tests
- Elevated serum AFP usually seen in yolk sac tumor
- Highly elevated serum hCG suggests choriocarcinoma; borderline hCG elevation is not uncommon in seminoma and in other GCTs with syncytiotrophoblasts
- Serum levels of LDH, AFP, and hCG are incorporated into TNM stage, anatomic stage/prognostic groups

Treatment
- Treatment options depend on whether tumor is seminoma or NSGCT and TNM stage
  - Stage I seminoma
    - Radical inguinal orchiectomy followed by surveillance protocol (serum markers, chest radiographs, and CT scan), or single-dose carboplatin adjuvant therapy/radiation therapy
  - Stage I NSGCT
    - Radical inguinal orchiectomy followed by either surveillance or retroperitoneal lymph node dissection (RPLND) for stage IA tumor
    - Radical inguinal orchiectomy followed by either nerve-sparing RPLND or adjuvant chemotherapy for stage IB tumor
  - Stage II seminoma
    - Radical inguinal orchiectomy followed by radiation (low-volume disease) or adjuvant chemotherapy
  - Stage II NSGCT
    - Radical inguinal orchiectomy followed by RPLND, RPLND and chemotherapy, or chemotherapy and delayed RPLND
  - Stage III seminoma or NSGCT
    - Radical inguinal orchiectomy followed by multidrug chemotherapy

Prognosis
- Depends on histologic type, stage, and treatment
- Most types have favorable prognosis and respond well to chemotherapy &/or radiation therapy, as appropriate for tumor type
- Overall 95% survival rate in USA
- Morphologic prognostic factors
  - Lymphovascular invasion (pathologic stage at least pT2)
  - Proportion of embryonal carcinoma (> 80% poor prognosis)
  - Proportion of teratoma component (> 50% favorable prognosis)
  - Others: Tumor size (> 4 cm) and rete testis invasion (for seminoma)

Imaging Findings
- General Features
  - Testicular ultrasound may detect testicular mass
  - Abdominopelvic CT scan may detect retroperitoneal lymph node metastasis
  - Chest radiograph and CT scan may detect lung metastasis
  - MR may detect metastasis to bone and brain

MACROSCOPIC

Anatomic Features
- Testes are paired ovoid organ with average weight of 15-19 g and dimension of 2 x 3 x 4 cm
- Surrounded by thick capsule composed of 3 layers: Tunica vaginalis (outer layer), albuginea (middle), and vasculosa (inner)
- Posterior mediastinum contains blood vessels, lymphatics, and rete testis
- Fibrous septa divide testis into ~ 250 lobules: Seminiferous tubules and interstitium
- GCTs replace normal structures and present with either tumoral (common) or interstitial pattern

General Features
- Testicular mass with variable appearance depending on histologic type and component

Specimen Handling
- Radical Resection
  - Orient specimen and ink appropriately, if necessary
  - Procure spermatic cord margin before specimen is opened/bivalved; prevents tumor carry over
  - Bivalve the testis
  - Submit tumor entirely if small (< 2 cm)
  - For large tumors, at least 1 section per cm tumor
    - Sections to include areas with different appearances
    - Sections to include hemorrhagic and necrotic areas (usually high-grade component is present, such as embryonal carcinoma or choriocarcinoma)
    - More sections may be required in pure seminoma to rule out other germ cell components, especially if there are areas of hemorrhage and necrosis or serum AFP levels are elevated
    - Sections to include rete testis and epididymis
    - Sections to include uninvolved testicular parenchyma adjacent to tumor
    - At least 1 section of uninvolved testicular parenchyma away from tumor
- Subtotal Resection
  - Orient specimen and ink resection margins appropriately
  - Perpendicular section of tumor with margin for possible frozen section for margin and diagnosis
  - Sections usually include entire tumor
  - Section to include uninvolved testicular parenchyma

MICROSCOPIC

Normal Anatomy and Histology
- Histologic compartments of testis
  - Testis is composed of seminiferous tubules and interstitium
- Seminiferous tubules and spermatogenesis
  - Composed of Sertoli cells and germ cells in varying stages of differentiation or maturation
  - Germ cells mature from base to center of lumen and are divided into different stages based on their levels of maturation

General Concepts, Germ Cell Tumors

- Spermatogonia: Situated adjacent to basement membrane; small, round, dense nuclei with finely granular and vesicular chromatin and small nucleolus, clear or basophilic cytoplasm
- Primary spermatocytes: More centrally located; largest cell type; variable nuclear appearance, clumped chromatin (spireme type), beaded cytoplasm
- Secondary spermatocytes: More centrally located; smaller and fewer than primary spermatocytes; coarsely granular chromatin; no nucleoli
- Spermatids: Located near lumen; small cells with darkly stained chromatin
- Spermatozoa: Located in lumen; elongated eccentric nucleus with long cytoplasmic tail
  - Sertoli cells: Elongated pyramidal cells attached to basal lamina (10-12 Sertoli cells/tubules; germ cells: Sertoli cells ~ 13:1)
- Interstitium is divided into intertubular and peritubular regions
  - Peritubular region contains basement membrane and thin lamina propria
  - Intertubular interstitium contains blood vessels, lymphatics, nerve, and Leydig cells

General Features

- WHO Histologic Classification of Testicular Germ Cell Tumors
  - Germ cell tumors derived from germ cell neoplasia in situ (GCNIS)
    - Tumor of 1 histologic type (pure forms)
      - Seminomatous tumor: Classic seminoma
      - Nonseminomatous germ cell tumor: Embryonal carcinoma, postpubertal-type yolk sac tumor, trophoblastic tumors (choriocarcinoma and nonchoriocarcinomatous tumors), postpubertal-type teratoma, and teratoma with somatic-type malignancies
    - Nonseminomatous germ cell tumors of more than 1 histologic type
      - Mixed germ cell tumor
      - Regressed germ cell tumor
  - Germ cell tumors unrelated to germ cell neoplasia in situ (GCNIS)
    - Spermatocytic tumor
    - Prepubertal-type teratoma (dermoid cyst, epidermoid cyst, carcinoid tumor)
    - Prepubertal type mixed teratoma

Cytologic Features

- Seminoma: Evenly spaced, large, uniform cells with no nuclear overlapping and distinct cell borders
- Embryonal carcinoma: Pleomorphic and anaplastic cells, nuclear overlapping and indistinct cell borders, prominent nucleoli, multiple nucleoli, and nucleolar pleomorphism are frequent
- Yolk sac tumor: Cuboidal to flattened cells with indistinct cell borders, cytoplasmic vacuoles, and eosinophilic globules; polymorphic tumor cell population from epithelial-appearing to spindled basement membrane material deposition, Schiller-Duval bodies
- Choriocarcinoma
  - 2 cell types: Large multinucleated cells with dense eosinophilic cytoplasm (syncytiotrophoblasts) and mononuclear cells with pale or clear cytoplasm (cytotrophoblasts) in hemorrhagic/necrotic background
- Teratoma: Multiple different types of tissues and cells

Predominant Pattern

- Tumoral/solid pattern (well- or ill-defined tumor mass)
  - Tumoral/solid pattern forms mass with replacement of seminiferous tubules and interstitium
  - Hemorrhage and necrosis are not uncommon, particularly in NSGCTs
  - Entities typically displaying tumoral/solid pattern
    - Seminoma, NSGCTs, sex cord-stromal tumor
- Interstitial pattern
  - Tumor cells infiltrate interstitium with relative preservation of seminiferous tubules
  - Distinct tumor nodule may not be grossly apparent
  - Entities typically displaying interstitial pattern
    - Intertubular seminoma, lymphoma, plasmacytoma and leukemia, metastatic carcinoma; infectious and inflammatory processes are also interstitial
- Intratubular pattern
  - Lesions predominantly seen within seminiferous tubules with relative preservation of interstitium
  - Distinct tumor nodule may not be seen grossly
  - Lesions typically with intratubular pattern
    - GCNIS or intratubular extension of germ cell tumor (e.g., intratubular seminoma, embryonal carcinoma, spermatocytic tumor, etc.)
    - Intratubular extension of lymphoma, metastatic carcinoma, or idiopathic granulomatous orchitis

IMMUNOHISTOCHEMISTRY

Placenta-Like Alkaline Phosphatase

- 120 kd membrane-bound enzyme present in placental syncytiotrophoblastic cells, germ cell tumors, and tumors of other tissue
- Positive in all germ cell tumors (seminoma, EC, YST, choriocarcinoma)
- Clinical utility has diminished due to availability of more specific and sensitive markers

α-Fetoprotein

- Fetal protein produced by fetal yolk sac and resembles albumin
- Positive in YST, variable in EC

Human Chorionic Gonadotropin

- Hormone (glycoprotein) produced by the syncytiotrophoblast
- Positive in choriocarcinoma

CD30 (BerH2)

- Member of tumor necrosis factor receptor superfamily limited to immune cells, decidual tissue, and human embryonal carcinoma
- Positive in embryonal carcinoma (membranous stain); may be focally positive in seminoma

General Concepts, Germ Cell Tumors

Human Placental Lactogen
- 22 kd cytoplasmic protein with homology to growth hormone
- Positive in choriocarcinoma (syncytiotrophoblastic cells) and placental site trophoblastic tumor

OCT3/OCT4
- POU-domain, octamer-binding transcription factor in neoplastic germ cells with pluripotent potential
- Positive in GCNIS, seminoma, and embryonal carcinoma (negative in spermatocytic tumor, yolk sac tumor, and choriocarcinoma)

SALL4
- Zinc finger transcription factor in human embryonic stem cells
- Positive in all germ cell tumors (seminoma, YST, EC, choriocarcinoma, and immature teratoma)

CD117
- Receptor tyrosine kinase important for proliferation, survival, and differentiation of primordial germ cells
- Positive in GCNIS, seminoma, and spermatocytic tumor

Glypican-3
- Heparin sulfate proteoglycan involving embryonic cell growth and differentiation
- Positive in YST, syncytiotrophoblasts, and immature teratoma

Podoplanin (D2-40)
- Monoclonal antibody against oncofetal membrane antigen (M2A) present in fetal germ cells, lymphatic endothelial cells, and mesothelial cells
- Positive for seminoma (diffuse membranous), GCNIS, and some EC (focal apical membrane)

SOX2
- Transcription factor expressed in embryonic stem cells
- Positive in embryonal carcinoma (nuclear)

SOX17
- Nuclear transcription factor (member of SOX family) involving embryonic development
- Positive for seminoma

LIN28
- miRNA binding protein that promotes proliferation and induces pluripotency
- Positive for all germ cell tumors (similar to SALL4)

NANOG
- Homeobox DNA binding transcription factor involving differentiation of embryonic stem cells
- Positive in GCNIS, seminoma, and embryonal carcinoma

REPORTING CRITERIA
Key Elements
- Histologic type (seminoma vs. NSGCT)
- For germ cell tumors, report whether tumor is pure or mixed
- For mixed germ cell tumors, report percentage of each germ cell tumor component, beginning with predominant type, including seminoma
- Lymphovascular invasion (should state even in cases with no vascular invasion)
- Tumor size and rete testis interstitial invasion
- Presence of GCNIS
- Presence of syncytiotrophoblasts
- Margin status
- Involvement of adjacent structures

TNM TUMOR STAGING
Primary Tumor (pT)
- pTX: Primary tumor cannot be assessed
- pT0: No evidence of primary tumor (e.g., histologic scar in testis)
- pTis: Germ cell neoplasia in situ
- pT1
  - Tumor limited to testis and epididymis without vascular/lymphatic invasion
  - Tumor may invade into tunica albuginea but not tunica vaginalis
- pT2
  - Tumor limited to testis and epididymis with vascular/lymphatic invasion or
  - Tumor extends through tunica albuginea with involvement of tunica vaginalis
- pT3: Tumor invades spermatic cord ± vascular/lymphatic invasion
- pT4: Tumor invades scrotum ± vascular/lymphatic invasion

Regional Lymph Node (pN)
- pNX: Regional lymph nodes cannot be assessed
- pN0: No regional lymph node metastasis
- pN1: Metastasis with lymph node mass ≤ 2 cm in greatest dimension; or multiple lymph nodes (≤ 5 lymph nodes), none > 2 cm in greatest dimension
- pN2: Metastasis with a lymph node mass, > 2 cm but ≤ 5 cm in greatest dimension; or > 5 lymph nodes, any 1 mass > 2 cm but ≤ 5 cm in greatest dimension; extranodal extension present
- pN3: Metastasis with a lymph node (nodes) mass > 5 cm in greatest dimension

Distant Metastasis (M)
- MX: Distant metastasis cannot be assessed
- M0: No distant metastasis
- M1a: Nonregional nodal or pulmonary metastasis
- M1b: Distant metastasis other than to nonregional lymph nodes and lungs

Serum Tumor Markers (S) (Postorchiectomy)
- SX: Marker studies not available or not performed
- S0: Marker study levels within normal limits
- S1: LDH < 1.5x upper normal limit and hCG < 5,000 mIu/mL and AFP < 1,000 ng/mL
- S2: LDH < 1.5-10x normal upper limit or hCG 5,000-50,000 mIu/mL or AFP < 1,000 ng/mL
- S3: LDH > 10x normal upper limit or hCG > 50,000 mIu/mL or AFP > 10,000 ng/mL

Differential Histologic Features of Pure Malignant Germ Cell Neoplasms

	Classic Seminoma	Spermatocytic Tumor	Embryonal Carcinoma	Yolk Sac Tumor	Choriocarcinoma
Growth pattern	Diffuse	Diffuse	Solid, glandular, papillary	Multiple patterns	Nodular
Lobular arrangement	Present	Uncommon	Variable	Absent	Variable
Fibrovascular septa	Present	Absent	Variable	Absent	Absent
Lymphocytes	Present	Absent	Variable	Variable	Absent
Granulomas	Present	Absent	Rare	Rare	Absent
Tumor cell nucleus	Polygonal/round	Polymorphous (3 cell types)	Very pleomorphic	Pleomorphic	2 cell populations
Nuclear chromatin	Fine	Variable	Coarse, vesicular	Fine	Variable
Nucleolus	Large, regular	Variable	Large, irregular, multiple	Usually small	Variable
Mitoses	Frequent	Infrequent	Brisk	Infrequent	Variable
Tumor cell spacing	Evenly spaced	Evenly spaced	Overlapping	Overlapping, variable	Overlapping
Cell boundary	Distinct	Indistinct	Indistinct	Variable	Distinct
Cytoplasm	Abundant, clear	Scant, dense acidophilic	Amphophilic	Variable	Variable
Specific cytoplasmic content	Glycogen	N/A	N/A	Eosinophilic globules	N/A

SELECTED REFERENCES

1. Berney DM et al: Handling and reporting of orchidectomy specimens with testicular cancer: areas of consensus and variation among 25 experts and 225 European pathologists. Histopathology. 67(3):313-24, 2015
2. Motzer RJ et al: Testicular Cancer, Version 2.2015. J Natl Compr Canc Netw. 13(6):772-99, 2015
3. Siegel RL et al: Cancer statistics, 2015. CA Cancer J Clin. 65(1):5-29, 2015
4. Ulbright TM et al: Best practices recommendations in the application of immunohistochemistry in testicular tumors: report from the International Society of Urological Pathology consensus conference. Am J Surg Pathol. 38(8):e50-9, 2014
5. Cao D et al: SALL4 is a novel sensitive and specific marker for metastatic germ cell tumors, with particular utility in detection of metastatic yolk sac tumors. Cancer. 115(12):2640-51, 2009
6. Gopalan A et al: Testicular mixed germ cell tumors: a morphological and immunohistochemical study using stem cell markers, OCT3/4, SOX2 and GDF3, with emphasis on morphologically difficult-to-classify areas. Mod Pathol. 22(8):1066-74, 2009
7. Jemal A et al: Cancer statistics, 2009. CA Cancer J Clin. 59(4):225-49, 2009
8. Large MC et al: Retroperitoneal lymph node dissection: reassessment of modified templates. BJU Int. 104(9 Pt B):1369-75, 2009
9. Looijenga LH: Human testicular (non)seminomatous germ cell tumours: the clinical implications of recent pathobiological insights. J Pathol. 218(2):146-62, 2009
10. Mai PL et al: The International Testicular Cancer Linkage Consortium: A clinicopathologic descriptive analysis of 461 familial malignant testicular germ cell tumor kindred. Urol Oncol. 28(5):492-9, 2009
11. Tarin TV et al: Estimating the risk of cancer associated with imaging related radiation during surveillance for stage I testicular cancer using computerized tomography. J Urol. 181(2):627-32; discussion 632-3, 2009
12. Westermann DH et al: High-risk clinical stage I nonseminomatous germ cell tumors: the case for chemotherapy. World J Urol. 27(4):455-61, 2009
13. de Jong J et al: Differential expression of SOX17 and SOX2 in germ cells and stem cells has biological and clinical implications. J Pathol. 215(1):21-30, 2008
14. Fléchon A et al: Management of advanced germ-cell tumors of the testis. Nat Clin Pract Urol. 5(5):262-76, 2008
15. Heidenreich A et al: Postchemotherapy retroperitoneal lymph node dissection in advanced germ cell tumours of the testis. Eur Urol. 53(2):260-72, 2008
16. Hersmus R et al: New insights into type II germ cell tumor pathogenesis based on studies of patients with various forms of disorders of sex development (DSD). Mol Cell Endocrinol. 291(1-2):1-10, 2008
17. Ponti G et al: The impact of histopathologic diagnosis on the proper management of testis neoplasms. Nat Clin Pract Oncol. 5(10):619-22, 2008
18. Taskinen S et al: Testicular tumors in children and adolescents. J Pediatr Urol. 4(2):134-7, 2008
19. Ulbright TM: The most common, clinically significant misdiagnoses in testicular tumor pathology, and how to avoid them. Adv Anat Pathol. 15(1):18-27, 2008
20. Young RH: Testicular tumors--some new and a few perennial problems. Arch Pathol Lab Med. 132(4):548-64, 2008
21. Emerson RE et al: Morphological approach to tumours of the testis and paratestis. J Clin Pathol. 60(8):866-80, 2007
22. Karellas ME et al: ITGCN of the testis, contralateral testicular biopsy and bilateral testicular cancer. Urol Clin North Am. 34(2):119-25; abstract vii, 2007
23. Looijenga LH et al: Chromosomes and expression in human testicular germ-cell tumors: insight into their cell of origin and pathogenesis. Ann N Y Acad Sci. 1120:187-214, 2007
24. Rajpert-de Meyts E et al: From gonocytes to testicular cancer: the role of impaired gonadal development. Ann N Y Acad Sci. 1120:168-80, 2007
25. del Vecchio MT et al: Intratubular germ cell neoplasia of unclassified type. Anal Quant Cytol Histol. 28(3):157-70, 2006
26. Carver BS et al: Germ cell tumors of the testis. Ann Surg Oncol. 12(11):871-80, 2005
27. di Pietro A et al: Testicular germ cell tumours: the paradigm of chemo-sensitive solid tumours. Int J Biochem Cell Biol. 37(12):2437-56, 2005
28. Emerson RE et al: The use of immunohistochemistry in the differential diagnosis of tumors of the testis and paratestis. Semin Diagn Pathol. 22(1):33-50, 2005
29. Hentrich M et al: Management and outcome of bilateral testicular germ cell tumors: Twenty-five year experience in Munich. Acta Oncol. 44(6):529-36, 2005
30. Hoei-Hansen CE et al: Carcinoma in situ testis, the progenitor of testicular germ cell tumours: a clinical review. Ann Oncol. 16(6):863-8, 2005
31. Parkin DM et al: Global cancer statistics, 2002. CA Cancer J Clin. 55(2):74-108, 2005
32. Ulbright TM: Germ cell tumors of the gonads: a selective review emphasizing problems in differential diagnosis, newly appreciated, and controversial issues. Mod Pathol. 18 Suppl 2:S61-79, 2005
33. Dieckmann KP et al: Clinical epidemiology of testicular germ cell tumors. World J Urol. 22(1):2-14, 2004
34. Honecker F et al: New insights into the pathology and molecular biology of human germ cell tumors. World J Urol. 22(1):15-24, 2004
35. Czene K et al: Environmental and heritable causes of cancer among 9.6 million individuals in the Swedish Family-Cancer Database. Int J Cancer. 99(2):260-6, 2002

General Concepts, Germ Cell Tumors

Seminiferous Tubules, Normal
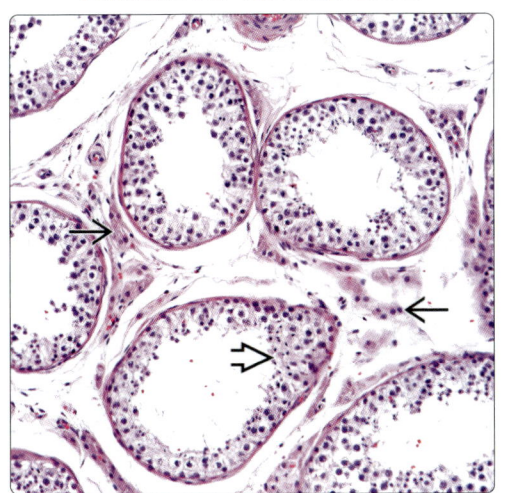

Normal Spermatogenesis
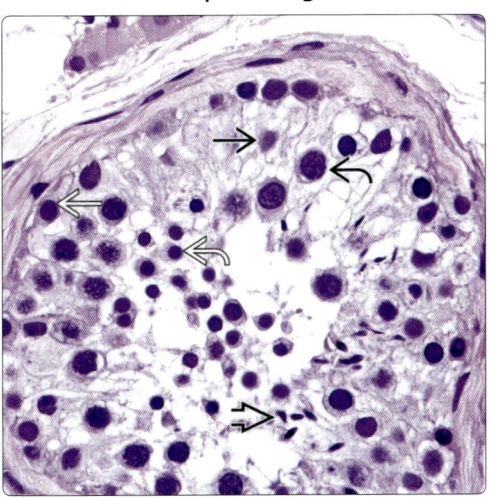

(Left) Low-power view of the testis shows seminiferous tubules with spermatogenesis ⇒ and the interstitium. The tubules are surrounded by a delicate basement membrane and a thin lamina propria. Scattered Leydig cells ⇒ are present within the interstitium. *(Right)* High-power view shows different stages of germ cells (spermatogonia ⇒, primary spermatocytes ⇒, spermatids ⇒, and spermatozoans ⇒) and Sertoli cell ⇒ within seminiferous tubule.

Seminoma
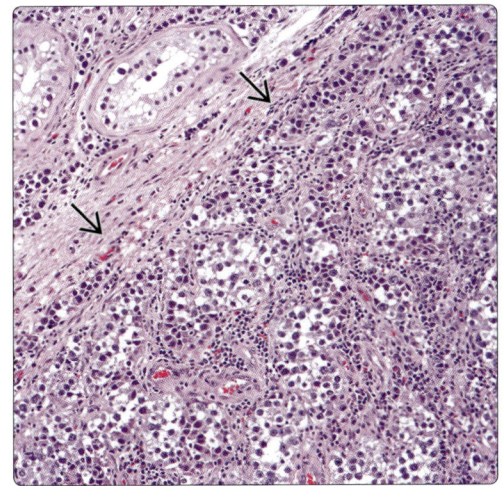

Embryonal Carcinoma
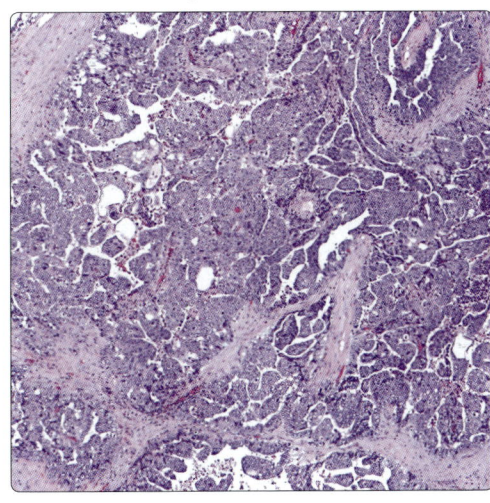

(Left) Testicular pathology may be approached as solid (tumoral), interstitial, and tubular patterns. This image shows the solid pattern ⇒ of seminoma forming a nodule with total effacement of seminiferous tubules. Adjacent to the tumor, the tubules and interstitium are discernible. *(Right)* H&E shows solid (tumoral) growth in embryonal carcinoma (EC). The tumor completely replaces the normal seminiferous tubules and interstitium. The papillary growth pattern and marked nuclear atypia in this case are diagnostic of EC.

Spermatocytic Tumor
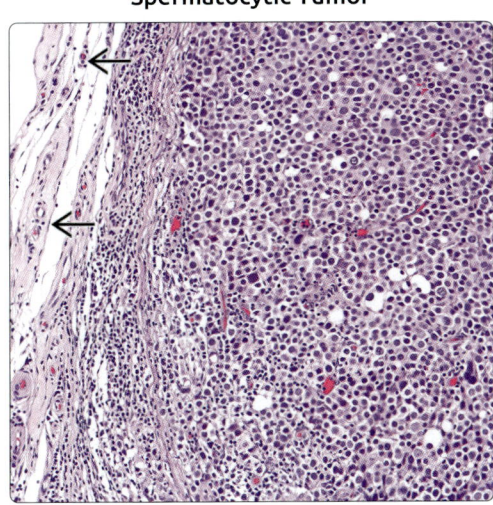

Seminoma: Interstitial Growth
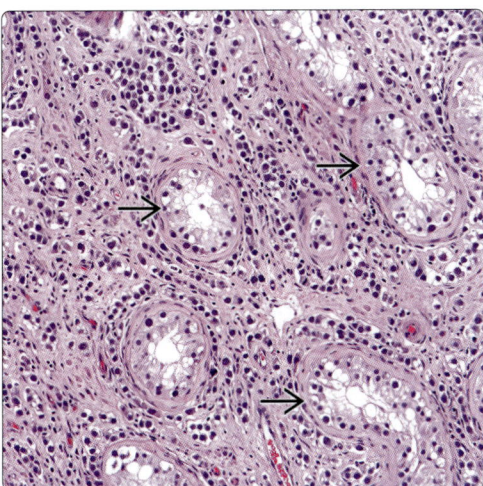

(Left) H&E shows solid (tumoral) pattern of spermatocytic tumor. Spermatocytic tumor cells replace the seminiferous tubules and interstitium, forming a well-circumscribed mass from the surrounding atrophic testis parenchyma ⇒. *(Right)* H&E shows interstitial growth pattern of seminoma. The tumor cells infiltrate the interstitium with architectural preservation of the seminiferous tubules ⇒ and interstitium. If this is the sole pattern, grossly, the tumor may not be evident.

General Concepts, Germ Cell Tumors

Malignant Lymphoma
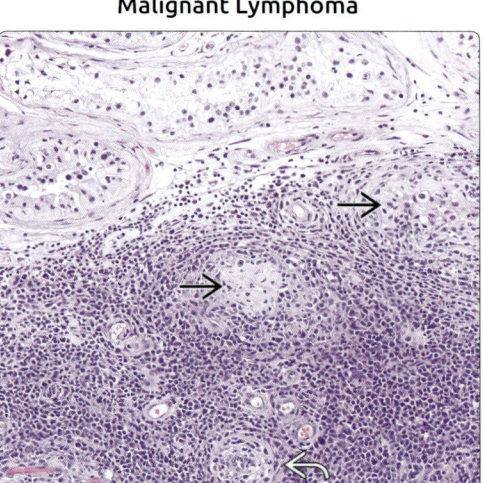

Intratubular Seminoma
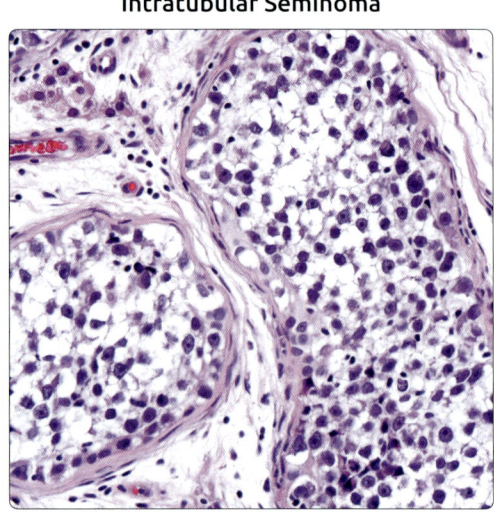

(Left) An interstitial growth pattern is characteristic of most lymphomas involving the testis. Tumor cells predominantly involve the interstitium with relative preservation of the tubules ⇒. The tubular wall and lumen are focally involved ⇒ and may occasionally be obliterated. (Right) H&E shows intratubular seminoma. In contrast to germ cell neoplasia in situ, the tubules are completely filled, replaced, and expanded by large monotonous clonal seminoma cells.

Seminoma
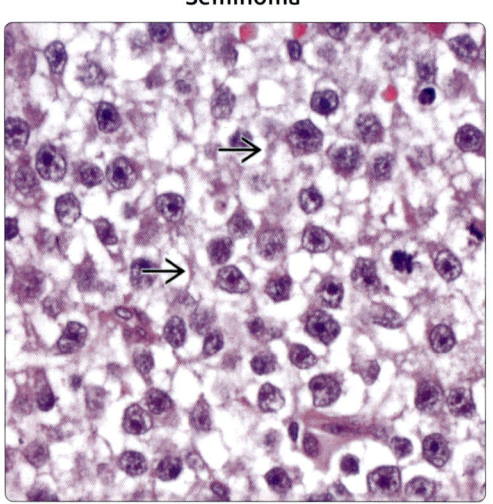

Yolk Sac Tumor
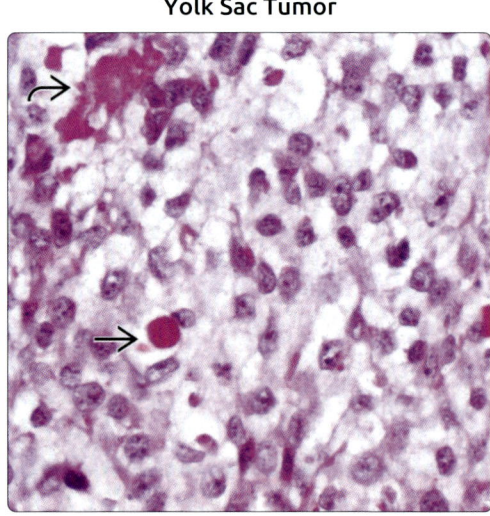

(Left) H&E shows seminoma with large uniform cells and prominent nucleoli. The cells are evenly spaced with abundant clear cytoplasm and distinct cell boundaries ⇒. These cytologic features are diagnostic of seminoma. (Right) H&E shows yolk sac tumor (YST) with solid pattern. The cells are cuboidal or flattened with uneven cellular distribution and no distinct cell boundaries. Eosinophilic hyaline globules ⇒ and basement membrane-like material ⇒ are important clues to the diagnosis.

Embryonal Carcinoma
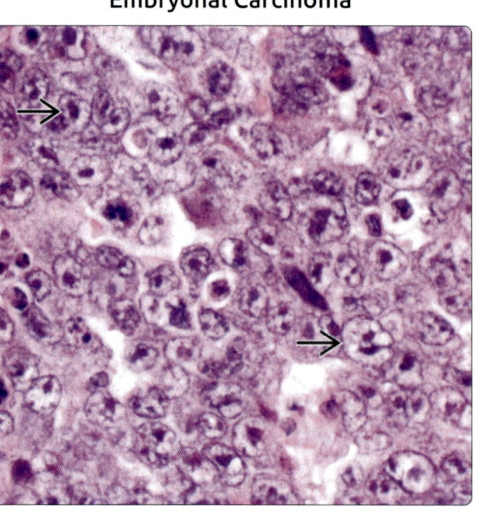

Choriocarcinoma
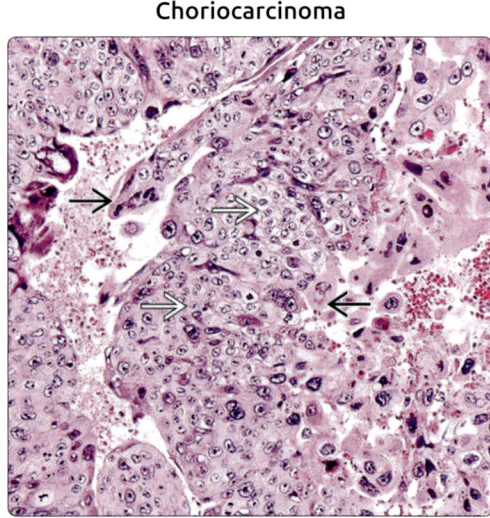

(Left) Anaplastic tumor cells and nuclear overlapping with indistinct cell boundaries are diagnostic features of embryonal carcinoma. The nucleoli ⇒ are much more prominent and irregular than in seminoma. (Right) Diagnostic triad for choriocarcinoma includes hemorrhage and necrosis, 2 cell populations with multinucleated cells ⇒ and mononuclear cells ⇒, and spatial relationship with multinucleated cells wrapping around mononuclear cells, forming villous configurations.

General Concepts, Germ Cell Tumors

Seminoma: PLAP

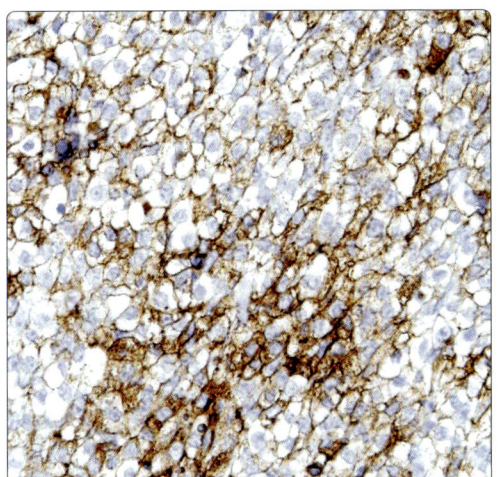

Embryonal Carcinoma: Cytokeratin

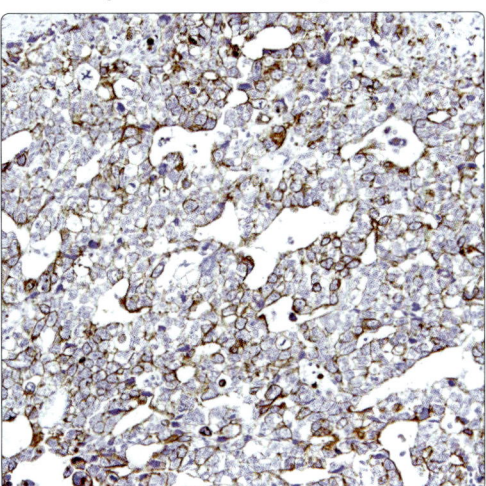

(Left) This image shows cytoplasmic and membranous staining of seminoma by PLAP. When the tumor has unusual features or is poorly preserved, immunostains with germ cell tumor markers (PLAP, podoplanin, OCT3/OCT4, and SALL4) may be necessary for the diagnosis. (Right) CK-PAN is helpful to distinguish seminoma from nonseminomatous tumors. Seminoma is often negative or focally weakly positive, but embryonal carcinoma (shown here) and other germ cell tumors are positive.

Seminoma: OCT3/OCT4

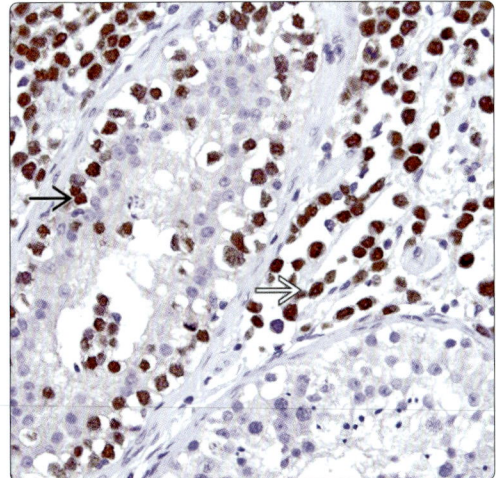

Seminoma: Podoplanin

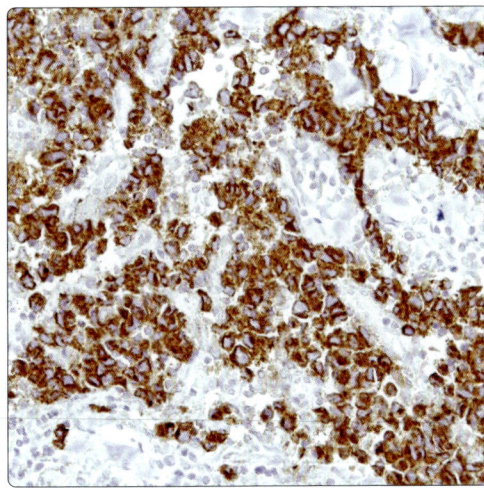

(Left) OCT3/OCT4 immunostain shows germ cell neoplasia in situ ➡ and interstitial seminoma ➡. Nuclear staining and high sensitivity makes OCT3/OCT4 a better marker than PLAP in diagnosing some germ cell tumor components. (Right) Strong membranous and cytoplasmic staining of seminoma with podoplanin is shown. In addition to seminoma, EC is also positive for podoplanin and OCT3/OCT4, but YST and choriocarcinoma are usually negative. SALL4 is positive in YST and choriocarcinoma.

Yolk Sac Tumor: Glypican-3

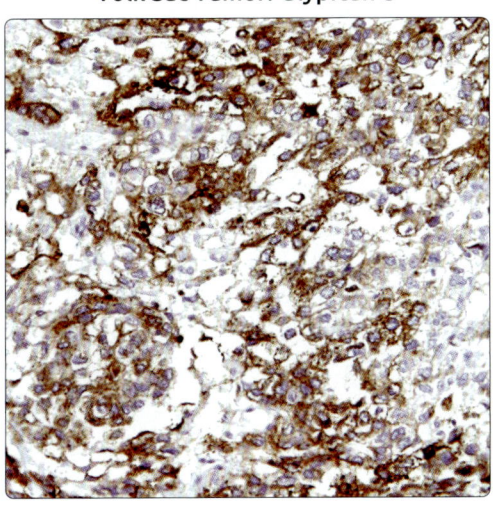

Yolk Sac Tumor: SAL4

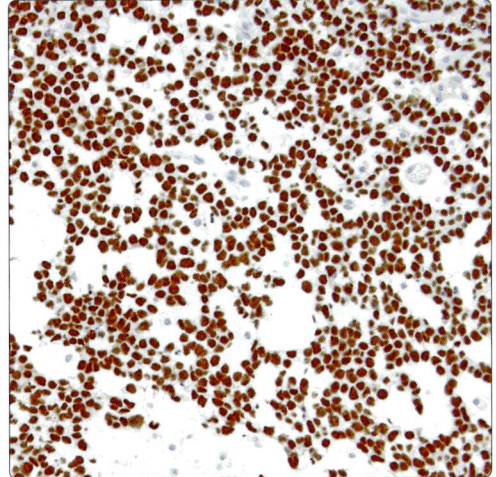

(Left) Besides AFP immunostaining, YST is strongly immunoreactive for glypican-3, whereas other germ cell tumors are usually negative. YST are negative for other germ cell tumor markers (podoplanin and OCT3/OCT4). (Right) Yolk sac tumor shows strong positivity for SALL4 (nuclear). Since SALL4 is positive in all germ cell tumor components, it is useful in distinguishing germ cell tumors from nongerm cell tumors, particularly at metastatic sites.

Germ Cell Neoplasia In Situ

KEY FACTS

TERMINOLOGY
- Proliferation of uncommitted neoplastic germ cells within atrophic seminiferous tubules located at periphery of tubules
  - Recent favored term germ cell neoplasia in situ (GCNIS)

CLINICAL ISSUES
- Often present in association with invasive malignant germ cell tumors or in cryptorchid testis
- May progress to malignant germ cell tumors in ~ 50% of cases within 5 years

MICROSCOPIC
- Intratubular proliferation of malignant germ cells distributed along periphery of atrophic tubules
- Large atypical cells with abundant clear to faintly eosinophilic cytoplasm, prominent cell borders, centrally located nucleus and prominent nucleolus, evenly distributed chromatin

- Pagetoid extension of GCNIS into rete testis may be seen; more frequent in nonseminomatous germ cell tumors than in seminoma

ANCILLARY TESTS
- Positive for PAS but sensitive to diastase
- Positive for D2-40, OCT3/4, and PLAP (CD117, SALL4, NANOG, and SOX17 positive, but nonspecific)
- Negative for cytokeratin, α-fetoprotein, CD30 (BerH2) (may be positive in intratubular embryonal carcinoma)

TOP DIFFERENTIAL DIAGNOSES
- Normal spermatogonia or spermatogenic arrest
- Spermatocytic seminoma (intratubular)
- Intratubular embryonal carcinoma
- Malignant lymphoma (intratubular)
- Metastatic carcinoma or melanoma (intratubular)

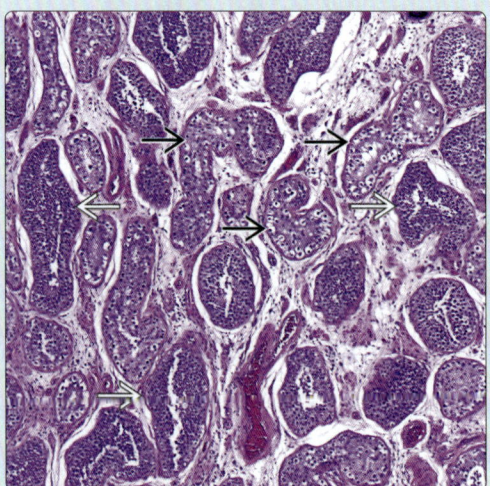

Germ Cell Neoplasia In Situ

(Left) The smaller tubules ➡ seen here exhibit large cells with abundant clear cytoplasm. The germ cell neoplasia in situ (GCNIS) cells are present at the periphery of tubules. The uninvolved tubules ➡ display active spermatogenesis with maturation sequence of germ cells. (Right) GCNIS is characterized by large atypical cells located along the periphery of the tubules ➡. The cells have centrally located nuclei, prominent nucleoli, and abundant clear cytoplasm.

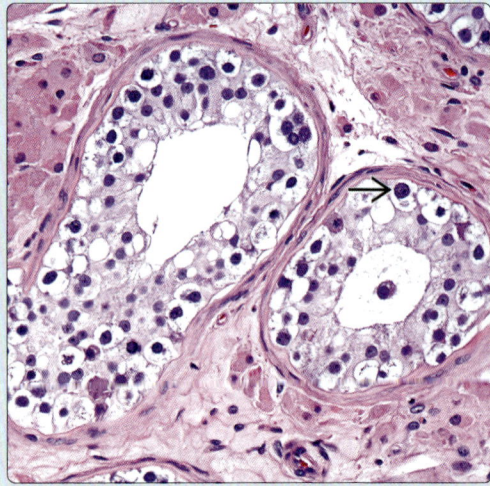

Germ Cell Neoplasia In Situ: Atypical Cells

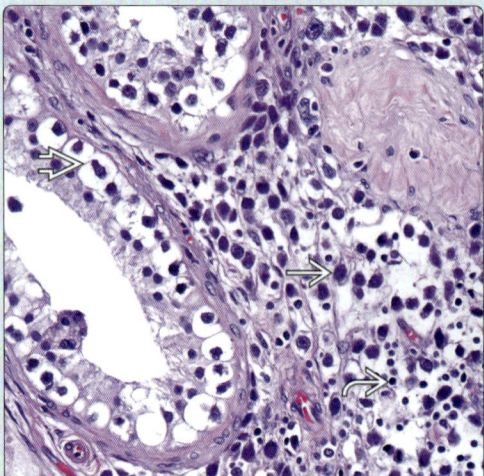

Germ Cell Neoplasia In Situ With Invasive Seminoma

(Left) This photomicrograph shows GCNIS ➡ with adjacent invasive seminoma ➡ and an associated lymphocytic infiltrate ➡. (Right) Immunohistochemical stain for OCT3/4 shows strong nuclear immunoreactivity in GCNIS cells ➡ within the seminiferous tubules. Normal germ cells are negative. CD117 often stains spermatogonia and hence is not as useful.

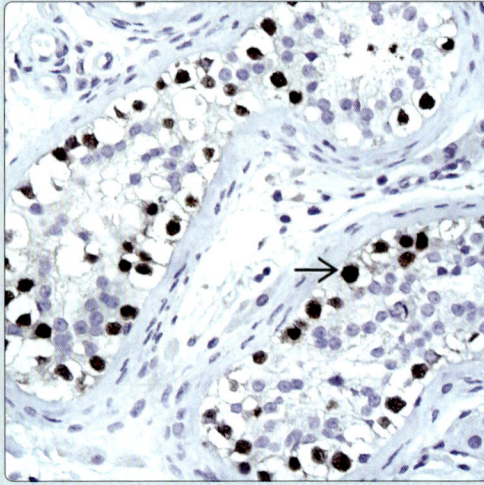

Germ Cell Neoplasia In Situ: OCT3/4 Stain

Germ Cell Neoplasia In Situ

TERMINOLOGY

Abbreviations
- Germ cell neoplasia in situ (GCNIS)

Synonyms
- Carcinoma in situ; intratubular germ cell neoplasia, unclassified type

Definitions
- Proliferation of uncommitted neoplastic germ cells within usually atrophic seminiferous tubules, aligned at periphery of tubules; may be associated with focal or absent spermatogenesis

CLINICAL ISSUES

Epidemiology
- Incidence
  - Present in ipsilateral uninvolved testis in 80-95% of patients with seminoma or nonseminomatous germ cell tumors
  - Present in contralateral testis in 5-8% of patients with malignant germ cell tumors

Presentation
- In cryptorchid testis or in association with malignant germ cell tumor
- Risk factors: Cryptorchidism, microlithiasis, gonadal dysgenesis with Y chromosome, family history (1st-degree male relative), androgen insensitivity syndrome

Treatment
- Unilateral GCNIS usually managed by active surveillance or orchiectomy
- Bilateral GCNIS may be treated by orchiectomy or radiation

Prognosis
- May progress to seminomatous or nonseminomatous germ cell tumors in ~ 50% of cases within 5 years

IMAGING

General Features
- Usually no abnormalities or microlithiasis on ultrasound

MACROSCOPIC

General Features
- No demonstrable testicular mass; testis size may be normal or smaller

MICROSCOPIC

Histologic Features
- Intratubular proliferation of malignant germ cells distributed along periphery of tubules
- Seminiferous tubules usually atrophic, decreased in diameter, and have thickened basement membrane
- Tubules with decreased or absent spermatogenesis
- May be associated with microlithiasis
- Pagetoid extension of GCNIS into rete testis may be seen; more frequent in nonseminomatous germ cell tumor than in seminoma
- May be associated with vascularized scar (regression)
- May be associated with microinvasive seminoma

Cytologic Features
- Large atypical cells with abundant clear to faintly eosinophilic cytoplasm, prominent cell borders, centrally located nucleus and prominent nucleolus, evenly distributed chromatin; mitoses may be seen

Predominant Pattern/Injury Type
- Intratubular growth pattern

Predominant Cell/Compartment Type
- Germ cells, uncommitted atypical germ cells, seminomatous/undifferentiated

ANCILLARY TESTS

Histochemistry
- Positive with PAS stain but disappear after diastase treatment

Immunohistochemistry
- Positive for D2-40, OCT3/4, PLAP, and germ cells (CD117, NANOG, SALL4, and SOX17 positive but nonspecific)
- Negative for cytokeratin, α-fetoprotein, and CD30 (BerH2)

DIFFERENTIAL DIAGNOSIS

Normal Spermatogonia or Spermatogenic Arrest
- Usually accompanied by mixture of spermatogonia, spermatocytes, spermatids, and spermatozoa
- Absence of tubular atrophy and thickening of peritubular basement membrane
- Negative for D2-40, OCT3/4, and PLAP; CD117 may be weakly positive

Spermatocytic Seminoma (Intratubular)
- Polymorphic cells (3 different cell types) in center of seminiferous tubules; no peripheral localization
- Negative for germ cell tumor markers: D2-40, OCT3/4, and PLAP

Intratubular Embryonal Carcinoma
- Intratubular tumor cells are far more pleomorphic with nuclear crowding, frequent necrosis, and apoptosis
- Positive for CK, OCT3/4, and CD30; negative for CD117

Intratubular Malignant Lymphoma, Carcinoma, or Melanoma
- Clinical history and histologic features of malignancy
- Positive for lymphoma, CD45(LCA), CD20 or CD3, metastatic carcinoma, CK, EMA/MUC, melanoma, S100, HMB-45
- Negative for germ cell tumor markers

SELECTED REFERENCES

1. Mitchell RT et al: Intratubular germ cell neoplasia of the human testis: heterogeneous protein expression and relation to invasive potential. Mod Pathol. 27(9):1255-66, 2014
2. Emerson RE et al: Intratubular germ cell neoplasia of the testis and its associated cancers: the use of novel biomarkers. Pathology. 42(4):344-55, 2010
3. Lau SK et al: Association of intratubular seminoma and intratubular embryonal carcinoma with invasive testicular germ cell tumors. Am J Surg Pathol. 31(7):1045-9, 2007

Germ Cell Neoplasia In Situ

(Left) This image shows comparison of a tubule involved by GCNIS ⇨ with adjacent seminiferous tubules with normal spermatogenesis ⇨. Clusters of Leydig cells ⇨ are seen within the interstitium. **(Right)** High-power photomicrograph shows a seminiferous tubule with large GCNIS cells at the periphery of the tubule ⇨ with centrally located nuclei, prominent nucleoli, and abundant clear cytoplasm. Spermatogenesis is absent.

Germ Cell Neoplasia In Situ and Leydig Cells
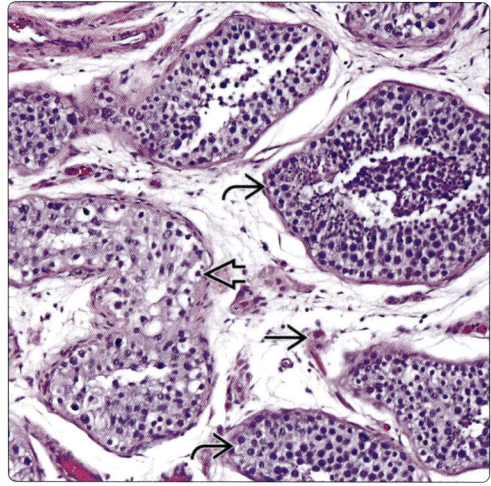

Large Germ Cell Neoplasia In Situ Cells
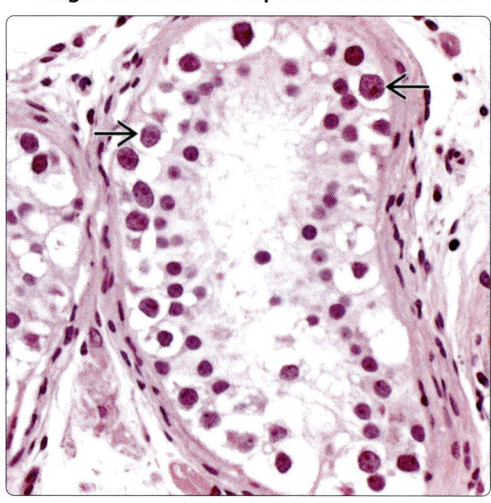

(Left) Hematoxylin & eosin stain shows the entire length of a seminiferous tubule containing GCNIS cells (large cells with clear cytoplasm and prominent nucleoli) along the periphery. **(Right)** High-power photomicrograph shows an atrophic tubule with prominent thickening of the peritubular tunica basement membrane and large atypical cells ⇨ at the periphery of the tubule.

Germ Cell Neoplasia In Situ
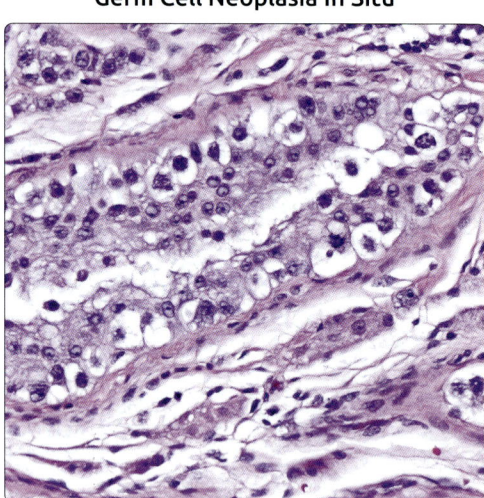

Atrophic Tubule
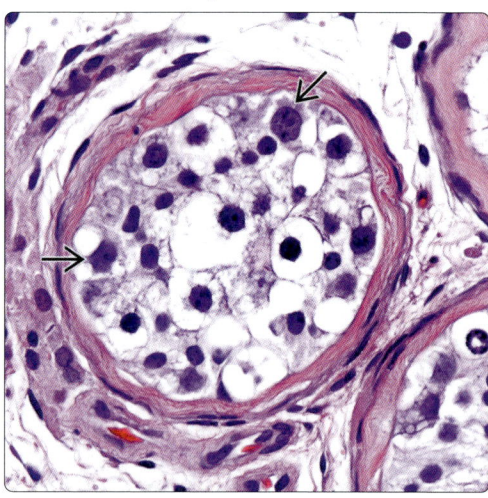

(Left) Low-power photomicrograph shows the testis with diffuse tubular atrophy and marked thickening of tubular walls. Some tubules are completely sclerotic; others are involved by GCNIS ⇨. In a cryptorchid testis, it is important to scrutinize lymphoid aggregates adjacent to GCNIS, as such foci may contain microinvasive seminoma. **(Right)** High-power photomicrograph shows atrophic and sclerotic tubules involved by GCNIS. Note the rare mitotic figure ⇨.

Testis
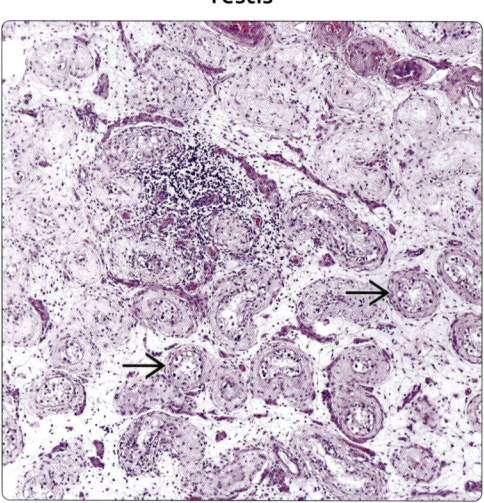

Atrophic and Sclerotic Tubules
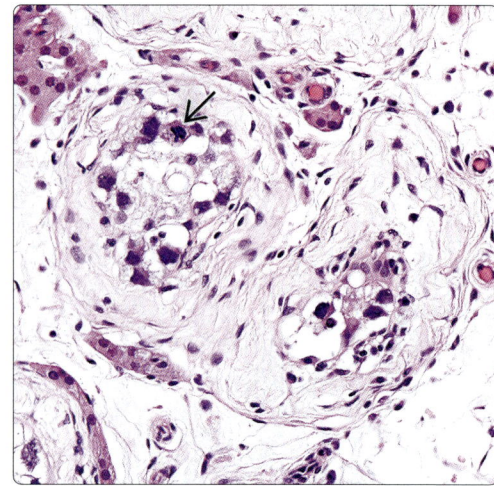

Germ Cell Neoplasia In Situ

Germ Cell Neoplasia In Situ Cells: Pagetoid
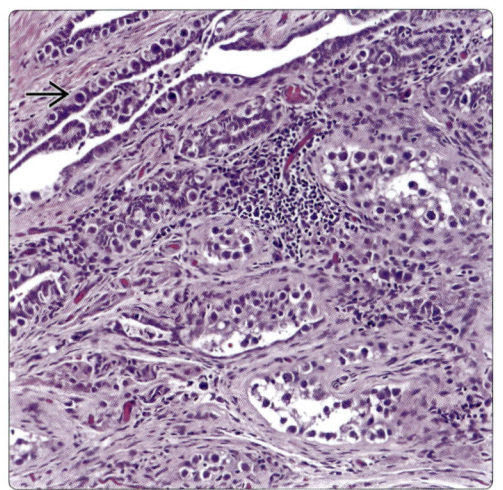

Rete Testis
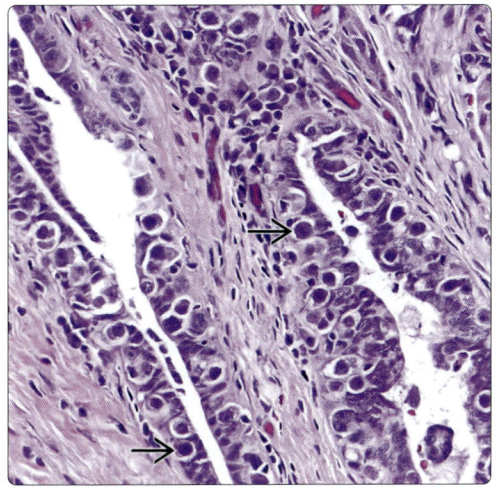

(Left) GCNIS cells involve several seminiferous tubules and extend to the rete testis in a pagetoid fashion ➡. This may occur in the absence of overt invasive seminoma. (Right) This high-power photomicrograph shows that the rete testis is involved by pagetoid extension of GCNIS ➡. The stroma adjacent to the rete testis shows no invasive germ cell tumor component. Immunostains for CD117 and OCT3/4 may be useful to confirm the diagnosis.

Germ Cell Neoplasia In Situ With Microinvasive Seminoma
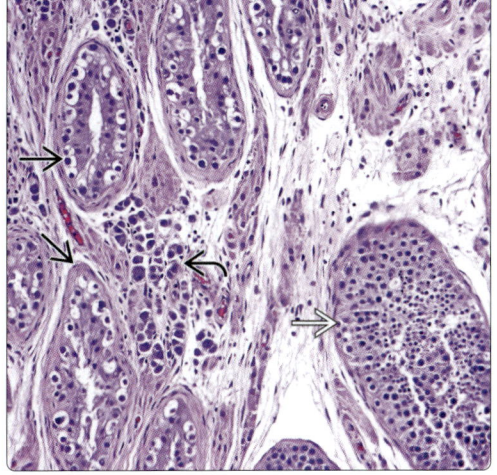

Embryonal Carcinoma With Germ Cell Neoplasia In Situ
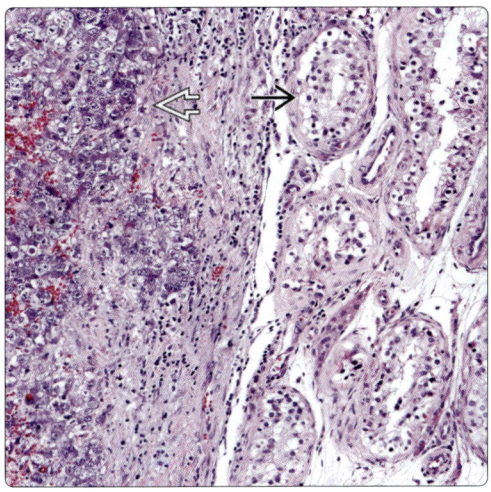

(Left) This photomicrograph shows microinvasive seminoma ➡ and multiple tubules involved by GCNIS ➡. One normal tubule ➡ with spermatogenesis is also present. It is important to look for GCNIS in all seminoma cases, as a malignant Sertoli cell tumor may very closely mimic invasive seminoma. (Right) This photomicrograph shows solid area of embryonal carcinoma ➡ with adjacent seminiferous tubules containing GCNIS ➡. No spermatogenesis is present in these tubules.

Germ Cell Neoplasia In Situ
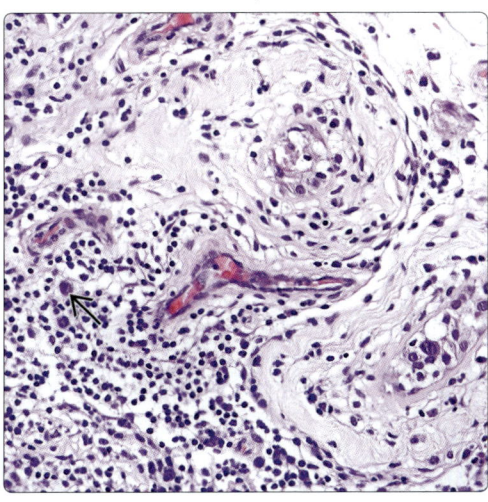

Microinvasive Seminoma
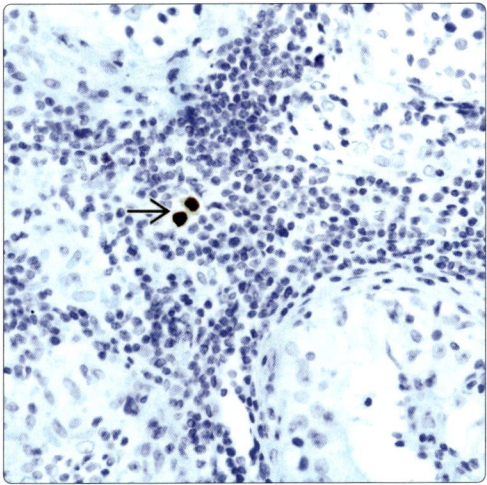

(Left) This photomicrograph focus shows intense chronic inflammation surrounding 2 atrophic seminiferous tubules with GCNIS. A single large atypical cell ➡, suspicious for invasive seminoma, is present. It is important to look for features of regression in an orchiectomy specimen in a young patient. (Right) This photomicrograph shows immunostain of OCT3/4. Two malignant cells exhibit intense nuclear staining for OCT3/4 ➡, which is very helpful to identify and confirm the rare invasive tumor cells in the interstitium.

Germ Cell Neoplasia In Situ

(Left) This photomicrograph shows GCNIS with intratubular calcification (microlithiasis) ⇾. Microlithiasis is frequently observed in cryptorchid, ex-cryptorchid testes, tubules adjacent to germ cell tumors, and infertile patients. (Right) PAS stain without diastase shows strong cytoplasmic positivity in GCNIS cells, reflecting a high content of cytoplasmic glycogen. This positivity is lost after diastase treatment. Sensitive and specific markers for GCNIS have minimized the use of PAS to confirm this finding in surgical pathology practice.

Germ Cell Neoplasia In Situ: Associated Microlith

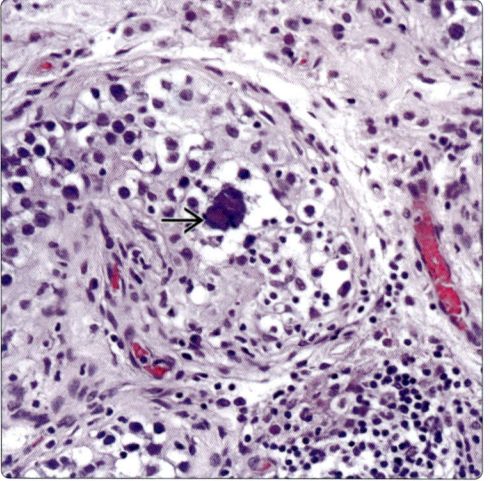

Germ Cell Neoplasia In Situ: PAS Stain

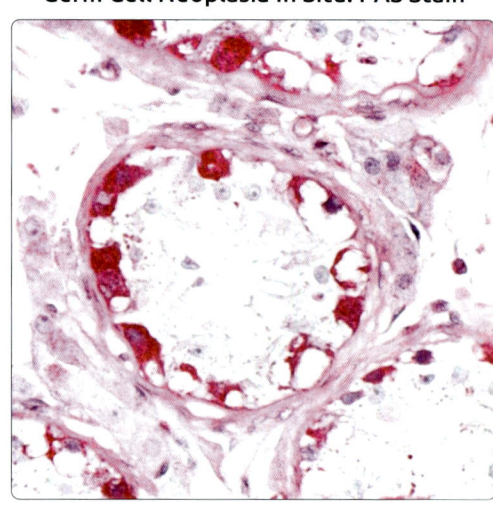

(Left) This is an example of intratubular seminoma with microinvasive seminoma ⇾. Early invasive seminoma is almost always associated with lymphocytic response, a sign of invasion. Such foci may occur in a cryptorchid testis or in a testis containing a germ cell tumor in the vicinity or distant from such foci. (Right) High-power photomicrograph shows an example of so-called intratubular seminoma. The seminiferous tubule is greatly distended by cells of classic seminoma.

Intratubular Seminoma

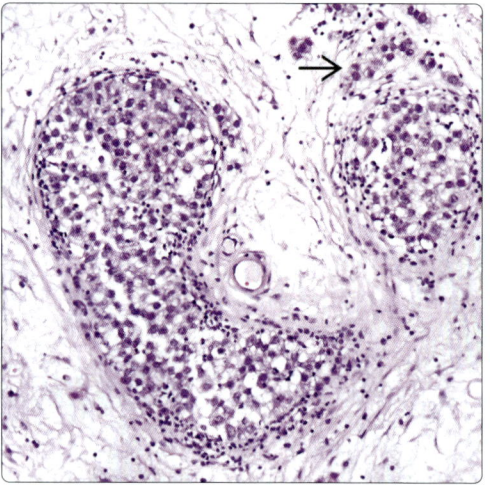

Intratubular Seminoma

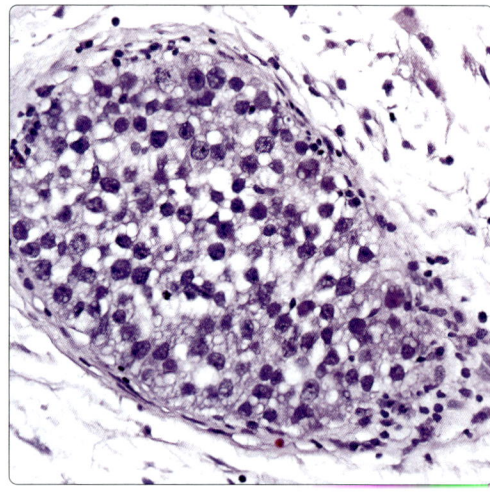

(Left) Two seminiferous tubules are involved by GCNIS ⇾ and other tubules are filled and greatly expanded by cells of classic seminoma (intratubular seminoma) ⇾. GCNIS is a precursor lesion for most germ cell tumors, whereas intratubular seminoma represents extension of seminoma into seminiferous tubules. (Right) This is another example of intratubular seminoma with focal microinvasive seminoma ⇾. The cytology of the intratubular and invasive component is identical.

Germ Cell Neoplasia In Situ and Intratubular Seminoma

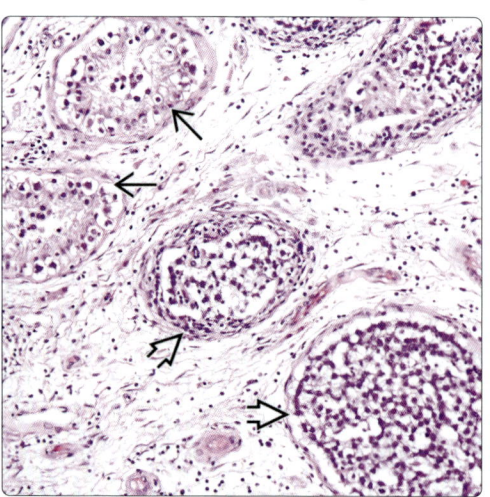

Intratubular and Microinvasive Seminoma

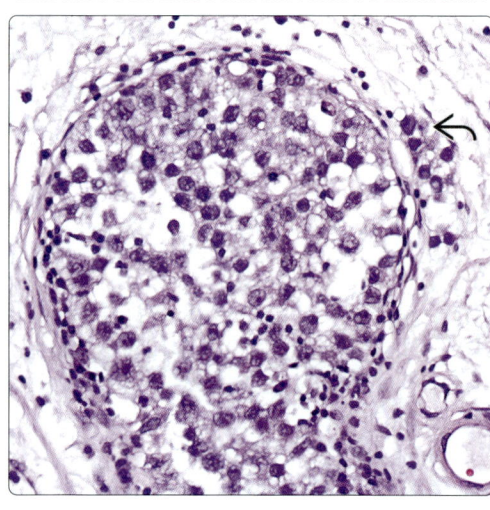

Germ Cell Neoplasia In Situ

Germ Cell Neoplasia In Situ: PLAP
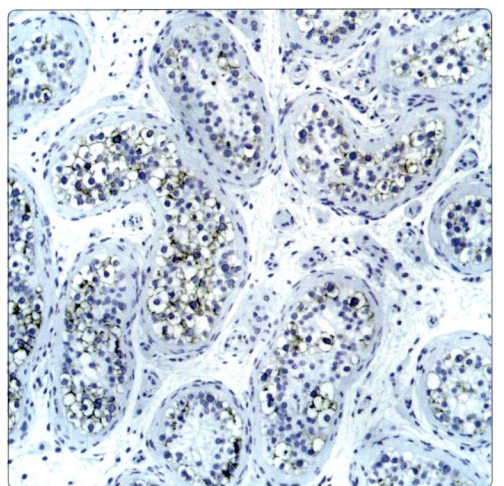

Germ Cell Neoplasia In Situ: Podoplanin
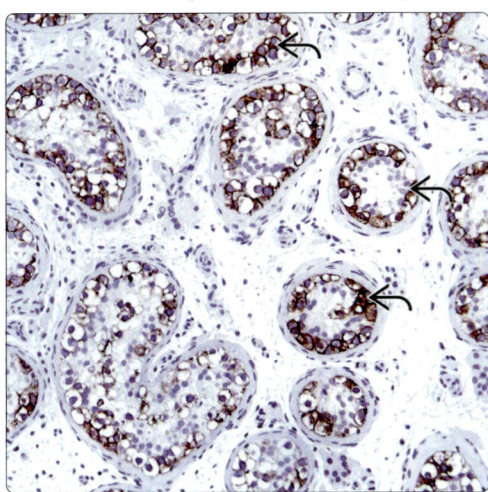

(Left) Immunohistochemical stain with PLAP highlights the tumor cells of GCNIS in a cytoplasmic membranous pattern. (Right) Podoplanin stains the cells of GCNIS in a cytoplasmic membranous pattern ➡. Podoplanin also stains background lymphatic endothelial cells; it is positive in classic seminoma but not in other germ cell components. The staining is typically membranous.

Spermatocytic Arrest
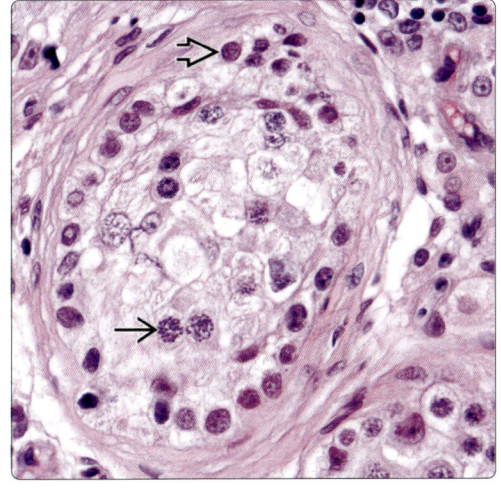

Intratubular Embryonal Carcinoma
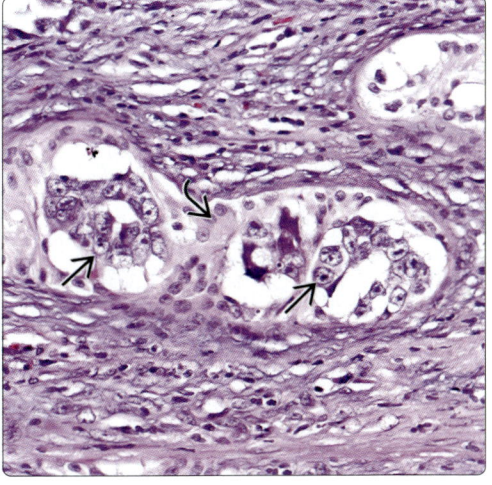

(Left) This is an example of spermatogenic arrest with a layer of spermatogonia ➡ and a few primary spermatocytes ➡. This may be mistaken as GCNIS because of the enlarged nuclei, clear cytoplasm, and prominent cell membrane. (Right) Pagetoid extension of embryonal carcinoma in seminiferous tubules is shown. The tumor cells have crowded and overlapping nuclei, vesicular chromatin, and prominent nucleoli ➡. Background nonneoplastic tubular elements ➡ are present.

Large B-Cell Lymphoma
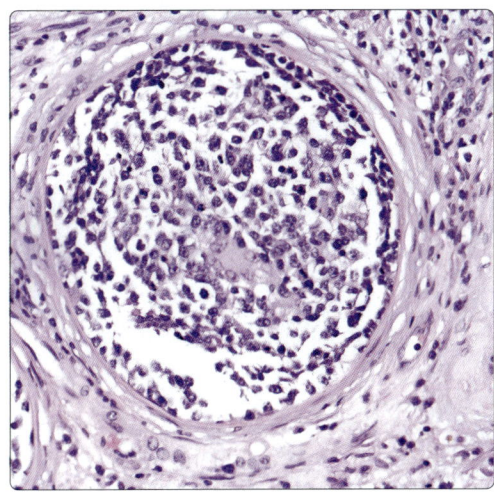

Metastatic Prostate Carcinoma
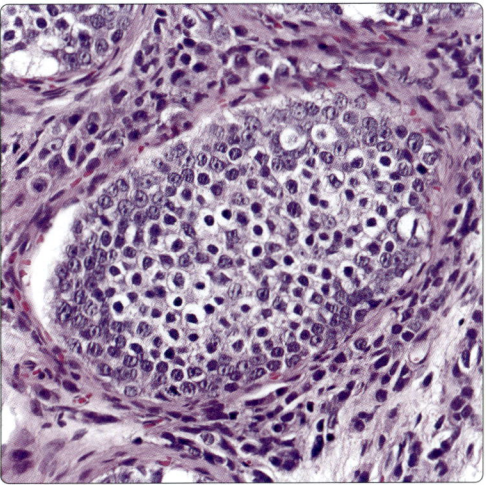

(Left) This is an example of intratubular large B-cell lymphoma admixed with a few small lymphocytes. Elsewhere within the testis, typical diffuse interstitial large B-cell lymphoma was present. Immunostains for CD45(LCA)(+) and OCT3/4(-) will confirm the diagnosis. (Right) Metastatic high-grade prostate carcinoma may also rarely have an intratubular growth pattern. The tumor cells are relatively uniform and have large nucleoli and prominent nucleoli. Invasive tumor cells are also present in the interstitium.

Seminoma

KEY FACTS

TERMINOLOGY
- Malignant germ cell tumor composed of relatively uniform cells with abundant clear cytoplasm, well-defined cell borders, and nuclei with 1 or more prominent nucleoli

CLINICAL ISSUES
- Most common malignant testicular germ cell tumor (~ 50%)

MACROSCOPIC
- Well circumscribed and homogeneous ± lobulation
- Gray-white, tan, creamy, fleshy or firm, often bulging cut surface; rare hemorrhage or necrosis

MICROSCOPIC
- Fibrous septa divide sheets or nests of tumor cells into lobules
- Large round-polygonal tumor cells with abundant clear cytoplasm
- Tumor cells are evenly spread without nuclear overlap in well-fixed tissues
- Prominent cytoplasmic membranes (distinct cell boundaries)
- Lymphoplasmacytic infiltrate, occasionally extensive with germinal centers in fibrous septa
- Ill-defined granuloma formation in ~ 50-60%; may be extensive, which may create diagnostic difficulty in recognizing tumor cells

ANCILLARY TESTS
- Positive for PLAP, OCT3/OCT4, CD117, Podoplanin (D2-40), vimentin, SALL4, NANOG, SOX17
- Negative for cytokeratin (may be focal or weak), EMA, α-fetoprotein, HCG, inhibin-α, CD30, glypican-3, SOX2

TOP DIFFERENTIAL DIAGNOSES
- Embryonal carcinoma, yolk sac tumor, monophasic choriocarcinoma, lymphoma, spermatocytic seminoma, Sertoli cell tumor, nonspecific granulomatous orchitis

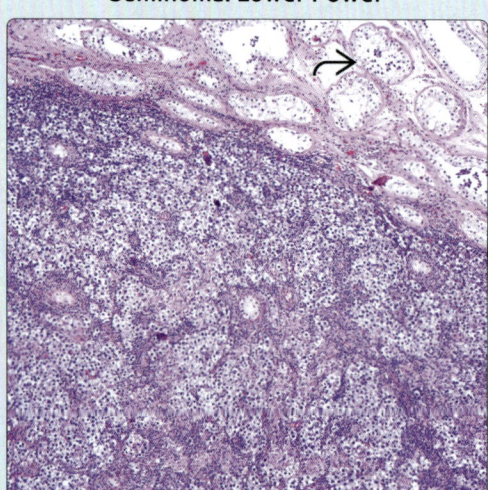

Seminoma: Lower Power

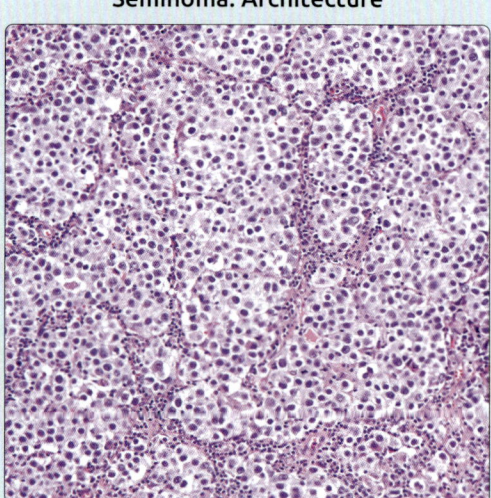

Seminoma: Architecture

(Left) Low-power photomicrograph shows a well-defined classic seminoma surrounded by nonneoplastic seminiferous tubules ⟹. Fibrovascular septa with small lymphocytic infiltrate divide the tumor into lobules. (Right) Diffuse sheets or nests of tumor cells are separated into lobules by fibrous septa containing small lymphocytes. The tumor cells in this example exhibit abundant eosinophilic cytoplasm.

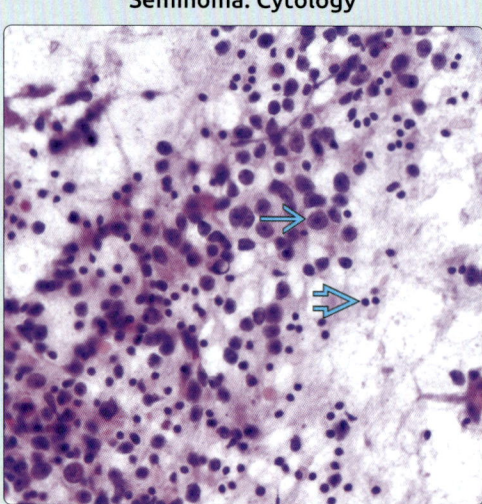

Seminoma: Cytology

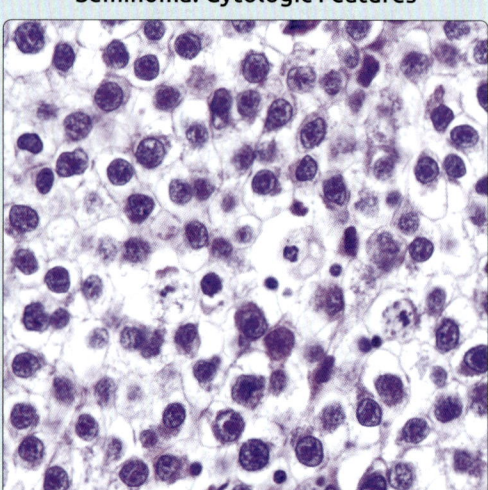

Seminoma: Cytologic Features

(Left) Touch preparation cytology of classic seminoma shows a dimorphic population of large seminomatous cells ⟹ with relatively uniform round nuclei, prominent nucleoli, and small dark lymphocytes ⟹. (Right) High-power photomicrograph of classic seminoma shows tumor cells with large nuclei, prominent nucleoli, abundant clear cytoplasm, distinct cell membranes, and even distribution of tumor cells.

Seminoma

TERMINOLOGY

Synonyms
- Germinoma in extragonadal sites
- Dysgerminoma in ovary

Definitions
- Malignant germ cell tumor composed of relatively uniform cells with abundant clear cytoplasm, well-defined cell borders, and nuclei with 1 or more prominent nucleoli

CLINICAL ISSUES

Epidemiology
- Incidence
  - Most common malignant testicular germ cell tumor (~ 50%)
- Age
  - Most common in men 35-45 yr old, uncommon in men over 50 yr, and rare in children; mean: 5-10 yr older than nonseminomatous germ cell tumors

Presentation
- Most commonly painless testicular mass (70%)
- Other presentations: Scrotal pain (10%), symptoms of metastasis (10%), asymptomatic (4%), gynecomastia and exophthalmos (rare)
- Mostly unilateral and rarely bilateral (~ 2%); bilaterality more common than in nonseminomatous germ cell tumors
- Spermatic cord involvement (rarer than in nonseminomatous germ cell tumors; < 5%)

Laboratory Tests
- Serum markers may be elevated
  - Serum lactate dehydrogenase (LDH)
  - Human chorionic gonadotropin (hCG)
- α-fetoprotein (AFP) should be normal for pure seminoma
  - AFP elevation in patient with pure seminoma is clinically treated as nonseminomatous germ cell tumor

Treatment
- For patients with stage I seminoma 3 options are available
  - Radical inguinal orchiectomy and surveillance with measurement of serum markers, chest x-ray, and CT of abdomen and pelvis
  - Radical inguinal orchiectomy with radiation therapy
  - Radical inguinal orchiectomy followed by either 1 or 2 doses of carboplatin adjuvant therapy
- For patients with stage II seminoma
  - Radical inguinal orchiectomy followed by radiation therapy to retroperitoneal and ipsilateral pelvic lymph nodes, or combination chemotherapy
- For patients with stage III seminoma
  - Radical inguinal orchiectomy followed by multidrug (bleomycin, etoposide, and cisplatin) chemotherapy

Prognosis
- Excellent prognosis with 98% cure rate for stage I or II seminoma
- Associated with pathologic stage, tumor size, rete testis invasion, and intertubular growth > 3 HPFs distance from main mass
- Lymphovascular invasion is important prognostic factor in univariate analysis but not independent prognostic factor
- Concept of anaplastic seminoma (> 3 mitoses per HPF) is not accepted as separate entity or adverse prognostic factor

MACROSCOPIC

General Features
- Well circumscribed and homogeneous ± lobulation; 90% confined to testis
- Gray-white, tan, creamy, fleshy or firm, often bulging cut surface; usually no hemorrhage or necrosis
  - Tumors with hemorrhage and necrosis often indicate nonseminomatous components or in large tumors
- May have geographic infarct-type necrosis (usually large tumors)
- Punctate hemorrhage (usually in areas of syncytiotrophoblasts)
- Small tumors may be difficult to see grossly; scar may be present in rare tumors
- Rare spermatic cord invasion (< 5%)

Size
- Average: 5 cm (range: 2-24 cm)

MICROSCOPIC

Histologic Features
- Main architectural growth patterns
  - Solid sheets or nests (most common)
  - Sclerotic or interstitial (in between seminiferous tubules; rare)
  - Tubular, alveolar, trabecular, or pseudoglandular (rare)
- Fibrous septa divide sheets or nests of tumor cells into lobules
- Tumor cells are evenly spread without nuclear overlap in well-fixed tissues
- Lymphoplasmacytic infiltrate, occasionally extensive, with germinal centers in fibrous septa
- Ill-defined granuloma formation in ~ 50-60%; may be extensive, which may create diagnostic difficulty in recognizing tumor cells
- Fibrosis, sclerosis, and scar formation may be prominent (burnt-out seminoma when no tumor cells present)
- Extensive hemorrhage and necrosis are rarely seen
- Syncytiotrophoblastic giant cells may be seen in areas of hemorrhage; present in ~ 10-20% of tumors
- Germ cell neoplasia in situ (GCNIS) in surrounding seminiferous tubules or pagetoid spread to rete testis

Cytologic Features
- Large round-polygonal tumor cells with abundant clear cytoplasm
- Prominent cytoplasmic membranes (distinct cell boundaries), no nuclear overlapping
- Relatively uniform, large central nuclei with 1-2 prominent nucleoli
- Mitotic figures range from few to frequent
- Some tumors can have larger cells, high N:C ratio, and more mitoses (> 3/HPF); known as anaplastic seminoma
- Rarely, tumor cells can have plasmacytoid, rhabdoid, or signet ring cell appearance

Seminoma

Predominant Pattern/Injury Type
- Neoplastic

Predominant Cell/Compartment Type
- Uncommitted large atypical malignant germ cells (primordial germ cells)

ANCILLARY TESTS

Histochemistry
- Positive for periodic acid-Schiff (PAS) without diastase

Immunohistochemistry
- Positive for PLAP, OCT3/OCT4, CD117, Podoplanin (D2-40), vimentin, SALL4, NANOG, SOX17
- Negative for cytokeratin (may be focal or weak), EMA, α-fetoprotein, hCG, inhibin-α, CD30, glypican-3, SOX2

DIFFERENTIAL DIAGNOSIS

Embryonal Carcinoma, Solid Pattern
- Usually admixed with glandular and papillary patterns
- Marked cellular pleomorphism, vesicular nuclei, nuclear crowding with overlapping and indistinct cell borders, irregularly shaped nucleoli, frequent mitoses or apoptoses
- Positive for cytokeratin and CD30 (BerH2)

Yolk Sac Tumor, Solid Pattern
- Variable growth patterns, most commonly microcystic and reticular
- Schiller-Duval bodies, basement membrane deposition, and hyaline globules are characteristic, if present
- Positive for cytokeratin, α-fetoprotein, and glypican-3

Malignant Lymphoma
- Usually older age group, history of lymphoma, frequent bilateral involvement, frequent spermatic cord involvement (> 40%)
- Predominantly interstitial pattern of tumor cells between seminiferous tubules
- Cytokeratin and germ cell markers negative; CD45 (LCA) and B- or T-cell markers positive (depending on type, B cell more common than T cell)

Spermatocytic Tumor
- Older age group (> 50 yr with average of 56 yr)
- Presence of 3 distinct types of tumor cells (small, intermediate, and large cells)
- Lack of lymphocytic infiltration or granulomatous reaction; no fibrous septa; no association with GCNIS
- Negative for PAS, germ cell tumor markers [PLAP, OCT3/OCT4, podoplanin (D2-40)]; SALL4 and CD117 may be positive

Monophasic Choriocarcinoma
- Extremely rare; primary or metastatic foci postchemotherapy
- Mononucleated tumor cells of variable sizes; more frequent associated hemorrhage and necrosis
- Positive for hCG and human placental lactogen (HPL)

Sertoli Cell Tumor
- Usually more prominent tubular or trabecular growth
- Usually lack fibrous septa with lymphoplasmacytic and granulomatous reaction
- Usually positive for α-inhibin, calretinin, and cytokeratin, negative for PLAP, podoplanin (D2-40), SALL4, and OCT3/OCT4

Nonspecific Granulomatous Orchitis
- Mixed population of inflammatory cells
- Predominantly involves seminiferous tubules

DIAGNOSTIC CHECKLIST

Pathologic Interpretation Pearls
- Relatively uniform tumor cells with abundant clear cytoplasm, distinct cell boundaries, evenly spaced tumor cells without nuclear overlapping
- Fibrous septa with lymphoplasmacytic infiltrates and granulomatous reaction
- Diagnostically difficult situations
  - Unusual growth patterns: Tubular, pseudoglandular, or interstitial
  - Extensive granulomatous reaction, sclerosis, or scar formation (regression)
  - GCNIS with microinvasion (microscopic invasion)
  - Poorly fixed tissue with artifact create more diagnostic problems

REPORTING

Key Elements to Report
- General information
  - Laterality, multifocality, tumor size
- Histologic type (pure, classic, or with other components)
- Pathologic stage (pTNM): Tumor extension, regional lymph node status, and distant metastasis
- Rete testis stromal invasion, not just pagetoid extension
- Margin status (spermatic cord and other)
- Venous/lymphatic vessel invasion
- Additional pathologic findings (GCNIS, syncytiotrophoblastic cells, scar, etc.), if present

SELECTED REFERENCES

1. Hanna NH et al: Testicular cancer–discoveries and updates. N Engl J Med. 371(21):2005-16, 2014
2. Ulbright TM et al: Best practices recommendations in the application of immunohistochemistry in testicular tumors: report from the International Society of Urological Pathology consensus conference. Am J Surg Pathol. 38(8):e50-9, 2014
3. Ye H et al: Difficult differential diagnoses in testicular pathology. Arch Pathol Lab Med. 136(4):435-46, 2012
4. Young RH: Testicular tumors–some new and a few perennial problems. Arch Pathol Lab Med. 132(4):548-64, 2008
5. Ulbright TM et al: Seminoma with tubular, microcystic, and related patterns: a study of 28 cases of unusual morphologic variants that often cause confusion with yolk sac tumor. Am J Surg Pathol. 29(4):500-5, 2005
6. Tickoo SK et al: Testicular seminoma: a clinicopathologic and immunohistochemical study of 105 cases with special reference to seminomas with atypical features. Int J Surg Pathol. 10(1):23-32, 2002
7. Warde P et al: Prognostic factors for relapse in stage I seminoma managed by surveillance: a pooled analysis. J Clin Oncol. 20(22):4448-52, 2002

Seminoma

Seminoma: Gross
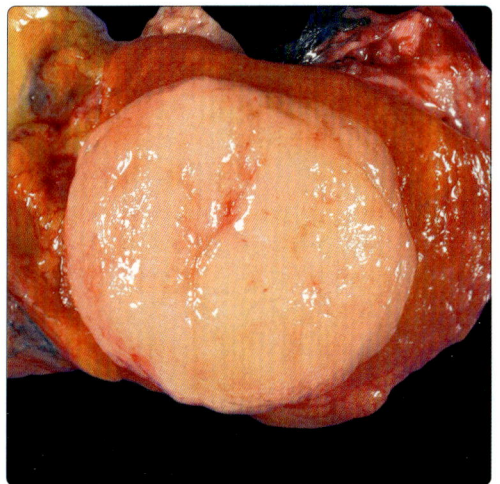

Seminoma: Necrosis
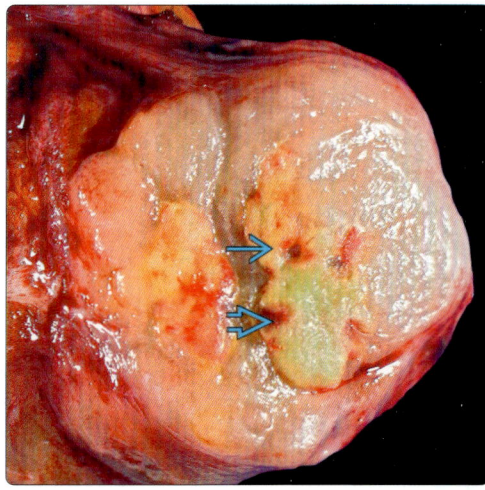

(Left) This photograph shows the typical gross appearance of a classic seminoma with a well-circumscribed mass with a tan, creamy, homogeneous cut surface. No hemorrhage or necrosis is present. (Right) Cut surface of a large classic seminoma shows focal necrosis ➡ and hemorrhage ➡. Necrosis and hemorrhage are much more commonly seen in embryonal carcinoma or mixed germ cell tumor. These areas should be sampled.

Large Seminoma
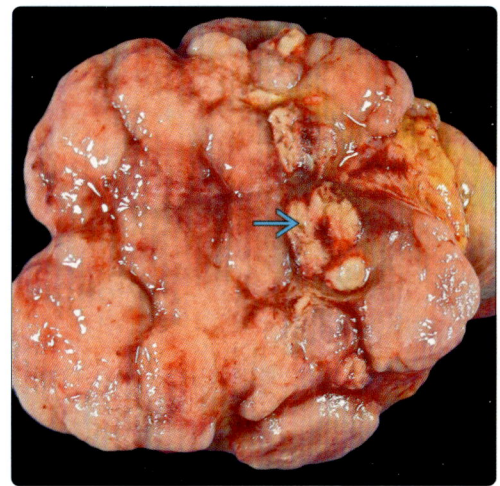

Multifocal Seminoma
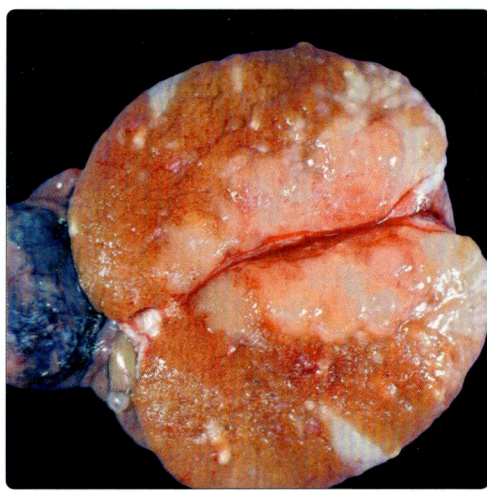

(Left) This classic seminoma shows prominent lobulation and focal necrosis ➡. The rete testis is also involved by tumor. (Right) Cut surface of a classic seminoma shows a multifocal and interstitial infiltrative tumor pattern. There is no well-defined tumor nodule as seen in other more typical examples. This appearance may be very similar to that of malignant lymphoma.

Seminoma: Architecture
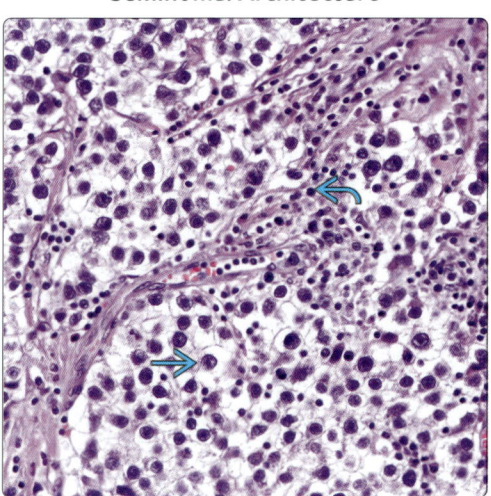

Seminoma: Architecture
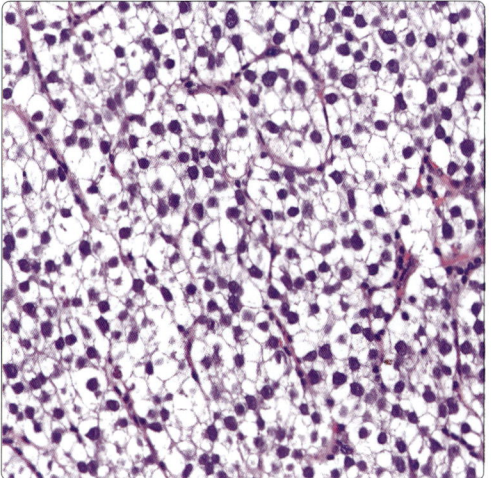

(Left) This photomicrograph shows nests of uniform seminomatous cells ➡ with abundant clear cytoplasm, centrally located nuclei, and distinct cells membranes. Fibrovascular septa with small lymphocytes ➡ are characteristic of seminoma. (Right) Solid sheets of clear seminomatous cells are separated by delicate fibrovascular septa with rare lymphocytes. The tumor cells are evenly distributed, and prominent cell boundaries are evident.

Seminoma

Seminoma: Lymphoid Follicle
Prominent Inflammation

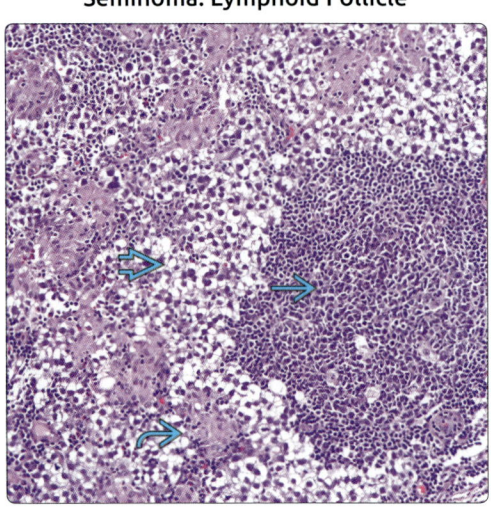

(Left) This image shows nests of seminomatous tumor cells ➡ with extensive granulomas ➡ and a lymphoid aggregate with germinal center ➡. The tumor cells contain abundant clear cytoplasm. (Right) This photomicrograph shows a classic seminoma with scattered large seminomatous germ cells ➡ with extensive lymphoplasmacytic infiltrates and vessels with plump endothelial cells. In some cases, the tumor cells may be sparse and difficult to find.

Seminoma: Granulomas
Seminoma: Prominent Inflammation

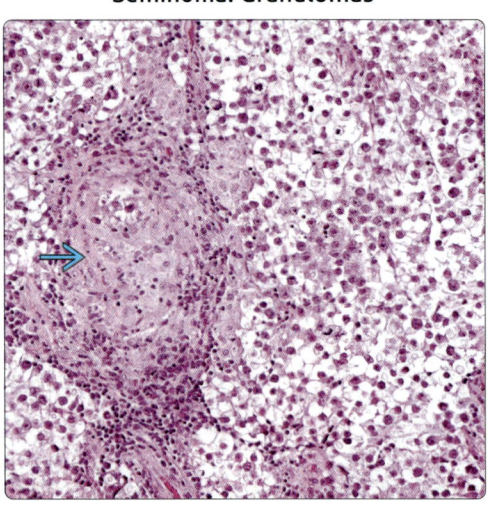
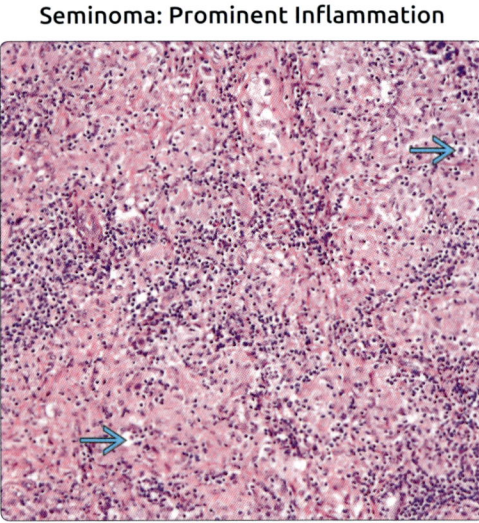

(Left) This image shows a classic seminoma with a large well-formed granuloma ➡ surrounded by small lymphocytes. The tumor cells have abundant clear cytoplasm and prominent cytoplasmic membranes. (Right) A classic seminoma with confluent granulomatous inflammation is shown. Only rare tumor cells ➡ may be seen. Elsewhere on the same slide, more characteristic tumor cells are present. In rare situations, immunostain with OCT3/OCT4 might be helpful to identify the tumor cells.

Tubular Seminoma
Tubular Seminoma

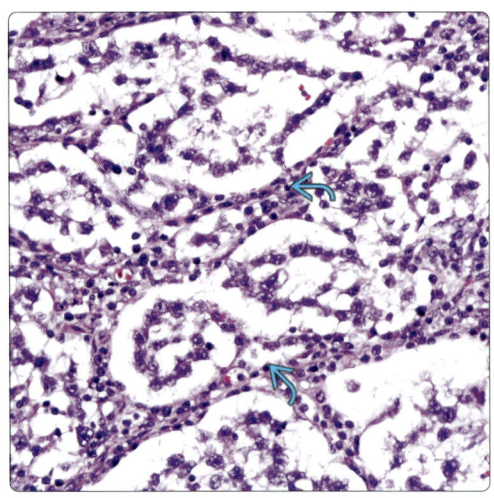
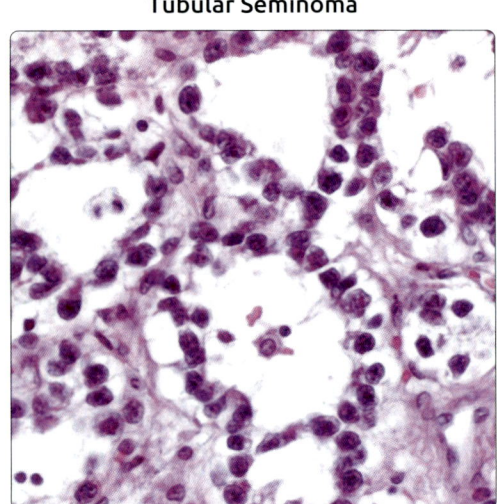

(Left) This photomicrograph shows seminoma with a tubular or pseudoglandular pattern. The cytologic features are those of classic seminoma with relatively uniform nuclei and clear cytoplasm. Also seen are fibrovascular septa with small lymphocytes ➡. (Right) This is a high-power photomicrograph of seminoma with tumor cells in a tubular growth pattern. The tumor cells have characteristic cytologic features of seminoma with relatively uniform nuclei and abundant clear cytoplasm.

Seminoma

Seminoma With Syncytiotrophoblasts
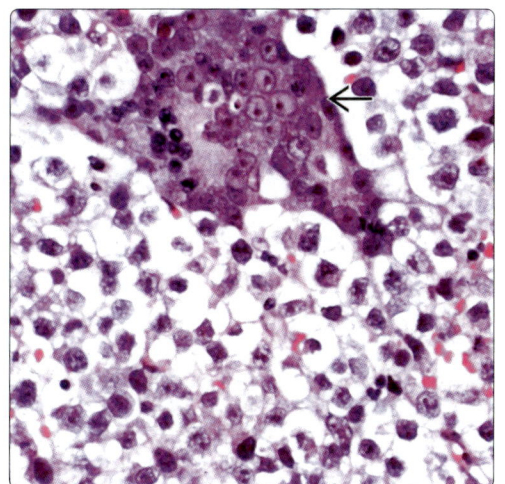

Seminoma: Cytokeratin Stain
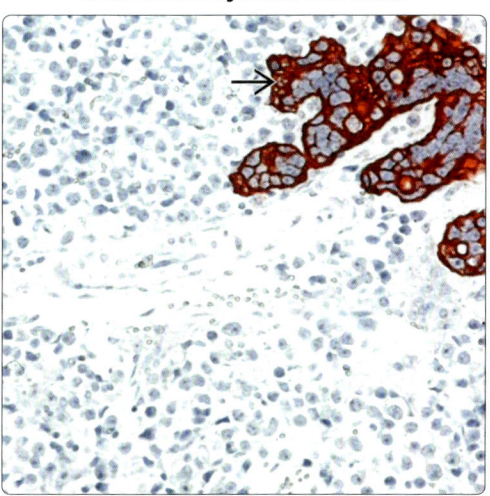

(Left) A classic seminoma with a multinucleated syncytiotrophoblastic giant cell ⇒ is shown. Approximately 30% of patients with pure seminoma have mild elevation of hCG (usually < 500 IU/mL). Presence of syncytiotrophoblasts is not an adverse prognostic feature. **(Right)** Cytokeratin immunostain strongly highlights the syncytiotrophoblasts ⇒, whereas seminoma tumor cells are negative.

Seminoma: Trabecular Growth
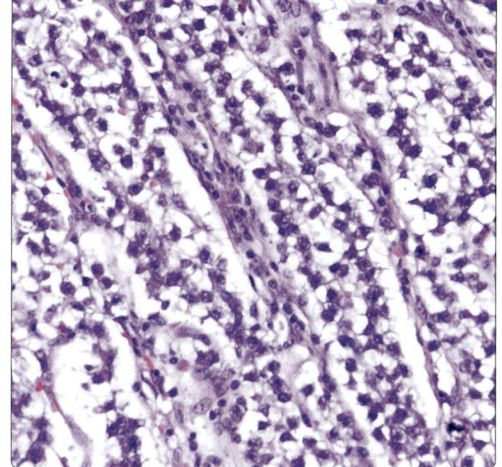

Seminoma: Cord-Like Growth
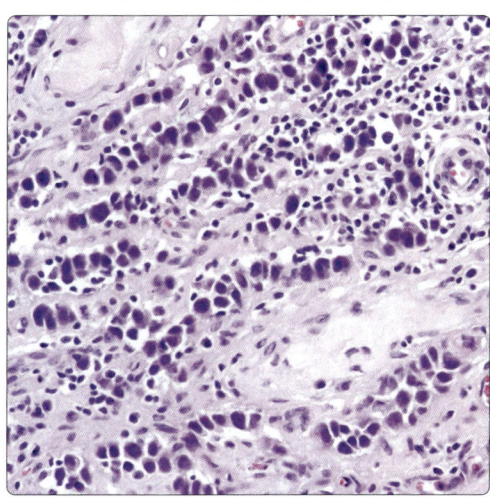

(Left) This image shows a classic seminoma with trabecular or elongated tubular growth pattern and fibrovascular septa. The tumor cells have relatively uniform nuclei with prominent nucleoli and abundant clear cytoplasm. Sertoli cell tumor is in the differential. **(Right)** This photomicrograph shows a seminoma with cord-like or trabecular growth pattern. There is interstitial fibrosis and a lymphoplasmacytic infiltrate also present.

Seminoma: Interstitial Growth
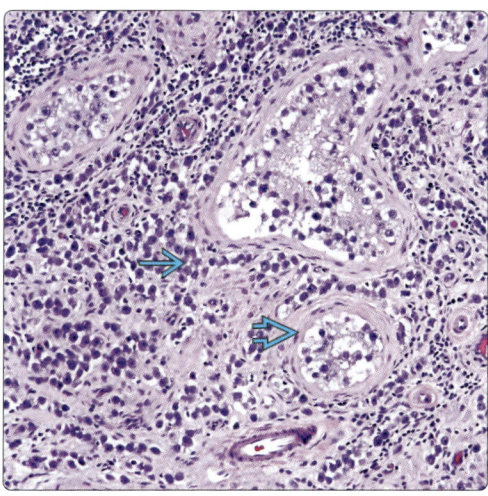

Seminoma: Prominent Sclerosis
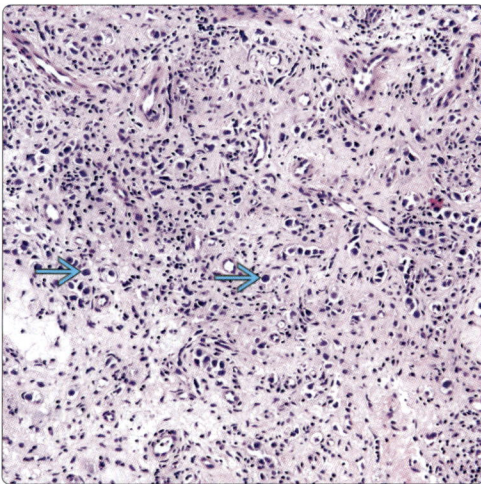

(Left) This photomicrograph shows an interstitial infiltrative pattern of seminomatous tumor cells ⇒ in between the atrophic seminiferous tubules involved by germ cell neoplasia in situ (GCNIS) ⇒. Also present are many small lymphocytes. **(Right)** This low-power image shows a seminoma with dense sclerotic stroma, scattered tumor cells ⇒, and small lymphocytes. In cases where tumor cells are difficult to identify by light microscopy, immunostain with OCT3/OCT4 can be very helpful.

Seminoma

Intratubular Seminoma

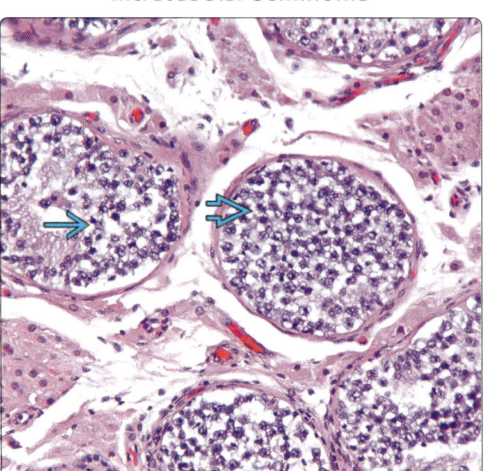

Intratubular Seminoma and GCNIS

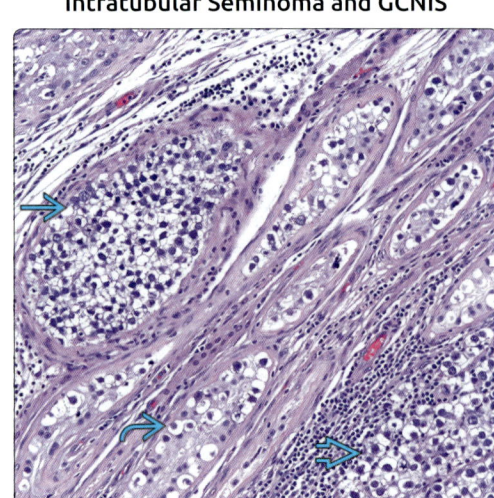

(Left) Intratubular seminoma is characterized by expansion of seminiferous tubules by monotonous seminomatous cells (complete ⇨ and partial ⇨). This is often present away from the main tumor mass and is usually not grossly evident. (Right) This photo shows invasive seminoma ⇨ with GCNIS ⇨ and intratubular seminoma ⇨. The tumor cells within different compartments have a similar morphologic appearance.

Rete Pagetoid Spread

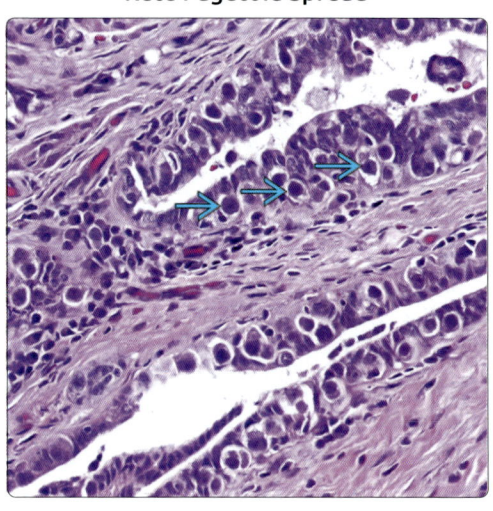

Rete Invasion

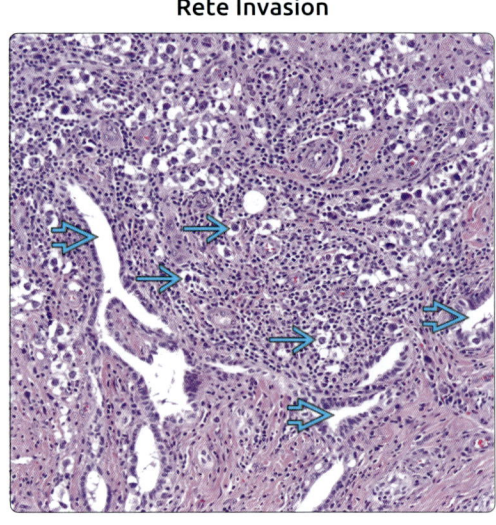

(Left) High-power photomicrograph of rete testis shows pagetoid spread of GCNIS. The tumor cells have large nuclei and abundant clear cytoplasm ⇨. (Right) An example of rete testis ⇨ extension by invasive seminoma is shown. The seminomatous tumor cells ⇨ have large nuclei and abundant clear cytoplasm. Prominent lymphoid infiltrate is also present. This is an adverse prognostic feature.

Anaplastic Seminoma

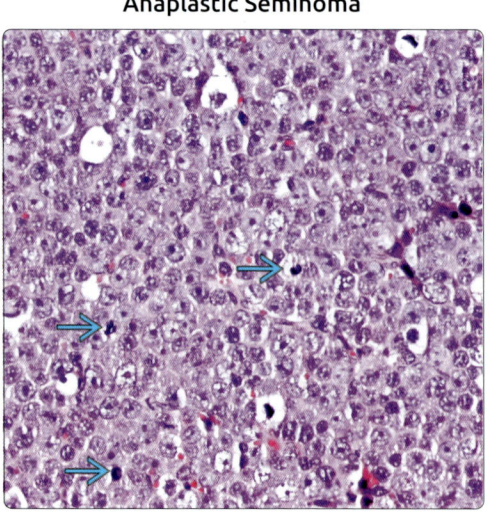

Seminoma: Necrosis

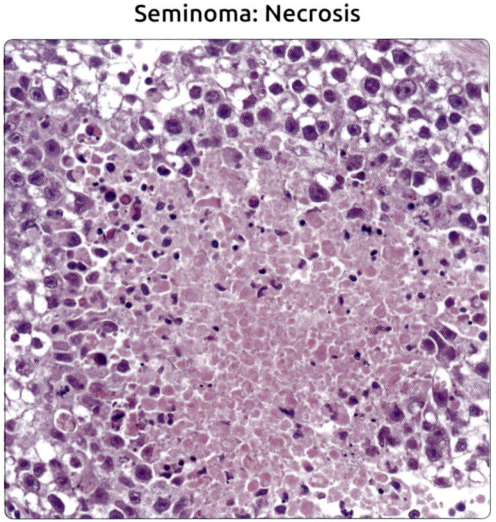

(Left) This is an example of so-called anaplastic seminoma. The tumor consists of solid tumor cells with larger nuclei, higher N:C ratio, and more cellular pleomorphism than typical seminoma. Frequent mitoses ⇨ are present. There is no clinical significance of anaplastic designation. (Right) An area of tumor cell necrosis (not common) is seen in this classic seminoma. The viable tumor cells have characteristic cytologic features of seminoma.

Seminoma

Seminoma: OCT3/OCT4
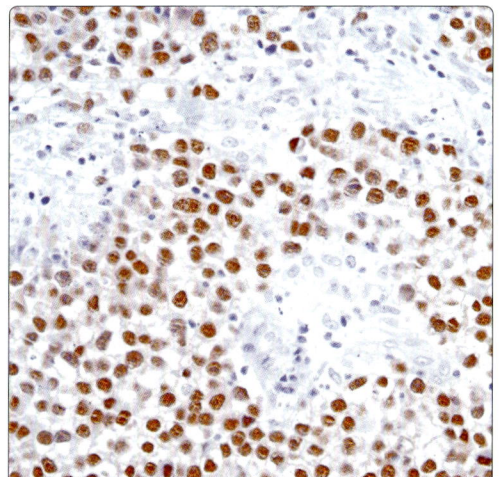

Seminoma: Podoplanin
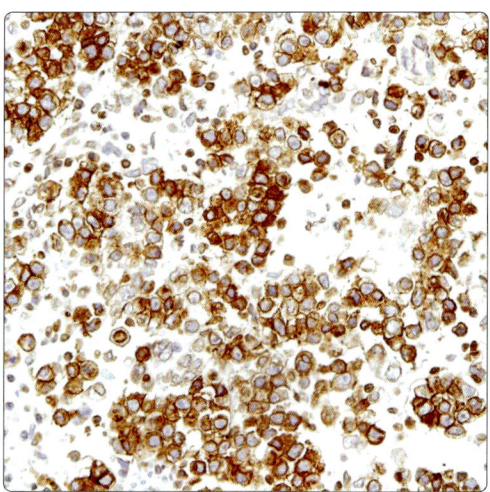

(Left) OCT3/OCT4 stains the seminoma in a strong nuclear pattern. OCT3/OCT4 is a very useful marker for identification of seminoma and embryonal carcinoma, particularly in a metastatic setting. **(Right)** Podoplanin (D2-40) stains the seminoma with a strong cytoplasmic and membranous pattern. Cytokeratin is useful to differentiate seminoma from embryonal carcinoma.

Seminoma
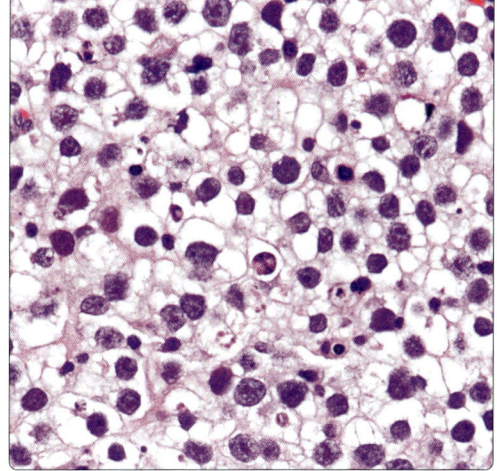

Yolk Sac Tumor
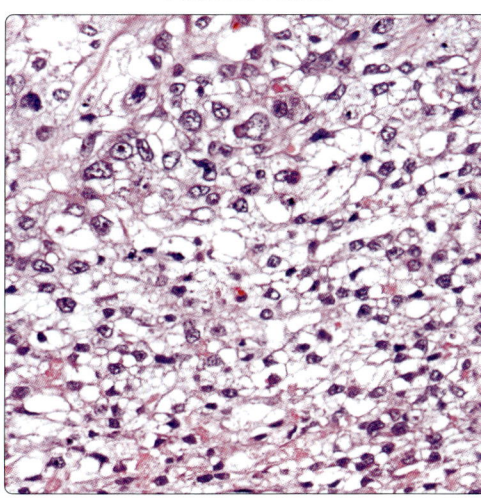

(Left) High-power photomicrograph shows a classic seminoma with a solid growth pattern. Note the relatively uniform and evenly distributed tumor cells with round nuclei, small nucleoli, and prominent cytoplasmic membrane boundaries. **(Right)** An example of a yolk sac tumor with a solid growth pattern is shown. The cytologic features are moderately pleomorphic cells with abundant clear or eosinophilic cytoplasm, cytoplasmic vacuoles, and microcyst formation.

Embryonal Carcinoma
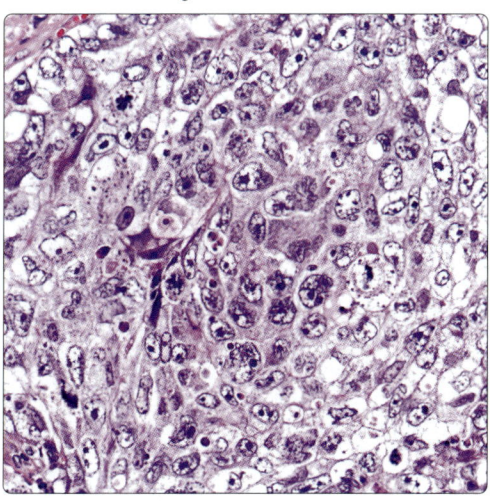

Sertoli Cell Tumor
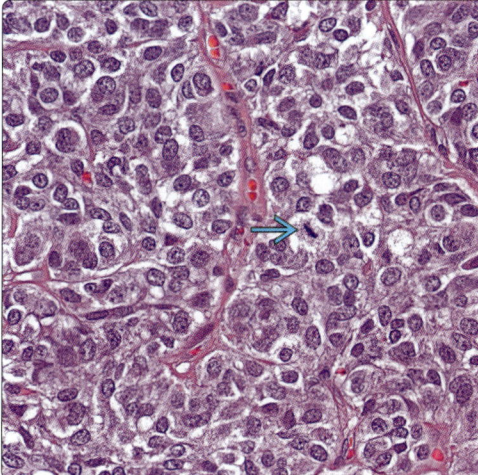

(Left) Solid embryonal carcinoma is composed of anaplastic tumor cells with nuclear overlapping. The tumor cells have coarse and vesicular chromatin, macro- and irregular nucleoli, and frequent mitoses and apoptotic bodies. **(Right)** A high-power photomicrograph of a solid Sertoli cell tumor is shown. The cytologic features show relatively uniform ovoid nuclei, prominent nucleoli, and abundant eosinophilic to clear cytoplasm. Rare mitoses may be seen ➔.

Embryonal Carcinoma

KEY FACTS

TERMINOLOGY
- Germ cell tumor composed of undifferentiated cells of epithelial appearance with marked cytologic anaplasia and variety of growth patterns

CLINICAL ISSUES
- 2nd most common pure testicular germ cell neoplasm after seminoma (~ 10%)
- Age ranges from 15-35 years (10 years younger than patients with seminoma)

MACROSCOPIC
- Often poorly circumscribed mass with more frequent extension to rete testis, epididymis, or spermatic cord (20%) than seminoma
- Variegated cut surface with large areas of hemorrhage and necrosis

MICROSCOPIC
- Pleomorphic tumor with 3 main growth patterns: Solid, glandular, and papillary
- Large cohesive, highly pleomorphic tumor cells with moderate amount of amphophilic cytoplasm and indistinct cell membranes
- Syncytial growth with nuclear overlapping with uneven cellular distribution, coarse or vesicular chromatin, prominent and irregular nucleoli
- Frequent mitoses and apoptoses
- Large areas of hemorrhage and necrosis common

ANCILLARY TESTS
- Positive for cytokeratin, CD30 (BerH2), OCT3/4, PLAP, SALL4, SOX2
- Negative for EMA/MUC1, CEA, CK20, SOX17, glypican-3, α-inhibin, and calretinin

Embryonal Carcinoma: Heterogenous

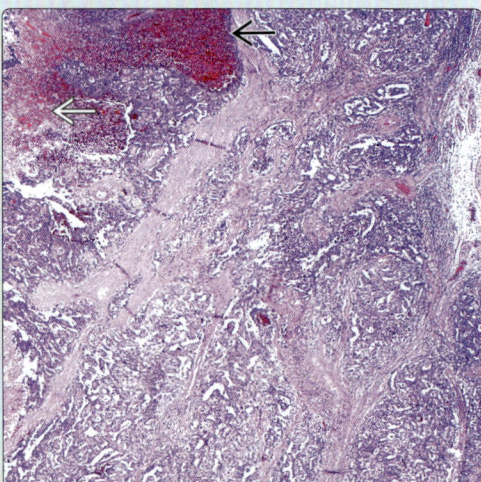

Embryonal Carcinoma: Solid Sheets

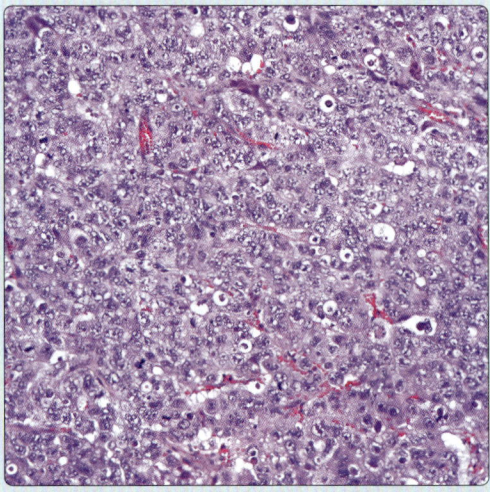

(Left) Low-power photomicrograph of embryonal carcinoma (EC) shows heterogeneous growth appearance with multiple patterns in the same tumor, including areas of glandular, papillary, and solid patterns. Areas of hemorrhage ➡ and necrosis ➡ are present. **(Right)** Solid EC shows sheets of large anaplastic cells with crowded nuclei, prominent nucleoli, and indistinct cell borders. In contrast, seminoma shows nonoverlapping cells with distinct cell borders; cells of yolk sac tumor (YST) are less atypical.

Embryonal Carcinoma: Papillary

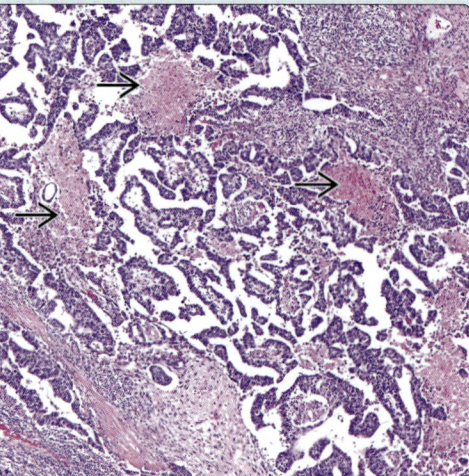

Embryonal Carcinoma: Glandular

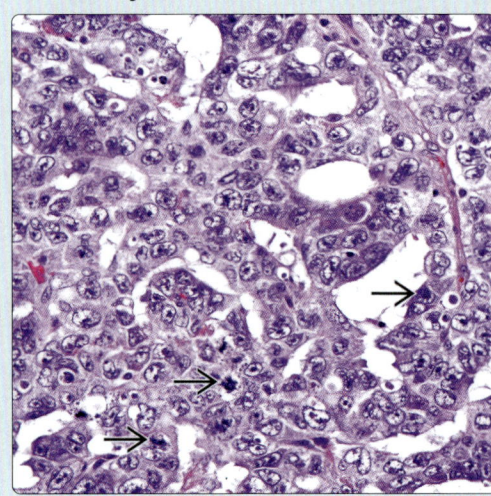

(Left) EC with papillary growth pattern and fibrovascular cores is shown. There are multiple foci of necrosis ➡. Although YST may be papillary, it has a much lesser degree of cytologic atypia and necrosis. **(Right)** EC with complex glandular pattern is shown. It is composed of anaplastic tumor cells with overlapping nuclei, vesicular chromatin, and frequent mitoses ➡.

Embryonal Carcinoma

TERMINOLOGY

Abbreviations
- Embryonal carcinoma (EC)

Definitions
- Germ cell tumor composed of undifferentiated cells of epithelial appearance with marked cytologic anaplasia and variety of growth patterns

CLINICAL ISSUES

Epidemiology
- Incidence
  - 2nd most common pure testicular germ cell neoplasm after seminoma (~ 10%)
  - More commonly seen as mixed with other germ cell tumor components (~ 80%)
- Age
  - 15-35 years (10 years younger than patients with seminoma)
  - Does not occur in infants or children; rare after 5th decade

Presentation
- Testicular mass or swelling
- Symptoms of metastasis, such as back pain, dyspnea, and neurologic symptoms
- Elevated serum lactate dehydrogenase, PLAP, and CA19-9 may be seen
- In pure EC, α-fetoprotein and β-hCG are not elevated

Treatment
- Similar to other nonseminomatous germ cell tumors; depends mainly on clinical stage

Prognosis
- Poorest among all germ cell tumors, worse than mixed germ cell tumor or seminoma
- Prognosis closely correlated to clinical and pathologic stage of tumor
  - Cure rate > 95% for stage I, 70-85% for bulky stage II and stage III disease
- More aggressive treatment with combined chemotherapy alone or in combination with retroperitoneal lymph node dissection following orchiectomy

IMAGING

General Features
- Ultrasonography may detect mass lesion (typically ill-defined and heterogeneous) in testis

MACROSCOPIC

General Features
- Often poorly circumscribed mass
- Variegated cut surface with large areas of hemorrhage and necrosis

Size
- Variable (mean tumor: 2.5 cm)
- Usually smaller than classic seminoma or mixed germ cell tumor

MICROSCOPIC

Histologic Features
- Pleomorphic tumor with variety of growth patterns and often mixed patterns
  - 3 main growth patterns
    - Solid, glandular, and papillary
  - Other less common patterns
    - Pseudopapillary, micropapillary, anastomosing/glandular, blastocyst-like
  - Appliqué pattern (central solid EC surrounded by peripheral degenerating tumor cells) may be seen
  - 2 rare distinctive patterns
    - Polyembryoma-like and diffuse embryoma-like (not pure, examples of mixed germ cell tumor)
- Hemorrhage and necrosis are common
- Lymphocytic infiltrates may be seen, but granulomatous reaction is rare
- More frequent lymphovascular invasion than seminoma
- More frequent rete testis, epididymis, and spermatic cord invasion than other germ cell tumors
- Germ cell neoplasia in situ (GCNIS) is commonly seen
- Intratubular EC with comedo-type necrosis and calcifications may be seen

Cytologic Features
- Large, cohesive, highly pleomorphic tumor cells with moderate amount of amphophilic cytoplasm and indistinct cell membranes
- Syncytial growth with nuclear overlapping with uneven cellular distribution, coarse or vesicular chromatin, prominent and irregular nucleoli
- Columnar cells with subnuclear or supranuclear cytoplasmic vacuoles in some glandular EC
- Frequent mitoses and apoptoses with geographic areas of necrosis

Predominant Pattern/Injury Type
- 3 main growth patterns
  - Solid, glandular, and papillary

Predominant Cell/Compartment Type
- Highly pleomorphic tumor cells with coarse or vesicular chromatin, prominent and irregular nucleoli

ANCILLARY TESTS

Immunohistochemistry
- Positive for cytokeratin, CD30 (BerH2), OCT3/4, PLAP, SALL4, SOX2
- May be focally positive for HCG or α-fetoprotein
- Negative for EMA/MUC1, CEA, CK20, SOX17, glypican-3, α-inhibin, and calretinin

DIFFERENTIAL DIAGNOSIS

Seminoma (Anaplastic Seminoma)
- Sheets or lobules of tumor cells with less cytologic atypia and distinct cell borders
- Presence of more prominent lymphoplasmacytic infiltrate or granulomas
- Positive for CD117, OCT3/4, SOX17

Embryonal Carcinoma

- Negative for CD30 (BerH2), SOX2, and cytokeratin (or focally positive)

Anaplastic Spermatocytic Tumor
- Occurs in older patients
- Associated with classic area of spermatocytic tumor
- Usually solid, occasionally micro- or macrocystic growth
- Negative for CD30, cytokeratin, podoplanin (D2-40), PLAP, and OCT3/4
- Positive for CD117 and SALL4 (variable)

Yolk Sac Tumor (Solid or Papillary)
- Less atypical cells with more abundant cytoplasm, eosinophilic globules, and basement membrane material
- Variety of growth patterns in same tumor
- Positive for α-fetoprotein and glypican-3
- Negative for CD30 (BerH2), OCT3/4, or podoplanin (D2-40)

Metastatic Carcinoma
- Occurs in older patients; clinical history of cancer
- More frequently bilateral
- Lack of GCNIS
- Positive for EMA/MUC1 and tissue-specific markers of metastatic origin
- Negative for germ cell markers (OCT3/4, SALL4)

Malignant Lymphoma
- Older age and more frequently bilateral (40%)
- Diffuse and interstitial growth patterns
- Tumor cells less cohesive and less pleomorphic than embryonal carcinoma
- Positive for leukocyte common antigen and B- and T-cell markers

Sex Cord-Stromal Tumors
- Tumor cells less pleomorphic, rare, or no mitoses
- Positive for inhibin, calretinin, Melan-A (MART-1), and SF1
- Negative for germ cell markers (OCT3/4, SALL4)

DIAGNOSTIC CHECKLIST

Pathologic Interpretation Pearls
- Heterogeneous, epithelial growth with frequent solid, glandular, papillary, or other rare patterns
- Highly anaplastic cytologic features of tumor cells
- Frequent hemorrhage and tumor necrosis
- Intratubular EC with comedonecrosis and coarse calcification

REPORTING

Key Elements To Report
- Pure or mixed with other germ cell tumor components (if mixed, indicate relative percentage of each component)
- Status of lymphovascular invasion
- Rete testis, spermatic cord, and tunica invasion
- Spermatic cord margin status
- Pathologic stage (pTNM)
- Presence of GCNIS, intratubular embryonal carcinoma, or syncytiotrophoblastic cells

SELECTED REFERENCES

1. Kao CS et al: Testicular embryonal carcinoma: a morphologic study of 180 cases highlighting unusual and unemphasized aspects. Am J Surg Pathol. 38(5):689-97, 2014
2. Giannatempo P et al: Persistent CD30 expression by embryonal carcinoma in the treatment time course: prognostic significance of a worthwhile target for personalized treatment. J Urol. 190(5):1919-24, 2013
3. Ye H et al: Difficult differential diagnoses in testicular pathology. Arch Pathol Lab Med. 136(4):435-46, 2012
4. de Jong J et al: Differential expression of SOX17 and SOX2 in germ cells and stem cells has biological and clinical implications. J Pathol. 215(1):21-30, 2008
5. Berney DM et al: The frequency of intratubular embryonal carcinoma: implications for the pathogenesis of germ cell tumours. Histopathology. 45(2):155-61, 2004
6. Albers P et al: Risk factors for relapse in clinical stage I nonseminomatous testicular germ cell tumors: results of the German Testicular Cancer Study Group Trial. J Clin Oncol. 21(8):1505-12, 2003
7. Leroy X et al: CD30 and CD117 (c-kit) used in combination are useful for distinguishing embryonal carcinoma from seminoma. J Histochem Cytochem. 50(2):283-5, 2002
8. Francis R et al: Surveillance for stage I testicular germ cell tumours: results and cost benefit analysis of management options. Eur J Cancer. 36(15):1925-32, 2000
9. Looijenga LH et al: Pathogenesis of testicular germ cell tumours. Rev Reprod. 4(2):90-100, 1999
10. van Echten J et al: No recurrent structural abnormalities apart from i(12p) in primary germ cell tumors of the adult testis. Genes Chromosomes Cancer. 14(2):133-44, 1995
11. Moul JW et al: Percentage of embryonal carcinoma and of vascular invasion predicts pathological stage in clinical stage I nonseminomatous testicular cancer. Cancer Res. 54(2):362-4, 1994
12. Jacobsen GK et al: Histopathological features in stage I non-seminomatous testicular germ cell tumours correlated to relapse. Danish Testicular Cancer Study Group. APMIS. 98(4):377-82, 1990
13. Wishnow KI et al: Identifying patients with low-risk clinical stage I nonseminomatous testicular tumors who should be treated by surveillance. Urology. 34(6):339-43, 1989
14. Mostofi FK et al: Developments in histopathology of testicular germ cell tumors. Semin Urol. 6(3):171-88, 1988
15. Rodriguez PN et al: Nonseminomatous germ cell tumor of the testicle: does extensive staging of the primary tumor predict the likelihood of metastatic disease? J Urol. 136(3):604-8, 1986
16. Krag Jacobsen G et al: Testicular germ cell tumours in Denmark 1976-1980. Pathology of 1058 consecutive cases. Acta Radiol Oncol. 23(4):239-47, 1984
17. von Hochstetter AR et al: The differential diagnosis of testicular germ cell tumors in theory and practice. A critical analysis of two major systems of classification and review of 389 cases. Virchows Arch A Pathol Anat Histol. 396(3):247-77, 1982
18. Bosl GJ et al: Tumor markers in advanced nonseminomatous testicular cancer. Cancer. 47(3):572-6, 1981

Embryonal Carcinoma

Embryonal Carcinoma: Gross
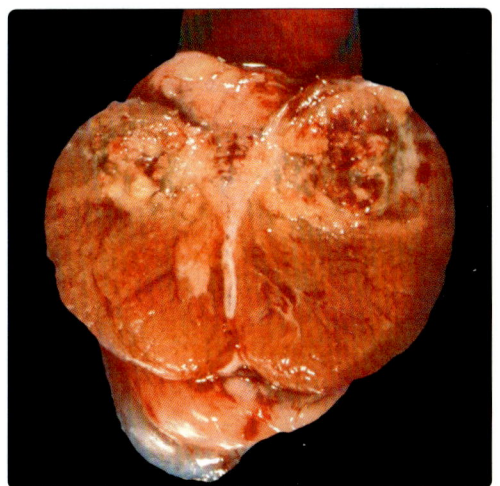

Embryonal Carcinoma: Gross
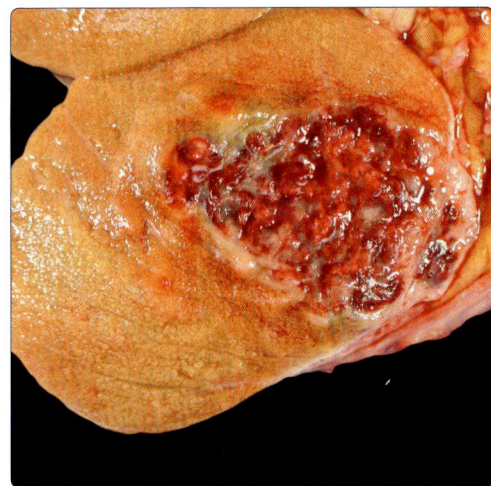

(Left) EC with a variegated cut surface, hemorrhage, and necrosis is shown. The tumor is poorly circumscribed. The rete testis and spermatic cord are more commonly involved in EC than in seminoma. (Right) This photo shows an EC with a variegated, hemorrhagic, and necrotic appearance and poorly demarcated borders. Hemorrhage and necrosis in a germ cell tumor often contain EC and choriocarcinoma components, such that sections should be taken from these areas when identified grossly.

Embryonal Carcinoma: Complex Glandular
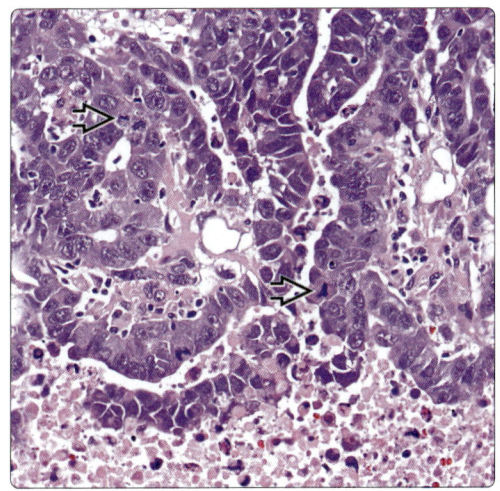

Embryonal Carcinoma: Solid
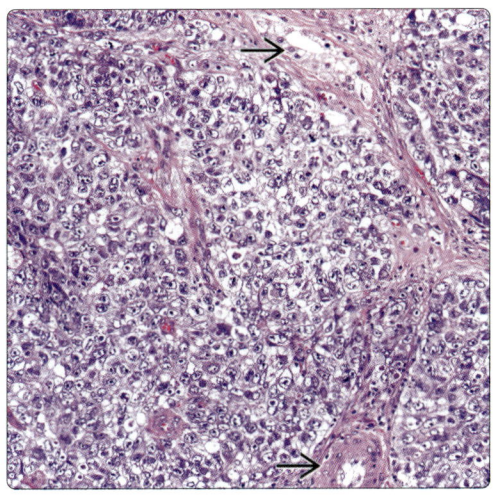

(Left) This image shows complex glandular growth of EC with highly pleomorphic cells with indistinct cell borders, overlapping nuclei, prominent nucleoli, and frequent mitoses ⇨. Tumor cell necrosis is also present. (Right) This image shows a solid EC with sheets of tumor cells divided by fibrous septa. Distinction from seminoma is based on cytologic features and absence of lymphocytic or granulomatous reaction. Also present are compressed atrophic seminiferous tubules ⇨.

Embryonal Carcinoma: Delicate Papillae
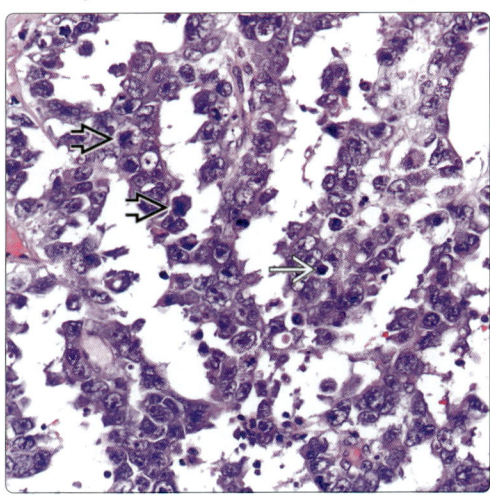

Embryonal Carcinoma: Papillary
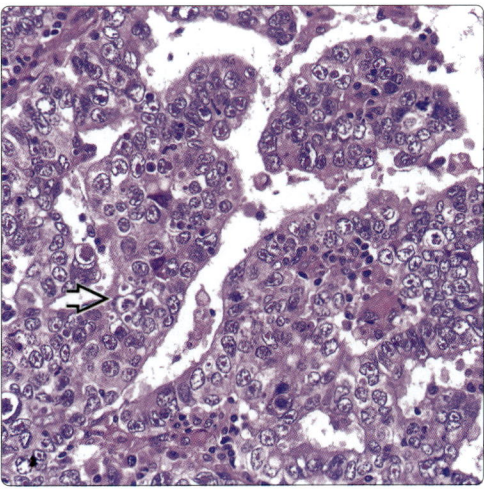

(Left) This EC has delicate papillae lined by highly pleomorphic tumor cells. The tumor cells exhibit nuclear overlapping (syncytial growth), macronucleoli, and frequent mitoses ⇨ and apoptosis ⇨. (Right) High-power photomicrograph shows papillary EC composed of cohesive anaplastic tumor cells with nuclear overlapping, uneven cellular distribution, large vesicular nuclei, macronucleoli, and frequent apoptoses ⇨. The cytoplasm is eosinophilic to amphophilic, and cell boundaries are indistinct.

Embryonal Carcinoma

(Left) *Papillary/glandular pattern of EC with columnar cells may mimic papillary YST, but YST has less pronounced cytologic atypia than EC. In difficult situations, immunostain with a panel of markers, CD30 and OCT3/4 for EC vs. α-fetoprotein and glypican-3 for YST, may be helpful.* **(Right)** *High-power image shows glandular EC with columnar cells and a brush border ➔ resembling YST with enteric/endometrioid pattern. Cytologic features are more pleomorphic than those of YST.*

Embryonal Carcinoma: Papillary/Glandular
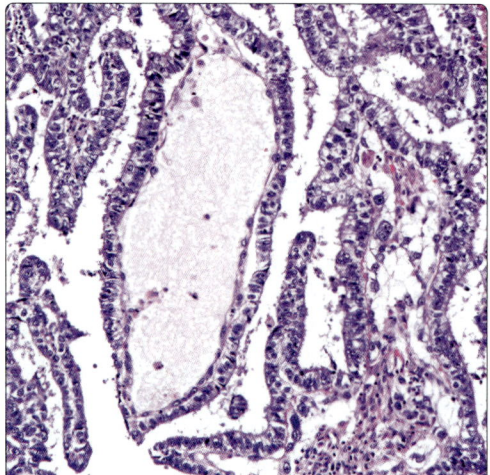

Embryonal Carcinoma: Glandular
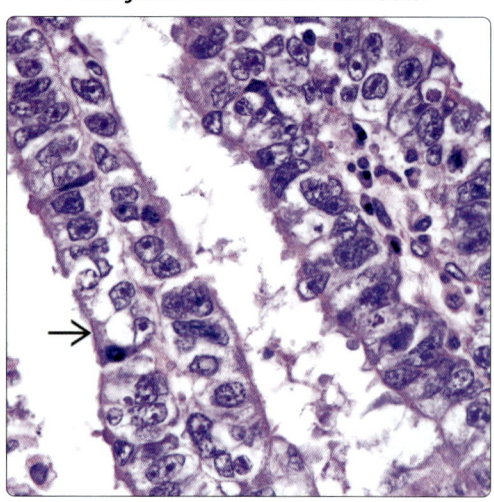

(Left) *EC with appliqué pattern shows central solid EC ➔ wrapped by degenerating cells ➔, which may mimic the biphasic pattern of choriocarcinoma. The lack of true syncytiotrophoblasts, hemorrhage, and villous configuration prevents the erroneous diagnosis of choriocarcinoma.* **(Right)** *This image shows EC with cribriform glands surrounded by desmoplastic stroma and retraction artifact, mimicking lymphovascular invasion. This pattern may raise the possibility of metastatic carcinoma.*

Embryonal Carcinoma: Appliqué Pattern
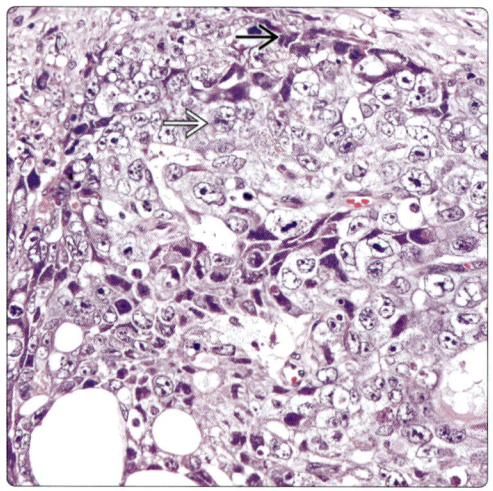

Embryonal Carcinoma: Cribriform
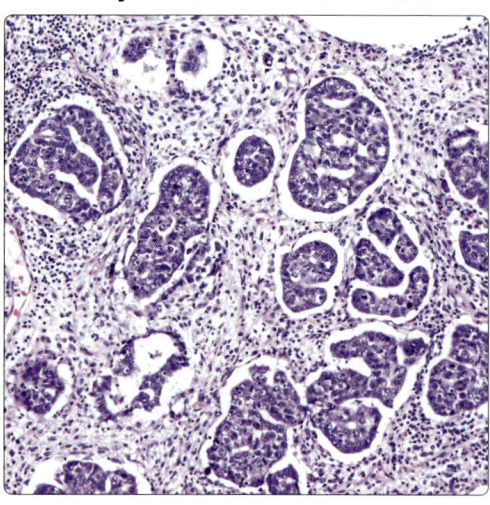

(Left) *EC with multifocal vascular invasion ➔ is shown. Features that confirm vascular invasion include peritumoral location ➔, tumor conforming to the shape of the vessels, and intravascular growth based on plump endothelial-lined spaces or attachment to the vascular wall. Vascular lymphatic invasion is an adverse prognostic factor and determines pathologic stage.* **(Right)** *Invasion of rete testis ➔ by solid EC ➔ is shown. Distinction from vascular invasion may be necessary by using immunostain with vascular markers.*

Embryonal Carcinoma: Vascular Invasion
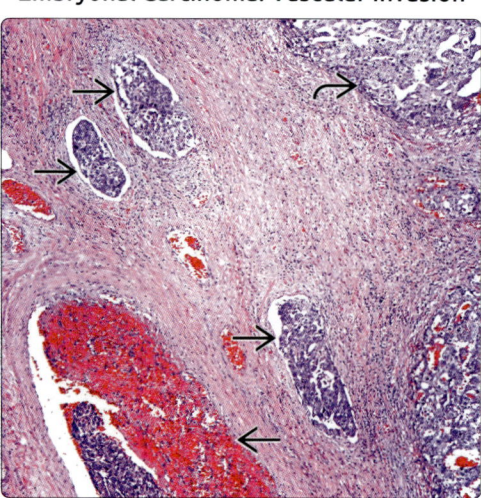

Embryonal Carcinoma: Rete Testis Invasion
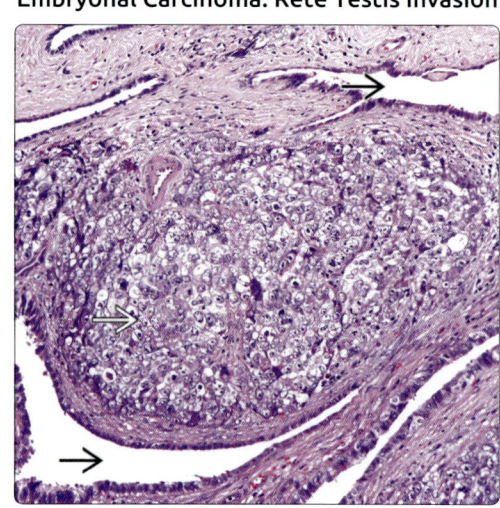

Embryonal Carcinoma

Intratubular Embryonal Carcinoma

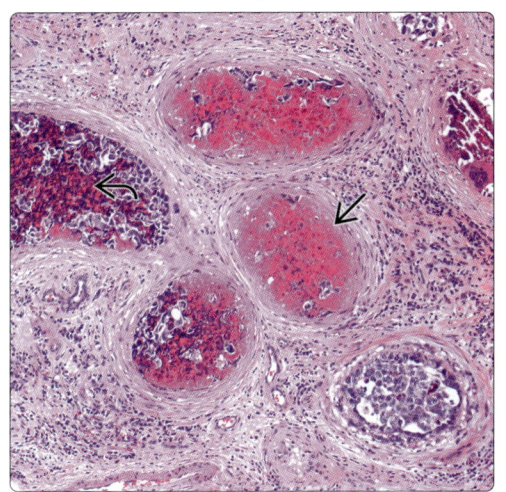

Intratubular Embryonal Carcinoma

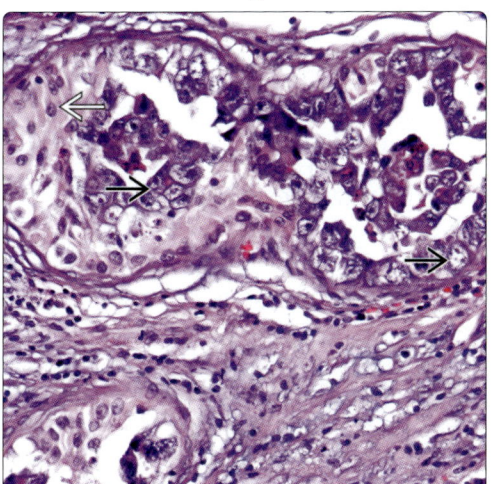

(Left) Intratubular EC may be seen within or at the edge of the tumor. Markedly atypical cells of EC within the seminiferous tubules, often with central comedo necrosis ⇨, are present. Necrotic tumor cell debris is often seen ⇨. (Right) This photomicrograph shows intratubular EC with anaplastic tumor cells ⇨ partially replacing the cellular constituents of the seminiferous tubules ⇨. The intratubular EC cells are identical to that of invasive EC cells.

Mixed Embryonal Carcinoma and YST

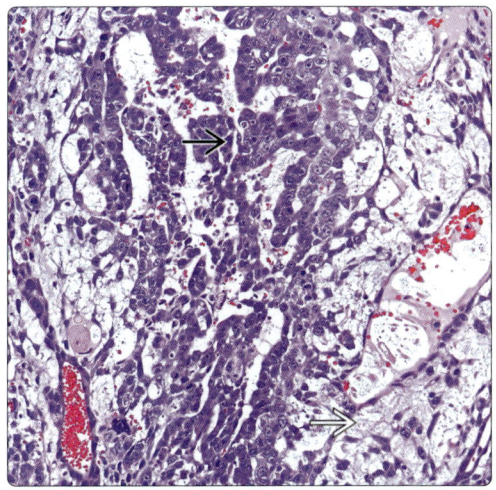

Embryonal Carcinoma: CK-PAN

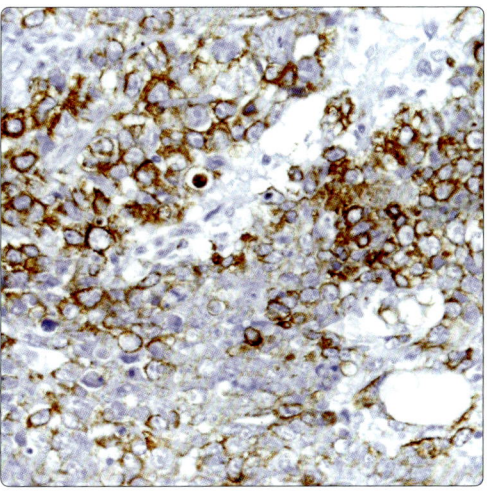

(Left) EC ⇨ admixed with YST ⇨ is a frequent finding of mixed germ cell tumor. The YST component is often seen at the edge of EC tumor cell nests. YST tumor cells may be deceptively benign with cuboidal or flattened cells. (Right) EC is often diffusely positive for CK-PAN, whereas seminoma is typically negative or only focally weakly positive. Thus, in any situation when EC and seminoma are serious differential diagnoses, cytokeratin and CD30 (BerH2) may be used for this purpose.

Embryonal Carcinoma: CD30

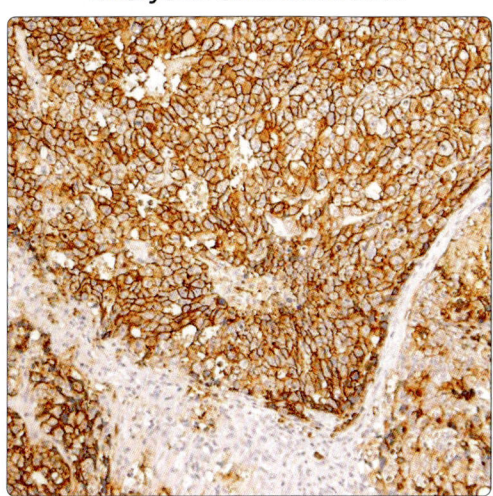

Embryonal Carcinoma: OCT3/4

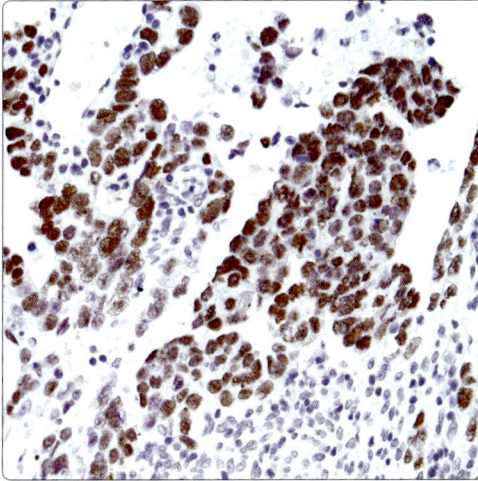

(Left) The tumor cells of EC are strongly positive for CD30 (BerH2) with membranous staining pattern. Such positivity with CD30 (BerH2) is not seen in YST or seminoma. (Right) The tumor cells of EC are positive for OCT3/4 in a nuclear pattern, similar to seminoma. The tumor cells of YST and choriocarcinoma are typically negative for OCT3/4. A combination of cytokeratin, OCT3/4, and CD30 (BerH2) is diagnostic of EC in the appropriate histologic context.

Yolk Sac Tumor

KEY FACTS

TERMINOLOGY
- Germ cell tumor characterized by variety of growth patterns that recapitulate yolk sac, allantois, and extraembryonic mesenchyme

CLINICAL ISSUES
- Most common germ cell tumor of infants and young children: No association with cryptorchidism (see separate chapter)
- Pure form extremely rare in adults; usually present as component of mixed germ cell tumors

MICROSCOPIC
- YST has multiple growth patterns with 1 or 2 dominant patterns or more frequently mixed patterns
  - Reticular or microcystic pattern most frequent (80%)
  - Other common patterns include endodermal sinus, solid, papillary, and glandular
- Relatively uniform cells with clear or vacuolated to lightly eosinophilic cytoplasm
- Bland cuboidal, columnar to flattened, or spindle cells
- Presence of small, spherical, intracellular, or extracellular hyaline globules
- Prominent basement membrane deposition

ANCILLARY TESTS
- Positive for cytokeratin, AFP, glypican-3, SALL4, PLAP (variable), SOX17 (variable)
- Negative for CD30(Ber-H2), podoplanin (D2-40), OCT3/4, CD117, hCG, NANOG, inhibin-α, calretinin

TOP DIFFERENTIAL DIAGNOSES
- Embryonal carcinoma
- Classic seminoma
- Leydig cell tumor (microcystic)
- Rete testis hyperplasia

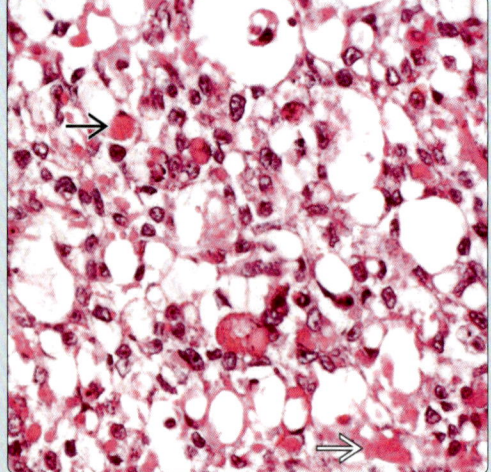

Yolk Sac Tumor: Microcystic and Reticular

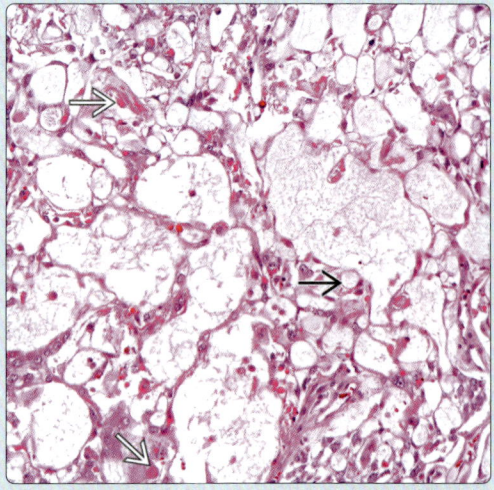

Yolk Sac Tumor: Microcystic

(Left) This image shows microcystic and reticular yolk sac tumor (YST) patterns in which tumor cells contain vacuolated cytoplasm, intercellular eosinophilic globules ⇒, and extracellular pink basement membrane-like material ⇒. (Right) This image shows typical microcystic, or a reticular pattern, of YST with tumor cells forming microcysts and a meshwork of spaces. Some cells contain intracytoplasmic vacuoles ⇒ resembling lipoblasts. Eosinophilic globules ⇒, which are a hallmark of YST, are present.

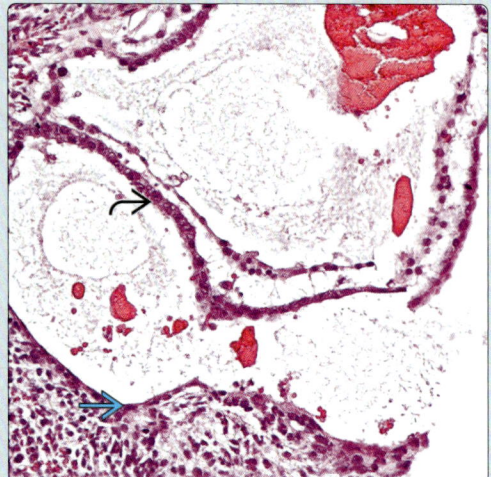

Yolk Sac Tumor: Macrocystic

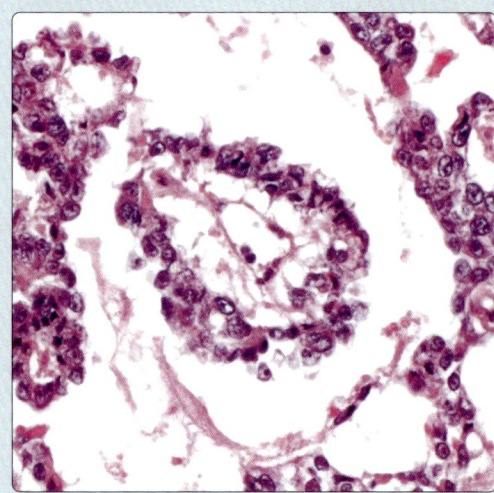

Yolk Sac Tumor: Schiller-Duval Body

(Left) A macrocystic YST results when multiple microcysts coalesce. A YST shows a spectrum of cytoplasmic features that vary from flattened ⇒ to cuboidal ⇒ to columnar. (Right) This image shows a Schiller-Duval body in a YST, which is characterized by a central vessel surrounded by a layer of tumor cells, a hollow space, and another layer of similar or more flattened cells, again set in an empty space.

Yolk Sac Tumor

TERMINOLOGY

Abbreviations
- Yolk sac tumor (YST)

Synonyms
- Endodermal sinus tumor (EST)

Definitions
- Germ cell tumor characterized by variety of growth patterns that recapitulate yolk sac, allantois, and extraembryonic mesenchyme

CLINICAL ISSUES

Epidemiology
- Incidence
  - Pure YST is most common testicular tumor of infants and young children (~ 75%)
    - No association with cryptorchidism or other germ cell tumor components
  - Pure YST is extremely rare (0.6%) in adult testes
    - At extragonadal sites, especially mediastinum, pure YST may occur
  - YST is frequent component of mixed germ cell tumors (in ~ 40%)
  - YST is frequent tumor component after chemotherapy
- Age
  - Mean: 16-18 months for pediatric YST
  - Mean: 25-35 years for adult YST
    - Generally 10 years younger than patients with seminoma

Presentation
- Nonsymptomatic, rapid testicular enlargement
- ~ 90% of patients with childhood YST have clinical stage I disease
- Presence of YST in adult patients with mixed germ cell tumor is frequently associated with lower stage presentation

Laboratory Tests
- More than 95% patients have elevated serum α-fetoprotein (AFP)
- Test for serum AFP is valuable tool in diagnosis and monitoring effectiveness of therapy

Treatment
- For infants and children with pure YST
  - Radical inguinal orchiectomy for stage I tumor with close follow-up protocol (surveillance)
  - Cisplatin-based therapy for relapse on surveillance, advanced stage disease, or metastasis
- For adult YST (usually mixed with other germ cell tumor)
  - Similar to other nonseminomatous germ cell tumor based on clinical stage
  - Radical inguinal orchiectomy ± retroperitoneal lymph node dissection
  - Cisplatin-based chemotherapy for metastatic disease

Prognosis
- Prognosis associated with clinical stage, lymphovascular invasion, level of serum AFP elevation
- Children have better prognosis than adults

IMAGING

General Features
- Ultrasonography may detect scrotal mass

MACROSCOPIC

General Features
- Nonencapsulated, gray-white, soft or firm, homogeneous mass with myxoid or gelatinous cut surface
- Tumors in adults are typically heterogeneous with other germ cell components and may have hemorrhage and necrosis

Size
- Range: 2-6 cm

MICROSCOPIC

Histologic Features
- YST frequently has multiple growth patterns with 1 or 2 dominant patterns
  - Microcystic or reticular pattern most frequent (80%)
    - Anastomosing thin cords forming round or irregular spaces or tubules of variable size
    - Characteristic intracellular vacuoles and merging of cells create sieve-like appearance
  - Endodermal sinus pattern
    - Composed of numerous Schiller-Duval bodies with central fibrovascular core lined by cuboidal to columnar tumor cells, which are surrounded by cystic spaces lined by another layer of flattened tumor cells
    - Labyrinthine spaces or perivascular arrangement of tumor cells are common
  - Solid pattern
    - Solid sheets of polygonal tumor cells with pale eosinophilic or clear cytoplasm, which lack fibrovascular septa, lymphocytes, or granulomas
    - Tumor cells with random pleomorphism and nuclear overlapping; slightly greater atypia than seminoma but less than embryonal carcinoma
  - Papillary and tubulopapillary
    - Papillae ± central fibrovascular cores
    - Tumor cells are often cuboidal and low columnar with hobnail appearance
  - Polyvesicular vitelline pattern
    - Large constricted vesicles lined by flattened to cuboidal cells
    - Often associated with abundant myxoid or loosely fibrous stroma
  - Glandular-alveolar pattern
    - Simple round to complex branching glands with intervening myxoid stroma
  - Parietal pattern
    - Epithelial cells surrounded by pink bands of basement membrane material
  - Enteric or endometrioid pattern
    - Glandular pattern with columnar cells, cytoplasmic clearing, subnuclear vacuoles, and smooth luminal surface
  - Hepatoid pattern

Yolk Sac Tumor

- Sheets of tumor cells with abundant eosinophilic cytoplasm and eosinophilic globules
  - Spindled cell or sarcomatoid pattern
    - Composed of spindle (or sarcomatoid) cells with myxoid stroma; variably cellular
  - Myxomatous pattern
    - Epithelioid to spindle cells dispersed in paucicellular light blue myxoid stroma
    - Frequently underrecognized due to innocuous appearance
  - Macrocystic pattern
    - Large cystic spaces due to coalescence of microcysts lined by flattened tumor cells
  - Mixed pattern
    - Mixture of any of above growth patterns
- Intra- and extracellular PAS(+) hyaline globules
  - More commonly seen in microcystic, reticular, solid, and hepatoid patterns

Cytologic Features
- Relatively uniform epithelioid cells with clear or vacuolated to pale eosinophilic cytoplasm
- Bland cuboidal, columnar to flattened, or frankly spindled cells with mild nuclear pleomorphism
- Slight nuclear overlapping with indistinct cell borders; frequently deceptively benign looking

Predominant Pattern/Injury Type
- Neoplastic

Predominant Cell/Compartment Type
- Germ cell

ANCILLARY TESTS

Histochemistry
- Positive PAS with diastase
  - Staining pattern: Hyaline globules

Immunohistochemistry
- Positive for cytokeratin, AFP, glypican-3, SALL4, PLAP (variable), SOX17 (variable)
- Negative for CD30(BerH2), podoplanin (D2-40), OCT3/4, CD117, hCG, NANOG, inhibin-α, calretinin

DIFFERENTIAL DIAGNOSIS

Embryonal Carcinoma
- Marked cytologic anaplasia, nuclear crowding, frequent mitoses and necrosis
- Positive for CD30(Ber-H2) and OCT3/4; negative for AFP and glypican-3

Seminoma (Tubular)
- Usually accompanied by typical sheets or lobules of more uniform tumor cells separated by fibrous septa with lymphoplasmacytic infiltrate and granulomas
- Distinct cell boundaries with no nuclear overlapping and abundant clear cytoplasm
- Positive for CD117, podoplanin (D2-40), and OCT3/4; negative for cytokeratin, AFP, and glypican-3

Leydig Cell Tumor (Microcystic)
- Well-circumscribed mass; solid growth with uniform cells and more prominent eosinophilic cytoplasm
- Positive for inhibin, calretinin, and SF1; negative for cytokeratin, AFP, SALL4, and glypican-3

Rete Testis Hyperplasia ± Hyaline Globules
- May occur in association ± germ cell tumor in testis
- Retiform proliferation of bland cuboidal cells with or without intracellular hyaline globules
- Lack of cytologic atypia or mitotic figures
- Positive for EMA/MUC1, pax-8; negative for germ cell markers (SALL4, AFP, and glypican-3)

DIAGNOSTIC CHECKLIST

Pathologic Interpretation Pearls
- Multiple different growth patterns
- Microcystic and reticular patterns are common
- Presence of Schiller-Duval bodies, hyaline globules, and basement membrane deposition

REPORTING

Key Elements to Report
- Pathologic stage
- Presence of lymphovascular invasion
- Involvement of rete testis, epididymis, spermatic cord, and tunica
- Status of spermatic cord margin
- Pathology of uninvolved testicular parenchyma

SELECTED REFERENCES

1. Ulbright TM: Gonadoblastoma and hepatoid and endometrioid-like yolk sac tumor: an update. Int J Gynecol Pathol. 33(4):365-73, 2014
2. Kao CS et al: Solid pattern yolk sac tumor: a morphologic and immunohistochemical study of 52 cases. Am J Surg Pathol. 36(3):360-7, 2012
3. Wang F et al: Diagnostic utility of SALL4 in extragonadal yolk sac tumors: an immunohistochemical study of 59 cases with comparison to placental-like alkaline phosphatase, alpha-fetoprotein, and glypican-3. Am J Surg Pathol. 33(10): 1529-39, 2009
4. McLean TW et al: Pediatric genitourinary tumors. Curr Opin Oncol. 20(3):315-20, 2008
5. Oottamasathien S et al: Testicular tumours in children: a single-institutional experience. BJU Int. 99(5):1123-6, 2007
6. Zynger DL et al: Glypican 3: a novel marker in testicular germ cell tumors. Am J Surg Pathol. 30(12):1570-5, 2006
7. Ciftci AO et al: Testicular tumors in children. J Pediatr Surg. 36(12):1796-801, 2001
8. Medica M et al: Adult testicular pure yolk sac tumor. Urol Int. 67(1):94-6, 2001
9. Foster RS et al: Clinical stage I pure yolk sac tumor of the testis in adults has different clinical behavior than juvenile yolk sac tumor. J Urol. 164(6):1943-4, 2000
10. Billings SD et al: Microcystic Leydig cell tumors mimicking yolk sac tumor: a report of four cases. Am J Surg Pathol. 23(5):546-51, 1999
11. Ulbright TM et al: Rete testis hyperplasia with hyaline globule formation. A lesion simulating yolk sac tumor. Am J Surg Pathol. 15(1):66-74, 1991
12. Krag Jacobsen G et al: Testicular germ cell tumours in Denmark 1976-1980. Pathology of 1058 consecutive cases. Acta Radiol Oncol. 23(4):239-47, 1984

Yolk Sac Tumor

Yolk Sac Tumor: Gross
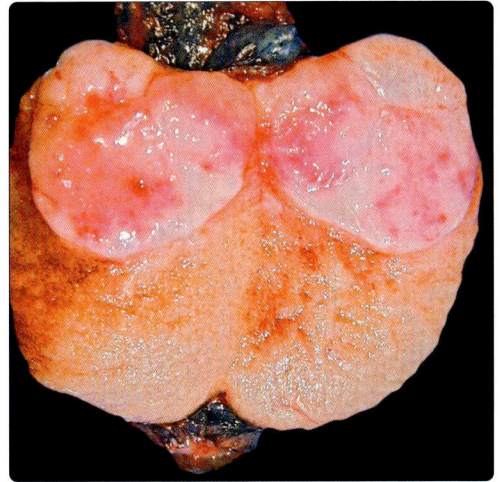

Yolk Sac Tumor: Gross
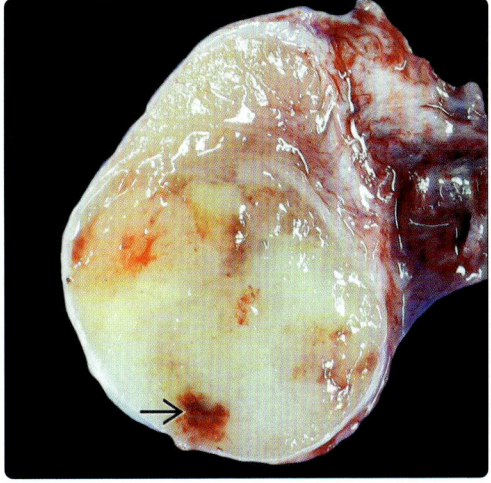

(Left) This is an adult pure YST, which has a homogeneous, mucoid cut surface. The finding of a pure YST in adults is extraordinarily rare. The relatively homogeneous appearance is in keeping with a pure histology under microscopy. (Courtesy Z. Qu, MD, PhD.) **(Right)** A large YST with a white, mucoid cut surface is shown. Focal hemorrhage is present ➡. Sampling heterogeneous-appearing areas in testicular tumors is important to identify different germ cell components.

Yolk Sac Tumor: Low Power
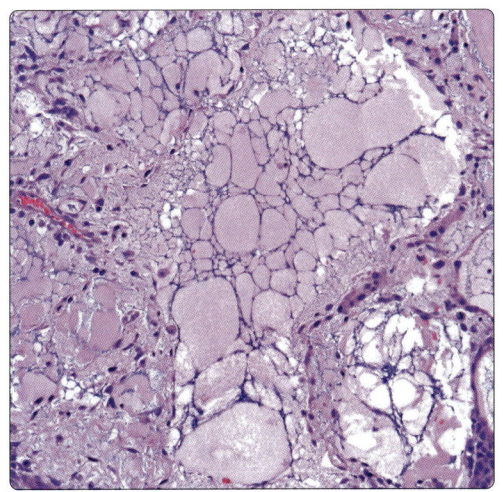

Yolk Sac Tumor: Microcystic and Reticular
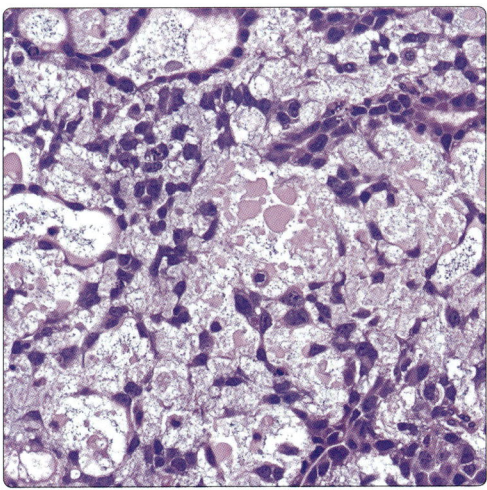

(Left) Low-power photomicrograph shows a microcystic and reticular pattern of YST with abundant eosinophilic (colloid-like) material. **(Right)** A microcystic and reticular pattern of a YST with abundant extracellular eosinophilic material is shown. The tumor cells vary in size and shape and are distinct from embryonal carcinoma cells, which show obvious nuclear atypia. In contrast, seminoma cells show abundant clear cytoplasm with well-defined cell borders.

Yolk Sac Tumor: Schiller-Duval Bodies
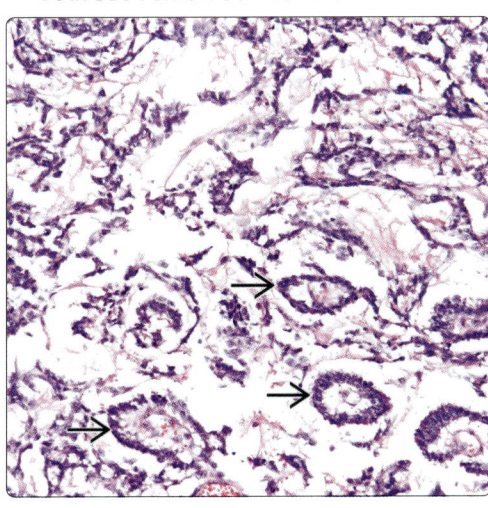

Yolk Sac Tumor: Schiller-Duval Bodies
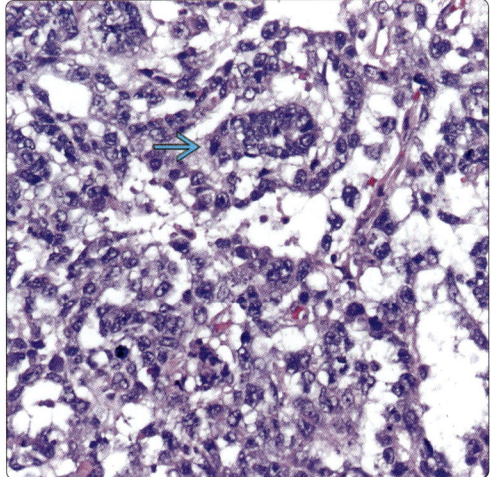

(Left) A YST with a typical endodermal sinus pattern is shown. Multiple Schiller-Duval bodies ➡, which are sectioned in variable planes, are distributed amidst a loose, myxoid stroma. A central blood vessel with a mantle of cells surrounded by space and another cellular layer are typical of this pattern. **(Right)** This image shows endodermal sinus pattern of a YST with a Schiller-Duval body ➡. The tumor cells are often unevenly distributed within edematous and myxoid stroma.

Yolk Sac Tumor

(Left) Solid (upper ➡) and microcystic (lower ➡) growth patterns of a YST are shown. The tumor cells are relatively uniform with ovoid to round nuclei and abundant pale eosinophilic cytoplasm. (Right) A solid growth pattern of a YST is shown. The cells contain abundant pale eosinophilic to clear cytoplasm, similar to that of seminoma, although a lobular configuration or an inflammatory infiltrate is absent. Distinction is possible based on the presence of multiple patterns elsewhere, and cell borders in a YST are usually not prominent.

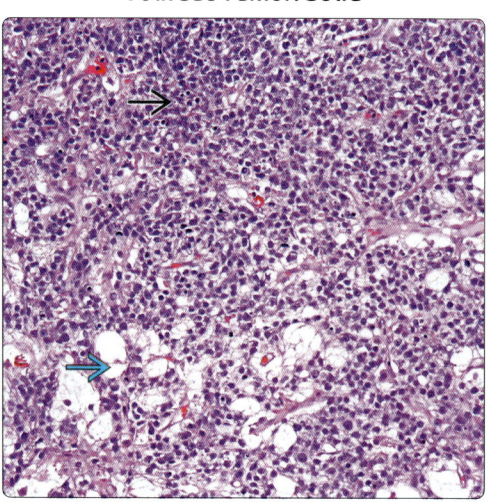

Yolk Sac Tumor: Solid

(Left) Low-power photomicrograph shows a YST with exuberant papillary growth pattern and central fibrovascular cores. The appearance of tumor cells is relatively low grade. (Right) High-power image shows a papillary YST with central fibrovascular cores lined by relatively uniform cuboidal to "hobnail" tumor cells. The bland cytologic features of this tumor are distinct from those of embryonal carcinoma with papillary growth, which have distinct high-grade nuclear atypia.

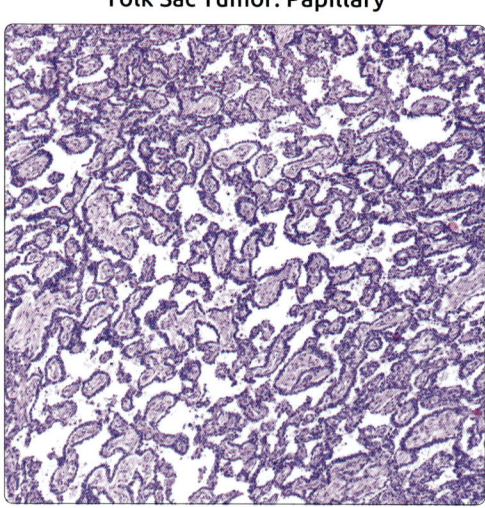 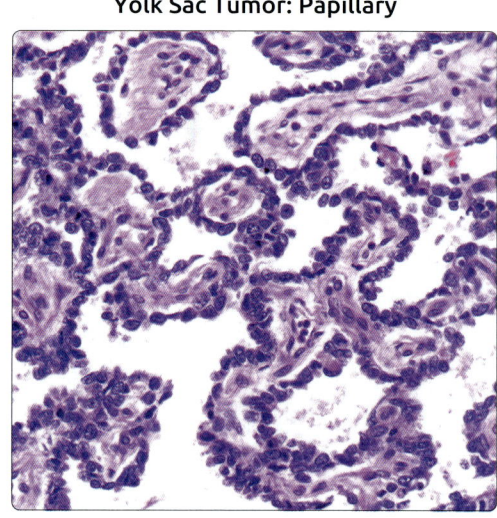

Yolk Sac Tumor: Papillary

(Left) This photomicrograph shows a polyvesicular vitelline pattern of a YST. It is composed of irregularly shaped cysts with central to eccentric constriction ➡ and loose myxoid stroma. The tumor cells are flattened and distributed in a variably cellular mesenchyme. (Right) A polyvesicular vitelline pattern of YST shows irregularly shaped cysts lined by flattened to cuboidal epithelium. The vesicles recapitulate embryonic subdivision of the primary yolk sac into the secondary yolk sac.

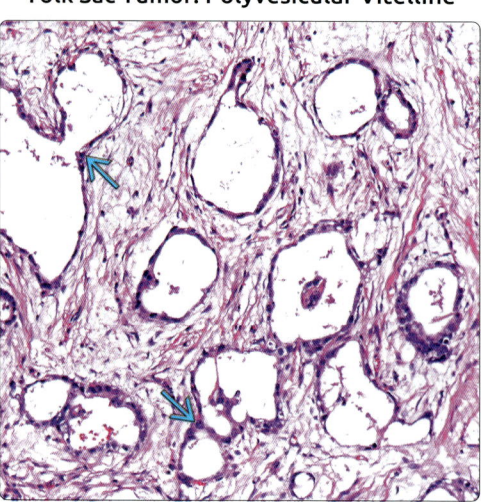 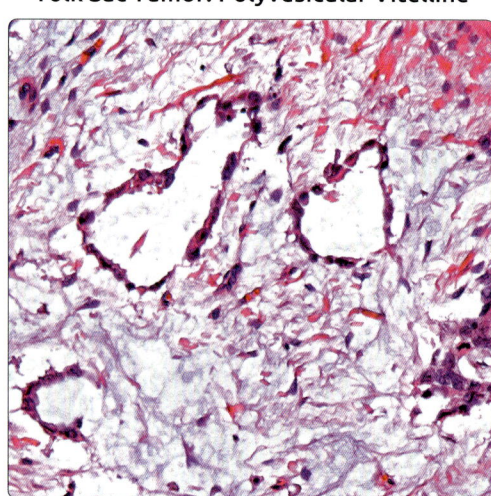

Yolk Sac Tumor: Polyvesicular Vitelline

Yolk Sac Tumor

Yolk Sac Tumor: Glandular
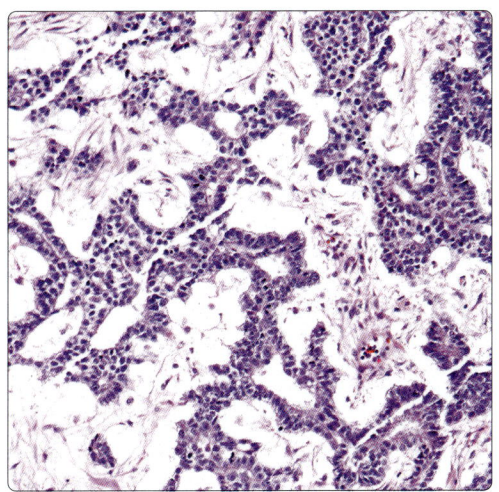

Yolk Sac Tumor: Glandular
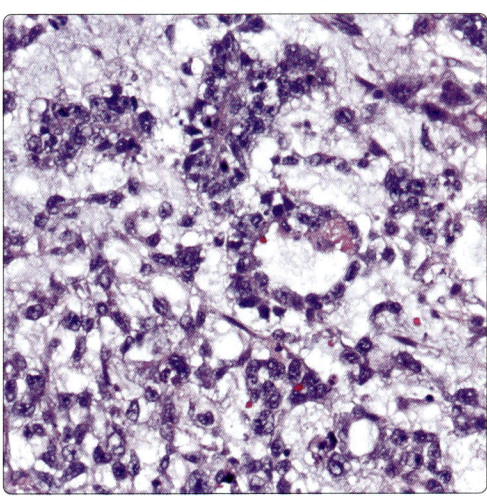

(Left) A glandular growth pattern of a YST with myxoid stroma is shown. The tumor cells are relatively uniform, a feature that is different from the glandular pattern in embryonal carcinoma or metastatic carcinoma. (Right) This image shows a glandular and reticular growth pattern of a YST with prominent myxoid stroma. A combination of multiple patterns within the same tumor is a key distinguishing feature in a YST and is also helpful in diagnosis at extragonadal sites.

Yolk Sac Tumor: Parietal
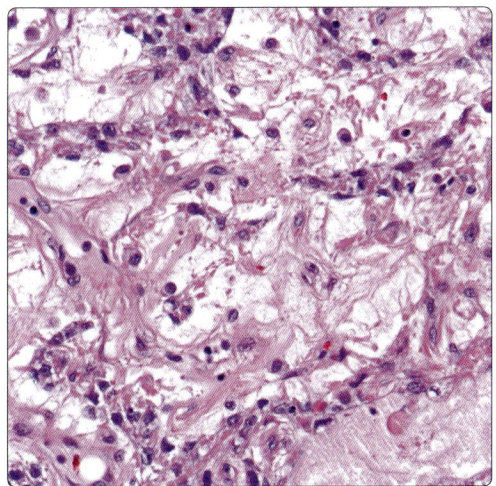

Yolk Sac Tumor: Parietal
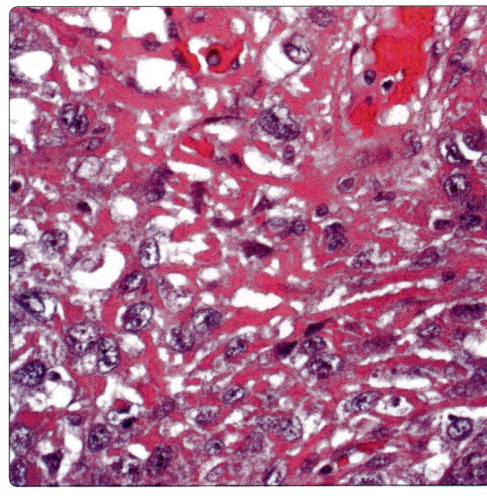

(Left) A parietal pattern of a YST is composed of tumor cells surrounded by abundant bands of pink basement membrane-like material. This pattern is typically associated with a microcystic or reticular pattern of a YST. (Right) High-power view of a parietal pattern of a YST shows tumor cells surrounded by dense pink-staining basement membrane-like material, which represents recapitulation of the parietal layer of the embryonic yolk sac of the rodent; it is usually negative for α-fetoprotein.

Yolk Sac Tumor: Endometrioid
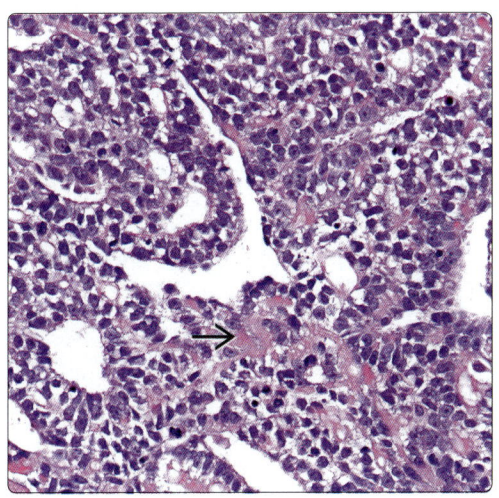

Yolk Sac Tumor: Endometrioid
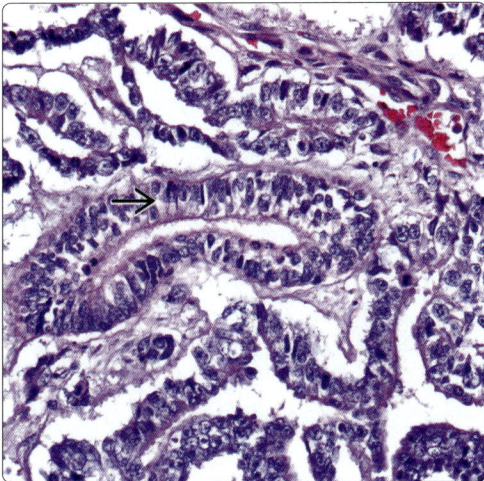

(Left) An enteric (endometrioid) pattern of a YST with columnar cells and subnuclear vacuoles is shown. Also note the focal presence of pink basement membrane-like material ➡. (Right) An enteric (endometrioid) pattern of a YST has tall columnar cells and supranuclear vacuoles ➡ resembling secretory phase endometrial glands. Although embryonal carcinoma may rarely demonstrate this pattern, cytologic features are discriminatory. Note that the luminal surface is smooth. Glypican-3 is positive.

Yolk Sac Tumor

(Left) A hepatoid pattern of a YST has solid sheets of tumor cells containing abundant pink cytoplasm and thin fibrovascular septa with sinusoidal arrangement. The tumor cells may occasionally demonstrate a bile canalicular pattern, although bile production is not present. (Right) A hepatoid pattern of a YST has solid sheets of tumor cells containing abundant pink cytoplasm and thin fibrovascular septa with sinusoidal arrangement. Hyaline globules are commonly seen in this pattern.

Yolk Sac Tumor: Hepatoid

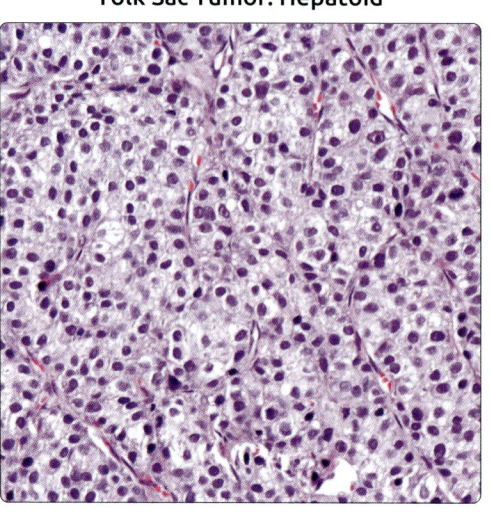

Yolk Sac Tumor: Hepatoid

(Left) An example of a spindle cell (sarcomatoid) area of a YST in a myxoid background is shown. Such foci are often seen in continuity with other classic patterns. Occasionally this pattern may predominate after chemotherapy. (Right) Complex glandular patterns of a YST composed of relatively uniform tumor cells with pseudostratification is shown. It can be differentiated from embryonal carcinoma by its positive immunoreactivity with AFP and glypican-3 and negative immunoreactivity with CD30 or OCT3/4.

Yolk Sac Tumor: Sarcomatoid

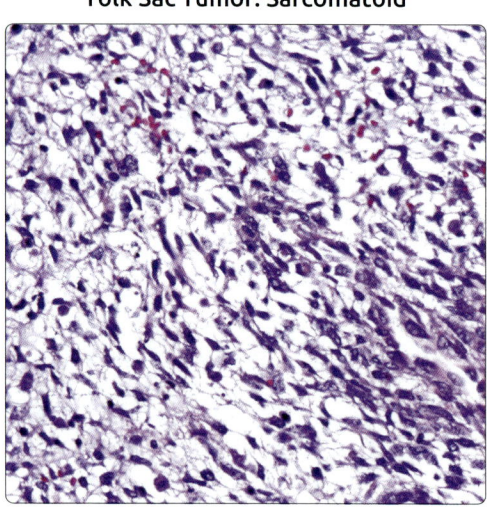

Yolk Sac Tumor: Complex Glandular

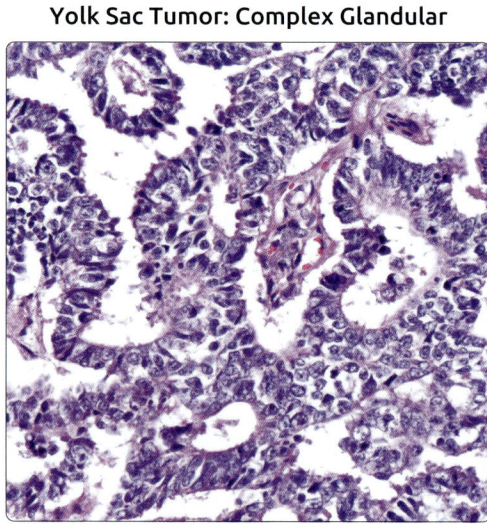

(Left) This photomicrograph shows a mixed germ cell tumor with a YST ➡ and embryonal carcinoma ➡. The different cytologic features between the 2 tumor types are key discriminators. (Right) Mixed germ cell tumor with a YST and embryonal carcinoma with differential staining for OCT3/4 is shown. The tumor cells of YST ➡ are negative, but embryonal carcinoma cells ➡ are positive (nuclear).

Mixed Germ Cell Tumor

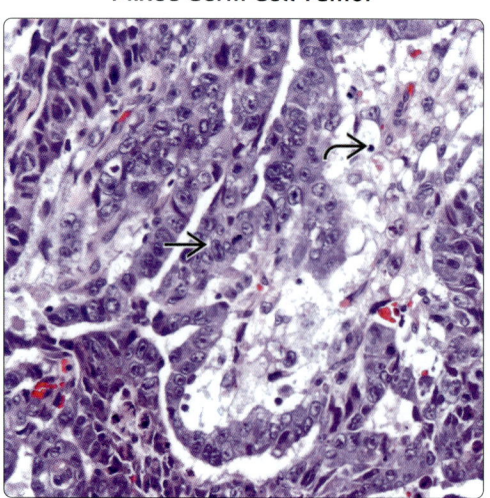

Mixed Germ Cell Tumor: OCT3/4

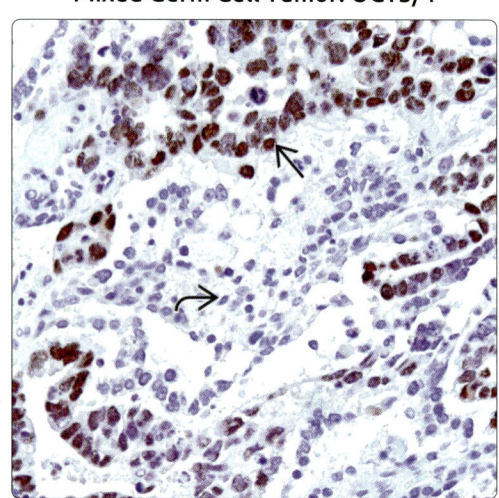

Yolk Sac Tumor

Yolk Sac Tumor: CK-PAN
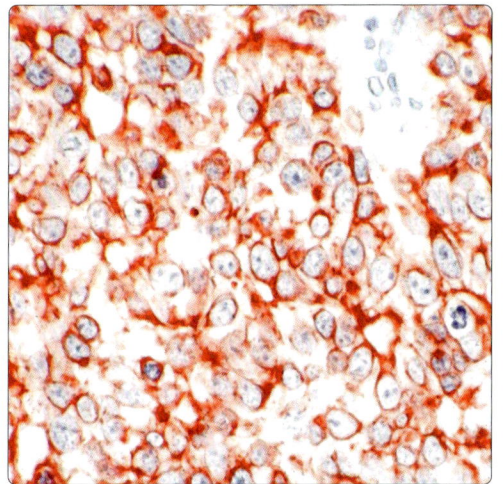

Yolk Sac Tumor: AFP
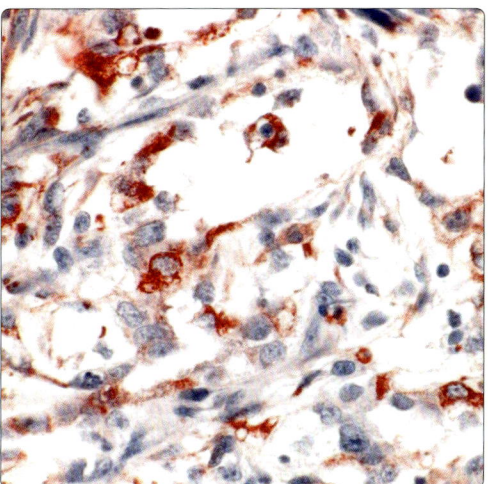

(Left) The tumor cells of YST are strongly positive for cytokeratin, a feature distinguishing it from seminoma. (Right) AFP staining in a YST is often quite variable, ranging between 55-100% in different studies. The staining may be focal and weak in some cases. Nonspecific staining in stroma and blood vessel contents may be seen due to high serum levels.

Yolk Sac Tumor: SALL4
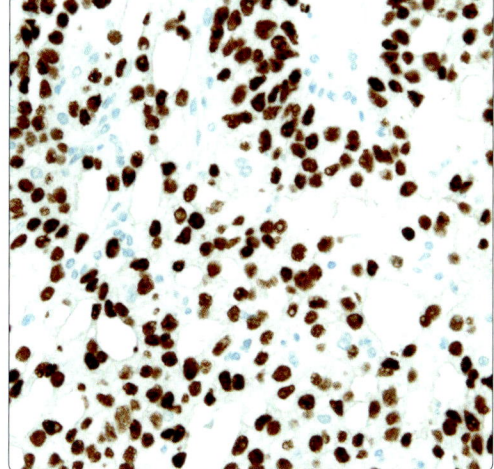

Yolk Sac Tumor: Glypican-3
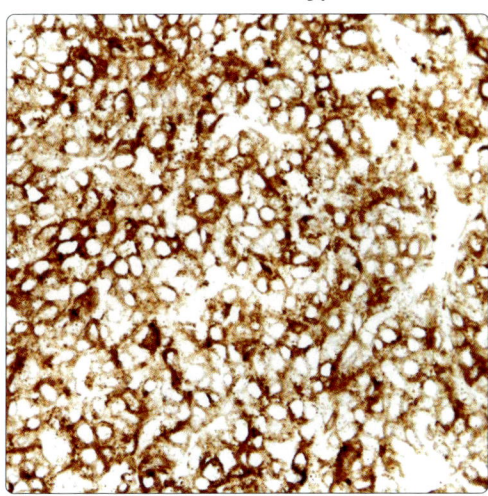

(Left) This image shows a diffuse nuclear stain of SALL4 in a YST, which is similar to seminoma and embryonal carcinoma. However, unlike seminoma and embryonal carcinoma, tumor cells of a YST are negative for OCT3/4. SALL4 is the most sensitive marker for a YST. (Right) The tumor cells of a YST are positive for glypican-3. Seminoma and embryonal carcinoma are typically negative for glypican-3, although syncytiotrophoblasts and, rarely, choriocarcinoma and teratoma, may be positive.

Seminoma: Differential
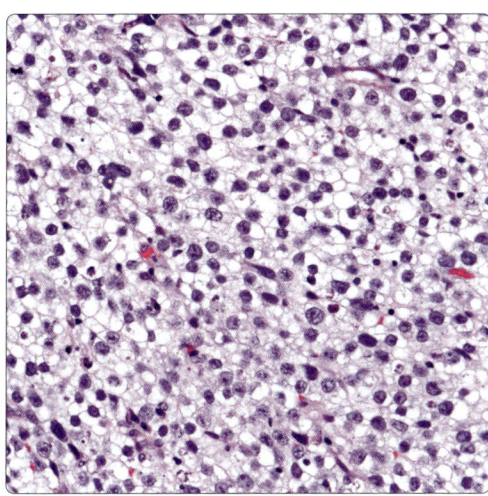

Leydig Cell Tumor: Differential
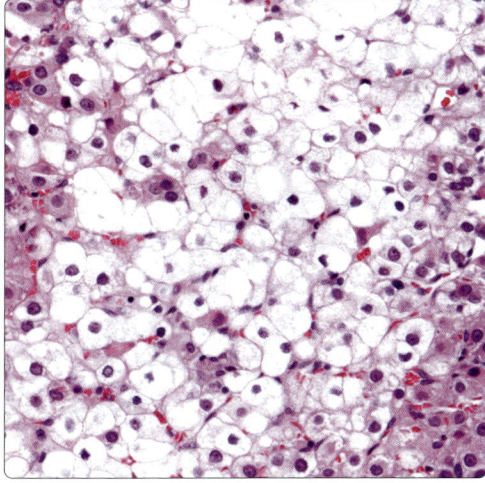

(Left) Typical solid growth pattern of a seminoma is shown. When the tumor lacks fibrovascular septa and lymphoplasmacytic infiltrate, it may be mistaken for a YST. Immunohistochemical stains are helpful to confirm the diagnosis. Unlike seminoma, a YST is positive for glypican-3 and AFP and negative for OCT3/4. (Right) This is a Leydig cell tumor, with a solid growth pattern of tumor cells with eosinophilic and clear cytoplasm. Unlike YST, the tumor cells are usually positive for inhibin or calretinin and negative for SALL4.

Choriocarcinoma and Variants

KEY FACTS

TERMINOLOGY
- Germ cell tumor composed of mixture of mononucleated trophoblastic cells and multinucleated syncytiotrophoblasts

CLINICAL ISSUES
- Pure choriocarcinoma (CC) comprises < 1% of germ cell tumor
- Known for early hematogeneous metastasis to lung, liver, and brain (cannonball metastasis)
- Patients typically have very high circulating human chorionic gonadotropin (usually > 100,000 mIU/mL)

MACROSCOPIC
- Hemorrhagic and necrotic mass with blood clot; ill-defined gray to tan tissue at periphery

MICROSCOPIC
- Classic CC consists of mixture of cytotrophoblasts and multinucleated syncytiotrophoblasts
- Syncytiotrophoblasts wrapping around mononuclear cytotrophoblastic cells and forming villous configuration
- Significant hemorrhage and necrosis
- Monophasic CC, a variant of CC, is usually seen in metastatic sites following chemotherapy
- Nonchoriocarcinomatous trophoblastic tumors (PSTT, ETT, and CTT) occurring in testis or metastatic sites have been reported

ANCILLARY TESTS
- Syncytiotrophoblasts are positive for cytokeratin, hCG, HPL, EMA/MUC1, inhibin, glypican-3, CEA, and SALL4
- Cytotrophoblasts are (+) for SALL4, GDF3, p63, and GATA3
- Negative for vimentin, CD30 (Ber-H2), podoplanin (D2-40), and OCT3/4

TOP DIFFERENTIAL DIAGNOSES
- Hemorrhage due to nonneoplastic process; other germ cell tumor with syncytiotrophoblasts, particularly seminoma; metastatic high-grade carcinoma

Choriocarcinoma: Gross
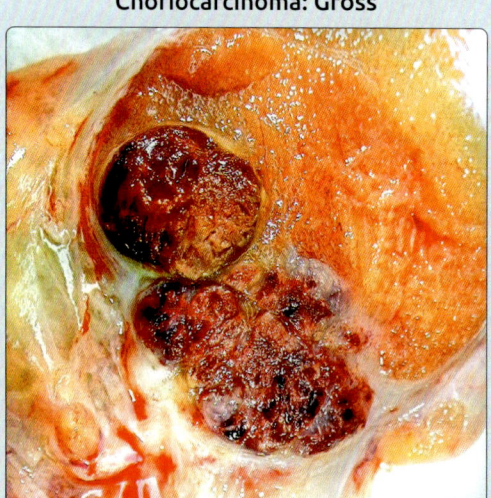

Choriocarcinoma: Low Power
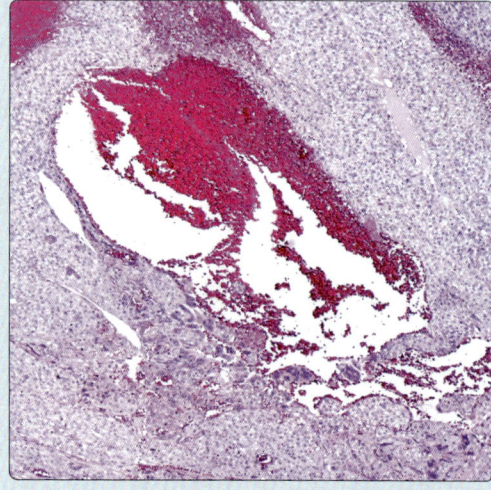

(Left) Gross photograph of CC shows typical hemorrhagic/necrotic cut surface. There are nodules of blood clot and tumor with cystic degenerative changes. (Courtesy T. Ulbright, MD.) (Right) Low-power photomicrograph shows CC with a central zone of hemorrhage and necrosis surrounded by a mixture of mononucleated cytotrophoblasts and multinucleated syncytiotrophoblasts. Gross or microscopic hemorrhage should always raise the possibility of a CC component.

Choriocarcinoma: Hemorrhage and Necrosis
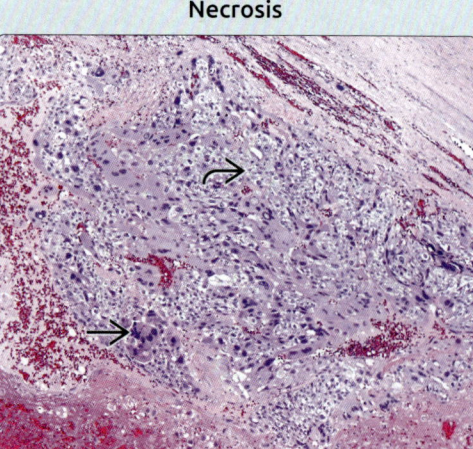

Choriocarcinoma: Cytology
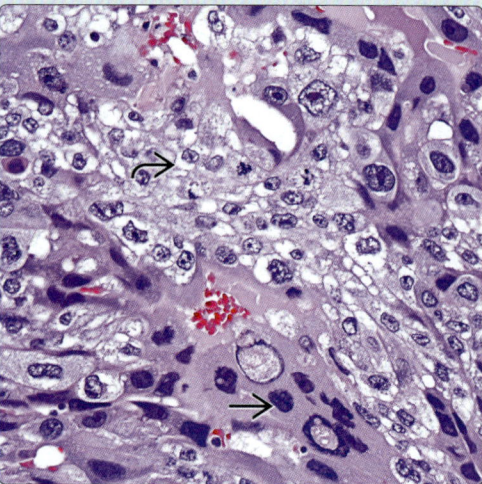

(Left) This photomicrograph shows the features of CC with large areas of hemorrhage and necrosis and 2 types of cells, i.e., syncytiotrophoblasts ⇥ and cytotrophoblasts ⇥. (Right) CC shows close spatial relationship of cytotrophoblasts ⇥ with clear cytoplasm and multinucleated syncytiotrophoblasts ⇥ with abundant eosinophilic cytoplasm and smudged nuclei.

Choriocarcinoma and Variants

TERMINOLOGY

Abbreviations
- Choriocarcinoma (CC)
- Placental site trophoblastic tumor (PSTT), epithelioid trophoblastic tumor (ETT), cystic trophoblastic tumor (CTT)

Synonyms
- Malignant teratoma, trophoblastic tumor, chorioepithelioma

Definitions
- Germ cell tumor composed of admixture of mononucleated cytotrophoblastic and multinucleated syncytiotrophoblastic cells
- Monophasic CC (rare, lacks syncytiotrophoblasts)
- PSTT (extremely rare; tumor of intermediate trophoblasts)

CLINICAL ISSUES

Epidemiology
- Incidence
  - Pure CC accounts only for 0.3% of germ cell tumors
  - Usually mixed with other germ cell tumor components (8% of mixed germ cell tumors)
- Age
  - 20-39 years (median: 29 years)

Presentation
- Testicular mass less often than other germ cell tumors
- Often presents with symptoms due to hematogeneous metastasis (hemoptysis, central nervous system dysfunction, hematemesis, melena, hypotension, anemia)
  - May present with metastasis with subsequent detection of primary
- May have gynecomastia (10% patients) or hyperthyroidism
- Some patients may present with so-called CC syndrome due to multiorgan involvement and high human chorionic gonadotropin (hCG) levels

Laboratory Tests
- Patients with CC typically have very high circulating hCG (usually > 100,000 mIU/mL)
- Patients with PSTT, ETT, and CTT may have elevation of hCG, but not as high as patients with CC

Treatment
- Radical orchiectomy and systemic chemotherapy

Prognosis
- Worse prognosis than other germ cell tumors, if pure
- Level of hCG correlates with prognosis, reflecting tumor burden
- Prognoses for PSTT, ETT, and CTT are likely not unfavorable, although data are relatively limited

IMAGING

General Features
- Similar to other nonseminomatous germ cell tumors, but mass is usually small or inapparent in pure CC

MACROSCOPIC

General Features
- For pure CC
  - Hemorrhagic and necrotic mass with blood clot; ill-defined gray to tan tissue at periphery
  - Primary site may be totally regressed with burnt-out focus

Size
- 1.5-10.0 cm (average: 7 cm)

MICROSCOPIC

Histologic Features
- Classic CC consists of mixture of cytotrophoblasts and multinucleated syncytiotrophoblasts
  - Cytotrophoblasts are round or polygonal cells with prominent cell borders, clear cytoplasm, and usually single bland nucleus
  - Syncytiotrophoblasts are large multinucleated cells, often degenerated-appearing, with abundant eosinophilic and vacuolated cytoplasm
  - These 2 cell populations exhibit spatial relationship with syncytiotrophoblasts, wrapping around mononuclear cytotrophoblastic cells
  - Villous configuration is occasionally seen and is typical for CC
  - Significant hemorrhage and necrosis is common finding
  - Frequent vascular invasion
  - Germ cell neoplasia in situ in adjacent testicular parenchyma
- Monophasic CC, variant of CC, is usually seen in metastatic sites following chemotherapy
  - Composed of predominantly mononucleated squamoid-appearing cytotrophoblasts with rare mitoses
- Nonchoriocarcinomatous trophoblastic tumors occurring in testis or metastatic sites after chemotherapy have been reported
  - PSTT
    - Composed of single or loosely cohesive implantation-type intermediate trophoblastic cells
      - Irregular, dense smudged nuclei, abundant eosinophilic cytoplasm
    - Often associated with invasion of muscular wall of vessels and fibrinoid changes
    - Typically positive for HPL
    - Negative for p63
  - ETT
    - Composed of solid nests or cords of squamoid, chorionic-type intermediate trophoblasts with eosinophilic or clear cytoplasm, distinct cell borders and hyaline matrix
    - Extracellular and intracellular eosinophilic globules with basophilic apoptotic nuclear debris are frequent findings
    - Usually negative or focally positive for HPL
    - Positive for p63
  - CTT
    - Characterized by multiple small cysts lined by layers of degenerated-appearing trophoblastic cells

Choriocarcinoma and Variants

- ▫ Smudged nuclei and abundant eosinophilic cytoplasm
  - Intracytoplasmic lacunae are often present in some lining cells of cysts
  - Cells may be really positive for hCG

Lymphatic/Vascular Invasion
- Vascular invasion is common for CC, but uncommon for PSTT, ETT, and CTT

Predominant Pattern/Injury Type
- Solid and villous pattern/neoplastic

Predominant Cell/Compartment Type
- CC is composed of mononucleated cytotrophoblasts and multinucleated syncytiotrophoblasts
- Each type of trophoblastic tumors has characteristic cellular morphology

ANCILLARY TESTS

Immunohistochemistry
- Cytotrophoblasts are positive for SALL4, GDF3, p63, and GATA3
- Intermediate trophoblasts are weakly positive for HPL
- Negative for vimentin, CD30 (Ber-H2), podoplanin (D2-40), and OCT3/4

DIFFERENTIAL DIAGNOSIS

Hemorrhage Due to Nonneoplastic Process
- Appropriate clinical history (testicular torsion, trauma)
- Coagulative necrosis with ghost outlines of seminiferous tubules; no malignant cells present

Other Germ Cell Tumor With Syncytiotrophoblasts, Particularly Seminoma
- Histologic features of other germ cell components
- Lack of diagnostic triad for CC
  - Hemorrhagic and necrotic background
  - 2 cell population with spatial relationship
  - Classic or vague villous configuration

Metastatic High-Grade Carcinoma
- Clinical history of carcinoma
- Histologic features of metastatic carcinoma
- Positive for tissue-specific markers, negative for germ cell markers

DIAGNOSTIC CHECKLIST

Clinically Relevant Pathologic Features
- May present with disseminated metastases without overt testicular mass
- Production of hCG by tumor may lead to serum hCG elevation, resulting in gynecomastia and thyrotoxicosis

Pathologic Interpretation Pearls
- Mixture of 2 cell types
- Frequent hemorrhage and necrosis
- Large multinucleate giant cells surrounding cytotrophoblasts with villous configuration

REPORTING

General Reporting Elements
- Type of CC and cell types and their percentage
- TNM stage
- Vascular invasion
- Immunoprofiles

SELECTED REFERENCES

1. Banet N et al: GATA-3 expression in trophoblastic tissues: an immunohistochemical study of 445 cases, including diagnostic utility. Am J Surg Pathol. 39(1):101-8, 2015
2. Idrees MT et al: Nonchoriocarcinomatous trophoblastic tumors of the testis: the widening wpectrum of trophoblastic neoplasia. Am J Surg Pathol. 39(11):1468-78, 2015
3. Alvarado-Cabrero I et al: Clinicopathologic analysis of choriocarcinoma as a pure or predominant component of germ cell tumor of the testis. Am J Surg Pathol. 38(1):111-8, 2014
4. Humphrey PA: Choriocarcinoma of the testis. J Urol. 192(3):934-5, 2014
5. Petersson F et al: Testicular germ cell tumor composed of placental site trophoblastic tumor and teratoma. Hum Pathol. 41(7):1046-50, 2010
6. Allan RW et al: Metastatic epithelioid trophoblastic tumor in a male patient with mixed germ-cell tumor of the testis. Am J Surg Pathol. 33(12):1902-5, 2009
7. Cao D et al: SALL4 is a novel diagnostic marker for testicular germ cell tumors. Am J Surg Pathol. 33(7): 1065-77, 2009
8. Gopalan A et al: Testicular mixed germ cell tumors: a morphological and immunohistochemical study using stem cell markers, OCT3/4, SOX2 and GDF3, with emphasis on morphologically difficult-to-classify areas. Mod Pathol. 22(8):1066-74, 2009
9. Lee SC et al: Mixed testicular germ cell tumor presenting as metastatic pure choriocarcinoma involving multiple lung metastases that was effectively treated with high-dose chemotherapy. Cancer Res Treat. 41(4):229-32, 2009
10. Ulbright TM: The most common, clinically significant misdiagnoses in testicular tumor pathology, and how to avoid them. Adv Anat Pathol. 15(1):18-27, 2008
11. Suurmeijer AJ et al: Placental site trophoblastic tumor in a late recurrence of a nonseminomatous germ cell tumor of the testis. Am J Surg Pathol. 28(6):830-3, 2004
12. Ulbright TM et al: Cystic trophoblastic tumor: a nonaggressive lesion in postchemotherapy resections of patients with testicular germ cell tumors. Am J Surg Pathol. 28(9):1212-6, 2004
13. Ulbright TM et al: Trophoblastic tumors of the testis other than classic choriocarcinoma: "monophasic" choriocarcinoma and placental site trophoblastic tumor: a report of two cases. Am J Surg Pathol. 21(3):282-8, 1997
14. Ulbright TM et al: Choriocarcinoma-like lesions in patients with testicular germ cell tumors. Two histologic variants. Am J Surg Pathol. 12(7):531-41, 1988
15. Manivel JC et al: Intermediate trophoblast in germ cell neoplasms. Am J Surg Pathol. 11(9):693-701, 1987
16. Henry SC et al: Choriocarcinoma of the testis. J Urol. 112(1):105-8, 1974

Choriocarcinoma and Variants

Choriocarcinoma: Fibrinoid Necrosis

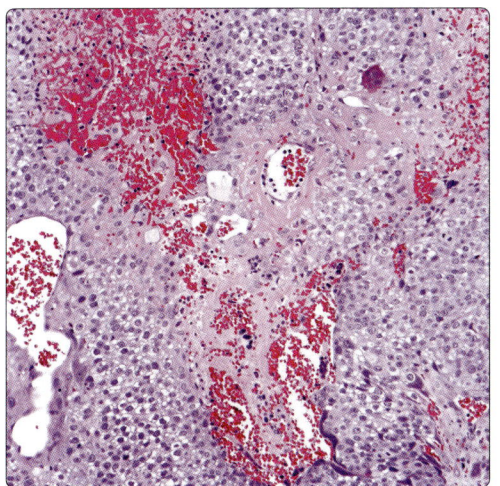

Choriocarcinoma: Necrosis

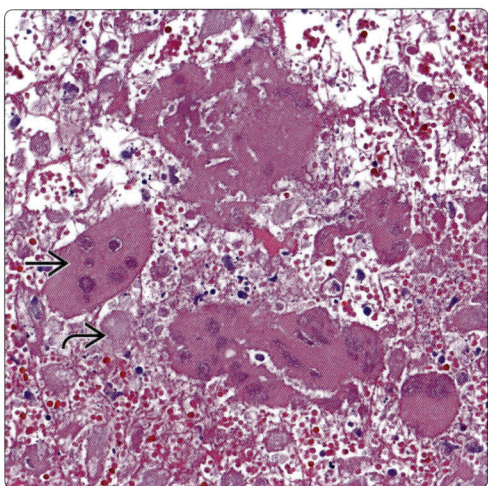

(Left) CC with typical syncytiotrophoblasts invading blood vessels is shown here. Fibrinoid necrosis and hemorrhage are present. Sheets of cytotrophoblasts are at the periphery of the hemorrhagic and necrotic zone. (Right) This photomicrograph shows necrotic tumor with ghost outlines of multinucleate syncytiotrophoblasts ➡ and mononuclear cytotrophoblasts ➡. Necrosis and hemorrhage are prominent features of a CC.

Choriocarcinoma: Cytology

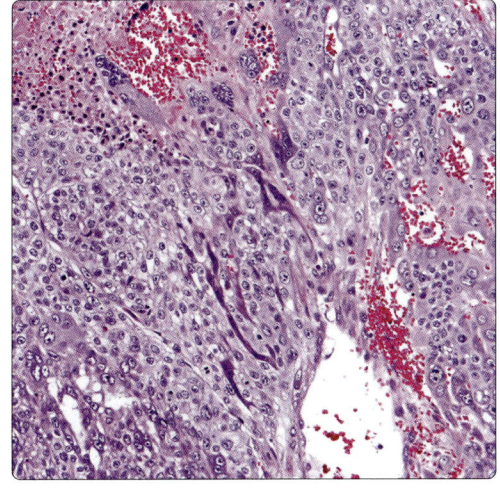

Choriocarcinoma: Cytology

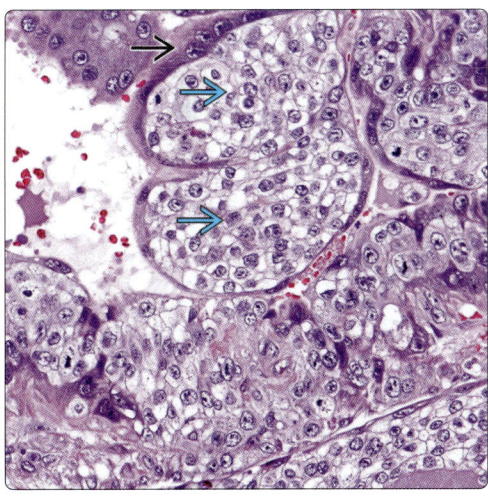

(Left) Intimate admixture of mononucleate cytotrophoblasts with clear cytoplasm and a few multinucleate syncytiotrophoblasts is typical for CC. Fibrinoid necrosis and hemorrhage are present. (Right) This photomicrograph shows CC with syncytiotrophoblastic ➡ capping of nests of cytotrophoblasts ➡, a feature reminiscent of immature placental villi.

Choriocarcinoma: Cytology

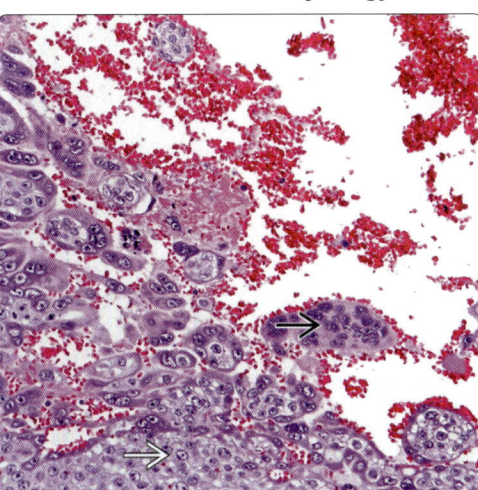

Choriocarcinoma: Cytology

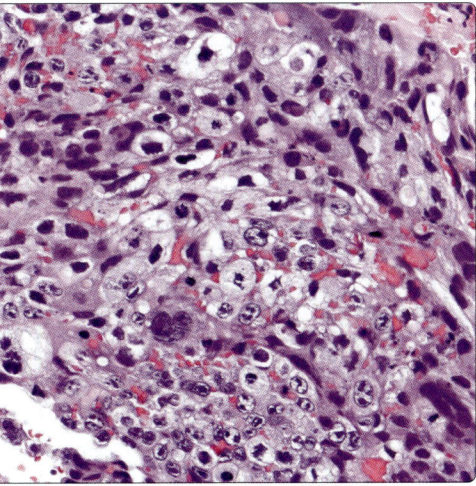

(Left) CC with a central zone of hemorrhage is shown. Pale cytotrophoblasts ➡ are surrounded by multinucleate syncytiotrophoblasts ➡ with dense eosinophilic cytoplasm. The close relationship of the 2 distinctive cell types is characteristic of CC. (Right) This photomicrograph of CC shows intimate admixture of mononucleate cytotrophoblasts with clear cytoplasm and a few multinucleate syncytiotrophoblasts with dense eosinophilic cytoplasm and smudged nuclei.

Choriocarcinoma and Variants

Choriocarcinoma: Cell Types

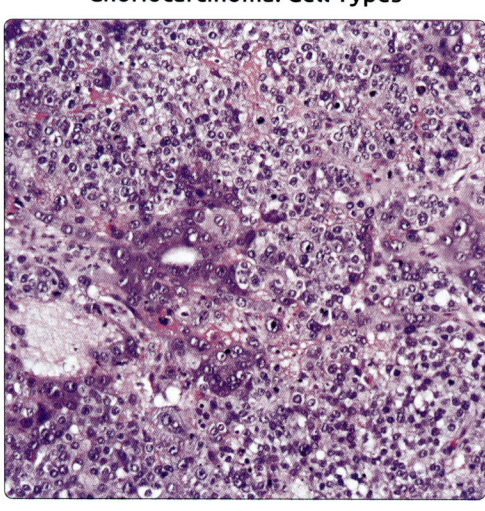

(Left) CC demonstrates a spectrum of malignant trophoblastic cells from relatively small to large mononucleate cells, as well as multinucleate syncytiotrophoblastic tumor cells. The arrangement of cytotrophoblasts is in sheets.

Choriocarcinoma: Cell Types

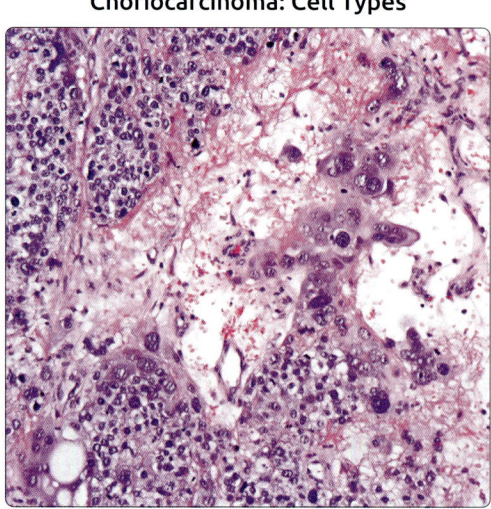

(Right) CC is shown in which the 2 cell types (syncytiotrophoblasts and cytotrophoblasts) are present but do not show the typical biphasic pattern. Syncytiotrophoblasts are more commonly seen at the periphery in most CC, as in this case.

Choriocarcinoma: Monophasic

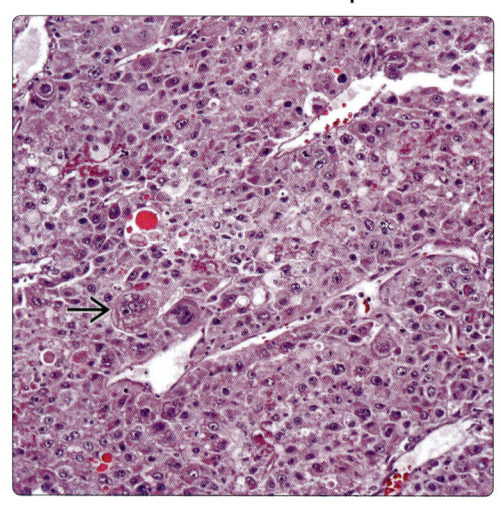

(Left) This is an example of monophasic CC with sheets of mononucleate epithelioid tumor cells with round to ovoid nuclei and abundant pale eosinophilic cytoplasm. Rare, scattered syncytiotrophoblasts ➡ are seen.

Choriocarcinoma: Monophasic

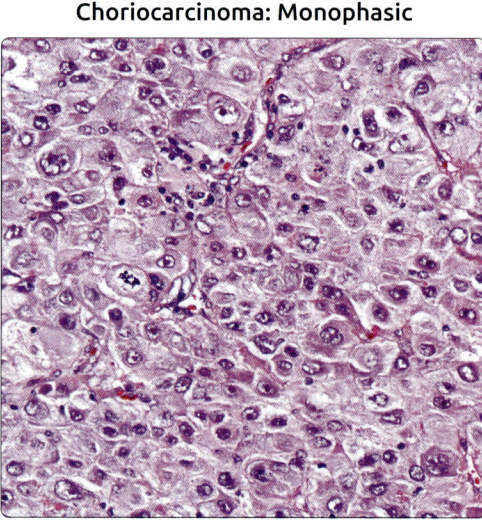

(Right) High-power photomicrograph shows a monophasic CC with sheets of mononucleated epithelioid or squamoid tumor cells with round to ovoid nuclei, prominent nucleoli, and abundant pale eosinophilic cytoplasm.

Choriocarcinoma: Monophasic

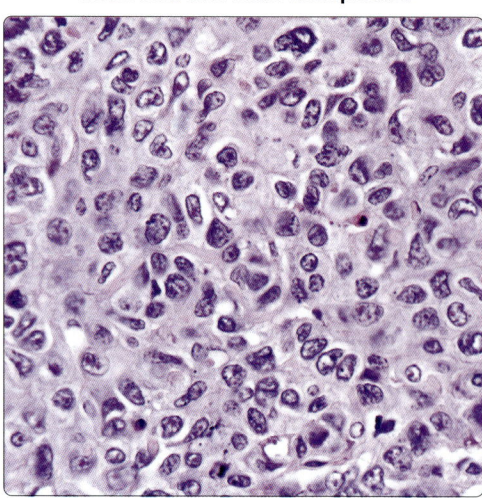

(Left) This is a metastatic monophasic CC to the lung in a patient with testicular mixed germ cell tumor after chemotherapy. The tumor is composed of sheets of cytotrophoblasts with clear to eosinophilic cells.

Monophasic Choriocarcinoma: β-hCG

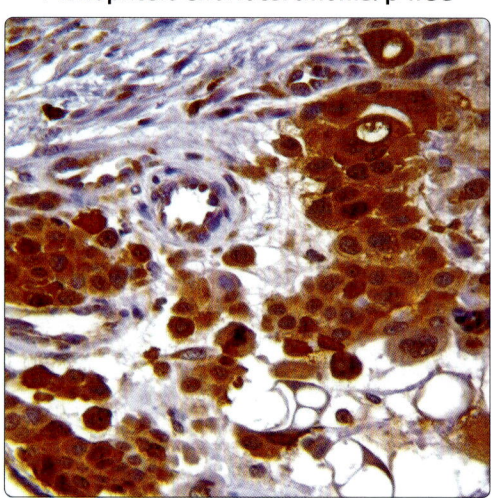

(Right) The tumor cells of monophasic CC are diffusely positive for β-hCG. Immunohistochemistry is necessary to confirm CC when syncytiotrophoblasts are scant to absent. The differential diagnosis includes other germ cell tumor components but most closely resembles a solid yolk sac tumor.

Choriocarcinoma and Variants

Placental Site Trophoblastic Tumor: Cytology

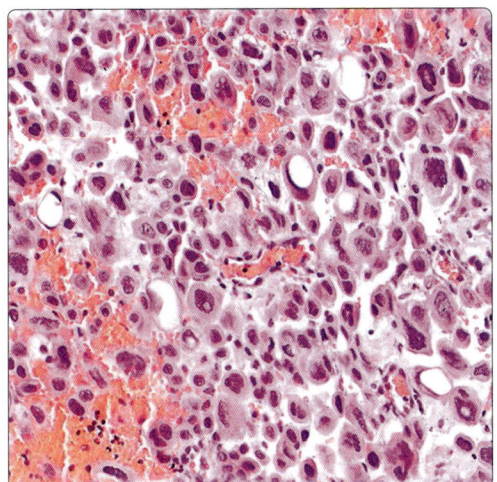

Placental Site Trophoblastic Tumor: β-hCG

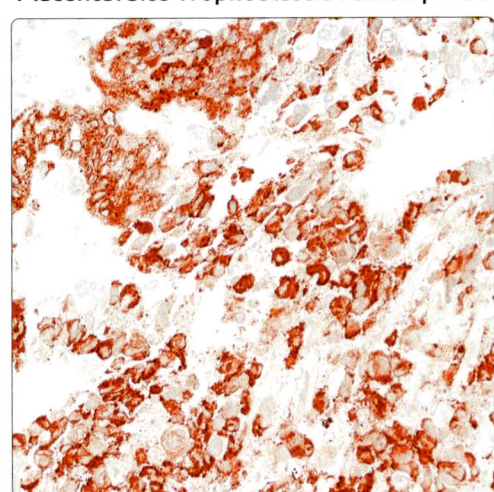

(Left) Placental site trophoblastic tumor (PSTT) is composed of intermediate trophoblastic cells that are large and mononucleated with abundant, dense eosinophilic cytoplasm. The nuclei are irregularly shaped and have smudged chromatin. *(Right)* The intermediate trophoblastic tumor cells of a PSTT are diffusely positive for β-hCG. These tumors are also strongly positive for HPL.

Epithelioid Trophoblastic Tumor: Cytology

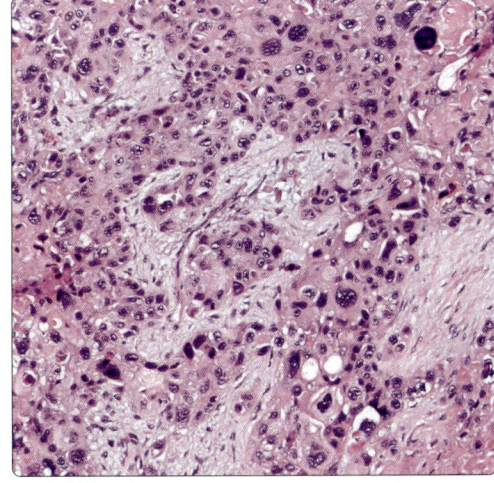

Epithelioid Trophoblastic Tumor: Cytology

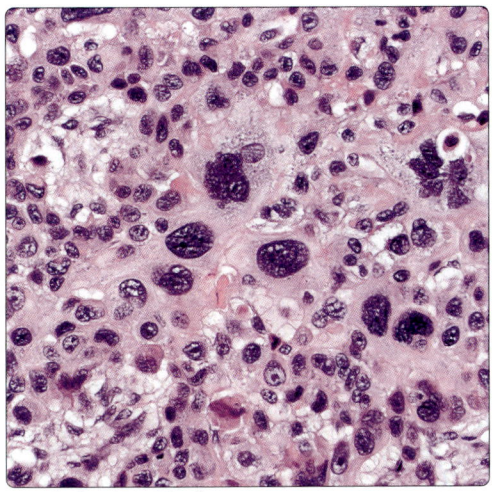

(Left) Epithelioid trophoblastic tumor is composed of solid sheets of squamoid cells with eosinophilic cytoplasm and dense hyalinized stroma. Nuclear pleomorphism is evident. (Courtesy M. Idrees, MBBS.) *(Right)* High-power view of epithelioid trophoblastic tumor shows squamoid tumor cells with eosinophilic cytoplasm, distinct cell borders. There is marked nuclear pleomorphism. (Courtesy M. Idrees, MBBS.)

Cystic Trophoblastic Tumor: Cystic

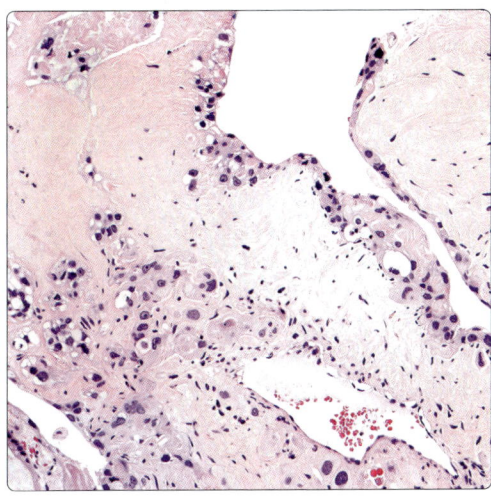

Cystic Trophoblastic Tumor: Cytology

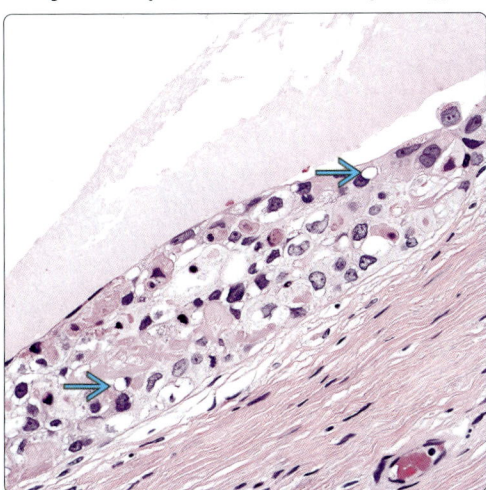

(Left) Cystic trophoblastic tumor is characterized by multiple small cysts lined by single or multiple layers of degenerated-appearing cells with abundant eosinophilic cytoplasm. (Courtesy M. Idrees, MBBS.) *(Right)* Cystic trophoblastic tumor is characterized by multiple cysts lined by layers of degenerated-appearing cells with smudged nuclei and abundant eosinophilic cytoplasm. In some cells, there are intracytoplasmic lacunar space ➡. (Courtesy M. Idrees, MBBS.)

Teratoma, Adult Type

KEY FACTS

TERMINOLOGY
- Tumors with somatic tissue of > 1 different germinal layers (ectoderm, mesoderm, or endoderm)

CLINICAL ISSUES
- Painless, firm, testicular mass
- Pure form is rare and constitutes 4-9% of all testicular tumors in adults
- Frequently mixed with other germ cell tumor types (more than 90%)
- Adult teratomas are considered malignant because of relatively high recurrence or metastasis (22-37%)

MACROSCOPIC
- Often well-circumscribed, nodular and firm mass with heterogeneous cut surface with solid and cystic areas

MICROSCOPIC
- Mature teratoma is composed of mixture of elements of ectoderm, endoderm, and mesoderm
- Most common components are different types of epithelia, cartilage, or nerve
- Respiratory and gastrointestinal epithelium, muscle, and cartilage are more commonly seen in testis than in ovary
- Frequent germ cell neoplasia in situ in adjacent uninvolved testicular parenchyma
- Immature teratoma is composed of undifferentiated spindle cells, primitive endoderm and primitive neuroectoderm tissue, blastomatous or embryonic rhabdomyoblastic tissue
- Highly variable and depends on tissue type and maturity

TOP DIFFERENTIAL DIAGNOSES
- Primary or metastatic sarcoma
- Metastatic carcinoma
- Mature dermoid and epidermoid cysts

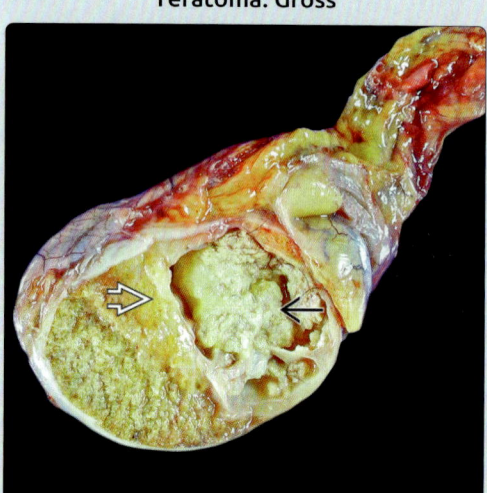

Teratoma: Gross

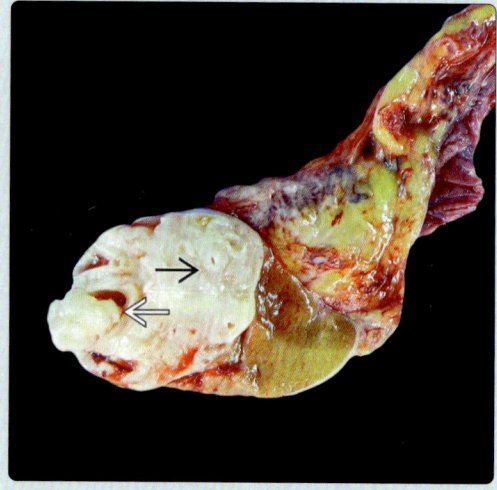

Teratoma: Gross

(Left) This mature teratoma shows a cystic mass with chalky keratin debris ➡. Solid mucoid and gelatinous components ➡ are also present, and these frequently correlate microscopically with immature teratomatous components. (Right) Mature teratoma with both solid ➡ and cystic ➡ components is shown. The cystic component contains chalky keratinous material. The solid areas are mucoid and gelatinous microscopically coinciding with glandular and cartilaginous tissue components.

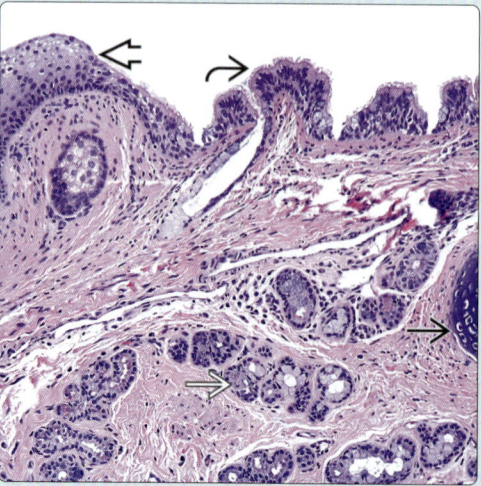

Teratoma: Adult Type

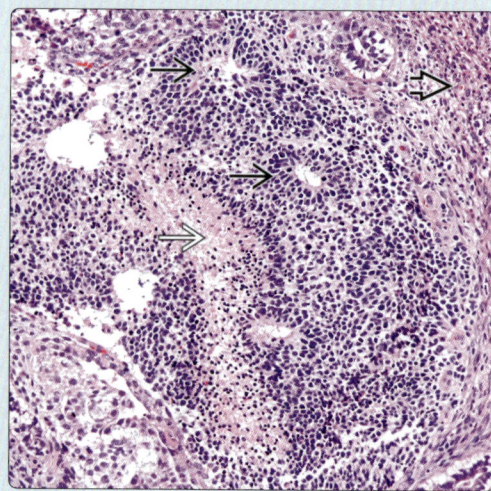

Teratoma: Adult Type (Immature)

(Left) This mature teratoma shows squamous ➡ and respiratory epithelium ➡, seromucinous glands ➡, and cartilage ➡. Virtually all somatic tissue types may be seen in a teratoma. (Right) Immature teratoma shows neuroectodermal cells and neural tube-like structures ➡. Focal necrosis ➡ and cellular spindle immature mesenchymal tissue ➡ are also present.

Teratoma, Adult Type

TERMINOLOGY

Definitions
- Tumors with somatic tissue of > 1 different germinal layers (ectoderm, mesoderm, or endoderm)

ETIOLOGY/PATHOGENESIS

Genetics
- Unlike prepubertal teratoma, adult teratomas are often aneuploid (hypotriploid) and associated with i (12p) and germ cell neoplasia in situ (GCNIS)

CLINICAL ISSUES

Epidemiology
- Incidence
  - Pure form is rare and constitutes 4-9% of all testicular tumors in adults
  - Frequently mixed with other germ cell tumor types (> 90%)
- Age
  - Similar to that of mixed germ cell tumor (3rd-4th decades)

Presentation
- Painless, firm, testicular mass

Treatment
- For teratoma in adults, regardless of maturation, radical orchiectomy with close follow-up

Prognosis
- Adult teratomas are considered malignant because of relatively high recurrence or metastasis (22-37%)

IMAGING

General Features
- Solid and cystic testicular mass by US

MACROSCOPIC

General Features
- Often well-circumscribed, nodular, and firm mass with heterogeneous cut surface with solid and cystic areas
- Cysts filled with clear, white, flaky, gelatinous or mucoid material
- Mature tissue with hair, cartilage, bone, or teeth may be seen

MICROSCOPIC

Histologic Features
- Adult type mature teratoma
  - Composed of mixture of elements of ectoderm, endoderm, and mesoderm
    - Ectoderm: Epidermis, neuronal tissue
    - Endoderm: Gastrointestinal or respiratory mucosa, other seromucous glands
    - Mesoderm: Bone, cartilage, muscle
  - Most common components are different types of epithelia, cartilage, or nerve
  - Respiratory and gastrointestinal epithelium, muscle, and cartilage are more commonly seen in testis than in ovary
  - Pancreatic, dental, renal, and thyroid tissue are less commonly seen in testis than in ovary
  - Frequent GCNIS in adjacent uninvolved testicular parenchyma
  - Scar, testicular atrophy and microlithiasis may be seen
- Immature teratoma
  - Primitive mesoderm: Undifferentiated spindle cell component (most common immature element in testis)
  - Primitive endoderm and primitive neuroectoderm (resembling neural tube and embryonic nervous system), PNET component
  - Blastomatous tissue (resembling blastema and embryonic tubules of developing lung or kidney), embryonic rhabdomyoblastic tissue
  - See chapter on Somatic Malignancy in Germ Cell Tumor for criteria of malignancy in epithelial or stromal elements

Cytologic Features
- Highly variable and depends on tissue type and maturity

ANCILLARY TESTS

Immunohistochemistry
- Highly variable and depends on component of teratoma (rarely necessary in clinical practice)
  - Cytokeratin, CEA, and EMA/MUC1: Positive in epithelial tissue or carcinoma of teratomatous type
  - Vimentin: Positive in mesenchymal tissue
  - Germ cell markers: May be positive for HCG (syncytiotrophoblastic cells) and α-fetoprotein (enteric and hepatoid tissue); negative for PLAP (some glandular tissue); OCT3/4, SOX2, CD30

DIFFERENTIAL DIAGNOSIS

Primary or Metastatic Sarcoma
- Usually involves the paratesticular structures
- More homogeneous population of pleomorphic spindle cells

Metastatic Carcinoma
- Older age and clinical history of carcinoma elsewhere
- Presence of pure carcinomatous component

Dermoid and Epidermoid Cysts
- Cyst with organoid arrangement of stratified squamous epithelium with or without skin adnexal structures
- Lack of GCNIS

SELECTED REFERENCES

1. Zhang C et al: Evidence supporting the existence of benign teratomas of the postpubertal testis: a clinical, histopathologic, and molecular genetic analysis of 25 cases. Am J Surg Pathol. 37(6):827-35, 2013
2. Ye H et al: Difficult differential diagnoses in testicular pathology. Arch Pathol Lab Med. 136(4):435-46, 2012
3. Ulbright TM: Gonadal teratomas: a review and speculation. Adv Anat Pathol. 11(1):10-23, 2004
4. Rabbani F et al: Clinical outcome after retroperitoneal lymphadenectomy of patients with pure testicular teratoma. Urology. 62(6):1092-6, 2003
5. Leibovitch I et al: Adult primary pure teratoma of the testis. The Indiana experience. Cancer. 75(9):2244-50, 1995

Teratoma, Adult Type

(Left) Mature teratoma shows skin and adnexal structure, including pilosebaceous units ⇒, cartilage ⇒, and focal intestinal epithelium with abundant lymphoid stroma ⇒. **(Right)** Mature teratoma is shown with ciliated respiratory epithelium. Focally, goblet cells ⇒ are present in the lining mucosa. There are scattered smooth muscle bundles in the wall of the cyst ⇒.

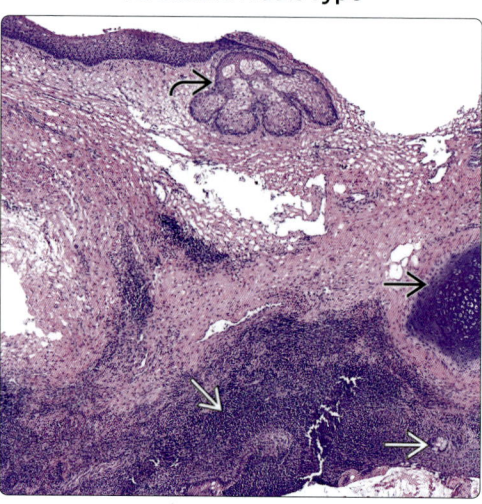

Teratoma: Adult Type (left) and Teratoma: Adult Type (right)

(Left) This mature teratoma shows ductal and glandular epithelium of pancreatic ⇒ and gastric type ⇒. The dilated glands are lined by attenuated flat epithelium and contain mucinous secretions. **(Right)** This mature teratoma has multiple somatic tissue components, including squamous ⇒ and glandular epithelium ⇒, and loose mesenchymal tissue component. Respiratory and gastrointestinal epithelium are the most frequent endodermal components in mature teratoma.

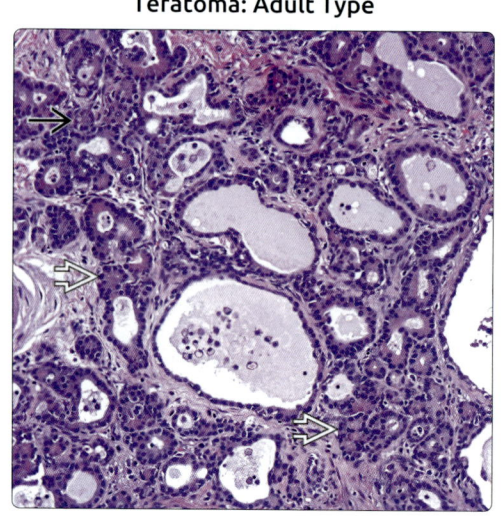
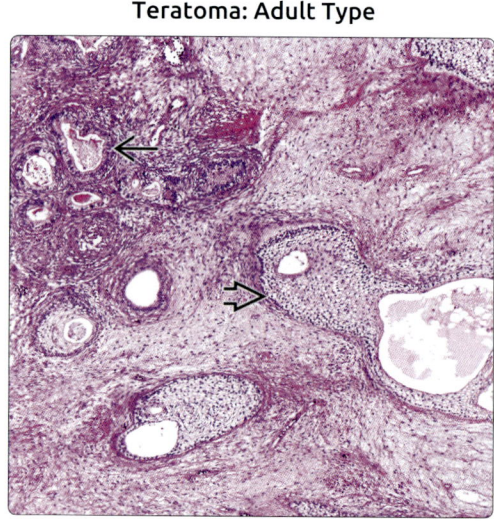

Teratoma: Adult Type (left) and Teratoma: Adult Type (right)

(Left) This mature teratoma is composed of squamous epithelium ⇒, glandular epithelium ⇒, and immature loosely arranged spindle cell mesenchymal tissue ⇒. **(Right)** Mature teratoma with mature glial tissue is shown. In adjacent areas (not shown), other mature teratomatous components, including bone, cartilage, glands, and squamous epithelium were seen.

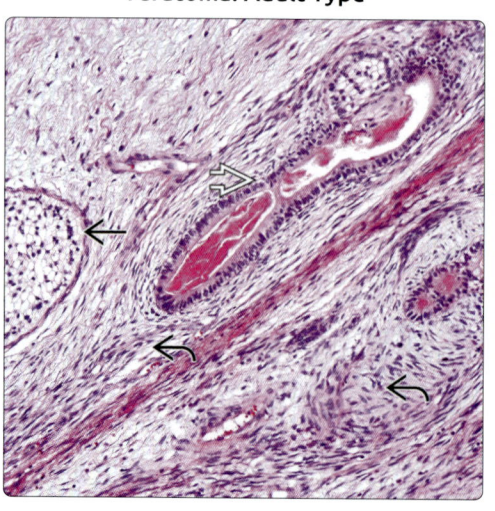
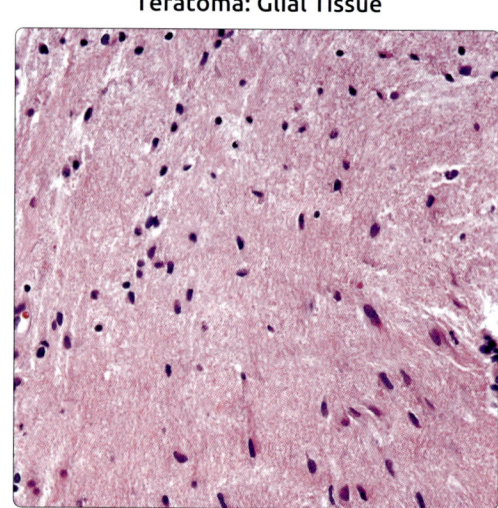

Teratoma: Adult Type (left) and Teratoma: Glial Tissue (right)

Teratoma, Adult Type

Teratoma: Adult Type
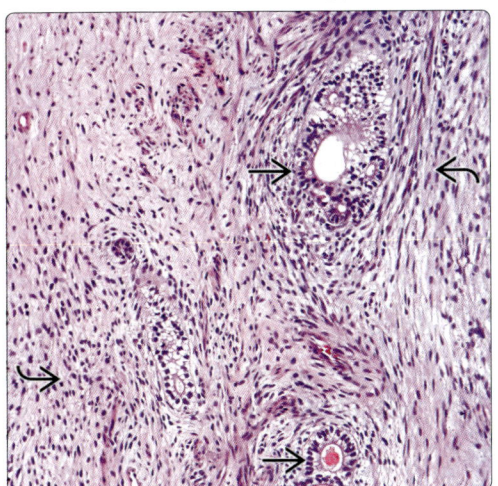

Teratoma: Adult Type (Immature)
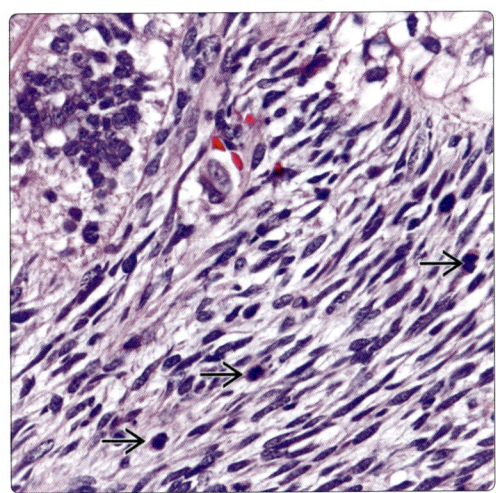

(Left) This teratoma shows mature glandular epithelium ➡ surrounded by immature cellular spindle cell mesenchymal tissue ➡ around the glands. The immature spindle component often encircles the glandular and squamous components. *(Right)* This image shows immature teratoma with glandular tissue surrounded by cellular spindle mesenchymal component with frequent mitoses ➡. The cellular spindle component is the most common element of immature teratoma in the testis.

Teratoma: Adult Type (Immature)
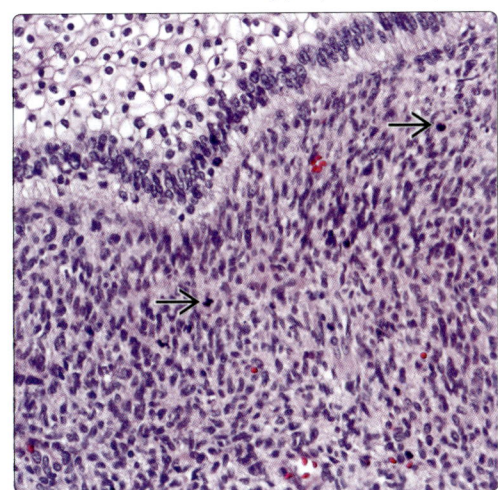

Teratoma: Adult Type (Immature)
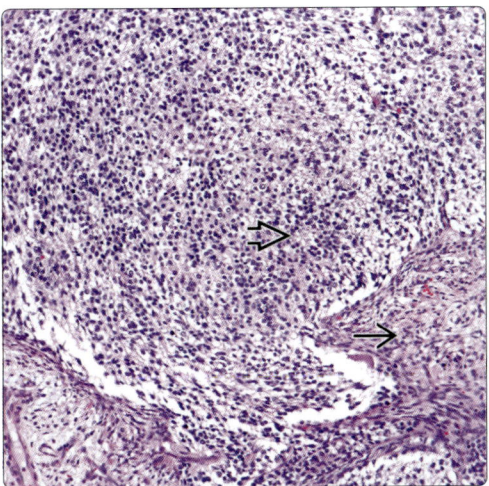

(Left) Immature teratoma shows squamous epithelium with clear cell change on the top and immature cellular spindle cells with frequent mitoses ➡. It is rare for this immature component to show sarcomatous overgrowth, as it is frequently interspersed with squamous or glandular teratomatous tissue. *(Right)* An immature teratoma shows cellular spindle mesenchymal tissue ➡ admixed with immature primitive neuroectodermal tissue composed, forming rosettes ➡.

Teratoma: Adult Type (Immature)
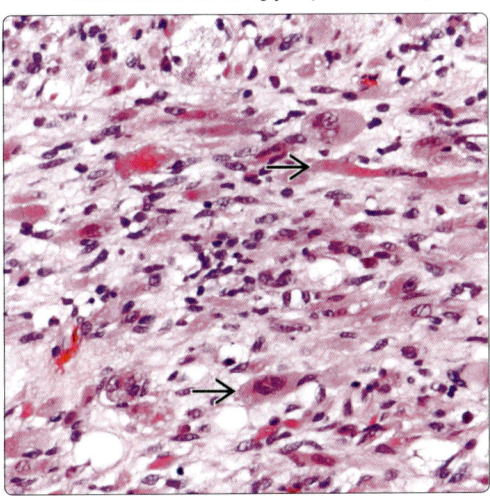

Teratoma: Adult Type (PNET)
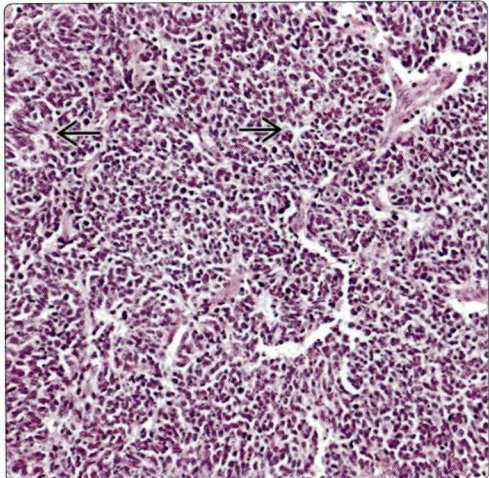

(Left) Immature teratoma with sarcomatous overgrowth shows an embryonal rhabdomyosarcoma with rhabdomyoblastic cells. Tadpole cells ➡ with vague cross striations are seen. These cells are positive for MYOD1 and myogenin. *(Right)* Primitive neuroectodermal tumor (PNET) component shows hypercellular small round blue cells with poorly formed rosettes ➡. In order to designate a sarcomatous malignant transformation in an immature teratoma, PNET growth should exceed > 1 low-power field (5 mm).

Mixed Germ Cell Tumors

KEY FACTS

TERMINOLOGY
- Germ cell tumor composed of > 1 histologic type of germ cell tumor, including seminoma

CLINICAL ISSUES
- Range: 20-40 years (10 years younger than seminoma)
- Accounts for 30-40% of all testicular germ cell tumors
- Prognosis depends on clinical stage, proportion of embryonal carcinoma component, and lymphovascular invasion

MACROSCOPIC
- Variegated cystic and solid mass with hemorrhage and necrosis
- Teratomatous components with bone, cartilage, and skin elements

MICROSCOPIC
- Variable combination and percentage of any 2 or more germ cell tumor components

- Most common combinations include embryonal carcinoma (EC) with yolk sac tumor (YST), teratoma (T), seminoma
- Areas of necrosis and hemorrhage are common
- Rare special variants include polyembryoma and diffuse embryoma

ANCILLARY TESTS
- Immunoprofile reflects histologic component of different germ cell tumors
- 1st-line germ cell markers: OCT3/4, PLAP, podoplanin (D2-40), CD30 (BerH2), glypican-3, HCG, cytokeratin
- Other useful germ cell markers: CD117, AFP, SALL4, LIN28, NANOG

TOP DIFFERENTIAL DIAGNOSES
- Pure germ cell tumor, such as EC, YST, or teratoma
- Metastatic carcinoma

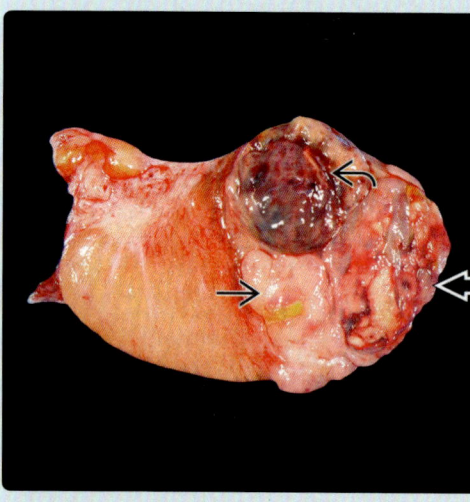

Mixed Germ Cell Tumor: Gross

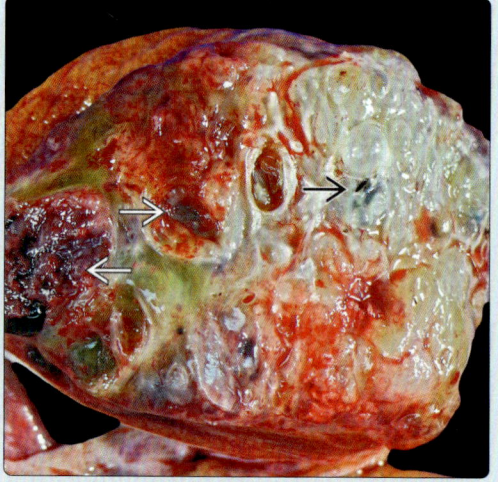

Mixed Germ Cell Tumor: Variegated Appearance

(Left) Mixed germ cell tumor (MGCT) usually shows an irregular mass with variegated cut surface. Creamy gray lobulated areas suggest seminoma ➔, mucoid areas suggest teratoma ➔, and hemorrhagic/necrotic areas suggest EC ➔. Gross appearances are not absolutely specific for histologic subtypes. (Right) Large MGCT with a variegated cut surface replaces entire testicular parenchyma. The tumor is predominantly teratoma ➔; other areas are solid, hemorrhagic, & necrotic EC and YST components ➔.

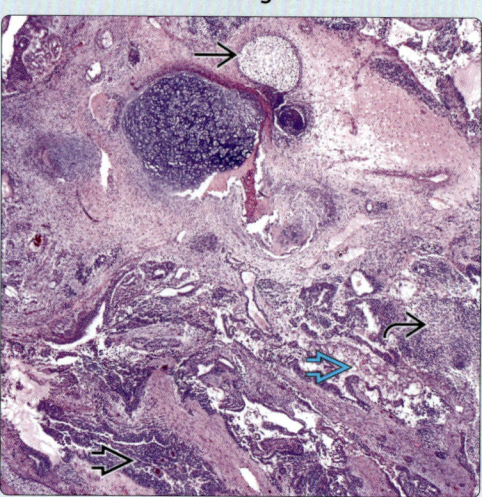

Mixed Germ Cell Tumor: Multiple Histologies

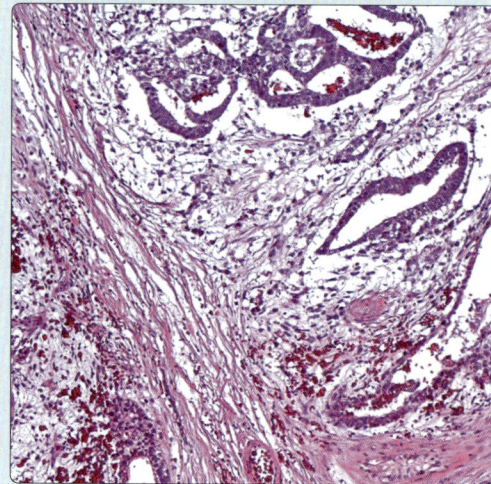

Mixed Germ Cell Tumor: Embryonal Carcinoma and Yolk Sac Tumor

(Left) A MGCT composed of variable germ cell tumor components includes mature teratoma (including cartilage, bone, and squamous nest ➔), immature teratoma with neuroectodermal element ➔, EC ➔, and YST ➔. (Right) MGCT shows glandular embryonal carcinoma component and microcystic/reticular, myxoid areas of more bland-appearing yolk sac tumor elements characterized by spindled cells with low nuclear grade. This component is often underdiagnosed.

Mixed Germ Cell Tumors

TERMINOLOGY

Abbreviations
- Mixed germ cell tumor (MGCT)

Definitions
- Germ cell tumor composed of > 1 histologic type of germ cell tumor, including seminoma

CLINICAL ISSUES

Epidemiology
- Incidence
  - Most common nonseminomatous germ cell tumor (NSGCT) (30-40%)
- Age
  - Range: 20-40 years (10 years younger than seminoma)
  - Rarely seen in prepubertal children and older adults (> 50 years)

Presentation
- Testicular mass or swelling ± pain

Treatment
- Similar to pure nonseminomatous germ cell tumor and depends on clinical stage
- Radical inguinal orchiectomy ± retroperitoneal lymph node dissection or adjuvant therapy

Prognosis
- Depends on clinical stage, proportion of embryonal carcinoma (unfavorable) and mature teratoma (favorable) component, rete testis interstitial invasion, and lymphovascular invasion
- Cure rate > 95% for stage I and stage II disease, 70-85% for stage III disease

IMAGING

Radiographic Findings
- Heterogeneous testicular mass on ultrasound examination
- May be accompanied by retroperitoneal lymph node enlargement

MACROSCOPIC

General Features
- Variegated cystic and solid mass with hemorrhage and necrosis
- Teratomatous components with bone, cartilage, and skin elements

Sections to Be Submitted
- Multiple sections of different areas of tumor and at least 1 section per cm tumor
- Should include necrotic and hemorrhagic areas
- Very important exercise to review gross

Size
- Variable; often large, bulky mass

MICROSCOPIC

Histologic Features
- Variable combination and percentage of any 2 or more germ cell tumor components
- Most common combinations include embryonal carcinoma (EC) with yolk sac tumor (YST), teratoma (T), seminoma
- Areas of necrosis and hemorrhage are common
- Rare variants include polyembryoma and diffuse embryoma
  - Polyembryoma is composed of entirely or predominantly embryoid bodies with embryonic disc, yolk sac, and surrounded by myxoid stroma
  - Diffuse embryoma is characterized by intimate admixture of EC and YST with YST wrapping around EC component

Cytologic Features
- Reflects histologic composition of each component

ANCILLARY TESTS

Immunohistochemistry
- Immunoprofile reflects histologic component of different germ cell tumors
- 1st-line germ cell markers: OCT3/4, PLAP, podoplanin (D2-40), CD30 (BerH2), glypican-3, hCG, cytokeratin
- Other useful germ cell markers: CD117, AFP, SALL4, LIN28, NANOG

DIFFERENTIAL DIAGNOSIS

Pure Germ Cell Tumor
- Single tumor component such as embryonal carcinoma, yolk sac tumor, or teratoma

Metastatic Carcinoma
- Older age, history, and bilaterality
- Interstitial pattern is frequently seen in metastatic carcinoma

REPORTING

Key Elements to Report
- Specific histologic types and percentage of each component
- Lymphovascular invasion
- Invasion of rete testis, epididymis, spermatic cord, and tunica
- Pathology of uninvolved testicular parenchyma

SELECTED REFERENCES

1. Yilmaz A et al: Testicular hilum and vascular invasion predict advanced clinical stage in nonseminomatous germ cell tumors. Mod Pathol. 26(4):579-86, 2013
2. Vogt AP et al: Rete testis invasion by malignant germ cell tumor and/or intratubular germ cell neoplasia: what is the significance of this finding? Hum Pathol. 41(9):1339-44, 2010
3. Gopalan A et al: Testicular mixed germ cell tumors: a morphological and immunohistochemical study using stem cell markers, OCT3/4, SOX2 and GDF3, with emphasis on morphologically difficult-to-classify areas. Mod Pathol. 22(8):1066-74, 2009
4. Mosharafa AA et al: Histology in mixed germ cell tumors. Is there a favorite pairing? J Urol. 171(4):1471-3, 2004
5. Sesterhenn IA et al: Pathology of germ cell tumors of the testis. Cancer Control. 11(6):374-87, 2004

Mixed Germ Cell Tumors

(Left) Image of MGCT shows intimate admixture of papillary and glandular histology of EC ⇨ and microcystic or reticular morphology of YST ⇨. This is one of the most common combinations of MGCT. (Right) This MGCT shows microcystic ⇨ and solid YST ⇨, admixed with mature teratoma with keratinizing squamous epithelial nests ⇨. The tumor cells of YST are sometimes deceptively bland and are frequently underdiagnosed.

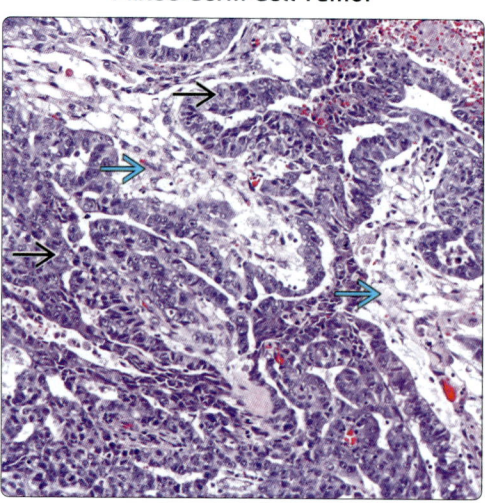
Mixed Germ Cell Tumor

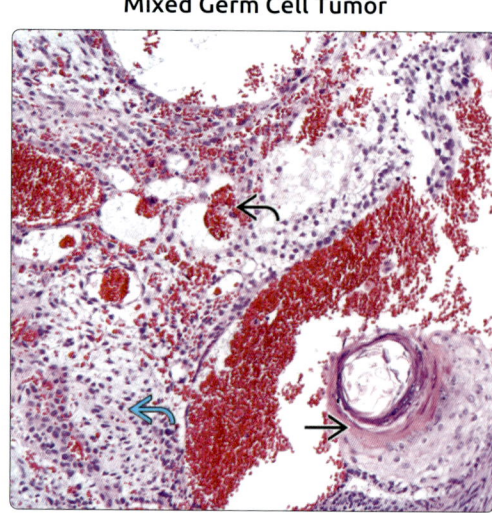
Mixed Germ Cell Tumor

(Left) A MGCT composed of EC ⇨ and seminoma ⇨ is shown. The 2 tumor types are contrasted from one another by the marked nuclear atypia and hyperchromasia of EC vs. the more monotonous appearance of seminoma. (Right) High-power photomicrograph of MGCT shows EC ⇨ admixed with seminoma ⇨. Seminoma cells are evenly spaced with abundant clear cytoplasm. EC cells are more cohesive with overlapping nuclei and marked nuclear pleomorphism.

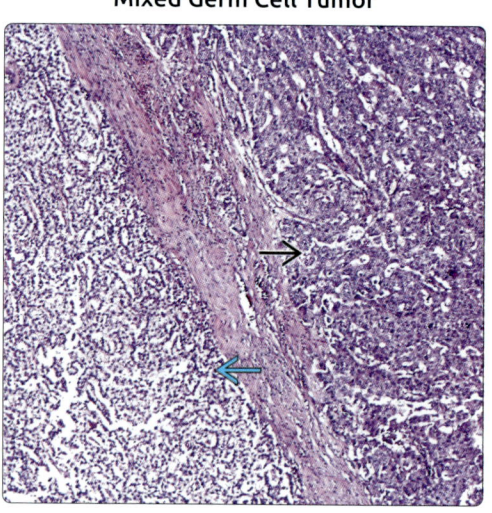
Mixed Germ Cell Tumor

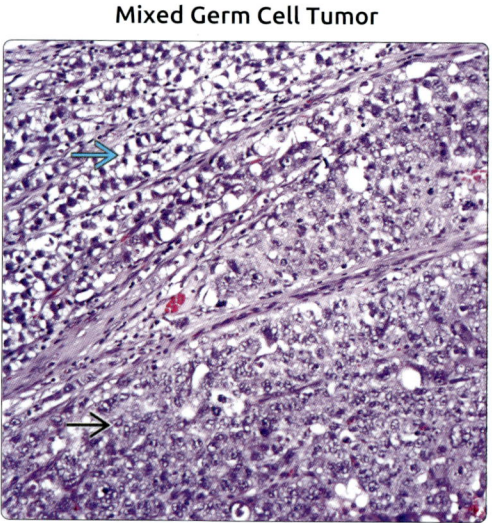
Mixed Germ Cell Tumor

(Left) This area of MGCT has a variety of germ cell tumor components, including EC with cohesive pleomorphic cells ⇨, reticular pattern of YST with bland-appearing cuboidal to flattened cells ⇨, teratomatous glands ⇨, and primitive neuroepithelial tissue ⇨. (Right) Teratomatous component of a MGCT includes cartilage, bone, and immature cellular spindle mesenchymal tissue ⇨. Focal glandular epithelium ⇨ is also present. In other areas (not shown), EC and YST components were present.

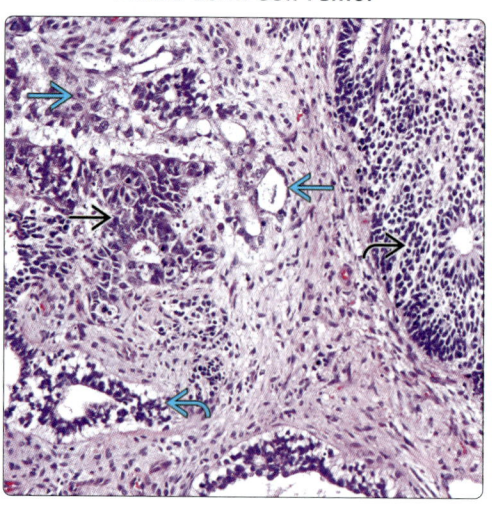
Mixed Germ Cell Tumor

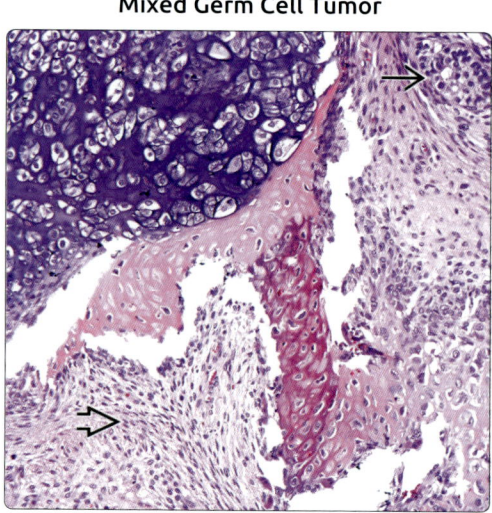
Mixed Germ Cell Tumor

Mixed Germ Cell Tumors

Mixed Germ Cell Tumor

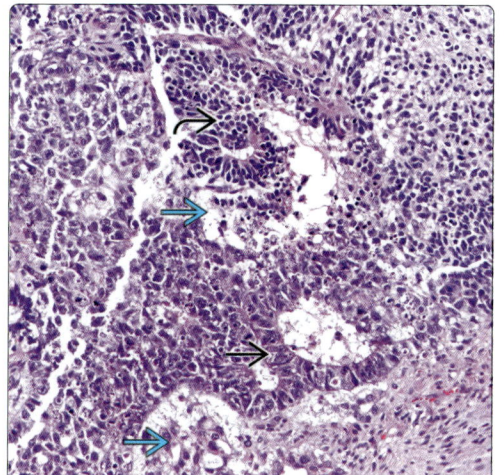

Mixed Germ Cell Tumor

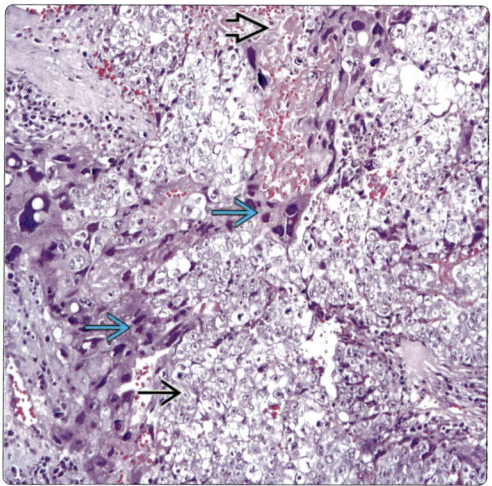

(Left) MGCT shows components of glandular EC with cohesive, pleomorphic cells and nuclear overlapping ⇒, microcystic and reticular YST ⇒, and immature neuroepithelial tissue with neurotubule formation ⇒. (Right) This MGCT shows a significant choriocarcinomatous component characterized by cytotrophoblasts ⇒ with clear cytoplasm surrounded by a layer of multinucleated syncytiotrophoblasts ⇒. Hemorrhage and necrosis ⇒ are present.

Mixed Germ Cell Tumor (Polyembryoma)

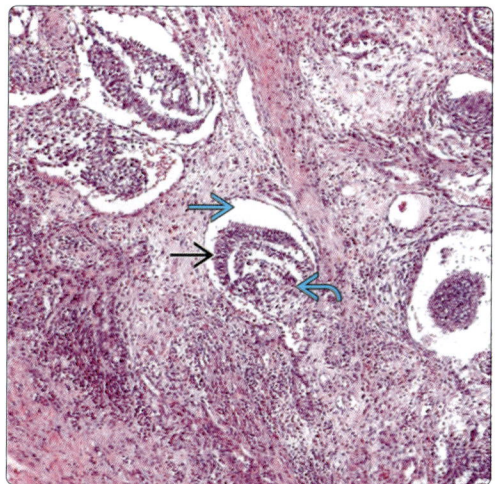

Mixed Germ Cell Tumor (Diffuse Embryoma)

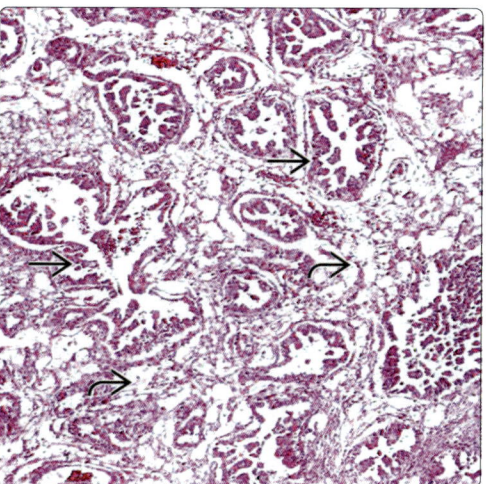

(Left) Polyembryoma, a special type of MGCT, is composed exclusively or predominantly of embryoid bodies in a myxoid stroma. The embryoid body is characterized by a central embryonic disc ⇒, amniotic sac ⇒, and yolk sac ⇒. (Right) Diffuse embryoma, the other special MGCT type, is composed of equal amounts of papillary/glandular EC ⇒ and microcystic and reticular patterns of YST ⇒. The EC component exhibits complex papillary infolding with a stellate lumen.

Mixed Germ Cell Tumor

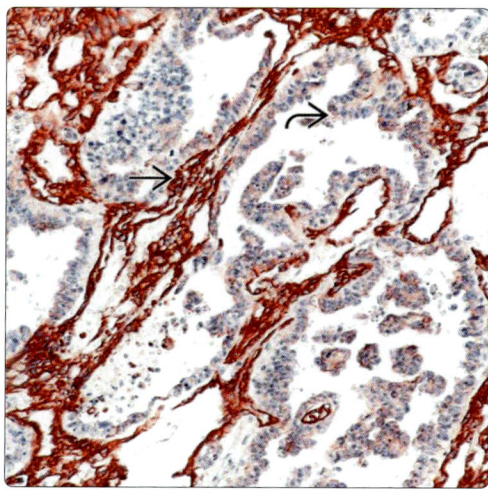

Mixed Germ Cell Tumor

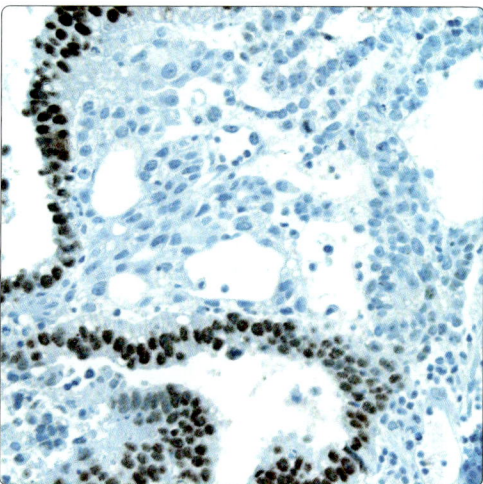

(Left) Cytokeratin immunostain shows differential staining intensity in YST ⇒ and EC ⇒. Immunohistochemistry is usually not necessary for the histologic diagnosis of germ cell tumors; however, it may be useful in situations when there is ambiguous histology or work-up for a metastasis. (Right) This photomicrograph shows differential OCT3/4 immunohistochemical staining of EC (positive) and YST (negative). Optimal fixation and appropriate sampling are very important.

Somatic-Type Malignancy in Germ Cell Tumor

KEY FACTS

TERMINOLOGY
- Carcinoma or sarcoma arising from preexisting teratoma or other germ cell tumor

CLINICAL ISSUES
- Occurs in 3-6% of testicular germ cell tumors
- Occurs only in postpubertal patients (age range: 15-68 years)
- Tumor occurs within primary testis tumor: More commonly in retroperitoneal lymph nodes or other metastatic sites
- For tumor in testis, treatment is same as nonseminomatous germ cell tumor
- Presence of somatic-type malignancy in testis does not appear to impact prognosis

MACROSCOPIC
- Similar to other nonseminomatous germ cell tumor

MICROSCOPIC
- Nodular/expansile or infiltrative growth of carcinomatous or sarcomatous component: Stromal overgrowth of sarcomatous components
- Mixed with teratomatous or other germ cell tumor components
- Most common carcinoma is adenocarcinoma of various growth patterns
- Rhabdomyosarcoma is most common (> 50%) sarcoma
- Other sarcomas include leiomyosarcoma, angiosarcoma, chondrosarcoma
- Other tumor type is primitive neuroendocrine carcinoma

TOP DIFFERENTIAL DIAGNOSES
- Mixed germ cell tumor
- Metastatic carcinoma
- Primary testicular/paratesticular sarcoma

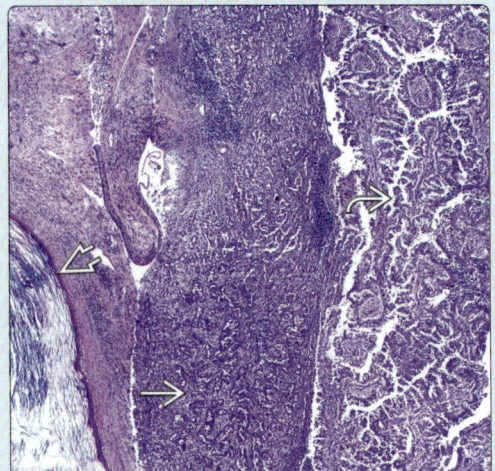

Somatic-Type Malignancy in Germ Cell Tumor: Adenocarcinoma

(Left) This photomicrograph shows a cystic teratoma component ⇨ with squamous lining and keratin debris adjacent to an adenocarcinoma with tubular ⇨ and papillary ⇨ growth patterns. (Right) This area of adenocarcinoma is composed of well- and poorly formed glands and single cells. Some glands contain intraluminal mucin. The carcinomatous overgrowth should occupy at least 1 low-power field (4x objective, 5 mm in diameter).

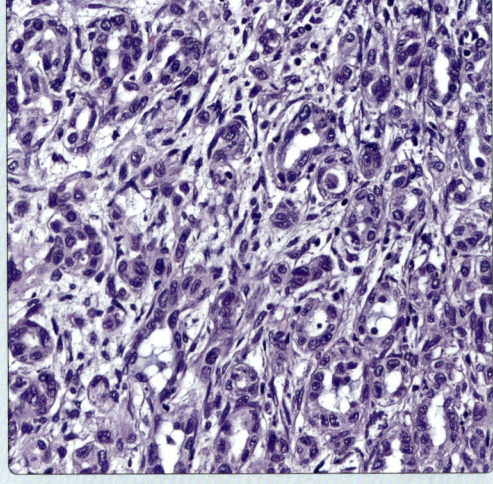

Somatic-Type Malignancy in Germ Cell Tumor: Adenocarcinoma

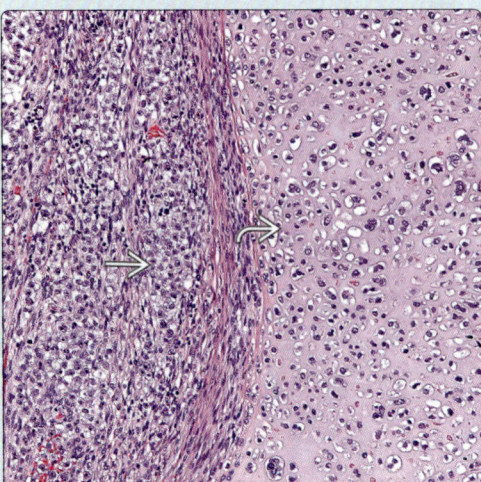

Somatic-Type Malignancy in Germ Cell Tumor: Chondrosarcomatous

(Left) This photomicrograph shows a chrondrosarcomatous component composed of hypercellular pleomorphic epithelioid cells in clear spaces ⇨ and adjacent seminomatous component ⇨. (Right) An example of a primitive neuroectodermal tumor (PNET) is shown. The tumor is composed of a vaguely lobular growth of small, round to oval, blue cells with minimal to modest pale eosinophilic cytoplasm. Focal rosettes with central solid eosinophilic, fibrillary material are present.

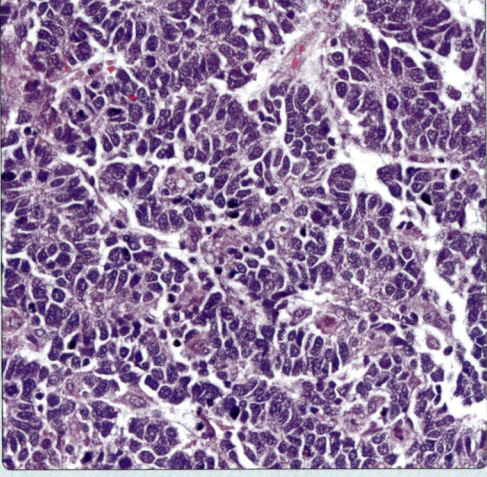

Somatic-Type Malignancy in Germ Cell Tumor: PNET

Somatic-Type Malignancy in Germ Cell Tumor

TERMINOLOGY

Abbreviations
- Somatic-type malignancy associated with teratomatous germ cell tumor

Synonyms
- Teratoma with malignant transformation, teratoma with secondary malignancy

Definitions
- Carcinoma or sarcoma arising from preexisting teratoma

CLINICAL ISSUES

Epidemiology
- Occurs in 3-6% of testicular germ cell tumors
- Occurs only in postpubertal patients (age range: 15-68 years)

Presentation
- Tumor may occur within testis and more commonly in retroperitoneal lymph node or other metastatic sites

Treatment
- Surgical approaches
  - For tumor in testis, treatment is same as nonseminomatous germ cell tumor
  - Surgical resection if possible for metastatic site
  - Chemotherapy and prognosis for somatic transformation are different in metastatic sites

Prognosis
- Presence of somatic-type malignancy in testis does not appear to impact prognosis
- Development of somatic-type malignancy in metastasis increases risk of death

IMAGING

Radiographic Findings
- Similar to other nonseminomatous germ cell tumor

MACROSCOPIC

General Features
- Similar to other nonseminomatous germ cell tumors

MICROSCOPIC

Histologic Features
- Nodular/expansile or infiltrative growth of carcinomatous or sarcomatous component
- Mixed with teratomatous or other germ cell tumor
- Most common carcinoma is adenocarcinoma of various growth pattern
- Carcinoma or sarcoma component should consist of pure expansile proliferation occupying at least 1 low-power field (4x objective, 5 mm in diameter)
- Other types of carcinoma include squamous cell carcinoma, neuroendocrine carcinoma, and poorly differentiated carcinoma
- Rhabdomyosarcoma is most common (> 50%)
- Other sarcomas include leiomyosarcoma, angiosarcoma, chondrosarcoma, and other sarcoma
- Other tumor type is primitive neuroendocrine carcinoma (PNET)

Cytologic Features
- Cellular features reflect type of malignancy

ANCILLARY TESTS

Immunohistochemistry
- Carcinomatous component positive for EMA, CK-PAN; negative for germ cell markers
- Sarcomatous component positive for markers of specific line of differentiation
- PNET positive for CD99, FLI-1, vimentin, and NSE

DIFFERENTIAL DIAGNOSIS

Mixed Germ Cell Tumor
- Histologic features of specific types of germ cell tumor
- Positive for germ cell tumor markers

Metastatic Carcinoma
- Occurs in older age group
- Clinical history of primary tumor
- Lack of teratoma or other germ cell tumor components
- Lack of germ cell neoplasia in situ

Primary Testicular/Paratesticular Sarcoma
- Homogenous sarcomatoid neoplasm
- Lack of teratoma or other germ cell tumor components
- Lack of germ cell neoplasia in situ

DIAGNOSTIC CHECKLIST

Pathologic Interpretation Pearls
- Presence of teratoma or germ cell tumor with carcinomatous or sarcomatous components

SELECTED REFERENCES

1. Howitt BE et al: Many postchemotherapy sarcomatous tumors in patients with testicular germ cell tumors are sarcomatoid yolk sac tumors: a study of 33 cases. Am J Surg Pathol. 39(2):251-9, 2015
2. Magers MJ et al: "Somatic-type" malignancies arising from testicular germ cell tumors: a clinicopathologic study of 124 cases with emphasis on glandular tumors supporting frequent yolk sac tumor origin. Am J Surg Pathol. 38(10):1396-409, 2014
3. Rice KR et al: Management of germ cell tumors with somatic type malignancy: pathological features, prognostic factors and survival outcomes. J Urol. 192(5):1403-9, 2014
4. Tarrant WP et al: Relationship between primary and metastatic testicular germ cell tumors: a clinicopathologic analysis of 100 cases. Hum Pathol. 44(10):2220-6, 2013
5. Colecchia M et al: Teratoma with somatic-type malignant components in germ cell tumors of the testis: a clinicopathologic analysis of 40 cases with outcome correlation. Int J Surg Pathol. 19(3):321-7, 2011
6. Necchi A et al: Towards the definition of the best management and prognostic factors of teratoma with malignant transformation: a single-institution case series and new proposal. BJU Int. 107(7):1088-94, 2011
7. Donadio AC et al: Chemotherapy for teratoma with malignant transformation. J Clin Oncol. 21(23):4285-91, 2003
8. Motzer RJ et al: Teratoma with malignant transformation: diverse malignant histologies arising in men with germ cell tumors. J Urol. 159(1):133-8, 1998

Burnt-Out (Regressed) Germ Cell Tumor

KEY FACTS

TERMINOLOGY
- Fibrotic nodule or scar ± residual malignant germ cell tumor in testis

CLINICAL ISSUES
- < 5% of testicular germ cell tumor have variable degrees of spontaneous regression
- Often 1st present with symptoms of retroperitoneal or distant metastasis
- Prognosis is usually worse than that of nonregressed germ cell tumor, as it often presents at advanced stage
- Radical orchiectomy is necessary to confirm diagnosis and eliminate relapse

MACROSCOPIC
- Well-demarcated, white to tan, solitary, or multiple nodules, less commonly band-like, stellate, or linear scar

MICROSCOPIC
- May be divided into: Scar only, scar with germ cell neoplasia in situ, scar with minor residual germ cell tumor components
- Well-demarcated vascularized, fibrotic scar is most common finding
- Lymphoplasmacytic infiltrate, hyalinized tubules, increased vascularity, and siderophages
- Presence of coarse intratubular calcifications
- Atrophy and sclerosis of seminiferous tubules
- Leydig cell hyperplasia and intratubular psammomatous-type calcifications

TOP DIFFERENTIAL DIAGNOSES
- Nonspecific, chronic, or granulomatous orchiditis
- Postinflammatory or ischemic scar

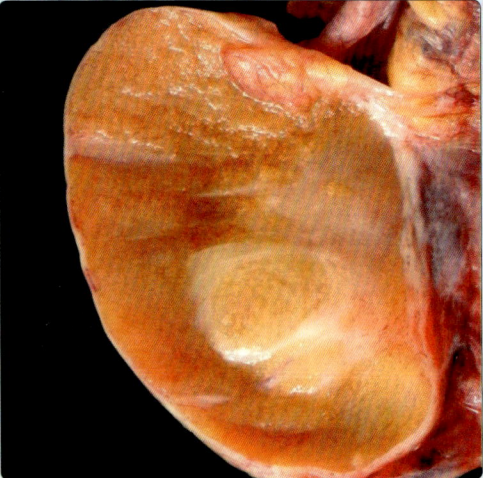
Burnt-Out Germ Cell Tumor: Gross

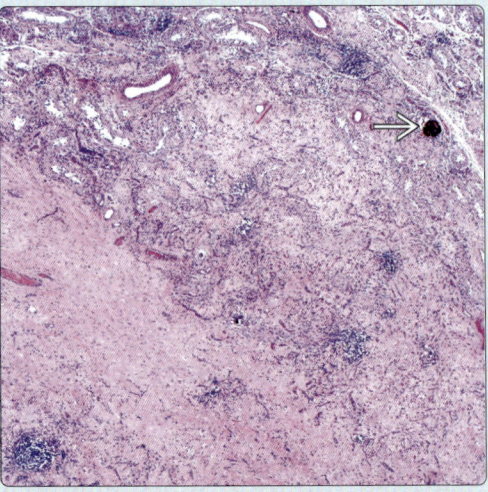
Burnt-Out Germ Cell Tumor: Fibrosis

(Left) This orchiectomy specimen shows a burnt-out germ cell tumor, which is characterized by a relatively well-demarcated, white to tan, solitary fibrotic scar area. *(Right)* Low power of burnt-out germ cell tumor shows zones of central dense fibrosis, increased vascular proliferation, and lymphoid aggregates. Focal coarse calcification ➡ is present. The background seminiferous tubules are atrophic. This finding in an orchiectomy should always raise concern for germ cell tumor.

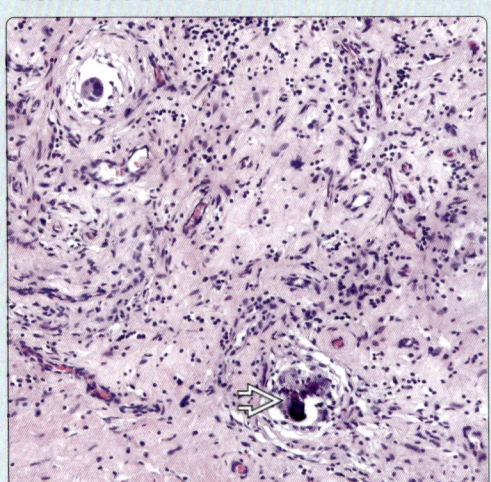
Burnt-Out Germ Cell Tumor: Calcification

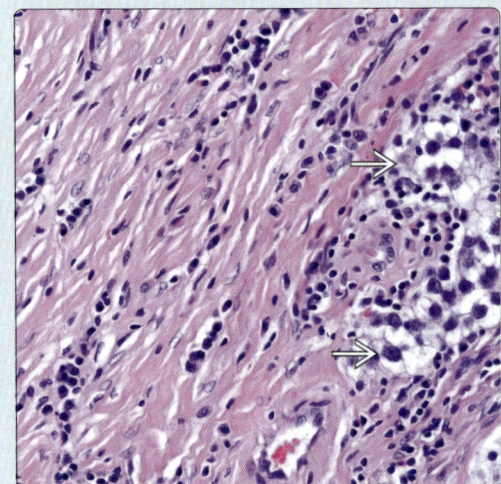
Burnt-Out Germ Cell Tumor: Seminoma

(Left) This example of burnt-out germ cell tumor shows fibrosis with increased vascularity and lymphoplasmacytic infiltrate. Focal coarse calcification ➡ associated with giant cell reaction is present. *(Right)* Burnt-out germ cell tumor shows residual small focus of seminoma ➡ with adjacent dense fibrosis and lymphoplasmacytic infiltrate. Extensive sampling is always necessary.

Burnt-Out (Regressed) Germ Cell Tumor

TERMINOLOGY

Synonyms
- Regressed germ cell tumor

Definitions
- Fibrotic nodule or scar ± residual malignant germ cell tumor in testis

CLINICAL ISSUES

Epidemiology
- < 5% of testicular germ cell tumors have variable degrees of spontaneous regression

Presentation
- Often 1st present with symptoms of retroperitoneal or distant metastasis
- Less commonly: Testicular enlargement or pain or elevated serum markers

Treatment
- Surgical approaches
  - Radical orchiectomy is necessary to confirm diagnosis and eliminate relapse
  - Nodal dissection and chemotherapy for metastatic disease

Prognosis
- Usually worse than that of nonregressed germ cell tumor, as it usually presents at advanced stage

IMAGING

Radiographic Findings
- Nonspecific, variable hyperechogenic or hypoechogenic areas in testis by ultrasound

MACROSCOPIC

General Features
- Testis may or may not be enlarged
- Well-demarcated, white to tan, solitary or multiple nodules, less commonly band-like, stellate, or linear scar

MICROSCOPIC

Histologic Features
- May be divided into: Scar only, scar with GCNIS, scar with minor residual germ cell tumor components
- Well-demarcated vascularized, fibrotic scar is most common finding
- Lymphoplasmacytic infiltrate, hyalinized tubules, increased vascularity, and siderophages
- Presence of coarse intratubular calcifications (intratubular microliths)
- Presence of GCNIS or intratubular embryonal carcinoma in adjacent seminiferous tubules
- Atrophy and sclerosis of seminiferous tubules
- Leydig cell hyperplasia and intratubular psammomatous-type calcifications
- Both seminomatous and nonseminomatous germ cell tumor undergo regression; very rare in spermatocytic tumor

Cytologic Features
- Minor component of seminomatous or nonseminomatous germ cell component may be present

ANCILLARY TESTS

Immunohistochemistry
- GCNIS cells positive for OCT4, PLAP, or D2-40 (do not use SALL4 or CD117 to detect GCNIS)
- Malignant germ cell tumor positive for SALL4, OCT4 (except yolk sac tumor and choriocarcinoma), PLAP

DIFFERENTIAL DIAGNOSIS

Nonspecific Chronic or Granulomatous Orchiditis
- Lack of GCNIS or germ cell tumor despite thorough sampling
- Lack of elevation of serum markers
- Immunohistochemistry using germ cell tumor-associated markers helpful to exclude germ cell neoplasia
- Extensive sampling is key to rule out germ cell tumor or GCNIS

Postinflammatory or Ischemic Scar
- Significant clinical history of infection or trauma

DIAGNOSTIC CHECKLIST

Clinically Relevant Pathologic Features
- Scar only, scar with germ cell neoplasia in situ (GCNIS), scar with minor residual germ cell tumor components

Pathologic Interpretation Pearls
- Presence of vascularized scar in adult (20-50 years) should make one suspect burnt-out germ cell tumor
- Extensive sampling necessary to identify residual in situ or malignant germ cell component
- Immunohistochemical stain using broad-spectrum germ cell tumor markers may be necessary

SELECTED REFERENCES

1. Qureshi JM et al: Metastatic "burned-out" germ cell tumor of the testis. J Urol. 192(3):936-7, 2014
2. Angulo JC et al: Clinicopathological study of regressed testicular tumors (apparent extragonadal germ cell neoplasms). J Urol. 182(5):2303-10, 2009
3. Miller JS et al: The utility of microscopic findings and immunohistochemistry in the classification of necrotic testicular tumors: a study of 11 cases. Am J Surg Pathol. 33(9):1293-8, 2009
4. Balzer BL et al: Spontaneous regression of testicular germ cell tumors: an analysis of 42 cases. Am J Surg Pathol. 30(7):858-65, 2006
5. Curigliano G et al: "Burned out" phenomenon of the testis in retroperitoneal seminoma. Acta Oncol. 45(3):335-6, 2006
6. Comiter CV et al: Burned-out primary testicular cancer: sonographic and pathological characteristics. J Urol. 156(1):85-8, 1996
7. Krag Jacobsen G et al: Testicular germ cell tumours in Denmark 1976-1980. Pathology of 1058 consecutive cases. Acta Radiol Oncol. 23(4):239-47, 1984

Spermatocytic Tumor

KEY FACTS

TERMINOLOGY
- Germ cell tumor composed of 3 cell types of variable sizes ranging 6-100 μm

CLINICAL ISSUES
- Rare testis germ cell tumor (1-2%)
- Average age of patients: 53.6 yr
- Painless testicular swelling and mass
- Serum tumor markers are not elevated
- Radical inguinal orchiectomy alone is curative

MACROSCOPIC
- Well-circumscribed, soft, friable, tan-gray mass with mucoid or gelatinous, bulging cut surface

MICROSCOPIC
- Diffuse or solid sheet-like pattern with scant fibrous or edematous stroma is most common finding
- Rare growth patterns include pseudoglandular, microcystic, trabecular, nests, or single cells
- Polymorphous cell population is hallmark of spermatocytic seminoma: Small lymphocyte-like cells, intermediate cells, and giant cells
- Lack cytoplasmic glycogen, fibrovascular septa, lymphoplasmacytic infiltrate, or granulomatous inflammation
- Lack association with germ cell neoplasia in situ

ANCILLARY TESTS
- Negative for most germ cell-associated markers [OCT3/OCT4, Podoplanin (D2-40), PLAP, α-fetoprotein, glypican-3, HCG, and CD30(BerH2)], cytokeratin, and vimentin
- Positive for SALL4, CD117, MAGE-A4, OCT2, SSX, SAGE1; often focal or patchy

TOP DIFFERENTIAL DIAGNOSES
- Classic seminoma
- Embryonal carcinoma
- Malignant lymphoma

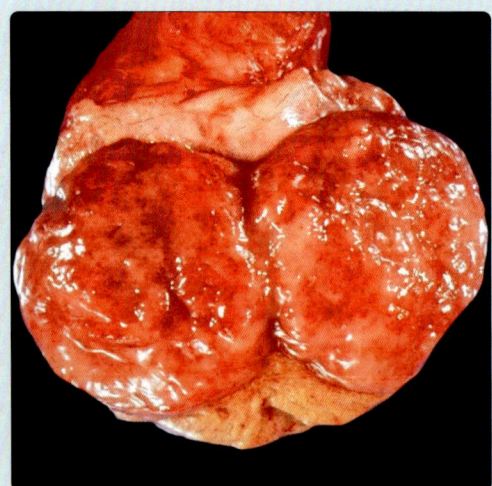

Spermatocytic Tumor: Gross

(Left) *Spermatocytic tumor has a bulging, nodular, soft, tan-gray, mucoid cut surface. Classic seminoma, spermatocytic seminoma, and lymphoma may have a similar gross appearance, but they differ in age, frequency of bilaterality, and spermatic cord involvement.* (Right) *Low-power view of diffuse growth pattern of spermatocytic tumor reveals no fibrovascular septa and no lymphocytic or granulomatous inflammation, typical features of classic seminoma.*

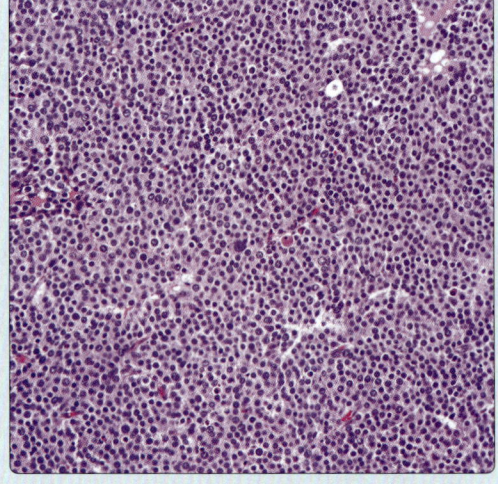

Spermatocytic Tumor: Solid

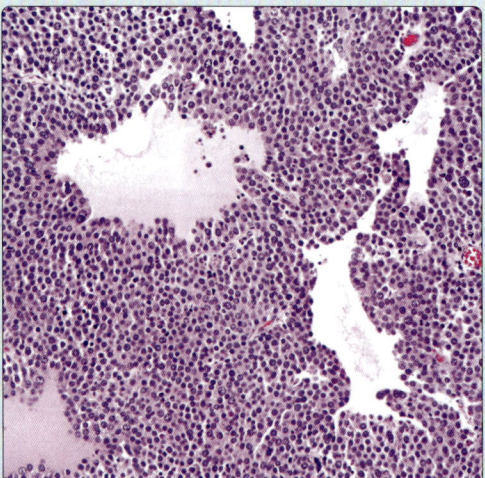

Spermatocytic Tumor: Stromal Edema

(Left) *Low-power photomicrograph of spermatocytic tumor shows cystic spaces due to accumulation of edema fluid and lack of stroma. The edematous fluid and lack of cell cohesion are helpful features of this tumor in making the distinction from seminoma.* (Right) *This high-power photomicrograph shows the characteristic 3 cell types in spermatocytic tumor: Small lymphocyte-like cells ➡ with darkly stained nuclei, intermediate ➡ and giant cells with spireme-type chromatin ➡.*

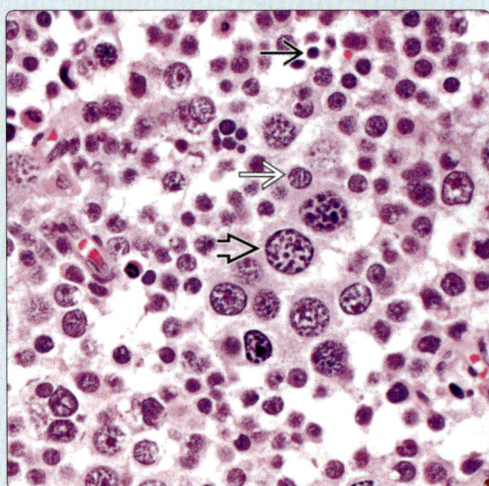

Spermatocytic Tumor: Cytology

Spermatocytic Tumor

TERMINOLOGY

Synonyms
- Spermatocytic seminoma

Definitions
- Germ cell tumor recapitulating spermatogenic sequence composed of 3 cell types of variable sizes, ranging 6-100 µm

ETIOLOGY/PATHOGENESIS

Cytogenetic Changes
- Diploid or near hypodiploid, different from that of seminoma
- Chromosomal numerical changes (most commonly gain of chromosome 9)
- Group of heterogenous tumors that originate from different types of spermatogonia

CLINICAL ISSUES

Epidemiology
- Incidence
  - Rare testis germ cell tumor (< 1%); bilaterality is more common (> 9%) than in seminoma
  - No ovarian or extragonadal counterpart of spermatocytic seminoma
  - Not associated with cryptorchidism; no race predilection as in other germ cell tumors
- Age
  - Range: 25-87 yr (average: 53.6 yr)

Presentation
- Painless testicular swelling and mass
- Serum tumor markers are not elevated

Treatment
- Radical inguinal orchiectomy alone is curative

Prognosis
- Excellent prognosis with rare malignant behavior (< 1%)
- Sarcomatoid transformation is rare but when present is associated with distant metastasis and death

MACROSCOPIC

General Features
- Well-circumscribed, soft, friable, tan-gray mass with mucoid or gelatinous, bulging cut surface
- Lobulation, cystic change, focal hemorrhage or necrosis may be seen

Size
- Range: 2-20 cm (average: 7 cm)

MICROSCOPIC

Histologic Features
- Diffuse or solid sheet-like pattern with scant fibrous or edematous stroma is most common finding
- Other rarer patterns include pseudoglandular, microcystic, trabecular, nests, or single cells
- Polymorphous cell population with 3 distinct cell types is hallmark of spermatocytic tumor
  - Small lymphocyte-like cells: 6-8 µm; densely hyperchromatic nuclei and scant amount of cytoplasm
  - Intermediate cells: 15-20 µm; most common cell type; round nuclei, finely granular chromatin, variable nucleoli, moderate amount of cytoplasm; occasional spireme-type chromatin
  - Giant cells: 50-100 µm; least common cell type; distinctive filamentous or spireme-type chromatin
- Lack cytoplasmic glycogen, fibrovascular septa, lymphoplasmacytic infiltrate, or granulomatous inflammation
- Intratubular spermatocytic seminoma with large, highly atypical cells expanding tubules may be seen
- Lack association with germ cell neoplasia in situ
- Anaplastic spermatocytic seminoma is characterized by predominantly monomorphous intermediate-sized cells with prominent nucleoli and brisk mitoses
- Sarcomatous transformation may rarely occur (6%) and is characterized by undifferentiated primitive spindle cell sarcoma; rhabdomyoblastic differentiation has been reported

ANCILLARY TESTS

Histochemistry
- Negative for PAS diastase

Immunohistochemistry
- Positive for SALL4, CD117, MAGE-A4, OCT2, SSX, SAGE1
- Negative for most germ cell-associated markers [OCT3/OCT4, Podoplanin (D2-40), PLAP, α-fetoprotein, glypican-3, HCG, and CD30(BerH2)], cytokeratin, and vimentin

DIFFERENTIAL DIAGNOSIS

Classic Seminoma
- Relatively monotonous cell population with fibrovascular septa, lymphoplasmacytic and granulomatous inflammation
- Positive for OCT3/OCT4, PLAP, D2-40

Embryonal Carcinoma (Solid Pattern)
- Greater extent of cytologic anaplasia with different concurrent growth patterns (solid, glandular, and papillary)
- Positive for cytokeratin and OCT3/OCT4, CD30

Malignant Lymphoma
- Typical interstitial growth pattern with uniform cell population
- Positive for CD45 (LCA), and CD20 or CD3

SELECTED REFERENCES

1. Kao CS et al: The utility of immunostaining for NUT, GAGE7 and NY-ESO-1 in the diagnosis of spermatocytic seminoma. Histopathology. 65(1):35-44, 2014
2. Sereno M et al: Squamous-cell carcinoma of the lungs: is it really so different? Crit Rev Oncol Hematol. 84(3):327-39, 2012
3. Lim J et al: OCT2, SSX and SAGE1 reveal the phenotypic heterogeneity of spermatocytic seminoma reflecting distinct subpopulations of spermatogonia. J Pathol. 224(4):473-83, 2011
4. Borneisl PE et al: Spermatocytic seminoma. J Urol. 177(2):734, 2007

Spermatocytic Tumor

Spermatocytic Tumor: Cell Types

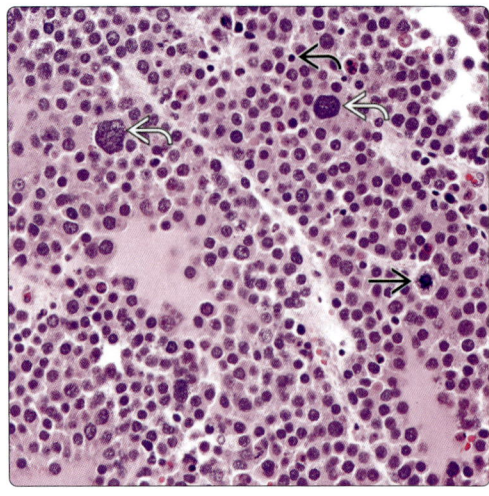

Spermatocytic Tumor: Cytology

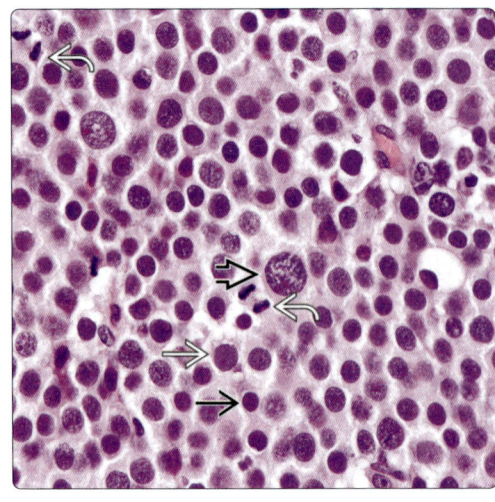

(Left) Cellular polymorphism is the hallmark of a spermatocytic tumor. The most common cell type is the intermediate-sized cell. There are few small cells ➡ and giant cells ➡ in this example. Mitoses ➡ may be brisk in some cases. **(Right)** This photomicrograph shows the cytologic features of the 3 cell types in spermatocytic tumor: Small lymphocyte-like cells ➡, intermediate ➡, and giant cells ➡. Mitoses ➡ are also seen. This degree of cellular polymorphism would be unusual in classic seminoma.

Spermatocytic Tumor: Stromal Edema

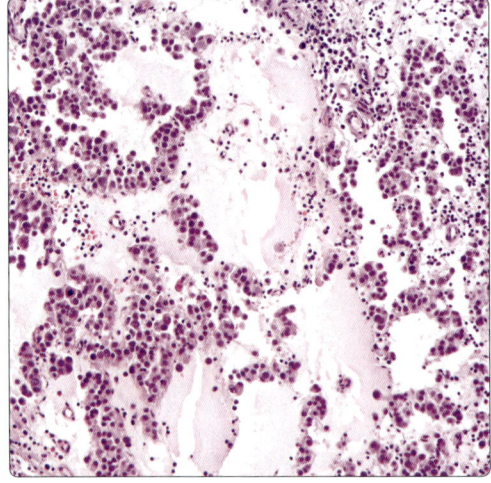

Spermatocytic Tumor: Solid Sheets

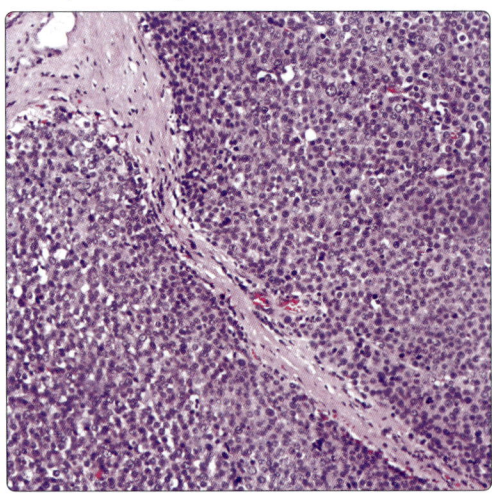

(Left) Spermatocytic tumor with extensive intercellular edema is shown. This results in a cystic and mucoid gross appearance. This pseudoglandular or cystic histology raises the possibility of other testicular tumors. **(Right)** Occasional fibrous bands separate diffuse sheets of spermatocytic tumor into lobules. There are no lymphocytic infiltrates or granulomas, features that are different from classic seminoma. The tumor cells do not show distinct cell boundaries and lack abundant clear cytoplasm.

Spermatocytic Tumor: Interstitial

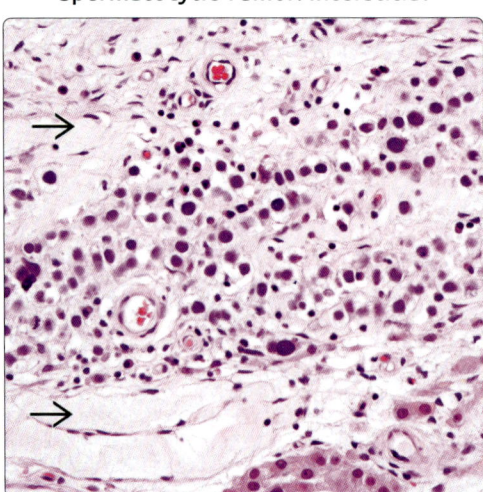

Spermatocytic Tumor: Intratubular

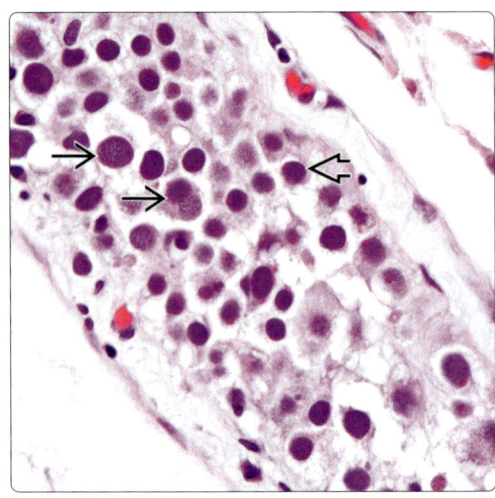

(Left) At the periphery of a spermatocytic tumor, an interstitial pattern between seminiferous tubules ➡ may be seen. Lymphocytic infiltrate, a feature seen in early invasive seminoma, is not present. **(Right)** Intratubular spermatocytic tumor is characterized by a polymorphic cell population with large atypical cells ➡ filling the lumen of a seminiferous tubule with few preserved germ cells ➡. This pattern is different from that of GCNIS in which neoplastic cells are typically located at the periphery.

Spermatocytic Tumor

Spermatocytic Tumor: Anaplastic

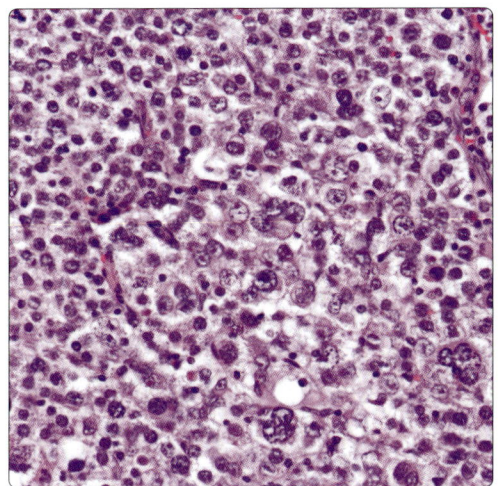

Spermatocytic Tumor: Rhabdomyoblastic Transformation

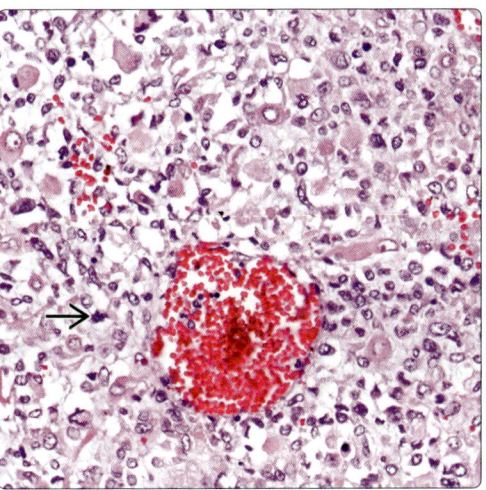

(Left) So-called anaplastic spermatocytic tumor is characterized by proliferation of predominantly intermediate cells with coarse chromatin and prominent nucleoli. Embryonal carcinoma and classic seminoma may be in the differential diagnosis. **(Right)** Rhabdomyoblastic sarcomatous transformation of spermatocytic tumor is shown. There is a proliferation of atypical spindle cells with abundant pink cytoplasm and frequent mitoses ➡. In other areas, a classic spermatocytic tumor histology was seen.

Spermatocytic Tumor: Hemorrhage

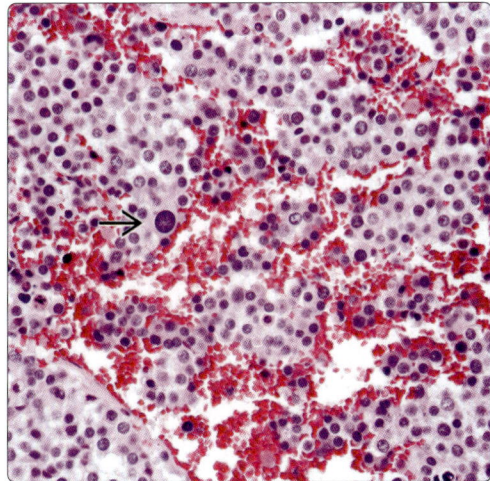

Spermatocytic Tumor: OCT3/4

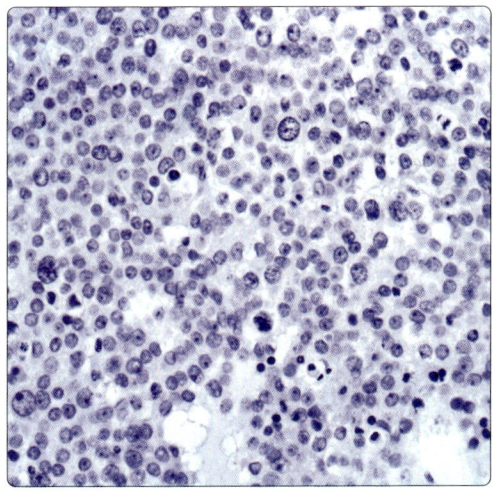

(Left) Spermatocytic tumor with cystic changes and hemorrhage is shown. The tumor is composed of a polymorphic population of cells composed of mainly intermediate size cells and abundant eosinophilic cytoplasm and occasional large tumor cells ➡. **(Right)** This image shows negative OCT3/4 immunoreactivity in a spermatocytic tumor. However, tumor cells are positive for markers expressed in spermatogonia (SALL4, CD117, MAGE-A4, etc.).

Classic Seminoma: Differential

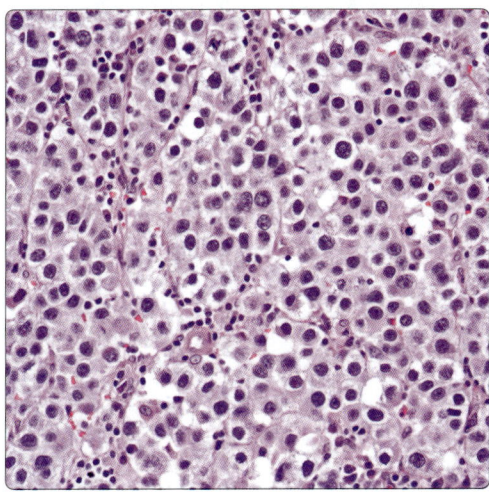

Spermatocytic Tumor: Polymorphous

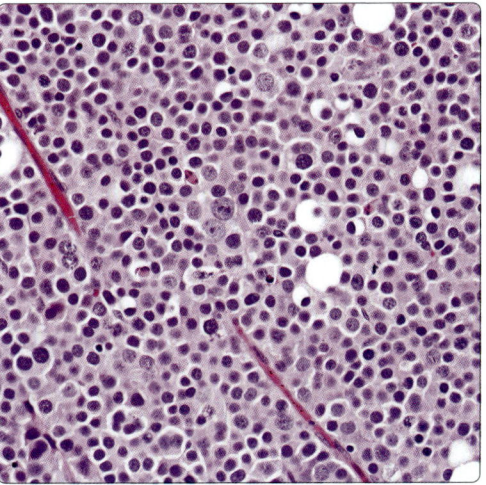

(Left) Classic seminoma is the major differential diagnosis of a spermatocytic tumor. In addition to the fibrovascular septa with small lymphocytes, the tumor cells have a uniform monomorphous population of tumor cells with distinct cell membranes. **(Right)** Compared with classic seminoma, this spermatocytic tumor has a polymorphous population of 3 cell types and lacks the features of fibrovascular septa, lymphocytes, and granulomas.

Teratoma, Prepubertal Type

KEY FACTS

TERMINOLOGY
- Prepubertal testicular tumor composed of elements resembling somatic tissues derived from 1 or more germinal layers (endoderm, mesoderm, and ectoderm)

ETIOLOGY/PATHOGENESIS
- Different from teratoma in older patients
- May be derived from nontransformed germ cells
- Isochromosome 12p abnormality is absent

CLINICAL ISSUES
- 2nd most common testicular tumor in prepubertal children
- Epidermoid cyst more common than dermoid cyst
- Testicular mass found incidentally by physical examination or imaging
- Serum tumor markers (LDH, AFP, and hCG) are not elevated
- Conservative, testicle-preserving surgery is appropriate

MICROSCOPIC
- Mature and immature teratoma components with ectodermal, mesodermal, and endodermal tissues
- Dermoid cyst is composed of unilocular cyst lined by epidermis and dermis containing skin adnexal structures (hair follicle, sebaceous, apocrine, or eccrine glands)
- Dermoid cyst has orderly arrangement of pilosebaceous units with epidermal surface resembling that of skin
- Epidermoid cyst is composed of unilocular cyst with keratinized squamous epithelial lining containing granular cell layer without skin adnexal structures
- Carcinoid tumor can be pure or associated with other teratoma elements
- Uninvolved testis lacks of significant atrophy or germ cell neoplasia in situ

TOP DIFFERENTIAL DIAGNOSES
- Postpubertal teratoma

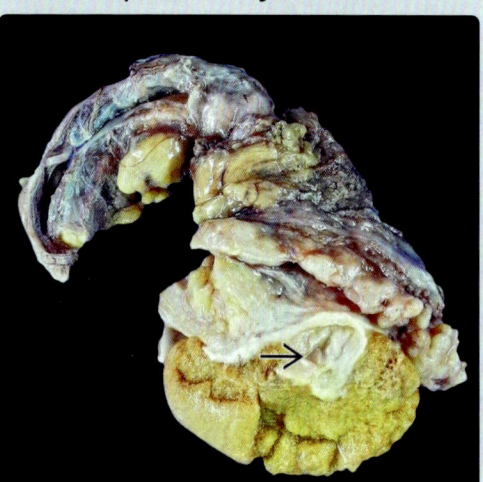

Epidermoid Cyst: Gross

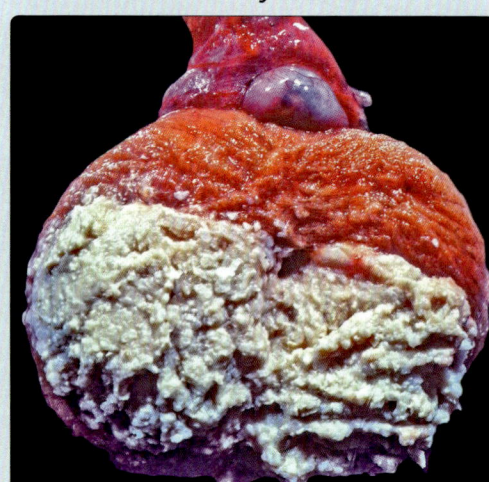

Dermoid Cyst: Gross

(Left) This well-defined unilocular cyst ➡ bulging from the testicular surface is an epidermoid cyst. The inner surface is smooth and lacks a solid component. The background testis is grossly unremarkable but needs extensive sampling to rule out germ cell neoplasia in situ (GCNIS). (Right) This gross photograph shows a large, well-circumscribed testicular dermoid cyst with a collection of granular, chalky keratin and sebaceous material. The surrounding testicular parenchyma is unremarkable.

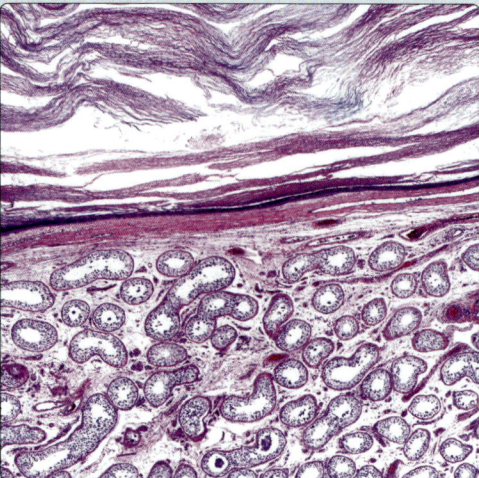

Epidermoid Cyst: Unilocular Cyst

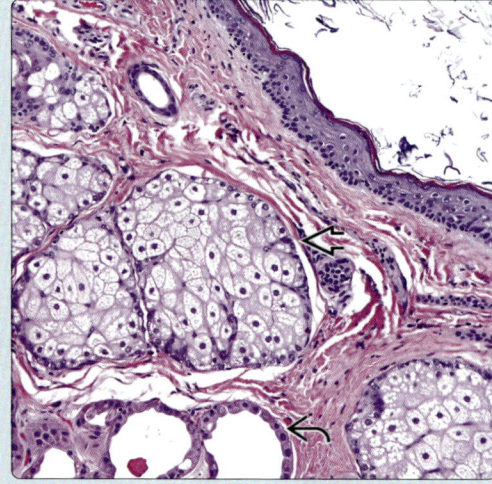

Dermoid Cyst: Skin and Adnexa

(Left) A testicular epidermoid cyst is composed of a unilocular cyst lined by keratinizing squamous epithelium and keratin debris. Note that there are no skin adnexal structures. GCNIS is not present in the surrounding testicular parenchyma. (Right) Dermoid cyst is characterized by keratinizing squamous epithelium and adnexal structures with well-organized sebaceous ➡ and apocrine ➡ glands. No GCNIS was present in the surrounding seminiferous tubules (not shown).

Teratoma, Prepubertal Type

TERMINOLOGY

Synonyms
- Epidermoid, dermoid cyst, prepubertal testicular teratoma, and carcinoid

Definitions
- Prepubertal testicular tumor composed of elements resembling somatic tissues derived from 1 or more germinal layers (endoderm, mesoderm, and ectoderm)

ETIOLOGY/PATHOGENESIS

Unknown
- Different from teratoma in postpubertal older patients; may be derived from nontransformed germ cells
- No association with germ cell neoplasia in situ (GCNIS)
- Isochromosome 12p abnormality is absent

CLINICAL ISSUES

Epidemiology
- 2nd most common testicular tumor in prepubertal children (median age: 13-14 months)
- Epidermoid cyst more common than dermoid cyst and rarely occur in adults

Presentation
- Testicular mass found incidentally by physical examination or imaging
- Serum tumor markers (LDH, AFP, and hCG) are not elevated

Treatment
- Surgical approaches
  - Conservative, testicle-preserving surgery is appropriate

Prognosis
- Benign behavior

IMAGING

Ultrasonographic Findings
- Intratesticular hypoechoic cystic mass
- May see onion ring appearance on US due to laminated keratin

MACROSCOPIC

General Features
- Intraparenchymal, well-defined fibrous-walled cystic lesion containing degenerating keratin debris
- Nodular and firm with variably cystic and solid cut surface
- Gray-white nodules representing cartilage; hair or melanin-containing tissue may be rarely seen

Size
- Variable

MICROSCOPIC

Histologic Features
- Prepubertal teratoma is composed of mixed ectodermal, mesodermal, and endodermal tissue
  - Squamous cysts with hair follicle and skin adnexal structures, ciliated epithelium and smooth muscle arranged in organoid fashion
  - Other common elements include meningothelium, fat, cartilage, bone, and muscle tissue; these tissues may be immature
  - All tissue elements show lack of significant atypia
- Dermoid cyst, specialized benign form of monodermal cystic teratoma
  - Usually unilocular cyst lined by epidermis and dermis containing skin adnexal structures (hair follicle, sebaceous, apocrine or eccrine glands)
  - Orderly arrangement of pilosebaceous units to epidermal surface resembling that of skin
  - Cystic wall with smooth muscle bundles may be present
  - Lipogranulomatous reaction to cyst contents may be seen when cyst ruptured
  - "Pilomatrixoma" as variant of dermoid cyst has been reported
- Epidermoid cyst, specialized benign cyst with keratinizing squamous lining without skin adnexal structures
  - Usually unilocular cyst with keratinized squamous epithelial lining containing granular cell layer without skin adnexal structures
  - Cystic wall may be calcified or ossified
- Carcinoid tumor (monodermal teratoma)
  - May be pure or associated with other teratoma elements
- Uninvolved testis shows lack of significant atrophy or GCNIS

DIFFERENTIAL DIAGNOSIS

Postpubertal Teratoma
- Disorganized elements of somatic tissue derived from different germinal layers
- Presence of GCNIS
- Occurs in postpubertal age

DIAGNOSTIC CHECKLIST

Clinically Relevant Pathologic Features
- Meticulous sampling and evaluation of background testis to search presence of GCNIS or other germ cell tumor component

SELECTED REFERENCES

1. Zhang C et al: Evidence supporting the existence of benign teratomas of the postpubertal testis: a clinical, histopathologic, and molecular genetic analysis of 25 cases. Am J Surg Pathol. 37(6):827-35, 2013
2. Xu Q et al: Incidence and survival for testicular germ cell tumor in young males: a report from the Northern Region Young Person's Malignant Disease Registry, United Kingdom. Urol Oncol. 25(1):32-7, 2007
3. Ross JH et al: Clinical behavior and a contemporary management algorithm for prepubertal testis tumors: a summary of the Prepubertal Testis Tumor Registry. J Urol. 168(4 Pt 2):1675-8; discussion 1678-9, 2002
4. Ulbright TM et al: Dermoid cyst of the testis: a study of five postpubertal cases, including a pilomatrixoma-like variant, with evidence supporting its separate classification from mature testicular teratoma. Am J Surg Pathol. 25(6):788-93, 2001
5. Hawkins E et al: The prepubertal testis (prenatal and postnatal): its relationship to intratubular germ cell neoplasia: a combined Pediatric Oncology Group and Children's Cancer Study Group. Hum Pathol. 28(4):404-10, 1997

Teratoma, Prepubertal Type

Prepubertal Teratoma: Glandular Component

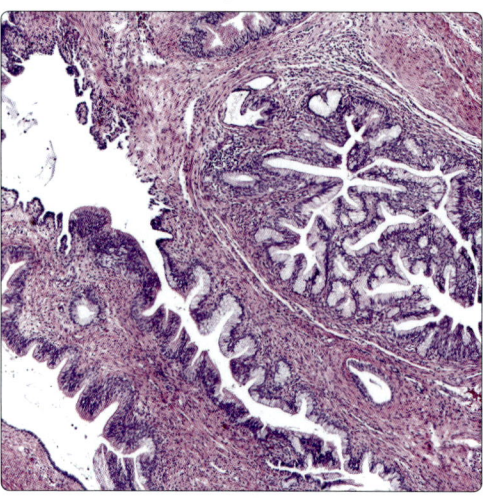

Prepubertal Teratoma: Immature Component

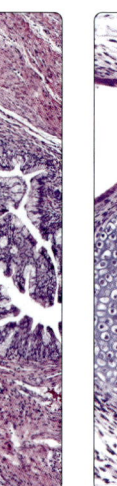

(Left) A prepubertal teratoma composed of mucinous and ciliated epithelium surrounded by smooth muscle is shown. The key difference from postpubertal teratoma is their organoid appearance and lack of background germ cell neoplasia in situ besides age of the patient. (Right) This prepubertal teratoma is composed of mature glandular epithelium, cartilage, and immature neuroepithelium ➡.

Prepubertal Teratoma: Intestinal Component

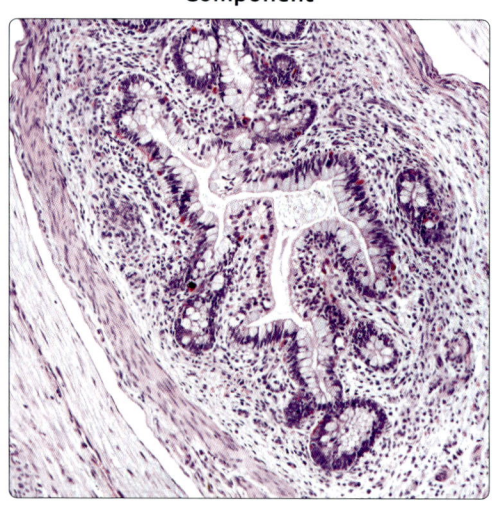

Prepubertal Teratoma: Immature Neuroepithelial Component

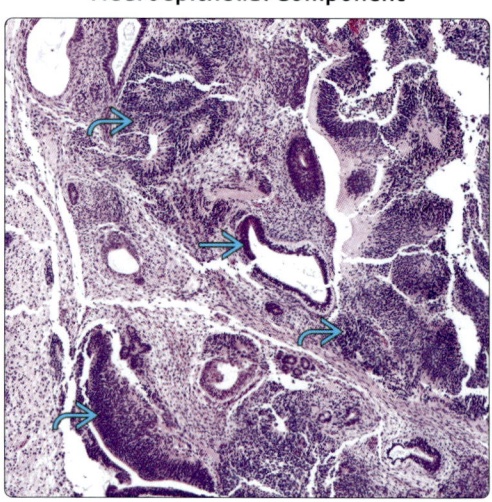

(Left) A prepubertal teratoma composed of intestinal-type epithelium with goblet cells surrounded by muscularis mucosae-type smooth muscle fibers is shown. (Right) Low-power photomicrograph shows a prepubertal teratoma composed of mixture of glandular epithelium ➡ and prominent immature neuroepithelial tissue ➡.

Epidermoid Cyst: Unilocular Cyst

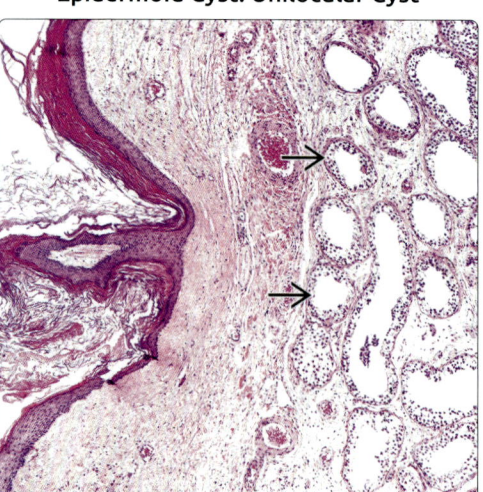

Epidermoid Cyst: Keratin Material

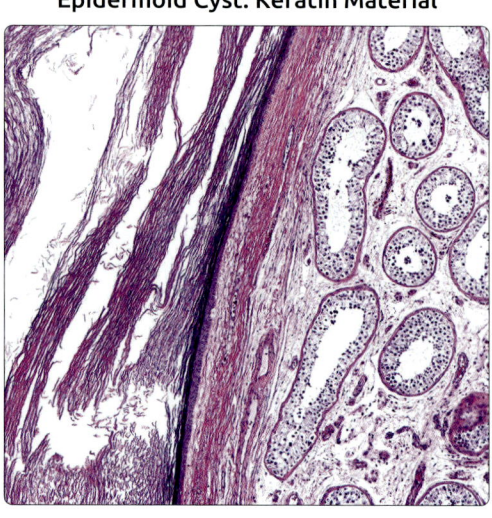

(Left) Unilocular epidermoid cyst is lined by keratinizing squamous epithelium and luminal keratin debris with no skin adnexal structures. The cyst is well demarcated from surrounding seminiferous tubules ➡. (Right) This epidermoid cyst shows that a part of the cyst wall is lined by mature squamous epithelium. There is laminated keratinous material on the luminal surface. No skin adnexal structures are seen. The adjacent seminiferous tubules lack GCNIS.

Teratoma, Prepubertal Type

Dermoid Cyst: Skin and Adnexa
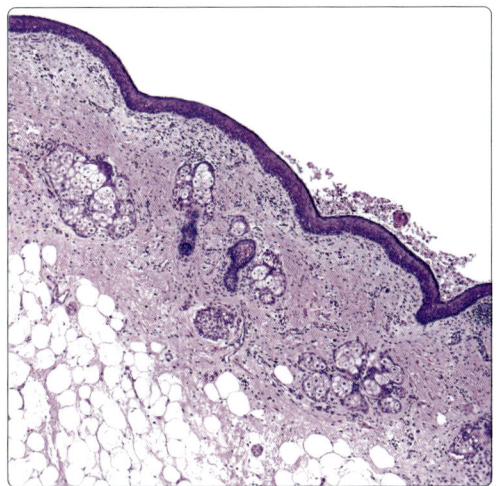

Dermoid Cyst: Unilocular
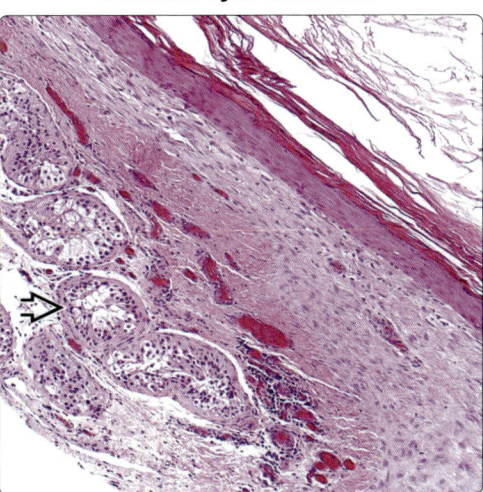

(Left) This dermoid cyst shows well-organized keratinizing squamous epithelium, pilosebaceous units, and adipose tissue. Ciliated epithelium or cartilage may be present, but these elements must maintain an organoid pattern. Haphazard presence of these structures indicates a mature teratoma. (Right) Low-power photomicrograph of dermoid cyst shows the interface of cyst wall and testicular parenchyma. Rare adnexal structures were present (not shown). The background testis ➔ lacks germ cell neoplasia in situ.

Dermoid Cyst: Histiocytes
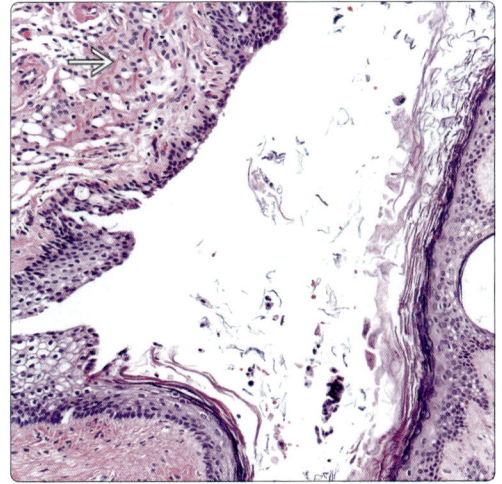

Dermoid Cyst: Organoid
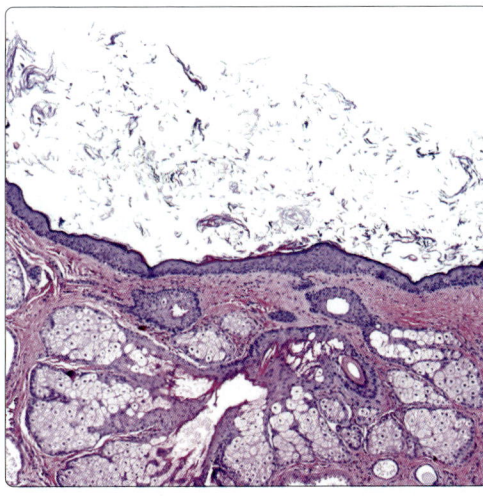

(Left) This dermoid cyst shows well-organized keratinizing squamous epithelium with keratin debris. Collection of foamy histiocytes ➔ are present indicating rupture of a cyst. Elsewhere, adnexal structures were present. (Right) This example of dermoid cyst shows extensive but organoid pilosebaceous units in the fibrotic cystic wall. Grossly, this lesion had grumous "cheesy" material within the cyst corresponding to the keratin material.

Dermoid Cyst: Inflammation
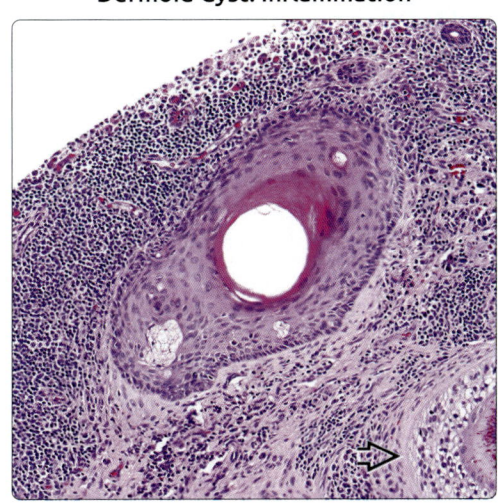

Dermoid Cyst: Lipogranulomatous Reaction
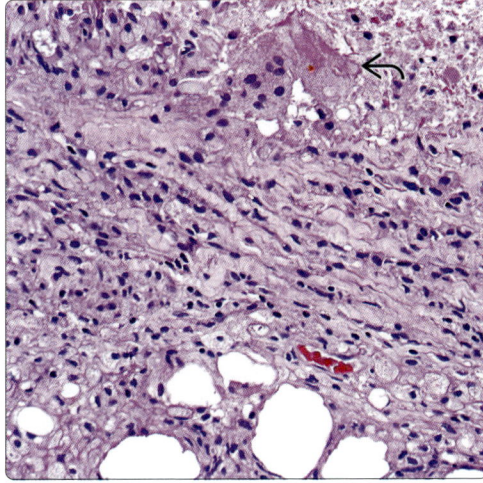

(Left) A dermoid cyst is shown in which the lining epithelium is denuded and associated with extensive chronic inflammation and granulation tissue. The diagnosis of dermoid cyst is tenable due to the presence of adnexal structures in the cyst wall with a pilosebaceous unit ➔. (Right) This dermoid cyst required multiple sections to identify keratin debris ➔ within a lipogranulomatous reaction as well as rare adnexal structures (not shown). Lipogranulomatous reaction is a characteristic finding in dermoid cysts.

Yolk Sac Tumor, Prepubertal Type

KEY FACTS

TERMINOLOGY
- Pediatric germ cell tumor that is not associated with germ cell neoplasia in situ

CLINICAL ISSUES
- Most common pediatric (> 12 years) pure germ cell tumor
- Yolk sac tumor accounts for 48-62% of prepubertal testicular tumors
- Amenable for testicular-preserving surgery
- Patients have excellent prognosis with nearly 100% survival

MACROSCOPIC
- Usually well-circumscribed, solid, gray to tan-yellow mass with mucoid cut surface

MICROSCOPIC
- Most common patterns: Micro- or macrocystic, reticular, glandular or alveolar, endodermal sinus, papillary, solid, myxomatous
- Parietal and polyvesicular vitelline patterns have rarely been reported
- No necrosis or germ cell neoplasia in situ in adjacent seminiferous tubules
- Tumor cells with mild to moderately pleomorphic, compressed nuclei, vacuolated cytoplasm
- Intracytoplasmic hyaline globules or extracellular, band-like deposits of basement membrane are frequent findings

ANCILLARY TESTS
- Positive for α-fetoprotein, cytokeratin, glypican-3, GATA3, SALL4
- Negative for EMA, OCT4

TOP DIFFERENTIAL DIAGNOSES
- Juvenile granulosa cell tumor
- Sex cord-stromal tumor

Prepubertal Yolk Sac Tumor

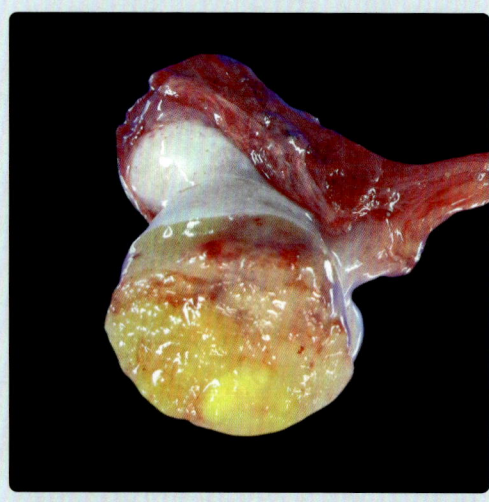

Prepubertal YST Involving Spermatic Cord

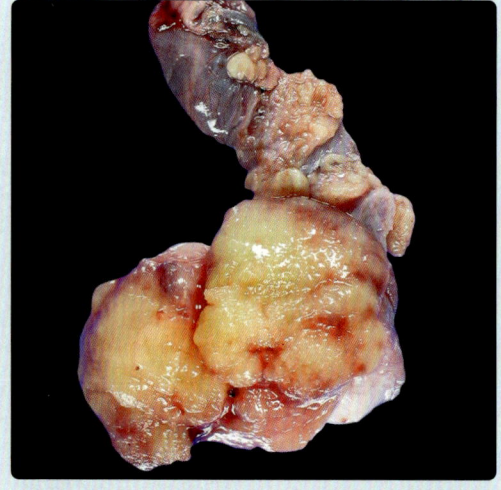

(Left) This photo shows a yolk sac tumor (YST) in a child. It has a bulging, white, myxoid, and yellow cut surface. Pure YST is the most common testicular tumor of infants and young children. *(Right)* YST in a child with a white and yellow myxoid cut surface is shown. The tumor involves the spermatic cord. Most pediatric YSTs present with a low clinical stage.

YST: Mixed Solid and Cystic Components

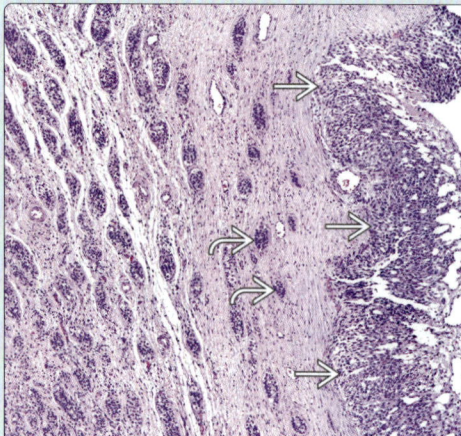

YST: Mixed Microcystic and Solid Patterns

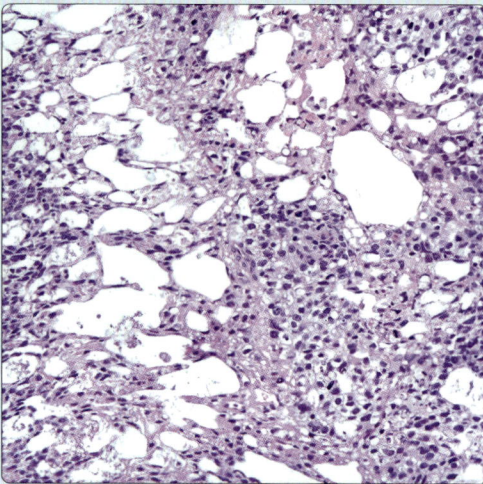

(Left) A YST is composed of mixed solid and cystic components ➡. The tumor is well demarcated from adjacent immature seminiferous tubules ➡. *(Right)* This image shows a typical YST with mixed microcystic and solid patterns. The tumor cells form microcysts and a meshwork of spaces.

Yolk Sac Tumor, Prepubertal Type

TERMINOLOGY

Abbreviations
- Yolk sac tumor (YST)

Synonyms
- Endodermal sinus tumor; type I germ cell tumor of testis

Definitions
- Pediatric germ cell tumor that is not associated with germ cell neoplasia in situ

ETIOLOGY/PATHOGENESIS

Cause Unknown
- Postulated that YST develops from teratoma through tumor progression

CLINICAL ISSUES

Epidemiology
- Most common pediatric (> 12 years) pure germ cell tumor
- Median age: 16-20 months
- YST accounts for 48-62% of prepubertal testicular tumors
- No racial or geographic predilection

Presentation
- Testicular swelling or mass
- Most patients have elevation of α-fetoprotein (AFP)
- Over 80% of patients present with stage I at presentation

Treatment
- Surgical approaches
  - Orchiectomy is curative
  - Amenable for testicular-preserving surgery
- Adjuvant therapy
  - Chemotherapy is usually not necessary

Prognosis
- Patients have excellent prognosis with nearly 100% survival

IMAGING

Ultrasonographic Findings
- Ultrasonography is sensitive in detecting scrotal mass

MACROSCOPIC

General Features
- Usually well-circumscribed, solid, gray to tan-yellow mass with mucoid cut surface

MICROSCOPIC

Histologic Features
- Similar to adult YST, has variety of morphologic growth patterns
- Most common patterns: Micro- or macrocystic, reticular, glandular or alveolar, endodermal sinus, papillary, solid, myxomatous
- Parietal and polyvesicular vitelline patterns have rarely been reported
- No necrosis or germ cell neoplasia in situ in adjacent seminiferous tubules

Cytologic Features
- Tumor cells with mild to moderately pleomorphic, compressed nuclei, vacuolated cytoplasm
- Mitotic figures are variable, but usually high
- Intracytoplasmic hyaline globules or extracellular, band-like deposits of basement membrane are frequent findings

ANCILLARY TESTS

Immunohistochemistry
- Positive for AFP, cytokeratin, glypican-3, GATA3, SALL4
- Negative for EMA, OCT4

DIFFERENTIAL DIAGNOSIS

Juvenile Granulosa Cell Tumor
- Lobular growth with cellular areas and follicles of variable sizes and shapes
- Positive for inhibin, calretinin, and CD99
- Negative for SALL4, AFP, or glypican-3

Sex Cord-Stromal Tumor
- Variable morphologic patterns with biphasic epithelioid and spindle cell components
- Positive for inhibin and calretinin
- Negative for SALL4, AFP, or glypican-3

DIAGNOSTIC CHECKLIST

Clinically Relevant Pathologic Features
- Testicular swelling or mass; elevation of AFP

Pathologic Interpretation Pearls
- Mixed growth patterns with moderately pleomorphic, compressed nuclei, and vacuolated cytoplasm
- Intracytoplasmic hyaline globules or extracellular basement membrane-like material
- Common pediatric germ cell tumor, pure (not mixed) histology, and absent germ cell neoplasia in situ

SELECTED REFERENCES

1. Cornejo KM et al: Yolk sac tumor of the testis in infants and children: a clinicopathologic analysis of 33 cases. Am J Surg Pathol. 39(8):1121-31, 2015
2. Ulbright TM et al: Testicular and paratesticular tumors and tumor-like lesions in the first 2 decades. Semin Diagn Pathol. 31(5):323-81, 2014
3. Wei Y et al: Testicular yolk sac tumors in children: a review of 61 patients over 19 years. World J Surg Oncol. 12:400, 2014
4. Bujons A et al: Prepubertal testicular tumours and efficacy of testicular preserving surgery. BJU Int. 107(11):1812-6, 2011
5. Hisamatsu E et al: Prepubertal testicular tumors: a 20-year experience with 40 cases. Int J Urol. 17(11):956-9, 2010
6. Marulaiah M et al: Testicular and paratesticular pathology in children: a 12-year histopathological review. World J Surg. 34(5):969-74, 2010

Yolk Sac Tumor, Prepubertal Type

YST: Mixed Papillary and Solid Growth Patterns

YST: Papillary and Solid Growth Pattern

(Left) Low-power photomicrograph shows a YST with mixed papillary and solid growth patterns. In some areas, a central fibrovascular core is present. (Right) High-power image shows a YST with a papillary and solid growth pattern. The central fibrovascular core is lined by relatively uniform cuboidal to hobnail tumor cells. The cytologic atypia is not as prominent as that of embryonal carcinoma.

Yolk Sac Tumor: Macrocystic Pattern

Yolk Sac Tumor: Cells Unevenly Distributed

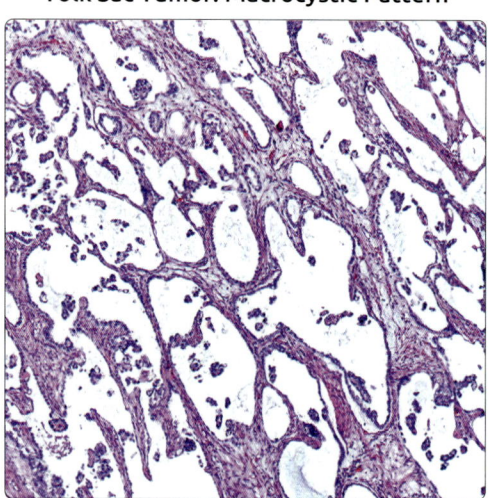

(Left) This photomicrograph shows a macrocystic pattern of a YST. It is composed of irregular cysts lined by a single layer of cuboidal to flattened tumor cells. (Right) This image shows a YST with microcystic, macrocystic, and reticulated patterns. The tumor cells are unevenly distributed and have abundant vacuolated and eosinophilic cytoplasm.

Yolk Sac Tumor: Sold Growth Pattern

Yolk Sac Tumor With Cytologic Atypia

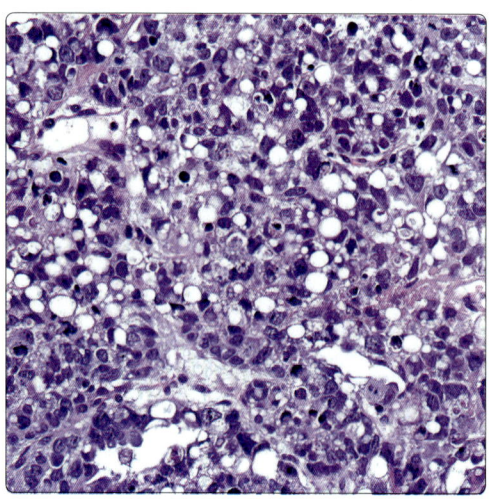
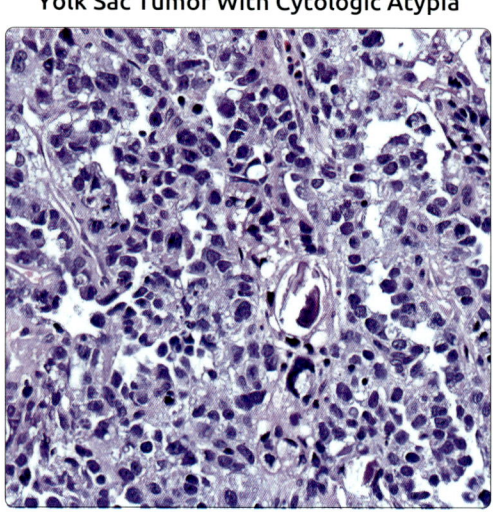

(Left) A solid growth patten of a YST is shown. The cells contain abundant clear and vacuolated cytoplasm, similar to that of seminoma. The tumor cells are moderately pleomorphic and have frequent mitotic figures. Unlike seminoma, there is no inflammatory infiltrate. (Right) A YST with a solid growth pattern is shown. There is cytologic atypia, but not to the degree of embryonal carcinoma. Focal psammoma body type calcification is present in the tumor.

Yolk Sac Tumor, Prepubertal Type

YST: Exuberant Papillary Growth Pattern

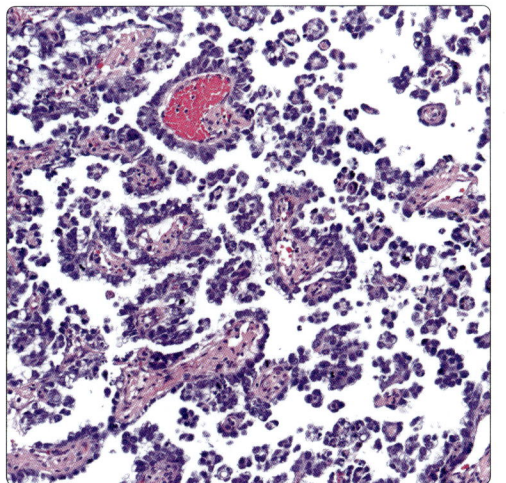

YST: Central Fibrovascular Cores

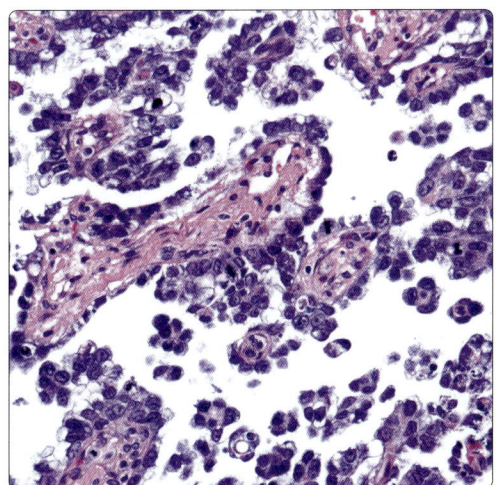

(Left) Low-power photomicrograph shows a YST with an exuberant papillary growth pattern and central fibrovascular cores. The appearance of tumor cells is relatively low grade. (Right) High-power photomicrograph shows a YST with exuberant papillary growth pattern and central fibrovascular cores. The appearance of tumor cells is relatively low grade. In the pediatric age group, this pattern is virtually diagnostic of the diagnosis.

Yolk Sac Tumor: Glandular Growth Pattern

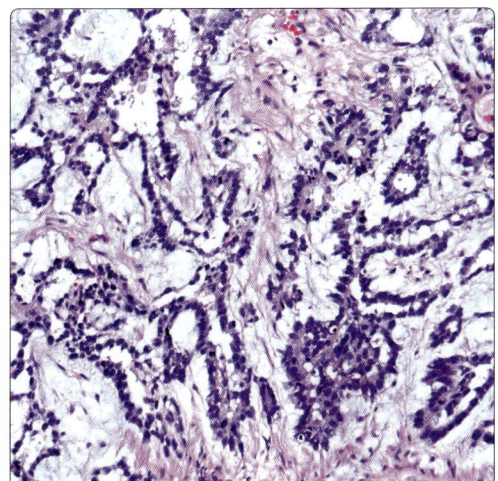

Yolk Sac Tumor: Glandular Growth Pattern

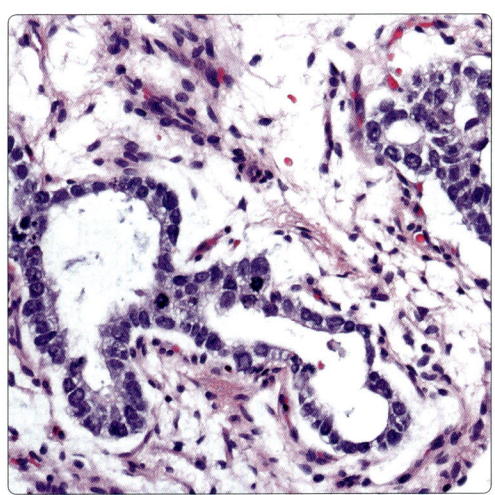

(Left) A glandular growth pattern of YST with myxoid stroma is shown. The tumor cells are relatively uniform, a feature that is different from the glandular pattern in embryonal carcinoma or metastatic carcinoma. (Right) A glandular growth pattern of a YST with myxoid stroma is shown at higher power. A Sertoli cell tumor is also in the differential diagnosis.

Yolk Sac Tumor: Parietal Pattern

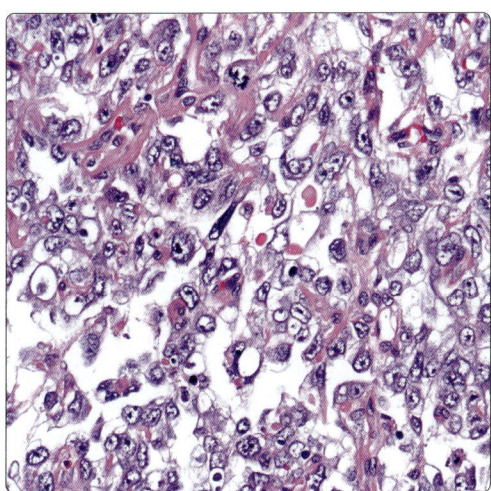

Yolk Sac Tumor: Parietal Pattern

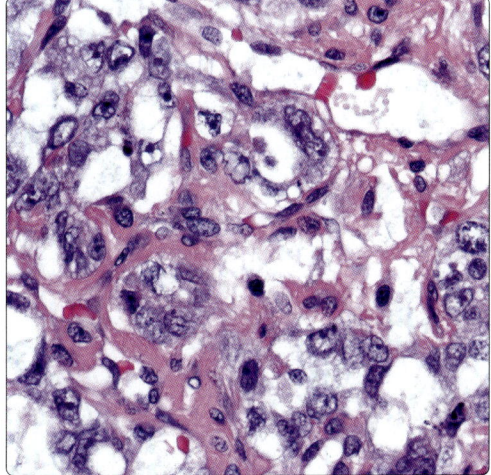

(Left) High-power view of a parietal pattern of a YST shows tumor cells surrounded by dense pink-staining basement membrane-like material, which represents recapitulation of the parietal layer of the embryonic yolk sac of the rodent; it is usually negative for AFP. (Right) A parietal pattern of a YST, rare in pediatric YSTs, shows tumor cells surrounded by dense pink-staining basement membrane-like material.

Carcinoid Tumor

KEY FACTS

TERMINOLOGY
- Well-differentiated tumor of testis with neuroendocrine differentiation

CLINICAL ISSUES
- Majority (> 70%) are pure carcinoid &/or associated with teratoma (20%)
- Testicular enlargement ± pain
- Prognosis is excellent for patients with localized testicular carcinoid

MACROSCOPIC
- Pure carcinoid tumors are usually solid, well-circumscribed masses with pale yellow to brown cut surface
- Cystic component usually indicates associated teratoma

MICROSCOPIC
- Growth patterns: Insular, solid nests, trabecular, or acinar
- Delicate fibrous to hyalinized stroma
- Tumor cells with round nuclei, coarse or salt and pepper chromatin
- Usually monotonous tumor cells with occasional large cells
- Abundant eosinophilic, granular cytoplasm
- Teratomatous component may be seen in some cases
- No associated germ cell neoplasia in situ in adjacent seminiferous tubules

ANCILLARY TESTS
- Positive for cytokeratin, synaptophysin, chromogranin, CD56, and hormones (serotonin, substance-P, gastrin, VIP)
- Negative for germ cell tumor markers and sex cord tumor markers

TOP DIFFERENTIAL DIAGNOSES
- Metastatic carcinoid
- Leydig or Sertoli cell tumor

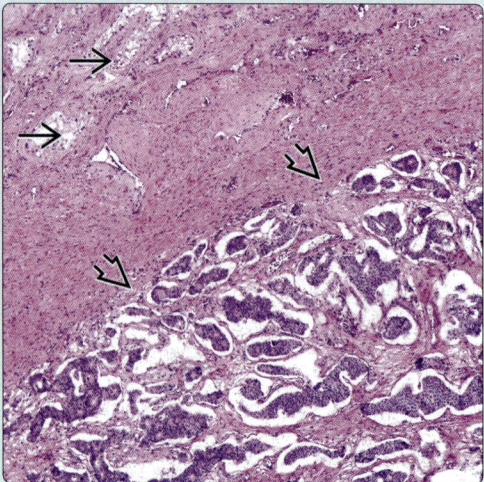

Carcinoid Tumor: Well Circumscribed

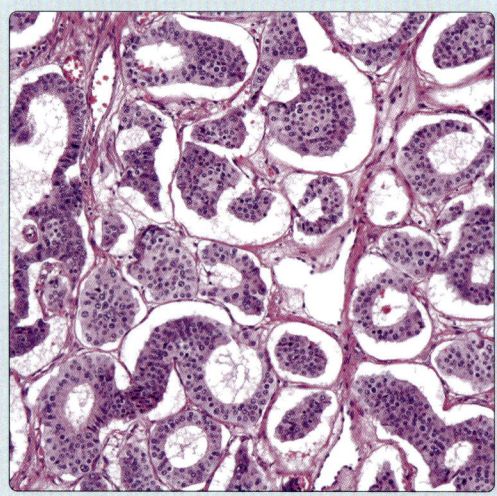

Carcinoid Tumor: Nested and Insular

(Left) Testicular carcinoid tumor ➔ shows a well-circumscribed nodule demarcated from the adjacent seminiferous tubules ➔. The tumor has nested, trabecular, and insular growth patterns with monotonous uniform cells. (Right) Testicular carcinoid tumor shows nested and insular growth patterns with delicate fibrovascular stroma. Artifactual retraction spaces are prominent in this carcinoid tumor.

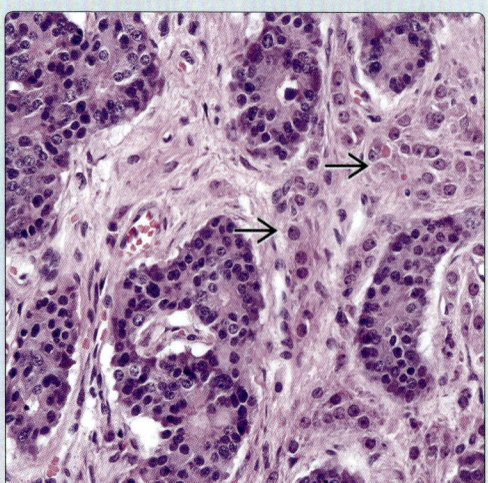

Carcinoid Tumor: Infiltrative

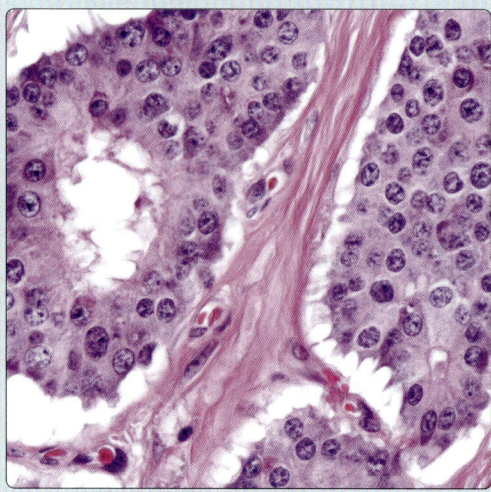

Carcinoid Tumor: Cytology

(Left) In the stroma of this carcinoid tumor, there are scattered Leydig cells ➔, indicating infiltrative growth of the tumor at the periphery. Notice the monotony of the tumor cells and peripheral nuclear palisading. (Right) High-power view shows a carcinoid tumor with relatively uniform cells, round to ovoid nuclei, salt and pepper chromatin, and abundant eosinophilic and granular cytoplasm.

Carcinoid Tumor

TERMINOLOGY

Synonyms
- Monodermal teratoma

Definitions
- Well-differentiated tumor with neuroendocrine differentiation, which may occur as pure tumor, as component associated with teratoma, or metastatic to testis

ETIOLOGY/PATHOGENESIS

Pathogenesis
- Considered to be monodermal form of teratoma

CLINICAL ISSUES

Epidemiology
- Incidence
  - Extremely rare (< 1% of all testicular tumors)
  - Majority (> 70%) are pure carcinoid &/or associated with teratoma (20%)
  - Rare cases of metastatic carcinoid (up to 10%) from lung or gastrointestinal tract have been reported
- Age
  - Range: 10-83 years (average: 46 years); primary carcinoid: 44 years; metastasis: 61 years; carcinoid within teratoma: 38 years
  - In general, occurs in older age group than most other types of germ cell tumor

Presentation
- Testicular enlargement ± pain
- May be associated with hydrocele (10%), carcinoid syndrome (12%)

Laboratory Tests
- 5-hydroxyindoleacetic acid or metabolite of serotonin may be elevated

Treatment
- Surgical approaches
  - Surgical excision is preferred, and other therapies (somatostatin analogues, interferon-α) may be used for symptom control

Prognosis
- Prognosis is excellent for patients with localized testicular carcinoid
- Neither tumor necrosis nor local tumor invasion (vascular invasion or tunica invasion, etc.) correlate with adverse prognosis

IMAGING

General Features
- Well-circumscribed hypervascular mass on ultrasonography

MACROSCOPIC

General Features
- Pure carcinoid tumor is usually solid, well-circumscribed mass with pale yellow to brown cut surface
- Cystic component usually indicates associated teratoma

Size
- 0.1-11.0 cm (mean: 3.5 cm) for pure carcinoid tumor
- Carcinoid tumor associated with teratoma is usually smaller than those occurring in pure form

MICROSCOPIC

Histologic Features
- Growth patterns: Insular, solid, nests, trabecular, or acinar
- Delicate fibrous to hyalinized stroma
- Predominantly monotonous tumor cells with occasional interspersed larger cells
- Abundant eosinophilic, granular cytoplasm
- Tumor cells with round nuclei, peripheral palisading, inconspicuous nucleoli, and coarse or salt and pepper chromatin
- Teratomatous component may be seen in some cases (20%)
- No associated germ cell neoplasia in situ in adjacent seminiferous tubules
- Other than tumor size (which has been correlated with malignant outcome), there are no other reliable histologic features predictive of malignancy

ANCILLARY TESTS

Immunohistochemistry
- Positive for cytokeratin, synaptophysin, chromogranin, CD56, and hormones (serotonin, substance-P, gastrin, VIP)
- Negative for germ cell tumor markers and sex cord tumor markers

DIFFERENTIAL DIAGNOSIS

Metastatic Carcinoid
- Clinical history and imaging studies for tumors occurring in locations where carcinoid tumor is known
- Presence of teratoma favors primary carcinoid
- Lymphovascular invasion, bilaterality, and multifocal involvement favor metastasis

Leydig or Sertoli Cell Tumor
- Less distinct insular or nested arrangement
- Lack of characteristic salt and pepper chromatin and presence of nucleoli
- Positive for inhibin, calretinin, and sometimes synaptophysin; negative for neuroendocrine markers

SELECTED REFERENCES

1. Wang WP et al: Primary carcinoid tumors of the testis: a clinicopathologic study of 29 cases. Am J Surg Pathol. 34(4):519-24, 2010
2. Abbosh PH et al: Germ cell origin of testicular carcinoid tumors. Clin Cancer Res. 14(5):1393-6, 2008
3. Stroosma OB et al: Carcinoid tumours of the testis. BJU Int. 101(9):1101-5, 2008
4. Fujita K et al: Primary carcinoid tumor of the testis with teratoma metastatic to the para-aortic lymph node. Int J Urol. 12(3):328-31, 2005
5. Merino J et al: Pure testicular carcinoid associated with intratubular germ cell neoplasia. J Clin Pathol. 58(12):1331-3, 2005
6. Ulbright TM et al: Carcinoid tumor of the testis. Am J Clin Pathol. 121(2):297; author reply 298, 2004

Carcinoid Tumor

(Left) Testicular carcinoid tumor is well demarcated from the uninvolved testicular parenchyma by thin fibrous tissue ⇒. The tumor shows neuroendocrine features with uniform cells forming nests. **(Right)** Another example shows testicular carcinoid with ill-defined border between tumor ⇒ and uninvolved testicular parenchyma.

Carcinoid Tumor: Well Circumscribed
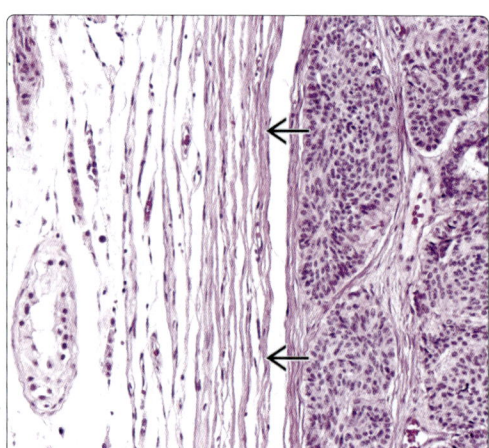

Carcinoid Tumor: Ill-Defined Border
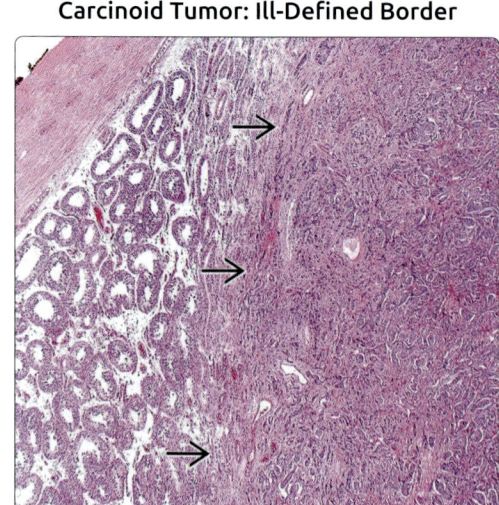

(Left) Solid nests of tumor cells are surrounded by prominent hyalinized fibrous stroma. Peritumoral artifactual spaces ⇒, as seen in this case, are among the helpful features to make the diagnosis of carcinoid. **(Right)** High-power photomicrograph shows classic cytology of carcinoid tumor with relatively uniform nuclei, salt and pepper chromatin, and abundant eosinophilic and granular cytoplasm. No mitosis or necrosis is seen.

Carcinoid Tumor: Hyalinized Stroma
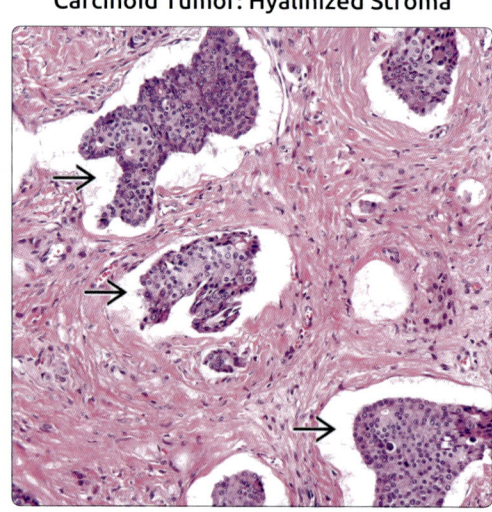

Carcinoid Tumor: Cytology
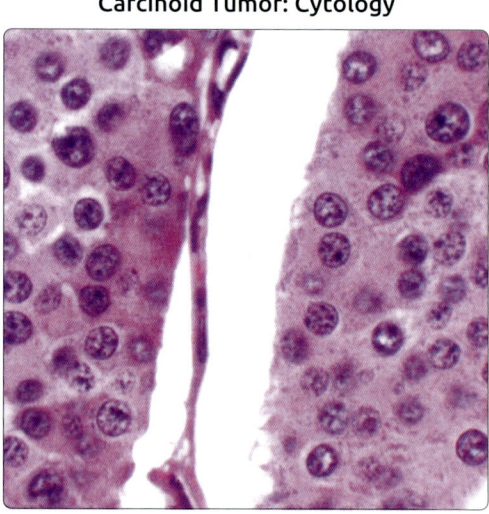

(Left) This carcinoid tumor shows cords of tumor cells with dense hyalinized stroma. The differential diagnoses include Sertoli cell or Leydig cell tumor, metastatic carcinoma, or cellular adenomatoid tumor. Neuroendocrine markers are required to make a definitive diagnosis. **(Right)** This image shows strong and diffuse immunoreactivity with CK-PAN(AE1/AE3) within a carcinoid tumor. Although sex cord-stromal tumor may be positive for cytokeratin, the positivity is usually less intense and diffuse.

Carcinoid Tumor: Hyalinized Stroma
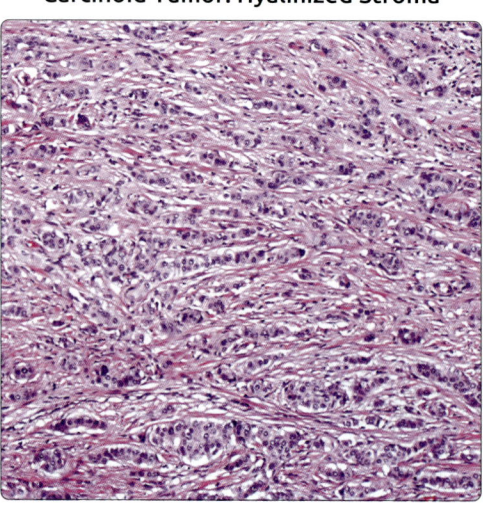

Carcinoid Tumor: CK-PAN
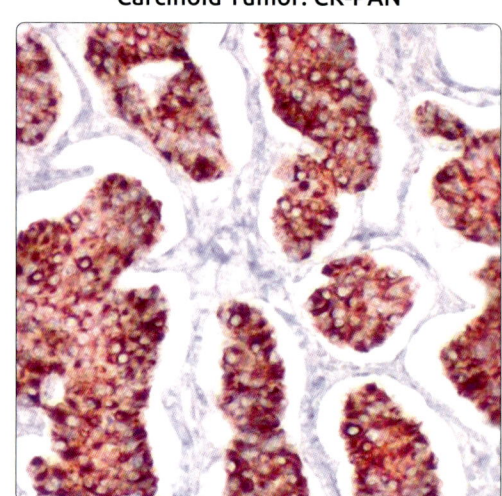

Carcinoid Tumor

Carcinoid Tumor: Synaptophysin

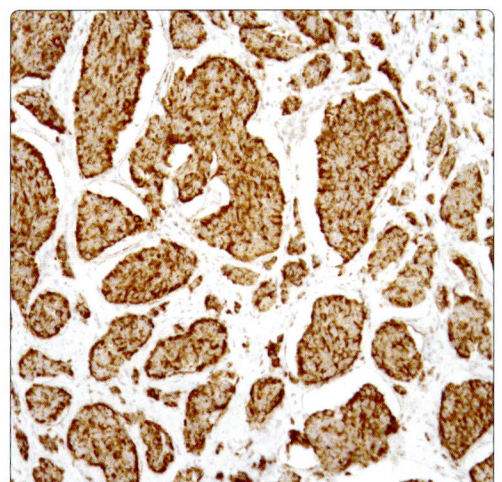

Carcinoid Tumor: Chromogranin

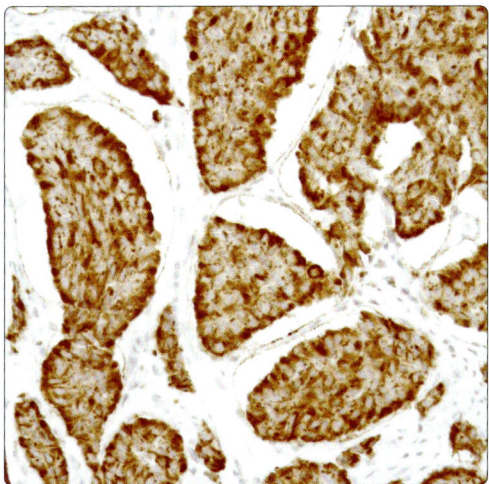

(Left) Synaptophysin shows carcinoid tumor with diffuse and strong cytoplasmic immunostaining, supporting the diagnosis of carcinoid tumor. **(Right)** Chromogranin stain shows diffuse cytoplasmic positivity within the tumor cells, further supporting the diagnosis of carcinoid tumor. Distinct from sex cord-stromal tumors, carcinoid tumors are negative for inhibin and calretinin. Sex cord tumors may occasionally be positive for synaptophysin.

Leydig Cell Tumor: Differential

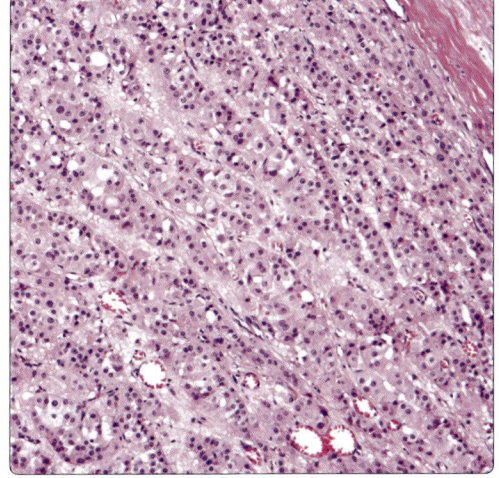

Leydig Cell Tumor: Differential

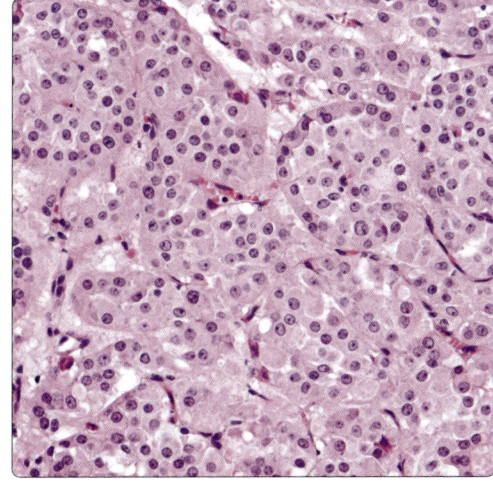

(Left) The nested and trabecular growth patterns of this Leydig cell tumor are similar to that of a carcinoid tumor. Immunohistochemical stains with inhibin and neuroendocrine markers are helpful in making a definitive diagnosis. **(Right)** Although the cytoplasmic features of this Leydig cell tumor are superficially similar to those of a carcinoid tumor, the prominent nucleoli and absence of salt and pepper chromatin favor the diagnosis of Leydig cell tumor.

Sertoli Cell Tumor: Differential

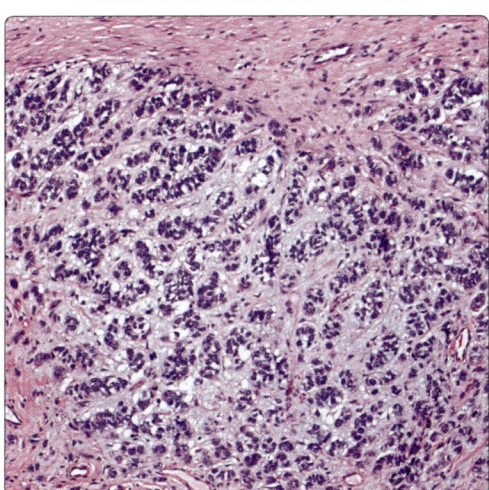

Sertoli Cell Tumor: Differential

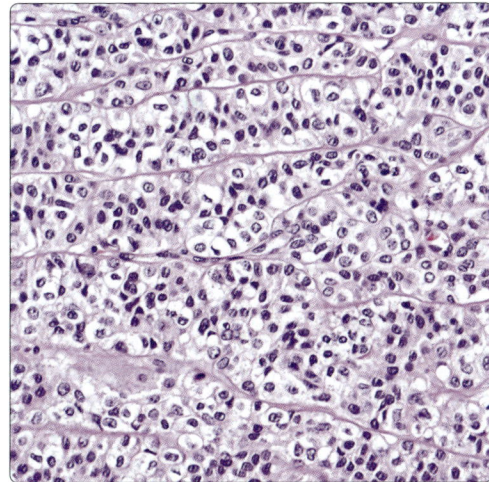

(Left) This Sertoli cell tumor shows nested growth and dense stroma, similar to that of a carcinoid tumor. Unlike carcinoid tumor, the tumor cells are positive for inhibin and negative for neuroendocrine markers. **(Right)** This image shows diffuse and trabecular growth of Sertoli cell tumor. In contrast to carcinoid tumor, the nucleoli are prominent and nuclei lack a salt and pepper appearance. Prominent clear cytoplasm also favors Sertoli cell tumor.

General Concepts, Sex Cord-/Gonadal Stromal Tumors

TERMINOLOGY

Definitions

- Neoplasms that have features of Leydig (interstitial) cells, Sertoli cells, granulosa cells, or rarely, theca cells
- Sex cord-stromal tumor (SCST) may be of mixed classifiable SCST or unclassifiable SCST
- Mixed germ cell and SCST (gonadoblastoma and unclassified type) have been reported

EPIDEMIOLOGY

Incidence

- 2-5% of adult testicular neoplasms
- 20-30% of testicular tumors in infants and children
- Unlike germ cell tumors, there is no racial difference in frequency

ETIOLOGY/PATHOGENESIS

Histogenesis

- Poorly understood in general
- May relate to disruption of hypothalamic-pituitary-testicular axis and hormonal disturbance
- No definitive association with cryptorchidism
- Specific types of sex cord-stromal tumor may be associated with genetic syndromes; e.g., large cell calcifying Sertoli cell tumor in Peutz-Jeghers syndrome and Sertoli cell tumors in testicular feminization syndrome
- Although testicular granulosa cell or theca cell tumors have been reported, no granulosa or theca cells are normally present in testis

CLINICAL IMPLICATIONS

Presentation

- Painless mass (rarely painful)
- Asymptomatic or rarely hormone-related symptoms
- Infants with Leydig cell tumor usually present with isosexual pseudoprecocity
- Some types may cause gynecomastia or impotence

Treatment

- Surgical approaches
  - Orchiectomy is curative; staging work-up required
  - Testis sparing resection possible

Prognosis

- 5%-10% of adult-type SCSTs are malignant and may metastasize
- Metastasis is only reliable criterion for malignancy; histologic factors alone may not predict malignancy
- Features that may be associated with disease progression include
  - Nuclear pleomorphism, frequent and abnormal mitoses (> 4/10 high-power fields), necrosis
  - Infiltrative growth, large size (> 5 cm), extension to paratesticular tissue, and vascular invasion
- Tumors occurring in infants and children are almost always benign with rare exception

Clinical Presentation

- Painless testicular swelling or mass
- Symptomatology of hormonal disturbance or genetic syndrome

MACROSCOPIC

General Features

- Size
  - Range from microscopic to several cm (malignant forms usually larger, > 5 cm)

Specimen Handling

- Total Resection
  - Procure cord margin before cutting into testis
  - Small tumors may be entirely embedded
  - Submit at least 1 section/cm tumor
    - Sections to include: Tumor with adjacent parenchyma
    - Sections to include: Rete testis, epididymis, and spermatic cord
    - At least 2 sections of grossly normal parenchyma
- Subtotal Resection

Leydig Cell Tumor

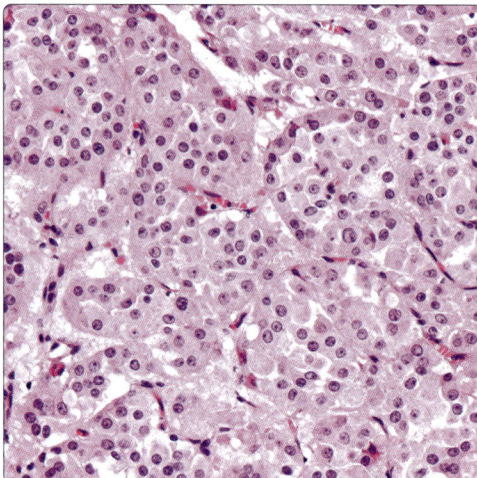

Sertoli Cell Tumor

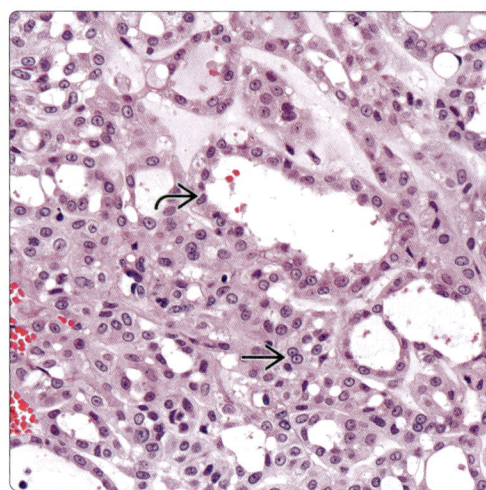

(Left) Leydig cell tumor (LCT) with solid and nested growth patterns is shown. The tumor cells are uniform, round, and have prominent nucleoli and abundant eosinophilic/granular cytoplasm. **(Right)** Sertoli cell tumor (SCT) with tubular ⊅ pattern is shown. The tumor cells have ovoid-to-round nuclei with occasional prominent nucleoli ⊅, pale eosinophilic and vacuolated cytoplasm.

General Concepts, Sex Cord-/Gonadal Stromal Tumors

- o Ink resection margin 1st
- o Take perpendicular sections of tumor with margin
- o Submit entire tumor, if appropriate
- o Sections to include: Normal parenchyma

MICROSCOPIC

Normal Histology

- Interstitial (Leydig) cells
  - o Present in interstitium as single cells or in clusters
  - o They may be also present in tunica albuginea, rete testis, epididymis, and spermatic cord (ectopic Leydig cells)
  - o Leydig cells have uniform, round nuclei, prominent nucleoli, and abundant eosinophilic cytoplasm
  - o Intracytoplasmic lipofuscin pigment may be seen, particularly in older men
  - o Reinke crystalloids (better demonstrated with trichrome stain)
  - o Immunoreactive with vimentin, inhibin, and calretinin, but not cytokeratin (may be focally and weakly positive)
- Sertoli cells
  - o Sertoli cells are located within seminiferous tubules and comprise ~ 10-15% of cells within tubules (germ cell:Sertoli cell is ~ 13:1)
  - o Located 1 or 2 cells away from basement membrane of tubules
  - o Pyramidal shaped-cells with round-to-ovoid nuclei, finely granular chromatin, often prominent nucleoli
  - o Cytoplasm is eosinophilic and granular with fine vacuoles
  - o Immunoreactive with vimentin, CAM5.2, CK19, inhibin, and calretinin
- Granulosa cells
  - o Probably represent precursor Sertoli cells in fetal seminiferous tubules
  - o These cells are cuboidal or columnar in shape and rest on tubular basement membrane
  - o Not found in normal adult testis
- Undifferentiated sex cord-stromal cells
  - o Present early in fetal gonadal development
  - o Primitive cells with potential for elaboration of steroid hormones
  - o Not found in normal adult testis

General Features

- WHO histologic classification of sex cord-stromal tumors of testis
  - o Leydig cell tumor (LCT)
    - Malignant LCT
  - o Sertoli cell tumor (SCT)
    - Sertoli cell carcinoma
    - Large cell calcifying SCT
    - Intratubular large cell hyalinizing SCT
    - Sclerosing SCT
  - o Granulosa cell tumor (GCT)
    - Adult type GCT
    - Juvenile GCT
  - o Tumor of thecoma/fibroma group
    - Thecoma
    - Fibroma
  - o Mixed and unclassified sex cord-/gonadal stromal tumor
    - Mixed SCST
    - Unclassified SCST
    - Myoid gonadal stromal tumor
  - o Tumors containing both germ cell and sex cord-/gonadal stromal elements
    - Gonadoblastoma

Cytologic Features

- Depends on tumor types

Predominant Pattern

- Solid or nested pattern
  - o Usually seen in LCTs, GCTs, unclassified SCST, fibroma-thecoma
- Pseudoglandular, trabecular, or tubular
  - o Usually seen in SCTs, may be seen in LCTs, GCTs
- Mixed growth patterns
  - o Often seen in unclassified or mixed SCSTs, or less commonly in LCTs or SCTs

Predominant Cell Type

- LCT
  - o Round-to-polygonal cells with abundant eosinophilic cytoplasm, lipofuscin pigment, and often prominent nucleoli
- SCT
  - o Uniform cuboidal or columnar cells with moderately pale-to-light eosinophilic cytoplasm and cytoplasmic vacuoles
- GCT
  - o Uniform round, ovoid, or carrot-shaped cells with scant, lightly staining cytoplasm and characteristic nuclear grooves
- Fibroma-thecoma
  - o Uniform spindle cells with scant cytoplasm
- Undifferentiated SCSTs
  - o Mixture of epithelioid cells with vesicular nuclei, prominent nucleoli, and nondescript undifferentiated spindle cells

IMMUNOHISTOCHEMISTRY

Inhibin

- 32 kD dimeric glycoprotein composed of α and β subunit
- Produced by ovarian granulosa cells and testicular Sertoli and Leydig cells
- Immunoreactive with LCT, SCT, large cell calcifying SCT, and GCT

Calretinin

- 29 kD intracellular calcium-binding protein expressed in variety of tumors, including mesothelioma
- Immunoreactive with LCT, SCT, and SCST, NOS

CK-PAN (AE1/AE3)

- SCT usually positive, GCT and mixed unclassified SCST often positive, LCT usually negative or focally positive

Vimentin

- Most SCSTs positive for vimentin

S100

- SCT usually positive, LCT may be positive (more nuclear positivity and weak cytoplasmic)
- Large cell calcifying Sertoli cell tumor is frequently positive

General Concepts, Sex Cord-/Gonadal Stromal Tumors

Immunohistochemistry of Sex Cord-Stromal Tumor

	Inhibin	Calretinin	Keratin	Vimentin	S100	Actin-sm	Melan-A	FOXL2	SF1
Leydig cell tumor	(+)	(+)	(-/+)	(+)	(-/+)	(-)	(+)	(+)	(+)
Sertoli cell tumor, NOS	(+/-)	(+/-)	(+)	(+)	(+/-)	(-/+)	(-)	(+/-)	(+/-)
Granulosa cell tumor	(+)	(+)	(-/+)	(+)	(+/-)	(-/+)	(-)	(+)	(+)
Sex cord-stromal tumor, NOS	(+/-)	(+/-)	(-/+)	(+)	(+)	(+)	(+/-)	(+/-)	(+/-)

Actin-sm
- Positive in unclassified SCST (shows myofibroblastic differentiation)

Melan-A (MART-1)
- All sex cord-stromal tumors may be positive for melan-A (MART-1); most frequently expressed in Leydig cell tumors

WT1
- Present in normal granulosa cells, expressed by majority of sex cord-stromal tumors

CD99
- Present in normal granulosa cells, expressed by majority of sex cord-stromal tumors, including adult and juvenile GCTs and Sertoli-Leydig cell tumors (focal)

SF1 (Steroidogenic Factor 1)
- Transcription factor regulating steroidogenesis and sexual differentiation
- Positive in most SCSTs

FOXL2
- Transcription factor involving granulosa cell function and ovarian follicle development
- Positive in most SCSTs

DIFFERENTIAL DIAGNOSIS

Germ Cell Tumors
- Usually more heterogeneous with different growth pattern; tumor cells more pleomorphic with increased mitoses
- Frequent hemorrhage and necrosis
- Negative for inhibin and calretinin; positive for germ cell markers (OCT3/OCT4, SALL4)

Metastatic Carcinoma or Melanoma
- Older age and clinical history
- Tumor cells have greater pleomorphism and more frequent mitoses
- Interstitial growth pattern and frequent vascular-lymphatic invasion and bilateral involvement
- Negative for inhibin and calretinin; positive for tissue-specific markers

Lymphoma/Leukemia
- Diffuse and interstitial infiltration of tumor cells
- Positive for LCA or B-cell and T-cell markers; negative for inhibin and calretinin

Adenomatoid Tumor (Cellular)
- Rarely intratesticular
- More prominent stroma and cytoplasmic vacuoles
- Depending on cytology and architecture, may mimic Leydig cell tumor or Sertoli cell tumor
- Negative for inhibin; positive for Podoplanin (D2-40), CK5/CK6, calretinin, WT1 (calretinin and WT1 staining overlap with sex cord-stromal tumor)

SELECTED REFERENCES

1. Kao CS et al: Sclerosing Sertoli cell tumor of the testis: a clinicopathologic study of 20 cases. Am J Surg Pathol. 38(4):510-7, 2014
2. Kao CS et al: Myoid gonadal stromal tumor: a clinicopathologic study of three cases of a distinctive testicular tumor. Am J Clin Pathol. 142(5):675-82, 2014
3. Ulbright TM et al: Best practices recommendations in the application of immunohistochemistry in testicular tumors: report from the International Society of Urological Pathology consensus conference. Am J Surg Pathol. 38(8):e50-9, 2014
4. Al-Agha OM et al: FOXL2 is a sensitive and specific marker for sex cord-stromal tumors of the ovary. Am J Surg Pathol. 35(4):484-94, 2011
5. Acar C et al: Current treatment of testicular sex cord-stromal tumors: critical review. Urology. 73(6):1165-71, 2009
6. Zhao C et al: SF-1 is a diagnostically useful immunohistochemical marker and comparable to other sex cord-stromal tumor markers for the differential diagnosis of ovarian sertoli cell tumor. Int J Gynecol Pathol. 27(4):507-14, 2008
7. Al-Agha OM et al: An in-depth look at Leydig cell tumor of the testis. Arch Pathol Lab Med. 131(2):311-7, 2007
8. Michal M et al: Mixed germ cell sex cord-stromal tumours of the testis. Virchows Arch. 451(6):1095-6, 2007
9. Ulbright TM et al: Intratubular large cell hyalinizing sertoli cell neoplasia of the testis: a report of 8 cases of a distinctive lesion of the Peutz-Jeghers syndrome. Am J Surg Pathol. 31(6):827-35, 2007
10. Michal M et al: Mixed germ cell sex cord-stromal tumors of the testis and ovary. Morphological, immunohistochemical, and molecular genetic study of seven cases. Virchows Arch. 448(5):612-22, 2006
11. Young RH: Sex cord-stromal tumors of the ovary and testis: their similarities and differences with consideration of selected problems. Mod Pathol. 18 Suppl 2:S81-98, 2005
12. Henley JD et al: Malignant Sertoli cell tumors of the testis: a study of 13 examples of a neoplasm frequently misinterpreted as seminoma. Am J Surg Pathol. 26(5):541-50, 2002
13. Ulbright TM et al: Leydig cell tumors of the testis with unusual features: adipose differentiation, calcification with ossification, and spindle-shaped tumor cells. Am J Surg Pathol. 26(11):1424-33, 2002
14. McCluggage WG et al: Immunohistochemical study of testicular sex cord-stromal tumors, including staining with anti-inhibin antibody. Am J Surg Pathol. 22(5):615-9, 1998
15. Young RH et al: Sertoli cell tumors of the testis, not otherwise specified: a clinicopathologic analysis of 60 cases. Am J Surg Pathol. 22(6):709-21, 1998

General Concepts, Sex Cord-/Gonadal Stromal Tumors

Seminiferous Tubule With Sertoli Cells

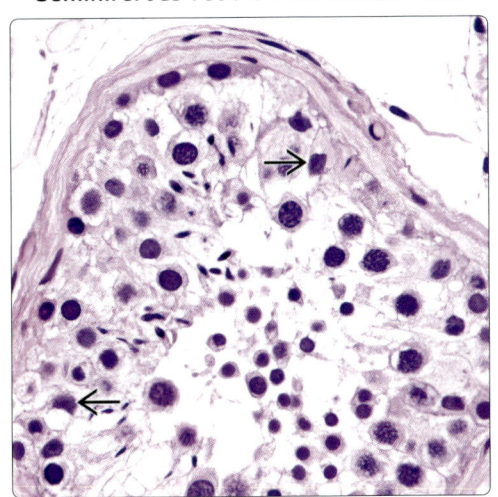

Interstitium With Leydig Cells

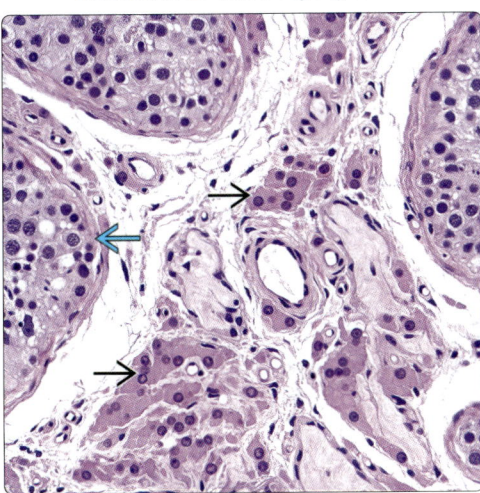

(Left) *This image shows a seminiferous tubule with germ cells in different stages of spermatogenesis. The Sertoli cells ➡ have a pyramidal shape and abundant, pale eosinophilic cytoplasm with prominent nucleoli.* **(Right)** *This image shows seminiferous tubules with spermatogenesis ➡. The interstitium contains several clusters of Leydig cells ➡ with abundant eosinophilic cytoplasm and round, central nuclei with occasional prominent nucleoli.*

Leydig Cell Tumor

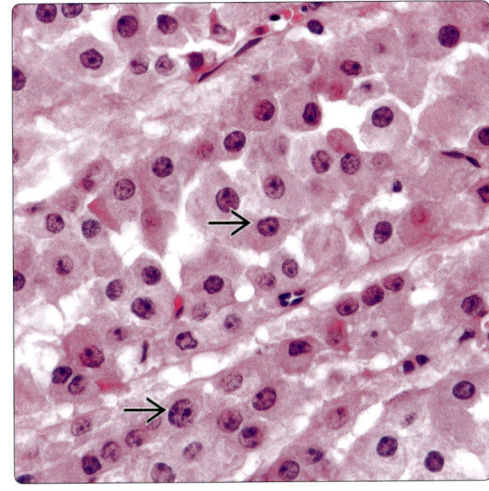

Sertoli Cell Tumor

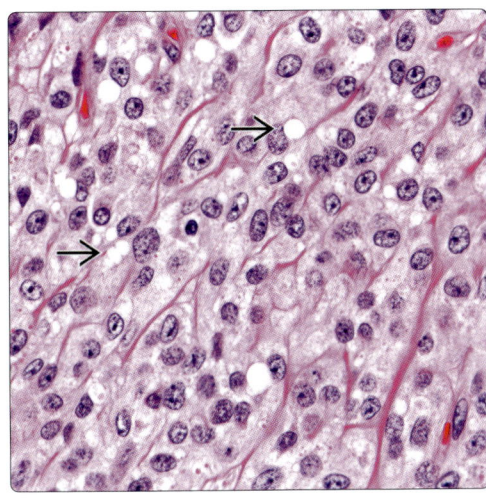

(Left) *A typical LCT shows solid sheets and trabeculae of tumor cells with voluminous eosinophilic cytoplasm, round nuclei, and prominent nucleoli ➡.* **(Right)** *The solid pattern of SCT may resemble LCT, but the nuclei are slightly irregular and have coarsely granular chromatin, pale eosinophilic cytoplasm with vacuoles ➡. SCT is usually positive for cytokeratin, whereas LCT is often negative or weakly positive.*

Sex Cord-Stromal Tumor, Unclassified

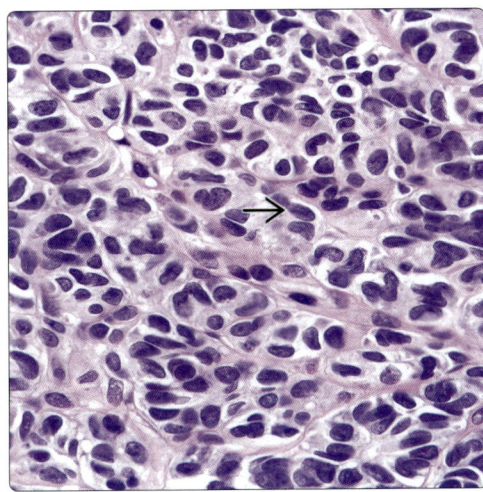

Fibroma-Thecoma

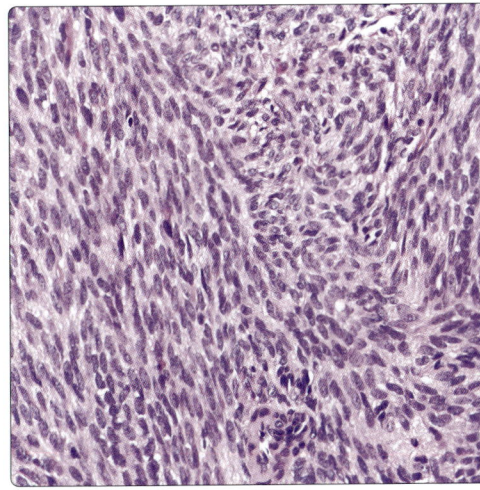

(Left) *This unclassified sex cord-stromal tumor is composed of short, oval-to-spindled tumor cells with nuclear grooves ➡ and moderate cytoplasm. The morphology may suggest granulosa cell differentiation, and the vaguely nested pattern may resemble SCT.* **(Right)** *Fibroma-thecoma shows fascicles of spindle cells with scant cytoplasm. Although rare, these may occur in the testis or paratestis. The tumor may be diagnosed as unclassified sex cord-stromal tumor by some.*

General Concepts, Sex Cord-/Gonadal Stromal Tumors

Leydig Cell Tumor: Adverse Histology
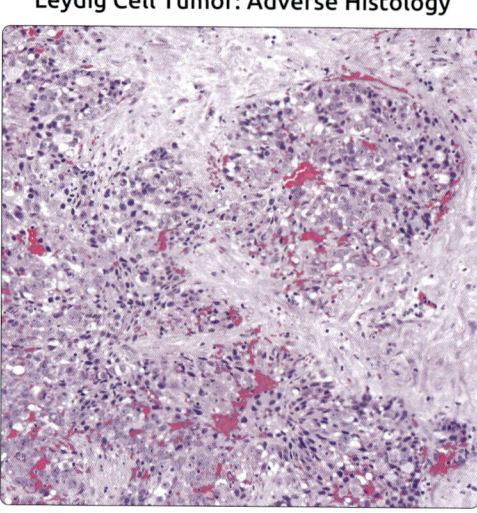

Leydig Cell Tumor: Adverse Histology
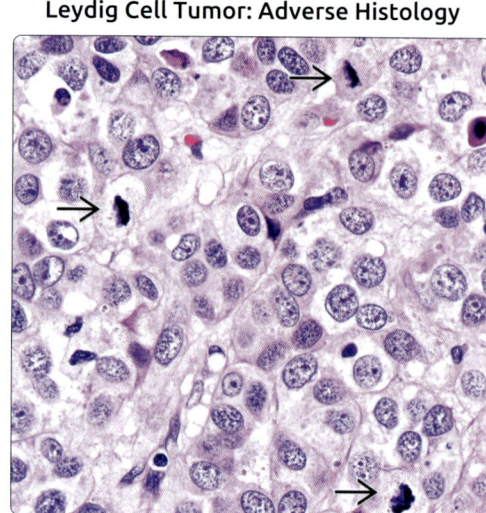

(Left) LCT with adverse histologic features is shown. The tumor has solid growth and invades through the tunica. Although there are no reliable histologic criteria to predict malignant behavior, invasive growth and high cellularity, as seen here, may often result in clinical metastasis. (Right) This LCT shows significant cytologic atypia and frequent mitoses ⇒. A combination of adverse features is predictive of malignancy.

Sertoli Cell Tumor: Adverse Histology
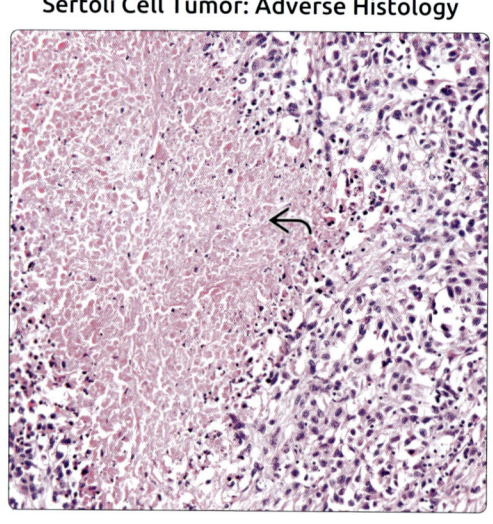

Sertoli Cell Tumor: Adverse Histology
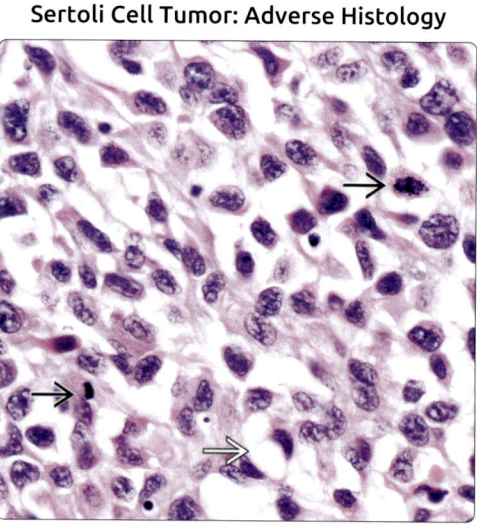

(Left) SCT with adverse histologic features is shown. There are large geographical areas of necrosis ⇒. Features that are associated with malignancy include invasive growth, vascular invasion, nuclear pleomorphism, increased mitoses (> 4/10 HPFs), and necrosis. (Right) In this SCT, there is marked nuclear pleomorphism and frequent mitoses ⇒. The cells contain clear cytoplasm and cytoplasmic vacuoles ⇒, features that are suggestive of SCT.

Leydig Cell Tumor: Inhibin
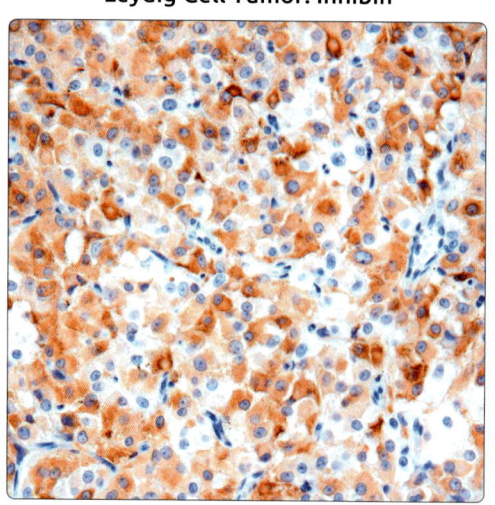

Granulosa Cell Tumor: Inhibin
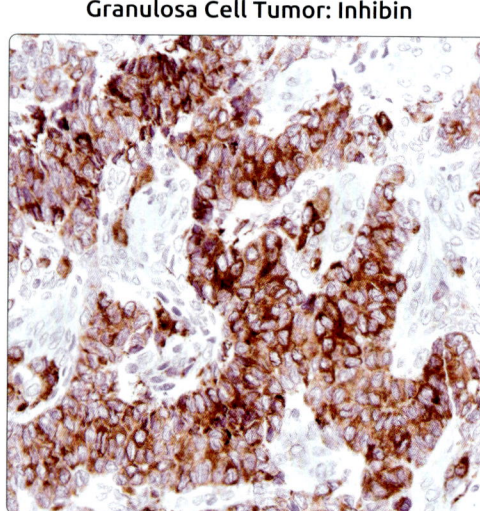

(Left) LCT shows strong positivity for inhibin. Inhibin is 1 of the most reliable markers for the diagnosis of sex cord-stromal tumor of testis. Other markers include Melan-A (MART-1), SF1, WT1, calretinin, and CD99. (Right) Inhibin immunostaining in a granulosa cell tumor (GCT) is shown. Among sex cord-stromal tumors, cytokeratin positivity is most typical in SCT; it is often negative to weak in LCT and variable in GCT.

General Concepts, Sex Cord-/Gonadal Stromal Tumors

Leydig Cell Tumor

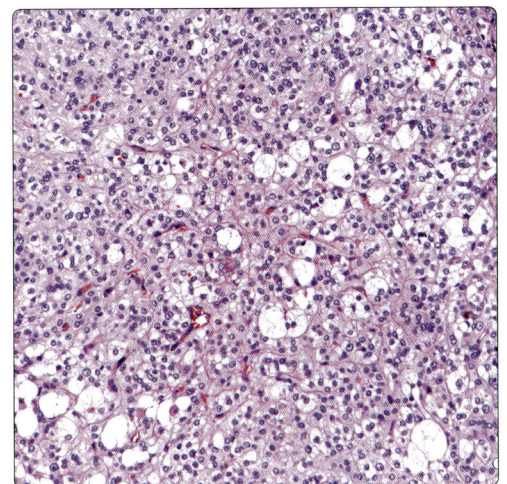

Yolk Sac Tumor

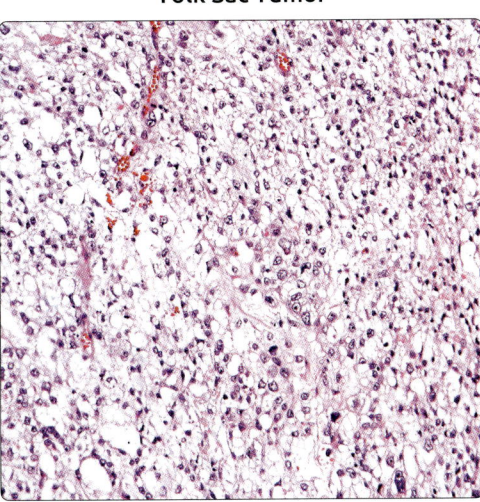

(Left) This LCT shows prominent cytoplasmic vacuoles and microcystic appearance, which resembles a yolk sac tumor. Multiple patterns, hyaline globules, basement membrane deposition, or Schiller-Duval bodies, as seen in yolk sac tumor, are not present. *(Right)* Yolk sac tumor with microcystic and solid growth patterns may mimic an LCT or SCT. α-fetoprotein, glypican-3, and SALL4 are positive, and inhibin and calretinin are negative in yolk sac tumor.

Sertoli Cell Tumor

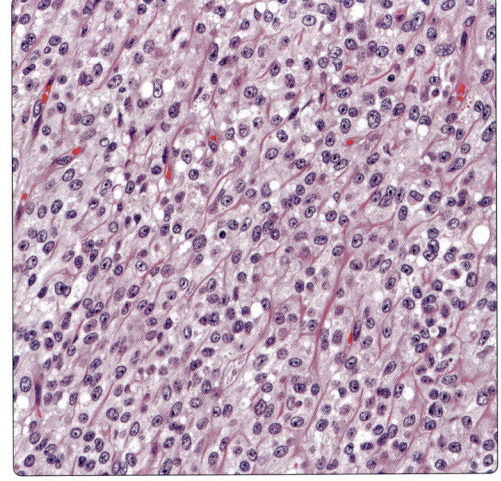

Seminoma

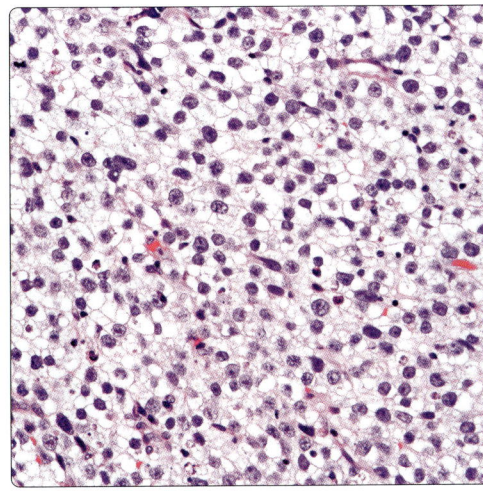

(Left) This image shows a solid SCT with delicate fibrous septa. The tumor cells are relatively uniform, with prominent nucleoli and pale eosinophilic cytoplasm with cytoplasmic vacuoles, superficially resembling a seminoma. *(Right)* This classic seminoma shows tumor cells with clear and pale eosinophilic cytoplasm. When there is a paucity of lymphocytes and fibrous septa, seminoma may resemble a solid pattern that is seen in SCT or LCT.

Plasmacytoma

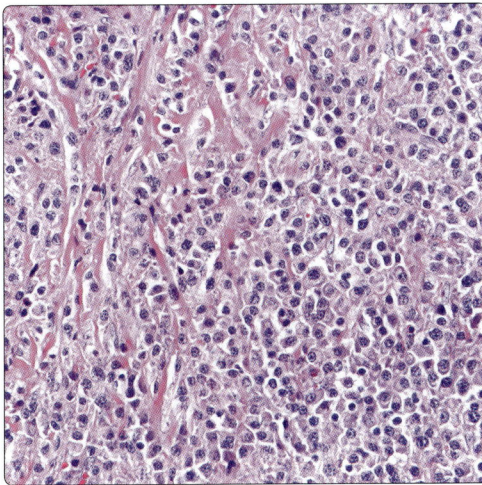

Adenomatoid Tumor

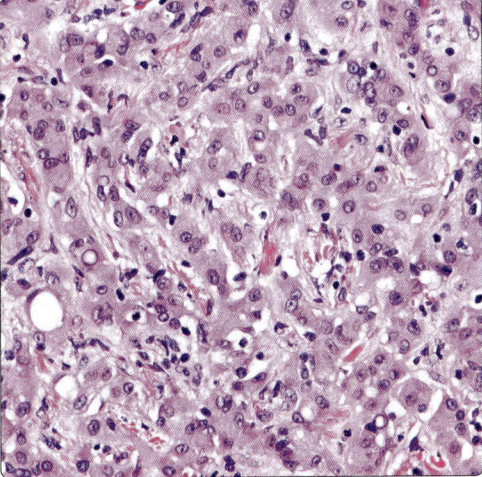

(Left) This plasmacytoma has a vaguely nested appearance, which may resemble an LCT. Closer examination shows that the tumor cells have plasmacytoid nuclear features and perinuclear halos. Inhibin and calretinin are negative. *(Right)* Cellular adenomatoid tumor may mimic an LCT. The tumor cells contain abundant eosinophilic cytoplasm and prominent nucleoli. Cytokeratin and podoplanin are strongly positive, and inhibin is negative in this paratesticular tumor.

Leydig Cell Tumors

KEY FACTS

TERMINOLOGY
- Pure testicular stromal tumor composed of cells that recapitulate normal interstitial (Leydig) cells

CLINICAL ISSUES
- Most common type of sex cord-stromal tumor (1-3% of testicular neoplasms)
- Majority have benign behavior; 5-10% malignant

MACROSCOPIC
- Well-circumscribed, intraparenchymal nodule with golden-brown to yellow, or gray-white homogeneous cut surface

MICROSCOPIC
- Growth patterns: Diffuse (most common), lobular, insular, tubular, ribbon-like, and pseudofollicular
- Large, round or polygonal cells with well-defined cell borders, eosinophilic or vacuolated cytoplasm
- Relatively uniform round or ovoid nuclei, prominent nucleoli; focal nuclear pleomorphism, binucleated or multinucleated cells may be seen
- Cytoplasmic vacuoles or foamy cytoplasm (lipid content), lipofuscin (15%), and Reinke crystals (30-40%) may be seen
- Other uncommon features: Fatty metaplasia; spindle, clear cell, or microcystic changes; myxoid degeneration; calcification or ossification; and rhabdoid features
- Metastasis is only criterion for malignancy

ANCILLARY TESTS
- Positive for inhibin-α, calretinin, Melan-A (MART-1), WT1, androgenic hormones (P450scc, 3β-HSD, etc.), CD99, steroidogenic factor (SF-1), and vimentin (strong and diffuse)
- Negative for cytokeratin, chromogranin, and synaptophysin (rarely focally positive for these 3 markers), S100 and PLAP (rarely positive for these 2 markers), nuclear beta-catenin, germ cell tumor markers

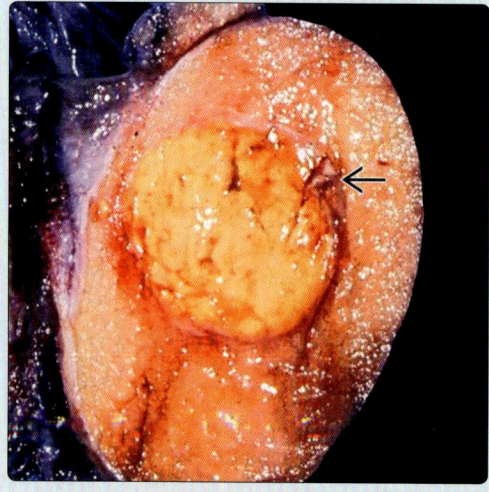

Leydig Cell Tumor: Gross

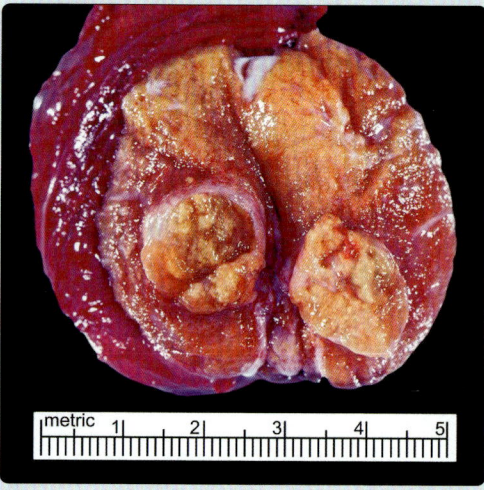

Leydig Cell Tumor: Gross

(Left) Leydig cell tumor is usually a well-circumscribed mass with a homogeneous, yellow-tan cut surface. Focal cystic change ➡ is present. Hemorrhage or necrosis is lacking. (Right) A well-circumscribed Leydig cell tumor is shown with solid, homogeneous, yellow-tan cut surface. There is minimal hemorrhage and no necrosis. The tumor is confined within the testis without extratesticular extension.

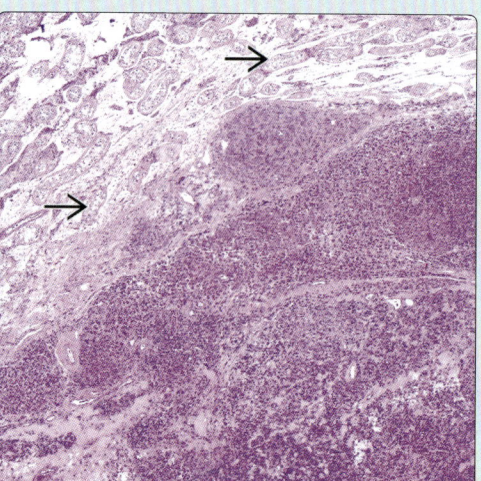

Leydig Cell Tumor: Low Power

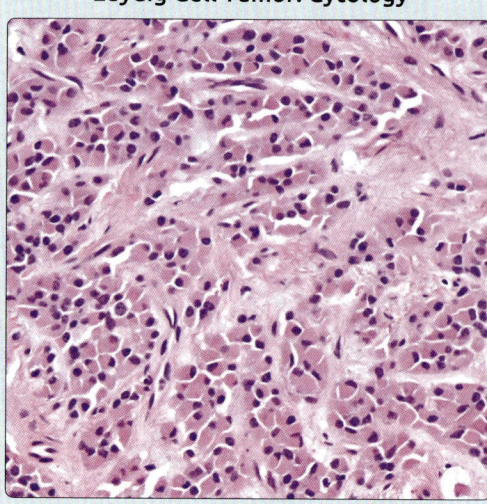

Leydig Cell Tumor: Cytology

(Left) Low-power image of Leydig cell tumor shows a nodular pattern of tumor cells with fibrous septa. Even at this low power, the eosinophilic cytoplasm of the tumor is appreciated. The tumor is demarcated from the seminiferous tubules ➡, which lack GCNIS. (Right) Leydig cell tumor is composed of broad cords of tumor cells separated by paucicellular and edematous fibrous stroma. The tumor cells have uniform, round to ovoid nuclei and abundant eosinophilic cytoplasm.

Leydig Cell Tumors

TERMINOLOGY

Abbreviations
- Leydig cell tumor (LCT)

Definitions
- Pure testicular stromal tumor composed of cells that recapitulate normal interstitial (Leydig) cells

CLINICAL ISSUES

Epidemiology
- Incidence
  - Most common type of sex cord-stromal tumor (1-3% of testicular tumors)
  - Rarely associated with Klinefelter syndrome
  - Rare association with the hereditary leiomyomatosis renal cell carcinoma (HLRCC) syndrome caused by germline mutations of fumarate hydratase (*FH*) gene
- Age
  - Any age with 2 peaks: 5-10 & 30-35 years

Presentation
- Testicular enlargement, usually painless, decreased libido (20%), gynecomastia (15%), undescended testis (10%), or precocious puberty
- May produce testosterone, androstenedione, and dehydroepiandrosterone
- May be associated with cryptorchidism, testicular atrophy, infertility
- Bilaterality in 3% of cases

Treatment
- Surgical approaches
  - Orchiectomy is curative in majority of tumors; baseline staging work-up is required
  - Retroperitoneal lymph node dissection may be required in older patients and those with tumors with unfavorable histology

Prognosis
- Majority have benign behavior
- ~ 5-10% are malignant and may metastasize

MACROSCOPIC

General Features
- Well-circumscribed, intraparenchymal mass with golden-brown to yellow, or gray-white homogeneous cut surface, lobulation may be seen
- Focal hemorrhage or necrosis may be seen (25%)
- Most confined within testis; extratesticular extension possible (10%)

Size
- Range: 0.5-5 cm (average: 3 cm)

MICROSCOPIC

Histologic Features
- Growth patterns: Diffuse (most common), lobular, insular, tubular, ribbon-like, and pseudofollicular
- Large, round or polygonal cells with well-defined cell borders, eosinophilic or vacuolated cytoplasm
- Relatively uniform round or ovoid nuclei, prominent nucleoli; focal nuclear pleomorphism (including endocrine-type), binucleated, or multinucleated cells may be seen
- Cytoplasmic vacuoles or foamy cytoplasm (lipid content), lipofuscin (15%), and Reinke crystals (30-40%) may be seen
- Frequent fibrous, hyalinized, edematous or myxoid stroma
- Other uncommon features: Fatty metaplasia; spindle, clear cell, or microcystic changes; myxoid degeneration; calcification or ossification; and rhabdoid features
- Features that tend to be seen more often in malignant tumors: Large tumor size (> 5 cm), infiltrative borders, vascular invasion, nuclear atypia, necrosis, high mitotic rate (> 3/10 HPF)
- Metastasis is only criterion for malignancy

ANCILLARY TESTS

Immunohistochemistry
- Positive for inhibin-α, calretinin, Melan-A (MART-1), WT1, androgenic hormones (P450scc, 3β-HSD, etc.), CD99, steroidogenic factor (SF-1), and vimentin (strong and diffuse)
- Negative for cytokeratin, chromogranin, and synaptophysin (rarely focally positive for these 3 markers), S100 and PLAP (rarely positive for these 2 markers), nuclear beta-catenin, germ cell tumor markers

Genetic Testing
- Most frequent changes including gains of chromosomes X, 19, and 19p and losses of chromosomes 8 and 16

DIFFERENTIAL DIAGNOSIS

Large Cell Calcifying Sertoli Cell Tumor
- More calcification, frequent bilaterality (40%), intratubular growth of tumor cells, nests or cords of growth

Testicular Tumors of Adrenogenital Syndrome
- Multinodular, bilaterality, pleomorphism, pigmentation, and hyalinized fibrous stroma, interstitial growth pattern with entrapped seminiferous tubules

Ectopic Leydig Cells Mimicking Extratesticular Extension
- Cytologically bland Leydig cell proliferation in extratesticular locations (tunica albuginea, epididymis, spermatic cord)
- Intraneural, perineural, perivascular locations

Leydig Cell Hyperplasia
- Small size (< 0.5 cm), multifocal, shows interstitial growth with intervening seminiferous tubules

SELECTED REFERENCES

1. Sangoi AR et al: Evaluation of SF-1 expression in testicular germ cell tumors: a tissue microarray study of 127 cases. Appl Immunohistochem Mol Morphol. 21(4):318-21, 2013
2. Jou P et al: Leydig cell tumor of the testis. J Urol. 181(5):2299-300, 2009
3. Loeser A et al: Testis-sparing surgery versus radical orchiectomy in patients with Leydig cell tumors. Urology. 74(2):370-2, 2009
4. Verdorfer I et al: Leydig cell tumors of the testis: a molecular-cytogenetic study based on a large series of patients. Oncol Rep. 17(3):585-9, 2007
5. Carvajal-Carmona LG et al: Adult leydig cell tumors of the testis caused by germline fumarate hydratase mutations. J Clin Endocrinol Metab. 91(8):3071-5, 2006

Leydig Cell Tumors

(Left) Lower power photomicrograph of Leydig cell tumor shows nests and cords of uniform oval to round tumor cells separated by sclerotic and myxoid stroma. (Right) Leydig cell tumor with uniform, oval to round tumor cells is shown. The tumor cells have abundant eosinophilic cytoplasm and distinct cell boundaries. Nucleoli ➡ are prominent. The tumor is vaguely divided into lobules by delicate sinusoidal vessels. There is absence of pleomorphism, necrosis, or mitosis.

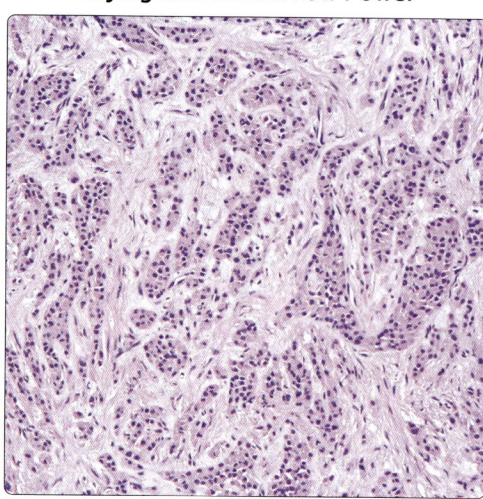
Leydig Cell Tumor: Low Power

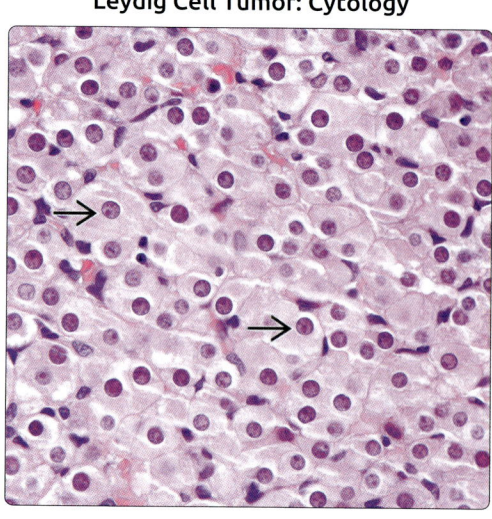
Leydig Cell Tumor: Cytology

(Left) Leydig cell tumor with intracytoplasmic lipofuscin pigment ➡ is shown. Mild degree of nuclear irregularity and prominent nucleoli ➡ are present. (Right) Leydig cell tumor with a rod-shaped intracytoplasmic Reinke crystal ➡ is seen. The crystalloid is detected in approximately 30-40% of this tumor and is typically a focal finding. It is not obligatory to find them, though when seen are diagnostic.

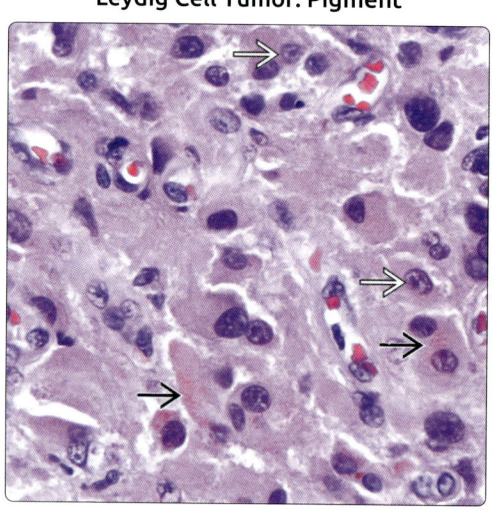
Leydig Cell Tumor: Pigment

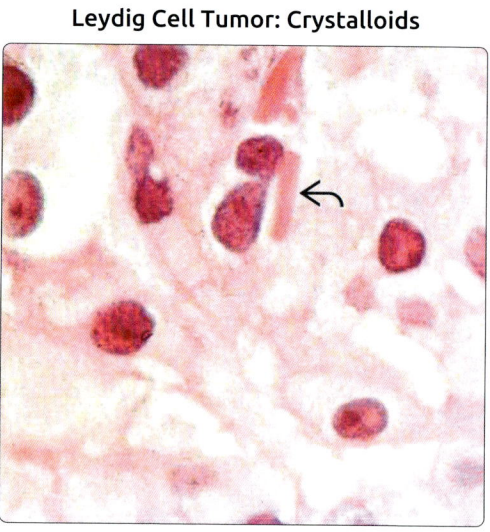
Leydig Cell Tumor: Crystalloids

(Left) Leydig cell tumor with rhabdoid features shows tumor cells with voluminous eosinophilic cytoplasm, eccentrically located nuclei, and prominent nucleoli. Besides other more common oncocytic tumors, the differential diagnoses include malignant melanoma and plasmacytoma. (Right) The tumor cells with rhabdoid features are strongly positive for inhibin and negative for cytokeratin. Other useful markers include Melan-A (MART-1), WT1, and calretinin, which are also positive in Leydig cell tumor.

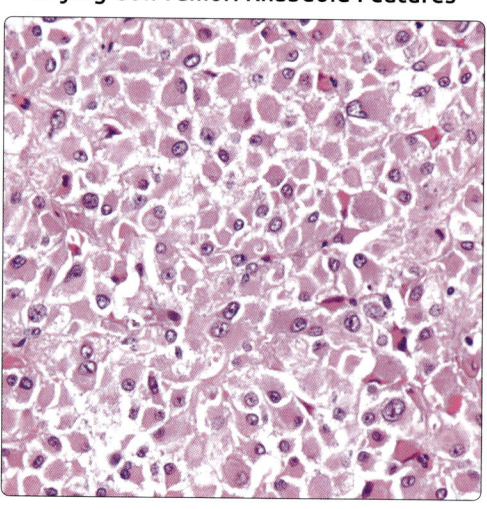
Leydig Cell Tumor: Rhabdoid Features

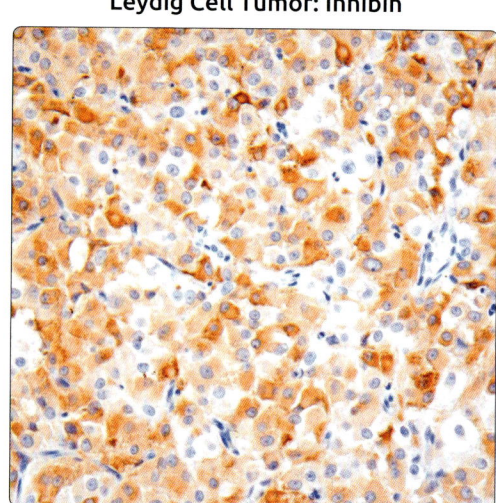
Leydig Cell Tumor: Inhibin

Leydig Cell Tumors

Leydig Cell Tumor: Clear Cells

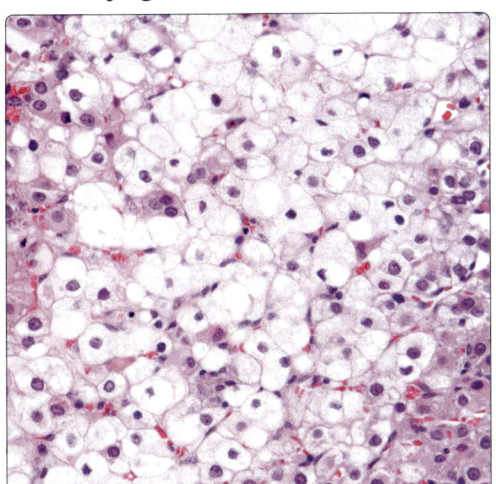

Leydig Cell Tumor: Ossification

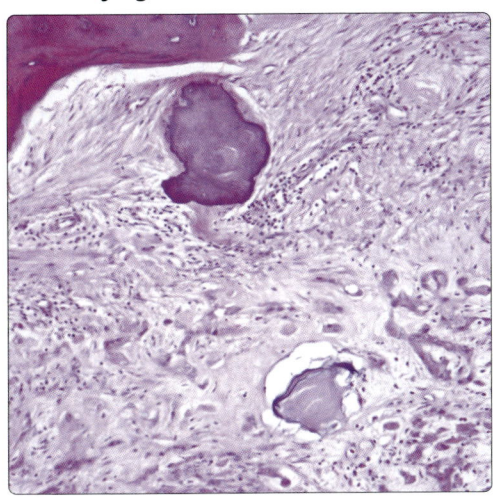

(Left) Leydig cell tumor may have prominent clear cells and abundant anastomosing capillary network resembling that of the zona fasciculata of the adrenal cortex. (Right) Leydig cell tumor with ossification is shown. The tumor cells are arranged in cords and trabeculae with fibrous tissue. The differential diagnosis from a large cell calcifying Sertoli cell tumor (LCCSCT) may be difficult. Bilaterality, association with syndromes, and keratin positivity in LCCSCT are helpful in favoring LCCSCT.

Leydig Cell Tumor: Vimentin

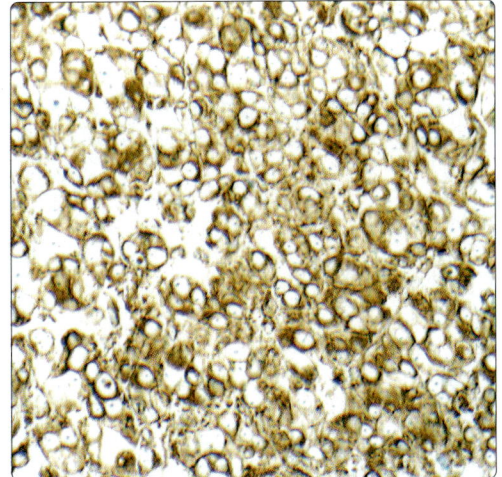

Leydig Cell Tumor: Inhibin

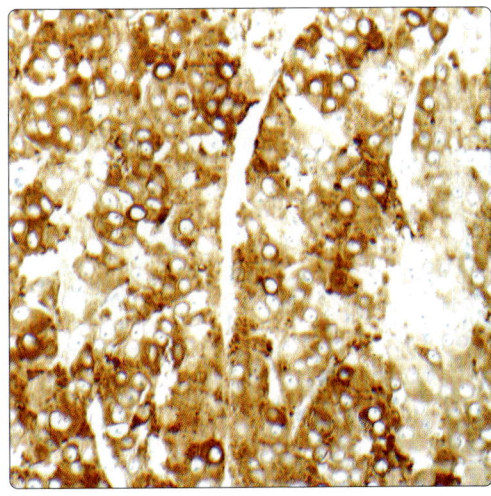

(Left) The tumor cells of Leydig cell tumor are diffusely positive for vimentin. All sex cord-stromal tumors are positive for vimentin. Cytokeratin, however, is negative or focal or weakly positive in Leydig cell tumor. (Right) Leydig cell tumors show diffuse cytoplasmic positivity for α-inhibin. Other useful markers include Melan-A (MART-1), calretinin, SF1, and WT1, which are positive in Leydig cell tumor. Androgenic hormones may be positive but are rarely necessary in clinical practice.

Leydig Cell Tumor: Atypia

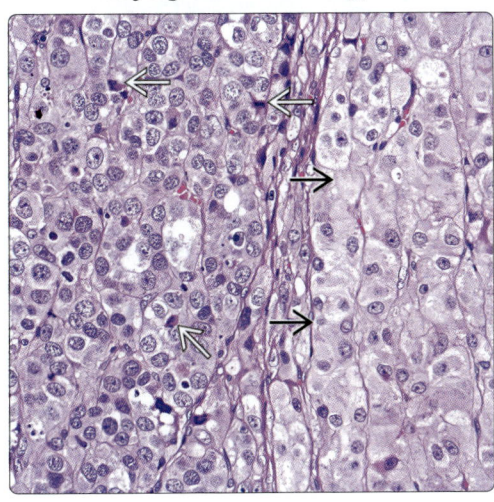

Leydig Cell Tumor: Atypia

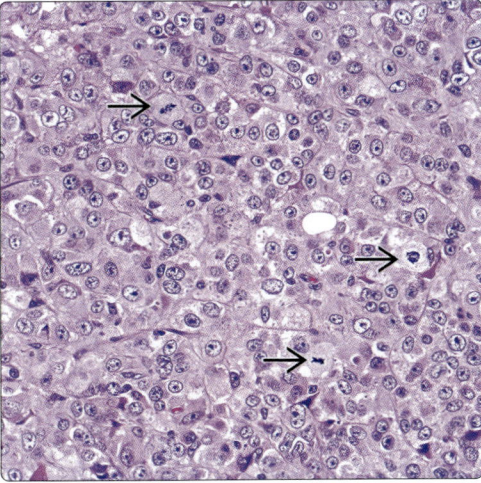

(Left) This image shows an area of typical Leydig cell tumor ⇨ juxtaposed with an area with histologically malignant features, such as increased cellularity, high N:C ratio, frequent mitoses and apoptoses ⇨. Approximately 5-10% of Leydig cell tumor are malignant. (Right) A malignant Leydig cell tumor with several mitoses ⇨ is shown. Features seen more commonly in tumors with malignant outcome include capsular or vascular invasion, mitoses > 3/10 HPF, significant pleomorphism, and necrosis.

Sertoli Cell Tumors

KEY FACTS

TERMINOLOGY
- Pure sex cord-stromal tumor composed of Sertoli cells

CLINICAL ISSUES
- < 1% of testicular tumors; most are sporadic
- All ages (average: 45 yr)
- Slowly enlarging testicular mass

MACROSCOPIC
- Small, well-circumscribed, homogeneous gray-white to yellow, firm mass

MICROSCOPIC
- Growth patterns: Tubules, microcystic, solid cords and nests, and rarely spindled (sarcomatoid)
- Most common pattern is tubule formation surrounded by basement membrane
- Uniform cuboidal or columnar cells with moderate pale to lightly eosinophilic cytoplasm, often prominent cytoplasmic vacuoles
- Bland round to ovoid nuclei, occasional centrally located nucleoli, and rare mitoses
- May have paucicellular, hyalinized, vascular fibrous stroma, or lymphoid aggregates
- Charcot-Böttcher filaments (perinuclear arrays of filaments) are considered pathognomonic of Sertoli cell differentiation by electron microscopy

ANCILLARY TESTS
- Positive for CK-PAN (AE1/AE3), EMA/MUC1, vimentin, α-inhibin, Melan-A (MART-1), WT1, SF1, CD99, calretinin, S100 (weak), SOX9, nuclear β-catenin (60-70%): synaptophysin may be positive
- Negative for PLAP, Podoplanin (D2-40), OCT3/OCT4, SALL4, α-fetoprotein, CD30 (BerH2), HCG

TOP DIFFERENTIAL DIAGNOSES
- Yolk sac tumor or seminoma (tubular) or malignant
- Adenomatoid tumor
- Sertoli cell nodule

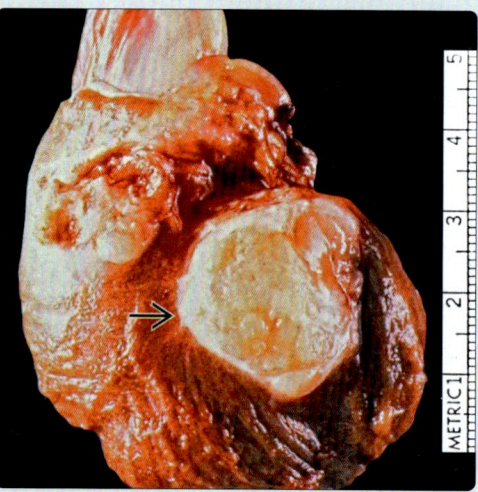

Sertoli Cell Tumor: Gross

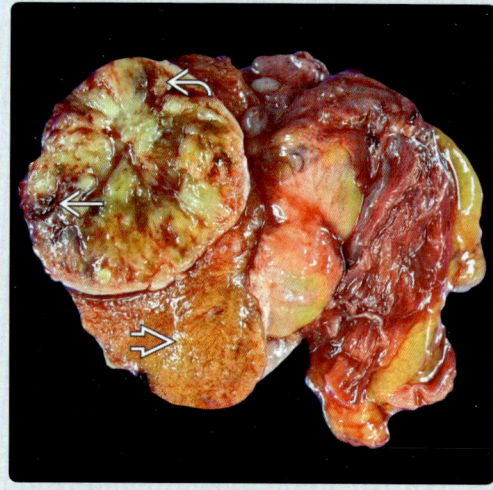

Sertoli Cell Tumor: Gross

(Left) A well-circumscribed Sertoli cell tumor (SCT) ➡ with a tan-white firm cut surface is shown. The gross finding is different from Leydig cell tumor, which usually is tan-brown to yellow due to high lipid content. (Right) An encapsulated SCT with a tan-white, variegated, and gelatinous cut surface is shown. There are cystic changes ➡ and focal hemorrhage ➡. The tumor is confined within the testis. Uninvolved testis is seen ➡.

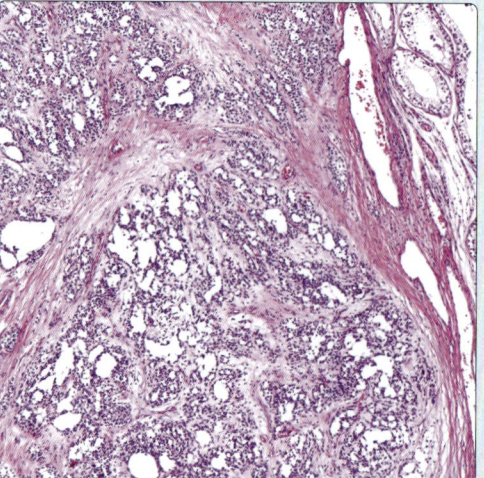

Sertoli Cell Tumor: Low Power

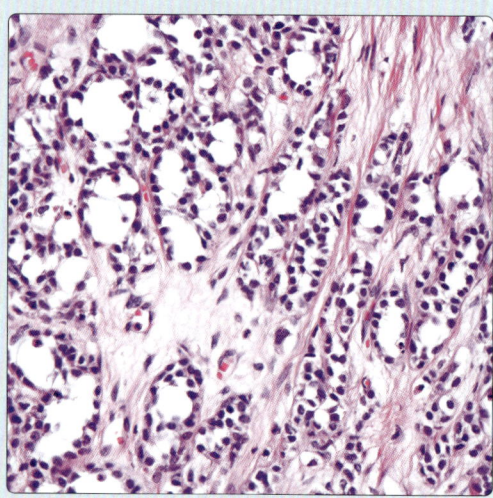

Sertoli Cell Tumor: Tubules

(Left) Low-power image shows a well-circumscribed SCT with a lobular growth pattern, tubular and microcystic architecture, and hyalinized stroma. Tubular differentiation is the hallmark of this neoplasm. (Right) High-power photomicrograph of SCT shows uniform cuboidal or ovoid tumor cells arranged in elongated or round tubules separated by a delicate fibrous stroma. The amount of cytoplasm varies between tumors and in different areas of the tumor.

Sertoli Cell Tumors

TERMINOLOGY

Definitions
- Pure sex cord-stromal tumor of Sertoli cell origin that shows variety of architectural patterns, including solid growth, but which shows at least focal tubular differentiation

CLINICAL ISSUES

Epidemiology
- Incidence
  - < 1% of testicular tumors; most are sporadic
  - May occur in patients with undescended testes, Peutz-Jeghers syndrome, Carney syndrome, androgen insensitivity, and testicular feminization syndromes
- Age
  - Occurs in any age with no age predilection (average: 45 yr)
  - Up to 30% occur in 1st decade of life

Presentation
- Asymptomatic, slowly enlarging testicular mass, most unilateral
- Hormone-related symptoms are unusual; may present with hyperestrinism (gynecomastia)

Treatment
- Surgical approaches
  - Surgical resection is often curative (radiation and chemotherapy have little effect)

Prognosis
- Up to 10% may be malignant
- Excellent prognosis unless metastasis occurs, usually involves retroperitoneal lymph nodes but may also be in hematogenous distribution

MACROSCOPIC

General Features
- Usually small, well-circumscribed, homogeneous gray-white to yellow, firm mass
- May be lobulated with focal cystic changes or hemorrhage

Size
- Range: Most 2-5 cm

MICROSCOPIC

Histologic Features
- Growth patterns: Tubules, microcystic, cords, nests, solid sheets, and rarely spindled (sarcomatoid)
  - Most common pattern is tubules, which are hollow, round, solid, or elongated
- Uniform cuboidal or columnar cells with moderate pale to lightly eosinophilic cytoplasm, often with prominent cytoplasmic vacuoles
- Bland, round to ovoid nuclei, occasionally centrally located nucleoli, and rare mitoses
- May have paucicellular, hyalinized, or vascular fibrous stroma; lymphoid aggregates may be present
- May have clear cells arranged in nests by fibrous septa and lymphoid infiltrates resembling that of seminoma
- Entrapped germ cells within Sertoli cell tumor (usually at periphery) may mimic mixed germ cell sex cord-stromal tumor
- Some tumors may have abundant cytoplasmic lipid (lipid-rich variant)
- Features seen more often in tumors with malignant outcome include
  - Large size (> 5 cm), lymphovascular invasion, and extratesticular extension
  - Marked nuclear pleomorphism, increased mitoses (> 5/10 high power fields), and necrosis
- Sclerosing Sertoli cell tumor
  - Characterized by markedly sclerotic fibrous stroma (comprising at least 50% of the tumor) containing cords, solid or hollow tubules, and nests of Sertoli cells

ANCILLARY TESTS

Immunohistochemistry
- Positive for CK-PAN (AE1/AE3), EMA/MUC1, vimentin, α-inhibin, Melan-A (MART-1), WT1, SF1, CD99, calretinin, S100 (weak), SOX9, nuclear β-catenin (60-70%); Synaptophysin may be positive
- Negative for PLAP, Podoplanin (D2-40), OCT3/OCT4, SALL4, α-fetoprotein, CD30 (BerH2), HCG

Genetic Testing
- Gain of chromosome X (~ 40%) and rarely deletion of entire or part of chromosomes 2 and 19
- CTNNB1 gene (encodes β-catenin) mutations in some tumors

Electron Microscopy
- Charcot-Böttcher filaments (perinuclear arrays of filaments) are pathognomonic of Sertoli cell differentiation

DIFFERENTIAL DIAGNOSIS

Yolk Sac Tumor or Seminoma (Tubular)
- Yolk sac tumor (microcystic or glandular) and seminoma (tubular) have larger tumor cells, prominent nucleoli, and abundant cytoplasm
- Positive for germ cell markers; negative for inhibin and calretinin
- Malignant Sertoli cell tumors may have fibrous septa but no germ cell neoplasia in situ

Adenomatoid Tumor
- Location usually in paratesticular site or epididymis
- Negative for inhibin, SF1

Sertoli Cell Nodule
- Microscopic, usually small size (< 0.5 cm)
- Tubules with thickened basement membranes and hyaline bodies lined by immature Sertoli cells

SELECTED REFERENCES

1. Kao CS et al: Sclerosing Sertoli cell tumor of the testis: a clinicopathologic study of 20 cases. Am J Surg Pathol. 38(4):510-7, 2014
2. Perrone F et al: Frequent mutation and nuclear localization of β-catenin in sertoli cell tumors of the testis. Am J Surg Pathol. 38(1):66-71, 2014
3. Adayener C et al: Sertoli cell tumor of the testis: a case with late metastasis. Int Urol Nephrol. 40(4):1005-8, 2008

Sertoli Cell Tumors

(Left) SCT typically have tubules ➡, microcysts ➡, and cords ➡ lined by bland ovoid to round tumor cells with scant clear to eosinophilic cytoplasm. There is no nuclear pleomorphism, tumor necrosis, or mitotic activity. (Right) High-power photomicrograph of SCT shows tubules ➡, microcysts ➡, and cords lined by bland ovoid to elongated tumor cells with clear to pale eosinophilic cytoplasm or cytoplasm with fine vacuolization ➡.

Sertoli Cell Tumor: Tubules and Microcysts
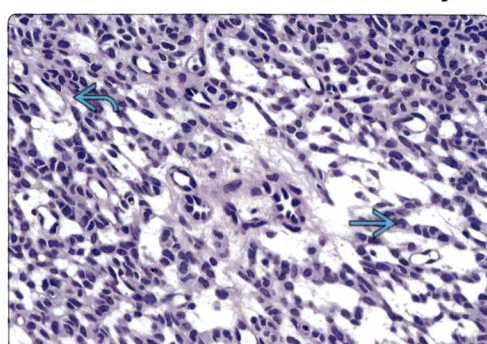

Sertoli Cell Tumor: Cytology
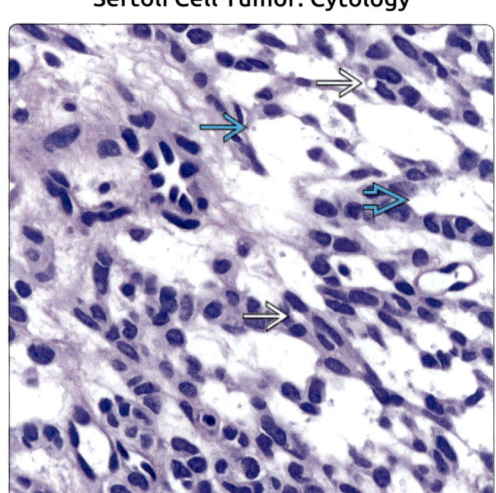

(Left) Microcystic ➡ and tubular ➡ patterns of SCT may superficially resemble that of a yolk sac tumor. SCT may rarely have lymphoid infiltrates, raising the differential diagnosis of seminoma with tubular growth pattern. (Right) SCTs are known to exhibit numerous architectural patterns. A high-power photomicrograph of SCT demonstrates tubules ➡ and cords ➡. The amount of stroma may vary and prominent areas of hyalinization are not uncommon.

Sertoli Cell Tumor: Tubules and Microcysts
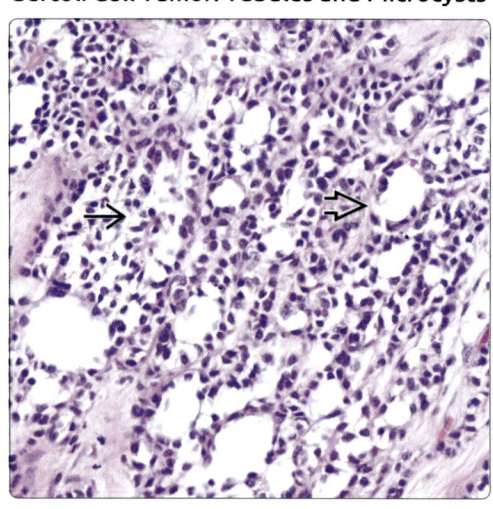

Sertoli Cell Tumor: Tubules and Cords
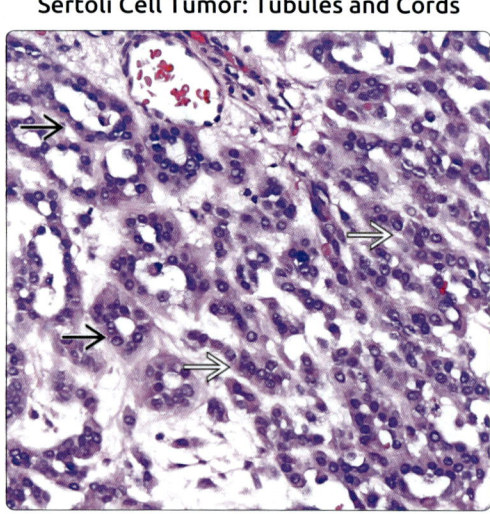

(Left) This SCT shows tubules of differing sizes lined by a single layer of monotonous cuboidal cells with clear cytoplasm. The background stroma is edematous and myxoid. Tubules lined by clear cells are one of the most helpful diagnostic features of SCT. (Right) This is an example of SCT with a focal retiform growth pattern characterized by irregularly elongated branching channels lined by bland cuboidal to flattened tumor cells.

Sertoli Cell Tumor: Tubules
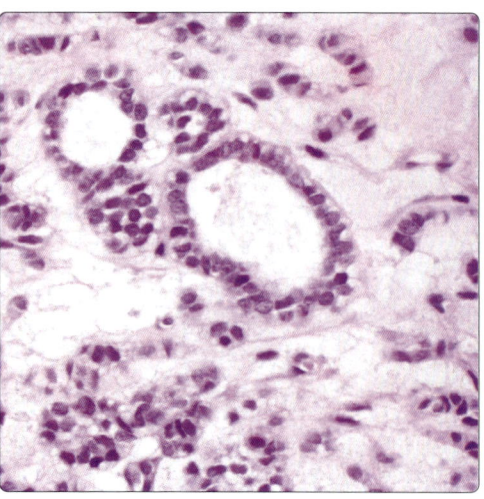

Sertoli Cell Tumor: Retiform
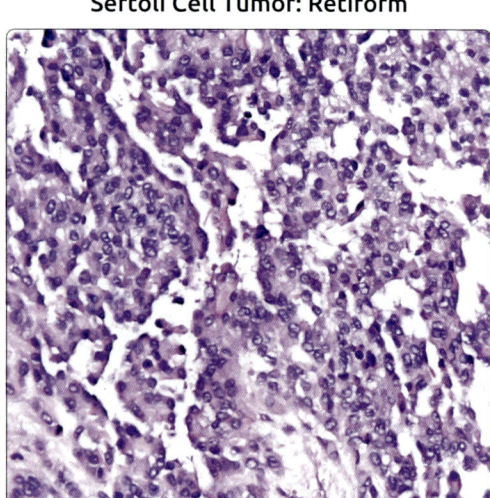

Sertoli Cell Tumors

Sertoli Cell Tumor: Mixed Patterns

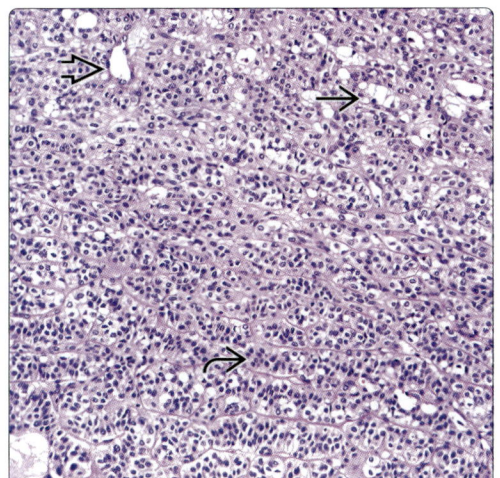

Sertoli Cell Tumor: Solid Tubular

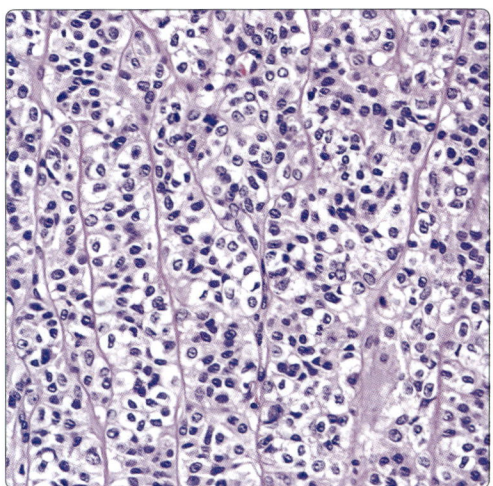

(Left) Low-power image of a SCT shows solid ⇨, tubular ⇨, and microcytic ⇨ areas. Although the tumor is fairly cellular, there is no significant cytologic atypia, increased mitoses, or necrosis. (Right) SCT shows a solid tubular growth pattern surrounded by thin, fibrous septa. The cells have bland, ovoid nuclei and abundant clear cytoplasm with vacuolization. Some SCT may have a variety of cytoplasmic features, including clear cells, eosinophilic cells, and lipid-rich cells.

Sertoli Cell Tumor: Cords

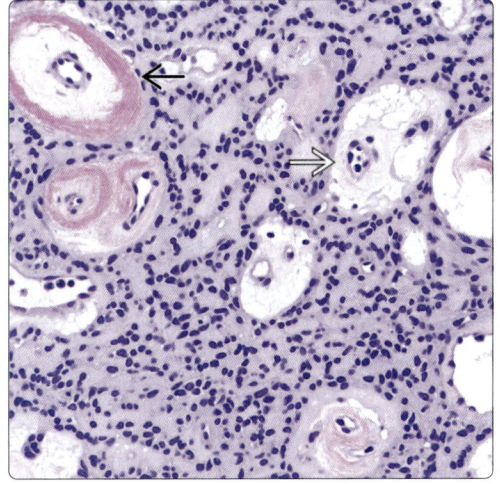

Sertoli Cell Tumor: Follicles

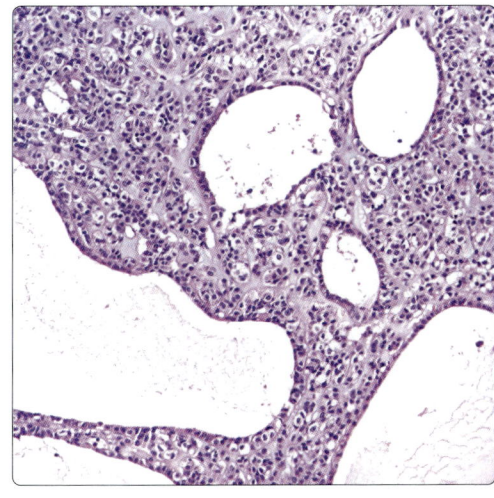

(Left) SCT is composed of cords of tumor cells embedded in a paucicellular hyalinized fibrous stroma. The blood vessels show hyalinization of the wall ⇨ and perivascular edema ⇨. (Right) This SCT has small and markedly dilated follicles lined by bland cuboidal or flattened tumor cells. Because of follicular features, juvenile granulosa cell tumor (JGCT) may be in the differential diagnosis. However, JGCT occurs almost exclusively in children younger than 6 months.

Sertoli Cell Tumor: Collagenized Stroma

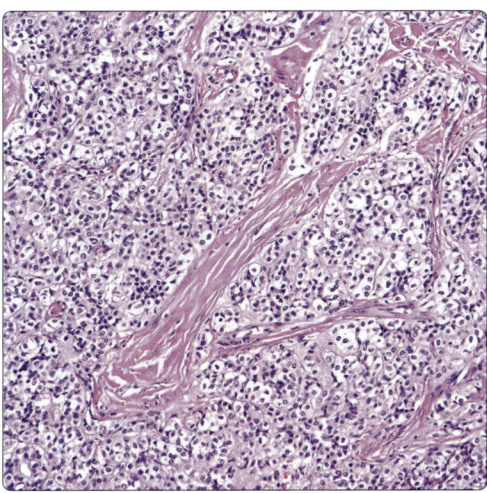

Sertoli Cell Tumor: Tubules and Microcysts

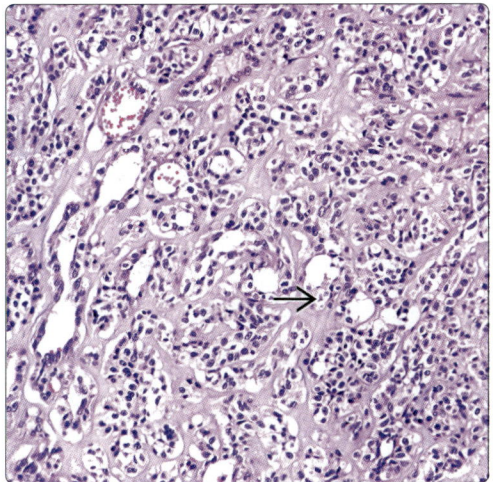

(Left) This SCT shows a solid growth pattern interspersed with variable collagenized stroma. The lobular appearance superficially resembles a seminoma; however, the cytologic features are key in the distinction. (Right) SCT can have tubules and microcysts ⇨ of variable sizes with prominent myxoid stroma, which may resemble a yolk sac tumor. However, the nuclear features are relatively bland, and there is absence of hyaline globules or basement membrane material.

Sertoli Cell Tumors

Sertoli Cell Tumor: Sheets and Nests

Sertoli Cell Tumor: Spindle Cells

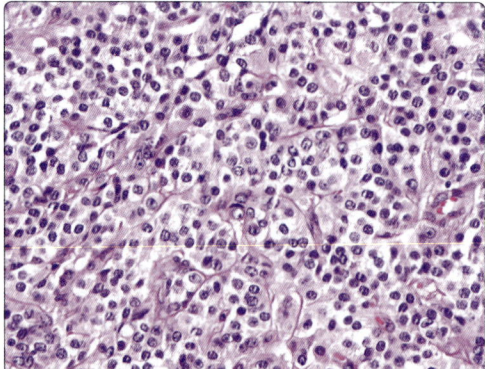

(Left) SCT may have diffuse, sheet-like, and nested growth and is composed of cells with clear to eosinophilic cytoplasm, which may mimic a Leydig cell tumor. However, in other areas, classic SCT with tubules were seen. (Right) SCT with prominent spindle cells (sarcomatoid growth) is shown. There is moderate clear to pale eosinophilic cytoplasm. The chief differential diagnosis is an unclassified sex cord-stromal tumor. In this case, there were areas of classic SCT, distinct and not admixed.

Sertoli Cell Tumor: Sclerosing

Sertoli Cell Tumor: Sclerosing

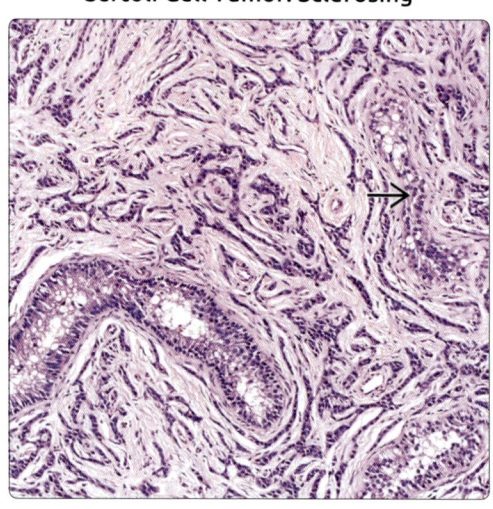

(Left) Low-power photomicrograph of a sclerosing SCT shows cord-like growth of tumor cells within a dense sclerotic stroma. Compressed entrapped seminiferous tubules are present ➡ and more frequently seen in this variant of SCT. (Right) Sclerosing SCT with a cord-like growth pattern and dense sclerotic stroma is shown. To date, metastasis has not been reported in the sclerosing variant of SCT. Carcinoid tumor and adenomatoid tumor are in the differential.

Malignant Sertoli Cell Tumor: Necrosis

Malignant Sertoli Cell Tumor: Vascular Invasion

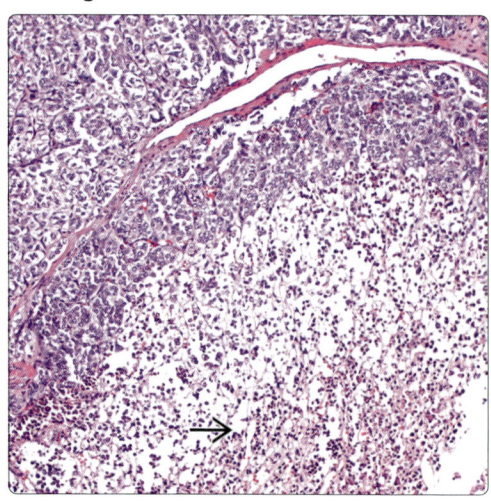
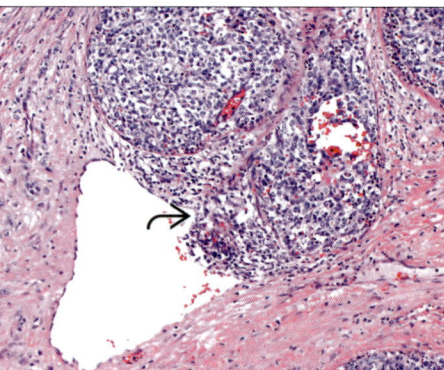

(Left) SCT with a malignant outcome shows solid sheets of tumor cells with hypercellularity, increased nuclear:cytoplasmic ratio, and a large area of necrosis ➡. There is no single diagnostic criterion for malignant SCT. Features that are seen more often in malignant SCT include pleomorphism, increased mitoses, necrosis, vascular invasion, and infiltrative growth pattern. (Right) A malignant SCT is composed of solid tumor nodules seen outside of the testis with focal vascular invasion ➡.

Sertoli Cell Tumors

Malignant Sertoli Cell Tumor

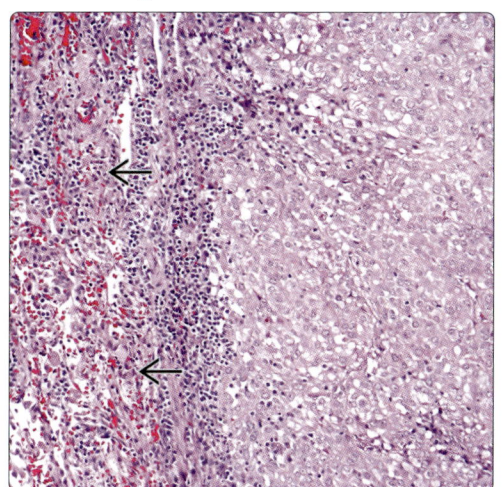

Metastatic Sertoli Cell Tumor

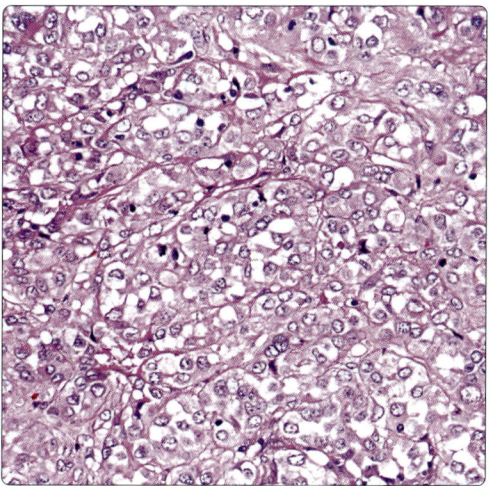

(Left) Metastatic SCT nodule to the lung ⇒ is composed of sheets of epithelioid cells with pale eosinophilic cytoplasm. The tumor in the testis showed more obvious Sertoli cell features. *(Right)* Metastatic SCT to the lung shows a solid tubular growth pattern with large tumor cells, prominent nucleoli, and abundant eosinophilic cytoplasm separated by delicate fibrovascular septa. Clinical history and immunoreactivity with inhibin and cytokeratin are helpful in making the diagnosis.

Sertoli Cell Tumor: Inhibin

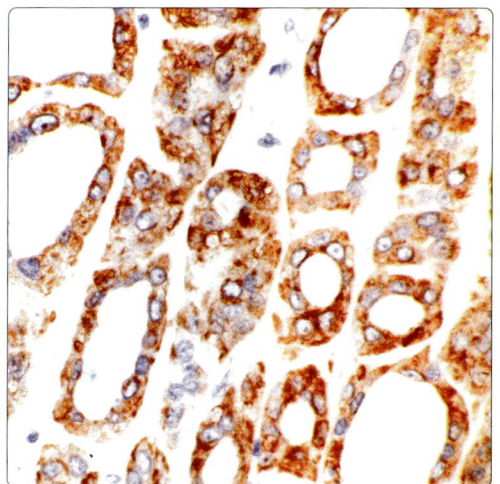

Sertoli Cell Tumor: CK-PAN

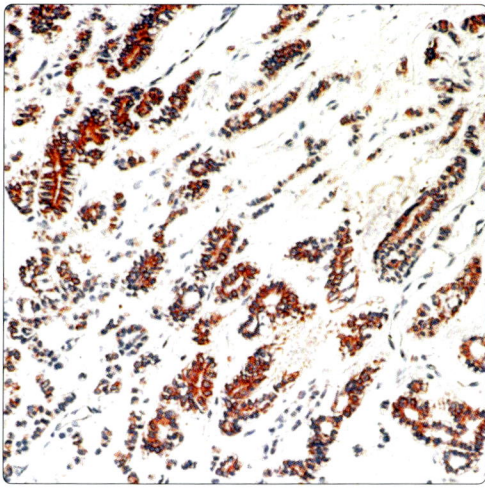

(Left) The tumor cells in this tubular SCT are strongly positive for inhibin. Positive immunoreactivity with SF1, inhibin, calretinin, WT1, CD99, and Melan-A (MART-1) are very helpful in establishing sex cord-stromal cell differentiation; all markers are not required. *(Right)* Tumor cells of SCT are strongly positive for CK-PAN (AE1/AE3), a helpful feature for the diagnosis of SCT. In contrast, Leydig cell tumors and granulosa cell tumors are often weakly or focally positive or negative for cytokeratin.

Yolk Sac Tumor: Differential

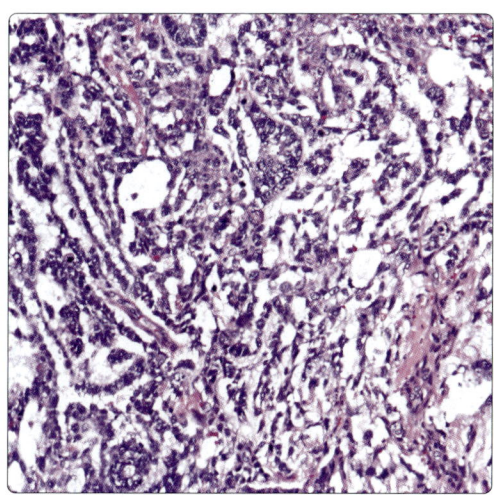

Adenomatoid Tumor: Differential

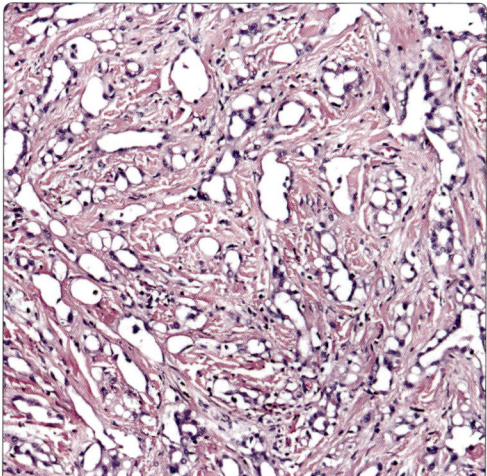

(Left) Yolk sac tumor consists of tumor cells arranged in microcystic and glandular patterns. The presence of teratoma or other germ cell tumors, as well as germ cell neoplasia in situ can distinguish it from Sertoli cell tumor. Immunostain with germ cell markers is helpful. *(Right)* Adenomatoid tumor is composed of gland-like spaces lined by flattened cells. Positive immunoreactivity with podoplanin, CK5/CK6, and thrombomodulin can distinguish it from Sertoli cell tumor.

Large Cell Calcifying Sertoli Cell Tumor

KEY FACTS

TERMINOLOGY
- Variant of Sertoli cell tumor with large epithelioid cells and peculiar calcifications, often associated with clinical syndromes

CLINICAL ISSUES
- Extremely rare; only ~ 50 cases have been reported
- Range: 1.5-48 years (average: 16 years)
- Sporadic (60%) or as component of Carney and Peutz-Jeghers syndromes

MACROSCOPIC
- Well-circumscribed, white-tan or yellow mass associated with granular or gritty calcifications
- Usually < 4 cm

MICROSCOPIC
- Common growth patterns include nests, cords or trabeculae, or solid tubules
- Large polygonal cells with abundant eosinophilic, ground-glass, or finely granular cytoplasm
- Tumor cells have vesicular nuclei and prominent nucleoli
- Fibrous or myxohyaline stroma with marked calcifications
- May have marked neutrophilic infiltration
- Some have intratubular growth

ANCILLARY TESTS
- Positive for Melan-A (MART-1), inhibin-α, S100, desmin, actin-sm, SF-1
- Negative for nuclear beta-catenin, cytokeratin (may be focally positive), α-fetoprotein, HCG, PLAP, podoplanin (D2-40), and OCT3/4

TOP DIFFERENTIAL DIAGNOSES
- Leydig cell tumor
- Tumor of adrenogenital syndrome
- Sertoli cell tumor

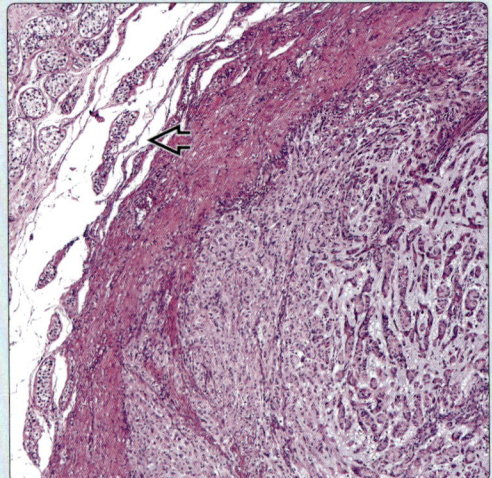

Large Cell Calcifying Sertoli Cell Tumor: Well Circumscribed

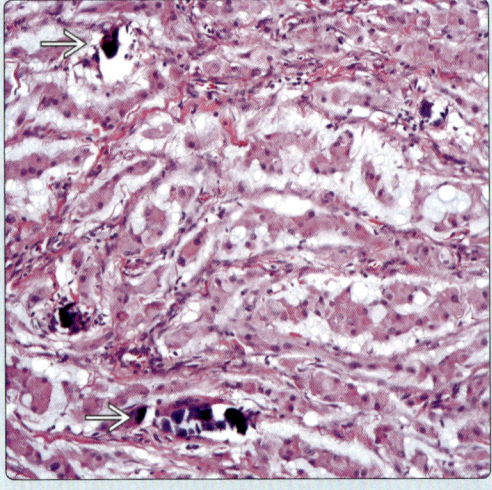

Large Cell Calcifying Sertoli Cell Tumor: Epithelioid Cell

(Left) Well-circumscribed large cell calcifying Sertoli cell tumor (LCCSCT) is demarcated from the adjacent testis ⇨ by a thick fibrous capsule. The tumor is composed of cords and nests of tumor cells with hyalinized or myxoid stroma. *(Right)* A LCCSCT shows cords of large epithelioid cells containing abundant eosinophilic cytoplasm. The hallmark of this tumor is the presence of scattered calcifications ⇨. This variant of Sertoli cell tumor has cells resembling Leydig cell tumor.

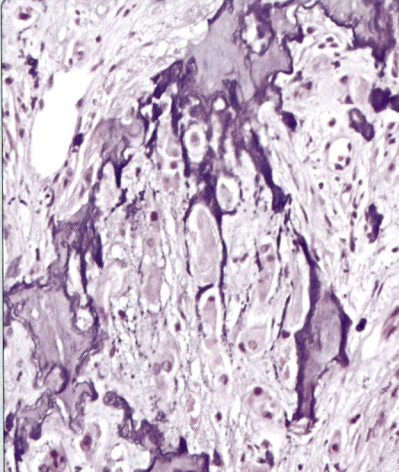

Large Cell Calcifying Sertoli Cell Tumor: Calcification

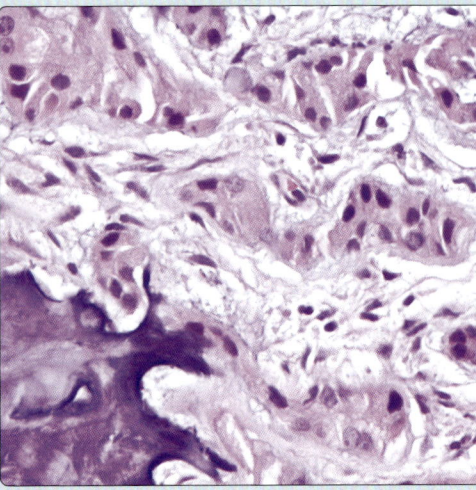

Large Cell Calcifying Sertoli Cell Tumor: Epithelioid Cells

(Left) LCCSCT is seen arranged singly or in groups of large epithelioid cells, surrounded by large areas of calcifications, which are often intercellular. A calcified or ossified Leydig cell tumor should also be included in the differential diagnosis. However, bilaterality and syndrome association favor the diagnosis of LCCSCT. *(Right)* LCCSCT is shown with nests of large epithelioid cells with abundant eosinophilic cytoplasm. A large area of calcification is seen in the loose fibromyxoid stroma.

Large Cell Calcifying Sertoli Cell Tumor

TERMINOLOGY

Abbreviations
- Large cell calcifying Sertoli cell tumor (LCCSCT)

Definitions
- Variant of Sertoli cell tumor with large epithelioid cells and peculiar calcifications, often associated with clinical syndromes

CLINICAL ISSUES

Epidemiology
- Incidence
  - Extremely rare
- Age
  - Range: 1.5-48 years (average: 16 years)

Presentation
- Slowly enlarging, painless testicular mass
- Sporadic (60%) or as component of Carney and Peutz-Jeghers syndromes
- May be associated with adrenocortical hyperplasia, hypercortisolemia, or testicular Leydig cell tumor
- Bilaterality (40%) and multifocality (60%), associated with Carney syndrome; unilateral and unifocal in sporadic cases
- Tumors occurring in Peutz-Jeghers syndrome are distinctive and called intratubular large cell hyalinizing Sertoli cell neoplasia
- Malignant form reported: Mean age: 39 years; more often unilateral and solitary compared to benign tumors

Treatment
- Surgical approaches
  - Orchiectomy is usually curative; long-term follow-up is necessary

Prognosis
- Excellent, but some (20%) may have malignant behavior

MACROSCOPIC

General Features
- Well-circumscribed, white-tan or yellow mass associated with granular or gritty calcifications

Size
- Usually < 4 cm; malignant tumor may be larger

MICROSCOPIC

Histologic Features
- Common growth patterns include nests, cords, trabeculae, or solid tubules
- Large polygonal cells with abundant eosinophilic, ground-glass, or finely granular cytoplasm
- Tumor cells have vesicular nuclei and prominent nucleoli
- Calcifications are a hallmark; large, wavy laminated nodules, sometimes small psammoma bodies and rare ossification
- Fibrous or myxohyaline stroma
- May have marked neutrophilic infiltration
- Intratubular large cell calcifying Sertoli cell tumor
  - Distinct morphologic variant of LCCSCT
  - Abnormal large seminiferous tubules filled with Sertoli cells and peritubular basement membrane material with psammoma body-type calcification
  - Sertoli cells often have abundant pale to eosinophilic, vacuolated cytoplasm with fibrillar quality; bland nuclei and no mitosis
- Features seen more often in malignant tumors: Size > 4 cm, ≥ 4 mitoses/10 HPF, marked cytologic atypia, necrosis, angiolymphatic invasion

ANCILLARY TESTS

Immunohistochemistry
- Positive for Melan-A (MART-1), inhibin-α, S100, desmin, actin-sm, SF-1
- Negative for nuclear beta-catenin, cytokeratin (may be focally positive), α-fetoprotein, HCG, PLAP, podoplanin (D2-40), and OCT3/4

Genetic Testing
- Mutations in the *PRKAR1A* gene on chromosome 17q22–24 in 60-70% of Carney syndrome associated cases and occasionally in sporadic tumors

DIFFERENTIAL DIAGNOSIS

Leydig Cell Tumor
- Usually lacks calcification and has a more solid growth pattern, although it may be rarely ossified
- No intratubular growth and bilaterally is less common
- Usually sporadic with no syndromic association

Tumor of Adrenogenital Syndrome
- Solid growth pattern is more frequent with no intratubular component
- Entrapped tubules frequently seen within tumor; lacks calcification
- Prominent fibrous bands and spotty nuclear atypia are common

Sertoli Cell Tumor
- Large epithelioid cells with eosinophilic cytoplasm are distinctly uncommon
- Calcification or neutrophilic infiltration is absent; uncommonly bilateral
- Usually positive for nuclear beta-catenin

SELECTED REFERENCES

1. Coleman S et al: Testicular sclerosing sertoli cell tumor: a case report and review of the literature. Rev Urol. 16(4):191-3, 2014
2. Gourgari E et al: Large-cell calcifying Sertoli cell tumors of the testes in pediatrics. Curr Opin Pediatr. 24(4):518-22, 2012
3. Petersson F et al: Large cell calcifying Sertoli cell tumor: a clinicopathologic study of 1 malignant and 3 benign tumors using histomorphology, immunohistochemistry, ultrastructure, comparative genomic hybridization, and polymerase chain reaction analysis of the PRKAR1A gene. Hum Pathol. 41(4):552-9, 2010
4. Halat SK et al: Large cell calcifying Sertoli cell tumor of testis. J Urol. 177(6):2338, 2007
5. Ulbright TM et al: Intratubular large cell hyalinizing sertoli cell neoplasia of the testis: a report of 8 cases of a distinctive lesion of the Peutz-Jeghers syndrome. Am J Surg Pathol. 31(6):827-35, 2007
6. Kratzer SS et al: Large cell calcifying Sertoli cell tumor of the testis: contrasting features of six malignant and six benign tumors and a review of the literature. Am J Surg Pathol. 21(11):1271-80, 1997

Large Cell Calcifying Sertoli Cell Tumor

Large Cell Calcifying Sertoli Cell Tumor: Cords and Tubules

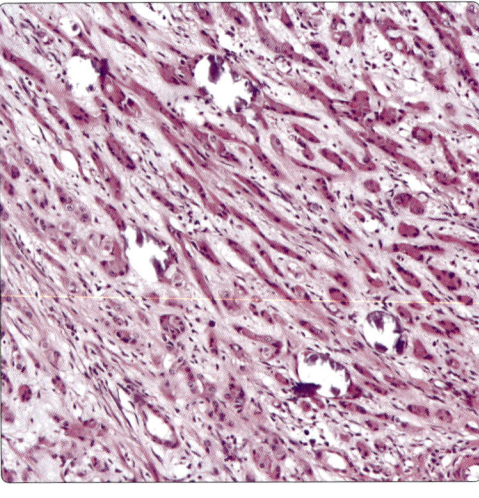

Large Cell Calcifying Sertoli Cell Tumor: Epithelioid Cells

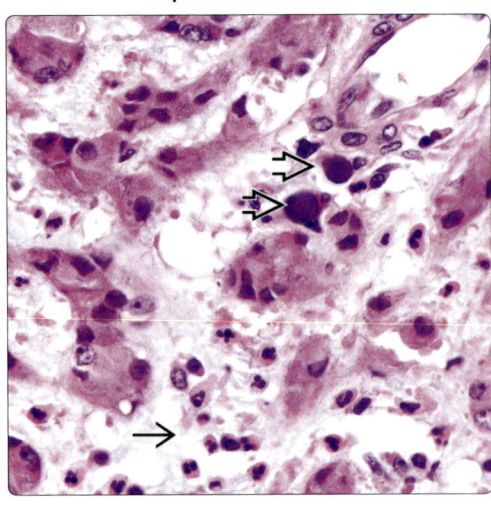

(Left) LCCSCT shows cords or tubules of large cells embedded in a fibromyxoid stroma. Multiple scattered calcifications are present. When one sees scattered calcifications in a sex cord-stromal tumor, LCCSCT should be the top diagnostic consideration. *(Right)* LCCSCT shows nests of large epithelioid cells with abundant eosinophilic cytoplasm and psammoma body-type calcifications ➡. Within the myxoid stroma, there are numerous neutrophils ➡.

Large Cell Calcifying Sertoli Cell Tumor: Neutrophilic Infiltrate

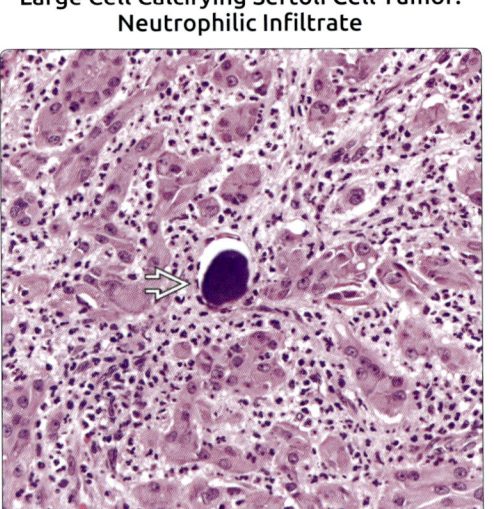

Large Cell Calcifying Sertoli Cell Tumor: Fibromyxoid Stroma

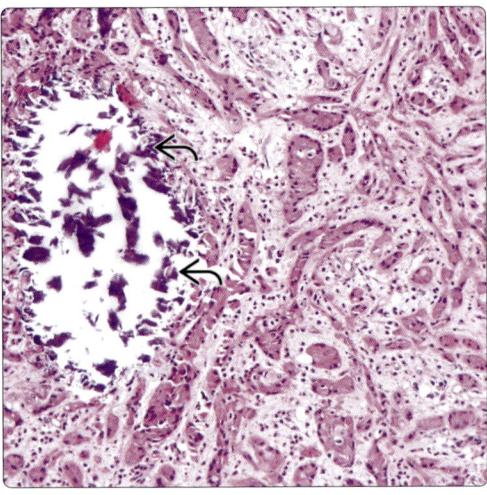

(Left) LCCSCT shows cords and small nests of large epithelioid cells embedded in a fibrous background with dense neutrophilic infiltrate and a psammoma body ➡. A neutrophilic background is an important diagnostic feature. *(Right)* Cords and trabeculae of large epithelioid cells embedded in a fibromyxoid background is typical for LCCSCT. A large area of calcification ➡ is present. There is marked morphologic overlap with Leydig cell tumor, which does not have an intratubular component.

Large Cell Calcifying Sertoli Cell Tumor: Tubules and Trabeculae

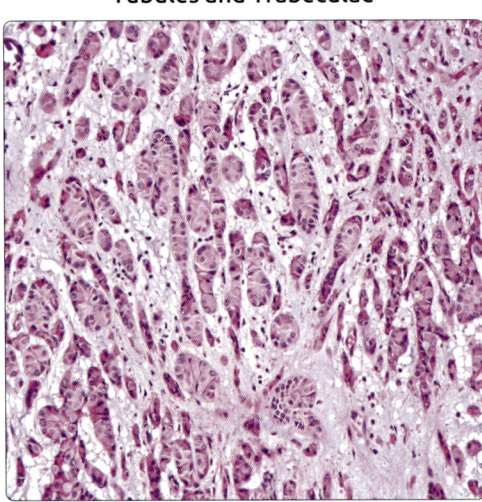

Large Cell Calcifying Sertoli Cell Tumor: Solid Tubules

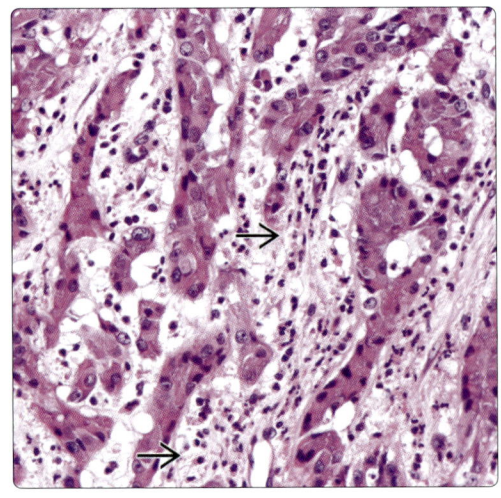

(Left) LCCSCT shows solid tubules and trabeculae of large epithelioid cells with abundant eosinophilic cytoplasm. In the absence of prominent calcification, Leydig cell tumor and testicular tumor of adrenogenital syndrome are in the differential. *(Right)* LCCSCT shows trabeculae or solid tubules of large epithelioid tumor cells with abundant eosinophilic cytoplasm and loose fibromyxoid stroma containing numerous neutrophils ➡.

Large Cell Calcifying Sertoli Cell Tumor

Large Cell Calcifying Sertoli Cell Tumor: Epithelioid Cells

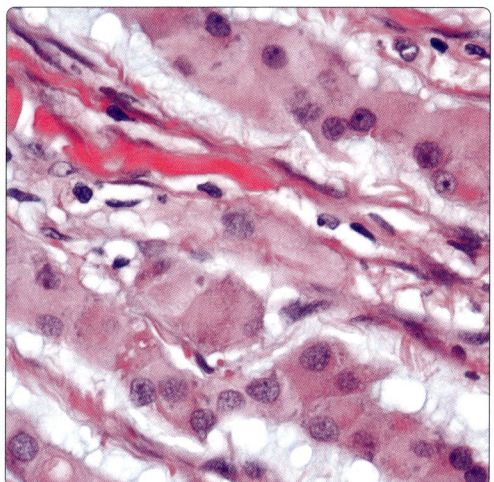

Large Cell Calcifying Sertoli Cell Tumor: Inhibin

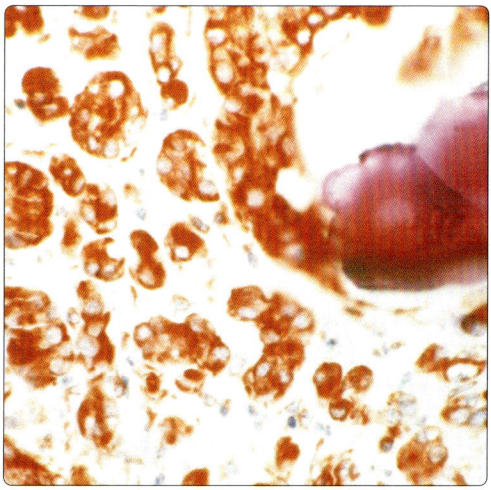

(Left) High power photomicrograph of LCCSCT shows large epithelioid cells with abundant dense eosinophilic cytoplasm, large ovoid to round nuclei, vesicular chromatin and prominent nucleoli. In between the cell nests is prominent myxoid stroma. *(Right)* Similar to other sex cord-stromal cell tumors, the tumor cells in an LCCSCT are strongly positive for inhibin by immunohistochemistry. S100 and keratin positivity are more common compared to Leydig cell tumor.

Large Cell Calcifying Sertoli Cell Tumor (Intratubular)

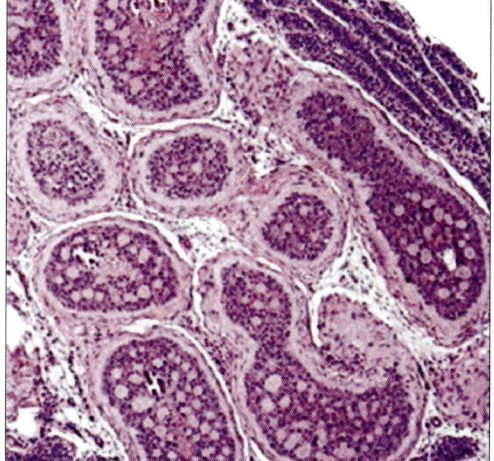

Large Cell Calcifying Sertoli Cell Tumor (Intratubular)

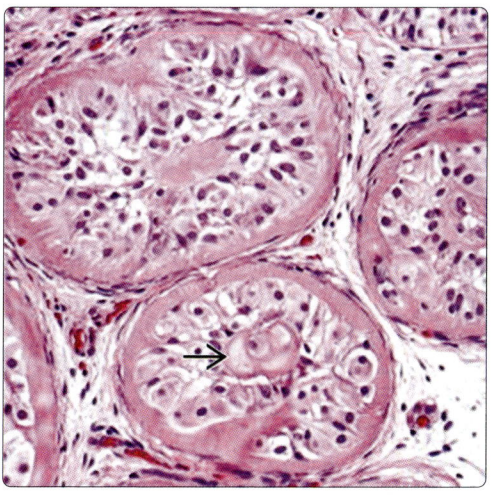

(Left) Testicular tumor occurring in a patient with Peutz-Jeghers syndrome is shown. There is prominent intratubular growth of cells resembling Sertoli cells and associated with peritubular and intratubular hyalinization. *(Right)* Intratubular large cell hyalinizing Sertoli cell tumor in a patient with Peutz-Jeghers syndrome. The cytoplasm of tumor cells has a fibrillary quality. Note the prominent peritubular and intratubular hyalinization and dystrophic calcification ➔.

Leydig Cell Tumor: Differential

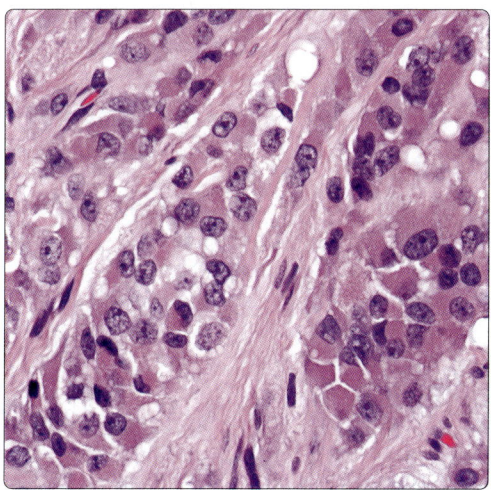

Sertoli Cell Tumor: Differential

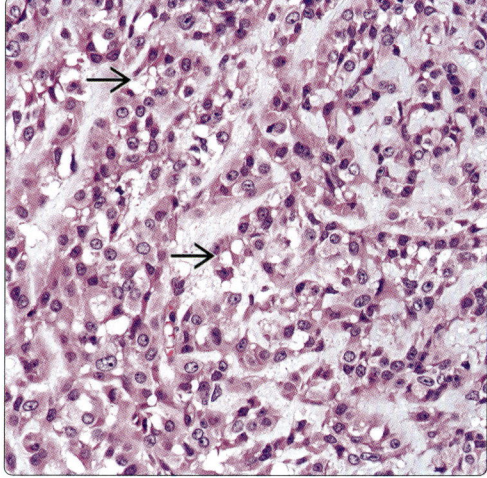

(Left) High-power photomicrograph of a Leydig cell tumor shows cords and nests of large epithelioid tumor cells with abundant eosinophilic cytoplasm. There are no calcifications or neutrophilic infiltrates, which are often seen in an LCCSCT. *(Right)* A Sertoli cell tumor is composed of nests of tumor cells with eosinophilic cytoplasm and myxoid stroma. There are cytoplasmic vacuoles ➔. Bilaterality and multifocality are rare and no calcifications in Sertoli cell tumors, NOS, compared to LCCSCT.

Granulosa Cell Tumor

KEY FACTS

TERMINOLOGY
- Adult testicular tumor of granulosa cell differentiation resembling ovarian counterpart

CLINICAL ISSUES
- Extremely rare in the testis; accounting for < 0.5% of all sex cord-stromal tumors
- Range: 16-76 years (average: 44 years)

MACROSCOPIC
- Well-circumscribed, sometimes encapsulated, homogeneous, yellow to gray, firm mass

MICROSCOPIC
- Growth patterns: Diffuse (most common), microfollicular, trabecular, insular, macrofollicular, gyriform, or cystic
- Presence of Call-Exner bodies (eosinophilic material surrounded by palisading granulosa cells)
- Relatively uniform round or ovoid cells (carrot-shaped) with scant, lightly staining cytoplasm
- Elongated or angular nuclei with grooves (coffee bean-shaped) and 1 or 2 peripherally located nucleoli
- Some show focal theca cell differentiation or have smooth muscle or osteoid differentiation
- Features seen more often in malignant tumors: Large size (> 7 cm), mitoses, necrosis, lymphovascular invasion

ANCILLARY TESTS
- Positive for vimentin, inhibin, calretinin, SMA, CD56, FOXL2, SF1, S100, and focally positive for CK-PAN (AE1/AE3)
- Negative for EMA, nuclear beta-catenin, PLAP, podoplanin (D2-40), OCT3/4, SALL4, AFP, HCG, CD30 (BerH2)

TOP DIFFERENTIAL DIAGNOSES
- Carcinoid tumor
- Sertoli cell tumor
- Leydig cell tumor
- Mixed germ cell and sex cord-stromal tumor (gonadoblastoma or unclassified)

Gross Pathology

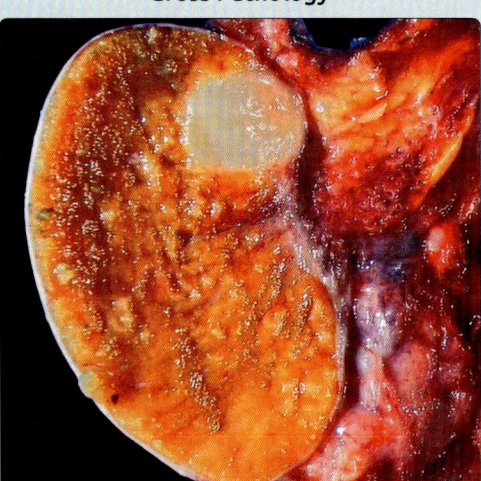

Low Power

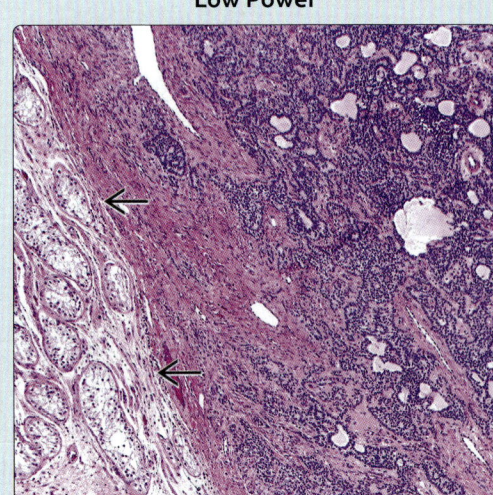

(Left) Granulosa cell tumor (GCT) shows a well-circumscribed, homogeneous, tan-white nodule. The tumor is small and, like many sex cord-stromal tumors, does not extensively involve the testis. Hemorrhage and necrosis are lacking. (Right) A well-circumscribed adult GCT with adjacent uninvolved testicular seminiferous tubules ➡ is shown. The tumor is arranged in solid nests, trabeculae, and micro- and macrofollicles.

Intermediate Power

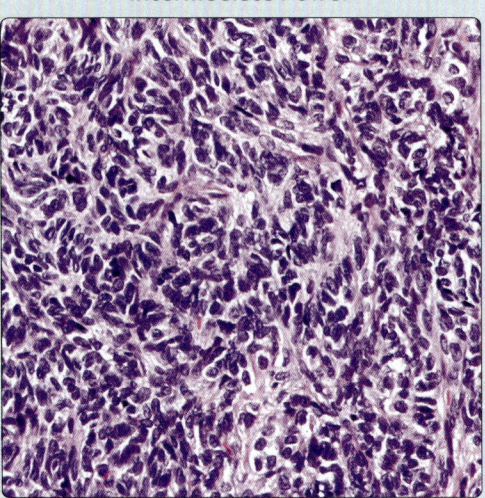

High Power

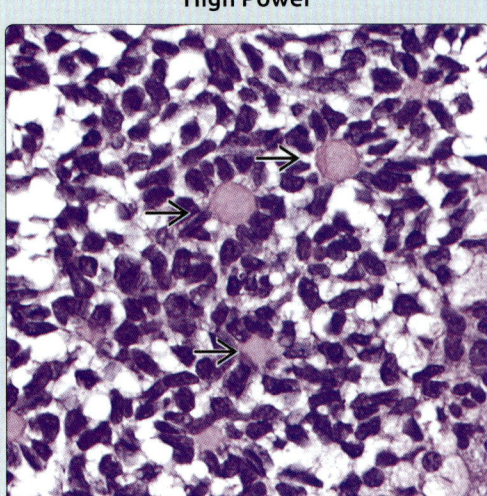

(Left) GCT shows diffuse growth pattern and focal palisading. The tumor is composed of carrot-shaped spindle cells with scant pale staining cytoplasm. No pleomorphism or necrosis is seen. When these cells predominate, unclassified sex cord stromal tumor should be included in the differential diagnosis. (Right) GCT shows typical Call-Exner bodies ➡ characterized by central eosinophilic material and palisading tumor cells resulting in a rosette appearance. The tumor cells have scant cytoplasm.

Granulosa Cell Tumor

TERMINOLOGY

Abbreviations
- Granulosa cell tumor (GCT)

Definitions
- Sex cord-stromal tumor of testis occurring in adults and resembling its counterpart of ovarian granulosa cell tumor

CLINICAL ISSUES

Epidemiology
- Incidence
  - Extremely rare; accounting for < 0.5% of all sex cord-stromal tumors
- Age
  - Range: 16-76 years (mean: 44 years)
  - Juvenile GCT occurs in 1st few months of life

Presentation
- Painless testicular mass
- May be associated with gynecomastia (~ 25%)

Treatment
- Surgical approaches
  - Curable by surgical resection in most cases
  - May be managed by partial orchiectomy

Prognosis
- Most have indolent clinical course but have malignant potential
- Metastasis has been reported (20% of cases), most frequently to retroperitoneal lymph nodes but may metastasize to liver, lungs, and bone
- Long-term follow-up is recommended for all patients

MACROSCOPIC

General Features
- Well-circumscribed, sometimes encapsulated, homogeneous, yellow to gray, firm, lobulated mass
- Cysts may be seen infrequently
- Hemorrhage or necrosis is unusual

Size
- Range: 0.5-10 cm (average: 5 cm)

MICROSCOPIC

Histologic Features
- Growth patterns: Diffuse (most common), microfollicular, trabecular, insular, macrofollicular, gyriform, or cystic
- Presence of Call-Exner bodies (eosinophilic material surrounded by palisading granulosa cells)
- Relatively uniform round or ovoid cells (carrot-shaped) with scant, lightly staining cytoplasm
- Elongated or angular nuclei with grooves (coffee bean-shaped) and 1 or 2 peripherally located nucleoli
- Focal cytologic atypia and rare mitoses; mitoses may be high with varying degree of nuclear pleomorphism
- May intermingle with seminiferous tubules and infiltrate tunica albuginea
- Some show focal theca cell differentiation or have smooth muscle or osteoid differentiation
- Rare hemorrhage, necrosis, or angiolymphatic invasion
- Features seen more often in tumors with malignant outcome: Large size (> 7 cm), frequent mitoses (> 4/10 HPF), hemorrhage, necrosis, lymphovascular invasion

ANCILLARY TESTS

Immunohistochemistry
- Positive for inhibin, Melan-A (MART-1), calretinin, actin-sm, CD56, CD99, vimentin, FOXL2, SF1, S100; focally positive for PAN-CK (AE1/AE3)
- Negative for EMA, nuclear beta-catenin, PLAP, podoplanin (D2-40), OCT3/4, LIN28, SALL4, AFP, HCG, CD30 (BerH2)

Genetic Testing
- Acquired FOXL2 mutations in a smaller proportion of these tumors

DIFFERENTIAL DIAGNOSIS

Carcinoid Tumor
- Typical organoid, insular, or trabecular growth patterns
- Diffusely positive for neuroendocrine markers, strong and diffuse CK-PAN (AE1/AE3) positive and negative for inhibin-α

Sertoli Cell Tumor
- More prominent well-formed tubules, cords, and nests
- Abundant clear or eosinophilic cytoplasm with large vesicular nuclei and prominent centrally located nucleoli
- Usually diffusely positive for CK-PAN (AE1/AE3)

Leydig Cell Tumor
- Solid growth with fine fibrous or fibromyxoid septa
- Abundant eosinophilic cytoplasm, often round nuclei and prominent nucleoli

Mixed Germ Cell and Sex Cord-Stromal Tumor (Gonadoblastoma or Unclassified)
- Prominent, rounded nests with large, seminoma-like cells
- Spindle cell or round cell unclassified stromal component or differentiated stromal component, including granulosa cell
- Positive for germ cell markers [OCT3/4, CD117, podoplanin (D2-40)] and sex cord-stromal markers [inhibin, Melan-A (MART-1), CD99] in respective cell types

DIAGNOSTIC CHECKLIST

Pathologic Interpretation Pearls
- Carrot-shaped cells with nuclear grooves and Call-Exner bodies resembling ovarian counterpart

SELECTED REFERENCES

1. Cornejo KM et al: Adult granulosa cell tumors of the testis: a report of 32 cases. Am J Surg Pathol. 38(9):1242-50, 2014
2. Lima JF et al: FOXL2 mutations in granulosa cell tumors occurring in males. Arch Pathol Lab Med. 136(7):825-8, 2012
3. Hammerich KH et al: Malignant advanced granulosa cell tumor of the adult testis: case report and review of the literature. Hum Pathol. 39(5):701-9, 2008
4. Suppiah A et al: Adult granulosa cell tumour of the testis and bony metastasis. A report of the first case of granulosa cell tumour of the testicle metastasising to bone. Urol Int. 75(1):91-3, 2005
5. Guzzo T et al: Granulosa cell tumor of the contralateral testis in a man with a history of cryptorchism. Urol Int. 72(1):85-7, 2004

Granulosa Cell Tumor

(Left) GCT with gyriform, trabecular, macro-, and microfollicular growth patterns is shown. The entire tumor should have similar cytologic features to be designated as GCT, as tumors may contain other sex cord-stromal elements, justifying the classification of a mixed sex cord-stromal tumor. **(Right)** The tumor cells of a GCT have angulated nuclei, pale staining chromatin, and clear to lightly eosinophilic cytoplasm. Occasional nuclear grooves ⇒ are present.

Architectural Features
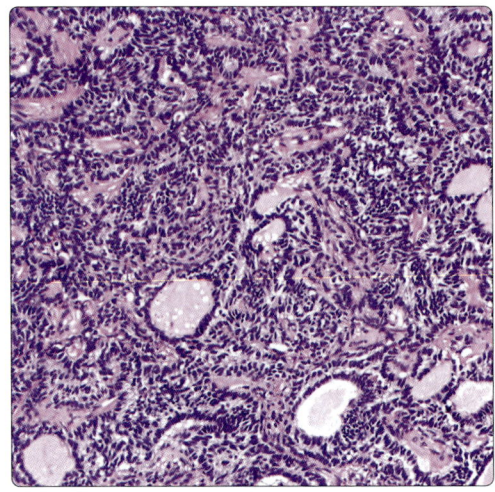

Cytologic Features
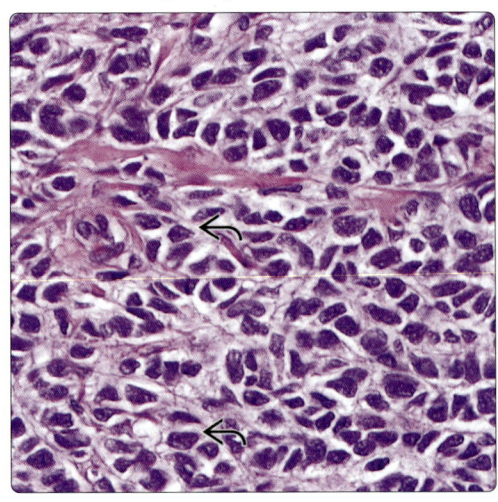

(Left) High-power view of GCT shows sheets of tumor cells and a Call-Exner body ⇒. The tumor cells have elongated or angulated nuclei with occasional nuclear grooves ⇒ and scant cytoplasm. GCT is positive for sex cord-stromal markers, including inhibin, Melan-A (MART-1), CD99, and WT1. **(Right)** High-power photomicrograph of GCT shows macrofollicles ⇒ with eosinophilic amorphous edematous fluid and microfollicles with central eosinophilic material (Call-Exner body ⇒).

Call-Exner Body
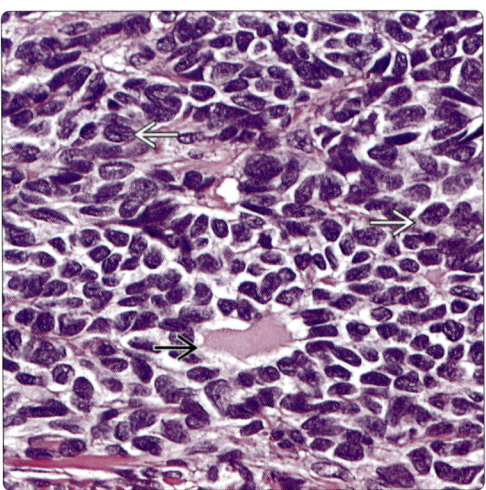

Macro- and Microfollicles
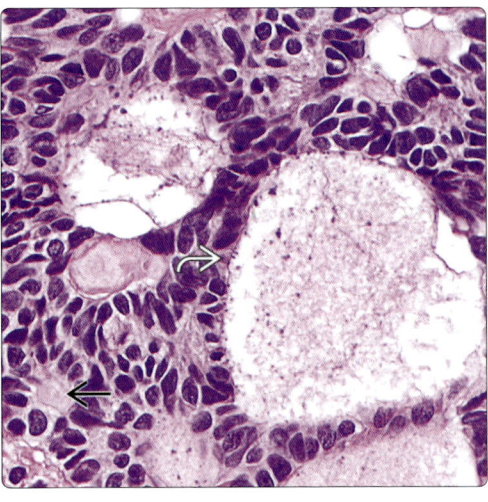

(Left) GCT shows epithelial growth pattern with nests or trabeculae composed of elongated hyperchromatic tumor cells. Although small follicular arrangement ⇒ is present, no well-defined Call-Exner bodies are seen. **(Right)** GCT shows nests ⇒ of tumor cells with ovoid to round nuclei, small nucleoli, and occasional nuclear grooves ⇒. Mitotic rate is generally low in these tumors and rarely a prominent fibrothecomatous pattern may be present.

Trabecular Architecture
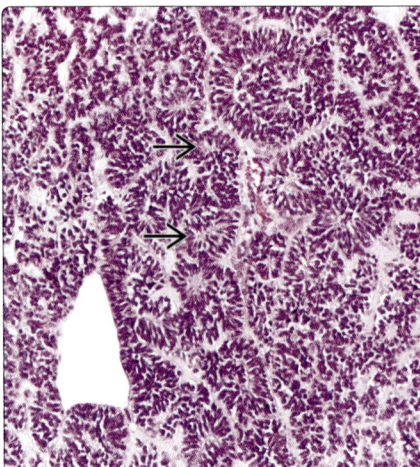

Cytologic Features
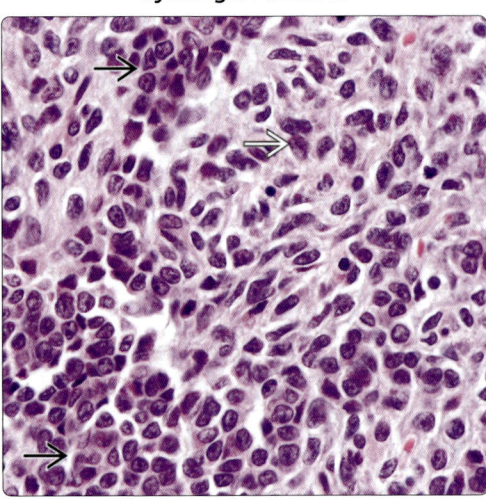

Granulosa Cell Tumor

Spindle Cell Morphology

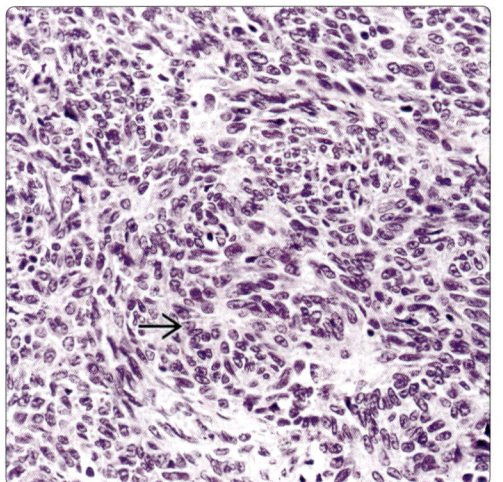

Call-Exner Bodies

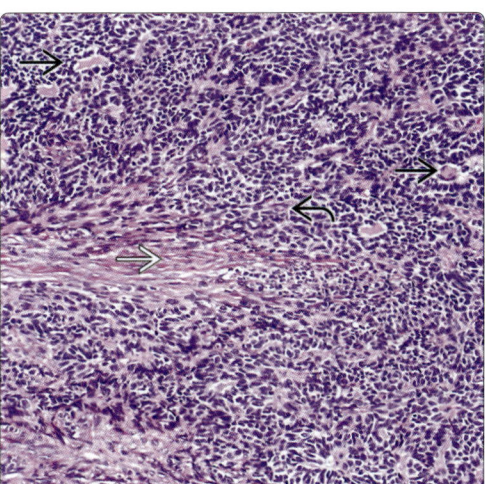

(Left) Some GCTs show a more prominent spindle cell appearance (pseudosarcomatous appearance). Vague follicular differentiation with rosette appearance ⇨ is discernible. *(Right)* GCT has numerous microfollicles (Call-Exner bodies ⇨) intermingled with spindle cells ⇨ and some of them with possible myogenic differentiation ⇨ showing fibrillar cytoplasm.

Cellular Atypia

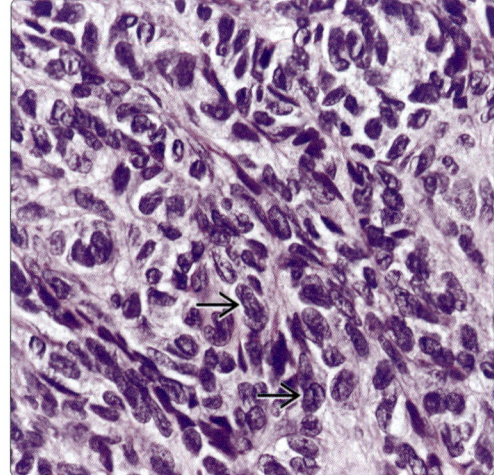

IHC: Inhibin-α

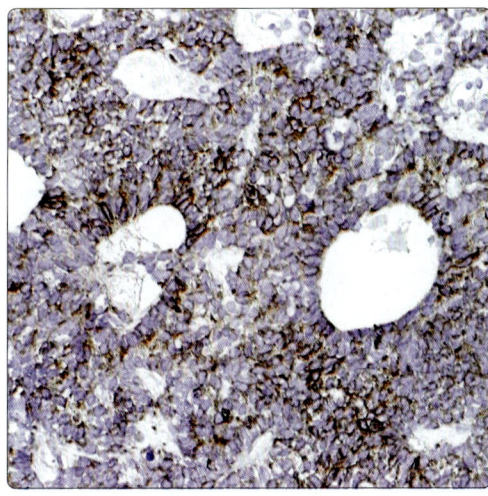

(Left) GCT with pseudosarcomatous appearance is shown. Random cellular pleomorphism and crowding are evident. The cells are carrot-shaped with occasional nuclear grooves ⇨, which are characteristic cytologic features of GCT. *(Right)* Tumor cells of GCT are diffusely positive for inhibin-α, a diagnostic immunostain for all sex cord-stromal tumors. GCT is positive for sex cord-stromal markers, including inhibin, Melan-A (MART-1), SF1, calretinin, CD99, and WT1. EMA/MUC1 and CK7 are usually negative.

Differential Diagnosis: Carcinoid Tumor

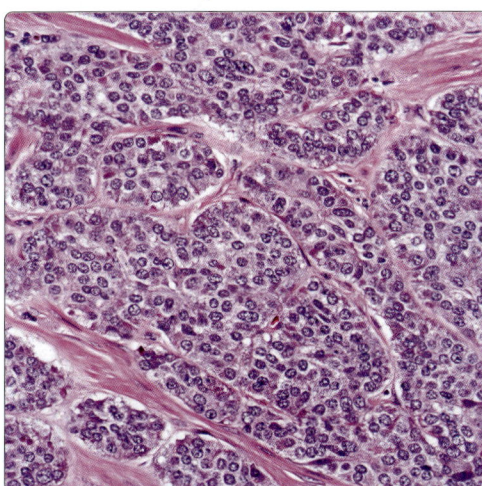

Differential Diagnosis: Leydig Cell Tumor

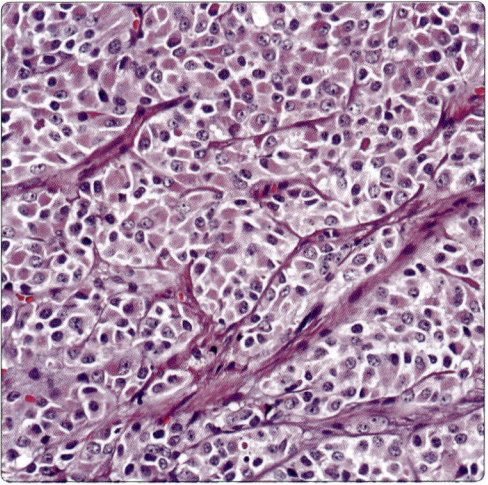

(Left) Carcinoid tumor has typical solid nests or trabecular growth pattern. Unlike granular cell tumor, the tumor cells are oval to round and have salt and pepper chromatin and abundant granular eosinophilic cytoplasm. *(Right)* This example of Leydig cell tumor shows solid sheets of tumor cells with prominent eosinophilic cytoplasm (rhabdoid appearance), round nuclei, and prominent nucleoli.

Juvenile Granulosa Cell Tumor

KEY FACTS

TERMINOLOGY
- Testicular tumor that is multicystic and composed of multiple follicles lined by granulosa and theca-like cells

CLINICAL ISSUES
- Rare, but is most common congenital testicular neoplasm (6.6% of all prepubertal testicular tumors)
- Infants younger than 2 years old; most common testis tumor in infants < 6 months

MACROSCOPIC
- Well-circumscribed or partially encapsulated multicystic mass with solid yellow and variable papillary areas

MICROSCOPIC
- Multiple irregular cystic areas interspersed with solid areas
- Variably sized follicles lined by bland-looking oval round cells arranged in single or multiple layers with outer layers resembling theca cells
- Granulosa cells have round to ovoid nuclei, inconspicuous nucleoli, and scant to vacuolated cytoplasm
- Mitotic activity is usually evident and often prominent
- Basophilic to faintly eosinophilic fluid within follicles
- Call-Exner bodies and nuclear grooves, often seen in adult granulosa cell tumor are absent

ANCILLARY TESTS
- Positive for CAM5.2, vimentin, S100, inhibin-α, calretinin, SOX9; focally positive for actin-sm, CK-PAN and CD99
- Negative for EMA/MUC1, α-fetoprotein, PLAP, podoplanin (D2-40), OCT3/4, SALL4, glypican-3, CD45 (LCA)

TOP DIFFERENTIAL DIAGNOSES
- Yolk sac tumor
- Sex cord-stromal tumor, unclassified
- Rhabdomyosarcoma

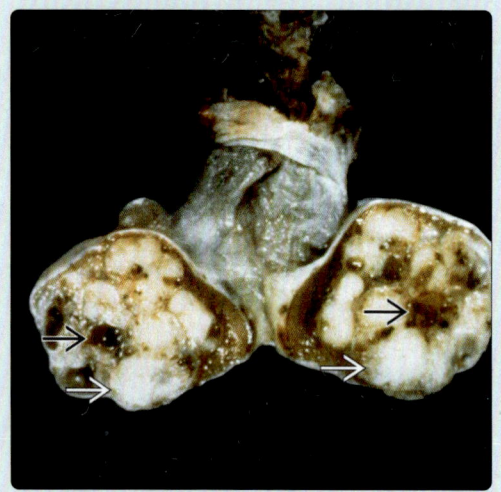

Juvenile Granulosa Cell Tumor: Gross

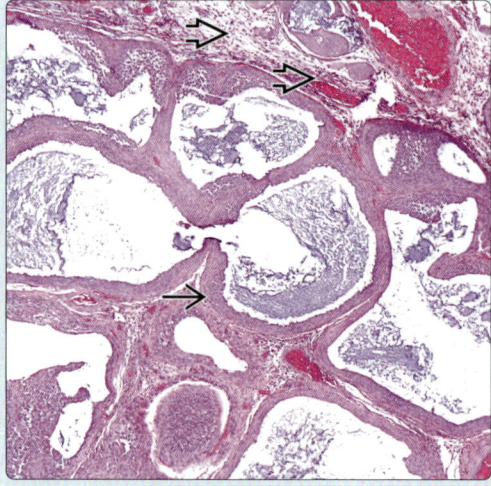

Juvenile Granulosa Cell Tumor: Multicystic

(Left) Juvenile granulosa cell tumor (JGCT) with lobulated, white-tan cut surface is shown. The tumor has cystic ➡ and solid areas with myxoid change ➡. Some JGCT may be predominantly cystic with gelatinous fluid. *(Right)* JGCT, which is relatively well circumscribed from the surrounding testis ➡, is composed of multicystic follicular spaces lined by multilayers of granulosa cells ➡ containing basophilic fluid. The age of patients (congenital or less than 2 years) is helpful.

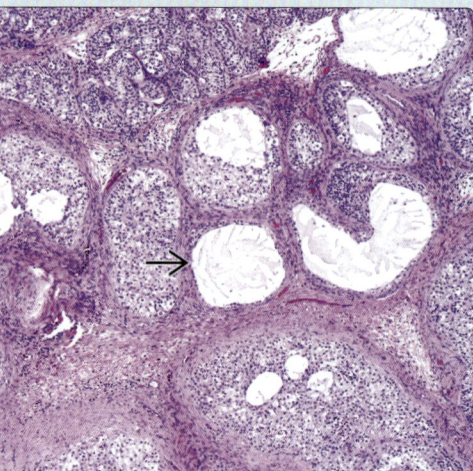

Juvenile Granulosa Cell Tumor: Cystic Follicles

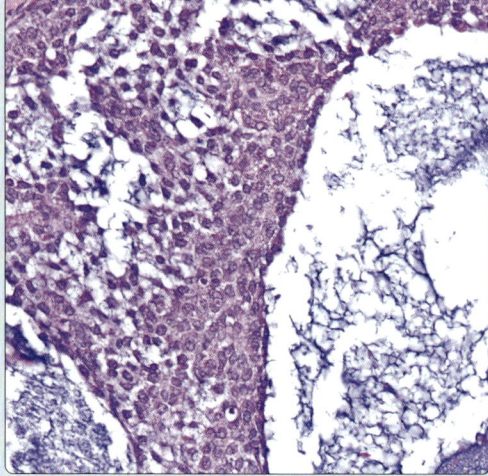

Juvenile Granulosa Cell Tumor: Cytology and Secretion

(Left) JGCT is composed of cystic/follicular structures ➡ and solid tumor component. The follicular/cystic lumen is filled with basophilic secretion characteristic of JGCT. *(Right)* JGCT has solid and follicular areas composed of cells with uniform round to oval nuclei and moderate cytoplasm. Prominent extracellular and intraluminal basophilic mucinous material is present.

Juvenile Granulosa Cell Tumor

TERMINOLOGY

Abbreviations
- Juvenile granulosa cell tumor (JGCT)

Definitions
- Testicular tumor that is multicystic and composed of multiple follicles lined by granulosa and theca-like cells occurring predominantly in infants

CLINICAL ISSUES

Epidemiology
- Incidence
  o Extremely rare in testis
  o Most common testicular tumor in infants
  o 6.6% of all prepubertal testicular tumors
- Age
  o Infants younger than 2 years (most younger than 6 months)
  o Rarely occurs in adults

Presentation
- Painless scrotal or abdominal mass, almost invariably unilateral
- Associations
  o Undescended testes
  o Gonadal dysgenesis with chromosomal abnormality affecting Y chromosome or 45X/46XY mosaicism (Denys-Drash syndrome)
- Contralateral testis is often undescended
- No known presentation with gynecomastia or endocrine disorders, unlike adult tumors

Treatment
- Surgical approaches
  o Orchiectomy is curative
  o Partial orchiectomy (testis sparing) may be option

Prognosis
- Clinically benign
- Malignant behavior or metastasis has not been reported

MACROSCOPIC

General Features
- Well-circumscribed or partially encapsulated multicystic mass with solid yellow and papillary areas

Size
- Range: 0.8-6.0 cm

MICROSCOPIC

Histologic Features
- Multiple irregular cystic areas interspersed with solid areas
- Variably sized follicles lined by oval to round cells arranged in single or multiple layers with outer layers resembling theca cells
- Granulosa cells have round to ovoid nuclei, inconspicuous nucleoli, and scant to vacuolated cytoplasm
- Mitotic activity is usually evident and often prominent
- Theca-like cells are elongated and have scant cytoplasm
- Basophilic to faintly eosinophilic fluid within follicles
- Call-Exner bodies and nuclear grooves that are often seen in adult GCT are absent
- Sarcomatoid transformation has not been reported, in contrast to ovarian counterpart

ANCILLARY TESTS

Immunohistochemistry
- Positive for CAM5.2, vimentin, S100, inhibin-α, calretinin, SOX9; focally positive for actin-sm, CK-PAN, and CD99
- Negative for EMA/MUC1, α-fetoprotein, podoplanin (D2-40), OCT3/4, glypican-3, SALL4, CD45 (LCA)

Genetic Testing
- Some patients may have abnormal karyotypes including mosaics (45, X/47XYY or 45, X/46X, r(Y)
- $FOXL2$ mutation has been tested in only one case and was negative

DIFFERENTIAL DIAGNOSIS

Yolk Sac Tumor
- Occurs more commonly in older age group (> 1 year)
- Variety of patterns, including microcystic and reticular, within same tumor
- Cysts are lined by single layer of cells with greater atypia
- Presence of intracellular or extracellular eosinophilic hyaline globules, basement membrane material and Schiller-Duval bodies
- Positive for germ cell markers (α-fetoprotein, SALL4, glypican-3) and cytokeratin
- Negative for S100 and inhibin-α, calretinin

Sex Cord-Stromal Tumor, Unclassified
- Variable morphologic patterns with biphasic epithelioid and spindle cell components
- Lack of cystic follicles

Rhabdomyosarcoma
- More typically in paratesticular location
- Lacks follicle formation; small round blue cells with rhabdomyoblasts
- Positive for desmin, MYOD1, and myogenin

SELECTED REFERENCES

1. Kao CS et al: Juvenile granulosa cell tumors of the testis: a clinicopathologic study of 70 cases with emphasis on its wide morphologic spectrum. Am J Surg Pathol. 39(9):1159-69, 2015
2. Lima JF et al: FOXL2 mutations in granulosa cell tumors occurring in males. Arch Pathol Lab Med. 136(7):825-8, 2012
3. Dudani R et al: Juvenile granulosa cell tumor of testis: case report and review of literature. Am J Perinatol. 25(4):229-31, 2008
4. Alexiev BA et al: Testicular juvenile granulosa cell tumor in a newborn: case report and review of the literature. Int J Surg Pathol. 15(3):321-5, 2007
5. Shukla AR et al: Juvenile granulosa cell tumor of the testis:: contemporary clinical management and pathological diagnosis. J Urol. 171(5):1900-2, 2004
6. Fagin R et al: Juvenile granulosa cell tumor of the testis. Urology. 62(2):351, 2003
7. Perez-Atayde AR et al: Juvenile granulosa cell tumor of the infantile testis. Evidence of a dual epithelial-smooth muscle differentiation. Am J Surg Pathol. 20(1):72-9, 1996
8. Groisman GM et al: Juvenile granulosa cell tumor of the testis: a comparative immunohistochemical study with normal infantile gonads. Pediatr Pathol. 13(4):389-400, 1993
9. Nistal M et al: Juvenile granulosa cell tumor of the testis. Arch Pathol Lab Med. 112(11):1129-32, 1988

Juvenile Granulosa Cell Tumor

(Left) JGCT is composed of follicular & solid components of tumor with fibrous stroma. The follicular lumen is filled with basophilic secretions. Also seen are spindle theca-like cells in the stroma ⇨. Separated from the tumor by a thin fibrous tissue are uninvolved immature seminiferous tubules ⇨. (Right) The tumor cells in both cystic/follicular and solid areas of JGCT are similar. Cellular theca-like spindle cells ⇨ are seen in the stroma. When myxoid areas are prominent, it has resemblance to yolk sac tumor.

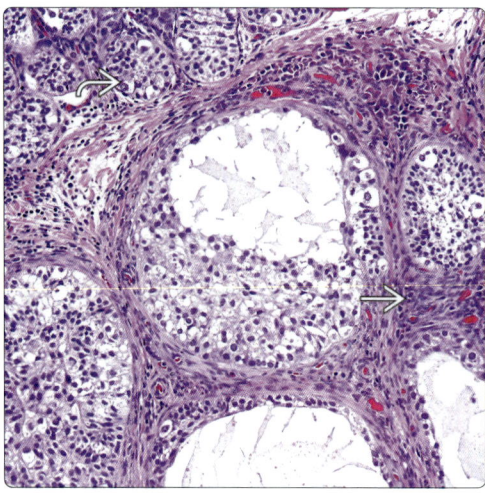
Juvenile Granulosa Cell Tumor: Stroma

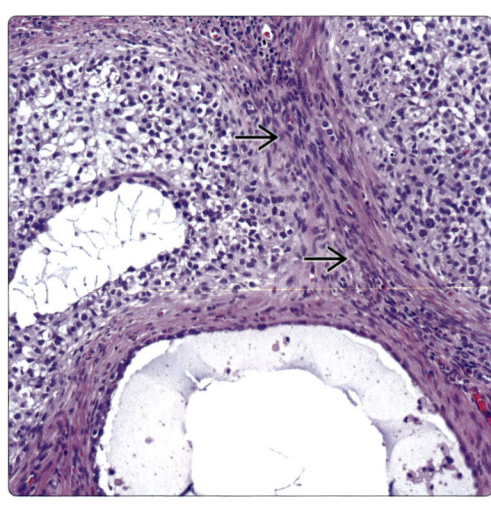
Juvenile Granulosa Cell Tumor: Stroma

(Left) JGCT with mixed solid and follicular patterns is shown. The tumor cells in both areas are similar and have round to ovoid nuclei, inconspicuous nucleoli, and eosinophilic to vacuolated cytoplasm. Mitotic activity is variable and frequently brisk (not shown here). (Right) High-power photomicrograph of JGCT shows a follicle lined by uniform tumor cells with oval to round nuclei and moderate amounts of pale eosinophilic and vacuolated cytoplasm. The basophilic material is positive for mucicarmine (if performed).

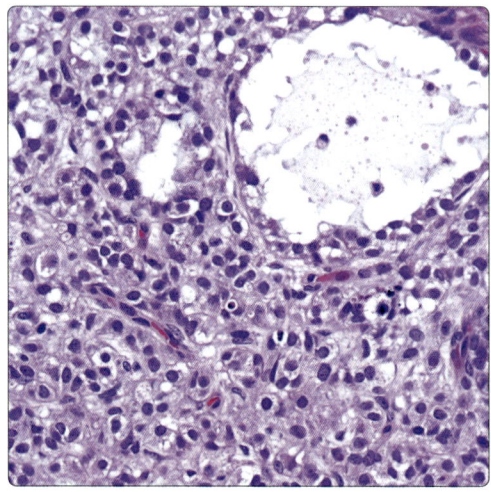
Juvenile Granulosa Cell Tumor: Solid

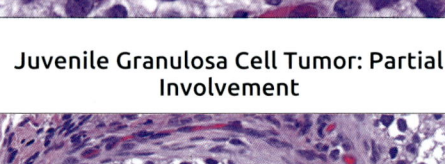
Juvenile Granulosa Cell Tumor: Basophilic Secretion

(Left) A large cystic follicle is partially involved by JGCT. Residual immature seminiferous tubules lined by Sertoli cells ⇨ are seen at the periphery. Basophilic secretions, a hallmark of the tumor, are a helpful feature. (Right) High-power photomicrograph shows a large cystic follicle partially involved by JGCT cells ⇨. Residual seminiferous tubule contains Sertoli cells ⇨ and immature germ cells with large nuclei ⇨. There is absence of germ cell neoplasia in situ.

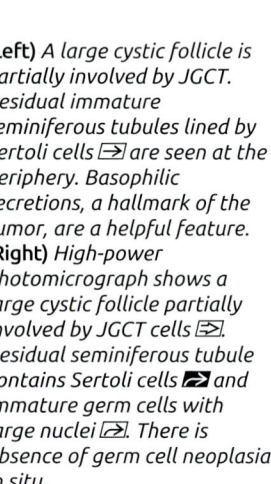

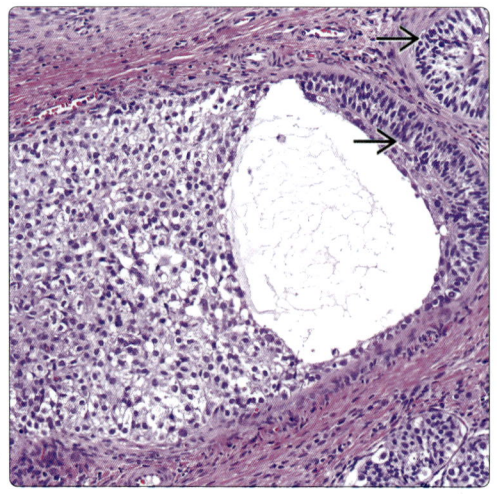
Juvenile Granulosa Cell Tumor: Partial Involvement

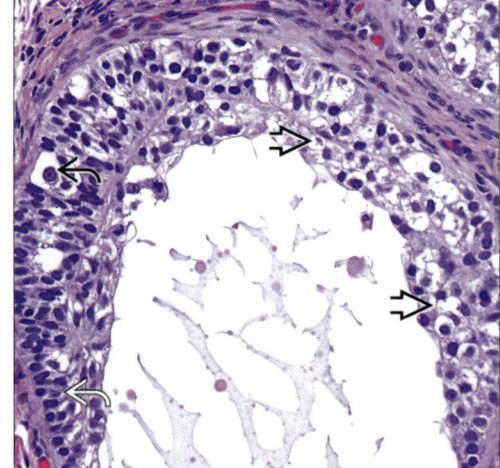
Juvenile Granulosa Cell Tumor: Partial Involvement

Juvenile Granulosa Cell Tumor

Juvenile Granulosa Cell Tumor: Degeneration

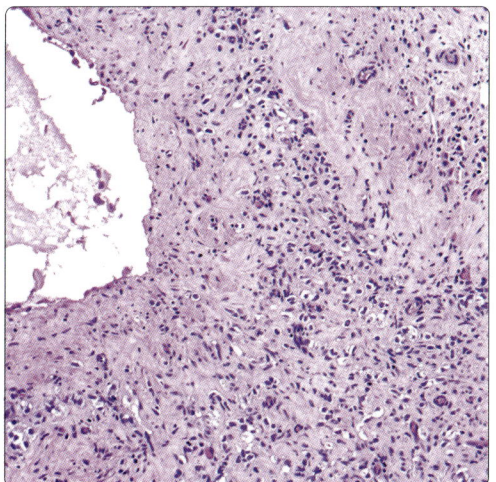

Juvenile Granulosa Cell Tumor: Mitoses

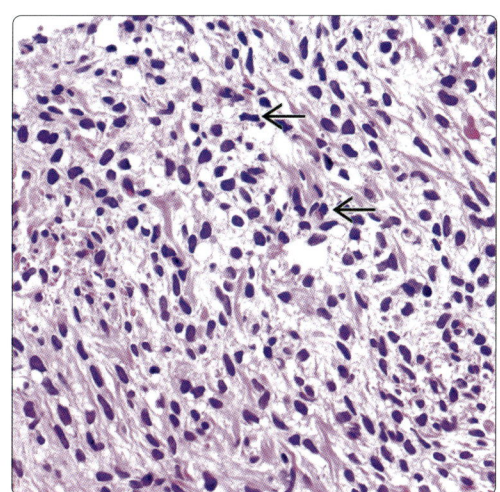

(Left) The cystic and solid components of JGCT show degeneration and fibrosis with paucity of tumor cells and stromal collagenization in the solid area. *(Right)* The solid area in a JGCT is shown. Medium- to large-sized tumor cells are arranged in sheets. The nuclei lack nuclear grooves and have numerous mitoses ➡. There is abundant clear to eosinophilic and vacuolated cytoplasm in the tumor shown in this focus.

Juvenile Granulosa Cell Tumor: Solid

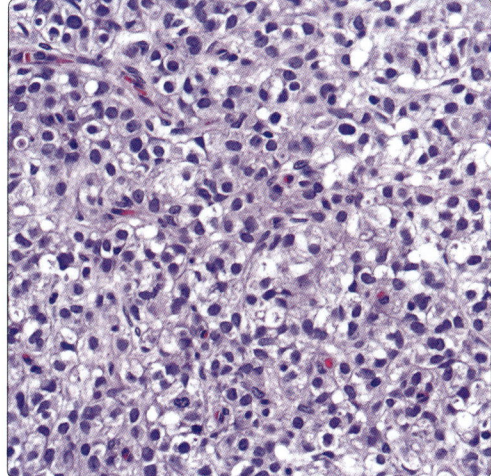

Juvenile Granulosa Cell Tumor: Solid

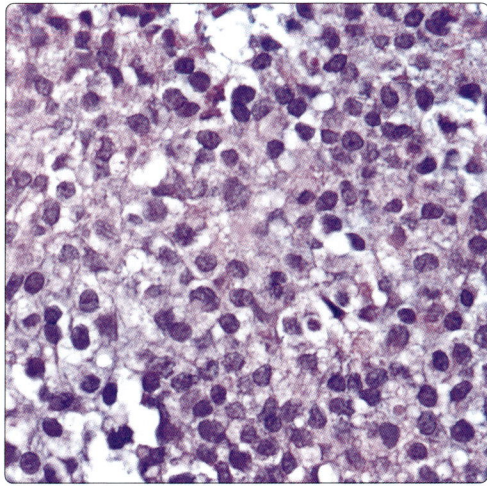

(Left) The solid area of JGCT shows uniform tumor cells. Nuclear pleomorphism or necrosis is not seen. *(Right)* A solid area of JGCT is shown with relatively uniform tumor cells with moderate amounts of pale eosinophilic and vacuolated cytoplasm, a feature that is not typically seen in adult GCT. Call-Exner-like structures and nuclear grooves are not present.

Juvenile Granulosa Cell Tumor: Vacuolated Cytoplasm

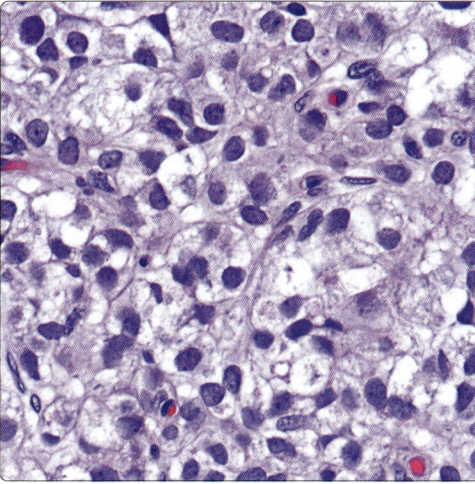

Juvenile Granulosa Cell Tumor: Reticular-Cystic

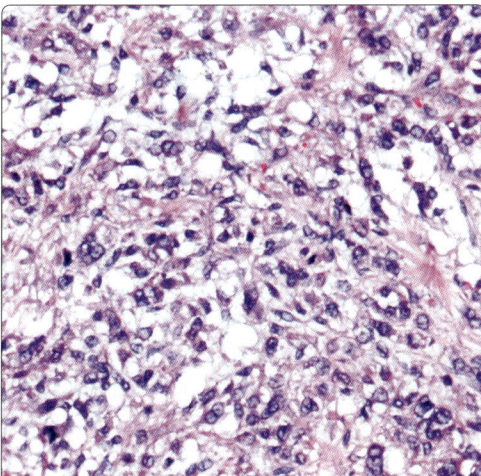

(Left) High-power photomicrograph of JGCT shows tumor cells that are relatively uniform with ovoid to round nuclei, occasional small nucleoli, and abundant pale eosinophilic and vacuolated cytoplasm. Mitotic activity may be brisk. The cells of JGCT are not carrot-shaped and lack nuclear grooves. *(Right)* High-power view of a JGCT shows reticular-cystic pattern of tumor cells with fibromyxoid stroma, mimicking yolk sac tumor.

Testicular Tumor of Adrenogenital Syndrome

KEY FACTS

TERMINOLOGY
- Benign bilateral testicular tumor in patients with congenital adrenal hyperplasia leading to growth of adrenal-like cells in testis that resembles Leydig cell tumor

CLINICAL ISSUES
- Age: Children to early adult (average: 22.5 yr)
- Presentation
  - Bilateral orchialgia (92%)
  - Testicular masses (2/3 palpable)
- Exogenous high-dose corticosteroids are standard medical treatment (pain control, regression of tumor)

MACROSCOPIC
- Well-circumscribed but not encapsulated, dark brown, lobulated mass with fibrous septa
- Often bilateral (83%), frequently multiple nodules

MICROSCOPIC
- Sheets, nests, cords, nodules, or diffuse proliferation of large cells separated by band of fibrous tissue
- Polyhedral or polygonal cells resembling Leydig cells
- Abundant eosinophilic cytoplasm with lipofuscin pigment
- Centrally located nuclei and prominent nucleoli
- Frequent nuclear pleomorphism, but no or rare mitoses
- Lack of Reinke crystalloid material
- Atrophic or sclerotic seminiferous tubules present within lesion

ANCILLARY TESTS
- Positive for inhibin, Melan-A (MART-1), CD56, and synaptophysin

TOP DIFFERENTIAL DIAGNOSES
- Leydig cell tumor
- Leydig cell hyperplasia
- Steroid cell nodules with other adrenal diseases

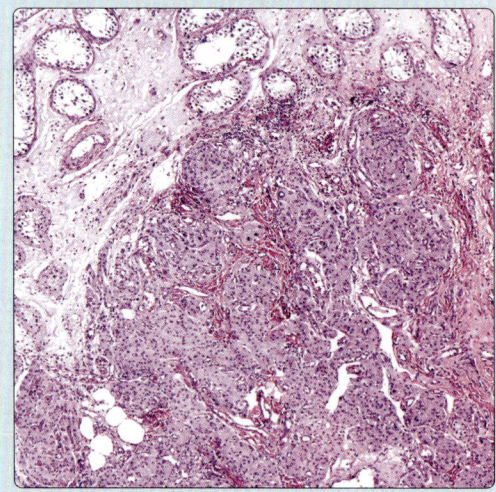

Testicular Tumor of Adrenogenital Syndrome: Well Circumscribed

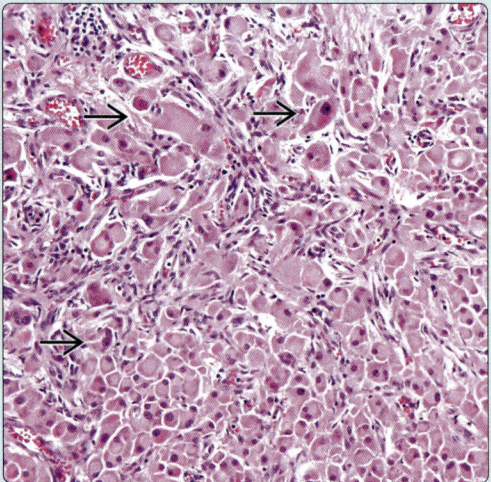

Testicular Tumor of Adrenogenital Syndrome: Cytology

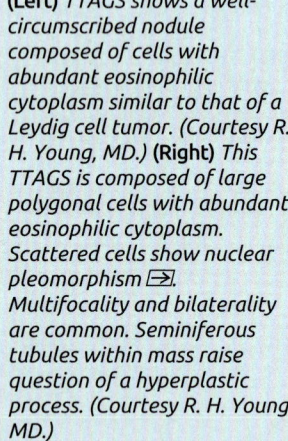

(Left) TTAGS shows a well-circumscribed nodule composed of cells with abundant eosinophilic cytoplasm similar to that of a Leydig cell tumor. (Courtesy R. H. Young, MD.) (Right) This TTAGS is composed of large polygonal cells with abundant eosinophilic cytoplasm. Scattered cells show nuclear pleomorphism ⇨. Multifocality and bilaterality are common. Seminiferous tubules within mass raise question of a hyperplastic process. (Courtesy R. H. Young, MD.)

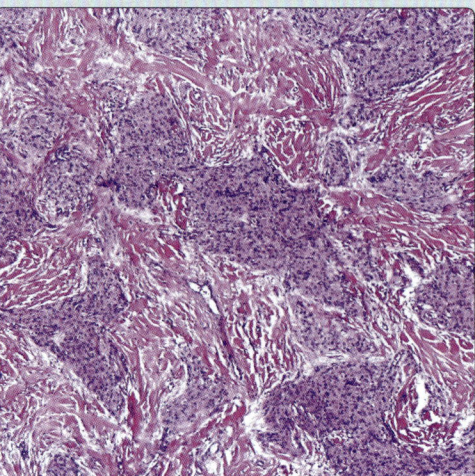

Testicular Tumor of Adrenogenital Syndrome: Collagenous Stroma

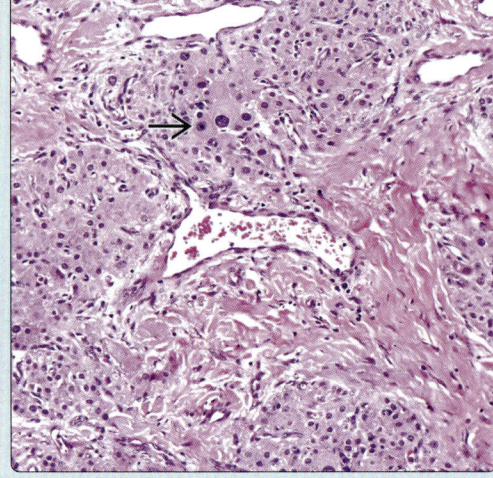

Testicular Tumor of Adrenogenital Syndrome: Nuclear Pleomorphism

(Left) This TTAGS shows nests of polygonal cells with abundant eosinophilic cytoplasm separated by broad bands of collagenous stroma. Viewed in isolation, the similarity with Leydig cell tumor is marked. (Right) This photomicrograph shows nodules of eosinophilic cells with dense hyalinization with dilated vascular channels. There are scattered cells with nuclear pleomorphism ⇨. Reinke crystals are absent in these tumors.

Testicular Tumor of Adrenogenital Syndrome

TERMINOLOGY

Definitions
- Benign bilateral testicular lesions in patients with congenital adrenal hyperplasia leading to growth of adrenal-like cells in testis that resemble Leydig cell tumor
- Bilaterality, multifocality, and response to medical treatment argue against this being neoplastic lesion

ETIOLOGY/PATHOGENESIS

Developmental Anomaly
- 21-hydroxylase deficiency (most common)
- Other associated conditions: 11-hydroxylase deficiency, Cushing disease, Addison disease, and other idiopathic enzyme defects
- Cellular origin uncertain; hilar pluripotential cells, adrenal cortical rest cells, Leydig cells are possible candidates

CLINICAL ISSUES

Epidemiology
- Incidence
  - Rare; few dozen cases reported in literature
- Age
  - Children to early adult (average: 22.5 yr)

Presentation
- Bilateral orchialgia (92%)
- Testicular masses (2/3 palpable)
- Symptoms related to steroid hormone deficiency
  - Salt-losing form of adrenal disorder in 2/3 and nonsalt-losing form in 1/3
- Isosexual precocious puberty

Laboratory Tests
- Steroid hormone evaluation (increased ACTH)
- Tumor markers (AFP, hCG, LDH) to exclude possible germ cell tumor

Treatment
- Drugs
  - Exogenous high-dose corticosteroids are mainstay of medical treatment (pain control and regression of tumor)
- Surgical approaches
  - Tumor enucleation or partial orchiectomy for persistently painful masses and steroid-unresponsive lesions in setting of bilaterality

Prognosis
- Benign lesion, symptoms relieved by steroid therapy or surgery
- Very rarely associated with seminoma and rare reported cases of malignant transformation

MACROSCOPIC

General Features
- Well-circumscribed but not encapsulated, dark brown, lobulated mass with fibrous septa
- Often bilateral (83%), frequently multiple nodules
- Most commonly present in hilar region (86%)

Size
- Range: 0.5-10 cm
- Larger size tumor usually seen in older patients

MICROSCOPIC

Histologic Features
- Sheets, nests, cords, nodules, or diffuse proliferation of large cells separated by bands of fibrous tissue
- Polyhedral or polygonal cells resembling Leydig cells
- Abundant eosinophilic cytoplasm with lipofuscin pigment, which may be prominent and diffuse
- Centrally located nuclei and prominent nucleoli
- Frequent nuclear pleomorphism but no or rare mitoses
- Crystalloids of Reinke are absent
- May have adipocytic metaplasia and lymphoid aggregates
- Extensive fibrosis may be present
- Atrophic or sclerotic seminiferous tubules present within lesion
- Myelolipomatous component has been reported

ANCILLARY TESTS

Immunohistochemistry
- Positive for inhibin, Melan-A (MART-1), CD56, and synaptophysin
- Negative for cytokeratin, androgen receptor

DIFFERENTIAL DIAGNOSIS

Leydig Cell Tumor
- Usually nonsymptomatic and unilateral
- Nuclear pleomorphism, fibrosis, lymphoid aggregates, and lipofuscin pigment less common
- Reinke crystals present in about 1/3 of tumors

Leydig Cell Hyperplasia
- Small nodules (< 0.5 cm)
- Crystalloids of Reinke are present

Steroid Cell Nodules With Other Adrenal Diseases
- Patients with bilateral adrenalectomy and rapidly growing pituitary adenoma
- Patients with Carney complex (not large cell calcifying Sertoli cell tumor)
- Clinical correlation important

SELECTED REFERENCES

1. Ulbright TM et al: Testicular and paratesticular tumors and tumor-like lesions in the first 2 decades. Semin Diagn Pathol. 31(5):323-81, 2014
2. Reisch N et al: Testicular adrenal rest tumors develop independently of long-term disease control: a longitudinal analysis of 50 adult men with congenital adrenal hyperplasia due to classic 21-hydroxylase deficiency. J Clin Endocrinol Metab. 98(11):E1820-6, 2013
3. Wang Z et al: Histopathological and immunophenotypic features of testicular tumour of the adrenogenital syndrome. Histopathology. 58(7):1013-8, 2011
4. Rutgers JL et al: The testicular "tumor" of the adrenogenital syndrome. A report of six cases and review of the literature on testicular masses in patients with adrenocortical disorders. Am J Surg Pathol. 12(7):503-13, 1988

Testicular Tumor of Adrenogenital Syndrome

(Left) Low-power view of a TTAGS with dense fibrosis at the periphery of the tumor shows a mild lymphocytic infiltrate ⇒. Atrophic and hyalinized seminiferous tubules ⇒ are seen outside the confines of the lesion. **(Right)** At the periphery of a TTAGS, nests or clusters of tumor cells are surrounded by fibrous stroma and foci of lymphoid infiltrates ⇒. Nuclear pleomorphism ⇒ is evident. The adjacent seminiferous tubules show lack of spermatogenesis.

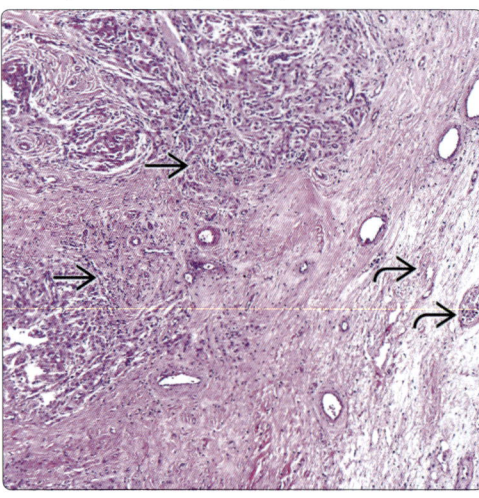
Testicular Tumor of Adrenogenital Syndrome: Lymphocytic Infiltrate

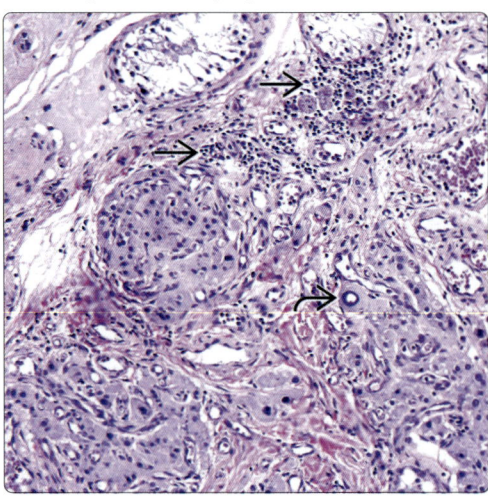
Testicular Tumor of Adrenogenital Syndrome: Lymphoid Infiltrate

(Left) This photomicrograph shows the cytologic features of TTAGS. The tumor cells are polygonal and have round to ovoid nuclei, prominent nucleoli, and characteristic abundant eosinophilic and granular cytoplasm. Lipofuscin pigment ⇒ is seen in some cells. **(Right)** TTAGS with clusters of tumor cells amidst prominent vascularity and stromal fibrosis is shown. The tumor cells ⇒ are distinguished by their round-to-ovoid nuclei, prominent nucleoli, and abundant eosinophilic cytoplasm.

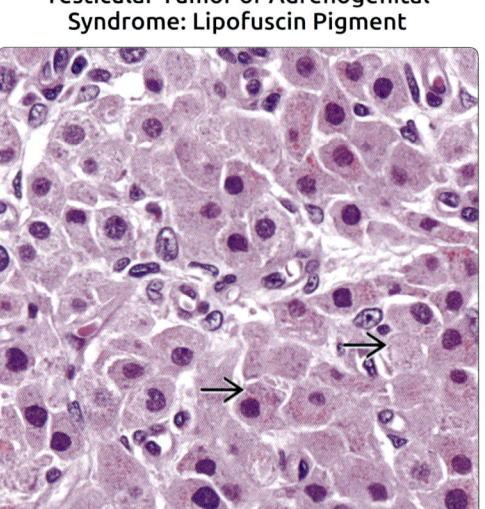
Testicular Tumor of Adrenogenital Syndrome: Lipofuscin Pigment

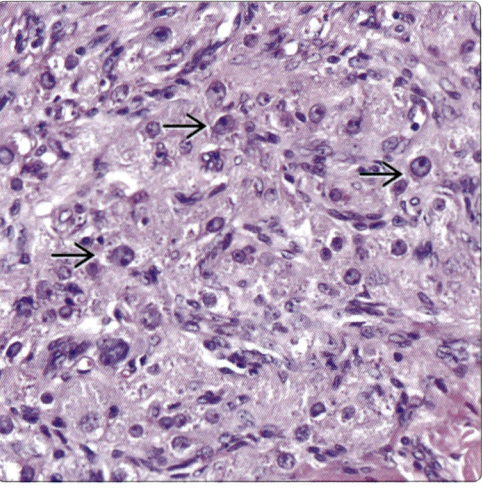
Testicular Tumor of Adrenogenital Syndrome: Vasculature

(Left) TTAGS shows marked nuclear pleomorphism, prominent nucleoli, and lipofuscin pigment. The atypia is usually random in nature, typical of endocrine atypia. Lipofuscin is more common in TTAGS than in Leydig cell tumors. **(Right)** Photomicrograph of TTAGS shows nuclear pleomorphism, irregular nuclear contours, and prominent nucleoli ⇒. The tumor cells are separated in this case by edematous stroma. There is intracytoplasmic lipofuscin and absence of Reinke crystals.

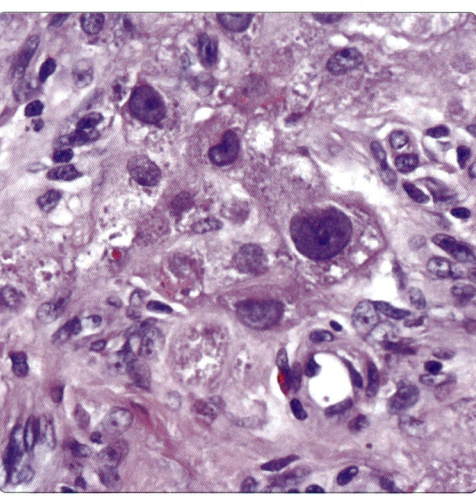
Testicular Tumor of Adrenogenital Syndrome: Nuclear Pleomorphism

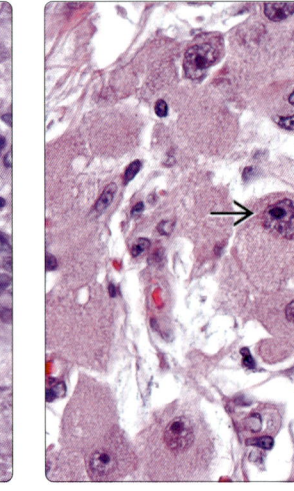
Testicular Tumor of Adrenogenital Syndrome: Prominent Nucleoli

Testicular Tumor of Adrenogenital Syndrome

Testicular Tumor of Adrenogenital Syndrome: Branching Cords

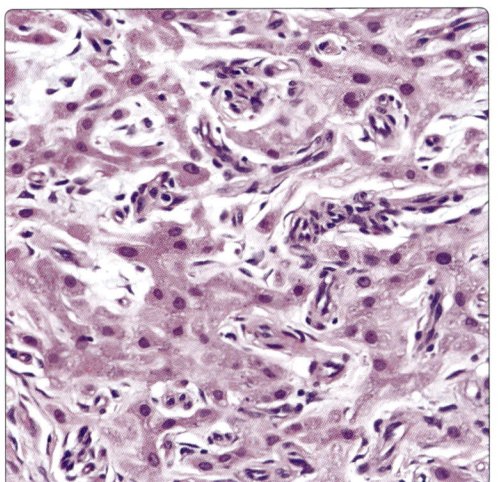

Testicular Tumor of Adrenogenital Syndrome: Fibrovascular Septa

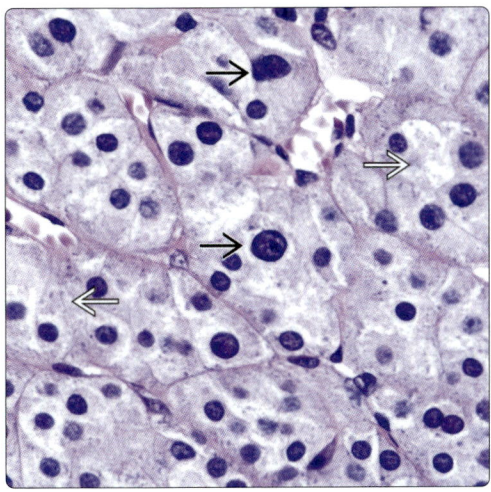

(Left) High-power photomicrograph of TTAGS shows irregularly branching cords of tumor cells separated by a fibromyxoid stroma with prominent vascularity. In this particular example, the cell borders are not well delineated. (Right) In this example, the TTAGS shows a prominent nested arrangement with delicate fibrovascular septa. The cells have a slightly clear appearance with spotty nuclear pleomorphism ⇨ and prominent nucleoli. Lipofuscin pigment ⇨ is also discernible.

Testicular Tumor of Adrenogenital Syndrome: Adipocytic Metaplasia

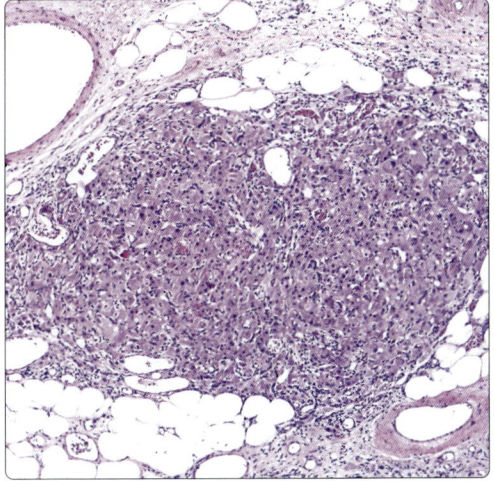

Testicular Tumor of Adrenogenital Syndrome: Adipocytic Metaplasia

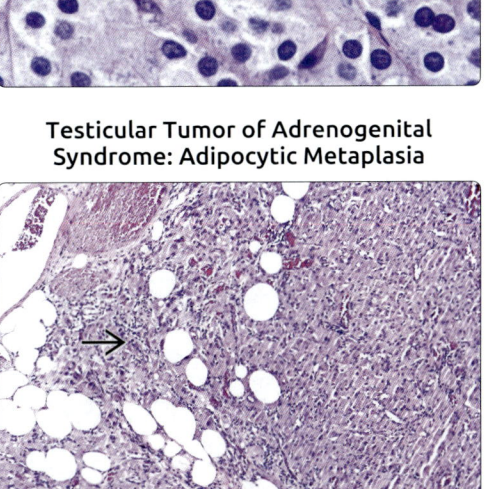

(Left) This photomicrograph shows a nodule of TTAGS with adipocytic metaplasia at the periphery as well as within the nodule. This finding is more common in TTAGS than in Leydig cell tumor but by itself is not discriminatory. (Right) This photomicrograph of TTAGS shows sheets of tumor cells with adipocytic metaplasia within the nodule. A lymphoid infiltrate ⇨ is also present within the fibrous septa.

Leydig Cell Tumor: Differential

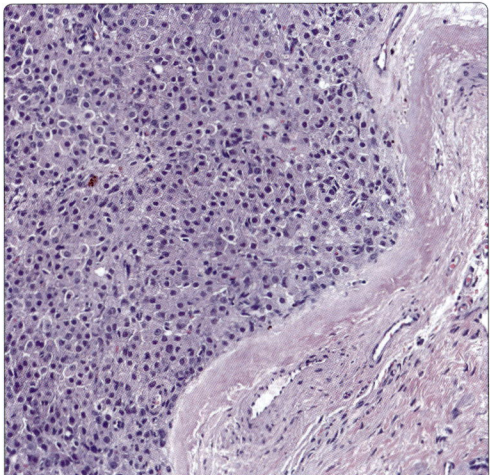

Leydig Cell Tumor: Differential

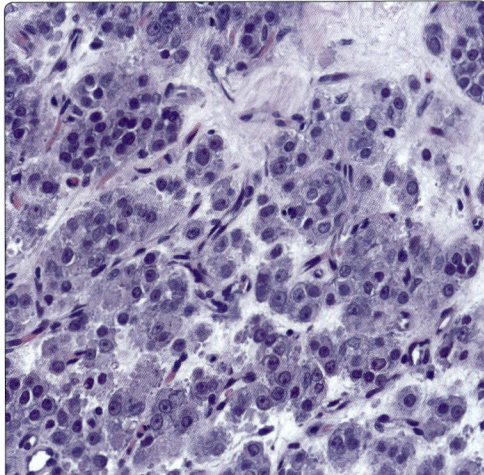

(Left) A well-circumscribed Leydig cell tumor is composed of relatively uniform cells with abundant eosinophilic cytoplasm with delicate sinusoidal vessels. (Right) Leydig cell tumor shows monomorphic population of tumor cells with abundant eosinophilic cytoplasm, round nuclei, and prominent nucleoli. Compared to TTAGS, Leydig cell tumor has less nuclear pleomorphism, fibrosis, lymphoid aggregates, and lipofuscin pigment. Clinical history is most important in helping to arrive at the correct diagnosis.

Sex Cord-Stromal Tumor, Mixed/Unclassified

KEY FACTS

TERMINOLOGY
- Group of sex cord-stromal tumor (SCST) with mixture of recognizable types
- SCST with incomplete differentiation or undifferentiated spindle cells or mixed spindle and epithelioid cells

CLINICAL ISSUES
- Extremely rare (< 1% of testicular neoplasms)

MACROSCOPIC
- Well-circumscribed, lobulated, white-yellow nodule

MICROSCOPIC
- Mixture of growth patterns and mixture of recognizable SCST components (LCT, SCT, or GCT)
- Mixture of epithelioid and undifferentiated spindle cell components
- Epithelioid component forms solid or hollow tubules, irregular aggregates, or anastomosing trabeculae
- Round to ovoid cells with eosinophilic, amphophilic, or vacuolated cytoplasm
- Undifferentiated stromal cell component is usually hypercellular spindle cells and merged with fibrous stroma
- Features that are seen more often in malignant tumors: Invasive growth, angiolymphatic invasion, nuclear atypia, increased mitoses (> 4/10 HPF), increased cellularity and areas of necrosis

ANCILLARY TESTS
- Positive for SF1, desmin, actin-sm, S100, CD99, cytokeratin (may be focal), inhibin and calretinin (focal)
- Negative for PLAP, OCT3/4, podoplanin (D2-40), SALL4, HMB-45

TOP DIFFERENTIAL DIAGNOSES
- Mixed germ cell tumor with prominent immature teratoma component
- Adult granulosa cell tumor
- Sertoli cell tumor

Sex Cord-Stromal Tumor, Unclassified

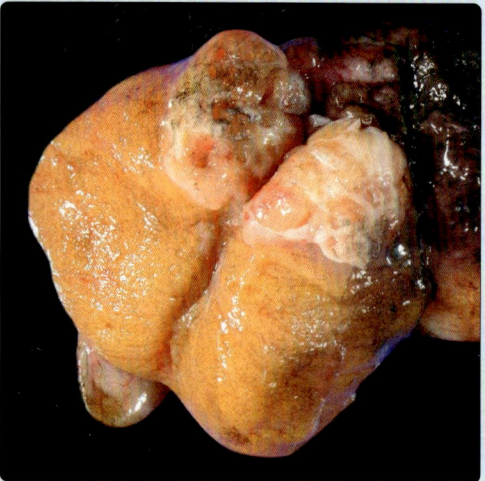

Sex Cord-Stromal Tumor, Unclassified

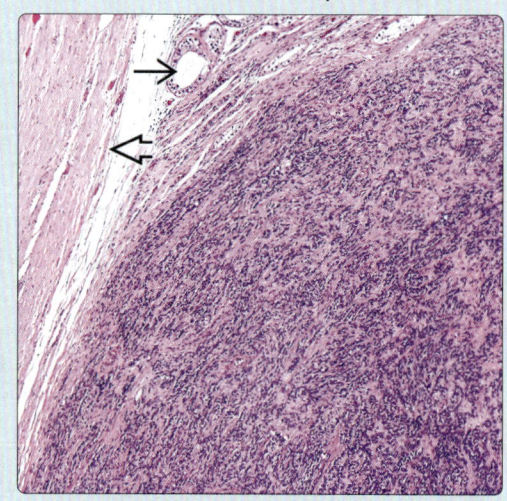

(Left) Gross photograph shows a well-circumscribed unclassified SCST. It has heterogeneous, soft, tan nodular areas with dense white fibrotic septa. SCSTs frequently do not replace the entire testis. (Right) A well-circumscribed unclassified SCST composed of cellular spindle cells is shown. No recognizable features of LCT, GCT, or SCT are seen. Note the relationship to the tunica ➡ and uninvolved testicular parenchyma ➡.

Sex Cord-Stromal Tumor, Mixed

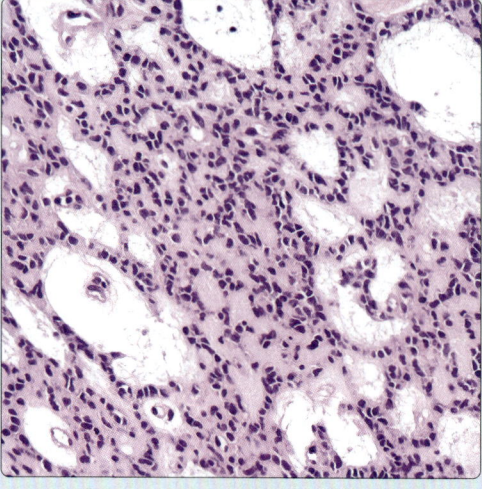

Sex Cord-Stromal Tumor, Unclassified

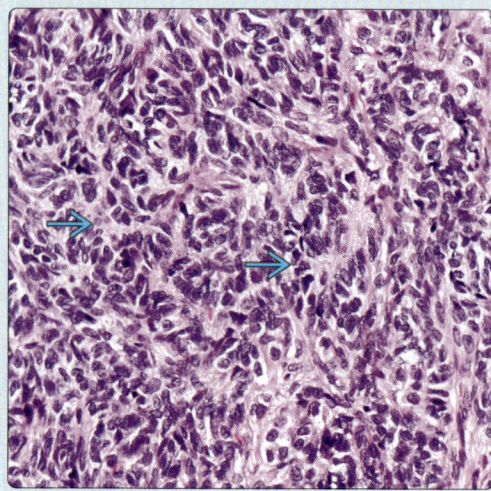

(Left) This photomicrograph shows an area of epithelial component in a mixed SCST with prominent microcystic and tubular patterns and cords of cells resembling those of Sertoli cell tumor. Other areas of the tumor had undifferentiated spindle cells, hence categorized as mixed/unclassified SCST. (Right) Unclassified SCST is shown with cellular proliferation of ovoid or elongated cells with scant, pale cytoplasm. No obvious differentiation is present. Vague rosette formation ➡ is seen.

Sex Cord-Stromal Tumor, Mixed/Unclassified

TERMINOLOGY

Abbreviations
- Sex cord-stromal tumor (SCST), Leydig cell tumor (LCT), Sertoli cell tumor (SCT), granulosa cell tumor (GCT)

Definitions
- Group of SCSTs with mixture of recognizable cell types or composed of incomplete or undifferentiated sex cord-stromal cells

CLINICAL ISSUES

Epidemiology
- Incidence
  - Extremely rare (< 1% of testicular neoplasms)
- Age
  - All ages
  - More commonly seen in children (30% < 1 year old)

Presentation
- Painless testicular enlargement
- 15% associated with gynecomastia

Treatment
- Surgical approaches
  - Surgical resection is usually curative

Prognosis
- Almost always benign in prepubertal children
- May be malignant in adults (20%)

MACROSCOPIC

General Features
- Well-circumscribed, lobulated, white-yellow, nodular mass; similar to other SCST with no unique gross features

MICROSCOPIC

Histologic Features
- Mixture of recognizable SCST components (Leydig cell, Sertoli cell, or granulosa cell, rarely theca cells)
- Mixture of undifferentiated or unclassifiable epithelioid and spindle sex cord-stromal cell components
- Epithelioid component
  - Solid or hollow tubules, irregular aggregates, or anastomosing trabeculae (SCT)
  - Round to ovoid cells with eosinophilic, amphophilic, or vacuolated cytoplasm and prominent nucleoli (LCT)
  - Oval round cells with nuclear grooves, Call-Exner-like bodies (GCT)
  - Mixture of above mentioned recognizable SCST
  - Unclassified epithelioid cells with vesicular nuclei, occasional prominent nucleoli, rare mitotic figures
  - Signet ring cell SCST has been reported
- Undifferentiated spindle cell component
  - Usually hypercellular spindle cells merged with fibrous stroma
  - Spindle cells may form fascicles
  - Spindle cells may have nuclear grooves
  - Cellular pleomorphism and mitotic figures are variable
  - Has been reported as variant of granulosa cell tumor because of its immunohistochemical similarities
- Features that are more commonly associated with malignant outcome: Invasive growth pattern, angiolymphatic invasion, nuclear atypia, increased mitoses (> 4/10 HPF), increased cellularity and areas of necrosis

ANCILLARY TESTS

Immunohistochemistry
- Positive for SF1, desmin, actin-sm, S100, CD99, cytokeratin (may be focal), inhibin and calretinin (focal)
- Negative for PLAP, OCT3/4, podoplanin (D2-40), SALL4, HMB-45

DIFFERENTIAL DIAGNOSIS

Mixed Germ Cell Tumor With Prominent Immature Teratoma Component
- High cellularity and increased mitoses
- Presence of various other germ cell tumor components
- Immature teratoma component may be positive for cytokeratin and CD34; negative for inhibin and calretinin
- Background germ cell neoplasia in situ

Adult Granulosa Cell Tumor
- More homogeneous neoplasm with well-formed Call-Exner bodies
- Immunohistochemical overlap with SCST

Sertoli Cell Tumor
- Usually demonstrates tubular morphology and is composed of single cell population
- Sarcomatoid variant of SCT may be challenging but usually has areas of more classic SCT

DIAGNOSTIC CHECKLIST

Pathologic Interpretation Pearls
- Purely undifferentiated spindle cell or mixed spindle and epithelioid proliferation or > 1 known SCST component

SELECTED REFERENCES

1. Kao CS et al: Myoid gonadal stromal tumor: a clinicopathologic study of three cases of a distinctive testicular tumor. Am J Clin Pathol. 142(5):675-82, 2014
2. Tarjàn M et al: Unclassified sex cord/gonadal stromal testis tumor with predominance of spindle cells. APMIS. 114(6):465-9, 2006
3. Young RH: Sex cord-stromal tumors of the ovary and testis: their similarities and differences with consideration of selected problems. Mod Pathol. 18 Suppl 2:S81-98, 2005
4. Ulbright TM et al: Sex cord-stromal tumors of the testis with entrapped germ cells: a lesion mimicking unclassified mixed germ cell sex cord-stromal tumors. Am J Surg Pathol. 24(4):535-42, 2000
5. Iczkowski KA et al: Inhibin A is a sensitive and specific marker for testicular sex cord-stromal tumors. Mod Pathol. 11(8):774-9, 1998
6. McCluggage WG et al: Immunohistochemical study of testicular sex cord-stromal tumors, including staining with anti-inhibin antibody. Am J Surg Pathol. 22(5):615-9, 1998
7. Renshaw AA et al: Immunohistochemistry of unclassified sex cord-stromal tumors of the testis with a predominance of spindle cells. Mod Pathol. 10(7):693-700, 1997
8. Goswitz JJ et al: Testicular sex cord-stromal tumors in children: clinicopathologic study of sixteen children with review of the literature. Pediatr Pathol Lab Med. 16(3):451-70, 1996

Sex Cord-Stromal Tumor, Mixed/Unclassified

(Left) Low-power photomicrograph of a mixed SCST shows poorly formed or compressed tubules of SCT ⮕ and a microscopic area of LCT with oval, round cells with abundant eosinophilic cytoplasm ⮕. **(Right)** Higher power photomicrograph of a mixed SCST shows nests and poorly formed tubules ⮕ lined by cells with ovoid or elongated nuclei and scant pale cytoplasm and clusters of Leydig cells ⮕ with abundant eosinophilic cytoplasm and prominent nucleoli.

Sex Cord-Stromal Tumor, Mixed

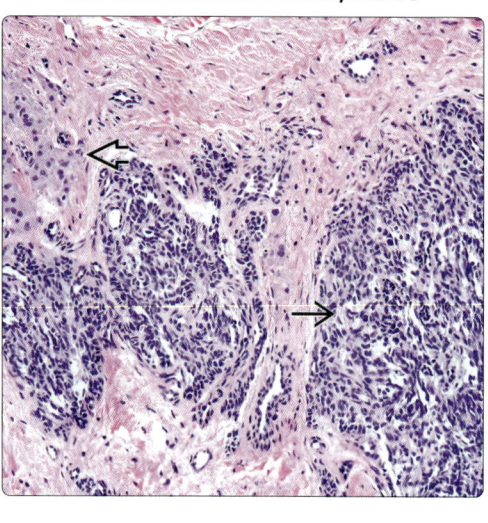

Sex Cord-Stromal Tumor, Mixed

(Left) An encapsulated unclassified SCST is shown. The tumor is composed of sheets of tumor cells with short spindle to ovoid nuclei and moderately abundant pale eosinophilic cytoplasm. No pleomorphism or necrosis is seen. **(Right)** High-power photomicrograph shows epithelioid cells with variable amounts of pale eosinophilic cytoplasm and indistinct cell boundaries. There is noticeable cellular pleomorphism ⮕ and occasional nuclear grooves ⮕.

Sex Cord-Stromal Tumor, Unclassified

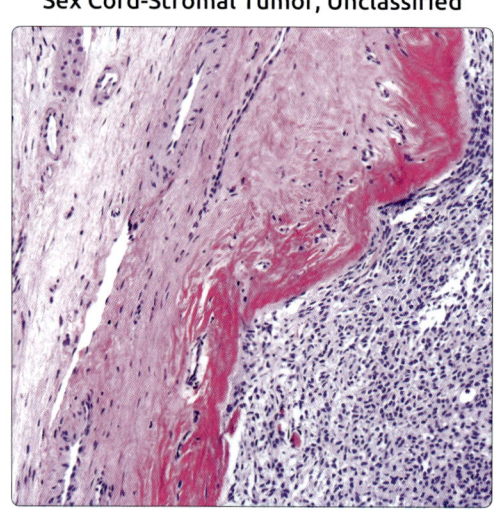

Sex Cord-Stromal Tumor, Unclassified

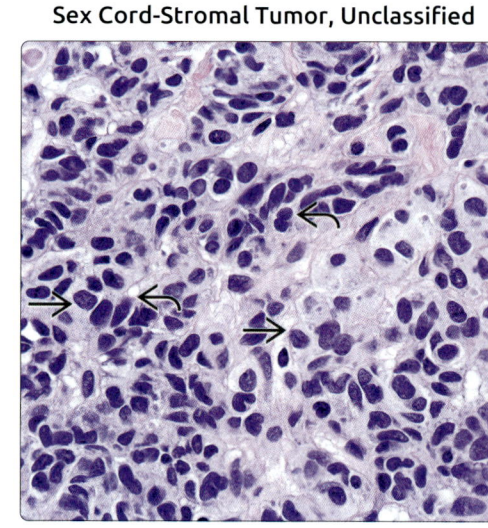

(Left) Unclassified SCST is shown with spindle-shaped tumor cells divided into lobules by paucicellular collagenized fibrous stroma. There is no specific line of differentiation. **(Right)** Unclassified SCST shows alternating density of spindle cell proliferation with resemblance of myofibroblastic cells. These cells were positive for inhibin and calretinin, indicating SCST. In contrast to intratesticular sarcomas, which are rare, anaplasia is not common.

Sex Cord-Stromal Tumor, Unclassified

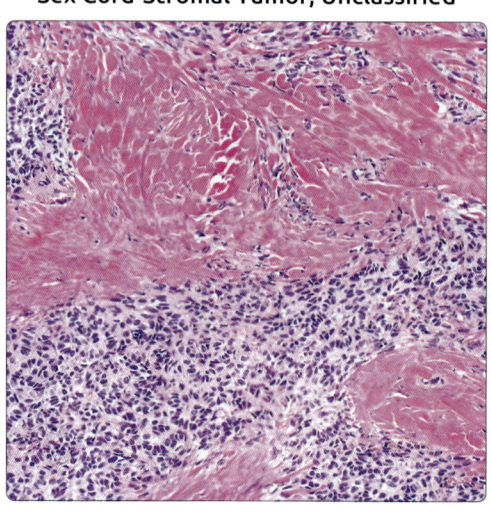

Sex Cord-Stromal Tumor, Unclassified

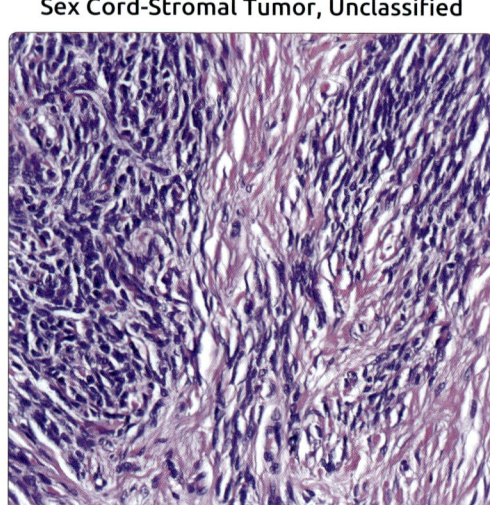

Sex Cord-Stromal Tumor, Mixed/Unclassified

Sex Cord-Stromal Tumor, Unclassified

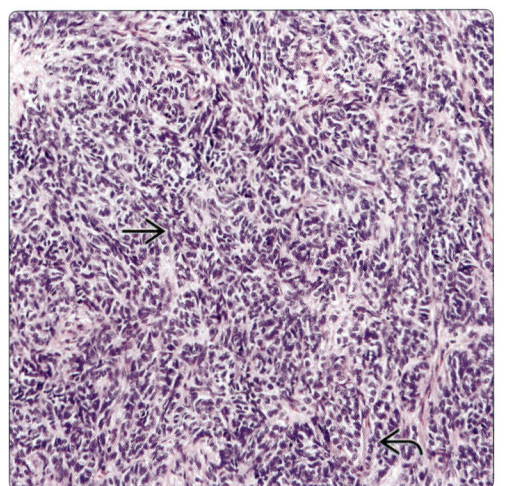

Sex Cord-Stromal Tumor, Unclassified

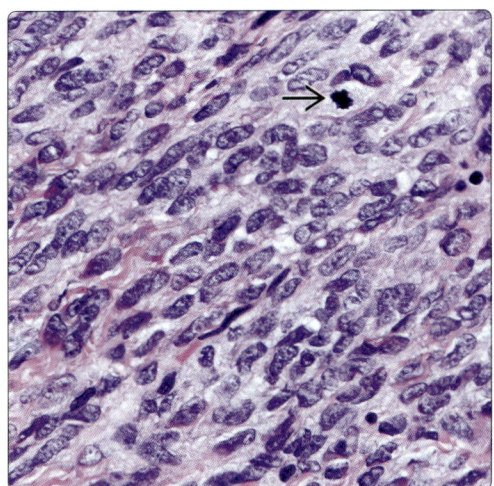

(Left) This photomicrograph of unclassified SCST shows compact growth of ovoid or spindle cells with focal, vague cord ➡ or tubule ➡ formation and focal storiform pattern. Tumor necrosis and pleomorphism are absent. *(Right)* Undifferentiated spindle cells of unclassified SCST have moderate nuclear pleomorphism and occasional mitoses ➡. Unclassified SCST is regarded as being potentially malignant except for small and cytologically innocuous tumors and those occurring in children.

Sex Cord-Stromal Tumor, Mixed

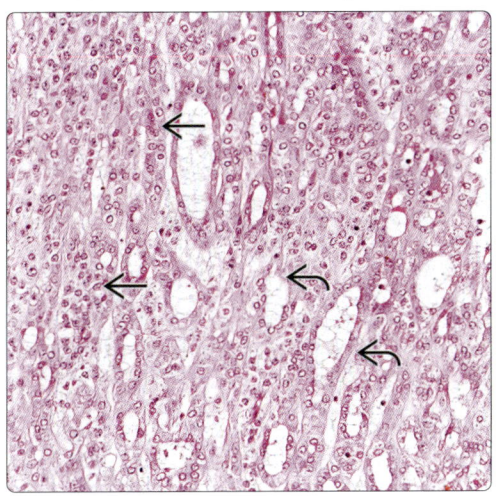

Sex Cord-Stromal Tumor, Mixed

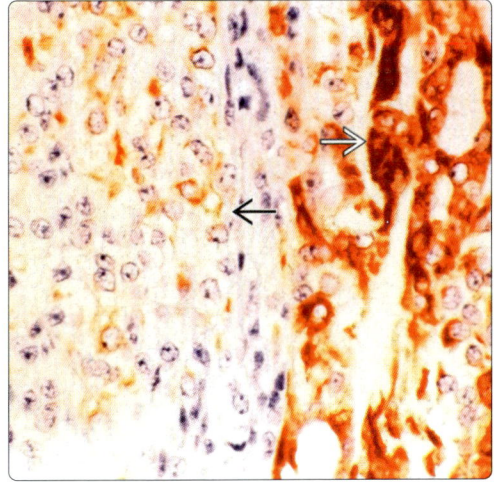

(Left) Mixed SCST is shown with solid growth of Leydig cell ➡ and Sertoli cell differentiation with tubule formation ➡. This combination of sex cord-stromal tumor histology is distinctly rare in the testis. *(Right)* The mixed SCST with Leydig cell ➡ and Sertoli cell differentiation ➡ may be supported by their differential immunohistochemical staining intensity with cytokeratin. The Sertoli cell component stains much stronger than the Leydig cell component.

Sex Cord-Stromal Tumor, Unclassified

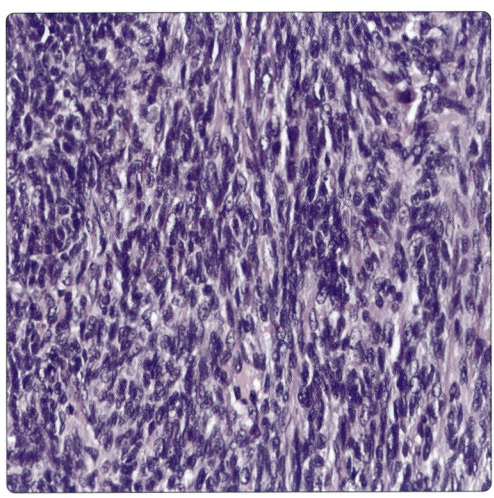

Sex Cord-Stromal Tumor, Unclassified

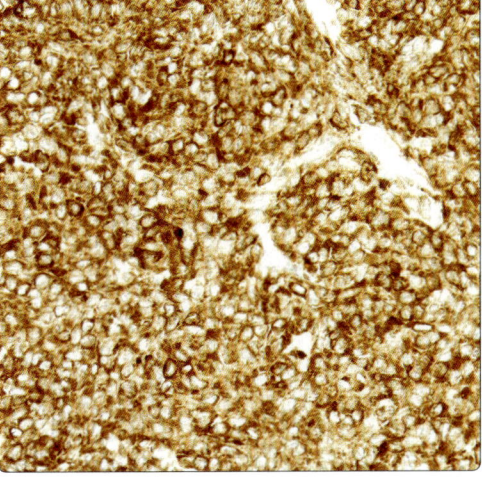

(Left) Unclassified SCST shows hypercellular proliferation of uncharacterized spindle cells with clear to pale eosinophilic cytoplasm. Although immature mesenchymal component of teratoma is mimicked, this component is never pure and admixed with other germ cell component. *(Right)* The diagnosis of this unclassified SCST is supported by its diffuse cytoplasmic inhibin stain.

Gonadoblastoma

KEY FACTS

TERMINOLOGY
- Tumor composed of mixture of seminomatous cells and immature sex cord tumor resembling Sertoli or granulosa cell tumors

CLINICAL ISSUES
- Extremely rare
- Occurs usually in patients with abnormal, dysgenetic gonads

MICROSCOPIC
- Nests of tumor cells composed of mixture of 2 types of cells (seminomatous germ cells and sex cord-stromal cells)
- Germ cells are large and round with vacuolated or clear cytoplasm, fine chromatin, and inconspicuous nucleoli
- Sex cord-stromal cells are usually immature Sertoli cells or granulosa cells, but rarely cells resemble Leydig cells or lutein-like cells

- Small, round-to-oval sex cord derivative forming Call-Exner bodies with central eosinophilic hyaline material
- Marked hyalinization or calcification present within nests or stroma
- Adjacent seminiferous tubules with germ cell neoplasia in situ may be seen
- Overgrowth of malignant germ cell tumor (usually seminoma) may obliterate gonadoblastomatous foci

ANCILLARY TESTS
- Germ cells positive for PLAP, podoplanin, OCT3, OCT4, CD117
- Gonadal stromal cells positive for inhibin, calretinin, Melan-A (MART-1), FOXL2, SF1, vimentin; focal weak or moderate positive for SOX9; may be positive for cytokeratin

Gonadoblastoma
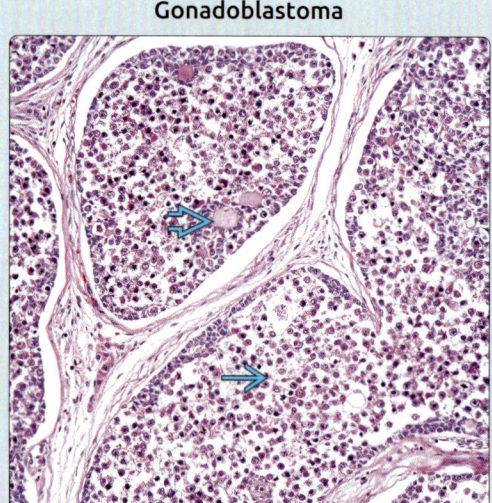

Call-Exner-Like Bodies
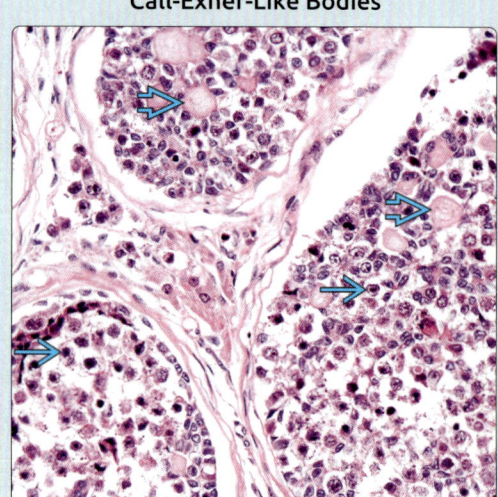

(Left) Gonadoblastoma is characterized by nests containing large seminomatous germ cells ➔ located in the center and sex cord-stromal cells, forming Call-Exner-like structures ➔ at the periphery of the nests. (Right) Gonadoblastoma is composed of nests containing population of large seminomatous germ cells ➔ and smaller sex cord-stromal cells forming Call-Exner-like structures ➔. The lesions may be microscopic only.

Call-Exner-Like bodies
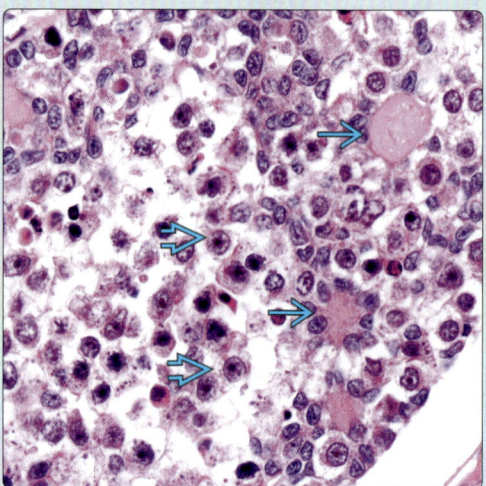

2 Cell Populations
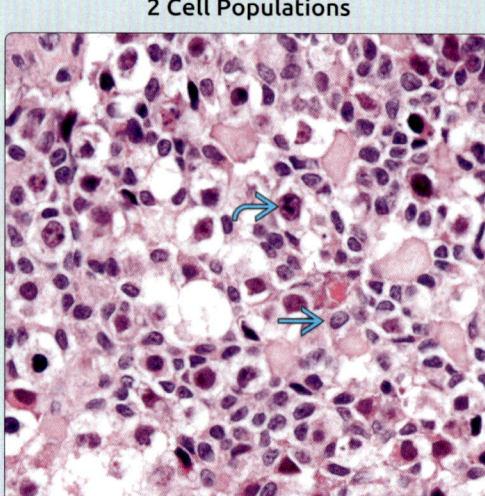

(Left) Gonadoblastoma shows smaller sex cord-stromal cells forming Call-Exner body-like structures ➔ and large seminomatous cells with abundant clear cytoplasm and prominent nucleolus ➔. (Right) High-power view of gonadoblastoma shows intimate admixture of larger seminomatous germ cells with prominent nucleolus and abundant clear cytoplasm ➔ and smaller sex cord-stromal cells ➔.

Gonadoblastoma

TERMINOLOGY

Definitions
- Tumor composed of mixture of seminomatous germ cells and immature sex cord tumor elements resembling Sertoli or granulosa cell tumor cells

CLINICAL ISSUES

Epidemiology
- Incidence
  - Extremely rare
  - Occurs usually in patients with abnormal, dysgenetic gonads
- Age
  - < 20 years old
- Sex
  - 20% phenotypically male, 80% phenotypically female (during early embryonic development, immature bipotential gonads fail to differentiate along male pathway)
  - XY gonadal dysgenesis or X0-XY mosaicism may be seen

Presentation
- Cryptorchidism, hypospadias or other ambiguous genitalia, and gynecomastia

Treatment
- Surgical approaches
  - Bilateral gonadectomy is recommended and curative

Prognosis
- Excellent if no associated invasive germ cell or malignant sex cord-stromal tumor components

MACROSCOPIC

General Features
- Gray to yellow-brown mass with soft, fleshy or firm, and gritty cut surface
- Streak gonads with incidental findings of very small-sized tumors
- Invasive malignant germ cell tumor component, usually seminoma, results in larger tumors

Size
- Range: Microscopic focus to 8 cm

MICROSCOPIC

Histologic Features
- Nests of tumor cells composed of mixture of 2 types of cells (seminomatous germ cells and sex cord-stromal cells)
- Germ cells are large and round with vacuolated or clear cytoplasm, central nuclei with fine chromatin, and prominent nucleoli seminoma-like)
- Sex cord-stromal cells are usually immature Sertoli cells or granulosa cells but rarely cells resemble Leydig cells or luteinizing theca-like cells
- Sex cord-stromal cells are located at periphery of nests
- Small, round-to-oval sex cord derivative cells form Call-Exner bodies with central eosinophilic hyaline material
- Marked hyalinization or calcifications present within nests or stroma
- Adjacent seminiferous tubules with germ cell neoplasia in situ may be seen
- Overgrowth of malignant germ cell tumor (usually seminoma) may obliterate gonadoblastomatous foci

ANCILLARY TESTS

Immunohistochemistry
- Germ cells positive for PLAP, podoplanin (D2-40), OCT3, OCT4, SALL4, CD117
- Gonadal stromal cells positive for inhibin, calretinin, Melan-A (MART-1), FOXL2, SF1, vimentin; focal weak or moderate positive for SOX9; may be positive for cytokeratin

DIFFERENTIAL DIAGNOSIS

Unclassified Mixed Germ Cell and Sex Cord-Stromal Tumors
- Occurs in patients with normal gonads and without cytogenetic abnormalities (normal XY chromosomes)
- Diffuse growth with no well-defined nodules
- Some authors argue about existence of this entity and classify this lesion under unclassified sex cord-stromal tumor with entrapped germ cells

Seminoma (Classic)
- No dysgenetic gonad; lack of sex cord-stromal tumor component or gonadoblastoma in background; often larger tumor size and older age (35-45 yr)

Sex Cord-Stromal Tumor With Annular Tubules
- Extremely rare in testis; associated with androgen insensitivity syndrome or Peutz-Jeghers syndrome; lack of germ cell tumor component

Sertoli Cell Nodule With Germ Cell Neoplasia In Situ
- Associated gonad is not dysgenetic; seminoma-like cells are not uniformly distributed throughout tumor

DIAGNOSTIC CHECKLIST

Pathologic Interpretation Pearls
- Dysgenetic gonad; well-defined nested growth with hyaline nodules and basement membranes; 2 cell populations with germ cells and sex cord-stromal cells

SELECTED REFERENCES

1. Kao CS et al: Gonadoblastoma: an immunohistochemical study and comparison to Sertoli cell nodule with intratubular germ cell neoplasia, with pathogenetic implications. Histopathology. 65(6):861-7, 2014
2. Ng SB et al: Gonadoblastoma-associated mixed germ cell tumour in 46,XY complete gonadal dysgenesis (Swyer syndrome): analysis of Y chromosomal genotype and OCT3/4 and TSPY expression profile. Histopathology. 52(5):644-6, 2008
3. Kersemaekers AM et al: Identification of germ cells at risk for neoplastic transformation in gonadoblastoma: an immunohistochemical study for OCT3/4 and TSPY. Hum Pathol. 36(5):512-21, 2005
4. Hussong J et al: Gonadoblastoma: immunohistochemical localization of Müllerian-inhibiting substance, inhibin, WT-1, and p53. Mod Pathol. 10(11):1101-5, 1997
5. Jørgensen N et al: Heterogeneity of gonadoblastoma germ cells: similarities with immature germ cells, spermatogonia and testicular carcinoma in situ cells. Histopathology. 30(2):177-86, 1997
6. Roth LM et al: Gonadoblastoma. Immunohistochemical and ultrastructural observations. Int J Gynecol Pathol. 8(1):72-81, 1989
7. Scully RE: Gonadoblastoma. A review of 74 cases. Cancer. 25(6):1340-56, 1970

Gonadoblastoma

Dysgenetic Gonad

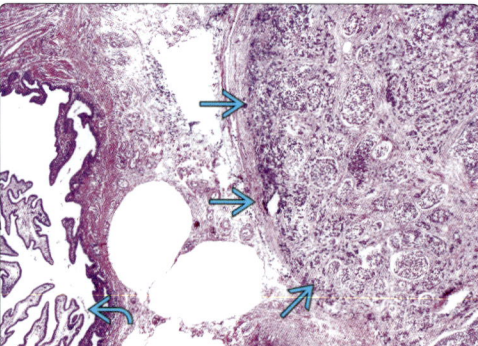

Dysgenetic Gonad

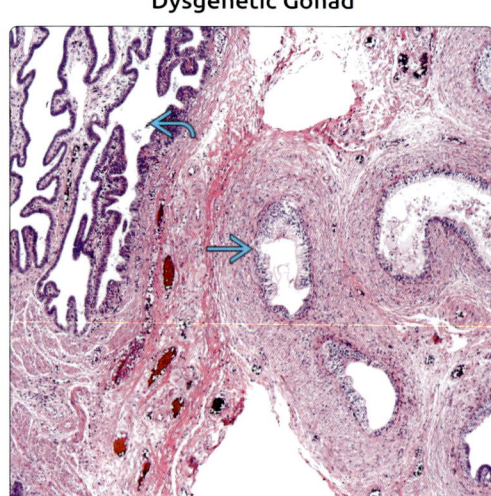

(Left) Low-power view shows a well-circumscribed gonadoblastoma ⇒ in the background of a streak dysgenetic gonad with epididymis ⇒ and fallopian tube ⇒. The tumor is cellular and shows a vague nodular configuration. (Right) This photomicrograph shows a streak dysgenetic gonad in a patient with gonadoblastoma. There are both epididymis with muscular wall ⇒ and adjacent fallopian tube tissue ⇒.

2 Cell Types

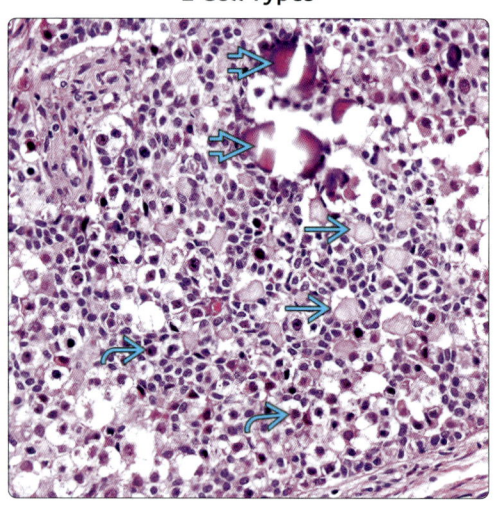

Calcification

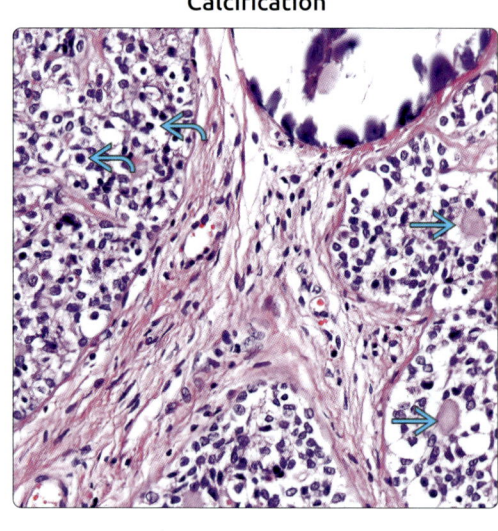

(Left) Gonadoblastoma is composed of an intimate mixture of larger seminomatous germ cells with large nuclei and abundant clear cytoplasm ⇒ and sex cord-stromal cells forming Call-Exner body-like structures ⇒. Focal scattered calcifications are present ⇒. (Right) A gonadoblastoma shows nests of seminomatous germ cells with clear cytoplasm ⇒ and sex cord-stromal cells with a lesser amount of cytoplasm. Call-Exner body-like structures ⇒ and a large area of calcification (top) are present.

Gonadoblastoma With Associated GCNIS

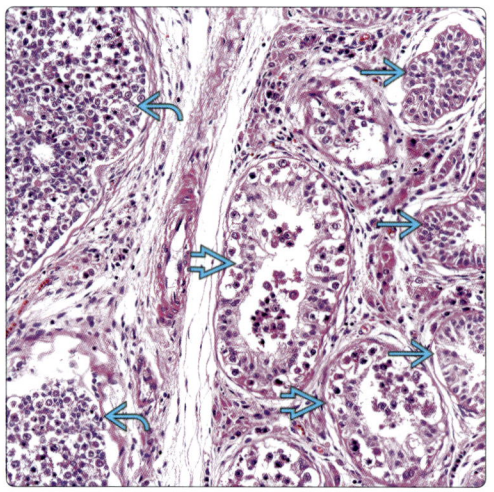

Gonadoblastoma With Associated GCNIS

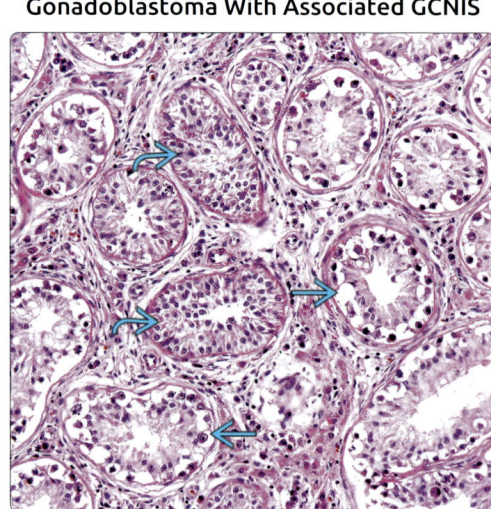

(Left) This image shows gonadoblastoma ⇒ with adjacent germ cell neoplasia in situ (GCNIS) characterized by large cells with abundant clear cytoplasm ⇒ and tubules containing only Sertoli cells ⇒. Gonadoblastoma with characteristic low-power features is seen on the left. (Right) The adjacent seminiferous tubules in a case of gonadoblastoma may show Sertoli cell-only features ⇒, while others tubules have extensive involvement by germ cell neoplasia in situ ⇒.

Gonadoblastoma

Gonadoblastoma With Intratubular Seminoma

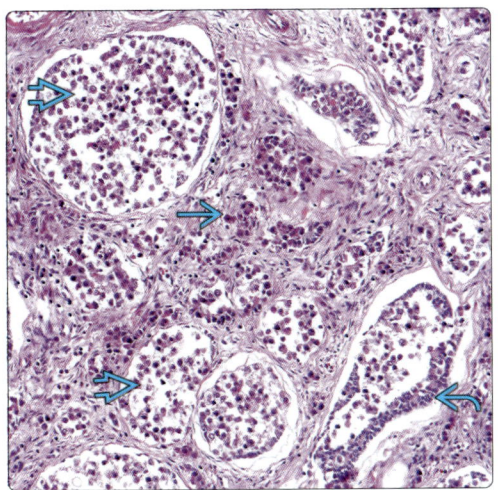

Gonadoblastoma With Seminoma

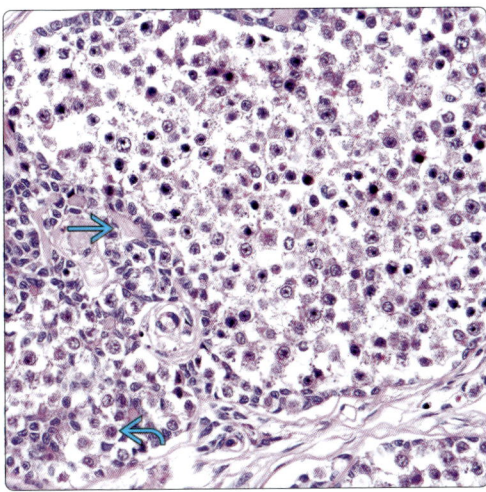

(Left) Gonadoblastoma with intratubular seminomatous overgrowth ⇨ coexists with microscopic foci of invasive seminoma associated with lymphocytes ⇨. Focal Call-Exner-like structures are seen at the periphery ⇨ of some tumor nests. (Right) One large nest of gonadoblastoma is juxtaposed by overgrowth of seminomatous germ cells with prominent nucleoli, abundant clear cytoplasm, and distinct cell boundaries. Adjacent to the seminomatous nodule, an area with mixture of germ cells ⇨ and sex cord-stromal cells ⇨ is seen.

Gonadoblastoma With Intratubular and Invasive Seminoma

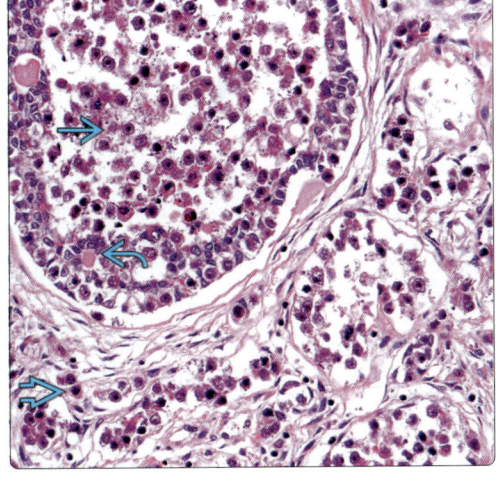

2 Cell Types

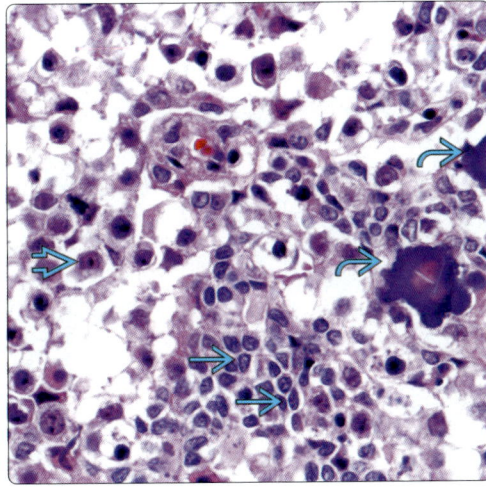

(Left) Gonadoblastoma with overgrowth of intratubular seminoma ⇨ and microscopic foci of invasive seminoma ⇨ is shown. Call-Exner-like structures ⇨ are still present at the periphery of the large tumor nest. (Right) High-power photomicrograph shows a gonadoblastoma composed of intratubular large seminoma tumor cells with prominent nucleoli and abundant clear cytoplasm ⇨ and clusters of smaller angulated sex cord-stromal cells ⇨ and calcifications ⇨.

Gonadoblastoma With Invasive Seminoma

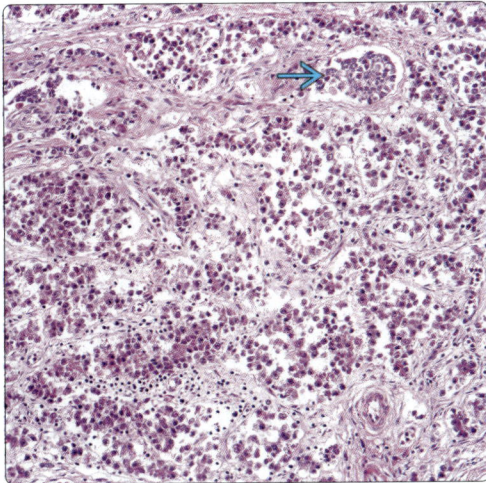

Mixed Germ Cell and Sex Cord-Stromal Tumor

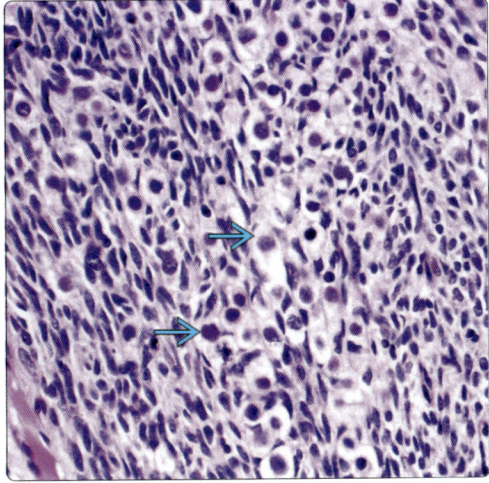

(Left) This photomicrograph shows overgrowth of invasive seminoma composed of nests of tumor cells within the fibrous stroma and scattered lymphocytic infiltrate and a small focus of gonadoblastoma ⇨. (Right) A mixed germ cell sex cord-stromal tumor shows unclassified sex cord-stromal elements and scattered large round cells, reminiscent of uncommitted germ cell tumor cells ⇨. Some authors classify this tumor under unclassified sex cord-stromal tumor with entrapped germ cells.

Lymphoma/Leukemia/Plasmacytoma

KEY FACTS

TERMINOLOGY
- Lymphoma and plasmacytoma of testis or paratesticular structures, which is either primary or secondary due to systemic spread
- Secondary leukemic infiltrates

CLINICAL ISSUES
- Malignant lymphoma accounts for 2-5% of all testicular neoplasms

MACROSCOPIC
- Lymphoma and plasmacytoma: Partial or complete replacement of testicular parenchyma by diffuse or lobulated mass
- Fleshy, creamy colored, tan, pale yellow or slightly pink homogeneous cut surface
- Leukemia: Most often no gross abnormalities and usually found by testicular biopsy

MICROSCOPIC
- Most common type of primary lymphoma is diffuse large B-cell lymphoma
- Diffuse interstitial pattern is most frequent finding
- Tumoral and intratubular replacement may also occur
- Effacement and infiltration of seminiferous tubules by lymphoma (onion skin appearance) may be seen
- Other lymphomas include MALT lymphomas, follicular lymphomas, extranodal NK/T-cell lymphomas, anaplastic large cell lymphoma, Burkitt lymphoma, and plasmablastic lymphoma
- Plasmacytoma is characterized by sheets of variably differentiated, monomorphic neoplastic plasma cells
- Leukemia (including granulocytic sarcoma) is similar to that of lymphoma microscopically

TOP DIFFERENTIAL DIAGNOSES
- Germ cell tumors, chronic orchitis, metastatic carcinoma, Leydig cell tumor

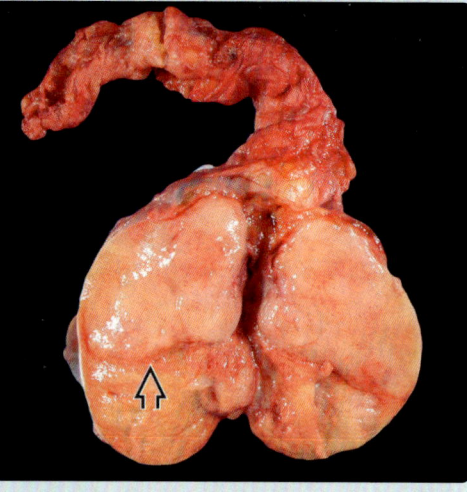

Malignant Lymphoma

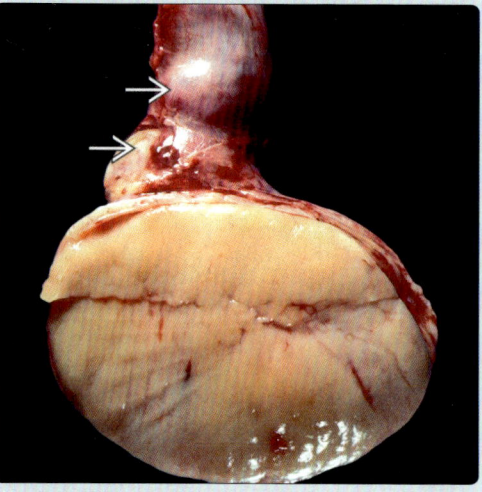

Spermatic Cord Involvement

(Left) Malignant lymphoma ➡ partially involves the testis and demonstrates sharp demarcation from the testicular parenchyma. It is relatively homogeneous, tan-white with a bulging cut surface, grossly similar to seminoma or spermatocytic seminoma. (Right) Malignant lymphoma of the testis shows a mass with homogeneous, tan-cream, bulging cut surface. The testicular parenchyma is completely replaced, and there is extension to the epididymis and spermatic cord ➡.

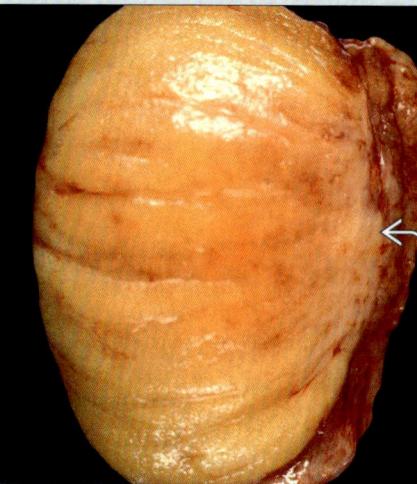

Burkitt Lymphoma

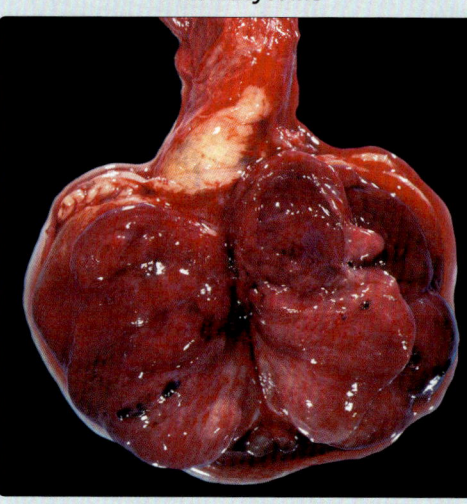

Plasmacytoma

(Left) Gross photograph shows Burkitt lymphoma involving the entire testis and rete testis ➡. The tumor is homogeneous, tan-gray with lobulation and a bulging cut surface. It usually involves the pediatric population and is known for rapid growth. (Right) Testicular plasmacytoma with extensive hemorrhage is shown here. Most plasmacytomas show a soft, tan to gray-white cut surface, similar to seminoma. Extensive hemorrhage may occur and obscure the typical features of the tumor, as seen in this case.

Lymphoma/Leukemia/Plasmacytoma

TERMINOLOGY

Definitions
- Lymphoma and plasmacytoma involve testis or paratesticular structures as either primary neoplasms or as secondary tumors due to systemic spread
- Leukemic involvement represents secondary spread to testis or paratesticular structures (testis is one of more common sanctuary sites)

CLINICAL ISSUES

Epidemiology
- Incidence
  - Malignant lymphoma accounts for 2-5% of all testicular neoplasms
    - Secondary involvement is more common than primary lymphoma
  - Primary plasmacytoma of testis is extremely rare (only handful of cases have been reported)
    - Secondary plasmacytoma occurs in 2% of patients with multiple myeloma at autopsy (clinically usually occult)
  - Frequent finding in patients with leukemia (at autopsy)
    - 40-65% of patients with acute leukemia have leukemic infiltrate
    - 20-35% of patients with chronic leukemia have leukemic infiltrate
- Age
  - Lymphoma and plasmacytoma: Average age 56-60 yr in different studies
    - 50% of testis tumors in patients over 60 yr are lymphomas
  - Leukemic infiltrates usually occur in children

Presentation
- Testicular mass or enlargement
- Systemic symptoms may occur such as fever, night sweats, weight loss
- Frequent bilaterality (20-38%); majority are metachronous
- Testicular lymphoma has predilection for widespread association with unusual sites, including CNS, Waldeyer ring, skin and lung lymphoma

Treatment
- Radical orchiectomy is often performed in older patients with primary testicular lymphoma or plasmacytoma
- Adjuvant therapy
  - Similar to that of nodal or other extranodal lymphomas
  - Doxorubicin- and rituximab-based chemotherapy with prophylactic intrathecal chemotherapy and radiation to contralateral testis

Prognosis
- Generally poor for adult testicular lymphoma
- The 5- and 10-yr overall survival is 37-48% and 19-27%, respectively, for all testicular lymphoma
- Prognostic factors include age, stage, epididymal or spermatic cord involvement, and histologic sclerosis
- Secondary lymphoma involvement in children often have excellent prognosis by chemotherapy alone
- Primary testicular plasmacytoma has favorable prognosis compared to multiple myeloma
- Leukemic involvement is predictive of subsequent systemic relapse

IMAGING

General Features
- Similar to and indistinguishable from testicular germ cell tumor on ultrasonography
- More frequent spermatic cord involvement than germ cell tumors
- There may be no imaging abnormalities or testicular enlargement in leukemic patients

MACROSCOPIC

General Features
- Lymphoma and plasmacytoma
  - Partial or complete replacement of testicular parenchyma by diffuse or lobulated mass
  - Fleshy, cream-colored, tan, pale yellow, or slightly pink homogeneous cut surface; similar to that of seminoma or spermatocytic seminoma
  - Focal hemorrhage and necrosis may be seen
  - Frequent epididymis (50%) or spermatic cord involvement and bilateral involvement
- Testicular leukemia
  - Usually no gross abnormalities with detection on surveillance biopsy
  - May rarely result in palpable mass, induration, or testicular enlargement

Size
- Lymphoma and plasmacytoma
  - Mean: 6 cm

MICROSCOPIC

Histologic Features
- Malignant lymphoma
  - Diffuse interstitial pattern is most frequent finding: Relative preservation of tubules
  - Tumoral (sheet-like) and intratubular growth may occur
  - Effacement and infiltration of seminiferous tubules by lymphoma (onion skin with reticulin stain) may be seen
  - Variable sclerosis: Presence of sclerosis is associated with more favorable prognosis
  - Most common type of primary lymphoma is diffuse large B-cell lymphoma (70-90%)
    - Composed of sheets of large atypical lymphoid cells of variable morphology (noncleaved, cleaved, multilobated, or immunoblastic)
    - Most belong to nongerminal center B-cell-like large cell lymphoma (CD10 and bcl-6 negative and MUM1 positive)
    - Has unique genetic changes with loss of chromosome 6p, gains of 19q13; t(14;18)
  - Other lymphomas include primary MALT lymphomas, follicular lymphomas, extranodal NK/T-cell lymphomas, CD30 (BER-H2) positive anaplastic large cell lymphoma, Burkitt lymphoma (children), plasmablastic lymphoma and rarely Hodgkin disease

Lymphoma/Leukemia/Plasmacytoma

- Features similar to that of nodal or other extranodal locations
- Plasmacytoma/myeloma
  - Composed of sheets of variably differentiated, monomorphic neoplastic plasma cells
- Leukemia (include granulocytic sarcoma)
  - Similar to that of lymphoma microscopically and may be misdiagnosed as lymphoma
  - Tumor cells usually have smaller, more evenly dispersed chromatin and less prominent nucleoli than that of lymphoma
  - Often prominent vessel wall invasion
  - Rare seminiferous tubule invasion

ANCILLARY TESTS

Immunohistochemistry

- Positive for CD45 (LCA), most are positive for CD20, CD79a
- May also be positive for bcl-2, CD10 (follicular)
- Plasmacytomas are positive for CD138 and monoclonal κ- or λ-light chain
- Leukemias are positive for lysozyme, MPO, CD117, CD68

DIFFERENTIAL DIAGNOSIS

Seminoma, Classic or Spermatocytic

- Younger age; bilaterality and spermatic cord invasion less frequent
- Usually diffuse tumoral pattern; interstitial pattern less prominent and commonly at periphery only
- Tumor cells are more monotonous with abundant clear cytoplasm and distinct cell boundaries compared to those of lymphoma
- Presence of germ cell neoplasia in situ (GCNIS)
- Positive for germ cell markers [PLAP, Podoplanin (D2-40), OCT3/OCT4, LIN28 and SALL4]; negative for CD45(LCA), CD20, and CD3

Embryonal Carcinoma

- Younger age (25-35 yr) and less frequently bilateral
- Hemorrhage and necrosis are more common
- Cohesive and epithelial growth patterns with solid, papillary, and tubular arrangement
- Anaplastic tumor cells with more numerous mitoses and irregular and prominent nucleoli
- Presence of GCNIS
- Positive for germ cell markers (PLAP, CD30, OCT3/OCT4, LIN28, and SALL4)
- Positivity for CD30 represents a pitfall, as both embryonal carcinoma and CD30(BerH2)-positive anaplastic large cell lymphoma are positive

Chronic Orchitis

- Cellular infiltrate is usually more patchy and lacks cytologic atypia
- Heterogeneous population of cells with lymphocytes, plasma cells, histiocytes, and neutrophils

Metastatic Tumors

- Clinical history of malignancy elsewhere
- Cohesive growth pattern in carcinoma
- Melanoma cells may be diffuse and dyscohesive, similar to that of lymphoma/plasmacytoma
- Positive for epithelial markers (cytokeratin, EMA/MUC1, etc.) in carcinoma
- Positive for S100, HMB-45, Melan-A (MART-1) in malignant melanoma
- Negative for lymphoma markers

Leydig Cell Tumor

- Neoplastic tumor cells have more abundant granular cytoplasm, lesser degree of cytologic atypia, and no or few mitoses
- Expansile mass without destruction of seminiferous tubules
- Positive for inhibin and calretinin; negative for lymphoma markers

STAGING

According to Ann Arbor Staging System Proposed for Hodgkin Lymphoma

- Staging evaluation includes: Physical, complete hematologic and biochemical examination, testicular ultrasound, CT scan, bone marrow biopsy, CSF examination, brain MR
- Staging subclassification system
  - Stage I: Involves unilateral testis only
  - Stage II: Involves bilateral testis and its regional lymph node (below diaphragm)
  - Stage III: Involves testis and lymph nodes of both sides of diaphragm or spleen
  - Stage IV: Disseminated (multifocal) involvement of 1 or more extralymphatic sites

SELECTED REFERENCES

1. Fonseca A et al: Testicular myeloid sarcoma: an unusual presentation of infant acute myeloid leukemia. J Pediatr Hematol Oncol. 36(3):e155-7, 2014
2. Ahmad SS et al: Primary testicular lymphoma. Clin Oncol (R Coll Radiol). 24(5):358-65, 2012
3. Liang DN et al: Extranodal nasal type natural killer/T-cell lymphoma of testis: report of seven cases with review of literature. Leuk Lymphoma. 53(6):1117-23, 2012
4. Lones MA et al: Primary follicular lymphoma of the testis in children and adolescents. J Pediatr Hematol Oncol. 34(1):68-71, 2012
5. Rosenberg S et al: Plasmacytoma of the testis in a patient with previous multiple myeloma: is the testis a sanctuary site? J Clin Oncol. 28(27):e456-8, 2010
6. Gundrum JD et al: Primary testicular diffuse large B-cell lymphoma: a population-based study on the incidence, natural history, and survival comparison with primary nodal counterpart before and after the introduction of rituximab. J Clin Oncol. 27(31):5227-32, 2009
7. Booman M et al: Genomic alterations and gene expression in primary diffuse large B-cell lymphomas of immune-privileged sites: the importance of apoptosis and immunomodulatory pathways. J Pathol. 216(2):209-17, 2008
8. Vitolo U et al: Primary testicular lymphoma. Crit Rev Oncol Hematol. 65(2):183-9, 2008
9. Bacon CM et al: Primary follicular lymphoma of the testis and epididymis in adults. Am J Surg Pathol. 31(7):1050-8, 2007
10. Vural F et al: Primary testicular lymphoma. J Natl Med Assoc. 99(11):1277-82, 2007
11. Darby S et al: Localised non-Hodgkin lymphoma of the testis: the Sheffield Lymphoma Group experience. Int J Oncol. 26(4):1093-9, 2005
12. Constantinou J et al: Testicular granulocytic sarcoma, a source of diagnostic confusion. Urology. 64(4):807-9, 2004
13. Lagrange JL et al: Non-Hodgkin's lymphoma of the testis: a retrospective study of 84 patients treated in the French anticancer centres. Ann Oncol. 12(9):1313-9, 2001
14. Ferry JA et al: Testicular and epididymal plasmacytoma: a report of 7 cases, including three that were the initial manifestation of plasma cell myeloma. Am J Surg Pathol. 21(5):590-8, 1997

Lymphoma/Leukemia/Plasmacytoma

Interstitial Growth
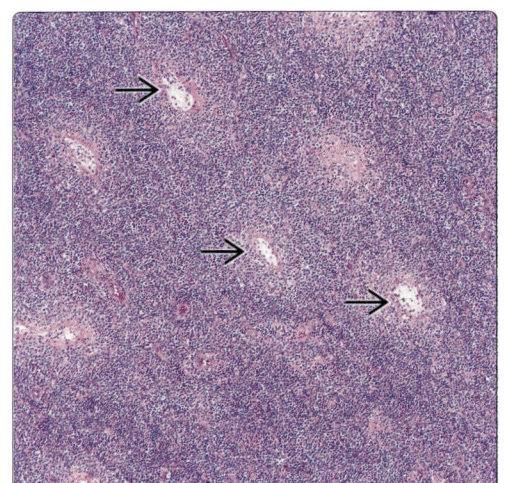

Interstitial Growth
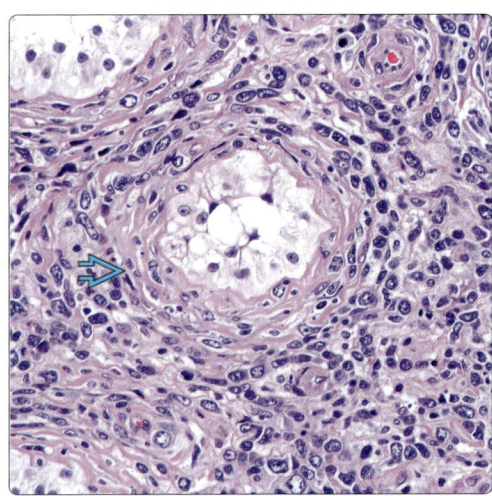

(Left) Testicular lymphoma with a diffuse interstitial infiltration of blue round cells with preserved but significantly effaced or atrophic seminiferous tubules ⇒ is shown here. (Right) High-power photomicrograph of lymphoma shows diffuse interstitial infiltration of large, cleaved, and noncleaved dyscohesive tumor cells, infiltrating the thickened wall of seminiferous tubules (onion skin pattern) ⇒.

Reticulin Stain
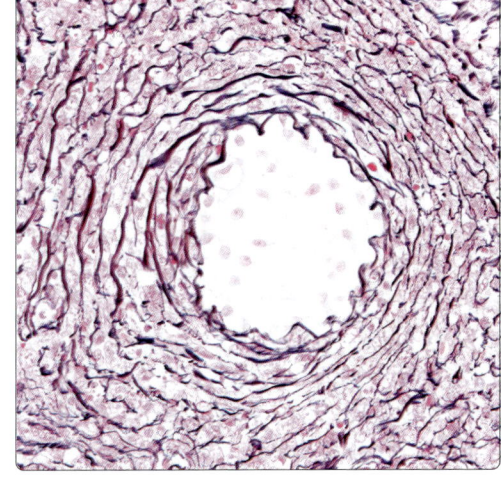

CD20
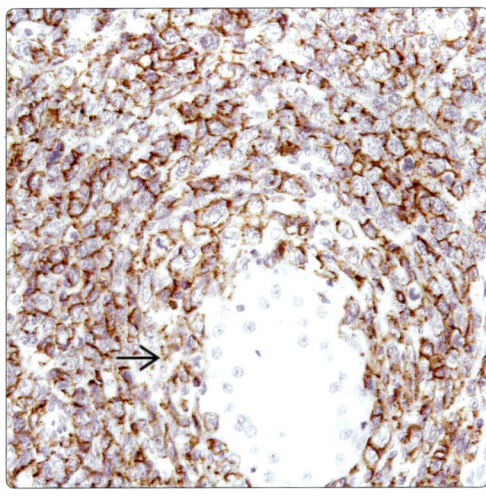

(Left) Reticulin stain of testicular lymphoma shows typical "onion skin" appearance around the seminiferous tubule. Reticulin staining is rarely required in current clinical practice, as immunophenotyping has more diagnostic, prognostic, and therapeutic relevance. (Right) This photomicrograph shows the immunostain of a large B-cell lymphoma with strong membranous staining by CD20. The tumor cells are seen in both the interstitium and the wall of a thickened seminiferous tubule ⇒.

Rete Testis Involvement
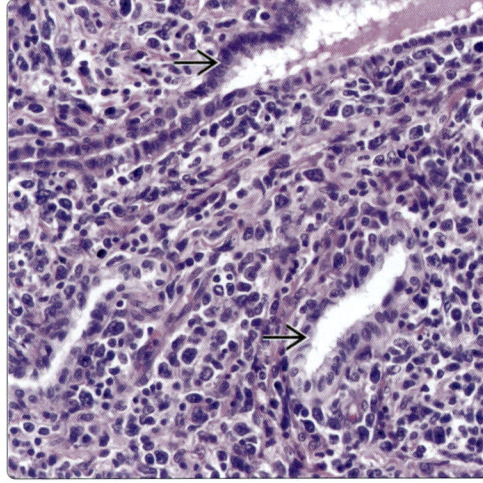

Involvement of Seminiferous Tubules
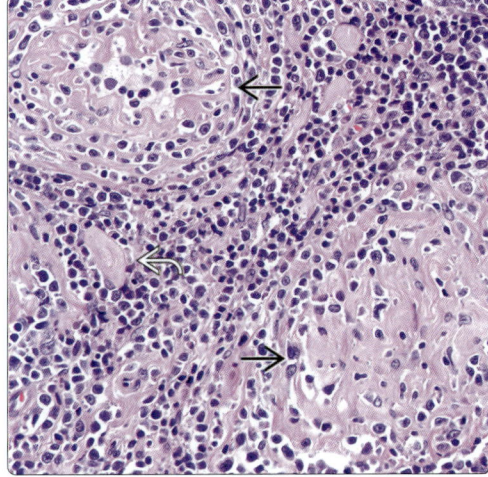

(Left) H&E shows involvement of the rete testis ⇒ by lymphoma. In contrast to seminoma, which usually exhibits intraepithelial pagetoid spread of tumor cells, the lymphoma cells show interstitial spread and are more pleomorphic, unevenly distributed with nuclear overlapping and indistinct cell boundaries. (Right) This photomicrograph shows partial to complete destruction of seminiferous tubules ⇒ by infiltrating lymphoma cells. Sclerosis of the interstitium may be seen ⇒.

Lymphoma/Leukemia/Plasmacytoma

(Left) In contrast to seminoma, this large B-cell lymphoma shows greater pleomorphism, uneven cellular distribution, and indistinct cell boundaries with lesser amounts of cytoplasm. Fibrous septa or granulomas are absent. **(Right)** This photomicrograph shows a large B-cell lymphoma with significant sclerosis in the interstitium ➡. The histologic finding of sclerosis in testicular lymphoma is one of the features associated with a favorable prognosis; other prognostic factors include age and stage of disease.

Large B-Cell Lymphoma
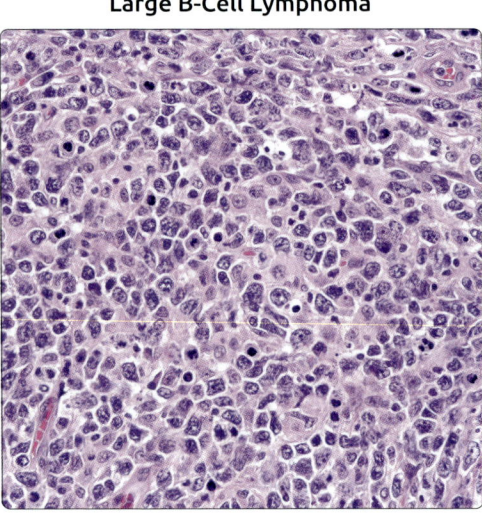

Sclerosis
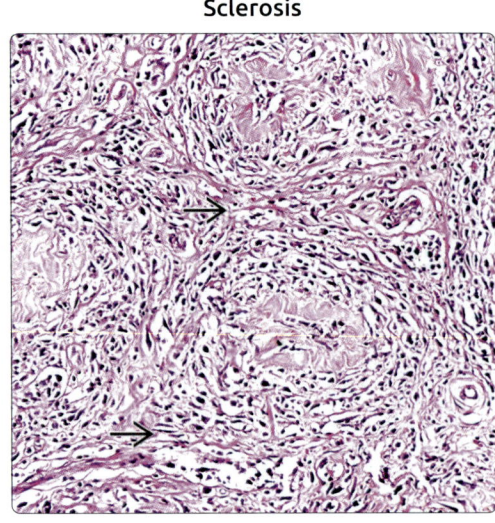

(Left) Seminiferous tubules involved by lymphoma cells (intratubular growth) may be easily confused with intratubular seminoma or embryonal carcinoma. In problematic cases, germ cell markers [podoplanin (D2-40), OCT3/OCT4, SALL4] and lymphoma markers will be discriminatory. **(Right)** Intratubular growth of lymphoma by anaplastic tumor cells with numerous mitoses ➡ and frequent apoptoses ➡; it should be noted that CD30 staining is seen in embryonal carcinoma and anaplastic lymphoma.

Intratubular Growth
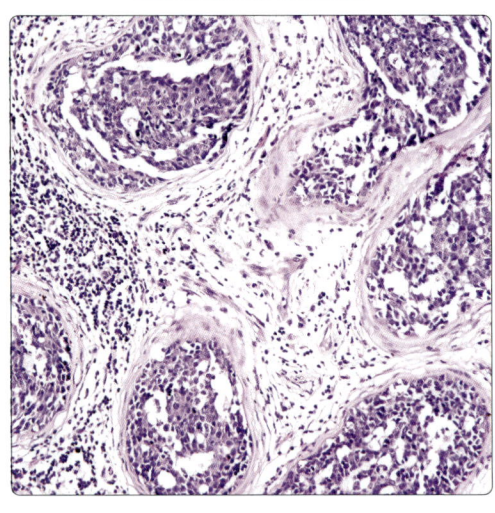

Intratubular Growth
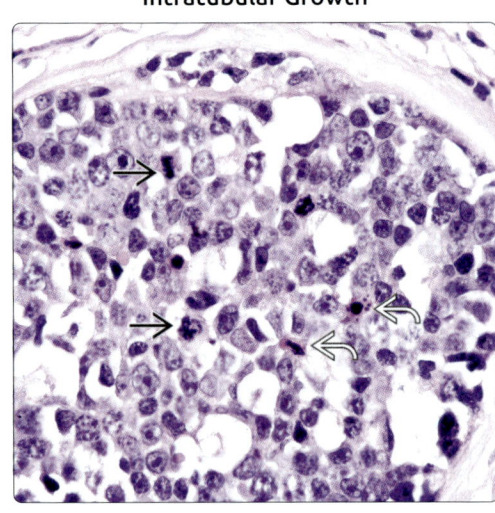

(Left) H&E shows Burkitt lymphoma of testis in a child. It is characterized by a diffuse interstitial infiltration of highly cellular lymphoid cells with a starry sky appearance. Note the relatively intact seminiferous tubules ➡. **(Right)** High-power photomicrograph of Burkitt lymphoma shows monotonous tumor cells with hyperchromatic nuclei, frequent mitoses and scant cytoplasm. Tingible body macrophages engulfing cell debris ➡ create the starry sky appearance.

Burkitt Lymphoma
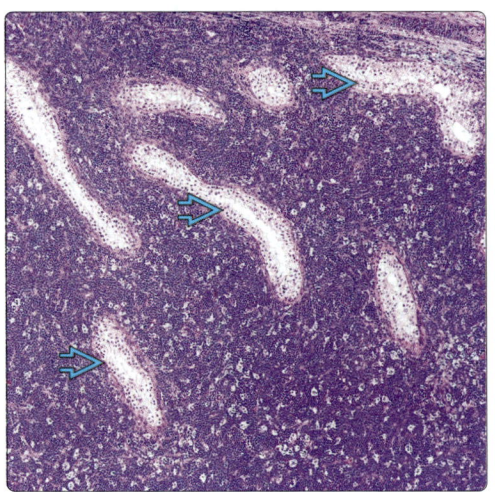

Burkitt Lymphoma
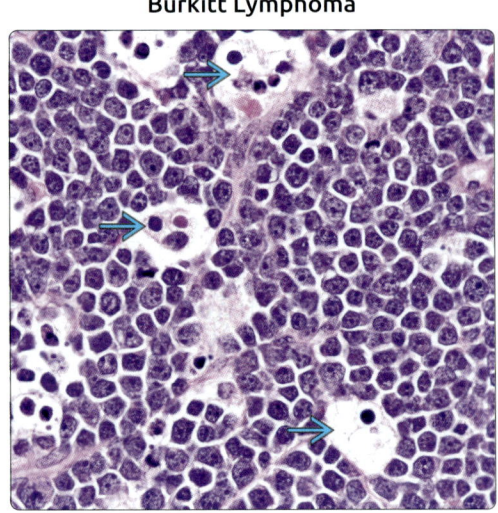

Lymphoma/Leukemia/Plasmacytoma

Plasmacytoma

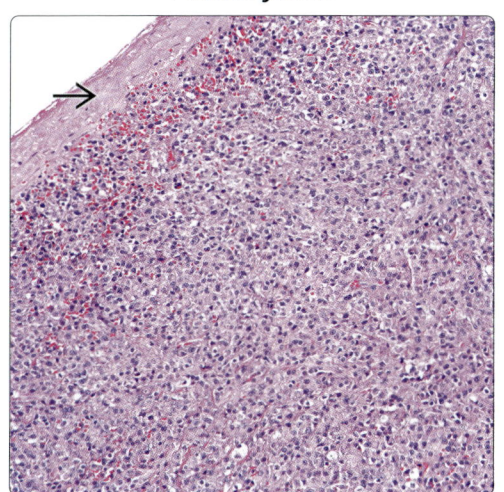

Plasmacytoma

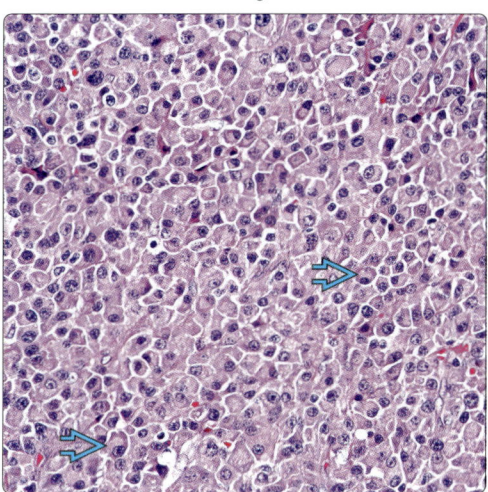

(Left) This is a low-power view of a plasmacytoma with sheets of atypical plasma cells. The tunica vaginalis and albuginea ⇨ are intact. The differential diagnosis includes non-Hodgkin lymphoma and spermatocytic tumor. **(Right)** Plasmacytoma shows atypical tumor cells with eccentric round-to-oval nuclei, abundant eosinophilic cytoplasm, and perinuclear clearing (halo) ⇨. Other differential diagnoses include rhabdoid type of Leydig cell tumor and chronic orchitis.

Interstitial Pattern of Seminoma

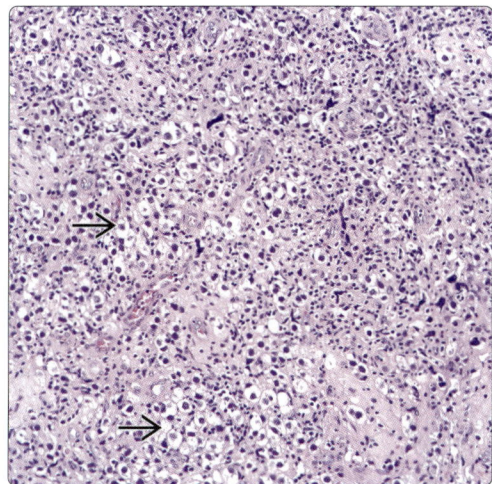

Spermatocytic Tumor

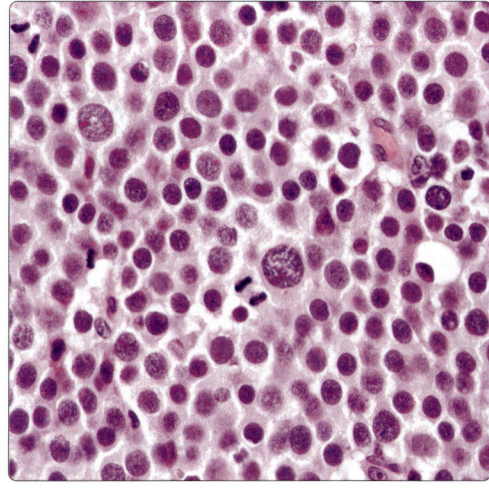

(Left) A classic seminoma with an interstitial pattern may simulate a malignant lymphoma. Helpful clues for the diagnosis for seminoma are 2 cell populations: Large tumor cells with abundant clear cytoplasm ⇨ and scattered small lymphocytes. **(Right)** An example of a spermatocytic tumor is shown. The key features distinguishing it from a lymphoma include 3 different cell populations with uniform round nuclei, fine or granular spireme-type chromatin, and more abundant cytoplasm.

Intratubular Seminoma

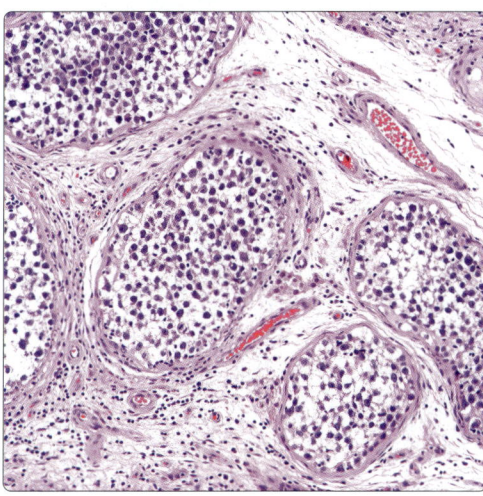

Intratubular Metastatic Carcinoma

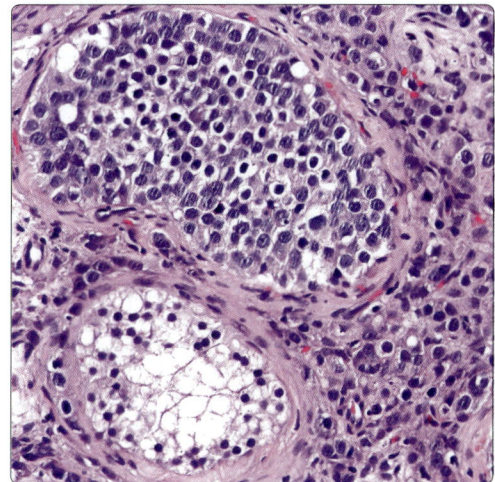

(Left) This intratubular seminoma may be similar to intratubular lymphoma. In contrast to lymphoma, the seminoma cells are evenly distributed and have abundant clear cytoplasm and distinct cell boundaries. **(Right)** This is an example of metastatic high-grade prostate carcinoma with intratubular and interstitial growth patterns, similar to that of a large cell lymphoma. Clinical history and immunostains are critical for the correct diagnosis.

Adenomatoid Tumor

KEY FACTS

TERMINOLOGY
- Benign paratesticular tumor of mesothelial cell origin, which has variety of growth patterns, including glands, cysts, tubules, cords, or isolated cells

CLINICAL ISSUES
- Most common tumor of testicular adnexa (32%)
- Usually asymptomatic, small and solid intrascrotal/extratesticular adnexal mass
- Most common in epididymis, also in tunica vaginalis, albuginea, and rete testis

MACROSCOPIC
- Small, well-circumscribed, white-tan, homogeneous, firm mass
- Size: < 5 cm (majority < 2 cm)

MICROSCOPIC
- Well-circumscribed, nonencapsulated mass
- Channels, gland-like or irregular cystic spaces, and nests and cords
- Cuboidal to flat or ovoid cells with round nuclei, abundant dense cytoplasm with vacuoles
- May show signet ring cell appearance
- Intervening fibrous stroma ± smooth muscle
- Lymphoid aggregates may be prominent within or at periphery of tumor
- Infarction or intratesticular parenchymal extension may occur

ANCILLARY TESTS
- Positive for cytokeratin, calretinin, podoplanin (D2-40), CK5/6, thrombomodulin, WT1

TOP DIFFERENTIAL DIAGNOSES
- Sex cord-stromal tumor, mesothelioma, metastatic carcinoma, epithelioid hemangioma/hemangioendothelioma, yolk sac tumor, leiomyoma/leiomyosarcoma and other sarcomas

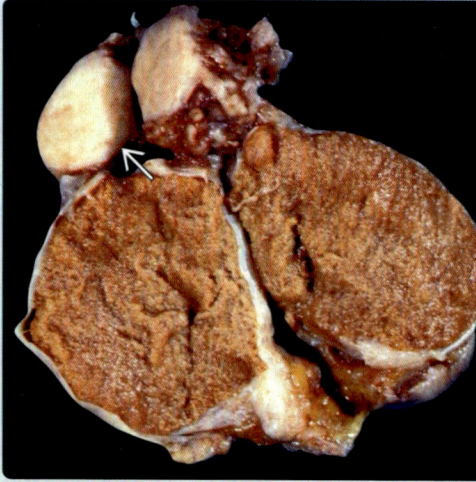

Adenomatoid Tumor: Gross

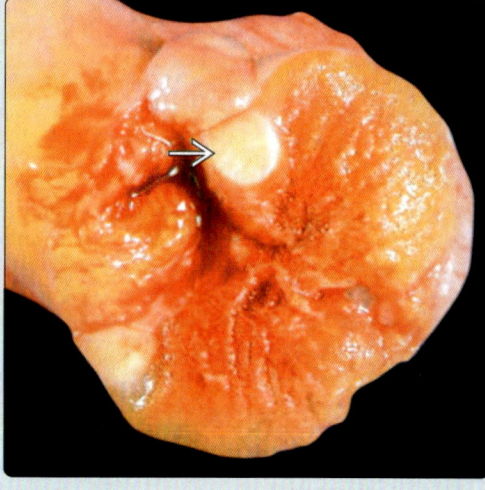

Adenomatoid Tumor: Gross

(Left) Adenomatoid tumor, the most common testicular adnexal tumor, presents as a well-demarcated, white-tan, firm mass ➡ in the epididymis. It lacks hemorrhage, necrosis, or infiltrative characteristics. (Right) A small, well-circumscribed, intraparenchymal adenomatoid tumor ➡ is shown. The tumor has a homogeneous, firm, tan-white cut surface. The main differential diagnosis based on gross examination is a sex cord-stromal tumor, which it may often grossly resemble.

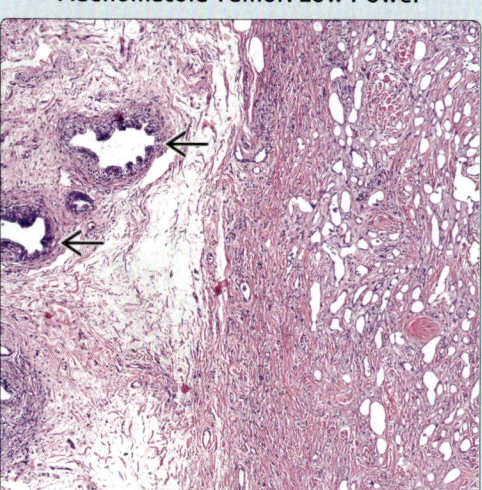

Adenomatoid Tumor: Low Power

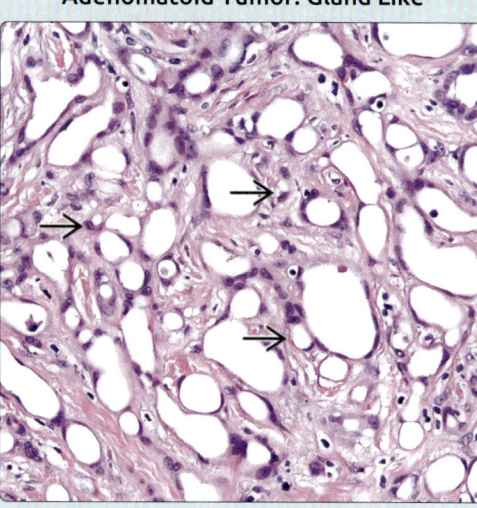

Adenomatoid Tumor: Gland Like

(Left) Low-power photomicrograph shows a typical adenomatoid tumor near the efferent ducts of rete testis ➡. The tumor is well demarcated and composed of variably sized tubules within a dense fibrous stroma. (Right) Adenomatoid tumor is characterized by irregularly shaped gland-like structures in a fibromyxoid stroma. The tumor cells are cuboidal to flattened and contain vacuolated cytoplasm ➡.

Adenomatoid Tumor

TERMINOLOGY

Definitions
- Benign paratesticular tumor of mesothelial cell origin, which has variety of growth patterns, including glands, cysts, tubules, cords, or isolated cells

CLINICAL ISSUES

Epidemiology
- Incidence
  - Most common tumor of testicular adnexa
- Age
  - Range: 18-79 years (average: 36 years)

Presentation
- Usually asymptomatic, small and solid intrascrotal mass
- Most commonly occurs in head of epididymis, although may occur in tunica vaginalis, albuginea, and rete testis
- Tumors may rarely be intratesticular and involve parietal tunica or spermatic cord

Treatment
- Surgical approaches
  - Surgical excision is curative

Prognosis
- Benign clinical course

MACROSCOPIC

General Features
- Small, well-circumscribed, white-tan, homogeneous, firm mass
- No hemorrhage or necrosis

Size
- < 5 cm (majority < 2 cm)

MICROSCOPIC

Histologic Features
- Well-circumscribed, unencapsulated mass
- Tubules; gland-like, irregular cystic spaces or channels
- Nests and cords; pure solid pattern rare
- Cuboidal, flat, or ovoid cells with round nuclei and abundant dense cytoplasm with vacuoles
- May show signet ring cell appearance
- May have prominent smooth muscle (leiomyomatous adenomatoid tumor)
- May be cellular or infarcted
- Lymphoid aggregates may be prominent within or at periphery of tumor
- Rare tumors may be infarcted

Cytologic Features
- Cuboidal, flat or ovoid, eosinophilic, vacuolated, signet ring

ANCILLARY TESTS

Histochemistry
- PAS-diastase: Negative
- Mucicarmine: Negative

Immunohistochemistry
- Positive for cytokeratin, calretinin, podoplanin (D2-40), CK5/6, thrombomodulin, WT1
- Negative for CEA, CD15, MOC-31, EpCAM/BER-EP4/CD326, S100, CD31, CD34, FLI-1

DIFFERENTIAL DIAGNOSIS

Sex Cord-Stromal Tumor
- Usually intraparenchymal tumor
- Positive for inhibin and Melan-A (MART-1)
- Usually negative for cytokeratin

Malignant Mesothelioma
- Larger tumor, destructive and infiltrative growth
- Greater cytologic atypia

Metastatic Signet Ring Cell Carcinoma
- Clinical history and older age
- Infiltrative growth, greater cytologic atypia, frequent mitoses
- Positive for CEA, CD15, EpCAM/BER-EP4/CD326, and MOC-31; negative for calretinin and podoplanin (D2-40)

Epithelioid Hemangioma/Hemangioendothelioma
- Vasoformative lesion composed of vacuolated cells
- Positive for vascular markers (CD31, CD34, FLI-1); negative or weakly/focally positive for cytokeratin

Germ Cell Tumors (Particularly Yolk Sac Tumor)
- Intraparenchymal mass with heterogeneous appearance
- Obvious malignant cytologic features
- Positive for OCT3/4, SALL4, and CD30 (BerH2); negative for calretinin

Leiomyosarcoma or Leiomyoma (vs. Leiomyomatous Adenomatoid Tumor)
- More compact cellular spindle cell proliferation with cytologic atypia and increased mitoses in leiomyosarcoma
- Lack of tubules or cystic spaces
- Negative or focally positive for cytokeratin

Liposarcoma
- Presence of lipoblasts and variable cells with adipocytic quality

SELECTED REFERENCES

1. Alexiev BA et al: Adenomatoid tumor of the testis with intratesticular growth: a case report and review of the literature. Int J Surg Pathol. 19(6):838-42, 2011
2. Pacheco AJ et al: Intraparenchymatous adenomatoid tumor dependent on the rete testis: A case report and review of literature. Indian J Urol. 25(1):126-8, 2009
3. Amin MB: Selected other problematic testicular and paratesticular lesions: rete testis neoplasms and pseudotumors, mesothelial lesions and secondary tumors. Mod Pathol. 18 Suppl 2:S131-45, 2005
4. Skinnider BF et al: Infarcted adenomatoid tumor: a report of five cases of a facet of a benign neoplasm that may cause diagnostic difficulty. Am J Surg Pathol. 28(1):77-83, 2004
5. Williams SB et al: Adenomatoid tumor of the testes. Urology. 63(4):779-81, 2004

Adenomatoid Tumor

Adenomatoid Tumor: Gland Like

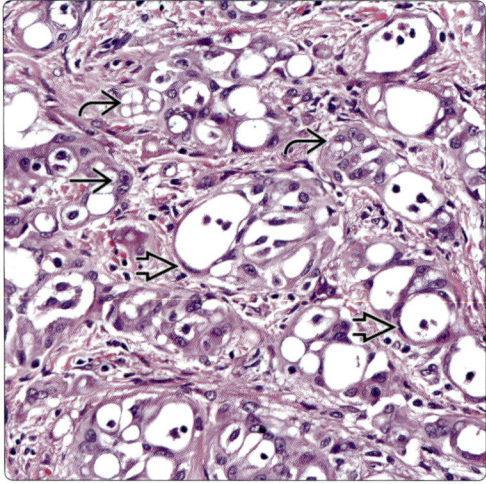

Adenomatoid Tumor: Cytology

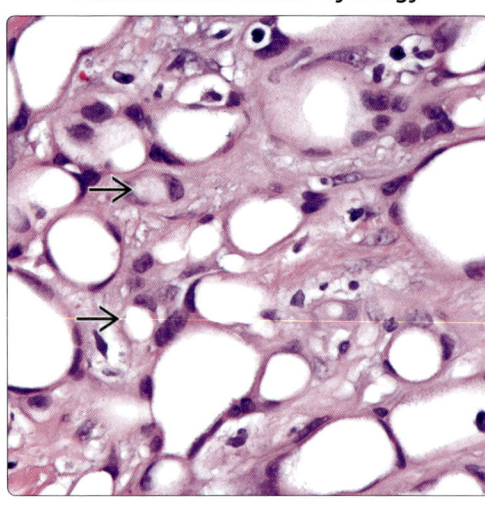

(Left) Adenomatoid tumor shows gland-like spaces of variable sizes lined by ovoid to cuboidal tumor cells with occasional prominent nucleoli ⇨ and vacuolated cytoplasm ⇨. Also seen are microcysts ⇨ lined by flattened lining cells. The amount of stroma is variable and often prominent. (Right) Adenomatoid tumor is composed of gland-like spaces lined by flattened cells. A few isolated cells with cytoplasmic vacuoles mimic signet ring cells ⇨. A variety of patterns is usually present and is a helpful feature to arrive at the correct diagnosis.

Adenomatoid Tumor: Intratesticular

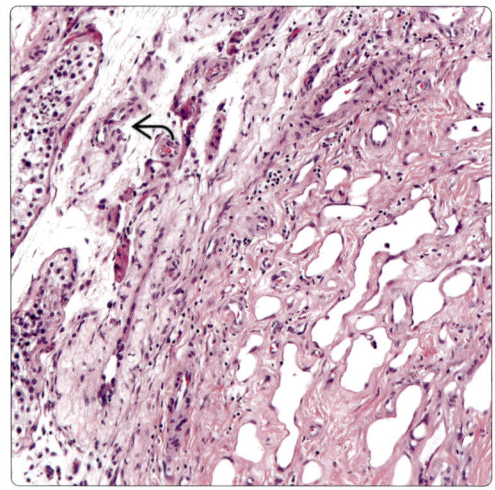

Adenomatoid Tumor: Solid Pattern

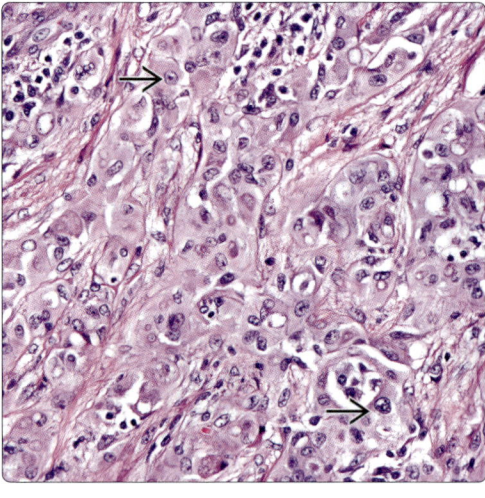

(Left) This image shows a well-circumscribed, intraparenchymal adenomatoid tumor with irregular tubules in a fibrous stroma. Atrophic ⇨ seminiferous tubules are present. (Right) High-power photomicrograph of a solid adenomatoid tumor shows proliferation of epithelioid tumor cells with occasional prominent nucleoli ⇨ and eosinophilic cytoplasm without forming tubules, which raises a possibility of Leydig cell tumor or mesothelioma.

Adenomatoid Tumor: Prominent Stroma

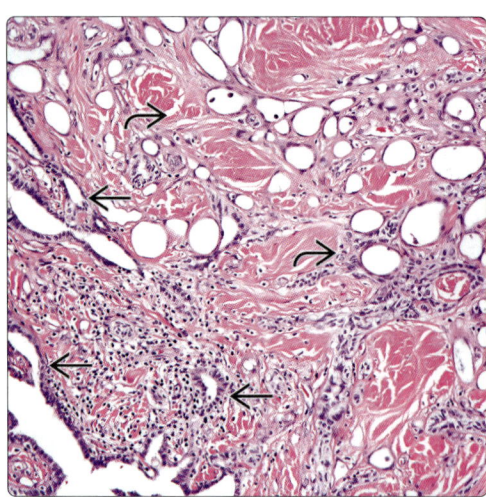

Adenomatoid Tumor: Leiomyomatous

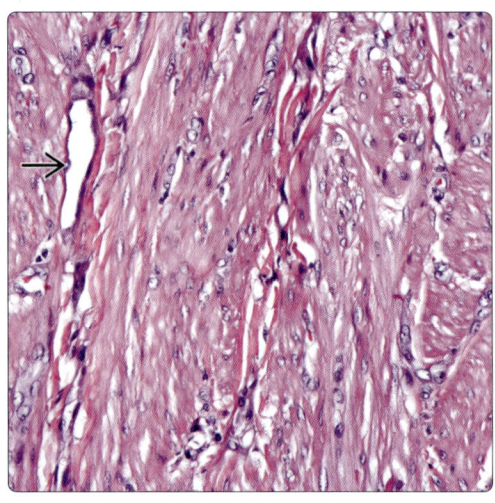

(Left) Adenomatoid tumor in the rete testis area ⇨ is shown. The tumor ⇨ shows variably sized tubules lined by cuboidal to flattened cells and accompanying dense, hyalinized, collagenous stroma and inflammatory cells. (Right) Stroma-rich adenomatoid tumor is shown with dense bundles of fibromuscular tissue with plump spindle cells, closely mimicking leiomyoma. A thin-walled space ⇨ looks like a vascular space. To prove mesothelial nature of the space, immunostaining is required.

Adenomatoid Tumor

Adenomatoid Tumor: Trabecular Pattern

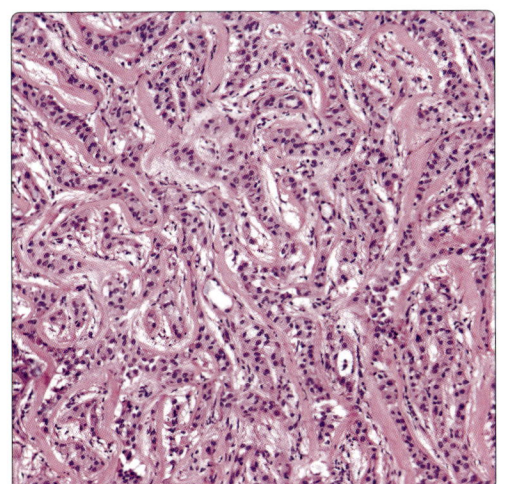

Adenomatoid Tumor: Lymphoid Infiltrate

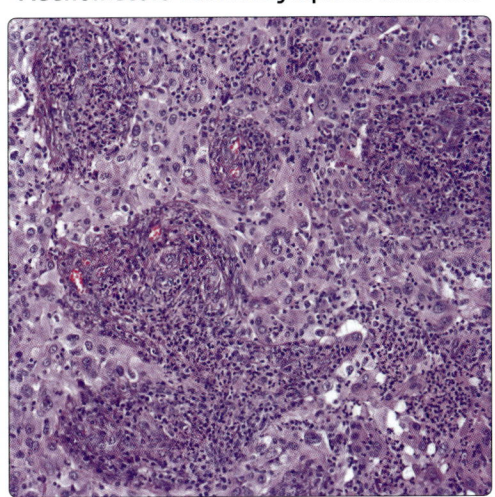

(Left) This adenomatoid tumor shows cords and trabeculae of cells within a hyalinized, fibrous stroma. Because of the extensive epithelial configuration, a misdiagnosis of carcinoma may be rendered in an older patient during frozen section evaluation. Leydig cell tumor is also in the differential diagnosis. *(Right)* This adenomatoid tumor has a prominent lymphoid infiltrate. Due to the intense lymphoid reaction, seminoma or inflammatory variant of liposarcoma is the differential diagnosis.

Adenomatoid Tumor: Cytokeratin

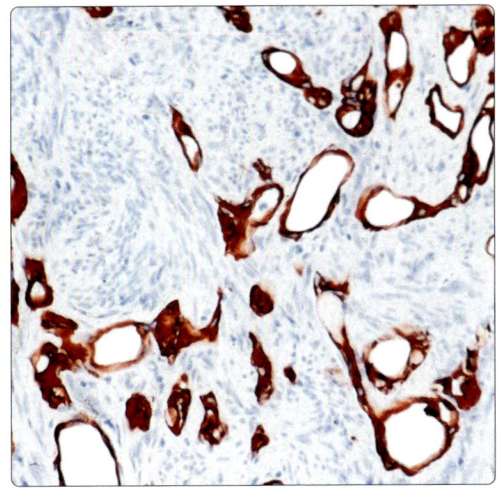

Adenomatoid Tumor: Calretinin

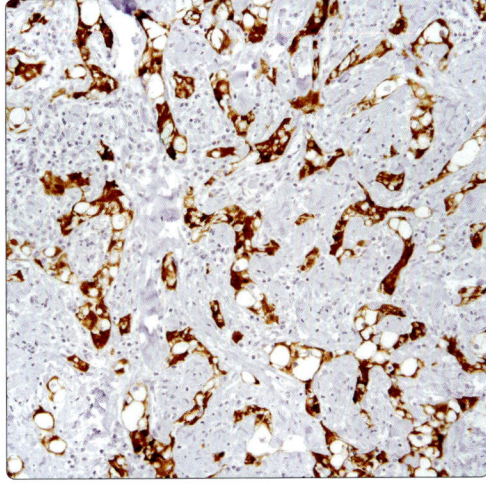

(Left) Cytokeratin stain is useful to define the nature of the vascular-like spaces or tubules in this adenomatoid tumor. The spaces or tubules are strongly positive for cytokeratin. It was also positive for calretinin, a mesothelial marker. *(Right)* Calretinin stain shows strong positivity in adenomatoid tumor. Since CK-PAN is (+) in both adenomatoid tumor & carcinoma, CK-PAN alone is not helpful. Other mesothelial cell-associated markers, including thrombomodulin, CK5/6, & podoplanin, are also (+) in adenomatoid tumors.

Malignant Mesothelioma: Differential

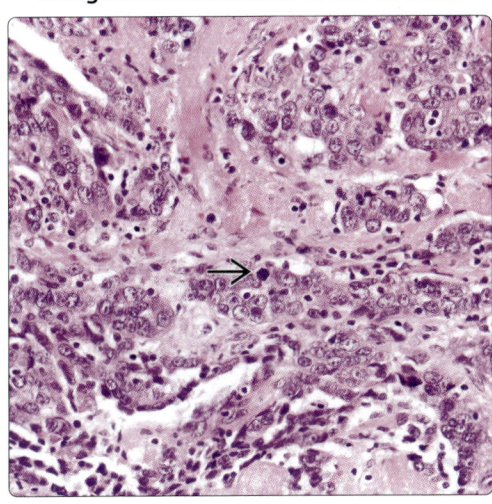

Metastatic Adenocarcinoma: Differential

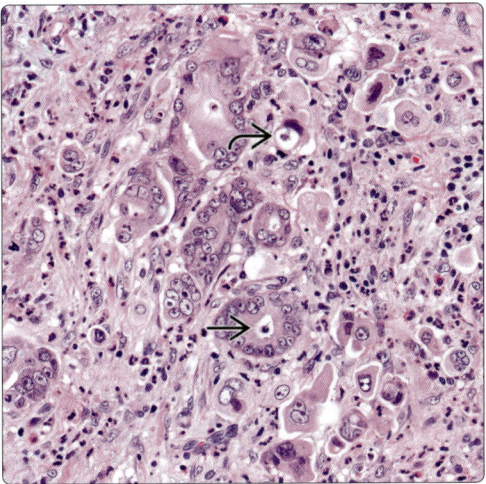

(Left) Malignant mesothelioma shows obvious cytologic atypia and increased mitotic activity ➡. Correlation with the gross findings is essential, as mesotheliomas are large, infiltrative, and associated with hemorrhage and necrosis. *(Right)* An example of metastatic adenocarcinoma to paratestis shows distinct glandular lumina ➡, greater cytologic atypia, and associated desmoplastic reaction with inflammation. Signet ring cells ➡ with marked nuclear atypia are present.

Malignant Mesothelioma

KEY FACTS

TERMINOLOGY
- Malignant tumor originating from mesothelial cells of tunica vaginalis

CLINICAL ISSUES
- Rare, but 2nd most common paratesticular malignancy after soft tissue sarcoma
- < 50% reported cases associated with asbestos exposure
- Age range: 6-90 yr (average: 54 yr)
- Paratesticular mass or associated with hydrocele

MICROSCOPIC
- Majority pure epithelial (60-70%) or biphasic type (30-40%)
- Common growth patterns: Papillary, tubulopapillary, glandular (well differentiated), or solid growth patterns (poorly differentiated)
- Rare sarcomatoid or desmoplastic types occur as well
- Round or cuboidal cells with mild or moderate cellular pleomorphism and often prominent nucleoli
- Dense hyperchromatic chromatin and frequent mitoses
- Foam cells, psammoma bodies may be seen
- Invasion is key diagnostic criterion

ANCILLARY TESTS
- Positive for CK-PAN (AE1/AE3), EMA/MUC1, vimentin, calretinin, podoplanin (D2-40), CK5/CK6, thrombomodulin, mesothelin, and WT1
- Negative for CEA, TAG72, CD15, EPCAM/BER-EP4/CD326

TOP DIFFERENTIAL DIAGNOSES
- Carcinoma of rete testis/epididymis
- Metastatic carcinoma
- Primary or metastatic sarcoma
- Papillary serous (müllerian) of tunica vaginalis
- Embryonal carcinoma
- Adenomatoid tumor
- Mesothelial hyperplasia

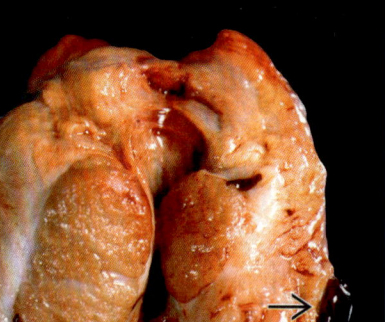
Gross Pathology

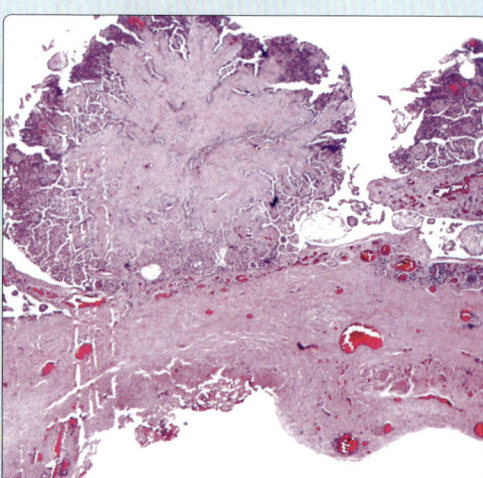
Low Power

(Left) Malignant mesothelioma demonstrates a large paratesticular nodular mass, arising in tunica and encasing the testis. The tumor shows hemorrhage ➡ and necrosis. (Right) Papillary mesothelioma with exophytic growth is shown. The main differential diagnosis is papillary mesothelial hyperplasia. Mesothelioma is usually large and shows a more complex growth pattern. However, the most important finding in mesothelioma is invasion.

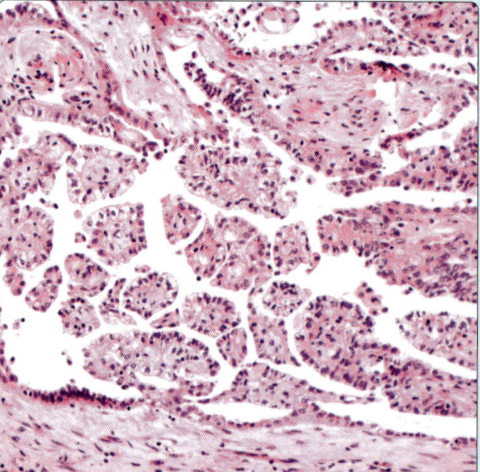
Papillary Architecture

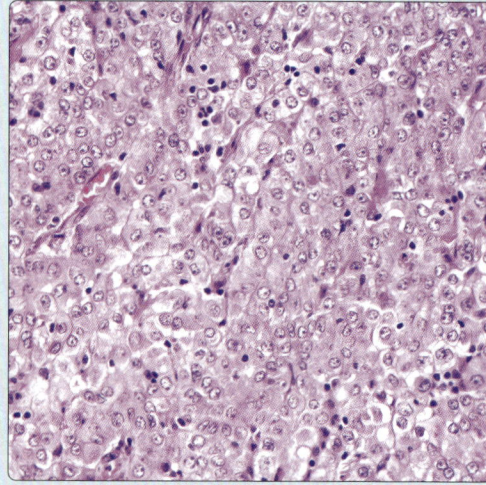
Poorly Differentiated Mesothelioma

(Left) Malignant mesothelioma with papillary growth is shown. Papillary mesothelial hyperplasia is the main differential diagnosis. In this case, formation of mass lesion and areas of tunica invasion were seen (not seen here). (Right) Poorly differentiated mesothelioma with solid growth pattern. Mesotheliomas demonstrate a range of different architectural patterns ranging from papillary to tubular to glandular and solid ± spindled (sarcomatoid) biphasic growth.

Malignant Mesothelioma

TERMINOLOGY

Definitions
- Malignant tumor arising from mesothelial cells in tunica vaginalis

ETIOLOGY/PATHOGENESIS

Pathogenesis
- Asbestos exposure is only known risk factor (associated with < 50% of cases in testicular mesothelioma)

CLINICAL ISSUES

Epidemiology
- Incidence
  o Rare, but 2nd most common paratesticular malignancy after soft tissue sarcoma
- Age
  o Range: 6-90 yr (average: 54 yr)
  o 10% of cases occur in patients younger than 25 yr

Presentation
- Paratesticular mass or associated with hydrocele

Treatment
- Surgical approaches
  o Surgical resection is treatment of choice
  o Adjuvant chemotherapy has been proved to have limited effect

Prognosis
- Variable depending on clinical stage; usually poor

MACROSCOPIC

General Features
- Variable, often diffuse thickening of tunica vaginalis with multiple friable nodules or excrescences
- Tumor may invade tunica albuginea, testis, epididymis, and spermatic cord

MICROSCOPIC

Histologic Features
- Majority pure epithelial (60-70%) or biphasic type (30-40%)
- Common growth patterns: Papillary, tubulopapillary, glandular (well differentiated), or solid growth patterns (poorly differentiated)
- Rare sarcomatoid or desmoplastic types may also occur
- Round or cuboidal cells with mild or moderate cellular pleomorphism and often prominent nucleoli
- Dense chromatin with variable mitotic activity
- Foam cells or psammoma bodies may be present
- Cytologic atypia or mesothelial proliferation alone may not be diagnostic for malignant mesothelioma
- Invasion beyond tunica is key diagnostic criterion

ANCILLARY TESTS

Immunohistochemistry
- Positive for CK-PAN (AE1/AE3), EMA/MUC1, vimentin, calretinin, Podoplanin(D2-40), CK5/CK6, thrombomodulin, mesothelin, WT1
- Negative for CEA, TAG72, CD15, EPCAM/BER-EP4/CD326, desmin (frequent)

DIFFERENTIAL DIAGNOSIS

Adenocarcinoma of Rete Testis/Epididymis
- More striking nuclear pleomorphism, significant desmoplasia, transition from rete testis epithelium
- Positive for pax-8, negative for calretinin, Podoplanin (D2-40), or CK5/CK6

Metastatic Carcinoma
- Clinical history of carcinoma elsewhere, usually greater cytologic atypia
- Negative for calretinin or Podoplanin (D2-40)

Embryonal Carcinoma
- Marked cytologic anaplasia, intratesticular mass, younger age
- Positive for CD30 (BerH2), PLAP, Podoplanin (D2-40), SALL4, and OCT3/OCT4

Primary or Metastatic Sarcoma vs. Sarcomatoid Carcinoma
- High-grade spindle cells with greater cytologic atypia
- Epicenter in spermatic cord; history of sarcoma elsewhere

Papillary Serous (Müllerian) Carcinoma of Tunica Vaginalis
- Morphologically, may be very similar with histology of mesothelioma
- Positive for WT1, p16, CD15, CA125, CEA; usually negative for calretinin, podoplanin (D2-40), or CK5/CK6

Adenomatoid Tumor
- Often asymptomatic, small size and well circumscribed, commonly seen in epididymis
- Bland cytologic features, no necrosis, no or few mitoses

Mesothelial Hyperplasia
- Overall less cytologic atypia and lack of architectural complexity and true invasion
- May be extremely difficult to distinguish from mesothelioma in small biopsy
- Desmin is more frequently positive in mesothelial hyperplasia than mesothelioma

SELECTED REFERENCES

1. Erdogan S et al: Well-differentiated papillary mesothelioma of the tunica vaginalis: a case study and review of the literature. Korean J Pathol. 48(3):225-8, 2014
2. Chekol SS et al: Malignant mesothelioma of the tunica vaginalis testis: diagnostic studies and differential diagnosis. Arch Pathol Lab Med. 136(1):113-7, 2012
3. Brimo F et al: Mesothelioma of the tunica vaginalis: a series of eight cases with uncertain malignant potential. Mod Pathol. 23:1165-72, 2010
4. Winstanley AM et al: The immunohistochemical profile of malignant mesotheliomas of the tunica vaginalis: a study of 20 cases. Am J Surg Pathol. 30(1):1-6, 2006
5. Amin MB: Selected other problematic testicular and paratesticular lesions: rete testis neoplasms and pseudotumors, mesothelial lesions and secondary tumors. Mod Pathol. 18 Suppl 2:S131-45, 2005

Malignant Mesothelioma

(Left) *Papillary mesothelioma shows complex papillae lined by relatively uniform mesothelial cells. Grossly, the tumor was large and encased the testis. Relationship with the tunica is important when other differential diagnoses, particularly mesothelial hyperplasia, are concerned. Hyperplasia rarely forms large masses.* (Right) *This is a papillary mesothelioma arising from the tunica vaginalis. The differential diagnoses includes ovarian-type papillary serous carcinoma.*

Malignant Mesothelioma
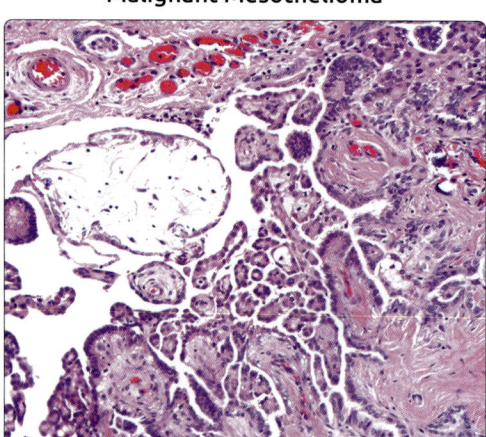

Malignant Mesothelioma
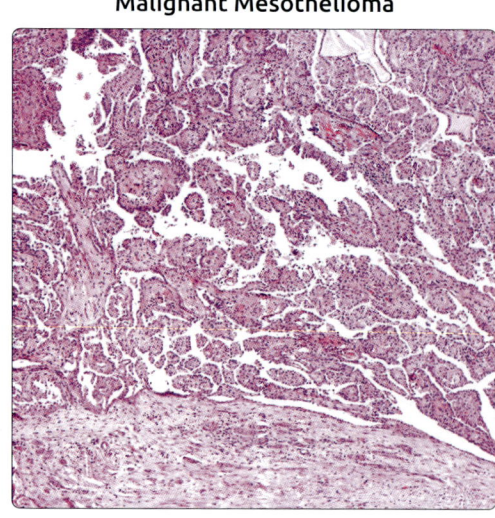

(Left) *This area of mesothelioma shows exophytic papillary and endophytic invasive growth of tumor cells. The tumor cells lining the papillae are relatively uniform. The nuclei of the invasive component are larger ➔ and have prominent nucleoli.* (Right) *Mesothelioma shows partly solid ➔ and well-formed glandular structures ➔ lined by relatively uniform neoplastic cells with prominent nucleoli. In contrast to most adenocarcinomas, mesotheliomas are lack of significant cytologic atypia.*

Malignant Mesothelioma: Invasion
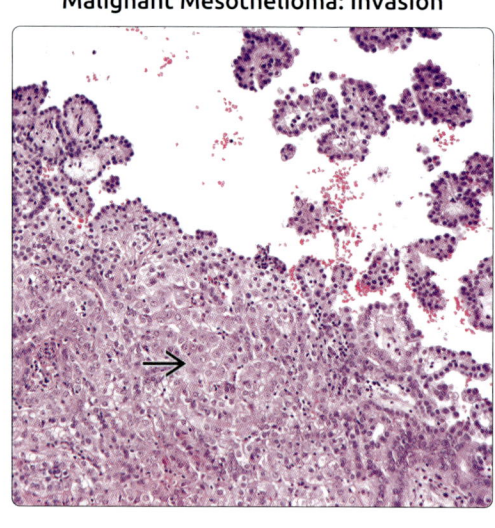

Malignant Mesothelioma: Cytology
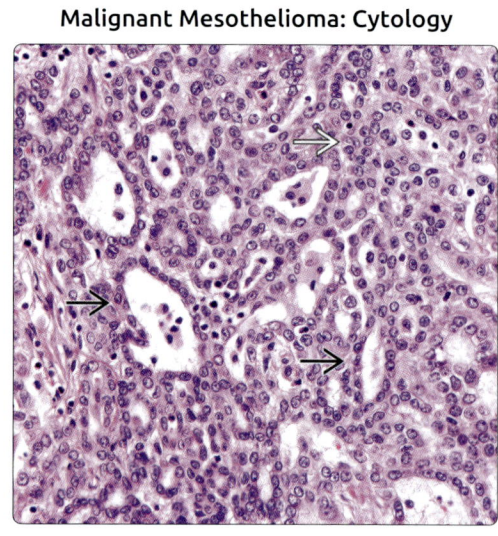

(Left) *Mesothelioma shows irregular anastomosing tubules and papillae lined by relatively uniform tumor cells with vesicular chromatin and prominent nucleoli. Psammoma body-type calcification is present ➔. A few foam cells ➔ are seen more frequently.* (Right) *Mesothelioma is composed of solid sheets of tumor cells with poor evidence of glandular differentiation ➔. Metastatic prostate carcinoma is in the differential diagnosis, although the latter is centered in the rete.*

Psammoma Body
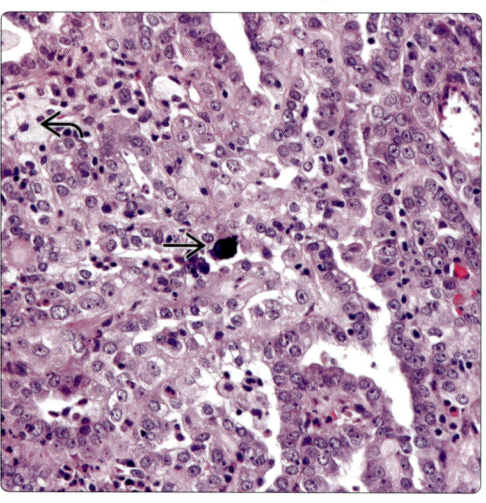

Malignant Mesothelioma
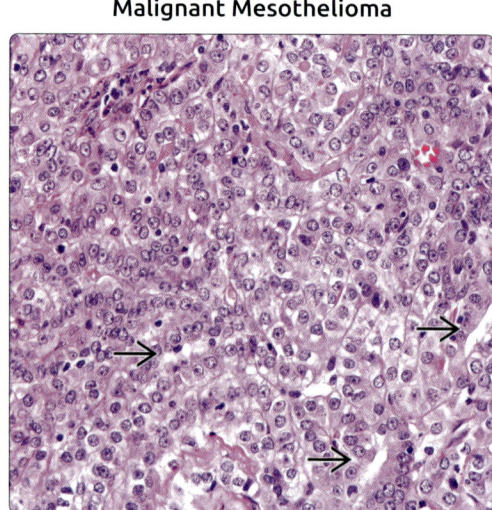

Malignant Mesothelioma

Papillary Mesothelial Hyperplasia

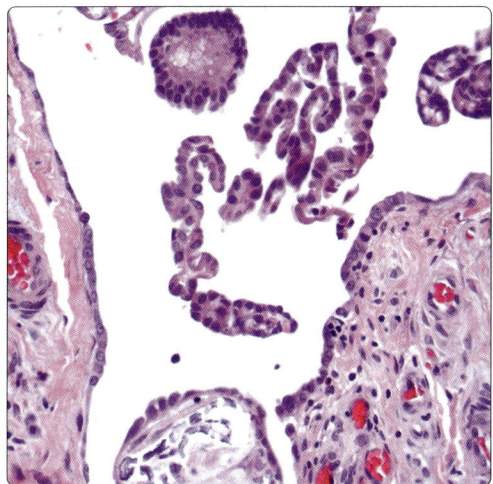

Well-Differentiated Papillary Mesothelioma

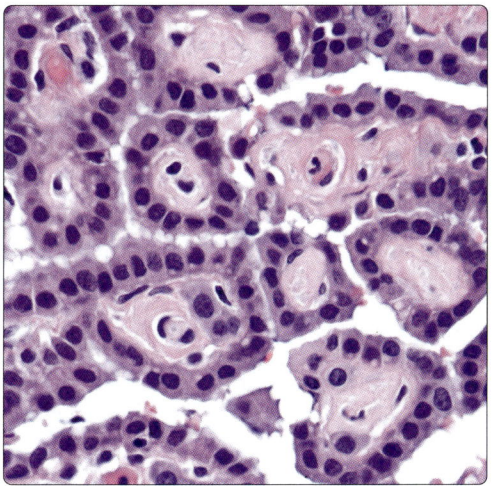

(**Left**) Papillary mesothelial hyperplasia composed of delicate papillae with monotonous mesothelial cells is shown. No significant cytologic atypia or invasion is present. (**Right**) Well-differentiated papillary mesothelioma shows delicate papillae lined by monotonous tumor cells. The distinction from papillary hyperplasia can be very difficult without demonstration of invasion. Sampling of the entire lesion is critical.

Malignant Mesothelioma: High-Grade Cytology

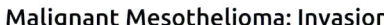

Malignant Mesothelioma: Invasion

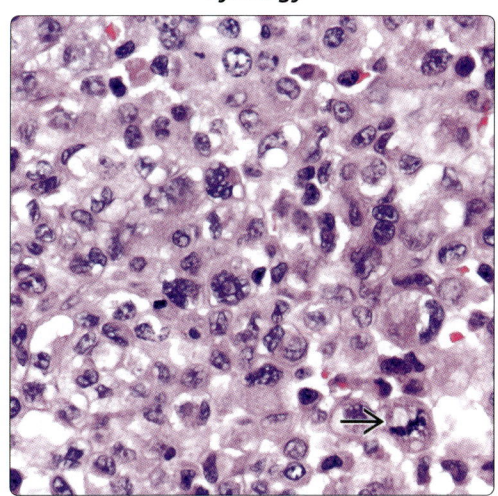

(**Left**) Although uncommon, mesothelioma may have marked nuclear pleomorphism, coarse chromatin, and increased mitoses ⇨. Immunostains with a mesothelioma-panel (including calretinin, Podoplanin (D2-40), CK5/CK6, CEA, Ber-Ep4, MOC31 or CD15) are mandatory. (**Right**) Mesothelioma with invasion into the tunica is shown. The hyalinized stroma and irregular anastomosing channels lined by uniform tumor cells are superficially reminiscent to that of adenomatoid tumor.

Deciduoid Morphology

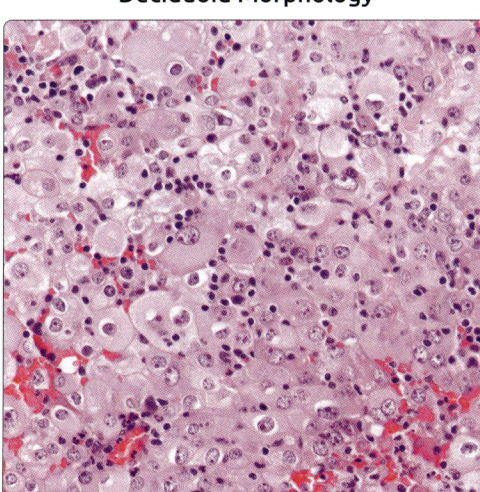

Calretinin Immunohistochemistry

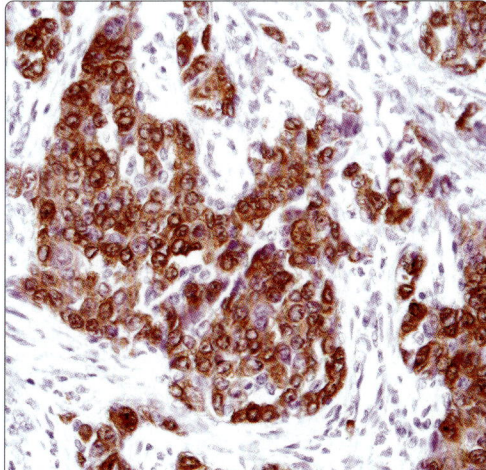

(**Left**) This mesothelioma is composed of sheets of large epithelioid cells with abundant eosinophilic cytoplasm and prominent nucleoli, which may be referred to as deciduoid or histiocytoid variant of mesothelioma. (**Right**) Mesothelioma is strongly positive (nuclear and cytoplasmic) for calretinin. A number of other markers [podoplanin (D2-40), CK5/CK6, WT1] are available for detection of mesothelial differentiation and are helpful to differentiate from adenocarcinoma.

Adenocarcinoma of Rete Testis/Epididymis

KEY FACTS

TERMINOLOGY
- Carcinoma with glandular differentiation arising from rete testis or epididymis

CLINICAL ISSUES
- Very rare
- Age range: 20-90 years (majority > 60 years)
- Large solid scrotal mass with pain

MACROSCOPIC
- Located in hilum of testis or epididymal area; white to gray, firm mass with hemorrhage or necrosis

MICROSCOPIC
- Solid, papillary, tubulopapillary, or tubular growth patterns with different degree of differentiation
- Invasive into surrounding tissue with desmoplasia
- Morphologic transition from nonneoplastic rete or epididymis to adenocarcinoma
- Nuclear stratification, incomplete gland formation, moderate to marked nuclear pleomorphism, frequent mitoses, apoptosis, and necrosis
- Intracytoplasmic or extracellular mucin may be seen

ANCILLARY TESTS
- Positive for cytokeratin, CEA, EMA/MUC1, MOC-31, CD15, EpCAM/BER-EP4/CD326, CK7, and pax-8
- Negative for PLAP, OCT3/4, SALL4, CD30 (BerH2), α-fetoprotein, glypican-3, HCG, calretinin, inhibin, and CK5/6

TOP DIFFERENTIAL DIAGNOSES
- Malignant mesothelioma
- Metastatic carcinoma
- Tumors of müllerian origin
- Embryonal carcinoma
- Rete testis hyperplasia
- Cystadenoma of epididymis

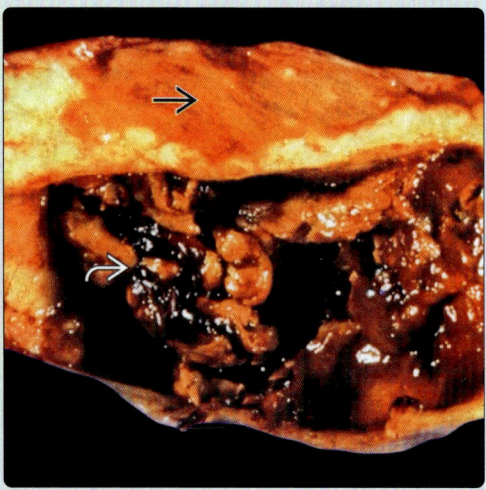

Carcinoma of Rete Testis

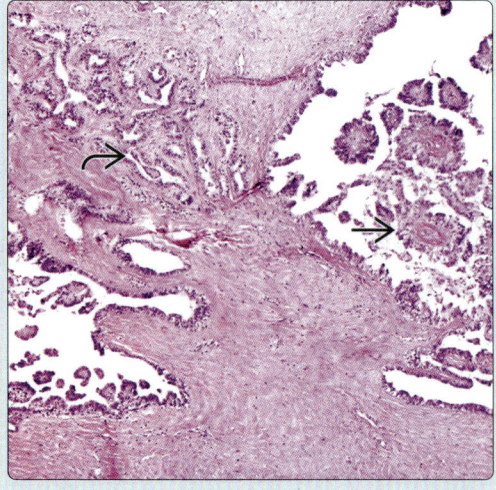

Carcinoma of Rete Testis

(Left) Carcinoma of rete testis with large hemorrhagic and cystic neoplasm in the hilum ⇨ is shown. The testicular parenchyma is uninvolved ⇨. Precise location of the mass is the key to determining the primary. (Right) Carcinoma of the rete testis shows a transition from normal-appearing rete ⇨ to a complex intracystic papillary architecture with abnormal cytology ⇨. Infiltrative growth was seen elsewhere.

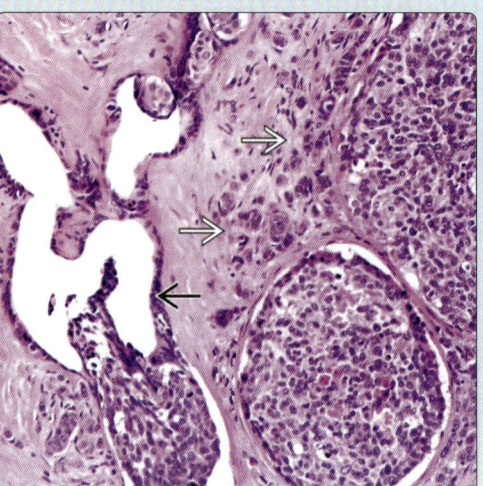

Carcinoma of Rete Testis

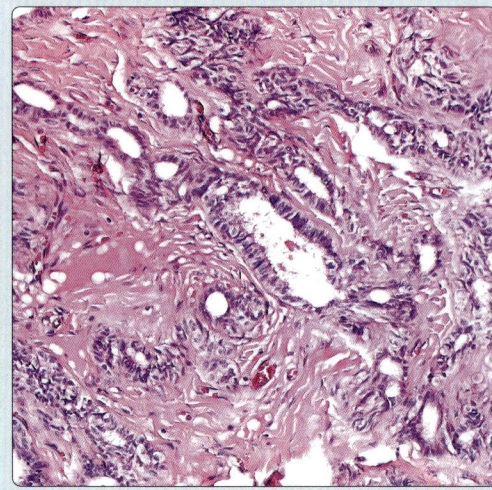

Rete Testis Hyperplasia

(Left) Carcinoma of rete testis shows nests of tumor cells with focal glandular lumina and infiltrative growth ⇨. The key diagnostic features include histologic transition ⇨ and epicenter in the rete testis area. (Right) Rete testis hyperplasia is characterized by proliferation of rete epithelium within dense fibromuscular stroma. Unlike carcinoma, there is no cytologic atypia, incomplete gland formation, desmoplastic reaction, or invasive growth. Hyperplasia rarely results in a large mass.

Adenocarcinoma of Rete Testis/Epididymis

TERMINOLOGY

Definitions
- Primary carcinoma with glandular differentiation arising from rete testis or epididymis
- Criteria for rete testis/epididymis adenocarcinoma include
  - Tumor centered in hilum or epididymis
  - Tumor incompatible with other testicular or paratesticular tumor by morphology and immunohistochemistry
  - Absence of similar extrascrotal tumor (need to rule out metastasis)

CLINICAL ISSUES

Epidemiology
- Incidence
  - Extremely rare; only handful of cases reported
- Age
  - Range: 20-90 years (majority > 60 years)

Presentation
- Large solid scrotal mass associated with pain
- ~ 25% are associated with hydrocele, inguinal hernia, or fistula

Treatment
- Surgical resection is treatment of choice
- Chemotherapy/radiation therapy in advanced and metastatic disease

Prognosis
- Generally poor when locally advanced or when distant metastasis occurs

IMAGING

General Features
- Large heterogeneous mass by ultrasonography

MACROSCOPIC

General Features
- White to gray, firm, rubbery, nonencapsulated infiltrative mass
- Hilar location (rete carcinoma) and epididymal location (epididymal carcinoma)

Size
- Range: 1-10 cm

MICROSCOPIC

Histologic Features
- Solid, papillary, or tubulopapillary growth with range of differentiation
- Invasive growth with desmoplasia
- Morphologic transition from nonneoplastic rete or epididymis to adenocarcinoma, including in situ changes
- Nuclear stratification, incomplete gland formation, moderate to marked nuclear pleomorphism with mitoses, apoptosis, and necrosis
- Intracytoplasmic or extracellular mucin may be seen; signet ring cells may be seen
- Sarcomatoid carcinoma has been reported

ANCILLARY TESTS

Histochemistry
- PAS-diastase: Diffuse positive (cytoplasmic)
- Mucicarmine and Alcian blue: Usually positive (cytoplasmic)

Immunohistochemistry
- Positive for cytokeratin, CEA, EMA/MUC1, MOC-31, CD15, EpCAM/BER-EP4/CD326, CK7, and pax-8
- Negative for PLAP, podoplanin (D2-40), OCT3/4, SALL4, CD30 (BerH2), α-fetoprotein, glypican-3, HCG, calretinin, inhibin, and CK5/6

DIFFERENTIAL DIAGNOSIS

Malignant Mesothelioma
- Epicenter in tunica vaginalis
- Histologic transition from mesothelial lining
- Positive for calretinin, podoplanin (D2-40), CK5/6; negative for MOC-31, CEA, CD15, EpCAM/BER-EP4/CD326

Metastatic Carcinoma
- History of carcinoma elsewhere, usually small size, lack of histologic transition from rete testis or epididymis
- Lymphovascular invasion and interstitial growth pattern commonly seen

Tumors of Müllerian Origin
- Lack of histologic transition from rete or epididymis, epicenter in tunica
- Papillary serous, endometrioid, clear cell, or mucinous morphology
- Borderline tumor may be seen

Embryonal Carcinoma
- Commonly seen in younger age group (25-35 years)
- Frequently associated with other germ cell tumor components and germ cell neoplasia in situ
- Positive for germ cell markers [PLAP, podoplanin (D2-40), OCT3/4, SALL4, and CD30 (BERH2)]; negative for EMA/MUC1

Rete Testis Hyperplasia
- Expands preexisting rete epithelium
- Intracytoplasmic and extracellular hyaline globules
- No cytologic atypia, invasive growth, or desmoplastic reaction; no large irregular gross mass

Cystadenoma of Epididymis
- Frequently associated with von Hippel-Lindau syndrome
- Usually occurs in young adults and frequently bilateral
- Small size with well-defined boundary
- Tumor cells have abundant clear cytoplasm and lack significant cytologic atypia

SELECTED REFERENCES

1. Peng Z et al: Advanced gastric cancer with brain metastasis effectively treated by arterial infusion chemotherapy: A case report. Oncol Lett. 7(2):449-451, 2014
2. Tong GX et al: PAX8 and PAX2 immunostaining facilitates the diagnosis of primary epithelial neoplasms of the male genital tract. Am J Surg Pathol. 35(10):1473-83, 2011

Papillary Serous Carcinoma, Müllerian Subtype

KEY FACTS

TERMINOLOGY
- Malignant müllerian-type epithelial neoplasms with serous differentiation, identical to ovarian counterpart
- Borderline serous tumor may also occur in testis

CLINICAL ISSUES
- Extremely rare; < 40 well-documented cases reported
- Range for patients with borderline tumors: 14-77 years (mean: 56 years)
- Range for patients with invasive tumors: 16-42 years (mean: 31 years)

MACROSCOPIC
- Serous carcinomas are usually firm, gritty masses with indistinct margins

MICROSCOPIC
- Invasive papillae lined by serous cuboidal or columnar cells with eosinophilic cytoplasm
- Cytologic atypia can range from bland to frankly anaplastic
- Micropapillary pattern with small clusters or nests of cells surrounded by lacunar spaces
- Abundant psammoma bodies are common
- Mucinous, endometrioid, Brenner, and clear cell-type invasive carcinoma as well as borderline tumor have rarely been reported

ANCILLARY TESTS
- Positive staining for pax-8, CK7, CA125, S100, EMA/MUC1, EpCAM/BER-EP4/CD326, CD15, TAG72, CEA

TOP DIFFERENTIAL DIAGNOSES
- Papillary cystadenoma of epididymis
- Malignant mesothelioma
- Carcinoma of rete testis or epididymis
- Metastatic adenocarcinoma

Gross Features

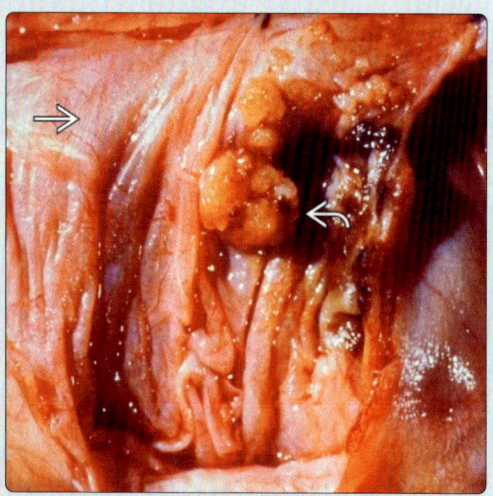

Papillary Serous Carcinoma: Focal Invasion

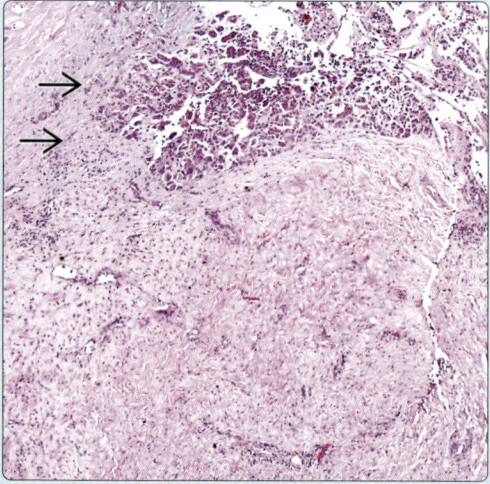

(Left) Gross image of a serous papillary tumor of borderline malignancy is shown. There is a large cystic component with a smooth wall ➡ interspersed with nodular and papillary excrescences ➡. (Right) Low-power photomicrograph of papillary serous carcinoma of paratestis shows focal invasion into the underlying tunica ➡ with accompanying desmoplastic reaction. Examination of cytologic features with immunostains is essential in the differential diagnosis from mesothelioma. (Courtesy R. Young, MD.)

Papillary Serous Carcinoma

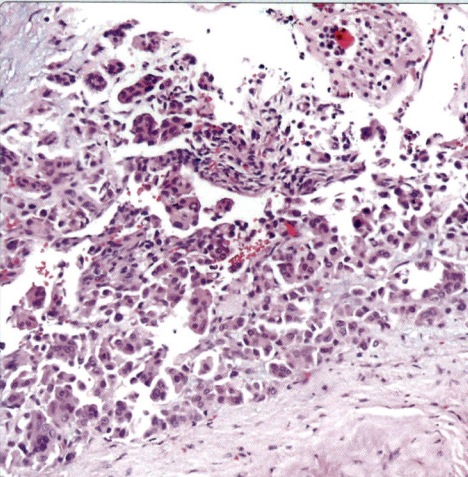

Papillary Serous Carcinoma: Micropapillary Histology

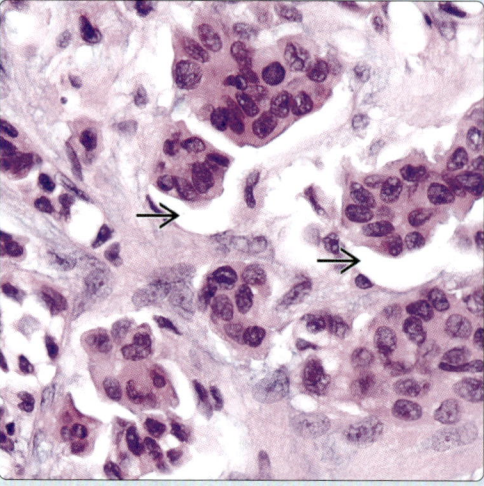

(Left) Papillary serous carcinoma of the paratestis arising from tunica vaginalis is composed of small papillae lined by uniform tumor cells with eosinophilic cytoplasm. (Courtesy R. Young, MD.) (Right) Invasive serous carcinoma (micropapillary features) is composed of clusters of tumor cells with eosinophilic cytoplasm in lacunar spaces ➡. This micropapillary pattern has also been described in carcinomas of lung, bladder, and other locations such that metastases should be ruled out.

Papillary Serous Carcinoma, Müllerian Subtype

TERMINOLOGY

Definitions
- Paratesticular homolog of ovarian malignant müllerian-type epithelial neoplasm with serous differentiation

ETIOLOGY/PATHOGENESIS

Pathogenesis Remains Speculative
- 2 possible theories
  - Müllerian metaplasia of tunica vaginalis or rarely intratesticular mesothelial inclusions
  - Müllerian rests in paratesticular soft tissue or of appendix testis

CLINICAL ISSUES

Epidemiology
- Incidence
  - Extremely rare; < 40 well-documented cases reported
- Age
  - Range for patients with borderline tumors: 14-77 years (mean: 56 years)
  - Range for patients with invasive tumors: 16-42 years (mean: 31 years)

Presentation
- Dull pain, swelling, palpable mass, hydrocele
- Mass located at testiculoepididymal groove, paratesticular soft tissues, rete testis, and tunica vaginalis

Laboratory Tests
- CA125 is elevated in some patients

Treatment
- Radical orchiectomy
- Chemotherapy or radiotherapy for locally advanced or metastatic disease

Prognosis
- Borderline tumors cured by radical orchiectomy
- Invasive carcinomas may recur or metastasize

MACROSCOPIC

General Features
- Borderline tumors typically cystic with papillary excrescences
- Serous carcinomas usually firm, gritty masses with indistinct margins, may have solid or cystic component
- Mucinous tumors predominantly cystic ± solid masses containing mucinous material
- May be associated with hydrocele

MICROSCOPIC

Histologic Features
- Histologic range includes serous borderline tumor, borderline tumor with microinvasion, and carcinoma
- Borderline tumors exhibit papillae with fibrovascular cores lined by stratified epithelium with varying atypia and mitotic activity
- Invasive clusters and papillae are lined by serous cuboidal or columnar cells with eosinophilic cytoplasm
- Cytologic atypia ranges from bland to anaplastic
- Micropapillary pattern with small clusters or nests of cells surrounded by lacunar spaces may be present
- Psammoma bodies, ciliated and hobnail cells are clues to serous differentiation
- Mucinous, endometrioid, Brenner, and clear cell-type invasive carcinoma as well as borderline tumors have been reported

ANCILLARY TESTS

Immunohistochemistry
- Positive staining for pax-8, CK7, WT1, CA125, EMA/MUC1, EpCAM/BER-EP4/CD326, CD15, TAG72, CEA, and S100
- May rarely be positive for PLAP and vimentin
- Negative for mesothelial-associated markers, such as podoplanin (D2-40), CK5/6, and calretinin; negative for CK20 (may be positive in mucinous tumor)

DIFFERENTIAL DIAGNOSIS

Papillary Cystadenoma of Epididymis
- Often associated with von Hippel-Lindau disease
- Well circumscribed, golden yellow, solid, and cystic
- Little or no atypia, no mitotic activity or stratification, may have bland clear cells

Malignant Mesothelioma
- Diffuse thickening of tunica vaginalis with multiple solid nodules
- Transition from normal to hyperplastic to atypical mesothelium and invasive growth
- Positive staining for podoplanin (D2-40) and calretinin

Carcinoma of Rete Testis or Epididymis
- Usually tubular, tubulocystic, or tubulopapillary high-grade adenocarcinomas
- Tumor epicenter in rete or epididymis determines primary site
- Histologic transition from rete or epididymal lining
- CD10 positive; negative for WT1, CA125

Metastatic Adenocarcinoma
- Clinical history of malignancy elsewhere
- Metastatic tumors usually small in size, often bilateral
- Positive for tissue-specific markers (TTF-1 for lung, PSA for prostate)

SELECTED REFERENCES

1. Narang V et al: Paratesticular papillary serous cystadenocarcinoma: a rare entity in Indian population. Indian J Pathol Microbiol. 57(4):614-6, 2014
2. Ibrahim AS et al: Borderline serous papillary tumour of the testis: a case report and review of the literature. Anticancer Res. 32(11):5011-3, 2012
3. Amin MB: Selected other problematic testicular and paratesticular lesions: rete testis neoplasms and pseudotumors, mesothelial lesions and secondary tumors. Mod Pathol. 18 Suppl 2:S131-45, 2005
4. Guarch R et al: Papillary serous carcinoma of ovarian type of the testis with borderline differentiation. Histopathology. 46(5):588-90, 2005
5. Tulunay O et al: Clear cell adenocarcinoma of the tunica vaginalis of the testis with an adjacent uterus-like tissue. Pathol Int. 54(8):641-7, 2004
6. Ulbright TM et al: Primary mucinous tumors of the testis and paratestis: a report of nine cases. Am J Surg Pathol. 27(9):1221-8, 2003
7. Becerra P et al: Papillary serous carcinoma of the tunica vaginalis testis. Pathol Res Pract. 196(11):781-782; discussion 780, 2000

Papillary Serous Carcinoma, Müllerian Subtype

(Left) Endometrioid carcinoma shows complex tubuloglandular architecture. The differential diagnosis includes carcinomas arising from the rete testis and epididymis as well as metastases, and hence correlation with gross and clinical history is important. (Right) Endometrioid adenocarcinoma arising from the tunica vaginalis is shown. Large, confluent cribriform glands are lined by stratified columnar cells, resembling its female counterpart: Endometrioid carcinoma of the uterus or ovary.

Endometrioid Carcinoma
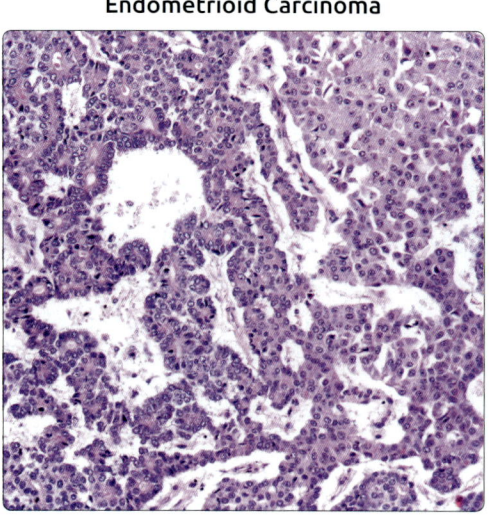

Endometrioid Carcinoma
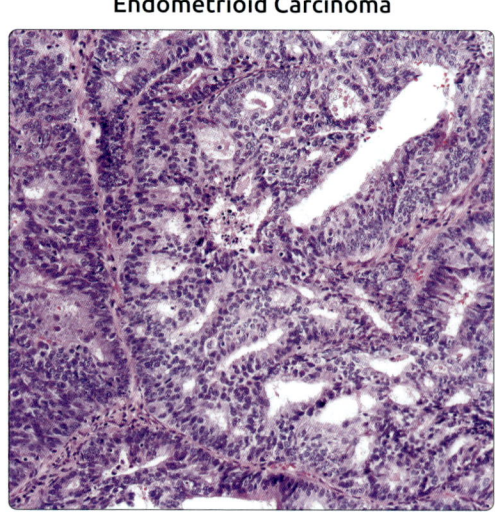

(Left) Clear cell carcinoma shows high-grade nuclear features with abundant clear cytoplasm and prominent nucleoli ⇨. Papillary growth and deposition of basement membrane-like material ⇨ are seen. Like its ovarian counterpart, a range of growth patterns, including papillary, tubular, and solid architecture may be seen. (Right) Clear cell carcinoma with solid growth is shown. Rete or epididymal carcinomas may show clear cell change as well.

Clear Cell Carcinoma
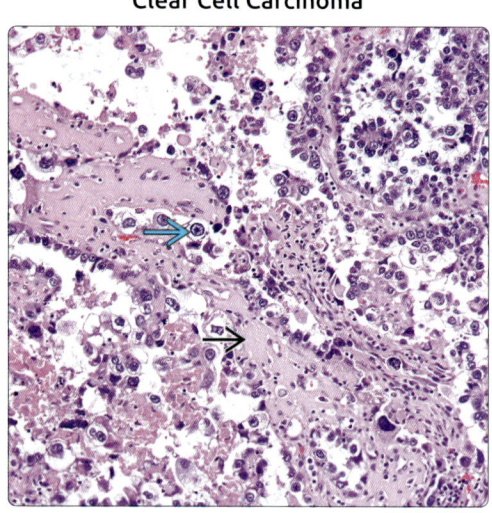

Clear Cell Carcinoma
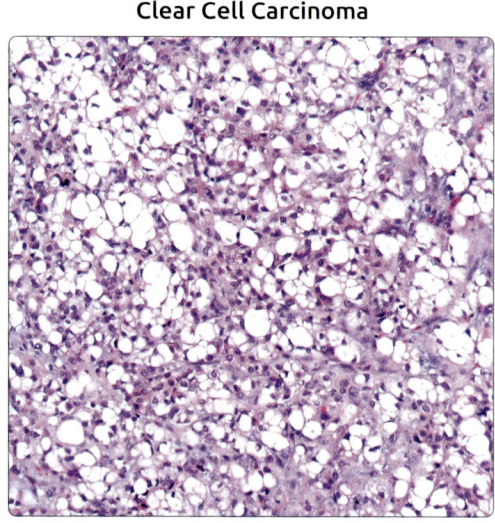

(Left) Clear cell carcinoma of müllerian type shows high-grade nuclear features with abundant clear cytoplasm and prominent nucleoli ⇨. Papillary growth, basement membrane-like material deposition ⇨, and areas of necrosis are seen. The tumor is similar to that seen in clear cell carcinoma of female counterpart. (Right) Brenner tumor of epididymis is characterized by nests of well-differentiated neoplastic urothelium surrounded by dense fibrous stroma. There is no significant cytologic atypia.

Clear Cell Carcinoma
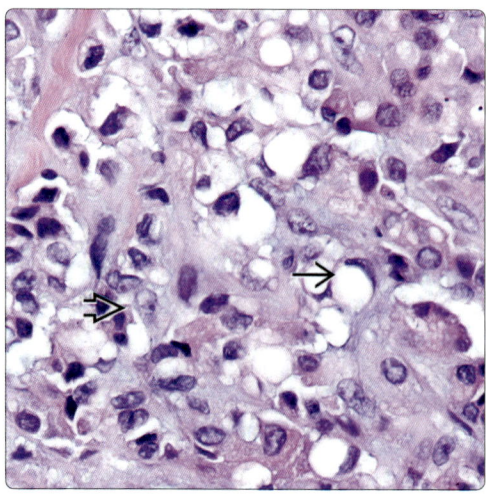

Brenner Tumor
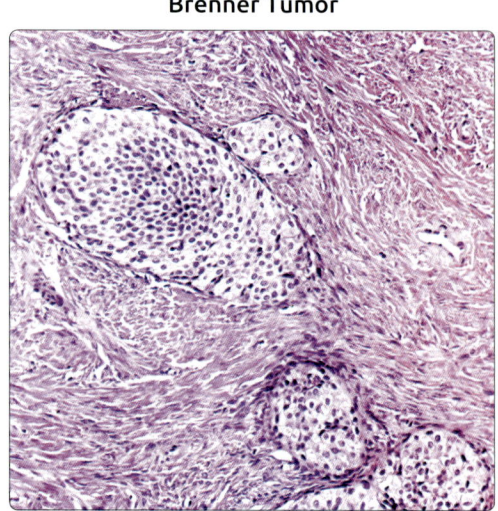

Papillary Serous Carcinoma, Müllerian Subtype

Papillary Serous Tumor: Borderline

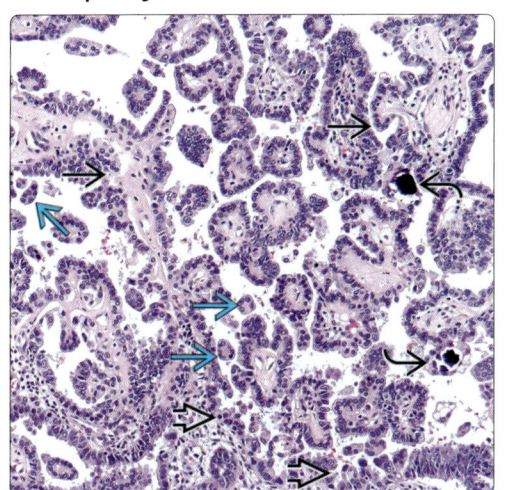

Papillary Serous Tumor: Borderline

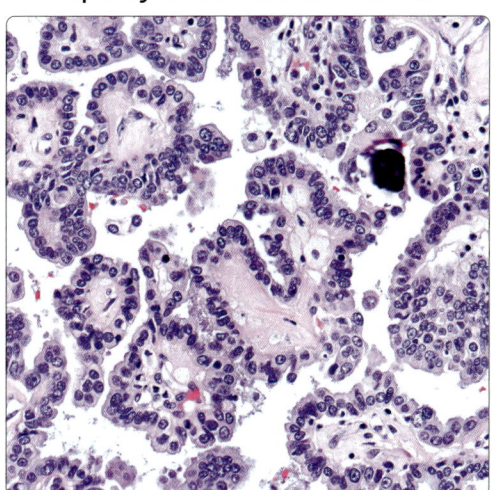

(Left) Papillary serous borderline tumor shows polypoid excrescences ⇨, micropapillae ⇨, stratified cells with budding ⇨, and psammoma bodies ⇨. There is no stromal invasion. (Right) High-power photomicrograph of borderline serous tumor shows an area with relatively bland nuclei and abundant cytoplasm. The main differential diagnosis is with a mesothelioma at the well-differentiated end of the spectrum.

Mucinous Tumor: Borderline

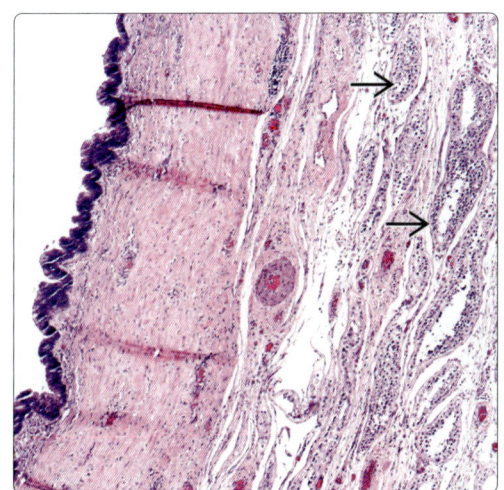

Mucinous Tumor: Borderline

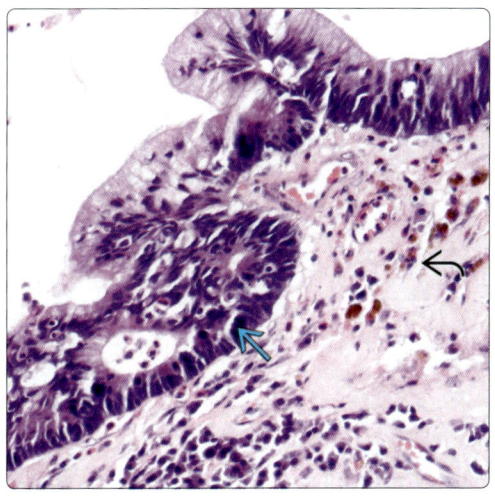

(Left) This image shows a borderline mucinous tumor arising from the tunica vaginalis. The tunica is replaced by stratified columnar mucinous epithelium. There is no stromal invasion. Uninvolved testis parenchyma ⇨ is on the right. (Right) Borderline mucinous tumor shows columnar epithelium with nuclear stratification and focal cribriform formation ⇨. The underlying stroma contains inflammatory cells and hemosiderin pigments ⇨, but there is no stromal invasion.

Paratesticular Mesothelioma

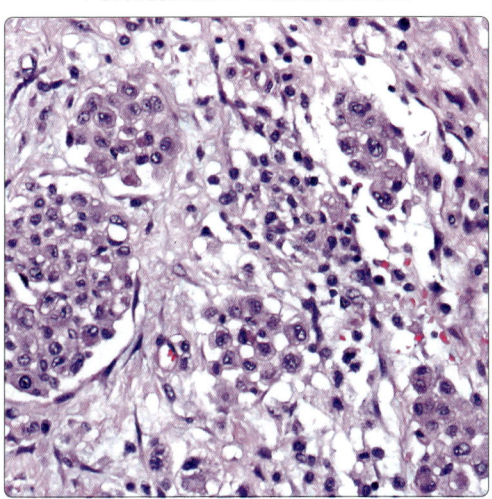

Metastatic Carcinoma

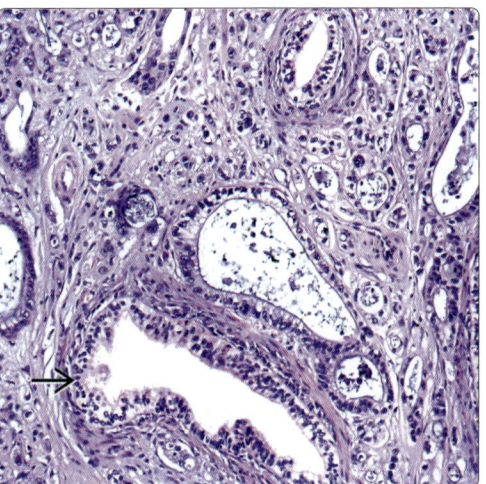

(Left) This is an image of paratesticular mesothelioma, which is one of the major differential diagnoses of müllerian-type papillary serous carcinoma. Immunohistochemistry with a panel of mesothelial- and adenocarcinoma-associated markers is often necessary to make a definitive diagnosis. (Right) This is an example of metastatic pancreatic adenocarcinoma involving epididymis ⇨. Before a diagnosis of primary müllerian carcinoma is made, a metastatic tumor has to be ruled out.

Liposarcoma

KEY FACTS

TERMINOLOGY
- Malignant neoplasm showing adipocytic differentiation

CLINICAL ISSUES
- Rare, but is most common sarcoma in paratesticular tissue in adults
- Range: 41-87 yr (average: 63 yr)
- Large scrotal mass
- Surgical resection is usually curative
- Unfavorable with dedifferentiation with metastasis

MACROSCOPIC
- Soft, homogeneous, multilobular, yellow-to-ivory mass
- Fleshy white/tan-to-tan/gray firm areas with hemorrhage or necrosis

MICROSCOPIC
- Mature adipose tissue of variable cellularity and fibrous tissue
- Marked variation in adipocyte size and shape
- Atypical cells with large, hyperchromatic nuclei
- Lipoblasts with multivacuolated or univacuolated cytoplasm may be present
- Dedifferentiated components, such as high-grade pleomorphic sarcoma or heterologous sarcoma components

ANCILLARY TESTS
- Positive for S100, CDK4, MDM2, p16

TOP DIFFERENTIAL DIAGNOSES
- Lipoma
- Adenomatoid tumor
- Sclerosing lipogranuloma
- Rhabdomyosarcoma
- Leiomyoma or leiomyosarcoma
- High-grade undifferentiated sarcoma (malignant fibrous histiocytoma)

Liposarcoma
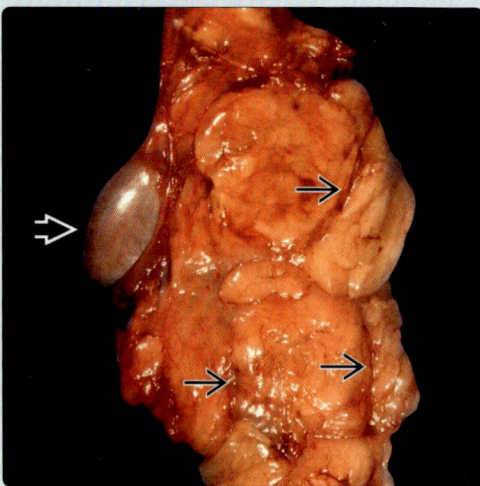

Liposarcoma With Dedifferentiation
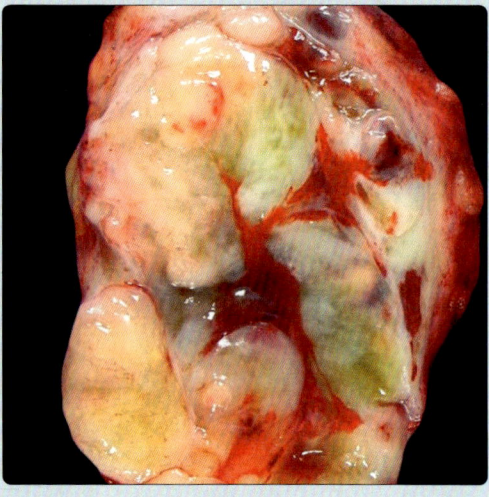

(Left) Bulky paratesticular mass with multilobulation due to fibrous bands ➡ and golden yellow appearance suggests an adipocytic tumor. Uninvolved testis ➡ is pushed to one side. (Right) Dedifferentiated liposarcoma shows nodular and fleshy white firm areas with hemorrhage. In other areas (not shown), there was yellow lobulated tissue of atypical lipomatous tumor (ALT) (WDL). Close gross examination and sampling of yellow areas is key to recognize ALT in a high-grade paratesticular sarcoma.

Atypical Lipomatous Tumor
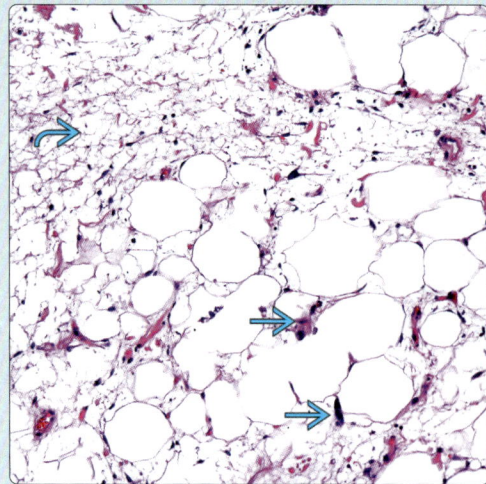

Atypical Lipomatous Tumor
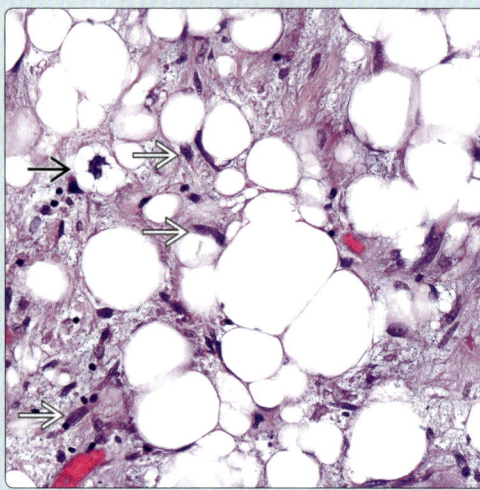

(Left) Lipoma-like ALT shows mature adipocytes of variable size and shape with fibrous bands ➡ and scattered atypical stromal cells ➡. Typical lipoblasts are not seen in this image. (Right) Lipoma-like subtype of ALT is shown. There is a significant variation in size and shape of adipocytes, increased fibrous tissue between adipocytes, and scattered atypical stromal cells ➡. A multivacuolated lipoblast ➡ is present.

Liposarcoma

TERMINOLOGY

Synonyms
- Atypical lipomatous tumor (ALT), well-differentiated liposarcoma (WDL)

Definitions
- Malignant neoplasm showing adipocytic differentiation

CLINICAL ISSUES

Epidemiology
- Incidence
  - Rare but is most common sarcoma in paratesticular tissue in adults
- Age
  - Range: 41-87 yr (average: 63 yr)

Presentation
- Large scrotal mass
- Usually involves spermatic cord, testicular tunica, or epididymis

Treatment
- Surgical approaches
  - Surgical resection is usually curative

Prognosis
- Favorable with complete excision
- Unfavorable with dedifferentiation with metastasis
- Local recurrence may occur

IMAGING

General Features
- Large hyperechoic mass by ultrasonography
- CT and MR more specific as may detect fat component

MACROSCOPIC

General Features
- Soft, homogeneous multilobular yellow-to-tan mass
- May be mistaken for lipoma except for its large size and fibrous bands
- Fleshy white-to-tan/gray firm areas with hemorrhage or necrosis indicate dedifferentiation

Size
- Range: 3-30 cm (average: 12 cm)

MICROSCOPIC

Histologic Features
- Mature adipose tissue of variable cellularity with variable fibrous bands
- Marked variation in adipocyte size and shape
- Lipoblasts should be present but may be few in numbers
- Atypical cells with large, hyperchromatic nuclei
- Dedifferentiated components, such as high-grade pleomorphic sarcoma or heterologous sarcoma components
- May have areas of low-grade leiomyosarcomatous dedifferentiation, which does not affect prognosis
- Myxoid variant of liposarcoma has rarely been associated

Predominant Pattern/Injury Type
- Lipomatous, sclerotic, or inflammatory

Predominant Cell/Compartment Type
- Mature adipose tissue and atypical pleomorphic nonlipogenic cells in dedifferentiated liposarcoma

ANCILLARY TESTS

Immunohistochemistry
- Positive for S100, CDK4, MDM2, p16
- Negative for HMB-45, actin-sm, desmin, MYOD1, or myogenin

DIFFERENTIAL DIAGNOSIS

Lipoma
- Mass usually small
- Uniform adipocytes with no irregular fibrous bands or atypical cells (lipoblasts)

Adenomatoid Tumor
- Small, well-circumscribed nodule
- Cytoplasmic vacuoles rather than true lipogenic differentiation
- Positive for calretinin, D2-40, WT1

Sclerosing Lipogranuloma
- Histiocytes, giant cells, and granulomatous reaction due to exogenous lipid
- Abundant inflammatory cells and absent lipoblasts

Rhabdomyosarcoma
- Occurs in children or young adults
- Composed of primitive cells and rhabdomyoblasts
- Positive for desmin, MYOD1, myogenin

Leiomyoma or Leiomyosarcoma
- Uniform spindle cells with eosinophilic cytoplasm
- Smooth muscle differentiation, including fascicles
- Lack of lipogenic differentiation
- Strong and uniformly positive for SMA and desmin

High-Grade Undifferentiated Sarcoma (Malignant Fibrous Histiocytoma)
- Lack of typical areas of well-differentiated liposarcoma
- No prior history of well-differentiated liposarcoma

SELECTED REFERENCES

1. Deyrup AT et al: Fibrosarcoma-like lipomatous neoplasm: a reappraisal of so-called spindle cell liposarcoma defining a unique lipomatous tumor unrelated to other liposarcomas. Am J Surg Pathol. 37(9):1373-8, 2013
2. Fitzgerald S et al: Paratesticular liposarcoma. J Urol. 181(1):331-2, 2009
3. Ghosh A et al: Unusual presentation of dedifferentiated liposarcoma as paratesticular mass. Indian J Pathol Microbiol. 51(1):42-4, 2008
4. Dotan ZA et al: Adult genitourinary sarcoma: the 25-year Memorial Sloan-Kettering experience. J Urol. 176(5):2033-8; discussion 2038-9, 2006
5. Ozkara H et al: Recurrent paratesticular myxoid liposarcoma in a young man. J Urol. 171(1):343, 2004
6. Montgomery E et al: Paratesticular liposarcoma: a clinicopathologic study. Am J Surg Pathol. 27(1):40-7, 2003
7. Folpe AL et al: Lipoleiomyosarcoma (well-differentiated liposarcoma with leiomyosarcomatous differentiation): a clinicopathologic study of nine cases including one with dedifferentiation. Am J Surg Pathol. 26(6):742-9, 2002
8. Laurino L et al: Well-differentiated liposarcoma (atypical lipomatous tumors). Semin Diagn Pathol. 18(4):258-62, 2001

Liposarcoma

Atypical Lipomatous Tumor

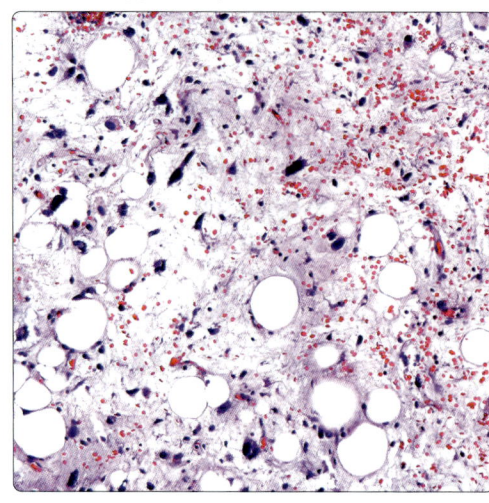

Sclerosing Atypical Lipomatous Tumor

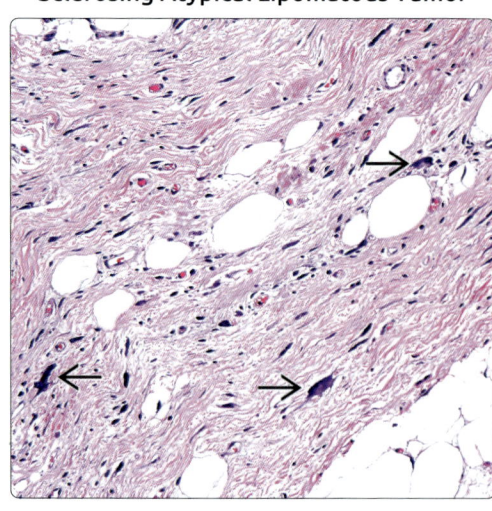

(Left) ALT shows irregularly shaped adipocytes, intervening loose fibrous tissue, and scattered atypical stromal cells. The tumor contrasts itself from a lipoma by large size, variation in size of adipocytes, and by presence of atypical stromal cells. **(Right)** Sclerosing variant of ALT shows sheets of dense mature collagen and fibrous tissue with irregularly sized and shaped adipocytes and scattered atypical stromal cells ➡. Sclerosing liposarcomas are more common in the inguinal region compared to other sites.

Sclerosing Atypical Lipomatous Tumor

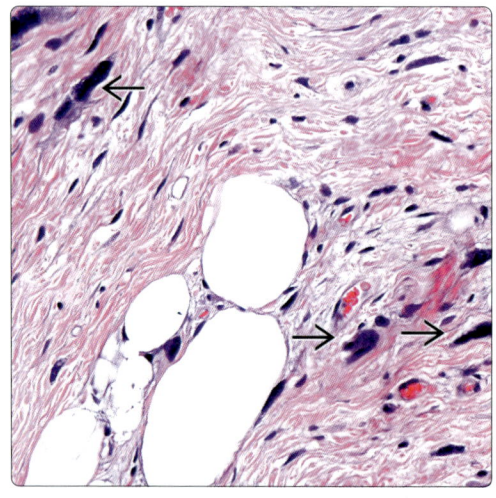

Dedifferentiation

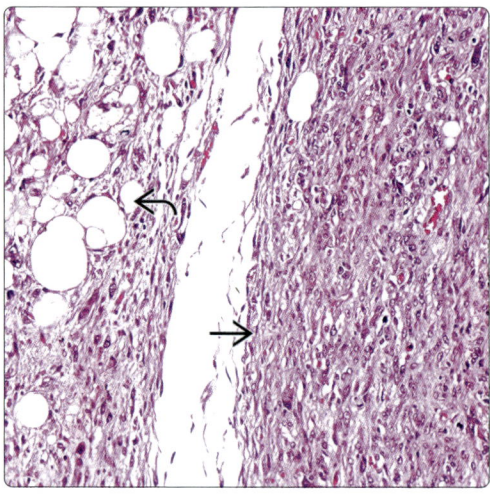

(Left) Sclerosing-type ALT shows irregular-sized adipocytes scattered in dense collagenous stroma and accompanied by markedly atypical stromal cells ➡. Atypical stromal cells are not present in sclerosing lipogranuloma. **(Right)** ALT ➡ with dedifferentiation ➡ is shown. In addition to typical ALT histology, there is an expansile area with highly atypical spindle cells of the nonlipogenic dedifferentiated component.

Dedifferentiation

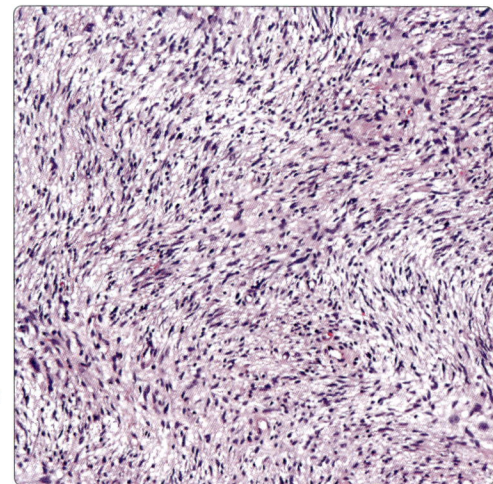

Dedifferentiation

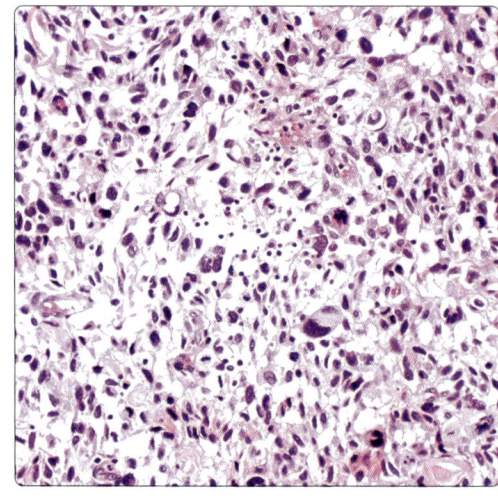

(Left) Dedifferentiated liposarcoma shows cellular spindle cell nonlipogenic tumor of high grade. In other areas of this tumor, lipoma-like ALT is seen (not shown). **(Right)** Dedifferentiated liposarcoma shows pleomorphic spindle-to-round cells with numerous mitoses, resembling malignant fibrous histiocytoma. To make a diagnosis of dedifferentiated liposarcoma, areas of ALT or prior history of ALT at the same site is required. Since this impacts prognosis, searching for an ALT is crucial.

Liposarcoma

Dedifferentiation
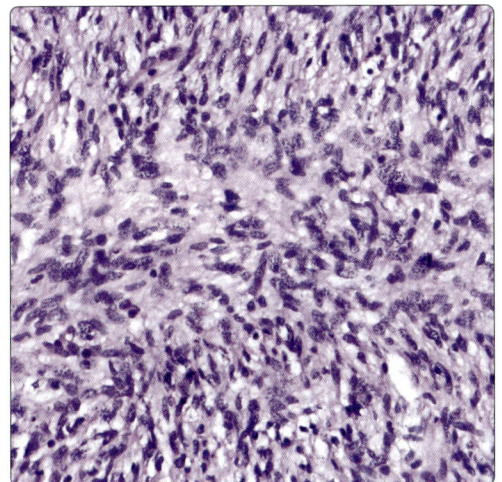

Dedifferentiation
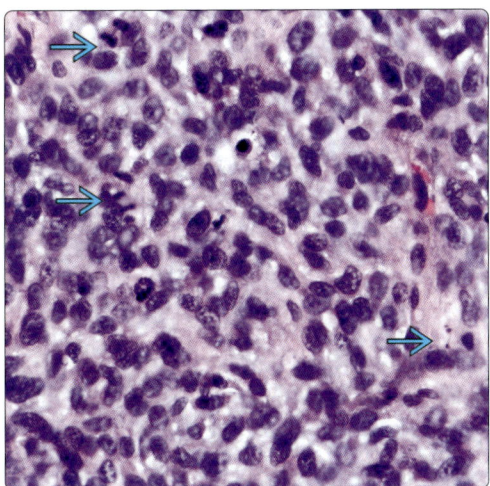

(Left) Differentiated liposarcoma is composed of fascicles of spindle cells resembling that of fibrosarcoma or leiomyosarcoma. To make a diagnosis, areas of ALT &/or history are required. (Right) This dedifferentiated liposarcoma is composed of cellular small round cells, suggesting Ewing sarcoma/peripheral neuroectodermal tumor or poorly differentiated synovial sarcoma. Mitoses ➔ are frequently seen.

Myxoid Liposarcoma
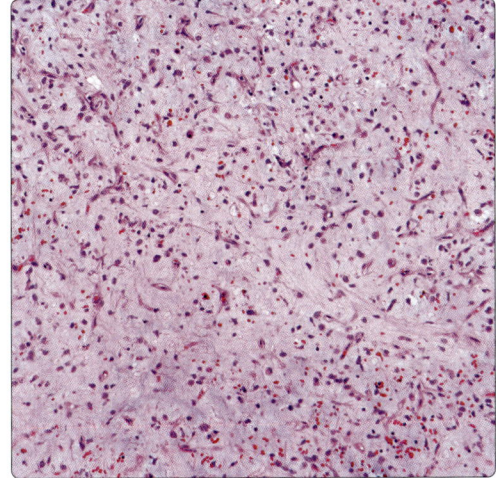

Myxoid/Round Cell Liposarcoma
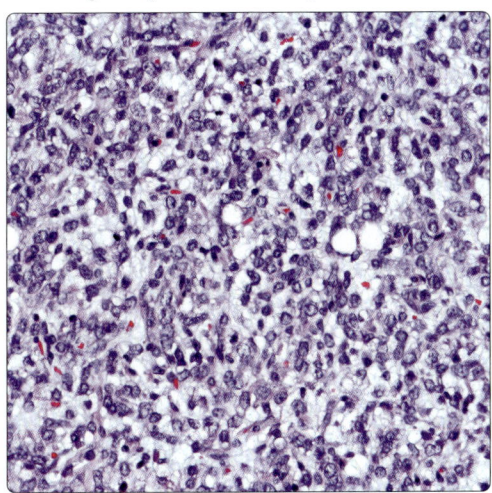

(Left) Myxoid liposarcoma shows myxoid stroma and characteristic "chicken wire" thin arborizing vasculature. At low power, myxoid malignant fibrous histiocytoma, embryonal rhabdomyosarcoma, and aggressive angiomyxoma are in the differential diagnosis. (Right) Myxoid/round cell liposarcoma with prominent round cell component is shown. The tumor cells have overlapping nuclei and myxoid stroma. It may be difficult to make a diagnosis of liposarcoma when there is no classic myxoid liposarcoma.

Sclerosing Lipogranuloma
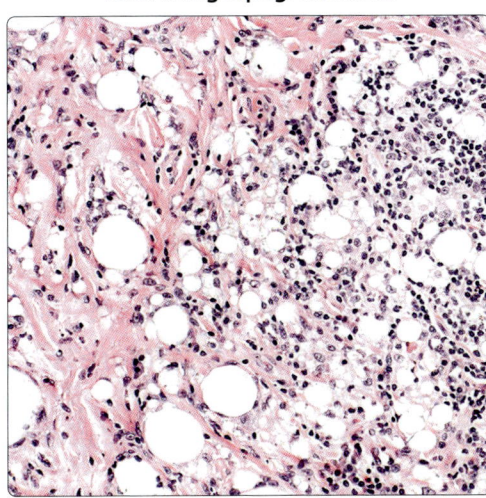

Adenomatoid Tumor
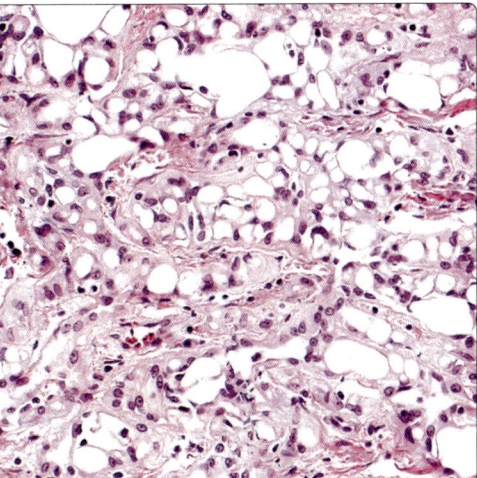

(Left) Sclerosing lipogranuloma is shown. Although there is a variation in size and shape of the adipose tissue with fibrous bands, the presence of an inflammatory infiltrate and absence of atypical stromal cells helps rule out ALT. (Right) Adenomatoid tumor with adipocytic morphology is shown. These tumors are rarely large-sized lesions and tend to be primarily paratesticular rather than centered in the spermatic cord or inguinal canal.

Melanotic Neuroectodermal Tumor

KEY FACTS

TERMINOLOGY
- Congenital melanocarcinoma, retinal anlage tumor, melanotic progonoma, melanotic hamartoma
- Rare paratesticular (usually epididymis) tumor of neural crest origin in infants and young children

CLINICAL ISSUES
- Extremely rare; < 12 cases reported involving testis or epididymis
- Range: 4 months to 8 years (80% < 1 year old)
- Firm mass in epididymis; may be associated with hydrocele

MACROSCOPIC
- Round to oval homogeneous white-gray to bluish firm nodule; may show areas of dark pigmentation

MICROSCOPIC
- Distinct biphasic tumor composed of 2 types of cells
  - Small neuroblast-like round cells with scant cytoplasm forming sheets or irregularly shaped nests
  - Large polygonal epithelioid cells with abundant eosinophilic cytoplasm, large vesicular nuclei, small nucleoli, and variable amounts of melanin pigment
- Large cells may form nests, cords, or gland-like structures
- Typically prominent fibrous and hyalinized stroma
- 2 cell components: Small cells, and large cells with melanin pigment

ANCILLARY TESTS
- Large cells positive for cytokeratin, vimentin, HMB-45, and S100
- Small cells positive for CD56, NSE, and synaptophysin; negative for keratin

TOP DIFFERENTIAL DIAGNOSES
- Other small blue cell tumors: Desmoplastic small round cell tumor, embryonal rhabdomyosarcoma, malignant lymphoma/leukemia, metastatic melanoma, neuroblastoma

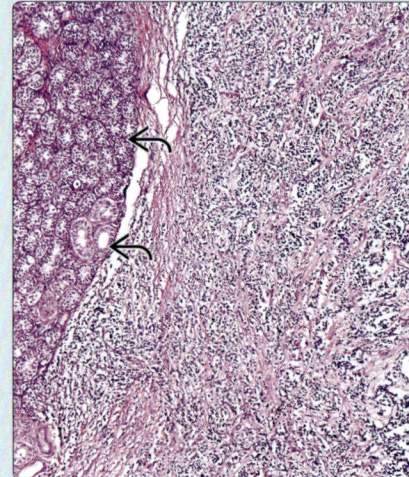

Melanotic Neuroectodermal Tumor: Well Demarcated

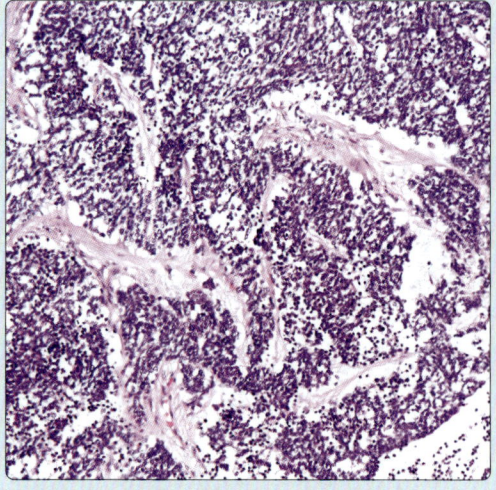

Melanotic Neuroectodermal Tumor: Small Blue Cells

(Left) Melanotic neuroectodermal tumor shows a paratesticular cellular tumor, which is well demarcated from the adjacent testis ⇨. It is characterized by sheets of small blue cells in a fibrous background. (Right) This area of melanotic neuroectodermal tumor exhibits sheets of small blue cells within dense fibrous stroma, similar to those of a desmoplastic small round cell tumor or other small blue cell tumors, such as Ewing sarcoma, rhabdomyosarcoma, or neuroblastoma.

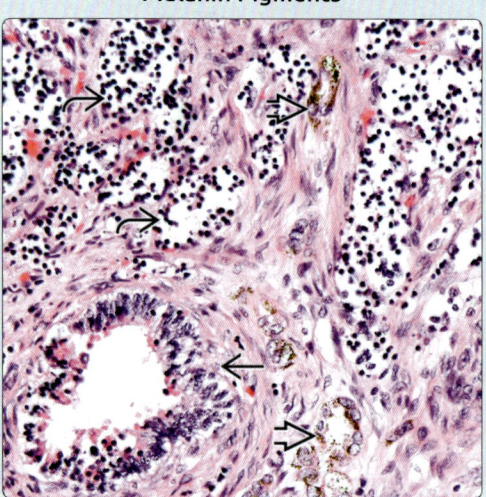

Melanotic Neuroectodermal Tumor: Melanin Pigments

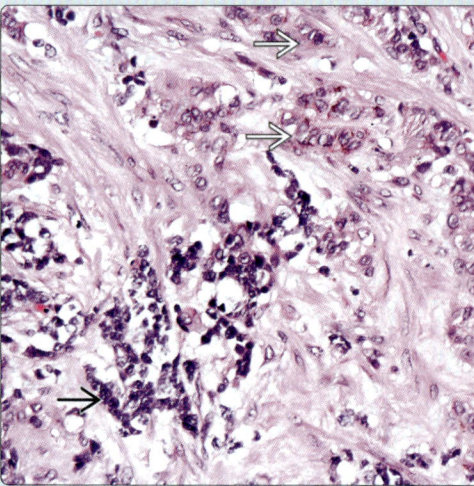

Melanotic Neuroectodermal Tumor: Small and Epithelioid Cells

(Left) Melanotic neuroectodermal tumor involves efferent ductules ⇨. The tumor is composed of the characteristic cellular components of small blue cells ⇨ and large epithelioid cells with brown melanin pigment ⇨ amidst a dense fibrous stroma. (Right) High-power photomicrograph shows a biphasic tumor composed of clusters of large epithelioid cells with melanin pigment ⇨ and nests of small blue cells ⇨. The degree of melanin may vary and may occasionally be inconspicuous.

Melanotic Neuroectodermal Tumor

TERMINOLOGY

Synonyms
- Congenital melanocarcinoma, retinal anlage tumor, melanotic progonoma, melanotic hamartoma

Definitions
- Rare paratesticular (usually epididymal) tumor of neural crest origin in infants and young children

CLINICAL ISSUES

Epidemiology
- Incidence
  - Extremely rare; < 12 cases reported in testis or epididymis
- Age
  - Range: 4 months to 8 years (80% < 1 year old)

Presentation
- Firm mass in epididymis; may be associated with hydrocele

Laboratory Tests
- Mild elevation of serum α-fetoprotein, urine vanillylmandelic acid (VMA), and homovanillic acid in some cases

Treatment
- Surgical resection, occasionally with adjuvant therapy (chemotherapy or radiotherapy)

Prognosis
- Generally behaves in benign fashion with rare recurrence and metastasis

MACROSCOPIC

General Features
- Round to oval homogeneous white-gray to bluish firm nodule
- May show dark brown or black areas due to pigmentation
- Closely apposed to, but usually does not involve, testicular parenchyma

Size
- Usually < 4 cm

MICROSCOPIC

Histologic Features
- Distinct biphasic tumor composed of 2 types of cells
  - Small neuroblast-like round cells with scant cytoplasm forming sheets or irregularly shaped nests
  - Large polygonal epithelioid cells with abundant eosinophilic cytoplasm, large vesicular nuclei, small nucleoli, and variable amounts of melanin pigments
- Large cells may form nests, cords, or gland-like structures
- Typically prominent fibrous and hyalinized stroma

ANCILLARY TESTS

Immunohistochemistry
- Large cells positive for cytokeratin, vimentin, HMB-45 and S100 (less common), synaptophysin, NSE, GFAP, and desmin; CD99 rarely positive
- Small cells positive for CD56, NSE, and synaptophysin; negative for cytokeratin

DIFFERENTIAL DIAGNOSIS

Desmoplastic Small Round Cell Tumor
- Occurs in older patients
- Tumor consists of only a small cell population and has more prominent desmoplasia
- Lack of large cells with melanin pigment
- Positive for cytokeratin and desmin

Embryonal Rhabdomyosarcoma
- Tumor with rhabdomyoblasts with variable degree of differentiation
- Small cells with minimal cytoplasm to fusiform cells with abundant cytoplasm and spindle cells with fibrillary background
- Positive for desmin, MYOD1, and myogenin

Malignant Lymphoma/Leukemia
- Diffuse interstitial infiltrative pattern and relatively uniform cell population
- Primarily testicular parenchymal involvement with secondary extension into paratesticular tissues
- Positive for CD45(LCA) and B- or T-cell related markers (depending on immunophenotype)

Metastatic Melanoma
- Occurs in older age patients and in those with history of primary tumor
- Prominent nucleoli, pseudonuclear inclusions, and numerous mitoses
- Most cells positive for melanocytic markers

Neuroblastoma
- Rare in paratesticular location
- Uniform single cell population
- NB84, neurofilament, synaptophysin, NSE, CD57 positive

SELECTED REFERENCES

1. Rachidi S et al: Melanotic neuroectodermal tumor of infancy: a systematic review. J Oral Maxillofac Surg. 73(10):1946-56, 2015
2. Ulbright TM et al: Testicular and paratesticular tumors and tumor-like lesions in the first 2 decades. Semin Diagn Pathol. 31(5):323-81, 2014
3. Desai S et al: Recurrent melanotic neuroectodermal tumour of infancy of the epididymis and testis: a case report. Indian J Pathol Microbiol. 48(3):363-4, 2005
4. Kobayashi T et al: Melanotic neuroectodermal tumor of infancy in the epididymis. Case report and literature review. Urol Int. 57(4):262-5, 1996
5. Calabrese F et al: Melanotic neuroectodermal tumor of the epididymis in infancy: case report and review of the literature. Urology. 46(3):415-8, 1995
6. Diamond DA et al: Melanotic neuroectodermal tumor of infancy: an important mimicker of paratesticular rhabdomyosarcoma. J Urol. 147(3):673-5, 1992
7. Pettinato G et al: Melanotic neuroectodermal tumor of infancy. A reexamination of a histogenetic problem based on immunohistochemical, flow cytometric, and ultrastructural study of 10 cases. Am J Surg Pathol. 15(3):233-45, 1991

Melanotic Neuroectodermal Tumor

(Left) This image shows a melanotic neuroectodermal tumor involving efferent ductules of the rete testis. There are large cells forming clusters ⇨ and scattered small blue cells ➡ in a dense fibrous stroma. (Right) High-power image shows a melanotic neuroectodermal tumor involving epididymis ➡. There are clusters of small blue cells ⇨ and large epithelioid cells with brown pigment ⇨.

Melanotic Neuroectodermal Tumor: Small and Epithelioid Cells
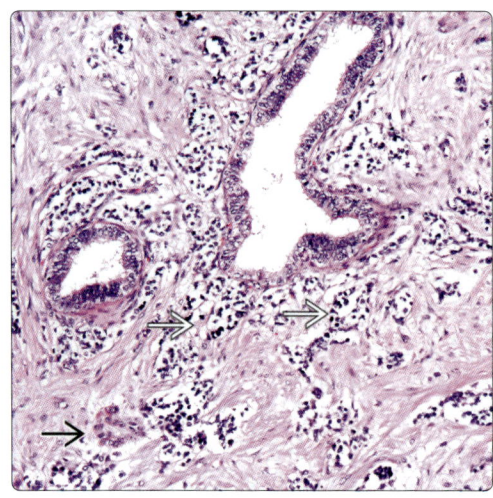

Melanotic Neuroectodermal Tumor: Melanin Pigments
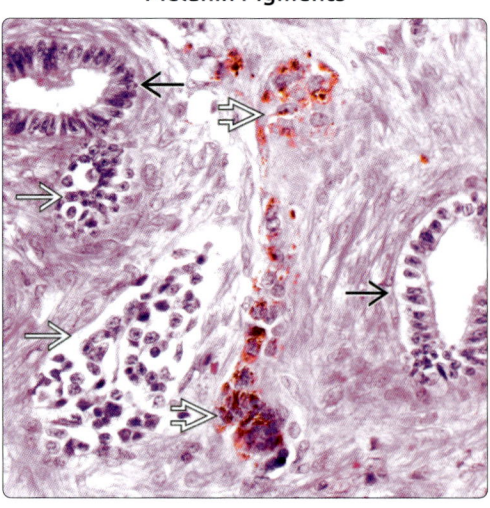

(Left) High-power view of melanotic neuroectodermal tumor shows nests of large epithelioid cells with vesicular nuclei, prominent nucleoli, and coarse melanin pigment ⇨. Also seen are scattered small blue cells ➡ and dense fibrous stroma. (Right) Typical biphasic appearance of melanotic neuroectodermal tumor is shown here. On the right is a sheet of small blue cells with hyperchromatic nuclei ➡, and on the left are epithelioid cells ⇨ with melanin pigment and glandular formation.

Melanotic Neuroectodermal Tumor: Epithelioid Cells and Melanin Pigments
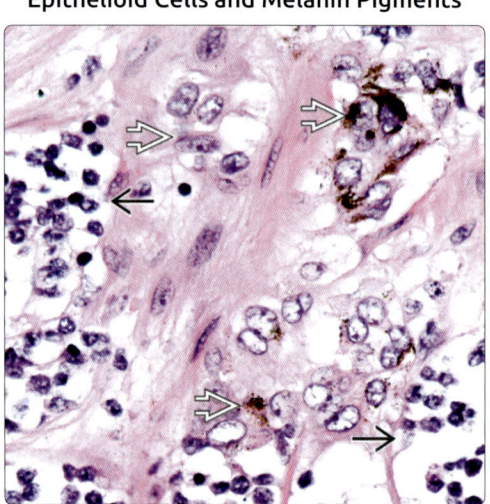

Melanotic Neuroectodermal Tumor: Small and Epithelioid Cells
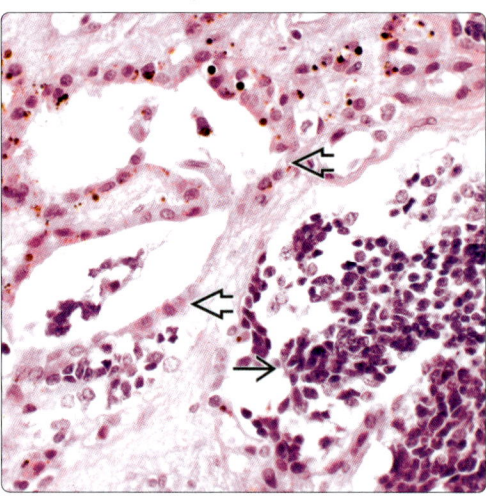

(Left) Melanotic neuroectodermal tumor shows nests of small blue cells ➡ within artifactual spaces, and large epithelioid cells with melanin pigment ⇨. The fibrous stromal response is a typical feature of the tumor. (Right) Melanotic neuroectodermal tumor shows nests of small blue cells ➡ surrounded by delicate fibrous septa. A few large epithelioid cells ⇨ are present. In this situation, the differential diagnosis from other small blue cell tumors in children may be difficult.

Melanotic Neuroectodermal Tumor: Small and Epithelioid Cells
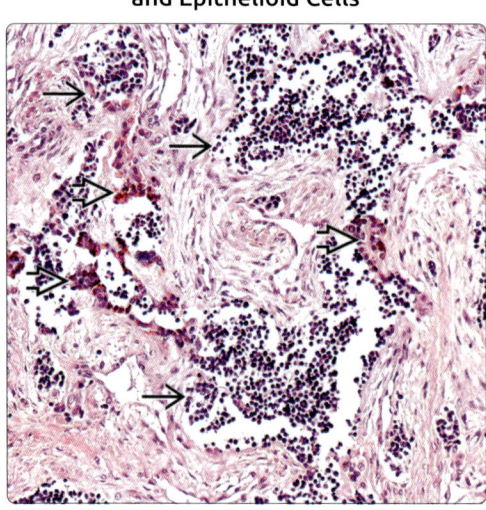

Melanotic Neuroectodermal Tumor: Small and Epithelioid Cells
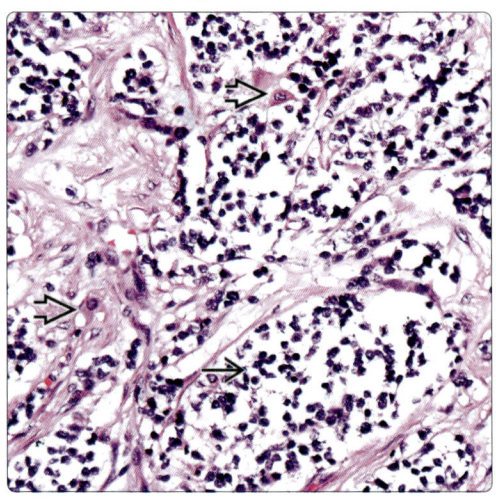

Melanotic Neuroectodermal Tumor

Melanotic Neuroectodermal Tumor: Small Blue Cells

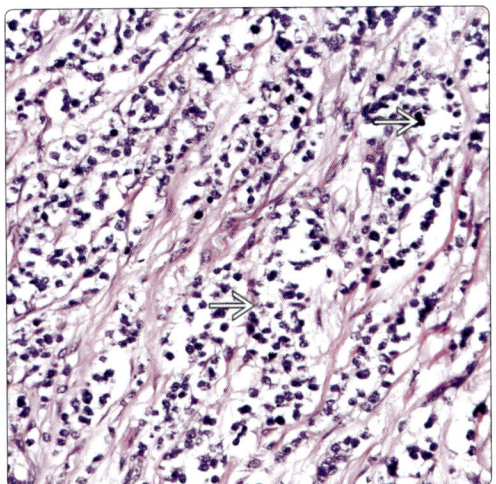

Melanotic Neuroectodermal Tumor: Small and Epithelioid Cells

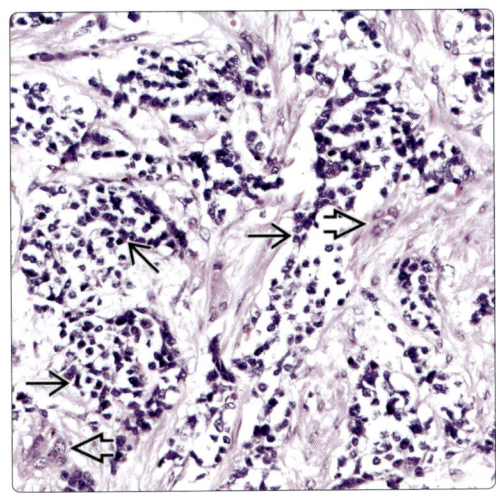

(Left) This area of a melanotic neuroectodermal tumor shows nests and sheets of small blue cells separated by delicate fibrous septa with pseudoglandular formation ➡. In other areas, not shown here, the other diagnostic component of large epithelioid cells with melanin pigment was observed. (Right) Cellular nests of small neuroblastoma-like blue cells ➡ are admixed with very few large epithelioid cells ➡. Homer Wright rosettes are not seen in this tumor and help in distinction from neuroblastoma and Ewing sarcoma PNET.

Desmoplastic Round Cell Tumor: Differential

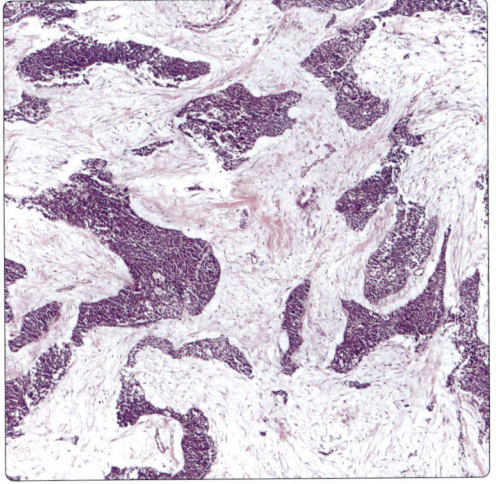

Desmoplastic Round Cell Tumor: Differential

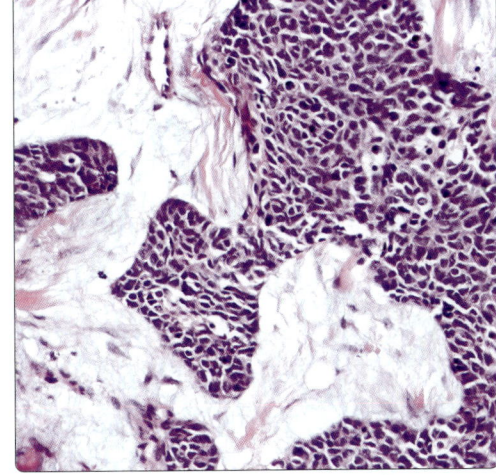

(Left) Low-power view of desmoplastic round cell tumor shows irregular solid nests of tumor cells and paucicellular desmoplastic stroma. It may be difficult to differentiate from melanotic neuroectodermal tumor. (Right) A desmoplastic round cell tumor has a similar appearance as that of small cell component of melanocytic neuroectodermal tumor. Age, identification of large epithelioid cells with melanin pigment, and typical immunostaining profile allow the distinction.

Rhabdomyosarcoma: Differential

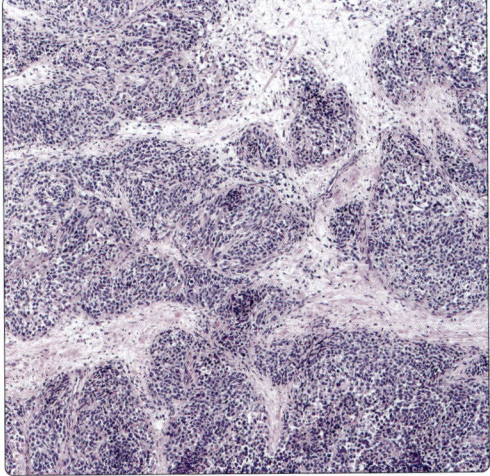

Rhabdomyosarcoma: Differential

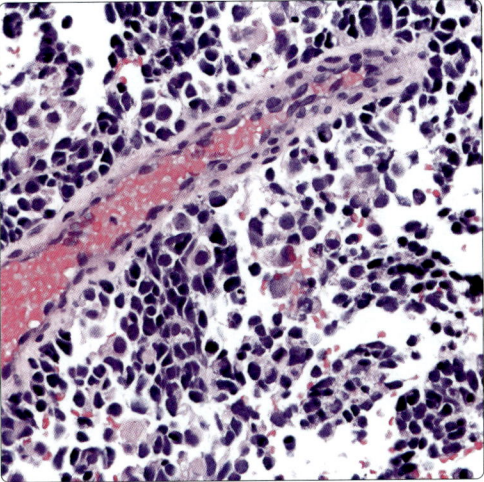

(Left) Low-power view of rhabdomyosarcoma is very similar to that of melanotic neuroectodermal tumor. It is composed of solid sheets of hypercellular tumor cells separated by dense fibrous stroma. (Right) High-power view of a rhabdomyosarcoma shows small blue cells with variable amount of cytoplasm, hyperchromatic nuclei with frequent mitoses and apoptosis. Immunostain with MYOD1 and myogenin is necessary to confirm the diagnosis.

Embryonal Rhabdomyosarcoma

KEY FACTS

TERMINOLOGY
- Malignant neoplasm with skeletal muscle differentiation that recapitulates embryogenesis of skeletal muscle and encompasses spindle cell and anaplastic variants

CLINICAL ISSUES
- Range: 7-36 years
- Paratesticular location is one of the more common sites of rhabdomyosarcoma (4% of all)

MACROSCOPIC
- Well-circumscribed, large paratesticular mass (average: 4-6 cm)
- Often multinodular with gelatinous, gray-white cut surface

MICROSCOPIC
- Mixture of primitive and variable proportion of well-differentiated rhabdomyosarcomatous component
- Alternating cellular and less cellular myxoid areas (embryonal rhabdomyosarcoma, not otherwise specified)
- Spindle cells with fascicular pattern, mimicking leiomyosarcoma (spindle leiomyomatous rhabdomyosarcoma)
- Primitive cells (blue cells) with small, round to oval, hyperchromatic cells or spindle cells
- Differentiating rhabdomyosarcoma cells with eosinophilic cytoplasm, fibrillary material, or cross striations

ANCILLARY TESTS
- Positive for desmin, actin-HHF-35, myoglobin, MYOD1, myogenin, and vimentin

TOP DIFFERENTIAL DIAGNOSES
- Leiomyosarcoma
- Dedifferentiated liposarcoma
- Malignant lymphoma/leukemia
- Other small blue cell tumors

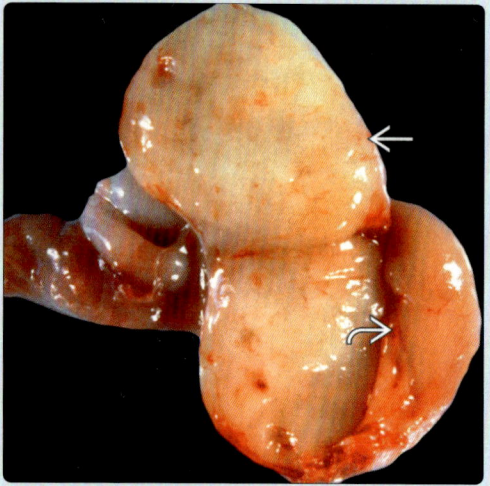

Embryonal Rhabdomyosarcoma: Gross

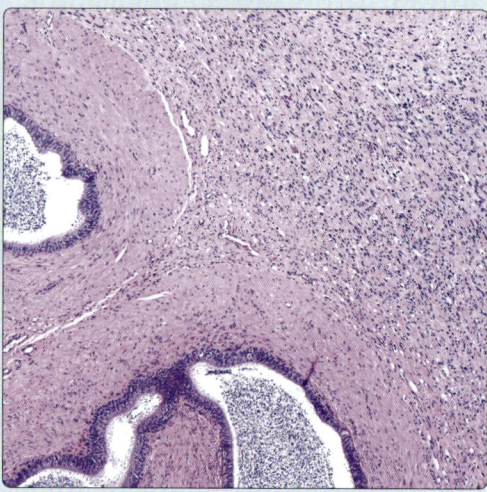

Embryonal Rhabdomyosarcoma: Low Power

(Left) Paratesticular embryonal rhabdomyosarcoma has a homogeneous, tan-white, gelatinous cut surface ➔. No necrosis or hemorrhage is seen. The testis ➔ is compressed but not involved. *(Right)* A low-power view of embryonal rhabdomyosarcoma involving proximal ductus deferens is shown. The tumor is composed of hypercellular spindle cell proliferation surrounding the muscular wall of ductus deferens.

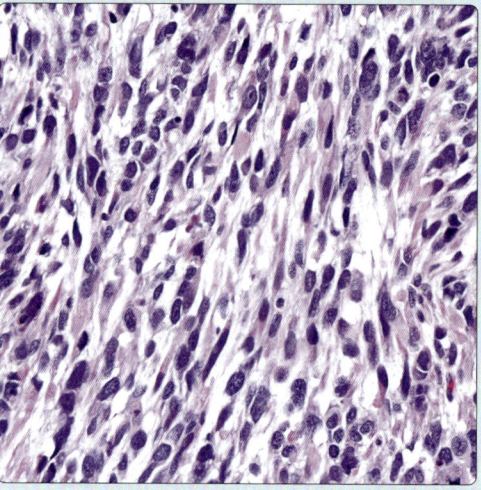

Embryonal Rhabdomyosarcoma: Spindle Cells

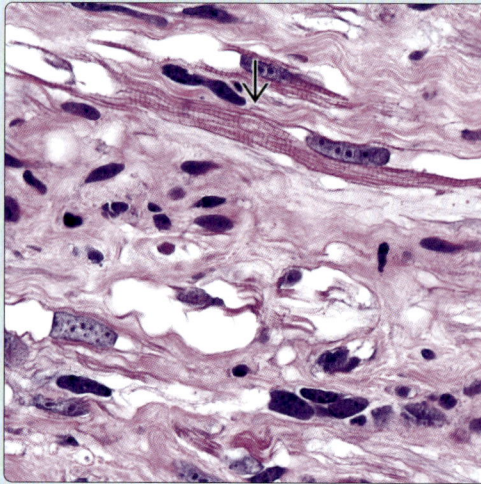

Embryonal Rhabdomyosarcoma: Cross Striations

(Left) Embryonal rhabdomyosarcoma of spindle type shows tumor is composed of spindle cells arranged in a vague fascicular pattern. Immunohistochemistry with MYOD1 and myogenin is necessary for a definitive diagnosis and to differentiate it from leiomyosarcoma. *(Right)* High-power photomicrograph of embryonal rhabdomyosarcoma shows well-differentiated rhabdomyoblasts (strap cells) with abundant eosinophilic cytoplasm & cross striations ➔. The stroma is myxoid.

Embryonal Rhabdomyosarcoma

TERMINOLOGY

Synonyms
- Embryonal rhabdomyosarcoma, not otherwise specified (NOS); spindle leiomyomatous rhabdomyosarcoma

Definitions
- Malignant neoplasm with skeletal muscle differentiation that recapitulates embryogenesis of skeletal muscle and encompasses spindle cell and anaplastic variants

CLINICAL ISSUES

Epidemiology
- Incidence
  o Most common sarcoma in children
  o Paratesticular location is one of more common sites of rhabdomyosarcoma (4% of all)
- Age
  o Range: 7-36 years

Presentation
- Paratesticular mass in young patients
- Gradual enlargement of scrotal sac with no acute onset symptoms
- Transillumination may be positive when lesion is associated with hydrocele
- May spread to paraaortic or paracaval lymph nodes and to bone and lung

Treatment
- Usually multimodal, surgical resection ± radiotherapy or chemotherapy

Prognosis
- Favorable prognosis in general with surgery, chemotherapy, and radiation therapy
- Prognosis associated with histologic type, age, tumor size and stage, and adequacy of resection
  o Embryonal, NOS, and spindle cell variants have excellent prognosis compared to anaplastic variant
  o Alveolar and pleomorphic types generally have poor prognosis (pleomorphic type occurs in adults)
  o Paratesticular rhabdomyosarcoma has significantly better prognosis than tumors occurring elsewhere in genitourinary tract because of early detection
  o Patients > 10 years of age and tumors > 5 cm have worse prognosis

MACROSCOPIC

General Features
- Well-circumscribed paratesticular mass
- Often multinodular with gelatinous, gray-white cut surface
- Patchy areas of necrosis, hemorrhage, or cystic change may be seen

Size
- Range: 1-18 cm (average: 4-6 cm)

MICROSCOPIC

Histologic Features
- Mixture of primitive and variable proportion of well-differentiated rhabdomyosarcomatous component
- Alternating cellular and less cellular myxoid areas (embryonal rhabdomyosarcoma, NOS)
- Spindle cells with fascicular pattern, mimicking leiomyosarcoma (spindle leiomyomatous rhabdomyosarcoma)
- Primitive cells (blue cells) with small, round to oval, hyperchromatic cells or spindle cells
- Differentiating rhabdomyosarcoma cells with eosinophilic cytoplasm, fibrillary material, or cross striations
- Diffuse anaplasia with atypical mitoses (anaplastic variant of embryonal rhabdomyosarcoma) may be seen
- Alveolar, pleomorphic, or botryoid types of rhabdomyosarcoma are extremely rare in paratesticular area

ANCILLARY TESTS

Immunohistochemistry
- Positive for desmin, actin-HHF-35, myoglobin, MYOD1, myogenin, and vimentin
- Negative for S100, cytokeratin, LCA

DIFFERENTIAL DIAGNOSIS

Leiomyosarcoma
- Occurs in older age group
- Uniform fascicular spindle cells with eosinophilic cytoplasm
- Diffusely positive for actin-sm and desmin; negative for myoglobin, MYOD1, and myogenin

Dedifferentiated Liposarcoma
- History of or current well-differentiated liposarcoma (atypical lipomatous tumor)
- Tumor with areas of atypical lipomatous component
- MDM2, CDK4 positive

Malignant Lymphoma/Leukemia
- Relatively uniform tumor cells and lack of cells with abundant eosinophilic cytoplasm, lack of myxoid background
- Primarily interstitial testicular involvement with paratesticular extension
- Positive for CD45(LCA) and CD20

Other Small Blue Cell Tumors
- Uniform small cell proliferation with lack of spindle cells and cells with eosinophilic cytoplasm
- Lack alternating cellular and myxoid areas
- Negative for desmin, myoglobin, MYOD1, and myogenin

SELECTED REFERENCES

1. Ulbright TM et al: Testicular and paratesticular tumors and tumor-like lesions in the first 2 decades. Semin Diagn Pathol. 31(5):323-81, 2014
2. Reeves HM et al: Paratesticular rhabdomyosarcoma. J Urol. 182(4):1578-9, 2009
3. Sugita Y et al: Testicular and paratesticular tumours in children: 30 years' experience. Aust N Z J Surg. 69(7):505-8, 1999
4. Stewart LH et al: Thirty-year review of intrascrotal rhabdomyosarcoma. Br J Urol. 68(4):418-20, 1991

Embryonal Rhabdomyosarcoma

Embryonal Rhabdomyosarcoma: Gross

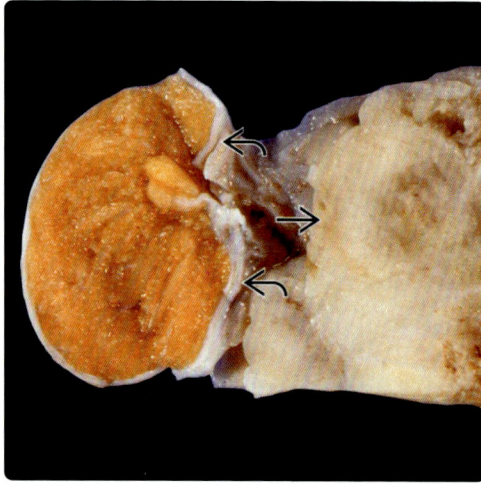

Embryonal Rhabdomyosarcoma: Gross

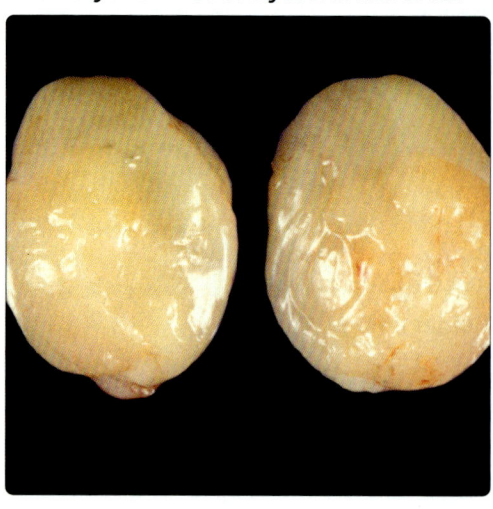

(Left) Paratesticular embryonal rhabdomyosarcoma with a tan-white, gelatinous cut surface ⇨, and lacking necrosis or hemorrhage is shown. The adjacent testicular parenchyma ⇨ is uninvolved. (Right) Gross photograph of a paratesticular rhabdomyosarcoma shows a homogeneous, fish-flesh appearance. A circumscribed, myxoid paratesticular mass in the child is most likely to be a rhabdomyosarcoma unless proved otherwise. (Courtesy H. Zhou, MD.)

Embryonal Rhabdomyosarcoma: Nodular

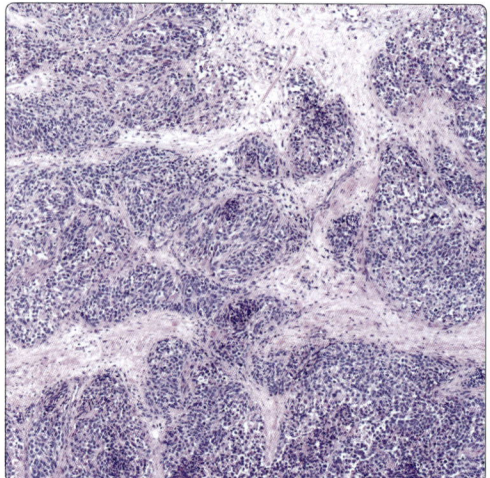

Embryonal Rhabdomyosarcoma: Small Blue Cells

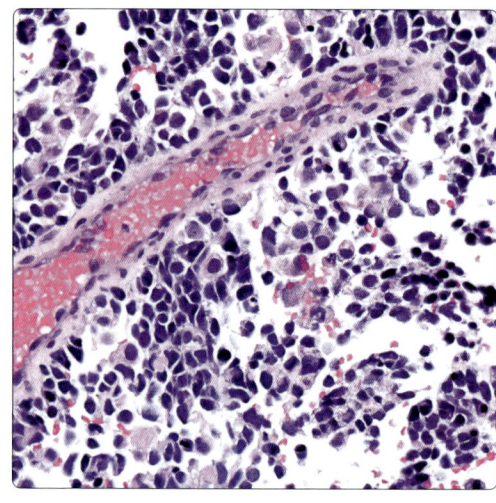

(Left) Low-power photomicrograph shows embryonal rhabdomyosarcoma, not otherwise specified (NOS) with nodules of tumor cells with foci of necrosis. There are dense fibrotic septa. (Courtesy H. Li, MD.) (Right) This paratesticular embryonal rhabdomyosarcoma, NOS is composed of small blue cells with hyperchromatic nuclei, variable amount of pink cytoplasm, and frequent apoptotic bodies. (Courtesy H. Li, MD.)

Embryonal Rhabdomyosarcoma: Spindle and Small Cells

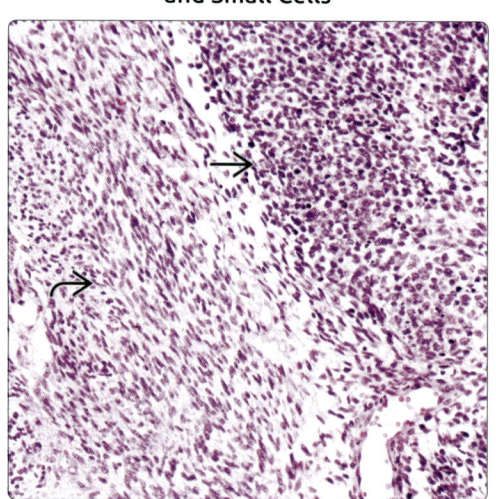

Embryonal Rhabdomyosarcoma: Rhabdomyoblasts

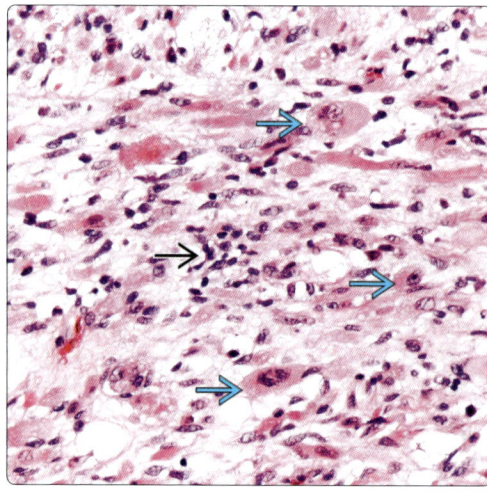

(Left) Embryonal rhabdomyosarcoma, NOS shows alternating cellular primitive ovoid small cells ⇨ and less cellular myxoid ⇨ areas composed of short spindle cells, characteristic of this tumor. (Right) Embryonal rhabdomyosarcoma shows small, primitive, ovoid cells ⇨ and numerous large elongated and ovoid cells with dense eosinophilic fibrillar cytoplasm (rhabdomyoblasts) ⇨.

Embryonal Rhabdomyosarcoma

Rhabdomyosarcoma: Leiomyomatous

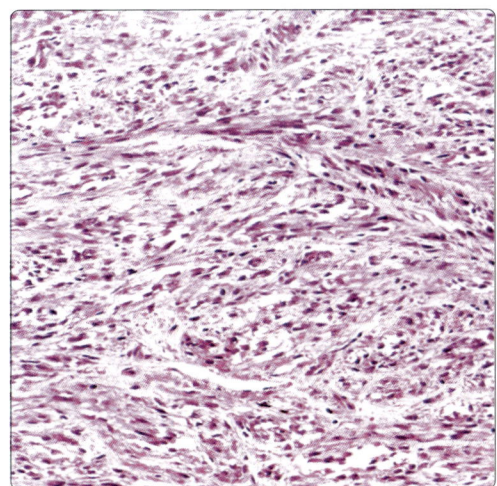

Rhabdomyosarcoma: Leiomyomatous

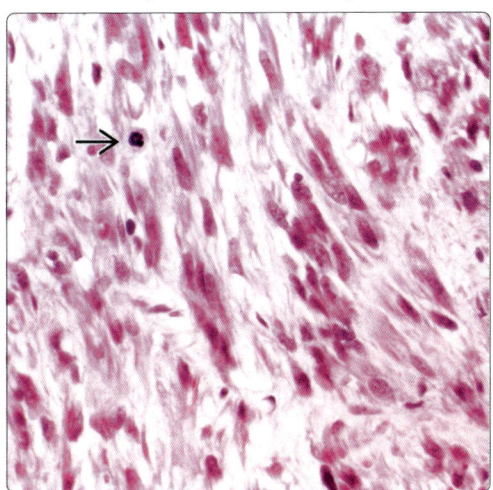

(Left) Leiomyomatous rhabdomyosarcoma shows relatively uniform spindle cells arranged in an irregular fascicular pattern, superficially resembling leiomyosarcoma. Immunostains (myoglobin, myogenin, and MYOD1) are essential to make the correct diagnosis. *(Right)* Spindle leiomyomatous rhabdomyosarcoma shows spindle tumor cells and a mitotic figure ➡. Occasionally, there may be prominent collagen with cells arranged in a storiform or whorled pattern.

Embryonal Rhabdomyosarcoma: Rhabdomyoblasts

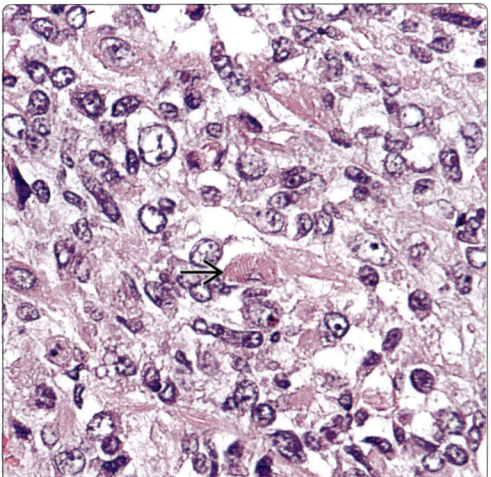

Embryonal Rhabdomyosarcoma: Anaplastic

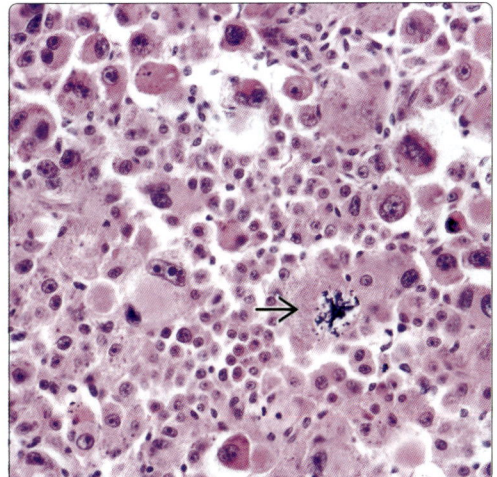

(Left) Embryonal rhabdomyosarcoma, NOS shows well-differentiated rhabdomyoblasts with prominent cross striations ➡. Manipulation of the condenser of the microscope is often helpful to appreciate cross striations. *(Right)* Higher power of anaplastic variant of embryonal rhabdomyosarcoma shows diffuse anaplasia with atypical mitosis ➡. It is similar to pleomorphic rhabdomyosarcoma but occurs in children and has more rhabdomyoblasts.

Embryonal Rhabdomyosarcoma: Actin-HHF-35

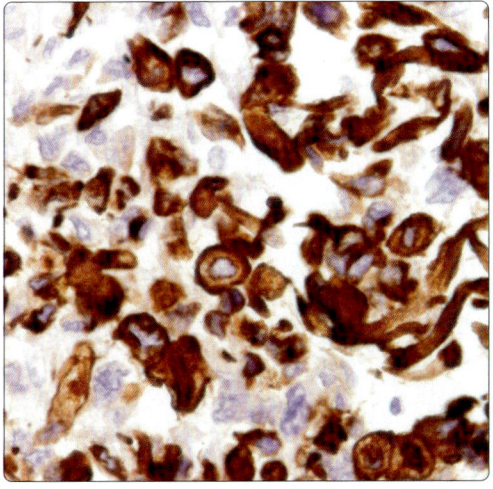

Embryonal Rhabdomyosarcoma: MYOD1

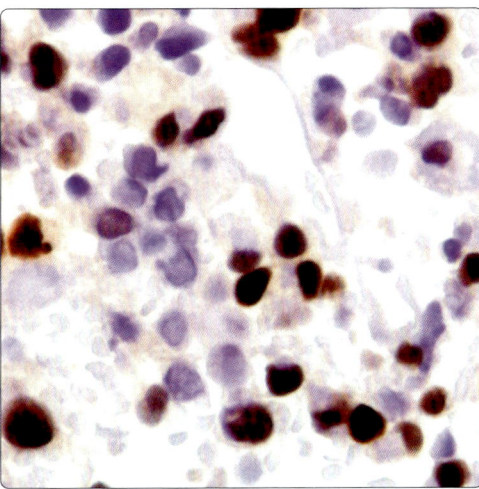

(Left) Immunohistochemical stain of rhabdomyosarcoma shows diffuse strong staining with desmin. Virtually all rhabdomyosarcomas are also positive for actin-HHF-35. *(Right)* Immunohistochemical stain of a embryonal rhabdomyosarcoma, NOS shows strong nuclear positivity of tumor cells for MYOD1, which is a specific marker for rhabdomyosarcomatous differentiation. Nonspecific cytoplasmic positivity for MYOD1 may also be seen in other tumors and has no diagnostic significance.

Other Sarcomas

KEY FACTS

TERMINOLOGY
- Malignant soft tissue tumors of paratesticular tissue origin other than more commonly occurring liposarcoma or rhabdomyosarcoma

CLINICAL ISSUES
- Range: 16-84 yr (average: 55 yr)
- Paratesticular (spermatic cord, tunics, and epididymis) mass
- Can be locally recurrent or metastatic
- Prognostic factors include histologic type, tumor grade, and stage at presentation

MACROSCOPIC
- Bulky mass with overall circumscription, tan-white, fleshy cut surface with hemorrhage or necrosis

MICROSCOPIC
- Liposarcoma is most common paratesticular sarcoma in adults
- Rhabdomyosarcoma is most common paratesticular sarcoma in children
- Leiomyosarcoma is 2nd most common sarcoma in adults
- Desmoplastic small round cell tumor may occur in this location and is histologically similar to abdominal/pelvic counterpart
- Other sarcomas (MFH, fibrosarcoma, MPNST, etc.) are much less common

ANCILLARY TESTS
- Immunoprofile similar to that of sarcomas in other more common locations

TOP DIFFERENTIAL DIAGNOSES
- Rhabdomyosarcoma
- Sarcoma arising in teratoma
- Sex cord-stromal tumor, mixed/unclassified
- Metastatic sarcomatoid carcinoma
- Other benign soft tissue tumors

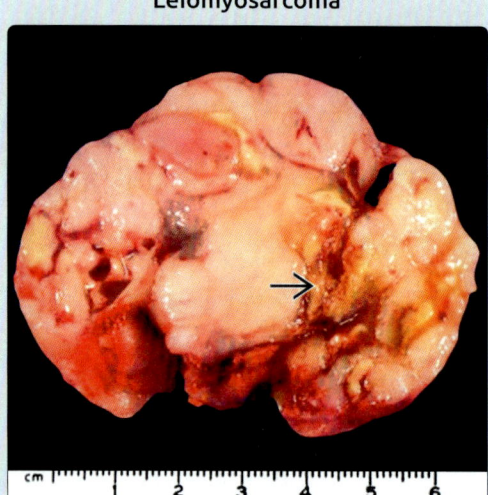
Leiomyosarcoma

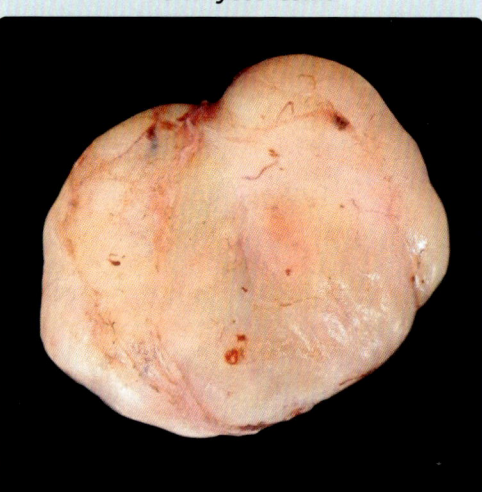
Leiomyosarcoma

(Left) Large, multinodular, tan paratesticular leiomyosarcoma with focal hemorrhage and necrosis ➡. The major differential diagnosis is a dedifferentiated liposarcoma in this location in adults. (Right) Large, tan paratesticular leiomyosarcoma with homogenous cut surface with focal hemorrhage is shown. The major differential diagnosis is a dedifferentiated liposarcoma in this location in adults.

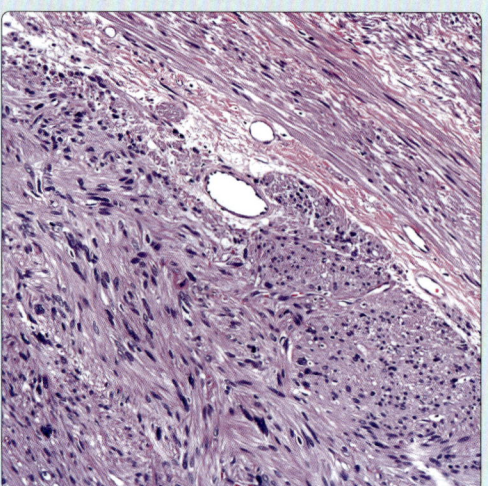
Leiomyosarcoma

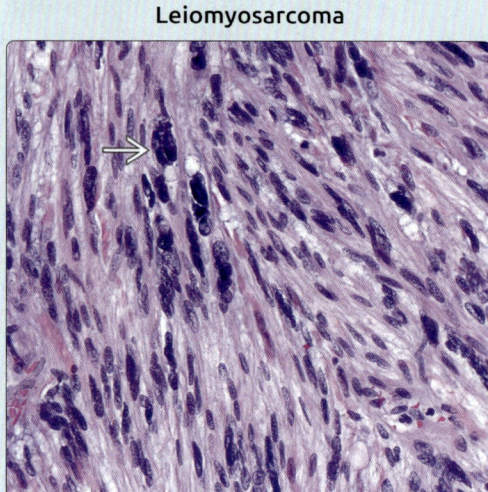
Leiomyosarcoma

(Left) Paratesticular leiomyosarcoma shows a well-circumscribed nodule composed of fascicular growth of spindle cells with eosinophilic cytoplasm and nuclear pleomorphism. (Right) Leiomyosarcoma is composed of a cellular spindle cell proliferation with bundles or fascicles. Cytologic atypia ➡ is evident. The main differential diagnosis is with leiomyomatous rhabdomyosarcoma.

Other Sarcomas

TERMINOLOGY

Definitions
- Malignant soft tissue tumors of paratesticular tissue origin other than more commonly occurring liposarcoma (adults) or rhabdomyosarcoma (children, young adults)

CLINICAL ISSUES

Epidemiology
- Incidence
  o Rare; < 1% of all soft tissue sarcomas
- Age
  o Range: 16-84 yr (average: 55 yr)

Presentation
- Paratesticular (spermatic cord, tunics, and epididymis) mass

Treatment
- Surgical approaches
  o Resection ± radiation or chemotherapy

Prognosis
- Local recurrence or metastasis; prognostic factors include histologic type, tumor grade, and stage at presentation

IMAGING

General Features
- Nonspecific hyperechoic mass by ultrasonography

MACROSCOPIC

General Features
- Bulky mass with overall circumscription, tan-white, fleshy cut surface with hemorrhage or necrosis

MICROSCOPIC

Histologic Features
- Liposarcoma is most common paratesticular sarcoma in adults
- Rhabdomyosarcoma is most common paratesticular sarcoma in children
- Leiomyosarcoma is 2nd most common paratesticular sarcoma in adults
  o Characterized by fascicles of spindle cells with eosinophilic fibrillar cytoplasm, hyperchromatic blunt-ended nuclei, and paranuclear vacuoles
  o May have prominent myxoid areas, pleomorphic component, inflammatory background, or epithelioid cells
- Desmoplastic small round cell tumor
  o Similar histology to those occurring in abdomen or pelvis
  o Characterized by epithelial-type nested growth of small blue cells in prominent desmoplastic stroma
- Other sarcomas are much less common
  o Malignant fibrous histiocytoma (MFH) and fibrosarcoma are diagnosis of exclusion
  o Malignant peripheral nerve sheath tumor (MPNST), osteosarcoma, Kaposi sarcoma, and angiosarcoma have been reported

ANCILLARY TESTS

Immunohistochemistry
- Immunoprofile similar to that of sarcomas in other more common locations
  o Leiomyosarcoma is positive for actin-sm, actin-HHF-35, and desmin; may be positive for CD34 and keratin
  o Desmoplastic small round cell tumor is positive for cytokeratin, EMA/MUC1, vimentin, desmin, and neuroendocrine markers (NSE, chromogranin, and synaptophysin)
  o Malignant fibrous histiocytoma may be focally positive for actin-sm, cytokeratin, and CD68- immunohistochemistry not diagnostic
  o Fibrosarcoma positive for actin-sm and vimentin

DIFFERENTIAL DIAGNOSIS

Rhabdomyosarcoma
- Embryonal rhabdomyosarcoma (spindle cell leiomyomatous histology) mimics leiomyosarcoma
- Positive for MYOD1, myogenin, and myoglobin

Sarcoma Arising in Teratoma
- Presence of mature or immature teratoma component
- Epicenter in testis parenchyma

Sex Cord-Stromal Tumor, Mixed/Unclassified
- Predominantly intratesticular mass; rarely paratesticular
- Sex cord-stromal differentiation in form of tubules or Call-Exner bodies may occur in background of predominantly spindle cell histology
- Positive for inhibin, calretinin, WT1, CD99, and variably for keratin and actin-sm

Metastatic Sarcomatoid Carcinoma
- Biphasic histology may be present
- Clinical history is important

Other Benign Soft Tissue Tumors
- Lipoma, leiomyoma, neurofibroma, granular cell tumor, angiomyofibroblastoma-like tumor, calcifying fibrous tumor, cellular angiofibroma, superficial angiomyxoma, aggressive angiomyxoma
- Usually small size, often well-circumscribed, bland cytologic features, and incidental findings

SELECTED REFERENCES

1. Deyrup AT et al: Fibrosarcoma-like lipomatous neoplasm: a reappraisal of so-called spindle cell liposarcoma defining a unique lipomatous tumor unrelated to other liposarcomas. Am J Surg Pathol. 37(9):1373-8, 2013
2. Fitzgerald S et al: Paratesticular liposarcoma. J Urol. 181(1):331-2, 2009
3. Korkes F et al: Paratesticular sarcomas in Brazil. Urol Int. 82(4):448-52, 2009
4. Al-Masri A et al: Primary paratesticular osteosarcoma: case report and a review of the literature. ScientificWorldJournal. 7:850-4, 2007
5. Dotan ZA et al: Adult genitourinary sarcoma: the 25-year Memorial Sloan-Kettering experience. J Urol. 176(5):2033-8; discussion 2038-9, 2006
6. Ozkan B et al: Adult paratesticular myxofibrosarcoma: report of a rare entity and review of the literature. Int Urol Nephrol. 38(1):5-7, 2006
7. Kalyvas KD et al: Paratesticular well-differentiated, adipocytic type liposarcoma presenting as inguinal hernia. Urol Int. 72(3):264-8, 2004
8. Montgomery E et al: Paratesticular liposarcoma: a clinicopathologic study. Am J Surg Pathol. 27(1):40-7, 2003
9. Fisher C et al: Leiomyosarcoma of the paratesticular region: a clinicopathologic study. Am J Surg Pathol. 25(9):1143-9, 2001

Other Sarcomas

(Left) Leiomyomatous rhabdomyosarcoma shows relatively uniform spindle cells arranged in an irregular fascicular pattern, superficially resembling leiomyosarcoma. Immunostains (myoglobin, myogenin, and MYOD1) are essential to make the correct diagnosis. **(Right)** Spindle leiomyomatous rhabdomyosarcoma shows spindle tumor cells and a mitotic figure ➡. Occasionally, there may be prominent collagen with cells arranged in a storiform or whorled pattern.

Rhabdomyosarcoma (Leiomyomatous)
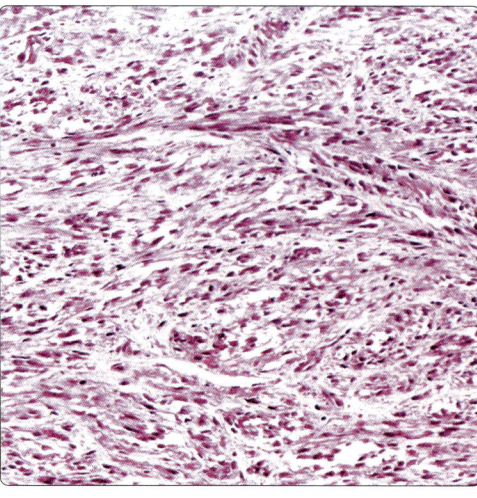

Rhabdomyosarcoma (Leiomyomatous)
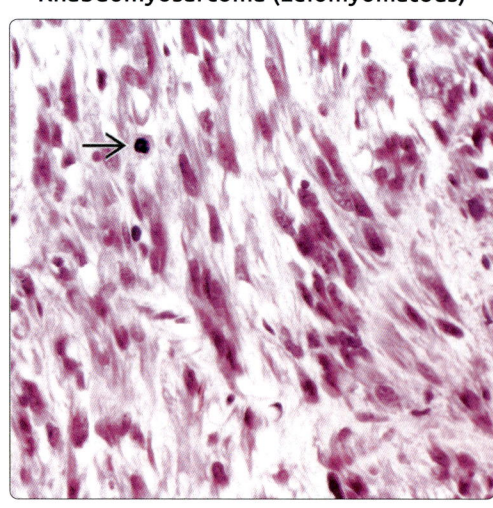

(Left) Leiomyosarcoma at high-power magnification exhibits pleomorphic spindle cells with abundant, fibrillary eosinophilic cytoplasm and occasional mitoses ➡. The nuclei are typically cigar shaped. **(Right)** Leiomyosarcoma is shown with scattered pleomorphic nuclei ➡ and fibrillary eosinophilic cytoplasm. There are prominent cytoplasmic vacuoles ➡. The age of the patient and immunohistochemistry are important in the distinction from rhabdomyosarcoma with leiomyomatous histology.

Leiomyosarcoma
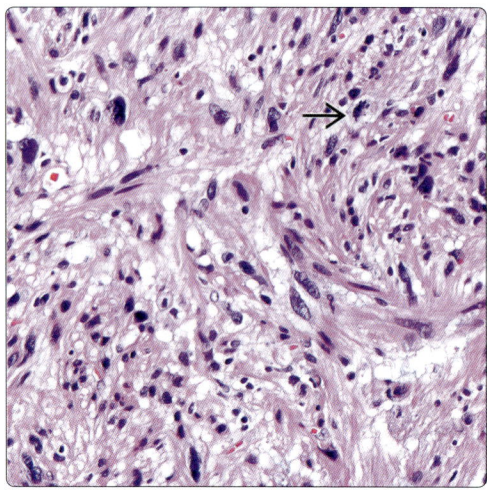

Leiomyosarcoma
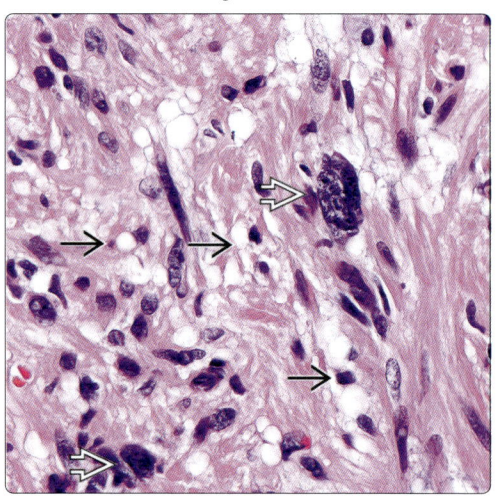

(Left) Malignant fibrous histiocytoma (MFH) with marked cytologic atypia and atypical mitoses ➡. The diagnosis of MFH is made only after exclusion of other pleomorphic high-grade sarcomas, i.e., dedifferentiated liposarcoma, rhabdomyosarcoma, leiomyosarcoma & MPNST, & sarcomatoid carcinoma using an appropriate panel of immunostains. **(Right)** This is another example of malignant fibrous histiocytoma with numerous bizarre tumor giant cells. There are scattered inflammatory cells as well.

Malignant Fibrous Histiocytoma
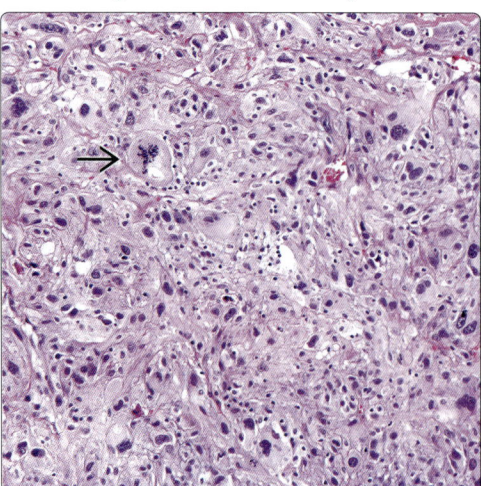

Malignant Fibrous Histiocytoma
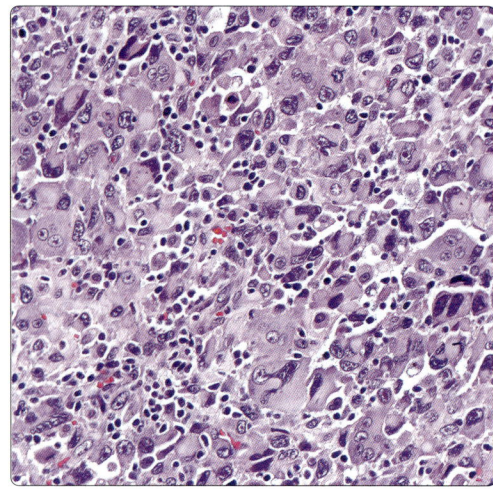

Other Sarcomas

Malignant Peripheral Nerve Sheath Tumor

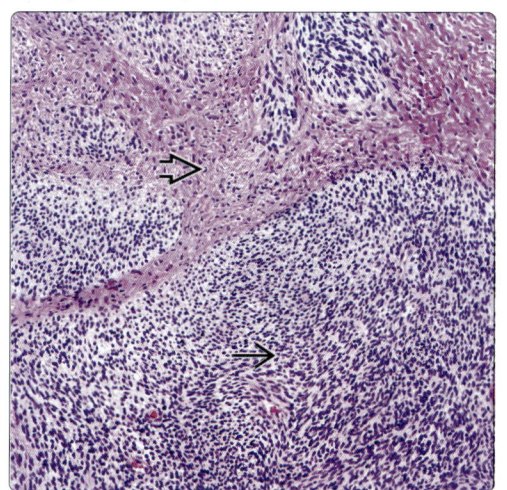

Malignant Peripheral Nerve Sheath Tumor

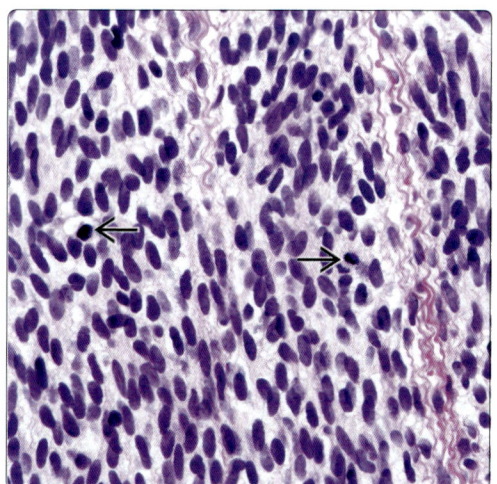

(Left) Malignant peripheral nerve sheath tumor (MPNST) is an extremely rare tumor in the paratesticular location. There are alternating hypo- ⇨ and hypercellular ⇨ spindle cell areas. (Right) MPNST shows hypercellular elongated ovoid tumor cells with fine nuclear chromatin. Mitoses are frequently seen ⇨. There is vague palisading of nuclei. The tumor cells were focally positive for S100 and negative for muscle markers, supporting the diagnosis of MPNST.

Desmoplastic Small Round Cell Tumor

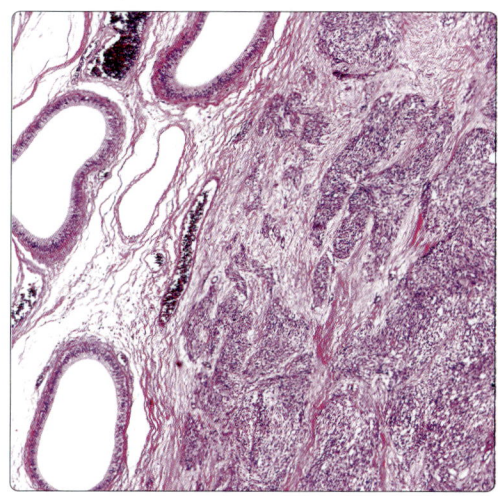

Desmoplastic Small Round Cell Tumor

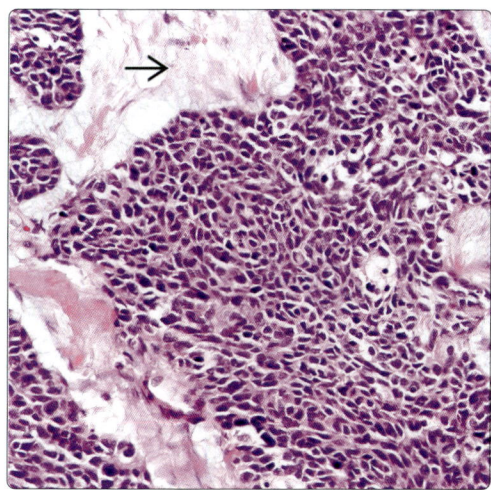

(Left) Desmoplastic small round cell tumor is seen involving the epididymis. It is characterized by nests of small blue cells surrounded by desmoplastic stroma. The tumor cells are positive for both epithelial markers and desmin, a diagnostic immunohistochemical panel. (Right) Desmoplastic small round cell tumor shows nests of small blue cells with scant cytoplasm, finely stippled chromatin, and inconspicuous nucleoli. Note also the prominent myxoid stroma in the background ⇨.

Angiosarcoma

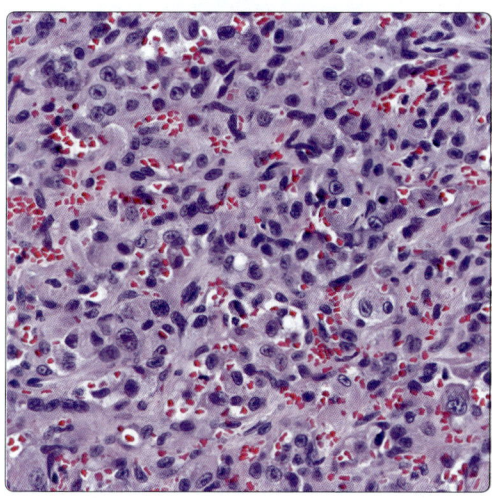

Angiomyofibroblastoma-Like Tumor

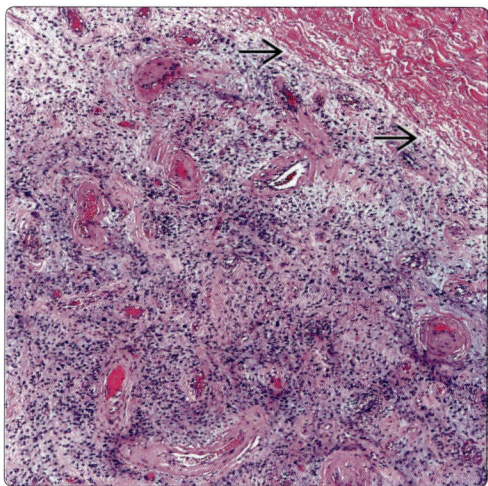

(Left) Paratesticular angiosarcoma has been described rarely and is composed of epithelioid tumor cells with prominent nucleoli and poorly formed vascular spaces. (Right) Angiomyofibroblastoma-like tumor is seen with a well-circumscribed border from uninvolved paratesticular tissue ⇨. There are abundant vascular channels with perivascular hyalinization. This is a rare benign tumor of the paratesticular region & should be differentiated from sarcoma.

Metastatic Tumors, Testis and Paratesticular Structures

KEY FACTS

TERMINOLOGY
- Tumors secondarily involving testis and paratesticular structures by hematogenous metastasis or intraperitoneal spread from distant sites; excludes hematopoietic tumors

CLINICAL ISSUES
- Metastatic tumors are rare in testis (compared to ovary) and occur in 0.68% of patients in autopsy studies
- Majority are > 50 years old
- Generally has poor prognosis

MACROSCOPIC
- Localized mass, multiple nodules, or diffuse enlargement of testis with no grossly apparent mass
- Usually unilateral and solitary (> 90%)

MICROSCOPIC
- Histologic, cytologic features recapitulate their site of origin
- Metastatic carcinomas are most common; prostate, lung, kidney, and gastrointestinal tract are frequent sites
- Histology not typical of germ cell tumor or sex cord-stromal tumor
- Interstitial infiltrative growth pattern between seminiferous tubules
- Prominent lymphovascular invasion

ANCILLARY TESTS
- Panel of stains should be based on differential diagnosis generated from clinical history, imaging, and histopathology

TOP DIFFERENTIAL DIAGNOSES
- Primary testicular germ cell tumor
- Primary testicular sex cord-stromal tumor
- Rete/epididymal carcinoma
- Malignant mesothelioma
- Malignant lymphoma
- Ovarian-type (müllerian) carcinoma

Metastatic Prostate Carcinoma
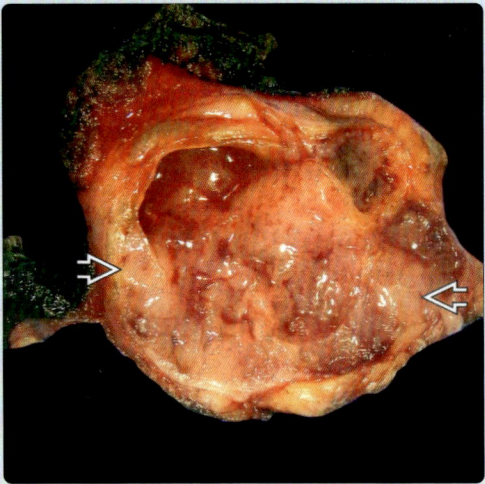

Metastatic Lung Adenocarcinoma
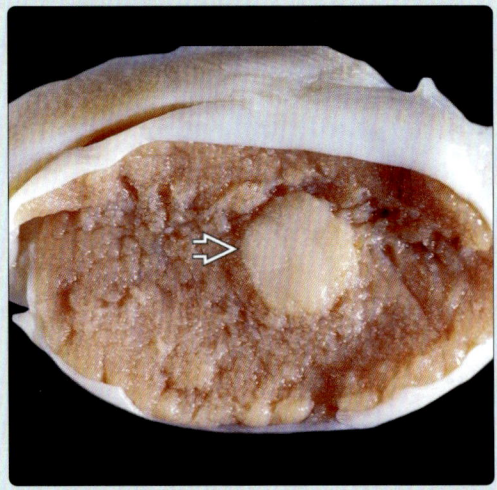

(Left) Metastatic prostatic carcinoma ⇨ is shown extensively involving the testis. The tumor is composed of a tan-pink, soft mass with focal cystic changes. This gross finding mimics a primary germ cell tumor. (Right) Metastatic adenocarcinoma from the lung is shown with a small solitary intraparenchymal, well-circumscribed, white-tan nodule ⇨ in an aged atrophic testis. Grossly, this tumor mimics a sex cord-stromal tumor.

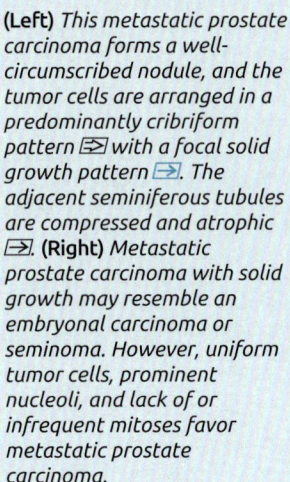

Metastatic Prostate Carcinoma
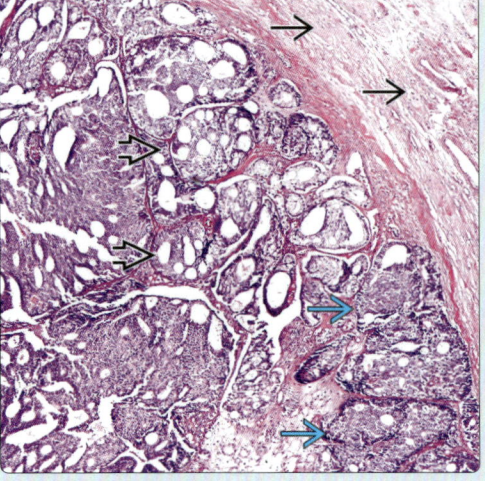

Metastatic Prostate Carcinoma
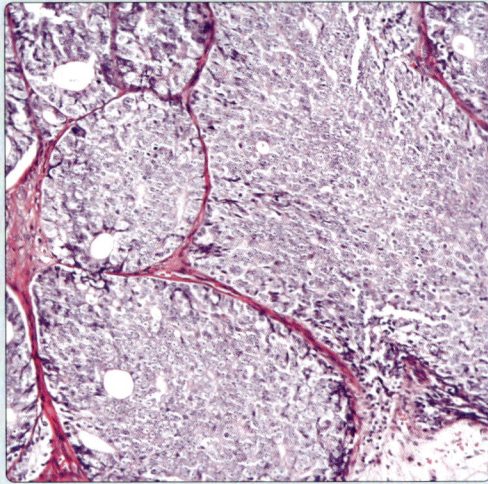

(Left) This metastatic prostate carcinoma forms a well-circumscribed nodule, and the tumor cells are arranged in a predominantly cribriform pattern ⇨ with a focal solid growth pattern ⇨. The adjacent seminiferous tubules are compressed and atrophic ⇨. (Right) Metastatic prostate carcinoma with solid growth may resemble an embryonal carcinoma or seminoma. However, uniform tumor cells, prominent nucleoli, and lack of or infrequent mitoses favor metastatic prostate carcinoma.

Metastatic Tumors, Testis and Paratesticular Structures

TERMINOLOGY

Definitions
- Tumors secondarily involving testis and paratesticular structures by hematogenous metastasis or intraperitoneal spread from distant sites; excludes hematopoietic tumors

CLINICAL ISSUES

Epidemiology
- Incidence
  - Metastases are rarer in testis than in ovary
  - Occur in 0.68% of patients with solid organ malignancies in autopsy studies
- Age
  - Majority are > 50 years old

Presentation
- Nonsymptomatic or incidental finding during hormonal ablation orchiectomy or autopsy for metastatic prostate cancer
- Symptomatic metastasis is rare and usually unilateral (> 90%) and solitary
- May present very rarely as carcinoma of unknown primary and mimic primary testicular or paratesticular tumors
- Rare metastasis to primary testicular germ cell tumor (tumor to tumor metastasis) is known to occur

Treatment
- Surgical resection for palliative pain control
- Adjuvant therapy based on primary site and histology

Prognosis
- Generally poor prognosis

IMAGING

General Features
- Radiologic studies are helpful in defining local extent of disease and primary site of tumor

MACROSCOPIC

General Features
- Localized mass, multiple nodules, or diffuse enlargement of testis with no grossly apparent mass
- Usually unilateral and solitary (> 90%)

MICROSCOPIC

Histologic Features
- Histologic features recapitulate their site of origin
  - Metastatic carcinomas are most common
    - Most common primary sites include prostate, lung, kidney, and gastrointestinal tract
    - Less common and rare sites include esophagus, bladder, pancreas
  - Metastatic melanoma or sarcoma to testis has been reported
  - Secondary involvement of testis by hematopoietic neoplasms is common (testis is sanctuary site)
- Histology not typical of germ cell tumor or sex cord-stromal tumor
  - Interstitial infiltrative growth pattern between seminiferous tubules
  - Discrete tumoral mass, nodules, or extensive infiltration of parenchyma
  - Intratubular growth pattern is rare and may mimic primary tumor
  - Prominent vascular invasion (~ 70%)

ANCILLARY TESTS

Immunohistochemistry
- Panel of stains should be based on differential diagnoses generated from clinical history, imaging, and histopathology
- Negative for germ cell tumor markers, positive for EMA/MUC1, HMCK(34βE12) and various tissue specific markers

DIFFERENTIAL DIAGNOSIS

Primary Testicular Germ Cell Tumor
- Usually occurs in younger age, rarely bilateral or multifocal
- Diffuse rather than interstitial growth pattern
- Positive for germ cell markers (OCT3/4, SALL4, LIN28, etc.)

Primary Testicular Sex Cord-Stromal Tumor
- Cytologically more banal-appearing tumor cells
- Leydig cell tumor may mimic malignant melanoma; Sertoli cell tumor may mimic carcinoma
- Positive for inhibin and calretinin; weakly positive or negative for cytokeratin

Rete/Epididymal Carcinoma
- Lack of clinical history of malignancy elsewhere
- Histologic transition from rete testis or epididymal epithelium is key feature
- Epicenter of mass in rete or epididymis

Malignant Mesothelioma
- Usually extensively and diffusely involves tunica
- Positive for mesothelial-associated markers [calretinin, podoplanin (D2-40), WT1, CK5/6]

Malignant Lymphoma
- Interstitial growth pattern of round blue cells
- Relative preservation of seminiferous tubules and intratubular infiltrative growth with onion skin appearance around tubules
- Positive for lymphoid markers; negative for cytokeratin, tissue-specific antibodies, or neuroendocrine markers

Ovarian-Type (Müllerian) Carcinoma
- Lack of clinical history of malignancy elsewhere
- Immunostains, including WT1, pax-8 and CA125

SELECTED REFERENCES

1. Moriyama S et al: Simultaneous bilateral testicular metastases from renal clear cell carcinoma: A case report and review of the literature. Oncol Lett. 7(4):1273-1275, 2014
2. Hatoum HA et al: Metastasis of colorectal carcinoma to the testes: clinical presentation and possible pathways. Int J Clin Oncol. 16(3):203-9, 2011
3. Ulbright TM et al: Metastatic carcinoma to the testis: a clinicopathologic analysis of 26 nonincidental cases with emphasis on deceptive features. Am J Surg Pathol. 32(11):1683-93, 2008

Metastatic Tumors, Testis and Paratesticular Structures

Metastatic Prostate Carcinoma

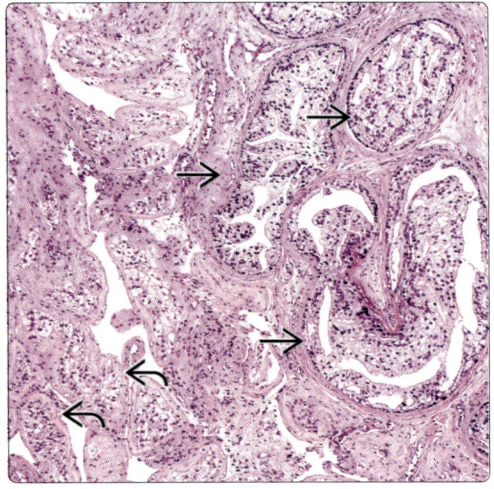

Metastatic Prostate Carcinoma

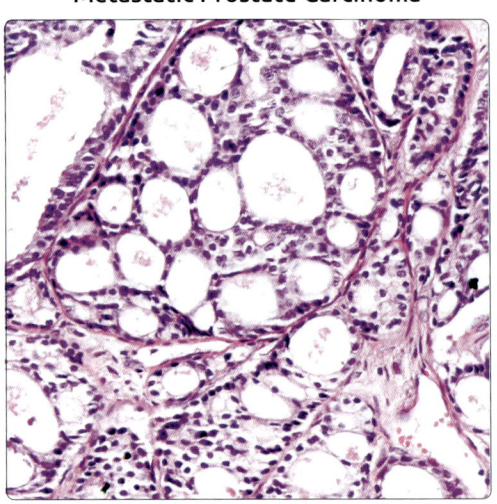

(Left) Metastatic prostate adenocarcinoma shows an interstitial growth pattern with a cribriform growth pattern of tumor cells that have abundant clear cytoplasm ⇒. The uninvolved tubules are atrophic ⇒ with no spermatogenesis. (Right) Metastatic prostate adenocarcinoma with a confluent cribriform glandular pattern is shown. The metastatic tumor maintains the classic histologic and cytologic features of prostate cancer. The background testis lacks germ cell neoplasia in situ.

Metastatic Prostate Carcinoma

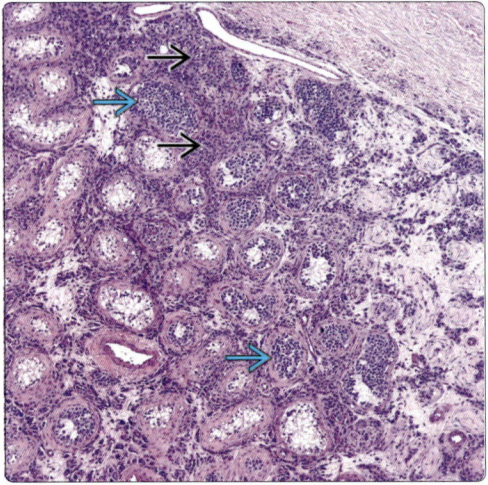

Metastatic Prostate Carcinoma

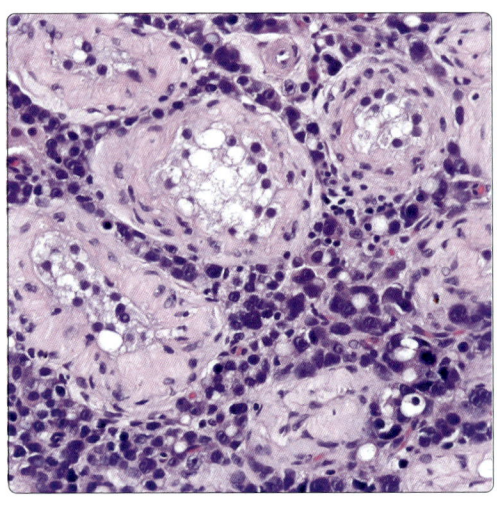

(Left) This image shows a metastatic prostate carcinoma with interstitial ⇒ and intratubular ⇒ growth patterns. The uninvolved testis parenchyma shows atrophic seminiferous tubules with thickening of the basement membrane. (Right) High-power view shows an interstitial infiltrative pattern of prostate carcinoma, closely simulating that of malignant lymphoma or interstitial seminoma. Features favoring prostate carcinoma include uniform nuclei and prominent nucleoli.

Metastatic Prostate Carcinoma

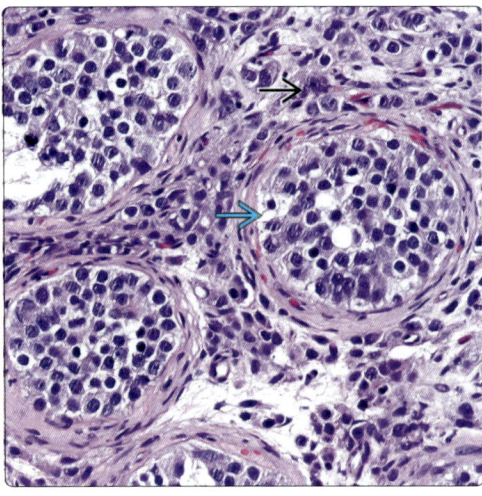

Metastatic Prostate Carcinoma

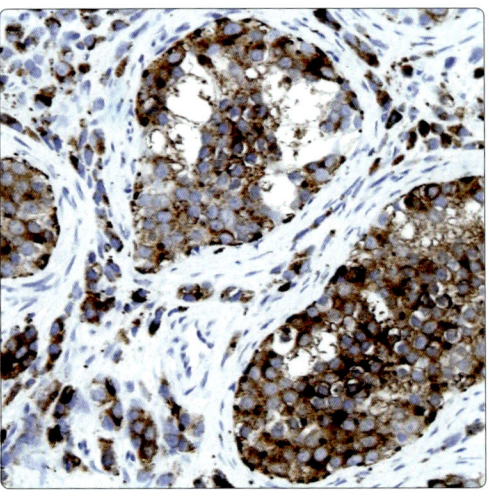

(Left) Metastatic prostate carcinoma is shown with intratubular ⇒ and interstitial ⇒ growth patterns in the testis. The tumor cells within and surrounding the tubules are similar and have relatively uniform cells with prominent nucleoli. (Right) PSA immunohistochemical stain shows that the tumor cells within or outside the tubules are strongly positive, confirming the diagnosis of metastatic prostate carcinoma.

Metastatic Tumors, Testis and Paratesticular Structures

Metastatic Renal Cell Carcinoma

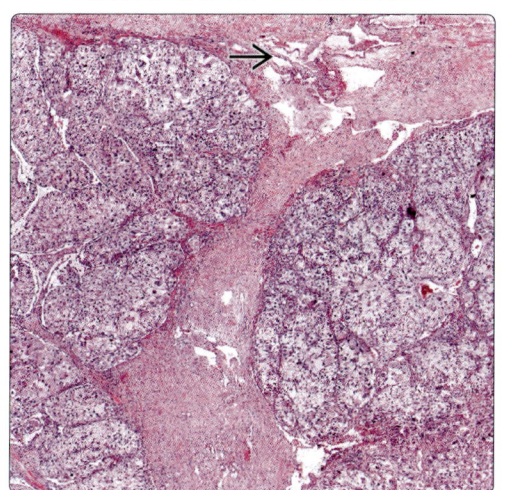

Metastatic Renal Cell Carcinoma

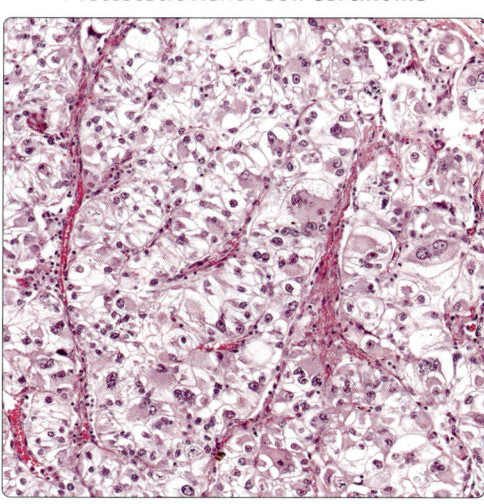

(Left) This metastatic carcinoma is a high-grade clear cell renal carcinoma near the rete testis ➡. The abundant sinusoidal vasculature and alveolar growth pattern are features of clear cell renal cell carcinoma. *(Right)* Metastatic clear cell renal cell carcinoma shows a distinct fibrovascular-supporting network between tumor cells containing abundant clear cytoplasm. It may mimic a seminoma but has a greater degree of nuclear pleomorphism and lacks a stromal lymphoid infiltrate.

Metastatic Lung Carcinoma

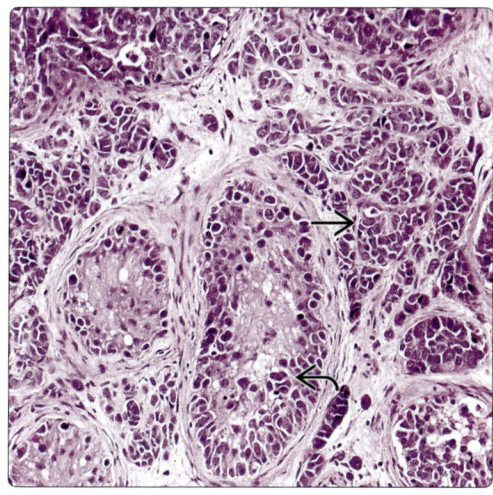

Metastatic Merkel Cell Carcinoma

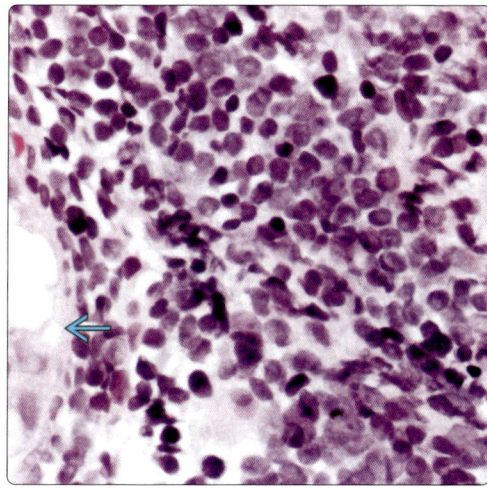

(Left) Metastatic poorly differentiated lung carcinoma with an interstitial ➡ growth pattern is shown. Tumor cells are also seen involving seminiferous tubules ➡. *(Right)* In this metastatic Merkel cell carcinoma to the testis, the tumor is composed of sheets of small blue cells with fine chromatin and scant cytoplasm. Malignant lymphoma is a major differential diagnosis. The tumor cells spare the seminiferous tubules ➡. Immunohistochemistry showed dot-like cytokeratin positivity.

Metastatic Melanoma

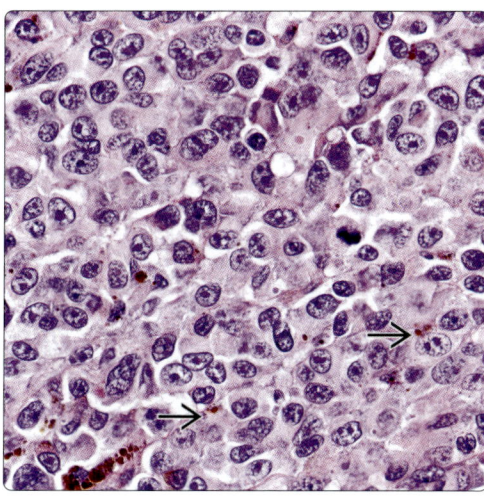

Large B-Cell Lymphoma

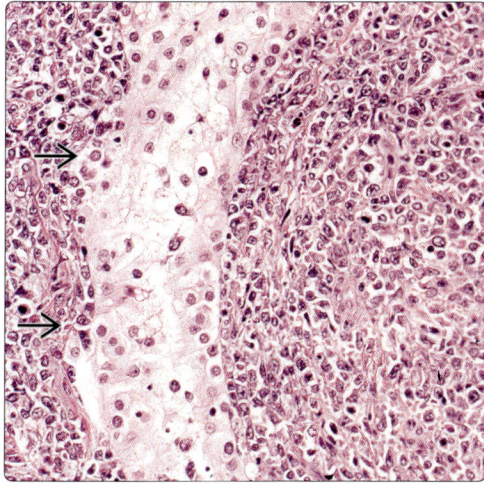

(Left) High-power image shows metastatic melanoma composed of large epithelioid cells with prominent nucleoli and melanin pigments ➡. In case of an amelanotic melanoma, differential diagnoses would include Leydig cell tumor, seminoma, embryonal carcinoma, and large B-cell lymphoma. *(Right)* In this large B-cell lymphoma involving the testis, the tumor has a diffuse interstitial pattern and spares the seminiferous tubules ➡.

Immunohistochemistry, Testis

Tumors With Diffuse Arrangement and Cells With Pale and Clear Cytoplasm

Antibody	Classic Seminoma	Spermatocytic Tumor	Embryonal Carcinoma	Yolk Sac Tumor	Sertoli Cell Tumor	Lymphoma	Renal Cell Carcinoma	Melanoma
CD117	(+)	(+)	(-)	V	(-)	(-/+)	V	V
POU5F1 (OCT3/OCT4)	(+)	(-)	(+)	(-)	(-)	(-)	(-)	(-)
CD30 (BerH2)	(-/+) rare focal cells	(-)	(+)	(-)	(-)	V	ND	(-)
α-fetoprotein	(-)	(-)	(-)	(+)	(-)	ND	(-)	(-)
Glypican-3	(-)	(-)	(-)	(+)	(-)	(-)	(-)	(-)
AE1/3 (CK-PAN)	(-)	(-)	(+)	(+)	(+/-)	(-)	(+)	(-)
CK7	V	ND	(+)	(-/+)	(-)	ND	V	(-)
EMA/MUC1	(-)	(-)	(+)	(-/+)	V/(+)	(-)	(+)	(-)
Inhibin	(-) (+) STC	ND	(-)	(-)	(+)	(-)	(-)	(-)
CD45 (LCA)	(-)	(-)	(-)	(-)	(-)	(+)	(-)	(-)
S100	(-)	(-)	(-)	(-)	(-/+)	(-)	(-)	(+)
RCC	(-)	ND	(V)	(-)	(-)	(-)	(+)	(-)
SALL4	(+)	(+) weak	(+)	(+)	(-)	(+/-)	(-)	(-)
PLAP	(+)	(-)	(+)	(-/+)	(-)	(-)	(-)	(-)
SOX17	(+)	(-)	(-)	(+/-)	(-)	ND	ND	V
SOX2	(-)	(-)	(+)	(-)	ND	(+/-)	ND	(+)
Podoplanin (D2-40)	(+)	(-)	(-/+)	(-)	(-)	(-/+)	(-)	(-)
LIN28	(+)	(-/+)	(+)	(+)	ND	ND	(-)	(-/+)
GATA3	(-)	(-)	(-/+)	(+)	(-)	(+/-)	(-)	(-)
SF1	(-)	(-)	(-)	(-)	(+)	ND	(-)	ND
β-catenin	(-)	(-)	(-)	(-)	(+)	V	(-)	(-)
pax-8	(-)	(-)	(-)	(-)	(-)	(-)	(+)	(-)

V = variable; ND = no data; STC = syncytiotrophoblast.

Tumors With Microcystic Pattern

Antibody	Yolk Sac Tumor	Seminoma	Leydig Cell Tumor	Sertoli Cell Tumor	Paratesticular Adenomatoid Tumor
α-fetoprotein	(+)	(-)	(-)	(-)	(-)
AE1/3 (CK-PAN)	(+)	(+) rare	(-/+)	(+/-)	(+)
POU5F1 (OCT3/OCT4)	(-)	(+)	(-)	(-)	(-)
CD117	(-)	(+)	(-)	(-)	V
Inhibin	(-)	(-)	(+)	(+)	(-)
Melan-A (MART-1)	(-)	(-)	(+)	(+)	(-)
Calretinin	(-)	(-)	(+)	(+)	(+)
WT1	(-)	(-)	(+)	(+)	(+)
SF1	(-)	(-)	(+)	(+)	(-)
Glypican-3	(+)	(-)	(-)	(-)	(-)

Immunohistochemistry, Testis

Tumors With Microcystic Pattern (Continued)

Antibody	Yolk Sac Tumor	Seminoma	Leydig Cell Tumor	Sertoli Cell Tumor	Paratesticular Adenomatoid Tumor
SALL4	(+)	(+)	(-)	(-)	(-)
Podoplanin (D2-40)	(-)	(+)	(-)	(-)	(+)
β-catenin	(-)	(-)	(-)	(+)	(-)

V = variable.

Tumors With Oxyphilic Cytoplasm

Antibody	Leydig Cell Tumor	Large-Cell Calcifying Sertoli Cell	Sertoli Cell Tumor, NOS	Carcinoid	Plasmacytoma
Inhibin	(+)	(+)	V	(-)	(-)
PLAP	(-)	(-)	(-)	(-)	(-)
CK-PAN (AE1/AE3)	(-/+)	(-/+)	(+/-)	(+)	(-)
Vimentin	(+)	(+)	V	V	V
S100	V	(+)	V	V	V
Synaptophysin	V	ND	V/(+)	(+)	(-)
SF1	(+)	(+)	(+)	(-)	(-)
Melan-A	(+)	(-)	(-)/V	(-)	(-)
Calretinin	(+)	(+/-)	(+)	(-)	(-)
WT1	(-)	(+)	(+)	(-)	(-)
β-catenin	(-)	(+/-)	(+)	(-)	(-)

V = variable; ND = no data.

Intratubular Atypical Cells: Pseudointratubular Germ Cell Neoplasm vs. Intratubular Germ Cell Neoplasm

Antibody	ITGCN	Pseudo-ITGCN
POU5F1 (OCT3/OCT4)	(+)	(-)
Podoplanin (D2-40)	(+)	(-)
PLAP	(+)	(-)
AE1/3 (CK-PAN)	(-)	(-)

ITGCN = intratubular germ cell neoplasm.

Tumors With Glandular/Tubular Pattern

Antibody	Embryonal Carcinoma	Seminoma	Yolk Sac Tumor	Sertoli Cell Tumor	Rete Testis Tumor	Metastatic Adenocarcinoma
POU5F1 (OCT3/OCT4)	(+)	(+)	(-)	(-)	(-)	(-)
CD30 (BerH2)	(+)	(-/+) rare focal cells	(+) rare	(-)	(-)	V
CD117	(-)	(+)	(-)	(-)	(-)	V
Inhibin	(-)	(-)	(-)	(+)	(-)	(-)
EMA/MUC1	(-)	(-)	(-/+)	(-/+)	V	(+)
SALL4	(+)	(+)	(+)	(-)	(-)	(+) gastric, ovarian, urothelial, lymphoma/leukemia

Tumors With Glandular/Tubular Pattern (Continued)

Antibody	Embryonal Carcinoma	Seminoma	Yolk Sac Tumor	Sertoli Cell Tumor	Rete Testis Tumor	Metastatic Adenocarcinoma
α-fetoprotein	(-)	(-)	(+)	(-)	(-)	(-)
Calretinin	(-)	(-)	(-)	(+)	(+)	(-/+)
Synaptophysin	(-)	(-)	(-)	V/(+)	(-)	(-)
Glypican-3	(-)	(-)	(+)	(-)	(-)	(-/+) in hepatocellular carcinoma
SF1	(-)	(-)	(-)	(+)	(+)	(-/+) in adrenal cortical tumors
GATA3	(-/+)	(-)	(+)	(-)	(-)	(+) breast, urothelial, squamous carcinoma
pax-8	(-)	(-)	(-)	(-)	(+/-)	(+) kidney, thyroid, neuroendocrine tumors of pancreas/GI tract
β-catenin	(-)	(-)	(-)	(+)	ND	(-/+) in colonic adenocarcinoma

V = variable; ND = no data.

Metastatic Poorly Differentiated Carcinoma in Young Adult Man vs. Germ Cell Tumor

Antibody	Germ Cell Tumor	Metastatic Carcinoma
SALL4	(+)	(+) Gastric, high-grade urothelial, hepatocellular carcinoma, lymphoma/leukemia
EMA/MUC1	(-)/V	(+)
POU5F1 (OCT3/OCT4)	(+)	(-)
S100	(-)	Melanoma
WT1	(-)	Mesothelioma, müllerian, sex cord-stromal tumors
CD45 (LCA)	(-)	Lymphoma
SF1	(-)	(+) Adrenal, sex cord-stromal tumors
pax-8	(-)	(+) Kidney, thyroid, neuroendocrine tumors of pancreas/GI tract

V = variable.

Immunohistochemistry, Testis

Paratesticular Tumors With Spindle Cell Morphology

Antibody	Leiomyosarcoma	Sarcomatoid Carcinoma	Melanoma	Mesothelioma	Unclassified Sex Cord-Stromal Tumor
AE1/3 (CK-PAN)	(-/+)	(+/-)	(-)	(+)	(-/+)
Inhibin	(-)	(-)	(-)	(-)	V
S100	(-)	(-)	(+)	(-)	(+)
Actin-sm	(+)	(-/+)	(-)	(-/+)	(+)
Calretinin	(-)	(-)	(-)	(+)	V
Melan-A (MART-1)	(-)	(-)	(+)	(-)	V
SF1	(-)	(-)	(-)	(-)	V/(+)

V = variable; ND = no data.

Paratesticular Tumors With Glandular/Tubular Pattern

Antibody	Metastatic Adenocarcinoma	Müllerian Epithelial Tumors	Sertoliform Cystadenoma of Rete Testis	Adenomatoid Tumor	Rete Adenocarcinoma	Mesothelioma	Paratesticular Sertoli Cell Tumor
AE1/3 (CK-PAN)	(+)	(+)	(+/-)	(+)	(+)	(+)	(+)
CD30 (BerH2)	(-)	(-/+)	(-)	(-)	(-)	(-)	(-)
ER	(-/+)	(+)	(-)	(-)	(-)	(-)	(-)
PR	(-/+)	(+)	(-)	(-)	(-)	(-)	(-)
CK7	(+/-)	(+)	(+/-)	(-/+)	(+)	(-/+)	(-)
Vimentin	(-/+)	(-/+)	(-)	(-)	(-)	(-)	(+)
Calretinin	(-)	(-)	(-)	(+)	(-)	(+)	(+)
WT1	(-)	(+)	(-)	(+)	(-)	(+)	(+)
Podoplanin (D2-40)	(-)	(-)	(-)	(+)	(-)	(+)	(-)
pax-8	(+) Kidney, thyroid, neuroendocrine tumors of pancreas and GI tract	(+)	ND	(-)	(+/-)	(-)	(-)
SF1	(-) (+) in adrenal cortical tumors	(-)	ND	(-)	ND	(-)	(+)
β-catenin	(-) (+) in colonic adenocarcinoma	(-)	ND	(-)	ND	(-)	(+)

ND = no data.

Paratesticular Papillary Tumors

Antibody	Müllerian Papillary Serous Carcinoma	Mesothelioma	Prostatic Adenocarcinoma
ER, PR	(+)	(-)	(-)/V
CK7	(+)	(-/+)	(-)
Calretinin	(-)	(+)	(-)
CK5/6	(-)	(+)	(-)
Podoplanin (D2-40)	(-)	(+)	(-)

Immunohistochemistry, Testis

Paratesticular Papillary Tumors (Continued)

Antibody	Müllerian Papillary Serous Carcinoma	Mesothelioma	Prostatic Adenocarcinoma
PSA, PAP	(-)	(-)	(+)
pax-8	(+)	(-)	(-)
WT1	(+)	(+)	(-)

V= variable.

Testicular Tumors vs. Metastasis

Müllerian	Mesothelial	Epithelial	Germ Cell	Sex Cord
CA125	Calretinin	EMA/MUC1	POU5F1 (OCT3/OCT4)	SF1
WT1	HMWK (34βE12)	CEA	PLAP	Inhibin
ER, PR	Podoplanin (D2-40)	CK7	SALL4	Calretinin
pax-8	Thrombomodulin	CK20	CD30	WT1
	Mesothelin	CDX-2 colorectal	CD117	Melan-A
	WT1	PSA prostate	Podoplanin (D2-40)	CD99
	CK5/CK6	TTF-1 lung and thyroid		β-catenin
		pax-8 kidney, thyroid, neuroendocrine tumors of pancreas/GI tract		Synaptophysin

Immunohistochemistry, Testis

Germ Cell Neoplasia In Situ
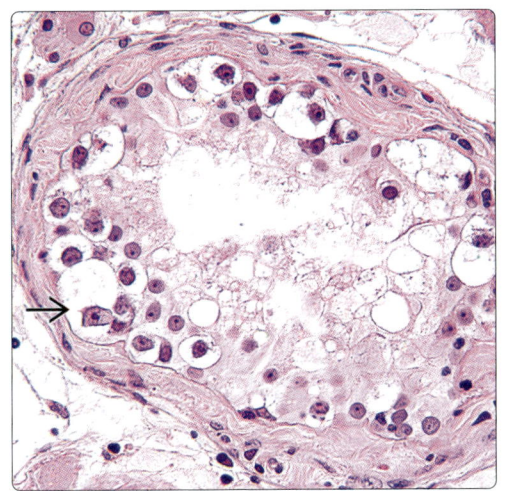

Germ Cell Neoplasia In Situ: POU5F1
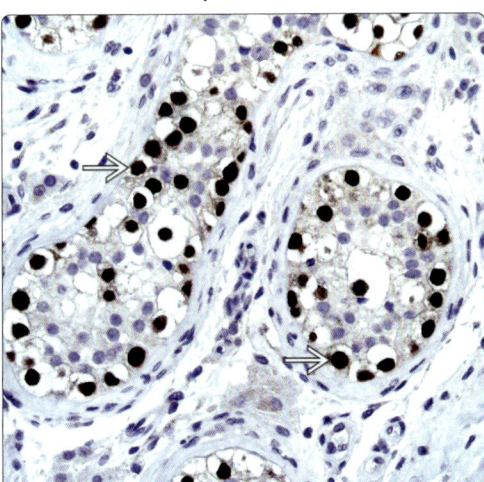

(Left) H&E shows germ cell neoplasia in situ composed of large atypical cells ⇢ situated at the periphery of an atrophic seminiferous tubule. The atypical cells have abundant clear cytoplasm and enlarged nuclei with prominent nucleoli. (Right) The tumor cells ⇢ of germ cell neoplasia in situ are highlighted by strong nuclear staining by POU5F1 (OCT3/OCT4). The nonneoplastic germ cells in the adjacent seminiferous tubule are negative. Immunostaining is useful in small biopsies in high-risk patients.

Seminoma
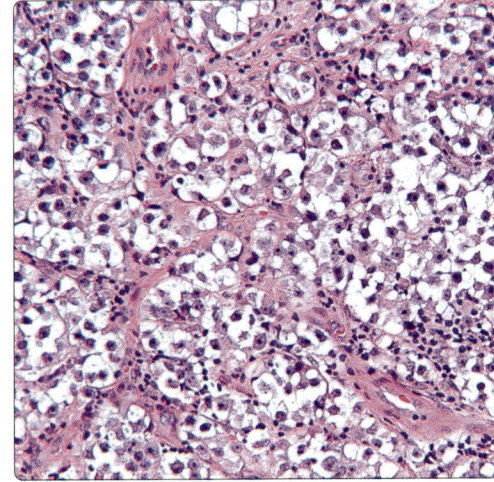

Seminoma: POU5F1
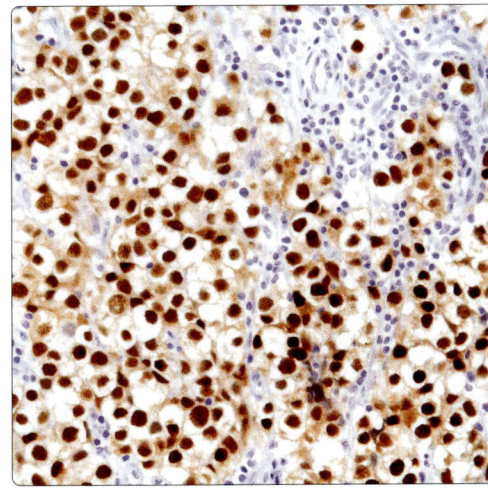

(Left) This is an example of classic seminoma with nests of seminomatous tumor cells separated by fibrous septa containing small lymphocytes. (Right) This image shows strong positive nuclear staining of seminoma cells by POU5F1 (OCT3/OCT4). The small lymphocytes are negative. POU5F1 is a useful marker for seminoma and embryonal carcinoma. It is also useful in metastatic setting or extragonadal germ cell tumors. Being a nuclear stain, it tends to be more reliable and easy to interpret.

Seminoma: CD117
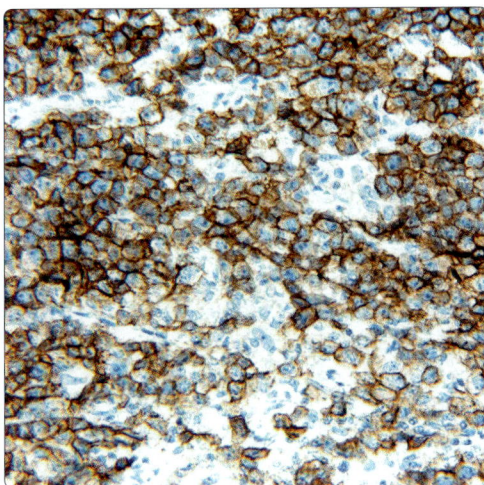

Seminoma: Podoplanin
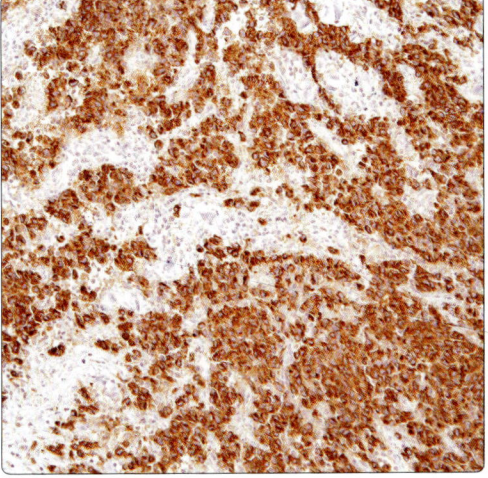

(Left) This image shows strong membranous staining of classic seminoma by CD117. It is also a sensitive marker for germ cell neoplasia in situ. Embryonal carcinoma is negative and yolk sac tumor (YST) may show rare and focal weak staining. (Right) This photomicrograph shows strong membranous and cytoplasmic staining of seminoma by podoplanin (D2-40). Podoplanin is an antibody against oncofetal protein M2A, which also stains lymphatic endothelial cells and mesothelial cells.

Immunohistochemistry, Testis

Embryonal Carcinoma

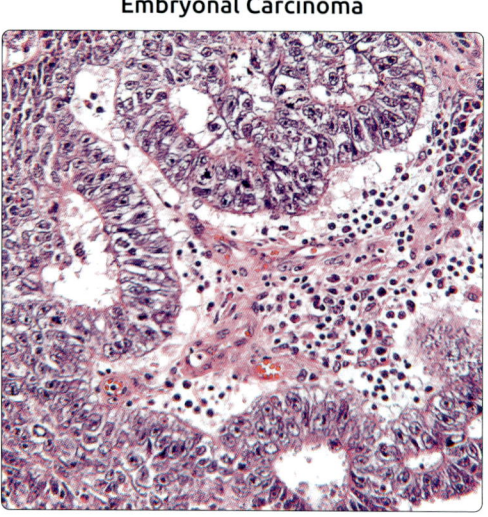

Mixed Cell Tumor

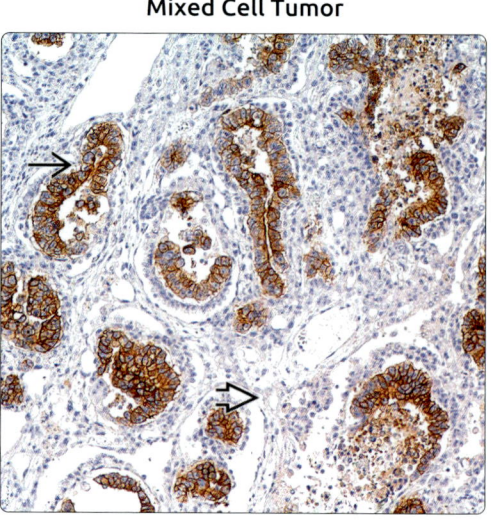

(Left) This image shows embryonal carcinoma with prominent glandular pattern. Important differential diagnoses include yolk sac tumor and metastatic carcinoma. (Right) Embryonal carcinoma shows membranous staining for CD30 (BER-H2) ⇨; the surrounding yolk cell tumor component is negative ⇨. Germ cell tumors are typically EMA/MUC1(-) compared to visceral epithelial malignancies. CD30 also stains anaplastic large cell lymphoma and hence should be used in a panel.

Mixed Germ Cell Tumor

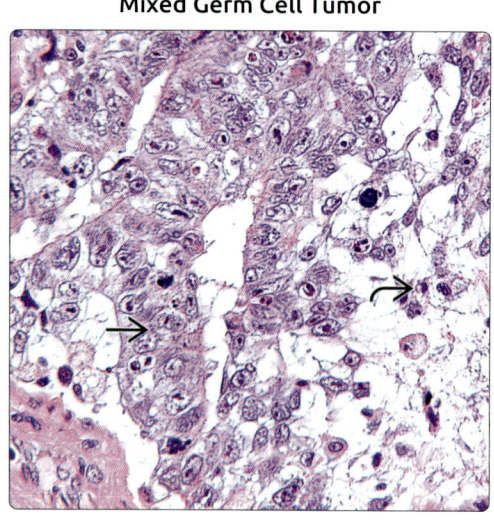

Mixed Germ Cell Tumor

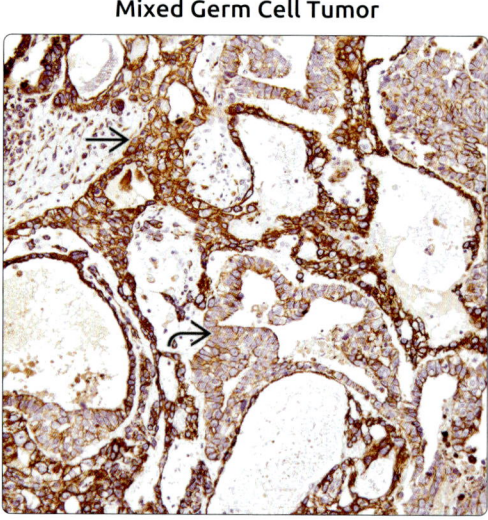

(Left) This image shows a mixed germ cell tumor, i.e., embryonal carcinoma ⇨ and YST ⇨. YST can be quite inconspicuous on H&E sections and is frequently underdiagnosed. (Right) This image shows embryonal carcinoma (EC) and YST stained by AE1/AE3 (CK-PAN). The differential staining in intensity is a helpful feature to identify the relative composition of EC and yolk sac tumor as the staining in yolk sac tumor ⇨ is much stronger than in the EC component ⇨.

Yolk Sac Tumor

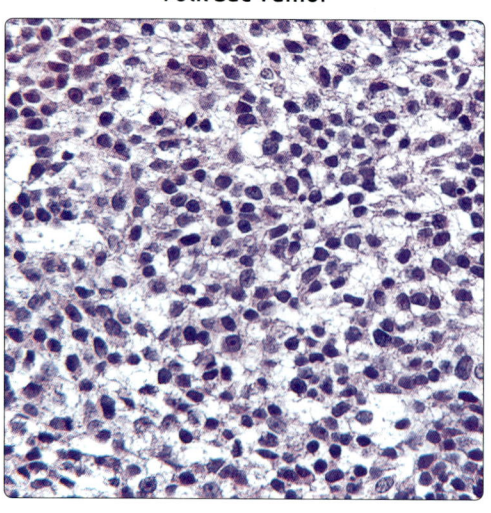

Yolk Sac Tumor: Glypican-3

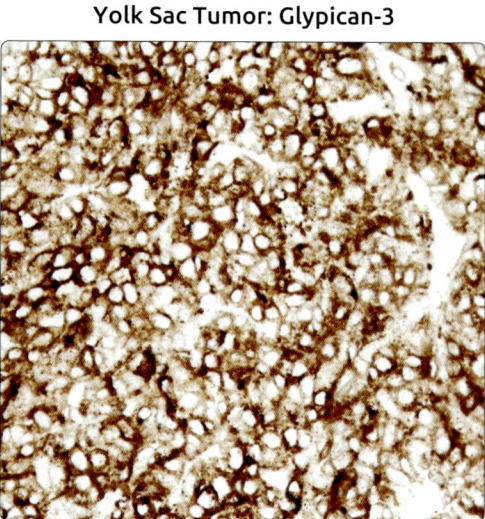

(Left) This is an example of YST with solid growth pattern. When predominant, the morphologic differential diagnoses would include seminoma, embryonal carcinoma, monophasic choriocarcinoma, and solid Leydig cell and Sertoli cell tumors. (Right) Positive membranous and cytoplasmic staining of the solid YST for glypican-3 is shown. Other germ cell tumor components are negative for glypican-3 except in syncytiotrophoblasts and rarely in immature teratoma.

Immunohistochemistry, Testis

Yolk Sac Tumor
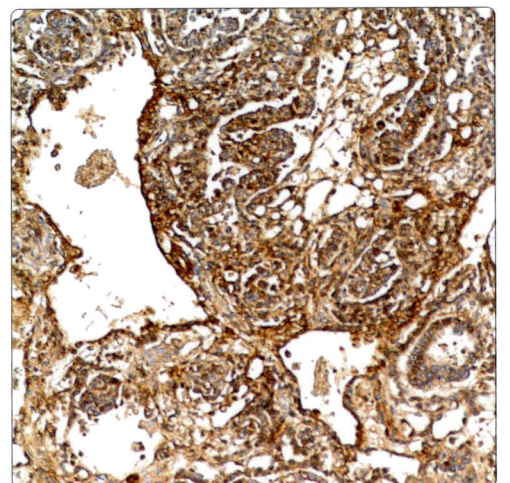

Yolk Sac Tumor: SALL4
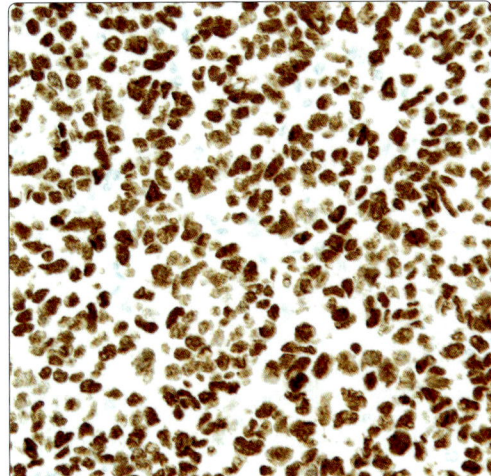

(Left) This image shows strong positive immunostaining of YST by α-fetoprotein is a time-honored marker, but it stains only 55-78% of YST and staining is often blotchy, frequently with nonspecific background staining. **(Right)** Strong nuclear staining of YST by SALL4 is shown, a zinc finger transcription factor expressed in human embryonic stem cells. SALL4 stains all germ cell tumor components and appears to be the most sensitive marker for YST.

Choriocarcinoma
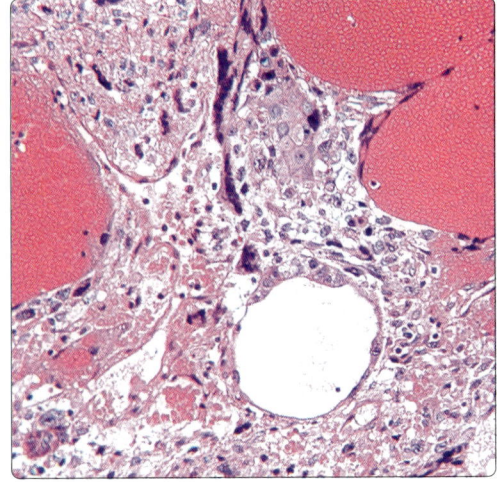

CC: HCG-β
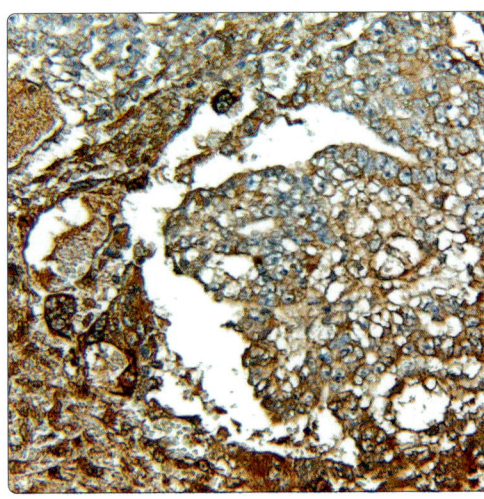

(Left) Choriocarcinoma (CC) shows prominent hemorrhage with intimate admixture of mononucleated cytotrophoblasts and multinucleated syncytiotrophoblasts. Presence of syncytiotrophoblasts with other germ cell components may be overdiagnosed as CC. **(Right)** CC shows strong cytoplasmic staining of mononucleated and multinucleated trophoblasts by HCG-β. Syncytiotrophoblasts are positive for cytokeratin and glypican-3.

Spermatocytic Tumor: CD117
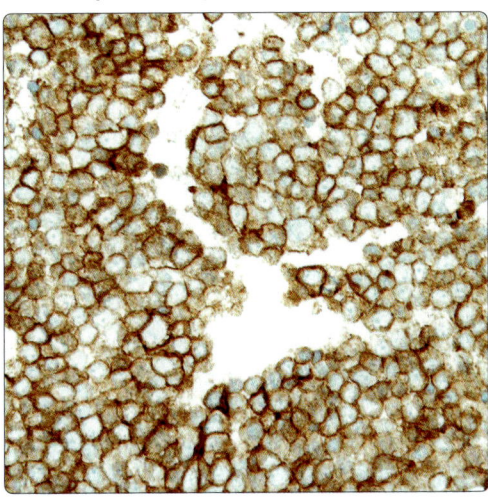

Spermatocytic Tumor: SALL4
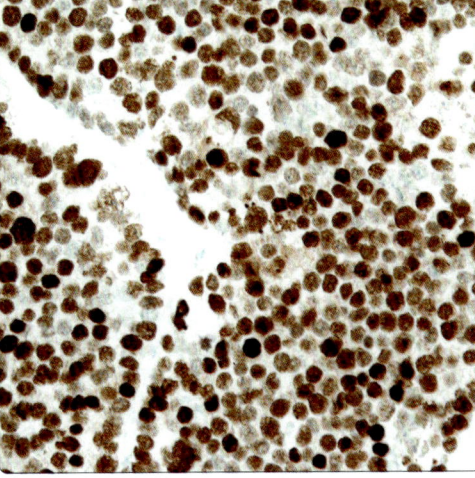

(Left) This image shows strong membranous staining of spermatocytic tumor by CD117. It is also a sensitive marker for classic seminoma and germ cell neoplasia in situ. **(Right)** This image shows strong nuclear stain of spermatocytic tumor by SALL4, a zinc finger transcription factor expressed in human embryonic stem cells. SALL4 stains all types of germ cell tumor including a spermatocytic tumor. Staining is often weak and focal.

SECTION 5
Penis and Scrotum

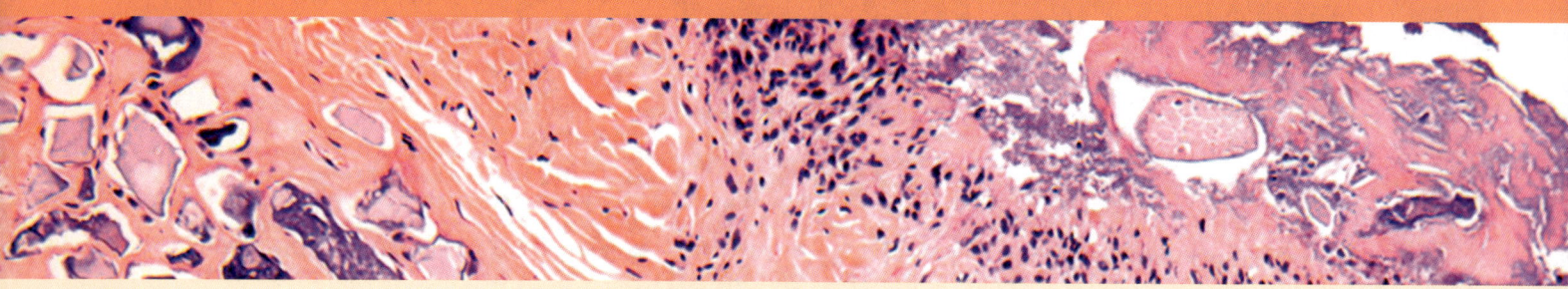

Frequent Lesions of Uncertain Relationship to Penile Neoplasia

Condylomas	**908**
Lichen Sclerosus et Atrophicus	**912**
Squamous Hyperplasia	**914**
Lipogranuloma	**918**
Scrotal Calcinosis	**920**

Penile Intraepithelial Neoplasia

Penile Intraepithelial Neoplasia	**922**

Primary Epithelial Tumors

General Concepts, Squamous Cell Carcinoma	**928**
Squamous Cell Carcinoma, Usual Type	**938**

Variants of Squamous Cell Carcinoma

Basaloid Squamous Cell Carcinoma	**942**
Basaloid Squamous Cell Carcinoma, Papillary Variant	**946**
Warty (Condylomatous) Squamous Cell Carcinoma	**948**
Warty-Basaloid Squamous Cell Carcinoma	**952**
Verrucous Squamous Cell Carcinoma	**954**
Papillary Squamous Cell Carcinoma, Not Otherwise Specified	**958**
Pseudoglandular Squamous Cell Carcinoma	**962**
Pseudohyperplastic Squamous Cell Carcinoma	**964**
Cuniculatum Squamous Cell Carcinoma	**966**
Sarcomatoid Squamous Cell Carcinoma	**970**
Mixed Squamous Cell Carcinoma	**974**
Lymphoepithelioma-Like Squamous Cell Carcinoma	**978**
Clear Cell Carcinoma	**980**

HPV- and Non-HPV-Related Tumors

Overview of HPV- and Non-HPV-Related Tumors	**982**

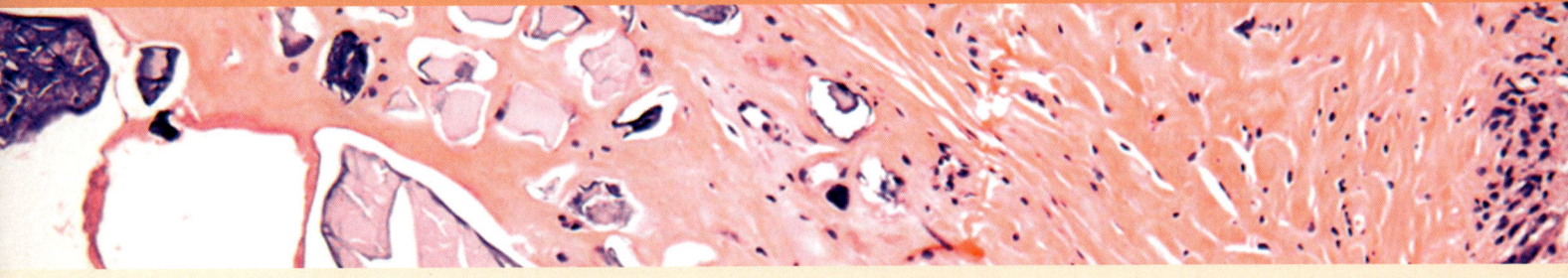

Other Neoplastic Conditions

Extramammary Paget Disease 986
Kaposi Sarcoma 990
Myointimoma 992

Metastatic Tumors

Metastatic Tumors, Penis 994

Immunohistochemical Profiles for Tumors Involving Penis

Immunohistochemistry, Penis 996

Condylomas

KEY FACTS

TERMINOLOGY
- Exophytic human papillomavirus (HPV)-related benign papillomatous proliferation of squamous epithelium
- Synonyms include condylomata acuminatum, benign condyloma, usual condyloma, flat condyloma, giant condyloma, genital wart

ETIOLOGY/PATHOGENESIS
- Majority of these lesions (85%) carry low-risk HPV6 and 11
- High-risk HPV16 and 18 may be identified in common condylomas in 15% of cases
- There may be history of multiple sexual partners (from 10 to 50) in 58% of cases
- Recurrent lesions are common, especially in men with multiple sexual partners

MACROSCOPIC
- Soft, exophytic cauliflower-like lesion from 1 mm to large tumors

MICROSCOPIC
- Arborescent condylomatous papillae with prominent central fibrovascular cores are characteristic
- Tip of papillae shows hyperkeratosis and parakeratosis
- Squamous cells are mature and nonatypical
- Atypia may be present, usually basal

TOP DIFFERENTIAL DIAGNOSES
- Early penile plaques
- Seborrheic keratosis
- Penile intraepithelial neoplasia
- Warty carcinoma
- Papillary carcinoma
- Verrucous carcinoma
- Condyloma with malignant transformation

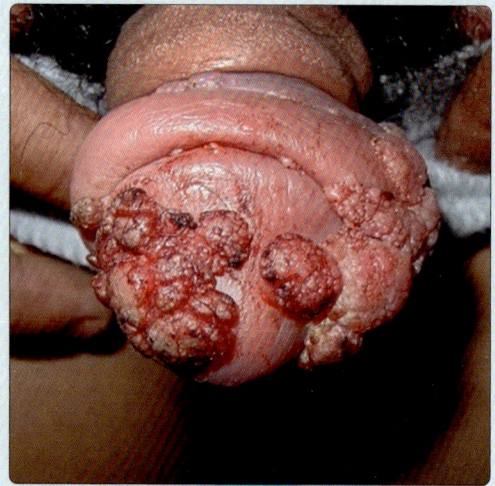

Genital Warts, Gross View

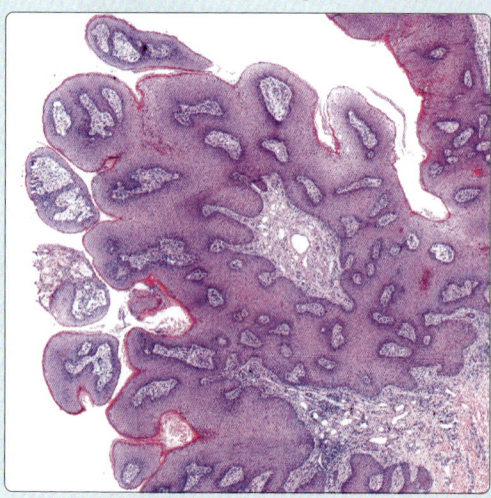

Condyloma, Low Magnification

(Left) Gross view shows multiple condylomatous lesions involving the glans, coronal sulcus, and foreskin. (Right) Papillomatous exophytic epithelial proliferation with arborescent cauliflower-like pattern is characteristic of fully developed lesions.

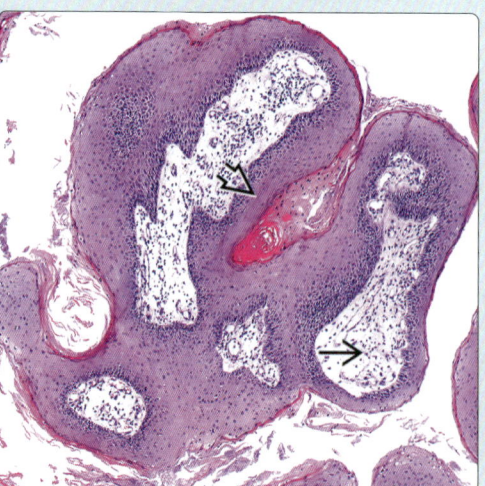

Condyloma, Architectural Features

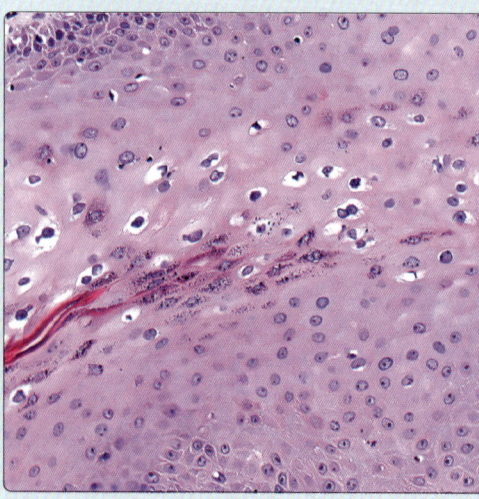

Condyloma, High-Power View

(Left) Medium magnification of this lesion shows papillomatosis with fibrovascular cores ⇨ composed of loose connective tissue and small vascular spaces. Acanthotic epithelium with hyperkeratosis and parakeratosis is shown ⇨. (Right) Koilocytes with dark wrinkled nuclei, occasional binucleation, and perinuclear halos are seen.

Condylomas

TERMINOLOGY

Synonyms
- Condylomata acuminatum, benign condyloma, usual condyloma, flat condyloma, giant condyloma, genital wart

Definitions
- Exophytic human papillomavirus (HPV)-related benign papillomatous proliferation of squamous epithelium

ETIOLOGY/PATHOGENESIS

Etiology
- Condylomas are causally related to HPV
- HPV is commonly present subclinically in penis in general population (15-50%)
- Conversion or progression of subclinical HPV infection to observable and pathologically diagnosed condylomas occurs in 5% of patients
- Majority of these lesions (85%) carry low-risk HPV 6 and 11
- Other low-risk HPV genotypes found in condylomas are 26, 40, 53, 54, 66, 71, 70, 73, and 82
- High-risk HPV may be identified in common condylomas in 15% of cases
- Other high-risk HPV in condylomas are 31, 33, 35, 39, 45, 51, 52, 56, 58, 59, and 68

Risk Factors
- Condylomas are contagious and transmitted through skin contact during oral, genital, or anal sex with infected partner
- Overall, patients with condylomas have less education than general population
- They are mostly uncircumcised, and few use condoms
- There is history of multiple sexual partners (from 10 to 50) in 58% of cases
- They are usually smokers or former smokers and alcohol abusers

CLINICAL ISSUES

Site
- Lesions are commonly multicentric affecting in this order of frequency glans, coronal sulcus, foreskin, and meatus, all within mucosal epithelial compartments of distal glans
- Unifocal lesions, usually large in size, may be present
- When long-standing lesion compromises most of distal penis and appears locally destructive, term giant condyloma may be utilized
- Nonmucosal compartments like skin of shaft, scrotum, or inguinal or pubic skin may also be affected

Presentation
- Clinically, condylomas may be confused with molluscum contagiosum
- Coexistence with other genital infections is not rare
- Majority of condylomas occur in sexually active younger men aged of 18 to 44 years (89%) and rarely in older patients
- Lesion usually present with verruciform papillomatous appearance
- Flat lesions may also be found, and they are usually confused with other lesions or penile intraepithelial neoplasia (PeIN)
- For flat lesions, which may be clinically inconspicuous, total acetic acid and peniscopy may be necessary for detection

Treatment
- Surgical approaches
  - Wide local excision or penectomy is recommended for large destructive giant condylomas
  - Surgical local excision is recommended for medium-sized lesions
  - For small lesions, cryosurgery, electrofulguration, laser ablation, and topical treatments are commonly used
- Drugs
  - Medical topical treatment may include imiquimod cream, 20% podophyllin antimitotic solution, 0.5% podofilox solution, 5% 5-FU cream, and trichloroacetic acid

Prognosis
- Overall prognosis of common condylomas is good, but there is high recurrent rate
- Surgical excision may remove warts, but HPV persists, so warts may recur after treatment in about 38–73% of cases
- Recurrence (or development of new lesions) occurs especially in younger men with multiple sexual partners
- Recurrent lesions are usually benign
- Condylomas may regress spontaneously
- Malignant transformation (high-grade dysplasia or invasive cancer) of small typical condyloma is very unusual
- Long-standing giant condylomas may harbor foci of carcinoma, intraepithelial or invasive
- Prognosis of carcinoma arising in condyloma is related to pathological features and prognostic factors of carcinoma

MACROSCOPIC

General Features
- Condylomas are soft reddish to gray, exophytic cauliflower-like lesions

Size
- Size ranges from 1 mm to large tumors
- Giant condyloma is arbitrary name for large lesions usually measuring 5-10 mm

MICROSCOPIC

Histologic Features
- Usual condylomas characteristically show arborescent condylomatous papillae with prominent central fibrovascular cores
- There is hyperkeratosis &/or parakeratosis at papillae surface
- Nonpleomorphic koilocytosis is present in upper 1/3 of epithelium
- 4 elements are required for diagnosis of koilocytosis: Clear cytoplasm, binucleation, wrinkled nuclei, and presence of keratinocytes
- Squamous cells are mature and nonatypical
- Above described features are typical of condylomatous papillae

Condylomas

- Pathological presentation of condylomas varies; most common is usual condyloma acuminatum detected in about 90% of cases
- Other pathological presentations are flat, focally atypical condyloma with malignant transformation or condyloma associated with invasive carcinoma
- Giant condylomas are identical to common condylomas but are larger and unicentric in older patients, with tendency for malignant transformation
- Differential diagnosis of flat condylomas with differentiated PeIN may be challenging, and HPV evaluation may be required
- Some condylomas may not show obvious koilocytes, and differential diagnosis with squamous hyperplasia or seborrheic keratosis may be considered
- Giant condylomas may be confused with penile verruciform carcinomas

DIFFERENTIAL DIAGNOSIS

Early Penile Plaques
- They are HPV(-) lesions with hyperkeratosis but no koilocytosis and no significant inflammation; more likely they represent hyperplastic lesions

Seborrheic Keratosis
- They show acanthosis, papillomatosis, and occasional hyperpigmentation
- Flat nonpapillary cases are also noted
- No koilocytosis is present, and p16 and HPV are usually negative

Papillomatosis of Glans Corona
- Also referred to as pearly penile papules, hirsutoid papillomas
- Occur in markedly sexually active younger patients
- They are common (30% of male patients)
- Always located in dorsum of glans corona
- Lesions are arranged in linear rows of 2 or 3 micronodules along corona
- Microscopically they are small fibroepithelial squamous papillomas
- p16 and HPV are negative

Penile Intraepithelial Neoplasia
- Flat lesions may be atypical and difficult to differentiate from differentiated PeIN
- Differentiated PeINs are negative for p16 and HPV
- Koilocytosis is diagnostic of condyloma, but in its absence lesion may still be condyloma, with HPV detection required
- p16 may be positive in some atypical condylomas

Warty Carcinoma
- Noninvasive warty carcinoma, with broad base, may simulate giant condylomas, which may also be atypical
- Warty carcinoma patients are usually older
- Atypical parakeratosis and pleomorphic koilocytosis are more frequent in warty carcinomas
- Immunostain p16 or high-risk HPV detection may be required, both positive in warty carcinomas but not in condylomas

Papillary Carcinoma, Not Otherwise Specified
- Papillary carcinomas may harbor condylomatous-like papillae, with central fibrovascular core
- However, in papillary carcinomas, there is no koilocytosis
- There is jagged infiltrative tumor base, not present in condylomas
- In problematic cases, negativity for p16 or HPV detection, typical of papillary carcinomas, may be required

Verrucous Carcinoma
- Rarely, verrucous carcinoma shows features simulating condylomatous papillae (pseudocondylomatous verrucous carcinomas)
- These papillae do not harbor koilocytes
- Like in condylomas, and different from papillary carcinomas not otherwise specified, base of tumor is broad or pushing
- p16 and HPV should be negative in verrucous carcinomas

Condylomas With Malignant Transformation
- Malignant transformation of common condyloma is extremely rare event
- When it occurs, it is usually within long-standing giant condyloma
- Histological type of malignant foci shows histology of usual squamous cell carcinoma
- Malignant foci tend to occur at tumor base or front
- Giant or large condylomas should be generously sampled to rule out foci of malignant transformation
- In some invasive squamous cell carcinomas, foci of residual condyloma may be present

DIAGNOSTIC CHECKLIST

Clinically Relevant Pathologic Features
- Multicentric mucosal lesions in sexually active younger patients should alert about possibility of condyloma
- Large cauliflower-like long-standing penile tumor in patients neglecting early medical attention should alert about possibility of giant condyloma with malignant transformation

Pathologic Interpretation Pearls
- Koilocytosis is not evident in some condylomas; if histological pattern is otherwise characteristic, it should be sufficient for diagnosis
- HPV detection in tissue may rarely be helpful
- If atypia is found in common or flat condylomas, consider ordering p16 stain to rule out high-risk HPV

SELECTED REFERENCES

1. Fernandez-Nestosa MJ et al: Detection of HPV genotypes according to subtypes of penile intraepithelial neoplasia (PeIN) – a study of 126 lesions in 43 patients using laser capture microdissection (LCM)-PCR. Mod. Pathol. 28: 219-220A, 2015
2. Ingles DJ et al: Human papillomavirus virus (HPV) genotype- and age-specific analyses of external genital lesions among men in the HPV Infection in Men (HIM) Study. J Infect Dis. 211(7):1060-7, 2015

Condylomas

Condyloma, Low Power
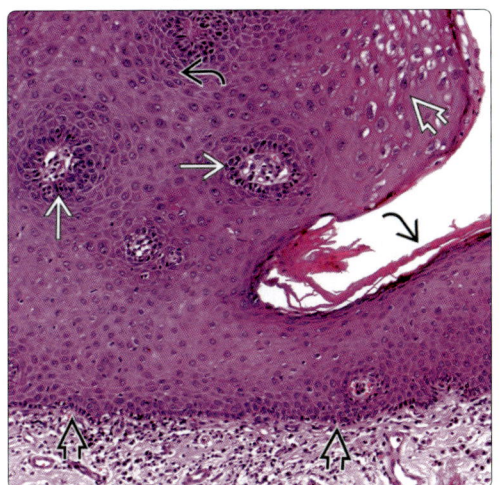

Condyloma, Intermediate Power
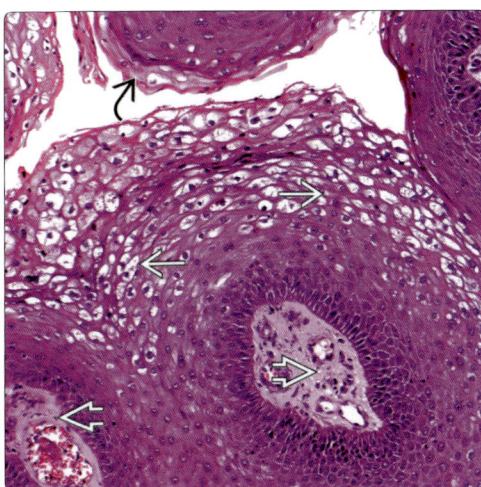

(Left) In condyloma acuminatum, the base ⇨ is broad and sharply defined, fibrovascular cores are prominent ⇨, and surface koilocytosis ⇨ and parakeratosis are easily found ⇨. (Right) Condyloma acuminatum is characterized by papillomatosis and prominent fibrovascular cores ⇨. Epithelium is acanthotic and exhibits squamous maturation. Koilocytes are easily found ⇨, and parakeratosis is common ⇨.

Koilocytosis
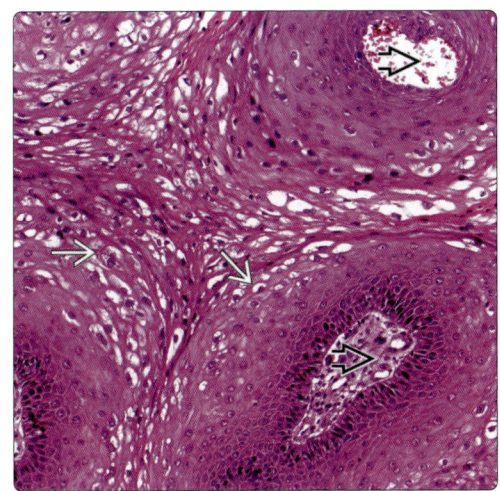

Giant Condyloma
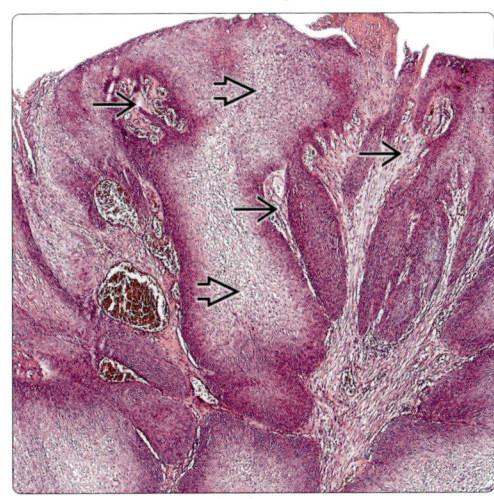

(Left) Papillomatosis with evident fibrovascular cores ⇨, surface koilocytosis ⇨, and absence of evident nuclear atypia are pathognomonic findings of usual condyloma acuminatum. (Right) Giant condyloma is characterized by marked acanthosis and an endophytic pattern of growth with bulbous extension of the base, prominent fibrovascular cores ⇨, and clear areas ⇨, which correspond to koilocytosis at higher power. Sampling of all tissue is necessary to rule out invasive carcinoma.

Koilocytosis
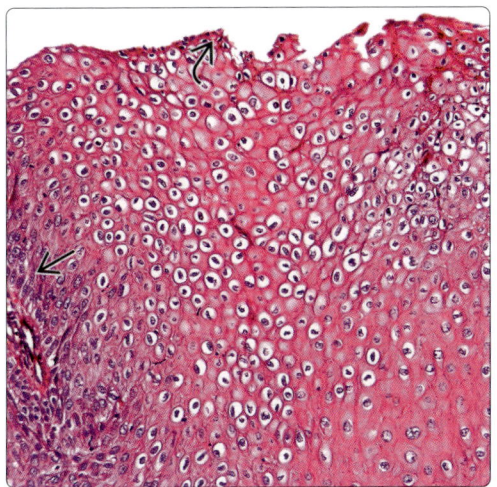

Koilocytosis
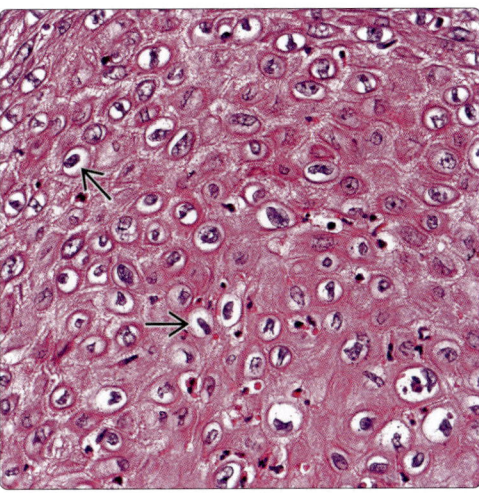

(Left) In both condyloma acuminatum and giant condyloma, koilocytes are easily found, subtle nuclear atypia may be present in cells of the basal layer ⇨, especially in the latter, and a thin parakeratotic layer ⇨ is commonly observed. (Right) Koilocytes are characterized by clear perinuclear halos ⇨ and wrinkled and hyperchromatic nuclei. The cytoplasm is eosinophilic, cellular borders are distinctive, and binucleation is common.

Lichen Sclerosus et Atrophicus

KEY FACTS

TERMINOLOGY
- Synonyms
  - Lichen sclerosus (LS); balanitis xerotica obliterans

CLINICAL ISSUES
- White atrophic patches with petechia affecting glans, coronal sulcus, &/or foreskin
- Hypertrophic/ hyperplastic foci need to be followed-up and biopsied if clinically indicated
- Differentiated penile intraepithelial neoplasia (PeIN) tends to arise in thick/hyperplastic foci
- ~ 9% of affected patients will develop penile squamous cell carcinoma (SCC)

MICROSCOPIC
- Hallmark of lesion is hyalinized/sclerotic band underneath epithelium
- Telangiectatic vessels are seen in this area of hyalinization
- Interface vacuolar alteration of basal layer
- Atrophic epithelium (often associated with at least focal hyperplastic areas)
- Variable degree of lymphoid infiltrate underneath sclerotic band
- Melanophages are present admixed with lymphoid cells

TOP DIFFERENTIAL DIAGNOSES
- Lichen planus
  - Lacks classical hyalinized band (hallmark of LS)
  - Early/inflammatory lesions of LS may be difficult to distinguish from LP
    - Deeper levels or additional sampling may be necessary to show classical foci of LS

REPORTING
- Important to report hyperplastic foci and atypical changes (differentiated PeIN arising in background of LS)

LS: Hyalinized Papillary Dermis
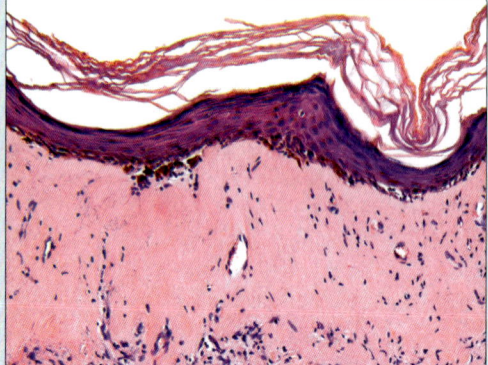

LS: Papillary Dermal Edema
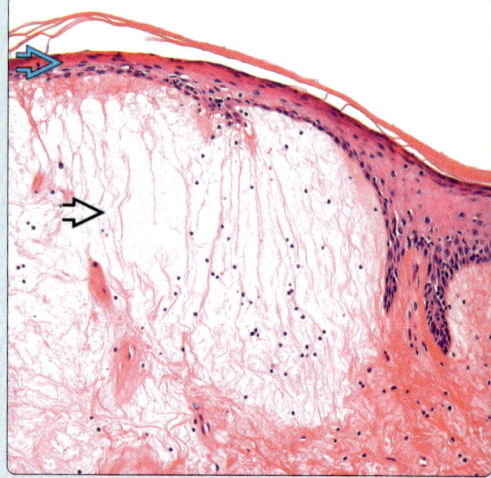

(Left) Note the atrophic epidermis associated with vacuolar alteration of the basal layer and a thick hyalinized connective tissue band in the papillary dermis in this case of lichen sclerosus (LS). (Right) Some cases of LS show prominent papillary dermal edema ➡. Note also the atrophic epidermis ➡.

LS: Hyperplastic Squamous Mucosa
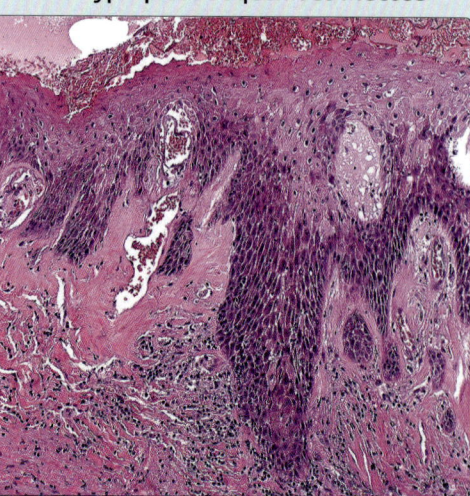

LS and Differentiated PeIN
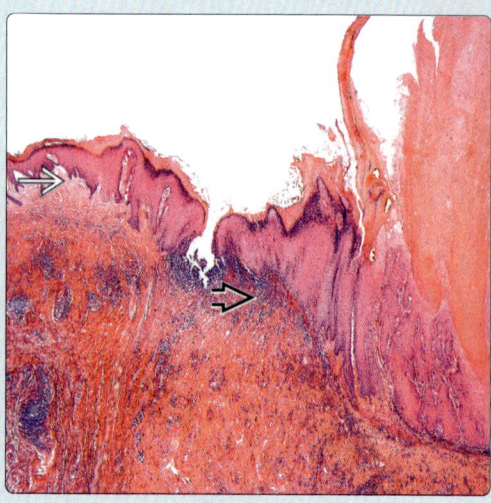

(Left) LS associated with hyperplastic squamous epithelium with atypia [differentiated, non-HPV-related, penile intraepithelial neoplasia (PeIN), and lichen LS] is shown. Usually, atypical/dysplastic changes arise in such hyperplastic foci. (Right) Low-power view shows LS ➡ with hyperplastic and mild atypical changes (differentiated, non-HPV-related, PeIN) adjacent to a verrucous carcinoma ➡.

Lichen Sclerosus et Atrophicus

TERMINOLOGY

Synonyms
- Lichen sclerosus (LS), balanitis xerotica obliterans

Definitions
- Interface vacuolar/lichenoid dermatitis with thickened papillary dermis/lamina propria showing band-like hyalinization (sclerosis)

ETIOLOGY/PATHOGENESIS

Pathogenesis
- Unknown

CLINICAL ISSUES

Presentation
- Early lesions appear as pink or purple macules that become papules
- Purpura and telangiectases are common
- Well-established lesions appear as white-gray, irregular geographic, and atrophic areas
- Erosion, ulceration may be present
- Elevated hyperkeratotic foci may also be seen
- Advanced cases may result in acquired phimosis or paraphimosis
- Lesions usually affect inner aspect of foreskin, glans, and perimeatal region; urethra may be involved
- Lesions tend to be broad and multifocal

Treatment
- Medical
- Circumcision (if only/predominantly affecting foreskin)

Prognosis
- Chronic condition
- Associated with squamous cell carcinoma (SCC) (~ 9% of affected patients will develop penile SCC)

MACROSCOPIC

Sections to Be Submitted
- When dealing with large specimen (such as circumcision), it is important to extensively sample thick, hyperkeratotic areas

MICROSCOPIC

Histologic Features
- Atrophic epithelium (early lesions)
  - Frequently intermixed with hyperplastic areas (chronic lesions)
- Vacuolar alteration of basal layer
- Thickened lamina propria/dermis with classic band-like hyalinization/sclerosis
- Telangiectasia within band of sclerosis
- Scattered melanophages in superficial dermis/lamina propria
- Band-like lymphoid infiltrate underneath band of sclerosis (well-established lesions)
  - Early lesions show more superficial lymphoid infiltrate underneath epithelium without well-formed sclerotic band
- Late lesions are sclerotic with minimal inflammation
- Sometimes prominent edema of papillary dermis/lamina propria
- Dermal-epidermal clefting or blisters may be seen secondary to marked basal cell vacuolar alteration
- Minority of cases of chronic LS may be associated with atypical foci in epithelium [differentiated, non-HPV-related, penile intraepithelial neoplasia (PeIN)]
- Minority of cases of LS will evolve to SCC
  - Most common types of SCC associated with LS are HPV unrelated variants of well-differentiated keratinizing SCC such as pseudohyperplastic SCC and verrucous carcinoma

Predominant Pattern/Injury Type
- Interface dermatitis with sclerosis

Predominant Cell/Compartment Type
- Epithelium and superficial dermis/lamina propria

DIFFERENTIAL DIAGNOSIS

Lichen Planus
- Denser and more superficial band-like lymphoid infiltrate obscuring dermal-epidermal junction
- Absence of classic hyalinized band in superficial dermis/lamina propria
- Wedge-shaped hypergranulosis

DIAGNOSTIC CHECKLIST

Clinically Relevant Pathologic Features
- Hyperplastic areas as seen in longstanding lesions may be associated with differentiated PeIN

Pathologic Interpretation Pearls
- Hallmark of LS is hyalinized (sclerotic) band in lamina propria/papillary dermis
  - Early lesions do not show classical band-like area of sclerosis/hyalinization
    - Thickened basement membrane and hyalinization around superficial blood vessels are clues to diagnosis of early lichen sclerosus

SELECTED REFERENCES

1. Philippou P et al: Genital lichen sclerosus/balanitis xerotica obliterans in men with penile carcinoma: a critical analysis. BJU Int. 111(6):970-6, 2013
2. Oertell J et al: Differentiated precursor lesions and low-grade variants of squamous cell carcinomas are frequent findings in foreskins of patients from a region of high penile cancer incidence. Histopathology. 58(6):925-33, 2011
3. Cubilla AL et al: Pseudohyperplastic squamous cell carcinoma of the penis associated with lichen sclerosus. An extremely well-differentiated, nonverruciform neoplasm that preferentially affects the foreskin and is frequently misdiagnosed: a report of 10 cases of a distinctive clinicopathologic entity. Am J Surg Pathol. 28(7):895-900, 2004
4. Velazquez EF et al: Lichen sclerosus in 68 patients with squamous cell carcinoma of the penis: frequent atypias and correlation with special carcinoma variants suggests a precancerous role. Am J Surg Pathol. 27(11):1448-53, 2003
5. Micali G et al: Lichen sclerosus of the glans is significantly associated with penile carcinoma. Sex Transm Infect. 77(3):226, 2001
6. Nasca MR et al: Penile cancer among patients with genital lichen sclerosus. J Am Acad Dermatol. 41(6):911-4, 1999

Squamous Hyperplasia

KEY FACTS

TERMINOLOGY
- Thickening of mucosal squamous epithelium without atypia
- Common epithelial alteration associated with penile cancer
- Frequently associated with dermatologic inflammatory conditions and differentiated penile intraepithelial neoplasia (PeIN)
- Found in association with usual, papillary, and verrucous SCC (HPV-unrelated variants of SCC)

MACROSCOPIC
- Whitish areas with irregular borders

MICROSCOPIC
- Acanthosis with hyperkeratosis
- Hypergranulosis
- Normal maturation with no cytologic atypia
- Parakeratosis is uncommon
- Koilocytes are absent

- Merging of SH with PeIN &/or invasive SCC is common finding
- Flat squamous hyperplasia is most common pattern
- Other subtypes include papillary, pseudoepitheliomatous, and verrucous

TOP DIFFERENTIAL DIAGNOSES
- Condyloma
- Seborrheic keratosis
- Differentiated PeIN
- Warty PeIN
- Warty-basaloid PeIN
- Pseudohyperplastic SCC
- Verruciform xanthoma
- Warty, papillary, and verrucous carcinoma

Clinical Presentation
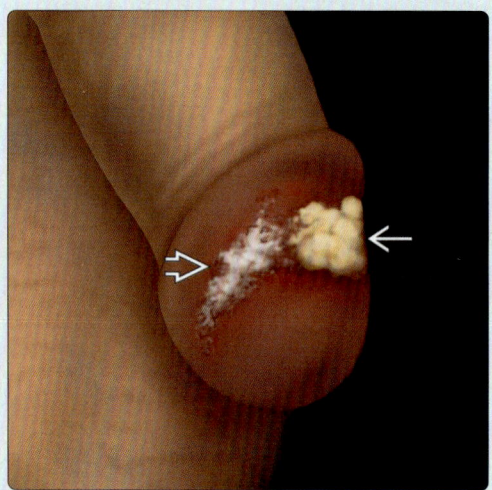

Flat Hyperplasia
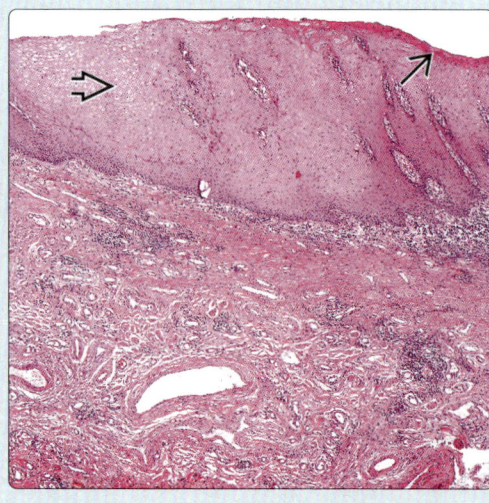

(Left) Squamous hyperplasia typically presents as whitish pearly areas ⇨ with irregular borders merging with an adjacent in situ or invasive component ⇨. (Right) Flat squamous hyperplasia is characterized by acanthosis ⇨, retained epithelial maturation, absence of cytologic atypia, hyperkeratosis ⇨, and a flat surface. Other patterns are papillary, verrucous, and pseudoepithelomatous.

Cytologic Features
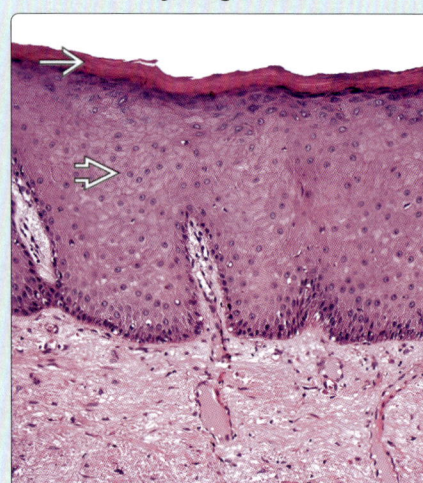

Papillary Hyperplasia
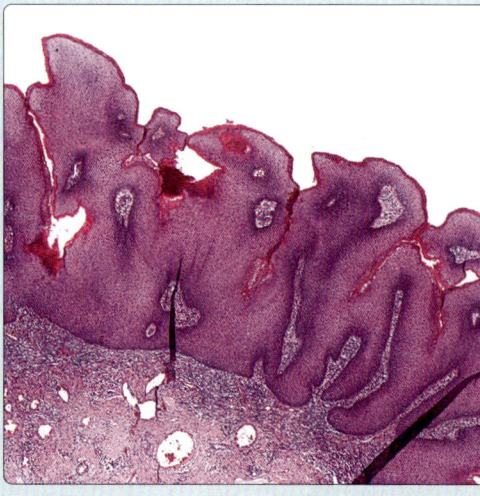

(Left) Hyperkeratosis ⇨ and acanthosis ⇨ in flat squamous hyperplasia. (Right) Papillary hyperplasia with hyperkeratosis and papillomatosis. There is absence of cytologic atypia by definition. Extensive sampling is necessary to rule out dysplastic changes.

Squamous Hyperplasia

TERMINOLOGY

Abbreviations
- Squamous hyperplasia (SH)

Definitions
- Thickening of mucosal squamous epithelium without cytologic atypia

ETIOLOGY/PATHOGENESIS

Pathogenesis
- Unknown
- Common epithelial change associated with penile cancer
- May be associated with, or part of, inflammatory condition, typically lichen sclerosus

CLINICAL ISSUES

Presentation
- Usually found in continuity or slightly distant from in situ or invasive squamous cell carcinoma (SCC)
- Distinction between SH and normal mucosa may be subtle
- Inapparent lesions may be better visualized with acetic acid (peniscopy)
- Clinically, it may be difficult to distinguish from penile intraepithelial neoplasia (PeIN)
- Micaceous balanitis and penile horn are clinically florid forms of SH with prominent hyperkeratosis

Treatment
- Benign epithelial change and usually no treatment is required

Prognosis
- May be precursor lesion of HPV-unrelated variants of SCC, but more studies are required to confirm this hypothesis

MACROSCOPIC

General Features
- Whitish areas with irregular borders
- Slightly raised areas with pearly appearance

MICROSCOPIC

Histologic Features
- Acanthosis with orthokeratotic hyperkeratosis and hypergranulosis
- Normal epithelial maturation
- Chronic inflammation may be present
- Absence of cytologic atypia
- Absent koilocytosis
- Absent intraepithelial keratin whorls (pearls)
- Associated with lichen sclerosus in some cases
- Frequently associated with differentiated PeIN
- Usually found in association with usual, papillary, and verrucous SCC (HPV-unrelated variants of SCC)

Histological Subtypes
- Flat
  - Most common subtype
  - Nonatypical acanthosis
  - Hyperkeratosis with orthokeratosis
  - Linear interface between basal layer and stroma
- Papillary
  - Represents minority of cases
  - Serrated appearance on low-power view
  - Jagged (noninvasive) interface with underlying stroma
  - Nonatypical acanthosis with short hyperkeratotic papillae
- Pseudoepitheliomatous
  - Unusual pattern of SH
  - Acanthosis
  - Downward elongated proliferation of narrow rete ridges that appear detached from epithelium
  - Regular epithelial nests with peripheral palisading
  - Stromal reaction is not prominent
  - Typically associated with papillary SH
- Verrucous
  - Present adjacent to verrucous carcinoma
  - Marked acanthosis with no atypia
  - Hyperkeratosis with hypergranulosis
  - Slight papillomatosis
- Mixed
  - 2nd most common type
  - Presence of mixed areas of flat and papillary SH

DIFFERENTIAL DIAGNOSIS

Differentiated PeIN
- Acanthosis, parakeratosis
- Aberrant keratinization with cytologic atypia
- Retained squamous maturation

Pseudohyperplastic SCC
- SCC-simulating pseudoepitheliomatous hyperplasia
- Minimal cytologic atypia
- Irregular epithelial nests
- Extension into lamina propria and superficial tissues
- Prominent stromal reaction

Verruciform Xanthoma
- Exophytic lesion with acanthosis and hyperkeratosis
- Xanthoma cells (foamy histocytes) in lamina propria

Verruciform SCC
- Includes warty, papillary, and verrucous carcinomas
- Evidence of destructive stromal invasion

SELECTED REFERENCES

1. Epstein JI et al: Tumors of the prostate gland, seminal vesicles, penis, and scrotum. In Atlas of Tumor Pathology, Tumors of The Penis. Washington, D.C.: Armed Forces Institute of Pathology, 2011
2. Velazquez EF et al: Epithelial abnormalities and precancerous lesions of anterior urethra in patients with penile carcinoma: a report of 89 cases. Mod Pathol. 18(7):917-23, 2005
3. Cubilla AL et al: Epithelial lesions associated with invasive penile squamous cell carcinoma: a pathologic study of 288 cases. Int J Surg Pathol. 12(4):351-64, 2004
4. Velazquez EF et al: Lichen sclerosus in 68 patients with squamous cell carcinoma of the penis: frequent atypias and correlation with special carcinoma variants suggests a precancerous role. Am J Surg Pathol. 27(11):1448-53, 2003
5. Cubilla AL et al: Morphological features of epithelial abnormalities and precancerous lesions of the penis. Scand J Urol Nephrol Suppl. (205):215-9, 2000

Squamous Hyperplasia

Schematic Representation and Distribution

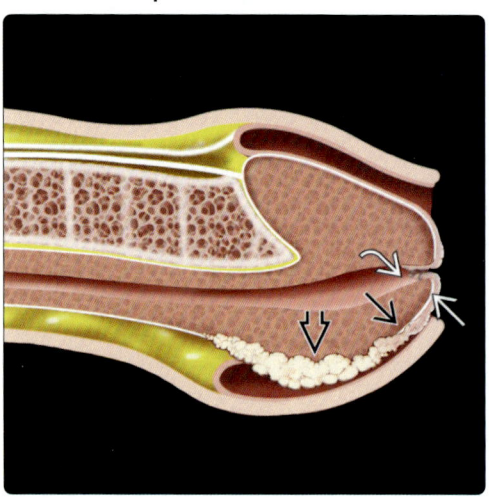

Flat Squamous Hyperplasia

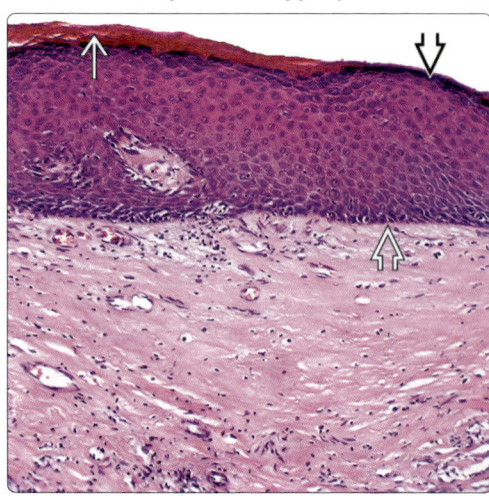

(Left) Squamous hyperplasia, noted as a thickening of the squamous mucosa ⇒, is frequently found in association with either in situ ⇒ or invasive ⇒ penile squamous cell carcinomas and can extend into the distal urethra ⇒. (Right) In flat squamous hyperplasia, the interface between the epithelium and lamina propria is regular and straight ⇒, surface is flat ⇒, acanthosis is prominent, but no cytologic atypia is seen, and hyperkeratosis ⇒ is commonly found.

Base of Lesion

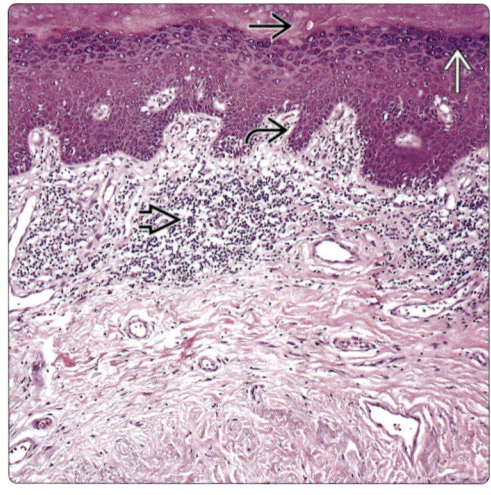

Papillary Squamous Hyperplasia

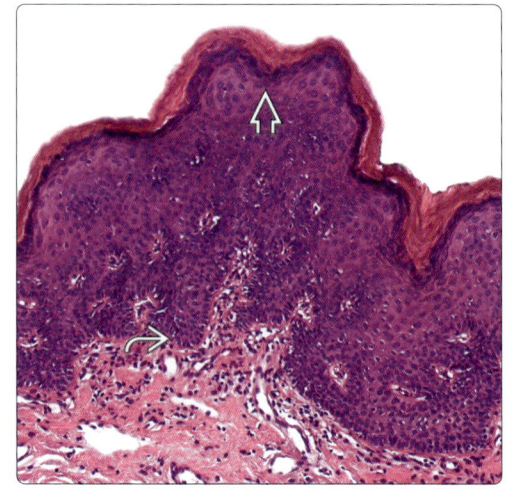

(Left) SH depicts hyperkeratosis ⇒, usually associated with hypergranulosis ⇒, rete ridges ⇒ slightly elongated with regular borders, no evidence of stromal invasion, and a mild-to-moderate chronic inflammatory infiltrate ⇒. (Right) Papillary squamous hyperplasia is shown with short papillae ⇒ and downward (pseudoepitheliomatous) proliferation of rete ridges ⇒, which may be prominent enough to raise the differential diagnosis of SCC.

Associated Lichen Sclerosus

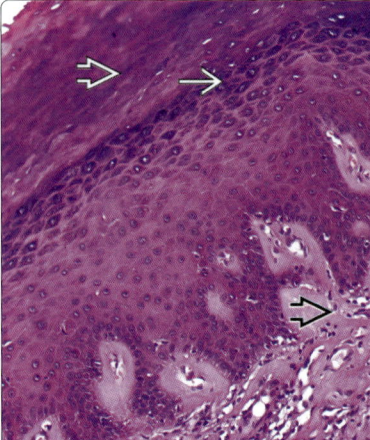

Lichen Sclerosus and Hyperplasia

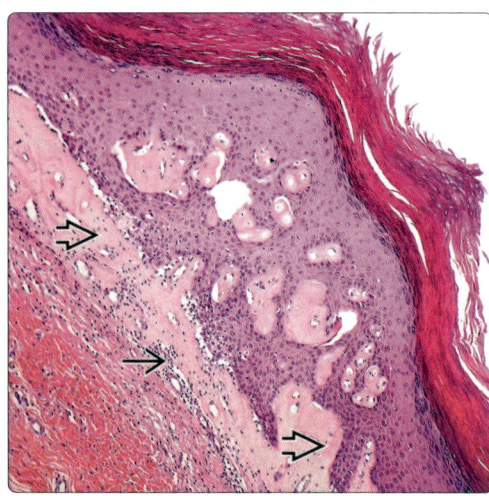

(Left) SH is shown here with prominent orthokeratotic hyperkeratosis ⇒ and hypergranulosis ⇒, retained epithelial maturation with no cytologic atypia, slightly elongated rete ridges ⇒, and changes of lichen sclerosus in the submucosa ⇒ with a mild inflammatory infiltrate. (Right) H&E shows SH associated with lichen sclerosus with evident acanthosis and hyperkeratosis in the epithelium and dense subepithelial sclerosis ⇒ with a band-like chronic inflammatory infiltrate ⇒.

Squamous Hyperplasia

Differentiated Penile Intraepithelial Neoplasia (PeIN)

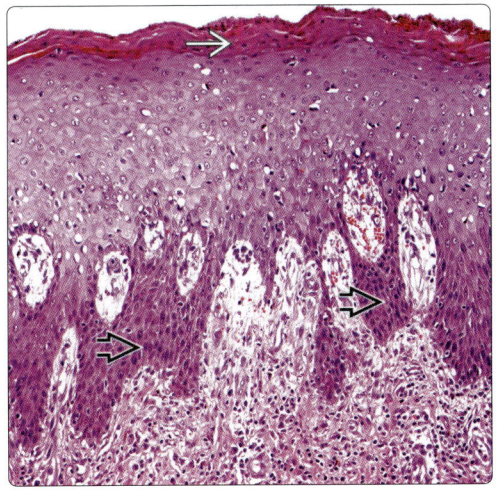

Basaloid PeIN

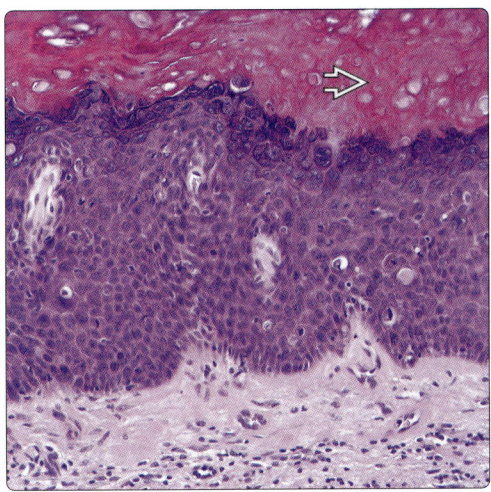

(Left) In differentiated PeIN, cytologic atypia is observed throughout the entire epithelium, although it is more prominent in the basal layer ➡. Parakeratosis ➡ is a common finding. (Right) In basaloid PeIN, the entire epithelium is replaced by a monotonous population of small- to intermediate-sized cells with scant cytoplasm and indistinct cellular borders. Note also a prominent hyperkeratosis ➡. Cytologic atypia distinguishes hyperplasia from all forms of PeIN.

Warty PeIN

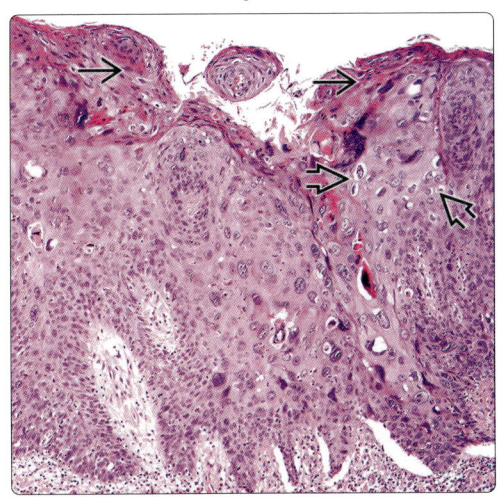

Pseudohyperplastic Carcinoma

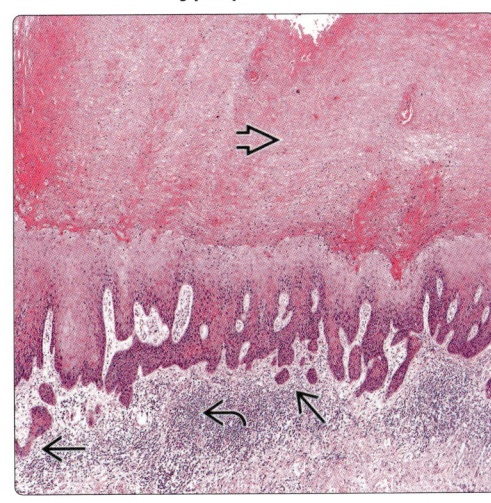

(Left) In warty PeIN, pleomorphic cells are seen throughout the entire epithelium, koilocytes ➡ are easily identified, surface is spiky, and parakeratosis ➡ is common. (Right) In pseudohyperplastic carcinoma there is acanthosis, slight cytological atypia, prominent hyperkeratosis ➡, with irregular infiltrative neoplastic nests ➡ at tumor base extending into the lamina propria, and a moderate stromal reaction ➡.

Verruciform Xanthoma

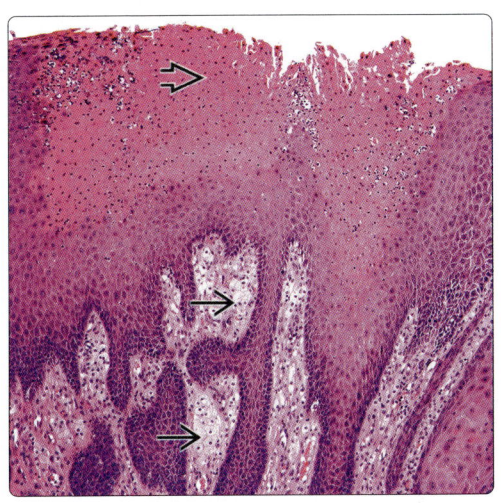

Verruciform Lesion

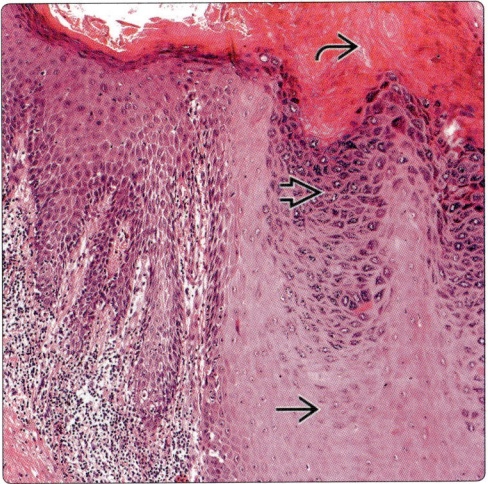

(Left) Verruciform xanthoma is characterized by prominent acanthosis, hyperkeratosis ➡, papillomatosis, absence of cytologic atypia, and foamy cells ➡ present in lamina propria between rete ridges. (Right) Some verruciform lesions showing acanthosis ➡, hypergranulosis ➡, and hyperkeratosis ➡ are sometimes difficult to classify. The differential diagnosis between verrucous SH and verrucous carcinoma is not always possible, especially in superficial biopsies.

Lipogranuloma

KEY FACTS

TERMINOLOGY
- Synonym: Paraffinoma

ETIOLOGY/PATHOGENESIS
- Most frequently secondary to injection of oil-based substances

CLINICAL ISSUES
- Indurated and sometimes tender plaque or tumor
  - Variable size (from few centimeters to massive replacement of genital area)
- Biopsy may be necessary to rule out neoplastic process

MICROSCOPIC
- Numerous lipid vacuoles of variable size embedded in sclerotic stroma
  - At low power, may mimic adipose tumor
  - At higher power, it is more obvious that many vacuoles are within mono- and multinucleated histiocytes
- Mixed-cell inflammatory infiltrate, including histiocytes, multinucleated giant cells, lymphoid cells, and eosinophils
  - Infiltrate may be multinodular or diffuse

ANCILLARY TESTS
- Immunohistochemical studies may be helpful to exclude neoplastic process
  - CD68 and CD163 confirm histiocytic nature of infiltrate
- Sections from frozen tissue showing positive staining with Oil Red O may be helpful

TOP DIFFERENTIAL DIAGNOSES
- Liposarcoma
- Metastatic carcinoma with clear/signet ring cells
- Adenomatoid tumor
- Lymphangioma

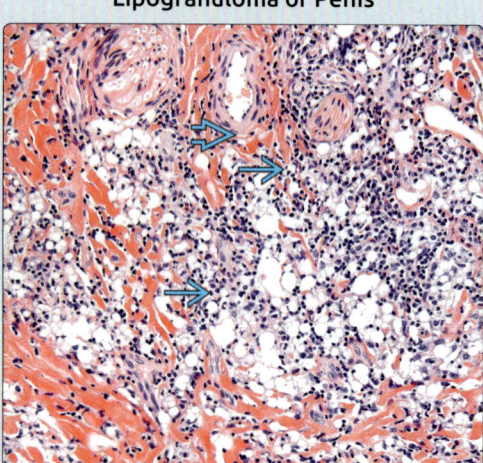

Lipogranuloma of Penis

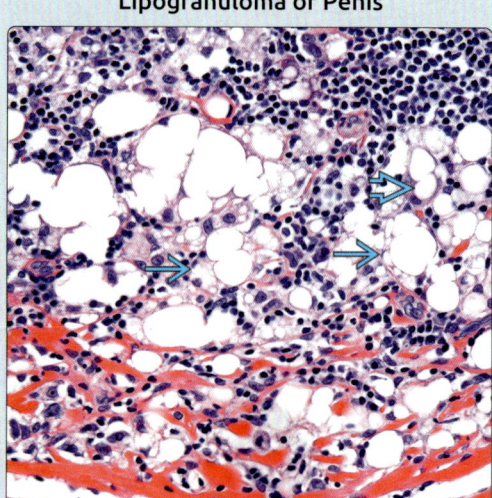

Lipogranuloma of Penis

(Left) Numerous vacuoles of different sizes are dispersed in a sclerotic stroma. Many of these vacuoles are within histiocytes. Some histiocytes are multivacuolated ⇒, and others show a signet ring ⇒ appearance. The lymphocytic-rich inflammatory infiltrate is prominent in this case. (Right) High-power view shows that many of the vacuoles are inside histiocytes. Note the multivacuolated ⇒ and signet ring ⇒ histiocytes. In addition to histiocytes, in this case, the inflammatory response is also rich in lymphocytes.

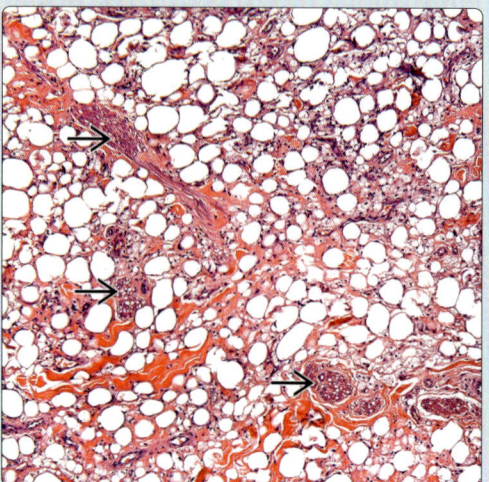

Sclerosing Lipogranuloma of Scrotum

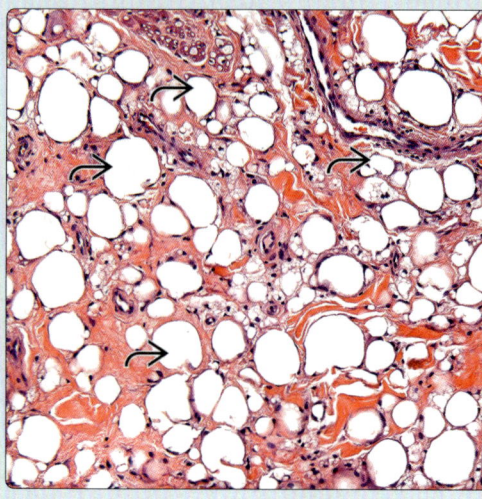

Sclerosing Lipogranuloma of Scrotum

(Left) Numerous lipid vacuoles of different sizes are apparent in the dermis and dartos. Note the dartos smooth muscle bundles ⇒ in the background. (Right) Higher power view shows numerous vacuoles ⇒ of different sizes embedded in a sclerotic stroma. This case shows prominent sclerosis and histiocytic infiltrate with very few lymphocytes.

Lipogranuloma

TERMINOLOGY

Synonyms
- Paraffinoma

Definitions
- Foreign body histiocytic/granulomatous and sclerotic reaction to oil-based substances

ETIOLOGY/PATHOGENESIS

Etiology
- Most cases are secondary to injection of oil-based substances, such as paraffin, silicone, or oil
- Less frequently secondary to topical application of oil-based substances
- Rarely, they may also be related to cold weather or trauma

Pathogenesis
- T-cell-mediated immune reaction appears to be important in its pathogenesis

CLINICAL ISSUES

Epidemiology
- Age
  - Usually patients younger than 40 years old

Site
- May affect penis &/or scrotum

Presentation
- Indurated and sometimes tender plaque or mass that varies in size from few centimeters to massive replacement of genital area
- Biopsy is necessary to exclude neoplasm, especially if there is no history of injection of exogenous material

MACROSCOPIC

General Features
- Specimen usually consists of firm, yellow to gray-white pieces of tissue with solid or multicystic appearance

MICROSCOPIC

Histologic Features
- Numerous lipid vacuoles of variable size embedded in sclerotic stroma
- Infiltrate of foamy histiocytes admixed with variable number of multinucleate giant cells
- Lymphoid cells and eosinophils are usually present
- Inflammatory infiltrate may be nodular or interspersed in sclerotic stroma
- Inflammatory infiltrate varies from mild to marked
- If necessary, sections from frozen tissue showing positive staining with Oil Red O may be helpful

Predominant Pattern/Injury Type
- Sclerotic and vacuolar

Predominant Cell/Compartment Type
- Hematopoietic, histiocytic

ANCILLARY TESTS

Immunohistochemistry
- Immunohistochemical studies have shown expression of lysozyme, α-1-antitrypsin, α-1-antichymotrypsin, CD68, and CD163 by multinucleated giant cells and epithelioid histiocytes
- Most of lymphocytes infiltrating lesions are CD3(+) T cells associated with some S100(+) dendritic cells

DIFFERENTIAL DIAGNOSIS

Liposarcoma
- Lobulated, bulky neoplasm in paratesticular soft tissue
- Well-differentiated or sclerosing type
- Presence of bizarre atypical cells
- If present, identification of lipoblasts may be helpful
- Absence of foreign body giant cell reaction and foamy histiocytes

Metastatic Carcinoma With Signet Ring or Clear Cell Changes
- Immunohistochemistry for keratin is positive in carcinoma and negative in lipogranuloma
- Atypical nuclei indented by intracytoplasmic mucin

Adenomatoid Tumor
- Benign mesothelial tumor
- Characterized by cystic and slit-like spaces lined by flattened or cuboidal cells
- Immunohistochemistry shows positivity with keratin and calretinin

Lymphangioma
- Benign proliferation of dilated lymphatic vessels
- If necessary, vascular markers (CD31) may help to clarify diagnosis

DIAGNOSTIC CHECKLIST

Clinically Relevant Pathologic Features
- Clinical correlation with injection of exogenous material is important to confirm diagnosis

Pathologic Interpretation Pearls
- Numerous vacuoles of different sizes in dermis/lamina propria and dartos
- At low power, they resemble adipose cells or lipoblasts
- Intimately associated at higher power; many are within histiocytes and multinucleated giant cells
- Sclerotic background with variable numbers of lymphoid cells and eosinophils
- Diagnosis usually not difficult, especially when there is good clinical history

SELECTED REFERENCES

1. Francis J et al: Ultrasound and MRI features of penile augmentation by "Jamaica Oil" injection. A case series. Med Ultrason. 16(4):372-6, 2014
2. Ohtsuki Y et al: Three cases of sclerosing lipogranuloma: an immunohistochemical study. Med Mol Morphol. 40(2):108-11, 2007
3. Watanabe K et al: Immunohistochemical profile of primary sclerosing lipogranuloma of the scrotum: report of five cases. Pathol Int. 45(11):854-9, 1995
4. Oertel YC et al: Sclerosing lipogranuloma of male genitalia. Review of 23 cases. Arch Pathol Lab Med. 101(6):321-6, 1977

Scrotal Calcinosis

KEY FACTS

ETIOLOGY/PATHOGENESIS
- Formerly considered idiopathic process
- Most cases represent ruptured and calcified cysts with eventual destruction of cyst wall

CLINICAL ISSUES
- Multiple hard calcified nodules on skin of scrotum
- Usually affects children and young adults

MACROSCOPIC
- Cut surface shows hard, white calcified deposits in dermis and dartos

MICROSCOPIC
- Basophilic granular and globular deposits
  - In dermis and upper part of dartos
- Usually surrounded by palisading histiocytes and multinucleated giant cells
- Remnants of preexisting cystic lesion or adnexal neoplasm may be identified

ANCILLARY TESTS
- Calcified material is positive with von Kossa stain

TOP DIFFERENTIAL DIAGNOSES
- Scrotal calcinosis has very distinctive appearance
  - Almost no histologic differential diagnosis
- Amyloidosis
  - Homogeneous and eosinophilic material
  - Positive with Congo red and crystal violet
  - Thioflavin T shows positive fluorescence
  - Negative with von Kossa

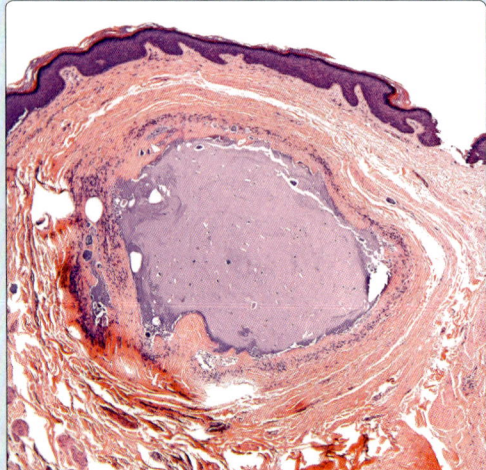
Scrotal Calcinosis

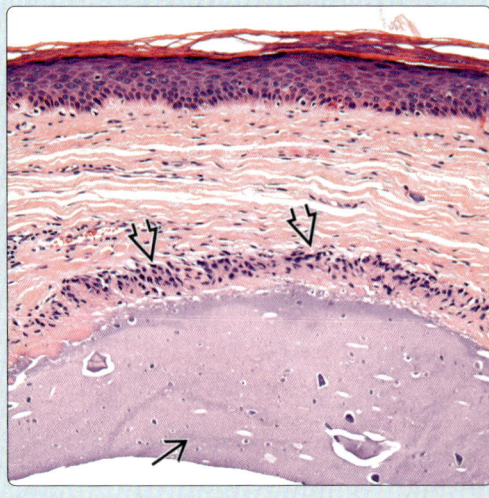
Scrotal Calcinosis

(Left) Large nodular aggregate of basophilic calcified material is seen in the dermis and dartos. (Right) Underneath a normal epidermis, there is a nodular basophilic homogeneous deposit ➡ surrounded by palisading histiocytic response ➡.

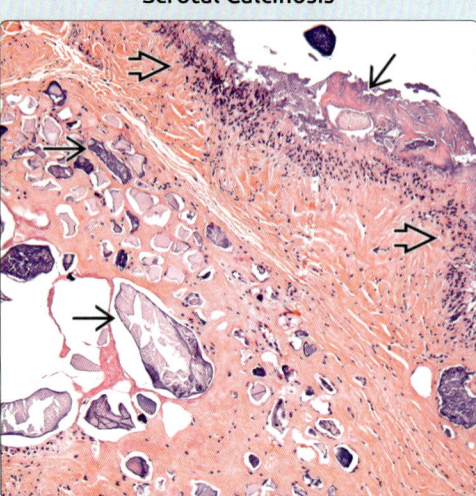
Scrotal Calcinosis

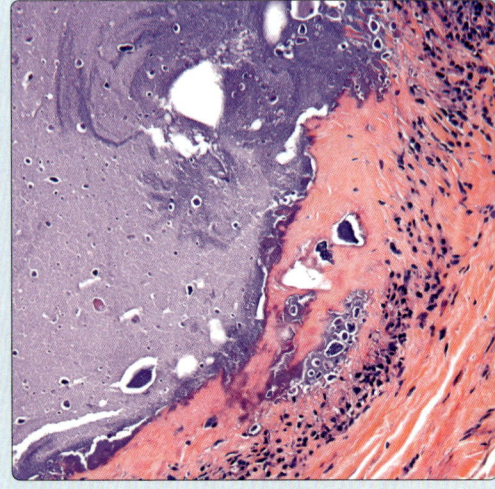
Scrotal Calcinosis

(Left) Homogeneous granular and globular pink and purple material ➡ is seen within the dermis admixed with sclerosis and palisading histiocytic inflammation ➡. (Right) Higher power view of the purple deposits of calcified material surrounded by a granulomatous response.

Scrotal Calcinosis

TERMINOLOGY

Synonyms
- Idiopathic calcinosis of scrotum

Definitions
- Benign, uncommon condition characterized by presence of single or multiple calcified nodules in scrotal skin

ETIOLOGY/PATHOGENESIS

Etiology
- Originally considered idiopathic condition
- Now accepted that majority of cases develop from dystrophic calcification of cyst contents

CLINICAL ISSUES

Epidemiology
- Incidence
  - Uncommon
- Age
  - Children and young adults

Site
- Scrotal skin

Presentation
- Single or multiple hard, marble-like nodules of varying size affecting scrotal skin
- Nodules vary in size from a few millimeters to a few centimeters
- Usually start to appear in childhood or early adult life
- Over time, nodules increase in number and size
- Nodules may break down and discharge chalky material
- Rarely, lesions may be polypoid
- Usually asymptomatic

Treatment
- Symptomatic single or grouped nodules can be excised surgically

Prognosis
- Benign condition
- Slow progression throughout life
- Lesions remain discrete and do not become confluent

IMAGING

Radiographic Findings
- Radiologic studies show calcified nodules

MICROSCOPIC

Histologic Features
- Granular and globular deposition of basophilic calcified material
- Histiocytic/giant cell granulomatous inflammatory response may be associated with deposits
- Process is located within dermis and may extend to dartos
- Early lesions start out as cysts, but they lose their cyst walls as they age and calcify
- Histologic remnants of preexisting epidermoid cyst or, even more rarely, partially cystic adnexal tumor (e.g., syringoma) may be identified
- Calcified material is positive with Von Kossa stain though staining is rarely necessary

Predominant Pattern/Injury Type
- Calcification

Predominant Cell/Compartment Type
- Dermis

DIFFERENTIAL DIAGNOSIS

Nodular Amyloidosis
- Eosinophilic (noncalcified) nodular deposits within dermis
- Usually associated with plasma cell-rich infiltrate
- Foreign body giant cell reaction may be present
- Amyloid deposits are positive for crystal violet and Congo red stains
  - Green birefringence under polarized light when stained with Congo red
- Positive fluorescence with thioflavin T
- von Kossa negative

DIAGNOSTIC CHECKLIST

Clinically Relevant Pathologic Features
- Lesions slowly progress throughout life
  - They slowly increase in number and size
- Nodules are mobile and do not attach to underlying structures

Pathologic Interpretation Pearls
- Globular and granular purple deposits within dermis surrounded by giant cell granulomatous reaction
- Sometimes remnants of cystic lesion can be identified
- Very distinctive appearance with almost no histologic differential diagnosis

SELECTED REFERENCES

1. Solanki A et al: Scrotal calcinosis: pathogenetic link with epidermal cyst. BMJ Case Rep. 2015, 2015
2. Gi N et al: Idiopathic scrotal calcinosis - a pedunculated rare variant. J Plast Reconstr Aesthet Surg. 61(4):466-7, 2008
3. Shah V et al: Scrotal calcinosis results from calcification of cysts derived from hair follicles: a series of 20 cases evaluating the spectrum of changes resulting in scrotal calcinosis. Am J Dermatopathol. 29(2):172-5, 2007
4. Ito A et al: Dystrophic scrotal calcinosis originating from benign eccrine epithelial cysts. Br J Dermatol. 144(1):146-50, 2001
5. Saad AG et al: Scrotal calcinosis: is it idiopathic? Urology. 57(2):365, 2001
6. Dini M et al: Should scrotal calcinosis still be termed idiopathic? Am J Dermatopathol. 20(4):399-402, 1998
7. Polk P et al: Polypoid scrotal calcinosis: an uncommon variant of scrotal calcinosis. South Med J. 89(9):896-7, 1996
8. Dave AJ: Scrotal calcinosis. J Am Acad Dermatol. 23(1):150-1, 1990
9. Song DH et al: Idiopathic calcinosis of the scrotum: histopathologic observations of fifty-one nodules. J Am Acad Dermatol. 19(6):1095-101, 1988
10. Moskovitz B et al: Idiopathic calcinosis of scrotum. Eur Urol. 13(1-2):130-1, 1987
11. Sarma DP et al: Scrotal calcinosis: calcification of epidermal cysts. J Surg Oncol. 27(2):76-9, 1984
12. Bhawan J et al: The so-called idiopathic scrotal calcinosis. Arch Dermatol. 119(9):709, 1983

Penile Intraepithelial Neoplasia

KEY FACTS

TERMINOLOGY

- Differentiated (simplex) penile intraepithelial neoplasia (PeIN) (HPV unrelated)
- Warty/basaloid PeIN (HPV related)
  - LAST Project recommends 2-tiered nomenclature system for HPV-related anogenital precancerous lesions
    - Low-grade squamous intraepithelial lesion (LGSIL)
    - High-grade squamous intraepithelial lesion (HGSIL)
      - Applies to all anogenital areas (further categorized with -IN)
      - In penis, further categorized as PeIN
    - Recommendations refer only to HPV-related precancerous conditions

MICROSCOPIC

- Differentiated (simplex) PeIN
  - Elongated and anastomosing rete ridges
  - Atypical basal cells with hyperchromatic nuclei
  - Subtle abnormal maturation (enlarged keratinocytes with abundant eosinophilic cytoplasm)
  - Whorling and keratin pearl formation
  - Usually associated with lichen sclerosus
- Basaloid PeIN
  - Basaloid cells replace most to full thickness of epithelium
  - Prominent apoptosis and mitosis
- Warty PeIN
  - Epithelium is replaced by pleomorphic cells with koilocytic changes (multinucleation, nuclei with irregular contours, perinuclear halo and dyskeratosis)
  - Undulated/spiky surface
  - Atypical parakeratosis
  - Numerous mitoses
- Warty-basaloid PeIN
  - Pleomorphic cells with koilocytic changes seen on upper epidermis
  - Basaloid cells replace lower epidermis
  - Usually undulated/spiky surface

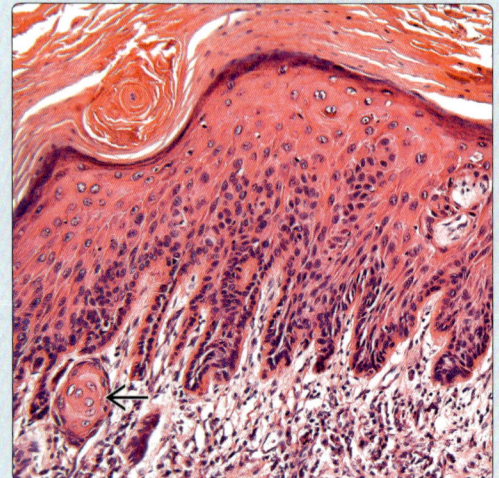

Differentiated Penile Intraepithelial Neoplasia

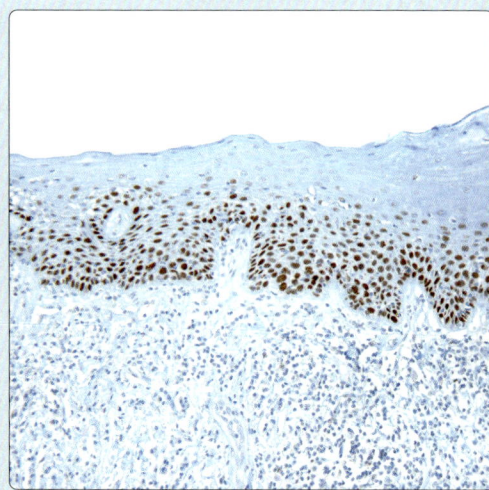

p53 in Differentiated Penile Intraepithelial Neoplasia

(Left) Note the elongated rete ridges and atypical basilar cells. There is mild spongiosis with abnormal maturation ➡, keratin pearl formation (usually in deep rete ridges), and parakeratosis. (Right) Differentiated penile intraepithelial neoplasia (PeIN) shows suprabasilar extension of p53 nuclear positivity.

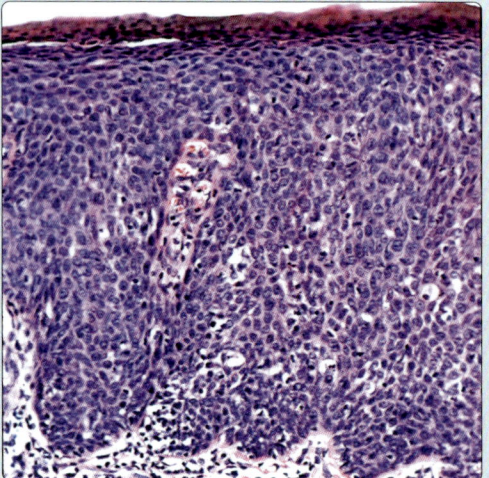

Basaloid Penile Intraepithelial Neoplasia

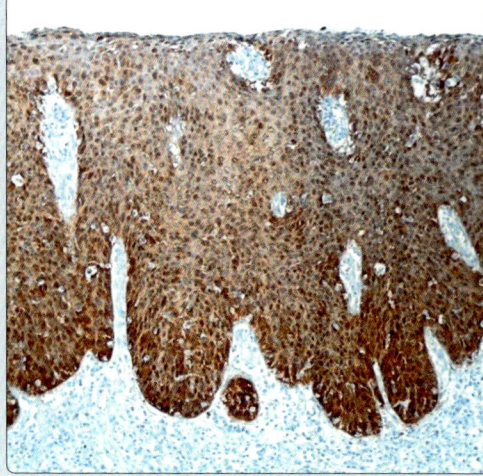

p16 Block Positivity in Basaloid Penile Intraepithelial Neoplasia

(Left) Proliferation of small round cells with high nuclear:cytoplasmic ratios and hyperchromatic nuclei replacing the entire thickness of the epithelium is seen in this case of basaloid PeIN. (Right) For p16 interpretation, block positivity (strong diffuse nuclear or nuclear and cytoplasmic staining of the basal layer with extension upward involving at least 1/3 the epithelial thickness) is considered positive. Any lesser staining should be considered p16 negative.

Penile Intraepithelial Neoplasia

TERMINOLOGY

Abbreviations
- Penile intraepithelial neoplasia (PeIN)

Synonyms
- Squamous cell carcinoma in situ (SCCIS), squamous intraepithelial lesion (SIL), erythroplasia of Queyrat, Bowen disease

Definitions
- PeIN is considered intraepithelial (in situ) precursor lesion of invasive squamous cell carcinoma (SCC)

ETIOLOGY/PATHOGENESIS

Pathogenesis
- Basaloid, warty and warty/basaloid PeIN are HPV related (especially HPV-16)
- Differentiated (simplex) PeIN is unrelated to HPV
- Lichen sclerosus may be implicated in pathogenesis of differentiated PeIN

CLINICAL ISSUES

Epidemiology
- Incidence
  - Real incidence is unknown
  - 2/3 associated with invasive SCC
  - When invasive SCC is associated with PeIN, 65% are differentiated PeIN and 35% are warty/basaloid PeIN
- Age
  - 4th and 6th decades

Presentation
- Differentiated PeIN
  - Older patients, frequently affects foreskin
  - Usually arises in setting of chronic scarring, inflammatory dermatosis, especially lichen sclerosus
- Warty/basaloid PeIN
  - Younger patients; usually affects glans, perimeatal region
  - Not associated with lichen sclerosus
  - May be associated with condyloma

Prognosis
- Unknown: Most studies are retrospective

MACROSCOPIC

General Features
- Heterogeneous gross appearance
  - Does not allow distinction between different types
- Unifocal (85%) or multifocal (15%)
- Flat to slightly elevated hyperkeratotic or even papillary lesions
- Sharp or ill-defined borders
- Pearly white, moist, erythematous, dark brown/black
- Macules, papules, or plaques
- Differentiated PeIN often arises in lichen sclerosus

MICROSCOPIC

Histologic Features
- Differentiated (simplex) PeIN (HPV unrelated)
  - Thickened epithelium
  - Elongated and anastomosing rete ridges
  - Atypical basal cells with hyperchromatic nuclei
  - Subtle abnormal maturation
  - Whorling and keratin pearl formation
  - Parakeratosis is frequent, absent koilocytosis
  - Usually associated with lichen sclerosus
  - Association with HPV-unrelated variants of invasive SCC
  - Pleomorphic variant of differentiated PeIN may exist
    - Exceptional and needs further characterization
  - Prominent intercellular bridges (spongiosis and sometimes acanthosis)
- HPV related
  - Warty PeIN (Bowenoid)
    - Undulating/spiky surface
    - Epithelium is replaced by pleomorphic cells with koilocytic changes
    - Numerous mitoses
  - Basaloid PeIN (undifferentiated)
    - Epithelium replaced by monotonous population of small immature cells with high nuclear:cytoplasmic ratios
    - Apoptosis and mitotic figures are numerous
  - Mixed PeIN (warty-basaloid)
    - Combined features of basaloid and warty types of PeIN
    - Lower part of epithelium is replaced by small basaloid cells
    - Upper portion of epithelium shows features of warty PeIN
    - Mitosis and apoptosis are prominent
  - Other less frequent variants: Pagetoid, clear cell, spindle cell
    - Exceptional
    - Most cases appear to be HPV related
    - Need further studies
  - Warty/basaloid PeIN is usually seen adjacent to HPV-related variants of invasive SCC

ANCILLARY TESTS

Immunohistochemistry
- PeIN basaloid/warty
  - Strong/diffuse block p16 positivity
    - Block p16 positivity supports presence of high-risk HPV
    - Block p16 positivity supports diagnosis of HPV-related precancerous lesion
  - Ki-67 suprabasal extension
  - p53 usually noncontributory
- Differentiated PeIN
  - Negative or non-block expression of p16
    - Negative or non-block p16 positivity may also be seen in
      - Non-precancerous reactive conditions (e.g. lichen simplex chronicus)

Penile Intraepithelial Neoplasia

Penile Intraepithelial Neoplasia

Characteristics	Differentiated PeIN	Warty/Basaloid PeIN
Location	Foreskin	Glans
Color	White	Red
Multifocality	Sometimes	Often
HPV related	No	Yes
p16	Negative	Positive
Association to lichen sclerosus	Yes	No
Associated invasive SCC	Usual/keratinizing, verrucous, pseudohyperplastic, papillary, sarcomatoid SCC	Warty, basaloid, mixed warty-basaloid SCC

- Ki-67 suprabasal extension
- p53 variable
  - Usually overexpression (suprabasal extension)
  - Sometimes absent (total lack of expression)
  - Sometimes basilar
- No good marker for differentiated PeIN

In Situ Hybridization

- Warty/basaloid PeIN
  - Usually positive for high-risk HPV
  - Negative for low-risk HPV
- Differentiated PeIN
  - Negative for low-risk and high-risk HPV

PCR

- Can be helpful to show association of warty/basaloid PeIN with high-risk HPV

DIFFERENTIAL DIAGNOSIS

Differentiated Penile Intraepithelial Neoplasia

- Squamous hyperplasia/lichen simplex chronicus
  - Reactive condition
  - None to minimal basilar atypia
  - Negative for HPV
  - Usually basilar expression of p53

Warty/Basaloid Penile Intraepithelial Neoplasia

- Condyloma
  - Koilocytosis confined to upper epithelium
  - Absence of nuclear pleomorphism
  - Mitoses are scant and confined to lower epithelium
    - Treated condylomas may show an increase in mitotic figures
- Bowenoid papulosis
  - Indistinguishable from warty/basaloid PeIN on histology alone
    - Usually associated to HPV-16
  - Clinical correlation is essential for this diagnosis
    - Younger patients
    - Small and multiple lesions
    - May regress spontaneously

DIAGNOSTIC CHECKLIST

Pathologic Interpretation Pearls

- Differentiated PeIN
  - At low power, atypia seems to be present only in lower levels of epidermis
  - At higher power, more clear that there is subtle but abnormal maturation in all levels of epithelium
- p16 can be helpful to support diagnosis of warty/basaloid PeIN
  - Only block diffuse p16 staining of epithelium should be interpreted as positive
- Negative result or non-block p16 positivity does not exclude precancerous condition
  - Differentiated PeIN shows p16 negativity or patchy weak staining

SELECTED REFERENCES

1. Amin A et al: Penile intraepithelial neoplasia with pagetoid features: report of an unusual variant mimicking Paget disease. Hum Pathol. 45(4):889-92, 2014
2. Darragh TM et al: The Lower Anogenital Squamous Terminology Standardization project for HPV-associated lesions: background and consensus recommendations from the College of American Pathologists and the American Society for Colposcopy and Cervical Pathology. Int J Gynecol Pathol. 32(1):76-115, 2013
3. Chaux A et al: Distribution and characterization of subtypes of penile intraepithelial neoplasia and their association with invasive carcinomas: a pathological study of 139 lesions in 121 patients. Hum Pathol. 43(7):1020-7, 2012
4. Velazquez EF et al: Histologic classification of penile intraepithelial neoplasia. Semin Diagn Pathol. 29(2):96-102, 2012
5. Chaux A et al: Distinctive immunohistochemical profile of penile intraepithelial lesions: a study of 74 cases. Am J Surg Pathol. 35(4):553-62, 2011
6. Oertell J et al: Differentiated precursor lesions and low-grade variants of squamous cell carcinomas are frequent findings in foreskins of patients from a region of high penile cancer incidence. Histopathology. 58(6):925-33, 2011
7. ABELL MR et al: Intraepithelial and infiltrative carcinoma of vulva: Bowen's type. Cancer. 14:318-29, 1961

Penile Intraepithelial Neoplasia

Differentiated Penile Intraepithelial Neoplasia

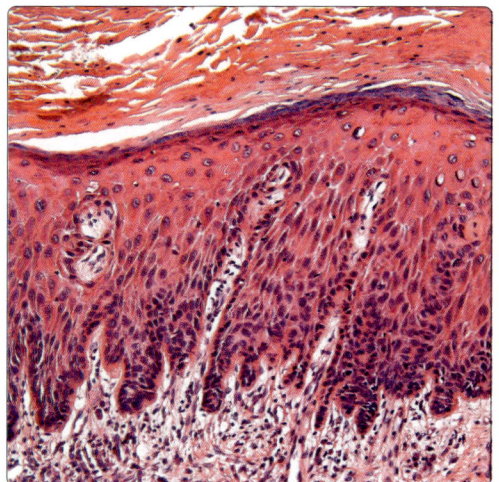

Differentiated Penile Intraepithelial Neoplasia

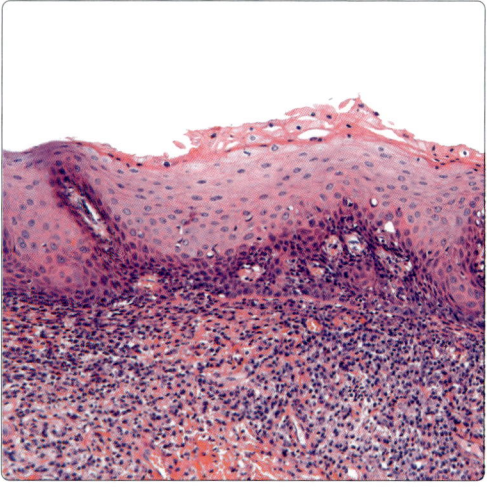

(Left) Acanthotic epithelium with subtle abnormal maturation and hyperchromatic atypical basilar cells are features of differentiated PeIN. Parakeratosis is seen on the surface. *(Right)* There are enlarged keratinocytes with plump vesicular nuclei and abundant eosinophilic cytoplasm. Atypia in the basilar/parabasal layer is easily recognized. Parakeratosis is seen on the surface.

Differentiated Penile Intraepithelial Neoplasia and Lichen Sclerosus

Differentiated Penile Intraepithelial Neoplasia and Lichen Sclerosus

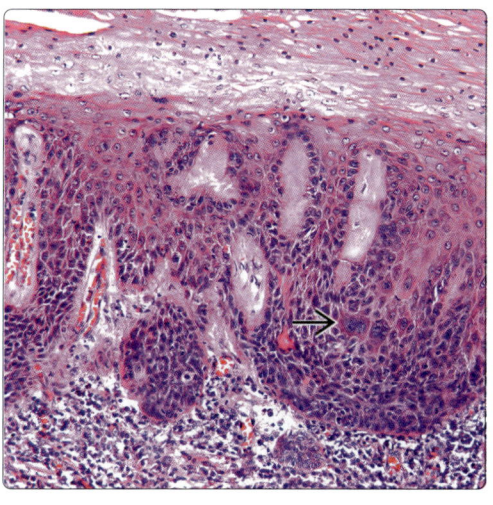

(Left) There is a markedly thickened epithelium with atypical basal and parabasal cells in this example of differentiated PeIN arising in a background of lichen sclerosus. *(Right)* The abnormal maturation is easily appreciated in this example. Some of the cells show marked atypia ➡. There is also a thickened basement membrane and hyalinization of the upper lamina propria corresponding to associated lichen sclerosus.

Differentiated Penile Intraepithelial Neoplasia and Squamous Cell Carcinoma

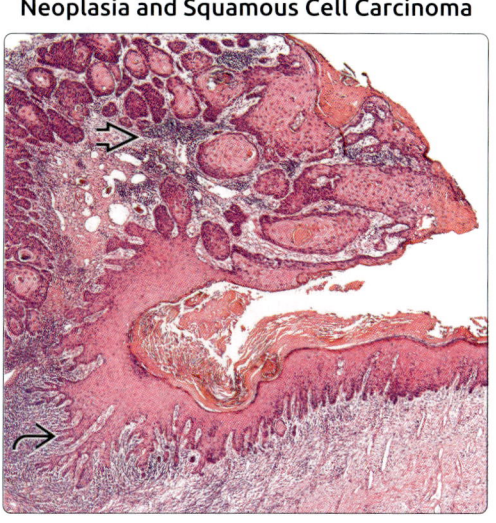

Differentiated Penile Intraepithelial Neoplasia and Squamous Cell Carcinoma

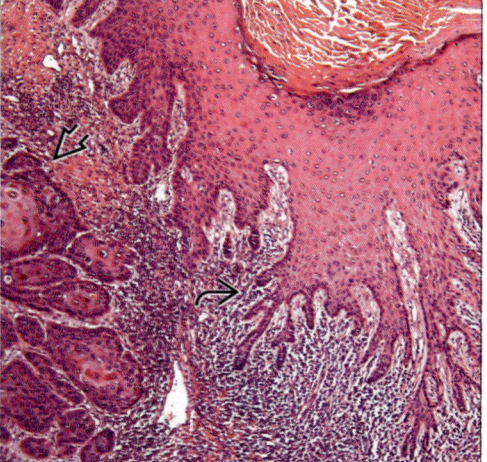

(Left) Differentiated PeIN ➡ is seen adjacent to an invasive SCC ➡. Note the characteristic elongation of the rete ridges and basilar hyperchromasia. In spite of the apparently subtle cytologic changes, juxtaposition to carcinoma argues for its premalignant potential. *(Right)* Differentiated PeIN ➡ is shown adjacent to an invasive squamous cell carcinoma (SCC) ➡. Note the elongation of the rete ridges and subtle abnormal maturation of the epithelium. Cytologic atypia is minimal.

Penile Intraepithelial Neoplasia

Warty Penile Intraepithelial Neoplasia

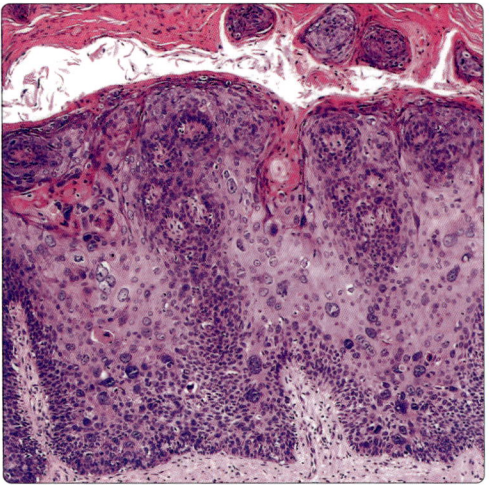

Warty-Basaloid Penile Intraepithelial Neoplasia

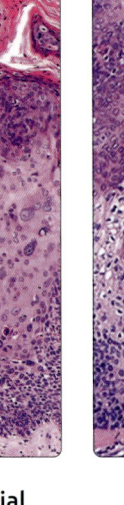

(Left) The epithelium is replaced by large pleomorphic and hyperchromatic nuclei in this example of warty PeIN. Irregular nuclear contours, bi- and multinucleation, and numerous mitoses are easily identified. (Right) There is full-thickness replacement of the epidermis by atypical cells. The lower part of the epidermis is replaced by small basaloid cells, and the upper part is replaced by larger cells showing koilocytotic changes. These features characterize PeIN of warty-basaloid type.

Warty-Basaloid Penile Intraepithelial Neoplasia

Basaloid Penile Intraepithelial Neoplasia

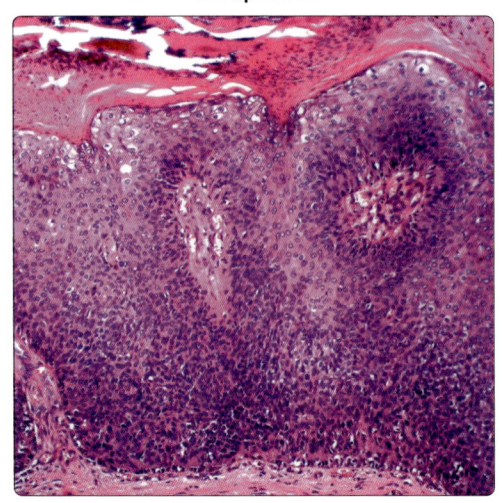

(Left) Spiky surface shows parakeratosis and atypical koilocytosis. The lower half of the epithelium shows basaloid cells. (Right) The epithelium is completely replaced by atypical cells with basaloid features. Numerous mitoses and apoptotic bodies are seen. The diagnosis of carcinoma in situ is easily achieved in high-grade basaloid PeIN.

Basaloid Penile Intraepithelial Neoplasia

p16 in Basaloid Penile Intraepithelial Neoplasia

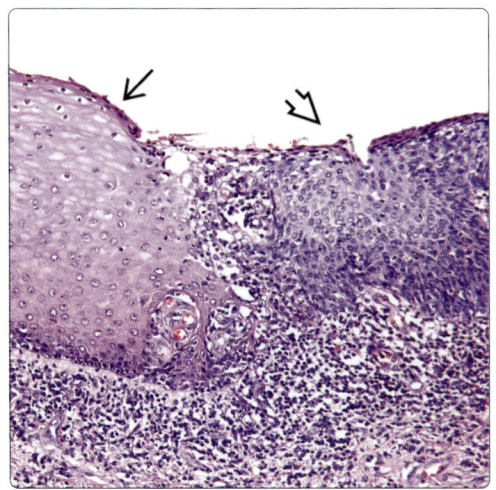
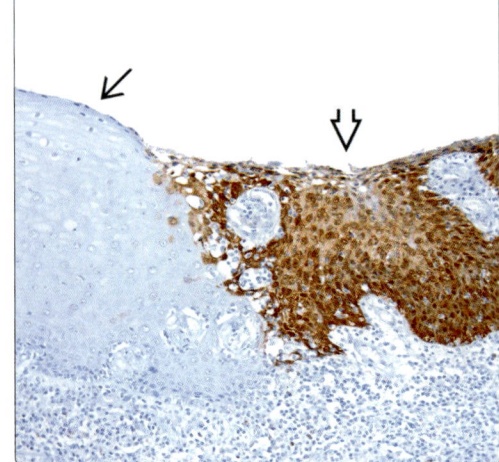

(Left) This picture illustrates a sharp demarcation between the basaloid PeIN ⇨ and hyperplastic squamous epithelium ⇨. (Right) Immunohistochemistry with p16 (surrogate marker for oncogenic HPV) is strongly positive in the area of basaloid PeIN ⇨. The hyperplastic epithelium is negative ⇨.

Penile Intraepithelial Neoplasia

Basaloid Penile Intraepithelial Neoplasia

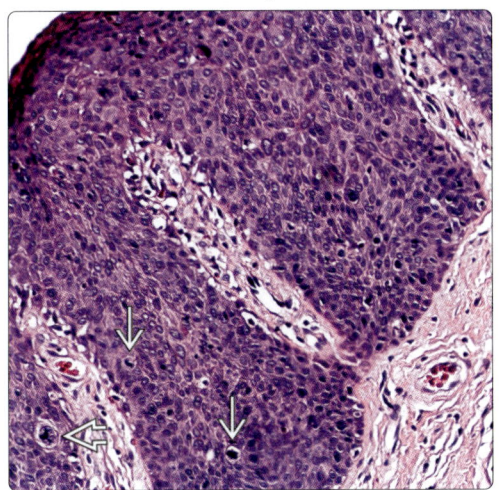

Warty Penile Intraepithelial Neoplasia

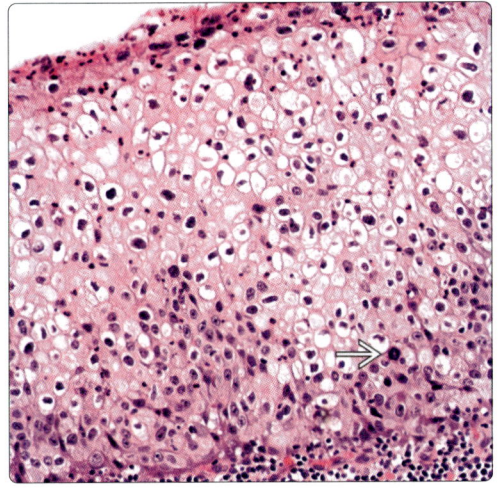

(Left) Uniform basaloid cells with atypia and numerous mitoses ➡, some of them atypical mitoses ➡, fill the epithelial lining. Parakeratosis is seen in the upper left corner. (Right) Clear cells with marked koilocytosis are replacing the full thickness of the epithelium. Note the wrinkled hyperchromatic nuclei. Some mitoses are presented mostly in the base of the lesion ➡.

Differentiated Penile Intraepithelial Neoplasia

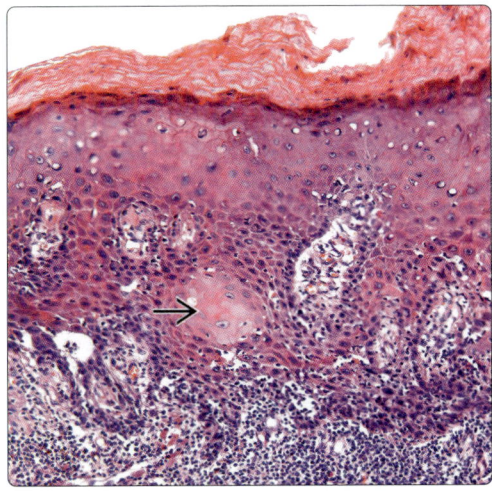

Differentiated Penile Intraepithelial Neoplasia and Lichen Sclerosus

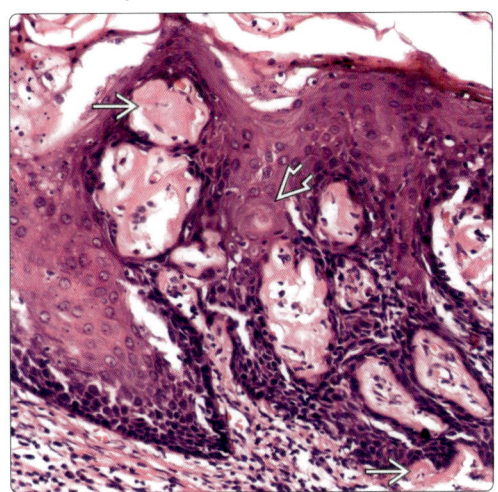

(Left) Note the enlarged keratinocytes with abundant eosinophilic cytoplasm throughout most of the epithelium in differentiated PeIN. Characteristic keratin pearl formation is present ➡. (Right) Hyperkeratosis, parakeratosis, and lichen sclerosus ➡ are common findings associated to differentiated PeIN. Note keratin pearl formation ➡ and atypia in the basal and parabasal layers.

Differentiated Penile Intraepithelial Neoplasia With Lichen Sclerosus

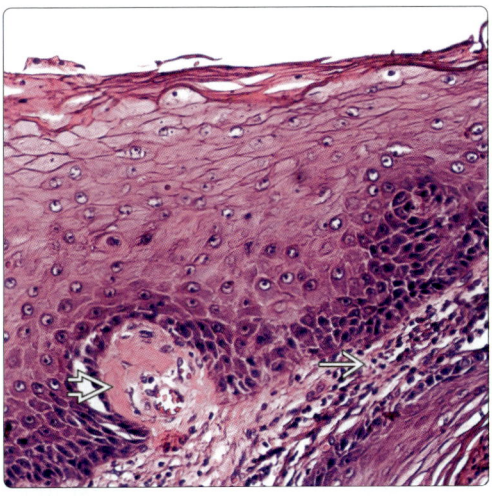

Squamous Hyperplasia and Lichen Sclerosus

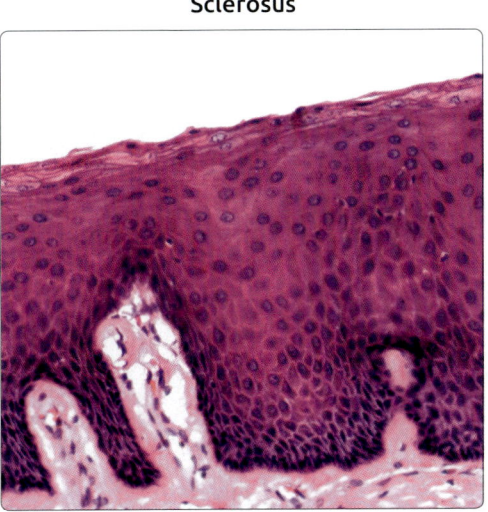

(Left) Hyperplasia of the squamous epithelium with atypia in the basal layer is diagnostic of this lesion. Chronic inflammatory infiltrate ➡ in the underlying stroma and lichen sclerosus ➡ are often associated with differentiated PeIN. (Right) Differential diagnosis of the low-grade differentiated PeIN with squamous hyperplasia could be challenging since both lesions have rise of epithelial thickness and they are often associated with lichen sclerosus, but as in this case squamous hyperplasia lacks of atypia and mitoses.

General Concepts, Squamous Cell Carcinoma

TERMINOLOGY

Abbreviations
- Squamous cell carcinoma (SCC)

Definitions
- Malignant epithelial neoplasia showing keratinocytic differentiation

ANATOMY AND HISTOLOGY

Anatomical Considerations
- Penile anatomical regions are glans, foreskin, and shaft
- Glans is cone-shaped, distal, and formed mainly by corpus spongiosum (CS) covered by squamous mucosa
  - Distal urethra open up into meatus, ventrally located slit-like orifice in glans
  - Glans corona separates glans from coronal sulcus
- Coronal sulcus is cul-de-sac between glans and foreskin
- Foreskin covers glans and presents mucosal (inner) and cutaneous (outer) surface
  - Frenulum connects foreskin to ventral portion of glans corona
- Penile shaft is composed mainly by ventral column of CS and 2 dorsal columns of corpora cavernosa (CC)
- Penile root anchors penis to perineal membrane and pubic arc

Histological Features
- Glans, coronal sulcus, and inner foreskin are covered by nonkeratinized squamous epithelium overlying loose lamina propria
- In glans, microscopic layers are lamina propria, CS, and CC
- In foreskin layers are lamina propria, dartos, and skin
- Vascular spaces of CS are more widely spaced and irregular when compared with CC
- CC presents more densely packed vascular spaces with less intervening stroma
- Tunica albuginea is composed of dense connective tissue and separates CS from CC
- Outer foreskin and shaft are covered by skin
- Bundles of dartos muscle extend underneath dermis throughout shaft and foreskin

EPIDEMIOLOGY

Age Range
- Most frequent in 6th-7th decades
- Average age: 60 years

Incidence
- SCC represents most common malignant tumor of penis
- Wide range of geographical variation
  - Low incidence in USA and Europe
  - High incidence in South America, Africa, and Asia

Natural History
- Local invasion of penile anatomical levels
- Extension to adjacent tissues
  - Scrotum, perineum, prostate
- Metastasis to inguinal lymph nodes
  - Sentinel node(s), superficial and deep nodes
- Metastasis to pelvic lymph nodes
- Systemic dissemination (nonregional lymph nodes, visceral, and bone involvement)
- Liver is most common site of metastatic dissemination followed by lungs and heart
- Systemic dissemination presents in up to 1/3 of patients in high-risk regions

ETIOLOGY/PATHOGENESIS

Human Papillomavirus Related
- 30-60% of all SCC are human papillomavirus (HPV) related
- High-risk HPV predominates
  - HPV-16 is most common genotype encountered
  - HPV-18 is 2nd most common type
  - Other reported genotypes include 45, 52, and 74
- Low-risk HPV infection is uncommon
  - Low-risk HPV reported are genotypes 6 and 11
- Striking correlation of HPV presence and tumor morphology

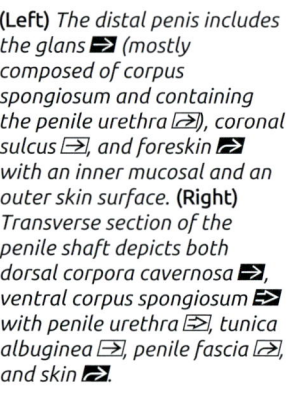

(Left) The distal penis includes the glans ➡ (mostly composed of corpus spongiosum and containing the penile urethra ➡), coronal sulcus ➡, and foreskin ➡ with an inner mucosal and an outer skin surface. (Right) Transverse section of the penile shaft depicts both dorsal corpora cavernosa ➡, ventral corpus spongiosum ➡ with penile urethra ➡, tunica albuginea ➡, penile fascia ➡, and skin ➡.

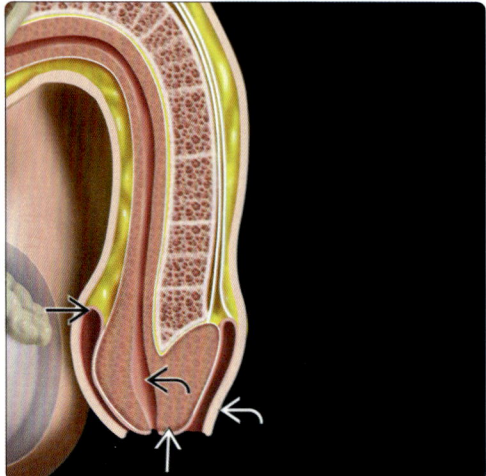

Anatomy

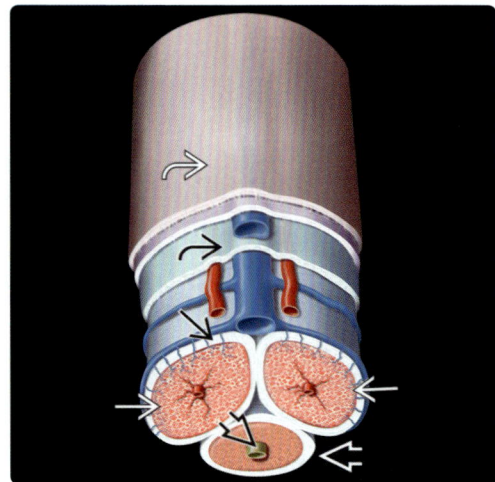

Penile Shaft: Transverse Section

General Concepts, Squamous Cell Carcinoma

- Basaloid and condylomatous (warty) SCC are HPV related in most cases

Human Papillomavirus Unrelated
- Verrucous, pseudohyperplasia, papillary not otherwise specified (NOS), and cuniculatum SCC are typically HPV(-) tumors
- Chronic inflammatory conditions (such as lichen sclerosus) are common in these cases

Risk Factors
- Phimosis is major risk factor for penile cancer
- Lack of neonatal circumcision
- HPV infection (especially by high-risk genotypes)
- History of genital warts
- Multiple sexual partners
- Poor hygiene
- Smoking
- Treatment with psoralen and ultraviolet A therapy

CLINICAL IMPLICATIONS

Clinical Presentation
- Glans is most common affected site followed by inner foreskin and coronal sulcus
- SCC of penile shaft are exceedingly rare
- Presence of painless tumoral mass is most frequent clinical presentation
- Ulceration may be present
- Urinary obstruction secondary to urethral tumoral extension is uncommon
- Phimosis is found in 50% of cases
- Some patients present with inguinal metastasis and primary tumor is occult

MACROSCOPIC

General Features
- Patterns of growth include superficial spreading, vertical, verruciform, and multicentric
  - **Superficial spreading**
    - Broad horizontal/superficial extension with involvement of 1 or more anatomical compartments
    - Extensive in situ component with tumoral invasion usually confined to lamina propria
  - **Vertical growth**
    - Deeply infiltrative tumor with frank invasion of CS or corpus cavernosum
  - **Verruciform**
    - Exophytic, cauliflower-like tumor mass usually invading only superficial anatomical levels
  - **Multicentric**
    - Presence of 2 or more independent foci of SCC
- Mixed/combinations of any aforementioned patterns may be seen
- Superficial spreading tumors show intermediate risk for inguinal metastasis
- Vertical growth tumors show higher rate of nodal involvement and poor outcome
- Verruciform tumors may reach large sizes but tend to be localized and metastatic rate is low
- In multicentric tumors, foci should be separately evaluated

Specimen Handling
- Wide local excision or glans resurfacing technique specimen
  - Fix in 10% buffered formalin, preferably overnight
  - Measure and describe specimen, identifying and describing tumor
  - Photograph or diagram specimen
  - Ink entire surgical margin of specimen
  - Section specimen transverse to longest axis
  - Submit tumor entirely if < 3-4 cm and section at least 1 per cm, including grossly apparent deepest penetration and all margins (if not entirely submitted)
- Circumcision specimen for tumor
  - Lightly stretch and pin specimen to flat surface
  - Fix in 10% buffered formalin, preferably overnight
  - Measure and describe specimen, identifying and describing tumor
  - Photograph or diagram specimen
  - Ink mucosal and cutaneous margins of resection with different colors
  - Section specimen transversally to its longest axis
  - Label each section from 1-12 clockwise
  - Submit entirely if < 3-4 cm, section at least 1 per cm, including grossly apparent deepest penetration and all margins (if not entirely submitted)
- Partial/total penectomy specimen
  - Fix entire specimen in 10% buffered formalin, preferably overnight
  - When fixed, section specimen in 2 halves using meatus and anterior urethra as guide
  - Do **not** probe urethra
  - If foreskin is not affected by tumor, separate leaving 3-mm margin from coronal sulcus and include as circumcision specimen
  - If foreskin is affected by tumor, do **not** remove
  - Photograph or diagram specimen, focusing on tumor invasion of anatomic levels
  - Section each 1/2 longitudinally to longest axis, at 3- to 5-mm intervals
  - Photograph (or diagram) and submit entire section, depicting deepest anatomic level infiltrated by tumor
  - If tumor affects multiple anatomic compartments, at least 3 sections of each affected compartment should be submitted
  - Sections should always include adjacent nontumoral mucosa
  - Resection margins in partial penectomies are urethra and periurethral tissues; CC and skin of shaft should be appropriately submitted
- Lymphadenectomy specimen
  - Fix in 10% buffered formalin, preferably overnight
  - Identify number and size of all lymph nodes
  - If feasible, record anatomic location of lymph nodes as upper inner quadrant, superficial and deep inguinal nodes
  - Submit all lymph nodes for histologic examination

MICROSCOPIC

General Features
- Most penile cancers are SCCs, but there are several histological subtypes/variants

General Concepts, Squamous Cell Carcinoma

- Each subtype is usually associated with defined clinical outcome and prognosis
- Subtyping helps in management of therapy
  o Some variants are often treated more aggressively than others

Histological Subtypes

- Subtyping should always be done following strict morphological criteria
- Histological subtypes of penile SCC include
  o Usual
  o Verrucous
  o Papillary, NOS
  o Warty (condylomatous)
  o Basaloid
  o Adenosquamous
  o Pseudoglandular (acantholytic, adenoid)
  o Cuniculatum
  o Pseudohyperplastic
  o Sarcomatoid
  o Mixed
  o Papillary basaloid
  o Warty/basaloid
  o Clear cell
  o Lymphoepithelioma-like

Ancillary Studies

- Immunohistochemistry (p16, p53, Ki-67, p63) optional
- Molecular studies for HPV typing (PCR, in situ hybridization)

PROGNOSTIC FACTORS

Growth Patterns

- Verruciform tumors include warty (condylomatous), verrucous, papillary NOS, and cuniculatum carcinomas; they are rarely associated with tumor spread
- Basaloid, high-grade usual type, and sarcomatoid SCCs (aggressive variants) usually present with vertical pattern of growth; they are frequently associated with tumor spread
- Superficial spreading growth pattern is characteristic of low-grade variants of SCC
- Multicentricity is more common in low-grade highly differentiated SCC variants, especially those located in foreskin (e.g., pseudohyperplastic SCC)

Histological Subtype

- Correlation of histological subtype, nodal metastasis, and patients outcome
- 3 risk groups: Low, intermediate, and high
  o In low risk category, there are verrucous, papillary NOS, pseudohyperplastic, and cuniculatum carcinomas
  o In high risk groups, there are sarcomatoid and basaloid carcinomas
  o Remaining subtypes are in intermediate risk category

Histological Grade

- Important predictive factor of inguinal lymph node metastasis and outcome
  o Grading should always be done following strict morphologic criteria
- Criteria for grading
  o Grade 1
    – Almost normal to slightly enlarged nuclei and abundant eosinophilic cytoplasm
    – Minimal basal/parabasal atypia and prominent keratinization
  o Grade 2
    – More disorganized growth compared to grade 1 lesions
    – Higher nuclear:cytoplasmic ratio, evident mitoses, and less prominent keratinization
  o Grade 3
    – Tumors composed of any proportion of anaplastic cells with evident nuclear pleomorphism
- Heterogeneous tumors showing areas with different histologic grades are seen in up to 1/2 of all cases
- Tumor grading should be performed considering highest grade component, regardless of its proportion

Depth of Invasion/Tumor Thickness

- Depth of invasion measured from basal cell layer of adjacent normal epithelia to deepest point of infiltration
- Thickness measured from nonnecrotic nonkeratinized tumor surface to its deepest point of infiltration
- Depth and thickness are equally useful, except for verruciform tumors, for which depth of invasion should be preferred
  o In tumors measuring < 5 mm, there is minimal risk for nodal metastasis
  o In tumors measuring > 10 mm, there is high risk for nodal involvement
  o In tumors measuring 5-10 mm, histological grade and perineural invasion are helpful to estimate potential for nodal metastasis

Anatomic Level of Invasion and Pathologic Stage

- Deepest anatomic level infiltrated by tumor should always be carefully determined
  o Anatomic levels in glans include
    – Squamous epithelium (level 0)
    – Lamina propria (level 1)
    – CS (level 2)
    – Corpus cavernosum, including tunica albuginea (level 3)
  o Anatomic levels in foreskin include
    – Squamous epithelium (level 0)
    – Lamina propria (level 1)
    – Dartos muscle layer (level 2)
    – Preputial skin (level 3)
- Superficial tumors invading lamina propria or superficial CS are associated with low risk for nodal metastasis
- Tumors invading deep CS or CC are at high risk for nodal metastasis
- Cancer specific mortality is 0%, 11%, and 20% for tumors invading lamina propria, CS, and CC, respectively

Tumor Site

- Tumors exclusive of foreskin show lower rate of nodal metastasis

Perineural Invasion

- Present in ~ 1/3 of SCCs
- Requires presence of tumoral cells in perineural space and not just surrounding neural bundles

General Concepts, Squamous Cell Carcinoma

- Should be reported since it is associated with increased risk for nodal metastasis and poor outcome

Vascular Invasion
- Requires presence of tumor cells in vascular spaces
  - Either lymphatic (more common) or venous (observed in more advance stages)
  - Tumor cells may be identified in erectile corpora (cavernosa or spongiosa) or nonerectile or nutritional (tumor neovascularity) vessels
- Independent pathologic factor related to nodal metastasis
- Present in ~ 1/3 of SCCs

Tumor Front of Invasion
- Infiltrating pattern vs. pushing infiltration of tumor cells into stroma
  - **Infiltrating pattern**: Small solid strands of tumor cells extensively and randomly infiltrate stroma
  - **Pushing infiltration**: Nests of tumor cells with well-defined tumor-stromal interface
- Infiltrating pattern is associated with higher metastatic rate

Resection Margins
- In penectomy specimen, tumor may be found in any of these sites
  - Urothelium/lamina propria of penile urethra
  - Corpus cavernosum/periurethral CS
  - Penile fascia (most common site of involvement)
  - Skin of penile shaft
- Each of these sites should be separately evaluated

Prognostic Index
- Useful for allocation of patients into risk groups for inguinal metastases and survival
- Uses combined power of histologic grade, anatomical level of infiltration, and perineural invasion to assess risk of nodal metastasis
  - Histologic grade categorized as well differentiated (1 point), moderately differentiated (2 points), or poorly differentiated (3 points)
  - Involved anatomic levels categorized as lamina propria (1 point), CS/preputial dartos (2 points), or CC/preputial skin (3 points)
  - Perineural invasion categorized as absent (0 points) or present (1 point)
- Numeric value of 2-7 is derived by adding values assigned to aforementioned variables
  - Patients with scores 2-3 are at low risk for nodal metastases
    - In absence of clinical evidence of nodal involvement, surveillance often suffices
  - Patients with scores 5-7 are at high risk for nodal metastasis
    - Patients may benefit from prophylactic inguinal lymphadenectomy even in absence of clinical evidence of nodal involvement
  - Patients with score 4 represent therapeutic dilemmas and need further evaluation
    - Ultrasound, TAC, PET scan, and MR may be useful and dynamic sentinel lymph node biopsy may be indicated

STAGING

Tumor Staging
- TNM staging is done considering deepest invasion of penile tissue (T), status of inguinal lymph nodes (N), and presence of distal metastasis (M)
- Broad pushing nondestructive penetration is permitted in noninvasive verrucous carcinoma
- Staging of inguinal lymph nodes may be done by clinical (palpation, imaging) or pathologic (based upon biopsy or surgery) means
- Distant metastases include lymph node metastases outside true pelvis in addition to visceral/bone sites

SELECTED REFERENCES

1. Corbishley CM et al: Glans resurfacing for precancerous and superficially invasive carcinomas of the glans penis: Pathological specimen handling and reporting. Semin Diagn Pathol. 32(3):232-7, 2015
2. Hernandez BY et al: Human papillomavirus genotype prevalence in invasive penile cancers from a registry-based United States population. Front Oncol. 4:9, 2014
3. Sanchez DF et al: Pathological factors, behavior, and histological prognostic risk groups in subtypes of penile squamous cell carcinomas (SCC). Semin Diagn Pathol. 32(3):222-31, 2014
4. Chaux A et al: Epidemiologic profile, sexual history, pathologic features, and human papillomavirus status of 103 patients with penile carcinoma. World J Urol. 31(4):861-7, 2013
5. Chaux A et al: Histologic grade in penile squamous cell carcinoma: visual estimation versus digital measurement of proportions of grades, adverse prognosis with any proportion of grade 3 and correlation of a Gleason-like system with nodal metastasis. Am J Surg Pathol. 33(7):1042-1048, 2009
6. Chaux A et al: The prognostic index: a useful pathologic guide for prediction of nodal metastases and survival in penile squamous cell carcinoma. Am J Surg Pathol. 33(7):1049-1057, 2009
7. Cubilla AL: The role of pathologic prognostic factors in squamous cell carcinoma of the penis. World J Urol. 27(2):169-77, 2009
8. Guimarães GC et al: Penile squamous cell carcinoma clinicopathological features, nodal metastasis and outcome in 333 cases. J Urol. 182(2):528-34; discussion 534, 2009
9. Velazquez EF et al: Histologic grade and perineural invasion are more important than tumor thickness as predictor of nodal metastasis in penile squamous cell carcinoma invading 5 to 10 mm. Am J Surg Pathol. 32(7):974-9, 2008

General Concepts, Squamous Cell Carcinoma

TNM Staging for Penile Carcinoma (2010)

Stage	Description
Primary Tumor (T)	
Tx	Primary tumor cannot be assessed
T0	No evidence of primary tumor
Tis	Carcinoma in situ
Ta	Noninvasive verrucous carcinoma
T1a	Tumor invades subepithelial connective tissue without vascular invasion and is not poorly differentiated
T1b	Tumor invades subepithelial connective tissue with vascular invasion or is poorly differentiated
T2	Tumor invades corpus spongiosum or cavernosum
T3	Tumor invades urethra
T4	Tumor invades other adjacent structures
Regional Lymph Nodes (N)	
Clinical stage definition	
cNx	Regional lymph nodes cannot be assessed
cN0	No palpable or visibly enlarged inguinal lymph nodes
cN1	Palpable mobile unilateral inguinal lymph node
cN2	Palpable mobile multiple or bilateral inguinal lymph nodes
cN3	Unilateral or bilateral palpable fixed inguinal nodal mass or pelvic lymphadenopathy
Pathologic stage definition	
pNx	Regional lymph nodes cannot be assessed
pN0	No regional lymph node metastasis
pN1	Metastasis in single inguinal lymph node
pN2	Metastasis in multiple or bilateral inguinal lymph nodes
pN3	Unilateral or bilateral extranodal extension of lymph node metastasis or pelvic lymph node(s)
Distant Metastasis (M)	
M0	No distant metastasis
M1	Distant metastasis

Anatomic Stage/Prognostic Groups (2009)

Stage	T	N	M
0	Tis	N0	M0
	Ta	N0	M0
I	T1a	N0	M0
II	T1b	N0	M0
	T2	N0	M0
	T3	N0	M0
IIIa	T1-T3	N1	M0
IIIb	T1-T3	N2	M0
IV	T4	Any N	M0
	Any T	N3	M0
	Any T	Any N	M1

General Concepts, Squamous Cell Carcinoma

Superficial Spreading Growth Pattern

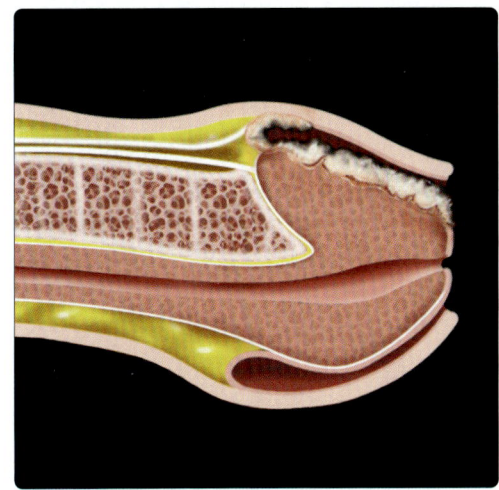

Superficial Spreading Growth Pattern

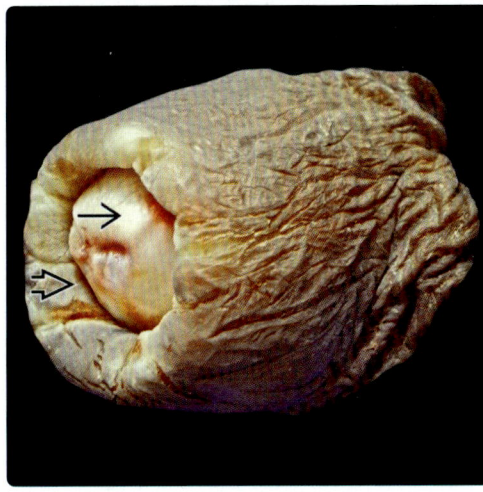

(Left) Superficial spreading growth pattern is characterized by a horizontal growth of tumor mass along the squamous mucosa of glans, coronal sulcus, and even inner foreskin with minimal infiltration of deeper tissues. *(Right)* Predominantly in situ penile squamous cell carcinoma (SCC) with isolated foci of infiltration in lamina propria depicts a superficial spreading growth pattern characterized by whitish and irregular areas extensively affecting the glans ➡ and extending to the foreskin ➡.

Vertical Growth Pattern

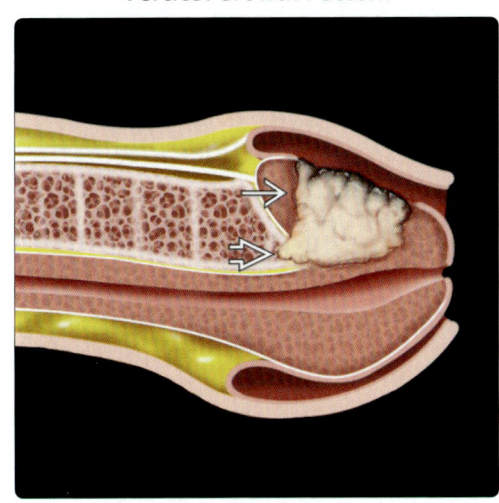

Vertical Growth Pattern

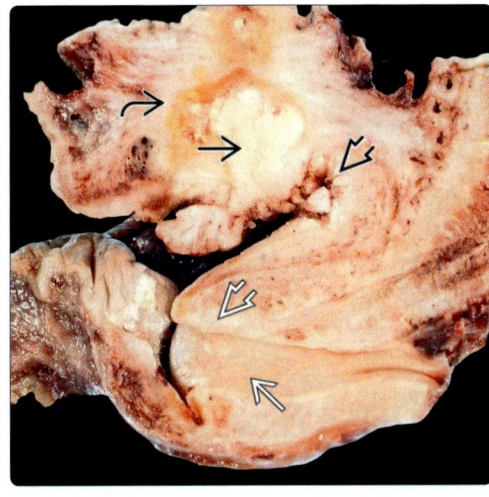

(Left) Tumors with a vertical growth pattern usually show an ulcerated surface and invade deep into penile erectile tissues, either corpus spongiosum ➡ or cavernosum ➡, and typically correspond to SCC variants, such as high-grade usual, basaloid, or sarcomatoid carcinomas. *(Right)* High-grade usual SCC ➡ located in the foreskin ➡ and extending to the coronal sulcus ➡ with a vertical growth pattern is shown invading into deep preputial levels and sparing the glans ➡ and distal urethra ➡.

Verruciform Growth Pattern

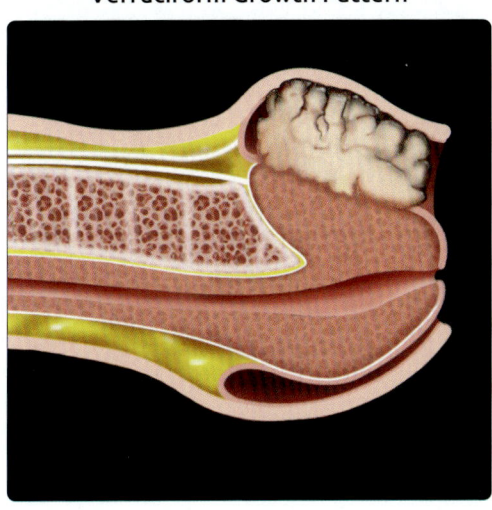

Verruciform Growth Pattern

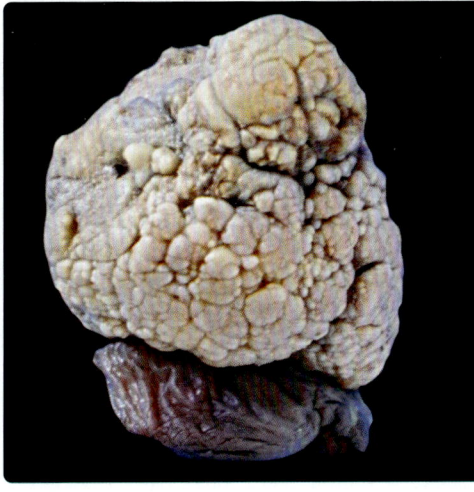

(Left) Penile verruciform tumors include warty, papillary, and verrucous carcinoma and are characterized by an exophytic papillomatous growth pattern, infiltration up to the lamina propria, or corpus spongiosum, and are associated with a relatively favorable prognosis. *(Right)* Gross photo shows a verruciform tumor corresponding to a warty carcinoma entirely replacing the glans and coronal sulcus in which, notwithstanding its large size, tumor invasion was limited to superficial corpus spongiosum.

General Concepts, Squamous Cell Carcinoma

Verruciform Growth Pattern

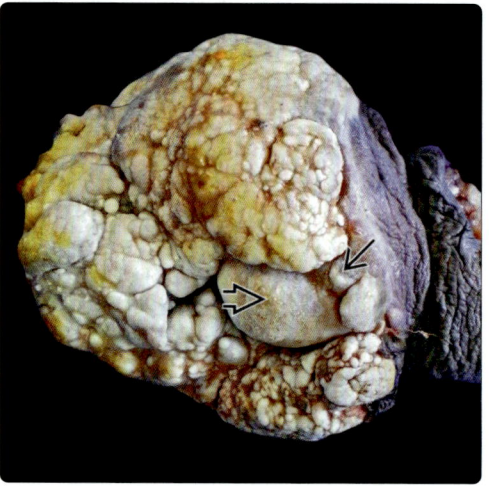

(Left) *Exophytic, cauliflower-like tumor with a verruciform growth pattern, histologically corresponding to a warty carcinoma, located in the foreskin and extending up to the coronal sulcus ⇒ without affecting the glans ⇒ is shown.* (Right) *Highly aggressive penile SCC histologically corresponds to a sarcomatoid carcinoma, with extensive areas of necrosis and hemorrhage located in the glans. The tumor deeply infiltrates the corpora cavernosa ⇒ and perforates the tunica albuginea ⇒.*

Sarcomatoid Carcinoma

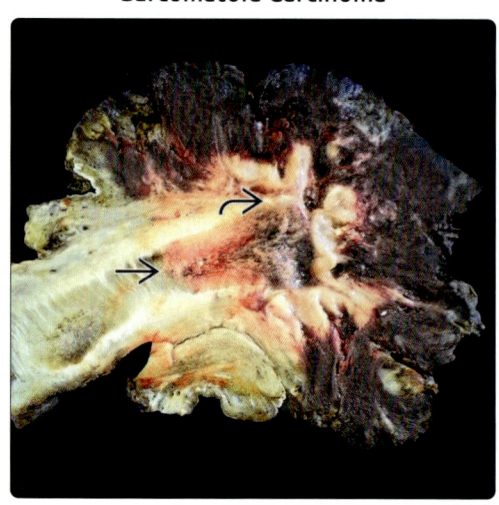

Squamous Cell Carcinoma: Usual Type

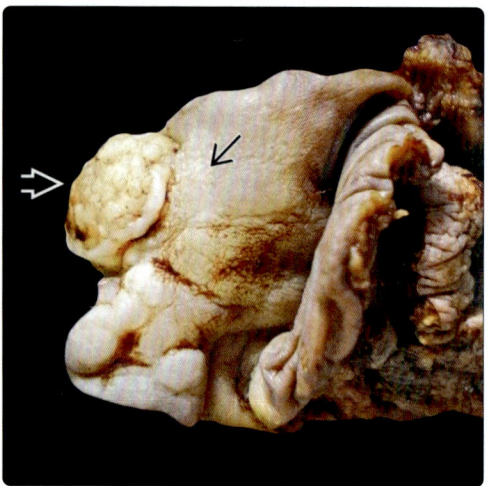

(Left) *Circumcision specimen shows an exophytic tumor ⇒ located in the inner foreskin mucosa ⇒ corresponding to a well-differentiated usual SCC with superficial infiltration of preputial tissues.* (Right) *In well-differentiated (grade 1) usual SCC, neoplastic cells in tumoral nests are almost indistinguishable from their normal counterparts, except for minimal basal/parabasal atypia, prominent keratinization ⇒, and infiltration of penile tissues with surrounding stromal reaction.*

Squamous Cell Carcinoma: Grade 1

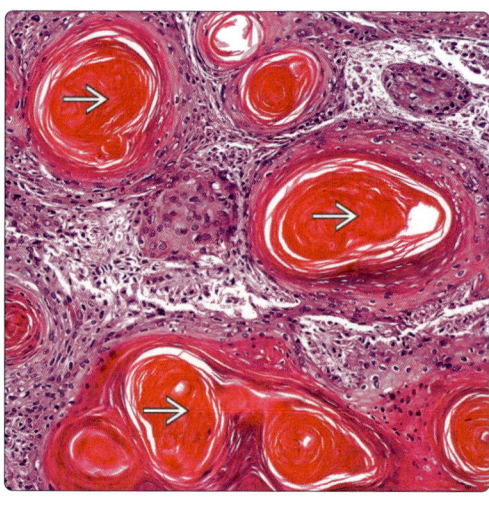

Squamous Cell Carcinoma: Grade 2

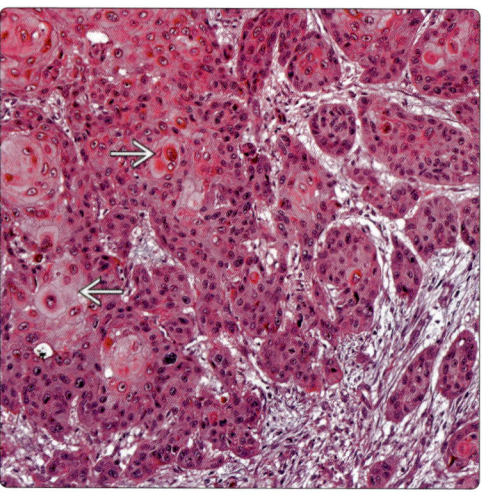

(Left) *In moderately differentiated (grade 2) usual SCC, cytologic atypia is more evident and pleomorphic cells are easily recognized; cytoplasm is ample and eosinophilic and epithelial maturation with keratinization ⇒ is retained.* (Right) *Solid tumoral nests composed of highly pleomorphic cells with anaplastic features ⇒ and ample eosinophilic cytoplasm indicate some degree of squamous differentiation and characterize poorly differentiated (grade 3) usual SCC.*

Squamous Cell Carcinoma: Grade 3

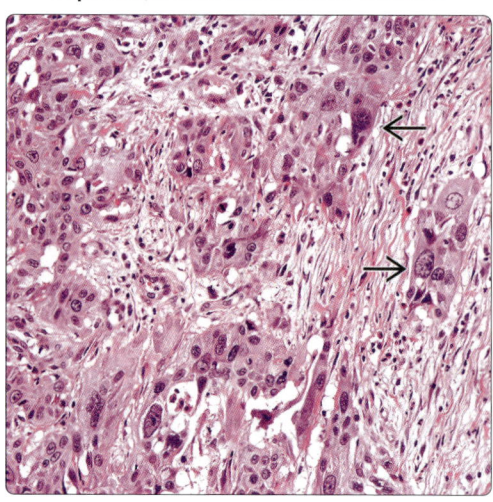

General Concepts, Squamous Cell Carcinoma

Warty Carcinoma

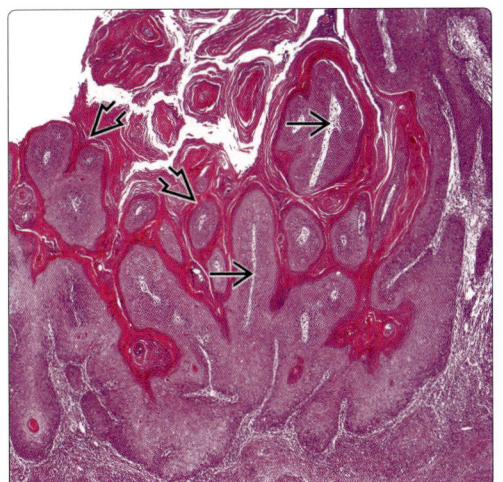

Warty Carcinoma

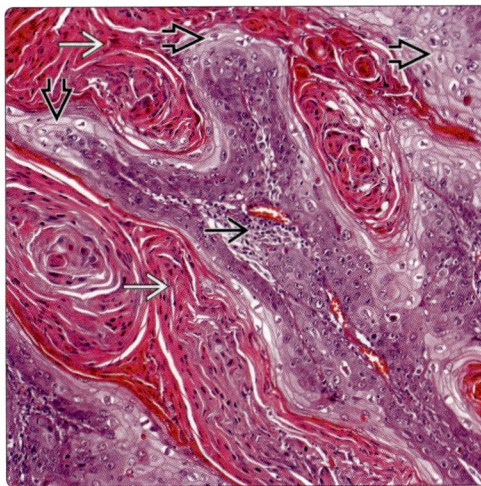

(Left) Warty (condylomatous) carcinoma is a verruciform tumor characterized by acanthosis, papillomatosis, and hyperkeratosis, with straight and spiky parakeratotic papillae ⇨, prominent and constant fibrovascular cores ⇨, and irregular and jagged tumor base. (Right) The papillae in warty carcinoma are elongated and spiky, show evident fibrovascular cores ⇨, mild to moderate acanthosis, and parakeratotic hyperkeratosis ⇨. Koilocytic changes with marked atypia ⇨ are easily found.

Warty Carcinoma

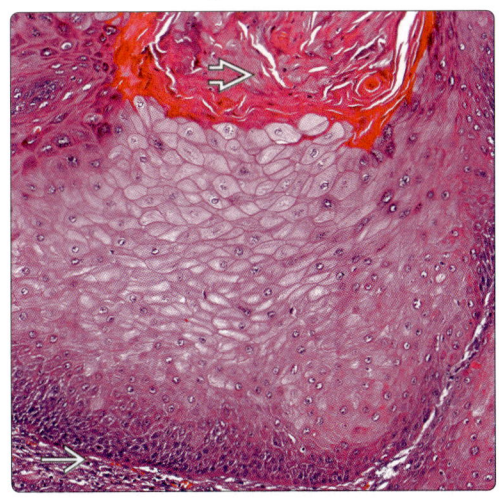

Papillary Carcinoma

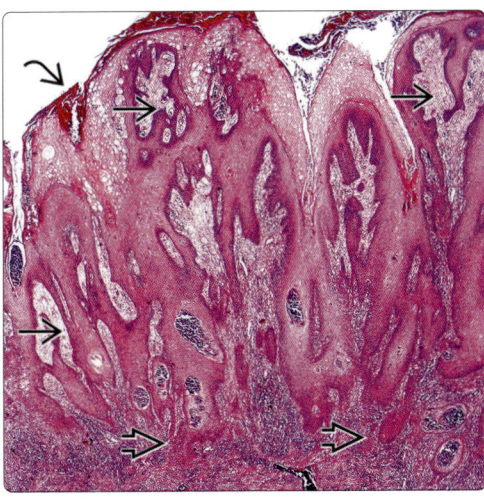

(Left) Verrucous carcinoma is characterized by papillomatosis, moderate to marked acanthosis, minimal cytological atypia, prominent hyperkeratosis ⇨ with absent or inconspicuous fibrovascular cores, and a broad, pushing tumor base ⇨. (Right) In papillary carcinoma, papillae are complex and fibrovascular cores ⇨ are irregular, tips are blunt, round, or spiky, hyperkeratosis ⇨ is commonly found, and the tumor base is irregular and jagged ⇨ with prominent stromal reaction.

Carcinoma Cuniculatum

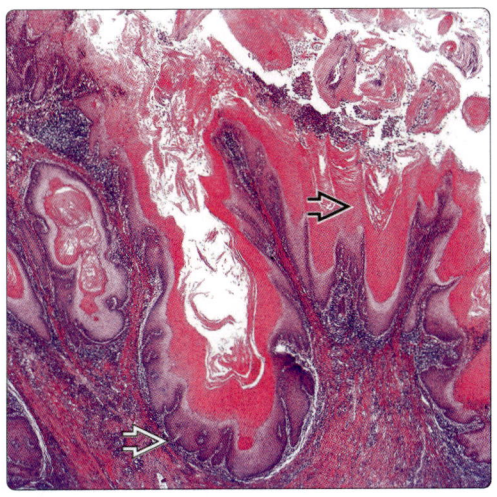

Basaloid Carcinoma

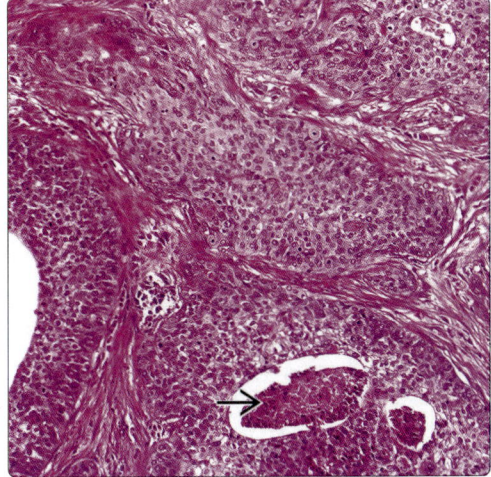

(Left) Carcinoma cuniculatum, a rare verruciform tumor, shows prominent acanthosis, papillomatosis and hyperkeratosis ⇨, broad and pushing tumor base ⇨, and a deeply infiltrating endophytic pattern of growth. (Right) Basaloid carcinoma is characterized by highly infiltrative tumor nests, with frequent central necrosis ⇨, composed of a monotonous population of small- to intermediate-sized cells with scant cytoplasm, abundant mitoses, and indistinct borders.

General Concepts, Squamous Cell Carcinoma

Basaloid Carcinoma

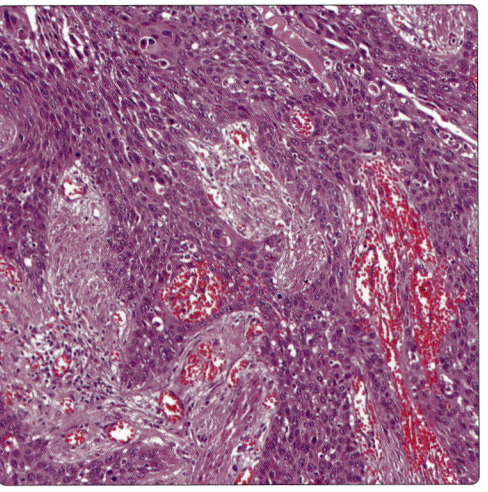

Adenosquamous Carcinoma

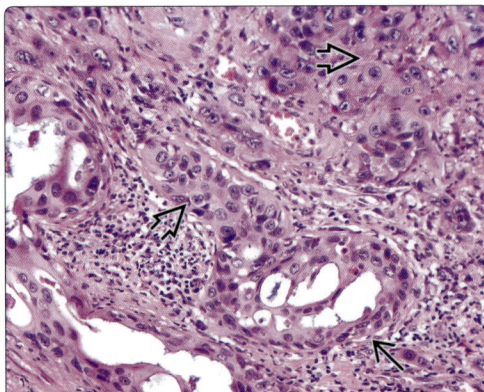

(Left) *Basaloid carcinomas may be composed of irregular tumor nests and greater nuclear pleomorphism but should not be confused with high-grade usual SCC, which is characterized by tumor cells with ample eosinophilic cytoplasm, distinctive borders, and intercellular bridges.* **(Right)** *Adenosquamous carcinoma is a biphasic SCC variant characterized by the presence of a solid, high-grade squamous component ⇒ intermingled with areas showing glandular differentiation ⇒.*

Pseudoglandular Squamous Cell Carcinoma

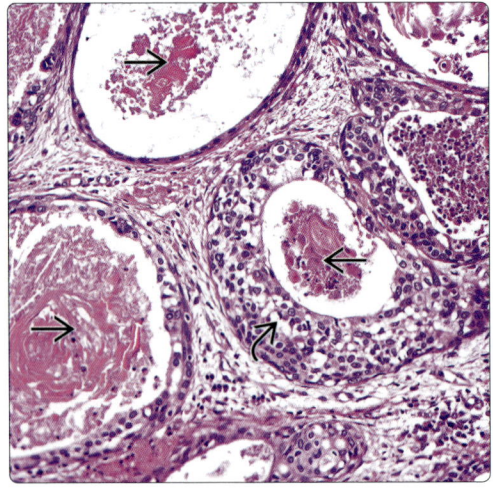

Pseudohyperplastic Carcinoma

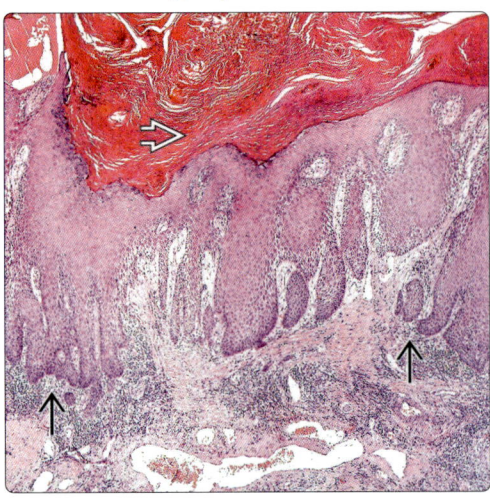

(Left) *In pseudoglandular SCC, solid tumor nests exhibit extensive central necrosis, intracytoplasmic vacuoles ⇒, and acantholysis ⇒, resulting in an appearance resembling glandular lumina.* **(Right)** *Pseudohyperplastic carcinoma, which may be difficult to distinguish from pseudoepitheliomatous hyperplasia, exhibits acanthosis and hyperkeratosis ⇒, downward proliferation of irregular epithelial nests ⇒ with infiltration of lamina propria, and prominent stromal reaction.*

Warty/Basaloid Mixed Squamous Cell Carcinoma

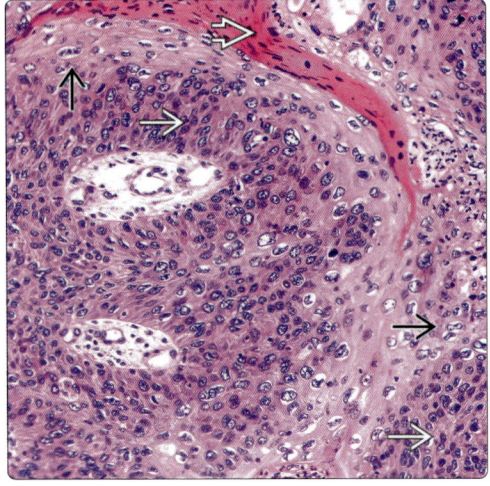

Sarcomatoid Carcinoma

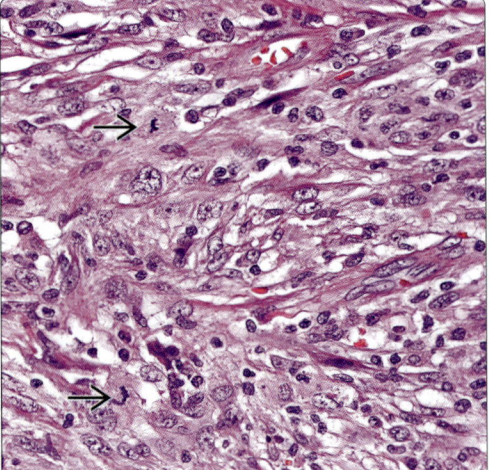

(Left) *Warty/basaloid carcinoma is a mixed SCC in which koilocytes ⇒, typical of warty carcinomas, are mingled with basaloid cells ⇒ either in superficial condylomatous papillae, frequently exhibiting parakeratosis ⇒, or in deeply infiltrative nests.* **(Right)** *Sarcomatoid carcinoma is a highly aggressive SCC variant composed of a predominant spindle cell component, with marked nuclear atypia and abundant mitoses ⇒ resembling leiomyosarcoma or fibrosarcoma.*

General Concepts, Squamous Cell Carcinoma

SCC: Clear Cell Change
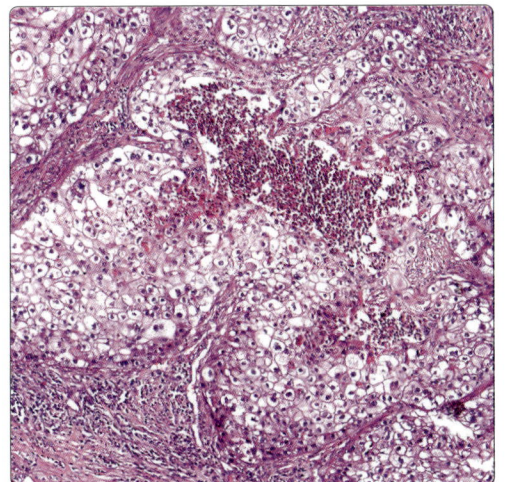

Differentiated PeIN
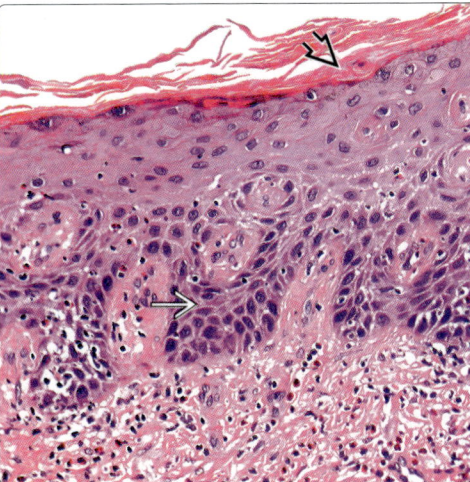

(Left) It is not unusual to find focal clear cell changes in an otherwise typical SCC, although in rare occasions this morphological aspect, usually due to abundant glycogen, may be the predominant histology and may be confused with clear cell carcinoma. **(Right)** Differentiated penile intraepithelial neoplasia (PeIN), frequently associated with keratinizing SCC variants, is characterized by atypical squamous cells, more prominent at bottom layers ➡, with a tendency to epithelial maturation and parakeratosis ➡.

Basaloid Penile Intraepithelial Neoplasia
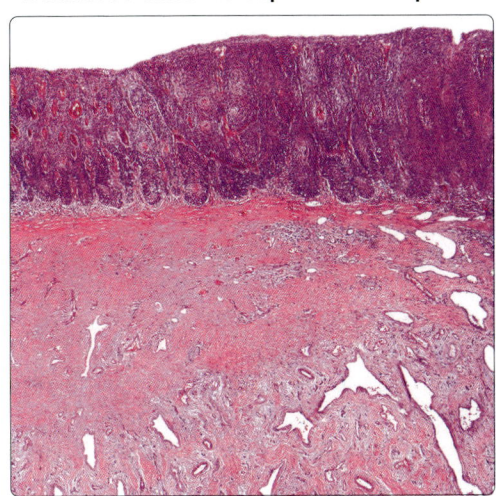

Warty Penile Intraepithelial Neoplasia
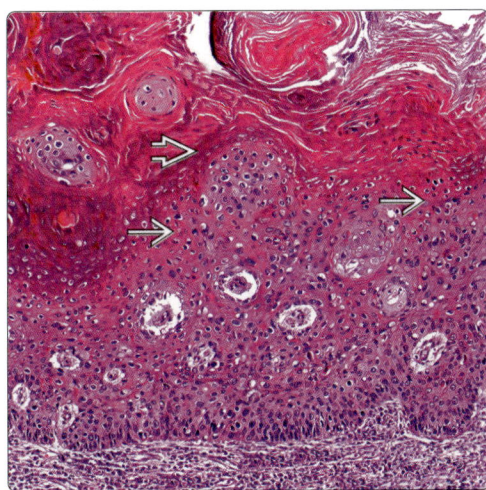

(Left) Basaloid PeIN found in association with warty/basaloid tumors, is characterized by replacement of the epithelium by a monotonous population of small- to intermediate-sized cells with high nuclear:cytoplasmic ratio, indistinct borders, abundant mitoses, and a flat surface. **(Right)** Warty PeIN, usually found adjacent to invasive carcinomas with warty/basaloid features, is characterized by acanthosis, a spiky and parakeratotic surface ➡, and conspicuous koilocytosis ➡.

Lichen Sclerosus
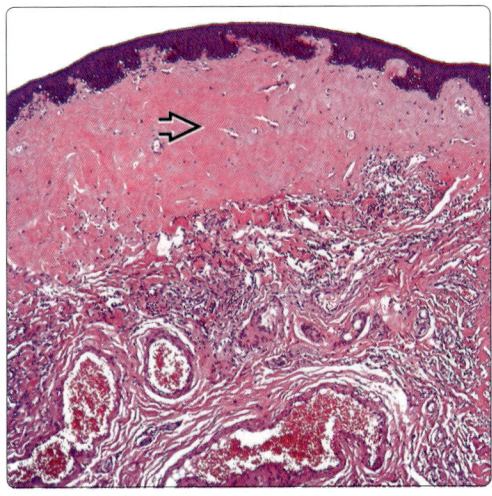

Verruciform Lesion: NOS
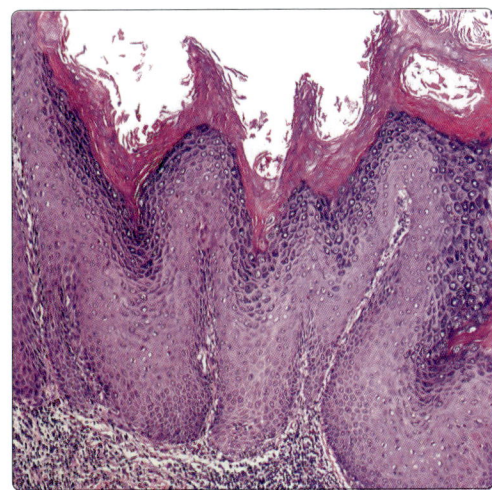

(Left) In lichen sclerosus, a dense area of collagenization ➡ is observed underneath the squamous epithelium, which shows atrophic, hyperplastic, or atypical changes. **(Right)** Well-differentiated verrucoid lesions are often difficult to classify, especially in small biopsies, and the differentials include verrucous squamous hyperplasia and verrucous carcinoma, the latter characterized by a clinically exophytic and large lesion when compared with the former.

Squamous Cell Carcinoma, Usual Type

KEY FACTS

TERMINOLOGY
- Squamous cell carcinoma (SCC)

ETIOLOGY/PATHOGENESIS
- HPV infection in up to 1/4 of cases

MACROSCOPIC
- Glans frequently affected
- Superficial growth pattern in most cases
- Gross features are nondistinctive

MICROSCOPIC
- Most common histological subtype of penile SCC
- Keratinization evident in most cases
- Mostly well to moderately differentiated
- Heterogeneous tumors and patterns in ~ 1/2 of all cases
- Focal presence of anaplastic cells is enough for grade 3
- Frequent invasion of penile erectile tissues
- Frequent extension to multiple compartments
- Squamous hyperplasia and differentiated penile intraepithelial neoplasia commonly found
- Most important prognostic factors
  - Histologic grade
  - Anatomical level of infiltration
  - Vascular invasion
  - Perineural invasion
- Inguinal nodal metastases in 1/3 of patients

TOP DIFFERENTIAL DIAGNOSES
- Pseudoepitheliomatous hyperplasia
- Pseudohyperplastic carcinoma
- Urothelial carcinoma of distal urethra
- Mixed SCC
- Metastatic SCC to penis

Gross Pathology
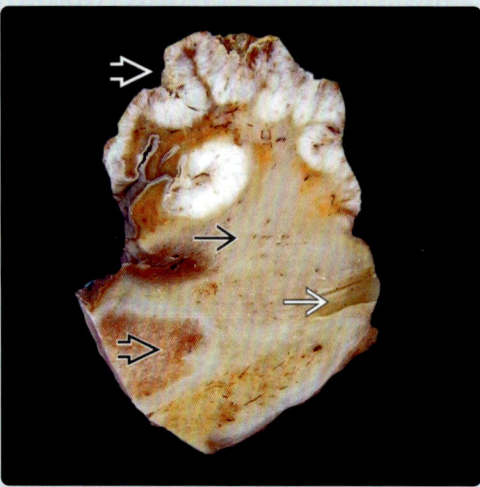

Well-Differentiated Carcinoma
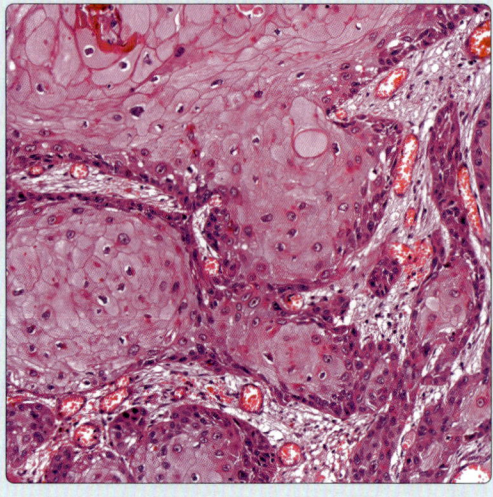

(Left) Gross photograph of a penile squamous cell carcinoma (SCC) ➡ with an exoendophytic growth pattern invades up to the corpus spongiosum ➡ of the glans but spares the urethra ➡ and corpus cavernosum ➡. **(Right)** Tumor nests of well-differentiated usual SCC are composed of neoplastic cells with ample, eosinophilic and keratinized cytoplasm, distinctive cellular borders, and retained epithelial maturation. An infiltrative architecture is also appreciated.

Moderately Differentiated Carcinoma
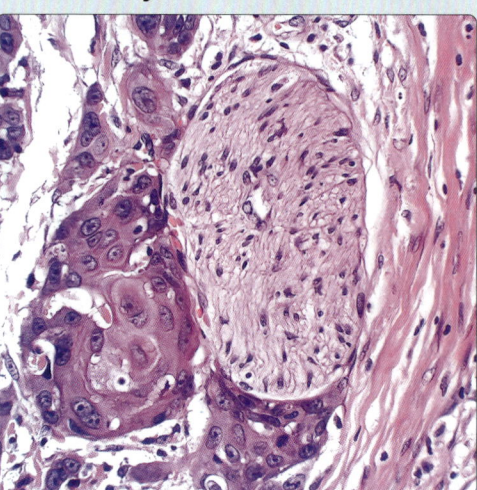

Poorly Differentiated Carcinoma
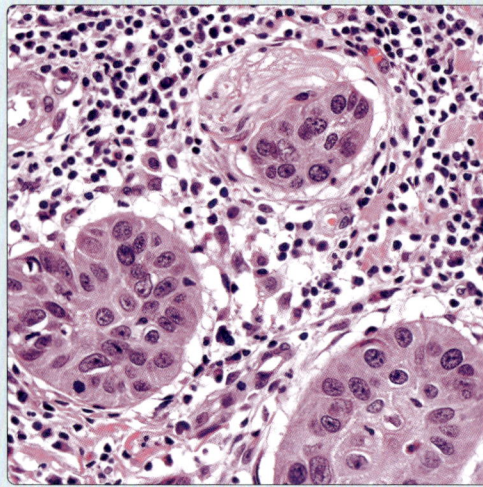

(Left) Moderately differentiated usual SCC with perineural invasion is shown. **(Right)** Poorly differentiated small nests of usual SCC are shown. Note the dense peritumoral inflammatory cells. Squamous differentiation is minimal to absent.

Squamous Cell Carcinoma, Usual Type

TERMINOLOGY

Abbreviations
- Squamous cell carcinoma (SCC)

Synonyms
- Conventional/typical SCC
- Epidermoid carcinoma
- SCC, not otherwise specified

Definitions
- Invasive carcinoma with features of keratinization (intracellular keratin pearls and intracellular bridges)

ETIOLOGY/PATHOGENESIS

Infectious Agents
- Human papillomavirus (HPV) infection in 10-25% of cases

CLINICAL ISSUES

Epidemiology
- Incidence
  ○ Most common histologic subtype of penile SCC (60-65%)
- Age
  ○ Average: 60 years

Presentation
- Solid mass usually affecting glans
- Ulceration, pain, bleeding, or erythema

Treatment
- Partial or total penectomy
- Penile-preserving therapy in low-grade superficial tumors
- Radiotherapy as adjuvant or neoadjuvant therapy
- Chemotherapy for advanced cases (unresectable primary tumor &/or regional involvement)
- Inguinal lymphadenectomy according to risk group

Prognosis
- Most important prognostic factors include
  ○ Histologic grade
  ○ Anatomic level of infiltration (pathologic stage)
  ○ Vascular, lymphatic, and perineural invasion
- Recurrences in 1/4 of cases
- Inguinal nodal metastases in 1/3 of patients

MACROSCOPIC

General Features
- Most tumors affect glans
- Tumors exclusive of foreskin are less common
- Average size: 2-5 cm

MICROSCOPIC

Histologic Features
- Squamous differentiation (keratinization)
- Most are well to moderately differentiated
- More than 1 histologic grade in ~ 1/2 of cases
  ○ Only highest grade is considered for tumor grading
- Focal areas of spindle, trabecular, solid, or clear cells in some cases
- Evident stromal reaction
- Vascular and perineural invasion in ~ 1/3 of cases
- Extension to distal urethra in almost 1/2 of cases
- Squamous hyperplasia (SH) and differentiated penile intraepithelial neoplasia (PeIN) commonly found in adjacent mucosa
- Basaloid and warty PeIN rarely found
- Lichen sclerosus in almost 1/2 of patients

DIFFERENTIAL DIAGNOSIS

Pseudoepitheliomatous Hyperplasia
- Pseudoinfiltrative growth pattern
- Epithelial nests orderly disposed
- No cytologic atypia, at most reactive appearing
- No stromal reaction

Pseudohyperplastic Carcinoma
- Extreme squamous differentiation
- Irregular tumor nests
- Prominent stromal reaction
- Multicentricity is common
- Lichen sclerosus frequently found

Urothelial Carcinoma of Distal Urethra
- Clinical antecedents of urothelial carcinoma
- Urothelial carcinoma in situ in adjacent areas
- CK20, uroplakin-2, and uroplakin-3 are positive in urothelial carcinoma and negative in SCC
  ○ p63 not helpful

Mixed Squamous Cell Carcinoma
- Foci of usual SCC intermingled with other subtypes
- Mostly with verrucous carcinoma
- Uncommon with HPV-related tumors

Metastatic Squamous Cell Carcinoma to Penis
- Prostatic adenocarcinomas and bladder urothelial carcinoma are most common
- Tumor located in penile shaft
- Tumor nests located mainly in vascular spaces of penile erectile tissues
- Clinical antecedent of primary malignancy elsewhere
- Priapism in 1/3-1/2 of patients

SELECTED REFERENCES

1. Sanchez DF et al: Pathological factors, behavior, and histological prognostic risk groups in subtypes of penile squamous cell carcinomas (SCC). Semin Diagn Pathol. 32(3):222-31, 2014
2. Epstein JI et al: Tumors of the prostate gland, seminal vesicles, penis, and scrotum. Washington DC: American Registry of Pathology and AFIP, 2011
3. Chaux A et al: Metastatic tumors to the penis: a report of 17 cases and review of the literature. Int J Surg Pathol 2011;19(5):597-606, 2010
4. Guimarães GC et al: Penile squamous cell carcinoma clinicopathological features, nodal metastasis and outcome in 333 cases. J Urol. 182(2):528-34; discussion 534, 2009
5. Chaux A et al: The prognostic index: a useful pathologic guide for prediction of nodal metastases and survival in penile squamous cell carcinoma. Am J Surg Pathol. 33(7):1049-1057, 2009
6. Chaux A et al: Histologic grade in penile squamous cell carcinoma: visual estimation versus digital measurement of proportions of grades, adverse prognosis with any proportion of grade 3 and correlation of a Gleason-like system with nodal metastasis. Am J Surg Pathol. 33(7):1042-1048, 2009

Squamous Cell Carcinoma, Usual Type

Gross Pathology

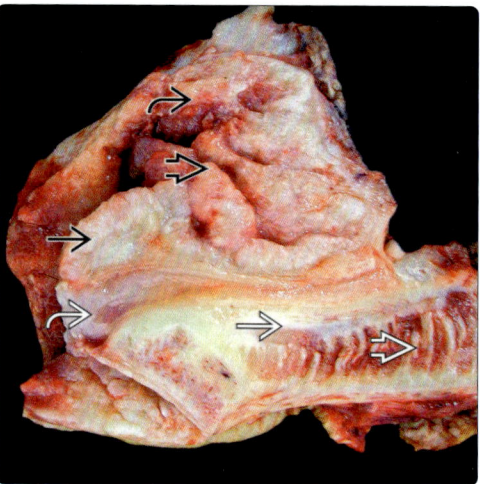

Schematic Representation

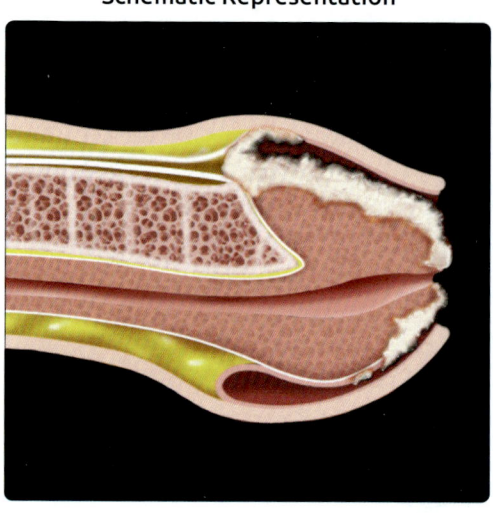

(Left) Usual SCC is shown affecting multiple anatomic compartments and extending through the glans ⇒, coronal sulcus ⇒, and foreskin ⇒, but sparing the distal urethra ⇒, tunica albuginea ⇒, and corpus cavernosum ⇒. (Right) Usual SCC tends to affect multiple anatomical compartments and extend through the glans, coronal sulcus, and inner foreskin, although invading only superficial anatomical levels, a pattern named superficial spreading may be occasionally seen.

Well Differentiated: Grade 1

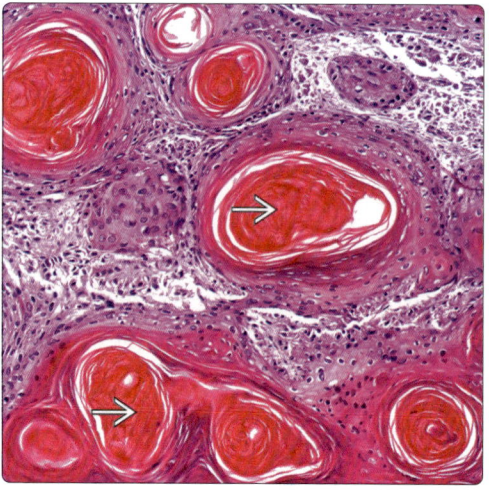

Moderately Differentiated: Grade 2

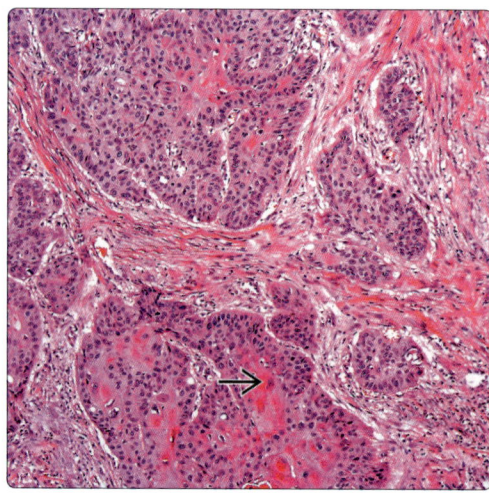

(Left) Tumor nests of grade 1 usual SCC show retained epithelial maturation, extensive keratinization with prominent keratin pearl formation ⇒, and minimal cytologic atypia limited to basal/parabasal layers. (Right) In grade 2 usual SCC, nuclear atypia is more evident and extensive, but neoplastic cells still exhibit features of squamous differentiation with ample eosinophilic cytoplasm, distinctive cellular borders, and foci of keratinization ⇒.

Poorly Differentiated: Grade 3

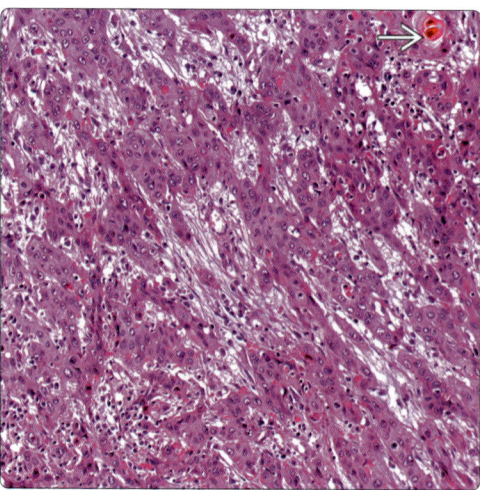

Poorly Differentiated: Anaplasia

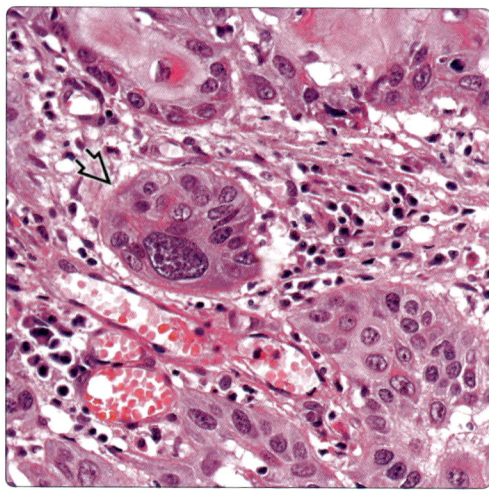

(Left) In grade 3 usual SCC, there is high-grade nuclear atypia and only minimal evidence of squamous differentiation ⇒, but cells retain the morphological features of squamous differentiation with ample, eosinophilic cytoplasm and distinctive cellular borders. (Right) Presence of focal areas of anaplastic cells ⇒, with nuclear pleomorphism, coarse chromatin, irregular nuclear outlines and evident nucleoli, in an otherwise low-grade usual SCC is sufficient to grade the tumor as grade 3.

Squamous Cell Carcinoma, Usual Type

Tumor Necrosis

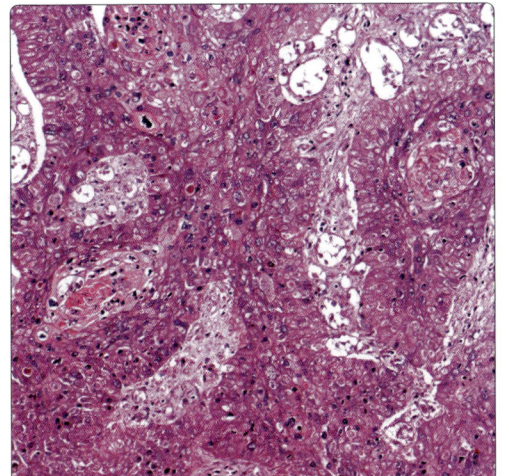

Clear Cell Change

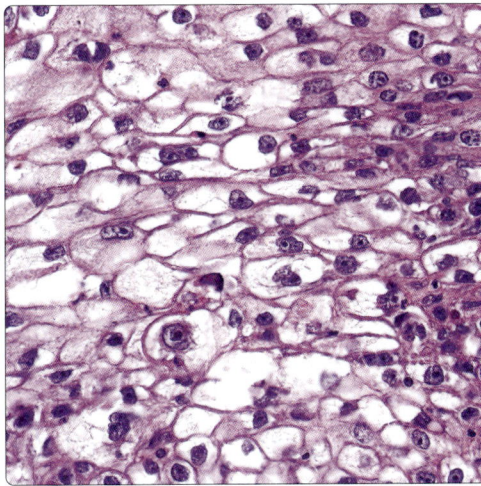

(Left) *Tumor necrosis is a common feature of high-grade carcinomas, and it is characterized by neoplastic cells with diffuse cytoplasmic eosinophilia, retained cell shape, and pyknotic to absent nuclei, intermingled with viable cells.* (Right) *Clear cells, showing ample and pale cytoplasm, distinctive cellular borders, and nuclear pleomorphism ranging from mild to moderate, may be observed in some cases of usual SCC, but they are usually focal and not prominent.*

Associated Precursor Lesion

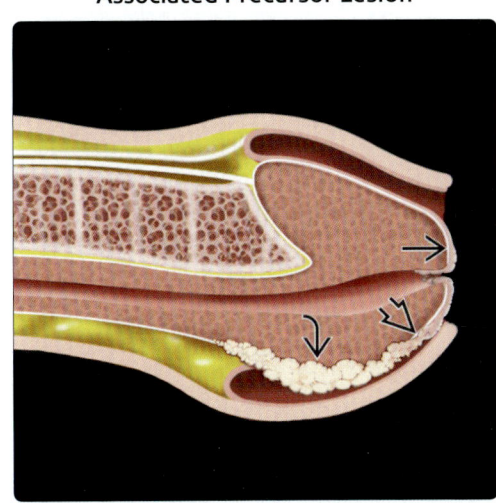

Differentiated PeIN

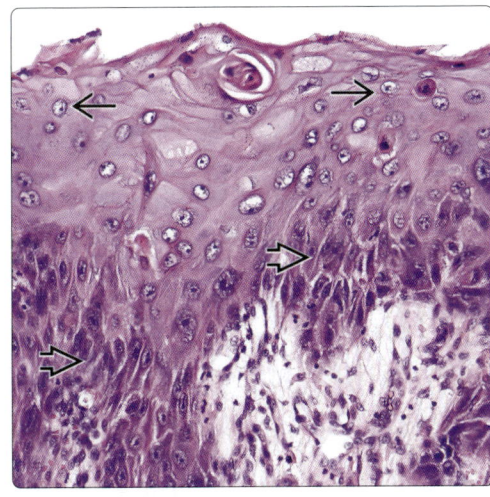

(Left) *Most invasive usual SCCs ➡ are topographically associated with areas of squamous hyperplasia ➡ and penile intraepithelial neoplasia (PeIN) ➡, either adjacent or in continuity with the main tumor mass.* (Right) *Differentiated PeIN is commonly found in areas adjacent to the invasive component, and it is characterized by atypical cells ➡ distributed throughout the entire epithelium ➡ with retained squamous differentiation and slight to moderate parakeratosis.*

Perineural Invasion

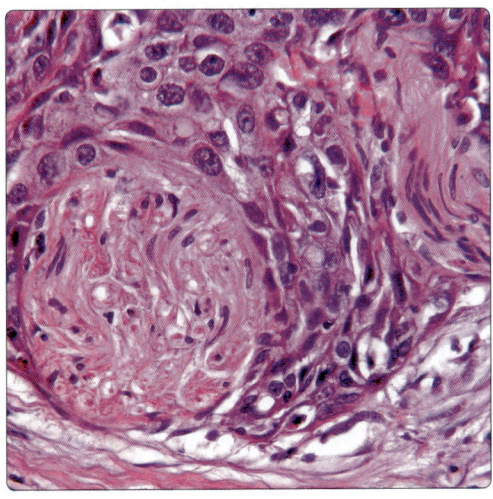

Vascular Invasion

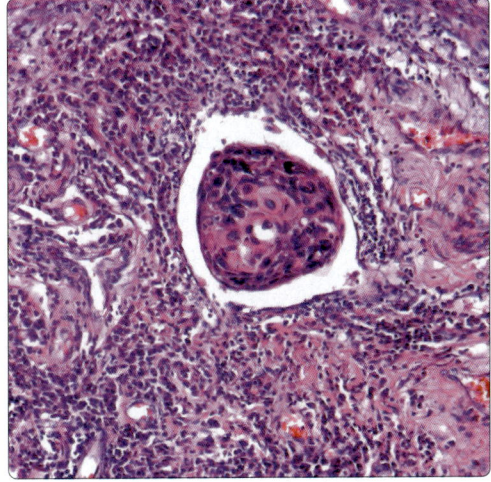

(Left) *Perineural invasion, an important pathological prognostic factor, is accurately defined as invasion of perineural space by neoplastic cells and not just extension of the tumor along nerve bundles (nerve entrapment).* (Right) *Vascular invasion, another important prognostic factor, is characterized by the presence of tumor emboli within vascular spaces, either within or in the periphery of the tumor, and may affect tumor neovasculature as well as the vascular penile erectile tissues.*

Basaloid Squamous Cell Carcinoma

KEY FACTS

ETIOLOGY/PATHOGENESIS
- Human papillomavirus (HPV) detected in most cases
- HPV-16 most common genotype

CLINICAL ISSUES
- 6th decade, 10 years younger than usual squamous cell carcinoma (SCC)
- 10-15% of all penile SCC
- Frequent metastases to inguinal lymph nodes at time of diagnosis

MACROSCOPIC
- Glans is most common site of origin
- Cut surface shows solid tan tumor with minute foci of necrosis
- Vertical growth pattern
- Frequently invades deeply into erectile tissues

MICROSCOPIC
- Sheets or nested pattern of invasive carcinoma
- Basaloid nests with central comedo or keratinous debris
- Retraction artifact common
- Numerous mitoses and apoptosis, starry-sky pattern
- Unusual adenoid, spindle, papillary, and clear cell patterns
- Adjacent basaloid &/or Warty-basaloid PeIN
- HPV positive by PCR or ISH, p16 positive

TOP DIFFERENTIAL DIAGNOSES
- Urothelial carcinoma of distal urethra
- Cutaneous basal cell carcinoma
- Neuroendocrine carcinoma

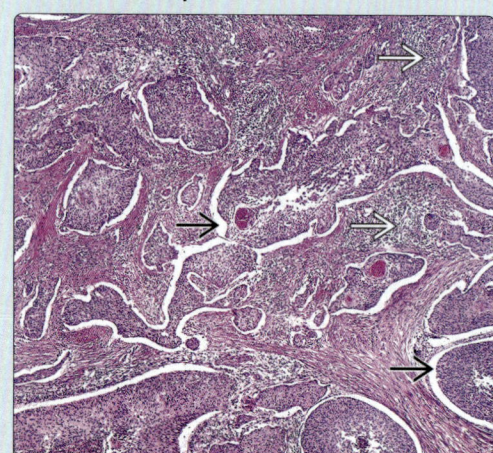

Basaloid Squamous Cell Carcinoma

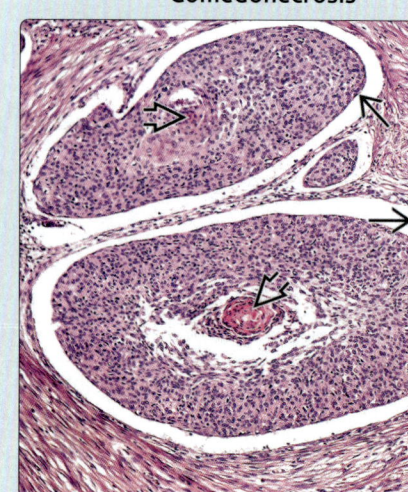

Comedonecrosis

(Left) Low-power view of basaloid carcinoma depicts the typical highly infiltrative pattern of nests composed of poorly differentiated cells with retraction artifact ➡ and intense stromal reaction ➡. (Right) Basaloid squamous cell carcinoma (SCC) nests of poorly differentiated carcinoma are seen with retraction spaces ➡ and central, abrupt foci of keratinization ➡. Keratinization is typically focal in the majority of cases.

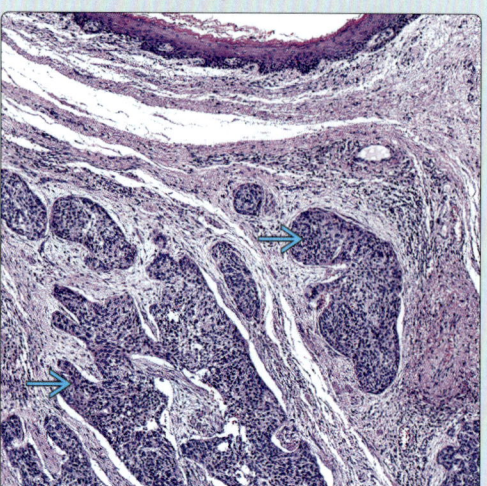

Deep Nests

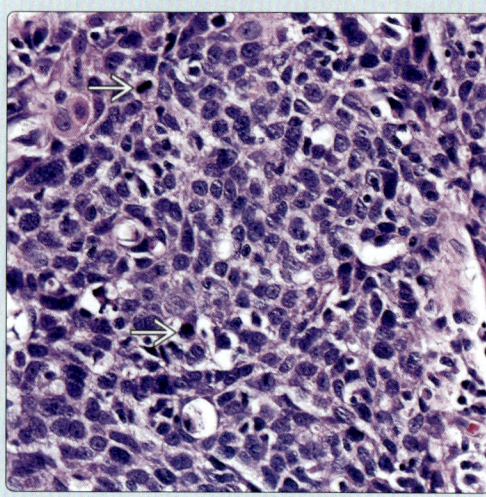

High-Power View

(Left) Note the nests of basaloid cells ➡. (Right) Note the basaloid cells with high nuclear:cytoplasmic ratio. Also, there are numerous mitoses ➡. The impression is of a poorly to undifferentiated, high-grade carcinoma with minimal evidence of squamous differentiation.

Basaloid Squamous Cell Carcinoma

TERMINOLOGY

Synonyms
- Basaloid squamous cell carcinoma (SCC)

Definitions
- Aggressive human papillomavirus (HPV)-related tumor composed of small to intermediate-sized uniform basaloid cells

ETIOLOGY/PATHOGENESIS

Infectious Agents
- HPV found in majority of cases
- HPV genotype 16 most prevalent

CLINICAL ISSUES

Epidemiology
- Incidence
  - 10-15% of all penile SCC
- Age
  - Most patients are in 6th decade

Presentation
- Distal penis tumor mass
- Nodal inguinal metastasis in ~ 1/2 of patients

Treatment
- Surgical approaches
  - Total penectomy in tumors invading corpora cavernosa
  - Partial penectomy in superficial tumors
  - Bilateral inguinal node dissection
- Adjuvant therapy
  - Chemotherapy for advanced cases
- Radiation
  - May be used in selected cases

Prognosis
- Local recurrence seen in 1/3 of cases
- Regional metastases present in 50% of cases
- Mortality varies from 25-45%

MACROSCOPIC

General Features
- Glans is most common site of origin
- Unicentric tumor
- May extend to coronal sulcus and foreskin
- Ulcerative firm lesion
- Cut surface shows tan, solid, deeply invasive tumor
- Punctate yellow foci of necrosis

MICROSCOPIC

Histologic Features
- Downward proliferation of sheets or nests
- Solid or necrotic tumor nests often surrounded by clear retraction artifact
- Peripheral palisading is rare
- Necrosis is central (comedonecrosis) ± keratin debris
- Central abrupt keratinization may be present
- Cells are small, uniform, and basophilic
- Mitoses are numerous
- Apoptosis is characteristic
- Vascular and perineural invasion are prevalent
- Stromal hyalinization may be present
- Unusual patterns are adenoid, papillary, spindle, pleomorphic, and clear cell
- Basaloid or warty-basaloid subtypes of penile intraepithelial neoplasia (PeIN) are frequently found in mucosa adjacent to tumor usually in continuity

ANCILLARY TESTS

Immunohistochemistry
- p16 is usually strongly positive

In Situ Hybridization
- High-risk HPV subtypes are positive

PCR
- High-risk HPV subtypes are present

DIFFERENTIAL DIAGNOSIS

Usual Squamous Cell Carcinoma With Nesting Pattern
- Cells are larger and pleomorphic
- Gradual and not abrupt keratinization
- Negative for p16
- Negative for HPV

Warty-Basaloid Carcinoma
- Mixed tumor with superficial warty and deep basaloid carcinoma features
- Presence of warty changes, usually papillomatous &/or prominent clear cell koilocytosis, excludes basaloid carcinoma

Cutaneous Basal Cell Carcinoma
- Usually arise in skin of shaft and not in penile mucosa
- Superficial tumors
- Distinct peripheral palisading and myxoid stromal changes

Neuroendocrine Carcinoma
- Extremely rare
- May be entirely composed of small, uniform, basophilic cells
- Organoid growth pattern
- Chromogranin and synaptophysin are usually positive

SELECTED REFERENCES

1. Guimarães GC et al: Penile squamous cell carcinoma clinicopathological features, nodal metastasis and outcome in 333 cases. J Urol. 182(2):528-34; discussion 534, 2009
2. Cubilla AL et al: Basaloid squamous cell carcinoma: a distinctive human papilloma virus-related penile neoplasm: a report of 20 cases. Am J Surg Pathol. 22(6):755-61, 1998
3. Gregoire L et al: Preferential association of human papillomavirus with high-grade histologic variants of penile-invasive squamous cell carcinoma. J Natl Cancer Inst. 87(22):1705-9, 1995

Basaloid Squamous Cell Carcinoma

Low-Power View

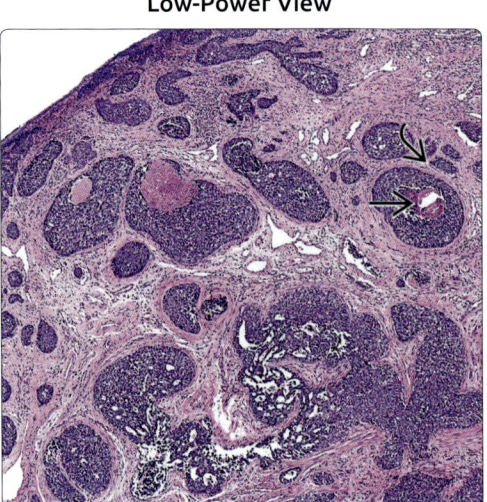

(Left) Tumor nests of basaloid carcinoma extensively infiltrate penile parenchyma. There is central comedonecrosis ⇨ and focal vascular lymphatic invasion ⇨. Peripheral palisading is inconspicuous. This carcinoma is frequently associated with vertical growth pattern of penile carcinoma. **(Right)** A tumor nest of basaloid carcinoma with central necrosis is seen containing keratinous debris ⇨. The retraction artifact ⇨ surrounding the tumor nest is a common feature.

Basaloid Nests

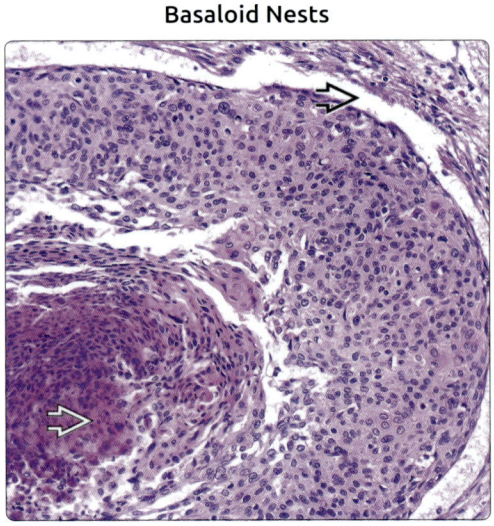

Mitotic Activity

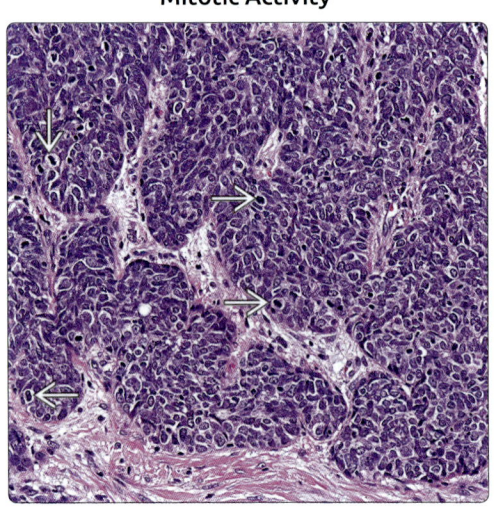

(Left) Neoplastic cells of basaloid carcinomas show moderate nuclear pleomorphism, indistinct cellular borders, and nonkeratinized cytoplasm. The cell population is monotonous and fairly uniform. There is an abundance of mitotic figures ⇨, which on low power may impart a starry-sky appearance. **(Right)** Focally, more pleomorphic and solid patterns may also be observed with greater degree of nuclear atypia and irregularly shaped tumor nests.

Pleomorphism

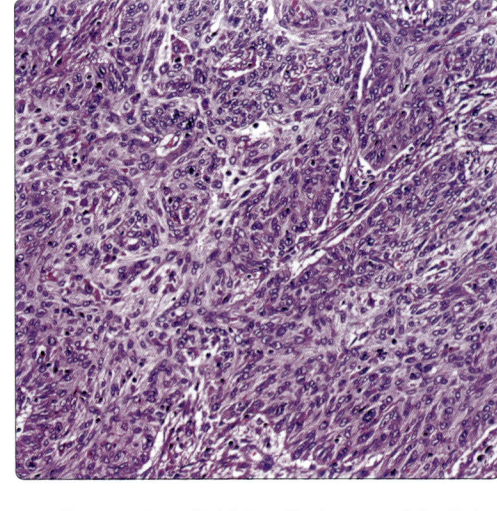

Spindled Areas

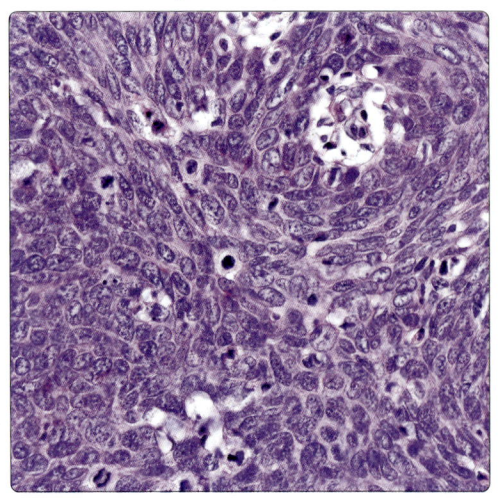

(Left) In this case of basaloid carcinoma, there are areas with greater pleomorphism and spindle cell morphology. Cytoplasm retains typical basaloid features with lack of keratinization, high nuclear:cytoplasmic ratios, and indistinct cellular borders. **(Right)** Basaloid (HPV-associated) penile intraepithelial neoplasm is frequently found adjacent to the invasive component. The entire epithelium is replaced by a monotonous population of basaloid cells. Parakeratosis ⇨ is a common finding.

Adjacent Basaloid Penile Intraepithelial Neoplasm

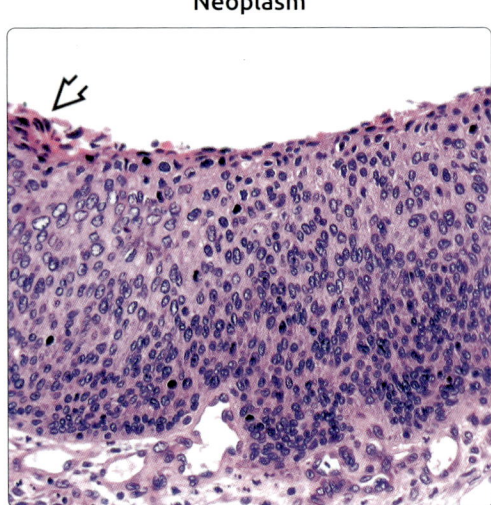

Basaloid Squamous Cell Carcinoma

Pseudoglandular Features

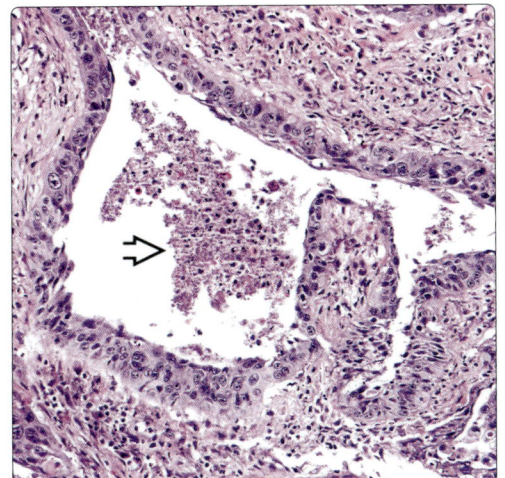

Adenoid Cystic-Like Pattern

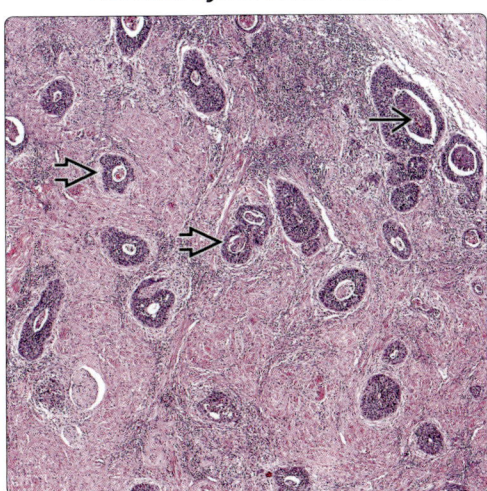

(Left) Tumor nests with extensive central necrosis ⇒ simulate pseudoglandular structures. When these features predominate throughout the tumor, the diagnosis of pseudoglandular (acantholytic) carcinoma may be appropriate. (Right) An adenoid cystic-like appearance may focally be observed, with highly infiltrative small & regular tumor nests ⇒ & central necrosis ⇒ simulating glandular lumina. Urothelial carcinomas, included in the differential diagnosis, are positive for GATA3 & uroplakin-2.

Starry-Sky Pattern

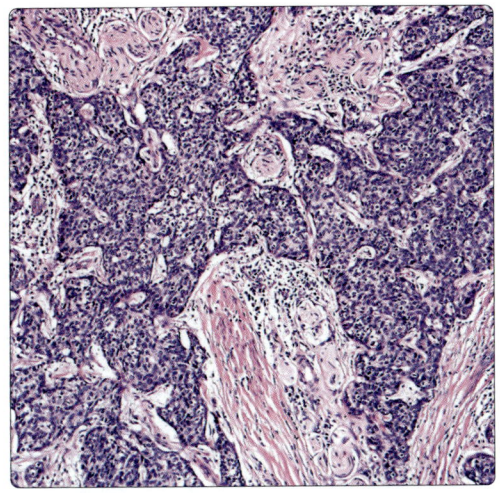

Differential Diagnosis

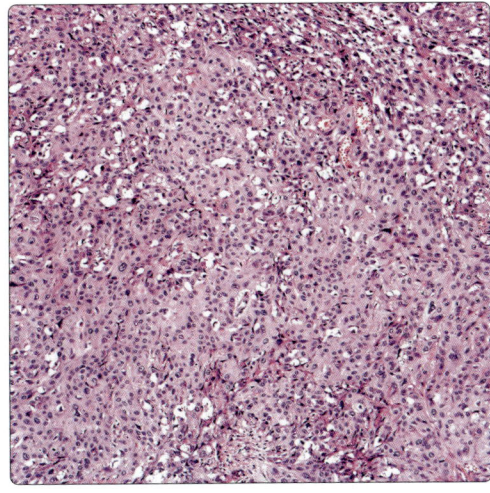

(Left) Solid deep sheets of small blue cells are shown with areas of starry-sky pattern of basaloid squamous cell carcinoma. (Right) High-grade usual SCC with a predominantly solid pattern of growth may simulate basaloid carcinoma; however, the neoplastic cells are typically more pleomorphic and retain squamous features, with ample and keratinized (eosinophilic) cytoplasm. In this setting, p16 immunohistochemistry may play a role.

Warty-Basaloid Squamous Cell Carcinoma

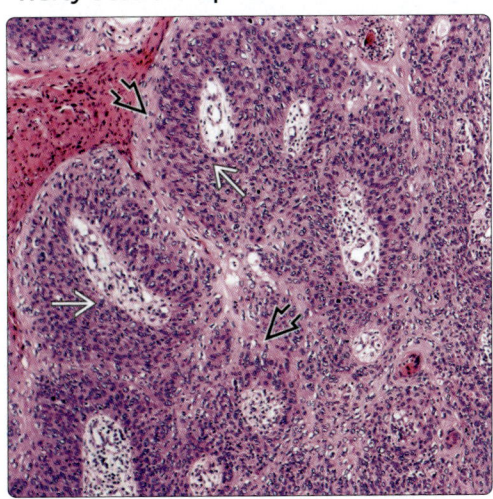

p16 Immunostaining

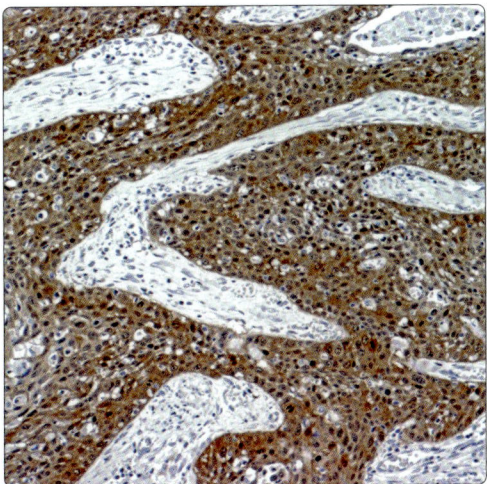

(Left) Warty/basaloid carcinoma is a mixed subtype of penile SCC with condylomatous papillae and tumor nests lined by pleomorphic koilocytes in the surface/periphery ⇒ and basaloid cells in the deep/central areas ⇒. (Right) In basaloid carcinomas, the neoplastic cells typically show strong and diffuse immunoreactivity for p16 overexpression.

Basaloid Squamous Cell Carcinoma, Papillary Variant

KEY FACTS

ETIOLOGY/PATHOGENESIS
- Most cases are human papillomavirus (HPV) related (> 90%)
- Serotype 16 is most common

CLINICAL ISSUES
- 1-2% of all SCC
- Large exoendophytic mass

MACROSCOPIC
- Unicentric papillary exophytic or endoexophytic tumor
- Level of invasion varies from superficially villiform lesions to deeply invasive solid tumors

MICROSCOPIC
- Papillae with central fibrovascular core lined by basophilic, poorly differentiated cells
- Resembles urothelial and condylomatous tumors
- Invasive component shows features indistinguishable from basaloid SCC
- Mitotic figures are numerous

ANCILLARY TESTS
- Positive for p16 immunostain

TOP DIFFERENTIAL DIAGNOSES
- Basaloid SCC
  - Shows no papillae
- Warty SCC
  - Abundant pleomorphic koilocytic cells
- Warty-basaloid SCC
  - Papillae are composed of both large clear and small basaloid cells
- Papillary NOS SCC
  - Papillae lined by well-differentiated cells with eosinophilic cytoplasm (pink cells)
- Urothelial carcinoma of distal urethra
  - Positive for uroplakin-2/-3, GATA3, and CK20 immunostains

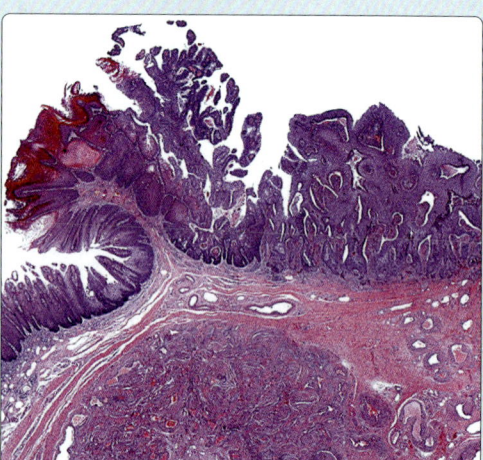

Low Power

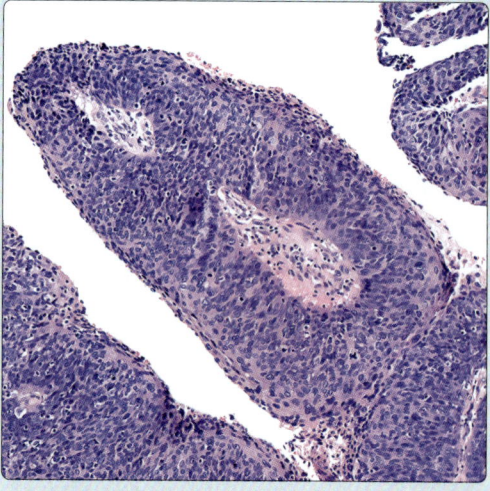

Intermediate Power

(Left) Low-power view of this tumor shows a basaloid exophytic papillary pattern of growth at the surface with a sharp, noninvasive tumor base. (Right) Medium magnification shows central fibrovascular cores lined by small, poorly differentiated basaloid cells with scanty cytoplasm. Cells boundaries are indistinct with abundant mitoses and apoptosis. Invasion should be evaluated in all lesions and sampling of all tissue is critical.

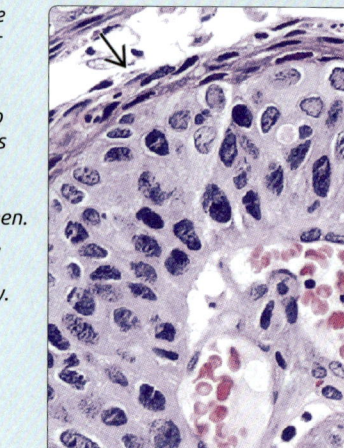

High Power

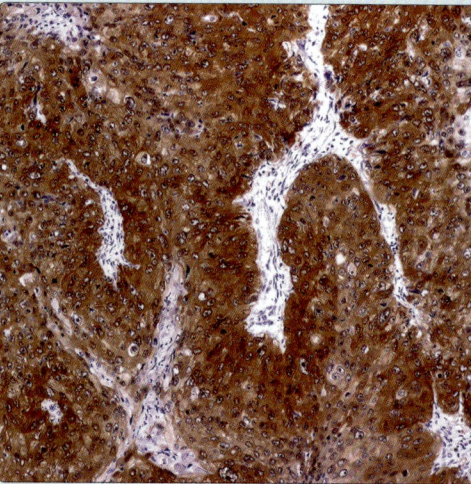

Immunohistochemistry

(Left) The papillae cores are composed of small vascular spaces surrounded by loose connective tissue. Tumoral nuclei vary from rounded to fusiform with inconspicuous nucleoli. Clear perinuclear artifact and atypical parakeratosis ➡ may be seen. (Right) Like in basaloid SCC, the neoplastic cells show diffuse and strong positivity.

Basaloid Squamous Cell Carcinoma, Papillary Variant

TERMINOLOGY

Synonyms
- Papillary basaloid squamous cell carcinoma (SCC)

Definitions
- Human papillomavirus (HPV)-related papillary tumor composed of small basophilic cells; variant of basaloid carcinoma

ETIOLOGY/PATHOGENESIS

Infectious Agents
- Most cases are HPV related (> 90%)
- Serotype 16 is most common

CLINICAL ISSUES

Epidemiology
- Incidence
  - 1-2% of all SCC
- Age
  - Average: 60-80 years (cases reported from 35-90)

Presentation
- Large exoendophytic mass
- > 1/2 of patients have positive inguinal nodes at diagnosis

Treatment
- Surgical approaches
  - Circumcision in tumors circumscribed to foreskin
  - Partial or total penectomy
  - Bilateral groin dissection in clinically evident compromised nodes or in tumors invading erectile corpora
- Adjuvant therapy
  - Limited experience for chemotherapy treatment

Prognosis
- Local recurrences are rare, it was reported in 1 of 12 cases
- Regional metastasis present in > 1/2 of patients
- High mortality rate but lower than classic basaloid SCC

MACROSCOPIC

General Features
- Unicentric papillary exophytic or endoexophytic tumor
- Usually located in glans
- Level of invasion varies from superficially villiform lesions to deeply invasive solid tumors
- Tan-gray papillary or spiky surface

MICROSCOPIC

Histologic Features
- Papillae with central fibrovascular core lined by basophilic poorly differentiated cells
- Basaloid cells are small, with scanty cytoplasm and round to ovoid nuclei with inconspicuous nucleoli
- Mitotic figures are numerous
- Keratinization is uncommon and when present is abrupt
- Resembles urothelial and atypical condylomatous tumors
- Invasive component shows features indistinguishable from basaloid SCC
- Cells with perinuclear halos and spindle cell features are rare
- Necrosis, lymphatic vascular invasion, and, less commonly, perineural invasion may be observed
- Undifferentiated penile intraepithelial neoplasm (PeIN) and rarely lichen sclerosus may be associated

ANCILLARY TESTS

Histochemistry
- Positive for p16 immunostain

DIFFERENTIAL DIAGNOSIS

Basaloid Squamous Cell Carcinoma
- Nesting pattern and shows no papillae

Warty Squamous Cell Carcinoma
- Large cells with eosinophilic cytoplasm (pink cells)
- Abundant pleomorphic koilocytic cells
- Cells with scant cytoplasm restricted to basal layer

Warty-Basaloid Squamous Cell Carcinoma
- Warty features on surface and basaloid features in deeper areas
- Papillae are composed of both large clear and small basaloid cells

Papillary Not Otherwise Specified Squamous Cell Carcinoma
- Papillae lined by well-differentiated cells with eosinophilic cytoplasm (pink cells)
- Usually associated with differentiated PeIN and lichen sclerosus
- Negative for p16, non-HPV-related tumor

Urothelial Carcinoma of Distal Urethra
- Adjacent flat urothelial carcinoma in situ or typical high-grade invasive urothelial carcinoma
- Sharper cellular delimitation
- Positive for uroplakin-2/-3, GATA3, and CK20 immunostains
- Non-HPV-related tumor

DIAGNOSTIC CHECKLIST

Pathologic Interpretation Pearls
- Papillae composed of homogeneous small basaloid cells with prominent central fibrovascular core
- Diffuse and strong positive p16 immunostain
- Invasive tumor component may be of warty-basaloid SCC subtype

SELECTED REFERENCES

1. Cubilla AL et al: Basaloid squamous cell carcinoma of the penis with papillary features: a clinicopathologic study of 12 cases. Am J Surg Pathol. 36(6):869-75, 2012
2. Chaux A et al: Diagnostic problems in precancerous lesions and invasive carcinomas of the penis. Semin Diagn Pathol. 29(2):72-82, 2012
3. Chaux A et al: The role of human papillomavirus infection in the pathogenesis of penile squamous cell carcinomas. Semin Diagn Pathol. 29(2):67-71, 2012

Warty (Condylomatous) Squamous Cell Carcinoma

KEY FACTS

TERMINOLOGY
- Condylomatous carcinoma

ETIOLOGY/PATHOGENESIS
- HPV-related tumor
  - Most commonly HPV-16

CLINICAL ISSUES
- Papillomatous tumor with cobblestone appearance
- Usually affecting glans
  - Often extends to other anatomical compartments

MACROSCOPIC
- Usually large, cauliflower-like tumor
- Exo- to endophytic neoplasm
- Papillomatous surface
- Variable (pushing or infiltrative) deep border
- Usually infiltrates corpus spongiosum

MICROSCOPIC
- Low-power view shows classical clear and dark pattern
- Arborescent/undulating papillae
- Pleomorphic cytology
- Numerous mitoses
- Atypical koilocytosis throughout neoplasm
- Variable (bulbous or infiltrative) deep borders
- Clear cell changes may be prominent
- Usually associated with undifferentiated PeIN (warty/basaloid)

TOP DIFFERENTIAL DIAGNOSES
- Condyloma acuminatum (including giant condyloma)
- Verrucous carcinoma
- Papillary carcinoma, not otherwise specified
- Mixed warty-basaloid carcinoma
- Papillary basaloid carcinoma
- Clear cell carcinoma
- Metastatic renal cell carcinoma

Penectomy Specimen

Schematic Representation

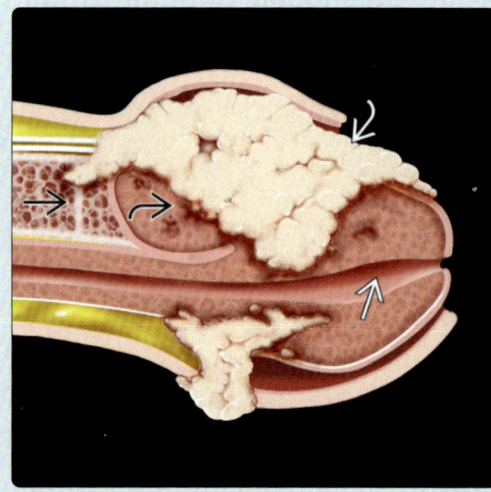

(Left) Cut section of a partial penectomy specimen shows a cauliflower-like, complex, papillomatous neoplasm deeply invading into corpus spongiosum, a warty (condylomatous) carcinoma (WC). (Right) Diagram shows a WC infiltrating the corpus spongiosum. Carcinoma ➡, corpus spongiosum ➡, corpus cavernosum ➡, and urethra ➡ is shown. Involvement of multiple compartments is common in large tumors.

Low Power

High Power

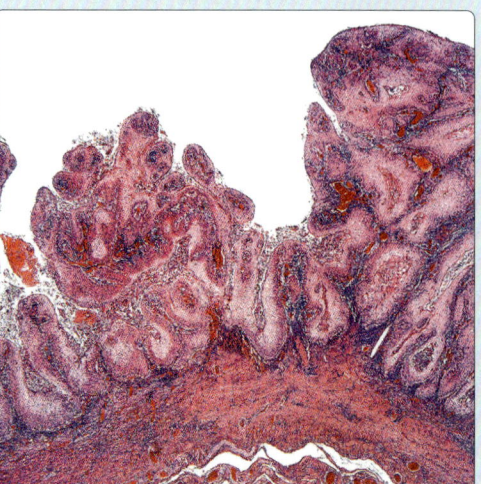
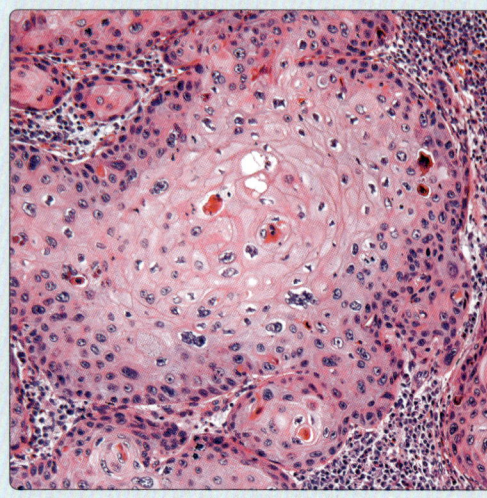

(Left) Low-power view of a WC illustrates condylomatous arborescent papillae with prominent fibrovascular cores. Note the dark (base) and clear (top) pattern. (Right) The deeper portion of this well-differentiated WC shows koilocytic atypia. Malignant cells with koilocytosis and infiltrative edge define malignancy.

Warty (Condylomatous) Squamous Cell Carcinoma

TERMINOLOGY

Abbreviations
- Warty carcinoma (WC)

Synonyms
- Condylomatous carcinoma

Definitions
- Tumor related to human papillomavirus (HPV)
  o Most commonly HPV-16
- Shares some gross and microscopic characteristics with condyloma
- Definitive malignant histology and metastatic potential

ETIOLOGY/PATHOGENESIS

Etiology
- HPV-related tumor
  o Most cases associated with HPV-16

Pathogenesis
- HPV oncoproteins E6 and E7 appear crucial in process of carcinogenesis
  o E6 interferes with p53 pathway, causing suppression of p53 normal inhibitory function of cell cycle
  o E7 targets retinoblastoma protein (pRB) interfering with p16/cyclin-D1/rb pathway

CLINICAL ISSUES

Epidemiology
- Incidence
  o 5-10% of penile squamous cell carcinoma (SCC)
- Age
  o 50-55 yr

Presentation
- Slow-growing verruciform/papillary tumor usually affecting glans
  o Coronal sulcus &/or foreskin may also be affected
- Usually presents as solid mass with papillary or cobblestone surface

Treatment
- Surgical

Prognosis
- Intermediate between that of other types of low-grade verruciform tumors (verrucous and papillary) and SCC of usual type
- It may be associated with inguinal nodal metastasis
- Worse prognosis associated with
  o Deeper invasion
  o Higher histological grade
  o Lymph node metastasis

MACROSCOPIC

General Features
- Verrucous exo- to endophytic cauliflower-like tumor
- Usually affects more than 1 anatomical compartment (glans, coronal sulcus, and foreskin)
- Cut sections show papillomatous surface
- Deep borders usually penetrate into corpus spongiosum &/or cavernosa
  o Deep border may be sharp or irregular/jagged

Size
- 5 cm in average diameter

MICROSCOPIC

Histologic Features
- Often long and undulating papillae with prominent central fibrovascular cores
- Sometimes rounded, arborescent papillae
- Atypical parakeratosis containing large nuclei is frequent
- Mixture of basaloid (lower epithelial layers) and koilocytotic cells (upper epithelial layers)
  o Gives classic light and dark low-power pattern
- Hallmark neoplastic cell represents koilocytotic cells with atypia
  o Enlarged nuclei with irregular contours
  o Frequent binucleation and multinucleation
  o Clear perinuclear halo
  o Dyskeratotic cells
- Atypical koilocytes present throughout tumor including deep nests
  o Not restricted to surface
- Cellular pleomorphism may be marked
- Clear cell changes may be prominent
- Numerous mitotic figures (including atypical ones) are frequent
- Variable deep borders: Pushing &/or jagged
  o Deep endophytic growth pattern may be seen
- Intraepithelial abscesses may be prominent
- p16 is positive in majority of cases
- Adjacent epithelium usually shows undifferentiated PeIN
  o Warty
  o Warty-basaloid
  o Basaloid

Predominant Pattern/Injury Type
- Papillary

Predominant Cell/Compartment Type
- Epithelial, squamous

DIFFERENTIAL DIAGNOSIS

Giant Condyloma
- Benign extremely well-differentiated lesion
- Papillary/arborescent surface
- Koilocytosis confined to surface
- No significant nuclear pleomorphism
- Bulbous sharp deep border confined to lamina propria
  o Presence of infiltrative border should raise suspicion of SCC arising in condyloma

Verrucous Carcinoma
- Extremely well-differentiated lesion with bulbous base
- Acanthotic papillae with thin fibrovascular cores
- Classical "piling-up" of orange keratin
- Lack of koilocytosis

Warty (Condylomatous) Squamous Cell Carcinoma

Papillary Carcinoma, Not Otherwise Specified
- Well-differentiated SCC
- HPV unrelated
  - Lack of koilocytosis
- Arborescent papillae
- Jagged infiltrative base

Mixed Warty-Basaloid Carcinoma
- Papillary surface showing features of WC
- Deep infiltrative base showing features of basaloid carcinoma
- Important to recognize because basaloid component has worse prognosis

Basaloid SCC With Papillary Features
- HPV related
- Papillary tumor
- Entirely composed of small basaloid cells
  - Resembling urothelial tumors
- Immunostains
  - p16 positive
  - Uroplakin-2, uroplakin-3, and GATA3 negative
- May represent papillary variant of basaloid carcinoma
- Better prognosis compared to basaloid carcinoma

Clear Cell Carcinoma
- HPV-associated tumor, very rare
- Affects penile mucosa
  - Inner portion of foreskin
  - Glans
- Solid and exophytic but no papillary
- Composed of large aggregates/nests of clear cells
- Comedonecrosis is common
- Often p16 positive
- Adjacent epithelium may show warty/basaloid PeIN
- High metastatic potential

Metastatic Carcinomas With Clear Cell Features (e.g., Renal Cell Carcinoma)
- Usually not connected to overlying epithelium
  - May show pagetoid intraepithelial extension of neoplastic cells
- Lack of papillomatous surface
- No true koilocytic changes
- Immunostains may be important to determine site of origin
- Multicentricity often present
- Involvement of corpus cavernosa vasculature
- Clinical history is important

DIAGNOSTIC CHECKLIST

Clinically Relevant Pathologic Features
- Most frequent penile carcinoma seen in HIV-positive patients

Pathologic Interpretation Pearls
- Clear and dark low-power pattern
- Arborescent undulating papillae
- Koilocytosis with atypical features throughout tumor

SELECTED REFERENCES

1. Sanchez DF et al: Pathological factors, behavior, and histological prognostic risk groups in subtypes of penile squamous cell carcinomas (SCC). Semin Diagn Pathol. 32(3):222-31, 2014
2. Chaux A et al: The role of human papillomavirus infection in the pathogenesis of penile squamous cell carcinomas. Semin Diagn Pathol. 29(2):67-71, 2012
3. Chaux A et al: New pathologic entities in penile carcinomas: an update of the 2004 world health organization classification. Semin Diagn Pathol. 29(2):59-66, 2012
4. Cubilla AL et al: Basaloid squamous cell carcinoma of the penis with papillary features: a clinicopathologic study of 12 cases. Am J Surg Pathol. 36(6):869-75, 2012
5. Soskin A et al: Warty/basaloid penile intraepithelial neoplasia is more prevalent than differentiated penile intraepithelial neoplasia in nonendemic regions for penile cancer when compared with endemic areas: a comparative study between pathologic series from Paris and Paraguay. Hum Pathol. 43(2):190-6, 2012
6. Chaux A et al: Warty-basaloid carcinoma: clinicopathological features of a distinctive penile neoplasm. Report of 45 cases. Mod Pathol. 23(6):896-904, 2010
7. Liegl B et al: Penile clear cell carcinoma: a report of 5 cases of a distinct entity. Am J Surg Pathol. 28(11):1513-7, 2004
8. Bezerra AL et al: Clinicopathologic features and human papillomavirus dna prevalence of warty and squamous cell carcinoma of the penis. Am J Surg Pathol. 25(5):673-8, 2001
9. Cubilla AL et al: Warty (condylomatous) squamous cell carcinoma of the penis: a report of 11 cases and proposed classification of 'verruciform' penile tumors. Am J Surg Pathol. 24(4):505-12, 2000

Warty (Condylomatous) Squamous Cell Carcinoma

Papillae in Warty Carcinoma
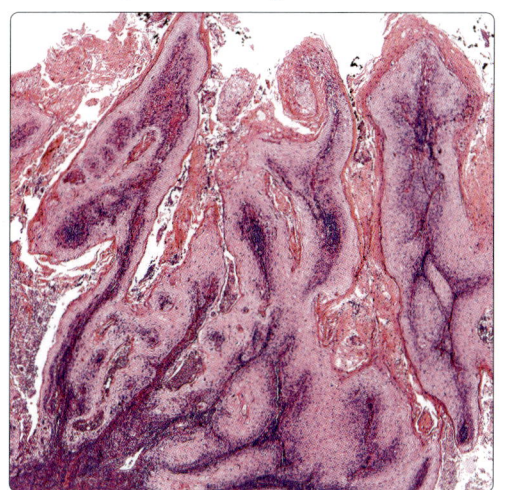

Cytologic Atypia
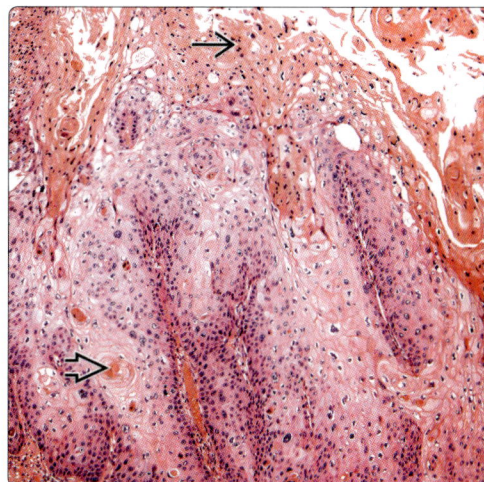

(Left) Another case of WC shows long and undulating papillae. As seen at low power, the key differential diagnosis is papillary carcinoma, not otherwise specified, although the dark and clear pattern is a helpful feature. (Right) Higher power view shows the papillae with prominent koilocytosis. There is marked parakeratosis ➡ and aberrant keratinization ➡.

Clear Cell Features
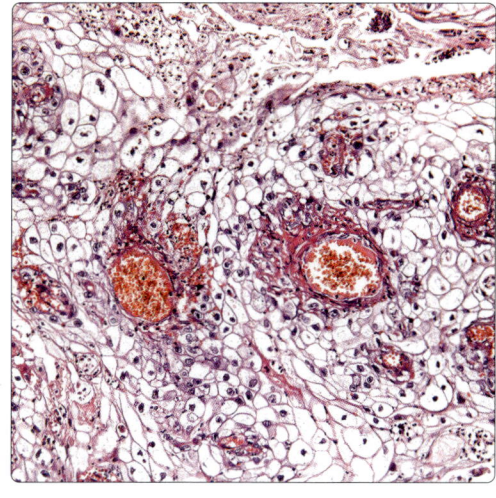

Invasive Front
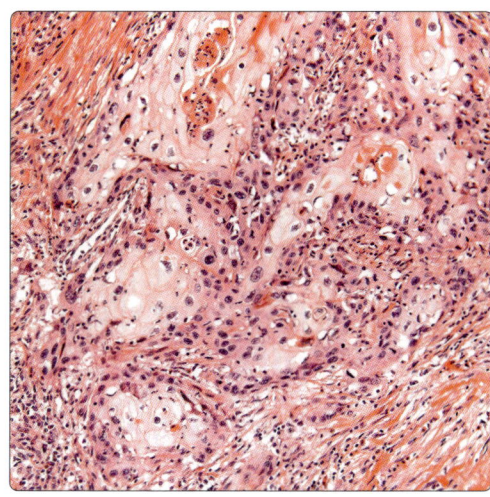

(Left) WC with prominent clear cell features is seen. The presence of papillae with prominent koilocytosis distinguishes this tumor from clear cell carcinoma of the penis, which is a solid tumor with confluent nests of clear cells often showing comedonecrosis. This tumor had associated foci of classical WC. (Right) WC with infiltrative and jagged deep borders is shown here. The tumor-stromal interface is irregular and signifies destructive invasion, a feature that is not expected in a giant condyloma.

Atypical Cells With Koilocytosis
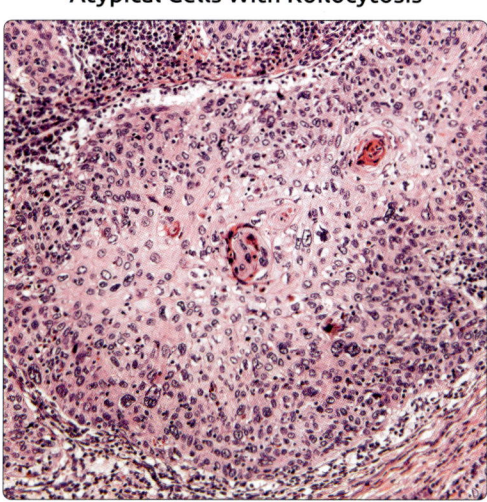

p16 IHC
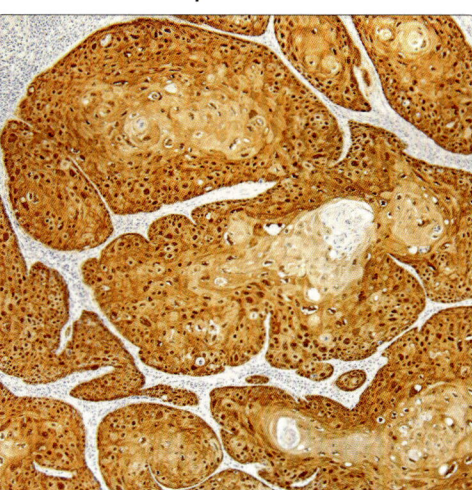

(Left) Koilocytosis is seen throughout the neoplasm. Note the obvious pleomorphic features of the neoplastic cells that are distributed randomly throughout. (Right) Immunohistochemistry with p16 shows diffuse positivity supporting the association of WC with high-risk HPV.

Warty-Basaloid Squamous Cell Carcinoma

KEY FACTS

TERMINOLOGY
- Mixed squamous tumor composed of condylomatous (warty) and basaloid features

ETIOLOGY/PATHOGENESIS
- Human papillomavirus (HPV)-related tumor
- HPV-16 most common genotype

CLINICAL ISSUES
- Large, aggressive exophytic tumor involving distal penis
- Regional metastasis present in ~ 1/2 of cases at diagnosis
- Mortality rate varies from 33-50%
- Represent 2-4% of all carcinomas

MACROSCOPIC
- Exoendophytic tumor
- Surface is villous papillomatous
- Cut surface shows papillomatous surface and solid deeply invasive tumor in erectile tissues

MICROSCOPIC
- There is combination of warty (clear) cells and basaloid (blue) cells
- Papillae are of condylomatous type, with central fibrovascular core lined by koilocytic cells
- There is invasive component with basaloid carcinoma features
- Vascular and perineural invasion are common

TOP DIFFERENTIAL DIAGNOSES
- Warty carcinoma
- Basaloid carcinoma
- Papillary variant of basaloid carcinoma

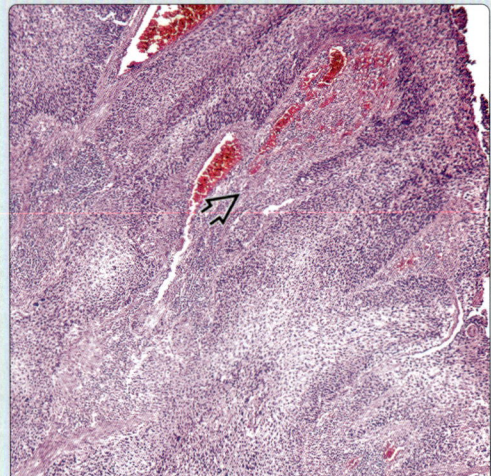

Warty-Basaloid Squamous Cell Carcinoma, Surface

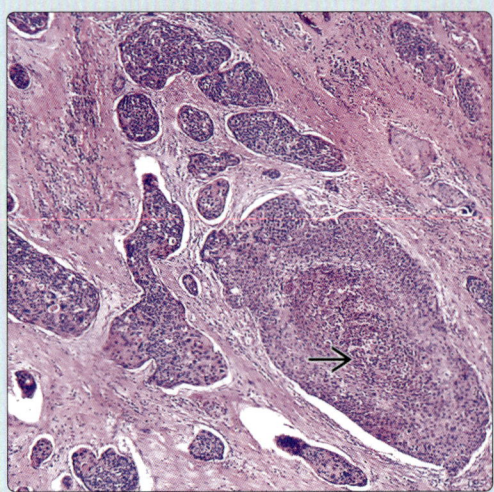

Warty-Basaloid Squamous Cell Carcinoma, Deep Basaloid Nests

(Left) Intermediate-power view shows a papillomatous invasive tumor. Note the central fibrovascular core ➡ and the clear and dark cell mixed pattern, typical of warty-basaloid carcinoma. (Right) The tumor shows a nesting pattern with comedo-like necrosis ➡, typical of basaloid carcinoma.

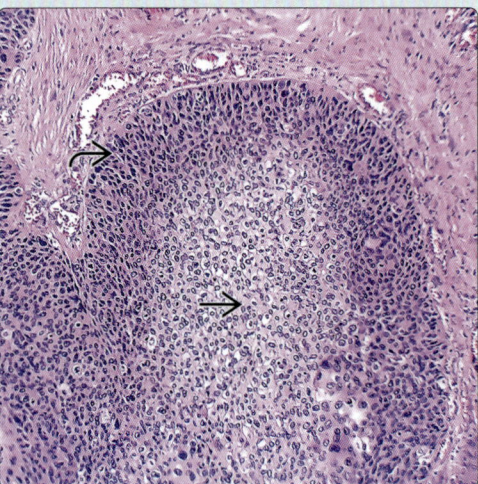

Warty-Basaloid Squamous Cell Carcinoma, Tumor-Stromal Interface

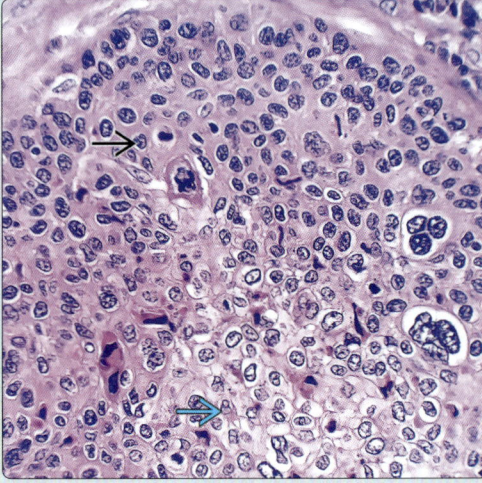

Warty-Basaloid Squamous Cell Carcinoma, Koilocytosis and Pleomorphism

(Left) Tumor nest with a biphasic central clear cell ➡ and peripheral small basaloid ➡ features is shown in the tumor-stromal interface. (Right) High-power view of the biphasic tumor. Central keratinizing cells show koilocytosis and are focally pleomorphic (warty component) ➡. Peripheral cells are small and uniform ➡ (basaloid component).

Warty-Basaloid Squamous Cell Carcinoma

TERMINOLOGY

Synonyms
- Warty-basaloid carcinoma

Definitions
- Mixed squamous tumor composed of malignant condylomatous (warty) and basaloid features

ETIOLOGY/PATHOGENESIS

Infectious Agents
- Majority of cases is associated with human papillomavirus (HPV)
- HPV-16 is most common genotype, but others may occur

CLINICAL ISSUES

Epidemiology
- Incidence
  - 2-4% of all penile carcinomas
- Age
  - Average: 65 years

Presentation
- Exophytic tumor mass in distal penis

Treatment
- Surgical approaches
  - Deeply invasive tumors; majority are treated with total penectomy
  - Tumors not invading corpus cavernosum are treated with partial penectomy
- Adjuvant therapy
  - Chemotherapy for cases with regional or systemic metastasis
- Radiation
  - There is no reported experience

Prognosis
- Regional metastasis present in ~ 1/2 of cases at diagnosis
- Mortality rate varies from 33-50%

MACROSCOPIC

General Features
- Large exophytic white-gray tumor
- Located in distal penis, glans, coronal sulcus, &/or foreskin
- Affects > 1 site
- Cut surface shows papillomatous surface and solid, deeply invasive tumor in erectile tissues

MICROSCOPIC

Histologic Features
- There is hyperkeratosis and papillomatosis at surface
- Papillae are of condylomatous type, with central fibrovascular core
- Clear cell koilocytotic changes are noted
- Features are indistinguishable from those of warty carcinoma
- There is invasive component with basaloid carcinoma features
- Prominent nesting pattern
- Central comedonecrosis
- Central abrupt keratinization
- Cells are small uniform and basophilic
- Vascular and perineural invasion are common
- In some cases, there is admixture of warty carcinoma (central) and basaloid carcinoma (peripheral) in same invasive tumor nests

ANCILLARY TESTS

Histochemistry
- p16 as surrogate of high-risk HPV

In Situ Hybridization
- High- and low-risk HPV detection

PCR
- Subtyping HPV

DIFFERENTIAL DIAGNOSIS

Warty Carcinoma
- No basaloid carcinoma component

Basaloid Carcinoma
- No warty (condylomatous) carcinoma component

Papillary Variant of Basaloid Carcinoma
- Papillae are condylomatous but composed of small basaloid cells; clear cells (malignant koilocytic change of warty carcinoma) are absent

DIAGNOSTIC CHECKLIST

Clinically Relevant Pathologic Features
- Exoendophytic tumor

Pathologic Interpretation Pearls
- Biphasic tumor composed of clear and blue cells

SELECTED REFERENCES

1. Sanchez DF et al: HPV- and non-HPV-related subtypes of penile squamous cell carcinoma (SCC): Morphological features and differential diagnosis according to the new WHO classification (2015). Semin Diagn Pathol. 32(3):198-221, 2015
2. Sanchez DF et al: Pathological factors, behavior, and histological prognostic risk groups in subtypes of penile squamous cell carcinomas (SCC). Semin Diagn Pathol. 32(3): 222-31, 2015
3. Chaux A et al: New pathologic entities in penile carcinomas: an update of the 2004 world health organization classification. Semin Diagn Pathol. 29(2):59-66, 2012
4. Chaux A et al: Diagnostic problems in precancerous lesions and invasive carcinomas of the penis. Semin Diagn Pathol. 29(2):72-82, 2012
5. Chaux A et al: Warty-basaloid carcinoma: clinicopathological features of a distinctive penile neoplasm. Report of 45 cases. Mod Pathol. 23(6):896-904, 2010

Verrucous Squamous Cell Carcinoma

KEY FACTS

CLINICAL ISSUES
- Usually unicentric
- Multicentric tumors may occur
- May be associated with longstanding lichen sclerosus

MACROSCOPIC
- Exophytic papillary tumor
- Broad and pushing base
- Usually confined to lamina propria
  - Rarely affects superficial corpus spongiosum
- Infiltrative base and foci of necrosis are not seen in verrucous carcinoma (VC)

MICROSCOPIC
- Acanthotic papillae
- Slender fibrovascular cores
- Prominent (orange) keratin craters between papillae
- Lack of koilocytosis
- Extremely well differentiated
- Epithelium of papillae and keratin predominate over fibrovascular core
- Pushing, club-shaped base
- Higher-grade areas &/or infiltrative borders are not features of pure VC
  - Such findings should raise consideration of hybrid/mixed variant of VC

TOP DIFFERENTIAL DIAGNOSES
- Condyloma acuminatum/giant condyloma
- Warty (condylomatous) carcinoma
- Papillary carcinoma, not otherwise specified
- Hybrid/mixed VC/squamous cell carcinoma (SCC) of usual type
  - VC with moderately and poorly differentiated foci and areas with infiltrative pattern
  - Hybrid VCs have more aggressive behavior
- Carcinoma cuniculatum
  - It is hybrid VC with peculiar burrowing pattern of growth

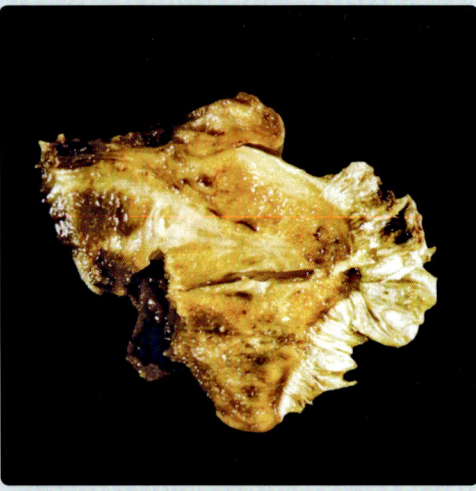

Verrucous Carcinoma: Gross Appearance

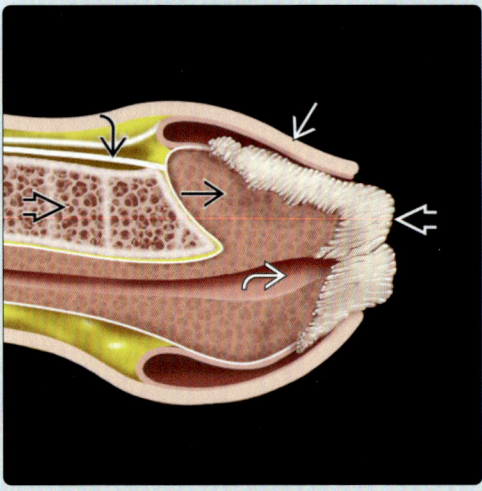

Verrucous Carcinoma: Schematic Representation

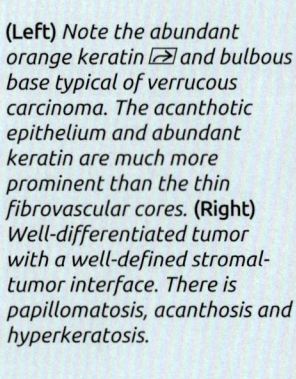

(Left) Cut section of a partial penectomy specimen shows a verruciform tumor with sharp bulbous base confined to the lamina propria. (Right) Graphic of a verrucous carcinoma (VC) (yellow) highlights the papillary, spiky surface and well-demarcated base. Note the VC ➡, corpus spongiosum ➡, foreskin ➡, albuginea ➡, corpus cavernosum ➡, and urethra ➡.

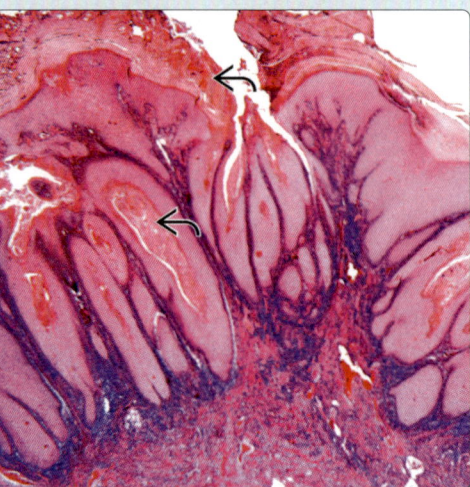

Verrucous Carcinoma: Low Power

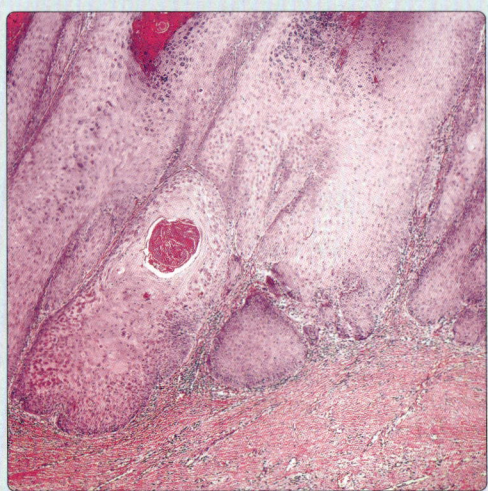

Verrucous Carcinoma: Broad Bulbous Prolongations

(Left) Note the abundant orange keratin ➡ and bulbous base typical of verrucous carcinoma. The acanthotic epithelium and abundant keratin are much more prominent than the thin fibrovascular cores. (Right) Well-differentiated tumor with a well-defined stromal-tumor interface. There is papillomatosis, acanthosis and hyperkeratosis.

Verrucous Squamous Cell Carcinoma

TERMINOLOGY

Abbreviations
- Verrucous carcinoma (VC)

Definitions
- Extremely well-differentiated verruciform squamous cell carcinoma (SCC) with bulbous deep borders and lack of koilocytosis

ETIOLOGY/PATHOGENESIS

Unknown Pathogenesis
- Likely human papillomavirus (HPV) unrelated
- Some cases are associated with lichen sclerosus
- p53 is believed to be involved in HPV-unrelated pathway of carcinogenesis

CLINICAL ISSUES

Epidemiology
- Incidence
  - Rare; ~ 4% of all penile carcinoma
- Age
  - Mean: 62 yr

Site
- Glans &/or foreskin
  - May be multicentric and affect > 1 anatomic site

Presentation
- Exophytic white-gray neoplasm
- 1-3 cm in diameter
- May affect glans, coronal sulcus, &/or foreskin

Treatment
- Surgical

Prognosis
- Pure VCs have excellent prognosis
- Pure tumors may recur but almost never metastasize
- Sporadic reports of sarcomatoid transformation after radiation therapy

MACROSCOPIC

General Features
- Exophytic white-gray neoplasms with papillary/spiky surface
- Cut sections reveal pushing (not infiltrative) deep border
- Tumors are usually confined to lamina propria
  - Involvement of deeper structures is less frequent

Size
- Average: 2 cm in diameter

MICROSCOPIC

Histologic Features
- Extremely well-differentiated neoplasm
- Thick acanthotic papillae with slender fibrovascular cores
- Papillae are separated by prominent keratin craters
- Orthokeratosis with presence of granular layer
- Parakeratosis may be occasional
- Absence of koilocytosis
- Pushing, broad club-shaped deep invaginations
- Adjacent epithelium often shows verrucous squamous hyperplasia &/or differentiated penile intraepithelial neoplasia
- Some cases associated with background of lichen sclerosus

Predominant Pattern/Injury Type
- Papillary

Predominant Cell/Compartment Type
- Epithelial, squamous

DIFFERENTIAL DIAGNOSIS

Giant Condyloma
- More rounded, arborescent papillae
- Koilocytosis on surface

Warty Carcinoma
- Higher histological grade
- Prominent koilocytosis with cytologic atypia throughout neoplasm
- May have infiltrative deep borders

Papillary Carcinoma
- Well to moderately differentiated, cytologic atypia
- Infiltrative borders

Mixed (Hybrid) Verrucous Carcinoma
- VC admixed with foci of SCC of usual type
- Focal infiltrative, jagged borders
- Focal higher-grade areas
- Prognosis is not as favorable as pure VC
  - 25% of cases associated with lymph node metastasis

Carcinoma Cuniculatum
- Hybrid (mixed) VC with higher grade foci
- Characteristic burrowing pattern

DIAGNOSTIC CHECKLIST

Pathologic Interpretation Pearls
- If entire lesion is not sampled, recommended diagnosis is well-differentiated SCC, verrucous histology
  - Acknowledges likelihood of unsampled moderately or poorly differentiated invasive conventional squamous carcinoma in definitive excision

SELECTED REFERENCES

1. Sanchez DF et al: Pathological factors, behavior, and histological prognostic risk groups in subtypes of penile squamous cell carcinomas (SCC). Semin Diagn Pathol. 32(3):222-31, 2015
2. Stankiewicz E et al: HPV infection and immunochemical detection of cell-cycle markers in verrucous carcinoma of the penis. Mod Pathol. 22(9):1160-8, 2009
3. Velazquez EF et al: Penile squamous cell carcinoma: anatomic, pathologic and viral studies in Paraguay (1993-2007). Anal Quant Cytol Histol. 29(4):185-98, 2007

Verrucous Squamous Cell Carcinoma

(Left) Low-power view of a verrucous carcinoma illustrates the thick acanthotic papillae, thin fibrovascular cores, and the classic piling up of keratin between papillae. **(Right)** Deep borders are bulbous and club-shaped in this case of pure verrucous carcinoma. Variable lymphoid infiltrate is present at the base.

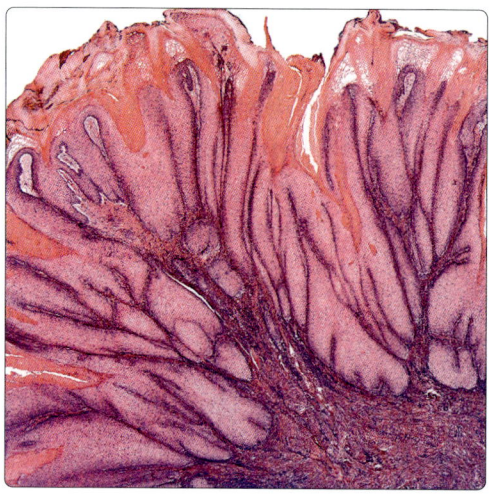
Verrucous Carcinoma: Exophytic Papillary Growth

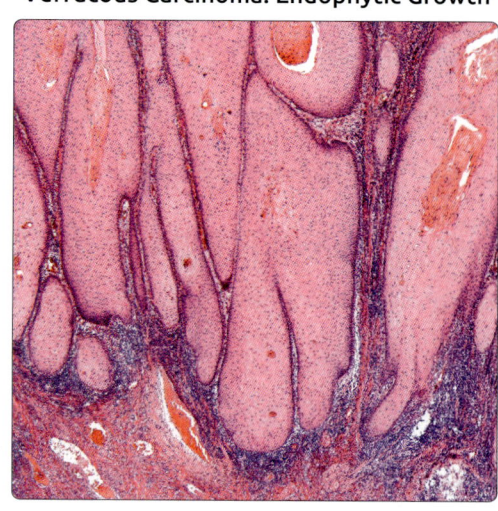
Verrucous Carcinoma: Endophytic Growth

(Left) Verrucous carcinoma shows extremely well-differentiated endophytic bulbous borders. **(Right)** Abundant keratin-filled craters are usually seen in verrucous carcinoma. In a superficial biopsy specimen in which the entire architecture cannot be appreciated, the diagnosis of malignancy may be challenging. Clinicopathologic correlation with the size of the lesion &/or additional sampling is necessary.

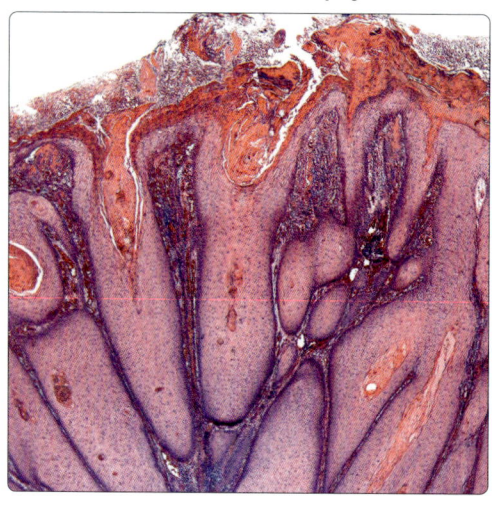
Verrucous Carcinoma: Endophytic Growth

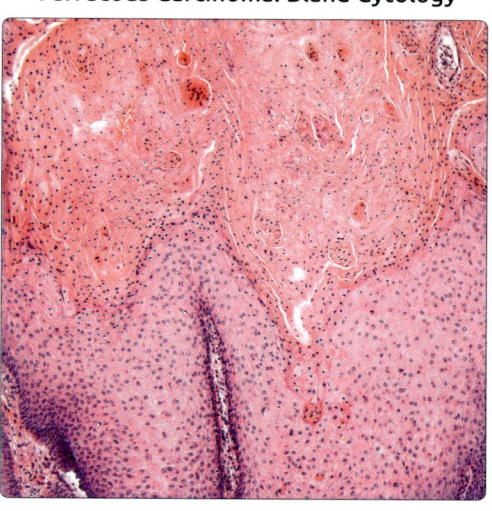
Verrucous Carcinoma: Bland Cytology

(Left) Extremely well-differentiated tumor with craters containing abundant (orange) keratin material ⇨ in this case of verrucous carcinoma. **(Right)** Note the club-shaped bulbous deep borders. Pure verrucous carcinoma is extremely well-differentiated, including its deep portion. The bulbous base is a key differentiating feature from pseudoepitheliomatous hyperplasia, which has narrow elongated rete ridges. The absence of koilocytic atypia helps distinguish it from a giant condyloma.

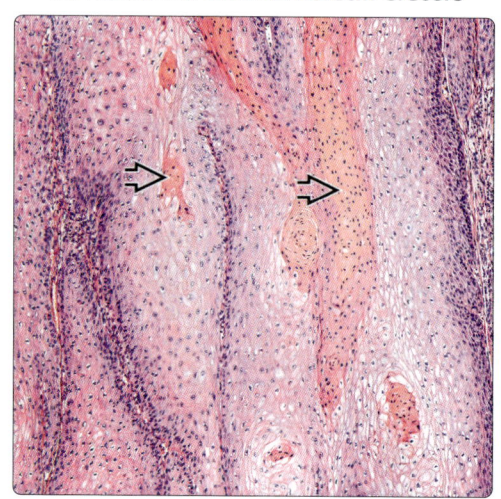
Verrucous Carcinoma: Keratin Craters

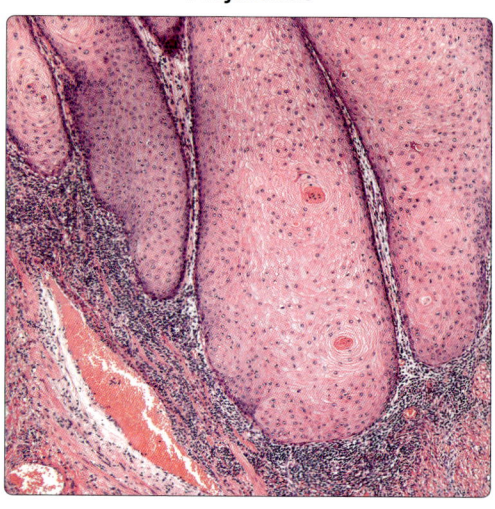
Verrucous Carcinoma: Broad Bulbous Projections

Verrucous Squamous Cell Carcinoma

Verrucous Carcinoma

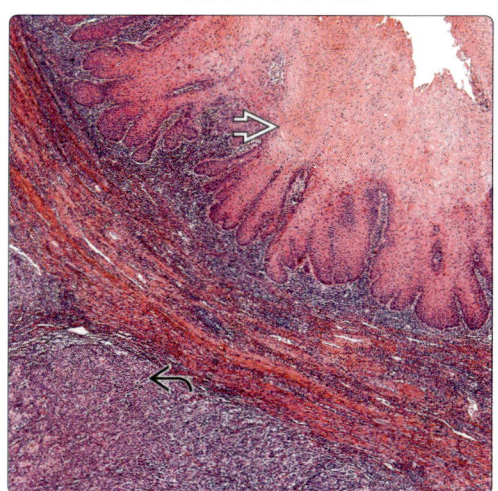

Hybrid Histology

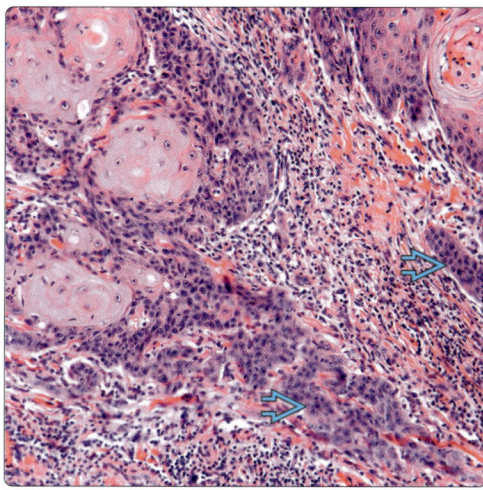

(Left) Hybrid (mixed) VC shows areas of classic VC ➡ associated with poorly differentiated areas ➡. If the entire lesion is not sampled, the recommended diagnosis is well-differentiated squamous cell carcinoma, verrucous histology. This acknowledges the likelihood that there may be unsampled moderately or poorly differentiated invasive conventional carcinoma in the definitive excision. *(Right)* Moderately differentiated foci with infiltrative pattern ➡ are incompatible with pure VC. They are usually seen in hybrid/mixed VC.

DD: Condyloma Acuminatum

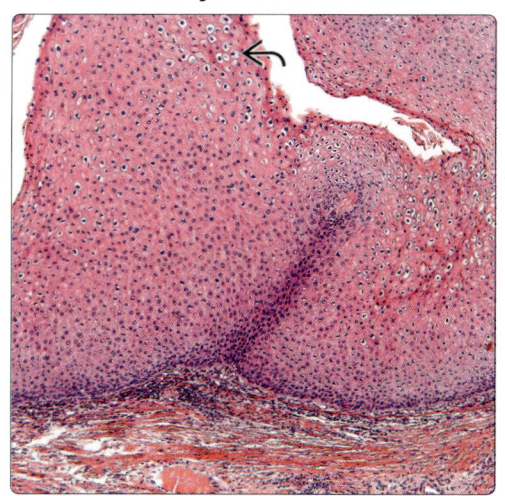

DD: Warty Carcinoma

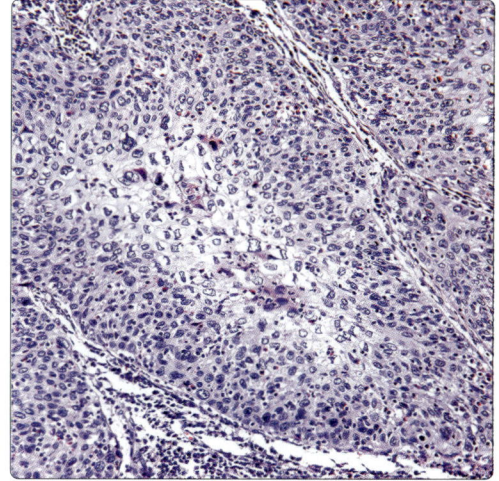

(Left) In this case of condyloma acuminatum, the lesion has some features reminiscent of verrucous carcinoma; however, there is koilocytosis on the surface ➡. *(Right)* Atypical koilocytic changes are seen throughout the tumor in this case of warty carcinoma. In addition to malignant cytologic features, this neoplasm demonstrates conventional destructive invasion at the base (not shown).

DD: Carcinoma Cuniculatum

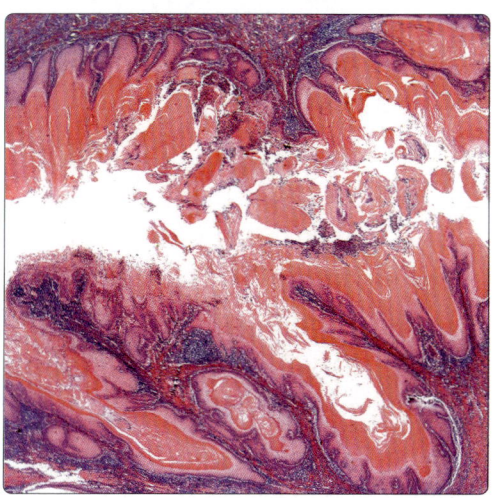

DD: Papillary Carcinoma, NOS

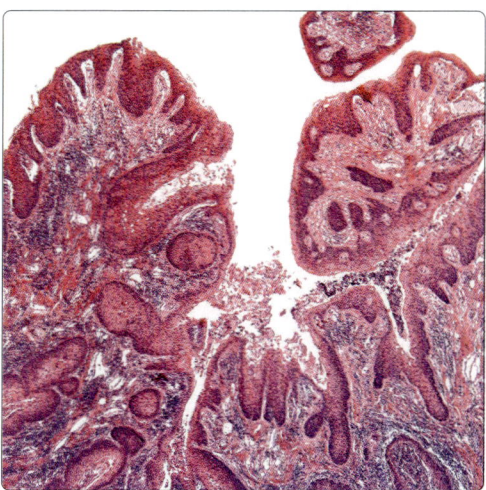

(Left) Carcinoma cuniculatum, the bulk of the tumor has features of verrucous carcinoma. The hallmark of the lesion is an endophytic and complex burrowing pattern; focal high-grade areas are usually present (not shown). *(Right)* Papillary carcinoma, not otherwise specified, shows arborescent papillae. Fibrovascular cores are more prominent than in VC. Papillary carcinoma, NOS, is less well differentiated than VC and shows infiltrative deep borders. It is distinguished from warty carcinoma by lack of atypical koilocytic changes.

Papillary Squamous Cell Carcinoma, Not Otherwise Specified

KEY FACTS

TERMINOLOGY
- Represents 5-15% of all penile squamous cell carcinoma (SCC)
- Accounts for 27-53% of all verruciform tumors

ETIOLOGY/PATHOGENESIS
- Unknown
- Frequently associated with lichen sclerosus

CLINICAL ISSUES
- Inguinal metastases are found in 0-12% of patients
- Cancer-specific mortality rate of 0-6%
- Less aggressive than usual SCC

MACROSCOPIC
- Exophytic verruciform pattern of growth
- Glans is most frequently affected compartment
- Extension to multiple compartments

MICROSCOPIC
- Papillae are architecturally complex
- Tips of papillae may be blunt or spiky
- Well to moderately differentiated carcinomas
- High-grade areas unusual; absent koilocytotic atypia
- Tumoral base irregular and jagged
- Squamous hyperplasia, differentiated penile intraepithelial neoplasia, and lichen sclerosus are frequently associated

TOP DIFFERENTIAL DIAGNOSES
- Warty (condylomatous) carcinoma
- Verrucous carcinoma
- Carcinoma cuniculatum
- Mixed usual-verrucous carcinoma
- Giant condyloma

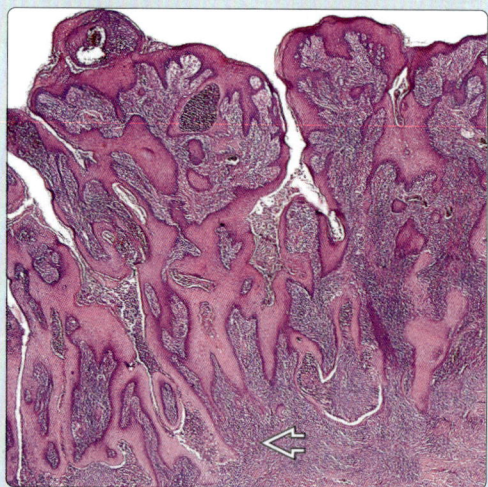

Papillary Carcinoma, Not Otherwise Specified (NOS)

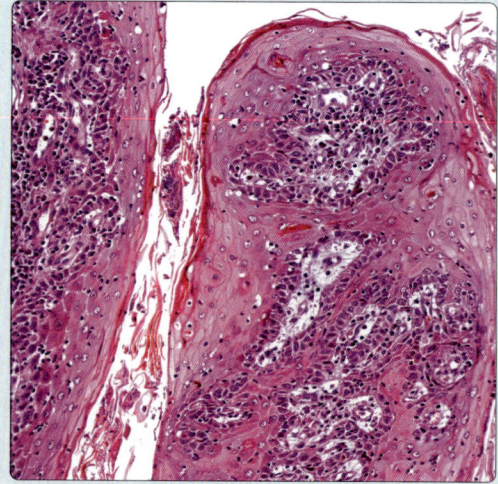

Papillary Carcinoma, Not Otherwise Specified

(Left) Low-power view of papillary squamous cell carcinoma (SCC) depicts the typical papillomatous pattern of growth with irregular and complex papillae and jagged tumor-stroma interface ➔ with a prominent stromal reaction. (Right) Histological features of the papillae include presence of mild acanthosis with moderate cytologic atypia, slight hyper- and parakeratosis, and no koilocytic changes in the epithelium.

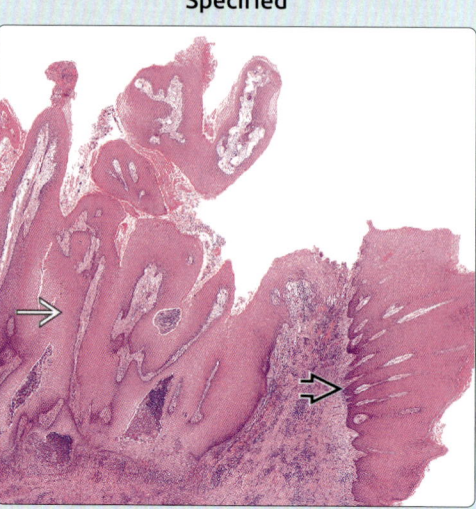

Papillary Carcinoma, Not Otherwise Specified

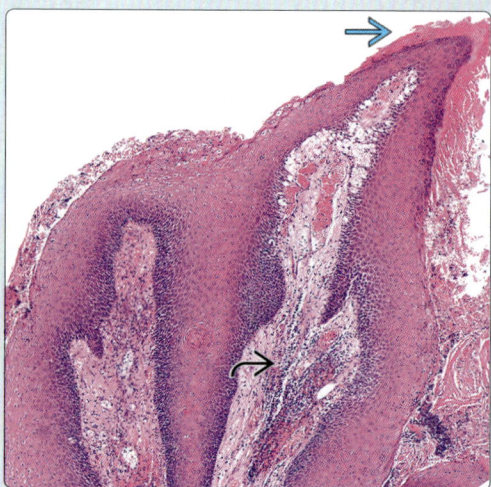

Papillary Carcinoma, Not Otherwise Specified

(Left) Low-power view of papillae ➔ shows the associated lesion, penile intraepithelial neoplasia (PeIN) ➔. (Courtesy Dr. Selina Bhattarai.) (Right) Intermediate-power view of papillae shows that there is a central fibrovascular core ➔ and hyper- and parakeratosis ➔. The base of the lesion (invasion) and cytologic atypia are important to recognize as carcinoma.

Papillary Squamous Cell Carcinoma, Not Otherwise Specified

TERMINOLOGY

Abbreviations
- Squamous cell carcinoma (SCC)

Synonyms
- Papillary carcinoma, not otherwise specified (NOS)

Definitions
- Low-grade tumor with exophytic pattern of growth
- Diagnosis is made only after exclusion of other verruciform tumors
- Represents 5-15% of all penile SCC

ETIOLOGY/PATHOGENESIS

Etiologic Factors
- Unknown but frequently associated with lichen sclerosus
- Nonhuman papillomavirus (HPV)-related carcinoma

CLINICAL ISSUES

Epidemiology
- Age
  - Average age: ~ 65 years

Presentation
- Granular and firm, cauliflower-like, large, exophytic tumor

Treatment
- Partial penectomy as primary treatment
- Inguinal lymphadenectomy according to risk group stratification

Prognosis
- Less aggressive than usual SCC
  - Inguinal metastases are found in ~ 1/10 of patients
  - Low mortality (0-6%)

MACROSCOPIC

General Features
- Exophytic verruciform pattern of growth
  - Glans is most frequently affected
- Average size: 4.5-5.8 cm
- Cut surface depicts serrated tumoral surface
- Poorly defined tumor-stroma interface

Anatomical Extension
- Affects multiple compartments
- Most tumors (65%) invade up to corpus spongiosum or dartos

MICROSCOPIC

Histologic Features
- Papillomatous pattern of growth
- Hyperkeratosis with parakeratosis
- Papillae are architecturally complex and may be short or elongated
  - Tips of papillae may be blunt or spiky
  - Central fibrovascular cores may be noted
- Most tumors are well to moderately differentiated SCC
  - High-grade areas are unusual and focal
- No koilocytotic atypia
- Tumoral base irregular and jagged
- Vascular and perineural invasion may be observed in some cases
- Presence in most cases of associated lesions in adjacent areas
  - Lichen sclerosus, differentiated penile intraepithelial neoplasia, and squamous hyperplasia

DIFFERENTIAL DIAGNOSIS

Warty (Condylomatous) Carcinoma
- More pleomorphic neoplastic cells
- Conspicuous koilocytotic atypia
- Jagged and irregular tumoral base
- HPV and p16 positive

Verrucous Carcinoma
- Less pleomorphic neoplastic cells
- Broad tumoral base with pushing borders
- Fibrovascular cores absent or very inconspicuous
- No koilocytic changes; HPV negative

Carcinoma Cuniculatum
- Less pleomorphic neoplastic cells
- Broad tumoral base with pushing borders
- Absence of koilocytosis; HPV negative
- Presence of cysts and sinus-like tracts connecting tumoral surface with deeper invaded areas

Mixed Usual-Verrucous Carcinoma
- Mixed pattern of growth
- Well-differentiated areas intermingled with more pleomorphic foci of neoplastic cells
- Irregular tumoral base due to presence of usual SCC
- High histological grade areas (usual SCC component)

Giant Condyloma
- Condylomatous papillae
- Conspicuous koilocytic changes
- Absence of pleomorphic or clearly malignant cells
- Broad tumoral base with pushing borders
- Low-risk HPV infection detected in most cases

SELECTED REFERENCES

1. Sanchez DF et al: HPV- and non-HPV-related subtypes of penile squamous cell carcinoma (SCC): Morphological features and differential diagnosis according to the new WHO classification (2015). Semin Diagn Pathol. 32(3):198-221, 2015
2. Guimarães GC et al: Penile squamous cell carcinoma clinicopathological features, nodal metastasis and outcome in 333 cases. J Urol. 182(2):528-34; discussion 534, 2009
3. Cubilla AL et al: Histologic classification of penile carcinoma and its relation to outcome in 61 patients with primary resection. Int J Surg Pathol. 9(2):111-20, 2001
4. Cubilla AL et al: Warty (condylomatous) squamous cell carcinoma of the penis: a report of 11 cases and proposed classification of 'verruciform' penile tumors. Am J Surg Pathol. 24(4):505-12, 2000
5. Gregoire L et al: Preferential association of human papillomavirus with high-grade histologic variants of penile-invasive squamous cell carcinoma. J Natl Cancer Inst. 87(22):1705-9, 1995

Papillary Squamous Cell Carcinoma, Not Otherwise Specified

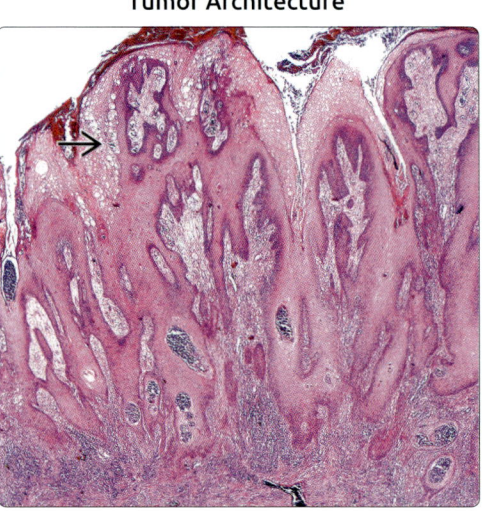
Tumor Architecture

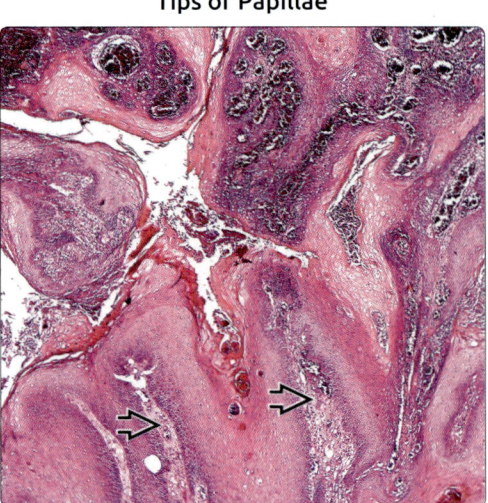
Tips of Papillae

(Left) Diagnostic clues include presence of papillomatosis with irregularly shaped papillae and occasional superficial clear cell changes ⇒, not to be confused with koilocytes, more or less prominent fibrovascular cores, and jagged tumor base. (Right) Papillae, short or elongated, depict a complex architecture; fibrovascular cores ⇒ are irregular, and, on low-power view, the histologic picture may simulate condylomatous features, resembling those of warty carcinoma. Koilocytosis is lacking.

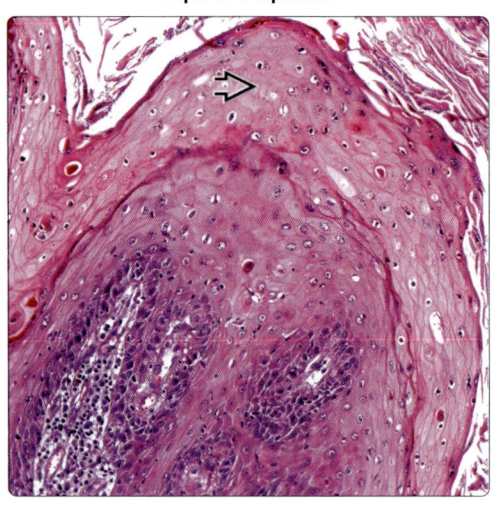
Tips of Papillae

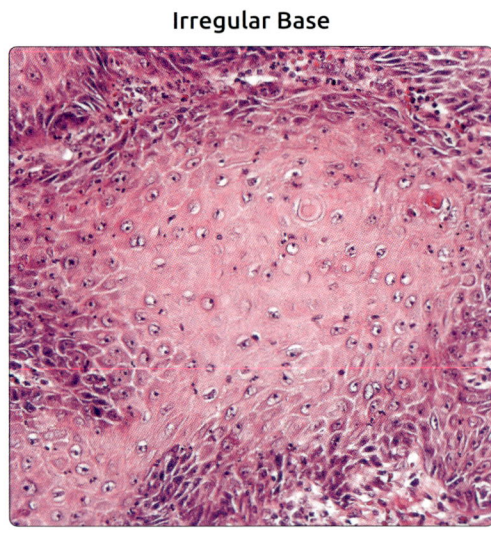
Irregular Base

(Left) Papillae usually show mild acanthosis with parakeratosis ⇒, and neoplastic cells are well to moderately differentiated with easily recognized cytologic atypia. (Right) Base of the papillae shows irregular nests of neoplastic cells with mild to moderate atypia, ample and acidophilic cytoplasm, distinctive cellular borders, and retained epithelial maturation. Cytologic atypia and invasion define malignancy.

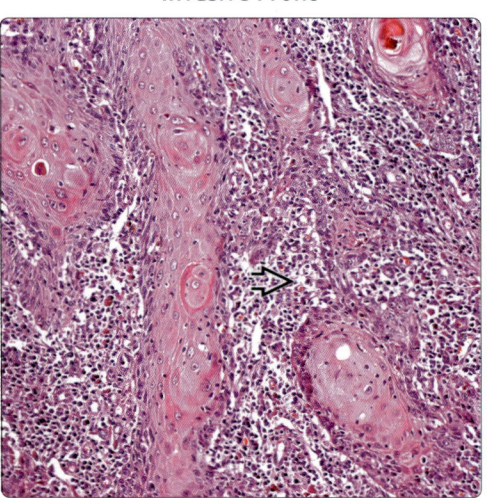
Invasive Front

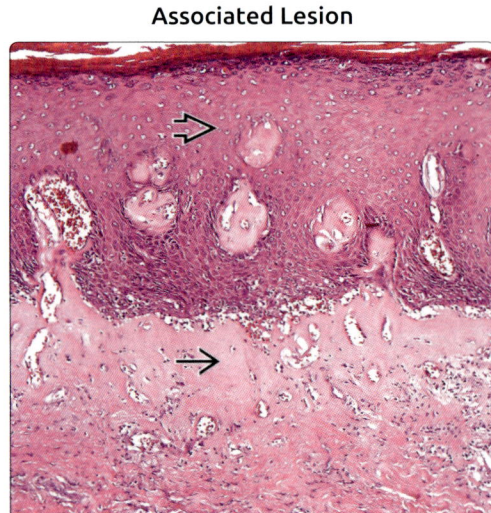
Associated Lesion

(Left) Front of invasion of papillary SCC with irregular nests of neoplastic cells imparts a jagged aspect to the tumoral base and an intense stromal reaction ⇒. (Right) Differentiated PeIN (low-grade intraepithelial lesion) ⇒, associated with underlying lichen sclerosus ⇒, is a common finding in papillary carcinoma.

Papillary Squamous Cell Carcinoma, Not Otherwise Specified

Warty Carcinoma, Low Power
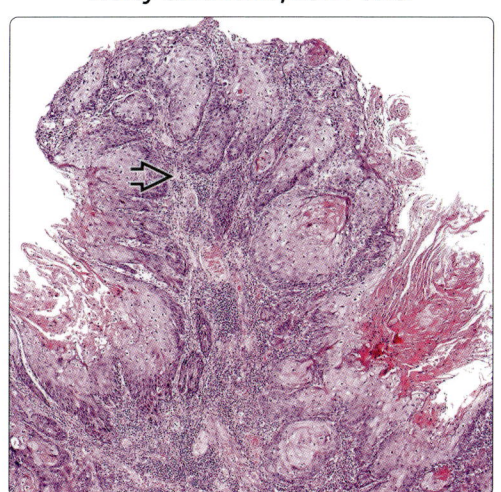

Warty Carcinoma, High Power
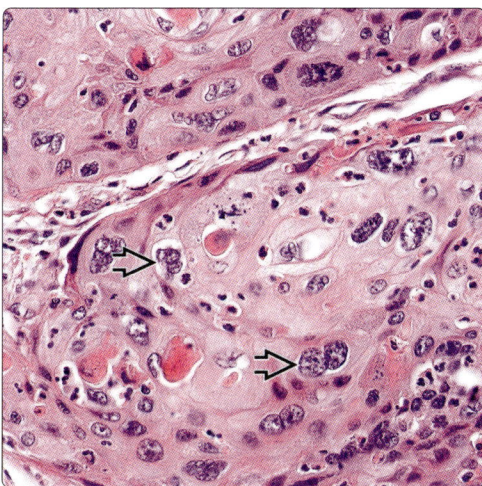

(Left) Warty carcinoma also shows a papillomatous pattern of growth and may be easily confused with papillary carcinoma; fibrovascular cores ⇨ are consistently present in the former, and most of the papillae are elongated and spiky. **(Right)** Warty carcinoma is defined by neoplastic cells with koilocytic atypia ⇨, sharing with papillary carcinoma a papillomatous architecture, keratinizing epithelium, and destructive stromal invasion.

Giant Condyloma
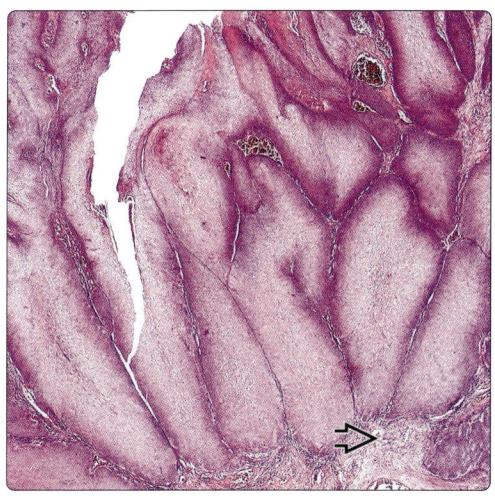

Verrucous Carcinoma
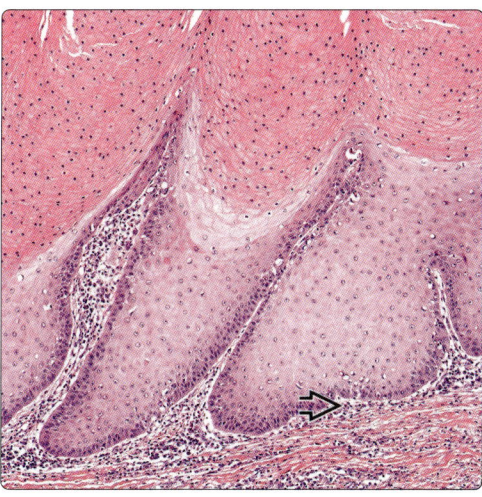

(Left) In giant condyloma, a verruciform tumor that may be confused with papillary carcinoma, koilocytes are easily found, although, marked cytologic atypia is absent and tumoral front ⇨ is broad and pushing. **(Right)** In verrucous carcinoma, the tumor front ⇨ is broad and pushing, fibrovascular cores are inconspicuous or absent, and neoplastic cells are extremely well differentiated.

Differential Diagnosis
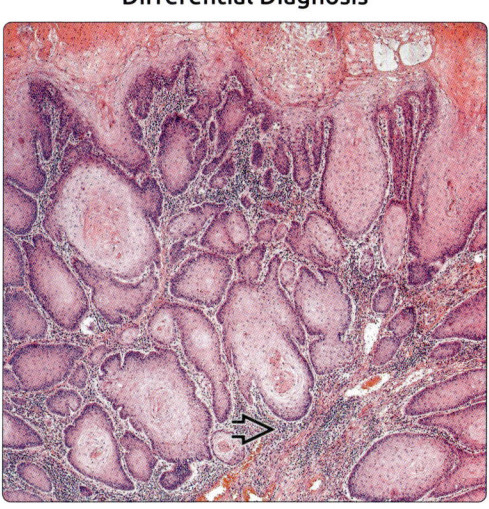

Papillary Carcinoma
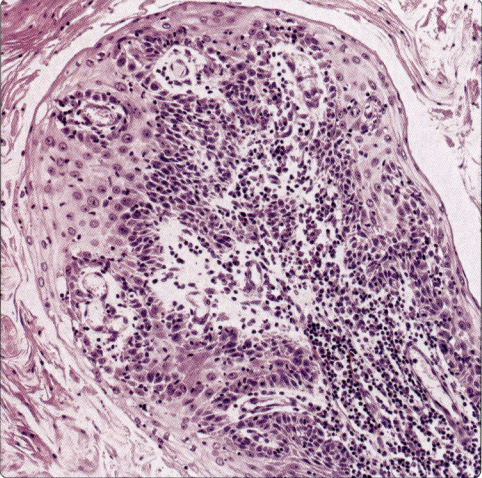

(Left) Carcinoma cuniculatum shows cytologic and architectural features similar to those of verrucous carcinoma but with extensive infiltration of deep anatomical levels ⇨ and formation of sinus tracks and cyst-like structures, findings that are absent in papillary carcinomas. **(Right)** Papillary carcinoma usually does not show overexpression of p16, a cell cycle-related protein that is used as a surrogate for high-risk human papillomavirus infection.

Pseudoglandular Squamous Cell Carcinoma

KEY FACTS

TERMINOLOGY
- Unusual high-grade carcinoma with prominent acantholysis and pseudoglandular features

CLINICAL ISSUES
- 1-2% of all squamous cell carcinoma (SCC)

MACROSCOPIC
- Unicentric large destructive and ulcerated tumor
- Deeply invasive carcinoma

MICROSCOPIC
- Honeycomb or multicystic appearance at low magnification
- Pseudoglandular features in 30-85% of specimen
- Open spaces are surrounded by high-grade cylindrical to flat squamous cells
- Cellular debris, microabscesses, keratin, or acantholytic cells fill central pseudoglandular spaces (comedocarcinoma-like pattern)

TOP DIFFERENTIAL DIAGNOSES
- Surface adenosquamous or mucoepidermoid SCC
  - True glandular differentiation and areas with squamous features
- Sarcomatoid SCC, angiosarcomatoid variant
  - Show typical sarcomatoid areas
  - Architecture shows presence of pseudovascular spaces (mimicking angiosarcoma)
- Urethral adenocarcinomas
  - Homogeneous glandular differentiation
  - Positive: Uroplakin-2 or uroplakin-3 and GATA3
  - In situ glandular changes may be present in urethra

Pseudoglandular Squamous Cell Carcinoma, Low Power

Pseudoglandular Squamous Cell Carcinoma, Medium Power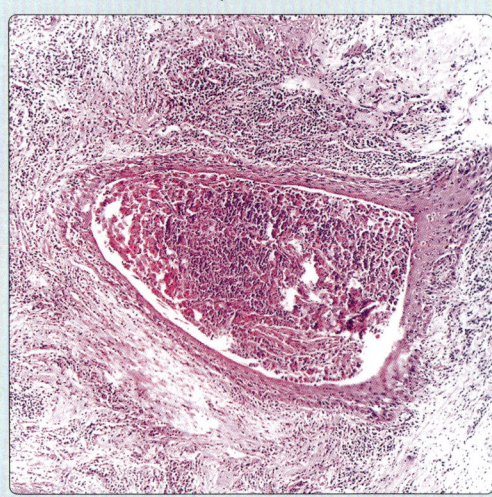

(Left) Low-power view shows tumor with multiple pseudocysts in a honeycomb pattern. (Right) Tumor nests with central acantholysis mimicking glands are characteristic features. The cytologic features are those of squamous cell carcinoma. The architectural acantholysis results in a pseudoglandular pattern.

Pseudoglandular Squamous Cell Carcinoma, High Power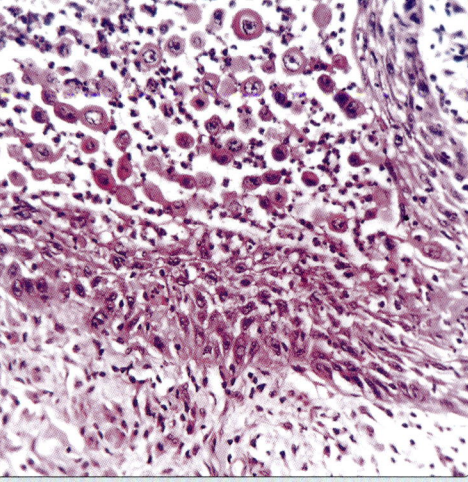

Pseudoglandular Squamous Cell Carcinoma, High Power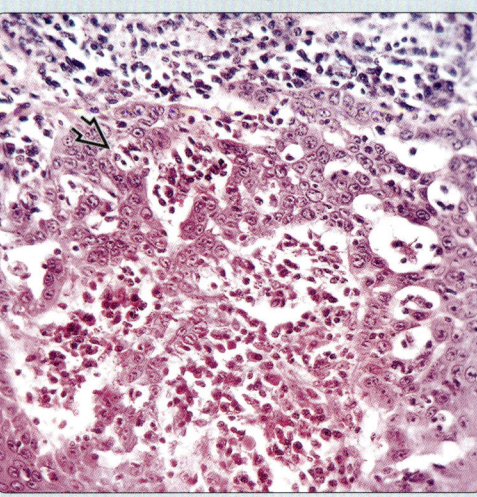

(Left) Pseudolumina are filled with amorphous eosinophilic material, keratin, neutrophils, and cellular debris. (Right) Pseudoglandular spaces are lined by single or multiple cell layers with severe atypia. Intracytoplasmic vacuoles ⇒ can cluster and form collarette structures in the wall of the pseudocyst. It is important to appreciate that background features are those of squamous carcinoma (not shown).

Pseudoglandular Squamous Cell Carcinoma

TERMINOLOGY

Abbreviations
- Squamous cell carcinoma (SCC)

Synonyms
- Acantholytic SCC
- Adenoid SCC

Definitions
- Unusual high-grade carcinoma with prominent acantholysis and pseudoglandular features

CLINICAL ISSUES

Epidemiology
- Incidence
  - 1-2% of all SCC
- Age
  - Average: 50-60 years (reported cases range in: 44-65 years)

Presentation
- Large ulcerated and destructive mass
- ~ 1/2 of patients have positive inguinal nodes at diagnosis

Treatment
- Surgical approaches
  - Partial or total penectomy
  - Bilateral groin dissection in clinically evident compromised nodes

Prognosis
- Local recurrence was reported in 2 of 7 cases
- Regional metastasis present in about 1/2 of patients
- Mortality rate, higher than usual SCC, is ~ 40%

MACROSCOPIC

General Features
- Unicentric large destructive and ulcerated tumor
- Average size: 4.6 cm
- Usually affects glans
- Secondary extension to multiple anatomic compartments
- Deeply invasive carcinoma
- Most of cases invade corpora cavernosa

MICROSCOPIC

Histologic Features
- Honeycomb (multicystic) appearance at low magnification
- Pseudoglands are mainly formed by solid nests with central acantholysis
- Cellular debris, microabscesses, keratin, or acantholytic cells fill central pseudoglandular spaces (comedocarcinoma pattern)
- Open spaces are surrounded by high-grade cylindrical to flat squamous cells
- Intracytoplasmic empty vacuoles in isolated or confluent arrangement (collarette) are seen in remaining cells
- Pseudoglandular features in 30-85% of specimen
- More solid nests or association with others SCC subtypes can be found
- Lymphatic-vascular invasion and perineural invasion are frequent
- Differentiated PeIN is present in > 1/2 of cases

ANCILLARY TESTS

Immunohistochemistry
- Some cases are positive for p16
- Negative for CEA

DIFFERENTIAL DIAGNOSIS

Surface Adenosquamous or Mucoepidermoid Squamous Cell Carcinoma
- True glandular differentiation associated with areas of squamous features
- Glandular lumen with clear or mucinous material
- Positive for mucin stains

Sarcomatoid Squamous Cell Carcinoma, Angiosarcomatoid Variant
- Epithelioid or spindle cells around pseudovascular spaces
- Typical sarcomatoid areas
- Positive: p63, CK5/6, HMCK
- Negative: FLI-1, ERG, CD31

Urethral Adenocarcinomas
- Adenocarcinoma in situ changes may be present in urethral mucosa
- Homogeneous glandular differentiation throughout tumor
- No squamous differentiation
- Positive: Uroplakin-2 or uroplakin-3 and GATA2

DIAGNOSTIC CHECKLIST

Pathologic Interpretation Pearls
- Hallmark of this tumor is presence of pseudoglandular structures
- Multiple histological areas associated with acantholytic features should suggest this subtype; at least > 30%
- Deep invasion is rule

SELECTED REFERENCES

1. Chaux A et al: New pathologic entities in penile carcinomas: an update of the 2004 world health organization classification. Semin Diagn Pathol. 29(2):59-66, 2012
2. Epstein JI et al: The penis. In Tumors of the Prostate Glade, Seminal Vesicles, Penis, and Scrotum. Washington, DC: American Registry of Pathology in collaboration with the Armed Forces Institute of Pathology, 2011
3. Cunha IW et al: Pseudoglandular (adenoid, acantholytic) penile squamous cell carcinoma: a clinicopathologic and outcome study of 7 patients. Am J Surg Pathol. 33(4):551-5, 2009
4. Colecchia M et al: Pseudoglandular (adenoid, acantholytic) penile squamous cell carcinoma. Am J Surg Pathol. 33(9):1421-2, 2009

Pseudohyperplastic Squamous Cell Carcinoma

KEY FACTS

ETIOLOGY/PATHOGENESIS
- Strong association with lichen sclerosus (LS)
- Non-HPV-related squamous cell carcinoma (SCC)

CLINICAL ISSUES
- Patients older than in usual SCC
- No inguinal nodes metastases
- Nonverruciform, hyperkeratotic tumor
- Surgical
- No cancer death reported

MACROSCOPIC
- Forms mass lesion
- Foreskin location
- Multicentricity
- Tumor with flat or slightly elevated hyperkeratotic surface

MICROSCOPIC
- Extremely well-differentiated carcinoma

- Infiltrative nests rarely beyond lamina propria in glans and dartos in foreskin
- Background of LS
- Adjacent epithelium shows hyperplasia &/or well differentiated penile intraepithelial neoplasia
- Superficially invasive
- Horn-pearl formation within infiltrating nests
- Lack of koilocytes

TOP DIFFERENTIAL DIAGNOSES
- Usual SCC, well differentiated
- Verrucous carcinoma
- Pseudoepitheliomatous hyperplasia

Pseudohyperplastic Carcinoma, Well Differentiated
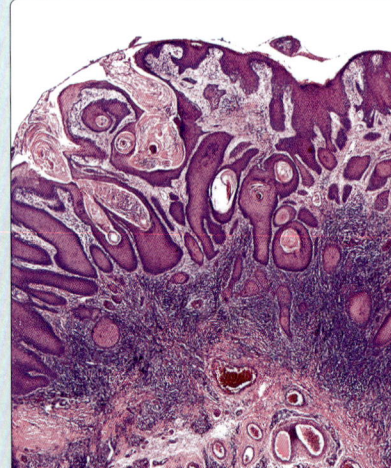

Pseudohyperplastic Carcinoma
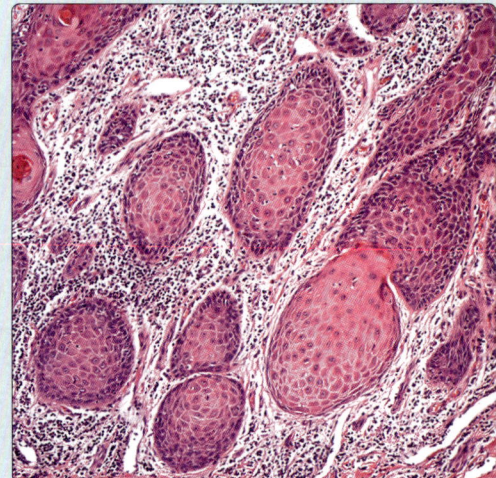

(Left) Well-differentiated pseudohyperplastic squamous cell carcinoma (SCC) is seen with a flat to polypoid surface and downward proliferation of irregular nests. The differential diagnosis is with pseudoepitheliomatous hyperplasia. **(Right)** Appreciation of infiltrative tongues of well-differentiated tumor that invade the subepithelial connective tissue helps distinguish pseudohyperplastic carcinoma from a pseudoneoplastic lesion.

Squamous Cell Carcinoma, Well Differentiated
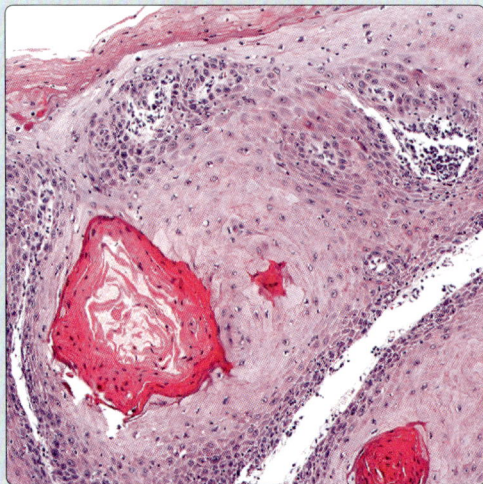

Pseudohyperplastic Carcinoma
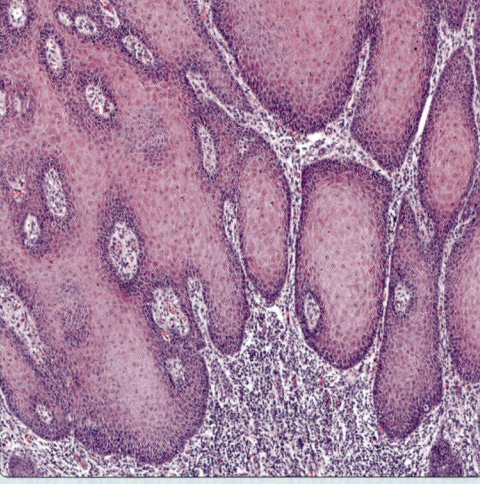

(Left) Well-differentiated SCC shows keratinizing nests with pearl formation. **(Right)** Orderly downward proliferation of squamous nests with mild basal atypia and reactive inflammatory stroma is shown.

Pseudohyperplastic Squamous Cell Carcinoma

TERMINOLOGY

Abbreviations
- Squamous cell carcinoma (SCC)
- Lichen sclerosus (LS)

Definitions
- Nonverruciform, low-grade, multicentric SCC preferentially affecting foreskin of older patients and strongly associated with LS

ETIOLOGY/PATHOGENESIS

Pathogenesis
- Unknown
- Strong association with LS
- Non-HPV related

CLINICAL ISSUES

Epidemiology
- Incidence
  - Only few cases reported in literature
- Age
  - 8th decade
  - Patients older than in usual SCC

Site
- Foreskin

Presentation
- Nonverruciform, hyperkeratotic tumor
- Usually affecting foreskin
- Often multicentric
- Slowly growing lesions usually arising in background of LS

Treatment
- Surgical

Prognosis
- No inguinal nodes metastases
- Minority of cases may recur showing higher grade areas
- There is no cancer death reported

MACROSCOPIC

General Features
- Hyperkeratotic, flat, or slightly elevated, nonverruciform tumors usually affecting foreskin
- Often multicentric
- Forms mass lesion

Sections to Be Submitted
- Due to multicentricity, careful examination of margins is advised

MICROSCOPIC

Histologic Features
- Extremely well-differentiated tumor
- Superficially invasive
- Confined to subepithelial connective tissue or infiltrate dartos in foreskin or rarely beyond lamina propria in glans
- Downward proliferation of keratinizing nests of squamous cells
- Horn-pearl formation within infiltrating nests
- Occasional individual cell keratinization and mild atypia of basal cells
- Lack of koilocytes
- Variable club-shaped and uneven/jagged infiltrative borders
- Asymmetrical infiltrative nests surrounded by reactive fibrous stroma
- Inflammation is usually mild
- Adjacent epithelium shows LS with hyperplasia
- May show differentiated penile intraepithelial neoplasia

DIFFERENTIAL DIAGNOSIS

Usual Squamous Cell Carcinoma, Well Differentiated
- Usually unicentric
- Most common in glans
- Histology of usual squamous carcinoma

Verrucous Squamous Cell Carcinoma
- Verruciform growth pattern with papillary architecture
- Elongated, broad, bulbous projections with pushing base

Pseudoepitheliomatous Hyperplasia
- Difficult differential diagnosis, especially in small biopsy specimens
- Limited to subepithelial connective tissue
- Infiltration of dartos or corpus spongiosum is not seen in hyperplasia
- Downward proliferation is more organized with elongated rete ridges
- Keratinization (keratin pearls) is less frequent
- Inflammation tends to be more prominent

DIAGNOSTIC CHECKLIST

Clinically Relevant Pathologic Features
- Often multicentric

Pathologic Interpretation Pearls
- It mimics pseudoepitheliomatous hyperplasia but deeper and more disorganized
  - Clinically, presence of mass favors carcinoma
- Diagnosis is difficult in small biopsies
- Pseudohyperplastic SCC is seen in elderly with longstanding LS
- Extreme caution is advised before making diagnosis of pseudohyperplastic SCC in young patients, especially in absence of LS

SELECTED REFERENCES

1. Sanchez DF et al: HPV- and non-HPV-related subtypes of penile squamous cell carcinoma (SCC): Morphological features and differential diagnosis according to the new WHO classification (2015). Semin Diagn Pathol. 32(3):198-221, 2015
2. Cubilla AL et al: Pseudohyperplastic squamous cell carcinoma of the penis associated with lichen sclerosus. An extremely well-differentiated, nonverruciform neoplasm that preferentially affects the foreskin and is frequently misdiagnosed: a report of 10 cases of a distinctive clinicopathologic entity. Am J Surg Pathol. 28(7):895-900, 2004

Cuniculatum Squamous Cell Carcinoma

KEY FACTS

TERMINOLOGY

- Squamous cell carcinoma, hybrid verrucous carcinoma
- Distinct variant of verrucous carcinoma characterized by deep burrowing growth pattern mimicking rabbit burrows (cuniculi); represents hybrid (mixed) verrucous carcinoma with unique growth pattern, sinus tracts

MACROSCOPIC

- Large exoendophytic tumor with cobblestone appearance
- Affects several anatomical compartments (glans, coronal sulcus, and foreskin)
- Hallmark of lesion is seen upon sectioning: Deep endophytic and interanastomosing pattern of sinus tracts mimicking rabbit burrows

MICROSCOPIC

- In most cases, carcinoma cuniculatum is hybrid (mixed) verrucous carcinoma with peculiar deep growth pattern
- Most of lesion is extremely well differentiated (verrucous carcinoma)
- Interanastomotic channels contain abundant keratin
- Sinus tracts are commonly seen
- Focal higher grade areas and infiltrative pattern are common (SCC of usual type)

TOP DIFFERENTIAL DIAGNOSES

- Verrucous carcinoma
  - Lacks higher grade areas and jagged borders
  - Lack of burrowing pattern
- Warty carcinoma
  - Prominent atypical koilocytosis
  - Overt infiltrative growth
- Papillary carcinoma
  - Lacks classic burrowing pattern
- Giant condyloma
  - Benign lesion with koilocytosis on surface

Carcinoma Cuniculatum, Cut Section

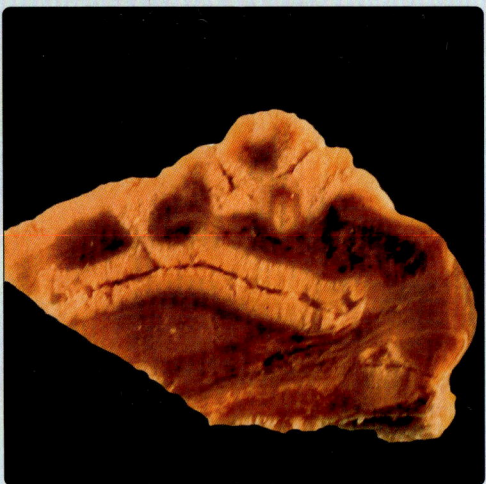

Carcinoma Cuniculatum, Low-Power View

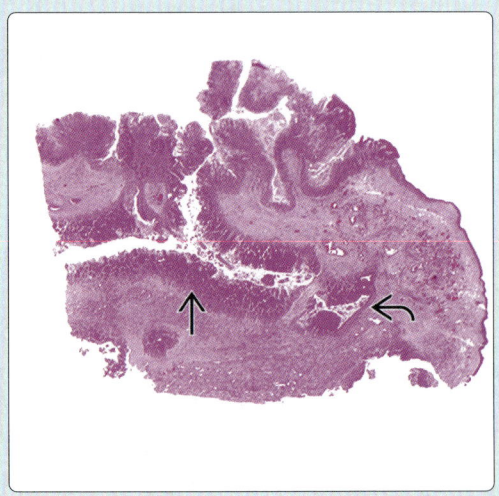

(Left) Cut section of a partial penectomy specimen shows a carcinoma cuniculatum. Note the deep tumoral invagination following the tunica albuginea and involving the corpus cavernosum. **(Right)** Low-power view of a cut section shows carcinoma cuniculatum. Note the endophytic burrowing channels ➡ and the deep pseudocystic space filled with keratin ➡.

Carcinoma Cuniculatum

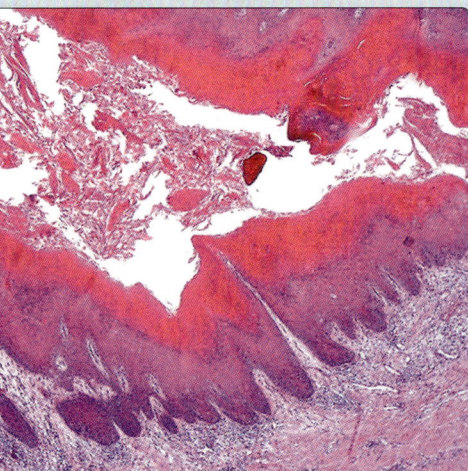

Carcinoma Cuniculatum

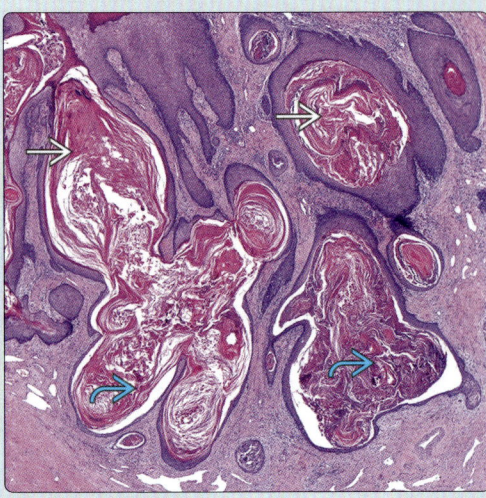

(Left) Tumor-stromal interface is well delineated. Here, the histology is of a verrucous carcinoma. **(Right)** Mid-power view shows the burrowing growth pattern ➡ and hyperkeratotic material ➡ filling the complex sinuses. Here, the histology is of a well-differentiated invasive squamous carcinoma.

Cuniculatum Squamous Cell Carcinoma

TERMINOLOGY

Synonyms
- Squamous cell carcinoma (SCC), hybrid verrucous carcinoma

Definitions
- Distinct variant of verrucous carcinoma characterized by deep burrowing growth pattern mimicking rabbit burrows (cuniculi)
- Represents hybrid (mixed) verrucous carcinoma with unique growth pattern with sinus tracts

ETIOLOGY/PATHOGENESIS

Pathogenesis
- Unknown
- Non-human papillomavirus related

CLINICAL ISSUES

Epidemiology
- Incidence
  - Very rare
- Age
  - Mean: 77 years

Site
- Usually affects glans and extending to coronal sulcus and foreskin

Presentation
- Large, papillomatous tumors with cobblestone appearance

Treatment
- Surgery

Prognosis
- Good prognosis
- No reported metastases

MACROSCOPIC

General Features
- Large, papillomatous lesion
- Cobblestone and sometimes spiky appearance
- Usually affects multiple compartments
  - Glans and extends to coronal sulcus and foreskin
- Cut sections reveal hallmark of neoplasm
  - Deeply endophytic tumoral invaginations mimicking rabbit burrows
- Deeply invasive keratin-filled pseudocysts or crypts are frequently seen

Size
- Average: 6.3 cm

MICROSCOPIC

Histologic Features
- Deep invaginations form interanastomosing channels and pseudocystic structures filled with keratin
- Interanastomosing channels and pseudocystic structures are lined by well-differentiated SCC
- Bulk of lesion has features of verrucous carcinoma
  - Extremely well-differentiated SCC
  - Acanthotic papillae with thin fibrovascular cores
  - Piling up of keratin among papillae
  - Bulbous deep borders
  - Lack of koilocytosis
  - Interface between tumor and stroma is sharply delineated
- Usually minor component showing features of SCC of usual type
  - Focal higher grade areas and infiltrative borders

Predominant Pattern/Injury Type
- Squamous

Predominant Cell/Compartment Type
- Epithelial, squamous

DIFFERENTIAL DIAGNOSIS

Verrucous Carcinoma
- Extremely well-differentiated verruciform tumor
- Lacks classic burrowing pattern
- Lack of focal higher grade areas and infiltrative pattern

Warty Carcinoma
- Prominent koilocytosis with malignant nuclear features
- Higher grade areas frequently with destructive invasion
- Lacks prominent burrowing pattern

Papillary Carcinoma
- Well-differentiated verruciform lesion with irregular, jagged, infiltrative borders and cytologic atypia
- Lacks classic burrowing pattern

Condyloma Acuminatum/Giant Condyloma
- Koilocytosis is seen on surface
- Lacks prominent burrowing pattern
- Lacks higher grade areas and infiltrative pattern

DIAGNOSTIC CHECKLIST

Pathologic Interpretation Pearls
- Well-differentiated tumor, similar to verrucous carcinoma
- Acanthotic papillae separated by abundant keratin
- Deep pushing borders
- Hallmark of lesion is deep and complex burrowing pattern
- Sinus tract formation is characteristic
- Focally, higher grade areas and jagged borders are frequent

SELECTED REFERENCES

1. Sanchez DF et al: HPV- and non-HPV-related subtypes of penile squamous cell carcinoma (SCC): Morphological features and differential diagnosis according to the new WHO classification (2015). Semin Diagn Pathol. 32(3):198-221, 2015
2. Chaux A et al: Comparison of morphologic features and outcome of resected recurrent and nonrecurrent squamous cell carcinoma of the penis: a study of 81 cases. Am J Surg Pathol. 33(9):1299-306, 2009
3. Barreto JE et al: Carcinoma cuniculatum: a distinctive variant of penile squamous cell carcinoma: report of 7 cases. Am J Surg Pathol. 31(1):71-5, 2007
4. Cubilla AL et al: Warty (condylomatous) squamous cell carcinoma of the penis: a report of 11 cases and proposed classification of 'verruciform' penile tumors. Am J Surg Pathol. 24(4):505-12, 2000

Cuniculatum Squamous Cell Carcinoma

(Left) The bulk of carcinoma cuniculatum has features of a verrucous carcinoma. Note the acanthotic papillae with prominent piling up of orange keratin ➡ between them. (Right) In most areas, carcinoma cuniculatum is indistinguishable from verrucous carcinoma. Note the deep, elongated, broad bulbous projections ➡ at the base of the tumor. Appreciation of deep growth and sinus tracts is important.

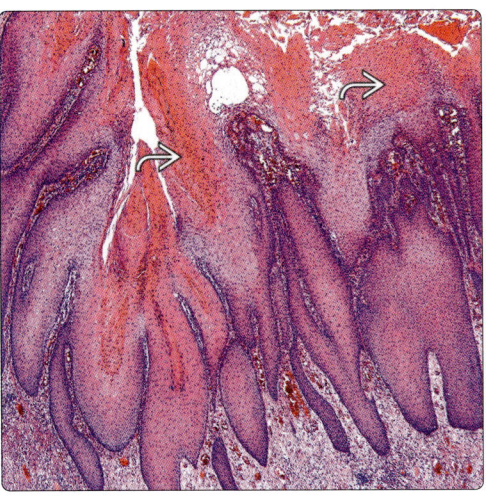
Carcinoma Cuniculatum

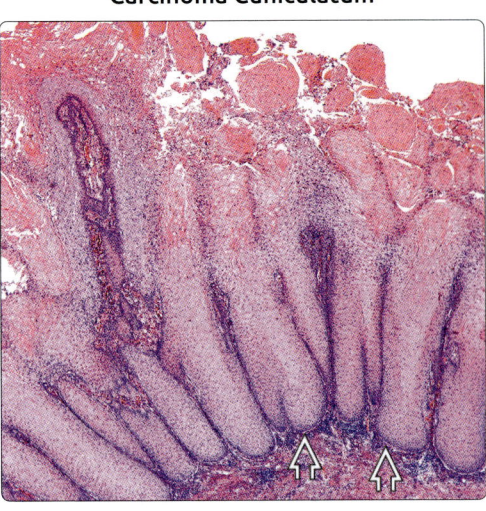
Carcinoma Cuniculatum

(Left) Bulbous deep borders and wide craters filled with abundant keratin ➡ are characteristic of the lesion. In a superficial biopsy, the presence of a well-differentiated epithelium with wide craters should raise the possibility of a verrucous carcinoma or carcinoma cuniculatum. Clinicopathologic correlation is necessary in such settings. (Right) Note the verruciform papillae with abundant interspersed orange keratin in this case of carcinoma cuniculatum.

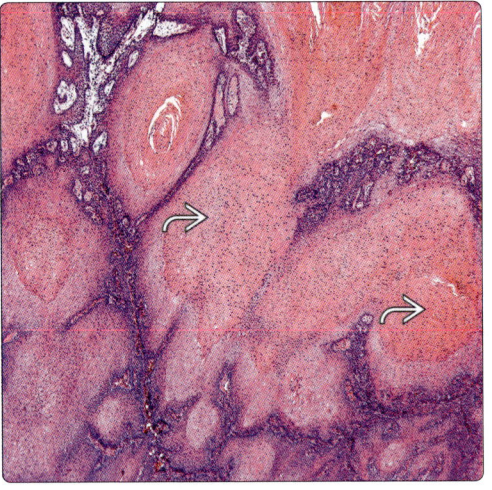
Well-Differentiated Carcinoma

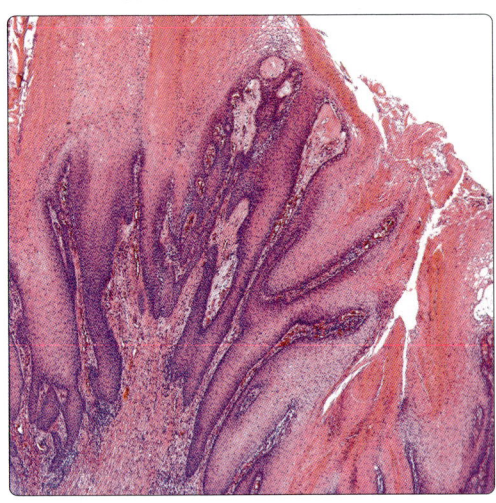
Carcinoma Cuniculatum

(Left) Complex tumor shows numerous irregular fistulae toward the surface. (Right) Sinus tracts communicating with the tumor surface are a frequent finding and a hallmark of this lesion. Note the opening of a sinus tract to the surface ➡. Areas of high-grade usual squamous carcinoma are focally present in most cases (not shown).

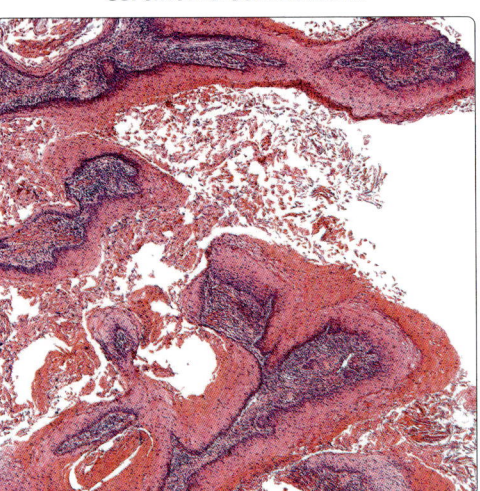
Carcinoma Cuniculatum

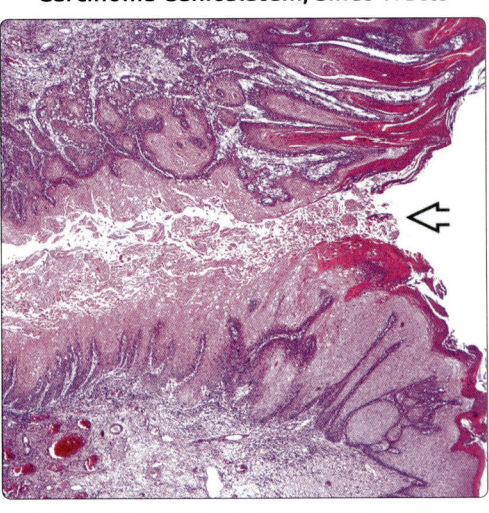
Carcinoma Cuniculatum, Sinus Tracts

Cuniculatum Squamous Cell Carcinoma

Carcinoma Cuniculatum
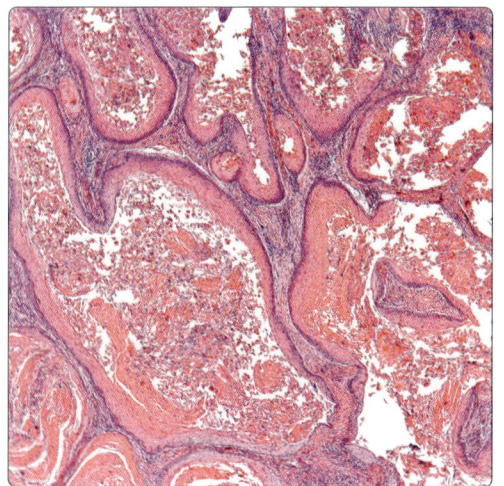

Carcinoma Cuniculatum
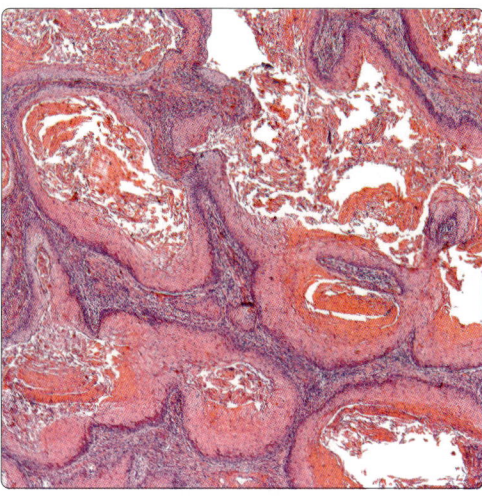

(Left) *Interanastomotic pattern, showing complex channels filled with keratin, is characteristic of the lesion.* (Right) *Interanastomosing and complex endophytic pattern is characteristic of carcinoma cuniculatum. The acanthotic epithelium is well differentiated and shows overall maintenance of polarity. Note the abundance of keratin within the endophytic channels.*

Carcinoma Cuniculatum, Low-Power View
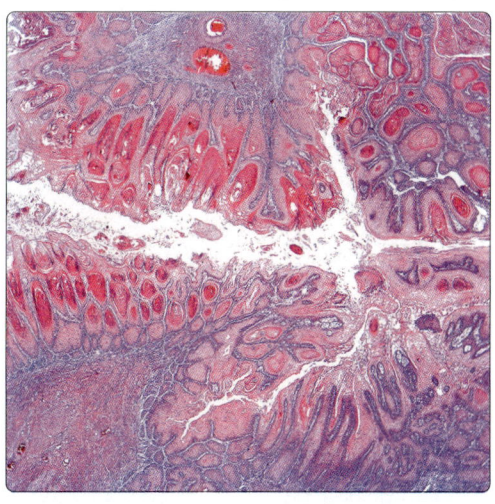

Carcinoma Cuniculatum
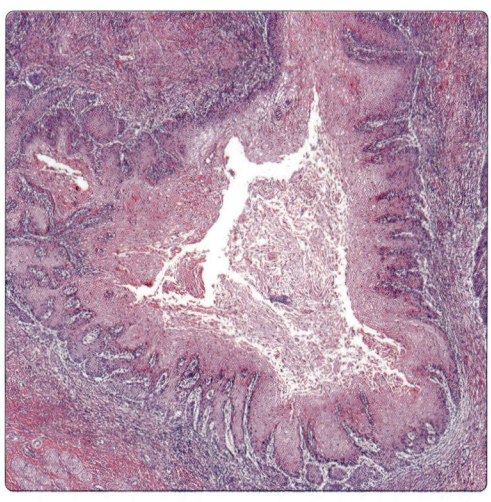

(Left) *Low-power view of carcinoma cuniculatum highlights the interanastomotic and complex pattern of this lesion. The deep burrowing pattern of well-differentiated epithelium mimicking rabbit burrows is the diagnostic hallmark.* (Right) *Carcinoma cuniculatum shows that deep tumoral invaginations may mimic cysts in some sections. This feature may be appreciated even at the macroscopic level. Note the orderly and well-differentiated nature of the epithelium.*

Carcinoma Cuniculatum
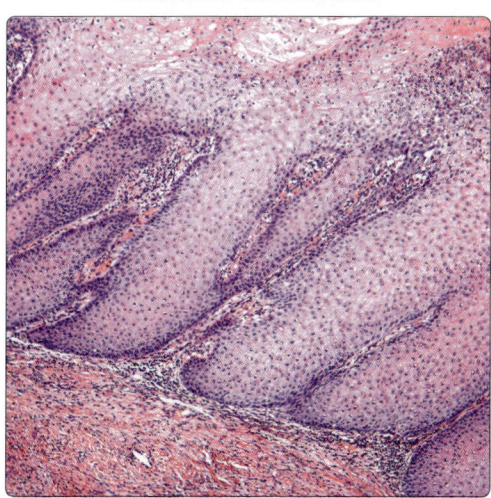

Carcinoma Cuniculatum
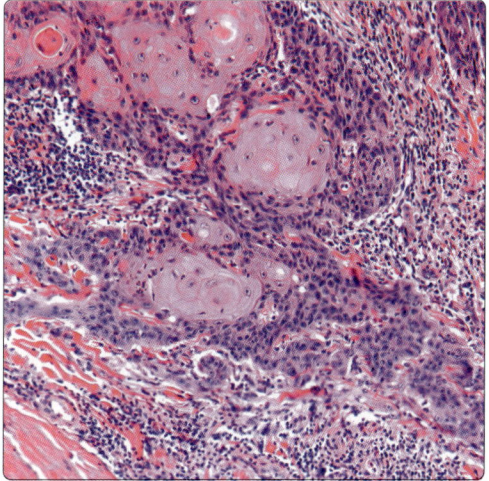

(Left) *The bulk of carcinoma cuniculatum is well differentiated. Note the sharp pushing borders similar to verrucous carcinoma.* (Right) *Higher grade areas and jagged borders are frequently a minor component of carcinoma cuniculatum. This feature clearly contrasts this tumor from verrucous carcinoma and underscores the importance of generous sampling and meticulous gross evaluation.*

Sarcomatoid Squamous Cell Carcinoma

KEY FACTS

TERMINOLOGY

- Synonyms
  - Spindle cell carcinoma, carcinosarcoma

MACROSCOPIC

- Large polyploid ulcerated mass
  - Usually affects glans, coronal sulcus, and foreskin
  - Deep invasion into corpora spongiosa and cavernosa
- Separate satellite nodules may be present

MICROSCOPIC

- Sarcomatoid squamous cell carcinoma (SCC) may be entirely composed of spindle cells
- Atypical spindle cells tend to arrange in interlacing fascicles
- Myxoid changes may be marked
- Pseudovascular spaces may be prominent, mimicking angiosarcoma
- Carcinoma in situ or clear-cut invasive SCC may be only very focally present

ANCILLARY TESTS

- Immunohistochemical studies are often necessary to make diagnosis
  - Spindle cells are positive for cytokeratins, p63, CK5/6, HMCK
  - Cytokeratin expression [especially CK-PAN (AE1/AE3) and CAM5.2)] by spindle cells may be only focal
  - CK-PAN (MNF116) and HMCK(34βE12) tend to be more diffusely expressed by spindle cells
  - Sarcomatoid SCC is negative for S100, desmin, CD34, and CD31
  - Spindle cells may be focally positive for SMA

TOP DIFFERENTIAL DIAGNOSES

- Spindle cell melanoma
- Sarcoma

Gross Appearance

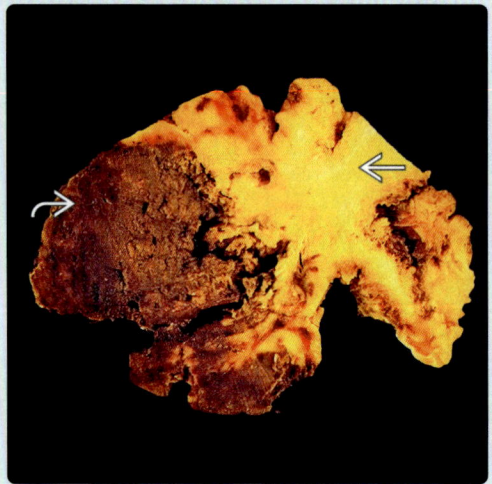

Gross Appearance: Schematic

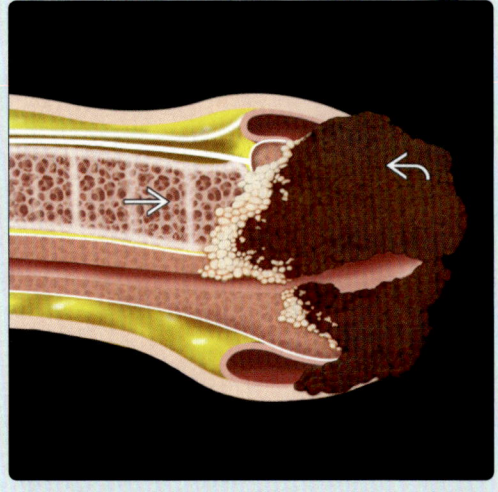

(Left) Partial penectomy specimen shows a large and hemorrhagic, deeply invasive tumor ➡ arising from the distal portion of the organ. The tumor extensively invades the corpora cavernosa ➡. Tumors are frequently fleshy and polypoid. (Right) Schematic representation shows a large and hemorrhagic sarcomatoid carcinoma ➡ deeply invading the corpora cavernosa ➡.

Sarcomatoid Carcinoma: Low Power

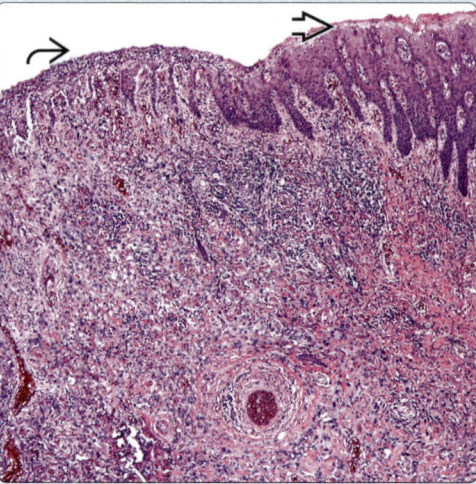

Sarcomatoid Carcinoma

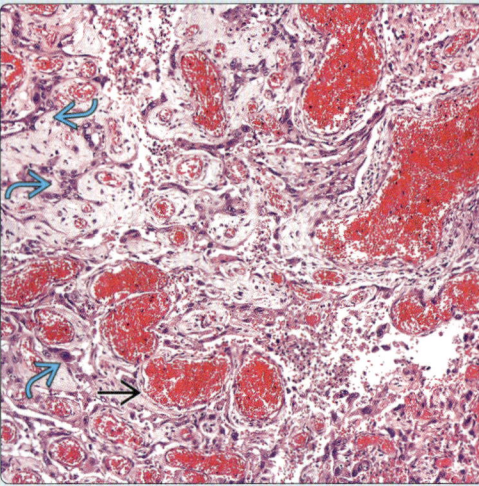

(Left) Low-power view illustrates an ulcerated tumor ➡ corresponding to a sarcomatoid carcinoma with pseudovascular features affecting the foreskin. The nonulcerated epithelium shows squamous hyperplasia ➡. (Right) Note the highly vascular ➡ and pseudovascular ➡ region with tumor cells simulating endothelium.

Sarcomatoid Squamous Cell Carcinoma

TERMINOLOGY

Abbreviations
- Sarcomatoid squamous cell carcinoma (SCC)

Synonyms
- Spindle cell carcinoma, carcinosarcoma, metaplastic carcinoma

Definitions
- Undifferentiated carcinoma arising from squamous epithelium composed of malignant spindle cells

ETIOLOGY/PATHOGENESIS

Pathogenesis
- Uncertain; human papillomavirus association unlikely

CLINICAL ISSUES

Epidemiology
- Incidence
  - ~ 4% of penile SCCs
- Age
  - Mean: 60 years

Site
- Often affect glands, coronal sulcus, and foreskin

Presentation
- Large, polypoid, and ulcerated tumor

Treatment
- Surgical or multimodal

Prognosis
- Poor; usually associated with lymph node metastasis

MACROSCOPIC

General Features
- Large, polypoid, and ulcerated tumor
- Usually involves > 1 anatomical compartment
  - Glans, coronal sulcus, &/or foreskin
- Cut surface shows solid white/gray to hemorrhagic or fleshy neoplasm
- Commonly invades corpora spongiosum and cavernosa
- Smaller satellite nodules may be present away from main mass

MICROSCOPIC

Histologic Features
- Composed of fascicles of atypical spindle cells
- Pleomorphic giant cells may be seen
- Myxoid changes may be prominent
- May show pseudovascular/angiosarcomatoid pattern
- Benign or malignant foci of bone/cartilage formation may be seen
- Mitotic figures are numerous, and necrosis may be prominent
- Lymphovascular and perineural invasion are common
- SCC in situ may be present on the surface
- Clear-cut squamous invasive tumor may be absent or represent minor component

ANCILLARY TESTS

Immunohistochemistry
- Often necessary to diagnose sarcomatoid SCC
- Spindle cells are positive cytokeratins, p63, CK5/6, and HMCK
  - CK-PAN (MNF116), HMCK (34βE12), and p63 tend to be more diffusely expressed by spindle cells
  - AE1/AE3 and CAM5.2 may be negative or focally positive
  - Not sufficient data available on utility of p40 (p63 isoform) in penile sarcomatoid SCCs
- Smooth muscle actin is usually negative (focal positivity may be present)
- S100, MART-1, SOX10, desmin, CD34, ERG, and CD31 are negative

DIFFERENTIAL DIAGNOSIS

Spindle Cell Melanoma
- Recognition of associated melanoma in situ is helpful
- Immunohistochemistry may be necessary
  - S100 and SOX10 positive
  - Melan-A (MART-1), HMB-45, and tyrosinase are usually negative
  - Cytokeratins and p63 are negative

Sarcomas
- Usually deeply located within corpus spongiosum or cavernosum with no connection to surface epithelium
  - Sarcomatoid SCC usually starts on the surface epithelium
- Absence of clear-cut squamous differentiation
- Immunohistochemistry may be necessary
  - Negative for cytokeratins and p63
  - Positive for mesenchymal markers
    - Leiomyosarcoma: Positive for SMA, desmin, calponin
    - Angiosarcoma: Positive for CD31, FLI-1, CD34, ERG
    - Malignant fibrous histiocytoma: Positive for vimentin, CD10; occasional positivity for SMA

DIAGNOSTIC CHECKLIST

Pathologic Interpretation Pearls
- Sarcomatoid carcinoma may be entirely composed of spindle cells
- Spindle cells may be negative for AE1/AE3 and CAM5.2

SELECTED REFERENCES

1. Ha Lan TT et al: Expression of the p40 isoform of p63 has high specificity for cutaneous sarcomatoid squamous cell carcinoma. J Cutan Pathol. 41(11):831-8, 2014
2. Katona TM et al: Soft tissue tumors of the penis: a review. Anal Quant Cytol Histol. 28(4):193-206, 2006
3. Sánchez-Ortiz R et al: Melanoma of the penis, scrotum and male urethra: a 40-year single institution experience. J Urol. 173(6):1958-65, 2005
4. Velazquez EF et al: Sarcomatoid carcinoma of the penis: a clinicopathologic study of 15 cases. Am J Surg Pathol. 29(9):1152-8, 2005
5. Lont AP et al: Sarcomatoid squamous cell carcinoma of the penis: a clinical and pathological study of 5 cases. J Urol. 172(3):932-5, 2004

Sarcomatoid Squamous Cell Carcinoma

(Left) This sarcomatoid carcinoma is predominantly composed of fascicles of atypical spindle cells with pleomorphic nuclei and mitoses. **(Right)** Sarcomatoid carcinoma composed of fascicles of spindle cells with scattered pleomorphic and hyperchromattic nuclei is shown. Cytologic atypia and features of malignancy are obvious.

Sarcomatoid Carcinoma: High Power
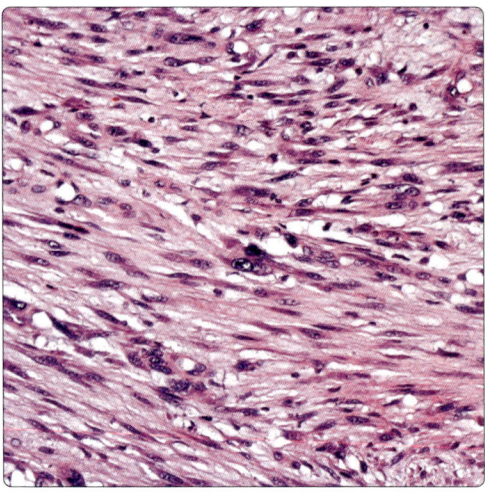

Sarcomatoid Carcinoma: Cytology
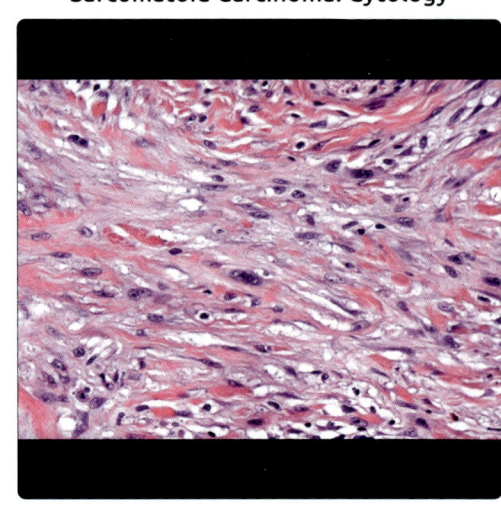

(Left) A storiform pattern is observed in this case of sarcomatoid carcinoma. Note the nuclear pleomorphism and scattered multinucleated giant cells. **(Right)** Sarcomatoid carcinoma shows prominent myxoid changes. Some tumors may be predominantly myxomatous. In the absence of an associated invasive SCC, the diagnosis may be confirmed by immunohistochemistry (keratin and p63 expression with negative muscle markers), previous history of SCC, or associated squamous cell carcinoma in situ (SCCIS).

Storiform Pattern
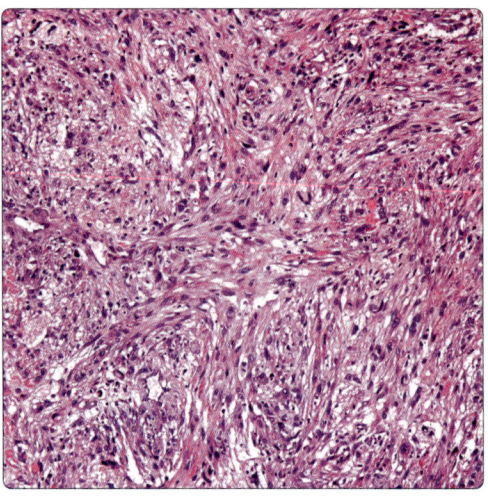

Myxoid Changes
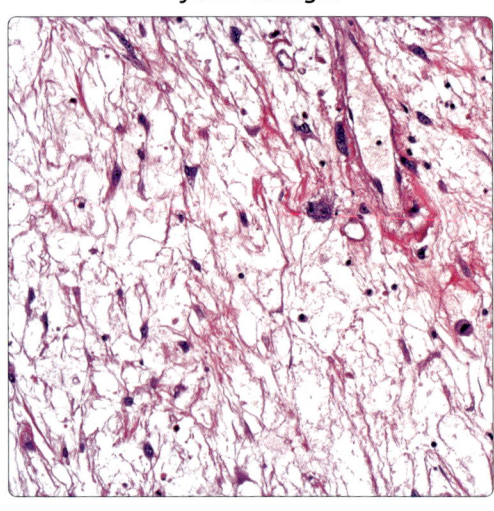

(Left) Sarcomatoid carcinoma predominantly composed of fascicles of spindle cells mimics a sarcoma. In the absence of a recognizable epithelial component, a sarcoma is in the differential diagnosis. Detailed morphologic evaluation and immunohistochemistry are helpful. **(Right)** Sarcomatoid carcinoma with pseudovascular features (angiosarcomatoid SCC) is predominantly composed of interanastomotic channels mimicking an angiosarcoma. The formation of such spaces is secondary to acantholysis.

Fascicles of Spindle Cells
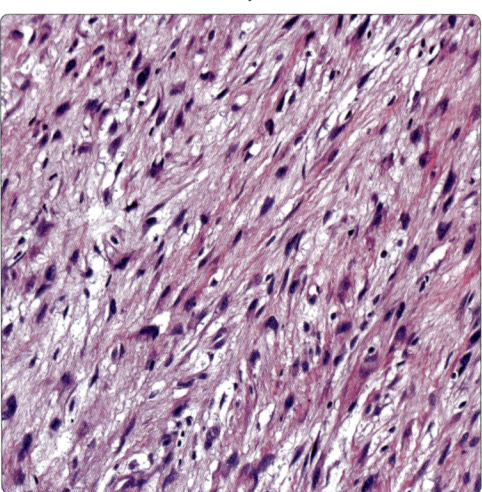

Pseudovascular Features
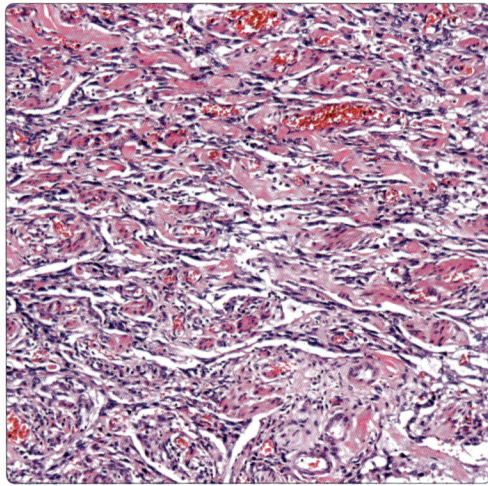

Sarcomatoid Squamous Cell Carcinoma

Pseudovascular Features

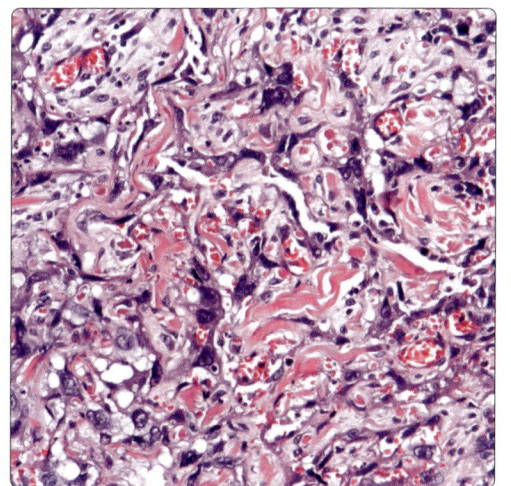

Metaplastic Bone

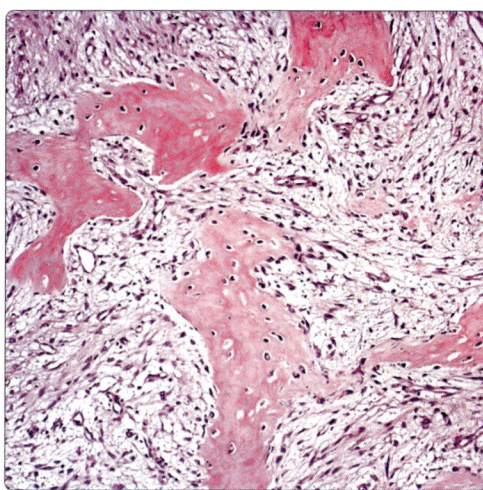

(Left) Sarcomatoid carcinoma with prominent pseudovascular spaces lined by large, atypical cells with pleomorphic nuclei may mimic angiosarcoma. Vascular markers (e.g., CD31) are negative in carcinomas. (Right) Spindle cell SCC shows bone formation. A tumor with sarcomatous histology affecting the distal penis is more likely to represent sarcomatoid carcinoma than true sarcoma.

Squamous Carcinoma In Situ

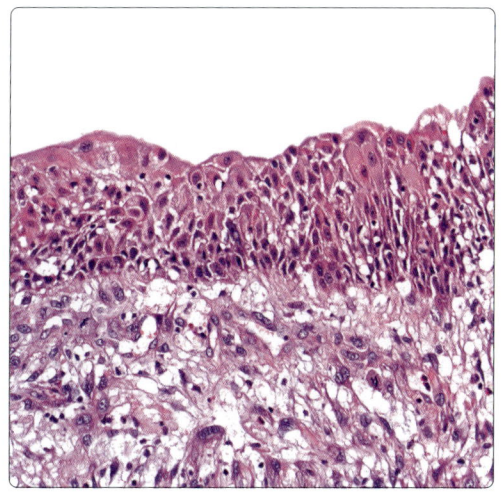

Associated Invasive Carcinoma

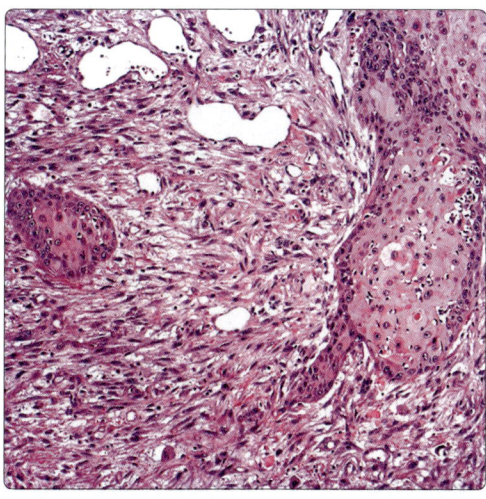

(Left) SCCIS may be only focally present in cases of sarcomatoid carcinoma. Strict criteria should be used to recognize SCCIS, as reactive changes may mimic dysplasia and overdiagnosis may result in misdiagnosis of the underlying tumor as a carcinoma. (Right) Clear-cut foci of invasive SCC are seen admixed with malignant spindle cells in this sarcomatoid carcinoma. Tumors may be almost entirely composed of spindle cells, and such squamous foci may be very difficult to identify.

HMCK IHC

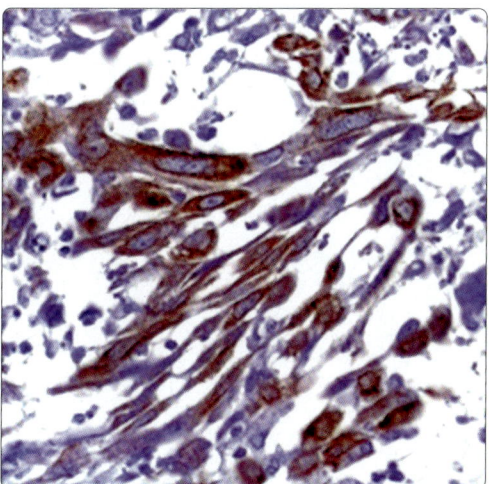

p63 IHC

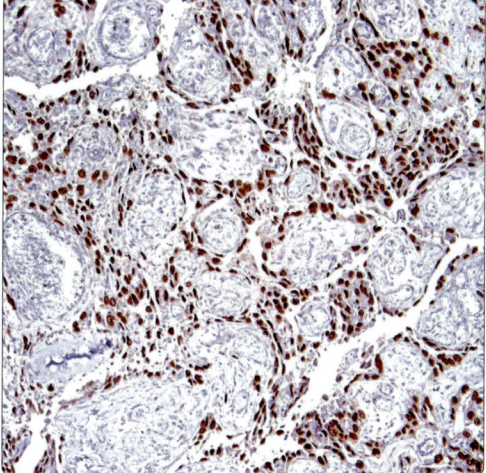

(Left) HMCK(34βE12) expression confirms the epithelial nature of this tumor. Expression of different cytokeratins (including CK5/6) and p63 is supportive of a diagnosis of sarcomatoid carcinoma. (Right) Diffuse p63 nuclear expression by the neoplastic cells in a case of sarcomatoid carcinoma with pseudovascular features (angiosarcomatoid carcinoma) supports the epithelial nature of this tumor.

Mixed Squamous Cell Carcinoma

KEY FACTS

TERMINOLOGY
- 2 or more histologic subtypes in same tumor
- 20% or more of at least 1 of histological components

CLINICAL ISSUES
- Prognosis is related to higher grade component

MACROSCOPIC
- Glans is most frequently affected site
- Mixed patterns of growth are common
- Verruciform and superficial spreading patterns correspond to low-grade tumors
- Vertical growth pattern is observed in high-grade tumors

MICROSCOPIC
- Coexistence of 2 or more histological subtypes
- Represents up to 1/3 of all penile squamous cell carcinoma (SCC)

- Histological grade distribution is variegated and depends on admixed subtypes
- Warty-basaloid is most frequent mixed SCC
- Hybrid verrucous represents 2nd most common type of mixed SCC
- Other less frequent patterns include usual-warty, usual-basaloid, and usual-papillary, and complex verruciform tumors
- Mixtures of differentiated and undifferentiated PeIN may also be identified
- Focal areas of usual SCC are observed in > 1/2 of sarcomatoid carcinoma cases
- Rare mixtures include adeno-basaloid SCC, mucoepidermoid SCC, and polymorphic variants

TOP DIFFERENTIAL DIAGNOSES
- Pure SCC variants
- Sarcomatoid carcinomas

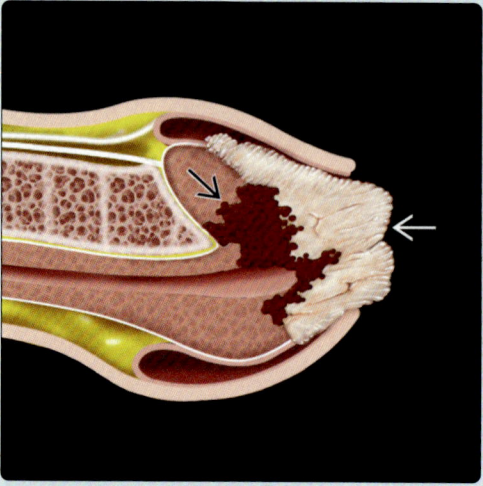

Mixed Penile Tumor

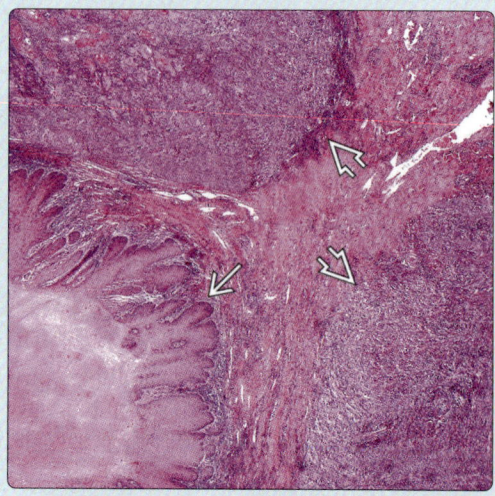

Hybrid Verrucous Carcinoma

(Left) Diagram of a mixed penile tumor depicts a low-grade superficial exophytic tumor ➡, corresponding to a verrucous carcinoma, and a focus of deeply infiltrating high-grade usual squamous cell carcinoma (SCC) ➡. (Right) Hybrid verrucous carcinoma shows concomitant presence of low-grade verrucous carcinoma with its typical bulbous tumor base ➡ intermingled with solid nests of a high-grade usual SCC ➡.

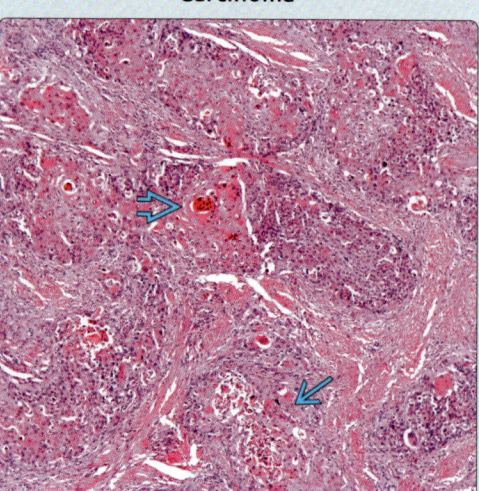

Mixed Usual-Basaloid Squamous Cell Carcinoma

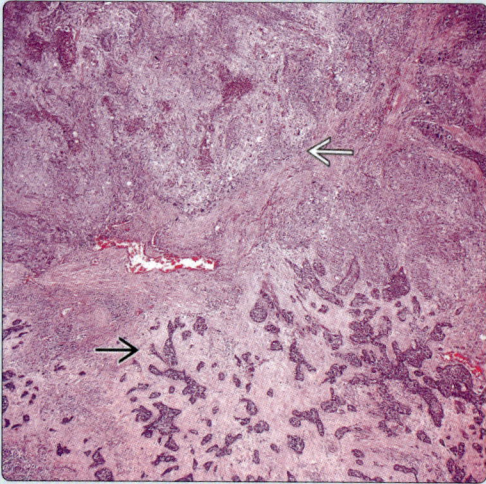

Mixed Warty-Basaloid Squamous Cell Carcinoma

(Left) In the upper left, one can appreciate a usual moderately differentiated SCC. Note the progressive keratinization ➡ with keratin pearls. In the bottom right, there is a classic basaloid SCC with abrupt keratinization ➡ and central cellular debris. (Right) In this pattern, the warty component is superficially located (nests of pink cells ➡) and separated from the deeply invasive basaloid component (nests of blue cells ➡).

Mixed Squamous Cell Carcinoma

TERMINOLOGY

Abbreviations
- Squamous cell carcinoma (SCC)

Definitions
- Coexistence of 2 or more histologic subtypes
- 20% or more of at least 1 of histologic components

CLINICAL ISSUES

Epidemiology
- Incidence
  - Represents 1/4-1/3 of all penile SCCs
- Age
  - 7th decade

Site
- Glans is most frequently affected site

Treatment
- Depends mainly on local extent and highest histologic grade of tumor
- Surgical approach should be considered for tumors invading beyond lamina propria
- Groin dissection should be performed based on risk group stratification

Prognosis
- Related to higher grade component
- Clinical behavior is variable in concordance with histologic picture and relative proportion of different components
- Local and regional recurrences may occur
- Inguinal nodal involvement is seen up to 40% of cases
- Cancer-specific mortality rate is similar to usual SCC

MACROSCOPIC

General Features
- Gross appearance is variable
- Mixed patterns of growth are common
- Verruciform and superficial spreading patterns correspond to low-grade tumors
- Vertical growth pattern is observed in high-grade tumors
- Average tumor size: 4.1 cm

MICROSCOPIC

Histologic Features
- Most frequent patterns include mixture of human papillomavirus (HPV)-related histologic subtypes
- Mixtures of usual SCC with other HPV-related and unrelated variants are also common
- Histologic grade distribution is variable and depends on subtypes present
- Vascular invasion, perineural invasion, and extension to distal urethra may be seen in ~ 1/3 of cases
- Mixtures of differentiated, basaloid, &/or warty penile intraepithelial neoplasia (PeIN) may be identified in adjacent overlying mucosa
- Warty-basaloid SCC is most frequent and it is classified as new entity
- Usual-verrucous carcinoma with other patterns
  - Represents ~ 1/4 of all mixed carcinomas
  - a.k.a. hybrid verrucous carcinoma
  - Admixture of usual SCC and verrucous carcinoma
  - Verrucous carcinoma is always low grade
  - Usual SCC may be well, moderately well, or poorly differentiated
  - Biological behavior is dictated by highest histologic grade
  - Even small foci of high-grade tumor impart metastatic potential, which is not the case in pure verrucous carcinoma
  - Pure verrucous SCC may locally recur as hybrid verrucous carcinoma (probably due to unsampled usual SCC in primary)
- SCC with mixed sarcomatoid features
  - At least focal areas of usual SCC are observed in > 1/2 of sarcomatoid carcinomas
  - In some cases, typical areas of verrucous, papillary, and basaloid SCC may be present
  - Regardless of presence of other histologic subtypes, all of these tumors are considered sarcomatoid carcinoma
- Other mixed patterns
  - Mixed usual-warty SCCs are unusual mixed penile carcinomas
  - Mixtures of basaloid SCC with usual SCC are also unusual
  - Papillary SCC admixed with usual SCC may be seen in minority of cases
  - Other mixtures include adenobasaloid SCC, mucoepidermoid SCC, and polymorphic variants
  - Complex verruciform tumors: Composed of variable proportions of benign condyloma, warty, verrucous and papillary SCCs

DIFFERENTIAL DIAGNOSIS

Pure Squamous Cell Carcinoma Variants
- Tumors should be adequately sampled in order to identify minor mixed areas, which may be of higher grade
- Strict criteria should be applied in histologic subtyping
- High-grade areas and variants may have random distribution
- Sampling is key in all verrucous carcinomas to identify areas of hybrid SCC pattern
- Mixed SCC with basaloid component behaves clinically better than pure basaloid SCC

Sarcomatoid Carcinoma
- In sarcomatoid carcinoma, presence of other intermingled SCC variants is not unusual
- Sarcomatoid carcinoma is clinically aggressive regardless of presence and extension of other morphological components

SELECTED REFERENCES

1. Sanchez DF et al: HPV- and non-HPV-related subtypes of penile squamous cell carcinoma (SCC): Morphological features and differential diagnosis according to the new WHO classification (2015). Semin Diagn Pathol. 32(3):198-221, 2015
2. Sanchez DF et al: Pathological factors, behavior, and histological prognostic risk groups in subtypes of penile squamous cell carcinomas (SCC). Semin Diagn Pathol. 32(3):222-31, 2014
3. Guimarães GC et al: Penile squamous cell carcinoma clinicopathological features, nodal metastasis and outcome in 333 cases. J Urol. 182(2):528-34; discussion 534, 2009

Mixed Squamous Cell Carcinoma

Warty-Basaloid Carcinoma

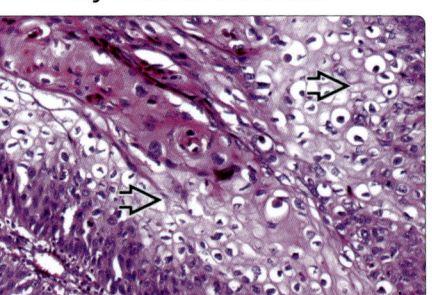

(Left) Warty-basaloid carcinomas are composed of a mixed cell population of pleomorphic cells with koilocytic changes at surface ⇨ and small basaloid cells at base of papillae ➡. **(Right)** Deep infiltrative nests of warty-basaloid carcinomas show a mixed population with a variable proportion of larger cells with koilocytotic atypia ➡ intermingled with smaller basaloid cells ➡.

Warty-Basaloid Penile Intraepithelial Neoplasia

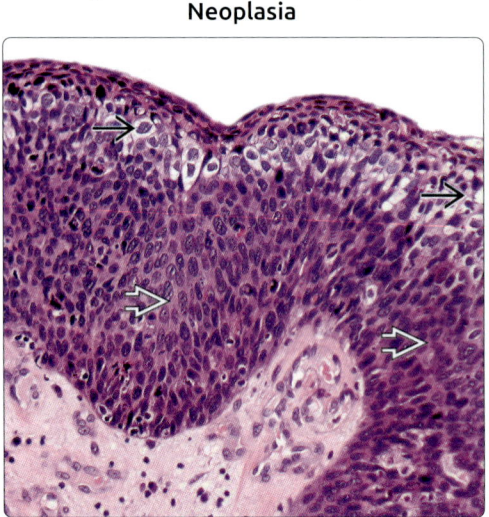

Hybrid Verrucous Carcinoma

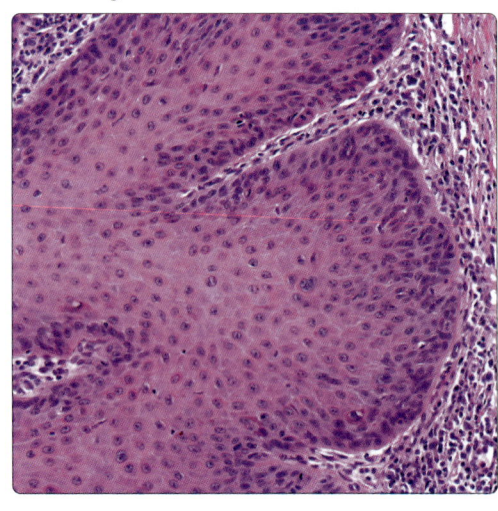

(Left) In warty-basaloid carcinoma, it is common to find associated areas of warty-basaloid penile intraepithelial neoplasia (PeIN) in which epithelium is replaced by basaloid cells in the lower 2/3 ➡ and by pleomorphic koilocytes on the surface ➡. **(Right)** Exophytic superficial area of a hybrid verrucous carcinoma shows the verrucous component, with its extremely well-developed squamous differentiation, broad tumor base, and chronic inflammatory reaction.

Hybrid Verrucous Carcinoma

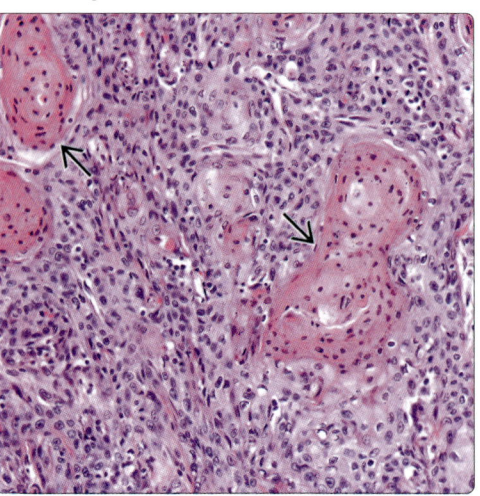

Hybrid Verrucous Carcinoma

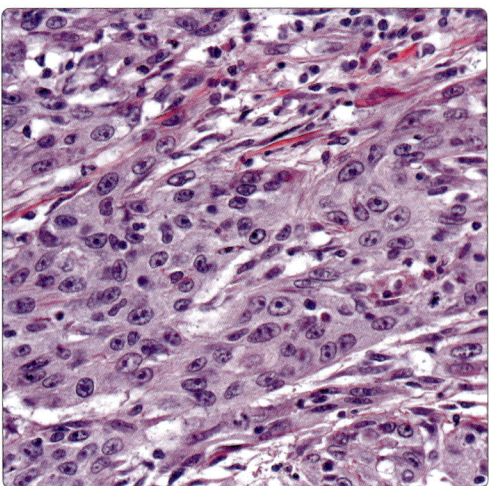

(Left) Infiltrative portion of a hybrid verrucous carcinoma with its usual squamous carcinoma component shows solid nests with moderate nuclear pleomorphism and foci of keratin pearl formation ➡, corresponding to a grade 2 usual SCC, located beneath the verrucous component (not shown). **(Right)** Deeply infiltrative portion of a hybrid verrucous carcinoma shows foci of poorly differentiated (grade 3) usual SCC composed of pleomorphic cells with ample and keratinized cytoplasm.

Mixed Squamous Cell Carcinoma

Hybrid Verrucous Carcinoma

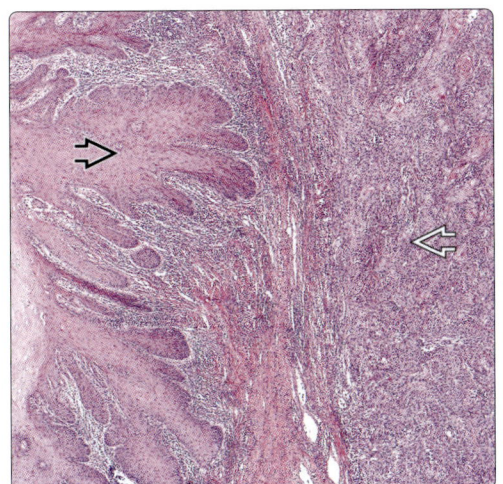

Hybrid Verrucous Carcinoma

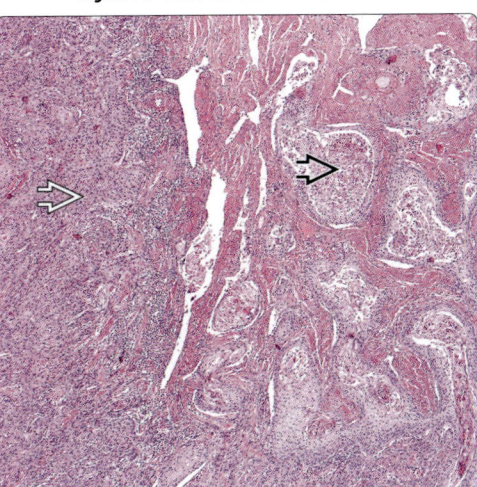

(Left) Hybrid verrucous carcinoma with extremely well-differentiated areas corresponds to the verrucous carcinoma component ⇨, and poorly differentiated foci corresponds to the high-grade SCC of usual type ⇨. *(Right)* Hybrid verrucous carcinoma shows solid areas of high-grade usual SCC ⇨ intermingled with highly infiltrative tumor nests having extensive central necrosis ⇨.

Sarcomatoid Carcinoma

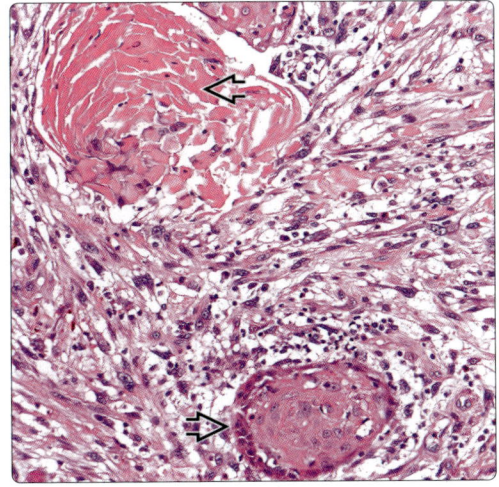

Sarcomatoid Carcinoma

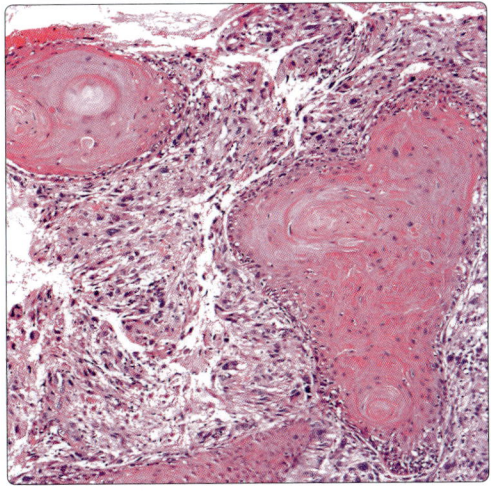

(Left) Isolated foci of squamous differentiation ⇨ are commonly observed in sarcomatoid carcinomas imparting a biphasic appearance to the tumor; although, in most cases, the spindle cell component usually predominates. *(Right)* The presence of well-differentiated atypical squamous nests surrounded by pleomorphic spindle cells helps identify the malignant spindle cell component as being sarcomatoid carcinoma over a high-grade sarcoma.

Adenosquamous Carcinoma

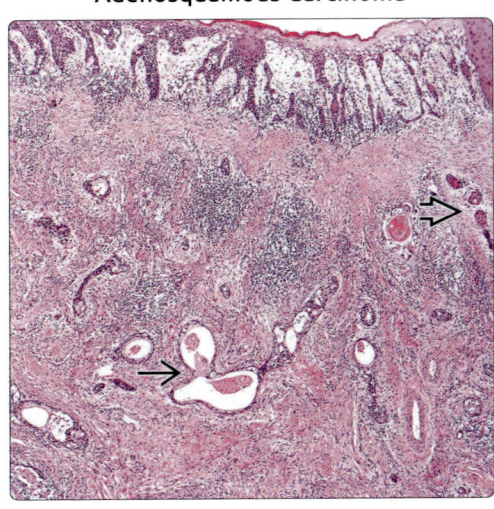

Adenosquamous Carcinoma

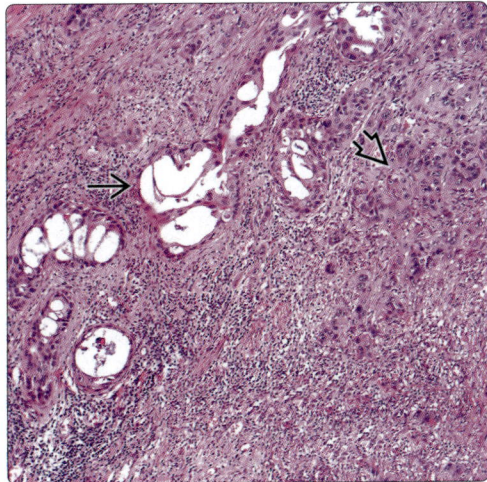

(Left) Adenosquamous carcinoma is a deeply infiltrative SCC variant in which foci of squamous ⇨ and glandular ⇨ differentiation coexist. *(Right)* Adenosquamous carcinoma shows the typical biphasic pattern in which irregularly shaped, high-grade, solid, neoplastic nests of usual SCC ⇨ are juxtaposed with areas of glandular differentiation ⇨.

Lymphoepithelioma-Like Squamous Cell Carcinoma

KEY FACTS

TERMINOLOGY
- Poorly differentiated invasive squamous cell carcinoma resembling lymphoepithelioma or undifferentiated nasopharyngeal carcinoma
- Rare subtype with few cases reported

CLINICAL ISSUES
- Uncircumcised men
- Large exophytic tumor located mainly in glans
- Perineural and vascular invasion
- Lymph node metastasis has been described

MICROSCOPIC
- Poorly differentiated squamous cells
- Invasive cords, trabeculae, nest, or sheets
- Indistinct cellular borders
- Heterogeneous nuclear size
- Prominent nucleoli

- Marked lymphoplasmacytic infiltrate associated with neoplastic squamous cells
- Undifferentiated penile intraepithelial neoplasia (PeIN) may be identified

ANCILLARY TESTS
- Immunohistochemistry positive for cytokeratins, p63, and p16
- In situ hybridization positive for high-risk human papillomavirus (HPV)
- Negative for EBV

TOP DIFFERENTIAL DIAGNOSES
- Lymphomas
- High-grade squamous cell carcinoma

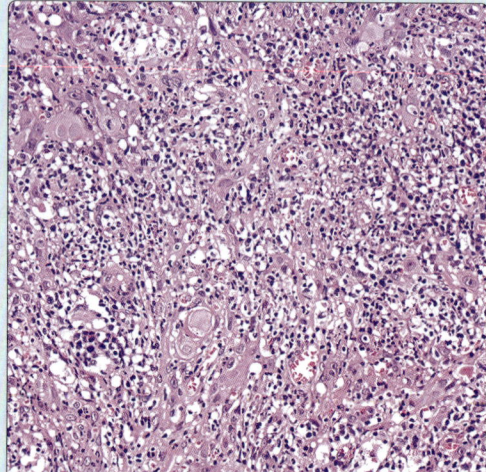

Lymphoepithelioma-Like Squamous Cell Carcinoma Middle-Power View

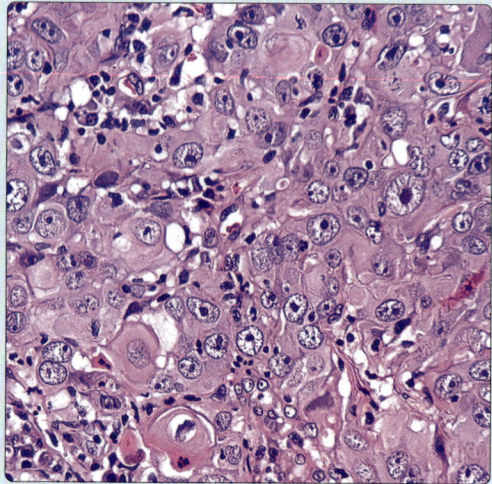

Lymphoepithelioma-Like Squamous Cell Carcinoma High-Power View, Nuclear Features

(Left) Dense inflammatory cell infiltrate is characteristic. Few eosinophilic neoplastic epithelial cells are less evident over the inflammatory background. (Right) Epithelial cells are poorly differentiated and nonkeratinizing. Nuclei are vesicular, heterogeneous in size, and with prominent nucleoli.

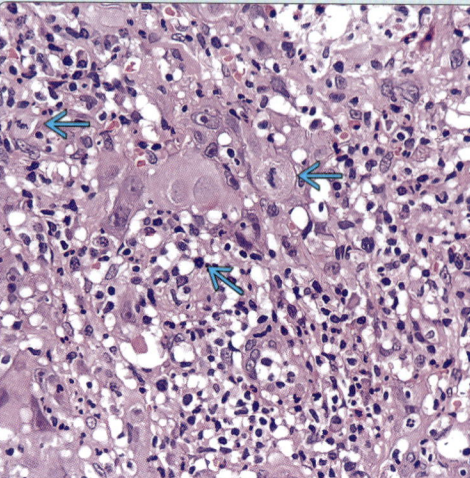

Lymphoepithelioma-Like Squamous Cell Carcinoma High-Power View

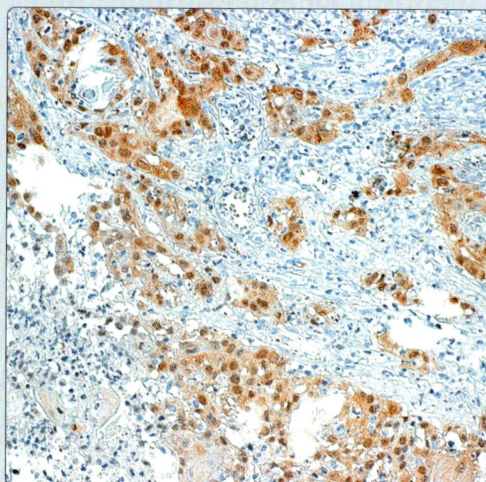

Lymphoepithelioma-Like Squamous Cell Carcinoma Immunohistochemical Stain

(Left) Scanty carcinoma cells with indistinct cellular borders are surrounded by dense inflammation. Some cells in mitosis can be seen ➡. (Right) A p16 immunostain emphasizes a syncytial growth pattern and highlights its relation with human papillomavirus.

Lymphoepithelioma-Like Squamous Cell Carcinoma

TERMINOLOGY

Definitions
- Poorly differentiated invasive squamous cell carcinoma with tumor cells obscured by marked lymphoplasmacytic inflammatory infiltrate

ETIOLOGY/PATHOGENESIS

Infectious Agents
- Most cases are human papillomavirus (HPV) related

CLINICAL ISSUES

Epidemiology
- Incidence
  - Extremely rare
- Age
  - Older men
  - Median: 66 years

Presentation
- Glans-based, large, exophytic tumor in uncircumcised men

Treatment
- Surgical approaches
  - Total penectomy
  - Bilateral groin dissection in clinically evident compromised nodes or in high-grade tumors invading erectile corpora
- Adjuvant therapy
  - Role unknown
- Radiation
  - Role unknown

Prognosis
- Perineural and vascular invasion were seen in reported cases
- Lymph node metastasis was described in 1 of 2 cases reported
- Patients died of other causes at 3 and 17 years of follow-up

MACROSCOPIC

General Features
- Exophytic, white-gray tumor located in glans
- Extension to coronal sulcus and foreskin
- Deeply invasive solid and firm tumor at cut surface

MICROSCOPIC

Histologic Features
- Poorly differentiated squamous cells
- Syncytial growth pattern
- Invasive cords, trabeculae, nest or sheets
- Indistinct cellular borders
- Heterogeneous nuclear size
- Irregular nuclear margins
- Prominent nucleoli
- Inflammatory (lymphoplasmacytic) infiltrate surrounding and sometimes obscuring neoplastic cells
- Dyscohesive areas and isolated neoplastic cells can be seen
- Abundant eosinophilic inflammatory infiltrate may be found
- Undifferentiated penile intraepithelial neoplasia (PeIN) may be identified in adjacent epithelium

ANCILLARY TESTS

Immunohistochemistry
- Positive for cytokeratins, p63, and p16
- Negative for p53 and cyclin-D1

In Situ Hybridization
- Positive for high-risk HPV
- Negative for Epstein-Barr virus

DIFFERENTIAL DIAGNOSIS

Lymphomas
- Mainly involve penile shaft
- Absence of squamous neoplastic cells
- Immunohistochemical studies may be necessary in some cases
- Eosinophils in background plus prominent nucleoli can simulate Hodgkin lymphoma

High-Grade Squamous Cell Carcinoma
- Prominent intercellular bridges or cellular borders
- Presence of focal keratinization

DIAGNOSTIC CHECKLIST

Pathologic Interpretation Pearls
- High-grade squamous cell carcinoma
- Close relationship of tumor cells with inflammatory cells is characteristic
- Syncytial growth pattern

SELECTED REFERENCES

1. Sanchez DF et al: HPV- and non-HPV-related subtypes of penile squamous cell carcinoma (SCC): Morphological features and differential diagnosis according to the new WHO classification (2015). Semin Diagn Pathol. 32(3):198-221, 2015
2. Sanchez DF et al: Pathological factors, behavior, and histological prognostic risk groups in subtypes of penile squamous cell carcinomas (SCC). Semin Diagn Pathol. 32(3): 222-31, 2015
3. Mentrikoski MJ et al: Lymphoepithelioma-like carcinoma of the penis: association with human papilloma virus infection. Histopathology. 64(2):312-5, 2014
4. Epstein JI et al. Tumors of the prostate gland, seminal vesicles, penis, and scrotum. In: Atlas of Tumor Pathology, Tumors of The Penis. Washington, D.C.: Armed Forces Institute of Pathology, 2011

Clear Cell Carcinoma

KEY FACTS

TERMINOLOGY
- Synonym: Clear cell squamous cell carcinoma
- Definition: Aggressive human papillomavirus (HPV)-related tumor arising in penile mucosal compartments

ETIOLOGY/PATHOGENESIS
- Presence of HPV

CLINICAL ISSUES
- Rare aggressive squamous cell carcinoma composed of clear cells

MACROSCOPIC
- Large, white-gray tumor mass replacing distal penis
- Affects mucosal compartments and sparing skin of shaft

MICROSCOPIC
- Nesting growth pattern
- Geographic and comedo-like central necrosis
- Prominent cytoplasmic clear cell features
- Vascular invasion
- Perineural invasion
- Presence of warty/basaloid penile intraepithelial neoplasia

ANCILLARY TESTS
- p16 immunostain positive
- HPV positive

TOP DIFFERENTIAL DIAGNOSES
- Warty carcinoma with prominent clear cells
- Basaloid carcinoma
- Sweat gland carcinoma
- Metastatic renal cell carcinoma

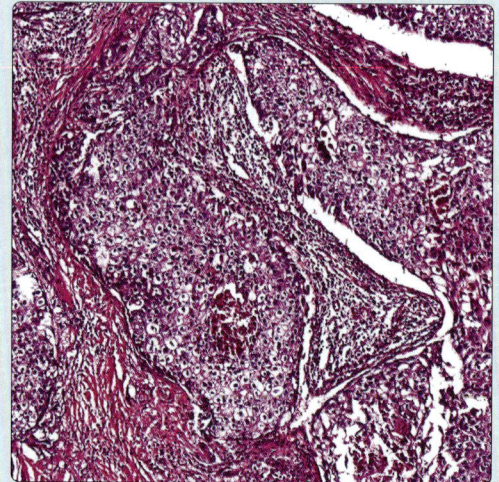

Nesting Pattern, H&E, Low Magnification

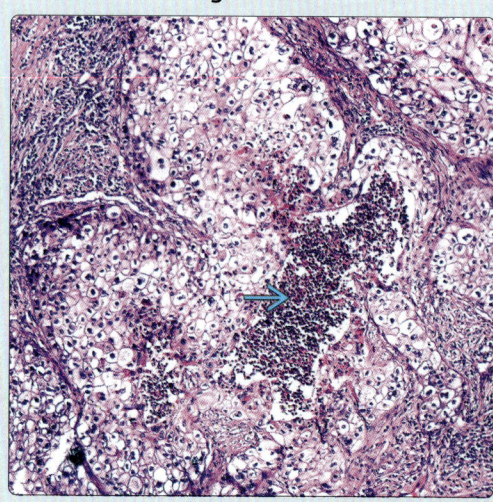

Central Necrosis, H&E, Medium Magnification

(Left) Low-power view shows an infiltrative solid tumor with confluent nests composed of clear cells and central necrosis pattern. (Right) There is an irregular nesting pattern with central necrosis ➡. Numerous differential diagnostic considerations are raised in this rare tumor. Note the marked inflammatory infiltrate surrounding the tumor.

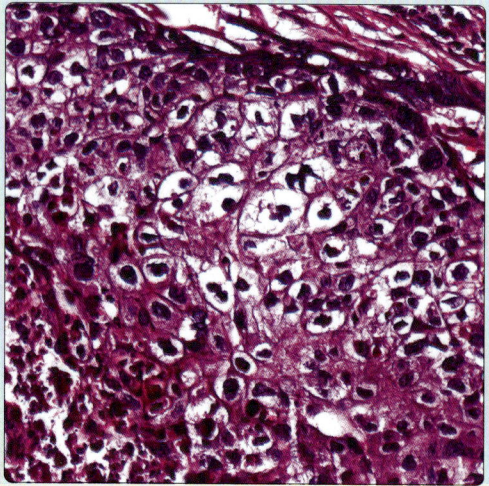

Clear Cell, H&E, High Magnification

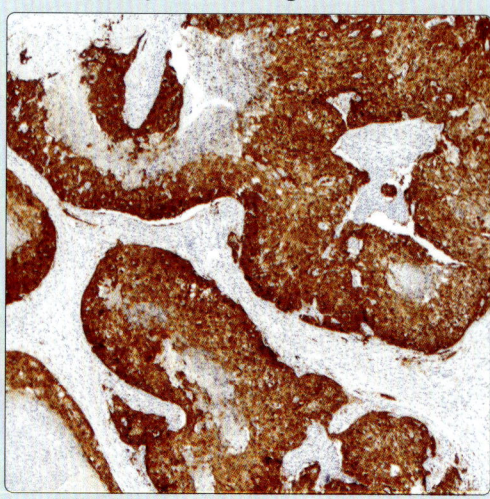

IHC, p16, Low Magnification

(Left) Cytoplasmic clear cell features are prominent. Some of the cells resemble koilocytes. Nuclei are irregular, hyperchromatic, and centrally located. There is no keratinization. (Right) p16 immunostain, a surrogate for high-risk HPV, shows strong and diffuse positivity.

Clear Cell Carcinoma

TERMINOLOGY

Synonyms
- Clear cell squamous cell carcinoma (SCC)

Definitions
- Aggressive human papillomavirus (HPV)-related tumor arising in penile mucosal compartments

ETIOLOGY/PATHOGENESIS

Infectious Agents
- All reported cases are positive for HPV

CLINICAL ISSUES

Epidemiology
- Extremely rare penile tumor

Presentation
- Large tumor mass affecting foreskin, coronal sulcus, or glans

Treatment
- Surgical approaches
  - Total penectomy and bilateral inguinal lymph node dissection
- Adjuvant therapy
  - Unknown
- Radiation
  - Unknown

Prognosis
- Locally destructive
- Adverse pathological prognostic factors present
  - Invasion of corpora cavernosa
  - High histological grade
  - Vascular and perineural invasion
- Frequent inguinal metastases
- 1/3 of patients die from tumor dissemination

MACROSCOPIC

General Features
- Large, white-gray, ulcerating tumor mass
- Affects distal penile mucosal epithelial compartments
- Probably arises from glans epithelial surface

MICROSCOPIC

Histologic Features
- Nesting growth pattern
- Without papillomatous architecture
- Confluent nests
- Geographical necrosis
- Comedonecrosis in central part of nest
- Clear cell features throughout tumor
- Presence of HPV
- Warty/basaloid penile intraepithelial neoplasia can be found adjacent to invasive carcinoma
- Minor component of warty or basaloid SCC nest can be found

Predominant Cell/Compartment Type
- Clear cells

ANCILLARY TESTS

Histochemistry
- PAS(+) cytoplasmic material

Immunohistochemistry
- p16(+)

DIFFERENTIAL DIAGNOSIS

Warty Carcinoma With Prominent Clear Cells
- Warty carcinoma is papillomatous
- Clear cell has a nonpapillary architecture

Basaloid Carcinoma
- Basaloid carcinoma also shows nesting pattern
- Cells are small, uniform, and basaloid
- Basaloid cells are not prominent in clear cell carcinoma

Sweat Gland Carcinoma
- Does not occur in penile mucosal compartments but in skin of the shaft
- p16 and HPV negative

Metastatic Renal Cell Carcinoma
- More common in corpus cavernosum
- p16 and HPV negative
- Positive for RCC markers (pax-8, RCC)
- Vascular lymphatic invasion

DIAGNOSTIC CHECKLIST

Pathologic Interpretation Pearls
- Nesting pattern composed of clear cells
- Comedonecrosis without basaloid cells

SELECTED REFERENCES

1. Sanchez DF et al: Clear cell carcinoma of the penis: an HPV-related variant of squamous cell carcinoma: a report of 3 cases. Am J Surg Pathol. ePub, 2016
2. Sanchez DF et al: HPV- and non-HPV-related subtypes of penile squamous cell carcinoma (SCC): Morphological features and differential diagnosis according to the new WHO classification (2015). Semin Diagn Pathol. 32(3):198-221, 2015
3. Sanchez DF et al: Pathological factors, behavior, and histological prognostic risk groups in subtypes of penile squamous cell carcinomas (SCC). Semin Diagn Pathol. 32(3): 222-31, 2015
4. Liegl B et al: Penile clear cell carcinoma: a report of 5 cases of a distinct entity. Am J Surg Pathol. 28(11):1513-7, 2004

Overview of HPV- and Non-HPV-Related Tumors

KEY FACTS

TERMINOLOGY
- Penile carcinoma: Uncommon malignant tumor with bimodal pathogenic pathway
  - One associated with and other unrelated to HPV infection

CLINICAL ISSUES
- HPV-related tumors affect younger patients and preferential location of tumor origin is in glans
- HPV-unrelated tumors are seen in older patients and preferential location of tumor origin is in foreskin
- HPV vaccine: Gardasil (Merck, Whitehouse Station, NJ) protects against infection from HPV types 6, 11, 16, and 18 and is recommended for men 9-26 years of age

MICROSCOPIC
- HPV frequently found in tumors with predominant basaloid cells (72%) and also in those with predominantly koilocytic cells (47%)
- Eosinophilic maturing keratinized cells are more common in HPV-negative tumors (81%)
- HPV-related carcinomas
  - Basaloid and warty and their mixtures
  - Lymphoepithelioma-like and clear cell carcinomas
- Non-HPV-related carcinomas
  - Verrucous carcinoma
  - Papillary NOS
  - Cuniculatum
  - Pseudohyperplastic
  - Pseudoglandular
  - Sarcomatoid

ANCILLARY TESTS
- Nucleic acid-hybridization assays
- Signal-amplification assays
- Nucleic acid-amplification methods
- p16 immunohistochemical stain

Undifferentiated Penile Intraepithelial Neoplasia

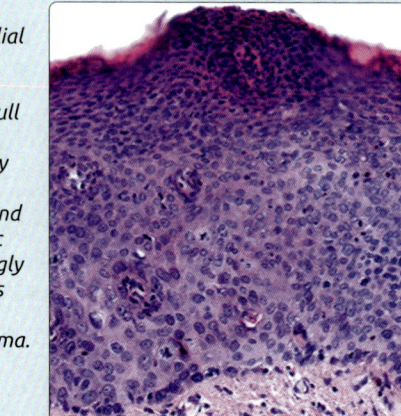

Basaloid Squamous Cell Carcinoma

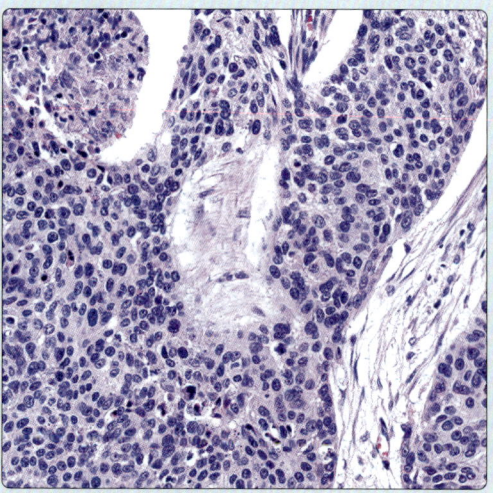

(Left) High-power view of basaloid penile intraepithelial neoplasia (PeIN) with a monotonous atypical blue cells population involving full epithelial thickness. (Right) High-grade cells with scanty cytoplasm, high nuclear:cytoplasmic ratio and small ovoid hyperchromatic nuclei (blue cells) are strongly associated with HPV. This is the typical histology of basaloid squamous carcinoma.

Differentiated Penile Intraepithelial Neoplasia

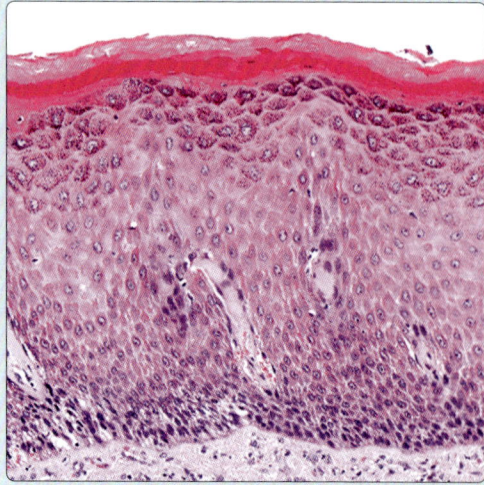

Usual Squamous Cell Carcinoma

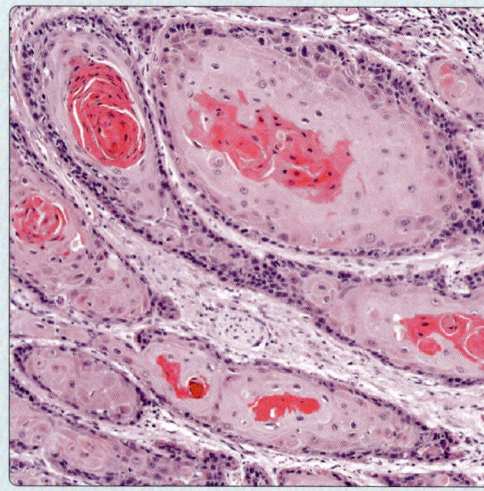

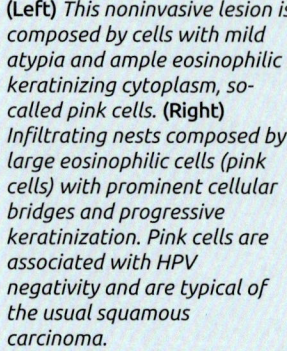

(Left) This noninvasive lesion is composed by cells with mild atypia and ample eosinophilic keratinizing cytoplasm, so-called pink cells. (Right) Infiltrating nests composed by large eosinophilic cells (pink cells) with prominent cellular bridges and progressive keratinization. Pink cells are associated with HPV negativity and are typical of the usual squamous carcinoma.

Overview of HPV- and Non-HPV-Related Tumors

TERMINOLOGY

Abbreviations
- Penile squamous cell carcinoma (SCC), penile carcinoma (PC), penile intraepithelial neoplasia (PeIN)

Definitions
- Penile carcinoma: Uncommon malignant tumor with heterogeneous etiology
  - Because of etiological and prognostic considerations, 2 morphologically and molecularly distinctive groups of subtypes of penile SCCs based on presence of HPV are currently recognized

ETIOLOGY/PATHOGENESIS

HPV Prevalence and Type Distribution
- Bimodal pathogenic pathway: One associated with and other unrelated to HPV infection
- Half of penile SCCs are related to HPV infection
- Most HPV infections are classified as high-risk genotypes and majority of these correspond to HPV-16, accounting for > 60% of HPV-attributable cases

CLINICAL ISSUES

Epidemiology
- Incidence
  - Geographic variation in incidence of penile cancer
    - In low-incidence regions (e.g., Europe and USA): 1 or less per 100,000 inhabitants
    - In high-frequency regions of Latin America, Africa, and Asia: 4 per 100,000 inhabitants
  - Associated risk factors
    - Phimosis
    - Long foreskin
    - Poor hygienic habits
    - Low socioeconomic condition
    - Poor educational level
    - Smoking
    - History of genital warts
    - History of multiple female partners
    - All factors are prevalent in HPV and non-HPV-related carcinomas; however, history of warts and of multiple female partners are significantly associated only with HPV-related carcinomas
  - HPV is detected in 30-50% of penile SCCs
    - Slightly more common in countries with low incidence of penile cancer
      - Exception is in regions of Africa, where HPV-positive tumors are frequent, and this phenomenon may be due to high concomitant incidence of HIV-positive patients more prone to developing HPV-related anogenital tumors
- Age
  - Most commonly affects men 50-70 years old
  - HPV-related tumors affect younger patients, whereas tumors unrelated to HPV are seen in older patients with phimosis (or unretractable foreskin), lichen sclerosus, or squamous hyperplasia

Presentation
- No particular differential clinical signs and symptoms in HPV-positive and -negative cases; in both groups, tumors may be exo- or endophytic, or of low or of high grade
  - In HPV-related carcinomas, preferential location of tumor origin is in glans
  - Non-HPV-related tumors occur in peripheral areas, foreskin and coronal sulcus, more frequently
  - Lichen sclerosus is significantly more common in non-HPV-related neoplasms

Clinical Risk Factors
- HPV unrelated
  - Chronic inflammatory conditions (lichen sclerosus)
  - Phimosis
  - Not being circumcised
  - Cigarette smoking
- HPV related
  - Multiple sexual partners
  - Genital warts or other sexually transmitted diseases
  - HPV infection

HPV Vaccine
- Gardasil (Merck, Whitehouse Station, NJ) vaccine has been approved by FDA in 2009 for prevention of penile cancer
- Recommended for men 9-26 years of age and men 27 years of age and older who have sex with men
- Protects against infection from HPV types 6, 11, 16, and 18
- Given in 3 doses over 6 months
- Most effective when given before 1st sexual contact; however, people who are sexually active may still benefit
- Protects against new HPV infections; does not treat or cure existing infections

MACROSCOPIC

General Features
- Gross features of non-HPV-related tumors are nonspecific, except 2 tumors
  - Verrucous carcinoma, which is distinctive exophytic papillomatous neoplasm with broadly based pushing border
  - Sarcomatoid carcinomas, with polypoid necrotic and hemorrhagic large neoplasm
- In HPV-related group, warty carcinoma show distinctive cobblestone surface, and basaloid carcinoma cut surface is characteristically tan, solid, homogeneous, and deeply invasive

Anatomic Features
- Poorly differentiated HPV-related carcinomas are more likely to develop around glans, where urethral-meatal mucosae merge (central tumors)
- Lower grade keratinizing HPV-unrelated carcinomas are more prevalent in foreskin (peripheral tumors)

MICROSCOPIC

Cytologic Features
- HPV is frequently found in tumors with predominant basaloid cells (72%) and also in those with predominantly koilocytic cells (47%)

Overview of HPV- and Non-HPV-Related Tumors

- Eosinophilic maturing keratinized cells are more common in HPV-negative tumors (81%)

HPV and Histologic Subtypes

- HPV is frequently found in
  - Basaloid and warty carcinomas and their mixtures
  - Lymphoepithelioma-like
  - Clear cell carcinomas
  - PeIN of similar basaloid or warty morphology is frequently identified in tissues adjacent to HPV-related invasive neoplasms
- HPV is usually negative in
  - Usual SCC
  - Pseudoglandular carcinoma
  - Sarcomatoid carcinoma
  - Pseudohyperplastic carcinomas
  - These tumors are frequently associated with differentiated PeIN and lichen sclerosus

ANCILLARY TESTS

HPV Detection and Genotyping

- Nucleic acid-hybridization assays
  - Southern blotting
  - In situ hybridization
  - Dot-blot hybridization
- Signal-amplification assays
  - Cervista HPV (Hologic, Inc., Marlborough, MA)
  - Hybrid Capture 2 system (hc2, Digene Corp., USA)
- Nucleic acid-amplification methods
  - Microarray analysis
  - PapilloCheck
  - Polymerase chain reaction (PCR)
  - Real-time PCR
  - Abbott real time
  - PCR-RFLP
  - HPV genome sequencing
  - INNO-LiPA (LiPA HBV GT; Innogenetics N.V., Ghent, Belgium)
  - COBAS 4800 HPV test
  - Linear Array HPV Genotyping (Roche Molecular Diagnostics, Pleasanton, CA)
  - CLART human papillomavirus 2
  - Microplate colorimetric hybridization assay (MCHA)
  - PreTect Proofer (HPV-mRNA detection)
  - APTIMA HPV assay (HPV-mRNA detection)
- p16 immunohistochemical stain is adequate, and less expensive, surrogate useful in routine practice of surgical pathology

SELECTED REFERENCES

1. Alemany L et al: Human papillomavirus DNA prevalence and type distribution in anal carcinomas worldwide. Int J Cancer. 136(1):98-107, 2015
2. Djajadiningrat RS et al: Human papillomavirus prevalence in invasive penile cancer and association with clinical outcome. J Urol. 193(2):526-31, 2015
3. Moch H, Humphrey PA, Ulbright TM, et al. WHO Classification of Tumours of the Urinary System and Male Genital Organs. Fourth Edition. IARC Press, 2015
4. Sanchez DF et al: HPV- and non-HPV-related subtypes of penile squamous cell carcinoma (SCC): Morphological features and differential diagnosis according to the new WHO classification (2015). Semin Diagn Pathol. 32(3):198-221, 2015
5. Steinestel J et al: The role of histologic subtype, p16(INK4a) expression, and presence of human papillomavirus DNA in penile squamous cell carcinoma. BMC Cancer. 15:220, 2015
6. Hernandez AL et al: Incidence of and risk factors for type-specific anal human papillomavirus infection among HIV-positive MSM. AIDS. 28(9):1341-9, 2014
7. Hernandez BY et al: Human papillomavirus genotype prevalence in invasive penile cancers from a registry-based United States population. Front Oncol. 4:9, 2014
8. Mentrikoski MJ et al: Lymphoepithelioma-like carcinoma of the penis: association with human papilloma virus infection. Histopathology. 64(2):312-5, 2014
9. Sanchez DF et al: Pathological factors, behavior, and histological prognostic risk groups in subtypes of penile squamous cell carcinomas (SCC). Semin Diagn Pathol. 32(3):222-31, 2014
10. Chaux A et al: Epidemiologic profile, sexual history, pathologic features, and human papillomavirus status of 103 patients with penile carcinoma. World J Urol. 31(4):861-7, 2013
11. Ferrándiz-Pulido C et al: Identification and genotyping of human papillomavirus in a Spanish cohort of penile squamous cell carcinomas: correlation with pathologic subtypes, p16(INK4a) expression, and prognosis. J Am Acad Dermatol. 68(1):73-82, 2013
12. Abreu AL et al: A review of methods for detect human Papillomavirus infection. Virol J. 9:262, 2012
13. Chaux A et al: Advances in the pathology of penile carcinomas. Hum Pathol. 43(6):771-89, 2012
14. Chaux A et al: Diagnostic problems in precancerous lesions and invasive carcinomas of the penis. Semin Diagn Pathol. 29(2):72-82, 2012
15. Chaux A et al: New pathologic entities in penile carcinomas: an update of the 2004 world health organization classification. Semin Diagn Pathol. 29(2):59-66, 2012
16. Cubilla AL et al: Basaloid squamous cell carcinoma of the penis with papillary features: a clinicopathologic study of 12 cases. Am J Surg Pathol. 36(6):869-75, 2012
17. Cubilla AL et al: Value of p16(INK)⁴(a) in the pathology of invasive penile squamous cell carcinomas: A report of 202 cases. Am J Surg Pathol. 35(2):253-61, 2011
18. Epstein JI et al: Tumors of the Prostate Gland, Seminal Vesicles, Penis, and Scrotum. Washington, DC: American Registry of Pathology and AFIP, 2011
19. Oertell J et al: Differentiated precursor lesions and low-grade variants of squamous cell carcinomas are frequent findings in foreskins of patients from a region of high penile cancer incidence. Histopathology. 58(6):925-33, 2011
20. Chaux A et al: Warty-basaloid carcinoma: clinicopathological features of a distinctive penile neoplasm. Report of 45 cases. Mod Pathol. 23(6):896-904, 2010
21. Cubilla AL et al: The basaloid cell is the best tissue marker for human papillomavirus in invasive penile squamous cell carcinoma: a study of 202 cases from Paraguay. Am J Surg Pathol. 34(1):104-14, 2010
22. de Sanjose S et al: Human papillomavirus genotype attribution in invasive cervical cancer: a retrospective cross-sectional worldwide study. Lancet Oncol. 11:1048-56, 2010
23. Backes DM et al: Systematic review of human papillomavirus prevalence in invasive penile cancer. Cancer Causes Control. 20(4):449-57, 2009
24. Miralles-Guri C et al: Human papillomavirus prevalence and type distribution in penile carcinoma. J Clin Pathol. 62(10):870-8, 2009
25. Cubilla AL et al: Pseudohyperplastic squamous cell carcinoma of the penis associated with lichen sclerosus. An extremely well-differentiated, nonverruciform neoplasm that preferentially affects the foreskin and is frequently misdiagnosed: a report of 10 cases of a distinctive clinicopathologic entity. Am J Surg Pathol. 28(7):895-900, 2004
26. Velazquez EF et al: Preputial variability and preferential association of long phimotic foreskins with penile cancer: an anatomic comparative study of types of foreskin in a general population and cancer patients. Am J Surg Pathol. 27(7):994-8, 2003
27. Bezerra AL et al: Clinicopathologic features and human papillomavirus dna prevalence of warty and squamous cell carcinomas of the penis. Am J Surg Pathol. 25(5):673-8, 2001
28. Rubin MA et al: Detection and typing of human papillomavirus DNA in penile carcinoma: evidence for multiple independent pathways of penile carcinogenesis. Am J Pathol. 159(4):1211-8, 2001
29. Cubilla AL, Reuter V, Velazquez E, et al: Histologic classification of penile carcinoma and its relation to outcome in 61 patients with primary resection. Int J Surg Pathol 2001;9:111-120, 2001
30. Gregoire L et al: Preferential association of human papillomavirus with high-grade histologic variants of penile-invasive squamous cell carcinoma. J Natl Cancer Inst. 87(22):1705-9, 1995

Overview of HPV- and Non-HPV-Related Tumors

HPV-Type Prevalence Distribution in Penile Carcinomas

Genotype	Frequency (%)	Relative Contribution Among HPV-Positive Cases (%)
HPV-16	18.3	60.23
HPV-18	6.3	13.35
HPV-6/11	3.8	8.13
HPV-31	0.5	1.16
HPV-45	0.5	1.16
HPV-33	0.4	0.87
HPV-52	0.3	0.58
Other types*	1.2	2.47
Any type	47.0	100

*Includes HPV-68 (0.2%), HPV-34 (0.14%), HPV-35 (0.14%), HPV-53 (0.14%), HPV-54 (0.14%), HPV-74 (0.14%), HPV-22 (0.07%), HPV-39 (0.07%), HPV-51 (0.07%), and HPV-70 (0.07%).

Modified from Miralles-Guri et al.

Variants of Penile Squamous Cell Carcinomas

Non-HPV Related	HPV Related	Others
Usual	Basaloid	Mixed
Verrucous	Warty	Unclassified
Papillary Not Otherwise Specified	Warty-basaloid	
Cuniculatum	Papillary basaloid	
Pseudoglandular	Clear cell	
Pseudohyperplastic	Lymphoepithelioma-like	
Sarcomatoid		
Adenosquamous		

Extramammary Paget Disease

KEY FACTS

TERMINOLOGY
- Extramammary Paget disease (EMPD)

CLINICAL ISSUES
- Erythematous patches or plaques with sharply defined borders
  - Pruritus is frequent
- May clinically mimic chronic eczema

MICROSCOPIC
- Round, large, pale cells in all levels of epidermis arranged as single units or confluent aggregates
  - May form true glandular lumina
  - May contain intracytoplasmic melanin
- Round vesicular nuclei with prominent nucleoli
- Abundant clear cytoplasm
- Absence of intercellular bridges
- Paget cells often extend to adnexal structures
- Flattened basal keratinocytes

ANCILLARY TESTS
- Paget cells positive for mucin
- Primary EMPD positive for CK7 and negative for CK20
- Secondary EMPD has more variable immunohistochemical profile
  - Secondary EMPD associated with urothelial carcinoma positive for CK7, CK20, GATA3
  - Secondary EMPD associated with anal/rectal carcinoma positive for CK20 and negative for CK7; positive for CDX2

TOP DIFFERENTIAL DIAGNOSES
- Melanoma in situ
- Squamous cell carcinoma in situ with pagetoid pattern
- Clear cell papulosis
- Benign mucinous metaplasia of penis

Primary Penile EMPD
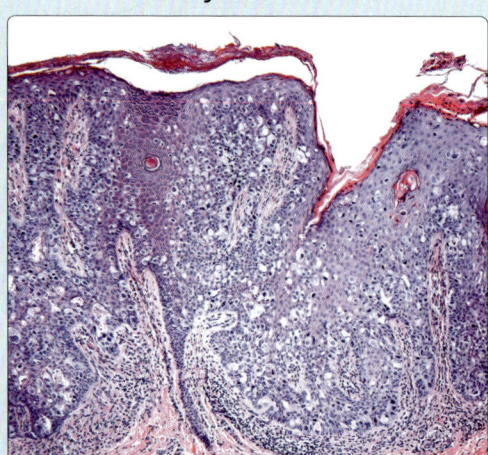

Primary Penile EMPD
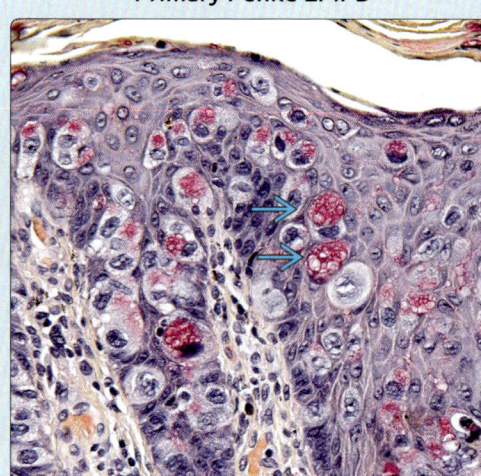

(Left) This section shows an intraepithelial proliferation of large atypical cells with pale cytoplasm within a hyperplastic squamous epithelium. EMPD = extramammary Paget disease. (Right) Mucicarmine stain shows red positive staining of the cytoplasm of Paget cells ➜.

Primary Penile EMPD
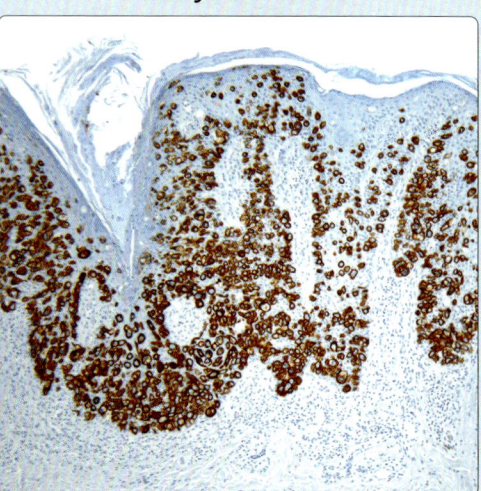

Immunohistochemistry: CK7
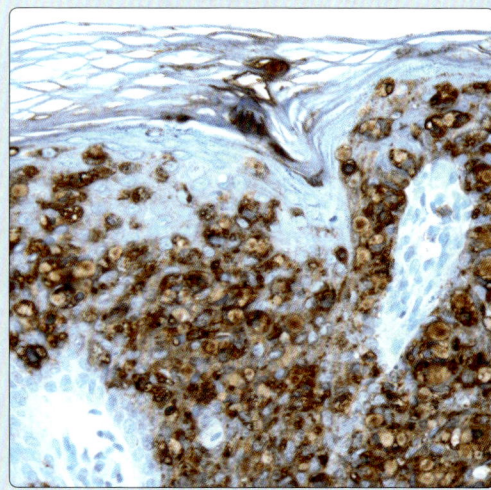

(Left) In this case of primary Paget disease of the penis, immunohistochemistry with CK7 highlights the neoplastic cells in all levels of the epidermis. (Right) CK7 immunohistochemistry highlights the cells of primary penile EMPD. CK20 positivity, if present, should raise the possibility of a secondary process.

Extramammary Paget Disease

TERMINOLOGY

Synonyms
- Extramammary Paget disease (EMPD)

Definitions
- Adenocarcinoma involving epidermis/squamous epithelium and commonly extending to epithelium of eccrine glands &/or hair follicles (adenocarcinoma in situ)
- May involve dermis/ lamina propria in minority of cases

ETIOLOGY/PATHOGENESIS

Pathogenesis
- Uncertain
- Cases limited to epidermis are postulated to originate from intraepidermal portion of sweat glands or from intraepidermal stem cells
- Heterogeneous condition: Classified as primary (cutaneous origin) and secondary (extracutaneous origin)
  - Rarely, primary EMPD is associated with underlying sweat gland adenocarcinoma
  - Secondary EMPD may represent extension from urethral, bladder, or anal/rectal carcinoma

CLINICAL ISSUES

Epidemiology
- Age
  - 6th or 7th decade

Site
- Skin regions rich in apocrine glands, such as anogenital area
- Primary EMPD
  - Scrotum and perineum with extension to adjacent areas is most frequent sites in primary lesions
  - Exclusive penile location is rare
    - Primary Paget disease may extend to urethral epithelium
- Secondary EMPD
  - Secondary Paget disease tends to affect glans and especially perimeatal region
  - May also affect perianal area extending to perineum and scrotum

Presentation
- Variable: Uni- or multifocal
  - Circinate or annular moist erythematous scaly patches or plaques
  - Gray-white eczematous patches
    - May be confused with eczema, delaying diagnosis
  - Hypopigmented macules, oozing, ulceration, crusting, or palpable tumor
- Pruritus, tenderness, and burning sensation can occur

Treatment
- Complete surgical excision is treatment of choice for primary EMPD
- Treatment in secondary lesions will depend on associated carcinoma

Prognosis
- Primary EMPD without invasion (in situ carcinoma) has good prognosis when completely excised
  - Dermal invasion is associated with worse prognosis
- Long-term follow-up is needed due to multifocal nature and high recurrence rate
- Prognosis in secondary Paget disease is related to underlying carcinoma and is usually poor

MACROSCOPIC

Sections to Be Submitted
- Important to carefully evaluate margins because neoplastic cells may extend beyond clinical borders

Size
- Few mm to large lesions that involve entire anogenital area

MICROSCOPIC

Histologic Features
- Intraepithelial proliferation of large round atypical cells (Paget cells)
  - Neoplastic cells have abundant pale or vacuolated cytoplasm
  - May contain intracytoplasmic melanin
  - Intercellular bridges are not appreciated between Paget cells on light microscopy
  - Large and vesicular nuclei with prominent nucleoli
  - Mitoses may be numerous
  - Early lesions may be subtle with only scattered Paget cells in epidermis
  - Established lesions show numerous Paget cells arranged as single units and confluent aggregates
    - May form true intraepidermal glandular structures
  - Paget cells compress squamous cells
    - Flattened basal keratinocytes lie between neoplastic cells and underlying dermis
  - Neoplastic cells often extend to epithelium of adnexal structures
- Epithelium varied from hyperplastic to atrophic
  - May be ulcerated and crusted
- Dermal mixed cell infiltrate is usually present
- Dermal involvement by tumoral cells may occur

ANCILLARY TESTS

Histochemistry
- Positive for mucicarmine

Immunohistochemistry
- Primary EMPD is positive for CEA, CK7, CAM5.2, EMA/MUC1, GCDFP-15, and BER-EP4
- Primary EMPD negative for melanocytic markers
- Immunohistochemical expression profile of secondary EMPD is related to associated carcinoma
  - Secondary EMPD associated with urothelial carcinoma
    - Positive for uroplakin-2/-3, GATA3, CK7, CK20
  - EMPD secondary to anal/rectal carcinomas
    - Expresses CK20, CDX-2, CEA

Extramammary Paget Disease

DIFFERENTIAL DIAGNOSIS

Melanoma In Situ
- Melanoma cells are present in all levels of epidermis, including basal layer
- No flattened basal cells are seen between melanoma cells and dermis
- Presence of melanin pigment in neoplastic cells does not indicate melanoma diagnosis
- Melanoma invades dermis much more frequently than Paget disease
- Immunohistochemical expression of melanocytic markers, such as S100, Melan-A(MART-1), and HMB-45

Squamous Cell Carcinoma In Situ With Pagetoid Pattern
- Presence of intercellular bridges among neoplastic cells
- Positive for HMCK (e.g., 34βE12), CK5/6, p63
- Negative for mucicarmine
- Negative for CEA, GCDFP-15, and CK20
- Usually negative for CK7 and BER-EP4
  - Subset of pagetoid squamous in situ cells may be positive

Clear Cell Papulosis
- Young children
- More often Asian
- Small macules or papules
- Lower part of trunk
- Predominantly milk line location
- Clear cells with pagetoid features in lower part of epidermis
- CK-PAN(AE1/AE3) and CEA (+)

Benign Mucinous Metaplasia of Penis
- Elderly patients
- Prepuce or glans
- Benign mucin containing cells in squamous epithelium
- Usually associated with chronic inflammatory conditions

Pagetoid Dyskeratosis
- Reactive process
- Intertriginous and genital area
- Lesional cells are keratinocytes showing early keratinization

Pagetoid Reticulosis
- Rare variant of cutaneous T-cell lymphoma
- Exclusive epidermal infiltration by medium- to large-sized T cells with abundant pale cytoplasm
- T cells are CD45(LCA) and CD3 (+)
- T cells may be either CD4 or CD8 (+), or double negative
- T cell gene rearrangement can be demonstrated

Merkel Cell Carcinoma
- May have prominent epidermotropic component
- Small round blue cells with scarce cytoplasm
- Not true glandular formation
- Characteristic dot-like pattern with CK20 and CK-PAN(AE1/AE3)
- In minority of cases may coexpress CK7
- Positive expression of neuroendocrine markers, such as chromogranin and synaptophysin

DIAGNOSTIC CHECKLIST

Clinically Relevant Pathologic Features
- Tissue distribution
  - Important to distinguish in situ lesions, in which Paget cells are confined within epidermis and epithelium of adnexal structures from tumors showing true dermal invasion
  - Important to recognize EMPD associated with underlying sweat gland carcinoma
  - Important clinically to rule out secondary EMPD

Pathologic Interpretation Pearls
- Large round cells with abundant pale cytoplasm in all levels of epidermis (Paget cells)
- Flattened basal keratinocytes lying between Paget cells and underlying basement membrane
- Presence of melanin and lack of glandular formation do not rule out Paget disease

SELECTED REFERENCES

1. Chang J et al: Diagnostic utility of p63 expression in the differential diagnosis of pagetoid squamous cell carcinoma in situ and extramammary Paget disease: a histopathologic study of 70 cases. Am J Dermatopathol. 36(1):49-53, 2014
2. De la Garza Bravo MM et al: Pigmented extramammary Paget disease of the thigh mimicking a melanocytic tumor: report of a case and review of the literature. J Cutan Pathol. 41(6):529-35, 2014
3. Sah SP et al: Diffuse CK7, CAM5.2 and BerEP4 positivity in pagetoid squamous cell carcinoma in situ (pagetoid Bowen's disease) of the perianal region: a mimic of extramammary Paget's disease. Histopathology. 62(3):511-4, 2013
4. Hegarty PK et al: Penoscrotal extramammary Paget's disease: the University of Texas M. D. Anderson Cancer Center contemporary experience. J Urol. 186(1):97-102, 2011
5. Wang Z et al: Penile and scrotal Paget's disease: 130 Chinese patients with long-term follow-up. BJU Int. 102(4):485-8, 2008
6. Liegl B et al: Mammary and extramammary Paget's disease: an immunohistochemical study of 83 cases. Histopathology. 50(4):439-47, 2007
7. De Nisi MC et al: Usefulness of CDX2 in the diagnosis of extramammary Paget disease associated with malignancies of intestinal type. Br J Dermatol. 153(3):677-9, 2005
8. Salamanca J et al: Paget's disease of the glans penis secondary to transitional cell carcinoma of the bladder: a report of two cases and review of the literature. J Cutan Pathol. 31(4):341-5, 2004
9. Brown HM et al: Uroplakin-III to distinguish primary vulvar Paget disease from Paget disease secondary to urothelial carcinoma. Hum Pathol. 33(5):545-8, 2002
10. van Randenborgh H et al: Extramammary Paget's disease of penis and scrotum. J Urol. 168(6):2540-1, 2002
11. Kuan SF et al: Differential expression of mucin genes in mammary and extramammary Paget's disease. Am J Surg Pathol. 25(12):1469-77, 2001
12. Ohnishi T et al: The use of cytokeratins 7 and 20 in the diagnosis of primary and secondary extramammary Paget's disease. Br J Dermatol. 142(2):243-7, 2000
13. Val-Bernal JF et al: Benign mucinous metaplasia of the penis. A lesion resembling extramammary Paget's disease. J Cutan Pathol. 27(2):76-9, 2000
14. Val-Bernal JF et al: Pagetoid dyskeratosis of the prepuce. An incidental histologic finding resembling extramammary Paget's disease. J Cutan Pathol. 27(8):387-91, 2000
15. Lee JY: Clear cell papulosis: a unique disorder in early childhood characterized by white macules in milk-line distribution. Pediatr Dermatol. 15(4):328-9, 1998

Extramammary Paget Disease

Paget Disease: Low Power
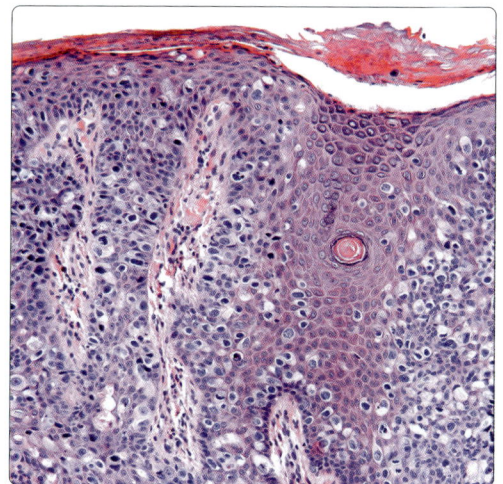

Paget Disease: High Power
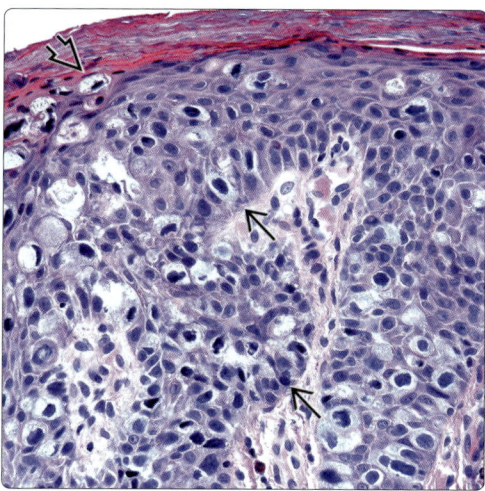

(Left) Note the numerous Paget cells in all levels of the epidermis, in this case of EMPD. The epidermis is hyperplastic. (Right) Numerous Paget cells arranged as confluent single units are seen in all levels of the epidermis, including the cornified layer ⇨. Note the slightly flattened preserved basal keratinocytes underneath the neoplastic cells ⇨.

Paget Disease: Dermal Interface
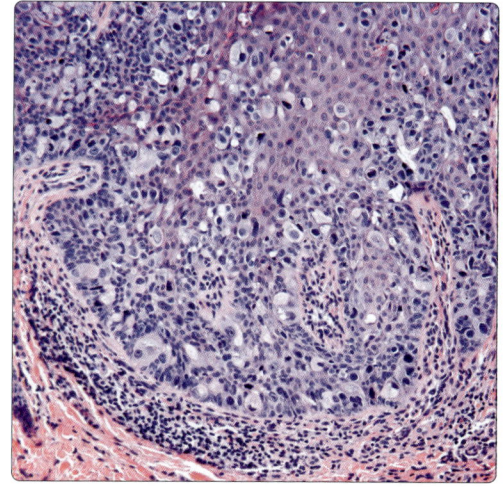

Primary EMPD of Penis
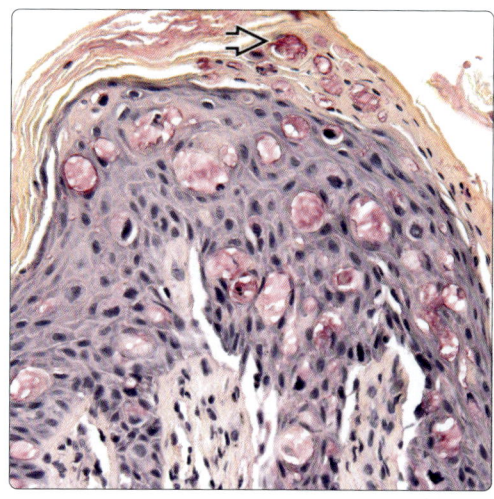

(Left) Paget cells are large, round to oval, and show ample pale cytoplasm. It is important to rule out invasion in cases of Paget disease, though it is not common. (Right) There is red intracytoplasmic positivity of the neoplastic cells with a mucicarmine stain. Note the presence of neoplastic cells at all levels of the epidermis including the cornified layer ⇨.

Secondary Paget Disease
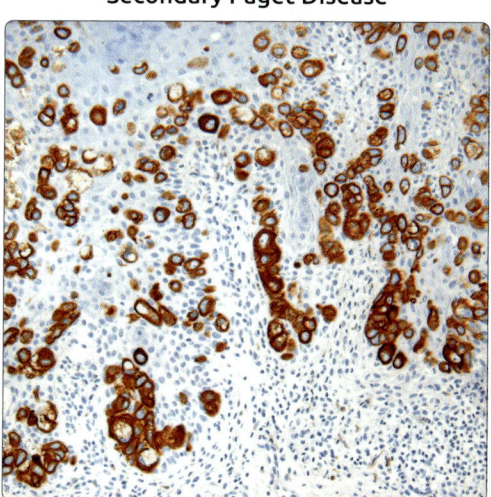

Penile Paget Disease Secondary to Anal/Rectal Carcinoma
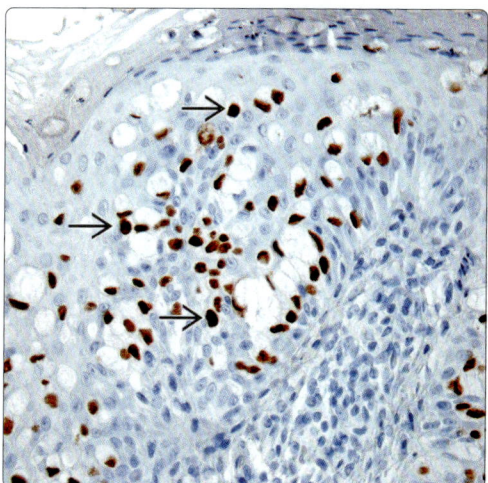

(Left) Note the CK20 expression of the neoplastic cells in this case of EMPD secondary to rectal/anal carcinoma. (Right) The neoplastic cells show nuclear positivity with CDX-2 ⇨ in EMPD secondary to anal/rectal carcinoma. Clinical history is key and should be ascertained in cases of Paget disease.

Kaposi Sarcoma

KEY FACTS

ETIOLOGY/PATHOGENESIS
- Human herpesvirus-8 (HHV-8)/Kaposi sarcoma (KS)-associated herpesvirus

MACROSCOPIC
- Specimens received are usually punch or incisional/excisional biopsies

MICROSCOPIC
- Early lesions show subtle proliferation of vessels around dermal sweat glands
- Well-established lesions show honeycomb-like network of blood-filled spaces/slits closely associated with spindle cell component

ANCILLARY TESTS
- Immunohistochemistry for HHV-8 is helpful to confirm diagnosis
- Positive for CD31, CD34, and podoplanin

TOP DIFFERENTIAL DIAGNOSES
- Angioma
  - Lacks jagged vascular pattern, promontory sign, and patchy infiltrate with plasma cells and siderophages characteristic of KS
- Angiosarcoma
  - Usually more pleomorphic cells lining vascular spaces
- Sarcomatoid carcinoma
  - Does not have slit-like spaces containing erythrocytes among spindle cells
- Sarcomatoid carcinoma
  - May be entirely composed of spindle cells; pseudovascular subtype has been described
  - Positive for keratins [especially CK-PAN(MNF116), HMWK(34βE12)] and p63/p40
  - Negative for HHV-8 and vascular markers

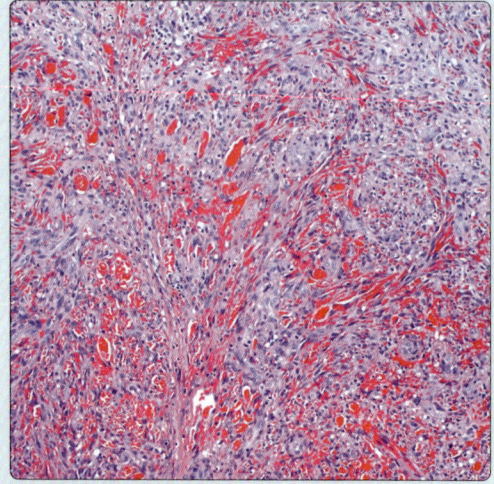

Well-Established Lesion of Kaposi Sarcoma

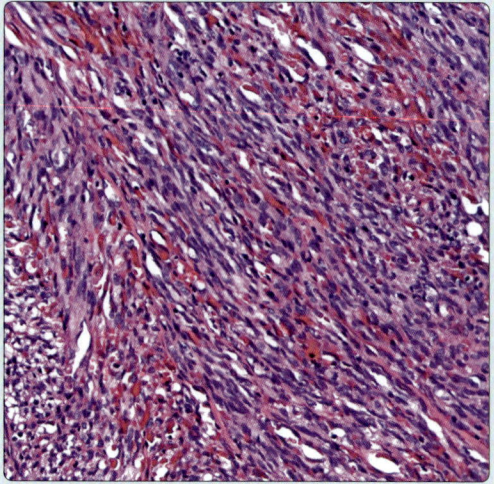

Spindle Cell Proliferation Admixed With Vascular Spaces

(Left) Low-power view in a well-established nodular lesion of Kaposi sarcoma shows a network of slit-like and slightly dilated vessels filled with red blood cells and a proliferation of relatively bland spindle cells. *(Right)* A well-established lesion of Kaposi sarcoma shows the characteristic honeycomb-like network of slit-like vascular spaces filled with erythrocytes separating the spindle cells.

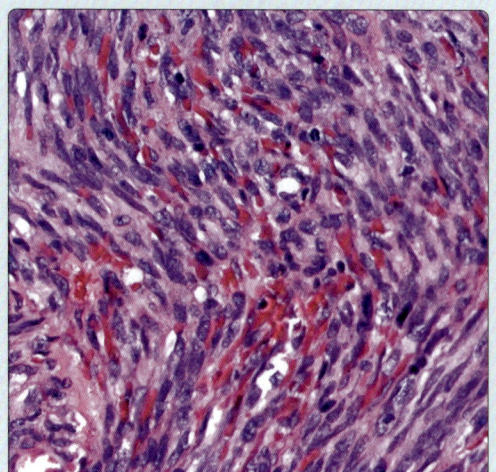

Slit-Like Spaces Containing Red Blood Cells

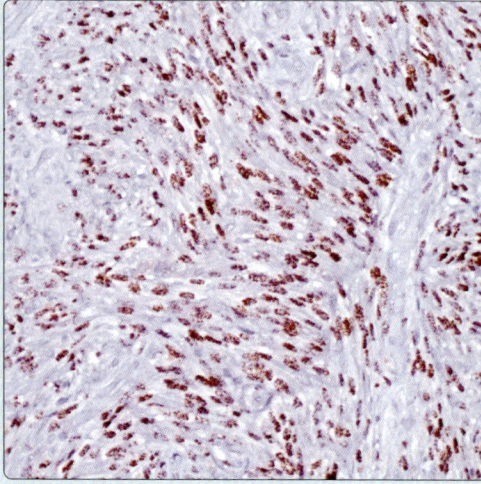

HHV-8 Nuclear Staining

(Left) Monomorphic spindle cells in ill-defined fascicles and arcs intimately admixed with slit-like vascular channels containing erythrocytes are a classic feature of Kaposi sarcoma. *(Right)* Immunohistochemical analysis with Kaposi sarcoma-associated herpesvirus/human herpesvirus-8 shows nuclear expression in Kaposi sarcoma.

Kaposi Sarcoma

TERMINOLOGY

Abbreviations
- Kaposi sarcoma (KS)

Definitions
- Virus-associated vascular tumor

ETIOLOGY/PATHOGENESIS

Etiology
- Human herpesvirus-8 (HHV-8), a.k.a. KS-associated herpesvirus (KSHV)

Pathogenesis
- Proliferating cell in KS appears to be lymphatic in origin
- KS may be classified into 4 main groups
  - Classic, endemic/African, AIDS-associated, and iatrogenic/transplantation-associated KS

CLINICAL ISSUES

Epidemiology
- Incidence
  - Penile and urogenital KS usually affects HIV(+) patients
    - Incidence has decreased with advent of antiretroviral therapy
  - May also be seen in patients affected by other forms of immunosuppression
  - Classic and endemic forms of KS affecting penis are extremely rare
- Age
  - AIDS-related KS and endemic forms affect younger patients
  - Classic KS and transplant-related KS tend to affect older patients

Site
- Most common location is glans
- May also affect coronal sulcus, foreskin, and skin of shaft

Presentation
- From ill-defined erythematous macules to violaceous plaques and nodules
- Frequently multifocal
- Tends to affect penis in setting of multiple disseminated lesions, especially in AIDS patients

Treatment
- Irradiation &/or chemotherapy

Prognosis
- Variable and dependent on different factors, such as immunologic host status and stage of disease
  - AIDS-related KS runs more rapid evolution than classical form

MACROSCOPIC

General Features
- Specimens received are usually punch or incisional/excisional biopsies

MICROSCOPIC

Histologic Features
- Patch stage
  - Subtle proliferation of slit-like &/or angulated/jagged vessels separating collagen bundles within dermis
  - Adnexal structures and preexisting vessels may protrude within newly formed vessels (promontory sign)
  - Extravasated red blood cells and siderophages
  - Patchy dermal infiltrate of lymphoid cells and plasma cells
- Plaque stage
  - Dermal vascular proliferation may extend to subcutis
  - Spindle cell component appears at this stage
  - Intra/extracellular PAS-D(+) hyaline globules
- Nodular stage
  - Spindle cell proliferation forms well-defined nodules, fascicles, and arcs
  - Spindle cells are intimately admixed/separated by slit-like spaces containing erythrocytes
  - Dilated blood vessels, inflammatory cells, and siderophages often seen at periphery of nodules

DIFFERENTIAL DIAGNOSIS

Angioma
- Lacks jagged vascular pattern, promontory sign, and patchy infiltrate with plasma cells and siderophages characteristic of KS

Angiosarcoma
- Usually more pleomorphic cells lining vascular spaces

Fibrosarcoma
- Does not have slit-like spaces containing erythrocytes among spindle cells

Sarcomatoid Carcinoma
- May be entirely composed of spindle cells; pseudovascular subtype has been described
- Positive for keratins [especially CK-PAN(MNF116), HMWK(34βE12)] and p63/p40
- Negative for HHV-8 and vascular markers

DIAGNOSTIC CHECKLIST

Pathologic Interpretation Pearls
- Low-power view in early lesions shows slender cords of cells among collagen bundles that may mimic histiocytes or stromal cells
  - Only closer view will reveal luminal differentiation or connection with preexisting blood vessels

SELECTED REFERENCES

1. Farshidpour M et al: Disseminated Kaposi's aarcoma with the involvement of penis in the setting of HIV infection. Indian J Dermatol. 60(1):104, 2015
2. Woldrich JM et al: Penile Kaposis sarcoma in the state of California. Can J Urol. 19(2):6178-82, 2012
3. Carroll PA et al: Kaposi's sarcoma-associated herpesvirus infection of blood endothelial cells induces lymphatic differentiation. Virology. 328(1):7-18, 2004
4. Micali G et al: Primary classic Kaposi's sarcoma of the penis: report of a case and review. J Eur Acad Dermatol Venereol. 17(3):320-3, 2003

Myointimoma

KEY FACTS

TERMINOLOGY
- Myointimal proliferation arising within corpus spongiosum of glans penis

CLINICAL ISSUES
- Small palpable nodular lesion on glans penis
- Simple conservative excision
- Benign, nonrecurring
- Rare tumor with few reported case series
- Affects children and adults

MICROSCOPIC
- Plexiform or multinodular growth
- Pure intravascular growth with extension along vessels of corpus spongiosum
- Individual cells have myofibroblast morphology
- Associated myxoid and fibrous stroma is characteristic
- Surrounding collarette of residual vascular wall smooth muscle generally present at periphery
- Intracytoplasmic juxtanuclear vacuoles are common

ANCILLARY TESTS
- Expresses smooth muscle actin
- Desmin highlights residual native smooth muscle of vessel walls
- Lesional cells are usually desmin negative

TOP DIFFERENTIAL DIAGNOSES
- Epithelioid hemangioendothelioma
  - Most clinically critical distinction
- Myofibroma
- Leiomyoma
- Plexiform fibrohistiocytic tumor
- Intravascular fasciitis
  - Myointimoma may be site-specific form of intravascular fasciitis

Myointimoma: Serpiginous Growth
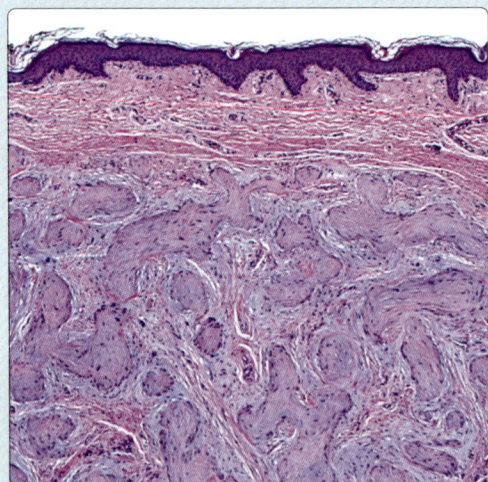

Myointimoma: Myofibroblastic Proliferation
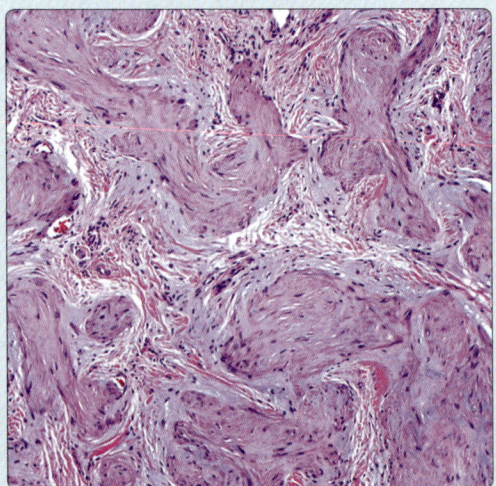

(Left) Penile myointimoma of the corpus spongiosum has a distinctive low-power serpiginous or nodular growth pattern secondary to extension along preexisting vascular channels. **(Right)** The lesional cells have a spindled myofibroblastic appearance and an associated fibrous and myxoid stroma. They expand the vascular spaces of the corpus spongiosum with atrophy of the vessel walls and loss of the lumen.

Myointimoma: Intravascular Growth
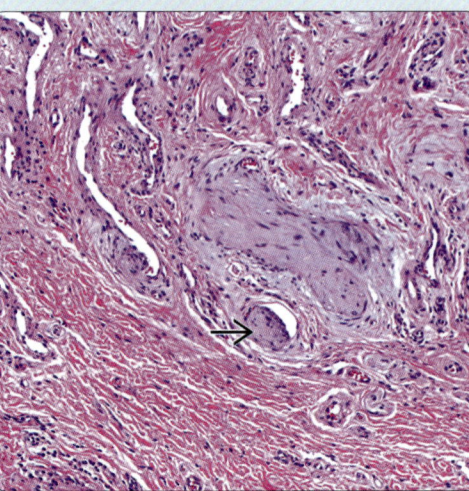

Myointimoma: Myxoid Stroma
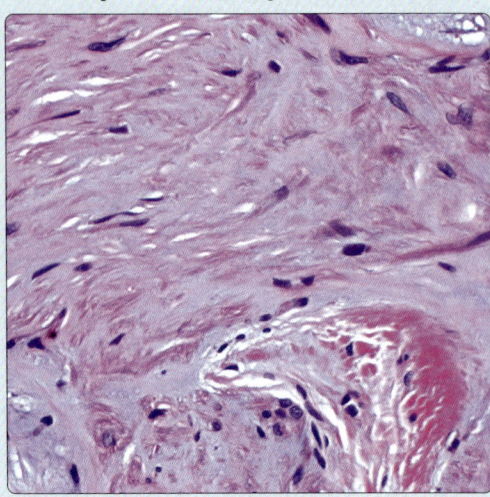

(Left) In these peripheral transition areas, there is partial filling of small vessel lumina by the lesional spindled cells with associated myxoid stroma ➡. Residual endothelial cells and smooth muscle collarettes are common in these foci. **(Right)** The lesional spindled cells of myointimoma are associated with a dense fibrous and myxoid stroma. They have tapered nuclei and elongated cytoplasmic processes. No significant nuclear atypia is seen.

Myointimoma

TERMINOLOGY

Definitions
- Benign myointimal proliferation occurring exclusively in corpus spongiosum of glans penis

CLINICAL ISSUES

Epidemiology
- Incidence
  - Rare tumor with few reported case series
- Age
  - Affects children and adults

Presentation
- Small palpable nodular lesion on glans penis

Treatment
- Simple conservative excision

Prognosis
- Benign
  - No recurrences reported and may spontaneously regress

MACROSCOPIC

Size
- Typically 0.5-2.0 cm

MICROSCOPIC

Histologic Features
- Plexiform or multinodular growth
  - Pure intravascular growth
  - Extension within preexisting vascular network of corpus spongiosum
- Individual cells have myofibroblastic features
- Associated myxoid and fibrous stroma is characteristic
- Intracytoplasmic juxtanuclear vacuoles are common
- Surrounding collarette of residual smooth muscle generally present at periphery

ANCILLARY TESTS

Immunohistochemistry
- Expresses smooth muscle markers
  - Smooth muscle actin
  - Calponin
- Desmin highlights residual native smooth muscle of vessel walls
  - Seen best at periphery of lesion
  - Lesional spindled cells are desmin negative
- S100 negative
- CD31 and CD34 highlight residual endothelial cells at periphery

DIFFERENTIAL DIAGNOSIS

Plexiform Fibrohistiocytic Tumor
- Similar plexiform/nodular growth
- Not described in penis and not intravascular
- Dimorphic morphology with myofibroblasts and nodules of histiocytic cells and scattered osteoclast-like cells

Myofibroma
- Often have classic biphasic appearance
  - Myoid nodules are similar in morphology to myointimoma cells
  - Hemangiopericytoma-like foci often admixed
- Myoid-predominant myofibromas do occur
- May involve vessels
  - Not exclusively confined to vascular lumina as in myointimoma

Leiomyoma
- Intersecting fascicular architecture
- Not typically multinodular/plexiform
- Lesional cells express desmin
- Not typically myxoid (more eosinophilic appearance)

Epithelioid Hemangioendothelioma
- Morphologically similar
  - Similar myxoid stroma
  - Usually more epithelioid but may be spindled
  - Intraluminal vacuoles common
- Rare in children
- Very uncommon in penis
  - Epithelioid hemangioma is more common in penis
    - However, less morphologic overlap with myointimoma
- Immunoreactivity for CD31, CD34, and ERG in spindled/epithelioid cell population

Nerve Sheath Tumors
- May have multinodular/plexiform growth pattern
  - Neurofibroma
  - Schwannoma
  - Nerve sheath myxoma
- Diffuse nuclear reactivity for S100
- Not common in penis

Intravascular Fasciitis
- May be same lesion

DIAGNOSTIC CHECKLIST

Clinically Relevant Pathologic Features
- Benign lesion does not require reexcision if transected

Pathologic Interpretation Pearls
- Anatomic site should alert pathologists to possibility of this diagnosis

SELECTED REFERENCES

1. Turner BM et al: Penile myointimoma. J Cutan Pathol. 36(7):817-9, 2009
2. McKenney JK et al: Penile myointimoma in children and adolescents: a clinicopathologic study of 5 cases supporting a distinct entity. Am J Surg Pathol. 31(10):1622-6, 2007
3. Vardar E et al: Myointimoma of the glans penis. Pathol Int. 57(3):158-61, 2007
4. Robbins JB et al: Penile nodule in a 54-year-old man: a case of a myointimoma. J Am Acad Dermatol. 53(6):1084-6, 2005
5. Fetsch et al: Mesenchymal tumours. In Eble JN et al: Pathology & Genetics of Tumours of the Urinary System and Male Genital Organs. Lyon: IARC Press, 294, 2004
6. Fetsch JF et al: A distinctive myointimal proliferation ('myointimoma') involving the corpus spongiosum of the glans penis: a clinicopathologic and immunohistochemical analysis of 10 cases. Am J Surg Pathol. 24(11):1524-30, 2000

Metastatic Tumors, Penis

KEY FACTS

TERMINOLOGY
- Genitourinary tumors are most common primary sites followed by gastrointestinal tumors
- Bladder urothelial carcinomas and prostatic adenocarcinomas account for most of cases
- Secondary involvement of penis by malignancy with predilection for erectile tissues of corpora cavernosa

ETIOLOGY/PATHOGENESIS
- Mostly by retrograde venous or lymphatic spread

CLINICAL ISSUES
- 1/3 are detected concurrently with primary neoplasm
- Symptoms include difficulty in urination, dysuria, urinary retention, and priapism
- Clinical history of primary tumor often available

MACROSCOPIC
- Corpora cavernosa are most frequent anatomic site affected
- Glans and foreskin are rarely involved

MICROSCOPIC
- Tumor cells mainly in vascular spaces of penile erectile tissues
- Multicentricity is the rule
- Histologic picture is consistent with that of primary tumor
- Perineural and vascular invasion are common
- Absence of in situ disease involving squamous mucosa or skin
- Immunohistochemical studies may be required to determine primary site

TOP DIFFERENTIAL DIAGNOSES
- Primary squamous cell carcinoma
- Primary penile sarcoma
- Urothelial carcinoma of urethra

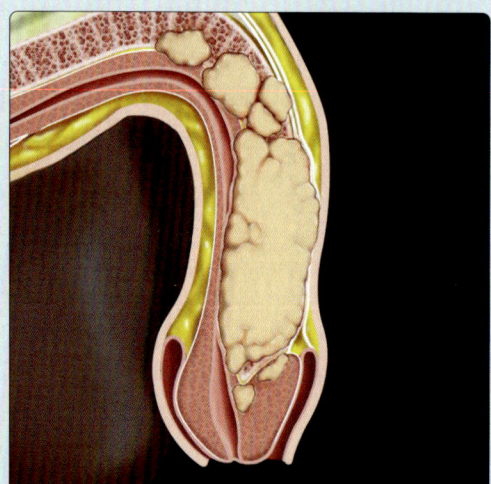

Metastatic Prostatic Adenosquamous Carcinoma to Penis

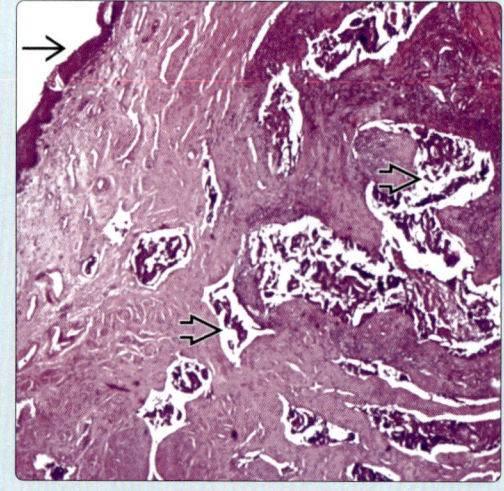

Metastatic Adenocarcinoma to Penis

(Left) Diagram of a secondary prostatic adenosquamous carcinoma shows multiple deep-seated metastatic nodules mainly located in corpora cavernosa of the penile shaft without affecting the glans surface. (Right) Metastatic adenocarcinoma from sigmoid colon extensively involving vascular spaces of penile erectile tissues ⮕ but with no involvement of penile shaft skin ⮕.

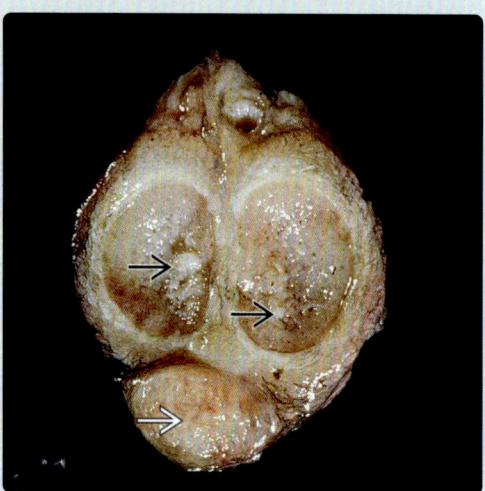

Metastatic Nodules in Penis

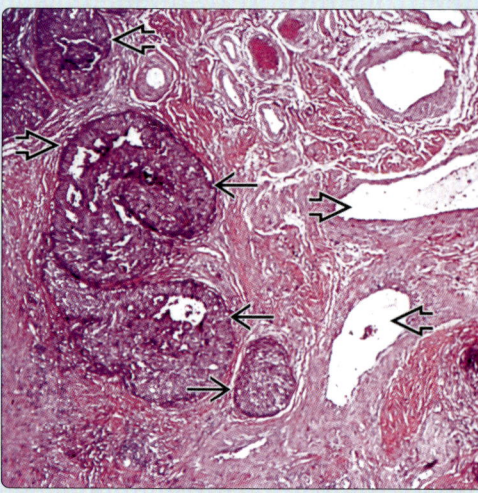

Urothelial Carcinoma Metastatic to Penis

(Left) Transverse section shows extensive involvement of both corpora cavernosa ⮕ as well as periurethral tissue ⮕. (Right) Urothelial carcinoma metastatic to the penis is shown with predilection of tumor nests ⮕ for vascular spaces ⮕ of the corpus cavernosum. Absence of in situ disease is an important observation.

Metastatic Tumors, Penis

TERMINOLOGY

Definitions
- Secondary involvement of penis by malignancy with predilection for erectile tissues of corpora cavernosa

ETIOLOGY/PATHOGENESIS

Routes of Spread
- Mostly by retrograde venous or lymphatic spread
- Arterial spread, direct extension from regional sites, and secondary embolization

CLINICAL ISSUES

Site
- Predilection for erectile tissues of corpora cavernosa
- Among tumors metastatic to penis, genitourinary (GU) tumors are most common (70%), although only minority of GU tumors metastasize to penis
  - Bladder urothelial carcinoma and prostatic adenocarcinomas account for most primary tumors
  - Other GU primary sites include kidney (renal cell carcinoma) and testis (seminoma)
- Gastrointestinal tumors are 2nd most frequent primary neoplasms (20%)
  - Colonic (sigmoid and rectal) adenocarcinomas are most common
  - Pancreatic, gastric, esophageal, and liver primaries have also been rarely reported
- Rare primary sites include melanoma, lung, thyroid gland, among others
- Malignant lymphomas may also secondarily affect penis due to systemic dissemination
- Range of sarcomas, including chondrosarcoma, synovial sarcoma, and angiosarcoma have been reported

Presentation
- Clinical history of primary tumor often available
- Very rarely penile metastasis is initial manifestation of disease
- 1/3 are detected concurrently with primary
- Common symptoms include difficulty in urination, dysuria, &/or urinary retention
- Priapism (malignant priapism) occurs in ~ 1/2 of cases due to massive erectile tissue involvement
- Painless mass is not infrequent clinical finding

Treatment
- Multidisciplinary approach is required

Prognosis
- Poor prognosis related to pathologic stage of primary
- Even with combined multimodal therapy, survival is poor (mean: 9 months)

IMAGING

General Features
- CT, MR, and ultrasound ± fine-needle aspiration
- Cavernosography is also useful but has relatively high complication rate

MACROSCOPIC

General Features
- Corpora cavernosa are most frequently involved
- Corpus spongiosum and glans are rarely involved
- Skin of shaft and foreskin are rarely involved

MICROSCOPIC

Histologic Features
- Tumor cells mainly in vascular spaces of penile erectile tissues
- Involvement may be extensive, from proximal to distal corpora cavernosa
- Histologic picture is consistent with morphology of primary tumor
- Pagetoid spread to urethra may be present in some urothelial carcinomas
- Perineural and vascular invasion are common findings
- Penile parenchymal involvement is rare and secondary to extensive vascular involvement
- Immunohistochemical studies may be required to determine primary site

Cytologic Features
- Identification of cercariform cells in aspiration cytology permits diagnosis of metastatic urothelial carcinoma

DIFFERENTIAL DIAGNOSIS

Primary Squamous Cell Carcinoma
- Glans affected in most cases and in situ changes in surface epithelium are commonly present
- Corpora cavernosa involvement is secondary to invasion of consecutive anatomic levels

Primary Penile Sarcoma
- Often considered in differential diagnosis as mucosa/skin is uninvolved
- Predilection for deep erectile tissues and parenchyma
- Histology and immunohistochemistry typical of primary sarcoma
- Metastatic sarcomas are vanishingly rare

Urothelial Carcinoma of Urethra
- Urothelial carcinoma in situ or papillary urothelial carcinoma involving urethra
- Secondary involvement of penile tissues, including corpus spongiosum, before cavernosa are involved
- Immunohistochemistry for urothelial markers (uroplakin-3, thrombomodulin)

DIAGNOSTIC CHECKLIST

Pathologic Interpretation Pearls
- Nonsquamous histology, multicentricity, and prominent vascular erectile tissue venous invasion

SELECTED REFERENCES

1. Ellis CL et al: Metastatic prostate adenocarcinoma to the penis: a series of 29 cases with predilection for ductal adenocarcinoma. Am J Surg Pathol. 39(1):67-74, 2015
2. Chaux A et al: Metastatic tumors to the penis: a report of 17 cases and review of the literature. Int J Surg Pathol 2011;19(5):597-606, 2010

Immunohistochemistry, Penis

Extramammary Paget Disease (EMPD)

Antibody	Primary EMPD	2° EMPD Associated With Urothelial Carcinoma	2° EMPD Associated With Anal/Rectal Carcinoma	Melanoma In Situ	Squamous Cell Carcinoma In Situ
CEA	(+)	(-)	(+)	(-)	(-)
CK7	(+)	(+)	(-)	(-)	(-)
CAM5.2	(+)	(-)	(+/-)	(-)	(-/+)
EMA/MUC1	(+)	(-)	(+/-)	(-)	(-)
GCDFP-15	(+)	(-)	(-)	(-)	(-)
CK20	(-)	(+/-)	(+)	(-)	(-)
S100	(-)	(-)	(-)	(+)	(-)
Melan-A (MART-1)	(-)	(-)	(-)	(+)	(-)
Tyrosinase	(-)	(-)	(-)	(+)	(-)
HMB-45	(-)	(-)	(-)	(+)	(-)
Uroplakin-2/-3	(-)	(+)	(-)	(-)	(-)
CDX-2	(-)	(-)	(+)	(-)	(-)

HPV-Associated Lesions

Antibody	Warty Carcinoma	Papillary Carcinoma NOS	Verrucous Carcinoma	Condyloma With Malignant Change
p16	(+)	(-)	(-)	(-/+)

Spindle Cell Lesions

Antibody	Sarcomatoid Carcinoma	Leiomyosarcoma	Angiosarcoma	Spindle Cell Melanoma
S100	(-)	(-)	(-)	(+)
Actin-sm	(-/+)	(+)	(-)	(-)
Desmin	(-)	(+)	(-)	(-)
Calponin	(-)	(+)	(-)	(-)
CK-PAN (AE1/AE3)	(+/-)	(-)/[(+) focal]	(-)/[(+); rare]	(-)
CAM5.2	(+/-)	(-)	(-)	(-)
HMCK (34βE12)	(+)	(-)	(-)	(-)
p63	(+)	(-)	(-)	(-)
Vimentin	(+)	(+)	(+)	(+)
FLI-1	(-)	(-)	(+)	(-)
CD31	(-)	(-)	(+)	(-)
CD34	(-)	(-)	(+)	(-)

Penile Intraepithelial Neoplasia and Squamous Hyperplasia

Antibody	D-PeIN	W/B-PeIN	Squamous Hyperplasia
p16	(-)	(+)	(-)
p53	(+/-)	(+/-)	(-)
Ki-67	(+)	(+)	(+/-)

Immunohistochemistry, Penis

Warty-Basaloid Carcinoma
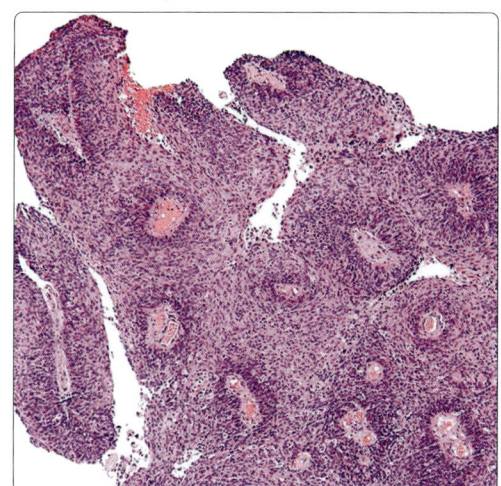

Warty-Basaloid Carcinoma, p16
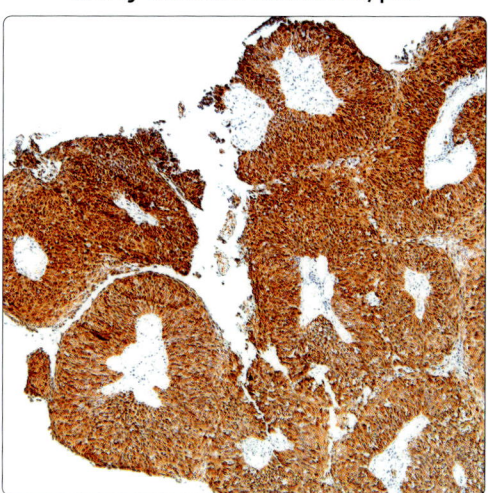

(Left) H&E shows the surface component of a warty-basaloid squamous cell carcinoma. The papillary surface of the tumor is lined by small basaloid cells at the center and larger pink cells with koilocytic changes at the periphery. Penile warty carcinoma, basaloid carcinoma, and mixed warty-basaloid carcinomas are usually associated with HPV. (Right) p16 immunohistochemical stain is strongly positive in this warty-basaloid squamous cell carcinoma, supporting its HPV-related etiopathogenesis.

Sarcomatoid Carcinoma
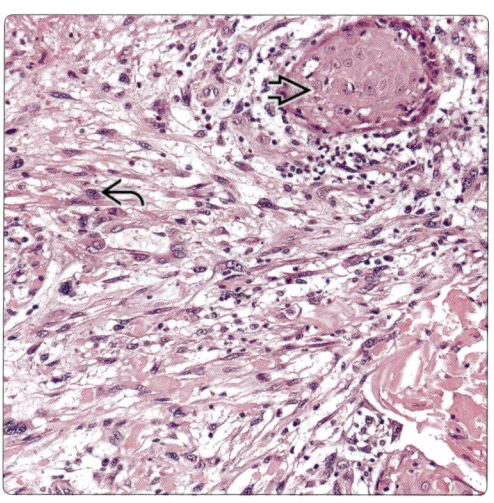

Sarcomatoid Carcinoma, CK-PAN
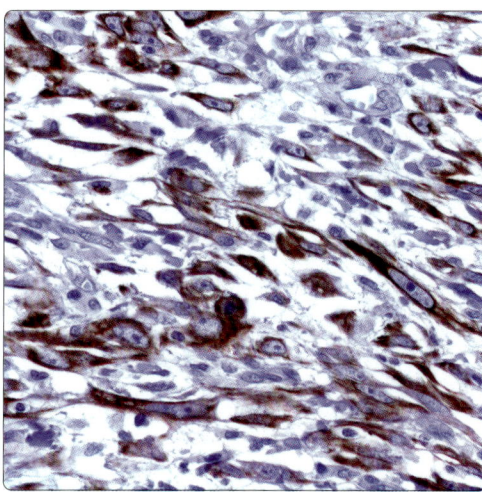

(Left) Sarcomatoid squamous cell carcinoma shows a predominant spindle cell component ⇨ and a focal but distinct component of invasive squamous cell carcinoma ⇨. Biphasic histology, presence of squamous cell carcinoma in situ, and previous history of squamous cell carcinoma support sarcomatoid differentiation. (Right) The focal positivity for CK-PAN in the spindle cell component of sarcomatoid carcinoma is further supportive of the diagnosis of sarcomatoid differentiation.

Kaposi Sarcoma
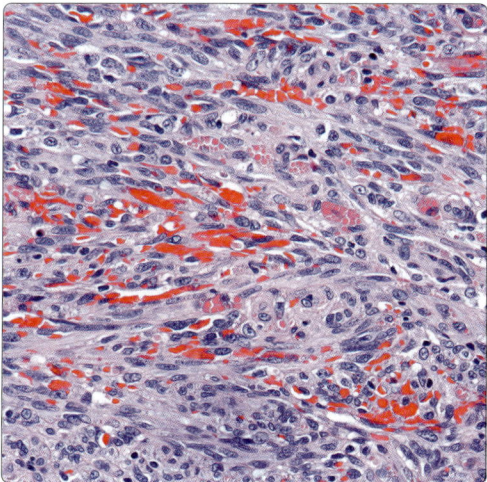

Kaposi Sarcoma, HHV-8
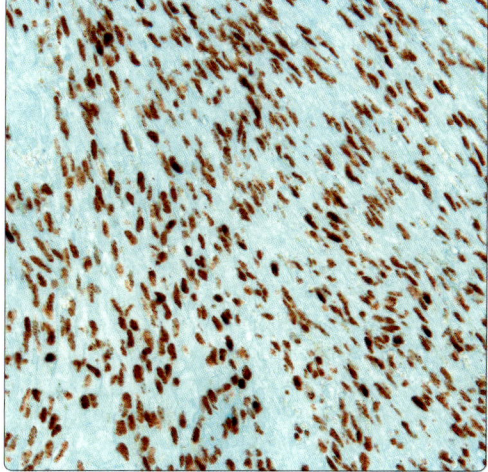

(Left) Kaposi sarcoma shows interlacing fascicles of spindle cells associated with slit-like vascular spaces. Leiomyosarcoma and sarcomatoid carcinoma are other spindle cell malignancies that more commonly involve the penis. (Right) The diagnosis of Kaposi sarcoma is supported by positive nuclear immunostaining for HHV-8. Leiomyosarcoma is typically positive for actin-sm and desmin; cytokeratin may be aberrantly expressed, although usually focal.

INDEX

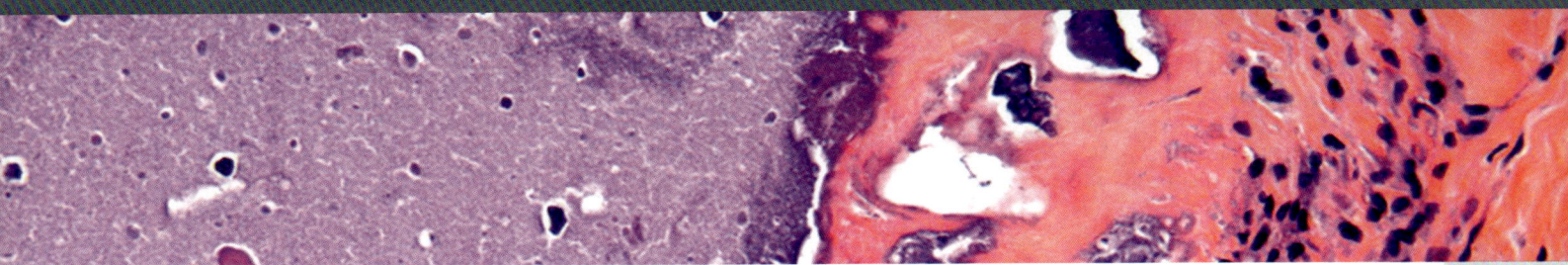

A

ABL1-BCR amplifications, **105**
Ablative techniques, for prostate carcinoma, **602**
Acantholytic squamous cell carcinoma. *See* Pseudoglandular squamous cell carcinoma.
Acinar adenocarcinoma, **536, 608–625**
- atrophy vs., **571**
- cribriform Gleason pattern 4 and 5, ductal adenocarcinoma vs., **652**
- high-grade, with cribriform pattern
    intraductal carcinoma vs., **646**
    prostatic intraepithelial neoplasia vs., **592**
- hyperplasia of mesonephric remnants vs., **577**
- low-grade
    adenosis vs., **567**
    prostatic intraepithelial neoplasia vs., **592**
    verumontanum mucosal gland hyperplasia vs., **581**
- poorly differentiated, prostate carcinoma with neuroendocrine differentiation vs., **667**
- prostatic
    with aberrant p63 expression, basal cell carcinoma vs., **674, 676**
    basal cell carcinoma vs., **674**
    cribriform pattern, basal cell carcinoma vs., **674**
    nephrogenic adenoma (metaplasia) of prostatic urethra vs., **584**
    poorly differentiated, basal cell carcinoma vs., **674**
- pseudohyperplastic variant of, prostate hyperplasia vs., **560**
- variants, **626–637**
    diagnostic checklist, **627–629**
Acinar proliferations, small
- atypical, **604**
    acinar adenocarcinoma vs., **611**
- benign, hyperplasia of mesonephric remnants vs., **577**
Acini, urothelial carcinoma involving, prostatic intraepithelial neoplasia vs., **593**
Acquired cystic disease-associated renal cell carcinoma, **132–137**
- diagnostic checklist, **134**
- differential diagnosis, **134**
- genetic testing, **134**
- predominant cell/compartment type, **134**
- predominant pattern/injury type, **134**
- prognosis, **133**
Actin-sm, sex cord-/gonadal stromal tumors, **820**
Adenoacanthoma. *See* Prostate carcinoma, with squamous differentiation.

Adenocarcinoma
- with aberrant p63 expression, **628, 637**
    Gleason grading of, **629**
- acinar. *See* Acinar adenocarcinoma.
- from adjacent anatomic site, carcinoma of urethra vs., **492**
- bladder
    invasive adenocarcinoma and, **413**
    prostatic adenocarcinoma vs., markers in differential of, **725**
    seminal vesicle adenocarcinoma vs., **723**
- clear cell, **416–421**
    clear cytoplasm and prominent nucleoli, **420**
    clear cytoplasm and stromal hyalinization, **420**
    dense stromal hyalinization, **420**
    diagnostic checklist, **417**
    differential diagnosis, **417**
    gynecologic tract, secondary involvement (direct extension) from, clear cell adenocarcinoma vs., **417**
    hyperchromasia and hobnail appearance, **420**
    morphologic similarity to gynecologic tract tumors, **420**
    nephrogenic adenoma (metaplasia) of prostatic urethra vs., **584**
    nuclear pleomorphism, **420**
    papillary, urothelial papilloma vs., **345**
    poorly differentiated carcinomas, **420**
    prognosis, **417**
    solid growth and clear cytoplasm, **420**
    tubulocystic patterns of, **420**
    of urinary bladder, nephrogenic adenoma vs., **296**
    urothelial carcinoma with clear cytoplasm vs., **385**
- colonic
    tumors of urachus vs., **524**
    villous adenoma vs., **409**
- colorectal, **471**
    metastatic, invasive adenocarcinoma vs., **411**
    seminal vesicle adenocarcinoma vs., **723**
- differential diagnosis of, **611**
- ductal, **612, 650–657**
    ancillary tests, **652**
    diagnostic checklist, **652**
    differential diagnosis, **652**
    genetics, **652**
    grading, **652**
    intraductal carcinoma vs., **646**
    prognosis, **651**
    prostatic intraepithelial neoplasia vs., **593**
- endometrioid of uterus, metastatic and secondary carcinomas and, **476**
- enteric-type, **471**
    involving bladder, markers in, **529**

i

INDEX

- gynecologic, **471**
- invasive, **410–415**
  - cystitis cystica and glandularis vs., **405**
  - diagnostic checklist, **411**
  - differential diagnosis, **410**
  - prognosis, **411**
- mesonephric. See Clear cell adenocarcinoma.
- metastatic
  - breast, metastatic and secondary carcinomas and, **477**
  - colorectal, metastatic and secondary carcinomas and, **475**
  - esophageal, metastatic and secondary carcinomas and, **475**
  - with glandular/tubular pattern, **899–900, 901**
  - invasive adenocarcinoma vs., **411**
  - papillary serous carcinoma vs., **875**
- papillary clear cell, urothelial papilloma vs., **345**
- PIN-like, prostatic intraepithelial neoplasia vs., **592**
- primary, of urinary bladder
  - invasive, müllerian lesions vs., **316**
  - tumors of urachus vs., **524**
- prostatic, **279, 471, 901–902**. See also Acinar adenocarcinoma.
  - with atrophic features, atrophy vs., **571**
  - bladder adenocarcinoma vs., markers in differential of, **725**
  - direct invasion by, invasive adenocarcinoma vs., **411**
  - high grade, paraganglioma vs., **464**
  - invasive adenocarcinoma and, **415**
  - involving bladder, **381**
  - ISUP grading system for, **612**
  - main mimics of variants, **629**
  - malakoplakia vs., **281**
  - markers for diagnosis, needle biopsy, **724**
  - markers used in metastatic setting to prove, **725**
  - metastatic and secondary carcinomas and, **474**
  - nephrogenic adenoma vs., **296**
  - papillary-polypoid cystitis vs., **274**
  - prostatic small cell carcinoma vs., markers for, **725–726**
  - seminal vesicle adenocarcinoma vs., **723**
  - urothelial carcinoma vs., markers in differential of, **724–725**
- rete testis/epididymis, **872–873**
  - ancillary tests, **873**
  - differential diagnosis, **873**
  - prognosis, **873**
- secondary involvement by
  - metastatic and secondary carcinomas and, **475**
  - Müllerian lesions vs., **316**
  - villous adenoma vs., **409**
- seminal vesicle, **722–723**
  - ancillary tests, **723**
  - differential diagnosis, **723**
  - natural history, **723**
- with squamous differentiation. See Prostate carcinoma, with squamous differentiation.
- tumor-like lesions of renal pelvis, **516**
- urachal, invasive adenocarcinoma and, **414**
- urethral, pseudoglandular squamous cell carcinoma vs., **963**

Adenofibroma, metanephric, mixed epithelial and stromal tumor (MEST) family tumors/pediatric cystic nephroma vs., **198**

Adenoid basal cell tumor. See Basal cell carcinoma.

Adenoid cystic carcinoma. See also Basal cell carcinoma.
- of Cowper glands, basal cell carcinoma vs., **674**
- prostatic intraepithelial neoplasia vs., **593**

Adenoid cystic-like tumor of prostate. See Basal cell carcinoma.

Adenoid squamous cell carcinoma. See Pseudoglandular squamous cell carcinoma.

Adenoma
- fibromyxoid nephrogenic, **439**
  - myofibroblastic proliferations vs., **434**
  - pseudocarcinomatous hyperplasia vs., **320**
- metanephric, **146–151**
  - diagnostic checklist, **148**
  - differential diagnosis, **148**
  - nephroblastoma (Wilms tumor) vs., **163**
  - with papillary or tubulopapillary architecture, **242–243**
  - papillary renal cell carcinoma vs., **83**
  - prognosis, **147**
- nephrogenic, **278, 294–301, 421, 495, 496, 497**
  - ancillary tests, **295–296**
  - atypical small acinar proliferations vs., **641**
  - carcinoma of urethra vs., **492**
  - clear cell adenocarcinoma vs., **417**
  - diagnostic checklist, **296**
  - differential diagnosis, **296**
  - diverticula and, **481**
  - hyperplasia of mesonephric remnants vs., **577, 579**
  - invasive urothelial carcinoma of bladder vs., **375, 376**
  - microcystic carcinoma vs., **383**
  - nested carcinoma vs., **383**
  - papillary urothelial carcinoma of low malignant potential vs., **351**
  - prognosis, **295**
  - prostatic-type polyp vs., **307**
  - of prostatic urethra, **582–589**
  - superficial biopsy mimicking, **421**
  - urothelial papilloma vs., **345**
  - verumontanum mucosal gland hyperplasia vs., **581**
- papillary, **44–47**
  - diagnostic checklist, **45**
  - differential diagnosis, **45**
  - genetic features, **45**
  - prognosis, **45**
  - renal, nephrogenic rests vs., **157**
- papillary nephrogenic
  - high-grade papillary urothelial carcinoma vs., **359**
  - papillary-polypoid cystitis vs., **274**
- tumor-like lesions of renal pelvis, **515**
- villous, **408–409**
  - of bladder, **408–409**
  - diagnostic checklist, **409**
  - differential diagnosis, **409**
  - tumor-like lesions of renal pelvis, **515**

INDEX

of urachus, tumors of urachus vs., **524**
Adenomatoid metaplasia. *See* Nephrogenic adenoma, of prostatic urethra.
Adenomatoid tumor, **864–867**
- ancillary tests, **865**
- cellular, sex cord-/gonadal stromal tumors vs., **820**
- differential diagnosis, **865**
- with glandular/tubular pattern, **901**
- lipogranuloma vs., **919**
- liposarcoma vs., **879**
- malignant mesothelioma vs., **869**
- paratesticular, with microcystic pattern, **898–899**
- prognosis, **865**
- Sertoli cell tumors vs., **829**

Adenomatous hyperplasia, atypical, **623**. *See also* Adenosis.
- atypical small acinar proliferations vs., **641**
- prostate hyperplasia vs., **560**

Adenosis, **566–569**
- diagnostic checklist of, **567**
- differential diagnosis of, **567**
- prognosis of, **567**
- sclerosing, **569, 625**
  - adenosis vs., **567**
  - atypical small acinar proliferations vs., **641**

Adenosquamous carcinoma, **936, 977**
Adipose tissue, **546–547**
- muscularis propria, **255**

Adrenal cortical lesions, immunohistochemistry, **232**
Adrenal cortical tumors, clear cell renal cell carcinoma vs., **57**
Adrenogenital syndrome
- testicular tumors of, **846–849**
  - ancillary tests, **847**
  - differential diagnosis, **847**
  - Leydig cell tumor vs., **825**
  - prognosis, **847**
- tumor of, large cell calcifying Sertoli cell tumor vs., **835**

Adult renal epithelial tumors, with predominant tubules and cysts, tubulocystic carcinoma vs., **125**
Adult rhabdomyosarcoma, **700–701**
Adventitia, **253**
- ureteral, **261**

Age, in prostate carcinoma, **600**
Allergic granulomatous prostatitis, **556**
Alveolar soft part sarcoma, paraganglioma vs., **464**
Amorphous secretions, eosinophilic, in acinar adenocarcinoma, **610**
Amyloid, papillary-polypoid cystitis vs., **274**
Amyloid tumor. *See* Amyloidosis, of bladder.
Amyloidosis, **495, 496**
- of bladder, **312–313**
  - ancillary tests, **313**
  - diagnostic checklist, **313**
  - differential diagnosis, **313**
  - diffuse, **313**
  - familial, **313**
  - localized, **313**
  - primary, **313**
  - prognosis, **313**
  - secondary, **313**

- nodular, scrotal calcinosis vs., **921**

Anal carcinoma, extramammary Paget disease associated with, immunohistochemistry, **996**
Anal cloacogenic carcinoma, basal cell carcinoma vs., **674**
Analgesics, in urothelial carcinoma of renal pelvis, **507**
Androgen deprivation therapy
- for intraductal carcinoma, **645**
- primary, for prostate carcinoma, **602**

Angioma, Kaposi sarcoma vs., **991**
Angiomyolipoma, **172–177, 702**
- ancillary tests, **174**
- diagnostic checklist, **174**
- differential diagnosis, **174**
- epithelioid, **178–183**
  - with clear-/light-staining cytoplasm, **242**
  - clear cell renal cell carcinoma vs., **57**
  - diagnostic checklist, **180**
  - differential diagnosis, **180**
  - with granular/eosinophilic cytoplasm, **243**
  - immunohistochemistry, **180, 183**
  - MiTF/TFE family translocation-associated carcinoma vs., **113**
  - prognosis, **179**
  - *TFE3* gene fusions, **179**
  - *TP53* mutations, **179**
- lymph nodes, **174**
- lymphatic/vascular invasion, **174, 176**
- mammalian target of rapamycin (mTOR) pathway, **173**
- oncocytoma-like, epithelioid chromophobe renal cell carcinoma vs., **93**
  - renal oncocytoma vs., **50**
- other rare tumors vs., **231–232**
- prognosis, **173**
- tumors with spindle cell morphology, **243–244**

Angiosarcoma, **701, 705**
- epithelioid, **459**
- immunohistochemistry, **232, 236–237, 996**
- Kaposi sarcoma vs., **991**
- mesenchymal tumors of bladder vs., **456**

Ann Arbor staging system, for Hodgkin lymphoma, **860**
Anterior fibromuscular stroma, **546**
Architectural patterns, in clear cell papillary renal cell carcinoma, **75, 76**
Asbestos exposure, malignant mesothelioma, **869**
Atrophic carcinoma, **628, 633–634**
- Gleason grading, **629**

Atrophic pattern, **612**
Atrophy, **536, 570–575, 624**
- differential diagnosis of, **571**
- diffuse, **571, 575**
- features of, prostate adenocarcinoma with, atrophy vs., **571**
- focal, **571**
- partial, **571, 573**
- prognosis of, **571**
- proliferative inflammatory, **575**
- sclerotic, **571, 574**
- simple, **571–572**
- variants, atypical small acinar proliferations vs., **641**

INDEX

Atypia
- reactive
    - prostate glands with, prostatic intraepithelial neoplasia vs., **592**
    - urothelial, flat urothelial lesions other than carcinoma in situ and, **341**
- with urethral flat urothelial lesions, nephrogenic adenoma (metaplasia) of prostatic urethra vs., **584**

Atypical adenomatous hyperplasia, **623**. *See also* Adenosis.
- atypical small acinar proliferations vs., **641**
- prostate hyperplasia vs., **560**

Atypical basal cell hyperplasia, prostatic intraepithelial neoplasia vs., **592**

Atypical large glandular proliferation, **612**

Atypical lipomatous tumor. *See* Liposarcoma.

Atypical mycobacterial spindle cell pseudotumor, malakoplakia vs., **281**

Atypical small acinar proliferations, **604, 638–643**
- acinar adenocarcinoma vs., **611**
- ancillary tests, **640**
- diagnostic checklist, **641**
- differential diagnosis, **640–641**
- grossing, histology protocols and diagnostic approach, **639**
- prognosis, **639**

Atypical stromal hyperplasia. *See* Stromal tumors.

B

B-cell lymphoma, **711**
- diffuse large, **712**

Bacillus Calmette-Guérin, **266**
- granuloma, **269**

Balanitis xerotica obliterans, **912–913**
- diagnostic checklist, **913**
- differential diagnosis, **913**
- predominant cell/compartment type, **913**
- predominant pattern/injury type, **913**
- prognosis, **913**

Balkan nephropathy, in urothelial carcinoma of renal pelvis, **507**

Basal cell carcinoma, **672–677**
- ancillary test, **673–674**
- cutaneous, basaloid squamous cell carcinoma vs., **943**
- diagnostic checklist, **674**
- differential diagnosis, **674**
- grading, **674**
- histologic features
    - ACC pattern, **673, 675**
    - BCC pattern, **673, 675**
    - combination, **673, 675**
- origin, **673**
- prostate carcinoma with neuroendocrine differentiation vs., **667**
- site of involvement, **673**

Basal cell hyperplasia, **560**
- adenoid cystic pattern, basal cell carcinoma vs., **674, 677**
- atypical, prostatic intraepithelial neoplasia vs., **592**
- atypical small acinar proliferations vs., **641**

Basal cell markers, **541**

Basal cells, **252, 260, 263**

Basaloid carcinoma, **935, 936**
- clear cell carcinoma vs., **981**
- papillary variant, warty-basaloid squamous cell carcinoma of penis vs., **953**
- warty-basaloid squamous cell carcinoma of penis vs., **953**

Basaloid mixed squamous cell carcinoma, **936**

Basaloid penile intraepithelial neoplasia, **937**
- differential diagnosis, **924**
    - ancillary tests, **923**

Basaloid squamous cell carcinoma, of penis, **942–945**
- ancillary tests, **943**
- differential diagnosis, **943, 945**
- papillary basaloid squamous cell carcinoma vs., **947**
- papillary variant, **946–947**
    - ancillary tests, **947**
    - diagnostic checklist, **947**
    - differential diagnosis, **947**
    - prognosis, **947**
    - warty squamous cell carcinoma of penis vs., **950**
- prognosis, **943**

Benign condyloma. *See* Condylomas.

Benign epithelial tumors/lesions, **536**
- renal pelvis, **515**
- ureter, **503–504**

Benign lymphoid aggregate, **713**

Benign mesenchymal tumors, **537**

Benign mucinous metaplasia, of penis, extramammary Paget disease vs., **988**

Benign multiloculated renal cortical cysts, multilocular cystic clear cell renal cell neoplasm of low malignant potential vs., **65**

Benign nonepithelial tumors/lesions
- renal pelvis, **516**
- ureter, **503–504**

Benign prostate hyperplasia nodule, with prominent papillary fronds, prostatic intraepithelial neoplasia vs., **592**

Benign prostatic epithelial polyp. *See* Prostatic-type polyp.

Benign prostatic hyperplasia
- adenosis vs., **567**
- prostatic-type polyp vs., **307**

Benign prostatic hypertrophy. *See* Prostatic hyperplasia.

Benign small acinar proliferations, hyperplasia of mesonephric remnants vs., **577**

Benign soft tissue tumors, other testicular and paratesticular sarcomas vs., **891**

Bilharziasis. *See* Schistosomiasis.

Biochemical recurrence, **604**

Biopsy, needle core, tumor volume in, **603**

Birt-Hogg-Dubé (BHD) syndrome, **16–19**
- diagnostic checklist, **18**
- diagnostic criteria, **17**
- differential diagnosis, **18**
- prognosis, **17**
- von Hippel-Lindau syndrome vs., **14**

INDEX

BK viral cytopathic effect, urothelial carcinoma in situ vs., **334**
Blackfoot disease, in urothelial carcinoma of ureter, **499**
Bladder
- enteric-type adenocarcinoma involving, markers in, **529**
- nephrogenic adenoma, **294–301**
    - ancillary tests, **295–296**
    - diagnostic checklist, **296**
    - differential diagnosis, **296**
- urothelial carcinoma of, urothelial carcinoma of ureter vs., **500**

Bladder adenocarcinoma
- clear cell, **416–421**
    - diagnostic checklist, **417**
    - differential diagnosis, **417**
    - prognosis, **417**
- invading prostate, **717**
- invasive, **410–415**
    - diagnostic checklist, **411**
    - differential diagnosis, **410**
    - prognosis, **411**
    - villous adenoma vs., **409**
- primary, tumors of urachus vs., **524**
- prostatic adenocarcinoma vs., markers in differential of, **725**
- seminal vesicle adenocarcinoma vs., **723**

Bladder cancer, tumor-like lesions of ureter, **503**
Bladder diverticula. *See also* Diverticula.
- cystitis cystica, **481**
- extensive inflammation, **481**
- fibrotic wall, **480**
- hypertrophic muscularis mucosae, **480**
- inflamed and denuded, **480**
- inflammation and fibrosis, **481**
- intestinal metaplasia, **481**
- muscularis propria, **480**
- near ostium, **480**
- nephrogenic adenoma (metaplasia), **481**
- squamous metaplasia, **481**

Bladder hamartoma, cystitis cystica and glandularis vs., **405**
Bladder neck, **252**
Bladder tumors and tumor-like lesions, classification of, **250–251**
Bladder wall, **254**
Blastema Wilms tumor
- predominant, clear cell sarcoma of kidney vs., **189**
- primitive neuroectodermal tumor vs., **213**
- synovial sarcoma vs., **205**

Blue mucin, in acinar adenocarcinoma, **610**
Blue nevus, **707**
- resection, **708**

Bone-metastasizing renal tumor of childhood. *See* Clear cell sarcoma, of kidney.
Botryoid fibroepithelial polyp. *See* Fibroepithelial polyp.
Bourneville disease. *See* Tuberous sclerosis complex.
Bowen disease. *See* Penile intraepithelial neoplasia.
Bowenoid papulosis, warty/basaloid PeIN vs., **924**
Brachytherapy, for prostate carcinoma, **602**

Branching tubules, in clear cell papillary renal cell carcinoma, **76**
Breast carcinoma, **471**
Brucellosis, nonspecific granulomatous orchitis vs., **745**
Bulbo-membranous urethra, **257**
Bullous cystitis. *See* Papillary-polypoid cystitis.
Burkitt lymphoma (BL), **217**

C

c-MET gene, mutations in, **33**
Calretinin, sex cord-/gonadal stromal tumors, **819**
Cancer, in bladder, tumor-like lesions of ureter, **503**
Carcinoid. *See also* Well-differentiated neuroendocrine tumor (carcinoid).
- with oxyphilic cytoplasm, **899**

Carcinoid tumor, **807, 814–817**
- ancillary tests, **815**
- differential diagnosis, **815**
- granulosa cell tumor vs., **839**
- hyalinized stroma, **816**
- ill-defined border, **816**
- inverted urothelial neoplasia vs., **366**
- von Brunn nests vs., **289**
- well circumscribed, **816**

Carcinoma. *See also* specific carcinoma.
- of collecting ducts of Bellini. *See* Collecting duct carcinoma.
- with stratified epithelium, **628, 636**
- undifferentiated, **612**

Carcinoma cuniculatum, **935**
- papillary squamous cell carcinoma vs., **959**
- verrucous squamous cell carcinoma vs., **955**

Carcinoma in situ. *See also* Germ cell neoplasia in situ.
- squamous cell. *See also* Penile intraepithelial neoplasia.
    - with pagetoid pattern, extramammary Paget disease vs., **988**
- urothelial, **330, 332–339**
    - ancillary tests, **333–334**
    - diagnostic checklist, **334**
    - differential diagnosis, **334**
    - flat urothelial lesions other than carcinoma in situ vs., **341**
    - intradiverticular, diverticular-associated neoplasia and, **484**
    - nephrogenic adenoma vs., **296**
    - prognosis, **333**
    - squamous proliferations other than carcinoma vs., **423**

Carcinosarcoma. *See* Sarcomatoid squamous cell carcinoma.
Caruncle, urethral, inflammatory lesions of urethra and, **487, 488, 489**
CD 30 (BerH2), germ cell tumors, **750**
CD99, sex cord-/gonadal stromal tumors, **820**
CD117, germ cell tumors, **751**
CDC73 gene, mutations in, **33**
Cell metaplasia, transitional, prostatic intraepithelial neoplasia vs., **592**

INDEX

Cell tumor
- granular, paraganglioma vs., **464**
- mixed, **904**

Cells, with pale and clear cytoplasm, **898**

Cellular mesoblastic nephroma
- plump cell variant, malignant rhabdoid tumor vs., **193**
- synovial sarcoma vs., **205**

Cellular schwannoma, smooth muscle tumors and, **447**

Central zone glands, prostate, prostatic intraepithelial neoplasia vs., **592**

Charcot-Böttcher filaments, **829**

Children's Oncology Group (COG), **161**
- staging of pediatric renal tumors, **163**

Chondrogenic tumors, **701**

Chordoma, myxoid stroma vs., **385**

Choriocarcinoma, **905**
- monophasic, seminoma vs., **764**
- and variants, **784–789**
    - ancillary tests, **786**
    - classic, **785**
    - diagnostic checklist, **786**
    - differential diagnosis, **786**
    - lymphatic/vascular invasion, **786**
    - monophasic, **785**
    - nonchoriocarcinomatous trophoblastic tumors, **785–786**
    - predominant cell/compartment type, **786**
    - predominant pattern/injury type, **786**
    - reporting, **786**

Chorioepithelioma. See Choriocarcinoma, and variants.

Chromophobe carcinoma, clear cell renal cell carcinoma vs., **57**

Chromophobe renal cell carcinoma, **89, 90–97**
- Birt-Hogg-Dubé syndrome vs., **18**
- classical, with clear-/light-staining cytoplasm, **242**
- diagnostic checklist, **93**
- differential diagnosis, **92–93, 127**
- eosinophilic
    - with granular/eosinophilic cytoplasm, **243**
        - renal oncocytoma vs., **50**
        - unclassified renal cell carcinoma vs., **143**
- epithelioid angiomyolipoma vs., **180**
- genetic features, **91**
- with papillary architecture, papillary renal cell carcinoma vs., **83**
- prognosis, **91**

Chromosome X, Sertoli cell tumors, **829**

Chronic inflammation, lymphoepithelioma-like carcinoma vs., **384**

Chronic orchitis, lymphoma/leukemia/plasmacytoma vs., **860**

Chronic prostatitis, hematopoietic neoplasms of prostate vs., **711**

Circumcision specimen, squamous cell carcinoma, of penis, **929**

CK-PAN, sex cord-/gonadal stromal tumors, **819**

Classic seminoma, spermatocytic tumor vs., **803, 805**

Clear cell adenocarcinoma, **416–421**
- diagnostic checklist, **417**
- differential diagnosis, **417**
- gynecologic tract, secondary involvement (direct extension) from, clear cell adenocarcinoma vs., **417**
- nephrogenic adenoma (metaplasia) of prostatic urethra vs., **584**
- papillary, urothelial papilloma vs., **345**
- prognosis, **417**
- of urinary bladder, nephrogenic adenoma vs., **296**
- urothelial carcinoma with clear cytoplasm vs., **385**

Clear cell carcinoma
- of penis, **980–981**
    - ancillary tests, **981**
    - diagnostic checklist, **981**
    - differential diagnosis, **981**
    - predominant cell/compartment type, **981**
    - prognosis, **981**
- warty squamous cell carcinoma of penis vs., **950**

Clear cell papillary carcinoma, clear cell renal cell carcinoma vs., **56–57**

Clear cell papillary-like areas, clear cell renal cell carcinoma, clear cell papillary renal cell carcinoma vs., **74, 78**

Clear cell papillary renal cell carcinoma, **72–79**
- with clear-/light-staining cytoplasm, **242**
- cystic, multilocular cystic clear cell renal cell neoplasm of low malignant potential vs., **65**
- differential diagnosis, **74**
- MiTF/TFE family translocation-associated carcinoma vs., **113**
- with papillary or tubulopapillary architecture, **242–243**
- papillary renal cell carcinoma vs., **83, 89**
- prognosis, **73**
- transcription elongation factor B-mutated renal cell carcinoma vs., **69**

Clear cell papulosis, extramammary Paget disease vs., **988**

Clear cell pattern, **612**

Clear cell renal cell carcinoma, **54–63**
- acquired cystic disease-associated renal cell carcinoma vs., **134**
- chromophobe renal cell carcinoma vs., **93**
- with clear-/light-staining cytoplasm, **242**
- with clear cell papillary-like areas, clear cell papillary renal cell carcinoma vs., **74, 78**
- cystic, with regression, multilocular cystic clear cell renal cell neoplasm of low malignant potential vs., **65**
- diagnostic checklist, **57**
- differential diagnosis, **56–57**
- end-stage kidney disease with, von Hippel-Lindau syndrome vs., **14**
- eosinophilic
    - with granular/eosinophilic cytoplasm, **243**
    - renal oncocytoma vs., **50**
- epithelioid angiomyolipoma vs., **180**
- exhibiting papillary or pseudopapillary growth, papillary renal cell carcinoma vs., **82**
- MiTF/TFE family translocation-associated carcinoma vs., **113**
- multifocal
    - bilateral, hereditary papillary renal cancer vs., **34**
    - nonsyndromic, von Hippel-Lindau syndrome vs., **14**
- other rare tumors vs., **232**

INDEX

- prognosis, **55**
- renal malakoplakia vs., **40**
- renal tuberculosis vs., **40**
- transcription elongation factor B-mutated renal cell carcinoma vs., **69**
- tuberous sclerosis complex vs., **26**
- xanthogranulomatous pyelonephritis vs., **40**

Clear cell sarcoma
- of kidney, **188–191**
  - classic pattern, **189**
  - congenital mesoblastic nephroma vs., **185**
  - diagnostic checklist, **189**
  - differential diagnosis, **189**
  - malignant rhabdoid tumor vs., **193, 195**
  - molecular genetics, **189**
  - prognosis, **189**
  - variant patterns, **189, 190–191**
- mesenchymal tumors of bladder vs., **456**

Clear cell squamous cell carcinoma, of penis. See Clear cell carcinoma, of penis.

CMN. See Congenital mesoblastic nephroma.

Collagen polyp, papillary-polypoid cystitis vs., **274**

Collagenization, amyloidosis vs., **313**

Collagenous micronodules, **610**

Collecting duct carcinoma, **98–103**
- diagnostic checklist, **100**
- differential diagnosis, **100**
- genetic features, **99**
- hereditary leiomyomatosis renal cell carcinoma syndrome vs., **22**
- metastatic tumors vs., **239**
- with papillary or tubulopapillary architecture, **242–243**
- papillary renal cell carcinoma vs., **82, 89**
- poorly differentiated carcinomas, **244**
- prognosis, **99**
- renal medullary carcinoma vs., **106**
- with TC-like areas, tubulocystic carcinoma vs., **125**
- unclassified renal cell carcinoma vs., **143**
- urothelial carcinoma of renal pelvis vs., **508**

Collecting tubules, **262**

Colliculus seminalis, **539**

Colonic adenocarcinoma
- tumors of urachus vs., **524**
- villous adenoma vs., **409**

Colorectal adenocarcinoma, **471**
- metastatic, invasive adenocarcinoma vs., **411**
- seminal vesicle adenocarcinoma vs., **723**

Comedonecrosis, invasive adenocarcinoma and, **412**

Condyloma acuminatum, **495, 496**
- cuniculatum squamous cell carcinoma vs., **967**
- invasive squamous cell carcinoma vs., **427**
- squamous proliferations other than carcinoma and, **423, 424**

Condylomas, **908–911**
- diagnostic checklist, **910**
- differential diagnosis, **910**
- giant
  - cuniculatum squamous cell carcinoma vs., **967**
  - papillary squamous cell carcinoma vs., **959**
  - verrucous squamous cell carcinoma vs., **955**
  - warty squamous cell carcinoma of penis vs., **949**
- with malignant change, immunohistochemistry, **996**
- with malignant transformation, condylomas vs., **910**
- prognosis, **909**
- warty/basaloid PeIN vs., **924**

Condylomata acuminatum. See Condylomas.

Condylomatous carcinoma. See Warty squamous cell carcinoma, of penis.

Congenital melanocarcinoma. See Melanotic neuroectodermal tumor.

Congenital mesoblastic nephroma, **184–187**
- cellular variant, **185**
- classical type, **185**
- diagnostic checklist, **185**
- differential diagnosis, **185**
- genetic features, **185**
- plump cell pattern, clear cell sarcoma of kidney vs., **189**
- prognosis, **185**

Congenital posterior urethral polyp. See Fibroepithelial polyp.

Conventional (clear cell) renal cell carcinoma. See Clear cell renal cell carcinoma.

Corpora amylacea, **545**
- in acinar adenocarcinoma, **610**

Cortex, **262**

Cowper gland duct cyst, urethral diverticula vs., **496**

Cowper gland hyperplasia, polypoid lesions vs., **496**

Cowper glands, **259, 546**
- adenoid cystic carcinoma of, basal cell carcinoma vs., **674**
- atypical small acinar proliferations vs., **640**

Cribriform Gleason patterns, **612**

Cribriform high-grade prostatic intraepithelial neoplasia, **623**

Cribriform hyperplasia, **560**
- ductal adenocarcinoma vs., **652**
- prostatic intraepithelial neoplasia vs., **592**

Cribriform pattern, high-grade acinar adenocarcinoma with, prostatic intraepithelial neoplasia vs., **592**

Cryptorchidism, **734–737**
- acquired, **735**
- developmental anomaly, **735**
- diagnostic checklist, **735**
- natural history, **735**

Crystalloids, in acinar adenocarcinoma, **610**

CTNNB1 gene, Sertoli cell tumors, **829**

Cuniculatum squamous cell carcinoma, of penis, **966–969**
- diagnostic checklist, **967**
- differential diagnosis, **967**
- predominant cell/compartment type, **967**
- predominant pattern/injury type, **967**
- prognosis, **967**

Cutaneous basal cell carcinoma, basaloid squamous cell carcinoma vs., **943**

Cystadenoleiomyofibroma. See Stromal tumors.

Cystadenoma, **718–721**
- ancillary test, **720**
- cystic neoplasm of glandular elements, **719**
- developmental anomaly, **719**
- diagnostic checklist, **720**
- differential diagnosis, **720**

INDEX

- of epididymis
    - adenocarcinoma of rete testis/epididymis vs., **873**
    - papillary, papillary serous carcinoma vs., **875**
- mixed epithelial-stromal tumor (MEST), proposed classification and criteria, **720**
- of seminal vesicle, seminal vesicle adenocarcinoma vs., **723**

Cystectomy
- partial, **479**
    - diverticular-associated neoplasia and, **483**
- radical, **479**
    - diverticular-associated neoplasia and, **483**

Cystic clear cell papillary renal cell carcinoma, multilocular cystic clear cell renal cell neoplasm of low malignant potential vs., **65**

Cystic clear cell renal cell carcinoma, with regression, multilocular cystic clear cell renal cell neoplasm of low malignant potential vs., **65**

Cystic epithelial stromal tumor. See Stromal tumors.

Cystic kidney disease, localized or segmental, cystic partially differentiated nephroblastoma vs., **171**

Cystic nephroma
- multilocular cystic clear cell renal cell neoplasm of low malignant potential vs., **65**
- pediatric, **196–203**
    - cystic partially differentiated nephroblastoma vs., **171**
    - diagnostic checklist, **198**
    - differential diagnosis, **198**
    - prognosis, **197**

Cystic partially differentiated nephroblastoma, **170–171**
- differential diagnosis, **171**
- histology vs. radiologic evaluation, **171**
- mixed epithelial and stromal tumor (MEST) family tumors/pediatric cystic nephroma vs., **198, 203**
- multilocular cystic clear cell renal cell neoplasm of low malignant potential vs., **65**
- prognosis, **171**

Cystic renal dysplasia, cystic partially differentiated nephroblastoma vs., **171**

Cystic trophoblastic tumor, **785–786, 789**

Cystic urachal tumors, mucinous, urachal remnants vs., **521**

Cystic Wilms tumor, cystic partially differentiated nephroblastoma vs., **171**

Cystitis
- emphysematous, **267**
- encrusted, **268, 270**
    - schistosomiasis vs., **287**
- eosinophilic, **266, 270**
- follicular, **266, 269**
- gangrenous, **268**
- giant cell, **268**
- granulomatous, **266**
- hemorrhagic, **268, 269**
- infectious, **267**
- interstitial, **267, 270**
- overview of, **266–271**
- papillary-polypoid, **272–279**
    - diagnostic checklist, **274**
    - differential diagnosis, **273–274**
    - fibroepithelial polyp vs., **303**
    - high-grade papillary urothelial carcinoma vs., **359**
    - low-grade papillary urothelial carcinoma vs., **355**
    - prognosis, **273**
    - prostatic-type polyp vs., **307**
    - urothelial papilloma vs., **345**
- proliferative. See von Brunn nests.
- radiation, **268, 271**
- radiation/chemotherapy. See Pseudocarcinomatous hyperplasia.
- subtypes, **266–268**

Cystitis cystica, **368, 404–407**
- diagnostic checklist, **405**
- differential diagnosis, **405**
- diverticula and, **481**
- florid, fibroepithelial polyp vs., **303**
- with intestinal metaplasia, **406**
    - and mucin extravasation, villous adenoma vs., **409**
- invasive urothelial carcinoma of bladder vs., **376**
- inverted urothelial neoplasia vs., **366**
- microcystic carcinoma vs., **383**
- with mucin extravasation, **405, 406**
- nested carcinoma vs., **382–383**
- prognosis, **405**
- prostatic-type polyp vs., **307**

Cystitis glandularis, **404–407**
- diagnostic checklist, **405**
- differential diagnosis, **405**
- extensive, invasive adenocarcinoma vs., **411**
- florid, fibroepithelial polyp vs., **303**
- hamartoma vs., **327**
- with intestinal metaplasia, **406**
    - invasive adenocarcinoma and, **415**
    - and mucin extravasation, villous adenoma vs., **409**
- invasive urothelial carcinoma of bladder vs., **376**
- microcystic carcinoma vs., **383**
- with mucin extravasation, **405, 406**
- nested carcinoma vs., **382–383**
- prognosis, **405**
- prostatic-type polyp vs., **307**

Cystomyoma. See Epithelial stromal tumors.

Cystosarcoma phyllodes. See Epithelial stromal tumors; Stromal tumors.

Cysts. See also specific cyst.
- adult renal epithelial tumors with, predominant tubules and, tubulocystic carcinoma vs., **125**
- formation of, simple atrophy with, **571–572**

Cytologic atypia, invasive adenocarcinoma and, **412**

Cytopathic effect, BK viral, urothelial carcinoma in situ vs., **334**

Cytoplasm
- cells with pale and clear, **898**
- glycogen rich, urothelial carcinoma with, **385**
    - differential diagnosis, **385**
- oxyphilic, tumors with, **899**

INDEX

D

Dedifferentiated liposarcoma, embryonal rhabdomyosarcoma vs., **887**
Del Castillo syndrome. *See* Sertoli cell-only syndrome.
Denonvilliers fascia, **547**
Dermoid cyst, **807**
- adult-type teratoma vs., **791**
- histiocytes, **809**
- inflammation, **809**
- lipogranulomatous reaction, **809**
- organoid, **809**
- skin and adnexa, **809**
- unilocular, **809**

Desmoplastic small round cell tumor, **891**
- melanotic neuroectodermal tumor vs., **883**
- small blue round cell tumors of kidney, **244**

Diet, in prostate carcinoma, **600**
Diffuse atrophy, **571, 575**
Diffuse embryoma, **795, 797**
Diffuse gastric carcinoma, metastatic and secondary carcinomas and, **475**
Diffuse large B-cell lymphoma, **217**
- testis, **860**

Distal urethra, penis or vulva with extension into, squamous cell carcinoma of, carcinoma of urethra vs., **492**

Distant metastasis, germ cell tumors, **751**
Diverticula, **478–481**
- prognosis, **479**

Diverticular-associated neoplasia, **482–485**
- prognosis, **483**

Diverticulectomy, **479**
- diverticular-associated neoplasia and, **483**

Dual chromogen antibody cocktails, **541**
Duct epithelium, ejaculatory, prostatic intraepithelial neoplasia vs., **592**
Ductal acinar unit, **544–545**
- basal cells, **544**
- ducts and acini, **544**
- endocrine-paracrine cells, **544**
- nonglandular or metaplastic cells, **544–545**
- secretory or acinar cells, **544**

Ductal adenocarcinoma, **612, 650–657**
- ancillary tests, **652**
- diagnostic checklist, **652**
- differential diagnosis, **652**
- genetics, **652**
- grading, **652**
- intraductal carcinoma vs., **646**
- prognosis, **651**
- prostatic intraepithelial neoplasia vs., **593**

Dysgerminoma in ovary. *See* Seminoma.
Dysplasia
- cystic renal, cystic partially differentiated nephroblastoma vs., **171**
- squamous
    keratinizing, **430**
    severe, **430**

squamous proliferations other than carcinoma vs., **423**
- urothelial
    and flat atypia of uncertain significance, urothelial carcinoma in situ vs., **334**
    flat urothelial lesions other than carcinoma in situ and, **341**

E

Ectopic adrenal tissue, **231, 237**
Ectopic prostate. *See* Prostatic-type polyp.
Ectopic prostate tissue, **495**
Ejaculatory duct epithelium
- atypical small acinar proliferations vs., **640**
- prostatic intraepithelial neoplasia vs., **592**

Ejaculatory ducts, **539, 546**
Electron microscopy
- in chromophobe renal cell carcinoma, **92**
- in metanephric adenoma, **148**
- in MiTF/TFE family translocation-associated carcinoma, **113**

Embryoma, diffuse, **795, 797**
Embryonal adenoma. *See* Metanephric adenoma.
Embryonal carcinoma, **770–775, 904**
- adenocarcinoma of rete testis/epididymis vs., **873**
- ancillary tests, **771**
- appliqué pattern, **774**
- CD30, **775**
- CK-PAN, **775**
- complex glandular, **773**
- cribriform, **774**
- delicate papillae, **773**
- diagnostic checklist, **772**
- differential diagnosis, **771–772**
- with diffuse arrangement, and cells with pale and clear cytoplasm, **898**
- glandular, **774**
- with glandular/tubular pattern, **899–900**
- gross, **773**
- intratubular, **775**
    germ cell neoplasia in situ vs., **757, 759, 761**
- lymphoma/leukemia/plasmacytoma vs., **860**
- malignant mesothelioma vs., **869**
- mixed, and YST, **775**
- OCT3/4, **775**
- papillary, **773, 774**
- predominant cell/compartment type, **771**
- predominant pattern/injury type, **771**
- reporting, **772**
- rete testis invasion, **774**
- solid pattern
    seminoma vs., **764, 769**
    spermatocytic tumor vs., **803**
- vascular invasion, **774**
- yolk sac tumor vs., **778**

Embryonal rhabdomyosarcoma, **886–889**
- ancillary tests, **887**
- differential diagnosis, **887**
- fibroepithelial polyp vs., **303**

INDEX

- hamartoma vs., **327**
- melanotic neuroectodermal tumor vs., **883**
- prognosis, **887**

Emerging prognostic system, for prostate carcinoma, **603**
Emphysematous cystitis, **267**
Encrusted cystitis, **268, 270**
- schistosomiasis vs., **287**

End-stage kidneys, **73**
Endocervicosis, **315**
Endodermal sinus tumor. See Yolk sac tumor; Yolk sac tumor, prepubertal type.
Endometrial adenocarcinoma, villous adenoma vs., **409**
Endometrial carcinoma, **471**
Endometrial stromal sarcoma, **461**
- mesenchymal tumors of bladder vs., **456**

Endometrioid carcinoma of prostate. See Ductal adenocarcinoma.
Endometriosis, **315**
- metastatic and secondary carcinoma vs., **472**

Endophytic neoplasia, urinary bladder neoplasms and, **329**
Endophytic urothelial lesions. See Urothelial neoplasia, of bladder.
Enteric-type adenocarcinoma, **471**
- involving bladder, markers in, **529**

Eosinophilic amorphous secretions, in acinar adenocarcinoma, **610**
Eosinophilic cystitis, **266, 270**
Eosinophilic variant chromophobe renal cell carcinoma, succinate dehydrogenase complex deficiency syndrome vs., **30**
Epidermoid carcinoma. See Prostate carcinoma, with squamous differentiation; Squamous cell carcinoma of penis, usual type.
Epidermoid cyst, **807**
- adult-type teratoma vs., **791**
- keratin material, **808**
- unilocular cyst, **808**

Epididymal tumors, classification, **732**
Epididymis
- adenocarcinoma of, **872–873**
  - ancillary tests, **873**
  - differential diagnosis, **873**
  - malignant mesothelioma vs., **869**
  - prognosis, **873**
- carcinoma of
  - metastatic tumors of testis and paratesticular structures vs., **895**
  - papillary serous carcinoma vs., **875**
- cystadenoma of, adenocarcinoma of rete testis/epididymis vs., **873**
- papillary cystadenoma of, papillary serous carcinoma vs., **875**

Epididymitis. See Nontuberculous infections.
Epididymo-orchitis, tuberculous, **746–747**
- ancillary tests, **747**
- differential diagnosis, **747**
- infectious agents, **747**

Epididymoorchitis. See Nontuberculous infections.
Epithelial components, nephroblastoma (Wilms tumor), **162, 164**

Epithelial differentiation, rare tumors of kidney with, **4**
Epithelial markers, **541**
Epithelial predominant hyperplasia, **559–560**
Epithelial predominant Wilms tumor, metanephric adenoma vs., **148**
Epithelial stromal tumors, **718–721**
- ancillary test, **720**
- developmental anomaly, **719**
- diagnostic checklist, **720**
- differential diagnosis, **720**
- epithelial component, **719–720**
- mixed epithelial-stromal tumor (MEST), proposed classification and criteria, **720**
- stromal component, **720**

Epithelial tumors/lesions
- benign, **536**
  - renal pelvis, **515**
  - ureter, **503–504**
- malignant
  - renal pelvis, **516**
  - ureter, **504**
- vs. metastasis, **902**

Epithelioid angiomyolipoma, **178–183**
- with clear-/light-staining cytoplasm, **242**
- clear cell renal cell carcinoma vs., **57**
- diagnostic checklist, **180**
- differential diagnosis, **180**
- with granular/eosinophilic cytoplasm, **243**
- immunohistochemistry, **180, 183**
- MiTF/TFE family translocation-associated carcinoma vs., **113**
- oncocytoma-like
  - chromophobe renal cell carcinoma vs., **93**
  - renal oncocytoma vs., **50**
- prognosis, **179**
- *TFE3* gene fusions, **179**
- *TP53* mutations, **179**

Epithelioid cell tumor, perivascular, MiTF/TFE family translocation-associated carcinoma vs., **113**
Epithelioid hemangioendothelioma, **701**
- myointimoma vs., **993**

Epithelioid hemangioma, adenomatoid tumor vs., **865**
Epithelioid perivascular epithelioid cell (PEC)oma (epithelioid PEComa). See Epithelioid angiomyolipoma.
Epithelioid trophoblastic tumor (ETT), **785, 789**
Erythroplasia of Queyrat. See Penile intraepithelial neoplasia.
Escherichia coli, malakoplakia, **281**
Ethnicity relationship, in prostate carcinoma, **600**
ETS gene fusion, TMPRSS2, **609**
Ewing sarcoma/PNET, small blue round cell tumors of kidney, **244**
Exophytic tumor, in renal pelvis, **509**
Exstrophy polyp, hamartoma vs., **327**
Extended biopsy, in prostate, **539**
Extensive cystitis glandularis, invasive adenocarcinoma vs., **411**
Extraadrenal pheochromocytoma. See Mesenchymal tumors, prostate.
Extragonadal sites, germinoma in. See Seminoma.

INDEX

Extramammary Paget disease, **986–989**
- ancillary tests, **987**
- diagnostic checklist, **988**
- differential diagnosis, **988**
- immunohistochemistry, **996**
- prognosis, **987**

Extranodal Rosai-Dorfman disease, malakoplakia vs., **281, 283**

Extraprostatic extension, **603**

Extrarenal or metastatic tumors, other rare tumors vs., **232**

Extratesticular extension, ectopic Leydig cells mimicking, Leydig cell tumor vs., **825**

F

Familial cancer syndromes, **12–37**
- Birt-Hogg-Dubé (BHD) syndrome, **16–19**
    - diagnostic checklist, **18**
    - diagnostic criteria, **17**
    - differential diagnosis, **18**
    - prognosis, **17**
- hereditary leiomyomatosis renal cell carcinoma syndrome, **20–23**
    - diagnostic checklist, **22**
    - differential diagnosis, **22**
    - genetic testing, **22**
    - prognosis, **21**
- hereditary papillary renal cancer syndrome, **32–37**
    - differential diagnosis, **34**
    - prognosis, **33**
- succinate dehydrogenase complex deficiency syndrome, **28–31**
    - diagnostic checklist, **30**
    - differential diagnosis, **30**
    - prognosis, **29**
- tuberous sclerosis complex, **24–27**
    - diagnostic checklist, **26**
    - differential diagnosis, **26**
    - genes, **25**
    - prognosis, **25**
- von Hippel-Lindau syndrome, **12–15**
    - differential diagnosis, **14**
    - gene alterations, **13**
    - prognosis, **13**

Familial prostate cancer, **601**

Familial syndromes, tumors associated with, **5**

Fasciitis, intravascular, myointimoma vs., **993**

Female urethra, **257**

α-fetoprotein, germ cell tumors, **750**

Fibroadenoma-like hyperplasia, **560**

Fibroepithelial polyp, **302–305, 495, 496**
- diagnostic checklist, **303**
- differential diagnosis, **303**
- papillary-polypoid cystitis vs., **274**
- prognosis, **303**
- skeletal muscle tumors vs., **449**
- tumor-like lesions of renal pelvis, **516**

Fibroepithelial tumor. See Epithelial stromal tumors.

Fibrohistiocytic tumor, plexiform, myointimoma vs., **993**

Fibroma, medullary. See Renomedullary interstitial cell tumor.

Fibromuscular stroma, renal tumors with
- clear cell papillary renal cell carcinoma vs., **74**
- transcription elongation factor B-mutated renal cell carcinoma vs., **69**

Fibroplasia, mucinous, **610**

Fibrosarcoma, Kaposi sarcoma vs., **991**

Fibrosis, amyloidosis vs., **313**

Fibrous cord, **521**

Fibrous histiocytoma, malignant, liposarcoma vs., **879**

Fine-needle aspiration biopsy, in prostate, **540**

FISH assays, in MiTF/TFE family translocation-associated carcinoma, **113**

Flat condyloma. See Condylomas.

Flat urothelial lesions, **250**
- markers used in, **528**
- urethral, with atypia, nephrogenic adenoma (metaplasia) of prostatic urethra vs., **584**

Florid von Brunn nests, inverted urothelial neoplasia vs., **366**

Foamy gland (xanthomatous) carcinoma, **628, 635**
- Gleason grading, **629**

Focal atrophy, **571**

Focal glandular atypia. See Atypical small acinar proliferations.

Focal therapy, for prostate carcinoma, **602**

Follicular carcinoma of kidney
- thyroid-like, **128–131**
    - diagnostic checklist, **129**
    - differential diagnosis, **129**
    - genetic features, **129**
    - prognosis, **129**

Follicular cystitis, **266, 269**

Follicular lymphoma (FL), **217, 219**

FOXL2 mutations
- granulosa cell tumor, **839**
- juvenile granulosa cell tumor, **843**

Fronds, papillary, prominent, benign prostate hyperplasia nodule with, prostatic intraepithelial neoplasia vs., **592**

Fumarate hydratase gene, germline inactivating mutations in, **21**

G

Gangrenous cystitis, **268**

Gardasil vaccine, **983**

Gastrointestinal stromal tumor
- involving prostate, **717**
- sarcomatoid carcinoma of prostate vs., **680**
- smooth muscle tumors vs., **442**
- stromal tumors vs., **693, 697**

Gene fusion, **609**

Genital wart. See Condylomas.

Germ cell aplasia. See Sertoli cell-only syndrome.

Germ cell neoplasia in situ, **756–761, 903**
- ancillary test, **757**
- associated microlith, **760**
- differential diagnosis, **757**

INDEX

- large, **758**
- Leydig cells, **758**
- with microinvasive seminoma, **759**
- pagetoid, **759**
- PAS stain, **760**
- PLAP, **761**
- podoplanin, **761**
- predominant cell/compartment type, **757**
- predominant pattern/injury type, **757**
- Sertoli cell nodule with, gonadoblastoma vs., **855**
- Sertoli cell-only syndrome vs., **739, 741**

Germ cell neoplasms
- intratubular, **899**
- nontuberculous infections vs., **743**
- pseudo intratubular, **899**

Germ cell tumors, **537**
- adenomatoid tumor vs., **865**
- age range, **748**
- anatomic features, **749**
- burnt-out (regressed), **800–801**
    - ancillary tests, **801**
    - diagnostic checklist, **801**
    - differential diagnosis, **801**
- classification, **732**
- cytogenetic changes, **748**
- cytologic features, **750**
- differential histologic features, **752**
- ethnicity, **748**
- general concepts, **748–755**
- immunohistochemistry, **750–751**
- metastatic poorly differentiated carcinoma, **900**
- mixed, **794–797, 904**
    - ancillary tests, **795**
    - differential diagnosis, **795**
    - granulosa cell tumor vs., **839**
    - prognosis, **795**
    - with prominent immature teratoma, mixed/unclassified sex cord-stromal tumor vs., **851**
    - reporting, **795**
    - somatic-type malignancy in germ cell tumor vs., **799**
    - unclassified, gonadoblastoma vs., **855**
- normal anatomy and histology, **749–750**
- predominant pattern, **750**
- pure, mixed germ cell tumors vs., **795**
- reporting criteria, **751**
- sex cord-/gonadal stromal tumors vs., **820**
- somatic-type malignancy in, **798–799**
    - ancillary tests, **799**
    - diagnostic checklist, **799**
    - differential diagnosis, **799**
- specimen handling, **749**
- with syncytiotrophoblasts, choriocarcinoma vs., **786**
- testicular, primary, metastatic tumors of testis and paratesticular structures vs., **895**
- TNM tumor staging, **751**
- vs. metastasis, **902**

Germinoma in extragonadal sites. *See* Seminoma.
Giant cell cystitis, **268**
Giant condyloma. *See* Condylomas.
Glandular differentiation, invasive urothelial carcinoma with, tumors of urachus vs., **524**
Glandular Gleason pattern 3, **612**
Glandular lesions of bladder
- clear cell adenocarcinoma, **416–421**
    - diagnostic checklist, **417**
    - differential diagnosis, **417**
    - gynecologic tract, secondary involvement (direct extension) from, clear cell adenocarcinoma vs., **417**
    - papillary, urothelial papilloma vs., **345**
    - prognosis, **417**
    - of urinary bladder, nephrogenic adenoma vs., **296**
    - urothelial carcinoma with clear cytoplasm vs., **385**
- cystitis cystica and glandularis, **404–407**
- invasive adenocarcinoma, **410–415**
    - cystitis cystica and glandularis vs., **405**
- villous adenoma, **408–409**

Glandular proliferation, **612**
Glans corona, papillomatosis of, condylomas vs., **910**
Glans resurfacing technique specimen, squamous cell carcinoma, of penis, **929**
Gleason grading system, **610**
Gleason pattern 1, **610**
Gleason pattern 2, **610, 618**
Gleason pattern 3, **610, 618**
- cribriform, **612**
- glandular, **612**
- tunneling, **619**
Gleason pattern 4, **610–612, 619**
- cribriform, **612**
- hypernephroid, **612**
Gleason pattern 5, **611, 620**
- cribriform, **612**
- single cell, **612**
- solid, **612**

Glomangiomas, **231, 233**
Glomangiomyomas, **231, 233**
Glomerulations, **610**
Glomus tumor, **231, 233**
- gross features, **230**
- juxtaglomerular cell tumor (reninoma) vs., **223, 225**

Glycogen-rich carcinoma, **472**
- urothelial, **396**

Glypican-3, germ cell tumors, **751**
Gonadoblastoma, **854–857**
- ancillary tests, **855**
- diagnostic checklist, **855**
- differential diagnosis, **855**
- granulosa cell tumor vs., **839**
- prognosis, **855**

Granular cell tumor, **455, 459**
- paraganglioma vs., **464**

Granuloma
- biopsy-related, **271**
- sperm
    - nonspecific granulomatous orchitis vs., **745**
    - tuberculous epididymo-orchitis vs., **747**

Granulomatous cystitis, **266**
Granulomatous inflammations
- renal malakoplakia vs., **40**
- renal tuberculosis vs., **40**
- xanthogranulomatous pyelonephritis vs., **40**

INDEX

Granulomatous orchiditis, burnt-out germ cell tumor vs., **801**
Granulomatous orchitis
- infectious, tuberculous epididymo-orchitis vs., **747**
- nonspecific, **744–745**
    - ancillary tests, **745**
    - differential diagnosis, **745**
    - seminoma vs., **764**
    - tuberculous epididymo-orchitis vs., **747**
    - unknown causes, **745**

Granulomatous prostatitis, **556**
- allergic, **556**
- infectious, **556**
- nonspecific, **555, 556**
- postprocedural, **555, 556**

Granulosa cell tumor, **819, 838–841**
- adult, mixed/unclassified sex cord-stromal tumor vs., **851**
- ancillary tests, **839**
- diagnostic checklist, **839**
- differential diagnosis, **839**
- juvenile, **842–845**
    - ancillary tests, **843**
    - differential diagnosis, **843**
    - prepubertal yolk sac tumor vs., **811**
    - prognosis, **843**
- prognosis, **839**

Granulosa cells, **819**

Gynecologic carcinoma, invasive urothelial carcinoma of bladder vs., **375**

Gynecologic tract clear cell adenocarcinoma, secondary involvement (direct extension) from, clear cell adenocarcinoma vs., **417**

H

Hamartoma, **326–327**
- ancillary tests, **327**
- bladder, fibroepithelial polyp vs., **303**
- diagnostic checklist, **327**
- differential diagnosis, **327**
- genetic, **327**
- melanotic. *See* Melanotic neuroectodermal tumor.
- papillary-polypoid cystitis vs., **274**
- prognosis, **327**

Hemangioendothelioma
- adenomatoid tumor vs., **865**
- epithelioid, **701**
    - myointimoma vs., **993**

Hemangioma, **231, 235, 459, 701**
- epithelioid, adenomatoid tumor vs., **865**
- mesenchymal tumors of bladder vs., **456**
- tumor-like lesions of renal pelvis, **516**

Hemangiopericytoma, juxtaglomerular cell tumor (reninoma) vs., **223**

Hematopoietic neoplasms
- amyloidosis vs., **313**
- prostate, **710–713**
    - ancillary tests, **711**
    - differential diagnosis, **711**

Hematopoietic tumors
- bladder, **251**
- kidney, **216–221**
    - classification, **5**
    - diagnostic checklist, **218**
    - genetic features, **217**
    - infectious agents, **217**
    - prognosis, **218**
- lymphoma/leukemia/plasmacytoma, **858–863**
    - ancillary tests, **860**
    - differential diagnosis, **860**
    - prognosis, **859**
    - staging, **860**
- prostate gland and seminal vesicle, **537**
- testis and paratesticular structures classification, **732**

Hemoglobinopathies, sickle cell, **105**

Hemorrhage, due to nonneoplastic process, choriocarcinoma vs., **786**

Hemorrhagic cystitis, **268, 269**

Hereditary leiomyomatosis and renal cell cancer-associated carcinoma, with TC-like areas, tubulocystic carcinoma vs., **125, 127**

Hereditary leiomyomatosis and renal cell cancer-associated renal cell carcinoma
- collecting duct carcinoma vs., **100**
- unclassified renal cell carcinoma vs., **143**

Hereditary leiomyomatosis and renal cell carcinoma-associated renal cell carcinoma
- with papillary or tubulopapillary architecture, **242–243**
- papillary renal cell carcinoma vs., **83, 89**
- succinate dehydrogenase complex deficiency syndrome vs., **30**

Hereditary leiomyomatosis renal cell carcinoma syndrome, **20–23**
- diagnostic checklist, **22**
- differential diagnosis, **22**
- genetic testing, **22**
- prognosis, **21**
- sarcomatoid features, **23**
- tubulocystic areas, **23**

Hereditary papillary renal cancer syndrome (HPRC), **32–37**
- differential diagnosis, **34**
- prognosis, **33**

Hereditary paraganglioma syndrome. *See* Succinate dehydrogenase complex deficiency syndrome.

Hereditary prostate cancer, **609**

Heterologous osteosarcoma, sarcomatoid urothelial carcinoma, **400**

High-grade acinar adenocarcinoma, with cribriform pattern, prostatic intraepithelial neoplasia vs., **592**

High-grade carcinoma, metastatic, choriocarcinoma vs., **786**

High-grade neuroendocrine carcinoma, **208–211, 231**
- developmental anomaly, **209**
- diagnostic checklist, **209**
- differential diagnosis, **209**
- prognosis, **209**

High-grade papillary urothelial carcinoma, **358–363**
- ancillary tests, **359**
- diagnostic checklist, **359**

xiii

INDEX

- differential diagnosis, **359**
- low-grade papillary urothelial carcinoma vs., **355**

High-grade prostatic intraepithelial neoplasia, **604**
- cribriform, **623**
- ductal adenocarcinoma vs., **652**
- intraductal carcinoma vs., **646**
- outpouching of, atypical small acinar proliferations vs., **641**

Histiocytic sarcoma, malakoplakia vs., **281**

Histiocytoma, malignant fibrous, **701**
- liposarcoma vs., **879**
- mesenchymal tumors of bladder vs., **456**

Histoanatomic structures, in prostate pathology, **548**

Histology, zonal variations in, **545**
- prostatic ducts and acini, **545**
- prostatic stroma, **545**

Hodgkin disease, **711**

Hormonal therapy, for acinar adenocarcinoma, **611, 622**

HSNF5/INI1/SMARCB1 tumor suppressor gene, malignant rhabdoid tumor, **193**

Human chorionic gonadotropin, germ cell tumors, **750**

Human papillomavirus (HPV)
- ancillary tests, **984**
- basaloid squamous cell carcinoma, **943**
- histologic subtypes, **984**
- infection, squamous cell carcinoma, of penis, **939**
- lesions associated with, immunohistochemistry, **996**
- in penile carcinomas, prevalence distribution, **985**
- squamous cell carcinoma, of penis, **928–929**
- tumors, of penis, **982–985**
- urinary bladder neoplasms and, **329**

Human placental lactogen, germ cell tumors, **751**

Hyaline globules, with or without rete testis hyperplasia, yolk sac tumor vs., **778**

Hyalinization, tubular, Sertoli cell-only syndrome vs., **739, 741**

Hybrid oncocytic tumors, **50**

Hybrid verrucous carcinoma, **976**. See also Cuniculatum squamous cell carcinoma.

Hypernephroid Gleason pattern 4, **612**

Hyperparathyroidism-jaw tumor syndrome (HPT-JT), **33**

Hyperplasia, **536**
- atypical adenomatous, **623**. See also Adenosis.
    - atypical small acinar proliferations vs., **641**
    - prostate hyperplasia vs., **560**
- atypical stromal. See Stromal tumors.
- basal cell, **560**
    - adenoid cystic pattern, basal cell carcinoma vs., **674, 677**
    - atypical, prostatic intraepithelial neoplasia vs., **592**
    - atypical small acinar proliferations vs., **641**
- benign, stromal tumors vs., **693**
- benign prostatic
    - adenosis vs., **567**
    - prostatic-type polyp vs., **307**
- Cowper gland, polypoid lesions vs., **496**
- cribriform, **560**
    - ductal adenocarcinoma vs., **652**
    - prostatic intraepithelial neoplasia vs., **592**
- epithelial predominant, **559–560**
- fibroadenoma-like, **560**
- Leydig cell, **740**
    - Leydig cell tumor vs., **825**
    - testicular tumor of adrenogenital syndrome vs., **847**
- mesonephric, verumontanum mucosal gland hyperplasia vs., **581**
- of mesonephric remnants, **576–579**
    - atypical small acinar proliferations vs., **641**
    - differential diagnosis of, **577**
- mesothelial, malignant mesothelioma vs., **869**
- mixed epithelial and stromal, **560**
- mucosal gland, verumontanum, **580–581**
    - diagnostic checklist of, **581**
    - differential diagnosis of, **581**
    - hyperplasia of mesonephric remnants vs., **577**
    - prognosis of, **581**
- nodule, prostate, benign, with prominent papillary fronds, prostatic intraepithelial neoplasia vs., **592**
- phyllodes type. See Stromal tumors.
- postatrophic, **571, 573–574, 624, 625**
    - atypical small acinar proliferations vs., **641**
- prostate, **558–565**
    - benign, adenosis vs., **567**
    - differential diagnosis of, **560**
    - prognosis, **559**
- prostatic stromal, with atypia (PSHA). See Stromal tumors.
- pseudocarcinomatous, **271, 318–325**
    - diagnostic checklist, **320**
    - differential diagnosis, **320**
    - invasive urothelial carcinoma of bladder vs., **376**
    - metastatic and secondary carcinomas vs., **472**
    - postchemotherapy. See Pseudocarcinomatous hyperplasia.
    - prognosis, **319**
    - radiation-induced. See Pseudocarcinomatous hyperplasia.
    - von Brunn nests vs., **289**
- pseudoepitheliomatous
    - pseudohyperplastic squamous cell carcinoma vs., **965**
    - squamous cell carcinoma of penis vs., **939**
- radiation-induced pseudocarcinomatous. See Pseudocarcinomatous hyperplasia.
- rete testis
    - adenocarcinoma of rete testis/epididymis vs., **873**
    - with or without hyaline globules, yolk sac tumor vs., **778**
- small glandular, **560**
- squamous, penis, **914–917**
    - differential diagnosis, **915**
    - prognosis, **915**
- stromal predominant, **560**
- verumontanum gland, **624**

Hyperreninemia, juxtaglomerular cell tumor (reninoma) and, **223**

Hypertension, juxtaglomerular cell tumor (reninoma) and, **223**

Hypertrophic muscularis mucosae, diverticula and, **480**

Hypertrophy, benign, prostatic. See Prostatic hyperplasia.

Hypospermatogenesis or maturation arrest, Sertoli cell-only syndrome vs., **739, 741**

INDEX

I

Iatrogenic soft tissue filler, myofibroblastic proliferations vs., **434**
Idiopathic calcinosis of scrotum. *See* Scrotal calcinosis.
Immature teratoma, nephroblastoma (Wilms tumor) vs., **163**
Immunohistochemistry
- kidney, **242–247**
  - poorly differentiated carcinomas, **244**
  - renal tumors with clear-/light-staining cytoplasm, **242**
  - renal tumors with granular/eosinophilic cytoplasm, **243**
  - renal tumors with papillary or tubulopapillary architecture, **242–243**
  - small blue round cell tumors of kidney, **244**
  - tumors with spindle cell morphology, **243–244**
- penis, **996–997**
- prostate, **541**
- testis, **898–905**
- urinary tract, **528–533**

Infarction, prostatic intraepithelial neoplasia vs., **592**
Infections
- nontuberculous, **742–743**
  - differential diagnosis, **743**
  - infectious agents, **743**
- repeated, tumor-like lesions of ureter, **503**

Infectious cystitis, **267**
Infectious granulomatous prostatitis, **556**
Infectious prostatitides, **555**
Infiltrative single cell pattern, **612**
Inflammations
- granulomatous
  - renal malakoplakia vs., **40**
  - renal tuberculosis vs., **40**
  - xanthogranulomatous pyelonephritis vs., **40**
- prostatic intraepithelial neoplasia vs., **592**
- xanthogranulomatous, malakoplakia vs., **281**

Inflammatory atrophy, proliferative, **575**
Inflammatory myofibroblastic tumor, **700, 703**. *See also* Myofibroblastic proliferations, of bladder; Urethra, inflammatory lesions of.
- skeletal muscle tumors vs., **449**
- smooth muscle tumors vs., **442**

Inflammatory pseudotumor. *See* Mesenchymal tumors, prostate; Myofibroblastic proliferations, of bladder.
Inflammatory/reactive lesions, atypical small acinar proliferations vs., **641**
Infundibulum, **263**
Inhibin, sex cord-/gonadal stromal tumors, **819**
Intermediate cells, **252, 260, 263**
International Society of Pediatric Oncology (SIOP), nephroblastoma classification, **161**
International Society of Urological Pathology, **610**
- grading system of, for prostatic adenocarcinoma, **612**

Interstitial cell tumor, renomedullary, **226–229**
- diagnostic checklist, **227**
- differential diagnosis, **227**
- electron microscopy, **227**
- immunohistochemistry, **227**
- prognosis, **227**

Interstitial cells, **819**
Interstitial cystitis, **267, 270**
Interstitium, **750**
Intestinal metaplasia
- cystitis glandularis with, **405**
- diverticula and, **481**

Intracystic growth, in clear cell papillary renal cell carcinoma, **75**
Intradiverticular high-grade urothelial carcinoma, diverticular-associated neoplasia and, **484**
Intradiverticular squamous cell carcinoma, diverticular-associated neoplasia and, **485**
Intradiverticular tumor, diverticular-associated neoplasia and, **484**
Intradiverticular urothelial carcinoma
- with glandular differentiation, diverticular-associated neoplasia and, **485**
- invasive into perivesical fat, diverticular-associated neoplasia and, **485**
- lymph node metastasis, diverticular-associated neoplasia and, **485**
- lymphovascular invasion, diverticular-associated neoplasia and, **485**
- superficial tumor, diverticular-associated neoplasia and, **485**

Intradiverticular urothelial carcinoma in situ, diverticular-associated neoplasia and, **484**
Intraductal carcinoma, **644–649**
- ancillary tests, **646**
- diagnostic checklist, **646**
- differential diagnosis, **646**
- genetics, **645**
- grade, **646**
- prognosis, **645**
- of prostate, prostatic intraepithelial neoplasia vs., **593**

Intraepithelial neoplasia
- high-grade, prostatic, **604**
  - cribriform, **623**
- penile, **922–927**
  - characteristics, **924**
  - condylomas vs., **910**
  - diagnostic checklist, **924**
  - differential diagnosis, **924**
  - prognosis, **923**
  - warty/basaloid, differential diagnosis, **924**
- prostatic, **590–599**
  - diagnostic checklist of, **593**
  - differential diagnosis of, **592–593**
  - genetics, **591**

Intraluminal crystalloids, **545**
Intraluminal secretions, **545**
Intratubular atypical cells, **899**
Intratubular germ cell neoplasia, unclassified type. *See* Germ cell neoplasia in situ.
Intratubular germ cell neoplasm, pseudo intratubular germ cell neoplasm vs., **899**
Intratubular large cell hyalinizing Sertoli cell neoplasia, **835**

INDEX

Intratubular malignant carcinoma, germ cell neoplasia in situ vs., **757**
Intratubular malignant lymphoma, germ cell neoplasia in situ vs., **757**
Intravascular fasciitis, myointimoma vs., **993**
Intravesical BCG, urothelial carcinoma in situ vs., **334**
Invasive adenocarcinoma, **410–415**
 - cystitis cystica and glandularis vs., **405**
 - diagnostic checklist, **411**
 - differential diagnosis, **410**
 - prognosis, **411**
Invasive carcinoma
 - subtypes, overview of, **382–403**
 - urinary bladder neoplasms and, **329**
Invasive neoplasms, **250**
Invasive squamous cell carcinoma, **426–431**
 - destructive invasion, **428**
 - diagnostic checklist, **427**
 - differential diagnosis, **427**
 - infiltration of, **428**
 - keratinous debris and calcification, **430**
 - prognosis, **427**
 - prominent keratinization, **428**
 - pseudocarcinomatous hyperplasia vs., **320, 321**
 - with pseudosarcomatous reaction, **428**
 - secondary, **431**
 - squamous differentiation, **428**
 - typical/classic type, **427**
 - verrucous, **427**
Invasive transitional cell carcinoma. *See* Urothelial carcinoma of bladder, invasive.
Invasive urothelial carcinoma, **330**
 - with glandular differentiation, tumors of urachus vs., **524**
 - of renal pelvis, **509**
 - with stromal retraction, micropapillary carcinoma vs., **383**
 - typical type, inverted urothelial neoplasia vs., **366**
Inverted (endophytic) urothelial neoplasms, noninvasive, **250**
Inverted growth, urothelial carcinoma with
 - tumor-like lesions of renal pelvis vs., **516**
 - tumor-like lesions of ureter vs., **504**
Inverted high-grade carcinoma, inverted urothelial neoplasia and, **366**
Inverted low-grade carcinoma, inverted urothelial neoplasia and, **365–366, 370**
Inverted neoplasia, analogy for application of WHO/ISUP system to, **330**
Inverted papilloma
 - fibroepithelial polyp vs., **303**
 - inverted urothelial neoplasia and, **365, 367**
 - tumor-like lesions of renal pelvis, **515**
 - von Brunn nests vs., **289**
Inverted urothelial neoplasia, pseudocarcinomatous hyperplasia vs., **320**
Inverted urothelial papilloma, with glandular feature, cystitis cystica and glandularis vs., **405**
Ischemic scar, burnt-out germ cell tumor vs., **801**

J

Juvenile granulosa cell tumor, **842–845**
 - ancillary tests, **843**
 - differential diagnosis, **843**
 - prepubertal yolk sac tumor vs., **811**
 - prognosis, **843**
Juxtaglomerular cell tumor, **222–225**
 - differential diagnosis, **223**
 - electron microscopy, **223**
 - genetic features, **223**
 - with papillary architecture, papillary renal cell carcinoma vs., **83**
 - prognosis, **223**

K

Kaposi sarcoma
 - immunohistochemistry, **997**
 - mesenchymal tumors of bladder vs., **456**
 - of penis, **990–991**
    diagnostic checklist, **991**
    differential diagnosis, **991**
    nodular stage, **991**
    patch stage, **991**
    plaque stage, **991**
    prognosis, **991**
Keratosis, seborrheic, condylomas vs., **910**
Kidney disease
 - cystic, localized or segmental, cystic partially differentiated nephroblastoma vs., **171**
 - end-stage, with clear cell renal cell carcinoma, von Hippel-Lindau syndrome vs., **14**
Kidney tumors and tumor-like conditions
 - acquired cystic disease-associated renal cell carcinoma, **132–137**
 - angiomyolipoma, **172–177**
 - Birt-Hogg-Dubé (BHD) syndrome, **16–19**
    von Hippel-Lindau syndrome vs., **14**
 - chromophobe renal cell carcinoma, **89, 90–97**
    Birt-Hogg-Dubé syndrome vs., **18**
    classical, with clear-/light-staining cytoplasm, **242**
    epithelioid angiomyolipoma vs., **180**
    with papillary architecture, papillary renal cell carcinoma vs., **83**
 - classification, **4–5**
 - clear cell papillary renal cell carcinoma, **72–79**
    with clear-/light-staining cytoplasm, **242**
    cystic, multilocular cystic clear cell renal cell neoplasm of low malignant potential vs., **65**
    MiTF/TFE family translocation-associated carcinoma vs., **113**
    with papillary or tubulopapillary architecture, **242–243**
    papillary renal cell carcinoma vs., **83, 89**
    transcription elongation factor B-mutated renal cell carcinoma vs., **69**

- clear cell renal cell carcinoma, 54–63
    - acquired cystic disease-associated renal cell carcinoma vs., 134
    - chromophobe renal cell carcinoma vs., 93
    - with clear-/light-staining cytoplasm, 242
    - with clear cell papillary-like areas, clear cell papillary renal cell carcinoma vs., 74, 78
    - cystic, with regression, multilocular cystic clear cell renal cell neoplasm of low malignant potential vs., 65
    - end-stage kidney disease with, von Hippel-Lindau syndrome vs., 14
    - epithelioid angiomyolipoma vs., 180
    - exhibiting papillary or pseudopapillary growth, papillary renal cell carcinoma vs., 82
    - MiTF/TFE family translocation-associated carcinoma vs., 113
    - other rare tumors vs., 232
    - renal malakoplakia vs., 40
    - renal tuberculosis vs., 40
    - transcription elongation factor B-mutated renal cell carcinoma vs., 69
    - tuberous sclerosis complex vs., 26
    - xanthogranulomatous pyelonephritis vs., 40
- clear cell sarcoma of kidney, 188–191
    - congenital mesoblastic nephroma vs., 185
    - malignant rhabdoid tumor vs., 193, 195
- collecting duct carcinoma, 98–103
    - hereditary leiomyomatosis renal cell carcinoma syndrome vs., 22
    - metastatic tumors vs., 239
    - with papillary or tubulopapillary architecture, 242–243
    - papillary renal cell carcinoma vs., 82, 89
    - poorly differentiated carcinomas, 244
    - renal medullary carcinoma vs., 106
    - with TC-like areas, tubulocystic carcinoma vs., 125
    - unclassified renal cell carcinoma vs., 143
    - urothelial carcinoma of renal pelvis vs., 508
- congenital mesoblastic nephroma, 184–187
    - plump cell pattern, clear cell sarcoma of kidney vs., 189
- cystic partially differentiated nephroblastoma, 170–171
    - mixed epithelial and stromal tumor (MEST) family tumors/pediatric cystic nephroma vs., 198, 203
    - multilocular cystic clear cell renal cell neoplasm of low malignant potential vs., 65
- epithelioid angiomyolipoma, 178–183
    - with clear-/light-staining cytoplasm, 242
    - clear cell renal cell carcinoma vs., 57
    - with granular/eosinophilic cytoplasm, 243
    - MiTF/TFE family translocation-associated carcinoma vs., 113
- hematopoietic tumors, 216–221
- hereditary leiomyomatosis renal cell carcinoma syndrome, 20–23
- hereditary papillary renal cancer syndrome, 32–37
- immunohistochemistry, 242–247
- introduction, 6–11
- juxtaglomerular cell tumor, 222–225
    - with papillary architecture, papillary renal cell carcinoma vs., 83
- malignant rhabdoid tumor, 192–195
- metanephric adenoma, 146–151
    - nephroblastoma (Wilms tumor) vs., 163
    - with papillary or tubulopapillary architecture, 242–243
    - papillary renal cell carcinoma vs., 83
- metanephric tumors other than metanephric adenoma, 152–155
- metastatic tumors, 238–241, 251
- MiTF/TFE family translocation-associated carcinoma, 110–117
- mixed epithelial and stromal tumor (MEST) family tumors and pediatric cystic nephroma, 196–203
- mucinous tubular and spindle cell carcinoma, 118–123
    - with papillary or tubulopapillary architecture, 242–243
    - papillary renal cell carcinoma vs., 83
    - tumors with spindle cell morphology, 243–244
- multilocular cystic renal cell neoplasm of low malignant potential, 64–67
- nephroblastoma, 160–169
- nephrogenic rests, 156–159
- other rare tumors, 230–237
    - classification, 4
- papillary adenoma, 44–47
    - renal, nephrogenic rests vs., 157
- papillary renal cell carcinoma, 80–89
    - acquired cystic disease-associated renal cell carcinoma vs., 134
    - clear cell papillary renal cell carcinoma vs., 74
    - clear cell renal cell carcinoma vs., 56
    - collecting duct carcinoma vs., 100
    - cystic clear cell, multilocular cystic clear cell renal cell neoplasm of low malignant potential vs., 65
    - metanephric adenoma vs., 148
    - MiTF/TFE family translocation-associated carcinoma vs., 113
    - mucinous tubular and spindle cell carcinoma vs., 119–120
    - multifocal sporadic, hereditary papillary renal cancer vs., 34
    - papillary adenoma vs., 45
    - with papillary or tubulopapillary architecture, 242–243
    - type 1, solid glomeruloid variant, nephroblastoma (Wilms tumor) vs., 163
    - type 2, hereditary leiomyomatosis renal cell carcinoma syndrome vs., 22
- primitive neuroectodermal tumor, 212–215
    - clear cell sarcoma of kidney vs., 189
    - synovial sarcoma vs., 205
- renal cell carcinoma, unclassified, 142–145
    - chromophobe renal cell carcinoma vs., 93
    - collecting duct carcinoma vs., 100
    - with medullary phenotype, renal medullary carcinoma vs., 106

INDEX

oncocytic type, succinate dehydrogenase complex deficiency syndrome vs., 30
poorly differentiated carcinomas, 244
renal oncocytoma vs., 50
urothelial carcinoma of renal pelvis vs., 508
- renal medullary carcinoma, 104–109
collecting duct carcinoma vs., 100
malignant rhabdoid tumor vs., 193
unclassified renal cell carcinoma vs., 143
- renal oncocytoma, 48–53
angiomyolipoma vs., 174
Birt-Hogg-Dubé syndrome vs., 18
chromophobe renal cell carcinoma vs., 92–93
succinate dehydrogenase complex deficiency syndrome vs., 30
unclassified renal cell carcinoma vs., 143
- renal tuberculosis, xanthogranulomatous pyelonephritis, renal malakoplakia, 38–43
- renomedullary interstitial cell tumor, 226–229
mixed epithelial and stromal tumor (MEST) family tumors/pediatric cystic nephroma vs., 198, 203
- subsequent second tumors, 138–141
- succinate dehydrogenase complex deficiency syndrome, 28–31
- synovial sarcoma, 204–207
- thyroid-like follicular carcinoma of kidney, 128–131
- transcription elongation factor B (*TCEB1*)-mutated renal cell carcinoma, 68–71
- tuberous sclerosis complex, 24–27
angiomyolipoma and, 173
epithelioid angiomyolipoma and, 179
von Hippel-Lindau syndrome vs., 14
- tubulocystic carcinoma, 124–127
mixed epithelial and stromal tumor (MEST) family tumors/ pediatric cystic nephroma vs., 198, 203
- von Hippel-Lindau syndrome, 12–15
- well-differentiated neuroendocrine tumor (carcinoid) and high-grade neuroendocrine carcinoma, 208–211
Kidneys, end-stage, 73
Klinefelter syndrome, 740

L

Lactogen, human placental, germ cell tumors, 751
Lamina propria, 257, 263, 264
- invasion, 328
- prostatic urethral carcinoma in situ with invasion of, 660
- ureter, 260, 261
- urinary bladder, 253
Large B-cell lymphoma, germ cell neoplasia in situ, 761
Large-cell calcifying Sertoli cell, with oxyphilic cytoplasm, 899
Large cell calcifying Sertoli cell tumor, 834–837
- ancillary tests, 835
- differential diagnosis, 835
- Leydig cell tumor vs., 825
- prognosis, 835
Large glandular proliferation, atypical, 612

Large nested carcinoma, 383, 389
- differential diagnosis, 383
- inverted urothelial neoplasia vs., 366
Lateral prostatic fascia, 547
Leiomyomas, 231, 699, 703
- angiomyolipoma vs., 174
- immunohistochemistry, 232, 234
- leiomyomatous adenomatoid tumor vs., 865
- liposarcoma vs., 879
- mesenchymal tumors of bladder vs., 456
- myointimoma vs., 993
- smooth muscle tumors and, 441, 443
- stromal tumors vs., 693, 697
Leiomyomatous nodule, 560
Leiomyomatous rhabdomyosarcoma, spindle. *See* Embryonal rhabdomyosarcoma.
Leiomyosarcoma, 234–235, 438, 528, 699, 703, 891
- angiomyolipoma vs., 174
- embryonal rhabdomyosarcoma vs., 887
- epithelioid, 703
smooth muscle actin, 703
- grading scheme, smooth muscle tumors and, 441
- immunohistochemistry, 996
- leiomyomatous adenomatoid tumor vs., 865
- liposarcoma vs., 879
- myofibroblastic proliferations vs., 434
- myxoid, 438
- primary, sarcomatoid UC vs., 384
- smooth muscle tumors and, 441, 443, 444
- with spindle cell morphology, 901
- stromal tumors vs., 693, 697
Lepromatous leprosy, 743
- nonspecific granulomatous orchitis vs., 745
Leprosy, lepromatous, 743
- nonspecific granulomatous orchitis vs., 745
Lesions
- in spindle cell, of bladder, 528, 531
- urothelial
flat, urethral, with atypia, nephrogenic adenoma (metaplasia) of prostatic urethra vs., 584
markers in, 529
Leukemia
- genetic features, 217
- histologic features, 218
- malignant
embryonal rhabdomyosarcoma vs., 887
melanotic neuroectodermal tumor vs., 883
- myeloid, 711
malakoplakia vs., 281
- sex cord-/gonadal stromal tumors vs., 820
- testis, 858–863
ancillary tests, 860
differential diagnosis, 860
prognosis, 859
staging, 860
Leydig cell hyperplasia, 740
- Leydig cell tumor vs., 825
- testicular tumor of adrenogenital syndrome vs., 847
Leydig cell tumors, 819, 824–827
- ancillary tests, 825
- atypia, 827

INDEX

- carcinoid tumor vs., **815, 817**
- clear cells, **827**
- crystalloids, **826**
- differential diagnosis, **825**
- granulosa cell tumor vs., **839**
- inhibin, **826, 827**
- large cell calcifying Sertoli cell tumor vs., **835**
- low power, **826**
- lymphoma/leukemia/plasmacytoma vs., **860**
- with microcystic pattern, **898–899**
- ossification, **827**
- with oxyphilic cytoplasm, **899**
- pigment, **826**
- rhabdoid features, **826**
- testicular tumor of adrenogenital syndrome vs., **847**
- vimentin, **827**
- yolk sac tumor vs., **778, 783**

Leydig cells, **819**
- ectopic, Leydig cell tumor vs., **825**
- germ cell neoplasia in situ, **758**

Lichen planus, lichen sclerosus et atrophicus vs., **913**
Lichen sclerosus, **937**
- differentiated penile intraepithelial neoplasia and, **925**

Lichen sclerosus et atrophicus, of penis, **912–913**
- diagnostic checklist, **913**
- differential diagnosis, **913**
- predominant cell/compartment type, **913**
- predominant pattern/injury type, **913**
- prognosis, **913**

LIN28, germ cell tumors, **751**

Lipofuscin
- in benign prostatic glands, **709**
- in seminal vesicle, **709**

Lipogranuloma, **918–919**
- ancillary tests, **919**
- differential diagnosis, **919**
- predominant cell/compartment type, **919**
- predominant pattern/injury type, **919**
- sclerosing, liposarcoma vs., **879**

Lipogranulomatous reaction, dermoid cyst, **809**

Lipomas, **231**
- liposarcoma vs., **879**
- mesenchymal tumors of bladder and, **458**

Lipomatous tumors, immunohistochemistry, **232**

Liposarcoma, **878–881, 891**
- adenomatoid tumor vs., **865**
- ancillary tests, **879**
- angiomyolipoma vs., **174**
- dedifferentiated, embryonal rhabdomyosarcoma vs., **887**
- differential diagnosis, **879**
- lipogranuloma vs., **919**
- predominant cell/compartment type, **879**
- predominant pattern/injury type, **879**
- primary, urothelial carcinoma with lipoid features vs., **385**
- prognosis, **879**

Littré glands, **257**

Low-grade acinar adenocarcinoma
- adenosis vs., **567**
- prostatic intraepithelial neoplasia vs., **592**
- verumontanum mucosal gland hyperplasia vs., **581**

Low-grade papillary urothelial carcinoma, **354–357**
- diagnostic checklist, **355**
- differential diagnosis, **355**
- prognosis, **355**

Low-grade urothelial carcinoma, high-grade papillary urothelial carcinoma vs., **359**

Luminal and cellular deposits, **545–546**
- corpora amylacea, **545**
- intraluminal crystalloids, **545**
- intraluminal secretions, **545**
- pigments, **545–546**

Lymph node, regional, germ cell tumors, **751**

Lymph node metastasis, urothelial carcinoma of renal pelvis, **512**

Lymphadenectomy specimen, squamous cell carcinoma, of penis, **929**

Lymphangioma, lipogranuloma vs., **919**

Lymphatic/vascular invasion, nephroblastoma (Wilms tumor), **162, 169**

Lymphoblastic lymphoma/leukemia, **711**

Lymphoepithelioma-like carcinoma, **383–384, 395, 453, 628**
- cytokeratin, **395**
- differential diagnosis, **384**

Lymphoepithelioma-like squamous cell carcinoma, of penis, **978–979**
- ancillary tests, **979**
- diagnostic checklist, **979**
- differential diagnosis, **979**
- prognosis, **979**

Lymphoid aggregate, benign, **713**

Lymphoma
- B-cell, **711**
    - diffuse large, **712**
- Burkitt, **217**
- with diffuse arrangement, and cells with pale and clear cytoplasm, **898**
- diffuse large B-cell, **217**
- follicular, **217, 219**
- intratubular malignant, germ cell neoplasia in situ vs., **757**
- intravascular. *See* Hematopoietic tumors.
- lymphoepithelioma-like carcinoma vs., **384**
- lymphoepithelioma-like squamous cell carcinoma vs., **979**
- malignant
    - embryonal carcinoma vs., **772**
    - embryonal rhabdomyosarcoma vs., **887**
    - melanotic neuroectodermal tumor vs., **883**
    - metastatic tumors of testis and paratesticular structures vs., **895**
    - nonspecific granulomatous orchitis vs., **745**
    - seminoma vs., **764**
    - spermatocytic tumor vs., **803**
- mantle cell, **217**
    - involving prostate, **713**
- plasmacytoid carcinoma vs., **383**
- poorly differentiated urothelial carcinoma vs., **385**
- sex cord-/gonadal stromal tumors vs., **820**

INDEX

- skeletal muscle tumors vs., **449**
- small blue round cell tumors of kidney, **244**
- small cell carcinoma vs., **384**
- small lymphocytic, **712**
    - involving prostate, **713**
    - pelvic lymph node, **713**
- T-cell, **711**

Lymphoma/leukemia/plasmacytoma, **858–863**
- ancillary tests, **860**
- differential diagnosis, **860**
- prognosis, **859**
- staging, **860**

Lymphovascular invasion, **604**
Lynch syndrome, urothelial carcinoma of renal pelvis in, **512**

M

Malacoplakia. *See* Malakoplakia.
Malakoplakia, **280–285**
- ancillary tests, **281**
- diagnostic checklist, **281**
- differential diagnosis, **281**
- inflammatory lesions of urethra and, **487, 488, 489**
- nonspecific granulomatous orchitis vs., **745**
- prostatitis vs., **556**
- renal, **38–43**
    - diagnostic checklist, **40**
    - differential diagnosis, **40**
    - prognosis, **39**
- tuberculous epididymo-orchitis vs., **747**

Male urethra, **256**
Malignant epithelial tumors
- renal pelvis, **516**
- ureter, **504**

Malignant fibrous histiocytoma, **701**
- liposarcoma vs., **879**
- mesenchymal tumors of bladder vs., **456**

Malignant glands, pathognomonic features for, **610**
Malignant lymphoma
- embryonal carcinoma vs., **772**
- embryonal rhabdomyosarcoma vs., **887**
- melanotic neuroectodermal tumor vs., **883**
- metastatic tumors of testis and paratesticular structures vs., **895**
- nonspecific granulomatous orchitis vs., **745**
- seminoma vs., **764**
- spermatocytic tumor vs., **803**

Malignant mesenchymal tumors, **537**
Malignant nonepithelial tumors, tumor-like lesions of renal pelvis, **516**
Malignant rhabdoid tumor, **192–195**
- diagnostic checklist, **193**
- differential diagnosis, **193**
- electron microscopy, **193**
- *HSNF5/INI1/SMARCB1* tumor suppressor gene, **193**
- immunohistochemistry, **193**
- prognosis, **193**
- *SMARCA4/BRG1* gene, **193**

Malignant teratoma. *See* Choriocarcinoma, and variants.

Mammalian target of rapamycin (mTOR) pathway, **173**
Mantle cell lymphoma, **217**
- involving prostate, **713**

Margin status, in prostate carcinoma, **603**
Maturation arrest or hypospermatogenesis, Sertoli cell-only syndrome vs., **739, 741**
Median umbilical ligament, **521**
Medulla, **262**
Medullary carcinoma, renal, **104–109**
- collecting duct carcinoma vs., **100**
- diagnostic checklist, **106**
- differential diagnosis, **106**
- predominant cell/compartment type, **106**
- predominant pattern/injury type, **106**
- prognosis, **105**
- unclassified renal cell carcinoma vs., **143**

Medullary fibroma. *See* Renomedullary interstitial cell tumor.
Medullary renal cell carcinoma. *See* Renal medullary carcinoma.
Melan-A (MART-1), sex cord-/gonadal stromal tumors, **820**
Melanocarcinoma, congenital. *See* Melanotic neuroectodermal tumor.
Melanocytic lesions of prostate, **706–709**
- ancillary tests, **707**
- differential diagnosis, **707**
- origin, **707**

Melanocytic tumors, **537**
Melanoma, **707**
- with diffuse arrangement, and cells with pale and clear cytoplasm, **898**
- intratubular malignant, germ cell neoplasia in situ vs., **757**
- malignant, paraganglioma vs., **464**
- mesenchymal tumors of bladder vs., **456**
- metastatic
    - melanotic neuroectodermal tumor vs., **883**
    - sex cord-/gonadal stromal tumors vs., **820**
- metastatic and secondary carcinomas and, **475**
- in situ, immunohistochemistry, **996**
- spindle cell
    - immunohistochemistry, **996**
    - sarcomatoid squamous cell carcinoma vs., **971**
- with spindle cell morphology, **901**
- urethra, **709**

Melanoma in situ, extramammary Paget disease vs., **988**
Melanosis, **707, 709**
- Fontana-Masson stain, **708**
- stromal, **708**

Melanotic hamartoma. *See* Melanotic neuroectodermal tumor.
Melanotic neuroectodermal tumor, **882–885**
- ancillary tests, **883**
- differential diagnosis, **883**
- prognosis, **883**

Melanotic progonoma. *See* Melanotic neuroectodermal tumor.
Membranous urethra, **257**
Merkel cell carcinoma, extramammary Paget disease vs., **988**

INDEX

Mesenchymal lesions of bladder
- myofibroblastic proliferations, **432–439**
- other tumors, **454–461**
  - differential diagnosis, **456**
- skeletal muscle tumors, **448–453**
- smooth muscle tumors, **440–447**

Mesenchymal neoplasms, **251**
- with myxoid features, mesenchymal tumors of bladder vs., **456**

Mesenchymal tumors
- benign, **537**
- malignant, **537**
- prostate, **698–705**
  - diagnostic checklist, **699–702**

Mesenchymal tumors of kidney
- angiomyolipoma, **172–177**
- benign, classification, **4**
- clear cell sarcoma, **188–191**
  - congenital mesoblastic nephroma vs., **185**
  - malignant rhabdoid tumor vs., **193**
- congenital mesoblastic nephroma, **184–187**
  - plump cell pattern, clear cell sarcoma of kidney vs., **189**
- epithelioid angiomyolipoma, **178–183**
- malignant or potentially malignant, classification, **4**
- malignant rhabdoid tumor, **192–195**
- synovial sarcoma, mesenchymal tumors of bladder vs., **456**

Mesenchymoma. See Epithelial stromal tumors.

Mesoblastic nephroma
- classical type, mixed epithelial and stromal tumor (MEST) family tumors/pediatric cystic nephroma vs., **198**
- congenital, classical variant, metanephric tumors other than metanephric adenoma vs., **153**

Mesonephric adenocarcinoma. See Clear cell adenocarcinoma.

Mesonephric hamartoma. See Epithelial stromal tumors.

Mesonephric hyperplasia, verumontanum mucosal gland hyperplasia vs., **581**

Mesonephric remnant hyperplasia, atypical small acinar proliferations vs., **641**

Mesonephric remnants
- adenosis vs., **567**
- hyperplasia of, **576–579**
  - differential diagnosis of, **577**

Mesothelial hyperplasia, malignant mesothelioma vs., **869**

Mesothelial tumors, vs. metastasis, **902**

Mesothelioma, **901–902**
- with glandular/tubular pattern, **901**
- malignant, **868–871**
  - adenocarcinoma of rete testis/epididymis vs., **873**
  - adenomatoid tumor vs., **865**
  - ancillary tests, **869**
  - differential diagnosis, **869**
  - metastatic tumors of testis and paratesticular structures vs., **895**
  - papillary serous carcinoma vs., **875**
  - prognosis, **869**
- with spindle cell morphology, **901**

Metanephric adenofibroma, mixed epithelial and stromal tumor (MEST) family tumors/pediatric cystic nephroma vs., **198**

Metanephric adenoma, **146–151**
- diagnostic checklist, **148**
- differential diagnosis, **148**
- nephroblastoma (Wilms tumor) vs., **163**
- with papillary or tubulopapillary architecture, **242–243**
- papillary renal cell carcinoma vs., **83**
- prognosis, **147**

Metanephric stromal tumor, congenital mesoblastic nephroma vs., **185**

Metanephric tumors other than metanephric adenoma, **152–155**
- ancillary tests, **153**
- *BRAF V600E* mutation, **153**
- diagnostic checklist, **153**
- differential diagnosis, **153**
- relationship with Wilms tumor, **153**

Metaplasia, **536**
- adenomatoid. See Nephrogenic adenoma, of prostatic urethra.
- intestinal, diverticula and, **481**
- nephrogenic. See also Nephrogenic adenoma, of prostatic urethra.
  - hypothesis, **583**
  - tumor-like lesions of renal pelvis, **515**
- squamous, **431**
  - benign prostatic glands with or without inflammation, prostate carcinoma with squamous differentiation vs., **686, 689**
  - diverticula and, **481**
  - keratinizing, invasive squamous cell carcinoma vs., **427**
  - squamous proliferations other than carcinoma and, **423, 424**
- transitional cell, prostatic intraepithelial neoplasia vs., **592**

Metaplastic carcinoma. See Sarcomatoid squamous cell carcinoma.

Metastasis
- distant, **328**
  - germ cell tumors, **751**
- in lymph node, urothelial carcinoma of renal pelvis, **512**
- testicular tumors vs., **902**

Metastatic adenocarcinoma
- breast, metastatic and secondary carcinomas and, **477**
- colonic, to bladder, invasive adenocarcinoma and, **414**
- colorectal, metastatic and secondary carcinomas and, **475**
- esophageal, metastatic and secondary carcinomas and, **475**
- with glandular/tubular pattern, **899–900, 901**
- invasive adenocarcinoma vs., **411**
- papillary serous carcinoma vs., **875**

Metastatic and secondary carcinomas, of bladder, **470–477**
- cribriform/acinar pattern, **472**
- diagnostic checklist, **472**
- differential diagnosis, **471–472**

- monotonous appearance, **472**
- prognosis, **471**
- pseudopapillary pattern, **472**
- solid pattern, **472**

Metastatic carcinoid, carcinoid tumor vs., **815**

Metastatic carcinoma
- adenocarcinoma of rete testis/epididymis vs., **873**
- adult-type teratoma vs., **791**
- collecting duct carcinoma vs., **100**
- embryonal carcinoma vs., **772**
- general features of, **471**
- high-grade, choriocarcinoma vs., **786**
- malignant mesothelioma vs., **869**
- mixed germ cell tumors vs., **795**
- papillary serous, **476**
- poorly differentiated, germ cell tumor vs., **900**
- sarcomatoid, other testicular and paratesticular sarcomas vs., **891**
- sex cord-/gonadal stromal tumors vs., **820**
- with signet ring or clear cell changes, lipogranuloma vs., **919**
- somatic-type malignancy in germ cell tumor vs., **799**
- unclassified renal cell carcinoma vs., **143**
- urothelial carcinoma of renal pelvis vs., **508**
- warty squamous cell carcinoma of penis vs., **950**

Metastatic melanoma
- malignant, epithelioid angiomyolipoma vs., **180**
- melanotic neuroectodermal tumor vs., **883**
- sex cord-/gonadal stromal tumors vs., **820**

Metastatic neoplasms, renal cell carcinoma, paraganglioma vs., **464**

Metastatic sarcoma
- adult-type teratoma vs., **791**
- malignant mesothelioma vs., **869**

Metastatic sarcomatoid carcinoma, other testicular and paratesticular sarcomas vs., **891**

Metastatic small cell carcinoma, small cell carcinoma vs., **384**

Metastatic squamous cell carcinoma, to penis, squamous cell carcinoma of penis vs., **939**

Metastatic thyroid carcinoma, thyroid-like follicular carcinoma of kidney vs., **129**

Metastatic tumors, **238–241, 251**
- diagnostic checklist, **238**
- differential diagnosis, **239**
- histologic features, **239**
- kidney, **5**
  - well-differentiated neuroendocrine tumor (carcinoid)/high-grade neuroendocrine carcinoma vs., **209**
- lymphoma/leukemia/plasmacytoma vs., **860**
- penis, **994–995**
  - diagnostic checklist, **995**
  - differential diagnosis, **995**
- testis and paratesticular structures, **894–897**
  - ancillary tests, **895**
  - differential diagnosis, **895**
  - prognosis, **895**
- tumor-like lesions of renal pelvis vs., **516**
- tumor-like lesions of ureter vs., **504**

a-methylacyl-CoA-racemase, **541**

Microanatomy, zonal variations and, **544–553**
- ductal acinar unit, **544–545**
- in histology, **545**
- luminal and cellular deposits, **545–546**
- nonglandular prostate, **546**
- nonprostatic structures, **546**
- periprostatic structures, **546–547**
- prostate anatomic zones, **545**
- seminal vesicle, **547**

Microcystic carcinoma, **383, 390**
- differential diagnosis, **383**
- urothelial, müllerian lesions vs., **316**

Micronodules, collagenous, **610**

Micropapillary carcinoma, **383, 393, 394**
- differential diagnosis, **383**
- in lymph node, **394**

Microscopy, electron
- in chromophobe renal cell carcinoma, **92**
- in metanephric adenoma, **148**
- in MiTF/TFE family translocation-associated carcinoma, **113**

MiTF/TFE family translocation-associated carcinoma, **110–117**
- with clear-/light-staining cytoplasm, **242**
- diagnostic checklist, **113**
- differential diagnosis, **113**
- with granular/eosinophilic cytoplasm, **243**
- prognosis, **111–112**

MiTF/TFE family translocation-associated renal cell carcinoma
- clear cell papillary renal cell carcinoma vs., **74**
- papillary renal cell carcinoma vs., **82–83, 89**

Mitomycin-associated changes, urothelial carcinoma in situ and, **334**

Mixed adenocarcinoma and SCC. See Prostate carcinoma, with squamous differentiation.

Mixed architectural patterns, well-differentiated neuroendocrine tumor (carcinoid)/high-grade neuroendocrine carcinoma, **209**

Mixed cell tumor, **904**

Mixed epithelial and stromal tumor
- renomedullary interstitial cell tumor vs., **227, 229**
- sporadic, hereditary papillary renal cancer vs., **34**

Mixed epithelial and stromal tumor (MEST) family tumors and pediatric cystic nephroma, **196–203**
- diagnostic checklist, **198**
- differential diagnosis, **198**
- prognosis, **197**

Mixed epithelial stromal neoplasm of seminal vesicle, müllerian lesions vs., **316**

Mixed germ cell tumors, **794–797, 904**. See also Germ cell tumors.
- ancillary tests, **795**
- differential diagnosis, **795**
- prognosis, **795**
- with prominent immature teratoma, mixed/unclassified sex cord-stromal tumor vs., **851**
- reporting, **795**
- somatic-type malignancy in germ cell tumor vs., **799**

INDEX

- unclassified, gonadoblastoma vs., **855**

Mixed squamous cell carcinoma, squamous cell carcinoma of penis vs., **939**

Monodermal teratoma. *See* Carcinoid tumor.

Monophasic choriocarcinoma, seminoma vs., **764**

Monophasic sarcomas, other, synovial sarcoma vs., **205**

MR-ultrasound (US) fusion biopsy, in prostate, **539**

mTOR pathway, epithelioid angiomyolipoma, **179**

Mucin, blue, in acinar adenocarcinoma, **610**

Mucinous carcinoma, **627, 630**
- Gleason grading of, **629**

Mucinous cystic urachal tumors, urachal remnants vs., **521**

Mucinous fibroplasia, **610**

Mucinous metaplasia, of penis, benign, extramammary Paget disease vs., **988**

Mucinous tubular and spindle cell carcinoma, **118–123**
- diagnostic checklist, **120**
- differential diagnosis, **119–120**
- with papillary or tubulopapillary architecture, **242–243**
- papillary renal cell carcinoma vs., **83**
- predominant cell/compartment type, **119**
- predominant pattern/injury type, **119**
- prognosis, **119**
- tumors with spindle cell morphology, **243–244**

Mucoepidermoid squamous cell carcinoma, pseudoglandular squamous cell carcinoma vs., **963**

Mucosa-associated lymphoid tissue (MALT), **217**. *See also* Hematopoietic tumors.

Mucosal epithelium, in male urethra, **257**

Mucosal gland hyperplasia, verumontanum, **580–581**
- diagnostic checklist of, **581**
- differential diagnosis of, **581**
- hyperplasia of mesonephric remnants vs., **577**
- prognosis of, **581**

Müllerian adenosarcoma-like tumor. *See* Epithelial stromal tumors.

Müllerian carcinoma
- ovarian-type, metastatic tumors of testis and paratesticular structures vs., **895**
- of tunica vaginalis, malignant mesothelioma vs., **869**

Müllerian duct cyst/remnant, **315**

Müllerian lesions, **314–317**
- ancillary tests, **316**
- diagnostic checklist, **316**
- differential diagnosis, **316**
- prognosis, **315**

Müllerian papillary serous carcinoma, **901–902**

Müllerian subtype, papillary serous carcinoma, **874–877**
- ancillary tests, **875**
- differential diagnosis, **875**
- prognosis, **875**

Müllerian tumors
- adenocarcinoma of rete testis/epididymis vs., **873**
- vs. metastasis, **902**

Müllerianosis, **315**
- of bladder, invasive adenocarcinoma and, **414**
- invasive adenocarcinoma vs., **411**
- metastatic and secondary carcinomas vs., **472**
- microcystic carcinoma vs., **383**

Multifocal bilateral clear cell renal cell carcinoma, hereditary papillary renal cancer vs., **34**

Multifocal clear cell renal cell carcinoma, von Hippel-Lindau syndrome vs., **14**

Multifocal sporadic papillary renal cell carcinoma, hereditary papillary renal cancer vs., **34**

Multilocular cyst. *See* Cystadenoma.

Multilocular cystic renal cell carcinoma (RCC). *See* Multilocular cystic renal cell neoplasm of low malignant potential.

Multilocular cystic renal cell neoplasm of low malignant potential, **64–67**
- differential diagnosis, **65**
- mixed epithelial and stromal tumor (MEST) family tumors/pediatric cystic nephroma vs., **198**
- prognosis, **65**

Multiloculated renal cortical cysts, benign, multilocular cystic clear cell renal cell neoplasm of low malignant potential vs., **65**

Multiparametric MR, in prostate carcinoma, **602**

Multiple myeloma, **711**

Mump orchitis, **743**

Muscle tumors, smooth, prostate hyperplasia vs., **560**

Muscularis mucosae muscle, **253, 254**

Muscularis propria, **253, 255, 263, 265**
- diverticula and, **480**
- invasion of, **328**
- ureter, **260, 261**

Mycobacterial spindle cell pseudotumor, atypical, malakoplakia vs., **281**

Myeloid leukemia, **711**
- malakoplakia vs., **281**

Myofibroblastic proliferations
- of bladder, **432–439**
    - actin, **436**
    - ALK1, **436**
    - associated with urothelial carcinoma, **437**
    - associations, **433**
    - cell variation, **435**
    - cytokeratin AE1/3, **436**
    - cytokeratin CAM5.2, **436**
    - diagnostic checklist, **434**
    - differential diagnosis, **433–434**
    - fine nuclear chromatin, **435**
    - infectious agents, **433**
    - loose fascicles, **435**
    - myometrial invasion, **435**
    - prognosis, **433**
    - prominent myxoid stroma and epithelioid cells, **435**
    - pseudosarcomatous, smooth muscle tumors vs., **442**
    - systemic disease, **433**
    - tapered cytoplasmic processes, **435**
- pseudosarcomatous, **528**
    - sarcomatoid urothelial carcinoma vs., **384**

Myofibroblastic tumor, inflammatory, **700, 703**
- skeletal muscle tumors vs., **449**
- smooth muscle tumors vs., **442**

Myofibroma, myointimoma vs., **993**

Myointimoma, **992–993**
- ancillary tests, **993**

INDEX

- diagnostic checklist, **993**
- differential diagnosis, **993**
- prognosis, **993**

Myxoid sarcoma, myxoid stroma vs., **385**

Myxoid stroma
- including chordoid, UC with, **384–385**
    - differential diagnosis, **385**
- renal cell carcinomas with, mucinous tubular and spindle cell carcinoma vs., **120**

N

NANOG, **751**
National Wilms Tumor Study (NWTS), **161**
NCCN guidelines 2015.1, in prostate carcinoma, **602**
Needle core biopsy
- in prostate, **539**
- tumor volume in, **603**

Neoplasia
- diverticular-associated, **482–485**
    - prognosis, **483**
- endophytic, urinary bladder neoplasms and, **329**
- inverted, analogy for application of WHO/ISUP system to, **330**
- Sertoli cell, intratubular large cell hyalinizing, **835**

Neoplasms, **250–251, 536–537**
- germ cell
    - intratubular, **899**
    - pseudo intratubular, **899**
- papillary, urethral, nephrogenic adenoma (metaplasia) of prostatic urethra vs., **584**
- smooth muscle, mesenchymal tumors of bladder vs., **456**
- urinary bladder, overview of, **328–331**

Nephroblastoma, **160–169**
- ancillary tests, **162**
- cystic partially differentiated, **170–171**
    - differential diagnosis, **171**
    - histology vs. radiologic evaluation, **171**
    - mixed epithelial and stromal tumor (MEST) family tumors/pediatric cystic nephroma vs., **198, 203**
    - multilocular cystic clear cell renal cell neoplasm of low malignant potential vs., **65**
    - prognosis, **171**
- developmental anomaly, **160–169**
- diagnostic checklist, **162–163**
- differential diagnosis, **162–163**
- lymphatic/vascular invasion, **162, 169**
- revised SIOP working classification of, after neoadjuvant therapy, **163**
- staging of pediatric renal tumors, **163**
- WT1 gene deletions or point mutations, **161**
- WT2 gene alterations, **161**

Nephroblastomatosis, **157**

Nephrogenic adenoma, **278, 294–301, 421, 495, 496, 497**
- ancillary tests, **295–296**
- atypical small acinar proliferations vs., **641**
- carcinoma of urethra vs., **492**
- clear cell adenocarcinoma vs., **417**
- diagnostic checklist, **296**
- differential diagnosis, **296**
- diverticula and, **481**
- fibromyxoid, **439**
    - myofibroblastic proliferations vs., **434**
    - pseudocarcinomatous hyperplasia vs., **320**
- hyperplasia of mesonephric remnants vs., **577, 579**
- invasive urothelial carcinoma of bladder vs., **375, 376**
- microcystic carcinoma vs., **383**
- nested carcinoma vs., **383**
- papillary
    - high-grade papillary urothelial carcinoma vs., **359**
    - papillary-polypoid cystitis vs., **274**
    - papillary urothelial carcinoma of low malignant potential vs., **351**
- prognosis, **295**
- prostatic-type polyp vs., **307**
- of prostatic urethra, **582–589**
    - diagnostic checklist of, **584**
    - differential diagnosis of, **584**
    - prognosis of, **583**
- superficial biopsy mimicking, **421**
- urothelial papilloma vs., **345**
- verumontanum mucosal gland hyperplasia vs., **581**

Nephrogenic metaplasia
- hypothesis, **583**
- tumor-like lesions of renal pelvis, **515**

Nephrogenic rests, **156–159**
- diagnostic checklist, **157**
- differential diagnosis, **157**
- intralobar, **157**
- molecular alterations, **157**
- perilobar, **157**
- prognosis, **157**

Nephrolithiasis, tumor-like lesions of ureter, **503**

Nephroma
- cellular mesoblastic
    - plump cell variant, malignant rhabdoid tumor vs., **193**
    - synovial sarcoma vs., **205**
- congenital mesoblastic, **184–187**
    - cellular variant, **185**
    - classical type, **185**
    - classical variant, metanephric tumors other than metanephric adenoma vs., **153**
    - diagnostic checklist, **185**
    - differential diagnosis, **185**
    - genetic features, **185**
    - plump cell pattern, clear cell sarcoma of kidney vs., **189**
    - prognosis, **185**
- cystic, multilocular cystic clear cell renal cell neoplasm of low malignant potential vs., **65**
- mesoblastic (classical type), mixed epithelial and stromal tumor (MEST) family tumors/ pediatric cystic nephroma vs., **198**
- pediatric cystic, **196–203**
    - cystic partially differentiated nephroblastoma vs., **171**
    - diagnostic checklist, **198**
    - differential diagnosis, **198**
    - prognosis, **197**

INDEX

Nephropathy, Balkan, in urothelial carcinoma of renal pelvis, **507**
Nerve sheath tumors
- benign, smooth muscle tumors vs., **442**
- myointimoma vs., **993**

Nested carcinoma, **382–383, 388**
- differential diagnosis, **382–383**
- large, **383, 389**

Nested urothelial carcinoma
- with associated tubules, cystitis cystica and glandularis vs., **405**
- of bladder, invasive, paraganglioma vs., **464**
- inverted urothelial neoplasia vs., **366**
- von Brunn nests vs., **289**

Neural differentiation, tumors with, **701**
Neural tumors, kidney, classification, **4–5**
Neuroblastoma, **139, 140**
- melanotic neuroectodermal tumor vs., **883**

Neuroectodermal tumor
- melanotic, **882–885**
    - ancillary tests, **883**
    - differential diagnosis, **883**
    - prognosis, **883**
- primitive, **212–215, 701–702, 705**
    - clear cell sarcoma of kidney vs., **189**
    - diagnostic checklist, **213**
    - differential diagnosis, **213**
    - prognosis, **213**
    - synovial sarcoma vs., **205**

Neuroendocrine carcinoma
- basaloid squamous cell carcinoma vs., **943**
- high-grade, **231**
- large cell, paraganglioma vs., **464**

Neuroendocrine neoplasm, low-grade, von Brunn nests vs., **289**

Neuroendocrine tumors
- kidney, classification, **4–5**
- primitive neuroectodermal tumor, **212–215, 701–702, 705**
    - clear cell sarcoma of kidney vs., **189**
    - diagnostic checklist, **213**
    - differential diagnosis, **213**
    - prognosis, **213**
    - synovial sarcoma vs., **205**
- well-differentiated (carcinoid), and high grade, **208–211**
    - developmental anomaly, **209**
    - diagnostic checklist, **209**
    - differential diagnosis, **209**
    - prognosis, **209**

Neurofibroma, **457**
- mesenchymal tumors of bladder vs., **456**
- myofibroblastic proliferations vs., **434**

Neurovascular bundle, **547**
Nodular amyloidosis, scrotal calcinosis vs., **921**
Nodules
- Sertoli cell, **737**
    - with germ cell neoplasia in situ, gonadoblastoma vs., **855**
    - Sertoli cell tumors vs., **829**
- steroid cell, with other adrenal diseases, testicular tumor of adrenogenital syndrome vs., **847**

Nonbladder sites, secondary carcinomas from, invasive carcinoma subtypes vs., **385**
Nonepithelial tumors/lesions
- benign
    - renal pelvis, **516**
    - ureter, **503–504**
- malignant, renal pelvis, **516**

Nonglandular prostate, **546**
- anterior fibromuscular stroma, **546**
- preprostatic sphincter, **546**
- prostatic "capsule," **546**
- striated sphincter, **546**

Noninvasive endophytic low-grade urothelial carcinoma, large nested carcinoma vs., **383**
Noninvasive inverted (endophytic) urothelial neoplasms, **250**
Noninvasive papillary tumors, **329**
Noninvasive papillary urothelial neoplasms, **250**
Noninvasive urothelial carcinoma, **511**
Nonneoplastic lesions, **250, 536**
Nonprostatic structures, **546**
- Cowper glands (bulbourethral glands), **546**
- ejaculatory duct, **546**
- prostatic urethra, **546**
- verumontanum (colliculus seminalis), **546**

Nonseminomatous germ cell tumor. *See* Germ cell tumors.
Nonspecific chronic orchiditis, burnt-out germ cell tumor vs., **801**
Nonspecific granulomatous orchitis, tuberculous epididymo-orchitis vs., **747**
Nonspecific granulomatous prostatitis, **555, 713**
Nonsyndromic clear cell renal cell carcinoma, von Hippel-Lindau syndrome vs., **14**
Nontuberculous infections, **742–743**
- differential diagnosis, **743**
- infectious agents, **743**

Nonurothelial neoplasms, other, invasive urothelial carcinoma of bladder vs., **375–376**
Normal urothelium, flat urothelial lesions other than carcinoma in situ vs., **341**
Nuclear beta-catenin, **471**
Nucleic acid-amplification methods, human papillomavirus, **984**
Nucleic acid-hybridization assays, human papillomavirus, **984**

Oat cell carcinoma. *See* Prostate carcinoma, with neuroendocrine differentiation.
OCT3/OCT 4, germ cell tumors, **751**
Oncocytic carcinoma, **628**
Oncocytic pattern, **612**
Oncocytic renal cell carcinoma, unclassified, Birt-Hogg-Dubé syndrome vs., **18**
Oncocytoma
- with granular/eosinophilic cytoplasm, **243**
- renal, **48–53**
    - angiomyolipoma vs., **174**

Birt-Hogg-Dubé syndrome vs., **18**
chromophobe renal cell carcinoma vs., **92–93**
diagnostic checklist, **50**
differential diagnosis, **50**
molecular abnormalities, **49**
prognosis, **49**
succinate dehydrogenase complex deficiency syndrome vs., **30**
unclassified renal cell carcinoma vs., **143**
Oncocytosis, renal, **49–50**
Orchiditis
- granulomatous, burnt-out germ cell tumor vs., **801**
- nonspecific chronic, burnt-out germ cell tumor vs., **801**
Orchitis. *See also* Nontuberculous infections.
- chronic, lymphoma/leukemia/plasmacytoma vs., **860**
- granulomatous, nonspecific, **744–745**
    ancillary tests, **745**
    differential diagnosis, **745**
    seminoma vs., **764**
    tuberculous epididymo-orchitis vs., **747**
    unknown causes, **745**
- infectious, nonspecific granulomatous orchitis vs., **745**
- mump, **743**
- syphilitic, **743**
- tuberculous epididymo-orchitis, **746–747**
    ancillary tests, **747**
    differential diagnosis, **747**
    infectious agents, **747**
Osteoclast-like giant cells, UC with, **384**
Osteogenic tumors, **701**
Other familial renal cell carcinoma syndromes, **33**
Other small round blue cell tumors, primitive neuroectodermal tumor vs., **213**
Ovarian carcinoma, **471**
Ovarian serous carcinoma, micropapillary carcinoma vs., **383**
Ovarian-type tumors, classification, **732**
Ovary
- dysgerminoma in. *See* Seminoma.
- Müllerian carcinoma, metastatic tumors of testis and paratesticular structures vs., **895**

P

p16 immunohistochemical stain, human papillomavirus, **984**
Paget disease, extramammary, **986–989**
- ancillary tests, **987**
- diagnostic checklist, **988**
- differential diagnosis, **988**
- immunohistochemistry, **996**
- prognosis, **987**
Pagetoid dyskeratosis, extramammary Paget disease vs., **988**
Pagetoid reticulosis, extramammary Paget disease vs., **988**
Papillae, **262, 264**
Papillary adenocarcinoma of seminal vesicle. *See* Seminal vesicle adenocarcinoma.
Papillary adenoma, **44–47**
- diagnostic checklist, **45**
- differential diagnosis, **45**
- genetic features, **45**
- prognosis, **45**
- renal, nephrogenic rests vs., **157**
Papillary architecture
- chromophobe renal cell carcinoma with, papillary renal cell carcinoma vs., **83**
- juxtaglomerular cell tumor with, papillary renal cell carcinoma vs., **83**
- tumors with, papillary renal cell carcinoma vs., **83**
Papillary carcinoma, **935**
- cuniculatum squamous cell carcinoma vs., **967**
- immunohistochemistry, **996**
- not otherwise specified
    condylomas vs., **910**
    warty squamous cell carcinoma of penis vs., **950**
- verrucous squamous cell carcinoma vs., **955**
Papillary clear cell adenocarcinoma, urothelial papilloma vs., **345**
Papillary cystadenoma, of epididymis, papillary serous carcinoma vs., **875**
Papillary cystitis. *See* Papillary-polypoid cystitis.
Papillary fronds, prominent, benign prostate hyperplasia nodule with, prostatic intraepithelial neoplasia vs., **592**
Papillary growth, clear cell renal cell carcinoma exhibiting, papillary renal cell carcinoma vs., **82**
Papillary neoplasms, urethral, nephrogenic adenoma (metaplasia) of prostatic urethra vs., **584**
Papillary nephrogenic adenoma
- high-grade papillary urothelial carcinoma vs., **359**
- papillary-polypoid cystitis vs., **274**
Papillary-polypoid cystitis, **272–279**
- diagnostic checklist, **274**
- differential diagnosis, **273–274**
- fibroepithelial polyp vs., **303**
- high-grade papillary urothelial carcinoma vs., **359**
- low-grade papillary urothelial carcinoma vs., **355**
- papillary urothelial carcinoma of low malignant potential vs., **351**
- prognosis, **273**
- prostatic-type polyp vs., **307**
- urothelial papilloma vs., **345**
Papillary/polypoid urethritis, inflammatory lesions of urethra and, **487, 488**
Papillary renal cell carcinoma, **80–89**
- acquired cystic disease-associated renal cell carcinoma vs., **134**
- clear cell, **72–79**
    differential diagnosis, **74**
    MiTF/TFE family translocation-associated carcinoma vs., **113**
    papillary renal cell carcinoma vs., **83, 89**
    prognosis, **73**
    transcription elongation factor B-mutated renal cell carcinoma vs., **69**
- clear cell papillary renal cell carcinoma vs., **74**
- clear cell renal cell carcinoma vs., **56**
- collecting duct carcinoma vs., **100**
- cystic clear cell, multilocular cystic clear cell renal cell neoplasm of low malignant potential vs., **65**

INDEX

- diagnostic checklist, **83**
- differential diagnosis, **82–83**
- metanephric adenoma vs., **148**
- MiTF/TFE family translocation-associated carcinoma vs., **113**
- mucinous tubular and spindle cell carcinoma vs., **119–120**
- multifocal sporadic, hereditary papillary renal cancer vs., **34**
- papillary adenoma vs., **45**
- with papillary or tubulopapillary architecture, **242–243**
- prognosis, **81**
- type 1, solid glomeruloid variant, nephroblastoma (Wilms tumor) vs., **163**
- type 2, hereditary leiomyomatosis renal cell carcinoma syndrome vs., **22**
- uncommon features, **88**

Papillary serous carcinoma
- Müllerian subtype, **874–877**
    - ancillary tests, **875**
    - differential diagnosis, **875**
    - prognosis, **875**
- of tunica vaginalis, malignant mesothelioma vs., **869**

Papillary squamous cell carcinoma
- not otherwise specified, papillary basaloid squamous cell carcinoma vs., **947**
- of penis, not otherwise specified, **958–961**
    - differential diagnosis, **959, 961**
    - prognosis, **959**

Papillary tumors
- noninvasive, **329–330**
- paratesticular, **901–902**

Papillary urothelial carcinoma
- of bladder, low-grade
    - diagnostic checklist, **355**
    - differential diagnosis, **355**
    - prognosis, **355**
- high-grade, **358**
    - ancillary tests, **359**
    - of bladder, low-grade papillary urothelial carcinoma vs., **355**
    - diagnostic checklist, **359**
    - differential diagnosis, **359**
- low-grade
    - papillary urothelial carcinoma of low malignant potential vs., **351**
    - urothelial papilloma vs., **345**
- nephrogenic adenoma vs., **296**
- of pelvicalyceal system, papillary renal cell carcinoma vs., **83**
- of renal pelvis, **509**
- urinary bladder neoplasms and, **329**

Papillary urothelial neoplasia, papillary-polypoid cystitis vs., **273–274**

Papillary urothelial neoplasm
- exophytic, **345**
- noninvasive, **250**
- prostatic-type polyp vs., **307**

Papillary urothelial neoplasm of low malignant potential, **350–353**
- diagnostic checklist, **351**
- differential diagnosis, **351**
- inverted, inverted urothelial neoplasia and, **365**
- low-grade papillary urothelial carcinoma vs., **355**
- prognosis, **351**
- urothelial papilloma vs., **345**

Papilloma
- inverted
    - fibroepithelial polyp vs., **303**
    - tumor-like lesions of renal pelvis, **515**
    - von Brunn nests vs., **289**
- squamous, squamous proliferations other than carcinoma and, **423**
- transitional cell. *See* Urothelial papilloma, of bladder.
- urothelial, **277, 352**
    - of bladder, **344–349**
    - fibroepithelial polyp vs., **303**
    - inverted, with glandular feature, cystitis cystica and glandularis vs., **405**
    - papillary urothelial carcinoma of low malignant potential vs., **351**

Papillomatosis, of glans corona, condylomas vs., **910**
Papulosis, clear cell, extramammary Paget disease vs., **988**
Paraganglia, **547**
Paraganglioma, **29, 700, 704**
- of bladder, **462–469**
    - associated normal urothelium, **466**
    - with basophilia, **465**
    - with biopsy artifact, **468**
    - with cautery artifact, **468**
    - chromogranin in, **469**
    - classic Zellballen, **465**
    - confounding prior biopsy site changes, **466**
    - diagnostic checklist, **464**
    - differential diagnosis, **464**
    - with endocrine atypia, **466**
    - fibrovascular septa, **465**
    - GATA3 in, **469**
    - with less-pronounced nests, **466**
    - to lymph node, **468**
    - with nuclear atypia, **466**
    - with nuclear inclusions, **465**
    - predominant cell/injury type, **463**
    - predominant pattern/injury type, **463**
    - prognosis, **463**
    - round nuclei, **465**
    - S100 protein in, **469**
    - SDHB loss in, **469**
    - small, incidental, **465**
    - with stromal retraction, **468**
    - synaptophysin in, **469**
    - synaptophysin in metastatic, **468**
    - with typical circumscription, **466**
    - with vascular invasion, **468**
- invasive urothelial carcinoma of bladder vs., **375**
- inverted urothelial neoplasia vs., **366**
- sclerosing, **467**
- von Brunn nests vs., **289**

Paraganglionic cells, normal, von Brunn nests vs., **289**

INDEX

Paramesonephric (müllerian) sinus, of urinary bladder, **315**
Paratesticular sarcoma, somatic-type malignancy in germ cell tumor vs., **799**
Paratesticular structures, tumors of, classification, **732**
Paratesticular tumors
- with glandular/tubular pattern, **901**
- papillary, **901–902**
- with spindle cell morphology, **901**

Parenchymal differentiation, rare tumors with, **4**
Parenchymal invasive urothelial carcinoma of renal pelvis, **509**
Partial atrophy, **571, 573, 624**
- atypical small acinar proliferations vs., **641**

Partial cystectomy, diverticula and, **479**
Partially differentiated nephroblastoma, cystic, multilocular cystic clear cell renal cell neoplasm of low malignant potential vs., **65**
Pediatric cystic nephroma, **196–203**
- cystic partially differentiated nephroblastoma vs., **171**
- diagnostic checklist, **198**
- differential diagnosis, **198**
- prognosis, **197**

Pelvicalyceal system, **262–263**
Pelvis, renal
- tumor-like lesions of, **514–519**
  - diagnostic checklist of, **516**
  - differential diagnosis of, **516**
  - prognosis of, **515**
- urothelial carcinoma of, **506–513**
  - diagnostic checklist of, **508**
  - differential diagnosis of, **508**
  - prognosis of, **507**
  - urothelial carcinoma of ureter vs., **500**

Penile carcinoma, related to human papillomavirus, **983**
- prevalence distribution, **985**

Penile intraepithelial neoplasia, **922–927**
- basaloid, **937**
- characteristics, **924**
- condylomas vs., **910**
- diagnostic checklist, **924**
- differential diagnosis, **924**
- differentiated, **937**
  - ancillary tests, **923–924**
  - differential diagnosis, **924**
  - squamous hyperplasia vs., **915**
- immunohistochemistry, **996**
- prognosis, **923**
- warty/basaloid, **976**
  - differential diagnosis, **924**

Penile (spongy) urethra, **257, 259**
Penis
- basaloid squamous cell carcinoma, **942–945**
  - ancillary tests, **943**
  - differential diagnosis, **943, 945**
  - papillary basaloid squamous cell carcinoma vs., **947**
  - papillary variant, **946–947**
  - prognosis, **943**
- clear cell carcinoma, **980–981**
  - ancillary tests, **981**
  - diagnostic checklist, **981**
  - differential diagnosis, **981**
  - predominant cell/compartment type, **981**
  - prognosis, **981**
- condylomas, **908–911**
  - warty/basaloid PeIN vs., **924**
- cuniculatum squamous cell carcinoma, **966–969**
  - diagnostic checklist, **967**
  - differential diagnosis, **967**
  - predominant cell/compartment type, **967**
  - predominant pattern/injury type, **967**
  - prognosis, **967**
- extramammary Paget disease, **986–989**
  - ancillary tests, **987**
  - diagnostic checklist, **988**
  - differential diagnosis, **988**
  - prognosis, **987**
- HPV- and non-HPV-related tumors
  - ancillary tests, **984**
  - overview, **982–985**
- immunohistochemistry, **996–997**
- Kaposi sarcoma, **990–991**
  - diagnostic checklist, **991**
  - differential diagnosis, **991**
  - nodular stage, **991**
  - patch stage, **991**
  - plaque stage, **991**
  - prognosis, **991**
- lichen sclerosus et atrophicus, **912–913**
  - diagnostic checklist, **913**
  - differential diagnosis, **913**
  - predominant cell/compartment type, **913**
  - predominant pattern/injury type, **913**
  - prognosis, **913**
- lipogranuloma, **918–919**
  - ancillary tests, **919**
  - differential diagnosis, **919**
  - predominant cell/compartment type, **919**
  - predominant pattern/injury type, **919**
- lymphoepithelioma-like squamous cell carcinoma, **978–979**
  - ancillary tests, **979**
  - diagnostic checklist, **979**
  - differential diagnosis, **979**
  - prognosis, **979**
- metastatic tumors, **994–995**
  - diagnostic checklist, **995**
  - differential diagnosis, **995**
- mixed squamous cell carcinoma, **974–977**
  - differential diagnosis, **975**
  - prognosis, **975**
- mucinous metaplasia of, benign, extramammary Paget disease vs., **988**
- myointimoma, **992–993**
  - ancillary tests, **993**
  - diagnostic checklist, **993**
  - differential diagnosis, **993**
  - prognosis, **993**
- papillary squamous cell carcinoma, not otherwise specified, **958–961**
  - differential diagnosis, **959, 961**
  - papillary basaloid squamous cell carcinoma vs., **947**
  - prognosis, **959**

INDEX

- pseudoglandular squamous cell carcinoma, **962–963**
    - ancillary tests, **963**
    - diagnostic checklist, **963**
    - differential diagnosis, **963**
    - prognosis, **963**
- pseudohyperplastic squamous cell carcinoma, **964–965**
    - diagnostic checklist, **965**
    - differential diagnosis, **965**
    - prognosis, **965**
    - squamous hyperplasia vs., **915**
- sarcoma of, primary, metastatic tumors vs., **995**
- sarcomatoid squamous cell carcinoma, **970–973**
    - ancillary tests, **971**
    - diagnostic checklist, **971**
    - differential diagnosis, **971**
    - prognosis, **971**
    - pseudoglandular squamous cell carcinoma vs., **963**
- scrotal calcinosis, **920–921**
    - diagnostic checklist, **921**
    - differential diagnosis, **921**
    - predominant cell/compartment type, **921**
    - predominant pattern/injury type, **921**
    - prognosis, **921**
- squamous cell carcinoma
    - anatomic level of invasion, **930**
    - anatomy and histology, **928**
    - ancillary studies, **930**
    - clear cell change, **937**
    - clinical implications, **929**
    - conventional. See Squamous cell carcinoma of penis, usual type.
    - depth of invasion, **930**
    - epidemiology, **928**
    - etiology/pathogenesis, **928–929**
    - with extension into distal urethra, carcinoma of urethra vs., **492**
    - general concepts, **928–937**
    - grade, **930, 934**
    - growth patterns, **930**
    - histological subtypes, **930**
    - multicentric, **929**
    - not otherwise specified. See Squamous cell carcinoma of penis, usual type.
    - pathologic stage, **930**
    - perineural invasion, **930–931**
    - primary, metastatic tumors vs., **995**
    - prognostic factors, **930–931**
    - prognostic index, **931**
    - resection margins, **931**
    - specimen handling, **929**
    - staging, **931**
    - superficial spreading, **929, 933**
    - tumor front of invasion, **931**
    - tumor site, **930**
    - tumor thickness, **930**
    - typical. See Squamous cell carcinoma of penis, usual type.
    - usual type, **938–941**
    - variants of, **985**
    - vascular invasion, **931**
    - verruciform, **929, 933, 934, 937**
    - vertical growth, **929, 933**
- squamous hyperplasia, **914–917**
    - differential diagnosis, **915**
    - differentiated PeIN vs., **924**
    - flat, **915**
    - mixed, **915**
    - papillary, **915**
    - prognosis, **915**
    - pseudoepitheliomatous, **915**
    - verrucous, **915**
- verrucous squamous cell carcinoma, **954–957**
    - diagnostic checklist, **955**
    - differential diagnosis, **955**
    - mixed (hybrid), verrucous squamous cell carcinoma vs., **955**
    - predominant cell/compartment type, **955**
    - predominant pattern/injury type, **955**
    - prognosis, **955**
    - pseudohyperplastic squamous cell carcinoma vs., **965**
- warty-basaloid squamous cell carcinoma, **952–953**
    - ancillary tests, **953**
    - diagnostic checklist, **953**
    - differential diagnosis, **953**
    - papillary basaloid squamous cell carcinoma vs., **947**
    - prognosis, **953**
- warty squamous cell carcinoma, **948–951**
    - diagnostic checklist, **950**
    - differential diagnosis, **949–950**
    - papillary basaloid squamous cell carcinoma vs., **947**
    - predominant cell/compartment type, **949**
    - predominant pattern/injury type, **949**
    - prognosis, **949**

Perineural invasion, **603–604**
Peripheral zone
- of prostate, **545**
- prostate cancer at, **613**

Periprostatic structures, **539, 546–547**
- adipose tissue, **546–547**
- Denonvilliers fascia, **547**
- lateral prostatic fascia, **547**
- neurovascular bundle, **547**
- paraganglia, **547**
- urinary bladder neck, **547**

Periurethral gland region, of prostate, **545**
Perivascular epithelioid cell neoplasm, **447, 460**
- epithelioid, **460**
- HMB45, **447**
- mesenchymal tumors of bladder vs., **456**
- smooth muscle tumors vs., **442**

Perivascular epithelioid cell tumor, **702**
- MiTF/TFE family translocation-associated carcinoma vs., **113**

Perivesical fat, diverticular-associated neoplasia and, **484**
Peutz-Jeghers syndrome, large cell calcifying Sertoli cell tumor, **835**
Pheochromocytoma, **29**
- of bladder. See Paraganglioma, of bladder.

Pheochromocytoma syndrome. See Succinate dehydrogenase complex deficiency syndrome.
Phyllodes tumor of prostate. See also Stromal tumors.
- cystadenoma vs., **720**

INDEX

- epithelial stromal tumor vs., **720**

Phyllodes type of hyperplasia. *See* Stromal tumors.

Pigmented melanocytosis. *See* Melanocytic lesions of prostate.

PIN-like adenocarcinoma, prostatic intraepithelial neoplasia vs., **592**

Placenta-like alkaline phosphatase, germ cell tumors, **750**

Placental site trophoblastic tumor (PSTT), **785, 789**

Plaques, penile, early, condylomas vs., **910**

Plasmacytoid carcinoma, **383, 391**
- differential diagnosis, **383**
- in fallopian tube, **392**
- in lymph node, **392**
- in periureteral tissue, **392**
- in seminal vesicle, **392**

Plasmacytoid invasive urothelial carcinoma of bladder, metastatic and secondary carcinomas vs., **472**

Plasmacytoma, **218, 220**
- with oxyphilic cytoplasm, **899**
- plasmacytoid carcinoma vs., **383**
- testis, **858–863**
    - ancillary tests, **860**
    - differential diagnosis, **860**
    - prognosis, **859**
    - staging, **860**

Pleomorphic giant cell adenocarcinoma, **628**

Plexiform fibrohistiocytic tumor, myointimoma vs., **993**

Podoplanin (D2-40), germ cell tumors, **751**

Point mutations, nephroblastoma (Wilms tumor), **161**

Polycystic kidney disease 1 (*PKD1*) gene deletions, **25**

Polyembryoma, **795, 797**

Polyomavirus, squamous proliferations other than carcinoma vs., **423**

Polyp
- exstrophy, hamartoma vs., **327**
- prostatic-type, **306–311, 495, 497**
    - ancillary tests, **307**
    - cystitis cystica and glandularis vs., **405**
    - differential diagnosis, **307**
    - fibroepithelial polyp vs., **303**
    - high-grade papillary urothelial carcinoma vs., **359**
    - papillary-polypoid cystitis vs., **274**
    - predominant cell/compartment type, **307**
    - urothelial papilloma vs., **345**

Polypoid cystitis. *See* Papillary-polypoid cystitis.

Polypoid prostatic adenocarcinoma involving urethra, **495**

Poorly differentiated carcinomas, **244**
- hematopoietic neoplasms of prostate vs., **711, 713**
- melanocytic lesions of prostate vs., **707**

Poorly differentiated neuroendocrine carcinoma. *See* Prostate carcinoma, with neuroendocrine differentiation.

Poorly differentiated urothelial carcinoma, **385**
- differential diagnosis, **385**

Postatrophic hyperplasia, **571, 573–574, 624, 625**
- atypical small acinar proliferations vs., **641**

Postchemotherapy, in MiTF/TFE family translocation-associated carcinoma, **111**

Postchemotherapy pseudocarcinomatous hyperplasia. *See* Pseudocarcinomatous hyperplasia.

Postinflammatory scar, burnt-out germ cell tumor vs., **801**

Postoperative spindle cell nodule. *See* Myofibroblastic proliferations, of bladder; Urethra, inflammatory lesions of.

Postoperative spindle cell nodule (PSCN). *See* Mesenchymal tumors, prostate.

Postprocedural granulomatous prostatitis, **555**

Postpubertal teratoma, prepubertal teratoma vs., **807**

Posttransplant lymphoproliferative disorders (PTLD)
- histologic features, **218**
- infectious agents, **217**

Posttreatment cancer, **612**

Posttreatment carcinoma, **612**

Predominant Wilms tumor, epithelial, metanephric adenoma vs., **148**

Preprostatic sphincter, **546**

Prepubertal teratoma, **806–809**
- diagnostic checklist, **807**
- differential diagnosis, **807**
- glandular component, **808**
- immature component, **808**
- immature neuroepithelial component, **808**
- intestinal component, **808**

Prepubertal testicular teratoma and carcinoid. *See* Teratoma, prepubertal type.

Prepubertal yolk sac tumor, **810–813**
- ancillary tests, **811**
- with cytologic atypia, **812**
- diagnostic checklist, **811**
- differential diagnosis, **811**
- exuberant papillary growth pattern, **813**
- glandular growth pattern, **813**
- macrocystic pattern, **812**
- papillary and solid growth pattern, **812**

Primary adenocarcinoma, of urinary bladder, tumors of urachus vs., **524**

Primary androgen deprivation therapy, for prostate carcinoma, **602**

Primary invasive adenocarcinoma of urinary bladder, müllerian lesions vs., **316**

Primary leiomyosarcoma, sarcomatoid UC vs., **384**

Primary liposarcoma, urothelial carcinoma with lipoid features vs., **385**

Primary sarcoma
- adult-type teratoma vs., **791**
- of kidney, **231**
- of prostate, sarcomatoid carcinoma of prostate vs., **680**

Primary testicular sarcoma, somatic-type malignancy in germ cell tumor vs., **799**

Primary vesical sarcoma, sarcomatoid UC vs., **384**

Primitive neuroectodermal tumor, **212–215, 701–702, 705**
- clear cell sarcoma of kidney vs., **189**
- diagnostic checklist, **213**
- differential diagnosis, **213**
- prognosis, **213**
- synovial sarcoma vs., **205**

PRKAR1A gene, **835**

Progonoma, melanotic. *See* Melanotic neuroectodermal tumor.

INDEX

Proliferations
- acinar, small, benign, hyperplasia of mesonephric remnants vs., **577**
- spindle cell, types of, marker positivity in, **528**

Proliferative cystitis. See von Brunn nests.

Proliferative inflammatory atrophy, **575**

Proliferative lesions, atypical small acinar proliferations vs., **641**

Proliferative pyelitis, **265**

Prominent papillary fronds, benign prostate hyperplasia nodule with, prostatic intraepithelial neoplasia vs., **592**

Prostate adenocarcinoma, **279, 471, 901–902**. See also Acinar adenocarcinoma.
- with atrophic features, atrophy vs., **571**
- bladder adenocarcinoma vs., markers in differential of, **725**
- direct invasion by, invasive adenocarcinoma vs., **411**
- high grade, paraganglioma vs., **464**
- invasive adenocarcinoma and, **415**
- involving bladder, **381**
  - invasive urothelial carcinoma of bladder vs., **375**
- ISUP grading system for, **612**
- main mimics of variants, **629**
- malakoplakia vs., **281**
- markers for diagnosis, needle biopsy, **724**
- markers used in metastatic setting to prove, **725**
- metastatic and secondary carcinomas and, **474**
- nephrogenic adenoma vs., **296**
- papillary-polypoid cystitis vs., **274**
- poorly differentiated, urothelial carcinoma involving prostate gland vs., **661**
- prostatic small cell carcinoma vs., markers for, **725–726**
- seminal vesicle adenocarcinoma vs., **723**
- urothelial carcinoma vs., markers in differential of, **724–725**
- variants, main mimics of, **629**
- work-up, minimal, **727**

Prostate carcinoma, **536–537**
- architecture, **614**
- atypical small acinar proliferations vs., **640**
- bladder urothelial carcinoma mimicking, **716**
- differential diagnosis for, **612**
- familial, **601**
- general concepts of, **600–607**
  - staging, **604**
- hereditary, **609**
- metastatic, germ cell neoplasia in situ vs., **761**
- with neuroendocrine differentiation, **664–671**
  - ancillary tests, **667**
  - carcinoid tumor, **665, 666–667**
  - classification, **665**
  - differential diagnosis, **667**
  - Gleason grading, **667**
  - large cell neuroendocrine carcinoma, **665, 667, 671**
  - markers, **670**
  - mixed neuroendocrine carcinoma/acinar adenocarcinoma, **665, 666, 668**
  - molecular pathology, **666**
  - origin, **665**
  - with overlapping features of SCC and acinar PCa, **665, 670–671**
  - Paneth cell-like, **665, 666, 668**
  - prognosis, **666**
  - reporting, **667**
  - small cell carcinoma, **665, 666, 669**
  - staging, **667**
- at peripheral zone, **613**
- prostatitis vs., **556**
- radiated, PIN4 in, **621**
- with radiotherapy effects, **621–622**
- with squamous differentiation, **684–689**
  - adenosquamous carcinoma, **685–686, 688, 689**
  - ancillary tests, **686**
  - diagnostic checklist, **686**
  - differential diagnosis, **686**
  - grading, **686**
  - origin, **685**
  - pure squamous cell carcinoma, **685, 687**
  - reporting, **686**
- staging, **604**
- with vacuolations, **620**
- variants, Gleason grading of, **629**

Prostate gland, **538–539**
- acinar adenocarcinoma variants, **626–637**
- adenosis, **566–569**
- anatomic features, **538–539**
- anatomic zones, **545**
  - central zone, **545**
  - peripheral zone, **545**
  - periurethral gland region, **545**
  - transition zone, **545**
- atrophy and its variants, **570–575**
- atypical small acinar proliferations, **604, 638–643**
  - acinar adenocarcinoma vs., **611**
- basal cell carcinoma, **672–677**
  - prostate carcinoma with neuroendocrine differentiation vs., **667**
- central zone glands, prostatic intraepithelial neoplasia vs., **592**
- cystadenoma and epithelial stromal tumor, **718–721**
- ductal adenocarcinoma, **650–657**
- ectopic. See Prostatic-type polyp.
- general concepts, **538–543**
  - prostate carcinoma, **600–607**
- hematopoietic neoplasms, **710–713**
- hyperplasia nodule, benign, with prominent papillary fronds, prostatic intraepithelial neoplasia vs., **592**
- hyperplasia of mesonephric remnants, **576–579**
- immunohistochemistry, **541, 724–729**
- intraductal carcinoma, **644–649**
  - prostatic intraepithelial neoplasia vs., **593**
- intraepithelial neoplasia, **590–599**
- lineage-specific markers, **541**
- mantle cell lymphoma involving, **713**
- melanocytic lesions, **706–709**
- mesenchymal tumors, **698–705**
- microanatomy and zonal variations, **544–553**
- nephrogenic adenoma of prostatic urethra, **582–589**
- pathology, histoanatomic structures in, **548**

INDEX

- phyllodes tumor
    - cystadenoma vs., **720**
    - epithelial stromal tumor vs., **720**
- primary sarcomas of, sarcomatoid carcinoma of prostate vs., **680**
- primary urothelial carcinoma, **659**
- prostatitis, **536, 554–557**
    - chronic, hematopoietic neoplasms of prostate vs., **711**
- pseudosarcomatous myofibroblastic proliferations of, sarcomatoid carcinoma of prostate vs., **680**
- with reactive atypia, prostatic intraepithelial neoplasia vs., **592**
- sarcomatoid carcinoma, **678–683**
    - ancillary tests, **680**
    - carcinomatous component, **679–680**
    - diagnostic checklist, **680**
    - differential diagnosis, **680**
    - heterologous elements, **681**
    - origin, **679**
    - predominant cell/compartment type, **680**
    - predominant pattern/injury type, **680**
    - sarcomatoid/sarcomatous component, **680**
- secondary tumors, **714–717**
    - ancillary tests, **715**
    - origin, **715**
    - pattern of spread, **715**
- small cell carcinoma secondarily involving, prostate carcinoma with neuroendocrine differentiation vs., **667**
- solitary fibrous tumor of, prostate hyperplasia vs., **560**
- specimen types and handling, **539–540**
- stromal tumors of, prostate hyperplasia vs., **560**
- transurethral resection of, **540**
- urothelial carcinoma involving, **658–663**
    - ancillary test, **661**
    - classification, **659**
    - differential diagnosis, **661**
    - grading, **661**
    - pattern of involvement, **660**
    - prevalence of involvement in reported series, **660**
    - staging, **661**
- verumontanum mucosal gland hyperplasia, **580–581**
    - atypical small acinar proliferations vs., **640**
    - hyperplasia of mesonephric remnants vs., **577**

Prostate tumors
- classifications of, **536–537**
- and tumor-like lesions, stromal tumors, **690–697**
    - chromosomal abnormality, **691**
    - clonality, **691**
    - diagnostic checklist, **693**
    - differential diagnosis, **693**
    - origin, **691**

Prostatectomy
- radical, **540**
    - for prostate carcinoma, **602**
- subtotal, **540**
    - tumor volume in, **603**

Prostatic acinar adenocarcinoma, **608–625**
- with aberrant p63 expression, basal cell carcinoma vs., **674, 676**
- basal cell carcinoma vs., **674**
- cribriform pattern, basal cell carcinoma vs., **674**
- nephrogenic adenoma (metaplasia) of prostatic urethra vs., **584**
- poorly differentiated
    - basal cell carcinoma vs., **674**
    - prostate carcinoma with neuroendocrine differentiation vs., **667**

Prostatic acini, urothelial carcinoma involving, **660–661**
Prostatic "capsule," **546**
Prostatic ductal adenocarcinoma, prostatic-type polyp vs., **307**
Prostatic ductal carcinoma, **279**
- high-grade papillary urothelial carcinoma vs., **359**
- urothelial papilloma vs., **345**

Prostatic ducts, **258**
- urothelial carcinoma involving, **660–661, 662**
    - prostatic intraepithelial neoplasia vs., **593**

Prostatic epithelial polyp, benign. *See* Prostatic-type polyp.
Prostatic histogenesis, markers, **728, 729**
Prostatic hyperplasia, **558–565**
- benign
    - adenosis vs., **567**
    - prostatic-type polyp vs., **307**
- differential diagnosis of, **560**
- prognosis, **559**

Prostatic hypertrophy, benign. *See* Prostatic hyperplasia.
Prostatic intraepithelial neoplasia, **590–599**
- diagnostic checklist of, **593**
- differential diagnosis of, **592–593**
- genetics, **591**
- Gleason grading of, **629**
- high-grade, **604**
    - cribriform, **623**
    - urothelial carcinoma involving prostate gland vs., **661**

Prostatic nevohyperplasia. *See* Melanocytic lesions of prostate.
Prostatic sarcoma, sarcomatoid carcinoma vs., markers, **726, 729**
Prostatic small cell carcinoma, prostatic adenocarcinoma vs., markers for, **725–726**
Prostatic stroma, tumors of, **537**
Prostatic stromal hyperplasia with atypia (PSHA). *See* Stromal tumors.
Prostatic stromal invasion, **661**
Prostatic stromal proliferations of uncertain malignant potential. *See* Stromal tumors.
Prostatic stromal sarcoma, **691**
- cellular atypia, **695**
- cystadenoma vs., **720**
- epithelial stromal tumor vs., **720**
- high grade, **692, 695–696**
- intermediate grade, **692**
- low grade, **692, 695**
- necrosis, **695**

Prostatic stromal tumor of uncertain malignant potential
- cystadenoma vs., **720**

INDEX

- epithelial stromal tumor vs., **720**

Prostatic tumors of uncertain malignant potential, **691, 694**
- degenerative atypia, **692, 694**
- hypercellular stroma, **692, 694**
- myxoid, **692, 694**
- phyllodes-type growth, **692**
- PR positivity, **697**

Prostatic-type polyp, **306–311, 495, 497**
- ancillary tests, **307**
- cystitis cystica and glandularis vs., **405**
- differential diagnosis, **307**
- fibroepithelial polyp vs., **303**
- high-grade papillary urothelial carcinoma vs., **359**
- papillary-polypoid cystitis vs., **274**
- predominant cell/compartment type, **307**
- urothelial papilloma vs., **345**

Prostatic urethra, **256, 256–257, 258, 539, 546**
- nephrogenic adenoma (metaplasia) of, **582–589**
   - diagnostic checklist of, **584**
   - differential diagnosis of, **584**
   - prognosis of, **583**
- noninvasive urothelial carcinoma, **660**

Prostatic urethral carcinoma in situ, **660**

Prostatic urethral polyp, ductal adenocarcinoma vs., **652**

Prostatic utricle, **258**

Prostatic utricle cyst, urethral diverticula vs., **496**

Prostatitis, **536, 554–557**
- allergic, **556**
- chronic, hematopoietic neoplasms of prostate vs., **711**
- diagnostic checklist of, **556**
- differential diagnosis, **556**
- granulomatous, **556**
   - nonspecific, **555, 556, 713**
   - postprocedural, **555, 556**
- xanthogranulomatous, **556**

Proximal/posterior urethra, **257**

Pseudo intratubular germ cell neoplasm, intratubular germ cell neoplasm vs., **899**

Pseudocarcinomatous hyperplasia, **271, 318–325**
- diagnostic checklist, **320**
- differential diagnosis, **320**
- invasive urothelial carcinoma of bladder vs., **376**
- metastatic and secondary carcinomas vs., **472**
- postchemotherapy. See Pseudocarcinomatous hyperplasia.
- prognosis, **319**
- radiation-induced. See Pseudocarcinomatous hyperplasia.
- von Brunn nests vs., **289**

Pseudocarcinomatous proliferation. See Pseudocarcinomatous hyperplasia.

Pseudoepitheliomatous hyperplasia
- pseudohyperplastic squamous cell carcinoma vs., **965**
- squamous cell carcinoma of penis vs., **939**

Pseudoglandular squamous cell carcinoma, **936**
- of penis, **962–963**
   - ancillary tests, **963**
   - diagnostic checklist, **963**
   - differential diagnosis, **963**
   - prognosis, **963**

Pseudohyperplastic carcinoma, **627, 632–633, 936**
- Gleason grading of, **629**
- squamous cell carcinoma of penis vs., **939**

Pseudohyperplastic pattern, **612**

Pseudohyperplastic squamous cell carcinoma
- of penis, **964–965**
   - diagnostic checklist, **965**
   - differential diagnosis, **965**
   - prognosis, **965**
- squamous hyperplasia vs., **915**

Pseudohyperplastic variant, of acinar adenocarcinoma, prostate hyperplasia vs., **560**

Pseudopapillary growth, clear cell renal cell carcinoma exhibiting, papillary renal cell carcinoma vs., **82**

Pseudopolyps, catheter-induced. See Papillary-polypoid cystitis.

Pseudosarcomatous fibromyxoid tumor. See Mesenchymal tumors, prostate; Myofibroblastic proliferations, of bladder; Urethra, inflammatory lesions of.

Pseudosarcomatous myofibroblastic proliferation, **487, 488, 489, 528, 700**. See also Mesenchymal tumors, prostate; Myofibroblastic proliferations, of bladder; Urethra, inflammatory lesions of.
- of prostate, sarcomatoid carcinoma of prostate vs., **680**
- sarcomatoid UC vs., **384**

PTEN, **609**

Putative premalignant lesions, **536**

Pyelonephritis, xanthogranulomatous, **38–43**
- diagnostic checklist, **40**
- differential diagnosis, **40**
- prognosis, **39**

R

Radiation, prostatic intraepithelial neoplasia vs., **592**

Radiation atypia, squamous proliferations other than carcinoma vs., **423**

Radiation/chemotherapy cystitis. See Pseudocarcinomatous hyperplasia.

Radiation/chemotherapy effect, urothelial carcinoma in situ vs., **334**

Radiation cystitis, **268, 271**

Radiation-induced pseudocarcinomatous hyperplasia. See Pseudocarcinomatous hyperplasia.

Radiation therapy, for acinar adenocarcinoma, **611**

Radiation therapy microspheres, selective internal, schistosomiasis vs., **287**

Radical cystectomy, diverticula and, **479**

Radical prostatectomy, **540**
- for intraductal carcinoma, **645**
- for prostate carcinoma, **602**

Radical resection, germ cell tumors, **749**

Rare tumors
- of kidney, with epithelial &/or parenchymal differentiation, classification, **4**
- other, **230–237**
   - differential diagnosis, **231–232**
   - immunohistochemistry, **232**

INDEX

Reactive atypia
- prostate glands with, prostatic intraepithelial neoplasia vs., **592**
- urothelial, flat urothelial lesions other than carcinoma in situ and, **341**

Rebiopsy, for intraductal carcinoma, **645**

Rectal adenocarcinoma, invading prostate, **717**
- beta-catenin, **717**
- CDX-2, **717**

Rectal carcinoma, extramammary Paget disease associated with, immunohistochemistry, **996**

Regional lymph node (pN), germ cell tumors, **751**

Regressed germ cell tumor. *See* Germ cell tumors, burnt-out (regressed).

Remnants, mesonephric
- adenosis vs., **567**
- hyperplasia of, **576–579**
  - differential diagnosis of, **577**

Renal-adrenal fusion, **231, 237**

Renal angiomyoadenomatous tumor (RAT)-like RCC, tuberous sclerosis complex vs., **26**

Renal calyces, **262**

Renal cell carcinoma, **6**
- acquired cystic disease-associated, **132–137**
  - diagnostic checklist, **134**
  - differential diagnosis, **134**
  - genetic testing, **134**
  - predominant cell/compartment type, **134**
  - predominant pattern/injury type, **134**
  - prognosis, **133**
- chromophobe, **89, 90–97**
  - Birt-Hogg-Dubé syndrome vs., **18**
  - diagnostic checklist, **93**
  - differential diagnosis, **92–93**
  - epithelioid angiomyolipoma vs., **180**
  - genetic features, **91**
  - with papillary architecture, papillary renal cell carcinoma vs., **83**
  - prognosis, **91**
- clear cell, **54–63**
  - acquired cystic disease-associated renal cell carcinoma vs., **134**
  - chromophobe renal cell carcinoma vs., **93**
  - with clear cell papillary-like areas, clear cell papillary renal cell carcinoma vs., **74, 78**
  - diagnostic checklist, **57**
  - differential diagnosis, **56–57**
  - end-stage kidney disease with, von Hippel-Lindau syndrome vs., **14**
  - eosinophilic variant, renal oncocytoma vs., **50**
  - epithelioid angiomyolipoma vs., **180**
  - exhibiting papillary or pseudopapillary growth, papillary renal cell carcinoma vs., **82**
  - MiTF/TFE family translocation-associated carcinoma vs., **113**
  - multifocal, nonsyndromic, von Hippel-Lindau syndrome vs., **14**
  - prognosis, **55**
  - renal malakoplakia vs., **40**
  - renal tuberculosis vs., **40**
  - transcription elongation factor B-mutated renal cell carcinoma vs., **69**
  - tuberous sclerosis complex vs., **26**
  - xanthogranulomatous pyelonephritis vs., **40**
- clear cell adenocarcinoma vs., **417**
- clear cell papillary, **72–79**
  - differential diagnosis, **74**
  - MiTF/TFE family translocation-associated carcinoma vs., **113**
  - papillary renal cell carcinoma vs., **83, 89**
  - prognosis, **73**
  - transcription elongation factor B-mutated renal cell carcinoma vs., **69**
- collecting duct carcinoma, **98–103**
  - diagnostic checklist, **100**
  - differential diagnosis, **100**
  - genetic features, **99**
  - hereditary leiomyomatosis renal cell carcinoma syndrome vs., **22**
  - metastatic tumors vs., **239**
  - with papillary or tubulopapillary architecture, **242–243**
  - papillary renal cell carcinoma vs., **82, 89**
  - poorly differentiated carcinomas, **244**
  - prognosis, **99**
  - renal medullary carcinoma vs., **106**
  - with TC-like areas, tubulocystic carcinoma vs., **125**
  - unclassified renal cell carcinoma vs., **143**
- cystic clear cell, with regression, multilocular cystic clear cell renal cell neoplasm of low malignant potential vs., **65**
- cystic clear cell papillary, multilocular cystic clear cell renal cell neoplasm of low malignant potential vs., **65**
- with diffuse arrangement, and cells with pale and clear cytoplasm, **898**
- eosinophilic variant chromophobe
  - renal oncocytoma vs., **50**
  - succinate dehydrogenase complex deficiency syndrome vs., **30**
  - unclassified renal cell carcinoma vs., **143**
- hereditary leiomyomatosis and renal cell cancer-associated
  - collecting duct carcinoma vs., **100**
  - unclassified renal cell carcinoma vs., **143**
- hereditary leiomyomatosis and renal cell carcinoma-associated
  - papillary renal cell carcinoma vs., **83, 89**
  - succinate dehydrogenase complex deficiency syndrome vs., **30**
- medullary carcinoma, **104–109**
  - collecting duct carcinoma vs., **100**
  - diagnostic checklist, **106**
  - differential diagnosis, **106**
  - malignant rhabdoid tumor vs., **193**
  - predominant cell/compartment type, **106**
  - predominant pattern/injury type, **106**
  - prognosis, **105**
  - unclassified renal cell carcinoma vs., **143**
- metastatic
  - clear cell carcinoma vs., **981**

INDEX

    paraganglioma vs., **464**
- MiTF/TFE family translocation-associated, **110–117**
  - with clear-/light-staining cytoplasm, **242**
  - clear cell papillary renal cell carcinoma vs., **74**
  - diagnostic checklist, **113**
  - differential diagnosis, **113**
  - with granular/eosinophilic cytoplasm, **243**
  - papillary renal cell carcinoma vs., **82–83, 89**
  - prognosis, **111–112**
- mucinous tubular and spindle cell carcinoma, **118–123**
  - diagnostic checklist, **120**
  - differential diagnosis, **119–120**
  - with papillary or tubulopapillary architecture, **242–243**
  - papillary renal cell carcinoma vs., **83**
  - predominant cell/compartment type, **119**
  - predominant pattern/injury type, **119**
  - prognosis, **119**
  - tumors with spindle cell morphology, **243–244**
- multifocal, bilateral clear cell, hereditary papillary renal cancer vs., **34**
- multifocal sporadic papillary, hereditary papillary renal cancer vs., **34**
- multilocular cystic renal cell neoplasm of low malignant potential, **64–67**
  - differential diagnosis, **65**
  - prognosis, **65**
- with myxoid stroma, mucinous tubular and spindle cell carcinoma vs., **120**
- oncocytic, unclassified, Birt-Hogg-Dubé syndrome vs., **18**
- papillary, **80–89**
  - acquired cystic disease-associated renal cell carcinoma vs., **134**
  - clear cell papillary renal cell carcinoma vs., **74**
  - clear cell renal cell carcinoma vs., **56**
  - collecting duct carcinoma vs., **100**
  - diagnostic checklist, **83**
  - differential diagnosis, **82–83**
  - metanephric adenoma vs., **148**
  - MiTF/TFE family translocation-associated carcinoma vs., **113**
  - mucinous tubular and spindle cell carcinoma vs., **119–120**
  - papillary adenoma vs., **45**
  - prognosis, **81**
  - uncommon features, **88**
- renal angiomyoadenomatous tumor (RAT)-like, tuberous sclerosis complex vs., **26**
- with sarcomatoid differentiation, angiomyolipoma vs., **174**
- SDHB-deficient
  - renal oncocytoma vs., **50**
  - unclassified renal cell carcinoma vs., **143**
- subsequent second tumors, **138–141**
  - autoimmune conditions, **139**
  - genetic features, **139**
  - prognosis, **139**
- TCEB1-mutated, **68–71**
  - clear cell renal cell carcinoma vs., **57**
  - differential diagnosis, **69**
  - genetic testing, **69**
  - papillary renal cell carcinoma vs., **83**
  - prognosis, **69**
  - tuberous sclerosis complex vs., **26**
- thyroid-like follicular carcinoma of kidney, **128–131**
  - diagnostic checklist, **129**
  - differential diagnosis, **129**
  - genetic features, **129**
  - prognosis, **129**
- translocation-associated, **139**
  - clear cell renal cell carcinoma vs., **56**
- tuberous sclerosis-associated
  - clear cell renal cell carcinoma vs., **57**
  - papillary renal cell carcinoma vs., **83, 89**
  - renal oncocytoma vs., **50**
  - transcription elongation factor B-mutated renal cell carcinoma vs., **69**
  - unclassified renal cell carcinoma vs., **143**
- tubulocystic, hereditary leiomyomatosis renal cell carcinoma syndrome vs., **22**
- tubulocystic carcinoma, **124–127**
  - differential diagnosis, **125**
  - mixed epithelial and stromal tumor (MEST) family tumors/ pediatric cystic nephroma vs., **198, 203**
  - prognosis, **125**
- type 2 papillary, hereditary leiomyomatosis renal cell carcinoma syndrome vs., **22**
- unclassified, **142–145**
  - chromophobe renal cell carcinoma vs., **93**
  - collecting duct carcinoma vs., **100**
  - differential diagnosis, **143**
  - with medullary phenotype, renal medullary carcinoma vs., **106**
  - oncocytic type, succinate dehydrogenase complex deficiency syndrome vs., **30**
  - poorly differentiated carcinomas, **244**
  - prognosis, **143**
  - renal oncocytoma vs., **50**
  - urothelial carcinoma of renal pelvis vs., **508**
- urothelial carcinoma with clear cytoplasm vs., **385**
- VCL-ALK, renal medullary carcinoma vs., **106**
- warty squamous cell carcinoma of penis vs., **950**

Renal cell carcinoma syndrome, hereditary leiomyomatosis, **20–23**
- diagnostic checklist, **22**
- differential diagnosis, **22**
- genetic testing, **22**
- prognosis, **21**

Renal cell tumors, **6–11**
- anatomic considerations, **6–7**
- benign. See Papillary adenoma; Renal oncocytoma.
- intraoperative (frozen-section) evaluation, **7**
- primary staging, **8**
- prognostic factors, **8**

Renal cortical adenoma. See Papillary adenoma.

Renal cortical cysts, benign multiloculated, multilocular cystic clear cell renal cell neoplasm of low malignant potential vs., **65**

INDEX

Renal cortical tumors
- grading issues, **7**
- specimen-handling issues, **7**
- staging issues, **7**

Renal epithelial tumors, adult, with predominant tubules and cysts, tubulocystic carcinoma vs., **125**

Renal hilum, **262**

Renal malakoplakia, **38–43**
- diagnostic checklist, **40**
- differential diagnosis, **40**
- prognosis, **39**

Renal medullary carcinoma, **104–109**
- collecting duct carcinoma vs., **100**
- diagnostic checklist, **106**
- differential diagnosis, **106**
- malignant rhabdoid tumor vs., **193**
- predominant cell/compartment type, **106**
- predominant pattern/injury type, **106**
- prognosis, **105**
- unclassified renal cell carcinoma vs., **143**

Renal medullary interstitial cell, **227**

Renal neoplasm, multilocular cystic, of low malignant potential, mixed epithelial and stromal tumor (MEST) family tumors/pediatric cystic nephroma vs., **198**

Renal oncocytoma, **48–53**
- angiomyolipoma vs., **174**
- Birt-Hogg-Dubé syndrome vs., **18**
- chromophobe renal cell carcinoma vs., **92–93**
- diagnostic checklist, **50**
- differential diagnosis, **50**
- molecular abnormalities, **49**
- prognosis, **49**
- succinate dehydrogenase complex deficiency syndrome vs., **30**
- unclassified renal cell carcinoma vs., **143**

Renal oncocytosis, **49–50**

Renal parenchyma, urothelial carcinoma of renal pelvis in, **509**

Renal pelvis
- exophytic tumor in, **509**
- microscopic anatomy, **262–265**
- tumor-like lesions of, **514–519**
   - diagnostic checklist of, **516**
   - differential diagnosis of, **516**
   - prognosis of, **515**
- urothelial carcinoma of, **506–513**
   - diagnostic checklist of, **508**
   - differential diagnosis of, **508**
   - prognosis of, **507**
   - urothelial carcinoma of ureter vs., **500**

Renal sinus, **262, 265**

Renal sinus invasion, urothelial carcinoma of renal pelvis with, **509**

Renal tuberculosis, **38–43**
- diagnostic checklist, **40**
- differential diagnosis, **40**
- prognosis, **39**

Renal tubular cell seeding hypothesis, **583**

Renal tumors
- CK7(+), with prominent fibromuscular stroma, clear cell papillary renal cell carcinoma vs., **74**
- with clear-/light-staining cytoplasm, **242**
- with fibromuscular stroma and CK7 positivity, transcription elongation factor B-mutated renal cell carcinoma vs., **69**
- with granular/eosinophilic cytoplasm, **243**
- with papillary or tubulopapillary architecture, **242–243**
- pediatric, staging of, **163**
- with spindle cell morphology, **243–244**

Reninoma, **222–225**
- differential diagnosis, **223**
- electron microscopy, **223**
- genetic features, **223**
- prognosis, **223**

Renomedullary interstitial cell tumor, **226–229**
- diagnostic checklist, **227**
- differential diagnosis, **227**
- electron microscopy, **227**
- immunohistochemistry, **227**
- keloid-like bands, **228**
- mixed epithelial and stromal tumor (MEST) family tumors/pediatric cystic nephroma vs., **198, 203**
- prognosis, **227**

Rete adenocarcinoma, with glandular/tubular pattern, **901**

Rete carcinoma, metastatic tumors of testis and paratesticular structures vs., **895**

Rete/epididymal carcinoma
- metastatic tumors of testis and paratesticular structures vs., **895**
- papillary serous carcinoma vs., **875**

Rete testis
- adenocarcinoma of, malignant mesothelioma vs., **869**
- carcinoma of, papillary serous carcinoma vs., **875**
- germ cell neoplasia in situ, **759**
- tumors of, classification, **732**

Rete testis/epididymis adenocarcinoma, **872–873**
- ancillary tests, **873**
- differential diagnosis, **873**
- prognosis, **873**

Rete testis hyperplasia
- adenocarcinoma of rete testis/epididymis vs., **873**
- with or without hyaline globules, yolk sac tumor vs., **778**

Rete testis tumor, with glandular/tubular pattern, **899–900**

Retinal anlage tumor. *See* Melanotic neuroectodermal tumor.

Revised SIOP working classification of nephroblastoma after neoadjuvant therapy, **163**

Rhabdoid tumor of kidney
- clear cell sarcoma of kidney vs., **189**
- congenital mesoblastic nephroma vs., **185**
- malignant, **192–195**
   - diagnostic checklist, **193**
   - differential diagnosis, **193**
   - electron microscopy, **193**
   - *HSNF5/INI1/SMARCB1* tumor suppressor gene, **193**
   - immunohistochemistry, **193**
   - prognosis, **193**

INDEX

SMARCA4/BRG1 gene, **193**
Rhabdomyosarcoma, **439, 528, 531**
- adult, **700–701, 704**
- alveolar, **451**
    - with anaplasia, **451**
- cellular foci in, **451**
- desmin, **452**
- embryonal, **886–889**
    - ancillary tests, **887**
    - differential diagnosis, **887**
    - fibroepithelial polyp vs., **303**
    - hamartoma vs., **327**
    - melanotic neuroectodermal tumor vs., **883**
    - prognosis, **887**
- juvenile granulosa cell tumor vs., **843**
- liposarcoma vs., **879**
- myofibroblastic proliferations vs., **434**
- myogenin, **452**
- nonspecific MYOD1 staining, **452**
- other testicular and paratesticular sarcomas vs., **891**
- small cell carcinoma vs., **384**
- smooth muscle tumors vs., **442**
- spindle leiomyomatous. *See* Embryonal rhabdomyosarcoma.
- synaptophysin, **452**

Ribbon-like architecture, well-differentiated neuroendocrine tumor (carcinoid)/high-grade neuroendocrine carcinoma, **209**
Rosai-Dorfman disease, extranodal, malakoplakia vs., **281, 283**
Round blue cell tumors, other small, primitive neuroectodermal tumor vs., **213**

S

S100, sex cord-/gonadal stromal tumors, **819**
SALL4, germ cell tumors, **751**
Sarcoidosis
 - nonspecific granulomatous orchitis vs., **745**
 - nontuberculous infections vs., **743**
Sarcomas, **231**
 - alveolar soft part, paraganglioma vs., **464**
 - arising in teratoma, other testicular and paratesticular sarcomas vs., **891**
 - clear cell
    - of kidney, congenital mesoblastic nephroma vs., **185**
    - mesenchymal tumors of bladder vs., **456**
 - high-grade
    - smooth muscle tumors vs., **442**
    - undifferentiated, liposarcoma vs., **879**
 - histiocytic, malakoplakia vs., **281**
 - Kaposi, of penis, **990–991**
    - diagnostic checklist, **991**
    - differential diagnosis, **991**
    - nodular stage, **991**
    - patch stage, **991**
    - plaque stage, **991**
    - prognosis, **991**
 - melanocytic lesions of prostate vs., **707**
 - metastatic, malignant mesothelioma vs., **869**
 - monophasic, other, synovial sarcoma vs., **205**
 - paratesticular, somatic-type malignancy in germ cell tumor vs., **799**
 - penile, primary, metastatic tumors vs., **995**
 - pleomorphic undifferentiated, mesenchymal tumors of bladder vs., **456**
 - postradiation, mesenchymal tumors of bladder vs., **456**
 - primary
    - malignant mesothelioma vs., **869**
    - of prostate, sarcomatoid carcinoma of prostate vs., **680**
 - primary or metastatic, adult-type teratoma vs., **791**
 - primary testicular, somatic-type malignancy in germ cell tumor vs., **799**
 - prostatic, sarcomatoid carcinoma vs., markers, **726, 729**
 - sarcomatoid squamous cell carcinoma vs., **971**
 - of specialized prostatic stroma. *See* Stromal tumors.
 - synovial, **204–207**
    - diagnostic checklist, **205**
    - differential diagnosis, **205**
    - genetic testing, **205**
    - molecular features, **205**
    - poorly differentiated, small blue round cell tumors of kidney, **244**
    - prognosis, **205**
 - testicular and paratesticular, other, **890–893**
    - ancillary tests, **891**
    - differential diagnosis, **891**
    - prognosis, **891**
 - tumors with spindle cell morphology, **243–244**
Sarcomatoid carcinoma, **612, 934, 936, 977**
 - HMWCK, smooth muscle tumors and, **445**
 - immunohistochemistry, **996, 997**
 - inflammatory lesions of urethra vs., **488**
 - Kaposi sarcoma vs., **991**
 - mesenchymal tumors of bladder vs., **456**
 - metastatic, other testicular and paratesticular sarcomas vs., **891**
 - mixed squamous cell carcinoma vs., **975**
 - other rare tumors vs., **232, 237**
 - of prostate, **678–683**
    - ancillary tests, **680**
    - carcinomatous component, **679–680**
    - diagnostic checklist, **680**
    - differential diagnosis, **680**
    - heterologous elements, **681**
    - origin, **679**
    - predominant cell/compartment type, **680**
    - predominant pattern/injury type, **680**
    - sarcomatoid/sarcomatous component, **680**
 - prostatic sarcoma vs., markers, **726, 729**
 - smooth muscle tumors and, **445**
 - with spindle cell morphology, **901**
 - stromal tumors vs., **693**
Sarcomatoid renal cell carcinoma, spindle cells in, tumors with spindle cell morphology, **243–244**
Sarcomatoid squamous cell carcinoma
 - of penis, **970–973**
    - ancillary tests, **971**
    - diagnostic checklist, **971**

INDEX

differential diagnosis, **971**
    prognosis, **971**
- pseudoglandular squamous cell carcinoma vs., **963**

Sarcomatoid urothelial carcinoma, **384, 398–399, 401, 439, 528**
- of bladder, in adults, skeletal muscle tumors vs., **449**
- differential diagnosis, **384**
- ERG, **400**
- with heterologous liposarcoma, urothelial carcinoma with lipoid features vs., **385**
- heterologous osteosarcoma, **400**
- mesenchymal tumors of bladder vs., **456**
- myofibroblastic proliferations vs., **433–434**
- pseudoangiosarcomatous, **400**
- smooth muscle tumors vs., **441–442**

Saturation biopsy, in prostate, **539**

Scar
- ischemic, burnt-out germ cell tumor vs., **801**
- postinflammatory, burnt-out germ cell tumor vs., **801**

Schiller-Duval bodies, yolk sac tumor, **779**

Schistosoma haematobium, **287**

Schistosoma japonicum, **287**

Schistosoma mansoni, **287**

Schistosomiasis, **429**
- of bladder, **286–287**
    diagnostic checklist, **287**
    differential diagnosis, **287**
    prognosis, **287**
- eggs, **430**
- urinary bladder neoplasms and, **329**

Schwannoma, **231**
- with ancient change, smooth muscle tumors and, **447**
- cellular, smooth muscle tumors and, **447**
- S100 protein, smooth muscle tumors and, **447**

Sclerosing adenosis, **569, 625**
- adenosis vs., **567**
- atypical small acinar proliferations vs., **641**

Sclerosing lipogranuloma, liposarcoma vs., **879**

Sclerosing paraganglioma, **467**

Sclerosing Sertoli cell tumor, **829**

Sclerotic atrophy, **571, 574**

Scrotal calcinosis, **920–921**
- diagnostic checklist, **921**
- differential diagnosis, **921**
- predominant cell/compartment type, **921**
- predominant pattern/injury type, **921**
- prognosis, **921**

Scrotum
- condylomas, **908–911**
- lipogranuloma, **918–919**
    ancillary tests, **919**
    differential diagnosis, **919**
    predominant cell/compartment type, **919**
    predominant pattern/injury type, **919**

SDHB-deficient renal cell carcinoma
- with granular/eosinophilic cytoplasm, **243**
- renal oncocytoma vs., **50**
- unclassified renal cell carcinoma vs., **143**

Seborrheic keratosis, condylomas vs., **910**

Second tumors, subsequent, renal, **138–141**
- autoimmune conditions, **139**
- genetic features, **139**
- prognosis, **139**

Secondary adenocarcinoma
- nephrogenic adenoma vs., **296**
- tumors of urachus vs., **524**

Secondary carcinoma, poorly differentiated urothelial carcinoma vs., **385**

Secondary tumors of prostate, **714–717**
- ancillary tests, **715**
- origin, **715**
- pattern of spread, **715**

Seeding hypothesis, tubular cell, renal, **583**

Selective internal radiation therapy (SIRT) microspheres, schistosomiasis vs., **287**

Seminal vesicle adenocarcinoma, **722–723**
- ancillary tests, **723**
- differential diagnosis, **723**
- natural history, **723**

Seminal vesicle cysts, congenital or developmental
- cystadenoma vs., **720**
- epithelial stromal tumor vs., **720**

Seminal vesicle epithelium, **624**

Seminal vesicle invasion, **604**

Seminal vesicles, **539, 547**
- atypical small acinar proliferations vs., **640**
- cystadenoma, **718–721**
- epithelial stromal tumors, **718–721**
    stromal tumors vs., **693**
- lipofuscin, **709**
- mixed epithelial stromal neoplasm of, müllerian lesions vs., **316**
- prostatic intraepithelial neoplasia vs., **592**
- tumors of, **537**

Seminiferous tubules, **741, 749**
- atrophic, **740**
    germ cell neoplasia in situ, **758**
- normal, **740**
- sclerotic, germ cell neoplasia in situ, **758**

Seminoma, **762–769, 903**. *See also* Germ cell tumors.
- anaplastic, **768**
    embryonal carcinoma vs., **771–772**
- ancillary tests, **764**
- architecture, **765**
- classic
    with diffuse arrangement, and cells with pale and clear cytoplasm, **898**
    gonadoblastoma vs., **855**
    lymphoma/leukemia/plasmacytoma vs., **860**
    spermatocytic tumor vs., **803, 805**
- cord-like growth, **767**
- cytokeratin stain, **767**
- diagnostic checklist, **764**
- differential diagnosis, **764**
- with extensive granulomatous inflammation, tuberculous epididymo-orchitis vs., **747**
- with glandular/tubular pattern, **899–900**
- granulomas, **766**
- gross, **765**
- interstitial growth, **767**
- intratubular, **768**
    germ cell neoplasia in situ, **760**

INDEX

- large, **765**
- lymphoid follicle, **766**
- with microcystic pattern, **898–899**
- microinvasive, germ cell neoplasia in situ with, **759, 760**
- multifocal, **765**
- necrosis, **765, 768**
- nonspecific granulomatous orchitis vs., **745**
- nontuberculous infections vs., **743**
- OCT3/OCT4, **769**
- podoplanin, **769**
- predominant cell/compartment type, **764**
- predominant pattern/injury type, **764**
- prominent inflammation, **766**
- prominent sclerosis, **767**
- reporting, **764**
- rete invasion, **768**
- rete pagetoid spread, **768**
- spermatocytic
    germ cell neoplasia in situ vs., **757**
    lymphoma/leukemia/plasmacytoma vs., **860**
- with syncytiotrophoblasts, **767**
    choriocarcinoma vs., **786**
- trabecular growth, **767**
- tubular, **766**
    Sertoli cell tumors vs., **829**
    yolk sac tumor vs., **778, 783**

Sertoli cell nodule, **737**
- with germ cell neoplasia in situ, gonadoblastoma vs., **855**
- Sertoli cell tumors vs., **829**

Sertoli cell-only syndrome, **738–741**
- developmental anomaly, **739**
- differential diagnosis, **739**
- environmental exposure, **739**

Sertoli cell tumors, **819, 828–833**
- ancillary tests, **829**
- carcinoid tumor vs., **815, 817**
- differential diagnosis, **829**
- with diffuse arrangement, and cells with pale and clear cytoplasm, **898**
- with glandular/tubular pattern, **899–900, 901**
- granulosa cell tumor vs., **839**
- large cell calcifying, **834–837**
    ancillary tests, **835**
    differential diagnosis, **835**
    Leydig cell tumor vs., **825**
    prognosis, **835**
- large cell calcifying Sertoli cell tumor vs., **835**
- with microcystic pattern, **898–899**
- mixed/unclassified sex cord-stromal tumor vs., **851**
- with oxyphilic cytoplasm, **899**
- prognosis, **829**
- sclerosing, **829**
- seminoma vs., **764, 769**

Sertoli cells, **750, 819**
- adult, **739**
- dedifferentiated, **739**
- dysgenetic, **739**
- immature, **739**
- involuting, **739**

Sertoliform cystadenoma, of rete testis, with glandular/tubular pattern, **901**

Serum tumor markers (S) (postorchiectomy), germ cell tumors, **751**

Sex cord-/gonadal stromal tumors
- classification, **732, 819**
- differential diagnosis, **820**
- general concepts, **818–823**
- gonadoblastoma, **854–857**
- granulosa cell tumor, **838–841**
- immunohistochemistry, **819–820**
- juvenile granulosa cell tumor, **842–845**
- large cell calcifying Sertoli cell tumor, **834–837**
    Leydig cell tumor vs., **825**
- Leydig cell tumors, **824–827**
    carcinoid tumor vs., **815, 817**
    granulosa cell tumor vs., **839**
    large cell calcifying Sertoli cell tumor vs., **835**
    lymphoma/leukemia/plasmacytoma vs., **860**
    testicular tumor of adrenogenital syndrome vs., **847**
    yolk sac tumor vs., **778, 783**
- mixed and unclassified, **819**
- mixed/unclassified, **850–853**
- predominant cell type, **819**
- predominant pattern, **819**
- Sertoli cell tumors, **828–833**
    carcinoid tumor vs., **815**
    large cell calcifying Sertoli cell tumor vs., **835**
    mixed/unclassified sex cord-stromal tumor vs., **851**
    seminoma vs., **764, 769**
- specimen handling, **818–819**
- testicular tumor of adrenogenital syndrome, **846–849**
    Leydig cell tumor vs., **825**

Sex cord-stromal cells, undifferentiated, **819**

Sex cord-stromal tumor
- adenomatoid tumor vs., **865**
- with annular tubules, gonadoblastoma vs., **855**
- embryonal carcinoma vs., **772**
- granulosa cell tumor vs., **839**
- mixed/unclassified, **850–853**
    ancillary tests, **851**
    diagnostic checklist, **851**
    differential diagnosis, **851**
    other testicular and paratesticular sarcomas vs., **891**
    prognosis, **851**
- prepubertal yolk sac tumor vs., **811**
- of Sertoli cell, **829**
- testicular, primary, metastatic tumors of testis and paratesticular structures vs., **895**
- unclassified
    gonadoblastoma vs., **855**
    juvenile granulosa cell tumor vs., **843**
    with spindle cell morphology, **901**

Sex cord tumors, vs. metastasis, **902**

Sextant biopsy, in prostate, **539**

SF1 (steroidogenic factor 1), sex cord-/gonadal stromal tumors, **820**

Sickle cell hemoglobinopathies, **105**

Signal-amplification assays, human papillomavirus, **984**

Signet ring cell adenocarcinoma, **413**
- plasmacytoid carcinoma vs., **383**

INDEX

- urothelial carcinoma with lipoid features vs., **385**
Signet ring cell carcinoma, **627, 631**
 - Gleason grading of, **629**
 - metastatic, adenomatoid tumor vs., **865**
Simple atrophy, **571–572**
 - atypical small acinar proliferations vs., **641**
 - with cyst formation, **571–572**
Single cell Gleason 5 pattern, **612**
Single cell pattern, infiltrative, **612**
Sinus fat, renal, urothelial carcinoma of renal pelvis in, **509**
Sinus invasion, renal, urothelial carcinoma of renal pelvis with, **509**
Skeletal muscle tumors, **251, 448–453**
 - alveolar rhabdomyosarcoma, **451**
 - cambium layer, **450**
 - cartilaginous differentiation, **450**
 - cellular foci in, **450**
 - diagnostic checklist, **449**
 - differential diagnosis, **449**
 - hypo- and hypercellular areas, **450**
 - ill-formed fascicles, **450**
 - myxoid background, **450**
 - pleomorphic rhabdomyosarcoma, **451**
 - prognosis, **449**
 - in situ hybridization, **449**
 - strap cells, **450**
Skene duct cyst, urethral diverticula vs., **496**
Small acinar proliferations
 - atypical, **604**
   acinar adenocarcinoma vs., **611**
 - benign, hyperplasia of mesonephric remnants vs., **577**
Small blue cell tumors
 - embryonal rhabdomyosarcoma vs., **887**
 - other, nephroblastoma (Wilms tumor) vs., **162**
Small blue round cell tumors of kidney, **244**
Small cell anaplastic carcinoma. *See* Prostate carcinoma, with neuroendocrine differentiation.
Small cell carcinoma, **384, 396, 612**
 - in adults, skeletal muscle tumors vs., **449**
 - basal cell carcinoma vs., **674**
 - differential diagnosis, **384**
 - lymphoepithelioma-like carcinoma vs., **384**
 - prostatic
   markers, **729**
   prostatic adenocarcinoma vs., markers for, **725–726**
 - secondarily involving prostate, prostate carcinoma with neuroendocrine differentiation vs., **667**
 - small blue round cell tumors of kidney, **244**
 - synaptophysin, **396**
Small cell neuroendocrine carcinoma. *See* Prostate carcinoma, with neuroendocrine differentiation.
Small cell pattern, **612**
Small glandular hyperplasia, **560**
Small glandular proliferation, **612**
Small lymphocytic lymphoma, **712**
 - involving prostate, **713**
 - pelvic lymph node, **713**
Small round blue cell tumors, other, primitive neuroectodermal tumor vs., **213**
Small round cell tumor, desmoplastic, **891**
 - melanotic neuroectodermal tumor vs., **883**

Small tubules, UC with, **383**
SMARCA4/BRG1 gene, malignant rhabdoid tumor, **193**
SMARCB1, **105**
Smooth muscle neoplasms, mesenchymal tumors of bladder vs., **456**
Smooth muscle tumors, **250, 440–447, 699–700**
 - diagnostic checklist, **442**
 - differential diagnosis, **441–442**
 - prognosis, **441**
 - prostate hyperplasia vs., **560**
 - stromal tumors vs., **693**
Soft tissue filler, **439**
 - iatrogenic, myofibroblastic proliferations vs., **434**
 - mesenchymal tumors of bladder and, **461**
Soft tissue tumors, benign, other testicular and paratesticular sarcomas vs., **891**
Solid Gleason pattern 5, **612**
Solid glomus tumors, **231**
Solitary fibrous tumor, **231, 446, 458, 700, 704**
 - immunohistochemistry, **232**
 - juxtaglomerular cell tumor (reninoma) vs., **223, 225**
 - mesenchymal tumors of bladder vs., **456**
 - of prostate, prostate hyperplasia vs., **560**
 - smooth muscle tumors vs., **442**
 - STAT6, **442**
   smooth muscle tumors and, **446**
 - stromal tumors of prostate vs., **693**
SOX2, germ cell tumors, **751**
SOX17, germ cell tumors, **751**
Specimen handling, squamous cell carcinoma, of penis, **929**
Sperm granuloma
 - nonspecific granulomatous orchitis vs., **745**
 - tuberculous epididymo-orchitis vs., **747**
Spermatic cord, **733**
Spermatids, **750**
Spermatocytes
 - primary, **750**
 - secondary, **750**
Spermatocytic seminoma
 - germ cell neoplasia in situ vs., **757**
 - lymphoma/leukemia/plasmacytoma vs., **860**
Spermatocytic tumor, **802–805, 905**
 - anaplastic, **805**
   embryonal carcinoma vs., **772**
 - ancillary test, **803**
 - cytogenetic changes, **803**
 - cytology, **804**
 - differential diagnosis, **803**
 - with diffuse arrangement, and cells with pale and clear cytoplasm, **898**
 - hemorrhage, **805**
 - interstitial, **804**
 - intratubular, **804**
 - OCT3/4, **805**
 - polymorphism, **804, 805**
 - rhabdomyoblastic transformation, **805**
 - seminoma vs., **764**
 - solid sheets, **804**
 - stromal edema, **804**
Spermatogenesis, **749**

INDEX

Spermatogenic arrest, germ cell neoplasia in situ vs., **757, 761**
Spermatogonia, **750**
- normal, germ cell neoplasia in situ vs., **757**

Spermatozoa, **750**
Spindle cell carcinoma. *See also* Sarcomatoid squamous cell carcinoma.
- mucinous tubular, papillary renal cell carcinoma vs., **83**

Spindle cell lesions
- differential diagnosis, **702**
- immunohistochemistry, **996**

Spindle cell melanoma
- immunohistochemistry, **996**
- sarcomatoid squamous cell carcinoma vs., **971**

Spindle cell nodule, postoperative. *See* Urethra, inflammatory lesions of.
Spindle cell pattern, **612**
Spindle cell pseudotumor, atypical mycobacterial, malakoplakia vs., **281**
Spindle cell tumor, immunohistochemical staining, **702**
Spindle cells
- markers in
    lesions in, of bladder, **528, 531**
    proliferations, types of, **528**
- in sarcomatoid RCC, tumors with spindle cell morphology, **243–244**

Spindle leiomyomatous rhabdomyosarcoma. *See* Embryonal rhabdomyosarcoma.
SPOP, **609**
Sporadic mixed epithelial and stromal tumor, hereditary papillary renal cancer vs., **34**
Squamous cell carcinoma
- cervical, metastatic and secondary carcinoma vs., **476**
- differentiated penile intraepithelial neoplasia and, **925**
- intradiverticular, diverticular-associated neoplasia and, **485**
- invasive, **426–431**
    destructive invasion, **428**
    diagnostic checklist, **427**
    differential diagnosis, **427**
    infiltration of, **428**
    keratinous debris and calcification, **430**
    prognosis, **427**
    prominent keratinization, **428**
    pseudocarcinomatous hyperplasia vs., **321**
    with pseudosarcomatous reaction, **428**
    secondary, **431**
    squamous differentiation, **428**
    typical/classic type, **427**
    verrucous, **427**
- keratinizing, diverticular-associated neoplasia and, **485**
- metastatic, squamous cell carcinoma of penis vs., **939**
- metastatic or secondary, invasive squamous cell carcinoma vs., **427**
- mixed, squamous cell carcinoma of penis vs., **939**
- primary, of bladder, metastatic and secondary carcinoma vs., **472**
- pseudohyperplastic, squamous hyperplasia vs., **915**
- secondary, involving prostate, prostate carcinomas with squamous differentiation vs., **686**
- squamous proliferations other than carcinoma and, **424, 425**
- tumor-like lesions of renal pelvis, **516**
- verruciform, squamous hyperplasia vs., **915**
- verrucous, of bladder, **427, 429**
- of vulva, with extension into distal urethra, carcinoma of urethra vs., **492**

Squamous cell carcinoma in situ. *See also* Penile intraepithelial neoplasia.
- with pagetoid pattern, extramammary Paget disease vs., **988**

Squamous cell carcinoma of penis
- anatomic level of invasion, **930**
- anatomy and histology, **928**
- ancillary studies, **930**
- basaloid, **942–945**
    ancillary tests, **943**
    differential diagnosis, **943, 945**
    papillary basaloid squamous cell carcinoma vs., **947**
    papillary variant, **946–947**
    prognosis, **943**
- clear cell. *See* Clear cell carcinoma, of penis.
- clear cell change, **937**
- clinical implications, **929**
- conventional. *See* Squamous cell carcinoma of penis, usual type.
- cuniculatum, **966–969**
    diagnostic checklist, **967**
    differential diagnosis, **967**
    predominant cell/compartment type, **967**
    predominant pattern/injury type, **967**
    prognosis, **967**
- depth of invasion, **930**
- epidemiology, **928**
- etiology/pathogenesis, **928–929**
- with extension into distal urethra, carcinoma of urethra vs., **492**
- general concepts, **928–937**
- grade, **930, 934**
- growth patterns, **930**
- high-grade, lymphoepithelioma-like squamous cell carcinoma vs., **979**
- histological subtypes, **930**
- lymphoepithelioma-like, **978–979**
    ancillary tests, **979**
    diagnostic checklist, **979**
    differential diagnosis, **979**
    prognosis, **979**
- mixed, **974–977**
    differential diagnosis, **975**
    prognosis, **975**
- multicentric, **929**
- not otherwise specified. *See* Squamous cell carcinoma of penis, usual type.
- papillary, not otherwise specified, **958–961**
    differential diagnosis, **959, 961**
    prognosis, **959**
- pathologic stage, **930**
- perineural invasion, **930–931**
- primary, metastatic tumors vs., **995**

- prognostic factors, **930–931**
- prognostic index, **931**
- pseudoglandular, **962–963**
    - ancillary tests, **963**
    - diagnostic checklist, **963**
    - differential diagnosis, **963**
    - prognosis, **963**
- pseudohyperplastic, **964–965**
    - diagnostic checklist, **965**
    - differential diagnosis, **965**
    - prognosis, **965**
- pure, mixed squamous cell carcinoma vs., **975**
- resection margins, **931**
- sarcomatoid, **970–973**
    - ancillary tests, **971**
    - diagnostic checklist, **971**
    - differential diagnosis, **971**
    - prognosis, **971**
- in situ, immunohistochemistry, **996**
- specimen handling, **929**
- staging, **931**
    - anatomic stage/prognostic groups, **932**
    - TNM, **932**
- superficial spreading, **929, 933**
- tumor front of invasion, **931**
- tumor site, **930**
- tumor thickness, **930**
- typical. See Squamous cell carcinoma of penis, usual type.
- usual type, **938–941**
    - differential diagnosis, **939**
    - with nesting pattern, basaloid squamous cell carcinoma vs., **943**
    - prognosis, **939**
    - pseudohyperplastic squamous cell carcinoma vs., **965**
- variants of, **985**
- vascular invasion, **931**
- verruciform, **929, 933, 934, 937**
- verrucous, **954–957**
    - diagnostic checklist, **955**
    - differential diagnosis, **955**
    - mixed (hybrid), verrucous squamous cell carcinoma vs., **955**
    - predominant cell/compartment type, **955**
    - predominant pattern/injury type, **955**
    - prognosis, **955**
- vertical growth, **929, 933**
- warty, **948–951**
    - diagnostic checklist, **950**
    - differential diagnosis, **949–950**
    - predominant cell/compartment type, **949**
    - predominant pattern/injury type, **949**
    - prognosis, **949**
- warty-basaloid, **952–953**
    - ancillary tests, **953**
    - diagnostic checklist, **953**
    - differential diagnosis, **953**
    - prognosis, **953**

Squamous differentiation, prostate carcinomas with, **684–689**
- adenosquamous carcinoma, **685–686, 688, 689**
- ancillary tests, **686**
- diagnostic checklist, **686**
- differential diagnosis, **686**
- grading, **686**
- origin, **685**
- pure squamous cell carcinoma, **685, 687**
- reporting, **686**

Squamous dysplasia
- keratinizing, **430**
- severe, **430**
- squamous proliferations other than carcinoma vs., **423**

Squamous hyperplasia
- differentiated PeIN vs., **924**
- immunohistochemistry, **996**
- penis, **914–917**
    - differential diagnosis, **915**
    - flat, **915**
    - mixed, **915**
    - papillary, **915**
    - prognosis, **915**
    - pseudoepitheliomatous, **915**
    - verrucous, **915**
- squamous proliferations other than carcinoma and, **423**

Squamous intraepithelial lesion. See Penile intraepithelial neoplasia.

Squamous lesions, **250**

Squamous metaplasia
- benign prostatic glands with or without inflammation, prostate carcinoma with squamous differentiation vs., **686, 689**
- diverticula and, **481**
- keratinizing
    - invasive squamous cell carcinoma vs., **427**
    - squamous proliferations other than carcinoma and, **424**
- squamous proliferations other than carcinoma and, **423, 424**

Squamous mucosa, nonkeratinizing, squamous proliferations other than carcinoma and, **424**

Squamous papilloma, squamous proliferations other than carcinoma and, **423**

Squamous proliferations other than carcinoma, of bladder, **422–425**
- diagnostic checklist, **423**
- differential diagnosis, **423**
- prognosis, **423**

Staging
- renal cell tumors, **8**
- renal cortical tumors, **7**

Steroid cell nodules, with other adrenal diseases, testicular tumor of adrenogenital syndrome vs., **847**

Striated sphincter, **546**

Stromal predominant hyperplasia, **560**

Stromal sarcoma, endometrial, mesenchymal tumors of bladder vs., **456**

Stromal tumors, **690–697**
- chromosomal abnormality, **691**
- clonality, **691**
- diagnostic checklist, **693**
- differential diagnosis, **693**

INDEX

- epithelial, **718–721**
    - ancillary test, **720**
    - developmental anomaly, **719**
    - diagnostic checklist, **720**
    - differential diagnosis, **720**
    - epithelial component, **719–720**
    - mixed epithelial-stromal tumor (MEST), proposed classification and criteria, **720**
    - stromal component, **720**
- gastrointestinal
    - sarcomatoid carcinoma of prostate vs., **680**
    - smooth muscle tumors vs., **442**
- metanephric, congenital mesoblastic nephroma vs., **185**
- mixed epithelial and, renomedullary interstitial cell tumor vs., **227**
- origin, **691**
- of prostate, prostate hyperplasia vs., **560**

Subsequent second tumors, renal, **138–141**
- autoimmune conditions, **139**
- genetic features, **139**
- prognosis, **139**

Subtotal prostatectomy, **540**
- tumor volume in, **603**

Subtotal resection, germ cell tumors, **749**
Succinate dehydrogenase complex deficiency syndrome, **28–31**
- diagnostic checklist, **30**
- differential diagnosis, **30**
- prognosis, **29**

Succinate dehydrogenase enzyme, genes encoding, **29**
Superficial (umbrella) cells, **252**
Surface adenosquamous carcinoma, pseudoglandular squamous cell carcinoma vs., **963**
Sweat gland carcinoma, clear cell carcinoma vs., **981**
Synaptophysin
- large cell neuroendocrine carcinoma, **670**
- markers of neuroendocrine differentiation, **670**

Syncytiotrophoblasts, germ cell tumors with, choriocarcinoma vs., **786**
Syndromal prostatitides, **555**
Synovial sarcoma, **204–207, 701, 705**
- diagnostic checklist, **205**
- differential diagnosis, **205**
- genetic testing, **205**
- molecular features, **205**
- poorly differentiated, small blue round cell tumors of kidney, **244**
- prognosis, **205**

Syphilis, nonspecific granulomatous orchitis vs., **745**
Syphilitic orchitis, **743**

T

T-cell lymphoma, **711**
t(6;11) renal carcinomas. *See* MiTF/TFE family translocation-associated carcinoma.
Tamm-Horsfall polyp, papillary-polypoid cystitis vs., **274**
TCEB1 gene, tumors with mutations in, **69**
TCEB1-mutated renal cell carcinoma
- with clear-/light-staining cytoplasm, **242**
- clear cell renal cell carcinoma vs., **57**
- papillary renal cell carcinoma vs., **83**
- tuberous sclerosis complex vs., **26**

Teratoma
- adult-type, **790–793**
    - ancillary tests, **791**
    - differential diagnosis, **791**
    - genetics, **791**
    - glial tissue, **792**
    - immature, **791, 793**
    - mature, **791**
    - PNET, **793**
- immature, nephroblastoma (Wilms tumor) vs., **163, 168**
- malignant. *See* Choriocarcinoma, and variants.
- with malignant transformation. *See* Germ cell tumors, somatic-type malignancy in.
- monodermal. *See* Carcinoid tumor.
- postpubertal, prepubertal teratoma vs., **807**
- prepubertal type, **806–809**
    - diagnostic checklist, **807**
    - differential diagnosis, **807**
    - glandular component, **808**
    - immature component, **808**
    - immature neuroepithelial component, **808**
    - intestinal component, **808**
- sarcoma arising in, other testicular and paratesticular sarcomas vs., **891**
- with secondary malignancy. *See* Germ cell tumors, somatic-type malignancy in.

Testicular sarcoma, primary, somatic-type malignancy in germ cell tumor vs., **799**
Testicular trauma or torsion, nontuberculous infections vs., **743**
Testicular tumors
- of adrenogenital syndrome, **846–849**
    - ancillary tests, **847**
    - differential diagnosis, **847**
    - Leydig cell tumor vs., **825**
    - prognosis, **847**
- vs. metastasis, **902**

Testis
- cryptorchid
    - atrophy, **736**
    - dysgenetic features, **737**
    - interstitial edema, **736**
    - Leydig cell hyperplasia, **737**
    - megatubules, **736**
    - microlith, **736**
    - paratesticular, **737**
    - Sertoli cells, **736**
- germ cell neoplasia in situ, **758**
- sex cord-stromal tumor of, **839**
- undescended. *See* Cryptorchidism.

Testis and paratesticular structures
- adenomatoid tumor, **864–867**
    - ancillary tests, **865**
    - differential diagnosis, **865**
    - prognosis, **865**
- burnt-out (regressed) germ cell tumor, **800–801**
- carcinoid tumor, **814–817**
- choriocarcinoma, monophasic, seminoma vs., **764**

INDEX

- choriocarcinoma and variants, 784–789
    - ancillary tests, 786
    - classic, 785
    - diagnostic checklist, 786
    - differential diagnosis, 786
    - lymphatic/vascular invasion, 786
    - monophasic, 785
    - nonchoriocarcinomatous trophoblastic tumors, 785–786
    - predominant cell/compartment type, 786
    - predominant pattern/injury type, 786
    - reporting, 786
- classification of, 732–733
- cryptorchidism, 734–737
    - acquired, 735
    - developmental anomaly, 735
    - diagnostic checklist, 735
    - natural history, 735
- embryonal carcinoma, 770–775
    - adenocarcinoma of rete testis/epididymis vs., 873
    - lymphoma/leukemia/plasmacytoma vs., 860
    - malignant mesothelioma vs., 869
    - solid pattern, spermatocytic tumor vs., 803
    - yolk sac tumor vs., 778
- embryonal rhabdomyosarcoma, 886–889
    - ancillary tests, 887
    - differential diagnosis, 887
    - prognosis, 887
- germ cell tumors, general concepts, 748–755
- gonadoblastoma, 854–857
    - ancillary tests, 855
    - diagnostic checklist, 855
    - differential diagnosis, 855
    - prognosis, 855
- granulomatous orchitis, nonspecific, 744–745
    - ancillary tests, 745
    - differential diagnosis, 745
    - seminoma vs., 764
    - unknown causes, 745
- granulosa cell tumor, 838–841
    - ancillary tests, 839
    - diagnostic checklist, 839
    - differential diagnosis, 839
    - prognosis, 839
- immunohistochemistry, 898–905
- juvenile granulosa cell tumor, 842–845
    - ancillary tests, 843
    - differential diagnosis, 843
    - prognosis, 843
- large cell calcifying Sertoli cell tumor, 834–837
    - Leydig cell tumor vs., 825
- Leydig cell tumors, 824–827
    - carcinoid tumor vs., 815, 817
    - granulosa cell tumor vs., 839
    - large cell calcifying Sertoli cell tumor vs., 835
    - lymphoma/leukemia/plasmacytoma vs., 860
    - testicular tumor of adrenogenital syndrome vs., 847
    - yolk sac tumor vs., 778, 783
- liposarcoma, 878–881
    - ancillary tests, 879
    - differential diagnosis, 879
    - predominant cell/compartment type, 879
    - predominant pattern/injury type, 879
    - prognosis, 879
- lymphoma/leukemia/plasmacytoma, 858–863
    - ancillary tests, 860
    - differential diagnosis, 860
    - prognosis, 859
    - staging, 860
- malignant mesothelioma, 868–871
    - ancillary tests, 869
    - differential diagnosis, 869
    - prognosis, 869
- melanotic neuroectodermal tumor, 882–885
    - ancillary tests, 883
    - differential diagnosis, 883
    - prognosis, 883
- metastatic tumors, 733, 894–897
    - ancillary tests, 895
    - differential diagnosis, 895
    - prognosis, 895
- mixed germ cell tumors, 794–797
    - somatic-type malignancy in germ cell tumor vs., 799
- nonspecific granulomatous orchitis, tuberculous epididymo-orchitis vs., 747
- nontuberculous infections, 742–743
- other sarcomas, 890–893
    - ancillary tests, 891
    - differential diagnosis, 891
    - prognosis, 891
- papillary serous carcinoma, müllerian subtype, 874–877
    - ancillary tests, 875
    - differential diagnosis, 875
    - prognosis, 875
- rete testis/epididymis adenocarcinoma, 872–873
    - ancillary tests, 873
    - differential diagnosis, 873
    - prognosis, 873
- seminoma, 762–769
- Sertoli cell-only syndrome, 738–741
    - developmental anomaly, 739
    - differential diagnosis, 739
    - environmental exposure, 739
- Sertoli cell tumors, 828–833
    - carcinoid tumor vs., 815
    - large cell calcifying Sertoli cell tumor vs., 835
    - mixed/unclassified sex cord-stromal tumor vs., 851
    - seminoma vs., 764, 769
- sex cord-/gonadal stromal tumors, general concepts, 818–823
- sex cord-stromal tumor, mixed/unclassified, 850–853
    - ancillary tests, 851
    - diagnostic checklist, 851
    - differential diagnosis, 851
    - prognosis, 851
- somatic-type malignancy in germ cell tumor, 798–799
- spermatocytic tumor, 802–805
- teratoma
    - adult-type, 790–793
    - prepubertal type, 806–809
- testicular tumor of adrenogenital syndrome, 846–849
    - ancillary tests, 847

INDEX

  differential diagnosis, **847**
  Leydig cell tumor vs., **825**
  prognosis, **847**
- tuberculous epididymo-orchitis, **746–747**
  ancillary tests, **747**
  differential diagnosis, **747**
  infectious agents, **747**
- yolk sac tumor, **776–783**
  prepubertal type, **810–813**

TFE3-associated renal cell carcinoma, mesenchymal tumors of bladder vs., **456**

TFE3 gene fusions, epithelioid angiomyolipoma, **179**

TFE3 (Xp11.2) carcinomas. See MiTF/TFE family translocation-associated carcinoma.

TFEB-associated renal cell carcinoma TFEB, mesenchymal tumors of bladder vs., **456**

TFEB [t(6;11)] carcinomas. See MiTF/TFE family translocation-associated carcinoma.

Thecoma/fibroma group, tumor of, **819**

Thyroid carcinoma, metastatic, thyroid-like follicular carcinoma of kidney vs., **129**

Thyroid-like follicular carcinoma of kidney, **128–131**
- diagnostic checklist, **129**
- differential diagnosis, **129**
- genetic features, **129**
- prognosis, **129**

TMPRSS2 gene fusion, ETS and, **609**

Tobacco smoking, in urothelial carcinoma
- of renal pelvis, **507**
- of ureter, **499**

Total penectomy specimen, squamous cell carcinoma, of penis, **929**

TP53 mutations, epithelioid angiomyolipoma, **179**

Transcription elongation factor B (TCEB1)-mutated renal cell carcinoma, **68–71**
- differential diagnosis, **69**
- genetic testing, **69**
- prognosis, **69**

Transition zone, of prostate, **545**

Transitional cell carcinoma
- grade 1. See Papillary urothelial neoplasm of low malignant potential.
- involving prostatic ducts and acini, prostatic intraepithelial neoplasia vs., **593**

Transitional cell metaplasia, prostatic intraepithelial neoplasia vs., **592**

Transitional cell papilloma. See Urothelial papilloma, of bladder.

Translocation-associated carcinoma. See MiTF/TFE family translocation-associated carcinoma.

Translocation-associated renal cell carcinoma, clear cell renal cell carcinoma vs., **56**

Transrectal ultrasound, in prostate carcinoma, **602**

Transurethral resection, **479, 483**

Transurethral resection of prostate, **540**

Trigone, **252, 254**

Trophoblastic tumor. See Choriocarcinoma, and variants.

Tuberculosis
- nonspecific granulomatous orchitis vs., **745**
- renal, **38–43**
  diagnostic checklist, **40**
  differential diagnosis, **40**
  prognosis, **39**

Tuberculous epididymo-orchitis, **746–747**
- ancillary tests, **747**
- differential diagnosis, **747**
- infectious agents, **747**

Tuberous sclerosis-associated renal cell carcinoma
- clear cell renal cell carcinoma vs., **57**
- papillary renal cell carcinoma vs., **83, 89**
- renal oncocytoma vs., **50**
- transcription elongation factor B-mutated renal cell carcinoma vs., **69**
- unclassified renal cell carcinoma vs., **143**

Tuberous sclerosis complex, **24–27**
- angiomyolipoma and, **173**
- diagnostic checklist, **26**
- differential diagnosis, **26**
- epithelioid angiomyolipoma and, **179**
- genes, **25**
- prognosis, **25**
- von Hippel-Lindau syndrome vs., **14**

Tubular cell seeding hypothesis, renal, **583**

Tubular hyalinization, Sertoli cell-only syndrome vs., **739, 741**

Tubular seminoma, yolk sac tumor vs., **778, 783**

Tubular spindle cell carcinoma, mucinous, **118–123**
- diagnostic checklist, **120**
- differential diagnosis, **119–120**
- papillary renal cell carcinoma vs., **83**
- predominant cell/compartment type, **119**
- predominant pattern/injury type, **119**
- prognosis, **119**

Tubules, adult renal epithelial tumors with, and cysts, tubulocystic carcinoma vs., **125**

Tubulocystic carcinoma, **124–127**
- differential diagnosis, **125**
- mixed epithelial and stromal tumor (MEST) family tumors/ pediatric cystic nephroma vs., **198, 203**
- prognosis, **125**

Tubulocystic renal cell carcinoma, hereditary leiomyomatosis renal cell carcinoma syndrome vs., **22**

Tumor-like lesions
- classification, **536–537, 732**
- of renal pelvis, **514–519**
  diagnostic checklist of, **516**
  differential diagnosis of, **516**
  prognosis of, **515**
- of ureter, **502–505**
  diagnostic checklist of, **504**
  differential diagnosis of, **504**
  prognosis of, **503**

Tumor necrosis, **30**

Tunica vaginalis, papillary serous carcinoma of, malignant mesothelioma vs., **869**

Type I germ cell tumor of testis. See Yolk sac tumor, prepubertal type.

INDEX

U

Ultrasonography, in prostate carcinoma, **602**
Umbilical ligament, median, **521**
Umbrella cells, **260, 263**
Unclassified renal cell carcinoma, urothelial carcinoma of renal pelvis vs., **508**
Undescended testis. *See* Cryptorchidism.
Urachal adenocarcinoma, **414**
- invasive adenocarcinoma vs., **411**

Urachal carcinoma, **523**
Urachal cysts, müllerian lesions vs., **316**
Urachal remnants, **520–521**
- differential diagnosis of, **521**

Urachus
- definition of, **521**
- mucinous cystic tumors of, **523**
- tumors of, **522–527**
  - cystic, mucinous, urachal remnants vs., **521**
  - differential diagnosis of, **524**
  - prognosis of, **523**

Ureter
- microscopic anatomy of, **260–261**
  - cross section at mid ureter, **261**
  - gross anatomy, **260**
  - segmental anatomy, **260**
- tumors and tumor-like lesions of, **502–505**
  - diagnostic checklist of, **504**
  - differential diagnosis of, **504**
  - prognosis of, **503**
- urothelial carcinoma of, **498–501**
  - differential diagnosis of, **500**
  - prognosis of, **499**

Ureteral adventitia, **261**
Ureteritis, papillary/polypoid, **261**
Ureterovesical junction, **479**
Urethra
- carcinoma of, **490–493**
  - differential diagnosis of, **492**
  - prognosis of, **491**
- distal
  - penis or vulva with extension into, squamous cell carcinoma of, carcinoma of urethra vs., **492**
  - urothelial carcinoma of, papillary basaloid squamous cell carcinoma vs., **947**
  - urothelial carcinoma of, squamous cell carcinoma of penis vs., **939**
- inflammatory lesions of, **486–489**
  - differential diagnosis, **488**
- internal sphincter of, **252**
- microscopic anatomy of, **256–259**
  - female, **257**
  - lamina propria, **257**
  - lymphatic drainage, **257**
  - male, **256**
  - microscopic, **257**
  - vascular supply, **257**
- prostatic, nephrogenic adenoma (metaplasia) of, **582–589**
  - diagnostic checklist of, **584**
  - differential diagnosis of, **584**
  - prognosis of, **583**
- tumors and tumor-like lesions of, **494–497**
  - differential diagnosis, **496**
  - prognosis, **495**
- urinary bladder with extension into, urothelial carcinoma of, carcinoma of urethra vs., **492**
- urothelial carcinoma of, metastatic tumors of penis vs., **995**

Urethral adenocarcinomas, pseudoglandular squamous cell carcinoma vs., **963**
Urethral carcinoma, inflammatory lesions of urethra vs., **488**
Urethral caruncle, inflammatory lesions of urethra and, **487, 488, 489**
Urethral diverticula, **495**
Urethral duplication, urethral diverticula vs., **496**
Urethral flat urothelial lesions, with atypia, nephrogenic adenoma (metaplasia) of prostatic urethra vs., **584**
Urethral papillary neoplasms, nephrogenic adenoma (metaplasia) of prostatic urethra vs., **584**
Urethral valves, **495**
Urethritis, inflammatory lesions of urethra and, **487, 488**
Urinary bladder, **471**
- amyloidosis, **312–313**
- carcinoma of urethra, **490–493**
- cervical squamous cell carcinoma, metastatic and secondary carcinoma and, **476**
- clear cell adenocarcinoma, **416–421**
  - gynecologic tract, secondary involvement (direct extension) from, clear cell adenocarcinoma vs., **417**
  - nephrogenic adenoma vs., **296**
  - papillary, urothelial papilloma vs., **345**
  - urothelial carcinoma with clear cytoplasm vs., **385**
- cystitis, **266–271**
- cystitis cystica and glandularis, **404–407**
- diverticula, **478–481**
- diverticular-associated neoplasia, **482–485**
- fibroepithelial polyp, **302–305, 495, 496**
  - papillary-polypoid cystitis vs., **274**
  - skeletal muscle tumors vs., **449**
  - tumor-like lesions of renal pelvis, **516**
- flat urothelial lesions other than carcinoma in situ, **340–343**
- hamartoma, **326–327**
  - bladder, fibroepithelial polyp vs., **303**
  - papillary-polypoid cystitis vs., **274**
- high-grade papillary urothelial carcinoma, **358–363**
  - low-grade papillary urothelial carcinoma vs., **355**
- immunohistochemistry, urinary tract, **528–533**
- inflammatory lesions of urethra, **486–489**
- invasive adenocarcinoma, **410–415**
  - cystitis cystica and glandularis vs., **405**
  - villous adenoma vs., **409**
- invasive carcinoma subtypes, overview of, **382–403**
- invasive squamous cell carcinoma, **426–431**
  - pseudocarcinomatous hyperplasia vs., **320, 321**

INDEX

- invasive urothelial carcinoma, 374–381
- inverted urothelial neoplasia, 364–373
- low-grade papillary urothelial carcinoma, 354–357
- malakoplakia, 280–285
    - inflammatory lesions of urethra and, 487, 488, 489
- metastatic and secondary carcinomas, 470–477
- microscopic anatomy of, 252–255
- Müllerian lesions, 314–317
- myofibroblastic proliferations, 432–439
- neoplasms, overview of, 328–331
- nephrogenic adenoma, 278, 294–301, 421, 495, 496, 497
    - carcinoma of urethra vs., 492
    - clear cell adenocarcinoma vs., 417
    - diverticula and, 481
    - invasive urothelial carcinoma of bladder vs., 375, 376
    - microcystic carcinoma vs., 383
    - nested carcinoma vs., 383
    - papillary urothelial carcinoma of low malignant potential vs., 351
    - prostatic-type polyp vs., 307
    - superficial biopsy mimicking, 421
    - urothelial papilloma vs., 345
- other mesenchymal tumors, 454–461
- papillary-polypoid cystitis, 272–279
    - fibroepithelial polyp vs., 303
    - high-grade papillary urothelial carcinoma vs., 359
    - low-grade papillary urothelial carcinoma vs., 355
    - papillary urothelial carcinoma of low malignant potential vs., 351
    - prostatic-type polyp vs., 307
    - urothelial papilloma vs., 345
- papillary urothelial neoplasm of low malignant potential, 350–353
    - low-grade papillary urothelial carcinoma vs., 355
    - urothelial papilloma vs., 345
- paraganglioma, 462–469
- primary adenocarcinoma of
    - invasive, müllerian lesions vs., 316
    - metastatic and secondary carcinoma vs., 471–472
    - tumors of urachus vs., 524
- primary sarcomas of, myofibroblastic proliferations vs., 434
- prostatic-type polyp, 306–311, 495, 497
    - cystitis cystica and glandularis vs., 405
    - fibroepithelial polyp vs., 303
    - high-grade papillary urothelial carcinoma vs., 359
    - papillary-polypoid cystitis vs., 274
    - urothelial papilloma vs., 345
- pseudocarcinomatous hyperplasia, 271, 318–325
    - invasive urothelial carcinoma of bladder vs., 376
    - metastatic and secondary carcinomas vs., 472
    - von Brunn nests vs., 289
- schistosomiasis, 286–287
- skeletal muscle tumors, 448–453
- smooth muscle tumors, 440–447
- squamous proliferations other than carcinoma, 422–425
- tumor-like lesions of renal pelvis, 514–519
- tumors and tumor-like lesions of ureter, 502–505
- tumors and tumor-like lesions of urethra, 494–497
- tumors of urachus, 522–527
    - cystic, mucinous, urachal remnants vs., 521
- urachal remnants, 520–521
- urothelial carcinoma in situ, 330, 332–339
    - flat urothelial lesions other than carcinoma in situ vs., 341
    - intradiverticular, diverticular-associated neoplasia and, 484
    - nephrogenic adenoma vs., 296
    - squamous proliferations other than carcinoma vs., 423
- urothelial carcinoma of, with extension into urethra, carcinoma of urethra vs., 492
- urothelial carcinoma of renal pelvis, 506–513
    - urothelial carcinoma of ureter vs., 500
- urothelial carcinoma of ureter, 498–501
- urothelial papilloma, 277, 344–349, 352
    - fibroepithelial polyp vs., 303
    - inverted, with glandular feature, cystitis cystica and glandularis vs., 405
    - papillary urothelial carcinoma of low malignant potential vs., 351
- villous adenoma, 408–409
- von Brunn nests, 288–293
    - cystitis cystica and glandularis and, 405
    - florid, pseudocarcinomatous hyperplasia vs., 320
    - nested carcinoma vs., 382

Urinary bladder neck, 547
Urinary tract, immunohistochemistry in, 528–533
Uroplakins, 263
Urothelial atypia
- reactive
    - flat urothelial lesions other than carcinoma in situ and, 341
    - urothelial carcinoma in situ vs., 334
- of unknown significance, flat urothelial lesions other than carcinoma in situ and, 341

Urothelial carcinoma
- with alternative/aberrant differentiation, 382
- carcinomatous component, 398
- with chordoid features, 402
- with clear cell features, 421
- with clear cytoplasm
    - clear cell adenocarcinoma vs., 417
    - metastatic and secondary carcinomas vs., 472
- with cytoplasm (glycogen rich), 385
    - differential diagnosis, 385
- of distal urethra
    - papillary basaloid squamous cell carcinoma vs., 947
    - squamous cell carcinoma of penis vs., 939
- extramammary Paget disease associated with, immunohistochemistry, 996
- with glandular differentiation
    - clear cell adenocarcinoma vs., 417
    - metastatic and secondary carcinomas vs., 472
    - microcystic carcinoma vs., 383
    - Müllerian lesions vs., 316
    - nephrogenic adenoma vs., 296
    - prostatic-type polyp vs., 307

- with glandular features, collecting duct carcinoma vs., **100**
- glycogen-rich, **396**
- intradiverticular
    - high-grade, diverticular-associated neoplasia and, **484**
    - invasive, diverticular-associated neoplasia and, **484**
- invasive
    - with glandular differentiation, tumors of urachus vs., **524**
    - with glandular differentiation or small tubules, invasive adenocarcinoma vs., **411**
    - nested carcinoma, paraganglioma vs., **464**
    - paraganglioma vs., **464**
- with inverted growth
    - tumor-like lesions of renal pelvis vs., **516**
    - tumor-like lesions of ureter vs., **504**
- involving prostate gland, **658–663**
    - ancillary test, **661**
    - classification, **659**
    - differential diagnosis, **661**
    - grading, **661**
    - pattern of involvement, **660**
    - prevalence of involvement in reported series, **660**
    - staging, **661**
- involving prostatic duct and acini, **660–661, 662**
    - prostatic intraepithelial neoplasia vs., **593**
- with large vacuolated clear cells, **421**
- lipid-rich (lipoid), **403**
- with lipoid features (lipid rich/lipid cell), **385**
    - differential diagnosis, **385**
- low-grade, high-grade papillary urothelial carcinoma vs., **359**
- malakoplakia vs., **281**
- markers in, **529**
- metastatic tumors vs., **239**
- microcystic, müllerian lesions vs., **316**
- micropapillary, metastatic and secondary carcinomas vs., **472**
- with myxoid stroma, myofibroblastic proliferations vs., **434**
- myxoid stroma (including chordoid), **384–385**
    - differential diagnosis, **385**
- nested
    - with associated tubules, cystitis cystica and glandularis vs., **405**
    - pseudocarcinomatous hyperplasia vs., **320, 321**
    - von Brunn nests vs., **289**
- nested or tubular or microcystic pattern variant of, nephrogenic adenoma vs., **296**
- noninvasive, **511**
    - involving prostatic urethra, **660**
- noninvasive papillary, **393**
    - squamous proliferations other than carcinoma vs., **423**
- osteoclast-like giant cells, **384**
- with osteoclast-type giant cells, **397**
- papillary
    - arising in periurethral ducts, **662**
    - with glandular differentiation, villous adenoma vs., **409**
    - high-grade, low-grade papillary urothelial carcinoma vs., **355**
    - low grade, urothelial papilloma vs., **345**
    - nephrogenic adenoma vs., **296**
- with papillary architecture, **421**
- of pelvicalyceal system, papillary, papillary renal cell carcinoma vs., **83**
- plasmacytoid, metastatic and secondary carcinomas vs., **472**
- poorly differentiated, **244, 397**
    - basal cell carcinoma vs., **674**
    - prostate carcinoma with neuroendocrine differentiation vs., **667**
    - small cell carcinoma vs., **384**
    - with syncytiotrophoblasts, metastatic and secondary carcinomas vs., **472**
- primary, of prostate, **659**
- with prominent lymphoid stroma, lymphoepithelioma-like carcinoma vs., **384**
- prostatic adenocarcinoma vs., markers in differential of, **724–725**
- with pseudoangiosarcomatous, sarcomatoid UC vs., **384**
- renal medullary carcinoma vs., **106**
- with retraction spaces, **394**
- with rhabdoid features, **384, 403**
- sarcomatoid, **398–399, 439, 528**
    - mesenchymal tumors of bladder vs., **456**
    - myofibroblastic proliferations vs., **433–434**
    - smooth muscle tumors vs., **441–442**
- secondary, with squamous differentiation, prostate carcinoma with squamous differentiation vs., **686**
- skeletal muscle tumors and, **453**
- with small tubules, **383, 390**
- specific variants of invasive, **472**
- with squamous differentiation, **431**
    - invasive squamous cell carcinoma vs., **427**
    - metastatic and secondary carcinomas vs., **472**
- with tubular features, **415**
- with tubular morphology, **415**
- typical invasive, pseudocarcinomatous hyperplasia vs., **320**
- of urethra, metastatic tumors of penis vs., **995**

Urothelial carcinoma in situ, **330, 332–339**
- ancillary tests, **333–334**
- diagnostic checklist, **334**
- differential diagnosis, **334**
- flat urothelial lesions other than carcinoma in situ vs., **341**
- intradiverticular, diverticular-associated neoplasia and, **484**
- nephrogenic adenoma vs., **296**
- prognosis, **333**
- squamous proliferations other than carcinoma vs., **423**

Urothelial carcinoma of bladder
- with extension into urethra, carcinoma of urethra vs., **492**
- invading prostate, **716**
- invading prostate stroma, **716**
- invasive, **374–381**
    - diagnostic checklist, **376**

INDEX

    differential diagnosis, 375–376
    patterns of, invasion, 375
    reporting, 376
    staging, 376
- mimicking prostate carcinoma, 716
- poorly differentiated, invading prostate, 716
- prostate carcinoma, 716
- secondarily involving bladder, 659
- urothelial carcinoma of ureter vs., 500

Urothelial carcinoma of renal pelvis, 506–513
- diagnostic checklist of, 508
- differential diagnosis of, 508
- prognosis of, 507
- urothelial carcinoma of ureter vs., 500

Urothelial carcinoma of ureter, 498–501
- differential diagnosis of, 500
- prognosis of, 499

Urothelial dysplasia
- and flat atypia of uncertain significance, urothelial carcinoma in situ vs., 334
- flat urothelial lesions other than carcinoma in situ and, 341

Urothelial lesions
- flat, urethral, with atypia, nephrogenic adenoma (metaplasia) of prostatic urethra vs., 584
- markers in, 529
    flat, 528
- other than carcinoma in situ, flat, 340–343
    diagnostic checklist, 341
    differential diagnosis, 341
- urothelial carcinoma in situ vs., 333

Urothelial markers, in UC vs. PCa differential, 529

Urothelial neoplasia
- of bladder, inverted, 364–373
    diagnostic checklist, 366
    differential diagnosis, 366
    prognosis, 365
- inverted, pseudocarcinomatous hyperplasia vs., 320
- papillary, papillary-polypoid cystitis vs., 273–274

Urothelial neoplasm, papillary
- exophytic, 345
- of low malignant potential, urothelial papilloma vs., 345
- prostatic-type polyp vs., 307

Urothelial papilloma, 277, 352
- of bladder, 344–349
    diagnostic checklist, 345
    differential diagnosis, 345
    prognosis, 345
- fibroepithelial polyp vs., 303
- inverted, with glandular feature, cystitis cystica and glandularis vs., 405
- papillary urothelial carcinoma of low malignant potential vs., 351

Urothelial (transitional cell) carcinoma, involving prostatic ducts and acini, intraductal carcinoma vs., 646

Urothelium, 252, 263, 264
- injury of, nephrogenic adenoma from, 295
- normal, flat urothelial lesions other than carcinoma in situ vs., 341
- ureter, 260, 261

V

Vaccine, for human papillomavirus, 983
Vascular malformation, mesenchymal tumors of bladder vs., 459
Vascular tumors, 701
VCL-ALK renal cell carcinoma, renal medullary carcinoma vs., 106
Verruciform squamous cell carcinoma, squamous hyperplasia vs., 915
Verruciform xanthoma, squamous hyperplasia vs., 915
Verrucous carcinoma, 425
- of bladder, 429
- condylomas vs., 910
- cuniculatum squamous cell carcinoma vs., 967
- hybrid, 976
- immunohistochemistry, 996
- mixed usual, papillary squamous cell carcinoma vs., 959
- papillary squamous cell carcinoma vs., 959
- of penis
    hybrid. *See* Cuniculatum squamous cell carcinoma.
    warty squamous cell carcinoma vs., 949
- pseudocarcinomatous hyperplasia vs., 320, 325
- squamous proliferations other than carcinoma vs., 423

Verrucous squamous cell carcinoma, 427
- of penis, 954–957
    diagnostic checklist, 955
    differential diagnosis, 955
    mixed (hybrid), verrucous squamous cell carcinoma vs., 955
    predominant cell/compartment type, 955
    predominant pattern/injury type, 955
    prognosis, 955
    pseudohyperplastic squamous cell carcinoma vs., 965

Verumontanum (colliculus seminalis), 539, 546
Verumontanum gland hyperplasia, 624
Verumontanum glands, 258
Verumontanum mucinous gland hyperplasia, polypoid lesions vs., 496
Verumontanum mucosal gland hyperplasia, 580–581
- atypical small acinar proliferations vs., 640
- diagnostic checklist of, 581
- differential diagnosis of, 581
- hyperplasia of mesonephric remnants vs., 577
- prognosis of, 581

Vesical diverticula. *See* Diverticula.
Vesical intradiverticular tumors, diverticular-associated neoplasia and, 483
Vesical sarcoma, primary, sarcomatoid UC vs., 384
Villous adenoma
- of bladder, 408–409
    diagnostic checklist, 409
    differential diagnosis, 409
- tumor-like lesions of renal pelvis, 515
- of urachus, tumors of urachus vs., 524

Vimentin, sex cord-/gonadal stromal tumors, 819
von Brunn nests, 288–293
- cystitis cystica and glandularis and, 405
- diagnostic checklist, 289

xlix

INDEX

- differential diagnosis, **289**
- florid, pseudocarcinomatous hyperplasia vs., **320**
- nested carcinoma vs., **382**
- prognosis, **289**

von Hippel-Lindau syndrome, **12–15**
- differential diagnosis, **14**
- gene alterations, **13**
- prognosis, **13**

Vulva, squamous cell carcinoma of, with extension into distal urethra, carcinoma of urethra vs., **492**

Wart, genital. *See* Condylomas.
Warty-basaloid carcinoma, **976**
- basaloid squamous cell carcinoma vs., **943, 945**
- immunohistochemistry, **997**

Warty/basaloid mixed squamous cell carcinoma, **936**
Warty/basaloid penile intraepithelial neoplasia, differential diagnosis, **924**
- ancillary tests, **923**

Warty-basaloid squamous cell carcinoma, of penis, **952–953**
- ancillary tests, **953**
- diagnostic checklist, **953**
- differential diagnosis, **953**
- papillary basaloid squamous cell carcinoma vs., **947**
- prognosis, **953**

Warty carcinoma, **935**
- condylomas vs., **910**
- cuniculatum squamous cell carcinoma vs., **967**
- immunohistochemistry, **996**
- papillary squamous cell carcinoma vs., **959**
- with prominent clear cells, clear cell carcinoma vs., **981**
- verrucous squamous cell carcinoma vs., **955**
- warty-basaloid squamous cell carcinoma of penis vs., **953**

Warty penile intraepithelial neoplasia, **937**
Warty squamous cell carcinoma, of penis, **948–951**
- diagnostic checklist, **950**
- differential diagnosis, **949–950**
- mixed warty-basaloid, differential diagnosis, **950**
- papillary basaloid squamous cell carcinoma vs., **947**
- predominant cell/compartment type, **949**
- predominant pattern/injury type, **949**
- prognosis, **949**

Well-differentiated liposarcoma (WDL). *See* Liposarcoma.
Well-differentiated neuroendocrine tumor (carcinoid), **208–211**
- developmental anomaly, **209**
- diagnostic checklist, **209**
- differential diagnosis, **209**
- prognosis, **209**

WHO/ISUP classification
- of flat lesions with atypia, **329**
- of papillary neoplasia, **329**

Wilms tumor, **160–169**
- ancillary tests, **162**
- blastema predominant, clear cell sarcoma of kidney vs., **189**
- blastemal
  primitive neuroectodermal tumor vs., **213**
  synovial sarcoma vs., **205**
- congenital mesoblastic nephroma vs., **185**
- cystic, cystic partially differentiated nephroblastoma vs., **171**
- developmental anomaly, **160–169**
- diagnostic checklist, **162–163**
- differential diagnosis, **162–163**
- epithelial predominant, metanephric adenoma vs., **148**
- lymphatic/vascular invasion, **162, 169**
- relationship with metanephric tumors other than metanephric adenoma, **153**
- revised SIOP working classification of, after neoadjuvant therapy, **163**
- small blue round cell tumors of kidney, **244**
- staging of pediatric renal tumors, **163**
- *WT1* gene deletions or point mutations, **161**
- *WT2* gene alterations, **161**

WT1, sex cord-/gonadal stromal tumors, **820**
WT1 gene deletions, nephroblastoma (Wilms tumor), **161**
WT2 gene alteration, nephroblastoma (Wilms tumor), **161**

Xanthogranulomatous inflammation, malakoplakia vs., **281**
Xanthogranulomatous prostatitis, **556**
Xanthogranulomatous pyelonephritis (XGP), **38–43**
- diagnostic checklist, **40**
- differential diagnosis, **40**
- prognosis, **39**

Xanthoma, verruciform, squamous hyperplasia vs., **915**
Xp11.2 renal carcinomas. *See* MiTF/TFE family translocation-associated carcinoma.

Y

Yolk sac tumor, **776–783, 904, 905**
- adenomatoid tumor vs., **865**
- AFP, **783**
- ancillary tests, **778**
- CK-PAN, **783**
- complex glandular, **782**
- diagnostic checklist, **778**
- differential diagnosis, **778**
- with diffuse arrangement, and cells with pale and clear cytoplasm, **898**
- embryonal carcinoma vs., **772**
- endometrioid, **781**
- glandular, **781**
- with glandular/tubular pattern, **899–900**
- glypican-3, **783**
- gross, **779**
- hepatoid, **782**
- juvenile granulosa cell tumor vs., **843**
- low power, **779**
- microcystic and reticular, **779**
- with microcystic pattern, **898–899**

INDEX

- mixed germ cell tumor, **782**
- papillary, **780**
- parietal, **781**
- polyvesicular vitelline, **780**
- predominant cell/compartment type, **778**
- predominant pattern/injury type, **778**
- prepubertal type, **810–813**
    - ancillary tests, **811**
    - with cytologic atypia, **812**
    - diagnostic checklist, **811**
    - differential diagnosis, **811**
    - exuberant papillary growth pattern, **813**
    - glandular growth pattern, **813**
    - macrocystic pattern, **812**
    - papillary and solid growth pattern, **812**
- reporting, **778**
- SALL 4, **783**
- sarcomatoid, **782**
- Schiller-Duval bodies, **779**
- Sertoli cell tumors vs., **829**
- solid, **780**
    - seminoma vs., **764, 769**

Z

Zonal variations, microanatomy and, **544–553**
- ductal acinar unit, **544–545**
- in histology, **545**
- luminal and cellular deposits, **545–546**
- nonglandular prostate, **546**
- nonprostatic structures, **546**
- periprostatic structures, **546–547**
- prostate anatomic zones, **545**

Zone glands, central, prostate, prostatic intraepithelial neoplasia vs., **592**